PRINCIPLES AND PRACTICE OF THE BIOLOGIC THERAPY OF CANCER

Third Edition

PRINCIPLES AND PRACTICE OF THE BIOLOGIC THERAPY OF CANCER

Third Edition

EDITED BY

Steven A. Rosenberg, M.D., Ph.D.

Chief of Surgery
National Cancer Institute
National Institutes of Health
Bethesda, Maryland
Professor of Surgery
Uniformed Services University of the Health Sciences
F. Hébert School of Medicine

with 131 contributing authors

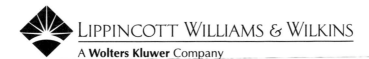

LIPPINCOTT WILLIAMS & WILKINS
A **Wolters Kluwer** Company

Philadelphia · Baltimore · New York · London
Buenos Aires · Hong Kong · Sydney · Tokyo

Developmental Editor: Stephanie Harris
Supervising Editor: Mary Ann McLaughlin
Production Editor: Alyson Langlois, Silverchair Science + Communications, Inc.
Manufacturing Manager: Kevin Watt
Cover Designer: Mark Lerner
Compositor: Silverchair Science + Communications
Printer: Courier Westford

© 2000 by LIPPINCOTT WILLIAMS & WILKINS
530 Walnut Street
Philadelphia, PA 19106 USA
LWW.com

Printed in the USA

Library of Congress Cataloging-in-Publication Data

Principles and practice of the biologic therapy of cancer / edited by Steven A. Rosenberg-- 3rd ed.
    p. ; cm.
  Includes bibliographical references and index.
  ISBN 0-7817-2272-1
  1. Biological response modifiers--Therapeutic use. 2. Cancer--Immunotherapy. 3.
Cancer--Gene therapy. I. Rosenberg, Steven A.
  [DNLM: 1. Neoplasms--therapy. 2. Biological Response Modifiers--immunology. 3.
Biological Response Modifiers--therapeutic use. 4. Immunotherapy. QZ 266 B6145 2000]
  RC271.B53 B55 2000
  616.99'406--dc21

                        99-059488

Care has been taken to confirm the accuracy of the information presented and to describe generally accepted practices. However, the authors, editors, and publisher are not responsible for errors or omissions or for any consequences from application of the information in this book and make no warranty, expressed or implied, with respect to the currency, completeness, or accuracy of the contents of the publication. Application of this information in a particular situation remains the professional responsibility of the practitioner.

The authors, editors, and publisher have exerted every effort to ensure that drug selection and dosage set forth in this text are in accordance with current recommendations and practice at the time of publication. However, in view of ongoing research, changes in government regulations, and the constant flow of information relating to drug therapy and drug reactions, the reader is urged to check the package insert for each drug for any change in indications and dosage and for added warnings and precautions. This is particularly important when the recommended agent is a new or infrequently employed drug.

Some drugs and medical devices presented in this publication have Food and Drug Administration (FDA) clearance for limited use in restricted research settings. It is the responsibility of health care providers to ascertain the FDA status of each drug or device planned for use in their clinical practice.

10 9 8 7 6 5 4 3 2 1

CONTENTS

CONTRIBUTING AUTHORS

Sanjiv S. Agarwala, M.D.
Assistant Professor of Medicine
Department of Hematology/Oncology
University of Pittsburgh Cancer Institute
University of Pittsburgh School of Medicine
Pittsburgh, Pennsylvania

H. Richard Alexander, Jr., M.D.
Head, Surgical Metabolism Section
Surgery Branch
National Cancer Institute
National Institutes of Health
Bethesda, Maryland

James P. Allison, Ph.D.
Investigator and Professor of Immunology
Department of Molecular and Cell Biology
Howard Hughes Medical Research Institute
University of California, Berkeley, School of Medicine
Berkeley, California

Michael B. Atkins, M.D.
Associate Professor of Medicine
Harvard Medical School
Director of Cutaneous Oncology and Biologic Therapy
    Programs
Division of Hematology/Oncology
Beth Israel Deaconess Medical Center
Boston, Massachusetts

John Barrett, M.D., F.R.C.P., F.R.C.Path.
Chief, Stem Cell Transplant Unit
Hematology Branch
National Heart, Lung and Blood Institute
National Institutes of Health
Bethesda, Maryland

Richard J. Barth, Jr., M.D.
Associate Professor
Department of Surgery
Dartmouth-Hitchcock Medical Center
Dartmouth Medical School
Lebanon, New Hampshire

David L. Bartlett, M.D.
Senior Investigator
Surgery Branch
National Cancer Institute
National Institutes of Health
Bethesda, Maryland

Jose Baselga, M.D.
Professor of Medicine
Medical Oncology Service
Vall d'Hebron University Hospital
Barcelona, Spain

Arie S. Belldegrun, M.D., F.A.C.S.
Professor of Urology
Chief, Division of Urologic Oncology
Director, Urologic Research
Department of Urology
University of California, Los Angeles, UCLA School of Medicine
Los Angeles, California

Jay A. Berzofsky, M.D., Ph.D.
Chief, Molecular Immunogenetics and Vaccine Research Section
Metabolism Branch
National Cancer Institute
National Institutes of Health
Bethesda, Maryland

Thierry Boon, Ph.D.
Professor
Ludwig Institute for Cancer Research
Université Catholique de Louvain
Brussels, Belgium

Malcolm K. Brenner, M.B., Ph.D.
Professor of Medicine
Center for Cell and Gene Therapy
Baylor College of Medicine
Houston, Texas

Allon Canaan, M.D.
Genetic Therapy Program
Yale Cancer Center
Medical Oncology Section
Yale University School of Medicine
New Haven, Connecticut

Andres Canova, M.D.
Genetic Therapy Program
Yale Cancer Center
Medical Oncology Section
Yale University School of Medicine
New Haven, Connecticut

Natasha J. Caplen, Ph.D.
Clinical Gene Therapy Branch
National Human Genome Research Institute
National Institutes of Health
Bethesda, Maryland

David P. Carbone, M.D., Ph.D.
Associate Professor of Medicine
Division of Hematology/Oncology
Vanderbilt University Medical School
Director, Experimental Therapeutics Program
Vanderbilt-Ingram Cancer Center
Vanderbilt Medical Center
Nashville, Tennessee

Paul B. Chapman, M.D.
Associate Attending Physician
Head, Melanoma Section
Department of Medicine
Memorial Sloan-Kettering Cancer Center
New York, New York

Yao-Tseng Chen, M.D., Ph.D.
Associate Professor of Pathology
Department of Pathology
Weill Medical College of Cornell University
New York, New York

Nai-Kong V. Cheung, M.D., Ph.D.
Member
Department of Pediatrics
Memorial Sloan-Kettering Cancer Center
New York, New York

Robert M. Conry, M.D.
Associate Professor of Medicine
Division of Hematology/Oncology
University of Alabama School of Medicine
Birmingham, Alabama

Kenneth G. Cornetta, M.D.
Associate Professor of Medicine
Bone Marrow and Stem Cell Transplantation
    Program
Indiana University School of Medicine
Indianapolis, Indiana

Ramsey M. Dallal, M.D.
Department of Surgical Oncology/Biological Therapy
University of Pittsburgh School of Medicine
Pittsburgh, Pennsylvania

Albert Deisseroth, M.D., Ph.D.
Director, Genetic Therapy Program
Yale Cancer Center
Ensign Professor of Medicine
Chief, Medical Oncology Section
Department of Internal Medicine
Yale University School of Medicine
New Haven, Connecticut

Chaitanya Divgi, M.D.
Associate Member
Nuclear Medicine Service
Department of Radiology
Memorial Sloan-Kettering Cancer Center
New York, New York

Mark E. Dudley, Ph.D.
Senior Staff Fellow
Surgery Branch
National Cancer Institute
National Institutes of Health
Bethesda, Maryland

Scott K. Durum, Ph.D.
Senior Investigator
Division of Basic Sciences
National Cancer Institute
National Institutes of Health
Frederick, Maryland

Marc S. Ernstoff, M.D.
Professor and Chief
Section of Hematology/Oncology
Stephen B. Currier Oncology Fellow
Dartmouth-Hitchcock Medical Center
Deputy Director
Norris Cotton Cancer Center
Lebanon, New Hampshire

Zeev Estrov, M.D.
Professor of Medicine
Department of Bioimmunotherapy
University of Texas M. D. Anderson Cancer Center
Houston, Texas

Bingliang Fang, M.D.
Section of Thoracic Molecular Oncology
Department of Thoracic and Cardiovascular Surgery
University of Texas M. D. Anderson Cancer Center
Houston, Texas

Alexander Fefer, M.D.
Professor of Medicine
University of Washington School of Medicine
Member
Fred Hutchinson Cancer Research Center
Seattle, Washington

Andrew L. Feldman, M.D.
Clinical Associate
Surgery Branch
National Cancer Institute
National Institutes of Health
Bethesda, Maryland

Robert A. Figlin, M.D.
University of California, Los Angeles, UCLA School
   of Medicine
Division of Hematology/Oncology
Los Angeles, California

Olivera J. Finn, Ph.D.
Professor
Department of Molecular Genetics and Biochemistry
University of Pittsburgh School of Medicine
Pittsburgh, Pennsylvania

Kenneth A. Foon, M.D.
Professor
Department of Internal Medicine
Director
Barrett Cancer Center for Prevention, Treatment
   and Research
Cincinnati, Ohio

Barbara Foster, Ph.D.
Department of Molecular and Cellular Biology
Baylor College of Medicine
Houston, Texas

Takuma Fujii, M.D.
Genetic Therapy Program
Yale Cancer Center
Medical Oncology Section
Yale University School of Medicine
New Haven, Connecticut

John A. Glaspy, M.D.
Associate Professor
Division of Hematology/Oncology
University of California, Los Angeles, UCLA School
   of Medicine
Los Angeles, California

Norman Greenberg, Ph.D.
Baylor College of Medicine
Houston, Texas

X. Y. David Guo, M.D.
Genetic Therapy Program
Yale Cancer Center
Medical Oncology Section
Yale University School of Medicine
New Haven, Connecticut

Lee J. Helman, M.D.
Chief
Pediatric Oncology Branch
National Cancer Institute
National Institutes of Health
Bethesda, Maryland

Helen E. Heslop, M.D.
Center for Cell and Gene Therapy
Baylor College of Medicine
Houston, Texas

Alan N. Houghton, M.D.
Professor
Department of Medicine and Immunology
Weill Medical School of Cornell University
Chairman, Immunology Program
Memorial Sloan-Kettering Cancer Center
New York, New York

Frank Hsieh, M.D.
Genetic Therapy Program
Yale Cancer Center
Medical Oncology Section
Yale University School of Medicine
New Haven, Connecticut

Arthur A. Hurwitz, M.D.
Cancer Research Laboratory
Department of Molecular and Cell Biology
University of California, Berkeley, School of Medicine
Berkeley, California

Patrick Hwu, M.D.
Senior Investigator
National Cancer Institute
National Institutes of Health
Bethesda, Maryland

Elizabeth M. Jaffee, M.D.
Associate Professor of Oncology and Pathology
Johns Hopkins University School of Medicine
Baltimore, Maryland

Rakesh K. Jain, Ph.D.
Andrew Werk Cook Professor of Tumor Biology
Department of Radiation Oncology
Massachusetts General Hospital
Harvard Medical School
Boston, Massachusetts

Hagop M. Kantarjian, M.D.
Chairman and Professor of Medicine
Department of Leukemia
University of Texas M. D. Anderson Cancer Center
Houston, Texas

Kenneth Kaushansky, M.D.
Professor of Medicine
Division of Hematology
University of Washington School of Medicine
Seattle, Washington

John M. Kirkwood, M.D.
Professor and Vice Chairman of Clinical Research
Director, Melanoma Center
Department of Medicine
Division of Hematology/Oncology
University of Pittsburgh Medical Center
University of Pittsburgh School of Medicine
Pittsburgh, Pennsylvania

Robert J. Kreitman, M.D.
Laboratory of Molecular Biology
National Cancer Institute
National Institutes of Health
Bethesda, Maryland

Susan E. Krown, M.D.
Professor of Medicine
Weill Medical College of Cornell University
Attending Physician and Member
Memorial Sloan-Kettering Cancer Center
New York, New York

Razelle Kurzrock, M.D.
Professor of Medicine
Department of Bioimmunotherapy
University of Texas M. D. Anderson Cancer Center
Houston, Texas

Eugene Kwon, M.D.
Assistant Professor of Urology
Department of Urology and Cancer Immunology
Loyola University of Chicago Stritch School
    of Medicine
Maywood, Illinois

Steven M. Larson, M.D.
Professor of Radiology
Chief, Nuclear Medicine Service
Weill Medical College of Cornell University
Memorial Sloan-Kettering Cancer Center
New York, New York

Irina Lebedeva, Ph.D.
Columbia University College of Physicians
    and Surgeons
New York, New York

Steven K. Libutti, M.D.
Senior Investigator
Surgery Branch
National Cancer Institute
National Institutes of Health
Bethesda, Maryland

Philip O. Livingston, M.D.
Professor of Medicine
Weill Medical College of Cornell University
Memorial Sloan-Kettering Cancer Center
New York, New York

Kenneth O. Lloyd, Ph.D.
Department of Immunology
Memorial Sloan-Kettering Cancer Center
New York, New York

Michael T. Lotze, M.D.
Professor and Chief
Division of Surgical Oncology
University of Pittsburgh Cancer Institute
Pittsburgh, Pennsylvania

Stewart D. Lyman, Ph.D.
Director, Extramural Research
Immunex Corporation
Seattle, Washington

David H. Lynch, Ph.D.
Immunex Corporation
Seattle, Washington

Robbie Mailliard, B.S.
Research Specialist and Laboratory Manager
Department of Surgery
University of Pittsburgh School of Medicine
Pittsburgh, Pennsylvania

Charles R. Maliszewski, Ph.D.
Senior Investigator
Department of Discovery Research
Immunex Corporation
Seattle, Washington

David G. Maloney, M.D., Ph.D.
Fred Hutchinson Cancer Research Center
University of Washington School of Medicine
Seattle, Washington

Eugene Maraskovsky, M.D.
Laboratory Head
Cancer Vaccine Laboratory
Ludwig Institute for Cancer Research
Austin and Repatriation Medical Centre
Melbourne, Australia

Francesco M. Marincola, M.D.
Senior Investigator
Surgery Branch
National Cancer Institute
National Institutes of Health
Bethesda, Maryland

J. Andrea McCart, M.D.
Surgical Oncology Fellow
Surgery Branch
National Cancer Institute
National Institutes of Health
Bethesda, Maryland

Cornelis J. M. Melief, M.D., Ph.D.
Professor of Medicine
Department of Immunohematology and Blood
   Transfusion
Leiden University Medical Center
Leiden, The Netherlands

John Mendelsohn, M.D.
President and Professor of Medicine
Department of Experimental Therapeutics
University of Texas M. D. Anderson Cancer Center
Houston, Texas

Malcolm A. S. Moore, Ph.D.
Professor of Medicine
Department of Cell Biology
Memorial Sloan-Kettering Cancer Center
New York, New York

Richard A. Morgan, Ph.D.
Clinical Gene Therapy Biologics
National Cancer Institute
National Institutes of Health
Bethesda, Maryland

James J. Mulé, Ph.D.
Maude T. Lane Professor of Surgical Immunology
Department of Surgery
University of Michigan Medical School
Ann Arbor, Michigan

Hyman B. Muss, M.D.
Professor of Medicine
Department of Hematology/Oncology
University of Vermont College of Medicine
Associate Director, Vermont Cancer Center
Fletcher Allen Health Care
Burlington, Vermont

Yuichi Obata, M.D.
Section Head
Laboratory of Immunology
Aichi Cancer Center Research Institute
Nagoya, Japan

Rienk Offringa, M.D.
Associate Professor
Department of Immunohematology and Blood
   Transfusion
Leiden University Medical Center
Leiden, The Netherlands

Hideho Okada, M.D., Ph.D.
Research Assistant Professor
Department of Neurological Surgery
University of Pittsburgh Medical Center
Pittsburgh, Pennsylvania

Lloyd J. Old, M.D.
Director
Ludwig Institute for Cancer Research
New York, New York

Michael S. O'Reilly, M.D.
Research Associate
Department of Surgical Research
Children's Hospital and Harvard Medical School
Boston, Massachusetts

Lee H. Pai-Scherf, M.D.
Clinical Investigator
Laboratory of Molecular Biology
National Cancer Institute
National Institutes of Health
Bethesda, Maryland

Dennis Panicali, Ph.D.
President and Chief Executive Officer
Therion Biologics Corporation
Cambridge, Massachusetts

Drew M. Pardoll, M.D., Ph.D.
Professor of Oncology, Medicine, Pathology, and Molecular
   Biology and Genetics
Department of Oncology
Johns Hopkins University School of Medicine
Baltimore, Maryland

Ira Pastan, M.D.
Laboratory of Molecular Biology
National Cancer Institute
National Institutes of Health
Bethesda, Maryland

Belur Patel, M.D.
Clinical Instructor
Department of Urology
University of California, Los Angeles, UCLA School of Medicine
Los Angeles, California

Xue Yuen Peng, Ph.D.
Postdoctoral Fellow
Department of Internal Medicine
Yale University School of Medicine
New Haven, Connecticut

James M. Pluda, M.D.
Senior Investigator
Investigational Drug Branch, Cancer Therapy Evaluation Program
National Cancer Institute
National Institutes of Health
Rockville, Maryland

Govindaswami Ragupathi, Ph.D.
Assistant Attending Immunologist
Assistant Laboratory Member
Department of Medicine, Clinical Immunology
    Service
Memorial Sloan-Kettering Cancer Center
New York, New York

Farhad Ravandi, M.B., B.S.
Junior Faculty Associate, Fellow
University of Texas M. D. Anderson Cancer Center
Houston, Texas

Nicholas P. Restifo, M.D.
Principal Investigator
National Cancer Institute
National Institutes of Health
Bethesda, Maryland

Paul F. Robbins, Ph.D.
Surgery Branch
National Cancer Institute
National Institutes of Health
Bethesda, Maryland

Bruce Roberts, Ph.D.
Senior Director, Cancer Gene Therapy
Genzyme Corporation
Framingham, Massachusetts

Michael J. Robertson, M.D.
Assistant Professor of Medicine
Bone Marrow and Stem Cell Transplantation Program
Indiana University School of Medicine
Indianapolis, Indiana

Cliona M. Rooney, Ph.D.
Associate Professor of Pediatrics
Center for Cell and Gene Therapy
Baylor College of Medicine
Houston, Texas

Steven A. Rosenberg, M.D., Ph.D.
Chief of Surgery
National Cancer Institute
National Institutes of Health
Bethesda, Maryland
Professor of Surgery
Uniformed Services University of the Health Sciences
    F. Hébert School of Medicine

Jack A. Roth, M.D.
Professor and Chairman
Section of Thoracic Molecular Oncology
Department of Thoracic and Cardiovascular Surgery
University of Texas M. D. Anderson Cancer Center
Houston, Texas

Michael L. Salgaller, Ph.D.
Director, Antigen Research and Discovery
Northwest Biotherapeutics, Inc.
Pacific Northwest Cancer Foundation
Seattle, Washington

Paul D. Savage, M.D.
Assistant Professor of Medicine
Molecular Genetics Program of Wake Forest University
Comprehensive Cancer Center of Wake Forest University
Wake Forest University School of Medicine
Winston-Salem, North Carolina

Matthew J. Scanlan, Ph.D.
Assistant Member
Ludwig Institute, New York Branch of Human Cancer
    Immunology
Memorial Sloan-Kettering Cancer Center
New York, New York

David A. Scheinberg, M.D., Ph.D.
Chief, Leukemia Service
Department of Medicine
Memorial Sloan-Kettering Cancer Center
New York, New York

Jeffrey Schlom, Ph.D.
Chief, Laboratory of Tumor Immunology and Biology
National Cancer Institute
National Institutes of Health
Bethesda, Maryland

Robert D. Schreiber, Ph.D.
Alumni Endowed Professor of Pathology
Department of Pathology
Washington University School of Medicine
St. Louis, Missouri

Scott M. Schuetze, M.D., Ph.D.
Research Associate
Clinical Research Division
Fred Hutchinson Cancer Research Center
Seattle, Washington

Douglas J. Schwartzentruber, M.D.
Senior Investigator
Surgery Branch
National Cancer Institute
National Institutes of Health
Division of Clinical Sciences
Bethesda, Maryland

George Sgouros, Ph.D.
Associate Member
Department of Medical Physics
Memorial Sloan-Kettering Cancer Center
New York, New York

Vijay Shankaran, A.B.
Graduate Student
Department of Pathology
Washington University School of Medicine
St. Louis, Missouri

Arun Shet, M.D.
Research Fellow
Division of Hematology/Oncology
Department of Internal Medicine
University of Illinois at Chicago College of Medicine
Chicago, Illinois

S. Shrimdkandada, M.D.
Genetic Therapy Program
Yale Cancer Center
Medical Oncology Section
Yale University School of Medicine
New Haven, Connecticut

Muthukumaran Sivanandham, M.D.
Research Manager
Assistant Professor
Surgical Research Laboratory
Saint Vincents Hospital and Medical Center
New York, New York

Jeffrey A. Sosman, M.D.
Associate Professor of Medicine
Director of Clinical Research
Department of Internal Medicine
University of Illinois at Chicago College of Medicine
Chicago, Illinois

Christos I. Stavropoulos, M.D.
Surgical Research Laboratory
Saint Vincents Hospital and Medical Center
New York, New York

C. A. Stein, M.D., Ph.D.
Associate Professor of Medicine and Pharmacology
Columbia University College of Physicians
   and Surgeons
New York, New York

Timothy Sullivan, B.A.
Department of Molecular and Cell Biology
University of California, Berkeley, School of Medicine
Berkeley, California

Mario Sznol
Head, Biologics Evaluation Section
Investigational Drug Branch
Cancer Therapy Evaluation Program
Division of Cancer Treatment and Diagnosis
National Cancer Institute
National Institutes of Health
Rockville, Maryland

Hideaki Tahara, M.D., Ph.D.
Department of Surgery
Institute of Medical Science
The University of Tokyo
Tokyo, Japan

Moshe Talpaz, M.D.
Professor of Medicine
Department of Bioimmunotherapy
University of Texas M. D. Anderson Cancer Center
Houston, Texas

Christopher Tretter, M.D.
Clinical Instructor
Department of Hematology/Oncology
Dartmouth-Hitchcock Medical Center
Lebanon, New Hampshire

Benoît J. Van den Eynde, M.D., Ph.D.
Ludwig Institute for Cancer Research
Université Catholique de Louvain
Brussels, Belgium

Sjoerd H. van der Burg, Ph.D.
Department of Immunohematology and Blood Transfusion
Leiden University Medical Center
Leiden, The Netherlands

Andrea van Elsas, M.D.
Department of Immunohematology and Blood Bank
Leiden University Medical Center
Leiden, The Netherlands

Margaret von Mehren, M.D.
Associate Member
Department of Medical Oncology
Fox Chase Cancer Center
Philadelphia, Pennsylvania

Thomas A. Waldmann, M.D.
Chief, Metabolism Branch
National Cancer Institute
National Institutes of Health
Bethesda, Maryland

Marc K. Wallack, M.D.
Professor of Surgery and Chairman
Department of Surgery
Saint Vincents Hospital and Medical Center
New York Medical College
New York, New York

Tao Wang, M.D.
Genetic Therapy Program
Yale Cancer Center
Medical Oncology Section
Yale University School of Medicine
New Haven, Connecticut

Louis M. Weiner, M.D.
Senior Member and Chairman
Department of Medical Oncology
Fox Chase Cancer Center
Philadelphia, Pennsylvania

Stephen A. White, M.D.
Hematology/Oncology Fellow
University of Alabama School of Medicine
Birmingham, Alabama

Bryan R. G. Williams, Ph.D.
Professor
Department of Cancer Biology
Lerner Research Institute
Cleveland Clinic Foundation
Cleveland, Ohio

Jo Hong Won, M.D.
Genetic Therapy Program
Yale Cancer Center
Medical Oncology Section
Yale University School of Medicine
New Haven, Connecticut

James Chung-Yin Yang, M.D.
Senior Investigator, Surgery Branch
National Cancer Institute
National Institutes of Health
Bethesda, Maryland

Lixin Zhang, M.D.
Genetic Therapy Program
Yale Cancer Center
Medical Oncology Section
Yale University School of Medicine
New Haven, Connecticut

Susan A. Zullo, Ph.D.
National Human Genome Research Institute
National Institutes of Health
Bethesda, Maryland

PREFACE

Progress in molecular biology and biotechnology has opened extraordinary opportunities for the development of new approaches to the treatment of patients with cancer. The molecular events underlying biologic processes are being increasingly understood. The application of recombinant DNA technology has made it possible to produce large amounts of biologic molecules previously available only in minute quantities. These developments have had a major impact on the treatment of patients with cancer, and this impact is likely to increase substantially in the near future.

This third edition of *Principles and Practice of the Biologic Therapy of Cancer* has been prepared to provide the scientific background and the practical information required to understand and apply developments in this emerging field. Leaders in the field of biologic therapy have provided their expertise for this text.

Each major area of biologic therapy is preceded by a chapter presenting the basic principles and preclinical studies that led to clinical applications. The clinical chapters present a comprehensive analysis of clinical data with an emphasis on the indications for treatment and the practical information necessary to safely apply these new approaches.

Since the first edition of this text was published in 1991, many biologic molecules, such as interleukin-2, α-interferon colony-stimulating factors, and a variety of monoclonal antibodies, have been approved for clinical use. Many other recombinant cytokines, antiangiogenic agents, monoclonal antibodies, and immunoregulatory molecules developed since that time are currently being evaluated in clinical trials. Technical developments have led to increased basic and applied studies in the fields of cancer vaccines and gene therapy, and each of these topics are presented in separate sections of the text.

Advances in biologic therapy will increasingly affect the practice of all oncologic specialties. This text has been designed to present state-of-the-art information to both research scientists and clinicians involved in the development and application of these new cancer treatments.

Steven A. Rosenberg, M.D., Ph.D.

PRINCIPLES AND PRACTICE OF THE BIOLOGIC THERAPY OF CANCER

Third Edition

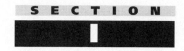

SECTION

I

PRINCIPLES AND PRACTICE OF CYTOKINE THERAPY

INTERLEUKINS: OVERVIEW

SCOTT K. DURUM

CYTOKINES

Nomenclature

Cytokines are proteins released by cells that react with receptors on other cells, triggering a response. Cytokines operate in all tissues, but some of the first to be studied and purified were involved in immune and inflammatory processes. In the late 1970s, a large committee of scientists created the interleukin (IL) terminology by applying "IL-1" and "IL-2" to two of the earliest cytokines. Since then, the discoverers of a new cytokine have sometimes pressed to term the protein an *interleukin*, which, although hard to remember, has never erred in being wildly optimistic [i.e., as in *tumor necrosis factor* (TNF), *oncostatin M,* or *leukemia inhibitory factor*]. Hundreds of cytokines are known, although this chapter covers only the 18 currently recognized interleukins. In the future, more cytokines will be discovered.

Clinical potential has driven cytokine research as much as scientific curiosity, judging from the proportion of cytokinology research performed in industry. Cytokines perform powerful activities, which, like those of hormones, are attractive as therapeutics. Cytokines have been difficult to harness, however, and not many have found a direct use in the clinic, except interferons (IFNs), colony-stimulating factors, and erythropoietin, which are not covered in this chapter. Small synthetic molecules that mimic or antagonize cytokines are a great hope. For each cytokine that has not been clinically used, I have tried to indicate some possibilities.

Preclinical and Clinical Studies

Cytokines have been extensively tested in rodents. In humans, IL-1, -2, -11, and -12 have been used in clinical trials. I am not able to summarize all of the preclinical therapeutic observations using the interleukins. When possible, I refer the reader to other reviews. *Ex vivo*, many cytokines have been used to expand human lymphocytes and hematopoietic stem cells, which then have been returned to the patient as a cellular therapy. This will undoubtedly be extended to *in vitro* growth of many other cell types and organs lost to pathologic processes, such as nerves, bones, liver, skin, and pancreas.

Pathologic Roles

Pathologic roles for some cytokines are implicated when their production is excessive or untimely or the reaction to the cytokines is excessive. Such pathology can derive from genetic proclivities or environmental circumstances. IL-1's production in excess is thought to be a key element in chronic inflammation, such as rheumatoid arthritis (RA), and possibly in septic shock. The IL-12 pathway is probably part of the pathology of parasitic diseases. IL-4 production is most likely part of allergy, whereas IL-5 production is probably part of asthma. Researchers strive to produce useful inhibitors of the cytokines. Several available inhibitors for blockade of receptors exist, such as IL-1RA, soluble forms of the cytokine receptors, and antibodies against ligands and receptors. In the future, researchers will create better inhibitors using rational drug design based on crystal structures of the cytokines, receptors, and signal transduction molecules. This same approach will also yield agonists.

Physiologic Roles

The physiologic roles of each cytokine are the primary focus in this chapter. Knockout mice have been produced for many of the interleukins and their receptors, and I have tried to cite papers that deal with this subject. These knockouts have been extremely informative in determining the physiologic roles of a cytokine. For example, knockouts showed that IL-7 is required for normal T-lymphocyte development, the basis of X-linked, severe combined immunodeficiency in man. Knockouts have been helpful in other ways when considering clinical problems. Knockouts showed that IL-4 is required to generate normal immunoglobulin (Ig) E levels, and because IL-4–deficient mice were otherwise fairly healthy, it supports the approach of blocking IL-4 in allergy. Another example is knockout of the IL-1 system, which affects susceptibility to inflammation of joints but has little ill effect on the health of mice, suggesting IL-1 blockade for treatment of arthritis.

Cytokines and Cancer

Two broad areas of cancer studies exist that have been impacted by cytokine research. Cytokine pathways can be involved in carcinogenesis and can be exploited in cancer therapy. I briefly discuss these areas.

Carcinogenesis

One major function of some cytokines is trophic: they are the signals from the microenvironment that tell a cell it is in the right place. Thus, when a normal cell is in the wrong place, it undergoes a kind of "atrophic" death. Trophic effects of cytokines are subverted by cancer cells, enabling them to live outside their normal microenvironments. In a few cases, tumor cells may make their own autocrines (e.g., IL-9 is implicated in Hodgkin's cells). Some cytokine receptors can mutate and become autosignaling, such as receptors for c-kit ligand, although none of the interleukin receptors seem to be capable of this. Some cytokine receptors normally suppress cell division or survival, which become inactivated in cancer; these include receptors for transforming growth-factor β and FasL, but, again, interleukin receptors are not among these.

Trophic mutations in cancer that are most relevant to the interleukins occur in their intracellular survival and death pathways. For example, Bcl-2, a mitochondrial protein that protects cells from death, is commonly induced by cytokines as part of their trophic activity and is commonly overexpressed in cancer cells. Moreover, blocking Bcl-2 production kills such cancer cells. Another example is Bax, a death protein that mediates death from cytokine withdrawal and is commonly inactivated by mutation in tumor cells. Thus, knowledge gained in understanding the trophic action of cytokines can have considerable bearing on the mechanisms of carcinogenesis.

Cancer Therapy

The following text covers the use of cytokines in cancer therapy. Here, I briefly mention that all the interleukins and many other cytokines have been tested on rodent tumors *in vitro* and *in vivo*. The types of antitumor effects include angiostasis, differentiation, and inflammation. Extending this research to humans has often produced toxicity and efficacy problems, although IFN is effective in treating hairy cell leukemia, and IL-2 has had positive effects in melanoma. Cytokines can be used to protect bone marrow and gut from the toxicity of radiation and chemotherapy. *Ex vivo* use of cytokines is widely used for expanding immune and hematopoietic cells before transfer into patients.

Omissions

For this extremely compressed review, I had to select a few cardinal points about each cytokine. I apologize for omitting many discoveries of probably equal importance. I particularly neglected to include studies in mice when human results were available. A major area I also neglected is the induction mechanisms of the cytokine genes because of its complexity. I have largely avoided discussing the promoters of these genes. Few mammalian genes exist, not just cytokines, whose induction is

understood. Although some proximal regulatory regions have been shown experimentally for most of these cytokine genes, these regions are usually shown to bind many interacting proteins and are influenced by distal regions. Major questions remain in understanding the accessibility of a gene, which is controlled by chromatin structure.

INTERLEUKIN-1

IL-1 (1,2) was among the earliest cytokines identified because it has so many potent activities. Many features of the IL-1 system, however, are not particularly representative of cytokines. IL-1 has an unusual mechanism of release from the cells that produce it. The two family members, α and β, are only distantly related but act on the same receptor. It has two dedicated inhibitors that block ligand-receptor interaction. IL-1 is a powerful inducer of inflammatory processes, both local and global, although knockout of the IL-1 system only modestly reduces these processes. Clinically, the main goals have been to block the IL-1 system in inflammatory states, such as RA and septic shock.

Proteins

Three members of the IL-1 family exist: α, β, and the receptor antagonist, encoded by a cluster of genes. IL-1α (3) and -β (4) have little homology to one another, but it is accurate to term them both *IL-1* because they act on the same receptor. Neither α nor β has a typical signal sequence, and both are released from the producing cell by an unusual mechanism. Mature 17-kd IL-1α is produced from a biologically inactive 31-kd precursor by cleavage (5) with caspase-1. Mature 17-kd IL-1α is also produced by cleavage from a different 31-kd precursor, which is biologically active. The receptor antagonist (6) is produced in two forms by alternative message splicing: one secreted form with a signal peptide and a second intracellular form lacking a signal peptide.

Producers

The most prolific IL-1–producing cells are macrophages following stimulation with a variety of microbial products or other agents, including cytokines. Many other cell types, such as keratinocytes, also produce IL-1. The IL-1 promoters are complex, perhaps accounting for the ability of these genes to respond to so many different stimuli in different cell types. In macrophages, the mechanism of IL-1 induction is partly based on the PU-1 transcription factor in cooperation with other nuclear factors (7,8). IL-1 production is also regulated by message stability, message translation, and the release mechanism. The receptor antagonist is produced concurrently with IL-1α and -β in many cell types, acting as a natural buffer to the action of IL-1.

Receptors and Cellular Response

Two IL-1 binding proteins exist: IL-1RI, which serves all known receptor function (9), and IL-1RII, which serves as a "decoy" receptor (10). These genes are also linked to the IL-1 gene cluster in humans, but not in mice. IL-1RI is a member of the "toll" family of receptors. After IL-1 binding, IL-1 receptor accessory proteins (11), a kinase [IL-2 receptor–associated kinase (IRAK)] (12) and TRAF6 (13), are recruited to the complex. IL-18 receptor forms a similar complex (see the section on IL-18). MyD88 serves as an adaptor protein, linking IRAK to the receptor complex (14). Intracellular cascades lead to activation of several types of transcription factors, including NFκB (15) and AP-1 (16). This results in the induction of many genes, including a number of other inflammatory cytokines, such as IL-6. A wide variety of cell types respond to IL-1. IL-18 signaling has many parallels with that of IL-1.

Activities

IL-1 is considered a key mediator of inflammation (2). It has a broad spectrum of inflammatory activities, including local effects, such as induction of prostaglandins, chemokines, and adhesion molecules. IL-1 also has global effects, such as fever, the acute-phase response, and hypotension. Knockout mice show deficiency in local inflammation and delayed-type hypersensitivity and are resistant to collagen-induced arthritis (17). The fact that IL-1 deficiency does not eliminate inflammation has been interpreted to mean that other cytokines with overlapping activities, such as TNF and IL-6, are equally important.

Clinical Use

Trials were performed in cancer patients (18) with some benefit in preventing thrombocytopenia induced by chemotherapy, but significant toxic side effects, such as hypotension, arrhythmia, and pulmonary-capillary leakage, occurred. Intratumoral injection in mouse cancers has shown promising responses. Blocking IL-1 activity via receptor antagonist, soluble receptors, or newly tailored drugs shows promise in controlling inflammatory diseases, such as RA and septic shock, probably most effectively if combined with blockade of other inflammatory cytokines, such as TNF and IL-6.

INTERLEUKIN-2

IL-2 was originally discovered as a growth factor for T cells *in vitro* and is one of the most extensively studied cytokines. Knockout of IL-2 in mice suggests complex regulatory roles, perhaps in programming T cells for death. The IL-2 receptor complex shares components with receptors for IL-4, -7, -9, and -15. IL-2 has been used clinically for acquired immunodeficiency syndrome, cancer, and for *ex vivo* expansion of T cells directed against tumors and viruses.

Protein

IL-2 (19,20) is 15 kd, contains one internal disulfide bond, and is a member of a family of cytokines (IL-4, -7, -9, and -15) containing α helixes.

Producers

IL-2 is produced by T lymphocytes after activation by antigen–major histocompatibility complexes (MHC) and costimulators on the surface of antigen-presenting cells. The T helper 1 (Th1) subset of memory T cells retains the capacity to produce IL-2, whereas the Th2 subset loses this capacity, producing IL-4 instead (21).

Receptor and Cellular Response

The IL-2 receptor comprises three chains: α (22), β (23), and γ$_c$ (24). The β and γ$_c$ chains are members of a cytokine receptor superfamily, whereas the α chain is related to IL-15Rα. The β and γ chains are essential for signaling, whereas the α chain increases affinity of the complex for IL-2 but is not required. After binding of IL-2, the janus kinase Jak3 (25,26), associated with the γ$_c$ chain, phosphorylates tyrosines on the β chain, which serve as docking sites for signal transducers and activators of transcription proteins (STATs) 3 and 5. The STATs (22,27) are then phosphorylated and translocate to the nucleus, where they serve as transcription factors. Many other intracellular second messenger pathways are also triggered by IL-2 (28) and involve lck, syk, ras, pI3 kinase, protein kinase C, and Akt. The γ$_c$ chain of the IL-2 receptor is shared by the receptors for IL-4, -7, -9, and -15. Jak3 is also a component of the signaling complex in these receptors.

Activities

The property that led to the discovery of IL-2 was its induction of activated T-cell proliferation (19). Thus, IL-2 is widely used for propagating T-cell lines. Knockout of IL-2 in mice (29), however, resulted in excessive, uncontrolled T-cell proliferation, leading to the concept that IL-2 is not essential for growth *in vivo*, but is essential for programming T cells to die. Other activities of IL-2 include stimulation of cytotoxicity in natural killer (NK) and T cells and acting as a cofactor in activating macrophages and B cells.

Clinical Use

IL-2 has been used clinically in several ways. Treatment of malignant melanoma renal cell carcinoma has shown efficacy (30,31). A significant side effect of IL-2 is the vascular leak syndrome (32). IL-2 has been used for *ex vivo* expansion of lymphokine-activated killer cells, tumor-infiltrating T cells (33), and antiviral T cells (34–36), which are then returned to the patient. Anti–IL-2 receptor shows promise in blocking rejection of organ transplants (37).

INTERLEUKIN-3

IL-3 is produced by activated T cells and induces hematopoiesis. Its receptor shares components with IL-5 and granulocyte-macrophage colony-stimulating factor (GM-CSF). It is used clinically to sustain explanted hematopoietic stem cells before reinfusion.

Proteins

IL-3 (38,39) is linked to IL-4, -5, -9, and -13 in humans.

Producers

Activated T cells are the major producers of IL-3 (40). Activated mast cells are also producers.

Receptors

Two chains that compose the IL-3 receptor exist in humans: IL-3Rα (41) and β$_c$ (42), which are shared by the receptors for GM-CSF and IL-5. In the mouse, two different β chains exist. Both α and β are members of the cytokine receptor superfamily. Cross-linking of the α to the β chain triggers receptor activation (43). The nature of this cross-linking process is thought to resemble that of the IL-2 and IL-4 receptors, in that the ligand directly binds one chain with intermediate affinity (see the sections on IL-2 and IL-4). The second receptor chain, which cannot bind ligand on its own, then recognizes some features of the complex formed by the ligand and the other receptor component. Jak2 is associated with the β chain (44) and activates STAT 5 (45). A number of other second messenger pathways are also activated (46). The cellular response includes survival, such as the pathway leading to disposal of BAD, the proapoptotic protein (46,47).

Activities

IL-3 stimulates production of macrophages, granulocytes, erythrocytes, and megakaryocytes from primitive pluripotential stem cells. Knockouts indicate that IL-3 is not required during normal hematopoiesis, indicating its importance probably lies in the hematopoietic stimulation during immune responses. Mature myelomonocytic-lineage cells also react to IL-3.

Clinical Use

IL-3 has been tested extensively for a variety of potential clinical uses (48). In individuals with normal hematopoiesis, IL-3 treatment increased platelets, reticulocytes, and leukocytes and showed only mild side effects (49). To increase hematopoiesis, IL-3 has been tested in myelodysplastic syndrome, aplastic anemia, Diamond-Blackfan anemia, chemotherapy, bone marrow transplantation, and stem-cell mobilization. Although responses were observed, it has not been adopted as a therapeutic. IL-3 is widely used as part of a cytokine cocktail to sustain hematopoietic stem cells *ex vivo*, however, for treatment after radiation or chemotherapy (i.e., promoting introduction of recombinant constructs for gene therapy) (50,51).

INTERLEUKIN-4

IL-4 is an important cofactor in B-lymphocyte activation, particularly for production of IgE. One type of IL-4 receptor incorporates γ$_c$, as do IL-2, -7, -9, and -15. IL-4 is closely related to IL-13 and can share some receptor components and signaling pathways. It is critical in directing activated T cells into the Th2 pathway. Overproduction is implicated in atopy.

Proteins

IL-4 (52–54) is 20 kd with six cysteines involved in intrachain disulfide bonds and forms four α helices. The human IL-4 gene is found in a cluster together with genes for IL-3, -5, -9, and -13.

Producers

Several types of T cells produce IL-4 after activation by antigen-MHC complexes and costimulators on the surface of antigen-presenting cells (21). IL-4 is a key member of the spectrum of cytokines produced by Th2 T cells. In mice, CD4 T cells that express NK1 are also producers, as are a subset of CD8 T cells. Mast cells and basophils also produce IL-4 (55). The induction of Th2 cell development is dependent on IL-4 produced by T cells themselves (56). Production of IL-4 requires the transcription factor GATA3 (57) and possibly c-maf (58).

Receptors

The primary binding chain, IL-4Rα (59), forms two types of receptor complexes: IL-4Rα + γ$_c$ and IL-4Rα + IL-13Rα. (60). These receptor chains are members of the cytokine receptor superfamily. IL-4 first binds to IL-4Rα; γ$_c$ is then recruited to the complex. The janus kinase Jak3, bound to the intracellular domain of γ$_c$, is required for many, but not all, IL-4 effects (61). STAT 6 is required for IL-4 signaling (62). IRS-1 is an important adaptor molecule, coupling the receptor to second messenger pathways other than the Jak–STAT pathway (60,63).

Activities

IL-4 was discovered as a growth factor for preactivated B cells and induces class II MHC expression on B cells. In macrophages, it suppresses production of inflammatory cytokines and it has effects on endothelial cells and fibroblasts. Knockout mice show major defects in Th2-cell generation and in IgE production (64), suggesting that the selective value of IL-4 may be immunity against parasitic infections.

Clinical Use

An overactive IL-4 pathway appears to be one component of atopy (65–67). Therefore, IL-4 presents a therapeutic target for allergy. IL-4 itself could be used to divert immunity away from autoimmune or inflammatory directions.

INTERLEUKIN-5

IL-5 induces production of eosinophils during immune responses, which probably contributes to protection against some kinds of parasites. It shares a receptor component with IL-3 and GM-CSF.

Proteins

IL-5 (68,69) is a disulfide-linked homodimer, which is unusual among the interleukins and is heavily glycosylated. Its crystal structure resembles that of two IL-4 molecules with two bundles, each with four α helices (70). It is genetically linked to IL-3, -4, -9, and -13 in humans (68).

Producers

IL-5 is produced by activated Th2 cells (21), as well as mast cells and eosinophils.

Receptors

The receptors for IL-5 consist of two chains: IL-5Rα (71) and β_c (42), which is shared by the receptors for GM-CSF and IL-3. Both chains are members of the cytokine receptor superfamily. Cross-linking principles are similar to IL-3, as are the ensuing Jak2–STAT5 pathways and other second messenger pathways (46).

Activities

IL-5 was initially identified as a T-cell factor that induced production of eosinophils (72). Knockout of IL-5 eliminated the eosinophilia induced by helminth infection (73), whereas baseline production of eosinophils was normal. IL-5 also promotes local accumulation (74) and sustains the lifespan and function of eosinophils in tissues, such as the lung and bowel. Evidence exists that IL-5, presumably via its eosinophil activities, contributes to protection from helminth infections (75,76).

Clinical Use

IL-5 has long been implicated in allergic asthma (77). Efforts are therefore being made to develop IL-5 antagonists (78).

INTERLEUKIN-6

IL-6 is a key inflammatory mediator produced by many cell types. It is the major inducer of the acute-phase response and fever. IL-6 receptor shares the gp130 chain with several other cytokine receptors.

Proteins

IL-6 is a glycoprotein of 21 to 28 kd.

Producers

IL-6 is produced after stimulation by many cell types, including T and B lymphocytes, macrophages, fibroblasts, and endothelial cells.

Receptors

Two components of the IL-6 receptor exist: a ligand-specific α chain (79) and a signal-transducing gp130 chain (80), which is shared by receptors for leukocyte inhibitory factor (LIF), oncostatin M (OSM), ciliary neurotrophic factor (CNTF), IL-11, and CT-1. The α chain binds IL-6. This complex then cross-links multiple gp130 chains, initiating signal transduction. Unlike many cytokine receptors, the α chain has no intracellular signaling function in this class of receptors. The janus kinases Jak1, Jak2, and Tyk2 are activated, as are the transcription factors STATs 1, 3, and 5, as well as other signal transduction pathways, such as the ras-MAP kinase pathway (81).

Activities

IL-6 (82,83) was originally characterized based on its activity in inducing Ig synthesis by activating B cells. Knockout of IL-6 (84,85) showed defects in a number of inflammatory processes, including production of acute-phase reactants and bone loss after estrogen depletion. Fever responses depend on IL-6 (86). Hematopoietic defects were also found in IL-6 knockouts (87).

Clinical Use

Blocking IL-6 may alleviate RA and may also be effective in other autoimmune, inflammatory, and bone-erosive diseases. In mice, IL-6 is required for development of oil-induced plasmacytomas (88) and is involved in tumor cachexia (89). In humans, IL-6 is a growth factor for myelomas (90), suggesting further applications of IL-6 blockers.

INTERLEUKIN-7

IL-7 is produced by stromal cells and is essential for T lymphopoiesis, partly because of a survival or "trophic" effect, a partial role in V(D)J recombination. This is the pathway deficient in X-linked, severe combined immunodeficiency in humans. IL-7 also has trophic effects on mature T and B lymphocytes and is therefore potentially useful in the clinic as an adjuvant.

Proteins

IL-7 is a 25-kd protein predicted to contain four α helices and an internal disulfide bond (91). After secretion, it binds to extracellular matrix via a glycosaminoglycan-binding site (92), which could be the form encountered by developing thymocytes.

Producers

Unlike most interleukins, IL-7 is produced constitutively by nonhematopoietic cells. In the thymus, the IL-7 producer resembles the cortical epithelial cell (93). In bone marrow, the producer is a reticular stromal cell (94). Other sources include the intestine (95), skin (96), and follicular dendritic cells (94).

Receptors

The primary binding chain for IL-7 is IL-7Rα (97). The IL-7–IL-7Rα complex then recruits γ_c (98,99), bearing Jak3 to the complex. TSLP, a homologue of IL-7, also binds the IL-7Rα chain but does not recruit γ_c and Jak3 (100). Jak1 and a number of other kinases are induced (101), including pI3 kinase. STATs 3 and 5 partly mediate the nuclear effects. Because γ_c is also a component of the receptors for IL-2, -4, -9, and -15, some similarities appear to exist in the signal transduction pathways.

Activities

IL-7 was discovered based on its activity in inducing proliferation of murine pro-B cells (91). B-cell development depends on IL-7 in mice, but not humans (102). Normal T-cell development requires IL-7 based on the knockout phenotypes for IL-7 (103) and its receptor (104), which show a severe block at an early stage in T-cell development. A related block is seen in X-linked, severe combined immunodeficiency in humans, which is in γ_c, a component of the IL-7 receptor. This requirement for IL-7 is partly attributed to its trophic activity on lymphoid progenitors (105) and its promotion of V(D)J recombination (106). In mice, the γσ lineage is particularly dependent on IL-7, perhaps not only during thymic generation, but also for survival in the intestine and skin. Pharmacologic activity of IL-7 has been observed in mice, inducing increases in B and T cells (107,108). Overexpression of IL-7 in mice can induce lymphomagenesis (109). In human skin, IL-7 may provide trophic support for the survival of lymphoma cells (110).

Clinical Use

IL-7 has not been tested clinically. Potential clinical uses of IL-7 include boosting immunity to infectious diseases or prolonging the life of lymphocytes, as in acquired immunodeficiency syndrome. Antagonists to IL-7 might be effective in treating autoimmune diseases, blocking rejection of allografted organs, or treating lymphoma.

INTERLEUKIN-8

IL-8 induces chemotaxis and activation of neutrophils. It is one of the chemokines, a large group of chemotactic cytokines. IL-8 signals through seven transmembrane G protein–coupled receptors that are related to other chemokine receptors.

Proteins

IL-8 (111–114) is a 6- to 8-kd glycoprotein containing two intrachain disulfide bonds. At high concentrations, IL-8 homodimerizes via hydrogen bonding. It is presented to neutrophils on endothelial cell surfaces (115). IL-8 was the first to be discovered of the family of cytokines known as *chemokines* (116). More than 50 members have been identified; only IL-8 has the interleukin terminology. IL-8 is one of a subgroup termed *CXC chemokines* and is linked to a group of these genes. Mice lack a close homologue to human IL-8. It is thought that its inflammatory roles are fulfilled in mice by other chemokines using the same receptor.

Producers

Many cell types produce IL-8 after stimulation with lipopolysaccharide, IL-1, or TNF (117), including macrophages, endothelial cells, and keratinocytes.

Receptors

Two functional IL-8 receptors exist: CXCR1 (118) and CXCR2 (119,120). They are both members of the seven-transmembrane family of receptors that includes rhodopsin. These receptors also respond to other chemokines. The two receptors induce some overlapping and distinct responses (121). Receptors are coupled to G proteins, including Gi2α (122), which trigger downstream events involving phospholipase C, diacylglycerol, inositol triphosphate, release of calcium from intracellular stores, RhoA, and the ras pathway.

Activities

IL-8 induces neutrophil chemotaxis, respiratory burst, and degranulation. In rabbits, blocking IL-8 with antibodies has potent inhibitory effects on some inflammatory processes, particularly of the lung (123–125). Knockouts in mice cannot directly address IL-8 function because no close IL-8 homologue exists in mice. Mice lack CXCR1. Knockout of the receptor CXCR2, however, greatly affects neutrophil attraction to inflamed peritoneum (126), which establishes that chemokines are involved in neutrophil accumulation *in vivo*. IL-8 also induces angiogenesis (127).

Clinical Use

Increased IL-8 is detected in a variety of human clinical conditions, ranging from myocardial infarction to RA (128), and suggests potential applications for IL-8 blockers. In rabbits, a number of studies have shown that anti–IL-8 inhibits inflammation of various tissues. Despite the numerous chemokines that exist, blocking IL-8 alone can be sufficient.

INTERLEUKIN-9

IL-9 is related to IL-2, -4, -7, and -15 and has some overlapping activities based most likely on sharing some receptor components. It is produced by T cells and acts on lymphocytes and mast cells, and may be involved in Hodgkin's disease and lymphoma.

Proteins

IL-9 (129,130) is predicted to have an α-helical topology like IL-2, -4, -7, and -15. The human IL-9 gene is found in a cluster together with genes for IL-3, -4, -5, -9, and -13. This does not apply to mice. Ten cysteines exist, implying extensive intrachain disulfide bonding, heavy *N*-linked glycosylation, and a high isoelectric point (approximately ten).

Producers

Memory-helper T cells produce IL-9 after activation (131). This induction involves a cascade of cytokines, including IL-2, -4, and -10, eventually leading to IL-9 production (132). Murine Th2 clones are producers (133).

Receptors

The IL-9 receptor α chain (134) is a member of the hematopoietin superfamily. In humans, the IL-9 receptor α chain is unusual because it is encoded on chromosomes X and Y (135). Four IL-9Rα pseudogenes also exist. The receptor complex shares the γ_c chain (136) with receptors for IL-2, -4, -7, and -15. After receptor ligation, Jak3 (γ_c-associated) and Jak1 (IL-9Rα–associated) increase their tyrosine kinase activity, phosphorylating the IL-9Rα chain, adaptor protein IRS-1 (137), and transcription factors STATs 1, 3, and 5 (138,139).

Activities

IL-9 was discovered as a growth factor for T-cell clones (129) and independently as a growth factor for mast-cell lines (130, 140). It is not clear, however, whether a normal T-cell growth role should be ascribed to IL-9 because normal T cells have not been found to proliferate in response to it until after 10 days or so of prior *in vitro* stimulation. Some transformed T cells, however, can respond to IL-9, and human T-cell leukemia–transformed T cells produce it (141); overexpression of IL-9 as a transgene induced T-cell transformation (142), suggesting possible autocrine function. This was also suggested for Hodgkin's disease (143). Mast cells and eosinophils, B lymphocytes (144), and hematopoietic stem cells (145) also respond to IL-9. Because its receptor is a member of the γ_c family, overlapping activities are expected to be present with other cytokines in this group.

Clinical Use

No extensive preclinical data on IL-9 are present. The possibility that it has autocrine activity in Hodgkin's disease and T lymphomas suggests potential uses for IL-9 antagonists.

INTERLEUKIN-10

IL-10 is a powerful inhibitor of inflammatory and immune responses, partly via its inhibition of some macrophage functions. It is produced by Th2 cells. Its receptor is related to IFN receptors.

Proteins

Human IL-10 is an 18-kd monomer with little glycosylation and two presumed intrachain disulfide bonds.

Producers

Activated Th2 cells were the originally described IL-10 producers. Other cell types, including macrophages and keratinocytes, however, also produce IL-10. Epstein-Barr virus encodes an active IL-10 homologue (146).

Receptors and Cellular Response

The first identified component of IL-10 receptor (147,148) is related to the IFN receptors. It is expressed by many types of hematopoietic cells. In mice, a second receptor component, CRF2-4, has been identified (149), which is related and linked to the IFN receptors. Jak1 and Tyk2 are activated by IL-10 (150). STAT 3 mediates some downstream effects in macrophages (151).

Activities

IL-10 was originally discovered and cloned (152) as an inhibitor of the ability of Th1 cells to synthesize IFN. This inhibition is largely via effects on antigen-presenting cells, such as macrophages, especially by inhibiting their IL-12 production. Other macrophage functions are also inhibited, such as synthesis of inflammatory cytokines (i.e., IL-1, IL-6, IL-8, and TNF) and phagocytosis. IL-10 knockout mice show extensive pathology, particularly in the gut, thought to arise from unattenuated immune responses to gut flora (153). Receptor knockout mice have similar pathology (149).

Clinical Use

IL-10 has been shown to inhibit some lipopolysaccharide-induced inflammatory responses in humans (154). Clinical trials are under way in inflammatory bowel disease, RA, thoracic-abdominal aortic surgery, acute lung injury, multiple sclerosis, psoriasis, and human immunodeficiency virus infection (155). Evidence exists that the Epstein-Barr virus IL-10 homologue acts as an autocrine in B lymphomas, suggesting benefit in blocking IL-10 (156,157).

INTERLEUKIN-11

IL-11 is a mesenchymal cell product with activity on hematopoietic cells. IL-11 has been used to promote hematopoiesis in patients. IL-11 receptor shares the gp130 component with IL-6, LIF, OSM, CNTF, and CT-1. IL-11 is required for embryonic implantation in the uterus.

Proteins

IL-11 (158) is a 19-kd protein with no intrachain disulfide bonds. IL-11 is slightly homologous to IL-6, OSM, and LIF.

Producers

IL-11 is produced by a variety of mesenchymal cells, including keratinocytes, chondrocytes, osteoblasts, fibroblasts, and bone marrow stromal cells (159).

Receptors and Cellular Response

The IL-11 receptor includes a ligand-specific α chain and gp130, which is common to IL-6, LIF, OSM, CNTF, and CT1. Two alternative α chains exist in the mouse. The ligand-binding chains of this family do not contribute to signaling, which is wholly performed by gp130. Thus, the intracellular cascades should be the same for all members (see the section on IL-6 for a discussion of gp130 signaling). As in the IL-6 system, soluble IL-11 receptor can capture its ligand and then associate with cell-bound gp130 and signal (160).

Activities

IL-11 was identified based on promoting growth of a plasmacytoma line (158,159). It stimulates multilineage hematopoiesis when administered to mice and humans and is particularly effective in stimulating thrombopoiesis by inducing production of megakaryocytes. Knockout of the major receptor did not show a requirement in hematopoiesis (161) but revealed an IL-11 requirement in the uterine response to implantation (162).

Clinical Use

Trials performed in breast cancer patients show that IL-11 can significantly restore suppressed hematopoiesis and alleviate thrombocytopenia induced by chemotherapy (163). In mice, IL-11 also protects intestinal cells from damage induced by chemo- and radiotherapy (164).

INTERLEUKIN-12

IL-12 is produced by antigen-presenting cells. IL-12 promotes Th1-cell development and IFN production. It is required for development of some types of autoimmunity in mice.

Proteins

IL-12 (165–167) is a heterodimer consisting of disulfide-linked 35-kd and 40-kd subunits encoded by distinct genes. Both subunits are glycosylated and have intrachain disulfide bonds. Homodimers of p40 are also observed (168) and in mice have receptor-antagonist activity. This does not apply to humans.

Producers

Macrophages, B lymphocytes, and dendritic cells are major producers of IL-12. In macrophages, this synthesis is stimulated by microbial products and during contact with T cells via CD40L–CD40 interaction (169). The two IL-12 chains associate intracellularly before secretion. The p35 subunit is expressed by a much wider range of cell types than the p40 subunit (166,170).

Receptors and Cellular Response

Two components comprise the IL-12 receptor, the β 1 and β 2 chains (171,172). Th2 cells fail to respond to IL-12 because they lack the β 2 chain (173). Many protein kinases are triggered by the IL-12 receptor, including the Janus kinases tyk2 and Jak2 (174), which are associated with the β 1 and β 2 chains, respectively (175). STAT 3, STAT 4, and IRF-1 are implicated in gene induction by IL-12 (176,177).

Activities

IL-12 was discovered as a factor promoting cytotoxic T cells and independently for promoting NK cells. These activities include proliferation, differentiation, and cytokine secretion, especially IFN. The IFN-γ–inducing activity of IL-12 is as a cofactor, such as with IL-18 (see the section on IL-18). IL-12 knockout mice (178) showed greatly suppressed IFN production and revealed a requirement for IL-12 in development of Th1 cells in some settings, but not in others (179).

Clinical Use

IL-12 has been tested in cancer patients in phase 1 trials with no major toxicity other than a decrease in circulating lymphocytes, which, nevertheless, showed increased activity (180). In preclinical studies, antitumor activity of IL-12 was detected (181), and increased effects were seen in combination with a pulse of IL-2 (182). In mice, IL-12 is a required component of some types of autoimmunity in tissues, including the bowel, joint, eye, pancreas, and central nervous system (183).

INTERLEUKIN-13

IL-13 is a T-cell product closely related to IL-4 and shares a receptor component. It elicits a subset of IL-4 responses and is implicated in Th2-cell generation and IgE synthesis. IL-13 is antiinflammatory.

Proteins

IL-13 (184) is 12 kd and structurally related to IL-4, although the homology is low (185,186). The gene is clustered together with IL-3, -4, -5, and -9.

Producers

IL-13 is expressed in Th2 cells after activation by antigen-MHC complexes and costimulators on the surface of antigen-presenting cells. Unlike IL-4, IL-13 expression is not strictly repressed in Th1 cells. IL-13 is also produced by dendritic cells.

Receptors and Cellular Response

The IL-13 receptor is comprised of IL-13Rα together with IL-4Rα. The same receptor complex also responds to IL-4. Two homologous IL-13Rα chains exist with different affinities for IL-13 in the absence of IL-4Rα: a high-affinity α2 chain (187) and a low-affinity α1 chain (188). Receptors are expressed on

88. Hilbert DM, Kopf M, Mock BA, Kohler G, Rudikoff S. Interleukin 6 is essential for *in vivo* development of B lineage neoplasms. *J Exp Med* 1995;182:243–248.

89. Strassmann G, Kambayashi T. Inhibition of experimental cancer cachexia by anti-cytokine and anti-cytokine-receptor therapy. *Cytokines Mol Ther* 1995;1:107–113.

90. Hawley RG, Berger LC. Growth control mechanisms in multiple myeloma. *Leuk Lymphoma* 1998;29:465–475.

91. Namen AE, Lupton S, Hjerrild K, et al. Stimulation of B-cell progenitors by cloned murine interleukin-7. *Nature* 1988;333:571–573.

92. Kitazawa H, Muegge K, Badolato R, et al. IL-7 activates $\alpha4\beta1$ integrin in murine thymocytes. *J Immunol* 1997;159:2259–2264.

93. Oosterwegel MA, Haks MC, Jeffry U, Murray R, Kruisbeek AM. Induction of TCR gene rearrangements in uncommitted stem cells by a subset of IL-7 producing, MHC class-II-expressing thymic stromal cells. *Immunity* 1997;6:351–360.

94. Funk PE, Stephan RP, Witte PL. Vascular cell adhesion molecule 1-positive reticular cells express interleukin-7 and stem cell factor in the bone marrow. *Blood* 1995;86:2661–2671.

95. Watanabe M, Ueno Y, Yajima T, et al. Interleukin-7 is produced by human intestinal epithelial cells and regulates the proliferation of intestinal mucosal lymphocytes. *J Clin Invest* 1995;95:2945–2953.

96. Kroncke R, Loppnow H, Flad HD, Gerdes J. Human follicular dendritic cells and vascular cells produce interleukin-7: a potential role for interleukin-7 in the germinal center reaction. *Eur J Immunol* 1996;26:2541–2544.

97. Goodwin RG, Friend D, Ziegler SF, et al. Cloning of the human and murine interleukin-7 receptors: demonstration of a soluble form and homology to a new receptor superfamily. *Cell* 1990;60:941–951.

98. Noguchi M, Nakamura Y, Russell SM, et al. Interleukin-2 receptor gamma chain: a functional component of the interleukin-7 receptor. *Science* 1993;262:1877–1880.

99. Kondo M, Takeshita T, Higuchi M, et al. Functional participation of the IL-2 receptor gamma chain in IL-7 receptor complexes. *Science* 1994;263:1453–1454.

100. Levin SD, Koelling RM, Friend SL, et al. Thymic stromal lymphopoietin: a cytokine that promotes the development of IgM+ B cells *in vitro* and signals via a novel mechanism. *J Immunol* 1999; 162:677–683.

101. Foxwell BM, Beadling C, Guschin D, Kerr I, Cantrell D. Interleukin-7 can induce the activation of Jak 1, Jak 3 and STAT 5 proteins in murine T cells. *Eur J Immunol* 1995;25:3041–3046.

102. Prieyl JA, LeBien TW. Interleukin 7 independent development of human B cells. *Proc Natl Acad Sci U S A* 1996;93:10348–10353.

103. von Freeden-Jeffry U, Vieira P, Lucian LA, McNeil T, Burdach SE, Murray R. Lymphopenia in interleukin 7 gene-deleted mice identifies IL-7 as a nonredundant cytokine. *J Exp Med* 1995;181: 1519–1526.

104. Peschon JJ, Morrissey PJ, Grabstein KH, et al. Early lymphocyte expansion is severely impaired in interleukin-7 receptor-deficient mice. *J Exp Med* 1994;180:1955–1960.

105. Kim K, Lee CK, Sayers TJ, Muegge K, Durum SK. The trophic action of IL-7 on pro-T cells: inhibition of apoptosis of pro-T1, -T2, -T3 cells correlates with Bcl-2 and Bax levels and is independent of Fas and p53 pathways. *J Immunol* 1998;160:5735–5741.

106. Muegge K, Vila MP, Durum SK. Interleukin-7: a cofactor for VDJ rearrangement of the T cell receptor beta gene. *Science* 1993;261:93–95.

107. Morrissey PJ, Conlon P, Charrier K, et al. Administration of IL-7 to normal mice stimulates B-lymphopoiesis and peripheral lymphadenopathy. *J Immunol* 1991;147:561–568.

108. Komschlies KL, Gregorio TA, Gruys ME, Back TC, Faltynek CR, Wiltrout RH. Administration of recombinant human IL-7 to mice alters the composition of B-lineage cells and T cell subsets, enhances T cell function, induces regression of established metastases. *J Immunol* 1994;152:5776–5784.

109. Rich BE, Campos-Torres J, Tepper RI, Moreadith RW, Leder P. Cutaneous lymphoproliferation and lymphomas in interleukin-7 transgenic mice. *J Exp Med* 1993;177:305–316.

110. Dalloul A, Laroche L, Bagot M, et al. Interleukin-7 is a growth factor for Sezary lymphoma cells. *J Clin Invest* 1992;90:1054–1060.

111. Yoshimura T, Matsushima K, Tanaka S, et al. Purification of a human monocyte-derived neutrophil chemotactic factor that has peptide sequence similarity to other host defense cytokines. *Proc Natl Acad Sci U S A* 1987;84:9233–9237.

112. Walz A, Peveri P, Aschauer H, Baggiolini M. Purification and amino acid sequencing of NAF, a novel neutrophil-activating factor produced by monocytes. *Biochem Biophys Res Commun* 1987;149: 755–761.

113. Schroder JM, Mrowietz U, Morita E, Christophers E. Purification and partial biochemical characterization of a human monocyte-derived, neutrophil-activating peptide that lacks interleukin-1 activity. *J Immunol* 1987;139:3474–3483.

114. Schmid J, Weissmann C. Induction of mRNA for a serine protease and a beta-thromboglobulin-like protein in mitogen-stimulated human leukocytes. *J Immunol* 1987;139:250–256.

115. Middleton J, Neil S, Wintle J, et al. Transcytosis and surface presentation of IL-8 by venularendothelial cells. *Cell* 1997;91:385–395.

116. Wang JM, Su S, Gong W, Oppenheim JJ. Chemokines, receptors, and their role in cardiovascular pathology. *Int J Clin Lab Res* 1998;28:83–90.

117. Baggiolini M, Dewald B, Moser B. Interleukin-8 and related chemotactic cytokines—CXC and CC chemokines. *Adv Immunol* 1994;55: 97–179.

118. Murphy PM, Tiffany HL. Cloning of complementary DNA encoding a functional human interleukin-8 receptor. *Science* 1991;253: 1280–1283.

119. Holmes WE, Lee J, Kuang WJ, Rice GC, Wood WI. Structure and functional expression of a human interleukin-8 receptor. *Science* 1991;253:1278–1280.

120. Murphy PM. Neutrophil receptors for interleukin-8 and related CXC chemokines. *Semin Hematol* 1997;34:311–318.

121. Jones SA, Wolf M, Qin S, Mackay CR, Baggiolini M. Different functions for the interleukin-8 receptors IL-8R of human neutrophil leukocytes: NADPH oxidase and phospholipase D are activated through IL-8R1 but not IL-8R2. *Proc Natl Acad Sci U S A* 1996;93:6682–6686.

122. Damaj BB, McColl SR, Mahana W, Crouch MF, Naccache PH. Physical association of Gi2alpha with interleukin-8 receptors. *J Biol Chem* 1996;271:12783–12789.

123. Sekido N, Mukaida N, Harada A, Nakanishi I, Watanabe Y, Matsushima K. Prevention of lung reperfusion injury in rabbits by a monoclonal antibody against interleukin-8. *Nature* 1993;365:654–657.

124. Broaddus VC, Boylan AM, Hoeffel JM, et al. Neutralization of IL-8 inhibits neutrophil influx in a rabbit model of endotoxin-induced pleurisy. *J Immunol* 1994;152:2960–2967.

125. Folkesson HG, Matthay MA, Hebert CA, Broaddus VC. Acid aspiration-induced lung injury in rabbits is mediated by interleukin-8-dependent mechanisms. *J Clin Invest* 1995;96:107–116.

126. Cacalano G, Lee J, Kikly K, et al. Neutrophil and B cell expansion in mice that lack the murine IL-8 receptor homolog. *Science* 1994;265: 682–684.

127. Moore BB, Arenberg DA, Addison CL, Keane MP, Strieter RM. Tumor angiogenesis is regulated by CXC chemokines. *J Lab Clin Med* 1998;132:97–103.

128. Harada A, Mukaida N, Matsushima K. Interleukin-8 as a novel target for intervention therapy in acute inflammatory diseases. *Mol Med Today* 1996;2:482–489.

129. Van Snick J, Goethals A, Renauld JC, et al. Cloning and characterization of a cDNA for a new mouse T cell growth factor P40. *J Exp Med* 1989;169:363–368.

130. Hultner L, Druez C, Moeller J, et al. Mast cell growth-enhancing activity MEA is structurally related and functionally identical to the novel mouse T cell growth factor P40/TCGFIII interleukin-9. *Eur J Immunol* 1990;20:1413–1416.

131. Renauld JC, Goethals A, Houssiau F, Merz H, Van Roost E, Van Snick J. Human P40/IL-9. Expression in activated CD4+ T cells, genomic organization, and comparison with the mouse gene. *J Immunol* 1990;144:4235–4241.

132. Houssiau FA, Renauld JC, Fibbe WE, Van Snick J. IL-2 dependence of IL-9 expression in human T lymphocytes. *J Immunol* 1992;148: 3147–3151.

133. Gessner A, Blum H, Rollinghoff M. Differential regulation of IL-9-expression after infection with Leishmania major in susceptible and resistant mice. *Immunobiology* 1993;189:419–435.

134. Renauld JC, Druez C, Kermouni A, et al. Expression cloning of the murine and human interleukin-9 receptor cDNAs. *Proc Natl Acad Sci U S A* 1992;89:5690–5694.

135. Vermeesch JR, Petit P, Kermouni A, Renauld JC, Van Den Berghe H, Marynen P. The IL-9 receptor gene, located in the Xq/Yq pseudoautosomal region, has an autosomal origin, escapes X inactivation and is expressed from the Y. *Hum Mol Genet* 1997;6:1–8.

136. Kimura Y, Takeshita T, Kondo M, et al. Sharing of the IL-2 receptor gamma chain with the functional IL-receptor complex. *Int Immunol* 1995;7:115–120.

137. Yin T, Tsang ML, Yang YC. JAK1 kinase forms complexes with interleukin-4 receptor and 4PS/insulin receptor substrate-1-like protein and is activated by interleukin-4 and interleukin-9 in T lymphocytes. *J Biol Chem* 1994;269:26614–26617.

138. Demoulin JB, Uyttenhove C, Van Roost E, et al. A single tyrosine of the interleukin-9 (IL-9) receptor is required for STAT activation, antiapoptotic activity, growth regulation by IL-9. *Mol Cell Biol* 1996;16:4710–4716.

139. Bauer JH, Liu KD, You Y, Lai SY, Goldsmith MA. Heteromerization of the gamma c chain with the interleukin-9 receptor alpha subunit leads to STAT activation and prevention of apoptosis. *J Biol Chem* 1998;273:9255–9260.

140. Yang YC, Ricciardi S, Ciarletta A, Calvetti J, Kelleher K, Clark SC. Expression cloning of cDNA encoding a novel human hematopoietic growth factor: human homologue of murine T-cell growth factor P40. *Blood* 1989;74:1880–1884.

141. Kelleher K, Bean K, Clark SC, et al. Human interleukin-9: genomic sequence, chromosomal location, sequences essential for its expression in human T-cell leukemia virus HTLV-I-transformed human T cells. *Blood* 1991;77:1436–1441.

142. Renauld JC, van der Lugt N, Vink A, et al. Thymic lymphomas in interleukin 9 transgenic mice. *Oncogene* 1994;9:1327–1332.

143. Merz H, Houssiau FA, Orscheschek K, et al. Interleukin-9 expression in human malignant lymphomas: unique association with Hodgkin's disease and large cell anaplastic lymphoma. *Blood* 1991;78:1311–1317.

144. Petit-Frere C, Dugas B, Braquet P, Mencia-Huerta JM. Interleukin-9 potentiates the interleukin-4-induced IgE and IgG1 release from murine B lymphocytes. *Immunology* 1993;79:146–151.

145. Donahue RE, Yang YC, Clark SC. Human P40 T-cell growth factor interleukin-9 supports erythroid colony formation. *Blood* 1990;75:2271–2275.

146. Hsu DH, de Waal M, Fiorentino DF, et al. Expression of interleukin-10 activity by Epstein-Barr virus protein BCRF1. *Science* 1990;250:830–832.

147. Ho AS, Liu Y, Khan TA, Hsu DH, Bazan JF, Moore KW. A receptor for interleukin 10 is related to interferon receptors. *Proc Natl Acad Sci U S A* 1993;90:11267–11271.

148. Liu Y, Wei SH, Ho AS, de Waal M, Moore KW. Expression cloning and characterization of a human IL-10 receptor. *J Immunol* 1994;152:1821–1829.

149. Spencer SD, Di Marco F, Hooley J, et al. The orphan receptor CRF2-4 is an essential subunit of the interleukin 10 receptor. *J Exp Med* 1998;187:571–578.

150. Finbloom DS, Winestock KD. IL-10 induces the tyrosine phosphorylation of tyk2 and Jak1 and the differential assembly of STAT1 alpha and STAT3 complexes in human T cells and monocytes. *J Immunol* 1995;155:1079–1090.

151. O'Farrell AM, Liu Y, Moore KW, Mui AL. IL-10 inhibits macrophage activation and proliferation by distinct signaling mechanisms: evidence for Stat3-dependent and -independent pathways. *EMBO J* 1998;17:1006–1018.

152. Moore KW, Vieira P, Fiorentino DF, Trounstine ML, Khan TA, Mosmann TR. Homology of cytokine synthesis inhibitory factor IL-10 to the Epstein-Barr virus gene BCRFI. *Science* 1990;248:1230–1234.

153. Kuhn R, Lohler J, Rennick D, Rajewsky K, Muller W. Interleukin-10-deficient mice develop chronic enterocolitis. *Cell* 1993;75:263–274.

154. Pajkrt D, Camoglio L, Tiel-van Buul MC, et al. Attenuation of proinflammatory response by recombinant human IL-10 in human endotoxemia: effect of timing of recombinant human IL-10 administration. *J Immunol* 1997;158:3971–3977.

155. Opal SM, Wherry JC, Grint P. Interleukin-10: potential benefits and possible risks in clinical infectious diseases. *Clin Infect Dis* 1998;27:1497–1507.

156. Beatty PR, Krams SM, Martinez OM. Involvement of IL-10 in the autonomous growth of EBV-transformed B cell lines. *J Immunol* 1997;158:4045–4051.

157. Khatri VP, Caligiuri MA. A review of the association between interleukin-10 and human B-cell malignancies. *Cancer Immunol Immunother* 1998;46:239–244.

158. Paul SR, Bennett F, Calvetti JA, et al. Molecular cloning of a cDNA encoding interleukin 11, a stromal cell-derived lymphopoietic and hematopoietic cytokine. *Proc Natl Acad Sci U S A* 1990;87:7512–7516.

159. Du X, Williams DA. Interleukin-11: review of molecular, cell biology, clinical use. *Blood* 1997;89:3897–3908.

160. Baumann H, Wang Y, Morella KK, et al. Complex of the soluble IL-11 receptor and IL-11 acts as IL-6-type cytokine in hepatic and non-hepatic cells. *J Immunol* 1996;157:284–290.

161. Nandurkar HH, Robb L, Tarlinton D, et al. Adult mice with targeted mutation of the interleukin-11 receptor IL11Ra display normal hematopoiesis. *Blood* 1997;90:2148–2159.

162. Robb L, Li R, Hartley L, Nandurkar HH, Koentgen F, Begley CG. Infertility in female mice lacking the receptor for interleukin-11 is due to a defective uterine response to implantation. *Nat Med* 1998;4:303–308.

163. Tepler I, Elias L, Smith JW, et al. A randomized placebo-controlled trial of recombinant human interleukin-11 in cancer patients with severe thrombocytopenia due to chemotherapy. *Blood* 1996;87:3607–3614.

164. Du XX, Williams DA. Interleukin-11: a multifunctional growth factor derived from the hematopoietic microenvironment. *Blood* 1994;83:2023–2030.

165. Gubler U, Chua AO, Schoenhaut DS, et al. Coexpression of two distinct genes is required to generate secreted bioactive cytotoxic lymphocyte maturation factor. *Proc Natl Acad Sci U S A* 1991;88:4143–4147.

166. Wolf SF, Temple PA, Kobayashi M, et al. Cloning of cDNA for natural killer cell stimulatory factor, a heterodimeric cytokine with multiple biologic effects on T and natural killer cells. *J Immunol* 1991;146:3074–3081.

167. Trinchieri G. Interleukin-12: a cytokine at the interface of inflammation and immunity. *Adv Immunol* 1998;70:83–243.

168. Mattner F, Fischer S, Guckes S, et al. The interleukin-12 subunit p40 specifically inhibits effects of the interleukin-12 heterodimer. *Eur J Immunol* 1993;23:2202–2208.

169. Shu U, Kiniwa M, Wu CY, et al. Activated T cells induce interleukin-12 production by monocytes via CD40-CD40 ligand interaction. *Eur J Immunol* 1995;25:1125–1128.

170. Schoenhaut DS, Chua AO, Wolitzky AG, et al. Cloning and expression of murine IL-12. *J Immunol* 1992;148:3433–3440.

171. Chua AO, Chizzonite R, Desai BB, et al. Expression cloning of a human IL-12 receptor component. A new member of the cytokine receptor superfamily with strong homology to gp130. *J Immunol* 1994;153:128–136.

172. Presky DH, Yang H, Minetti LJ, et al. A functional interleukin 12 receptor complex is composed of two beta-type cytokine receptor subunits. *Proc Natl Acad Sci U S A* 1996;93:14002–14007.

173. Szabo SJ, Dighe AS, Gubler U, Murphy KM. Regulation of the interleukin IL-12R beta 2 subunit expression in developing T helper 1 Th1 and Th2 cells. *J Exp Med* 1997;185:817–824.

174. Bacon CM, McVicar DW, Ortaldo JR, Rees RC, O'Shea JJ, Johnston JA. Interleukin 12 IL-12 induces tyrosine phosphorylation of JAK2 and TYK2: differential use of Janus family tyrosine kinases by IL-2 and IL-12. *J Exp Med* 1995;181:399–404.

175. Zou J, Presky DH, Wu CY, Gubler U. Differential associations between the cytoplasmic regions of the interleukin-12 receptor subunits beta1 and beta2 and JAK kinases. *J Biol Chem* 1997;272: 6073–6077.

176. Jacobson NG, Szabo SJ, Weber-Nordt RM, et al. Interleukin 12 signaling in T helper type 1 Th1 cells involves tyrosine phosphorylation of signal transducer and activator of transcription Stat3 and Stat4. *J Exp Med* 1995;181:1755–1762.

177. Coccia EM, Passini N, Battistini A, Pini C, Sinigaglia F, Rogge L. Interleukin-12 induces expression of interferon regulatory factor-1 via signal transducer and activator of transcription-4 in human T helper type 1 cells. *J Biol Chem* 1999;274:6698–6703.

178. Magram J, Connaughton SE, Warrier RR, et al. IL-12-deficient mice are defective in IFN gamma production and type 1 cytokine responses. *Immunity* 1996;4:471–481.

179. Piccotti JR, Li K, Chan SY, Ferrante J, Magram J, Eichwald EJ, Bishop DK. Alloantigen-reactive Th1 development in IL-12-deficient mice. *J Immunol* 1998;160:1132–1138.

180. Robertson MJ, Cameron C, Atkins MB, et al. Immunological effects of interleukin 12 administered by bolus intravenous injection to patients with cancer. *Clin Cancer Res* 1999;5:9–16.

181. Brunda MJ, Luistro L, Warrier RR, et al. Antitumor and antimetastatic activity of interleukin 12 against murine tumors. *J Exp Med* 1993;178:1223–1230.

182. Wigginton JM, Komschlies KL, Back TC, Franco JL, Brunda MJ, Wiltrout RH. Administration of interleukin-12 with pulse interleukin-2 and the rapid and complete eradication of murine renal carcinoma. *J Natl Cancer Inst* 1996;88:38–43.

183. Caspi RR. IL-12 in autoimmunity. *Clin Immunol Immunopathol* 1998;88:4–13.

184. de Vries JE. The role of IL-13 and its receptor in allergy and inflammatory responses. *J Allergy Clin Immunol* 1998;102:165–169.

185. Brown KD, Zurawski SM, Mosmann TR, Zurawski G. A family of small inducible proteins secreted by leukocytes are members of a new superfamily that includes leukocyte and fibroblast-derived inflammatory agents, growth factors, indicators of various activation processes. *J Immunol* 1989;142:679–687.

186. McKenzie AN, Culpepper JA, de Waal M, et al. Interleukin-13, a T-cell-derived cytokine that regulates human monocyte and B-cell function. *Proc Natl Acad Sci U S A* 1993;90:3735–3739.

187. Aman MJ, Tayebi N, Obiri NI, Puri RK, Modi WS, Leonard WJ. cDNA cloning and characterization of the human interleukin-13 receptor alpha chain. *J Biol Chem* 1996;271:29265–29270.

188. Hilton DJ, Zhang JG, Metcalf D, Alexander WS, Nicola NA, Willson TA. Cloning and characterization of a binding subunit of the interleukin-13 receptor that is also a component of the interleukin-4 receptor. *Proc Natl Acad Sci U S A* 1996;93:497–501.

189. Keegan AD, Johnston JA, Tortolani PJ, et al. Similarities and differences in signal transduction by interleukin-4 and interleukin-13: analysis of Janus kinase activation. *Proc Natl Acad Sci U S A* 1995;92:7681–7685.

190. McKenzie GJ, Emson CL, Bell SE, et al. Impaired development of Th2 cells in IL-13-deficient mice. *Immunity* 1998;9:423–432.

191. Grabstein KH, Eisenman J, Shanebeck K, et al. Cloning of a T cell growth factor that interacts with the beta chain of the interleukin-2 receptor. *Science* 1994;264:965–968.

192. Burton JD, Bamford RN, Peters C, et al. A lymphokine, provisionally designated interleukin T and produced by a human adult T-cell leukemia line, stimulates T-cell proliferation and the induction of lymphokine-activated killer cells. *Proc Natl Acad Sci U S A* 1994;91:4935–4939.

193. Cosman D, Kumaki S, Anderson D, Kennedy M, Eisenman J, Park L. Interleukin 15. *Biochem Soc Trans* 1997;25:371–374.

194. Bamford RN, DeFilippis AP, Azimi N, Kurys G, Waldmann TA. The 5' untranslated region, signal peptide, the coding sequence of the carboxyl terminus of IL-15 participate in its multifaceted translational control. *J Immunol* 1998;160:4418–4426.

195. Giri JG, Ahdieh M, Eisenman J, et al. Utilization of the beta and gamma chains of the IL-2 receptor by the novel cytokine IL-15. *EMBO J* 1994;13:2822–2830.

196. Giri JG, Kumaki S, Ahdieh M, et al. Identification and cloning of a novel IL-15 binding protein that is structurally related to the alpha chain of the IL-2 receptor. *EMBO J* 1995;14:3654–3663.

197. Tagaya Y, Burton JD, Miyamoto Y, Waldmann TA. Identification of a novel receptor/signal transduction pathway for IL-15/T in mast cells. *EMBO J* 1996;15:4928–4939.

198. Williams NS, Klem J, Puzanov IJ, et al. Natural killer cell differentiation: insights from knockout and transgenic mouse models and *in vitro* systems. *Immunol Rev* 1998;165:47–61.

199. Lodolce JP, Boone DL, Chai S, et al. IL-15 receptor maintains lymphoid homeostasis by supporting lymphocyte homing and proliferation. *Immunity* 1998;9:669–676.

200. Center DM, Cruikshank W. Modulation of lymphocyte migration by human lymphokines. I. Identification and characterization of chemoattractant activity for lymphocytes from mitogen-stimulated mononuclear cells. *J Immunol* 1982;128:2563–2568.

201. Cruikshank W, Center DM. Modulation of lymphocyte migration by human lymphokines. II. Purification of a lymphotactic factor LCF. *J Immunol* 1982;128:2569–2574.

202. Cruikshank WW, Kornfeld H, Center DM. Signaling and functional properties of interleukin-16. *Int Rev Immunol* 1998;16:523–540.

203. Zhang Y, Center DM, Wu DM, et al. Processing and activation of pro-interleukin-16 by caspase-3. *J Biol Chem* 1998;273:1144–1149.

204. Muhlhahn P, Zweckstetter M, Georgescu J, et al. Structure of interleukin-16 resembles a PDZ domain with an occluded peptide binding site. *Nat Struct Biol* 1998;5:682–686.

205. Laberge S, Cruikshank WW, Kornfeld H, Center MD. Histamine-induced secretion of lymphocyte chemoattractant factor from CD8+ T cells is independent of transcription and translation. Evidence for constitutive protein synthesis and storage. *J Immunol* 1995;155:2902–2910.

206. Lim KG, Wan HC, Bozza PT, et al. Human eosinophils elaborate the lymphocyte chemoattractants. IL-16 lymphocyte chemoattractant factor and RANTES. *J Immunol* 1996;156:2566–2570.

207. Bellini A, Yoshimura H, Vittori E, Marini M, Mattoli S. Bronchial epithelial cells of patients with asthma release chemoattractant factors for T lymphocytes. *J Allergy Clin Immunol* 1993;92:412–424.

208. Cruikshank WW, Greenstein JL, Theodore AC, Center DM. Lymphocyte chemoattractant factor induces CD4-dependent intracytoplasmic signaling in lymphocytes. *J Immunol* 1991;146:2928–2934.

209. Theodore AC, Center DM, Nicoll J, Fine G, Kornfeld H, Cruikshank WW. CD4 ligand IL-16 inhibits the mixed lymphocyte reaction. *J Immunol* 1996;157:1958–1964.

210. Maciaszek JW, Parada NA, Cruikshank WW, Center DM, Kornfeld H, Viglianti GA. IL-16 represses HIV-1 promoter activity. *J Immunol* 1997;158:5–8.

211. Rouvier E, Luciani MF, Mattei MG, Denizot F, Golstein P. CTLA-8, cloned from an activated T cell, bearing AU-rich messenger RNA instability sequences, and homologous to a herpesvirus saimiri gene. *J Immunol* 1993;150:5445–5456.

212. Yao Z, Painter SL, Fanslow WC, et al. Human IL-17: a novel cytokine derived from T cells. *J Immunol* 1995;155:5483–5486.

213. Yao Z, Timour M, Painter S, Fanslow W, Spriggs M. Complete nucleotide sequence of the mouse CTLA8 gene. *Gene* 1996;168: 223–225.

214. Fossiez F, Djossou O, Chomarat P, et al. T cell interleukin-17 induces stromal cells to produce proinflammatory and hematopoietic cytokines. *J Exp Med* 1996;183:2593–2603.

215. Yao Z, Fanslow WC, Seldin MF, et al. Herpesvirus Saimiri encodes a new cytokine, IL-17, which binds to a novel cytokine receptor. *Immunity* 1995;3:811–821.

216. Antonysamy MA, Fanslow WC, Fu F, et al. Evidence for a role of IL-17 in organ allograft rejection: IL-17 promotes the functional differentiation of dendritic cell progenitors. *J Immunol* 1999;162: 577–584.

217. Spriggs MK. Interleukin-17 and its receptor. *J Clin Immunol* 1997;17:366–369.

218. Okamura H, Tsutsi H, Komatsu T, et al. Cloning of a new cytokine that induces IFN-gamma production by T cells. *Nature* 1995;378: 88–91.

219. Fantuzzi G, Dinarello CA. Interleukin-18 and interleukin-1 beta:

two cytokine substrates for ICE caspase-1. *J Clin Immunol* 1999;19: 1–11.

220. Gu Y, Kuida K, Tsutsui H, et al. Activation of interferon-gamma inducing factor mediated by interleukin-1beta converting enzyme. *Science* 1997;275:206–209.

221. Ghayur T, Banerjee S, Hugunin M, et al. Caspase-1 processes IFN-gamma-inducing factor and regulates Lps-induced IFN-gamma production. *Nature* 1997;386:619–623.

222. Puren AJ, Fantuzzi G, Dinarello CA. Gene expression, synthesis, secretion of interleukin-18 and interleukin-1 beta are differentially regulated in human blood mononuclear cells and mouse spleen cells. *Proc Natl Acad Sci U S A* 1999;96:2256–2261.

223. Parnet P, Garka KE, Bonnert TP, Dower SK, Sims JE. IL-1Rrp is a novel receptor-like molecule similar to the type I interleukin-1 receptor and its homologues T1/ST2 and IL-1R AcP. *J Biol Chem* 1996;271:3967–3970.

224. Torigoe K, Ushio S, Okura T, et al. Purification and characterization of the human interleukin-18 receptor. *J Biol Chem* 1997;272: 25737–25742.

225. Dale M, Nicklin MJ. Interleukin-1 receptor cluster: gene organization of IL-1R2, IL-1R1, IL-1RL2 IL-1Rrp2, IL-1RL1 T1/ST2, IL-18R1 IL-1Rrp on human chromosome 2q. *Genomics* 1999;57: 177–179.

226. Born TL, Thomassen E, Bird TA, Sims JE. Cloning of a novel receptor subunit, AcPL, required for interleukin-18 signaling. *J Biol Chem* 1998;273:29445–29450.

227. Novick D, Kim SH, Fantuzzi G, Reznikov LL, Dinarello CA, Rubinstein M. Interleukin-18 binding protein: a novel modulator of the Th1 cytokine response. *Immunity* 1999;10:127–136.

228. Kojima H, Takeuchi M, Ohta T, et al. Interleukin-18 activates the IRAK-TRAF6 pathway in mouse EL-4 cells. *Biochem Biophys Res Commun* 1998;244:183–186.

229. Xu D, Chan WL, Leung BP, et al. Selective expression and functions of interleukin-18 receptor on T helper Th type 1 but not Th2 cells. *J Exp Med* 1998;188:1485–1492.

230. Takeda K, Tsutsui H, Yoshimoto T, et al. Defective NK cell activity and Th1 response in IL-18-deficient mice. *Immunity* 1998;8: 383–390.

2

INTERLEUKIN-2: PRECLINICAL TRIALS

RICHARD J. BARTH, JR.
JAMES J. MULÉ

Interleukin-2 (IL-2) was first described in 1976 as a factor produced by mitogen-stimulated human T cells that mediated selective expansion of T cells from normal human bone marrow *in vitro* (1). Large amounts of highly purified recombinant IL-2 (rIL-2) with full biological activity have become available for *in vivo* studies through the cloning of the gene for IL-2 and its insertion and expression in *Escherichia coli* (2,3). IL-2 exerts potent effects on immune cells that can mediate tumor regressions *in vivo*; it is particularly important in the antigen-specific clonal expansion of T cells, but also for the stimulation of nonspecific effectors, such as natural killer (NK) and lymphokine-activated killer (LAK) cells. This chapter reviews the pharmacokinetics, antitumor effects, and mechanisms of activity and toxicity of systemically administered IL-2. This chapter also examines the antitumor effects and mechanism of action of IL-2 delivered locally to the tumor site, whether it be in the form of injected-soluble cytokine, the cytokine gene, tumor cells gene-modified to express IL-2, or IL-2 monoclonal antibody (MAb) fusion protein. Many preclinical investigations have focused on the combination of IL-2 with other cancer therapies. Therefore, this chapter reviews studies that evaluate the role of IL-2 when combined with other cytokines, cytotoxic chemotherapy, radiation therapy, adoptive immunotherapy, and vaccines.

INTERLEUKIN-2: SYSTEMIC ADMINISTRATION

Pharmacokinetics

Initial pharmacokinetic studies tested native IL-2 derived from a mitogen-stimulated EL-4–thymoma cell line in C57BL/6 mice (4). IL-2 had a serum half-life of 3.7 ± 0.8 minutes after intravenous (i.v.) injection, with a titer of 2 U per mL detectable for less than 30 minutes. More prolonged serum levels of IL-2 could be achieved by intraperitoneal (i.p.) or subcutaneous (s.c.) administration: after i.p. and s.c. injection, titers remained higher than 2 U per mL for 2 and 6 hours, respectively. Similar results were obtained when rIL-2 was studied. Chang et al. measured a serum half-life of 1.6 ± 0.3 minutes in mice after an i.v. bolus injection of 20,000 U rIL-2, with i.p. and s.c. administration resulting in IL-2 serum levels of more than 1 U per mL for 3 to 5 hours after 10,000 U rIL-2 (5). Rapid clearance from the

kidney accounted for the short serum half-life after an i.v. injection (4). Biodistribution studies of radiolabeled rIL-2 indicated that the liver and kidney were the organs of greatest cytokine uptake (6). Chemical modification by forming an ester with polyethylene glycol (PEG-IL-2) prolonged the half-life of i.v.-administered cytokine to 4.5 hours (7).

Antitumor Effects of Systemic Interleukin-2 Administration

Rosenberg and colleagues studied the effect of systemic administration of rIL-2 at escalating doses on established pulmonary metastases from a weakly immunogenic sarcoma, MCA-105 (8). Mice bearing 3-day-old metastases were treated with doses ranging from 3,000 to 170,000 U rIL-2 i.p. t.i.d. for 5 days. When compared with control mice who received saline, mice who received between 3,000 and 8,000 U rIL-2 had 5 ± 5% reductions in metastases. Mice who received between 20,000 and 50,000 U rIL-2 had 22 ± 9% reductions, whereas mice who received between 100,000 and 170,000 U rIL-2 experienced 79 ± 7% reductions in pulmonary metastases. Reductions of 10-day-old pulmonary macrometastases could also be achieved with rIL-2 therapy. Pulmonary macrometastases were reduced by 34 ± 13% with 1,000 to 6,000 U rIL-2, whereas 20,000 to 50,000 U and 100,000 to 200,000 U rIL-2 reduced 10-day-old metastases by 89 ± 4% and 80 ± 5%, respectively. Of note, doses of 50,000 U rIL-2 i.p. t.i.d. were effective in reducing the numbers of 3-day-old pulmonary metastases, whereas lower doses (20,000 U rIL-2 t.i.d.) were effective in the treatment of larger, 10-day-old metastases. As shown in Figure 1, the systemic administration of rIL-2 was also effective in the treatment of 3-day-old pulmonary metastases from several other murine tumors, including the nonimmunogenic MCA-101 sarcoma, MC-38 colon adenocarcinoma, and M3 melanoma (9). For each tumor, higher doses resulted in greater antitumor effects.

Using the 3-day-old MCA-105 pulmonary metastasis model, Ettinghausen and Rosenberg evaluated different routes and schedules of rIL-2 administration (10). The same cumulative daily doses of rIL-2 administered intravenously or intraperitoneally once daily or intraperitoneally t.i.d. were compared. The i.p. t.i.d. protocol resulted in the most effective reduction in pulmonary metastases, indicating that sustained lower levels of rIL-

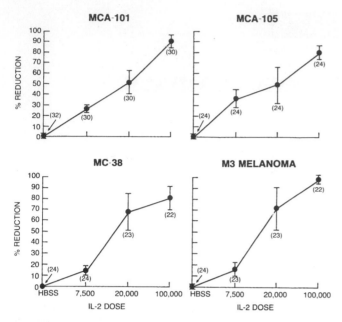

FIGURE 1. Effects of dose titration of recombinant interleukin-2 (rIL-2) on experimentally induced pulmonary metastases from multiple murine tumors. The effect of rIL-2 is demonstrated for two murine sarcomas (MCA-105, MCA-101), a murine adenosarcoma (MC-38), and a murine melanoma (M3). Numbers in parentheses indicate total number of mice. Increasing doses of rIL-2 led to a reduction in the number of pulmonary metastases. Each point reflects the mean percentage reduction for all experiments performed. (Hanks' balanced salt solution.) (From Papa MZ et al. The anti-tumor efficacy of lymphokine-activated killer cells and recombinant interleukin-2 *in vivo*: successful immunotherapy of established pulmonary metastases from weakly- and non-immunogenic murine tumors of three distinct histologic types. *Cancer Res* 1986;46:4973–4978, with permission.)

2 were more effective than brief, high-peak levels for antitumor activity. It was also shown that the duration of IL-2 administration was crucial because 6 consecutive days of rIL-2 injections resulted in a greater antitumor effect compared with 1 or 3 days.

Systemic immunotherapy with rIL-2 has also been effective in the treatment of s.c. and hepatic tumors, and disseminated leukemia and lymphomas. Initiation of rIL-2 therapy (200,000 U i.p. t.i.d.) 10 days after the s.c. injection of MCA-105 sarcoma, when palpable nodules with a diameter of 2 to 4 mm are present, resulted in a complete response in one-half of the mice; the rest had a marked reduction in tumor growth (8). Treatment with rIL-2 demonstrated modest effectiveness against 3-day-old metastases from a variety of murine tumors established in the liver (11,12). For example, treatment of mice harboring MCA-105 hepatic metastases with 10,000 U rIL-2 i.p. t.i.d. for 8 days caused a significant decrease in the number of hepatic metastases from a mean of 242 hepatic metastases in control mice to 61 in treated mice. Thompson et al. evaluated the therapeutic efficacy of systemically administered rIL-2 against the disseminated murine leukemia FBL-3 (13). As shown in Figure 2, doses of rIL-2 (48,000 U per day) administered on days 5 to 9 after tumor injection cured 50% of the mice. As observed in the treatment of MCA-105 pulmonary metastases, delaying the injections of rIL-2 to treat more established leukemia (i.e., on days 5 to 9) was far more effective than the treatment of early disease (i.e., on days 0 to 4). Everse et al. also evaluated the timing of IL-2 therapy in a disseminated SL-2 lymphoma model (14). Initiation of 5 days of treatment with rIL-2 on days 1 to 6 after tumor initiation was completely ineffective, whereas therapy begun on days 7 to 12 was effective. Maximal effectiveness was seen when rIL-2 therapy was begun on day 9 or 10, which resulted in cures of 80% of the mice.

Multiple investigators have compared the therapeutic effectiveness of rIL-2 with PEG-IL-2, which has a significantly longer serum half-life. Whereas some investigators found that systemically (15) or intratumorally (16) administered PEG-IL-2 was therapeutically superior to free cytokine, others (7,17) concluded that the therapeutic effectiveness of the two preparations was approximately equivalent; the main advantage of PEG-IL-2 was that less frequent dosing was required.

Mechanisms by which Systemic Interleukin-2 Administration Mediates Tumor Regressions

A strong indication that the antitumor effect of rIL-2 *in vivo* was immune mediated came from the histologic assessment of

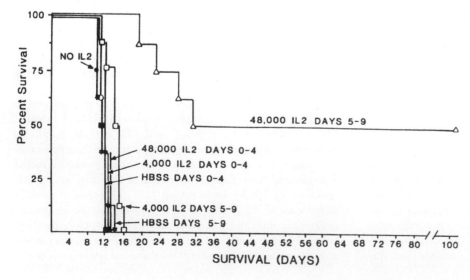

FIGURE 2. High-dose recombinant interleukin-2 (rIL-2) can cure disseminated FBL-3 *in vivo*. C57BL/6 mice inoculated intraperitoneally with 5 × 106 FBL-3 received either no therapy, no IL-2, or treatment with rIL-2 injected intraperitoneally at a dose of 48,000 U or 4,000 U per day (in three equivalent doses) on days 0 to 4 or 5 to 9 with Hanks' balanced salt solution. (From Thompson JA et al. Eradication of disseminated murine leukemia by treatment with high-dose interleukin-2. *J Immunol* 1986;137:3675–3680, with permission.)

TABLE 1. LYT-2 CELLS[a] MEDIATE REDUCTION OF ESTABLISHED 10-DAY-OLD PULMONARY MACROMETASTASES FROM WEAKLY IMMUNOGENIC SARCOMAS BY HIGH-DOSE INTERLEUKIN-2 (IL-2)

Tumor	Treatment[b]				No. of Metastases at Day 18	Mean	p[c]
	HBSS	IL-2	Anti-L3T4	Anti-Lyt-2			
MCA-105	+	–	–	–	250, 250, 250, 250, 206	241	—
	–	+	–	–	14, 36, 70, 7, 62	38	<.01
	–	+	+	–	80, 16, 41, 49, 39	45	<.01
	–	+	–	+	250, 250, 250, 213, 149	222	NS
MCA-106	+	–	–	–	250, 250, 250, 250, 250, 250	250	—
	–	+	–	–	20, 66, 53, 151, 33, 66	65	<.005
	–	+	–	+	250, 250, 250, 250, 250, 250	250	NS

HBSS; Hanks' balanced salt solution; NS, not significant; +, received treatment; –, did not receive treatment.
[a]Number of tumor cells injected was 6×10^5 and 2×10^5 for MCA-105 and MCA-106, respectively.
[b]IL-2 or HBSS was injected i.p. three times per d for 5 (MCA-105; 50,000 U per injection) or 4 (MCA-106; 100,000 U per injection) consecutive d, starting on d 10 after tumor injection. Antibody was injected i.v. 2 hr before the onset of IL-2 injection.
[c]Wilcoxon rank sum test of treated groups compared with groups receiving HBSS alone (two-sided).
From Mulé JJ et al. Identification of cellular mechanisms operational *in vivo* during the regression of established pulmonary metastases by the systemic administration of high-dose recombinant interleukin-2. *J Immunol* 1987;139:285–294, with permission.

regressing pulmonary metastases (8). By 2 days after the injection of rIL-2 into mice bearing 10-day-old pulmonary metastases, lymphocytes were seen infiltrating the periphery of the tumor. At later time points, lymphocyte infiltration progressed as the tumors underwent regression. Evidence that IL-2 was acting through a radiation-sensitive host-immune component came from the observations that the antitumor effect of rIL-2 was eliminated if mice received a prior dose of 500 cGy total-body irradiation (8,11).

Definitive identification of the immune cells involved in rIL-2–mediated tumor regressions came from studies by Mulé et al., who used selective depletion of lymphocyte subsets *in vivo* (18). In the course of these studies, an interesting difference emerged when comparing the treatment of weakly immunogenic (MCA-105 and MCA-106) tumors with that of nonimmunogenic (MCA-101 and MCA-102) sarcomas. The systemic administration of high-dose rIL-2 mediated a significant reduction in established 3-day-old pulmonary micrometastases from weakly immunogenic and nonimmunogenic sarcomas. When 10-day-old pulmonary metastases were treated, however, only those established from weakly immunogenic sarcomas remained susceptible. Ten-day-old pulmonary metastases from nonimmunogenic sarcomas were refractory to IL-2 therapy. Cells with potent LAK activity *in vitro* were identified in the lungs of rIL-2-treated mice. By flow cytometry, the majority of these effector cells were Thy-1[+], L3T4[−] (CD4[−]), Lyt-2[−] (CD8[−]), and ASGM-1[+]. Depletion *in vivo* of ASGM-1[+] cells eliminated the ability of high-dose rIL-2 therapy to decrease 3-day-old pulmonary metastases from nonimmunogenic sarcomas and also eliminated recoverable LAK cell activity in the lungs. In mice with 3-day-old pulmonary metastases from weakly immunogenic sarcomas (MCA-105 and MCA-106), both Lyt-2[+] cells and ASGM-1[+] cells were involved in rIL-2–mediated tumor regression. Lyt-2[+] cells appeared to be the more potent mediators in the response. Depletion of L3T4[+] cells had no effect on tumor regression. Because high-dose rIL-2 administration resulted in significant reductions in 10-day-old metastases from weakly immunogenic sarcomas,

the effector cell responsible for this effective therapy was also characterized. As shown in Table 1, Lyt-2[+] cells were mediators of rIL-2–induced regression of 10-day-old pulmonary macrometastases from the weakly immunogenic sarcomas.

Although LAK effectors derived from ASGM-1[+] precursors eliminated 3-day-old pulmonary micrometastases regardless of tumor immunogenicity, Lyt-2[+] cells were involved in the elimination of 3-day-old pulmonary micrometastases and 10-day-old macrometastases from weakly immunogenic tumors. These results imply that the effect of high-dose rIL-2 administration may be twofold. One effect is the stimulation of LAK cell activity against small tumor burdens from weakly immunogenic and nonimmunogenic tumors. A second effect may be the stimulation of specific host antitumor responses directed against tumor-associated antigens.

Peace and Cheever used a similar approach to identify the cells responsible for rIL-2–induced tumor regressions in the FBL-3 leukemia system (19). In this model, the therapeutic efficacy of high-dose rIL-2 was dramatically reduced by infusion of MAb to Lyt-2 and L3T4, but not NK-1.1.

Toxicity of Systemic Interleukin-2 Administration

The adverse effects of rIL-2 treatment in mice include: (a) a vascular leak syndrome (manifested as pulmonary edema, pleural effusions, and ascites), (b) hepatocyte necrosis, (c) prerenal azotemia, (d) splenomegaly, (e) anemia, and (f) thrombocytopenia (20). Pulmonary edema and systemic vascular leakage are the cause of mortality. Studies by Rosenstein et al., who used radiolabeled albumin in mice, revealed that rIL-2 induced increases in vascular permeability that were directly related to the dose of rIL-2 and the duration of administration (21). In rats, mortality occurred after 12 daily doses of more than 2.7×10^6 U per kg per day as a consequence of hepatocellular necrosis and anemia (20). The manifestations of rIL-2 toxicity in monkeys were similar to those in mice. Repeated doses of more than 2.3×10^6 U per kg per day resulted in death from vascular leak-

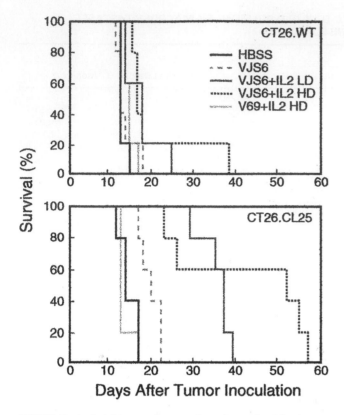

FIGURE 3. Active immunotherapy is enhanced with exogenous recombinant interleukin-2 (rIL-2) and rubella vaccine–like virus given in concert. BALB/c mice (five per group) were challenged intravenously with 5×10^6 CT26.WT or CT26.CL25 tumor cells. After 3 days, they received a single intravenous injection of medium alone (HBSS, Hanks' balanced salt solution) or medium containing 5×10^6 plaque-forming units of different TK rubella vaccine–like virus expressing (VJS6) or not expressing (V69) γ-galactosidase. Two different regimens of rIL-2 administration were started 12 hours after rubella vaccine–like virus injection: high dose (100,000 Cetus U, twice a day, intraperitoneally for 3 days) or low dose (15,000 Cetus U, twice a day, intraperitoneally for 5 days). Mice were checked twice a day for survival. (From Bronte V et al. IL-2 enhances the function of recombinant poxvirus-based vaccines in the treatment of established pulmonary metastases. *J Immunol* 1995;154:5282–5291, with permission.)

age, pulmonary edema, renal and hepatic failure, and hypotension (20).

In vivo immune-cell subset depletions were performed to determine the cells responsible for rIL-2–mediated toxicity. Gately and colleagues showed that the rIL-2 dosage regimens required to produce large granular lymphocytes with LAK activity in the pleural cavities and livers of mice correlated with the induction of pleural effusions and hepatotoxicity (22). Treatment of mice with anti–ASGM-1 antiserum *in vivo* concurrent with IL-2 greatly reduced the severity of pulmonary edema and hepatotoxicity and prolonged mouse survival. Studies by Mulé et al., however, showed that this antiserum treatment severely diminished the therapeutic efficacy of rIL-2 in mice bearing 3-day-old pulmonary metastases (18). Peace and Cheever, using specific MAb to selectively deplete L3T4[+], Lyt-2[+], or NK-1.1[+] cells in mice with FBL-3 leukemia, showed that elimination of NK-1.1[+] (but not L3T4[+] or Lyt-2[+]) cells attenuated rIL-2 toxicity without compromising therapeutic efficacy (19). These stud-

ies clearly show that ASGM-1[+] and NK-1.1[+] cells are responsible for rIL-2 toxicity.

Since these initial studies, several agents have been identified that appear to inhibit rIL-2 toxicity without compromising antitumor effects. These include pentoxifylline (23), methotrexate (24), and CNI-1493 (25). Tumor necrosis factor–α (TNF-α) has been implicated in the pathogenesis of rIL-2–induced capillary leak by studies that showed the following:

1. IL-2 induces macrophage–TNF-α production.
2. TNF-α expression is increased in rIL-2–treated mouse lungs (26).
3. Treatment of mice with neutralizing-soluble TNF receptor (26,27) or anti-TNF antibody (Ab) (28) significantly diminished vascular leak.

Anti-TNF Ab, however, also inhibited therapeutic efficacy (28). In one study, pentoxifylline, which suppresses macrophage-TNF gene transcription, inhibited many of the toxic effects of rIL-2 without reducing the therapeutic effect of rIL-2 on MCA-105 pulmonary metastases (23).

DeJoy et al. have shown that methotrexate inhibits rIL-2 vascular leak syndrome and improves the survival of mice receiving high-dose rIL-2 without compromising the efficacy of rIL-2 in the treatment of pulmonary metastases (24). The mechanism by which methotrexate inhibits rIL-2 toxicity is under study.

Kemeny et al. have shown that CNI-1493, a tetravalent guanylhydrazone that inhibits macrophage-cytokine production, conferred complete protection against fatal rIL-2 toxicity at rIL-2 doses ten times higher than the maximum tolerated dose in rats (Fig. 3) (25). Two of eight hepatoma-bearing rats treated with the maximum tolerated dose (3×10^6 U per m^2 per day) of rIL-2 alone developed tumor regressions. When rats were treated with tenfold higher doses of rIL-2 plus CNI-1493, one-half of the treated rats had no detectable tumor. The remaining one-half had substantial reduction of the tumor mass. CNI-1493 has been shown to inhibit the production of several inflammatory cytokines by monocytes and macrophages, including TNF-α. It remains to be determined whether this inhibition is directly responsible for the observed reduction of rIL-2 toxicity in the treated rats.

LOCAL DELIVERY OF INTERLEUKIN-2 AT SITES OF TUMORS

To avoid the toxicity of systemic administration of IL-2, several investigators have evaluated ways to locally deliver IL-2 to the tumor site. Direct injection of IL-2 into tumors has been shown to decrease the growth rate or cause regressions of different tumors, including (a) CE-2 sarcoma (29), (b) MC-2 mammary adenocarcinoma (30), (c) line 1 alveolar carcinoma cells (31), (d) MBT2 transitional cell bladder carcinoma (32), (e) SL-2 lymphoma and a mastocytoma (33), and (f) B16 melanoma (34). This effect is dose dependent. On histologic evaluation, this effect is associated with an increased accumulation of macrophages and T cells in the tumor. Dubinett et al. showed that intratumoral IL-2 therapy was also effective in decreasing tumor growth in athymic, splenectomized mice who had received cyclophosphamide, indicating that a non–T cell immune effector is responsible for tumor regression (31). Similar findings were reported by Sacchi et al., who found that intratumoral IL-2 therapy was effective in the treatment of human tumor xenografts in an athymic mouse model (35).

Although nonspecific effectors, such as macrophages or NK cells, may be responsible for the initial tumor destruction induced by directly injected IL-2, antigen-specific T cell–mediated immunity is then generated. For example, Maas et al. treated i.p. SL-2 lymphomas with i.p. injections of IL-2 and found that 75% of the primary tumors regressed. Fifty percent of s.c. tumors at a distance also regressed (33). No significant regression of an antigenically distinct s.c. tumor was observed. Vaage also observed that local intratumor injection of IL-2 caused regression of the primary tumor and was able to induce systemic immunity, which resulted in complete regressions of MC-2 mammary carcinomas at a distant s.c. site (30). Of note, Yeung et al. showed that peritumoral IL-2 injection was more effective than systemic IL-2 in retarding distant tumor growth and prolonging survival of the treated mice (34).

Investigators have tried to improve the therapeutic effectiveness of locally administered IL-2 by prolonging its release. Egilmez et al. have loaded IL-2 into biodegradable polylactic acid microspheres (36). When IL-2–loaded microspheres were coinjected s.c. with tumor cells, tumor growth was suppressed in 80% of mice. In contrast, bolus injections of PEG-IL-2 were ineffective. NK cells were demonstrated to mediate tumor destruction in this human tumor and severe combined immunodeficiency disease mouse model. Others have shown that IL-2–loaded liposomes can cause reduction of tumor growth in mice bearing hepatic micrometastases (37) and slow-release preparations of IL-2 injected into sc-prostatic carcinomas in rats can cause reductions in tumor growth rates without systemic toxicity (38).

Injection of Interleukin-2–Expressing Adenoviral Vectors into Tumors

Another promising vehicle for local delivery of IL-2 to the tumor site is by direct injection of adenoviral vectors expressing IL-2 into a tumor. Using this approach, Levraud and Kourilsky showed that 70% of 10-day-old, 2- to 5-mm–diameter s.c. P815 tumors underwent complete regression (39). By using a transgenic adenoviral vector that expressed murine and human IL-2, Levraud and Kourilsky showed by polymerase chain reaction that expression of IL-2 was detectable at the tumor site 10 days after vector injection. These investigators made several interesting observations on the mechanism of IL-2–induced tumor regression. It had been postulated that locally injected IL-2 was effective because it induced an immune response by fostering proliferation of antigen-specific cytoxic T-lymphocyte (CTL) precursors or reactivating anergized CTL (40). Levraud et al. did not detect any increase in tumor-specific T cells, using polymerase chain reactions with primers for specific Vβ T-cell reactivity rear-

rangements particular for P815 antigens in the regressing primary tumors. Instead, these investigators found polyclonal T-cell expansion, as well as a marked increase in interferon-γ (IFN-γ) expression, in the regressing primary tumors and at the site of challenge tumors injected into immunized mice. The cell type responsible for IL-2–induced IFN-γ expression in the primary tumors is unclear. At the challenge tumor site, it is likely that IFN-γ is secreted by tumor-reactive CD4+ or CD8+ lymphocytes. We have shown that IFN-γ secretion by adoptively transferred tumor-infiltrating lymphocytes (TIL) was critical for their effectiveness in the immunotherapy of established micrometastases (41). These observations support the concept that tumor destruction induced by local expression of IL-2 in primary tumors and T lymphocytes in challenge tumors is mediated largely by IFN-γ–stimulated nonspecific effectors, such as macrophages.

Successful treatment of a murine hepatocellular carcinoma, MH134, using a recombinant adenovirus vector expressing IL-2 has also been reported (42). Fifty percent of mice whose liver tumors were injected with Ad-IL-2 completely regressed. Regression was accompanied by massive infiltration with T cells and macrophages. Mice in whom tumors regressed were immune to repeat tumor challenge at different sites.

Gene Modification of Tumor Cells to Express Interleukin-2

Perhaps the most intensively studied mechanism for the local expression of IL-2 at the tumor site in experimental animal models has been through genetic modification of tumor cells to express IL-2. For most tumors studied, the local secretion of IL-2 by gene-modified tumor cells resulted in their rejection by syngeneic-immunocompetent hosts. Rejected primary tumors included: (a) the CMS-5 murine sarcoma (43), (b) CT26 colon adenocarcinoma (40), (c) P815 plasmacytoma (44), (d) TS/A mammary adenocarcinoma (45), (e) Lewis lung carcinoma (46), (f) MCA-102 sarcoma (47), and (g) J558L plasmacytoma (48). Expression of IL-2 by rat glioblastoma cells inhibited the growth of these tumors when subcutaneously injected, but not when injected intracranially (49).

The mechanism of rejection of the primary tumor was investigated by examining the histologic composition of the regressing tumor, host-cellular subset-Ab depletion studies, and the growth of the tumors in immunodeficient mice. In regressing MCA-102 and J558L tumors, progressive lymphocytic infiltration was observed. Regressing TS/A tumors were noted to be predominantly infiltrated by polymorphonuclear lymphocytes (45). In three reports, selective depletion of CD8+ T lymphocytes enabled a significant fraction of tumors to grow (45,47,48), indicating that CD8+ T cells play an important role in the rejection of IL-2–secreting tumors. It has been hypothesized that tumor IL-2 expression will bypass the need for CD4+ T-cell help in the generation of CTLs. In accord with this hypothesis, Ab depletion of CD4+ T lymphocytes did not affect tumor rejection (41,46,48,49). The growth of J558L tumors in nude mice was delayed compared with wild-type mice, supporting a role for a non–T-effector cell in tumor growth inhibition (48). Depletion of NK cells impaired the ability of mice to

TABLE 2. TREATMENT OF ESTABLISHED RODENT TUMORS BY INTERLEUKIN-2 GENE–MODIFIED TUMOR CELLS

Tumor System	Tumor Establishment	Treatment	Result	Reference
Lewis lung carcinoma	Footpad inoculation 11 d, 2×10^5	6 weekly i.p. XRT 2×10^6	Decreased number of lung metastases	Porgador et al. (46)
R3327-MatLyLu prostate cancer	a. s.c. 3 d, 10^4 b. Intraprostatic 3 d, 10^4	3 doses 10^6, XRT ID 3 d apart	a. 60% to 100% survival b. Prolonged survival	Vieweg et al. (53)
TS/A mammary adenocarcinoma	s.c. or i.v., 1 d, 7 d, 14 d	1 dose s.c. 10^5 weekly $\times$ 3 or biweekly $\times$ 3	20% survival with d 7 or d 14 s.c., d 7 i.v.	Cavallo et al. (51)
MBT-2 bladder cancer	Bladder wall implant 7 d, 2×10^4	3 weekly i.p. XRT 5×10^6	50% survival	Saito et al. (54)

ID, individual dose; XRT, x-ray therapy.

reject an IL-2–secreting, nonimmunogenic MCA-102 sarcoma (47). Therefore, evidence supports a role for CD8$^+$ T lymphocytes, NK cells, and polymorphonuclear neutrophils in the rejection of IL-2 gene-modified tumor cells.

In many cases, regression of the primary IL-2–secreting tumor generates a systemic immune response capable of rejecting a secondary parental tumor challenge. For example, rejection of IL-2–secreting CMS-5 sarcomas, CT26 colon adenocarcinomas, and P815 plasmacytomas elicits splenic CTL activity and protects the treated mice from a secondary tumor challenge. In these systems, a causal role for IL-2 in the generation of systemic immunity was not proved because irradiated, nonmodified parental tumor cells could also effectively prevent tumor growth from the secondary challenge. Irradiated IL-2–secreting B16 melanoma provided no better protection than irradiated parental tumor (50). Of note, regression of IL-2–secreting Lewis lung carcinoma did not protect mice significantly from secondary challenge unless the mice were also vaccinated with two boosts of irradiated tumor cells (46). In another study, regression of the nonimmunogenic, but major histocompatibility complex (MHC) class I–expressing, IL-2–secreting MCA-102 sarcoma did not confer resistance to rechallenge (47).

Other work has shown that the development of protective immunity is caused by IL-2 secretion. Studies of the TS/A adenocarcinoma are particularly interesting. A single immunizing dose of mitomycin-C–inactivated TS/A tumor afforded no protection, whereas vaccination with five different IL-2–secreting TS/A tumors protected 50% to 70% of mice from a secondary tumor challenge (45,51). Although multiple vaccinations with mitomycin-C–inactivated TS/A tumors could protect mice, IL-2–secreting tumors provided more potent immunity (51). Histologic analyses of the regressing tumor challenge sites revealed a preponderance of lymphocytes and macrophages. Host-cell subset-depletion studies revealed that this protective immunity was caused by CD4$^+$ T lymphocytes, not CD8$^+$ or ASGM-1$^+$ cells. In fact, little CTL activity was detected in a 4-hour (51) chromium-release assay using splenocytes from immune mice against TS/A targets. Therefore, studies in the TS/A tumor system revealed that genetic modification of tumor cells to secrete IL-2 could induce systemic immunity mediated largely by CD4$^+$ T lymphocytes. Using a murine melanoma model, it was shown that M-3 melanoma cells gene-modified to express IL-2 could induce protective immunity, whereas mock-transfected tumors were ineffective (52). Both CD4$^+$ and CD8$^+$ T cells

were required for the generation of protective immunity. Of note, the dose of IL-2 expressed by the tumor cells influenced the ability to achieve protective immunity. Expression of 1,000 to 3,000 U IL-2 per 10^5 cells per day was more effective than lower rates of expression of IL-2. Doses higher than 5,000 U IL-2 per 10^5 cells per day, however, led to the loss of ability to generate protective immunity. The reason for the ineffectiveness of high expression rates of IL-2 was unclear: No toxic effects or vascular leak was observed.

IL-2 gene-modified tumor cells have also been used to treat established tumors in rodents. In one study, when IL-2–expressing tumors were directly injected multiple times into 7-day-old TS/A tumors, 60% of mice were cured (51). Multiple injections led to rejections of 14-day-old tumors in 30% of mice. Other studies have shown that IL-2–expressing tumor vaccines could cause regressions of established tumors at distant sites, as summarized in Table 2. In each of these studies, the IL-2–secreting tumor vaccine was superior to irradiated or inactivated control tumor vaccines.

Some investigators have gene-modified tumor cells to express multiple cytokines or costimulatory molecules in addition to IL-2. For example, Rosenthal et al. cotransfected IL-2–expressing tumor cells with IFN-γ or granulocyte-macrophage colony-stimulating factor (GM-CSF) (55). In this model, CMS-5 fibrosarcomas transfected with IL-2, IFN-γ, and GM-CSF alone, and with the combination of IL-2 and GM-CSF progressively grew, whereas tumors expressing IL-2 and IFN-γ were rejected. It was postulated that this enhanced effect was secondary to IFN-γ–induced upregulation of MHC class I molecules on the tumor cell surface. Induction of protective immunity was not assessed in this study. In another report, it was shown that murine pancreatic carcinoma cells, which coexpressed IFN-γ and IL-2, were more effective than tumors expressing either IFN-γ or IL-2 alone in the treatment of 3-day-old established micrometastases (56).

Strome et al. have evaluated tumor cells that were modified to coexpress IL-2 and IL-4 (57). Coexpression led to rejection of primary tumor challenges and induced systemic immunity more effectively than tumor cells mixed with *Corynebacterium parvum*. Of interest, these investigators and Rosenthal and colleagues found that, although coexpression of two cytokines by a single tumor cell did lead to tumor regression, a mixture of tumor cells expressing only one cytokine did not. Rejection of IL-4– and IL-2–secreting tumors was not dependent on CD4$^+$

or CD8[+] T cells. CD4[+] T cells, however, were required for the generation of protective immunity.

Multiple investigative groups have double gene-modified tumor cells to express the costimulatory molecule B7.1 plus IL-2. The rationale for this approach is an attempt to induce tumor cells to act as their own antigen-presenting cells by presenting tumor antigens in the context of MHC class I and providing costimulation to T cells. Thus, the induction of T-cell anergy is avoided. For example, Emtage and colleagues directly injected an adenoviral vector containing B7.1 and IL-2 genes into established s.c. polyoma middle T-transformed breast adenocarcinoma tumors (58). Whereas 100% of the tumors injected with the B7.1/IL-2 vector completely regressed, only 38% and 42% of the tumors injected with vectors containing B7.1 or IL-2 alone, respectively, regressed. All mice in whom the tumor regressed were protected from secondary tumor challenges. In addition, Gaken et al. have shown that irradiated B7.1 and IL-2 gene-modified adenocarcinomas are more effective than tumors expressing B7.1 or IL-2 alone in the therapy of small s.c. tumors at a distance from the vaccine site (59). Although these antitumor results are potentially important, it is unclear from these experiments whether antigen presentation was accomplished by the transfected tumor cells per se, or by host-derived, antigen-presenting cells.

Another approach to deliver IL-2 locally to the tumor site consists of the injection of IL-2–secreting fibroblasts directly into a tumor. In a murine leukemia model, mice immunized with parental tumor cells plus gene-modified fibroblasts secreting IL-2 were able to prevent challenge tumor growth in 60% of cases, comparing favorably with tumors modified to express the gene encoding for GM-CSF (20% protection) (60). The combination of irradiated tumor cells plus IL-2–secreting fibroblasts, however, did not prolong the survival of mice given an i.v. injection of leukemia cells 3 days before the vaccine. In contrast, when IL-2–secreting fibroblasts were mixed with irradiated CT26 colorectal carcinoma cells, protective immunity was induced in 65% of mice (compared with 33% of mice protected with irradiated tumor cells alone) (61). In therapy experiments, some regressions of established CT26 tumors were seen. IL-2–secreting fibroblasts have also been used to treat intracerebral gliomas, resulting in a small, but statistically significant, improvement in survival (62). Interesting studies by Sun and Cohen have demonstrated that DNA from various tumors can be transfected into fibroblasts, which had previously been gene modified to express IL-2. In this manner, immunologic specificity was purportedly transferred to a cell line designed to produce IL-2 with modest antitumor effect (63).

Interleukin-2 Fusion Proteins

Another promising method for delivering IL-2 to the local tumor site is by using Ab-IL-2 fusion proteins. Becker and Reisfeld transfected B16 melanoma cells with the gene for ganglioside GD2, forming a cell line B78-D14 (64,65). They constructed a fusion protein containing an Ab to GD2 and human IL-2. When 50-mm^3 s.c. tumor nodules were treated with an i.v. injection of fusion protein, 37% of tumors completely regressed, and 63% partially regressed. This fusion protein was also used to treat 1-week-old pulmonary metastases induced by the i.v. injection of a mixture of B78-D14 and B16 (GD2-negative) tumor cells at a 5:1 ratio. Treatment with this IL-2 fusion protein was ineffective against B16 melanoma but effectively decreased the number of pulmonary metastases in mice injected with the mixture of B78-D14 and B16 tumors. The authors postulated that bystander killing of GD2-negative B16 tumors was induced and suggested that this strategy might be useful in the treatment of antigenically heterogeneous tumors. Of note, treatment with the IL-2 fusion protein was clearly more effective than concomitant treatment with the anti-GD2 Ab and systemic IL-2 or treatment with a nonspecific MAb–IL-2 fusion protein. IL-2 fusion protein treatment was effective in C57BL/6 beige/beige mice, indicating that NK cells were not involved in tumor destruction, but was only marginally effective in T-cell–deficient C57BL/6 severe combined immunodeficiency disease mice. In addition, Ab plus complement depletion of CD8+ T cells decreased the effectiveness of this fusion protein, indicating that CD8+ T cells were involved in IL-2 fusion protein–induced primary tumor regressions. These authors speculated that IL-2 fusion proteins may be operative by activating naïve T cells that were not previously activated, because peptide MHC or costimulatory molecules were at low levels, or by enhancing antigen-presenting cells phagocytosis of tumor cells. Long lived, tumor-specific protective immunity was established in mice that were cured of their tumors by IL-2 fusion protein therapy. Further experiments have shown that IL-2 fusion proteins can also effectively treat gene-modified, GD2-expressing neuroblastoma-hepatic metastases (66).

Other investigators have evaluated the efficacy of fusion protein–targeted IL-2 therapy. Melani et al. demonstrated that treatment with a fusion protein composed of IL-2 plus a single-chain Fv to α-folate receptor was able to reduce the volume of s.c. tumors (67). Liu and colleagues formed a fusion protein with IL-2 and an antiidiotype Ab that recognized the murine B-cell lymphoma 38C13. The IL-2 fusion protein inhibited lymphoma growth *in vivo* to a greater extent than combined therapy with anti-Id Ab plus systemic IL-2 (68). Using the same tumor system, Penichet et al. demonstrated that multiple injections with an IL-2–anti-Id fusion protein were effective in preventing tumor growth in the majority of animals but were ineffective in generating protective immunologic memory (69). Taking a different approach, Epstein et al. used IL-2 fusion proteins to selectively alter tumor vascular permeability in an attempt to deliver greater doses of Iodine 125–labeled MAbs to the tumor site (70). They found that pretreatment with a fusion protein consisting of IL-2 and an antifibronectin Ab, TV-1, led to a threefold higher uptake of radiolabeled Ab in the tumor compared with control mice treated with MAb TV-1 alone.

INTERLEUKIN-2: COMBINATION THERAPY

Interleukin-2 and Other Systemic Cytokines

Systemic IL-2 therapy has been combined with other systemically administered cytokines in an attempt to enhance antitumor effectiveness and decrease dose-limiting toxicity. In a series of preclinical murine tumor studies conducted in Rosenberg's laboratory, synergistic antitumor effects of immunotherapy were obtained by the combined administration of rIL-2 with TNF-α alone or with TNF-α plus IFN-α (71,72). Although enhanced therapeutic efficacy of the combination was achieved against the weakly immunogenic MCA-106 sarcoma at both s.c. and visceral sites, no significant antitumor effects were observed against the nonimmunogenic MCA-102 sarcoma. Wigginton and colleagues evaluated combination therapy with IL-2 and IL-12 (73). Whereas daily IL-2 therapy (300,000 IU per day) was prohibitively toxic, pulse treatment with IL-2 once per week combined with low-dose daily IL-12 injections was well tolerated and cured 60% of mice with established s.c. renal cell carcinoma (RenCa). This treatment strategy was also used in the adjuvant setting to treat metastatic disease after nephrectomy to remove the primary RenCa tumor. IL-2 or IL-12 alone had limited effectiveness, whereas the combination of low-dose IL-12 and pulse IL-2 resulted in cure for nearly all the mice.

Vallera et al. demonstrated that the combination of M-CSF and IL-2 delivered continuously by a pump protected approximately 80% of mice from a challenge with EL-4 lymphoma cells; this was significantly better than the protection elicited by either cytokine alone (74).

Interleukin-2 and Chemotherapy

Systemic IL-2 has also been combined with chemotherapy. In most of these studies, cytotoxic chemotherapeutic agents were administered first, followed by IL-2, with the rationale that lymphocytes would recover from cytotoxic chemotherapy sooner than the tumor cells. Papa and colleagues demonstrated that cyclophosphamide increased the effectiveness of IL-2 in the treatment of 10-day-old pulmonary metastases formed by two different tumors: the MCA-106 sarcoma and MC-38 adenocarcinoma (75). In similar experiments, doxorubicin hydrochloride (Adriamycin) and bischloroethylnitrosourea did not enhance the effectiveness of IL-2 therapy. Gautam et al. also evaluated the combination of IL-2 and doxorubicin hydrochloride (76). RenCa tumors treated with doxorubicin hydrochloride 14 days after implantation completely regressed in 90% of the mice but then recurred within 2 weeks in all mice. If mice were treated with doxorubicin hydrochloride, then followed by IL-2 daily for 10 days, tumor recurrence was delayed, and 25% of mice remained tumor free for 4 months. Treatment with IL-2 alone, in contrast, produced no antitumor responses. Mice rendered tumor free by treatment with doxorubicin hydrochloride and IL-2 were resistant to secondary tumor challenge.

Studies by other investigators of the combination of doxorubicin hydrochloride plus IL-2 (77); DTIC plus IL-2 (77); and cyclophosphamide, etoposide, and cisplatin plus IL-2 (78) have also demonstrated enhanced antitumor effects using the combination approach.

Interleukin-2 and Radiation Therapy

Seminal observations on the ability of IL-2 to enhance local tumor responses to radiation therapy were provided by Cameron, Spiess, and Rosenberg (79). Mice bearing 6-day-old hepatic metastases induced by an intrasplenic injection of the MC-38 colon adenocarcinoma were treated with saline, rIL-2 (50,000 U rIL-2 i.p. t.i.d. for 5 days), 750 cGy irradiation to the liver, or radiation plus IL-2. Although IL-2 alone did not improve survival, irradiation was associated with a median survival time of 20 days versus 11 days in control mice (p <.0001). The addition of IL-2 to local radiation therapy further improved the median survival time to 38 days (p <.0001 compared with radiation therapy alone). Hunter et al. showed a similar IL-2–induced enhancement of the effects of radiation therapy on lung metastases, although no improvement was seen in the treatment of the same tumor in an intramuscular site (80).

Younes and Haas investigated whether the combination of radiation therapy and IL-2 would enhance systemic immunity (81). In a RenCa pulmonary metastasis model in mice, treatment of the left lung with radiation therapy decreased the number of metastases present in a dose-dependent fashion but had no effect on the number of metastases in the opposite lung. Addition of IL-2 both decreased the number of metastases in the irradiated (left) lung and also caused a marked decrease in metastases in the right lung. These authors postulated that this systemic effect was caused by a radiation-induced increase in tumor MHC class I expression and showed that depletion of either ASGM1+, CD4+, or CD8+ cells abrogated the antitumor effect.

In s.c. SL-2 lymphoma and M8013 adenocarcinoma models in mice, Everse and colleagues showed that the combination of IL-2 with radiation therapy improved local tumor responses and disease-free survival, compared with treatment with either modality alone (82). For example, treatment of M8013 tumors with IL-2 or radiation therapy alone resulted in some partial responses, but tumors progressed in all mice. Treatment with radiation and 10 days of IL-2 resulted in cures of 50% of mice. To test for induction of systemic immunity, tumors were injected subcutaneously on both flanks. Only one side was treated with radiation and intratumoral IL-2. Systemic immune effects of the combination therapy were modest: only 30% of contralateral tumors achieved a partial or complete regression, and all of these mice died as a result of progressive tumor growth.

Interleukin-2 and Adoptive Immunotherapy

Before the identification of IL-2, adoptive immunotherapy was largely limited to the transfer of splenocytes from immunized mice. The recognition of IL-2 as a T-cell growth factor and its purification broadened the methods by which T cells with antitumor reactivity could be generated. Incubation of lymphoid cells in high-dose IL-2 resulted in the formation of LAK cells, which were characterized by their ability to lyse tumor cells, but not normal cells, *in vitro*. When LAK cells were adoptively transferred to tumor-bearing mice, the marked tumor regressions that were obtained were dependent on the systemic coadministration of IL-2 (11,83). rIL-2 has also made possible the growth of lymphocytes from viable tumor preparations, called *TILs*. Culture of TIL from tumors in high doses of IL-2 (1,000 U per mL) resulted in TIL with nonspecific cytolytic activity, whereas culture in lower doses of IL-2 (10–20 U per mL) generated TIL that exhibited immune specificity (84) and were more potent effectors in adoptive therapy of established tumors (85). Although high doses of TIL administered without IL-2 could mediate regressions of 3-day-old established pulmonary metastases, coadministration of systemic IL-2 significantly enhanced their therapeutic effectiveness (86), presumably by stimulating their proliferation *in vivo*.

Chang and Shu used a technique termed *in vitro sensitization* (IVS), whereby lymph node cells from tumor-bearing mice were cultured in the presence of IL-2 and irradiated tumor cells to generate cells that caused tumor regression on adoptive transfer to mice. As with TIL, IVS cells grown in low-dose IL-2 were more potent than IVS cells cultured in high-dose IL-2 when used to treat tumor-bearing mice (87). Furthermore, their effectiveness *in vivo* was also enhanced at least threefold by the concomitant administration of systemic IL-2 (88). These IVS effectors derived from tumor-draining lymph nodes were a mixture of CD4+ and CD8+ T lymphocytes, and Ab depletion studies have shown that both cell types were required for effective adoptive immunotherapy of tumor micrometastases (89). Of interest, administration of systemic IL-2 to CD4+ T cell depleted, activated tumor-draining lymph node cells restored the therapeutic effectiveness of the CD8+ T cells. It was postulated that IL-2 was able to substitute for CD4+ T-cell mediated "help" for CTLs *in vivo*. (Exogenous administration of IL-2 did not restore the antitumor efficacy of the adoptively transferred, CD8+ T-cell depleted cells.) Similar observations were made with CD8+, CD4– TIL cultures: coadministration of TIL with IL-2 resulted in potent antitumor effects (41). Of note, TIL cultured in low-dose IL-2 and injected intravenously could provide protection against subsequent tumor challenge for as long as 6 weeks, even in the absence of exogenous IL-2 (90).

Various strategies involving IL-2 have been used in an attempt to improve the efficacy of adoptive immunotherapy. Loeffler and Ochoa demonstrated that treatment of hepatic metastases using *in vitro*–stimulated splenocytes from tumor-bearing mice was more effective when IL-2 is delivered in liposomes rather than as free cytokine (91). Ohno et al. attempted to improve the potency of lymph node–derived effector cells by immunizing mice with an IL-2 gene-modified MCA-205 sarcoma (92). Tumor-draining lymph node cells harvested from mice bearing the IL-2 secreting tumors and activated *in vitro* were approximately threefold more effective than cells harvested from lymph nodes draining the control parental tumor. In similarly designed experiments with the poorly immunogenic B16-BL6 melanoma, Arca and colleagues demonstrated that tumors modified to express GM-CSF were more effective than IL-2–secreting tumors for priming lymph node cells for the generation of antitumor effectors (93). Finally, Nakamura et al. used an adenoviral vector to gene modify murine TIL to secrete IL-2 (94). These TIL were slightly more effective than nontransduced TIL in a B16 melanoma lung metastasis model.

Interleukin-2 and Vaccines

In 1982, Rosenberg et al. demonstrated that IL-2 administration *in vivo* could enhance the generation of cytotoxic cells directed against alloantigens (95). In these experiments, both normal and previously immunized C57BL/6 mice were injected with irradiated allogeneic P815 tumor cells, then treated with IL-2 for 3 days starting the day after tumor challenge. At 7 days, the antigen-specific cytotoxicity of splenocytes was greatly increased in mice that received IL-2. No enhanced activity was noted when IL-2 was given before or concurrently with antigen challenge.

Numerous subsequent investigators have confirmed the finding that IL-2 can enhance the effectiveness of tumor vaccines. O'Donnell et al. immunized mice with 3 s.c. injections of irradiated line 1 (L1) alveolar carcinoma cells (96). IL-2 was administered by different routes and schedules after each immunization. Mice were then challenged with live L1 tumors. The addition of IL-2 markedly increased the percentage of mice surviving the tumor challenge; its daily administration for 7 days was more effective than shorter courses. The antitumor effect required that IL-2 be injected adjacent to the site of the L1 vaccine; s.c. injection at a distant site or i.p. injections were not effective. Similar experiments using irradiated B16 melanoma as a vaccine also showed that IL-2 could enhance the development of protective antitumor immunity (97).

Arroyo et al. evaluated the value of IL-2 in combination with a vaccinia colon cancer oncolysate vaccine (98). Mice bearing 4-day-old CC-36 colon carcinoma hepatic metastases were treated with vaccinia oncolysate with or without IL-2. Although the vaccine alone had no effect on the number of hepatic tumor nodules and only a slight effect on survival, the combination of vaccinia plus IL-2 markedly decreased the number of hepatic metastases and resulted in survival of 67% of the treated mice (98,99). Similar results were obtained when a vaccinia virus IL-2 construct was used in place of free IL-2 (99). Bronte and colleagues also demonstrated that IL-2 could enhance the antitumor effectiveness of a vaccinia-virus vaccine. These investigators treated mice bearing 3-day-old pulmonary metastases from a β-galactosidase–expressing CT26 carcinoma with a β-galactosidase–expressing recombinant vaccinia virus (100). Results showed negligible survival benefit from the vaccine alone or when the vaccine was administered with GM-CSF, TNF, or IFN-γ. Marked improvement in survival occurred, however, with the systemic injection of IL-2 in conjunction with vaccine (see Fig. 3). Furthermore, insertion of the copy DNA encoding IL-2 into the vaccinia virus enhanced vaccine effectiveness, whereas GM-CSF, TNF, and IFN-γ gene insertion did not. In similar experiments, McLaughlin and associates showed that IL-2 could enhance the effectiveness of a recombinant vaccinia virus carcinoembryonic antigen (rV-CEA) vaccine (101). Seventy percent of mice bearing palpable CEA-expressing MC-38 tumors were cured by treatment with rV-CEA plus IL-2, compared with no long-term survivors when treated with rV-CEA alone or with control virus plus IL-2. Splenocytes from mice treated with rV-CEA plus IL-2 showed enhanced antigen-specific proliferation, cytotoxicity, and IFN-γ secretion.

The efficacy of combination therapy with IL-2 and a herpes simplex virus thymidine kinase vector "suicide" gene has also been evaluated. Chen and colleagues showed that hepatic metastases could be induced to undergo necrosis by direct injection of an adenoviral vector containing the herpes simplex virus

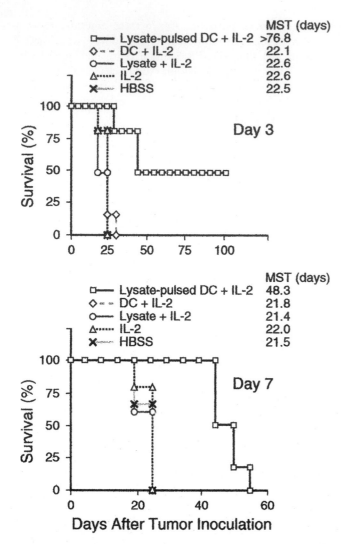

FIGURE 4. Treatment with the combination of tumor lysate–pulsed DC and interleukin-2 (IL-2) can prolong survival and result in cures of mice bearing established pulmonary metastases. Mice harboring MCA-207 lung metastases were immunized three times on days 3, 7, and 11 (*upper graph*) or days 7, 10, and 13 (*lower graph*) after tumor injection. IL-2 was given intraperitoneally twice daily at 20,000 IU per dose (*upper*) or 40,000 IU per dose (*lower*) for 3 consecutive days after each immunization. Control groups of mice received Hanks' balanced salt solution (HBSS) tumor lysate plus IL-2, unpulsed DC plus IL-2, or IL-2 alone. Survival was monitored over time after tumor injection, and the mean survival time (MST) in days was determined. (From Shimuzu K et al. Systematic administration of interleukin 2 enhances the therapeutic efficacy of dendritic cell-based tumor vaccines. *Proc Natl Acad Sci U S A* 1999;96:2268–2273, with permission.)

thymidine kinase vector gene, followed by treatment with ganciclovir (102). Protective immunity against subsequent challenge, however, only developed in mice infected concurrently with an adenoviral IL-2 vector.

Shimuzu et al. demonstrated that low-dose IL-2 could enhance protective and therapeutic immunity resulting from tumor lysate-pulsed dendritic cell (DC) vaccines (103). Mice harboring 3-day-old MCA-207 sarcoma pulmonary metastases were immunized with DC on days 3 and 7 and treated with

low-dose IL-2 on days 3 to 10. Fifty percent of the mice treated with DC plus IL-2 were cured of tumor. Immunization of mice bearing 7-day-old tumors with DC vaccine followed by IL-2 administration resulted in a greater reduction in pulmonary metastases than that obtained with DC vaccines treatment alone (Fig. 4). Furthermore, when IL-2 was combined with three DC immunizations in the treatment of 14-day-old s.c. MCA-207 tumors, 80% of mice could be rendered disease free.

CONCLUSION

The lymphokine IL-2 is a glycoprotein secreted predominantly by Th1 cells that mediates a variety of immunologic effects *in vitro* and *in vivo*. Large quantities of rIL-2 became available in the early 1980s through DNA technology. In addition, the advent of new technologies to efficiently insert, by recombinant, viral, or other means, the copy DNA encoding for IL-2 into a variety of mammalian target cells has allowed for the local production of IL-2 at tumor sites. As described in this chapter, extensive preclinical studies of IL-2, alone or combined with other biotherapeutic agents, in the immunotherapy of established cancer have been conducted in a variety of animal models. When administered systemically to mice, IL-2 can mediate substantial regressions of s.c. tumors, as well as visceral metastases. Importantly, the antitumor efficacy of IL-2 can be enhanced by its combination with other therapies, allowing for lower effective doses with reduced toxicity. Preclinical animal studies have also provided important insight into the characteristics of tumor cells that determine sensitivity or resistance to IL-2–based immunotherapies, particularly with respect to the expression of MHC molecules and relative tumor immunogenicity *in vivo*. Moreover, the dissection of the *in vivo* mechanisms underlying IL-2–mediated tumor regression, as well as toxic side effects in animal models, has shown that it may be possible to selectively inhibit IL-2 toxicity while maintaining (or increasing) therapeutic efficacy. Lastly, the combination of IL-2 with new vaccine strategies that use either potent DCs or recombinant viral vectors have provided new promising applications of IL-2 for cancer treatment.

REFERENCES

1. Morgan DA, Ruscetti FW, Gallo RC. Selective *in vitro* growth of T lymphocytes from normal human bone marrow. *Science* 1976;193: 1007–1008.
2. Taniguchi T, Matsui H, Fujita T, et al. Structure and expression of a cloned cDNA for human interleukin-1. *Nature* 1983;302:305–309.
3. Rosenberg SA, Grimm EA, McGrogan M, et al. Biological activity of recombinant human interleukin-2 produced *E coli. Science* 1984;223:1412–1414.
4. Donohue JH, Rosenbert SA. The fate of interleukin-2 after *in vivo* administration. *J Immunol* 1983;130:2203–2208.
5. Chang AE, Hyatt CL, Rosenberg SA. Systemic administration of recombinant human interleukin-2 in mice. *J Biol Response Mod* 1984;3:561–572.
6. Gennuso R, Spigelman MK, Vallabhajosula S, et al. Systemic biodistribution of radio-iodinated interleukin-2 in the rat. *J Biol Response Mod* 1989;8:375–384.

7. Yang JC, Schwarz Sl, Perry-Lalley DM, et al. Murine studies using polyethylene glycol-modified recombinant human interleukin-2 (PEG-IL-2): antitumor effects of PEG-IL-2 alone and in combination with adoptive cellular transfer. *Lymphokine Cytokine Res* 1991;10:475–480.

8. Rosenberg SA, Mulé JJ, Spiess PJ, et al. Regression of established pulmonary metastases and subcutaneous tumor mediated by the systemic administration of high-dose recombinant interleukin-2. *J Exp Med* 1985;161:1169–1188.

9. Papa MZ, Mulé JJ, Rosenberg SA. The anti-tumor efficacy of lymphokine-activated killer cells and recombinant interleukin-2 *in vivo*: successful immunotherapy of established pulmonary metastases from weakly- and non-immunogenic murine tumors of three distinct histologic types. *Cancer Res* 1986;46:4973–4978.

10. Ettinghausen SE, Rosenberg SA. Immunotherapy of murine sarcomas using lymphokine-activated killer cells: optimization of the schedule and route of administration of recombinant interleukin-2. *Cancer Res* 1986;46:2784–2792.

11. Lafreniere R, Rosenberg SA. Successful immunotherapy of murine experimental hepatic metastases with lymphokine-activated killer cells and recombinant interleukin-2. *Cancer Res* 1985;45:3735–3741.

12. Lafreniere R, Rosenberg SA. Adoptive immunotherapy of murine hepatic metastases with lymphokine-activated killer (LAK) cells and recombinant interleukin-2 (rIL-2) can mediate the regression of both immunogenic and nonimmunogenic sarcomas and an adenocarcinoma. *J Immunol* 1985;135:4273–4280.

13. Thompson JA, Peace DJ, Klarnet JP, et al. Eradication of disseminated murine leukemia by treatment with high-dose interleukin-2. *J Immunol* 1986;137:3675–3680.

14. Everse LA, Bernsen MR, Dullens HF, et al. The success of locoregional, low-dose recombinant interleukin-2 therapy in tumor-bearing mice is dependent on the time of rIL-2 administration. *J Exp Ther Oncol* 1996;1:231–236.

15. Kedar E, Braun E, Rutkowski Y, et al. Delivery of cytokines by liposomes. II. Interleukin-2 encapsulated in long-circulating sterically stabilized liposomes: immunomodulatory and anti-tumor activity in mice. *J Immunol* 1994;16:115–124.

16. Mattijssen V, Balemans LT, Steerenberg PA, et al. Polyethylene-glycol-modified interleukin-2 is superior to interleukin-2 in locoregional immunotherapy of established guinea-pig tumors. *Int J Cancer* 1992;51:812–817.

17. Bernsen MR, Dullens HFJ, Den Otter W, et al. Re-evaluation of the superiority of polyethylene glycol-modified interleukin-2 over regular recombinant interleukin-2. *J Interferon Cytokine Res* 1995;15:641–645.

18. Mulé JJ, Yang JC, Lafreniere RL, et al. Identification of cellular mechanisms operational *in vivo* during the regression of established pulmonary metastases by the systemic administration of high-dose recombinant interleukin-2. *J Immunol* 1987;139:285–294.

19. Peace DJ, Cheever MA. Toxicity and therapeutic efficacy of high-dose interleukin-1: *in vivo* infusion of antibody to NK-1.1 attenuates toxicity without compromising efficacy against murine leukemia. *J Exp Med* 1989;169:161–173.

20. Anderson TD, Hayes TJ, Powers GD, et al. Comparative toxicity and pathology associated with administration of recombinant IL-2 to animals. *Int Rev Exp Pathol* 1993;34:57–77.

21. Rosenstein M, Ettinghausen SE, Rosenberg SA. Extravasation of intravascular fluid mediated by the systemic administration of recombinant interleukin-2. *J Immunol* 1986;137:1735–1742.

22. Gately MK, Anderson TD, Hayes TJ. Role of asialo-GM1-positive lymphoid cells in mediating the toxic effects of recombinant IL-2 in mice. *J Immunol* 1988;14:189–200.

23. Edwards MJ, Heniford BT, Klar FA, et al. Pentoxifylline inhibits interleukin-2-induced toxicity in C57BL/6 mice but preserves antitumor efficacy. *J Clin Invest* 1992;90:637–641.

24. DeJoy SQ, Jeyaseelan R, Torley LW, et al. Attenuation of interleukin-2 induced pulmonary vascular leak syndrome by low doses of oral methotrexate. *Cancer Res* 1995;55:4929–4935.

25. Kemeny MM, Botchkina GI, Ochani M, et al. The tetravalent guanylhydrazone CNI-1493 blocks the toxic effects of interleukin-2 without diminishing antitumor efficacy. *Proc Natl Acad Sci U S A* 1998;95:4561–4566.

26. Dubinett SM, Huang M, Lichtenstein A, et al. Tumor necrosis factor-alpha plays a central role in interleukin-2 induced pulmonary vascular leak and lymphocyte accumulation. *Cell Immunol* 1994;157:170–180.

27. Quinn TD, Miller FN, Wilson MA, et al. Interleukin-2 induced lymphocyte infiltration of multiple organs is differentially suppressed by soluble tumor necrosis factor receptor. *J Surg Res* 1994;56:117–122.

28. Fraker DL, Thom AK, Doherty GM, et al. Tumour necrosis factor mediates the survival benefit of interleukin-2 in a murine pulmonary metastases model. *Surg Oncol* 1992;1:1–9.

29. Forni G, Gioivarelli M, Santoni A. Lymphokine-activated tumor inhibition *in vivo*. *J Immunol* 1985;134:1305–1311.

30. Vaage J. Local and systemic effects during interleukin-2 therapy of mouse mammary tumors. *Cancer Res* 1987;47:4296–4298.

31. Dubinett SM, Patrone L, Tobias J, et al. Intratumoral interleukin-2 immunotherapy: activation of tumor-infiltrating and splenic lymphocytes *in vivo*. *Cancer Immunol Immunother* 1993;36:156–162.

32. Sosnowski JT, DeHaven JI, Riggs DR, et al. Treatment of murine transitional cell carcinoma with intralesional interleukin-2 and murine interferon gamma. *J Urol* 1991;146:1164–1167.

33. Maas RA, Henk D, Weering JV, et al. Intratumoral low-dose interleukin-2 induces rejection of distant solid tumour. *Cancer Immunol Immunother* 1991;33:389–394.

34. Yeung RS, Vollmer C, Taylor DD, et al. Intratumoral rIL-2-based immunotherapy in B16 melanoma. *J Surg Res* 1992;53:203–210.

35. Sacchi M, Snyderman CH, Heo DS, et al. Local adoptive immunotherapy of human head and neck cancer xenografts in nude mice with lymphokine-activated killer cells and interleukin 2. *Cancer Res* 1990;50:3113–3118.

36. Egilnez NK, Jong YS, Iwanuma Y, et al. Cytokine immunotherapy of cancer with controlled release biodegradable microspheres in a human tumor xenograft/SCID mouse model. *Cancer Immunol Immunother* 1998;46:21–24.

37. Okuno K, Nakamura K, Tanaka A, et al. Hepatic immunopotentiation by galactose-entrapped liposomal IL-2 compound in the treatment of liver metastases. *Surg Today* 1998;28:64–69.

38. Hautmann S, Huland E, Huland H. Intratumoral depot interleukin-2 therapy inhibits tumor growth in Dunning adenocarcinoma of the prostate implanted subcutaneously in rats. *J Cancer Res Clin Oncol* 1997;123:614–618.

39. Levraud JP, Duffour MT, Cordier L, et al. IL-2 gene delivery within an established murine tumor causes its regression without proliferation of pre-existing antitumor-specific CTL. *J Immunol* 1997;158:3335–3342.

40. Fearon ER, Pardoll DM, Itaya T, et al. Interleukin-2 production by tumor cells bypasses T helper function in the generation of an antitumor response *Cell* 1990;60:397.

41. Barth RJ, Mulé JJ, Spiess PJ, et al. Interferon and tumor necrosis factor have a role in tumor regressions mediated by murine CD8+ tumor-infiltrating lymphocytes. *J Exp Med* 1991;173:647–658.

42. Huang H, Chen SH, Kosai K, et al. Gene therapy for hepatocellular carcinoma: long-term remission of primary and metastatic tumors in mice by interleukin-2 gene therapy *in vivo*. *Gene Therapy* 1996;3:980–987.

43. Gansbacher B, Zier K, Daniels B, et al. Interleukin-2 gene transfer into tumor cells abrogates tumorigenicity and induces protective immunity. *J Exp Med* 1990;172:1217–1224.

44. Ley VP, Langlade-Demoyen P, Kourilsky P, et al. Interleukin-2-dependent activation of tumor-specific cytotoxic T lymphocytes *in vivo*. *Eur J Immunol* 1991;21:851–854.

45. Cavallo F, Gioivarelli M, Gulino A, et al. Role of neutrophils and CD4+ T lymphocytes in the primary and memory response to nonimmunogenic murine mammary adenocarcinoma made immunogenic by IL-2 gene transfection. *J Immunol* 1992;149:3627–3635.

46. Porgador A, Gansbacher B, Bannerji R, et al. Antimetastatic vaccination of tumor-bearing mice with IL-2 gene-inserted tumor cells. *Int J Cancer* 1993;53:471–477.

47. Karp SE, Farber A, Salo JC, et al. Cytokine secretion by genetically modified nonimmunogenic murine fibrosarcoma. *J Immunol* 1993; 150:896–908.

48. Hock H, Dorsch M, Kunzendorf U, et al. Mechanisms of rejection induced by tumor cell-targeted gene transfer of interleukin-2, interleukin-4, interleukin-7, tumor necrosis factor or interferon γ. *Immunology* 1993;90:2774–2778.

49. Ram Z, Walbridge S, Heiss J, et al. In vivo transfer of the human interleukin-2 gene: negative tumoricidal results in experimental brain tumors. *J Neurosurg* 1994;80:535–540.

50. Dranoff G, Jaffee E, Lazenby A, et al. Vaccination with irradiated tumor cells engineered to secrete murine granulocyte-macrophage colony-stimulating factor stimulates potent, specific and long-standing antitumor immunity. *Proc Natl Acad Sci U S A* 1993;90:3539–3543.

51. Cavallo F, Di Pierro F, Giovarelli M, et al. Protective and curative potential of vaccination with interleukin-2 gene-transfected cells from a spontaneous mouse mammary adenocarcinoma. *Cancer Res* 1993;53:5067–5070.

52. Schmidt W, Schweighoffer T, Herbst E, et al. Cancer vaccines: the interleukin-2 dosage effect. *Proc Natl Acad Sci U S A* 1995;92: 4711–4714.

53. Vieweg J, Rosenthal FM, Bannerji R, et al. Immunotherapy of prostate cancer in the Dunning rat model: use of cytokine gene modified tumor vaccines. *Cancer Res* 1994;54:1760–1765.

54. Saito S, Bannerji R, Gansbacher B, et al. Immunotherapy of bladder cancer with cytokine gene-modified tumor vaccines. *Cancer Res* 1994;54:3516–3520.

55. Rosenthal FM, Cronin K, Bannerji R, et al. Augmentation of antitumor immunity by tumor cells transduced with retroviral vector carrying the interleukin-2 and interferon-γ c DNAs. *Blood* 1994;83: 1289–1298.

56. Clary BM, Coveney EC, Blazer DG, et al. Active immunotherapy of pancreatic cancer with tumor cells genetically engineered to secrete multiple cytokines. *Surgery* 1996;120:174–181.

57. Strome SE, Chang AE, Shu S, et al. Secretion of both IL-2 and IL-4 by tumor cells results in rejection and immunity. *J Immunother* 1996;19:21–23.

58. Emtage P, Yonghong W, Bramson JL, et al. A double recombinant adenovirus expressing the costimulatory molecule B7-1 (murine) and human IL2 induces complete tumor regression in a murine breast adenocarcinoma model. *J Immunol* 1998;160:2533–2538.

59. Gaken JA, Hollingsworth SJ, Hirst WJ, et al. Irradiated NC adenocarcinoma cells transduced with both B7.1 and interleukin-2 induce CD4+-mediated rejection of establishing tumors. *Hum Gene Ther* 1997;8:477–488.

60. De Vos S, Kohn DB, Cho SK, et al. Immunotherapy against murine leukemia. *Leukemia* 1998;12:401–405.

61. Faljrao J, Shawler DL, Gjerset R, et al. Cytokine gene therapy with interleukin-2-transduced fibroblasts: effects of IL-2 dose on antitumor therapy. *Hum Gene Ther* 1995;6:591–601.

62. Glick RP, Lichtor T, Mogharbel A, et al. Intracerebral versus subcutaneous immunization with allogeneic fibroblasts genetically engineered to secrete interleukin-2 in the treatment of central nervous system glioma and melanoma. *Neurosurgery* 1997;41:898–906.

63. Sun T, Kim TS, Waltz MR, et al. Interleukin-2-secreting mouse fibroblasts transfected with genomic DNA from murine neoplasms induce tumor-specific immune responses that prolong the lives of tumor-bearing mice. *Cancer Gene Ther* 1995;2:183–190.

64. Becker JC, Varki N, Gillies SD, et al. An antibody-interleukin-2 fusion protein overcomes tumor heterogeneity by induction of a cellular immune response. *Immunology* 1996;93:7826–7831.

65. Becker JC, Pancook JD, Gillies SD, et al. T cell-mediated eradication of murine metastatic melanoma induced by targeted interleukin 2 therapy. *J Exp Med* 1996;183:2361–2366.

66. Lode HN, Xiang R, Varki NM, et al. Targeted interleukin-2 therapy for spontaneous neuroblastoma metastases to bone marrow. *J Natl Cancer Inst* 1997;89:1586–1594.

67. Melani C, Figini M, Nicosia D, et al. Targeting of interleukin-2 to human ovarian carcinoma by fusion with a single-chain Fv of anti-folate receptor antibody. *Cancer Res* 1998;58:4146–4154.

68. Liu SJ, Sher YP, Ting CC, et al. Treatment of B-cell lymphoma with chimeric IgG and single-chain Fv antibody-interleukin-2 fusion proteins. *Blood* 1998;92:2103–2112.

69. Penichet ML, Harvill ET, Morrison SL. An IgG3-IL-2 fusion protein recognizing a murine B cell lymphoma exhibits effective tumor imaging and antitumor activity. *J Interferon Cytokine Res* 1998;18: 597–607.

70. Epstein AI, Khawli LA, Hornick JL, et al. Identification of a monoclonal antibody, TV-1 directed against the basement membrane of tumor vessels, and its use to enhance the delivery of macromolecules to tumors after conjugation with interleukin-2. *Cancer Res* 1995; 55:2673–2680.

71. McIntosh JK, Mule JJ, Merino MJ, et al. Synergistic antitumor effects of immunotherapy with recombinant IL-2 and recombinant TNF. *Cancer Res* 1988;48:4011–4017.

72. McIntosh JK, Mule JJ, Krosnick JA, et al. Combination cytokine immunotherapy with TNF, IL-2 and IFN and its synergistic antitumor effects in mice. *Cancer Res* 1989;49:1408–1414.

73. Wigginton JM, Komschlies KL, Back TC, et al. Administration of interleukin-12 with pulse interleukin-2 and the rapid and complete eradication of murine renal carcinoma. *J Natl Cancer Inst* 1996;88: 38–42.

74. Vallera DA, Taylor PA, Aukerman SL, et al. Antitumor protection from the murine T-cell leukemia/lymphoma EL4 by the continuous subcutaneous coadministration of recombinant macrophage-colony stimulating factor and interleukin-2. *Cancer Res* 1993;53:4273–4280.

75. Papa MZ, Yang JC, Vetto JT, et al. Combined effects of chemotherapy and interleukin-2 in the therapy of mice with advanced pulmonary tumors. *Cancer Res* 1988;48:122–129.

76. Gautam SC, Chikkala NF, Ganapathi R, et al. Combination therapy with adriamycin and interleukin-2 augments immunity against murine renal cell carcinoma. *Cancer Res* 1991;51:6133–6137.

77. LoRusso PM, Aukerman SL, Polin L, et al. Antitumor efficacy of interleukin-2 alone and in combination with adriamycin and dacarbazine in murine solid tumor systems. *Cancer Res* 1990;50:5876–5882.

78. Rinehart JJ, Triozzi PL, Lee MH, et al. Modulation of hematologic and immunologic effects of high dose chemotherapy by interleukin-2 in a murine tumor model. *Mol Biother* 1992;4:77–82.

79. Cameron RB, Spiess PJ, Rosenberg SA. Synergistic antitumor activity of tumor-infiltrating lymphocytes, interleukin-2, and local tumor irradiation. *J Exp Med* 1990;171:249.

80. Hunter N, Nakayama T, Ito H, et al. Combination of interleukin-2 and irradiation in therapy of murine tumors. *Clin Exp Metastasis* 1992;10:431–436.

81. Younes E, Haas GB, Dezso B, et al. Local tumor irradiation augments the response to IL-2 therapy in a murine renal adenocarcinoma. *Cell Immunol* 1995;165:243–251.

82. Everse LA, Renes IB, Jurgenliemk-Schultz IM, et al. Local low-dose interleukin-2 induces systemic immunity when combined with radiotherapy of cancer. A pre-clinical study. *Int J Cancer* 1997;72: 1003–1007.

83. Mulé JJ, Shu S, Schwarz SL, et al. Adoptive immunotherapy of established pulmonary metastases with LAK cells and recombinant IL-2. *Science* 1984;225:1487–1489.

84. Barth RJ, Bock SN, Mulé JJ, et al. Unique murine tumor-associated antigens identified by tumor infiltrating lymphocytes. *J Immunol* 1990;144:1531–1537.

85. Yang JC, Perry-Lalley D, Rosenberg SA. An improved method for growing murine tumor-infiltrating lymphocytes with in vivo antitumor activity. *J Bio Resp Mod* 1990;9:149–159.

86. Spiess PJ, Yang JC, Rosenberg SA. In vivo antitumor activity of tumor-infiltrating lymphocytes expanded in recombinant interleukin-2. *J Natl Cancer Inst* 1987;79:1067–1075.

87. Chou T, Bertera S, Chang AE, et al. Adoptive immunotherapy of microscopic and advanced visceral metastases with in vitro sensitized lymphoid cells from mice bearing progressive tumors. *J Immunol* 1988;141:1775–1781.

88. Yoshizawa H, Chang AE, Shu S. Specific adoptive immunotherapy mediated by tumor-draining lymph node cells sequentially activated with anti-CD3 and IL-2. *J Immunol* 1991;147:729–737.

89. Yoshizawa H, Chang AE, Shu S. Cellular interactions in effector cell generation and tumor regression mediated by anti-CD3/interleukin 2-activated tumor-draining lymph node cells. *Cancer Res* 1992;52:1129–1136.

90. Alexander RB, Rosenberg SA. Long term survival of adoptively transferred tumor infiltrating lymphocytes in mice. *J Immunol* 1990;145:1615–1620.

91. Loeffler CM, Platt JL, Anderson PM, et al. Antitumor effects of interleukin 2 liposomes and anti-CD3-stimulated T-cells against murine MC-38 hepatic metastases. *Cancer Res* 1991;51:2127–2132.

92. Ohno K, Yoshizawa H, Tsukada H, et al. Adoptive immunotherapy with tumor-specific T lymphocytes generated from cytokine gene-modified tumor-primed lymph node cells. *J Immunol* 1996;156:3875–3881.

93. Arca MJ, Krauss JC, Strome SE, et al. Diverse manifestations of tumorigenicity and immunogenicity displayed by the poorly immunogenic B16-BL6 melanoma transduced with cytokine genes. *Cancer Immunol Immunother* 1996;42:237–245.

94. Nakamura Y, Wakimoto H, Abe J, et al. Adoptive immunotherapy with murine tumor-specific T lymphocytes engineered to secrete interleukin 2. *Cancer Res* 1994;54:5757–5760.

95. Rosenberg SA, Spiess PJ, Schwarz SL. *In vivo* administration of interleukin-2 enhances specific alloimmune responses. *Transplantation* 1983;35:631–634.

96. O'Donnell RW, Marquis DM, Mudholkar GS, et al. *In vivo* enhancement of antitumor immunity by interleukin-2-rich lymphokines. *Cancer Res* 1986;46:3273–3278.

97. Stidham KR, Ricci WM, Vervaert C, et al. Modulation of specific active immunization against murine melanoma using recombinant cytokines. *Surg Oncol* 1996;5:221–229.

98. Arroyo PJ, Bash JA, Wallack MK. Active specific immunotherapy with vaccinia colon oncolysate enhances the immunomodulatory and antitumor effects of interleukin-2 and interferon in a murine hepatic metastasis model. *Cancer Immunol Immunother* 1990;31:305–311.

99. Tanaka N, Sivanandham M, Wallack MK. Immunotherapy of a vaccinia colon oncolysate prepared with interleukin-2 gene-encoded vaccinia virus and interferon-alpha increases the survival of mice bearing syngeneic colon adenocarcinoma. *J Immunother* 1994;16: 283–293.

100. Bronte V, Tsung K, Rao JB, et al. IL-2 enhances the function of recombinant poxvirus-based vaccines in the treatment of established pulmonary metastases. *J Immunol* 1995;154:5282–5291.

101. McLaughlin JP, Schlom J, Kanter JA, et al. Improved immunotherapy of a recombinant carcinoembryonic antigen vaccinia vaccine when given in combination with interleukin-2. *Cancer Res* 1996;56: 2361–2367.

102. Chen SH, Chen XH, Wang Y, et al. Combination gene therapy for liver metastasis of colon carcinoma *in vivo. Med Sci* 1995;92:2577–2581.

103. Shimizu K, Fields RC, Giedlin M, et al. Systemic administration of interleukin 2 enhances the therapeutic efficacy of dendritic cell-based tumor vaccines. *Proc Natl Acad Sci U S A* 1999;96: 2268–2273.

INTERLEUKIN-2: CLINICAL APPLICATIONS

Principles of Administration and Management of Side Effects

DOUGLAS J. SCHWARTZENTRUBER

INTERLEUKIN-2

Interleukin-2 (IL-2) is a hormone that was first described as a T-cell growth factor in 1976 (1). The many immune-modulating properties of IL-2 led to its use in the treatment of cancer patients. The first reported use was in 1983 by Bindon and colleagues (2), who treated two melanoma patients with natural IL-2 derived from stimulated normal lymphocytes. Shortly after, Lotze and colleagues treated acquired immunodeficiency syndrome and cancer patients with IL-2 that was derived from the Jurkat cell line, a human T-cell tumor (3,4). Patients treated with this preparation had measurable changes in various immunologic parameters. No antitumor responses were observed, however, because small doses were used. Large-scale use of IL-2 was not feasible until recombinant IL-2 (rIL-2) became available. This was made possible when the gene for IL-2 was discovered (5) and subsequently expressed in the bacteria *Escherichia coli*. This new molecule was shown to be biologically and functionally similar to natural IL-2 (6,7).

A variety of doses and routes of administration of rIL-2 and Jurkat-derived IL-2 were explored (4,8,9). These studies defined the maximal tolerated doses and toxicities of IL-2. Initially, tumor regressions were not seen until rIL-2 was combined with lymphokine-activated killer (LAK) cells (10). The first patient to respond to this treatment was a woman with widely metastatic cutaneous melanoma who experienced a complete disappearance of tumors. Shortly after, responses to rIL-2 administered alone were observed (11). Randomized studies demonstrated that IL-2 was as effective alone as when combined with LAK cells in patients with metastatic renal cell cancer and melanoma (12) (SA Rosenberg, *personal communication*).

The use of high-dose bolus intravenous IL-2 regimens, as developed by Rosenberg et al. (10), was based on laboratory models, indicating that tumor responses correlated with dose intensity (13). Many studies using this regimen of IL-2 alone have described partial or complete tumor regression in 14% to 20% of patients with metastatic melanoma or renal carcinoma (14–18). These conditions are reviewed in other chapters. Based on such

studies, the U.S. Food and Drug Administration approved the use of IL-2 for the treatment of metastatic renal carcinoma in 1992 and for metastatic melanoma in 1998.

rIL-2 has also been used by continuous intravenous infusion: one day a week (19,20), 4 to 5 days per week (21–28), or for 21 to 90 days (9,29,30) (Table 1). The most common regimens in the United States and Europe consist of daily subcutaneous IL-2 administration (31–37) (see Table 1). The various routes, doses, and schedules of IL-2 administration have resulted in different toxicities and immunomodulatory effects (8,20,30,38–41). Comparative studies to define the optimal regimen are needed. One such study is currently under way (42). Other less frequent routes of IL-2 administration have included intraperitoneal (43–46), intrapleural (47–49), intralesional (50,51), intracranial (52–57), intravesical (58,59), intraarterial (60,61), perilymphatic (62), intralymphatic (63), continuous subcutaneous (64), intramuscular (40), and by inhalation (65) (see Table 1).

Many unique and diverse side effects can be associated with the various routes and regimens of IL-2 administration. This chapter focuses on the side effects associated with the most intense form of administration—high-dose intravenous therapy in adult patients. Low-dose IL-2 administered as an outpatient generally manifests a lesser degree of toxicity but can affect the same organ systems as high-dose IL-2 and is potentially as severe (66). Interest in the use of IL-2 to treat pediatric malignancies is growing (67–70). The role of IL-2 in the treatment of this patient population remains to be defined.

Pharmacology

Proleukin(R) (Aldesleukin) is presently the only commercially available rIL-2 that is approved for human use in the United States. This preparation, produced by Cetus Oncology Division of Chiron Corporation, varies from natural IL-2 because it is nonglycosylated, the cysteine at amino acid position 125 has been replaced by serine, and it lacks the N-terminal alanine. rIL-2 has been shown to be biologically and functionally similar to

TABLE 1. ROUTES OF INTERLEUKIN-2 ADMINISTRATION

Daily subcutaneous (31–37)
Bolus intravenous every 8 h
  High dose (14–18)
  Low dose (42)
Continuous intravenous infusion
  1 d/wk (19,20)
  4–5 d/wk (21–28)
  21–90 d (9,29,30)
Infrequent routes of interleukin-2 administration
  Intraperitoneal (43–46)
  Intrapleural (47–49)
  Intralesional (50,51)
  Intracranial (52–57)
  Intravesical (58,59)
  Intraarterial (60,61)
  Perilymphatic (62)
  Intralymphatic (63)
  Continuous subcutaneous (64)
  Intramuscular (40)
  Inhalation (65)

natural IL-2 (6,7). Other companies (i.e., Hoffmann-LaRoche, Ortho, and Biogen) have supplied IL-2 with comparable biologic activity and toxicities in clinical trials. All preparations vary according to unit system and are administered according to body weight or body surface area. To help standardize the use of IL-2, the World Health Organization defined international units based on an international standard (71). This standard replaced the interim reference reagent previously established by the biologic response modifiers program of the National Cancer Institute (72). One Cetus (Chiron) unit is equivalent to 6 international units and is approximately 2.3 Hoffmann-La Roche units.

IL-2 is rapidly cleared from the circulation after intravenous administration. Initial clearance (α distribution) of rIL-2 is rapid, with a half-life of 7 to 13 minutes, followed by a longer β clearance with a half-life of 60 to 85 minutes (8,73). The later delayed clearance is consistent with a two-compartment model of rapid initial egress of IL-2 into the extravascular space, then a slower return into the plasma. With subcutaneous administration, lower peak serum levels of IL-2 are achieved than with intravenous administration, and levels remain fairly constant for 8 hours (73,74). IL-2 is eliminated from the body primarily by metabolism in the kidneys, as demonstrated in a murine model (75).

Immunologic Activity

Immunologic changes are among the earliest measurable consequences of the systemic administration of IL-2 to the human body. Lymphopenia develops within minutes of a single dose of IL-2 (8,23,38,41,76,77). With ongoing therapy, whether bolus or continuous infusion, the lymphopenia is profound and persistent. This phenomenon is thought to occur secondary to margination and egress of lymphocytes into the extravascular space. Twenty-four to 36 hours after discontinuation of IL-2, a rebound lymphocytosis of 2- to 70-fold above baseline occurs, which persists for 2 to 7 days; this rebound is dose and schedule dependent (23,38,41,77).

Paralleling the rapid lymphopenia is the acute loss of LAK precursors and natural killer activity from the circulation, occurring within 15 minutes of a single (bolus) dose of intravenous IL-2 (8,78); cytolytic activity is recovered in 24 to 72 hours. During continuous infusion of IL-2, peripheral blood mononuclear cells regain cytolytic activity by 5 to 7 days (8,79). One to 2 days after discontinuation of bolus or continuous IL-2, cytolysis of Daudi and K562 rebounds above baseline in a dose- and schedule-dependent fashion (8,38,39,41,79). When IL-2 is given subcutaneously and the dose escalated weekly, natural killer and LAK killing by fresh peripheral blood mononuclear cells at day twenty-eight is increased when compared with baseline (80). Phenotypically, increases in CD56+ cells can be measured during or after continuous or prolonged therapy with IL-2, as well as increased CD2 expression on CD56+ cells (27,81–83).

Peripheral blood mononuclear cells display decreased proliferative responses to IL-2, mitogens, and soluble antigens during IL-2 therapy (8,79,84,85), responses that rebound after IL-2 discontinuation. With repetitive IL-2 administration, lymphocytes become activated, as demonstrated by the expression of the IL-2 receptor (CD25) on the cell surface (8,27,38,39,86). Soluble IL-2 receptors shed from the cell surface are increased in the serum (40,86–89); soluble CD8 increases as well (88). Other activation markers, such as HLA-DR expression, increase on CD3+ and CD56+ cells (38,39,90). The expression of the adhesion molecule ICAM-1 increases on large granular lymphocytes after beginning IL-2 (91). At the tissue level, profound lymphocytic infiltrates have been documented in a variety of organs and tumors (92–94). After IL-2 therapy, patients can develop immediate hypersensitivity to skin test recall antigens (85). Delayed-type hypersensitivity responses, however, are depressed (84,85).

The effects of IL-2 on B cells and their function have been less well characterized. B-cell numbers decrease with IL-2 infusion (20,84,95,96). Several days after discontinuation of IL-2, B cells return to baseline but do not rebound to the same extent as T cells (84). B-cell products, immunoglobulin (Ig) G, IgM, and IgA, are moderately decreased during IL-2 infusion (79,84,85,96) but return to normal or higher levels after stopping IL-2. This phenomenon may be partly a result of redistribution changes secondary to fluid shifts characteristic of vascular leak syndrome (VLS). Tetanus-specific IgG is increased during IL-2 therapy after tetanus reimmunization, suggesting that B-cell function is preserved (79). Markedly depressed tetanus- and KLH-specific Igs were noted, however, after vaccination of patients receiving IL-2 within 3 weeks of intensive chemotherapy or bone marrow transplantation when compared with non–IL-2 recipients (96). This suggests that B-cell function may be impaired by IL-2 therapy in the setting of recent chemotherapy.

Neutrophil counts have generally been unaffected by IL-2. Severe neutropenia during or shortly after IL-2 therapy is rare (15,16,41,97). In fact, increased neutrophils are noted in the first 24 hours of IL-2, along with a shift to immature forms (77,98). Transient neutrophil dysfunction occurs, however, as noted by decreased Fc-receptor expression and decreased chemotaxis while bacterial phagocytosis is preserved (98,99).

TABLE 2. TOXICITY ASSOCIATED WITH THE ADMINISTRATION OF HIGH-DOSE INTERLEUKIN-2 ALONE IN 447 CONSECUTIVE TREATMENT COURSES

Category	Toxicity (% of Courses)
Systemic	Malaise[a] (14.5), chills[a] (18.3), pruritus[a] (8.9), weight gain >5% body weight (70.9), edema causing neurovascular compression (0.9)
Hemodynamic	Hypotension requiring pressors (52.1)
Cardiac	Arrhythmia (6.5), angina (1.1), myocardial infarction (0.4)
Pulmonary	Respiratory distress (4.0), intubation (2.9), pleural effusion requiring thoracentesis (1.1)
Renal	Oliguria (26.1), elevated creatinine (2.1 mg/dL–6.0 mg/dL = 62.0; >6.0 mg/dL = 6.3)
Gastrointestinal	Mucositis[a] (0.4), nausea/vomiting[a] (38.0), diarrhea[a] (30.2)
Hepatic	Hyperbilirubinemia (2.1 mg/dL–6.0 mg/dL = 62.4; >6.0 mg/dL = 21.9)
Neurologic	Disorientation (13.9), somnolence (4.9), coma (2.2)
Hematologic	Anemia requiring transfusion (21.0), thrombocytopenia (20,000/mm^3–60,000/mm^3 = 29.3; ≤20,000/mm^3 = 3.6)
Infectious	Infection (4.0), line sepsis (2.0)
Death	Treatment related (0.7)

[a]Grade 3 and 4 toxicity only.
From Rosenberg SA et al. Treatment of 283 consecutive patients with metastatic melanoma or renal cell cancer using high-dose bolus interleukin-2. *JAMA* 1994;271:907–913, with permission.

Many cytokines, including tumor necrosis factor–α (TNF-α), interferon-γ (IFN-γ), granulocyte-macrophage colony-stimulating factor, macrophage colony-stimulating factor, granulocyte colony-stimulating factor, IL-4, IL-5, IL-6, IL-8, and IL-10, have been measured in the serum after IL-2 administration (23,78,100–110). Serum IL-2 levels have been measured primarily in the context of pharmacokinetic studies and are proportional to the treatment dose. IL-2 levels with successive cycles of treatment have not been well studied. IL-2 levels progressively decreased, whereas the secondary production of TNF-α increased during four consecutive cycles of treatment (23). This phenomenon was not attributed to the development of antibodies to IL-2. Anti–IL-2 antibodies are frequent after intravenous IL-2 (20,63,111) and are generally nonneutralizing. In contrast, neutralizing antibodies have developed after subcutaneous IL-2 administration (32,112). Serum sickness has not been observed (63,113). The implications of anti–IL-2 antibodies are unknown.

SYSTEMIC EFFECTS OF INTERLEUKIN-2 TREATMENT AND MANAGEMENT OF TOXICITIES

IL-2 has systemic effects that depend on route, dose, and schedule of administration and variably impact every organ system in the body. High-dose bolus intravenous IL-2, as developed by Rosenberg and colleagues in the Surgery Branch of the National Cancer Institute, has been associated with the most frequent and intense side effects (Table 2). Less toxic regimens using lower doses of IL-2 administered intravenously or subcutaneously, however, have the potential to result in significant toxicity (Table 3).

In many studies, a variety of cytokines and cellular therapies have been combined with IL-2. When possible, this review focuses primarily on IL-2 without the concomitant use of biologic agents, which may add to the toxicity profile. Interest exists in developing less toxic treatment regimens that maximize immunologic and clinical response. No good *in vitro* predictors of clini-

TABLE 3. GRADE 3 OR 4 TOXICITY IN PATIENTS RANDOMIZED TO THREE DIFFERENT INTERLEUKIN-2 REGIMENS

Toxicity	High-Dose i.v. IL-2[a]	Low-Dose i.v. IL-2[b]	Subcutaneous IL-2[c]
Total courses	102	94	119
Platelets <50,000/mm^3	10	3	0
Bilirubin >7.5 mg/dL	2	0	0
Nausea/Vomiting	7	2	5
Diarrhea	7	2	2
Creatinine >8.0 mg/dL	1	0	0
Urine <80 mL/8 h	8	3	2
Pulmonary	11	1	0
Malaise	19	10	14
Infection	7	2	1
Arrhythmia (atrial)	8	0	0
Hypotension	36	5	0
Level of consciousness	2	0	0
Disorientation	15	0	2

IL-2, interleukin-2
[a]720,000 IU/kg every 8 hr, up to 15 consecutive doses and repeated in 10–14 d.
[b]72,000 IU/kg every 8 hr, up to 15 consecutive doses and repeated in 10–14 d.
[c]250,000 IU/kg/d for 5 of 7 d in wk 1 and 125,000 IU/kg/d in wks 2 to 6.
From Yang JC, Rosenberg SA. An ongoing prospective randomized comparison of interleukin-2 regimens for the treatment of metastatic renal cell cancer. *Cancer J Sci Am* 1997;3:S79–S84.

TABLE 4. GUIDELINES FOR MONITORING PATIENTS RECEIVING INTERLEUKIN-2 THERAPY

	Frequency		
	Inpatient		
Parameter to Monitor	Not Requiring Vasopressors	Requiring Intensive Care Unit/ Vasopressors	Outpatient
Vital signs	Every 4 h	Every 1 h	As needed
Intake and output	Every 8 h	Every 1 h	Not strictly measured
Weight	Daily	Daily	Daily
Mental status	Every 8 h	Every 4 h	Daily
Intravenous site/injection site	Every 8 h[a]	Every 8 h[a]	Daily
Complete blood cell count and differential	Daily	Twice daily	Weekly
Electrolytes, blood urea nitrogen, creatinine, glucose	Daily	Twice daily	Weekly
AST, ALT, alkaline phosphates and bilirubin	Daily	Daily	Weekly
Albumin, CA^{2+}, Mg^{2+}, and phosphorus	Daily	Daily	Each course
Creatinine phosphokinase	Daily	Daily	Weekly
Prothrombin time, partial thromboplastin time	Every 3 d	Every 3 d	Weekly
Thyroid-stimulating hormone and free T_4	Each cycle	Each cycle	Each course
Urinalysis	Each cycle	Each cycle	Each course
Electrocardiogram	Each cycle	Each cycle	Each course
Chest x-ray	Each cycle	Each cycle	Each course

ALT, alanine aminotransferase; AST, aspartate aminotransferase.
[a]Change peripheral i.v. every 3 d.

cal response to IL-2 alone have been identified (114). Although various clinical and treatment-related parameters have been associated with higher clinical responses (100,115), none have been useful in selecting patients for therapy.

Before initiating therapy with IL-2, patients should be carefully screened with histories, physical examinations, and laboratory measurements. The extent of tumor involvement should be assessed with magnetic resonance imaging of the brain; computed tomography of the chest, abdomen, and pelvis; and a bone scan. The presence of brain or spinal cord metastases has generally excluded patients from high-dose IL-2 therapy. Patients with abnormal renal, hepatic, cardiac, or pulmonary function are not candidates for high-dose therapy and should be considered for less aggressive regimens. Suggested screening guidelines for high-dose IL-2 include a serum creatinine less than or equal to 1.6 mg per dL, bilirubin less than 1.6 mg per dL, and pulmonary function tests higher than 65% of that predicted. Mandatory cardiac stress testing for patients older than 50 years and the exclusion of those with silent coronary artery disease have reduced the cardiac toxicity of high-dose IL-2 (116,117). The intensity of patient monitoring during therapy depends on the dose, route, and schedule used and must be tailored to each individual (Table 4). Assessment of tumor response should be performed approximately 2 months after IL-2 therapy. Therapy should be discontinued if the disease has progressed. Patients with stable or regressing disease are candidates for additional therapy.

The toxicities of IL-2 administration have been reviewed (118–123) and can involve virtually every organ system in the body. The maximal tolerated dose of IL-2 is 7.2×10^6 IU per kg when given by intravenous bolus and 2.16×10^4 IU per kg per hour when given by continuous infusion (8). For a given dose, continuous-infusion IL-2 (i.e., over 24 hours) is more toxic than the same dose given by bolus infusion (38). Thus, greater total quantities of IL-2 can be given when adminis-

tered by intermittent bolus. The typical clinical course of patients receiving high-dose IL-2 (i.e., 7.2×10^5 IU per kg every 8 hours) begins with fever and chills. Moderate hypotension and tachycardia develop soon after and are initially asymptomatic. Oliguria may manifest within 24 hours of starting IL-2 and generally responds to fluid administration. As treatment progresses, hypotension and oliguria may worsen and require pharmacologic intervention. Nausea, vomiting, and diarrhea are most prominent as therapy nears completion. Peripheral edema, pulmonary congestion, and weight gain are common. Transient thrombocytopenia and elevated serum creatinine can be measured. Most side effects resolve within 2 to 3 days of IL-2 discontinuation.

A variety of concomitant medications have been useful in diminishing the side effects of IL-2 and are listed in Table 5. Many of the toxicities of IL-2, including TNF induction, can be ameliorated with steroids (124,125), but these are not currently used because of the possibility of interfering with therapeutic response. In murine studies, corticosteroids abrogate the side effects of IL-2 and also eliminate antitumor responses (126). As experience has been gained with high-dose IL-2, the safety profile has improved (117). Treatment-related mortality in the Surgery Branch of the National Cancer Institute was 0.7% in 1,241 patients and occurred primarily during early experience with high-dose IL-2 (117). Despite the many systemic effects of high-dose IL-2, this therapy is safe when administered by experienced physicians.

Outpatient therapy with subcutaneous or intravenous IL-2 uses much smaller doses than the inpatient regimen. The most common side effects associated with outpatient therapy include fever, chills, skin changes, fatigue, diarrhea, nausea, vomiting, anorexia, hypotension, myalgia, arthralgia, stomatitis, and pain and swelling at the injection site (66). Particularly common with subcutaneous IL-2 administration are generalized fatigue and local

TABLE 5. CONCOMITANT MEDICATIONS USED DURING INTERLEUKIN-2 THERAPY

Medication	Dose/Frequency/Route	Side Effect Treated
Acetaminophen	650 mg q4h, p.o./p.r.	Fever, myalgia
Indomethacin	50–75 mg q8h, p.o./p.r.	Fever, myalgia
Meperidine hydrochloride	25–50 mg q1h, i.v. prn	Chills
Ranitidine hydrochloride	50 mg q8h, i.v.	Gastritis
Aluminum hydroxide, 200 mg; magnesium hydroxide, 200 mg; simethicone, 20 mg	30 mL q3h, p.o. prn	Gastric upset
Droperidol	1 mg q4–6h, i.v. prn	Nausea
Prochlorperazine	25 mg q4h, p.r. prn or 10 mg q6h, i.v. prn	Nausea
Ondansetron hydrochloride	10 mg q8h, i.v. prn	Nausea
Granisetron hydrochloride	0.01mg/kg daily, prn	Nausea
Lorazepam	0.5–1.0 mg q6h, p.o./i.v. prn	Nausea, anxiety
Haloperidol	1–5 mg q1h, i.v./i.m. prn	Agitation, combativeness
Loperamide	2 mg q3h, p.o. prn	Diarrhea
Diphenoxylate hydrochloride 2.5 mg, atropine sulfate 25 μg	q3h, p.o. prn	Diarrhea
Atropine sulfate	25 μg	—
Codeine sulfate	30–60 mg q4h, p.o. prn	Diarrhea
Tucks	Apply locally, prn	Perianal discomfort
Hydroxyzine hydrochloride	10–20 mg q6h, p.o. prn	Pruritus
Diphenhydramine hydrochloride	25–50 mg q4h, p.o. prn	Pruritus
Oatmeal powder/baths	Apply locally prn	Pruritus
Lubriderm, 8 oz with 0.25% camphor and 0.25% menthol	Apply locally prn	Pruritus
Sodium bicarbonate 6 tsp/1,500 mL	Swish and swallow prn	Mucositis
Lidobenalox oral	5 mL q3h, p.o. prn	Mucositis
Pseudoephedrine hydrochloride	30 mg q6h, p.o. prn	Sinus congestion
Temazepam	15–30 mg qhs, p.o. prn	Insomnia
Zolpidem	5–10 mg qhs, p.o. prn	Insomnia
Normal saline	250–500 mL i.v. prn	Oliguria, hypotension
Dopamine hydrochloride	100 mg/250 mL, i.v. prn (2 μg/kg/min)	Oliguria
Phenylephrine	40 mg/100 mL, titrate i.v. (0.1–2.0 μg/kg/min)	Hypotension
Calcium gluconate 10%	1 g (over 1 h), i.v. prn	Hypocalcemia
Magnesium sulfate	1 g (over 1 h), i.v. prn	Hypomagnesemia
Potassium phosphate	10–15 mmol (over 6h), i.v. prn	Hypophosphatemia
Potassium chloride	10 mg (over 1h), i.v. prn	Hypokalemia
Cefazolin	1 g q6h, i.v.	Prevent central line sepsis
Clindamycin	900 mg q8h, i.v.	Prevent central line sepsis

prn, as needed.

pain and induration at the site of injection. The subcutaneous induration at injection sites slowly resolves over several months (31). Guidelines for the management of IL-2 side effects in non-hospitalized patients have been published (66). This chapter focuses on the management of side effects of IL-2 as they pertain to each body system and to patients receiving high-dose therapy.

Pathophysiology (Vascular Leak Syndrome)

The toxicities of IL-2 are believed to result in part from lymphoid infiltration, which is seen in many organs (92), as well as VLS (127). VLS has been documented by the rapid disappearance of radiolabeled albumin from the circulation (128,129). Mechanisms of VLS include (a) the induction of circulating cytokines, such as TNF-α (125) and IL-5 (leading to eosinophilia and extravascular degranulation) (110); (b) generation of complement-activation product C5a (130); (c) neutrophil activation (131); and (d) activation of endothelial-cell antigens (132).

Manifestations of VLS include generalized edema, weight gain, pulmonary congestion, hypotension, oliguria, pleural effusions, and ascites (9). Organ edema is difficult to quantify but is likely respon-

sible for many of the observed toxicities. Patient weight gain greater than 5% above baseline occurs in 71% of courses with high-dose IL-2 (15); this gain is dependent on the intensity of therapy and the amount of additional fluids used to correct hypotension. In a randomized study comparing the efficacy of colloid versus crystalloid for fluid resuscitation during IL-2 therapy, patients receiving saline boluses experienced more oliguria than colloid recipients and had lower albumin levels (133). These patients experienced no difference in weight gain or other parameters, including hypotension. The current practice is to use saline (as opposed to colloid) when additional fluids are needed, judiciously balanced with the use of vasopressors. After stopping IL-2, the fluid shift reverses rapidly and the majority of patients are discharged at or below admission weight in a median of 3 days (134). Despite improved safety and reduction in multiple treatment-related toxicities, maximal weight gain during IL-2 has remained constant in a 12-year-period review (117).

Fever and Chills

Without premedication, shaking chills develop 1 to 2 hours after bolus intravenous IL-2 and are followed by fevers up to 40.5°C

1 to 2 hours later (8,9,11,113,135,136). It was learned in these early studies that fevers, myalgias, arthralgias, and malaise could be ameliorated by pretreatment with acetaminophen and nonsteroidal antiinflammatory agents, such as indomethacin (Indocin). These agents should be started at least 8 hours before IL-2 and continued for 8 to 24 hours after the last IL-2 dose (see Table 5). The occurrence of fevers at times other than after the first or second dose of IL-2 should arouse the suspicion of infection and prompt a diligent search for a source.

Induction of circulating TNF-α has been postulated as a mechanism for the febrile response to IL-2 (103). TNF-α induction can be completely eliminated with the use of steroids (125), but the use of steroids may be contraindicated. Chills occur primarily after the first and second doses of IL-2; they can be treated with warm blankets and repeated doses of intravenous meperidine hydrochloride (Demerol). Malignant hyperthermia is extremely rare but has resulted in one death (121).

Hemodynamic and Cardiovascular Toxicity

Two hours after administration of high-dose IL-2, a drop in systemic blood pressure and a rise in heart rate can be measured (128). Invasive monitoring also reveals a decrease in systemic vascular resistance and an increase in cardiac index (Fig. 1). These effects persist during therapy (128,137–140) and reverse within 24 to 48 hours of IL-2 discontinuation. For that reason, hypertensive patients should discontinue antihypertensive medications during IL-2 therapy. β-blocking agents should be weaned before initiating treatment. At the time of hospital discharge, all medications should be resumed because IL-2 does not have long-term antihypertensive effects (141).

Intravenous fluid administration is the initial therapy for hypotension. Cautious use of fluids is necessary because they may compound the edema and pulmonary toxicity associated with VLS. Systolic blood pressure of less than 90 mm Hg that is not responsive to fluids (up to 1.5 L per day above maintenance) indicate the need for vasopressor support (phenylephrine, up to 2.0 μg per kg per minute) via a central line. Hypotension requiring vasopressors occurs in approximately 50% of treatments (116), although the incidence has decreased to 31% (117). Hypotension is usually preceded by oliguria. Renal-perfusion doses of dopamine (2 μg per kg per minute) should be initiated as well. As therapy nears completion, higher doses of vasopressors may be needed to maintain the systolic blood pressure, which is most labile 4 to 6 hours after each IL-2 dose. When the peak effects have passed and phenylephrine can be weaned to 0.5 μg per kg per minute, additional IL-2 dosing can be considered.

Central venous pressures and pulmonary capillary wedge pressures can decrease during therapy and should be cautiously interpreted. Fluid resuscitation based on the goal of correcting low central-venous pressures can lead to excessive hydration. As a choice of fluids, crystalloid is favored over colloid based on a randomized study that demonstrated both were equally effective in supporting blood pressure (133).

Nitric oxide is a potent vasodilator that has been implicated in the etiology of hypotension associated with IL-2 therapy. Plasma nitrate and nitrite (oxidation products of nitric oxide)

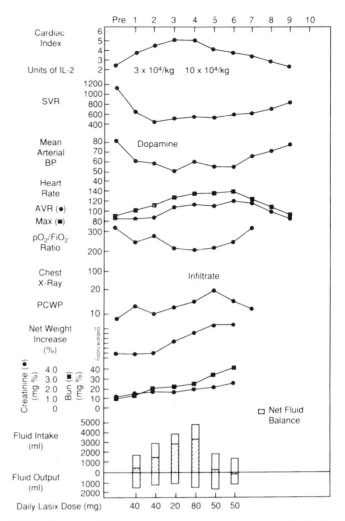

FIGURE 1. Sequential hemodynamic measurements in a patient who received interleukin-2 (IL-2) (30,000 U per kg) administered three times daily on days 1 through 3, and 100,000 U on days 3 through 6. Systematic vascular resistance (SVR) (dyne·s·cm⁻⁵) and mean arterial blood pressure (BP) (mm Hg) decreased. The cardiac index (L per min per m²) increased. The pulmonary capillary wedge pressure (PCWP) (mm Hg) and net weight increased during both cycles. A rapid return to normal was noted after discontinuation of treatment. (AVR, accelerated ventricular rhythm; FiO₂, fraction of inspired oxygen.) (Adapted from Lee RE et al. Cardiorespiratory effects of immunotherapy with interleukin-2. *J Clin Oncol* 1989;7:7–20)

levels increase during IL-2 administration (142–145). In preliminary clinical studies, *N*-methyl-L-arginine (inhibitor of nitric oxide synthase) reverses IL-2–induced hypotension (146). Studies are under way to confirm this finding. Another agent that may work through the nitric oxide pathway is melatonin. In one randomized study of patients, melatonin reduced grades 1 and 2 hypotension associated with subcutaneous IL-2 therapy (147).

Left ventricular ejection fraction or stroke-work index decreases significantly during high-dose IL-2 therapy and generally returns to baseline on follow-up (116,128,137,138, 148,149). Lower doses of IL-2 that do not result in ventricular wall motion abnormalities impair left ventricular filling rate as measured by echocardiography or radionuclide scans (150,151). The observed cardiac dysfunction may be mediated by circulating myocardial depressant factors, cytokines, or lymphoid cell infiltration in the heart. Myocarditis owing to lymphocyte and eosinophil infiltration has been described (152–154). Creatine kinase isoenzymes with MB-band elevations have been noted, suggesting myocardial injury or inflammation as a consequence of IL-2 administration (116,138,148,153–155). MB-band elevations were observed in 2.5% of 199 patients (156) and occurred 1 to 2 days after the last dose of IL-2. These elevations, which were generally asymptomatic and detected by routine creatine kinase screening, returned to normal in 1 to 2 days. Accompanying electrocardiogram, echocardiogram, and thallium tests revealed transient abnormalities that generally reversed by follow-up. One patient had persistent dysfunction as long as 6 months after IL-2. Cardiac catheterizations performed in patients with cardiac toxicity have generally shown normal coronary arteries. Some patients have been uneventfully retreated with IL-2 after documenting normalization of cardiac function. Decisions to retreat patients that sustain cardiac toxicity must be carefully individualized.

Myocardial infarctions, occurring in 2.5% of patients receiving high-dose IL-2 alone in early trials (14), have been virtually eliminated with aggressive cardiac screening and patient selection, including mandatory stress thallium screening for patients older than 50 years or anyone suspected of having a prior cardiac event (117). Such screening may not be necessary for low-dose IL-2 regimens because hemodynamic changes are not common (157). A history of cardiovascular disease has not been an exclusion criteria for subcutaneous IL-2.

Arrhythmias, which occur during 6% of treatment courses (15,116), are primarily supraventricular (atrial fibrillation and tachycardia), of short duration, and rarely hemodynamically compromising. Usually, they occur at the peak of systemic toxicities and in the presence of multiple electrolyte and metabolic abnormalities. The treatment includes (a) discontinuation of IL-2, (b) correction of serum abnormalities (i.e., hypokalemia), (c) maintenance of proper oxygenation, and (d) diuretics if intravascular fluid overload exists. Acute intervention, with agents such as digoxin, verapamil, diltiazem, or adenosine, is frequently used. Digoxin is generally not continued after a successful loading dose. Future retreatment is safe because only a minority of patients develop arrhythmias again.

Ventricular tachycardia is rare, usually of short duration, and generally does not require intervention except for discontinuation of IL-2. Unifocal premature ventricular contractions are not infrequent and do not require treatment with antiarrhythmics. Patients experiencing premature ventricular contractions should receive IL-2 in a monitored setting. If premature ventricular contractions become multifocal or frequent (i.e., bigemini), IL-2 therapy should probably be terminated.

Pulmonary Toxicity

High-dose IL-2 administration can result in the progressive development of interstitial pulmonary edema (128,158–162), principally caused by VLS. Transient cardiac dysfunction may compound the problem. In early series of patients receiving IL-2 and LAK cells, dyspnea at rest occurred in as many as 30% of patients. Intubation was required in 5% to 7% of patients

(118,128,158). Patients receiving high-dose IL-2 alone develop severe respiratory distress in 3% of treatment courses and require intubation in less than 1% (116). The need for pulmonary intubation has diminished over time as greater experience with IL-2 has been obtained (117).

Selective transcutaneous monitoring of oxygen (O_2) saturation for patients experiencing shortness of breath during treatment has been extremely helpful. O_2 should be delivered by nasal cannula to maintain saturation above 95%. If this level is not met with 4 L per minute by nasal cannula or 40% O_2 by mask, IL-2 dosing should be discontinued. The auscultation of rales as high as the midlung fields or a markedly abnormal chest x-ray should also caution against further IL-2 dosing. Radiographic evaluation of the chest is performed selectively and the results are used to supplement the clinical examination. Although 42% to 52% of patients may develop pleural effusions radiographically (158–161), pleural effusions requiring aspiration are rare (<1%) (116). Chest tube drainage during IL-2 therapy should be avoided because of the concern for infectious complications. After stopping IL-2, pulmonary congestion rapidly improves if diuresis can be achieved. Nasal congestion is not uncommon during IL-2 therapy (10). Symptomatic relief can be obtained with room vaporizers and pseudoephedrine.

Pretherapy screening should include pulmonary function testing for patients with smoking histories or those with large tumor burdens in the lung. High-dose IL-2 therapy should be declined if forced vital capacity or forced expiratory volume is less than 65% of that predicted. Smokers are strongly advised to quit smoking 2 weeks before therapy. Patients experiencing hemoptysis should undergo bronchoscopy. The presence of endobronchial lesions causing significant airway obstruction have generally been an exclusion criteria for high-dose IL-2 therapy because of the concern for postobstructive pneumonia.

Renal Toxicity

Most of the effects of IL-2 on kidney function have been described as prerenal (134,156,163–169). Hypotension, impaired cardiac function, and decreased intravascular volume lead to decreased renal perfusion and prerenal azotemia. Renal carcinoma patients, by virtue of prior nephrectomy, are at greater risk for dysfunction (134,170). Oliguria, elevated serum creatinine, and low fractional excretion of sodium occur in the majority of patients receiving high-dose IL-2 therapy and resolve promptly after IL-2 discontinuation. Severe oliguria has occurred in 26% of treatment courses with high-dose IL-2 alone (15). Creatinine values higher than 2.0 mg per dL were observed in 68% of courses.

In a series of 199 patients (134), the highest mean peak creatinine value during therapy with high-dose IL-2 was 2.7 mg per dL (Fig. 2). After stopping IL-2, creatinine values returned promptly to baseline. Elevation in creatinine was dose limiting in 11% of courses. In all studies, the creatinine values returned to baseline in the majority of patients by 7 to 14 days. The use of hemodialysis has been extremely rare.

Oliguria during therapy is initially treated with fluids. If 1.0 to 1.5 total L of crystalloid fluid boluses, in addition to maintenance fluids, do not result in improved urine output, a urinary

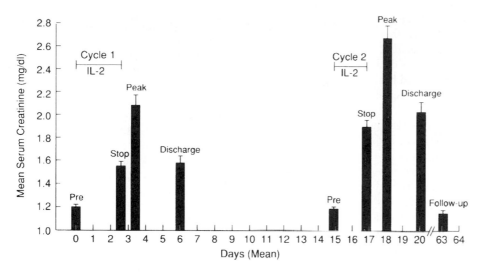

FIGURE 2. Mean serum creatinine for 199 patients during course 1 of high-dose interleukin-2 (IL-2) therapy. Mean creatinine values (± SEM) are plotted against the mean number of days when they occurred. (Discharge, day when patient went home; Follow-up, clinic visit or last available follow-up; Peak, highest creatinine value; Pre, before IL-2; Stop, when IL-2 dosing was discontinued.)

catheter should be inserted and dopamine (2 µg per kg per minute) should be started. Although low-dose dopamine appears to be effective in improving IL-2–induced oliguria (171), the routine use of prophylactic low-dose dopamine to prevent oliguria is not justified (172). Urine output higher than 10 to 20 mL per hour should be established before additional IL-2 dosing. The development of pulmonary insufficiency during IL-2 therapy should encourage less aggressive fluid replacement to correct oliguria (and earlier use of vasopressors in hypotensive patients). Generally, when serum creatinine values reach 3.0 mg per dL, high-dose IL-2 therapy should be discontinued. Diuretics are rarely effective at the peak of renal dysfunction. After stopping IL-2 (and vasopressors, if used), diuretics should be liberally administered to initiate diuresis and promote the rapid return to normal fluid balance.

Urinalyses during therapy reveal proteinuria and bilirubinuria, as well as granular casts, which resolve completely on follow-up (134). Transient increases in white and red blood cells are also observed in urinalyses and may be attributed to the use of indwelling urinary catheters.

Other changes observed during IL-2 therapy include hypomagnesemia, hypocalcemia, hypophosphatemia, and decreased serum bicarbonate (163,164). These have not been attributed to altered renal function and have been accompanied by hypoalbuminemia. Minerals are generally replaced to achieve serum levels in the lower range of normal and bicarbonate is corrected to achieve values of greater than 19 mEq per L; albumin is generally not replaced.

Pretherapy screening for high-dose IL-2 has generally excluded patients with hypercalcemia or serum creatinine values greater than 1.6 mg per dL. Patients with ureteral stents have also been generally excluded because of the presumed risk of increased infection and stent occlusion during therapy.

Gastrointestinal Toxicity

Anorexia, nausea, vomiting, and diarrhea occur to some degree in most patients receiving IL-2 (14,118) and may be dose limiting. Many antiemetics are available to treat nausea (see Table 5)

and should generally be alternated until the most effective agent is found. Droperidol is one of the most effective agents. It is equivalent to ondansetron in controlling emesis caused by high-dose IL-2 (173). At the first sign of loose or frequent bowel movements, antidiarrheals are initiated (see Table 5). Antidiarrheals are used cautiously because many patients experience abdominal distention, principally attributable to intestinal ileus, which may be aggravated by these medications. The etiology of IL-2–induced diarrhea is not clearly understood; one study observed that gut permeability does not significantly increase after 48 hours of high-dose IL-2 therapy (174). Although the incidence of severe diarrhea (grade 3–4) has diminished to approximately 20% (117), additional studies are needed to understand its cause and develop more effective therapies.

Ascites can develop and is generally not clinically compromising. Glossitis (10,175), xerostomia and stomatitis (118,176) are frequent and treated with mouth washes and nystatin if a yeast infection is suspected (see Table 5). Gastritis has been largely prevented with antihistamines, which have been used since early studies (11). Ranitidine (or an antihistamine other than cimetidine) is initiated 8 hours before IL-2 administration and continued for 8 to 24 hours after the last dose of IL-2. Gastrointestinal symptoms largely resolve 2 to 3 days after IL-2 discontinuation. Appetite is regained by 5 to 7 days. As a consequence of these side effects, a loss in lean body mass is common. Parenteral nutrition during IL-2 therapy has not been used.

Colonic necrosis and perforation is a rare complication of IL-2, occurring in 1% to 5% of patients in early series (177,178) and has not been reported recently. Bowel perforation, which may be more frequent in patients receiving IL-2 with IFN-α (179), must be addressed promptly and surgically. Small bowel mucosal ulceration and necrosis is extremely rare but must be considered in the differential diagnosis (121,178). Exacerbation of Crohn's disease during IL-2 therapy may prompt surgical intervention as well (180). The diagnosis of bowel perforation can be difficult because the symptoms can be masked by the common side effects of IL-2. Plain abdominal x-rays revealing free intraperitoneal air are diagnostic and should be performed frequently in patients experiencing abdominal pain. After successful surgical treatment and recovery from bowel perforation, patients can be safely retreated with IL-2. Extreme caution must be used, however, to exclude residual infection with the aid of computed tomography scans and barium studies before initiating therapy. Patients with active Crohn's disease should not receive IL-2 therapy.

A rare cause of abdominal pain has been pancreatitis (181). The diagnosis can be made by computed tomography scan and elevated serum amylase or lipase. The treatment includes discontinuation of IL-2, gastrointestinal rest, and supportive measures. Retreatment with subsequent courses of IL-2 should proceed with caution. Other causes of abdominal pain may include hepatic capsular distention secondary to parenchymal congestion or hemorrhage into metastases. Splenomegaly can occur and is generally not associated with abdominal pain (182). Gastrointestinal hemorrhage is extremely rare (16,118), although occult blood in the stool is not uncommon in patients with severe diarrhea. Frank rectal bleeding during IL-2 should lead to discontinuation of IL-2 and a gastrointestinal evaluation. If bleeding is self-limited, this evaluation may be performed after recovery from IL-2 side effects and before the next cycle of therapy.

Hepatic Toxicity

Hepatic toxicity is primarily manifested as reversible cholestasis (183). Elevations in serum bilirubin and alkaline phosphatase are accompanied by more modest elevations in asparate aminotransferase and alanine aminotransferase (183,184). Only mild elevations in prothrombin time and small decreases in albumin are noted (Fig. 3). Bilirubin levels return to a normal mean of 5.6 days after stopping high-dose IL-2 (183). In a large series of patients, bilirubin values greater than 2.0 mg per dL occurred in 84% of treatment courses (see Table 2). In general, IL-2 therapy is not discontinued because of jaundice, unless the bilirubin reaches approximately 8.0 to 10 mg per dL. Hepatitis or long-lasting sequelae have not been reported; one death caused by hepatic necrosis occurred in a patient receiving continuous IL-2 (26). Because of the transient hepatic dysfunction occurring during IL-2 therapy, caution must be used when administering concomitant medications that are metabolized by the liver. Patients with diminished hepatic reserve (i.e., more than 50% of the liver replaced by tumor), are generally not eligible for high-dose IL-2 therapy.

Neurologic Toxicity

High-dose IL-2 therapy may result in disorientation (14% of courses), somnolence (5%), or coma (2%) (15). Symptoms usually occur at the end of treatment and resolve completely within hours or several days of IL-2 discontinuation. Careful cognitive testing has documented full recovery (185).

Behavioral changes range from mild agitation to combativeness, which may require medication with haloperidol and occasional restraints (185). The preferred agent for agitation is haloperidol because it has not been accompanied by the

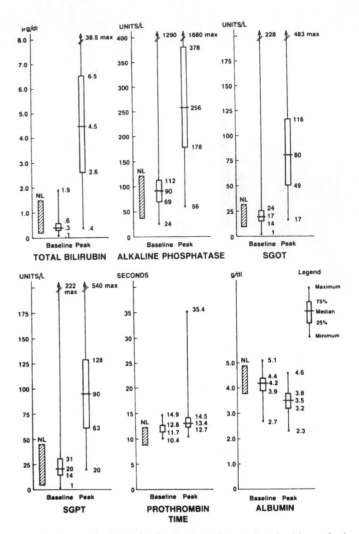

FIGURE 3. Interleukin-2 (IL-2) treatment is associated with marked increases in bilirubin. Shown for each measured chemical analyte is the normal range, as well as the baseline and peak (or trough) values for the 261 patients receiving IL-2 therapy. (SGOT, serum glutamic-oxaloacetic transaminase; SGPT, serum glutamic-pyruvic transaminase.)

secondary side effects of many other sedatives. IL-2 should be stopped at the first sign of neuropsychiatric toxicity. Premonitory signs include lethargy; impaired memory; responses that are slow, vague, or incoherent; impaired attention; irritability; mild aphasia or paraphrasia; "picking" motion; and insistence on getting out of bed (185). Symptoms of neurologic toxicity generally worsen after stopping IL-2. If severe obtundation develops, endotracheal intubation is advised to protect the airway.

Sleep disturbances and vivid dreams are not uncommon during therapy and may persist for several days after stopping IL-2. IL-2 dosing should be discontinued if these dreams become disturbing or if patients hallucinate. Fatigue is frequent (185) and may be due in part to altered sleep patterns. Paranoia or emotional lability manifested by frequent crying may also occur. Patients and their families must be extensively assured that all neuropsychiatric symptoms are transient. It is important to provide a safe physical environment and increased patient supervision during periods of altered mental status to prevent accidental injury.

The mechanism of neurologic toxicity is unclear. It is known that IL-2 penetrates the blood–brain barrier (186) and results in increased brain-water content as measured by magnetic resonance imaging (187). Magnetic resonance imaging performed in eight patients with cancer or human immunodeficiency virus infection who experienced severe neurologic toxicity during IL-2 therapy, including coma, ataxia, hemiparesis, seizures, aphasia, apraxia, and cortical blindness, has revealed multiple white- and gray-matter lesions (188). The exact nature of these lesions is unknown, but the lesions resolved as neurologic function improved with the cessation of IL-2. Transient vision loss resembling transient ischemic attacks have been described in two patients (189). Fatal leukoencephalopathy (190) and stroke in one patient (37) have also been reported. The causal relationship of these severe central nervous system toxicities to IL-2 is unclear.

The fear of increased intracranial pressure from edema, as well as the potential for hemorrhage into lesions, has led to the exclusion of patients with brain metastasis from most high-dose IL-2 protocols. Carefully selected patients with small brain metastases and little edema have been treated without added morbidity (191).

Extremity paresthesias (192) and peripheral neuropathy (31) may result from soft tissue edema. Extremity elevation, diuretics, and use of compression garments provides symptomatic relief. Carpal tunnel syndrome requiring surgical decompression (193) and brachial plexopathy (194) are extremely infrequent.

Musculoskeletal Toxicity

Myalgias and arthralgias are frequent during IL-2 therapy (192,195). The shoulder area is a common site of symptoms and can show increased radionuclide activity on bone scan (196). Symptoms are generally controlled with acetaminophen (Tylenol) and nonsteroidal antiinflammatory agents. Symptoms may persist for several weeks, but rarely last for prolonged periods (197). One patient developed severe muscle pain and weakness after IL-2 and tumor-BCG vaccination, leading to a biopsy that revealed necrotizing myositis (198). Reactivation of rheumatoid arthritis has been described (199).

Dermatologic Toxicity

Cutaneous macular erythema begins in the face and neck 1 to 3 days after starting IL-2, and generally progresses to the trunk and extremities (175,200). Erythema is accompanied by generalized skin burning and itching and begins to resolve with mild, dry, scaly desquamation within 1 to 3 days of IL-2 discontinuation. Skin from the palms and soles may exfoliate as confluent sheets in some patients. Petechial purpura may occasionally develop in the extremities and is not clearly associated with thrombocytopenia. Skin biopsies have shown mild dermal papillary edema and perivascular infiltration of T cells expressing HLA-DR (175,200), as well as increased expression of adhesion molecules on endothelial cells (132,200).

Pruritus and desquamation, which may persist for 3 to 6 weeks in some patients, can be treated with a variety of oral or topical agents (see Table 5). Steroids are rarely required and should be avoided. Patients are advised to protect against heavy sun exposure because of increased skin sensitivity. Infrequently, IL-2 therapy results in skin blisters and moist desquamation (200–202), which can be treated with silver sulfadiazine and oral antibiotic prophylaxis. One case of fatal pemphigus vulgaris has occurred after IL-2 and IFN-β (203). Moist desquamation of the intertriginous areas of the perineum requires vigorous local hygiene. Fournier gangrene after high-dose IL-2 (204) is extremely rare and requires prompt surgical débridement and aggressive antibiotic therapy.

Glossitis (10,175), xerostomia, and stomatitis (118,176) frequently occur during therapy and are treated with topical agents (see Table 5). Angioneurotic edema of the face is extremely rare (205) and may require discontinuation of IL-2 therapy. Diffuse hair loss and thinning may occur (175) but is generally mild and does not require the use of prosthesis. Subcutaneous IL-2 administration commonly results in self-limiting pain and inflammation at the injection site (31). Subcutaneous IL-2 administration has rarely resulted in skin necrosis (33). One patient developed lobular panniculitis at a subcutaneous injection site, which was exacerbated with subsequent intravenous IL-2 (206). IL-2–based regimens have also been implicated in the development of erythema nodosum (207) and exacerbation of preexisting psoriasis (208).

Vitiligo has been noted in 15% to 45% of patients with metastatic melanoma who receive IL-2–based therapy, and has been associated with clinical response (209,210). Vitiligo is manifested as the appearance of white patches of hair on the scalp, mustache, or beard; patches of depigmented skin on the trunk or extremities; and halo depigmentation around nevi or cutaneous tumors.

Endocrine and Metabolic Effects

Intravenous or subcutaneous IL-2 alters the circadian rhythm of stress-related hormones. β-endorphin, adrenocorticotrophic hormone, cortisol, and corticotrophic-releasing hormone increase 4 to 12 hours after IL-2 is administered (211–214). The magnitude of these changes may be increased on reexposure to IL-2 (214). Epinephrine and norepinephrine levels have increased 2 hours after bolus IL-2 (136). Melatonin decreases acutely, whereas growth hormone, prolactin, follicle-stimulating hormone, and luteinizing hormone are mildly affected or not affected at all (212,213). Men receiving high-dose IL-2 experience transient decreases in plasma testosterone and increases in estradiol levels (215). Serum acute-phase reactants, such as C-reactive protein, increase within 24 hours of IL-2 administration and remain elevated during therapy (113,184,216).

Acute adrenal insufficiency during IL-2 therapy is uncommon but has been reported in one patient after presumed hemorrhage into one of bilateral adrenal metastases (217). This scenario is extremely rare. The fear of adrenal insufficiency should not preclude IL-2 treatment in patients with adrenal metastases. Bilateral adrenalectomy has generally been considered a contraindication for therapy with IL-2 because of the immunosuppressive effects that may or may not be experienced with replacement doses of steroids. One patient received high-dose IL-2 after bilateral adrenalectomy and experienced the usual side effects of this therapy (218). No series demonstrating the efficacy of therapy in such patients, however, have been performed.

Thyroid dysfunction occurs in 13% to 41% of patients receiving IL-2 alone (219–221). A similar incidence is seen in patients receiving IL-2 with LAK cells or IFN (219,222–228). Hypothyroidism is the most common abnormality and occurs in 35% of patients receiving high-dose IL-2 alone (221). The majority of these cases are subclinical, which highlights the importance of routine testing of thyroid function during immunotherapy. Nine percent of patients received thyroid hormone replacement for moderate or severe hypothyroidism (221). The incidence of hypothyroidism increases with multiple courses or duration of IL-2 treatment. Contrary to some reports, hypothyroidism is most likely not associated with clinical response (219–221,224,227). Studies claiming an association with clinical response (222,223,226) have generally not accounted for duration of treatment or the bias that continued therapy is offered to responders. Hyperthyroidism is less frequent than hypothyroidism, occurs in 7% of patients, and is generally transient (221). Most of the time, hyperthyroidism is diagnosed on routine testing and has not resulted in symptoms or alteration of the treatment plan.

Symptoms of thyroid dysfunction may be difficult to distinguish from those of IL-2 when patients are in active treatment; routine screening of thyroid-stimulating hormone and FT4 is necessary with each course of therapy. Routine measurements of T3 and T4 are not necessary because they fluctuate widely in the majority of patients receiving IL-2 and are not useful in making clinical decisions (221). Moderate or severe hypothyroidism should be treated with levothyroxine as soon as the diagnosis is made. IL-2 dosing is generally not interrupted for the diagnosis of hypothyroidism; if the diagnosis is made before initiating IL-2, it is prudent to delay IL-2 therapy for several days while starting hormone replacement. Thyroid dysfunction is reversible but may persist for many months. The current practice is to wean levothyroxine after 1 year of replacement.

Transient decreases in serum cholesterol are common during IL-2 therapy (229,230). The significance of this finding is unknown and no intervention is required. Similarly, transient decreases in serum ferritin and increases in transferrin have been reported (231). Low serum levels of potassium, calcium, magnesium, and phosphorus are frequent (164,165) and should be repleted to achieve serum levels in the lower range of normal (see Table 5). Transient vitamin C deficiency has been reported (232) and is not commonly treated.

Hematologic Toxicity

Anemia develops with IL-2 therapy, partly because of the frequent blood draws required for treatment monitoring, and partly because of bone marrow suppression. Decreased circulating erythroid and granulocyte and macrophage progenitors have been noted during therapy (97,106). These progenitors rapidly rebound after stopping IL-2. Red blood cell transfusions were required in 14% of treatment courses in 199 patients receiving high-dose IL-2 alone (77), although a majority of patients (>70%) have required transfusions in studies of IL-2 with LAK cells (12,118). For inpatient regimens, the hematocrit is generally maintained above 28% to 30% if the patient is hemodynamically unstable.

Neutrophil counts have generally been little affected by IL-2. Increases in neutrophils are noted in the first 24 hours of IL-2, along with a shift to immature forms (77,98). Severe neutropenia during or shortly after IL-2 therapy is rare (15,16,41,97). Transient declines in neutrophils to less than 500 per μL occur in 3% of patients or less (38,99,233). Transient neutrophil dysfunction occurs as noted by decreased Fc receptor expression and decreased chemotaxis while preserving bacterial phagocytosis (98,99). These findings may explain the occurrence of infections during IL-2 therapy. During IL-2 therapy, evidence of neutrophil activation (hydrogen peroxide and hypochlorous acid production) exists, which may relate to the development of VLS (131).

Eosinophilia is common with various doses and schedules of IL-2 (eosinophil counts may reach 40,000 per μL) (9,38,39,41,77,97,110,234,235). It is progressive with continued or repetitive treatments, and counts return to baseline within 3 to 14 days after discontinuation of IL-2. It is proposed that eosinophilia is mediated by IL-5 (110,236). IL-2 infusion leads to elevated plasma levels of IL-5, which is a growth factor for eosinophils (110). Major basic protein, a product of eosinophil degranulation, increases in the circulation and is deposited in the dermis, suggesting a mechanism for the vascular leak associated with IL-2 (110).

Lymphocytopenia develops rapidly and persists during IL-2 treatment (8,23,38,41,76,77). One to 2 days after discontinuation of IL-2, lymphocytes rebound manyfold above baseline and are elevated for 3 to 7 days before returning to normal levels.

Progressive thrombocytopenia develops with repeated IL-2 infusion (15,16,77,97,237,238) and is dependent on intensity of therapy. Platelet counts may continue to drop for 1 to 2 days after IL-2 discontinuation but then return promptly to baseline. With high-dose IL-2 alone, platelet counts less than 60,000 per μL occurred in one-third of treatment courses and less than 20,000 per μL in 4% of courses (15), resulting in platelet transfusions in 2% of courses (77). Platelet counts less than 25,000 per μL have been seen in as many as 16% of patients receiving constant infusion IL-2 (237). Those patients had increased megakaryocytes observed in bone marrow biopsies, suggesting peripheral platelet loss or sequestration. Thrombocytopenia is more severe when IL-2 is combined with chemotherapy (210,239,240).

Bolus IL-2 dosing is generally discontinued when platelet counts reach 30,000 to 40,000 per μL. Hemorrhage has been extremely rare (77,121), despite low platelet counts, mildly elevated prothrombin time (77,183,241), elevated partial thromboplastin time (77,242), and decreased levels of clotting factors (238,241,242). The remaining platelet pool consists of larger, more viable and activated platelets (243). Patients are generally transfused with platelets when counts fall below 20,000 per μL, or in the presence of bleeding. Vitamin K may be administered prophylactically to patients with significantly prolonged prothrombin time (241).

Infectious Complications

The incidence of infection in patients receiving a variety of IL-2–based therapies has ranged from 0 to 45% when reviewed by Pockaj et al. (244). With high-dose IL-2 therapy, bacterial infections occur in 13% to 19% of treatment courses (244,245) and are primarily venous catheter or urinary associated. The predominant infectious organisms are *Staphylococcus aureus, Staphylococcus epidermidis,* and *E. coli.* Surveillance blood cultures during continuous infusion IL-2 drawn from an implanted central venous catheter port have been positive in as many as 56% of patients, of which nearly one-half were symptomatic (246). Proper treatment of infections includes discontinuation of IL-2, catheter removal or surgical intervention when indicated, and prompt antibiotic coverage. Opportunistic infections have generally not occurred (15), and empiric therapy for such is generally not warranted. Resumption of IL-2 therapy is possible when all evidence of infection is resolved.

Patients receiving IL-2 have experienced more frequent infections than patients receiving IFN-γ (247) or parenteral nutrition (245) in similar environments. The vigilant monitoring for infection, the liberal use of antibiotics for suspected infection, and the use of prophylactic antibiotics have resulted in decreased infectious episodes (117,244). Careful attention to prevention of infections is mandatory because IL-2 induces neutrophil dysfunction (98,99). Peripheral intravenous catheters should be changed routinely every 3 days; prophylactic antibiotics in this setting have not been commonly used. Patients with temporary or indwelling central venous catheters should receive antibiotic prophylaxis during IL-2 therapy. Central catheter sepsis has been almost completely prevented by the concomitant use of oxacillin or a first-generation cephalosporin (117,248,249). Those patients allergic to these antibiotics may be treated with clindamycin (see Table 5). Ciprofloxacin prophylaxis was not effective in preventing bacteremia in one study (16).

Fevers occurring after the first or second doses of IL-2 can usually be attributed to IL-2. Fevers occurring at other times, however, should prompt a search for an infectious etiology. Empiric broad-spectrum antibiotic therapy should be initiated after blood and urine cultures are obtained. If no source of infection is found and cultures remain negative for 3 days, the antibiotics may be discontinued. Antibiotics selected for use during IL-2 therapy should have low risk of nephrotoxicity.

Perineal hygiene is important during IL-2 therapy to prevent secondary infection. Skin edema and breakdown may have contributed to the development of Fournier's gangrene in one patient (204).

Hypersensitivity Reactions

One manifestation of immunologic "toxicity" is the development of hypersensitivity reactions to radiographic contrast agents (ionic > nonionic) after prior treatment with IL-2. Ten percent to 28% of patients develop reactions that include fever, chills, emesis, diarrhea, rash, wheezing, hypotension, edema, and oliguria within hours of intravenous contrast (59,61,250–253). Hospitalization for these reactions is required in as many as 10% of patients. Patients experiencing these reactions should be treated with supportive measures, including antihistamines. Planned IL-2 administration should be delayed until all clinical and laboratory abnormalities (i.e., elevated creatinine) are resolved. Steroids should be avoided because of the possibility of interfering with the antitumor response. Contrast agents have not generally been used in patients with prior reactions. Five of six patients who previously experienced reactions did not do so, however, with later reexposure to contrast (250).

Allergic reactions to chemotherapy agents in patients receiving high-dose IL-2 have been reported (254). These reactions generally occur after two courses of prior chemoimmunotherapy and 2 to 4 hours after the chemotherapy infusion. They manifest as cutaneous erythema, pruritus, hypotension, oliguria, and edema, and generally resolve in 24 to 48 hours with the aid of antihistamines and intravenous fluids.

SURGERY AND IMMUNOTHERAPY

Renal carcinoma patients who present with metastatic disease have traditionally undergone nephrectomy before initiating IL-2 therapy. The role and timing of nephrectomy in patients with metastatic disease is unclear. Forty percent of patients undergoing nephrectomy before IL-2 therapy could not subsequently receive the intended IL-2, because of disease progression (255), highlighting the pitfalls of this approach.

Patients with metastatic melanoma or renal carcinoma who have recurrent disease after achieving a partial or complete response to IL-2 therapy may derive limited benefit from surgical resection (256,257). This treatment option is worthy of consideration because retreatment with IL-2 in this context is unlikely to result in clinical responses (257).

Emergent surgery during or shortly after IL-2 has been performed primarily to treat infectious complications of therapy (177,178,204). After appropriate patient resuscitation, prompt surgical intervention has been safe.

Planned IL-2 treatment at the time of surgery for the purpose of preventing surgically induced immune suppression has also been done in limited studies. Preoperative or perioperative IL-2 has been given to patients undergoing surgery for colorectal cancer (258–261), gastric cancer (261), pancreatic cancer (261), non–small cell lung cancer (262), and hepatic tumors (261,263). Most of these studies have used low doses of IL-2. No major added morbidity has been noted.

APPROACHES TO REDUCE INTERLEUKIN-2 SIDE EFFECTS

The side effects of high-dose IL-2 therapy have diminished as experience with its administration has increased (117). Despite the improved safety, less toxic regimens or the discovery of agents that ameliorate side effects and preserve efficacy are needed. Lower doses of IL-2 with reduced side effects are currently being tested in a prospective randomized study in patients with metastatic renal carcinoma (42). Various agents expected to reduce vascular leak or hypotension during IL-2 have been studied. Agents that have not been clearly established as beneficial in reducing side effects of IL-2 include pentoxifylline and ciprofloxacin (264,265), soluble p75 TNF-receptor IgG chimera (266), lisofylline (267), and C1 esterase inhibitor (268). Melatonin has reduced the incidence of hypotension (while increasing clinical responses) in a randomized study of 91 patients receiving subcutaneous IL-2 (147). Further studies are needed, however, to confirm these findings. N-methyl-L-arginine has reversed hypotension in early clinical studies (146,269) and is currently undergoing clinical testing in patients receiving high-dose IL-2. Perhaps the most efficacious approach to reduce IL-2 side effects is the simultaneous use of steroids. Many of the toxicities of IL-2 can be ameliorated with steroids (124,125), but these are not currently used clinically because of the possibility of interfering with therapeutic response.

As new antigens expressed on the surface of tumors are identified, therapies with IL-2 are beginning to focus on its administration in conjunction with vaccines targeted against these antigens (191). It is hoped that as understanding of immune responses to tumors increases, specific therapies can be applied that do not have the undesirable side effects frequently associated with nonspecific immune stimulation.

REFERENCES

1. Morgan DA, Ruscetti FW, Gallo R. Selective in vitro growth of T lymphocytes from normal human bone marrows. *Science* 1976;193:1007–1008.
2. Bindon C, Czerniecki M, Ruell P, et al. Clearance rates and systemic effects of intravenously administered interleukin-2 (IL-2) containing preparations in human subjects. *Br J Cancer* 1983;47:123–133.
3. Lotze MT, Robb RJ, Sharrow SO, Frana LW, Rosenberg SA. Systemic administration of interleukin-2 in humans. *J Biol Response Mod* 1984;3:475–482.
4. Lotze MT, Frana LW, Sharrow SO, Robb RJ, Rosenberg SA. In vivo administration of purified human interleukin-2. I. Half life and immunologic effects of the Jurkat cell line-derived interleukin-2. *J Immunol* 1985;134:157–166.
5. Taniguchi T, Matsui H, Fujita T, et al. Structure and expression of a cloned cDNA for human interleukin-2. *Nature* 1983;302:305–310.
6. Rosenberg SA, Grimm EA, McGrogan M, et al. Biological activity of recombinant human interleukin-2 produced in *Escherichia coli*. *Science* 1984;223:1412–1415.
7. Doyle MV, Lee MT, Fong S. Comparison of the biological activities of human recombinant interleukin-2(125) and native interleukin-2. *J Biol Response Mod* 1985;4:96–109.
8. Lotze MT, Matory YL, Ettinghausen SE, et al. In vivo administration of purified human interleukin-2. II. Half life, immunologic effects, and expansion of peripheral lymphoid cells in vivo with recombinant IL-2. *J Immunol* 1985;135:2865–2875.
9. Lotze MT, Matory YL, Rayner AA, et al. Clinical effects and toxicity of interleukin-2 in patients with cancer. *Cancer* 1986;58:2764–2772.
10. Rosenberg SA, Lotze MT, Muul LM, et al. Observations on the systemic administration of autologous lymphokine-activated killer cells and recombinant interleukin-2 to patients with metastatic cancer. *N Engl J Med* 1985;313:1485–1492.
11. Lotze MT, Chang AE, Seipp CA, Simpson C, Vetto JT, Rosenberg SA. High-dose recombinant interleukin-2 in the treatment of patients with disseminated cancer. *JAMA* 1986;256:3117–3124.
12. Rosenberg SA, Lotze MT, Yang JC, et al. Prospective randomized trial of high-dose interleukin-2 alone or in conjunction with lymphokine-activated killer cells for the treatment of patients with advanced cancer. *J Natl Cancer Inst* 1993;85:622–632.
13. Papa MZ, Mulé JJ, Rosenberg SA. Antitumor efficacy of lymphokine-activated killer cells and recombinant interleukin-2 *in vivo*: successful immunotherapy of established pulmonary metastases from weakly immunogenic and nonimmunogenic murine tumors of three distinct histological types. *Cancer Res* 1986;46:4973–4978.
14. Rosenberg SA, Lotze MT, Yang JC, et al. Experience with the use of high-dose interleukin-2 in the treatment of 652 cancer patients. *Ann Surg* 1989;210:474–485.
15. Rosenberg SA, Yang JC, Topalian SL, et al. Treatment of 283 consecutive patients with metastatic melanoma or renal cell cancer using high-dose bolus interleukin-2. *JAMA* 1994;271:907–913.
16. Atkins MB, Sparano J, Fisher RI, et al. Randomized Phase II trial of high-dose interleukin-2 either alone or in combination with interferon alpha-2b in advanced renal cell carcinoma. *J Clin Oncol* 1993;11:661–670.
17. Fyfe G, Fisher RI, Rosenberg SA, Sznol M, Parkinson DR, Louie AC. Results of treatment of 255 patients with metastatic renal cell carcinoma who received high-dose recombinant interleukin-2 therapy. *J Clin Oncol* 1995;13:688–696.
18. Rosenberg SA, Yang JC, White DE, Steinberg SM. Durability of complete responses in patients with metastatic cancer treated with high-dose interleukin-2: identification of the antigens mediating response. *Ann Surg* 1998;228:307–319.
19. Creekmore SP, Harris JE, Ellis TM, et al. A phase I clinical trial of recombinant interleukin-2 by periodic 24 hour intravenous infusions. *J Clin Oncol* 1989;7:276–284.
20. Thompson JA, Lee DJ, Cox WW, et al. Recombinant interleukin-2 toxicity, pharmacokinetics, and immunomodulatory effects in a Phase I trial. *Cancer Res* 1987;47:4202–4207.
21. West WH, Tauer KW, Yannelli JR, et al. Constant-infusion recombinant interleukin-2 in adoptive immunotherapy of advanced cancer. *N Engl J Med* 1987;316:898–905.
22. Geertsen PF, Hermann GG, von der Maase H, Steven K. Treatment of metastatic renal cell carcinoma by continuous intravenous infusion of recombinant interleukin-2: a single-center phase II study. *J Clin Oncol* 1992;10:753–759.
23. Punt KCJA, Jansen RLH, De Mulder PHM, et al. Repetitive weekly cycles of 4-day continuous infusion of recombinant interleukin-2: a phase I study. *J Immunother* 1992;12:277–284.
24. Négrier S, Mercatello A, Bret M, et al. Intravenous interleukin-2 in patients over 65 with metastatic renal carcinoma. *Br J Cancer* 1992;65:723–726.
25. Gold PJ, Thompson JA, Markowitz DR, Neumann S, Fefer A. Metastatic renal cell carcinoma: long-term survival after therapy with high-dose continuous-infusion interleukin-2. *Cancer J Sci Am* 1997;3[Suppl 1]:S85–S91.
26. Legha SS, Gianan MA, Plager C, Eton OE, Papadopoulous NEJ. Evaluation of interleukin-2 administered by continuous infusion in patients with metastatic melanoma. *Cancer* 1996;77:89–96.
27. Hermann GG, Geertsen PF, von der Maase H, Zeuthen J. Interleukin-2 dose, blood monocyte and CD25+ lymphocyte counts as predictors of clinical response to interleukin-2 therapy in patients with renal cell carcinoma. *Cancer Immunol Immunother* 1991;34:111–114.
28. Whitehead RP, Wolf MK, Solanki DL, et al. A phase II trial of continuous-infusion recombinant interleukin-2 in patients with advanced renal cell carcinoma: a Southwest Oncology Group study. *J Immunother Emphasis Tumor Immunol* 1995;18:104–114.
29. Vlasveld LT, Rankin EM, Hekman A, et al. A phase I study of prolonged continuous infusion of low dose recombinant interleukin-2 in melanoma and renal cell cancer. Part I: clinical aspects. *Br J Cancer* 1992;65:744–750.
30. Caligiuri MA, Murray C, Soiffer RJ, et al. Extended continuous infusion low-dose recombinant interleukin-2 in advanced cancer: prolonged immunomodulation without significant toxicity. *J Clin Oncol* 1991;9:2110–2119.
31. Buter J, Sleijfer DT, van der Graaf WTA, de Vries EGE, Willemse PHB, Mulder NH. A progress report on the outpatient treatment of patients with advanced renal cell carcinoma using subcutaneous recombinant interleukin-2. *Semin Oncol* 1993;20:16–21.
32. Whitehead RP, Ward D, Hemingway L, Hemstreet GP III, Bradley E, Konrad M. Subcutaneous recombinant interleukin-2 in a dose

escalating regimen in patients with metastatic renal cell adenocarcinoma. *Cancer Res* 1990;50:6708–6715.

33. Atzpodien J, Körfer A, Evers P, et al. Low-dose subcutaneous recombinant interleukin-2 in advanced human malignancy: a phase II outpatient study. *Mol Biother* 1990;2:18–26.

34. Lissoni P, Barni S, Ardizzoia A, et al. Prognostic factors of the clinical response to subcutaneous immunotherapy with interleukin-2 alone in patients with metastatic renal cell carcinoma. *Oncology* 1994; 51:59–62.

35. Angevin E, Valteau-Couanet D, Farace F, et al. Phase I study of prolonged low-dose subcutaneous recombinant interleukin-2 (IL-2) in patients with advanced cancer. *J Immunol* 1995;18:188–195.

36. Tagliaferri P, Barile C, Caraglia M, et al. Daily low-dose subcutaneous recombinant interleukin-2 by alternate weekly administration: antitumor activity and immunomodulatory effects. *Am J Clin Oncol* 1998;21:48–53.

37. Tourani JM, Lucas V, Mayeur D, et al. Subcutaneous recombinant interleukin-2 (rIL-2) in out-patients with metastatic renal cell carcinoma. Results of a multicenter SCAPP1 trial. *Ann Oncol* 1996;7:525–528.

38. Thompson JA, Lee DJ, Lindgren CG, et al. Influence of dose and duration of infusion of interleukin-2 on toxicity and immunomodulation. *J Clin Oncol* 1988;6:669–678.

39. Gratama JW, Bruin RJ, Lamers CHJ, et al. Activation of the immune system of cancer patients by continuous i.v. recombinant IL-2 (rIL-2) therapy is dependent on dose and schedule of rIL-2. *Clin Exp Immunol* 1993;92:185–193.

40. Urba WJ, Steis RG, Longo DL, et al. Immunomodulatory properties and toxicity of interleukin-2 in patients with cancer. *Cancer Res* 1990;50:185–192.

41. Sosman JA, Kohler PC, Hank JA, et al. Repetitive weekly cycles of interleukin-2. II. Clinical and immunologic effects of dose, schedule, and addition of indomethacin. *J Natl Cancer Inst* 1988;80:1451–1461.

42. Yang JC, Rosenberg SA. An ongoing prospective randomized comparison of interleukin-2 regimens for the treatment of metastatic renal cell cancer. *Cancer J Sci Am* 1997;3:S79–S84.

43. Lotze MT, Custer MC, Rosenberg SA. Intraperitoneal administration of interleukin-2 in patients with cancer. *Arch Surg* 1986;121: 1373–1379.

44. Urba WJ, Clark JW, Steis RG, et al. Intraperitoneal lymphokine-activated killer cell/interleukin-2 therapy in patients with intra-abdominal cancer: immunologic considerations. *J Natl Cancer Inst* 1989;81:602–611.

45. Melioli G, Sertoli MR, Bruzzone M, et al. A phase I study of recombinant interleukin-2 intraperitoneal infusion in patients with neoplastic ascites: toxic effects and immunologic results. *Am J Clin Oncol* 1991;14:231–237.

46. Edwards RP, Gooding W, Lembersky BC, et al. Comparison of toxicity and survival following intraperitoneal recombinant interleukin-2 for persistent ovarian cancer after platinum: twenty-four-hour versus 7-day infusion. *J Clin Oncol* 1997;15:3399–3407.

47. Yasumoto K, Miyazaki K, Nagashima A, et al. Induction of lymphokine-activated killer cells by intrapleural instillations of recombinant interleukin-2 in patients with malignant pleurisy due to lung cancer. *Cancer Res* 1987;47:2184–2187.

48. Astoul P, Picat-Joossen D, Viallat JR, Boutin C. Intrapleural administration of interleukin-2 for the treatment of patients with malignant pleural mesothelioma, a Phase II study. *Cancer* 1998;83:2099–2104.

49. Goey SH, Eggermont AMM, Punt CJA, et al. Intrapleural administration of interleukin-2 in pleural mesothelioma: a phase I-II study. *Br J Cancer* 1995;72:1283–1288.

50. Pizza G, Severini G, Menniti D, De Vinci C, Corrado F. Tumour regression after intralesional injection of interleukin-2 (IL-2) in bladder cancer. Preliminary report. *Int J Cancer* 1984;34:359–367.

51. Ferlazzo G, Scisca C, Iemmo R, et al. Intralesional sonographically guided injections of lymphokine-activated killer cells and recombinant interleukin-2 for the treatment of liver tumors: a pilot study. *J Immunother* 1997;20:158–163.

52. Merchant RE, Grant AJ, Merchant LH, Young HF. Adoptive immunotherapy for recurrent glioblastoma multiforme using lymphokine activated killer cells and recombinant interleukin-2. *Cancer* 1988;62:665–671.

53. Jacobs SK, Wilson DJ, Kornblith PL, Grimm EA. Interleukin-2 and autologous lymphokine-activated killer cells in the treatment of malignant glioma. *J Neurosurg* 1986;64:743–749.

54. Barba D, Saris SC, Holder C, Rosenberg SA, Oldfield EH. Intratumoral LAK cell and interleukin-2 therapy of human gliomas. *J Neurosurg* 1989;70:175–182.

55. Yoshida S, Tanaka R, Takai N, Ono K. Local administration of autologous lymphokine-activated killer cells and recombinant interleukin-2 to patients with malignant brain tumors. *Cancer Res* 1988;48:5011–5016.

56. List J, Moser RP, Steuer M, Loudon WG, Blacklock JB, Grimm EA. Cytokine responses to intraventricular injection of interleukin-2 into patients with leptomeningeal carcinomatosis: rapid induction of tumor necrosis factor alpha, interleukin-1beta, interleukin-6, gamma-interferon, and soluble interleukin-2 receptor (M_r 55,000 protein). *Cancer Res* 1992;52:1123–1128.

57. Hayes RL, Koslow M, Hiesiger EM, et al. Improved long term survival after intracavitary interleukin-2 and lymphokine-activated killer cells for adults with recurrent malignant glioma. *Cancer* 1995;76:840–852.

58. Tubaro A, Stoppacciaro A, Velotti F, et al. Local immunotherapy of superficial bladder cancer by intravesical instillation of recombinant interleukin-2. *Eur Urol* 1995;28:297–303.

59. Schwaibold H, Huland E, Heinzer H, Schwulera U, Huland H. Toxicity of local, continuous and cyclic, high-dose bladder perfusion with recombinant and natural interleukin-2 in advanced cancer of the urinary bladder. *J Cancer Res Clin Oncol* 1995;121:239–246.

60. Thatcher N, Dazzi H, Johnson RJ, et al. Recombinant interleukin-2 (rIL-2) given intrasplenically and intravenously for advanced malignant melanoma. A phase I and II study. *Br J Cancer* 1989;60:770–774.

61. Zukiwski AA, David CL, Coan J, Wallace S, Gutterman JU, Mavligit GM. Increased incidence of hypersensitivity to iodine-containing radiographic contrast media after interleukin-2 administration. *Cancer* 1990;65:1521–1524.

62. Cortesina G, de Stefani A, Giovarelli M, et al. Treatment of recurrent squamous cell carcinoma of the head and neck with low doses of interleukin-2 injected perilymphatically. *Cancer* 1988;62:2482–2485.

63. Sarna G, Machleder H, Collins J, et al. A comparative study of intravenous versus intralymphatic interleukin-2, with assessment of effects of interleukin-2 on both peripheral blood and thoracic-duct lymph. *J Immunother* 1994;15:140–146.

64. Leahy MG, Pitfield D, Popert S, Gallagher CJ, Oliver RTD. Phase I study comparing continuous infusion of recombinant interleukin-2 by subcutaneous or intravenous administration. *Eur J Cancer* 1992;28A:1049–1051.

65. Huland E, Heinzer H, Mir TS, Huland H. Inhaled interleukin-2 therapy in pulmonary metastatic renal cell carcinoma: six years of experience. *Cancer J Sci Am* 1997;3[Suppl 1]:S98–S105.

66. Viele CS, Moran TA. Nursing management of the nonhospitalized patient receiving recombinant interleukin-2. *Semin Oncol Nurs* 1993;9:20–24.

67. Pais RC, Abdel-Mageed A, Ghim TT, et al. Phase I study of recombinant human interleukin-2 for pediatric malignancies: feasibility of outpatient therapy. A Pediatric Oncology Group Study. *J Immunother* 1992;12:138–146.

68. Ribeiro RC, Rill D, Roberson PK, et al. Continuous infusion of interleukin-2 in children with refractory malignancies. *Cancer* 1993;72:623–628.

69. Truitt RL, Piaskowski V, Kirchner P, McOlash L, Camitta BM, Casper JT. Immunological evaluation of pediatric cancer patients receiving recombinant interleukin-2 in a Phase I trial. *J Immunother* 1992;11:274–285.

70. Sievers EL, Lange BJ, Sondel PM, et al. Feasibility, toxicity, and biologic response of interleukin-2 after consolidation chemotherapy for acute myelogenous leukemia: a report from the Children's Cancer Group. *J Clin Oncol* 1998;16:914–919.

71. Gearing AJH, Thorpe R. The international standard for human interleukin-2. *J Immunol Methods* 1988;114:3–9.

72. Rossio JL, Thurman GB, Long C, Vargosko A, Pinsky C. The BRMP IL-2 reference reagent. *Lymphokine Res* 1986;5:S13–S18.

46 *Biologic Therapy of Cancer*

73. Konrad MW, Hemstreet G, Hersh EM, et al. Pharmacokinetics of recombinant interleukin-2 in humans. *Cancer Res* 1990;50:2009–2017.

74. Gustavson LE, Nadeau RW, Oldfield NF. Pharmacokinetics of Teceleukin (recombinant human interleukin-2) after intravenous or subcutaneous administration to patients with cancer. *J Biol Response Mod* 1989;8:440–449.

75. Donohue JH, Rosenberg SA. The fate of interleukin-2 after in vivo administration. *J Immunol* 1983;130:2203–2208.

76. Boldt DH, Mills BJ, Gemlo BT, et al. Laboratory correlates of adoptive immunotherapy with recombinant interleukin-2 and lymphokine-activated killer cells in humans. *Cancer Res* 1988;48:4409–4416.

77. MacFarlane MP, White RL Jr, Seipp CA, Einhorn JH, White DE, Rosenberg SA. The hematologic toxicity of interleukin-2 in patients with metastatic melanoma and renal cell carcinoma. *Cancer* 1995;75:1030–1037.

78. Salvo G, Samoggia P, Masciulli R, et al. Interleukin-2 bolus therapy induces immediate and selective disappearance from peripheral blood of all lymphocyte subpopulations displaying natural killer activity: role of cell adhesion to endothelium. *Eur J Cancer* 1992;28A:818–825.

79. Rosenthal NS, Hank JA, Kohler PC, et al. The in vitro function of lymphocytes from 25 cancer patients receiving four to seven consecutive days of recombinant IL-2. *J Biol Response Mod* 1988;7:123–139.

80. Schomburg A, Menzel T, Körfer A, et al. In vivo and ex vivo antitumor activity in patients receiving low-dose subcutaneous recombinant interleukin-2. *Nat Immun* 1992;11:133–143.

81. Weil-Hillman G, Fisch P, Prieve AF, Sosman JA, Hank JA, Sondel PM. Lymphokine-activated killer activity induced by in vivo interleukin-2 therapy: predominant role for lymphocytes with increased expression of CD2 and Leu19 antigens but negative expression of CD16 antigens. *Cancer Res* 1989;49:3680–3688.

82. Ellis TM, Creekmore SP, McMannis JD, Braun DP, Harris JA, Fisher RI. Appearance and phenotypic characterization of circulating leu 19+ cells in cancer patients receiving recombinant interleukin-2. *Cancer Res* 1988;48:6597–6602.

83. Caligiuri MA, Murray C, Robertson MJ, et al. Selective modulation of human natural killer cells in vivo after prolonged infusion of low dose recombinant interleukin-2. *J Clin Invest* 1993;91:123–132.

84. Wiebke EA, Rosenberg SA, Lotze MT. Acute immunologic effects of interleukin-2 therapy in cancer patients: decreased delayed type hypersensitivity response and decreased proliferative response to soluble antigens. *J Clin Oncol* 1988;6:1440–1449.

85. Kradin RL, Kurnick JT, Preffer FI, Dubinett SM, Dickersin GR, Pinto C. Adoptive immunotherapy with IL-2 results in the loss of delayed-type hypersensitivity responses and the development of immediate hypersensitivity to recall antigens. *Clin Immunol Immunopathol* 1989;50:184–195.

86. Lotze MT, Custer MC, Sharrow SO, Rubin LA, Nelson DL, Rosenberg SA. In vivo administration of purified human interleukin-2 to patients with cancer: development of interleukin-2 receptor positive cells and circulating soluble interleukin 2 receptors following interleukin-2 administration. *Cancer Res* 1987;47:2188–2195.

87. Viviani S, Salvini PM, Bidoli P, et al. Chronic effects of subcutaneous interleukin-2 therapy on soluble interleukin-2 receptors in advanced small cell lung cancer. *Int J Biol Markers* 1993;8:21–24.

88. Martens A, Janssen RAJ, Sleijfer DT, et al. Early sCD8 plasma levels during subcutaneous rIl-2 therapy in patients with renal cell carcinoma correlate with response. *Br J Cancer* 1993;67:1118–1121.

89. Lissoni P, Tisi E, Brivio F, et al. Increase in soluble interleukin-2 receptor and neopterin serum levels during immunotherapy of cancer with interleukin-2. *Eur J Cancer* 1991;27:1014–1016.

90. Janssen RAJ, Sleijfer DT, Heijn AA, Mulder NH, The TH, de Leij L. Peripheral blood lymphocyte number and phenotype prior to therapy correlate with response in subcutaneously applied rIL-2 therapy of renal cell carcinoma. *Br J Cancer* 1992;66:1177–1179.

91. Triozzi PL, Eicher DM, Rinehart JJ. Modulation of adhesion molecules on human large granular lymphocytes by interleukin-2 *in vivo* and *in vitro*. *Cell Immunol* 1992;140:295–303.

92. Kragel AH, Travis WD, Feinberg L, et al. Pathologic findings associated with interleukin-2-based immunotherapy for cancer: a postmortem study of 19 patients. *Hum Pathol* 1990;21:493–502.

93. Rubin JT, Elwood LJ, Rosenberg SA, Lotze MT. Immunohistochemical correlates of response to recombinant interleukin-2-based immunotherapy in humans. *Cancer Res* 1989;49:7086–7092.

94. Cohen PJ, Lotze MT, Roberts JR, Rosenberg SA, Jaffe ES. The immunopathology of sequential tumor biopsies in patients treated with interleukin-2. Correlation of response with T-cell infiltration and HLA-DR expression. *Am J Pathol* 1987;129:208–216.

95. Sondel PM, Kohler PC, Hank JA, et al. Clinical and immunological effects of recombinant interleukin-2 given by repetitive weekly cycles to patients with cancer. *Cancer Res* 1988;48:2561–2567.

96. Gottlieb DJ, Prentice HG, Heslop HE, Bello C, Brenner MK. IL-2 infusion abrogates humoral immune responses in humans. *Clin Exp Immunol* 1992;87:493–498.

97. Ettinghausen SE, Moore JG, White DE, Platanias L, Young NS, Rosenberg SA. Hematologic effects of immunotherapy with lymphokine-activated killer cells and recombinant interleukin-2 in cancer patients. *Blood* 1987;69:1654–1660.

98. Jablons D, Bolton E, Mertins S, et al. Il-2-based immunotherapy alters circulating neutrophil Fc receptor expression and chemotaxis. *J Immunol* 1990;144:3630–3636.

99. Klempner MS, Noring R, Mier JW, Atkins MB. An acquired chemotactic defect in neutrophils from patients receiving interleukin-2 immunotherapy. *N Engl J Med* 1990;322:959–965.

100. Blay J-Y, Favrot MC, Negrier S, et al. Correlation between clinical response to interleukin-2 therapy and sustained production of tumor necrosis factor. *Cancer Res* 1990;50:2371–2374.

101. Konrad MW, DeWitt SK, Bradley EC, et al. Interferon-gamma induced by administration of recombinant interleukin-2 to patients with cancer: kinetics, dose dependence, and correlation with physiological and therapeutic response. *J Immunother* 1992;12:55–63.

102. Weidmann E, Bergmann L, Stock J, Kirsten R, Mitrou PS. Rapid cytokine release in cancer patients treated with interleukin-2. *J Immunother* 1992;12:123–131.

103. Mier JW, Vachino G, van der Meer JWM, et al. Induction of circulating tumor necrosis factor (TNF alpha) as the mechanism for the febrile response to interleukin-2 (IL-2) in cancer patients. *J Clin Immunol* 1988;8:426–436.

104. Jablons DM, Mulé JJ, McIntosh JK, et al. IL-6/IFN-beta-2 as a circulating hormone. Induction by cytokine administration in humans. *J Immunol* 1989;142:1542–1547.

105. Gemlo BT, Palladino MA Jr, Jaffe HS, Espevik TP, Rayner AA. Circulating cytokines in patients with metastatic cancer treated with recombinant interleukin-2 and lymphokine-activated killer cells. *Cancer Res* 1988;48:5864–5867.

106. Tritarelli E, Rocca E, Testa U, et al. Adoptive immunotherapy with high-dose interleukin-2: kinetics of circulating progenitors correlate with interleukin-6, granulocyte colony-stimulating factor level. *Blood* 1991;77:741–749.

107. Schaafsma MR, Falkenburg JHF, Landegent JE, et al. In vivo production of interleukin-5, granulocyte-macrophage colony-stimulating factor, macrophage colony-stimulating factor, and interleukin-6 during intravenous administration of high-dose interleukin-2 in cancer patients. *Blood* 1991;78:1981–1987.

108. Tilg H, Atkins MB, Dinarello CA, Mier JW. Induction of circulating interleukin-10 by interleukin-1 and interleukin-2, but not interleukin-6 immunotherapy. *Cytokine* 1995;7:734–739.

109. Tilg H, Shapiro L, Atkins MB, Dinarello CA, Mier JW. Induction of circulating and erythrocyte-bound IL-8 by IL-2 immunotherapy and suppression of its in vitro production by IL-1 receptor antagonist and soluble tumor necrosis factor receptor (p75) chimera. *J Immunol* 1993;151:3299–3307.

110. van Haelst Pisani C, Kovach JS, Kita H, et al. Administration of interleukin-2 (IL-2) results in increased plasma concentrations of IL-5 and eosinophilia in patients with cancer. *Blood* 1991;78:1538–1544.

111. Allegretta M, Atkins MB, Dempsey RA, et al. The development of anti-interleukin-2 antibodies in patients treated with recombinant human interleukin-2 (IL-2). *J Clin Immunol* 1986;6:481–490.

112. Krigel RL, Padavic-Shaller KA, Rudolph AR, et al. A phase I study of recombinant interleukin-2 plus recombinant b-interferon. *Cancer Res* 1988;48:3875–3881.

113. Atkins MB, Gould JA, Allegretta M, et al. Phase I evaluation of recombinant interleukin-2 in patients with advanced malignant disease. *J Clin Oncol* 1986;4:1380–1391.

114. Schwartzentruber DJ. In vitro predictors of clinical response in patients receiving interleukin-2-based immunotherapy. *Curr Opin Oncol* 1993;5:1055–1058.

115. Royal RE, Steinberg SM, Krouse RS, et al. Correlates of response to IL-2 therapy in patients treated for metastatic renal cancer and melanoma. *Cancer J Sci Am* 1996;2:91–98.

116. White RL Jr, Schwartzentruber DJ, Guleria A, et al. Cardiopulmonary toxicity of treatment with high-dose interleukin-2 in 199 consecutive patients with metastatic melanoma or renal cell carcinoma. *Cancer* 1994;74:3212–3222.

117. Kammula US, White DE, Rosenberg SA. Trends in the safety of high dose bolus interleukin-2 administration in patients with metastatic cancer. *Cancer* 1998;83:797–805.

118. Margolin KA, Rayner AA, Hawkins MJ, et al. Interleukin-2 and lymphokine-activated killer cell therapy of solid tumors: analysis of toxicity and management guidelines. *J Clin Oncol* 1989;7:486–498.

119. Siegel JP, Puri RK. Interleukin-2 toxicity. *J Clin Oncol* 1991;9:694–704.

120. Parkinson DR. Interleukin-2 in cancer therapy. *Semin Oncol* 1988;15:10–26.

121. Mier JW, Aronson FR, Numerof RP, Vachino G, Atkins MB. Toxicity of immunotherapy with interleukin-2 and lymphokine-activated killer cells. *Pathol Immunopathol Res* 1988;7:459–476.

122. Whittington R, Faulds D. Interleukin-2. A review of its pharmacological properties and therapeutic use in patients with cancer. *Drugs* 1993;46:446–514.

123. Vial T, Descotes J. Clinical toxicity of interleukin-2. *Drug Safety* 1992;7:417–433.

124. Vetto JT, Papa MZ, Lotze MT, Chang AE, Rosenberg SA. Reduction of toxicity of interleukin-2 and lymphokine-activated killer cells in humans by the administration of corticosteroids. *J Clin Oncol* 1987;5:496–503.

125. Mier JW, Vachino G, Klempner MS, et al. Inhibition of interleukin-2-induced tumor necrosis factor release by dexamethasone: prevention of an acquired neutrophil chemotaxis defect and differential suppression of interleukin-2-associated side effects. *Blood* 1990;76:1933–1940.

126. Papa MZ, Vetto JT, Ettinghausn SE, Mulé JJ, Rosenberg SA. Effect of corticosteroid on the antitumor activity of lymphokine-activated killer cells and interleukin-2 in mice. *Cancer Res* 1986;46:5618–5623.

127. Baluna R, Vitetta ES. Vascular leak syndrome: a side effect of immunotherapy. *Immunopharmacology* 1997;37:117–132.

128. Lee RE, Lotze MT, Skibber JM, et al. Cardiorespiratory effects of immunotherapy with interleukin-2. *J Clin Oncol* 1989;7:7–20.

129. Ballmer-Weber BK, Dummer R, Küng E, Burg G, Ballmer PE. Interleukin-2-induced increase of vascular permeability without decrease of the intravascular albumin pool. *Br J Cancer* 1995;71:78–82.

130. Nurnberger W, Holthausen S, Michelmann I, Jurgens H, Burdach S, Gobel U. Generation of the complement activation product C5a precedes interleukin-2-induced capillary leakage syndrome. *J Immunother* 1996;19:45–49.

131. Carey PD, Wakefield CH, Guillou PJ. Neutrophil activation, vascular leak toxicity, and cytolysis during interleukin-2 infusion in human cancer. *Surgery* 1997;122:918–926.

132. Cotran RS, Pober JS, Gimbrone MA Jr, et al. Endothelial activation during interleukin-2 immunotherapy. A possible mechanism for the vascular leak syndrome. *J Immunol* 1987;139:1883–1888.

133. Pockaj BA, Yang JC, Lotze MT, et al. A prospective randomized trial evaluating colloid versus crystalloid resuscitation in the treatment of the vascular leak syndrome associated with interleukin-2 therapy. *J Immunother* 1994;15:22–28.

134. Guleria AS, Yang JC, Topalian SL, et al. Renal dysfunction associated with the administration of high-dose interleukin-2 in 199 consecutive patients with metastatic melanoma or renal cell carcinoma. *J Clin Oncol* 1994;12:2714–2722.

135. Eberlein TJ, Schoof DD, Michie HR, et al. Ibuprofen causes reduced toxic effects of interleukin-2 administration in patients with metastatic cancer. *Arch Surg* 1989;124:542–547.

136. Michie HR, Eberlein TJ, Spriggs DR, Manogue KR, Cerami A, Wilmore DW. Interleukin-2 initiates metabolic responses associated with critical illness in humans. *Ann Surg* 1988;208:493–503.

137. Ognibene FP, Rosenberg SA, Lotze M, et al. Interleukin-2 administration causes reversible hemodynamic changes and left ventricular dysfunction similar to those seen in septic shock. *Chest* 1988;94:750–754.

138. Nora R, Abrams JS, Tait NS, Hiponia DJ, Silverman HJ. Myocardial toxic effects during recombinant interleukin-2 therapy. *J Natl Cancer Inst* 1989;81:59–63.

139. Gaynor ER, Vitek L, Sticklin L, et al. The hemodynamic effects of treatment with interleukin-2 and lymphokine-activated killer cells. *Ann Intern Med* 1988;109:953–958.

140. Diana D, Sculier JP. Haemodynamic effects induced by intravenous administration of high doses of r-Met Hu IL-2 [ala-125] in patients with advanced cancer. *Intensive Care Med* 1990;16:167–170.

141. Pockaj BA, Rosenberg SA. Lack of antihypertensive effect of interleukin-2 administration in humans. *J Immunother* 1991;10:456–459.

142. Hibbs JB Jr, Westenfelder C, Taintor R, et al. Evidence for cytokine-inducible nitric oxide synthesis from L-arginine in patients receiving interleukin-2 therapy. *J Clin Invest* 1992;89:867–877.

143. Ochoa JB, Curti B, Peitzman AB, et al. Increased circulating nitrogen oxides after human tumor immunotherapy: correlation with toxic hemodynamic changes. *J Natl Cancer Inst* 1992;84:864–867.

144. Miles D, Thomsen L, Balkwill F, Thavasu P, Moncada S. Association between biosynthesis of nitric oxide and changes in immunological and vascular parameters in patients treated with interleukin-2. *Eur J Clin Invest* 1994;24:287–290.

145. Citterio G, Pellegatta F, Di Lucca G, et al. Plasma nitrate plus nitrite changes during continuous intravenous infusion interleukin-2. *Br J Cancer* 1996;74:1297–1301.

146. Kilbourn RG, Fonseca GA, Griffith OW, et al. NG-methyl-L-arginine, an inhibitor of nitric oxide synthase, reverses interleukin-2-induced hypotension. *Crit Care Med* 1995;23:1018–1024.

147. Lissoni P, Pittalis S, Ardizzoia A, et al. Prevention of cytokine-induced hypotension in cancer patients by the pineal hormone melatonin. *Support Care Cancer* 1996;4:313–316.

148. Goel M, Flaherty L, Lavine S, Redman BG. Reversible cardiomyopathy after high-dose interleukin-2 therapy. *J Immunother* 1992;11:225–229.

149. Du Bois JS, Udelson JE, Atkins MB. Severe reversible global and regional ventricular dysfunction associated with high-dose interleukin-2 immunotherapy. *J Immunother* 1995;18:119–123.

150. Citterio G, Fragasso G, Rossetti E, et al. Isolated left ventricular filling abnormalities may predict interleukin-2-induced cardiovascular toxicity. *J Immunother Emphasis Tumor Immunol* 1996;19:134–141.

151. Fragasso G, Tresoldi M, Benti R, et al. Impaired left ventricular filling rate induced by treatment with recombinant interleukin-2 for advanced cancer. *Br Heart J* 1994;71:166–169.

152. Kragel AH, Travis WD, Steis RG, Rosenberg SA, Roberts WC. Myocarditis or acute myocardial infarction associated with interleukin-2 therapy for cancer. *Cancer* 1990;66:1513–1516.

153. Samlowski WE, Ward JH, Craven CM, Freedman RA. Severe myocarditis following high-dose interleukin-2 administration. *Arch Pathol Lab Med* 1989;113:838–841.

154. Schuchter LM, Hendricks CB, Holland KH, et al. Eosinophilic myocarditis associated with high-dose interleukin-2 therapy. *Am J Med* 1990;88:439–440.

155. Osanto S, Cluitmans FHM, Franks CR, Bosker HA, Cleton FJ. Myocardial injury after interleukin 2 therapy. *Lancet* 1988;2:48–49.

156. Textor SC, Margolin K, Blayney D, Carlson J, Doroshow J. Renal, volume, and hormonal changes during therapeutic administration of recombinant interleukin-2 in man. *Am J Med* 1987;83:1055–1061.

157. Groeger JS, Bajorin D, Reichman B, Kopec I, Atiq O, Pierri MK. Haemodynamic effects of recombinant interleukin-2 administered by constant infusion. *Eur J Cancer* 1991;27:1613–1616.

158. Saxon RR, Klein JS, Bar MH, et al. Pathogenesis of pulmonary edema during interleukin-2 therapy: correlation of chest radiographic and clinical findings in 54 patients. *AJR Am J Roentgenol* 1991;156:281–285.

159. Mann H, Ward JH, Samlowski WE. Vascular leak syndrome associated with interleukin-2: chest radiographic manifestations. *Radiology* 1990;176:191–194.

160. Vogelzang PJ, Bloom SM, Mier JW, Atkins MB. Chest roentgenographic abnormalities in IL-2 recipients. *Chest* 1992;101:746–752.

161. Davis SD, Berkmen YM, Wang JCL. Interleukin-2 therapy for advanced renal cell carcinoma: radiographic evaluation of response and complications. *Radiology* 1990;177:127–131.

162. Berthiaume Y, Boiteau P, Fick G, et al. Pulmonary edema during Il-2 therapy: combined effect of increased permeability and hydrostatic pressure. *Am J Respir Crit Care Med* 1995;152:329–335.

163. Belldegrun A, Webb DE, Austin HA III, et al. Effects of interleukin-2 on renal function in patients receiving immunotherapy for advanced cancer. *Ann Intern Med* 1987;106:817–822.

164. Webb DE, Austin HA III, Belldegrun A, Vaughan E, Linehan WM, Rosenberg SA. Metabolic and renal effects of interleukin-2 immunotherapy for metastatic cancer. *Clin Nephrol* 1988;30:141–145.

165. Kozeny GA, Nicolas JD, Creekmore S, Sticklin L, Hano JE, Fisher RI. Effects of interleukin-2 immunotherapy on renal function. *J Clin Oncol* 1988;6:1170–1176.

166. Shalmi CL, Dutcher JP, Feinfeld DA, et al. Acute renal dysfunction during interleukin-2 treatment: suggestion of an intrinsic renal lesion. *J Clin Oncol* 1990;8:1839–1846.

167. Christiansen NP, Skubitz KM, Nath K, Ochoa A, Kennedy BJ. Nephrotoxicity of continuous intravenous infusion of recombinant interleukin-2. *Am J Med* 1988;84:1072–1075.

168. Ponce P, Cruz J, Travassos J, et al. Renal toxicity mediated by continuous infusion of recombinant interleukin-2. *Nephron* 1993;64:114–118.

169. Heys SD, Eremin O, Franks CR, Broom J, Whiting PH. Lithium clearance measurements during recombinant interleukin-2 treatment: tubular dysfunction in man. *Ren Fail* 1993;15:195–201.

170. Belldegrun A, Webb DE, Austin HA III, Steinberg SM, Linehan WM, Rosenberg SA. Renal toxicity of interleukin-2 administration in patients with metastatic renal cell cancer: effect of pre-therapy nephrectomy. *J Urol* 1989;141:499–503.

171. Memoli B, De Nicola L, Libetta C, et al. Interleukin-2–induced renal dysfunction in cancer patients is reversed by low-dose dopamine infusion. *Am J Kidney Dis* 1995;26:27–33.

172. Cormier JN, Hurst R, Vasselli J, et al. A prospective randomized evaluation of the prophylactic use of low-dose dopamine in cancer patients receiving interleukin-2. *J Immunol* 1997;20:292–300.

173. Kim H, Rosenberg SA, Steinberg SM, Cole DJ, Weber JS. A randomized double-blinded comparison of the antiemetic efficacy of ondansetron and droperidol in patients receiving high-dose interleukin-2. *J Immunol* 1994;16:60–65.

174. Ryan CM, Atkins MB, Mier JW, Gelfand JA, Tompkins RG. Effects of malignancy and interleukin-2 infusion on gut macromolecular permeability. *Crit Care Med* 1995;23:1801–1806.

175. Gaspari AA, Lotze MT, Rosenberg SA, Stern JB, Katz SI. Dermatologic changes associated with interleukin-2 administration. *JAMA* 1987;258:1624–1629.

176. Marmary Y, Shiloni E, Katz J. Oral changes in interleukin-2 treated patients: a preliminary report. *J Oral Pathol Med* 1992;21:230–231.

177. Schwartzentruber D, Lotze MT, Rosenberg SA. Colonic perforation. An unusual complication of therapy with high-dose interleukin-2. *Cancer* 1988;62:2350–2353.

178. Rahman R, Bernstein Z, Vaickus L, et al. Unusual gastrointestinal complications of interleukin-2 therapy. *J Immunother* 1991;10:221–225.

179. Sparano JA, Dutcher JP, Kaleya R, et al. Colonic ischemia complicating immunotherapy with interleukin-2 and interferon-α. *Cancer* 1991;68:1538–1544.

180. Sparano JA, Brandt LJ, Dutcher JP, DuBois JS, Atkins MB. Symptomatic exacerbation of Crohn disease after treatment with high-dose interleukin-2. *Ann Intern Med* 1993;118:617–618.

181. Birchfield GR, Ward JH, Redman BG, Flaherty L, Samlowski WE. Acute pancreatitis associated with high-dose interleukin-2 immunotherapy for malignant melanoma. *West J Med* 1990;152:714–716.

182. Ratcliffe MA, Roditi G, Adamson DJA. Interleukin-2 and splenic enlargement. *J Natl Cancer Inst* 1992;84:810–811.

183. Fisher B, Keenan AM, Garra BS, et al. Interleukin-2 induces profound reversible cholestasis: a detailed analysis in treated cancer patients. *J Clin Oncol* 1989;7:1852–1862.

184. Huang CM, Elin RJ, Ruddel M, Sliva C, Lotze MT, Rosenberg SA. Changes in laboratory results for cancer patients treated with interleukin-2. *Clin Chem* 1990;36:431–434.

185. Denicoff KD, Rubinow DR, Papa MZ, et al. The neuropsychiatric effects of treatment with interleukin-2 and lymphokine-activated killer cells. *Ann Intern Med* 1987;107:293–300.

186. Saris SC, Rosenberg SA, Friedman RB, Rubin JT, Barba D, Oldfield EH. Penetration of recombinant interleukin-2 across the blood-cerebrospinal fluid barrier. *J Neurosurg* 1988;69:29–34.

187. Saris SC, Patronas NJ, Rosenberg SA, et al. The effect of intravenous interleukin-2 on brain water content. *J Neurosurg* 1989;71:169–174.

188. Karp BI, Yang JC, Khorsand M, Wood R, Merigan TC. Multiple cerebral lesions complicating therapy with interleukin-2. *Neurology* 1996;47:417–424.

189. Bernard JT, Ameriso S, Kempf RA, Rosen P, Mitchell MS, Fisher M. Transient focal neurologic deficits complicating interleukin-2 therapy. *Neurology* 1990;40:154–155.

190. Vecht CJ, Keohane C, Menon RS, Henzen-Logmans SC, Punt CJA, Stoter G. Acute fatal leukoencephalopathy after interleukin-2 therapy. *N Engl J Med* 1990;323:1146–1147.

191. Rosenberg SA, Yang JC, Schwartzentruber DJ, et al. Immunologic and therapeutic evaluation of a synthetic peptide vaccine for the treatment of patients with metastatic melanoma. *Nat Med* 1998;4:321–327.

192. Sarna GP, Figlin RA, Pertcheck M, Altrock B, Kradjian SA. Systemic administration of recombinant methionyl human interleukin-2 (Ala 125) to cancer patients: clinical results. *J Biol Response Mod* 1989;8:16–24.

193. Heys SD, Mills KLG, Eremin O. Bilateral carpal tunnel syndrome associated with interleukin-2 therapy. *Postgrad Med J* 1992;68:587–588.

194. Loh FL, Herskovitz S, Berger AR, Swerdlow ML. Brachial plexopathy associated with interleukin-2 therapy. *Neurology* 1992;42:462–463.

195. Wallace DJ, Margolin K, Waller P. Fibromyalgia and interleukin-2 therapy for malignancy. *Ann Intern Med* 1988;108:909.

196. Baron NW, Davis LP, Flaherty LE, Muz J, Valdivieso M, Kling GA. Scintigraphic findings in patients with shoulder pain caused by interleukin-2. *AJR Am J Roentgenol* 1990;154:327–330.

197. Massarotti EM, Liu NY, Mier J, Atkins MB. Chronic inflammatory arthritis after treatment with high-dose interleukin-2 for malignancy. *Am J Med* 1992;92:693–697.

198. Esteva-Lorenzo FJ, Janik JE, Fenton RG, Emslie-Smith A, Engel AG, Longo DL. Myositis associated with interleukin-2 therapy in a patient with metastatic renal cell carcinoma. *Cancer* 1995;76:1219–1223.

199. Lavelle-Jones M, Al-Hadrani A, Spiers EM, Campbell FC, Cuschieri A. Reactivation of rheumatoid arthritis during continuous infusion of interleukin-2: evidence of lymphocytic control of rheumatoid disease. *BMJ* 1990;301:97.

200. Wolkenstein P, Chosidow O, Wechsler J, et al. Cutaneous side effects associated with interleukin-2 administration for metastatic melanoma. *J Am Acad Dermatol* 1993;28:66–70.

201. Staunton MR, Scully MC, Le Boit PE, Aronson FR. Life-threatening bullous skin eruptions during interleukin-2 therapy. *J Natl Cancer Inst* 1991;83:56–57.

202. Wiener JS, Tucker JA Jr, Walther PJ. Interleukin-2-induced dermatotoxicity resembling toxic epidermal necrolysis. *South Med J* 1992;85:656–659.

203. Ramseur WL, Richards F II, Duggan DB. A case of fatal *Pemphigus vulgaris* in association with beta interferon and interleukin-2 therapy. *Cancer* 1989;63:2005–2007.

204. Begley MG, Shawker TH, Robertson CN, Bock SN, Wei JP, Lotze MT. Fournier gangrene: diagnosis with scrotal US. *Radiology* 1988;169:387–389.

205. Baars JW, Wagstaff J, Hack CE, Wolbink G-J, Eerenberg-Belmer AJM, Pinedo HM. Angioneurotic oedema and urticaria during therapy with interleukin-2 (IL-2). *Ann Oncol* 1992;3:243–244.

206. Baars JW, Coenen JLLM, Wagstaff J, van der Valk P, Pinedo HM. Lobular panniculitis after subcutaneous administration of interleukin-2 (IL-2), and its exacerbation during intravenous therapy with IL-2. *Br J Cancer* 1992;66:698–699.

207. Weinstein A, Bujak D, Mittelman A, Davidian M. Erythema nodosum in a patient with renal cell carcinoma treated with interleukin-2 and lymphokine-activated killer cells. *JAMA* 1987;258:3120–3121.

208. Lee RE, Gaspari AA, Lotze MT, Chang AE, Rosenberg SA. Interleukin-2 and psoriasis. *Arch Dermatol* 1988;124:1811–1815.

209. Rosenberg SA, White DE. Vitiligo in patients with melanoma: normal tissue antigens can be targets for cancer immunotherapy. *J Immunother* 1996;19:81–84.

210. Richards JM, Gale D, Mehta N, Lestingi T. Combination of chemotherapy with interleukin-2 and interferon alfa for the treatment of metastatic melanoma. *J Clin Oncol* 1999;17:651 657.

211. Spinazze S, Viviani S, Bidoli P, et al. Effect of prolonged subcutaneous administration of interleukin-2 on the circadian rhythms of cortisol and beta-endorphin in advanced small cell lung cancer patients. *Tumori* 1991;77:496–499.

212. Lissoni P, Barni S, Rovelli F, et al. Neuroendocrine effects of subcutaneous interleukin-2 injection in cancer patients. *Tumori* 1991; 77:212–215.

213. Lissoni P, Barni S, Archili C, et al. Endocrine effects of a 24-hour intravenous infusion of interleukin-2 in the immunotherapy of cancer. *Anticancer Res* 1990;10:753–758.

214. Denicoff KD, Durkin TM, Lotze MT, et al. The neuroendocrine effects of interleukin-2 treatment. *J Clin Endocrinol Metab* 1989;69:402–410.

215. Meikle AW, Cardoso de Sousa JC, Ward JH, Woodward M, Samloswki WE. Reduction of testosterone synthesis after high dose interleukin-2 therapy of metastatic cancer. *J Clin Endocrinol Metab* 1991; 73:931–935.

216. Broom J, Heys SD, Whiting PH, et al. Interleukin-2 therapy in cancer: identification of responders. *Br J Cancer* 1992;66:1185–1187.

217. VanderMolen LA, Smith JW II, Longo DL, Steis RG, Kremers P, Sznol M. Adrenal insufficiency and interleukin-2 therapy [Letter]. *Ann Intern Med* 1989;111:185.

218. Deshpande H, Dutcher JP, Novik Y, Oleksowicz L. Successful treatment of a patient on adrenal steroid replacement therapy with high-dose bolus interleukin-2 for metastatic renal cell carcinoma [Letter]. *Cancer J Sci Am* 1999;5:52–53.

219. Kruit WHJ, Bolhuis RLH, Goey SH, et al. Interleukin-2-induced thyroid dysfunction is correlated with treatment duration but not with tumor response. *J Clin Oncol* 1993;11:921–924.

220. Vialettes B, Guillerand MA, Viens P, et al. Incidence rate and risk factors for thyroid dysfunction during recombinant interleukin-2 therapy in advanced malignancies. *Acta Endocrinol* 1993;129:31–38.

221. Krouse RS, Royal RE, Heywood G, et al. Thyroid dysfunction in 281 patients with metastatic melanoma or renal carcinoma treated with interleukin-2 alone. *J Immunother* 1996;18:272–278.

222. Atkins MB, Mier JW, Parkinson DR, Gould JA, Berkman EM, Kaplan MM. Hypothyroidism after treatment with interleukin-2 and lymphokine-activated killer cells. *N Engl J Med* 1988;318: 1557–1563.

223. Weijl NI, van der Harst D, Brand A, et al. Hypothyroidism during immunotherapy with interleukin-2 is associated with antithyroid antibodies and response to treatment. *J Clin Oncol* 1993;11:1376–1383.

224. Schwartzentruber DJ, White DE, Zweig MH, Weintraub BD, Rosenberg SA. Thyroid dysfunction associated with immunotherapy for patients with cancer. *Cancer* 1991;68:2384–2390.

225. Scalzo S, Gengaro A, Boccoli G, et al. Primary hypothyroidism associated with interleukin-2 and interferon α-2 therapy of melanoma and renal carcinoma. *Eur J Cancer* 1990;26:1152–1156.

226. Reid I, Sharpe I, McDevitt J, et al. Thyroid dysfunction can predict response to immunotherapy with interleukin-2 and interferon-2a. *Br J Cancer* 1991;64:915–918.

227. Jacobs EL, Clare-Salzler MJ, Chopra IJ, Figlin RA. Thyroid function abnormalities associated with the chronic outpatient administration

of recombinant interleukin-2 and recombinant interferon-α. *J Immunother* 1991;10:448–455.

228. Pichert G, Jost LM, Zobeli L, Odermatt B, Pedio G, Stahel RA. Thyroiditis after treatment with interleukin-2 and interferon α-2a. *Br J Cancer* 1990;62:100–104.

229. Wilson DE, Birchfield GR, Hejazi JS, Ward JH, Samlowski WE. Hypocholesterolemia in patients treated with recombinant interleukin-2: appearance of remnant-like lipoproteins. *J Clin Oncol* 1989;7:1573–1578.

230. Lissoni P, Brivio F, Pittalis S, et al. Decrease in cholesterol levels during the immunotherapy of cancer with interleukin-2. *Br J Cancer* 1991;64:956–958.

231. Lissoni P, Cazzaniga M, Ardizzoia A, et al. Cytokine regulation of iron metabolism: effect of low-dose interleukin-2 subcutaneous therapy on ferritin, transferrin and iron blood concentrations in cancer patients. *J Biol Regul Homeost Agents* 1993;7:31–33.

232. Marcus SL, Dutcher JP, Paietta E, et al. Severe hypovitaminosis C occurring as the result of adoptive immunotherapy with high dose interleukin-2 and lymphokine-activated killer cells. *Cancer Res* 1987;47:4208–4212.

233. Weiss GR, Margolin KA, Aronson FR, et al. A randomized phase II trial of continuous infusion interleukin-2 or bolus injection interleukin-2 plus lymphokine-activated killer cells for advanced renal cell carcinoma. *J Clin Oncol* 1992;10:275–281.

234. Bukowski RM, Goodman P, Crawford ED, Sergi JS, Redman BG, Whitehead RP. Phase II trial of high-dose intermittent interleukin-2 in metastatic renal cell carcinoma: a Southwest Oncology Group Study. *J Natl Cancer Inst* 1990;82:143–146.

235. Silberstein DS, Schoof DD, Rodrick ML, et al. Activation of eosinophils in cancer patients treated with IL-2 and IL-2-generated lymphokine-activated killer cells. *J Immunol* 1989;142:2162–2167.

236. Macdonald D, Gordon AA, Kajitani H, Enokihara H, Barrett AJ. Interleukin-2 treatment-associated eosinophilia is mediated by interleukin-5 production. *Br J Haematol* 1990;76:168–173.

237. Paciucci PA, Mandeli J, Oleksowicz L, Ameglio F, Holland JF. Thrombocytopenia during immunotherapy with interleukin-2 by constant infusion. *Am J Med* 1990;89:308–312.

238. Fleischmann JD, Shingleton WB, Gallagher C, Ratnoff OD, Chahine A. Fibrinolysis, thrombocytopenia, and coagulation abnormalities complicating high-dose interleukin-2 immunotherapy. *J Lab Clin Med* 1991;117:76–82.

239. Legha SS, Ring S, Eton O, et al. Development of a biochemotherapy regimen with concurrent administration of cisplatin, vinblastine, dacarbazine, inteferon-α, and interleukin-2 for patients with metastatic melanoma. *J Clin Oncol* 1998;16:1752–1759.

240. Rosenberg SA, Yang JC, Schwartzentruber DJ, et al. Prospective randomized trial of the treatment of patients with metastatic melanoma using chemotherapy with cisplatin, dacarbazine, and tamoxifen alone or in combination with interleukin-2 and interferon α-2b. *J Clin Oncol* 1999;17:968–975.

241. Birchfield GR, Rodgers GM, Girodias KW, Ward JH, Samlowski WE. Hypoprothrombinemia associated with interleukin-2 therapy: correction with vitamin K. *J Immunother* 1992;11:71–75.

242. Oleksowicz L, Strack M, Dutcher JP, et al. A distinct coagulopathy associated with interleukin-2 therapy. *Br J Haematol* 1994;88:892–894.

243. Oleksowicz L, Zuckerman D, Mrowiec Z, Puszkin E, Dutcher JP. Effects of interleukin-2 administration on platelet function in cancer patients. *Am J Hematol* 1994;45:224–231.

244. Pockaj BA, Topalian SL, Steinberg SM, White DE, Rosenberg SA. Infectious complications associated with interleukin-2 administration: a retrospective review of 935 treatment courses. *J Clin Oncol* 1993;11:136–147.

245. Snydman DR, Sullivan B, Gill M, Gould JA, Parkinson DR, Atkins MB. Nosocomial sepsis associated with interleukin-2. *Ann Intern Med* 1990;112:102–107.

246. Vlasveld LT, Rodenhuis S, Rutgers EJT, et al. Catheter-related complications in 52 patients treated with continuous infusion of low dose recombinant interleukin-2 via an implanted central venous catheter. *Eur J Surg Oncol* 1994;20:122–129.

247. Murphy PM, Lane HC, Gallin JI, Fauci AS. Marked disparity in incidence of bacterial infections in patients with the acquired immu-

nodeficiency syndrome receiving interleukin-2 or interferon-gamma. *Ann Intern Med* 1988;108:36–41.

248. Bock SN, Lee RE, Fisher B, et al. A prospective randomized trial evaluating prophylactic antibiotics to prevent triple-lumen catheter-related sepsis in patients treated with immunotherapy. *J Clin Oncol* 1990;8:161–169.

249. Hartmann LC, Urba WJ, Steis RG, et al. Use of prophylactic antibiotics for prevention of intravascular catheter-related infections in interleukin-2-treated patients. *J Natl Cancer Inst* 1989;81:1190–1193.

250. Shulman KL, Thompson JA, Benyunes MC, Winter TC, Fefer A. Adverse reactions to intravenous contrast media in patients treated with interleukin-2. *J Immunother* 1993;13:208–212.

251. Abi-Aad AS, Figlin RA, Belldegrun A, deKernion JB. Metastatic renal cell cancer: interleukin-2 toxicity induced by contrast agent injection. *J Immunother* 1991;10:292–295.

252. Choyke PL, Miller DL, Lotze MT, Whiteis JM, Ebbitt B, Rosenberg SA. Delayed reactions to contrast media after interleukin-2 immunotherapy. *Radiology* 1992;183:111–114.

253. Oldham RK, Brogley J, Braud E. Contrast medium "recalls" interleukin-2 toxicity. *J Clin Oncol* 1990;8:942–943.

254. Heywood GR, Rosenberg SA, Weber JS. Hypersensitivity reactions to chemotherapy agents in patients receiving chemoimmunotherapy with high-dose interleukin-2. *J Natl Cancer Inst* 1995;87:915–922.

255. Walther MM, Alexander RB, Weiss GH, et al. Cytoreductive surgery prior to interleukin-2-based therapy in patients with metastatic renal cell carcinoma. *Urology* 1993;42:250–258.

256. Kim B, Louie AC. Surgical resection following interleukin-2 therapy for metastatic renal cell carcinoma prolongs remission. *Arch Surg* 1992;127:1343–1349.

257. Lee DS, White DE, Hurst R, Rosenberg SA, Yang JC. Patterns of relapse and response to retreatment in patients with metastatic melanoma or renal cell carcinoma who responded to interleukin-2-based immunotherapy. *Cancer J Sci Am* 1998;4:86–93.

258. Brivio F, Lissoni P, Barni S, et al. Effects of a preoperative course of interleukin-2 on surgical and immunobiological variables in patients with colorectal cancer: a phase 2 study. *Eur J Surg* 1993;159:43–47.

259. Nichols PH, Ramsden CW, Ward U, Sedman PC, Primrose JN. Perioperative immunotherapy with recombinant interleukin-2 in patients undergoing surgery for colorectal cancer. *Cancer Res* 1992;52:5765–5769.

260. Deehan DJ, Heys SD, Ashby J, Eremin O. Interleukin-2 (IL-2) augments host cellular immune reactivity in the perioperative period in patients with malignant disease. *Eur J Surg Oncol* 1995;21:16–22.

261. Lissoni P, Brivio F, Brivio O, et al. Immune effects of preoperative immunotherapy with high-dose subcutaneous interleukin-2 versus neuroimmunotherapy with low-dose interleukin-2 plus the neurohormone melatonin in gastrointestinal tract tumor patients. *J Biol Regul Homeost Agents* 1995;9:31–33.

262. Masotti A, Morandini G, Ortolani R, Fumagalli L. Phase-II randomized study of pre-operative IL-2 administration in operable NSCLC. *Lung Cancer* 1998;20:191–202.

263. Elias D, Farace F, Triebel F, et al. Phase I-II randomized study on prehepatectomy recombinant interleukin-2 immunotherapy in patients with metastatic carcinoma of the colon and rectum. *J Am Coll Surg* 1995;181:303–310.

264. Thompson JA, Bianco JA, Benyunes MC, Neubauer MA, Slattery JT, Fefer A. Phase Ib trial of pentoxifylline and ciprofloxacin in patients treated with interleukin-2 and lymphokine-activated killer cell therapy for metastatic renal cell carcinoma. *Cancer Res* 1994; 54:3436–3441.

265. Anderson JA, Woodcock TM, Harty JI, Knott AW, Edwards MJ. The effects of oral pentoxifylline on interleukin-2 toxicity in patients with metastatic renal cell carcinoma. *Eur J Cancer* 1995;31A:714–717.

266. Du BJS, Trehu EG, Mier JW, et al. Randomized placebo-controlled clinical trial of high-dose interleukin-2 in combination with a soluble p75 tumor necrosis factor receptor immunoglobulin G chimera in patients with advanced melanoma and renal cell carcinoma. *J Clin Oncol* 1997;15:1052–1062.

267. Margolin K, Atkins M, Sparano J, et al. Prospective randomized trial of lisofylline for the prevention of toxicities of high-dose interleukin-2 therapy in advanced renal cancer and malignant melanoma. *Clin Cancer Res* 1997;3:565–572.

268. Ogilvie AC, Baars JW, Erenberg AJM, et al. A pilot study to evaluate the effects of C1 esterase inhibitor on the toxicity of high-dose interleukin-2. *Br J Cancer* 1994;69:596–598.

269. Shahidi H, Kilbourn RG. The role of nitric oxide in interleukin-2 therapy induced hypotension. *Cancer Metastasis Rev* 1998;17:119–126.

3.2

INTERLEUKIN-2: CLINICAL APPLICATIONS

Melanoma

MICHAEL B. ATKINS
ARUN SHET
JEFFREY A. SOSMAN

Melanoma poses an increasingly important health problem. It is estimated that in 2000, 1 in 75 people in the United States will run the risk of developing a malignant melanoma in their lifetimes. Although surgery with or without adjuvant therapy can be curative in early-stage disease, the outlook for patients with distant metastases remains bleak. Median survival in most series ranges from 6 to 9 months with 5-year survival rates of less than 4% (1). An estimated 7,300 Americans are expected to die of melanoma in 1999 (2). Many of these patients are young (median age, 46 to 50 years); therefore, their loss represents a societal burden in excess of their actual numbers. Although a variety of cytotoxic chemotherapy agents used either alone or in combination possess activity against metastatic melanoma, responses to these agents are usually partial and of short duration. In particular, combination cytotoxic chemotherapy results in 5-year durable responses in only 1% to 2% of patients (3), and has yet to be shown superior to single-agent dacarbazine in a randomized phase 3 trial (4–6). Similarly, although the addition of either tamoxifen or interferon-α (IFN-α) to cytotoxic chemotherapy has also been reported to improve results in phase 2 and small phase 3 trials (7–12), such benefits have not borne out in larger phase 3 trials (4,13–15). Thus, new approaches to the treatment of metastatic melanoma are clearly necessary.

Clinical and laboratory observations have suggested that host immunologic responses may occasionally influence the course of melanoma and have stimulated interest in the use of biologic response modifiers in melanoma. Virtually the entire repertoire of immunotherapeutic approaches have been explored; many have shown some antitumor and/or immunomodulatory activity (16). Areas of active investigation include: recombinant cytokines, either alone or in combination with adoptive immunotherapy, toxicity reduction agents, or cytotoxic chemotherapy; vaccines; monoclonal antibodies or antibody conjugates; and gene therapy. These various approaches are detailed throughout this textbook. This chapter focuses on clinical investigations using the cytokine interleukin-2 (IL-2) in melanoma.

IL-2 was first identified in 1976 as a T-cell growth factor (17); isolation of the complementary DNA clone was described in 1983 (18). Subsequently, recombinant IL-2 was shown to have potent immunomodulatory and antitumor activity in a number of murine tumor models (19). Clinical investigations with recombinant IL-2 showed that this agent possessed significant antitumor activity, producing durable complete responses (CRs) in a small percentage of patients with either metastatic melanoma or renal cell carcinoma. The high-dose intravenous (i.v.) bolus IL-2 regimen, developed at the National Cancer Institute (NCI) Surgery Branch, received U.S. Food and Drug Administration (FDA) approval for the treatment of metastatic renal cell carcinoma in 1992. FDA approval for the treatment of metastatic melanoma was granted in 1998. This section reviews the clinical investigations involving IL-2 administered as a single agent, either by the high-dose i.v. bolus route or by alternative administration schedules in patients with metastatic melanoma. It also describes results of clinical trials using IL-2 in combination with IFN-α, other cytokines, monoclonal antibodies, vaccines, cellular therapy, or chemotherapy in patients with melanoma. Finally, it also details results of various strategies aimed at dissociating the toxicity of IL-2 from its antitumor effects. As in previous reviews, doses of IL-2 are reported as international units (IU) when they are described by authors or when a conversion factor is provided by an author within the same reference. Otherwise, doses are reported in the text and tables as they are described by authors, followed by an annotation that includes the estimated IU to facilitate comparisons between treatment regimens. Per convention (20), the following conversion factors are used: 1.0 Cetus Unit = 6 IU, 1.0 Hoffman-LaRoche (HLR) Unit = 1.0 Biologic Response Modifier Program (BRMP) Unit =

2.6 IU. It must be noted, however, that other differences may exist between these various preparations (21); therefore, these simple conversions may not be entirely valid.

APPROACHES USING INTERLEUKIN-2 ALONE

Interleukin-2 Administered as a High-Dose Intravenous Bolus

The high-dose i.v. bolus IL-2 regimen was developed at the NCI Surgery Branch in the mid-1980s. Its development was based on murine experiments indicating that intraperitoneal administration of IL-2 could induce regression of established pulmonary and hepatic metastases from a variety of tumors, including the B16 melanoma (19–23). These studies showed that the tumor response to IL-2 was dose-dependent and was enhanced when the daily dosage of IL-2 was divided over three daily doses, or when IL-2 was combined with syngeneic lymphokine-activated killer (LAK) cells. Early clinical trials performed with natural and recombinant human IL-2 at the NCI Surgery Branch established toxicity and management guidelines and a maximum tolerated dose for the high-dose bolus regimen, administered either alone or in combination with autologous LAK cells (24–26). In this regimen, IL-2 (Cetus or Chiron) was administered at 600,000 to 720,000 IU per kg intravenously every 8 hours days 1 to 5 and 15 to 19 of a treatment course. A maximum of 28 to 30 IL-2 doses per course was administered; doses were frequently withheld for excessive toxicity, however. Treatment courses were repeated at 8- to 12-week intervals in responding patients. This IL-2 regimen, administered either alone or in combination with LAK cells, produced overall tumor responses in 15% to 20% of patients with metastatic melanoma in clinical trials conducted at the NCI Surgery Branch or within the Cytokine Working Group (CWG) (formerly the Extramural IL-2 and LAK Working Group). CRs were noted in 4% to 6% of patients and were frequently durable (27–30). Even though studies in animal models indicated that antitumor activity was optimal when IL-2 was combined with LAK cells, randomized and sequential clinical trials comparing IL-2 plus LAK with high-dose IL-2 alone failed to show a sufficient benefit for the addition of LAK cells to justify their continued use (31–33). Studies involving IL-2 and cellular therapy (adoptive immunotherapy) are described in detail in Chapter 13.1.

Long-term follow-up data on metastatic melanoma patients treated in early high-dose bolus IL-2 trials is now available. This data, which comes from several sources, confirms that IL-2 produces significant clinical benefits for a minority of patients. Atkins and colleagues reported a retrospective analysis of 270 patients treated on all eight trials involving high-dose bolus IL-2 conducted between 1985 and 1993 (34). Data was analyzed through fall 1996 (median follow-up, 62 months; range, 3 to 11 years). Although this population was highly selected for excellent organ function and absence of central nervous system (CNS) metastases or significant comorbidities, it included a large percentage of individuals with poor prognostic features, such as visceral metastases, multiple metastatic sites, previous systemic therapy, or a combination of these. Objective responses were seen in 43 patients (16%) [95% confidence interval (CI): 12% to 21%], including 17 CRs (6%) and 26 partial responses

TABLE 1. HIGH-DOSE INTRAVENOUS BOLUS INTERLEUKIN-2 ALONE THERAPY

Author (Reference)	Dose	Patients (No. Evaluable)	Response		Total (%)	Comments
			CR	PR		
Atkins et al. (34)	IL-2 (Chiron), 600,000–720,000 IU/kg i.v. every 8 h, d 1–5 and 15–19	270	17 (6%)	26 (10%)	43/270 (16)	5 patients received IL-2, 360,000–540,000 IU/kg
Rosenberg (37)	IL-2 (Chiron), 720,000 IU/kg i.v. every 8 h, d 1–5 and 15–19	Total (182)	12 (7%)	15 (8%)	27/182 (15)	
		Unique (35)	2 (6%)	2 (6%)	4/35 (11)	147 patients were also included in reference (34)
Total		305	19 (6%)	28 (9%)	47/305 (15)	

CR, complete response; IL-2, interleukin-2; PR, partial response.

(PRs) (10%) (Table 1). Responses occurred in all disease sites, including lung, liver, lymph nodes, soft tissue, adrenal, bone, and subcutaneous nodules and in patients with large tumor burdens or bulky individual lesions (Fig. 1). The median duration of response for all responders was 8.9 months (range, 2.5 months to more than 96.0 months), with 59% of complete

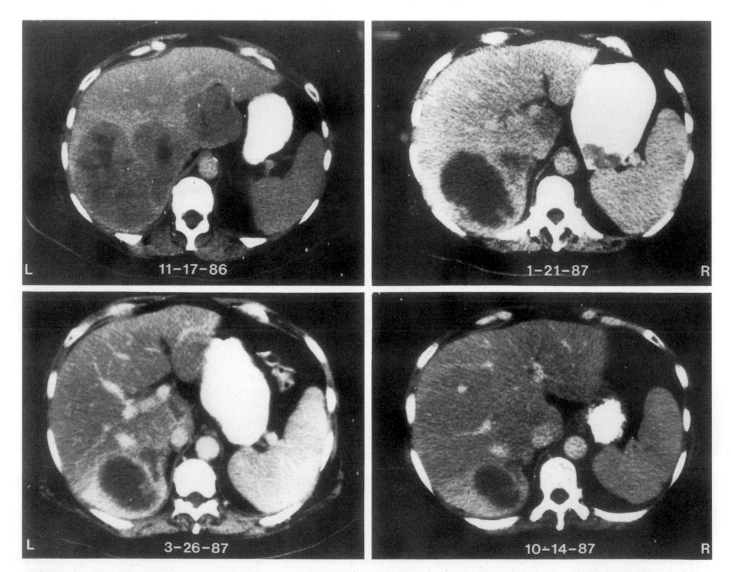

FIGURE 1. Sequential computed tomographic scans show response of large hepatic melanoma metastases to two courses of high-dose intravenous bolus interleukin-2 administered in December 1986 and February 1987. No melanoma was present on biopsy of the residual radiographic abnormality seen on the October 1997 scan. The patient developed central nervous system recurrence in 1988, ultimately leading to her death. No progression of hepatic disease was ever documented. (From Parkinson D et al. Interleukin-2 therapy in patients with metastatic malignant melanoma: a phase II study. *J Clin Oncol* 1989;7:477–485, with permission.)

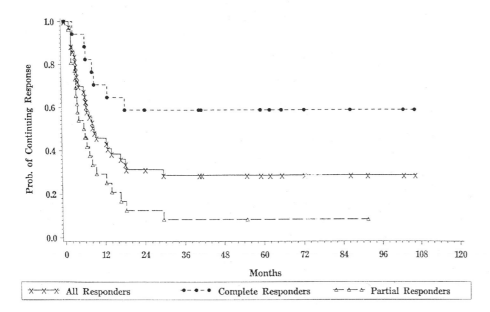

FIGURE 2. Kaplan-Meier plots of response durations for complete responses, partial responses, and all responders in U.S. Food and Drug Administration submission for high-dose interleukin-2 in melanoma. Updated November 1996. (Prob., probability.) (From Atkins MB et al. High-dose recombinant interleukin-2 therapy for patients with metastatic melanoma: analysis of 270 patients treated from 1985–1993. *J Clin Oncol* 1999;17:2105–2116, with permission.)

responders and 28% of all responders remaining long-term progression-free (Fig. 2). In addition, no patient responding longer than 30 months had progressed, suggesting that some patients actually may be "cured." Responses were less frequent in patients with baseline Eastern Cooperative Oncology Group (ECOG) performance status 1 or greater or in those patients who had received previous systemic therapy; responses were seen in equal frequency in those patients with multiple organ sites involved or visceral metastases. Fifteen responding patients had surgery or radiation therapy after IL-2 treatment; five of these remained long-term disease-free, suggesting a role for regional salvage treatment in patients who develop isolated site relapse after a response to IL-2 therapy. Forty-two patients (15.5%) were alive at last contact; the median Kaplan-Meier survival curve for the entire treated population was 11.4 months (Fig. 3). Twenty of the responding patients (47%) remained

alive; 15 had survived longer than 5 years. Toxicity was typical for high-dose bolus IL-2 regimens and was largely reversible (see Chapter 3.1). Six deaths (2.2%) all were related to infection (35). No treatment-related deaths occurred in the 88 patients treated after 1991, the period when antibiotic prophylaxis became a routine component of the treatment protocol. These encouraging results led to FDA approval of this high-dose IL-2 regimen for patients with metastatic melanoma.

Follow-up data on this population was collected through December 1998 (36). Eighteen responding patients remained alive; 13 were continually disease- or progression-free.

Rosenberg et al. reported long-term follow-up data on 409 patients (182 with metastatic melanoma, 217 with renal cell carcinoma) treated with high-dose i.v. bolus IL-2 alone at the NCI Surgery Branch (37). Patients were treated between September 1985 and November 1996. All patients received 720,000 IU of IL-2

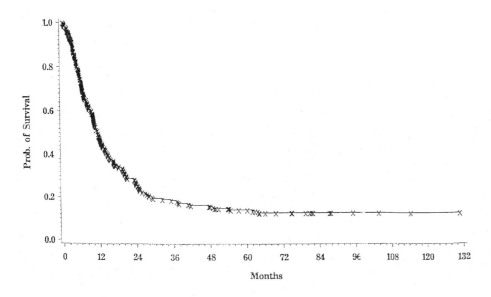

FIGURE 3. Kaplan-Meier plot of survival for the whole 270-patient population in U.S. Food and Drug Administration submission for high-dose interleukin-2 in melanoma. Updated November 1996. (Prob., probability.) (From Atkins MB et al. High-dose recombinant interleukin-2 therapy for patients with metastatic melanoma: analysis of 270 patients treated from 1985–1993. *J Clin Oncol* 1999;17:2105–2116, with permission.)

TABLE 2. ALTERNATE SCHEDULE AND LOW-DOSE INTERLEUKIN-2 ALONE REGIMENS

Author (Reference)	Dose	Patients (No. Evaluable)	Response		Total (%)
			CR	PR	
Dillman et al. (45)	18 MIU/m^2/day, c.i.v. × 5 d	188	33 (CR + PR)		33/188 (18)
Dillman et al. (46)	90 MIU/m^2 bolus + c.i.v., administered over 3 d	18	2	2	4/18 (22)
Legha et al. (47)	12 MIU/m^2/d, c.i.v. × 4 d/wk for 4 wks	31	1	6	7/31 (22)
Richards et al. (194)	3.0 MU/m^2/d (3.0–10.0)	16	0	0	0
Vlasveld et al. (50)	0.18–9 × 10^6 IU/m^2/d	13	0	1	9
Vlasveld et al. (51)	1.8 × 10^6 IU/m^2/d	15	0	0	0
Alzpodien et al. (195)	0.3 MU/m^2/d (maximum dose of 2.4 MU/m^2/d)	14	0	0	0
Hanninen et al. (196)	Variable dosing schedule	12	0	0	0
Tagliaferri et al. (197)	Pulse dose × 5 d	25	0	0	0

c.i.v., continuous intravenous infusion; CR, complete remission; IL-2, interleukin-2; PR, partial remission.

(Cetus or Chiron) every 8 hours, for a maximum of 15 doses per cycle as clinically tolerated. Some patients received polyethylene glycol (PEG)-IL-2 during the second treatment cycle; a randomized comparison showed that these patients fared no differently than those receiving high-dose bolus IL-2 alone, however (38). All but 35 of these patients were included in the 270 patient (Ref. 34) data set described above (see Table 1). Complete regression was observed in 12 of the 182 patients (6.6%) with metastatic melanoma; partial regression occurred in 15 patients (8%). Ten patients (6%) with melanoma exhibited ongoing continuous CRs from onset of treatment for 70 to more than 148 months. In this population, CRs were significantly more frequent in patients who had not received previous immunotherapy. Only 2% of previously treated patients exhibited CRs. In addition, the chance of achieving a CR was favorably associated with the amount of IL-2 administered during the first treatment course and the maximal lymphocyte count (rebound lymphocytosis) after the first cycle of IL-2.

Interleukin-2 Administered at Lower Doses or by Alternative Schedules

Due to significant toxicity associated with the high-dose i.v. bolus IL-2 regimen and the expense involved with necessary hospitalization and intensive monitoring, various investigators have attempted to establish active regimens using lower doses of IL-2. In these regimens, IL-2 is administered either by lower-dose i.v. bolus, continuous infusion, or subcutaneous injection in an effort to maintain or enhance antitumor effects while decreasing toxicity. Lower IL-2 doses also enable prolonged IL-2 treatment. Such prolonged treatment schedules were able to further expand the number and enhance the function of circulating natural killer (NK) cells (39–41). Clinical and experimental evidence demonstrated that antibody-dependent cellular cytotoxicity (ADCC) and NK/LAK cell activity were able to be increased by relatively low and considerably less toxic doses of IL-2 (39–43). However, these biologic parameters did not correlate consistently with the observed antitumor effect. The results of these treatment approaches in patients with metastatic melanoma are presented in Table 2.

The most widely used alternative IL-2 regimen was first reported in 1987 by West and colleagues (44). This treatment con-

sists of IL-2 administered at 18 MIU per m^2 per day by continuous i.v. infusion on days 1 to 5 and 11 to 15, with or without LAK cells. In their first report, this schedule of IL-2 administration together with LAK cells produced tumor responses in 5 of 10 (50%) evaluable patients with melanoma (44). Toxicity was still significant, but generally considered more predictable and manageable than with the high-dose i.v. bolus IL-2 schedule. The National Biotherapy Study Group (NBSG) studied this continuous infusion IL-2 regimen, omitting the LAK cells. Objective responses were seen in 33 of 188 patients (18%) with melanoma (45). Dillman and his colleagues in the NBSG subsequently explored an alternative schedule that combined bolus and continuous infusion IL-2. In this schedule, a total of 90 MIU per m^2 of IL-2 was administered over 3 instead of 5 days (46). Treatment was administered every 2 weeks for 2 months. Twenty-two patients with melanoma were enrolled, of whom 18 had measurable disease. Two CRs and two PRs occurred 22% overall response rate (RR); (6% to 48%; 95% CI). Additional studies of this regimen and long-term follow-up data on these initial patients have not yet been reported. Legha et al. reported their results with a treatment regimen that used a slightly lower dose IL-2 (12 MIU per m^2 per day) administered by continuous infusion for 4 days on 4 consecutive weeks (47). Out of 31 patients, they observed one CR and six PRs, for a 22% RR (10% to 41%; 95% CI). Toxicity was manageable on a general hospital ward. Responses lasted from 4 to more than 18 months. Finally, Dorval et al. investigated a regimen using a slightly higher dose of IL-2. Patients received IL-2 at 20 MIU per m^2 days 1 to 5, 15 to 18, and 29 to 31. Although significant toxicity occurred, eight responses were reported among 24 patients with metastatic melanoma (48). However, four of these responses were transient, lasting less than a month. Based on available data, the possibility exists that this continuous infusion regimen may possess antitumor activity roughly equivalent to that of high-dose bolus IL-2. The long-term follow-up experience with this regimen, however, raises concerns about the durability of these responses. In one study, only 10 of 175 patients (6%) with melanoma and 25% of the complete responders survived more than 3 years (49).

Several investigators have studied much lower doses of IL-2 that are safely administered in outpatient settings. Vlasveld and colleagues investigated a low-dose outpatient regimen in which

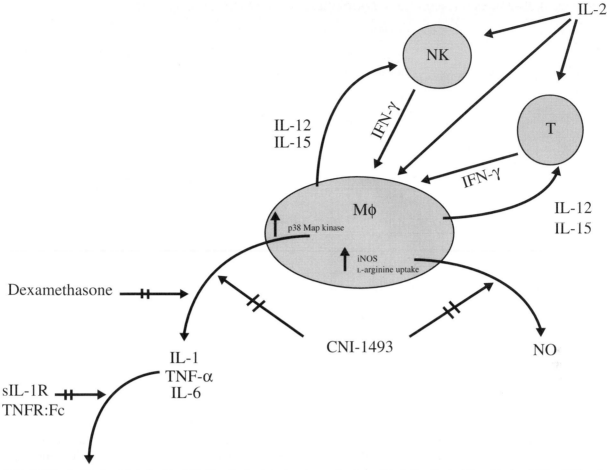

FIGURE 4. Model illustrating how interleukin-2 (IL-2) activates lymphocytes and monocytes. IL-2–activated T and natural killer (NK) cells produce interferon-γ (IFN-γ), which in turn activates monocytes leading to interleukin-12 and -15 production, further stimulating T and NK cells. Monocytes also make nitric oxide (NO) and proinflammatory cytokines, such as interleukin-1, tumor necrosis factor–α (TNF-α), and IL-6, all of which contribute to the toxicity of IL-2. Agents that block IL-1, TNF-α, and NO, such as CNI-1493, may block IL-2 toxic manifestations without interfering with T- and NK-cell activation. (iNOS, inducible nitric oxide synthase; MΦ, macrophage; sIL-1R, soluble interleukin-1 receptor; sTNFR:Fc, soluble TNF receptor Fc chimera.) (From Gollob JA, Atkins MB. Treatment of metastatic RCCA with high-dose IL-2. In: Vogelzang NJ, Scardino PT, Shipley WU, and Coffey DS, eds. *Comprehensive textbook of genitourinary oncology*, 2nd ed. Philadelphia: Lippincott Williams & Wilkins, 2000, with permission.)

IL-2 was administered at 1.8 MIU per m^2 per day by continuous infusion, 24 hours per day for 21 consecutive days (50). Although toxicity was quite manageable, no responses were observed in the 15 melanoma patients included in their phase 2 study (51). Whitehead explored a weekly bolus regimen of IL-2 in metastatic melanoma within the Southwest Oncology Group (52). This regimen produced significant short-term side effects and virtually no antitumor activity. Together, these results suggest that maximal antitumor activity likely requires dose-intensive IL-2 regimens that necessitate inpatient support. In particular, very low-dose, outpatient IL-2 regimens appear to be largely inactive in metastatic melanoma. Although no randomized comparisons with high-dose bolus IL-2 have been performed, the frequency, durability, and quality of responses to these less intensive regimens make such large-scale phase 3 trials unappealing.

Interleukin-2 Toxicity Reduction Strategies

The utility of high dose IL-2 has been limited by toxicity, many features of which resemble bacterial sepsis. Side effects

include hypotension, cardiac arrhythmias, pulmonary edema, fever, increased capillary permeability, catheter-related sepsis, and, rarely, death (34,53,54). These side effects and their management are described in more detail in Chapter 3.1. Given the limited benefits of regimens that use lower doses of IL-2 in metastatic melanoma, considerable effort has been focused on reducing the toxicity associated with high-dose IL-2 administration.

IL-2 is a potent inducer of proinflammatory cytokines, such as IL-1, tumor necrosis factor–α (TNF-α) and IFN-γ (25,55–57). These substances and others, including nitric oxide (58), likely play major roles in IL-2 toxicity. Tumor response, however, is thought to be mediated by cellular immune reactions, raising the possibility of enhancing the therapeutic index of IL-2 by dissociating its toxic effects from its antitumor effects.

A number of such toxicity dissociation approaches have been tried with limited success (Fig. 4). Most of these approaches used the high-dose i.v. bolus IL-2 schedule. The addition of dexamethasone prevented the usual induction of circulating TNF by IL-2 and was shown to significantly reduce treatment-

TABLE 3. INTERLEUKIN-2 TOXICITY REDUCTION STRATEGIES: MELANOMA RESPONSE RATE

Trial Design	Regimen		N	CR/PR	RR (%)	Author (Reference)
	IL-2[a]	Other Agent				
IL-2 + CT 1501R	High-dose bolus	1–5 mg/kg i.v., q6h	12	1/0	8	Margolin et al. (63)
IL-2 + sTNFR:FC						
Phase I	High-dose bolus	1–60 mg/m² 10 mg/m² d 1, 3, 5, 15, 17, and 19	7	2/1	43	Trehu et al. (61)
Phase III	High-dose bolus	10 mg/m², d 1 and 15 5 mg/m², d 3, 5, 17, and 19	8	1/1	25	Dubois et al. (62)
IL-2 + sIL-1R	High-dose bolus	1–55 mg/m², d 1 and 15	18	1/2	17	McDermott et al. (64)
IL-2 + CNI-1493	High-dose bolus	Escalating dose, d 1–5 and 15–19	—	—	—	In progress
Total response			**45**	**5/4**	**20**	

CR, complete response; IL-2; interleukin-2; PR, partial response; RR, response rate; sIL-1R, soluble interleukin-1 receptor; sTNFR:FC, soluble tumor necrosis factor receptor chimera.

[a]IL-2 (Chiron) 600,000 IU/kg, i.v., every 8 h, d 1–5 and 15–19.

From Atkins MB. Immunotherapy and experimental approaches for metastatic melanoma. *Hematol Oncol Clin North Am* 1998;12:877–902, with permission.

related toxicity, including fever and hypotension, allowing for a threefold increase in the maximum tolerated dose (59). Potential interference with antitumor efficacy limited this approach, however, (59,60) and highlighted the need for more selective ways of inhibiting the effects of secondary cytokines released in response to IL-2.

More recent investigations have involved the coadministration of IL-2 with soluble receptors to TNF (soluble TNF receptor: immunoglobulin Fc), IL-1 (soluble IL-1 receptor), methylxanthine-derived TNF, or IL-1 signal transduction inhibitors (pentoxifylline or CT1501R) (61–64). Several of these approaches showed significant promise in animal models and inhibited some of the biologic effects associated with high-dose IL-2 in patients, without interfering with antitumor effects. In fact, responses (five CRs and four PRs) were seen in 9 out of 45 patients (20%) with metastatic melanoma who were treated as part of these largely phase 1 trials (Table 3). However, none of these agents were able to significantly block IL-2 toxicity as measured by an ability to administer more therapy with a given toxicity or the induction of less toxicity with a given amount of therapy. These results probably indicate that multiple factors, including a variety of proinflammatory cytokines, nitric oxide, and, perhaps, direct interactions of activated lymphocytes with the vascular endothelium, are responsible for the major side effects of IL-2. If this is the case, the neutralization of just one element is unlikely to abrogate toxicity. Future exploration of this approach requires a combination of cytokine antagonists or use of novel antagonists of secondary cytokines with more pluripotent inhibitory effects.

Two potentially promising approaches involve the use of either *N*-methyl-L-arginine or CNI-1493. *N*-methyl-L-arginine is an inhibitor of nitric oxide synthase. Kilbourn and colleagues have shown that its administration is able to rapidly reverse the hypotension associated with high-dose-IL-2 in patients with metastatic renal cell carcinoma (65). Additional clinical trials of this agent in combination with IL-2 are in progress. CNI-1493 is a tetravalent guanylhydrazone compound that blocks the synthesis of proinflammatory cytokines, such as TNF and IL-1, through the inhibition of the p38

MAP kinase signaling pathway. It also has been shown to inhibit lipopolysaccharide and IFN-γ–induced nitric oxide production by blocking the upregulation of L-arginine uptake and inducible nitric oxide synthase activity (66,67). This compound is selectively taken up by monocytes; therefore, it has no effect on lymphocyte function or activation. Preclinical experiments suggest that CNI-1493 can broadly block the byproducts of macrophage activation (which may contribute significantly to the toxicity of IL-2) without interfering directly with lymphocyte activation by IL-2. In a rat hepatoma model, the use of CNI-1493 allowed administration of IL-2 at doses tenfold higher than the maximum tolerated dose and protected the animals from toxicity while enhancing the antitumor effects of IL-2 (68). These findings have formed the basis of an ongoing clinical trial of this agent in conjunction with high-dose i.v. bolus IL-2.

Potential Correlates of Response and Resistance

Various factors possibly contributing to response to IL-2 therapy are listed in Table 4. As mentioned in the first section of this chapter, in the 270-patient database presented to the FDA, tumor response was significantly associated with a baseline ECOG performance status of 0 and an absence of previous systemic therapy (34). No association of response with number of metastatic sites or amount of therapy administered was observed. In contrast, in the NCI Surgery Branch database, achievement of CR correlated with the absence of previous immunotherapy, total dose of IL-2 administered, and degree of rebound lymphocytosis after cessation of IL-2 (37). A previous analysis also found tumor response occurred more frequently in patients who developed vitiligo and whose metastases were limited to subcutaneous tissue (69). For the past 9 years, high-dose IL-2 treatment at the NCI Surgery Branch has involved much less IL-2 administration than in previous years. Patients treated after 1991 received an average of seven (rather than 13) doses of IL-2 per cycle (70). Despite a previous observation that tumor response correlated with the amount of IL-2 adminis-

TABLE 4. FACTORS ASSOCIATED WITH RESPONSE TO HIGH-DOSE INTERLEUKIN-2 (IL-2)

Factor	Author (Reference)
Pretreatment	
No prior therapy	
Any	Atkins et al. (34)
Immunotherapy	Rosenberg (37)
Performance status	Atkins et al. (34), Keilholz (72)
Subcutaneous metastases	Royal et al. (69)
Absence of visceral involvement	Tartour et al. (71)
Low serum IL-6 level	Tartour et al. (71)
Low serum CRP level	Tartour et al. (71)
Low serum LDH	Keillholz (72)
HLA-A11	Marincola et al. (76)
HLA-A19	Marincola et al. (76)
HLA-DQ1	Rubin et al. (78)
HLA- CW7	Scheibenbogen et al. (79)
HLA-A1	Scheibenbogen et al. (79)
During/post treatment	
Amount of IL-2 during first course	Royal et al. (69), Rosenberg (37)
Rebound lymphocytosis	Rosenberg (37)
Vitiligo	Rosenberg (37)
Autoimmune thyroiditis	Atkins (74)

CRP, cyclic adenosine monophosphate receptor protein; IL-6, interleukin-6; LDH, lactate dehydrogenase.

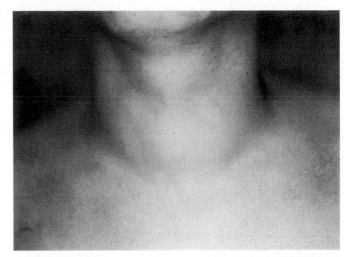

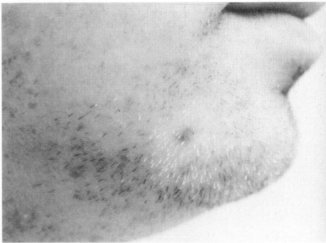

FIGURE 5. Diffuse goiter **(A)** and hypopigmentation of skin and facial hair surrounding a resolving cutaneous melanoma metastasis **(B)** in a patient exhibiting autoimmune thyroiditis and vitiligo associated with a complete response to high-dose interleukin-2 and lymphokine-activated killer cell therapy. Patient has remained in continuous complete remission since 1986. (From Atkins MB et al. Thyroid dysfunction after high-dose IL-2 therapy: an update. In: Scherbaum WA, Boqner U, Weinheimer B, Bottazzo GF, eds. *Autoimmune thyroiditis: approaches towards its etiobiological differentiation.* Berlin: Springer-Verlag, 1991;271–283, with permission.)

tered, no discernible decrement in RR has occurred for patients treated more recently.

A French multicenter analysis of 19 patients treated with IL-2 alone, 29 patients treated with IL-2 plus IFN-α, and 30 patients treated with *cis*-diaminedichloroplatinum/IL-2/IFN-α, correlated tumor response with pretreatment levels of IL-6, C-reactive protein (CRP), and lactate dehydrogenase (LDH) (71). In a multivariate analysis, serum CRP levels and diseases confined to skin, subcutaneous tissue, or lymph nodes (Mla or Mlb) were most predictive of response and survival. In another analysis of 65 patients treated with IL-2 and IFN-α, high serum LDH, poor performance status, and large tumor burdens were associated with poor responses to treatment and poor overall survival (72).

Other analyses correlated response with development of vitiligo (73) and other autoimmune phenomenon, such as thyroid dysfunction (Fig. 5) (74). Vitiligo has been the most extensively studied. Vitiligo was documented in 11 of 74 patients with melanoma who were followed for more than a year after receiving high-dose IL-2 alone (73); it was only seen in patients exhibiting objective tumor responses. None of 27 nonresponding patients with melanoma followed for a year or more developed vitiligo (*p* = .0002); likewise, vitiligo did not occur in patients receiving IL-2 for metastatic renal cell cancer. This data suggests that specific T-cell immunity may be responsible for the antitumor effects of IL-2, and that the presence of melanoma antigens are necessary to break down existing tolerance to normal host structures, such as melanocytes.

Many groups have attempted to correlate responses with specific host HLA alleles. The NCI Surgery Branch reported an association of tumor response with the HLA-A11 allele, especially in patients receiving tumor-infiltrating lymphocyte (TIL) and IL-2 therapy (75,76). HLA-A19 was also expressed more frequently among those melanoma patients responding to TIL/IL-2 (76). HLA-DR4

expression was associated with increased IL-2 toxicity (76). These associations were not as strong and convincing in later analyses that included larger numbers of patients (77). Another study correlated HLA-DQI expression with tumor response (*p* = .0017) and survival (*p* = .026) (78). Finally, Scheibenbogen et al. noted that HLA-CW7 and HLA-A1 phenotypes were more frequent in patients who responded to an IL-2 and IFN regimen (79). However, it has been difficult to confirm the contributions of these various phenotypes to antitumor response or toxicity, or to use such parameters to restrict this toxic therapy to those patients most likely to benefit.

Resistance to IL-2 therapy has been postulated to be owing to a number of factors, including tumor-induced immune suppression via the FAS/fas ligand interactions (80) or T-cell receptor dysfunction mediated via diminished zeta chain expression

TABLE 5. INTERLEUKIN-2 COMBINED WITH INTERFERON-α 2A OR 2B

Author (Reference)	Dose		IL-2 Route	Schedule (IL-2/IFN-α)	Patients (Total/ Evaluation)	Response		Total (%)
	IL-2	IFN-α				CR	PR	
IL-2 as bolus								
Rosenberg et al. (87)	1.0–4.5 MU/m^2	3–6 MU i.v.	i.v.	t.i.d.	39	3	10	33
Marincola (88)	2.6–15.6 × 10^6 IU/m^2	3–6 × 10^6 IU/m^2	i.v.	t.i.d./qd	82	6	14	24
Budd (198)	4–26% MU/m^2	10 MU i.m.	i.v.	qd	17	2	3	29
Sparano et al. (89)	4.5 mu/m^2	3.0 MU i.v.	i.v.	t.i.d./qd	41	0	4	10
Karp (90)	60,000 IU/m^2	10 MU s.q.	i.v.	t.i.d./qd	38	1	5	15
IL-2 as continuous infusion								
Lee (199)	3 × 10^6 IU/m^2	6 MU s.q.	c.i.v.	qd	15	1	2	20
Mittelman (200)	0.5–7.0 MU/m^2	6–12 MU i.m.	i.v.	qd	14	0	0	0
Keilholz et al. (91)	1 mg/m^2	10 MU/m^2 s.q.	c.i.v.	qd × 5	27	1	4	18
Kruit (94)	3 MU/m^2	6 MU s.q.	c.i.v.	pd	51	1	7	16
Oldham et al. (201)	18 MU/m^2	3 MU/m^2 s.q.	c.i.v.	qd	66	0	7	10
Whitehead et al. (95)	2 MU/m^2	6 MU/m^2 s.q.	c.i.v.	qd	14	0	0	0
Eton et al. (93)	9 MIU/m^2	5 MU/m^2/d i.m.	c.i.v.	qd	23	0	2	8
Hidalgo et al. (202)	18 × 10^6 IU/m^2	3 × 10^6 IU/m^2 s.q.	c.i.v.	5 d/wk × 2wk	22	CR + PR = 3		13.3
IL-2 as subcutaneous injection								
Castello et al. (96)	6 MIU/m^2	3 MIU i.m.	s.q.	qd	15	0	0	0
Hidalgo et al. (202)	4.8 × 10^6 IU/m^2	3 × 10^6 IU/m^2 s.q.	s.q.	5 d/wk × 3 wk	24		3	12.5
Gause et al. (203)	1.5 or 3 × 10^6 MU/m^2	1.5 or 3 × 10^6 MU/ m^2 s.q.	s.q.	Daily × 4 wk	12[a]	0	0	0

c.i.v., continuous intravenous infusion; CR, complete response; IFN-α, interferon-α; IL-2, interleukin-2; PR, partial response.
[a]Total of 53 patients with metastatic malignancy, of which only melanoma is shown.

(81). Of note, Rabinowich et al. have shown that these T-cell receptor abnormalities can be reversed by IL-2 immunotherapy and that such reversal may correlate with tumor response (82). Additional correlative laboratory studies performed in conjunction with current and future clinical trials are necessary to sort out the significance of these various molecular phenomena to the antitumor effects of IL-2.

INTERLEUKIN-2 IN COMBINATION WITH OTHER BIOLOGIC RESPONSE MODIFIERS

Interleukin-2 in Combination with Interferon-α

Preclinical laboratory and animal studies provide a strong rationale for clinical investigations involving the combination of IL-2 with IFN-α (83–86). In 1989, Rosenberg and colleagues reported promising results from a dose-escalation phase 1/2 trial using high-dose i.v. bolus IL-2 and i.v. IFN-α, both supplied by Hoffman LaRoche (87). They examined IFN α at 3 6 MU per m^2 and IL-2 at 2.6–12.0 MIU per m^2 per dose, each administered every 8 hours on days 1 to 5 and 15 to 19. Of 91 evaluable patients, 39 had metastatic melanoma. Tumor responses were seen in 25 patients (seven CRs, 18 PRs), including 13 patients with metastatic melanoma (three CRs, ten PRs). The RR was as high as 41% among the 27 patients treated at the highest doses of IL-2 (12 MIU/m^2) and IFN-α (6 MU). Toxicity was similar to that seen with regimens of high-dose IL-2 alone; a higher than anticipated incidence of cardiac and neurologic toxicity was observed, however. In 1995, Marincola and colleagues pub-

lished a long-term follow-up of the NCI Surgery Branch experience using the combination of IL-2 and IFN-α. They reported on 189 patients, of whom 82 had melanoma (88). The overall RR was 25% (43/189) and the RR in patients with melanoma was 24% (20/82). Only one patient treated for melanoma was a long-term progression-free survivor, however. They concluded that this combined regimen provided no obvious benefit relative to high-dose bolus IL-2 alone.

The CWG performed a randomized phase 3 comparison of i.v. bolus IL-2 with or without IFN-α. IL-2 was administered either alone at 6 MU per m^2 per dose (16 MIU/m^2) or at 4.5 MU per m^2 per dose (12.6 MIU/m^2) in combination with IFN-α at 3 MU per m^2 per dose (89). As with the NCI Surgery Branch study, both the IL-2 and IFN-α were supplied by Hoffmann-LaRoche. The toxicities of these regimens were essentially equivalent and resembled that of high-dose bolus IL-2 alone. Eighty-five patients were enrolled, with 44 patients randomized to IL-2 alone and 41 to IL-2 plus IFN-α, respectively. Responses were seen in only six patients, two of whom (5%) received IL-2 alone and four of whom (10%) received both IL-2 and IFN-α. No complete responses occurred on either arm. The study was terminated early due to disappointing results on both arms and the low likelihood that the addition of IFN-α would result in a meaningful improvement over standard regimens involving IL-2 alone.

Other investigations involving combinations of IL-2 and IFN-α are listed in Table 5. Karp combined thrice weekly IFN-α with low-dose IL-2 (60,000 IU/kg) administered as an i.v. bolus injection every 8 hours for up to 14 doses on days 1 to 5

TABLE 6. INTERLEUKIN-2 WITH OTHER IMMUNE ACTIVATING AGENTS

Author (Reference)	IL-2		Other Agent	Response			
	Dose	Route		Melanoma	CR	PR	Percentage
Viens et al. (98)	8×10^6 IU/m^2	i.v. q8h	IFN-γ (1×10^6 IU/m^2 escalating doses)	11	1	1	8
Thatcher et al. (108)	11×10^6 U/m2	i.v. qod[a]	FAA (4.8 gm/m^2)	34	1	4	15
O'Reilly et al. (109)	$6{-}18 \times 10^6$/m^2/day	c.i.v.	FAA (4.8 gm/m^2)	21	1	2	14
Kim et al. (97)	720,000 IU/kg	i.v. q8h	IFN-γ (in 20 patients);	20	1	1	10
			IFN-γ + TIL (in five patients)	5	0	0	
Ahmed et al. (106)[b]	3×10^6 IU/m^2/day	s.q.	Levamisole 50 t.i.d.	18	—	1	11.8
	5.4×10^6 IU/m^2/day, escalating doses	s.q.	Levamisole 50 t.i.d.	21	—	1	11.8
Olenki et al. (100)	3, 12, 48×10^6 IU/m^2	i.v., $3 \times$ wk	IL-4, 40, 120, 400 (μg/m^2)	39	0	2	5
Creagan et al. (103)	3×10^6 IU/m^2/d	s.q.	Levamisole, 50/m^2, t.i.d. p.o.	19	0	0	0
Hellerstrand et al. (110)[c]	18 MIU/m^2/d	c.i.v.	IFN-α 2a	7	0	1	14
			±	9	2	2	45
	2.4 MIU/m^2/b.i.d.	s.q.	Histamine	11	1	3	36

c.i.v., continuous intravenous infusion; IFN-α, interferon-α; IFN-γ, interferon-γ; IL-2, interleukin-2; IL-4; interleukin-4; FAA, folic acid antagonist; TIL, tumor-infiltrating lymphocyte.
[a]Patients initially received intrasplenic local IL-2 therapy followed by i.v. infusion.
[b]Two sequential randomized dose escalation studies of subcutaneous IL-2, with and without levamisole.
[c]Randomized study with IL-2 and IFN-α, with or without histamine; last two rows represent patients receiving IL-2, IFN-α 2, and histamine.

and 15 to 19 (90). He observed six responses (one CR and five PRs) among 38 evaluable patients (15% RR: 4% to 27%, 95% CI). Three of the six responses endured over 12 months, with two responses ongoing more than 26 and 40 months.

Keilholz and his colleagues explored two alternative regimens. Patients either received IFN-α 10 MU per m^2 per day subcutaneously for 5 days, followed by IL-2 (18 MIU/m^2/day) administered by continuous infusion for 5 days, or the same schedule of IFN-α followed by a decrescendo schedule of IL-2. This decrescendo schedule required IL-2 to be administered at 18 MIU per m^2 over 6 hours, followed by 18 MIU per m^2 over 12 hours, 18 MIU per m^2 over 24 hours, and, finally, a maintenance dose of 4.5 MIU per m^2 per day for 72 hours (92). This decrescendo regimen was designed to induce optimal IL-2 receptor expression and minimize toxicity by avoiding the induction of high circulating levels of secondary cytokines. The continuous-infusion IL-2 schedule produced five responses in 27 patients (one CR and four PRs; 18% RR; 6% to 36%; 95% CI), whereas the decrescendo IL-2 schedule yielded 11 responses, also in 27 patients (three CRs, eight PRs; 41% RR; 22% to 61%; 95% CI). The decrescendo IL-2 and IFN-α regimen produced tumor responses in 22% of patients whose disease had progressed after (dimethyltriazeno)imidazole carboxamide (DTIC) chemotherapy, and had an impressive 17-month median survival (91). In addition to encouraging antitumor activity, this regimen had a more favorable toxicity profile than the more conventional schedule. This decrescendo IL-2 and IFN-α schedule has been compared to the same schedule plus cisplatin in a large-scale phase 3 randomized trial conducted within the European Organization for Research on Treatment of Cancer (EORTC) (92). Sixty-six eligible patients were randomized to the IL-2/IFN-α arm, with responses observed in 18% of patients (four CRs and eight PRs). Although the RR was less than that seen with the cisplatin IL-2/IFN-α combination arm, overall and progression-free survival were equivalent (see Interleukin-2–Based Biochemotherapy).

Investigators at the M. D. Anderson Cancer Center added IFN-α to their continuous infusion IL-2 regimen. They observed only two PRs out of 23 patients (8% RR; 1% to 28%; 95% CI) (93). Kruit and his colleagues enrolled 57 patients with melanoma in a phase 2 multicenter Netherlands-based trial of IL-2 at 7.8 MIU per m^2 per day (HLR) by continuous infusion, and IFN-α at 6 MU, administered subcutaneously on days 1 to 4 every 2 weeks. Responses were seen in 16% of the 51 evaluable patients (eight responses; one CR, seven PRs) (94). Whitehead et al. explored a similar regimen, 2 MU per m^2 per day of IL-2 (HLR) plus IFN-α, with no responses occurring in 14 melanoma patients (95). Castello and colleagues also demonstrated no responses among 15 patients with melanoma who were treated with a similar regimen (except IL-2 was administered as a subcutaneous injection) (96).

Despite promising preclinical investigations and encouraging clinical results from a few regimens, there is no convincing evidence supporting the benefit of the IL-2 and IFN-α combination over high-dose IL-2 alone. Nonetheless, because some IL-2 and IFN-α combinations have produced tumor responses at doses of IL-2 that are inactive when used alone, this combination has served as a building block for clinical trials in which other biologic agents or cytotoxic chemotherapies have been added.

Interleukin-2 in Combination with Other Immune-Activating Agents

IL-2 is an attractive agent to combine with other cytokines or immunomodulatory molecules. Its multiple immunomodulatory properties create many opportunities for potential additive or synergistic antitumor effects. A variety of clinical trials with such combinations have been performed (Table 6).

A few trials have examined combinations of IFN-γ and IL-2. IFN γ is a cytokine with potent immune-enhancing activ-

TABLE 7. INTERLEUKIN-2 COMBINED WITH MONOCLONAL ANTIBODIES

Author (Reference)	IL-2 Dose	Monoclonal Lab	Other Agents	No. of Patients	Response CR	PR	Percentage
Barjorin et al. (128)	Cetus, 5 MIU/m^2, c.i.v.	Anti-GD3-R24[a]		20	0	1	5
Soiffer et al. (129)	Amgen (Thousand Oaks, CA), 4.5 × 10^5 U/m^2/d	Anti-GD3-R24		28	0	1	4
Nasi et al. (204)	0.5 MU/m^2/d	Anti-GD3-R24		12[d]	0	0	0
	1.0 MU/m/d			9[d]	0	0	
Alpaugh et al. (130)	3 MIU/d, s.q.	Anti-GD3-R24	IFN-α 2a	21	0	0	0
Sosman et al. (134)	0.45–1.3mg/m^2/8 h						
	Cetus, escalating dose	Anti-CD3 Ab[b]		16	0	1	6
Hank et al. (135)	3 × 10^6 U/m^2 HLR, c.i.v.	Anti-CD3 Ab	Pentoxifylline (for four patients)	15[e]	0	0	0
Albertini et al. (132)	1.5x10^6 IU/m^2, c.i.v.	CH 14.18 Ab[c]		24	1	1	4

Cetus, IL-2 from Cetus-Oncology Division of Chiron Corporation; c.i.v., continuous intravenous infusion; HLR, Hoffman-LaRoche Units; IFN-α, interferon-α; IL-2, interleukin-2.
[a]Anti-GD3-R24 monoclonal antibody.
[b]Anti-CD3 monoclonal antibody.
[c]Anti–CH 14.18 chimeric monoclonal antibody.
[d]Both groups of patients received IL-2 for 7 wk.
[e]Number of patients with metastatic melanoma: 15 out of 29.

ity. It induces macrophage and granulocyte activation, enhancement of major histocompatibility complex (MHC) class I and II, expression and tumor antigen expression. The NCI Surgery Branch studied IFN-γ administration before standard high-dose i.v. bolus IL-2 (97). Some of these patients also received TIL cells. Only 2 of 20 patients exhibited tumor responses; none of the five patients receiving IFN-γ, IL-2, and TIL responded. Other phase 1 trials combined IFN-γ with lower dose, more protracted IL-2 administration schedules but did not produce definitive clinical antitumor activity in any patients with melanoma (98,99).

Several investigators have explored IL-2 in combination with IL-4 (100,101). One rationale for this combination was enhancing tumor-specific T-cell responses and nonspecific NK/LAK cell-mediated cytotoxicities. These studies have been disappointing, however, with few tumor responses and minimal enhancement of IL-2 immunomodulatory effects observed. Although IL-4 continues to be of interest as a potential *ex vivo* dendritic cell (DC) growth factor in combination with granulocyte-macrophage colony-stimulating factor (102), combinations with IL-2 have not been pursued further.

Creagan and his colleagues at the Mayo Clinic investigated the combination of IL-2 and levamisole, an antiparasitic agent purported to have immunostimulatory properties (103). Levamisole has shown some potential benefit as an adjuvant to surgical resection in patients with high-risk melanoma (104,105). Creagan performed a phase 2 trial of subcutaneous IL-2 and levamisole that demonstrated no objective responses in 19 patients with melanoma (103). Ahmed and his colleagues at the Royal Marsden Hospital explored a combination of IL-2 at 3 and 5.4 MIU per m^2 per day, subcutaneously, with or without levamisole (106). Responses were seen only in patients receiving IL-2 alone.

Flavone-8-acetic acid (FAA) potentially enhances NK cell activity and synergizes with IL-2 in animal tumor models (107). Thatcher and colleagues performed a phase 2 trial of IL-2 combined with FAA in patients with metastatic melanoma (108).

IL-2 was first administered intrasplenically via femoral catheter, then by i.v. bolus on alternate days; FAA was administered intravenously as a 6-hour infusion before the IL-2. Five responses occurred in 34 patients, including one CR. Responses occurred mainly in nonvisceral sites. Thatcher et al. thought that this RR was not significantly better than that of IL-2 alone. O'Reilly explored FAA combined with continuous infusion IL-2, observing three responses (one CR, two PRs) in 21 patients (overall RR of 14%) (109).

Interest has been generated in the combination of IL-2 with histamine (110). Histamine, a biogenic amine, can inhibit monocyte-derived oxygen–free radical formation. Some investigators believe that monocyte free radical formation inhibits T-cell and NK-cell tumoricidal activity. Randomized trials are currently exploring the value of adding histamine to IL-2 in patients with metastatic melanoma or acute leukemia. One must conclude from the evidence above that no convincing information currently exists that any immunologic agent can add to the antitumor activity of IL-2 alone in metastatic melanoma.

Interleukin-2 and Monoclonal Antibodies

A variety of rationales have been proposed for combining IL-2 with monoclonal antibodies (MAbs) in the treatment of melanoma. Antibodies can bind to relatively unique tumor antigens, making the tumor cells more receptive to clearance by activated immune cells and IL-2 has been shown to enhance such antibody-dependent clearance (ADCC) (42,43,111–114). Alternatively, antibodies may be directed at molecules on the surfaces of host effector cells (e.g., CD3, CD2, CD16), which may activate them or make effector cell populations more receptive to IL-2–mediated expansion, or both (115–118). Furthermore, biotechnology advances have facilitated the creation of bispecific monoclonal antibodies that are capable of binding to effector and tumor cells and antibody:cytokine conjugates. These constructs may facilitate delivery of effector cells or cytokines to tumor cell surfaces (119,120). Clinical trials involving IL-2 and MAbs are displayed in Table 7.

The largest amount of clinical research activity has focused on ganglioside-specific MAbs. Gangliosides are glycolipid molecules composed of oligosaccharide chains linked to ceramide fatty acid cores. Melanoma cells are rich in gangliosides, two of which, GD2 and GD3, appear to be upregulated by the transformation of melanocytes (121,122). Ganglioside structures, which can trigger T-cell activation when bound, are also present on the surface of certain T cells (115). Phase 1 clinical trials of unconjugated ganglioside-specific monoclonal antibodies have shown they can reach tumor sites after systemic administration. Some tumor responses have been observed with R24 (anti-GD3), 3F8 (anti-GD2), and other murine MAbs (122–127).

The anti-GD3 ganglioside antibody, R24, has been the MAb most actively investigated in combination with IL-2. The initial study was performed by Bajorin and colleagues at the Memorial Sloan-Kettering Cancer Center (128). In this study, IL-2 was administered at 6 MIU per m^2, intravenously, over 6 hours on days 1 to 5 and 8 to 12, whereas R24 was given at one of four dose levels between 1 and 12 mg per m^2 daily on days 8 to 12. T-cell activation and the magnitude of the rebound lymphocytosis seemed to correlate with R24 dose level. Of the 20 treated patients, there was one PR and two minor responses. Human antimouse antibody (HAMA) formation was noted to occur surprisingly early—in less than 7 days—in some patients. In a study by Soiffer et al., R24 MAb was combined with very low dose, continuous-infusion IL-2 (129). IL-2 was administered for the entire 8-week period; R24 was administered during weeks 5 and 6. Twenty-eight patients with metastatic melanoma were enrolled, with only one PR (regression of liver metastases from an ocular primary melanoma) observed. Alpaugh et al. reported the results of a phase 1b trial that used a 5-day continuous infusion of R24 followed by 3 weeks of subcutaneous IL-2 and IFN-α (130). Twenty melanoma patients were enrolled. Tumor biopsies obtained on days 8 (before the initiation of IL-2 and IFN-α) and 29 showed chronic inflammation relative to pretreatment samples; it is difficult to determine to what extent the R24 may have contributed to this inflammatory reaction, however. In any event, no objective responses were seen in the 18 evaluable patients.

In an effort to avoid HAMA responses and potentiate ADCC, Albertini and his colleagues at the University of Wisconsin performed a phase 1 clinical trial using continuous-infusion IL-2 and the chimeric anti-GD2 ganglioside antibody 14.18 (131). This chimeric human/mouse antibody combines the antigen-binding Fab fragment of mouse 3F8 MAb with the heavy and light chains of a human immunoglobulin molecule. The combination of the chimeric 14.18 antibody and IL-2 led to enhanced ADCC and LAK activity and reduced human antichimera antibody (HACA) formation. Antitumor activity was observed in 2 of 24 patients (one CR, one PR). One case of peripheral neuropathy was observed; nerve pain was the dose-limiting toxicity. Concomitant laboratory evaluations suggested that the addition of IL-2 to the 14.18 antibody might have suppressed antiidiotypic antibody formation (132).

Although some tumor responses have been observed with combinations of IL-2 and antibodies directed against gangliosides, the limited antitumor activity seen with this approach

does not justify further clinical investigation of this strategy in patients with metastatic melanoma. Either more potent MAbs or additional information on how to optimally combine MAbs with IL-2 are necessary for this approach to be pursued further.

The use of IL-2 in combination with MAbs directed against T-cell antigens also has been explored. Preclinical studies support the concept that anti-CD3 MAb administered at low doses can activate T cells to release cytokines, proliferate, and mediate antitumor effects (116–118,133). Sosman and colleagues explored doses of anti-CD3 antibody OKT3 from 10 mg to 600 mg, followed by low-dose i.v. infusion of IL-2, subcutaneous IL-2, or high-dose bolus IL-2 (134–137). However, these trials failed to demonstrate that activated T cells (those expressing CD25, the high-affinity IL-2 receptor) could be expanded *in vivo*. Furthermore, when OKT3 was combined with high-dose IL-2, only one objective response was observed in 16 patients with melanoma (137). Although this approach has been disappointing, it is possible that this strategy may produce better results if bispecific MAbs or fusion antibodies that are able to activate effector cells directly at tumor cell surfaces can be developed.

In an effort to enhance ADCC at the tumor site, Gillies et al. linked IL-2 to the carboxy-terminus of the ch14.18 molecule (138). This fusion protein binds to GD2-expressing tumor cells *in vitro* as avidly as the native ch14.18 antibody, mediating ADCC against GD2-expressing melanoma cells by stimulating both cytotoxic T cells and NK cells that express IL-2 receptors, regardless of whether they express Fc receptors. Animal models using this fusion protein show it to be superior to IL-2 or ch14.18 alone (or both combined at comparable doses) (119,139,140). Phase 1 trials of this fusion protein in melanoma patients have recently been initiated.

Interleukin-2 and Tumor Vaccines

It has long been evident that melanomas possess tumor antigens that can be recognized by the host immune system (141); consequently, vaccination therapy with a variety of crude melanoma cell preparations has been pursued since the 1970s. Whereas some of these approaches appear promising, their beneficial effects have yet to be confirmed in phase 3 trials (141–147). Efforts to develop an effective vaccine have been hindered by a combination of poor immunogenicity of relevant antigens, tumor-reinforced tolerance, antigen shedding, and tumor heterogeneity. Nonetheless, any successful induction of T-cell immunity to a tumor through vaccination could be enhanced, theoretically, by subsequent IL-2 administration. As a consequence, several investigators have examined their vaccines in combination with IL-2 (Table 8).

Adler and colleagues have investigated an allogeneic liposomal melanoma vaccine with or without systemic or regional low-dose IL-2 administration (148). Nine of 24 patients with melanoma experienced objective responses, including six responses (three CRs, three PRs) in the ten patients who received the vaccine plus low-dose regional IL-2. However, follow-up reports or confirmatory studies on these results have not been forthcoming. Oratz and colleagues encapsulated their polyvalent shed-melanoma-antigen vaccine into liposomes combined with IL-2 in an effort to increase its

TABLE 8. INTERLEUKIN-2 COMBINED WITH VACCINES

Author (Reference)	IL-2			Type of Vaccine	No. of Doses	Additional Therapy	N	Response		Total Response (%)
	Dose	Route	Schedule					CR	PR	
Adler et al. (148)	Variable	i.v. bolus or regional	Every 8 h	Allogeneic liposomal melanoma vaccine	s.q. injection at two sites, every wk for 10 wk	Cimetidine, 800 mg, p.o. b.i.d., × 4 wk	24[a]	3	6	50
Oratz et al. (149)	0–5 × 105 IU	Liposome-encapsulated IL-2		Polyvalent melanoma vaccine encapsulated in IL-2 containing liposomes	i.d., q2wk × 4 and monthly × 3	None	8[b]	1	1	25
Rosenberg et al. (161)	720,000 U/kg	i.v. bolus	q8h × 5 d for 2 cycles	Modified peptide vaccine gp100:209-2M	1.0 mg, s.q. into thigh; two to six immunizations at 3-wk intervals	None	31	1	12	42

CR, complete remission; IL-2, interleukin-2; PR, partial response.
[a]Study included four arms, of which responses were seen only in the IL-2 + vaccine arms.
[b]Only 8 out of 36 patients studied had measurable disease.

immunogenicity (149). Thirty-six patients with stage IV melanoma received this combination vaccine, followed by daily low-dose IL-2 injections ($2–5 \times 10^5$ IU) for 2 weeks. The addition of IL-2 was perceived to induce a marked increase in frequency and duration of vaccine-induced delayed-type hypersensitivity responses relative to historical controls who received the vaccine alone (149). Of 28 patients whose metastatic disease had been completely resected at entry, 12 have been followed up for 2 years, nine of whom (75%) remained alive, compared to only 15% to 30% of "matched" historical controls. Two tumor responses (one CR, one PR) were observed in the eight patients with measurable disease. Longer follow-up and randomized controlled studies are necessary to determine the true value of this combination.

With advances in molecular biology and better understandings of immune recognition, efforts have shifted toward the study of defined-antigen vaccines. A number of melanoma-specific proteins that represent targets for cytotoxic, tumor-specific T cells have been cloned and characterized (150–152). The protein antigens and peptides include embryonic proteins (MAGE family), as well as tissue-restricted (melanocyte) proteins such as tyrosinase, MART-1, and gp100 (153–159). Rosenberg and colleagues investigated the immunologic and clinical effects of an 9–amino-acid peptide from the gp100 protein (residues 209–217) and a mutated version of this peptide (gp100 peptide 209-2M), which binds HLA-A2.1 more effectively in combination with incomplete Freund's adjuvant (160). Rosenberg also studied the mutant gp100:209-2M peptide in combination with high-dose IL-2 (161). Whereas the mutated peptide (gp100:209-2M) alone was quite effective in inducing specific T-cell responses (10 of 11 patients), few antitumor effects were observed. In contrast, 13 of 31 patients (42%) who received the peptide together with high-dose IL-2 experienced objective tumor responses. A confirmatory trial of this combination is currently under way within the CWG, and a phase 3 trial randomizing patients to either high-dose IL-2 alone or in combination with the gp100:209-2M peptide is contemplated.

Efforts to define additional peptide antigens and antigen-presenting strategies may yield more potent and broad-spectrum vaccines to be tested in combination with IL-2. Mulé diacritical and colleagues, for example, have demonstrated in animal models that low-dose IL-2 can enhance the antitumor effects of DC-based vaccines that utilize tumor lysates as sources of tumor antigens (102). These effects provide a rationale for combining IL-2 with DC-based vaccine approaches in melanoma.

INTERLEUKIN-2–BASED BIOCHEMOTHERAPY

Many investigators have studied the effects of combinations of IL-2–based immunotherapy and cytotoxic chemotherapy on melanoma. IL-2 plus DTIC combinations have produced considerable toxicity while yielding RRs of only 13% to 33% (4,20,162,163). More encouraging results have been observed with studies that combine cisplatin-based chemotherapy with high-dose IL-2 alone or lower doses of IL-2 combined with IFN-α (164–169). Composite results from a variety of inpatient regimens show a RR of approximately 50%, with 10% to 20% CR (Fig. 6) and a median survival of approximately 11 to 12 months (Table 9). PRs were frequently of short duration (median, 4 to 6 months in most studies) and were not associated with prolonged survival. In some studies, up to 60% of patients who obtained CRs remained long-term progression-free (169). Overall, approximately 10% of all patients appear to be disease-free for more than 2 years (4). As with high-dose IL-2 alone regimens, relapses beyond 2 years are extremely uncommon (169). In contrast to chemotherapy or immunotherapy alone, responses were seen in all disease sites with equal frequencies and no clear dose–response relationship for IL-2 was apparent. Although some investigators reported partial regressions of preexisting small CNS metastases (164,170), most trials excluded such patients, and the CNS was actually a common

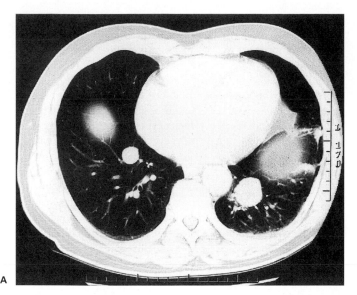 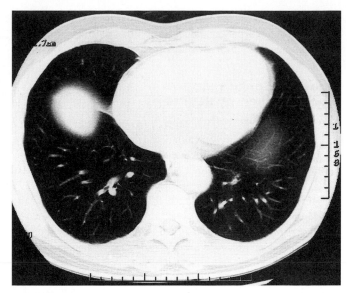

A

B

FIGURE 6. A, B: Serial chest computed tomographic scans documenting complete regression of pulmonary metastases in a patient after treatment with interleukin-2 and cisplatin-based biochemotherapy.

site of initial relapse (167). Responses were seen in patients with previous chemotherapy (168), and appeared to be associated with the frequent development of vitiligo (164). Cisplatin appeared to be required for synergy (168), and activity appeared greatest when chemotherapy was administered first (165). Early studies documented that cytotoxic chemotherapy did not interfere with ongoing responses to immunotherapy, enabling closer integration of these two modalities (166). The apparent higher RR and 10% durable, unmaintained CR rate suggests that these combination regimens may be superior to either chemotherapy or immunotherapy alone, and that synergistic interactions between the IL-2 and cisplatin-based chemotherapy may contribute to these improved results. Furthermore, two compilations of data from large numbers of patients seem to indicate

that biochemotherapy produces RRs superior to those of chemotherapy or immunotherapy alone. Keilholz et al. collected data on 631 patients treated with IL-2 alone or in combination with IFN-α or cytotoxic drugs (171). In this analysis, patients receiving IL-2, IFN-α, and chemotherapy experienced an RR of 44.8%, compared with RRs of 20.8% and 14.9%, respectively, for IL-2 and IFN-α and IL-2 alone. Median survival, however, was not significantly improved. Allen et al. performed a metaanalysis of 168 published trials involving 7,711 patients with metastatic melanoma treated with either chemotherapy, IL-2–based immunotherapy, or biochemotherapy (172). Once again, patients treated with a combination of IL-2, IFN-α, and cytotoxic chemotherapy experienced a significantly greater RR (p <.0001). However, these early biochemotherapy regimens

TABLE 9. PHASE 2 INPATIENT INTERLEUKIN-2/CISPLATIN–BASED BIOCHEMOTHERAPY TRIALS

Author (Reference)	Regimen/Dose	Evaluation	Response CR (%)	Response PR (%)	Total (%)	Comments
Antoine et al. (168)	C/IL-2 IFN ± tamoxifen	127	13 (10)	49 (39)	49	80% of patients had prior chemotherapy; tamoxifen-increased toxicity without increasing response
Legha et al. (165), Legha et al. (169)	Alternating CVD/bio	39	2 (5)	11 (28)	33	Sequential better than alternating; CVD first better than bio first; only CRs had prolonged survival
	Sequential bio/CVD	30	3 (10)	12 (40)	50	
	Sequential CVD/bio	31	10 (32)	11 (35)	68	
Richards (164)	CBDT/IL-2/IFN	83	12 (14)	34 (41)	55	Vitiligo seen in responders; some patients had brain metastases
Demchak et al. (166),	IL-2 (bolus)/C/Amifostine	27	3 (11)	7 (26)	37	Responses to IL-2 continued during C; much toxicity from HD bolus IL-2 and high-dose C
Atkins et al. (167)	C/DTIC/tam/IL-2 (bolus)[a]	38	3 (8)	13 (34)	42	
Total		375	46 (12)	137 (36)	48	Median response durations, 5–7 mo; median survivals, 10–12 mo

bio, continuous intravenous infusion interleukin-2 + subcutaneous interferon; C, cisplatin; CBDT, cisplatin, carmustine, dacarbazine, tamoxifen; CR, complete response; CVD, cisplatin, vinblastine, dacarbazine; DTIC, dacarbazine; HD, high dose; IFN-α, interferon-α; IL-2, interleukin-2; PR, partial response; tam, tamoxifen.
[a]Multicenter trial.

(see Table 9) involved extensive inpatient treatment and substantial toxicity, expense, and patient time commitments, making widespread use or phase 3 investigation impractical.

Inpatient Concurrent Biochemotherapy Regimens

Several investigators have endeavored to enhance the practicality and tolerability of inpatient biochemotherapy. The most promising of these approaches are displayed in Table 10. Legha et al. developed a regimen in which cisplatin, vinblastine, and DTIC (CVD) chemotherapy was administered concurrently with IL-2 and IFN-α immunotherapy (169,173). Therapy was administered in an inpatient setting over 5 days every 3 weeks. A maximum of six cycles was administered to responding patients. This regimen produced responses in 34 out of 53 patients (11 CRs, 23 PRs; RR 64%), with a median response duration of 6.5 months. The median time to disease progression and median survival for all patients were 5.0 months and 11.8 months, respectively. Five patients (9%) remained in continuous CR for 50 to 61 or more months. The principal side effects consisted of myelosuppression with 64% incidence of febrile neutropenia and 48% incidence of bacteremia. Other common side effects included nausea, vomiting, and anorexia, fluid retention, and hypotension. Hypotension, infections and severe thrombocytopenia were more common in patients who received three or more cycles of therapy. Neurologic, renal, and cardiopulmonary toxicities were uncommon. Antitumor activity appeared equivalent to the other biochemotherapy combinations, whereas the toxicity was considerably more manageable.

McDermott et al. completed a phase 2 pilot trial of a version of the Legha concurrent regimen that was modified slightly to further reduce toxicity and enhance convenience (174). Modifications included using antibiotic and granulocyte colony-stimulating factor (G-CSF) prophylaxis and more aggressive antiemetics, prohibiting long-term central venous access, and restricting therapy to a maximum of four cycles. A total of 131 treatment cycles was administered to 44 patients. These patients displayed inordinate amounts of poor prognostic features—82% of patients had visceral metastases and 75% had more than

one site of metastasis. In addition, 75% of patients received previous systemic therapy, including 53% who received previous IFN-α. Significant toxicities necessitating dose reductions were limited primarily to gastrointestinal toxicity (nausea and vomiting) and myelosuppression. The frequency of these toxicities was reduced with the incorporation of serotonin receptor-blocking antiemetics and G-CSF into the treatment regimen. Hypotension and renal insufficiency were uncommon, occurring in 11% and 3% of treatment cycles, respectively; significant cardiopulmonary toxicity was not observed. Hypotension was transient; all episodes resolved in less than 24 hours and were not associated with any symptoms or clinical sequelae. Neurotoxicity was only observed in two patients with resected brain metastases who had received previous cranial irradiation. Tumor responses were observed in 19 of 40 (48%) evaluable patients (eight CRs, 11 PRs). Responses occurred in all disease sites, including liver and bones. Responses were seen in 11 of 23 patients (48%) who had previously received IFN-α therapy. The median response duration was 6.5 months (range 2 to more than 22 months), with two patients remaining progression-free. Eleven responders (including four patients who had achieved CRs) had their initial relapses in the CNS. This high frequency of isolated or initial CNS relapse was believed to be the major explanation for the relative lack of durable responses. The observation by Moussieu et al. that small CNS metastases may respond as well as systemic metastases to biochemotherapy (170), however, questions this explanation. The extent to which poor prognostic characteristics of study patients, their heavy previous exposure to IFN-α, or any modification of treatment regimen impacted on the number of durable complete responses observed, remains speculative.

O'Day et al. (175) modified Legha's concurrent biochemotherapy regimen by adding tamoxifen and administering IL-2 in a decrescendo fashion similar to that described by Kielholz et al. (176). G-CSF was also added to prevent febrile neutropenia and infection. They have reported the results of their first 35 patients. Thirty-four percent of patients had received previous chemotherapy, 91% had multiple visceral sites of metastases, and 17% had small brain metastases. Treatment was well tolerated, with the majority of patients being discharged on day 5

TABLE 10. PHASE 2 CONCURRENT INTERLEUKIN-2/CISPLATIN–BASED BIOCHEMOTHERAPY TRIALS

Author (Reference)	Regimen/Dose	Evaluation	CR (%)	PR (%)	Total (%)	Comments
Legha et al. (173)	Concurrent CVD/bio	53	11 (21)	23 (43)	64	Survival for concurrent and sequential therapy equivalent
McDermott et al. (174)	Modified concurrent CVD/bio	40	8 (20)	11 (28)	48	RR equivalent in patients with previous IFN Frequent CNS relapse
O'Day et al. (175, 177)	Concurrent CVD/tam Decrescendo IL-2/IFN-α	35	7 (20)	13 (37)	57	No CRs in the 12 patients who had received previous chemotherapy
	Concurrent CVD/tam (HD) Decrescendo IL-2/IFN-α	27	2 (7)	10 (37)	44	Escalating dose tam; 17% of patients with CNS disease
Total		155	28 (18)	57 (37)	55	Median response durations, 5–7 mo; median survivals, 10–12 mo

bio, continuous infusion IL-2 + subcutaneous interferon; CNS, central nervous system; CR, complete response; CVD, cisplatin, vinblastine, dacarbazine; HD, high dose; IL-2, interleukin-2; IFN-α, interferon-α; PR, partial response; RR, response rate; tam, tamoxifen.

TABLE 11. PHASE 2 OUTPATIENT INTERLEUKIN-2/CISPLATIN–BASED BIOCHEMOTHERAPY TRIALS

Author (Reference)	Regimen/Dose	Evaluation	CR (%)	PR (%)	Total (%)	Comments
Flaherty et al. (178)	CDDP/DTIC/IL-2 (bolus)	32	5 (16)	8 (25)	41	First outpatient regimen; used only IL-2 alone
Atzpodien et al. (181)	CBDT/ IL-2 (s.q.)/IFN-α	27	3 (11)	12 (45)	55	
	Carboplatin/D/IL-2 (s.q.)/IFN-α	40	3 (7.5)	11 (27.5)	35	
Thompson et al. (180)	CBDT / IL-2 (s.q.)/IFN-α	53	10 (19)	12 (23)	42	Two CR ongoing >2 yr
Flaherty et al. (179)	CD / IL-2 (s.q.)/ IFN-α	38	1 (3)	6 (16)	19	
	CD / IL-2 (IV) / IFN-α	44	5 (12)	11 (25)	37	Randomized phase II CWG study; results better with i.v. IL-2
Richards (205)	CBDT/IL-2 (c.i.v.)/ IFN-α	27	3 (11)	4 (15)	26	2 wk c.i.v. of IL-2; frequent central line infections
Andreas (206)	CDDP/IL-2 (s.q.)/IFN-α	33	3 (9)	7 (21)	30	Multicenter trial
Hoffmann et al. (207)	CDBT/IL-2/IFN-α	69	7 (10)	20 (29)	39	
Honeycutt et al. (208)	CBDT/IL-2 (s.q.)/IFN-α	19	1 (5)	4 (20)	26	Short follow-up
Romanini et al. (209)	CDDP/DTIC/tam/IL-2 (i.v.)	17	2 (12)	2 (12)	24	Median survival, 8 mo
Guida et al. (210)	CDDP/DTIC/IL-2 (s.q.)	24	2 (8)	8 (33)	42	One durable CR
Bernengo et al. (211)	CDDP/tam/IL-2 (s.q.)/IFN-α	36	5 (14)	12 (33)	47	Median survival, 10 mo
Total		459	50 (11)	107 (23)	34	

CBDT, cisplatin, carmustine, dacarbazine, tamoxifen; CDDP, cisplatin; c.i.v., continuous intravenous infusion; CR, complete response; CWG, Cytokine Working Group; DTIC, dacarbazine; IL-2, interleukin-2; IFN-α, interferon-α; PR, partial response; tam, tamoxifen.

and readmission being required in only 6% of cycles. One treatment-related death occurred due to a CNS bleed. Responses were seen in 57% of patients (20% CR) with all CRs confined to 23 patients in the chemotherapy naïve population. Five patients underwent surgical resection of residual low-volume disease. Although these results are encouraging, the median follow-up of 8.7 months was too short to assess either long-term efficacy of this approach or the value of salvage surgery in this population. In a follow-up trial, escalating doses of tamoxifen were added to the regimen. Tumor responses were seen in 12 of 27 patients (177).

Outpatient Biochemotherapy Regimens

The observation that the activity of cisplatin and IL-2–based regimens may be more related to the proximity of biologic and cytotoxic components rather than actual doses of individual agents has raised the possibility of developing regimens suitable for outpatient administration (Table 11). With this in mind, Flaherty et al. developed a regimen in which patients received cisplatin and DTIC on day 1 and i.v. IL-2 (24 MIU/kg) on days 4 to 8 of a 21-day cycle (178). Responses were seen in 41% of patients. A similar regimen (except that IFN-α was added) was tested by the CWG. In this randomized phase 2 trial, patients were assigned to receive IL-2 either by subcutaneous or i.v. injection (179). Eighty-two patients were enrolled. Forty-four patients were randomized to the i.v. IL-2 arm and 38 to the subcutaneous IL-2 arm. The two arms were well-balanced for performance status, extent of disease, and previous IFN-α therapy. Seventy-six percent of all patients had visceral metastases and 23% had received IFN-α therapy before. Tumor responses were observed in 37% of patients (12% CRs, 25% PRs) on the i.v. IL-2 arm and 19% of patients (3% CRs, 16% PRs) on the subcutaneous IL-2 arm. Toxicity was compa-

rable, except a higher incidence of neutropenia occurred on the i.v. IL-2 arm.

Thompson et al. (180) evaluated a regimen involving cisplatin, carmustine, DTIC, chemotherapy on day 1, daily tamoxifen (CBDT), and subcutaneous IL-2 and IFN-α on days 3 to 9. Grade 3 and 4 nausea occurred in 32% of patients; hospitalization for supplemental i.v. hydration was necessary in 11% of treatment cycles. An overall RR of 42% (ten CRs, twelve PRs) was observed in 53 patients, with a median overall survival of 11 months.

Atzpodien et al. (181) reported on outpatient regimens involving carboplatin and DTIC or cisplatin, carmustine, dacarbazine, and tamoxifen (CBDT) for several cycles, followed by subcutaneous IL-2 and IFN-α. These regimens produced responses in 35% and 55% of patients, respectively, with minimal reported toxicity. Of note, a phase 2 trial of outpatient CBDT chemotherapy (days 1 to 3) with IL-2 administered for 3 days before chemotherapy and IFN-α administered concurrently (days 1 to 3) produced an RR of only 23% and more thrombocytopenia and nausea than were observed with chemotherapy alone (182). Whether these regimens are truly suitable for routine outpatient use and how they compare with either chemotherapy alone or more thoroughly tested inpatient biochemotherapy regimens remains to be determined.

Randomized Trials Involving Interleukin-2–Based Biochemotherapy

Several randomized phase 3 trials comparing biochemotherapy regimens to immunotherapy or chemotherapy alone have been initiated (Table 12). Initial results have been disappointing, however. The EORTC Melanoma Group has examined the value of adding cisplatin to decrescendo IL-2 and IFN-α in a randomized phase 3 trial. Although the cisplatin-containing

TABLE 12. PHASE 3 INTERLEUKIN-2/CISPLATIN–BASED BIOCHEMOTHERAPY TRIALS

Protocol/Principal Investigator(s) (Reference)	Design	Status
EORTC Kielholz et al. (92)	IL-2/ IFN-α^a vs. IL-2/IFN-α^a+ CDDP	Completed: RR higher for IL-2/IFN-α + CDDP, but no overall survival difference
NCI Surgery Branch Rosenberg et al. (183)	CDDP/ DTIC/tam vs. CDDP/DTIC/tam + HD IL-2/ IFN-α	Completed: no significant difference in RR or survival between the two groups
EORTC Keilholz et al. (184)	CDDP/DTIC/IFN-α vs. CDDP/DTIC/IFN-α + IL-2^a	In progress
M. D. Anderson Cancer Center Legha et al. (169)	CVD vs. sequential CVD + IL-2/IFN-α^b	Completed accrual
ECOG/SWOG 3695 Atkins/Flaherty (185)	CVD vs. concurrent CVD + IL-2/IFN-α^b	In progress

CDDP, cisplatin; CVD, cisplatin, vinblastine, dacarbazine; DTIC, dacarbazine; ECOG, Eastern Cooperative Oncology Group; EORTC, European Oncology Research Trial Council; HD, high dose; IFN-α, interferon-α; IL-2, interleukin-2; NCI, National Cancer Institute; RR, response rate; SWOG, Southwest Oncology Group; tam, tamoxifen.
^{a}Decrescendo IL-2 regimen.
^{b}IL-2, 9 MU/m^2 by c.i.v. for 96 h.
From Atkins MB, Gollob JA. Chemotherapy and cytokine-based immunotherapy for high-risk and metastatic melanoma. *Adv Oncol* 1999;15:22–29, with permission.

arm produced a significantly higher RR (35%) than IL-2/IFN alone (15%), responses were of shorter duration and no increase in the number of durable CRs or overall survivals occurred (192). The NCI Surgery Branch has pursued a different approach, reporting the results of a study comparing the combination of cisplatin, DTIC, and tamoxifen and high-dose bolus i.v. IL-2 plus subcutaneous IFN-α to cisplatin, DTIC, and tamoxifen alone (183). Chemotherapy was administered on days 2 to 4, and IL-2 and IFN-α were administered on days 5 to 8 on the biochemotherapy arm. Tamoxifen was administered throughout. Cycles were repeated at 21-day intervals, with up to 4 cycles administered to responding patients. One hundred two patients were enrolled, with 52 randomized to receive chemotherapy and 50 randomized to receive biochemotherapy. The two arms were balanced for most parameters, although twice as many patients with performance status 1 or 2 were enrolled on the biochemotherapy arm. The biochemotherapy regimen produced a slightly higher objective RR than the chemotherapy alone (44% vs. 27%, p = .071). Responses were generally of short duration in each treatment group, however; as a consequence, the improved RR did not translate into an improvement in number of durable CRs or overall survival rates for patients on the biochemotherapy arm. A trend toward survival advantage occurred in patients receiving chemotherapy alone (median survival, 15.8 months vs. 10.7 months; p = .052). These discouraging survival results and the low number of durable CRs (especially for a regimen containing high-dose bolus IL-2) raised concerns that chemotherapy may have diminished activity of immunotherapy in this combination. With only approximately 50 patients enrolled in each arm and the slight imbalance in performance status noted, however, this study was too small to definitively eliminate a benefit for biochemotherapy in melanoma.

Although confirmation is required, the lack of survival benefit in these two studies calls into question the value of biochemotherapy combinations relative to chemotherapy or IL-2 alone. Clearly, additional phase 3 trials comparing biochemotherapy to chemotherapy or immunotherapy alone are necessary to clearly establish a role for this approach. Legha and colleagues

at the M. D. Anderson Cancer Center have recently completed accrual for a similar study that compares their sequential CVD/IL-2/IFN regimen to CVD alone (169). The EORTC is conducting a study comparing cisplatin, DTIC, and IFN-α to the same regimen with decrescendo IL-2 (184). Finally, a phase 3 Intergroup trial (E3695) comparing the modified concurrent biochemotherapy regimen of McDermott et al. (174) to CVD chemotherapy alone was initiated within ECOG and the Southwest Oncology Group in early 1998.

Potential Mechanisms of Synergy for Biochemotherapy Regimens

Regardless of the overall benefits of biochemotherapy in melanoma, almost all studies have shown a higher RR exists for biochemotherapy than that anticipated for chemotherapy or immunotherapy alone. Mechanisms underlying this apparent synergy have been the focus of active investigation. Schmittel et al. examined T-cell responses to various peptides derived from tyrosinase in serial blood samples obtained from patients receiving cisplatin, DTIC, and IFN-α therapy with or without IL-2 (186). They were able to document the induction of tyrosinase–reactive T cells after therapy in four of seven patients. All four of these patients exhibited tumor responses. T-cell reactivity was lost in two patients at times of relapse. These data suggest that cytotoxic chemotherapy, possibly because it causes tumor cell death and releases apoptotic bodies, may lead to enhanced tumor–antigen presentation to the IL-2–activated immune system. Alternatively, others have suggested a potential role exists for either macrophage products or nitrous oxide in the tumor destruction produced by biochemotherapy regimens. Scheibogen et al. reported a correlation between neopterin (a protein predominantly released by activated macrophages) levels at day 8 of a treatment cycle and response to biochemotherapy (187). Anderson et al., however, were unable to confirm this observation in their biochemotherapy population (188). Anderson did observe, however, a weak correlation between day 5 serum nitrite levels, a product of enzymatic reduction of nitrous oxide, and tumor response. A potential mechanism for nitric oxide may be in enhancing the amount of DNA damage produced by cytotoxic chemotherapy, either directly or through the depletion of intracellular glutathione levels. In this regard, Buzaid and colleagues investigated the relationship between cisplatin-induced DNA damage *in vitro* and response to biochemotherapy (189). They examined cisplatin-induced damage to the glutathione *S*-transferase-π gene in peripheral blood mononuclear cells (pretreatment) and found a strong correlation between degree of damage and subsequent response to therapy. Attempts to confirm this finding in a larger patient population are currently under way. If confirmed, this observation may provide insight into mechanisms of antitumor responses to biochemotherapy and a tool for selecting the patients most likely to benefit from such treatments. Efforts to determine whether biochemotherapy-induced DNA damage *in vivo* in lymphocytes or tumor cells correlates with tumor response are also under way. These studies, together with an assessment of whether DNA damage is enhanced with biochemotherapy relative to cisplatin-based chemotherapy alone, are critical to our understanding of mechanisms underlying the improved RR observed in biochemotherapy. Understanding such mechanisms will aid the subsequent development of biochemotherapy regimens, including potential applications of biochemotherapy to other cisplatin-sensitive tumors.

Future Applications of Biochemotherapy in Metastatic Melanoma

Efforts to reduce incidences of CNS relapse associated with biochemotherapy combinations have focused on the drug temozolomide. Temozolomide is an oral derivative of DTIC that appears to be able to cross the blood–brain barrier. Phase 2 and 3 trials of temozolomide have shown it to possess systemic antitumor activity similar to that of DTIC (190). In addition, single-agent temozolomide occasionally produced regressions of CNS metastases in patients. The possibility exists, therefore, that a substitution of this agent for DTIC in biochemotherapy regimens may reduce the high incidence of CNS relapses observed in major responders. Studies involving temozolomide-containing biochemotherapy regimens are under way at several institutions.

Other studies have focused on moving biochemotherapy into neoadjuvant or adjuvant settings. In addition to less tumor burden, these earlier disease settings offer the potential advantage of a lowered likelihood of CNS involvement *a priori*. Buzaid et al. at the M. D. Anderson Cancer Center administered their concurrent biochemotherapy regimen neoadjuvantly to patients with bulky local regional metastases (191). Patients received two to four courses of therapy, depending on tumor response assessment after two cycles of therapy, then underwent definitive surgery. Sixty-four patients were enrolled, 63 of whom were evaluable for histologic response. Four patients (6%) experienced a pathologic CR; ten patients (16%) exhibited a major PR (<95% cytoreduction in tumor mass). The overall RR was in excess of 50%. At a median follow-up of 13 months, only 1 of the 14 patients achieving a pathologic CR or major PR recurred, compared with 25 out of 49 patients who achieved less than a major PR. These results highlight the critical need that exists for achieving a major response during or shortly after therapy to receive clinical benefit from biochemotherapy; it also raises concerns about the value of surgery in patients not exhibiting such major responses (192). Miller et al. examined the activity of biochemotherapy in the adjuvant setting (193). They performed a phase 2 trial of subcutaneous IL-2 (9 MIU/day, days 1–4) and i.v. DTIC (750 mg/m², day 1) administered every 4 weeks for six cycles to patients with stage IIB and III disease. They observed a promising 2-year relapse-free survival of 62%, a result that compares favorably to that achieved with high-dose IFN-α in a similar patient population. Considering the small patient numbers, short follow-up, and hazards of using historic controls in the adjuvant therapy of metastatic melanoma, however, these results should be viewed with extreme caution. Nonetheless, data such as these lend support to formally examining the role of biochemotherapy relative to IFN-α in the high-risk adjuvant setting.

CONCLUSIONS

Modest progress has been made in the treatment of metastatic melanoma over the past decade. With the advent of high-dose IL-2, a "cure," albeit in a minority of patients, is possible. Combinations of IL-2 and IFN-α along with chemotherapy may produce responses in as many as one-half of the patients treated; it is unclear, however, whether these combinations are going to increase the number of patients who survive long-term disease-free. Strong preclinical rationales for the combination of IL-2 with other cytokines, toxicity blocking agents, or various monoclonal antibodies or vaccines exist; however, these approaches have not been fully tested clinically. The wealth of promising potential treatment strategies that exists offers hope that "cures" for more than the rare patient with metastatic melanoma will be achieved within the near future. Whatever promising approach is developed, the likelihood exists that its activity can be enhanced by coadministration of IL-2.

ACKNOWLEDGMENT

The authors are indebted to Karen Soprych for her assistance in preparing this manuscript.

REFERENCES

1. Ahmed I. Malignant melanoma: prognostic indicators. *Mayo Clin Proc* 1997;72:356.
2. Landy SH, Murray T, Bolden S, Wingo PA. Cancer Statistics, 1999. *CA Cancer J Clin* 1999;49:3.
3. Hill GJ, Krementz ET, Hill HZ. Dimethyl triazeno imidazole carboxamide and combination therapy for melanoma. IV. Late results after complete response to chemotherapy (Central Oncology Group protocols 7130, 7131, and 7131A). *Cancer* 1984;53:1299.
4. Atkins MB. The role of cytotoxic chemotherapeutic agents either alone or in combination with biological response modifiers. In: Kirkwood JM, ed. *Molecular diagnosis, prevention and therapy of melanoma*. New York: Marcel Dekker, Inc, 1998:219–251.
5. Buzaid AD, Legha S, Winn R, et al. Cisplatin (C), Vinblastine (V),

and dacarbazine (D) versus dacarbazine alone in metastatic melanoma: preliminary results of a phase II Cancer Community Oncology Program (CCOP) Trial. *Proc ASCO* 1993;12:389.

6. Chapman PB, Einhorn LH, Meyers ML, et al. Phase III multicenter randomized trial of the Dartmouth Regimen Versus dacarbazine in patients with metastatic melanoma. *J Clin Oncol* 1999; 17:2745–2751.

7. Falkson CI, Falkson G, Falkson HC. Improved results with the addition of interferon alpha-2b to dacarbazine in the treatment of patients with metastatic malignant melanoma. *J Clin Oncol* 1991;9:1403–1408.

8. Thompson D, Adena M, McLeod GRC. Interferon alfa-2a does not improve response or survival when combined with dacarbazine in metastatic malignant melanoma: results of a multi-institutional Australian randomized trial, QMP8704. *Melanoma Res* 1993:3: 133–138.

9. Bajetta E, DiLeo A, Zampino M, et al. Multicenter randomized trial of dacarbazine alone or in combination with two different doses and schedules of interferon alfa-2a in the treatment of advanced melanoma. *J Clin Oncol* 1994;12:806–811.

10. Kirkwood JM, Ernstoff MS, Giuliano A, et al. Interferon α-2a and dacarbazine in melanoma. *J Natl Cancer Inst* 1990;82:1062–1063.

11. Cocconi G, Bella M, Calabresi F, et al. Treatment of metastatic malignant melanoma with dacarbazine plus tamoxifen. *N Engl J Med* 1992, 327:516–523.

12. McClay EF, Mastrangelo MJ, Berd D, Bellet RE. Effective combination chemo/hormonal therapy for malignant melanoma: experience with three clinical trials. *Int J Cancer* 1992;50:553–556.

13. Falkson CI, Ibrahim J, Kirkwood J, Coates AS, Atkins MB, Blum R. Phase III trial of dacarbazine versus dacarbazine with interferon a 2b versus dacarbazine with tamoxifen (TMX) versus dacarbazine with interferon a 2b and tamoxifen in patients with metastatic malignant melanoma: an Eastern Cooperative Oncology Group Study (E3690). *J Clin Oncol* 1998;16:1743–1751.

14. Rhusthoven JJ, Quirt IC, Iscoe NA, et al. Randomized, double-blind placebo-controlled trial comparing the response rates of carmustine, dacarbazine, and cisplatin with and without tamoxifen in patients with metastatic melanoma. National Cancer Institute of Canada Clinical Trials Group. *J Clin Oncol* 1996;14:2083–2090.

15. Atkins MB. The Treatment of Metastatic Melanoma with Chemotherapy and Biologics. *Curr Opin Oncol* 1997;9:205–213.

16. Atkins MB. Immunotherapy and experimental approaches for metastatic melanoma. *Hematol Oncol Clin North Am* 1998;12:877–902.

17. Morgan DA, Ruscetti FW, Gallo R. Selective in vitro growth of T lymphocytes for normal human bone marrows. *Science* 1976;1993: 1007–1008.

18. Taniguchi T, Matsui H, Fujita T, et al. Structure and expression of cloned cDNA for human interleukin-2. *Nature* 1983;302:305–310.

19. Rosenberg SA, Mulé JJ, Speiss PJ, et al. Regression of established pulmonary metastases and subcutaneous tumor mediated by the systemic administration of high-dose recombinant interleukin 2. *J Exp Med* 1985;161:1169–1188.

20. Marincola FM, Rosenberg SA. Interleukin 2: clinical applications: melanoma. In: DeVita VT, Hellman S, Rosenberg SA, eds. *Biologic therapy of cancer*, 2nd ed. Philadelphia: JB Lippincott Co, 1995:250.

21. Hank JA, Surfus J, Gan J, et al. Distinct clinical and laboratory activity of two recombinant interleukin-2 preparations. *Clin Cancer Res* 1999;5:281–289.

22. Ettinghausen SE, Rosenberg SA. Immunotherapy of murine sarcomas using lymphokine activated killer cells: optimization of the schedule and route of administration or recombinant interleukin-2. *Cancer Res* 1986;46:27–84.

23. Papa MZ, Mulé JJ, Rosenberg SA. Antitumor efficacy of lymphokine-activated killer cells and recombinant interleukin 2 in vivo: successful immunotherapy of established pulmonary metastases from weakly immunogenic and nonimmunogenic murine tumors of three distinct histologic types. *Cancer Res* 1986;46:49–73.

24. Lotze MT, Frana LW, Sharrow SO, et al. *In vivo* administration of purified human interleukin 2. I. Half-life and immunologic effects of the Jurkat cell line-derived interleukin 2. *J Immunol* 1985; 134:157.

25. Lotze MT, Matory YL, Ettinghausen, et al. *In vivo* administration of purified human interleukin 2. II. Half-life, immunologic effects and expansion of peripheral lymphoid celll *in vivo* with recombinant IL 2. *J Immunol* 1985;135:28–65.

26. Rosenberg SA, Lotze MT, Muul LM, et al. Observations on the systemic administration of autologous lymphokine-activated killer cells and recombinant interleukin-2 to patients with metastatic cancer. *N Engl J Med* 1985;313:1485–1492.

27. Rosenberg SA, Yang JC,Topalian SL, et al. Treatment of 283 consecutive patients with metastatic melanoma or renal cell cancer using high-dose bolus interleukin-2. *JAMA* 1994;271:907–913.

28. Dutcher JP, Creekmore S, Weiss GR, et al. A phase II study of interleukin-2 and Lymphokine Activated Killer (LAK) cells in patients with metastatic malignant melanoma. *J Clin Oncol* 1989;7:477–485.

29. Parkinson D, Abrams J, Wiernik P, et al. Interleukin-2 therapy in patients with metastatic malignant melanoma: a phase II study. *J Clin Oncol* 1990;8:1650–1656.

30. Sznol M, Dutcher JP, Atkins MB, et al. Review of interleukin-2 alone and interleukin-2/LAK clinical trials in metastatic malignant melanoma. *Cancer Treat Rev* 1989;16[Suppl A]:29–38.

31. Rosenberg SA, Lotze MT, Muul LM, et al. A progress report on the treatment of 157 patients with advanced cancer using lymphokine-activated killer cells and interleukin-2 or high dose interleukin-2 alone. *N Engl J Med* 1987;316:889.

32. McCabe MS, Stablein D, Hawkins MJ, et al. The modified group C experience—phase III randomized trials of IL-2 vs. IL-2/LAK in advanced renal cell carcinoma and advanced melanoma (abstract). *Proc Am Soc Clin Oncol* 1991;10:213.

33. Rosenberg SA, Lotze MT, Yanf JC, et al. Prospective randomized trial of high-dose interleukin-2 alone or in conjunction with lymphokine-activated killer cells for the treatment of patients with advanced cancer. *J Natl Cancer Inst* 1993;8:622.

34. Atkins MB, Lotze M, Dutcher JP, et al. High-dose recombinant interleukin-2 therapy for patients with metastatic melanoma: analysis of 270 patients treated from 1985–1993. *J Clin Oncol* 1999;17: 2105–2116.

35. Klempner MS, Snydman DR. Infectious complications associated with interleukin-2. In: Atkins MB, Mier JW, eds. *Therapeutic application of interleukin-2*, 1st ed. New York: Marcel Dekker, 1993:409–424.

36. Atkins MB, Kunkel L, Sznol M, Rosenbuerg SA. High-dose aldesleukin therapy in patients with metastatic melanoma: long-term survival update. *Cancer J Sci Am*, 2000 *(in press)*.

37. Rosenberg SA, Yang JC, White DE, Steinberg SM. Durability of complete responses in patients with metastatic cancer treated with high-dose interleukin-2: identification of the antigens mediating response. *Ann Surg* 1998;228:307–319.

38. Yang JC, Topalian SL, Schwartzentruber DJ, et al. The use of polyethylene glycol-modified interleukin-s (PEG-IL-2) in the treatment of patients with metastatic renal cell carcinoma and melanoma. A phase I study and a randomized prospective study comparing IL-2 alone versus IL-2 combined with PEG-IL-2. *Cancer* 1995;76:687–694.

39. Talmadge JE, Phillips H, Schindler J, et al. Systemic preclinical study on the therapeutic properties of IL-2 for the treatment of metastatic disease. *Cancer Res* 1987;47:5725–5732.

40. Sondel PM, Kohler PC, Hank JA, et al. Clinical and immunological effects of recombinant interleukin 2 given by repetitive weekly cycles to patients with cancer. *Cancer Res* 1988;48:2561–2567.

41. Thompson JA, Lee DJ, Lindgren CG, et al. Influence of dose and duration of infusion of interleukin-2 on toxicity and immunomodulation. *J Clin Oncol* 1988;6:669–678.

42. Hank JA, Robinson RR, Surfus J, et al. Augmentation of antibody dependent cell mediated cytotoxicity following *in vivo* therapy with interleukin-2. *Cancer Res* 1990;50:5234–5239.

43. Munn DH, Cheung NK. Interleukin-2 enhancement of monoclonal antibody-mediated cellular cytotoxicity against human melanoma. *Cancer Res* 1987;47:6600–6605.

44. West WH, Tauer KW, Yannelli JR, et al. Constant-infusion recombinant interleukin-2 in adoptive immunotherapy of advanced cancer. *N Engl J Med* 987;16:898–905.

45. Dillman RO, Church C, Oldham RK, et al. In-patient continuous infusion IL-2 in 788 patients with cancer. The National Biotherapy Study Group experience. *Cancer* 1993;71:2358–2370.

46. Dillman RO, Wiemann MC, VanderMolen LA, et al. Hybrid high-dose bolus/continuous infusion interleukin-2 in patients with metastatic melanoma: a phase II trial of the cancer biotherapy research group (formerly the National Biotherapy Study Group). *Cancer Biother Radiopharm* 1997;12:249–255.

47. Legha SS, Gianan MA, Plager C, et al. Evaluation of interleukin-2 administered by continuous infusion in patients with metastatic melanoma. *Cancer* 1996;77:89–96.

48. Dorval T, Mathiot C, Chosidow O, et al. IL-2 phase II trial in metastatic melanoma: analysis of clinical and immunological parameters. *Biotechnol Ther* 1992;3:63–79.

49. Dillman RO, Church C, Barth NM, et al. Long-term survival after continuous infusion interleukin-2. *Cancer Biother Radiopharm* 1997;12:243–248.

50. Vlasveld LT, Rankin EM, Heckman A, et al. A phase I study of prolonged continuous infusion of low dose recombinant IL-2 in melanoma and renal cell cancer. Part I clinical aspect. *Br J Cancer* 1992;65:744–750.

51. Vlasveld LT, Horenblas S, Hekman A, et al. Phase II study of intermittent continuous infusion of low-dose recombinant interleukin-2 in advanced melanoma and renal cell cancer. *Ann Oncol* 1994;5: 179–181.

52. Whitehead RP, Kopecky KJ, Samson MK, et al. Phase II study of intravenous bolus recombinant interleukin-2 in advanced malignant melanoma: Southwest Oncology Group study. *J Natl Cancer Inst* 1991;83:1250–1252.

53. Margolin K. The clinical toxicities of high-dose interleukin-2. In: Atkins MB, Mier JW, eds. *Therapeutic applications of Interleukin-2.* New York: Marcel Dekker, 1993:331–362.

54. Schwartzentruber DJ. Biologic therapy with interleukin-2: clinical applications: principles of administration and management of side effects. In: DeVita V, Hellman S, Rosenberg SA, eds. *Biologic therapy of cancer*, 2nd ed. Philadelphia: JB Lippincott Co, 1995:235–249.

55. Numerof RP, Aronson FR, Mier JW. IL-2 stimulates the production of IL-1 alpha and IL-1 beta by human peripheral blood mononuclear cells. *J Immunol* 1988;141:4250–4257.

56. Mier J, Vachino G, Van der Meer J, et al. Induction of circulating tumor necrosis factor (TNF) as the mechanism for the febrile response to interleukin-2 (IL-2) in cancer patients. *J Clin Immunol* 1988;8:426–436.

57. Gemlo BT, Pallidino MA, Jaffe HS, Espevik TP, Rayner AA. Circulation cytokines in patients with metastatic cancer treated with interleukin-2 and lymphokine-activated killer cells. *Cancer Res* 1988;48: 58–64.

58. Hibbs JB, Westenfelder C, Taintor R, et al. Evidence for cytokine inducible nitric oxide synthesis from L-arginine in patients receiving interleukin-2 therapy. *J Clin Invest* 1992;89:867–877.

59. Mier JW, Vachino G, Klempner MS, et al. Inhibition of interleukin-2 induced tumor necrosis factor release by dexamethasone: prevention of an acquired neutrophil chemotactic defect and differential suppression of interleukin-2 associated side effects. *Blood* 1990;76: 1933–1940.

60. Vetto JT, Papa MZ, Lotze MT, et al. Reduction of toxicity of interleukin-2 and lymphokine-activated killer cells in humans by the administration of corticosteroids. *J Clin Oncol* 1987;5:496.

61. Trehu EG, Mier JW, Shapiro L, et al. A Phase I trial of interleukin-2 in combination with the soluble tumor necrosis factor receptor p75 IgG chimera (TNFR:Fc). *Clin Cancer Res* 1996;2:1341–1351.

62. DuBois J, Trehu EG, Mier JW, et al. Randomized placebo-controlled clinical trial of high dose interleukin-2 (IL-2) in combination with the soluble TNF receptor IgG chimera (TNFR:Fc). *J Clin Oncol* 1997;15:1052–1062.

63. Margolin K, Weiss G, Dutcher J, et al. Prospective randomized trial of lisophylline (CT1501R) for the modulation of interleukin-2 (IL-2) toxicity. *Clin Cancer Res* 1997;3:565–572.

64. McDermott D, Trehu E, DuBois J, et al. Phase I clinical trial of the soluble IL-1 receptor either alone or in combination with high-dose

IL-2 in patients with advanced malignancies. *Clin Cancer Res* 1998;5:1203–1213.

65. Kilbourn RG, Fonseca GA, Griffith OW, et al. NG-methyl-L-arginine, an inhibitor of nitric oxide synthase, reverses interleukin-2-induced hypotension. *Crit Care Med* 1995;23:10–18.

66. Bianchi M, Bloom O, Raabe T, et al. Suppression of proinflammatory cytokines in monocytes by a tetravalent guanylhydrazone. *J Exp Med* 1996;183:927–936.

67. Bianchi M, Ulrich P, Bloom O. An inhibitor of macrophage arginine transport and nitric oxide production (CNI-1493) prevents acute inflammation and endotoxin lethality. *Mol Med* 1995:1:254–266.

68. Kemeny MM, Botchkina GI, Ochani M, Urmacher C, Tracey KJ. The tetravalent guanylhydrazone CNI-1493 blocks the toxic effects of interleukin-2 without diminishing antitumor activity. *Proc Natl Acad Sci U S A* 1998;95:4561–4566.

69. Royal RE, Steinberg SM, White D, et al. Correlates of response to IL-2 therapy in patients treated for metastatic renal cancer and melanoma. *Cancer J Sci Am* 1996;6:91.

70. Kammula US, White DE, Rosenberg SA. Trends in the safety of high dose bolus interleukin-2 administration in patients with metastatic cancer. *Cancer* 1998;83:797–805.

71. Tartour E, Blay JY, Dorval T, et al. Predictors of clinical response to interleukin-2 based immunotherapy in melanoma patients: a French multiinstitutional study. *J Clin Oncol* 1996;14:1697–1703.

72. Keilholz U, Scheibogen C, Sommer M, Pritsch M, Geuke AM. Prognostic factors for response and survival in patients with metastatic melanoma receiving immunotherapy. *Melanoma Res* 1996;6: 173–178.

73. Rosenberg SA, White DE. Vitiligo in patients with melanoma: normal tissue antigens can be targets for cancer immunotherapy. *J Immunother* 1996;19:81.

74. Atkins MB. Autoimmune disorders induced by interleukin-2 therapy. In: Atkins MB, Mier JW, eds. *Therapeutic applications of interleukin-2.* New York: Marcel Dekker, Inc, 1993;389–408.

75. Schwartzentruber DJ, Hom SS, Dadmarz R, et al. In vitro predictors of therapeutic response in melanoma patients receiving tumor-infiltrating lymphocytes and interleukin-2. *J Clin Oncol* 1994;12:1475–1483.

76. Marincola FM, Venzon D, White D, et al. HLA association with response and toxicity in melanoma patients treated with interleukin-2-based immunotherapy. Cancer Res 1992;52:6561–6566.

77. Marincola FM, Shamamian P, Rivoltini L, et al. HLA associations in the anti-tumor response against malignant melanoma. *J Immunol* 1996;18:242–252.

78. Rubin JT, Day R, Duquesnoy R, et al. HLA-DQ1 is associated with clinical response and survival of patients with melanoma who are treated with interleukin-2. *Ther Immunol* 1995;2:1–6.

79. Scheibenbogen C, Keilholz U, Mytilineos J, et al. HLA class I alleles and responsiveness of melanoma to immunotherapy with interferon-alpha (INF-alpha) and interleukin-2 (IL-2). *Melanoma Res* 1994; 4:191.

80. Hahne M, Rimoldi D, Schroter M, et al. Melanoma cell expression of Fas (Apo 1/CD95) ligand: implications for tumor immune escape. *Science* 1996;274:1363–1366.

81. Zea AH, Curti BD, Longo DL, et al. Alterations in T cell receptor and signal transduction molecules in melanoma patients. *Clin Cancer Res* 1995;1:1327–1335.

82. Rabinowich H, Banks M, Reichert TE, et al. Expression and activity of signaling molecules in T lymphocytes obtained from patients with metastatic melanoma before and after interleukin 2 therapy. *Clin Cancer Res* 1996;2:1263–1274.

83. Iigo M, Sakurai M, Tamura T, et al. In vivo anti-tumor activity of multiple injections of recombinant interleukin-2, alone and in combination with three different types of recombinant interferon, on various syngeneic murine tumors. *Cancer Res* 1988;48:260.

84. Rosenberg SA, Schwartz SL, Spiess PJ. Combination immunotherapy for cancer: synergistic antitumor interactions of interleukin-2, alfa interferon, and tumor-infiltrating lymphocytes. *J Natl Cancer Inst* 1988;80:13–93.

85. Brunda MJ, Bellantoni D, Sulich V. In vivo antitumor activity of combinations of interferon alpha and interleukin-2 in murine

model. Correlation of efficacy with the induction of cytotoxic cells resembling natural killer cells. *Int J Cancer* 1987;40:365–371.

86. Cameron RB, McIntosh JK, Rosenberg SA. Synergistic anti-tumor effects of combination immunotherapy with recombinant interleukin-2 and a recombinant hybrid alpha-interferon in the treatment of established murine hepatic metastases. *Cancer Res* 1988;48:5810.

87. Rosenberg SA, Lotze MT, Yang JC, et al. Combination therapy with interleukin-2 and alpha-interferon for the treatment of patients with advanced cancer. *J Clin Oncol* 1989;7:1863–1874.

88. Marincola FM, White DE, Wise AP, Rosenberg SA. Combination therapy with interferon alfa-2a and interleukin-2 for the treatment of metastatic cancer. *J Clin Oncol* 1995;13:1110–1122.

89. Sparano JA, Fisher RI, Sunderland M, et al. Randomized phase III trial of treatment with high-dose interleukin-2 either alone or in combination with alfa-2a in patients with advanced melanoma. *J Clin Oncol* 1993;11:1969–1977.

90. Karp SE. Low-dose intravenous bolus interleukin-2 with interferon-alpha therapy for metastatic melanoma and renal cell carcinoma. *J Immunother* 1998;21:56–61.

91. Keilholz U, Scheibenbogen C, Tilgen W, et al. Interferon-α and interleukin-2 in the treatment of metastatic melanoma: comparison of two phase II trials. *Cancer* 1993;72:607–614.

92. Keilholz U, Goey SH, Punt CJ, et al. Interferon alfa-2a and interleukin-2 with or without cisplatin in metastatic melanoma: a randomized trial of the European organization for research and treatment of cancer melanoma cooperative group. *J Clin Oncol* 1997;15:2579–2588.

93. Eton O, Talpaz M, Lee KH, et al. Phase II trial of recombinant human interleukin-2 and interferon-alpha 2a. *Cancer* 1996;77:893–899.

94. Kruit WHJ, Goey SH, Calabresi F, et al. Final report of a phase II study of interleukin-2 and interferon-alpha in patients with metastatic melanoma. *Br J Cancer* 1995;71:1319–1321.

95. Whitehead RP, Figlin R, Citron ML, et al. A phase II trial of concomitant human interleukin-2 and interferon-alpha-2a in patients with disseminated malignant melanoma. *J Immunother* 1993;13:117–121.

96. Castello G, Comella P, Manzo T, et al. Immunological and clinical effects of intramuscular rIFNα-2a and low-dose subcutaneous rIL-2 in patients with advanced malignant melanoma. *Melanoma Res* 1993;3:43–49.

97. Kim CJ, Taubenberger JK, Simonis TB, et al. Combination therapy with interferon-α and interleukin-2 for the treatment of metastatic melanoma. *J Immunol* 1996;19:50–58.

98. Viens P, Blaise D, Stoppa AM, et al. Interleukin-2 in association with increasing doses of interferon-gamma in patients with advanced cancer. *J Immunother* 1992;11:218–224.

99. Reddy SP, Harwood RM, Moore DF, et al. Recombinant interleukin-2 in combination with recombinant interferon-gamma in patients with advanced malignancy: a phase I study. *J Immunother* 1997;20:79–87.

100. Olencki T, Finke J, Tubbs R, et al. Immunomodulatory effects on interleukin-2 and interleukin-4 in patients with malignancy. *J Immunother* 1996;19:69–80.

101. Sosman JA, Fisher SG, Kefer C, et al. A phase I trial of continuous infusion interleukin-4 (IL-4) alone and following interleukin-2 (IL-2) in cancer patients. *Ann Oncol* 1994;5:447–452.

102. Shimizu K, Fields RC, Giedlin M, Mulé JJ. Systemic administration of interleukin 2 enhances the therapeutic efficacy of dendritic cell-based tumor vaccines. *Proc Natl Acad Sci U S A* 1999;96(5):2268–2273.

103. Creagan ET, Rowlan KM Jr, Suman VJ, et al. Phase II study of combined levamisole with recombinant interleukin-2 in patients with advanced malignant melanoma. *Am J Clin Oncol* 1997;20:490–492.

104. Quirt IC, Shelley WE, Pater JL, et al. Improved survival in patients with poor-prognosis malignant melanoma treated with adjuvant levamisole: a phase III study by the National Cancer Institute of Canada clinical trials group. *J Clin Oncol* 1991;9:729–735.

105. Spitler LE. A randomized trial of levamisole versus placebo as adjuvant therapy in malignant melanoma. *J Clin Oncol* 1991;9:736–740.

106. Ahmed FY, Leonard GA, A'Hern R, et al. A randomized dose escalation study of subcutaneous interleukin-2 with and without levami-

sole in patients with metastatic renal cell carcinoma or malignant melanoma. *Br J Cancer* 1996;74:1109–1113.

107. Salup RR, Sicker DC, Wolmark N, et al. Chemoimmunotherapy of metastatic murine renal cell carcinoma using flavone acetic acid and interleukin 2. *J Urol* 1992;147:1120–1123.

108. Thatcher N, Dazzi H, Mellor M, et al. Recombinant IL-2 with flavone acetic acid in advanced malignant melanoma: a phase II study. *Br J Cancer* 1990;61:618–621.

109. O'Reilly SM, Rustin GJ, Farmer K, et al. Flavone acetic acid (FAA) with recombinant interleukin-2 (rIL-2) in advanced malignant melanoma: I. Clinical and vascular studies. *Br J Cancer* 1993;67:1342–1345.

110. Hellstrand K, Hermodsson S, Noredi P, et al. Histamine and cytokine therapy. *Acta Oncologica* 1998;37:347–353.

111. Vuist WMJ, v. Buitenen F, de Rie MA, et al. Potentiation by interleukin-2 of Burkitt's lymphoma therapy with anti-pan B (anti-CD19) monoclonal antibodies in a mouse xenotransplantation model. *Cancer Res* 1989;49:37–83.

112. Gill I, Agab R, Hu E, Mazumder A. Synergistic anti-tumor effects of interleukin-2 and the monoclonal Lym-1 against human Burkitt lymphoma cells in vivo and in vitro. *Cancer Res* 1989;49:53–77.

113. Schultz KR, Klarnet JP, Peace DJ, et al. Monoclonal antibody therapy of murine lymphoma: enhanced efficacy by concurrent administration of interleukin-2 or lymphokine-activated killer cells. *Cancer Res* 1990;50:5421.

114. Eisenthal A, Lafreniere R, Lefor AT, Rosenberg SA. Effect of anti-B16 melanoma monoclonal antibody on established murine B16 melanoma liver metastases. *Cancer Res* 1987;47:27–71.

115. Welte K, Miller G, Chapman PB, et al. Stimulation of T lymphocyte proliferation by monoclonal antibodies against GD3 ganglioside. *J Immunol* 1987;139:1763–1771.

116. Hirsh R, Gress RE, Pluznile DH, et al. Effects of *in vivo* administration of anti CD3 monoclonal antibody on T cell function in mice. II. In vivo activation of T cells. *J Immunol* 1989;142:737–742.

117. Hirsh R, Eckhans M, Auchincloss H, et al. Effects of in vivo administration of anti CD3 monoclonal antibodies on T cell function in mice I. Immunosuppression or transplantation response. *J Immunol* 1988;140:3766–3772.

118. Ellen Horn JDI, Hirsh R, Scherber H, et al. In vivo administration of anti CD3 prevents progressive tumor growth. *Science* 1988;242:569–571.

119. Reisfeld RA, Gillies SD. Antibody-interleukin 2 fusion proteins: a new approach to cancer therapy. *J Clin Lab Anal* 1996;10:160–166.

120. Sondel PM, Hank JA. Combination therapy with interleukin-2 and antitumor monoclonal antibodies. *Cancer J Sci Am* 1997;3:S121–S127.

121. Albino AP, Houghton AN, Eisinger M, et al. Class II histocompatibility antigen expression in human melanocytes transformed by Harvey murine sarcoma virus (Ha-MSV) and Kirsten MSV retroviruses. *J Exp Med* 1986;164:1710–1722.

122. Thurin J, Thurin M, Elder DE, et al. GD2 ganglioside biosynthesis is a distinct biochemical event in human melanoma tumor progession. *FEBS Letts* 1982;107:357–361.

123. Bajorin DF, Chapman PB, Wong GY, et al. Treatment with high-dose mouse monoclonal (anti-GD3) antibody R24 in patients with metastatic melanoma. *Melanoma Res* 1992;2:355.

124. Cheung NV, Lazarus H, Miraldi FD, et al. Ganglioside GD2 specific monoclonal antibody 3F8: a phase I study in patients with neuroblastoma and malignant melanoma (published erratum appears in 10:671, 1992). *J Clin Oncol* 1987;5:1430–1440.

125. Saleh MN, Khazaeli MB, Wheeler RH, et al. Phase I trial of mouse monoclonal anti-GD2 antibody 14G2a in metastatic melanoma. *Cancer Res* 1992;52:4342.

126. Coit D, Houghton AN, Cordon-Cardo C, et al. Isolated limb perfusion with monoclonal antibody R24 in patients with malignant melanoma. *Proc Am Soc Clin Oncol* 1988;7:248.

127. Dippold WG, Bernhard H, Meyer zum Bushenfelde K-H. Immunological response to intrathecal GD3-ganglioside antibody treatment in cerebrospinal fluid melanosis. In: Oettgen HF, ed. *Gangliosides and cancer.* Weinheim: VCH, 1989:241–247.

128. Bajorin DF, Chapman PB, Dimaggio J, et al. Phase I evaluation of a combination of monoclonal antibody R24 and interleukin 2

in patients with metastatic melanoma. *Cancer Res* 1990;50: 7490–7495.

129. Soiffer RJ, Chapman PB, Murray C, et al. Administration of R24 monoclonal antibody and low-dose interleukin-2 for malignant melanoma. *Clin Cancer Res* 1997;3:17–24.

130. Alpaugh RK, von Mehren M, Palazzo I, et al. Phase IB trial for malignant melanoma using R24 monoclonal antibody, interleukin-2/alpha-interferon. *Med Oncol* 1998;15:191–198.

131. Albertini MR, Hank JA, Schuller JH, et al. Phase IB trial of chimeric antidisialoganglioside antibody interleukin-2 for melanoma patients. *Clin Cancer Res* 1997;3:1277–1288.

132. Albertini MR, Gan J, Jaeger P, et al. Systemic interleukin-2 modulates the anti-idiotypic response to chimeric anti-GD2 antibody in patients with melanoma. *J Immunother Emphasis Tumor Immunol* 1996;19:278–295.

133. Hoskins DW, Stankova J, Anderson SK, et al. Ameloriation of experimental lung metastases in mice by therapy with anti CD3 monoclonal antibodies. *Cancer Immunol Immunother* 1989;29:226–230.

134. Sosman JA, Weiss GR, Margolin KA, et al. Phase IB clinical trial of anti-CD3 followed by high-dose bolus interleukin-2 in patients with metastatic melanoma and advanced renal cell carcinoma: clinical and immunologic effects. *J Clin Oncol* 1993;11:1496–1505.

135. Hank JA, Albertini M, Wesley OH, et al. Clinical and immunological effects of treatment with murine anti-CD3 monoclonal antibody along with interleukin-2 in patients with cancer. *Clin Cancer Res* 1995;1:481–491.

136. Buter J, Janssen RA, Martens A, et al. Phase I/II study of low-dose intravenous OKT3 and subcutaneous interleukin-2 in metastatic cancer. *Eur J Cancer* 1993;29A:2108–2113.

137. Sosman JA, Kefer C, Fisher RI, et al. A phase IA/IB trial of anti-CD3 murine monoclonal antibody plus low-dose continuous-infusion interleukin-2 in advanced cancer patients. *J Immunother* 1995;17:171–180.

138. Gillies SD, Reilly EB, Lo KM, et al. Antibody targeted interleukin 2 stimulates T cell killing of autologous tumor cells PNAS. *Proc Natl Acad Sci U S A* 1992;89:1428–1432.

139. Becker JC, Pancook JD, Gillies SD, et al. T cell mediated eradication of murine metastatic melanoma induced by targeted interleukin 2 therapy. *J Exp Med* 1996;183:2361–2366.

140. Becker JC, Pancook JD, Gillies SD, et al. Eradication of human hepatic and pulmonary melanoma metastases in SCID mice by anti-body-interleukin fusion proteins. *Proc Natl Acad Sci U S A* 1996;93:2702–2707.

141. Livingston P, Sznol M. Vaccine Therapy. In: Balch CM, Houghton AN, Sober AJ, Soong S, eds. *Cutaneous melanoma*, 3rd ed. St. Louis: Quality Medical Publishing, Inc, 1998:437–450.

142. Morton DL, Foshag LJ, Hoon DS, et al. Prolongation of survival in metastatic melanoma after active specific immunotherapy with a new polyvalent melanoma vaccine. *Ann Surg* 1992;216:463. (published erratum appears in *Ann Surg* 1993;217:3091).

143. Bystryn JC. Clinical activity of a polyvalent melanoma antigen vaccine. *Recent Results Cancer Res* 1995;139:337.

144. Berd D, Murphy G, Magurie HC Jr, et al. Treatment of metastatic melanoma with an autologous tumor-cell vaccine: clinical and immunologic results in 64 patients. *J Clin Oncol* 1990;8:18–58.

145. Mitchell MS, Harel W, Kempf RA, et al. Active-specific immunotherapy for melanoma. *J Clin Oncol* 1990;8:856.

146. Jones PC, Sze LL, Liu PY, et al. Prolonged survival for melanoma patients with elevated IgM antibody to oncofetal antigen. *J Natl Cancer Inst* 1981;66:249.

147. Livingston PO, Wong GY, Adhuri S, et al. Improved survival in stage II melanoma patients with GM2 antibodies: a randomized trial of adjuvant vaccination with GM2 antibodies: a randomized trial of adjuvant vaccination with GM2 ganglioside. *J Clin Oncol* 1994;12.10–36.

148. Adler A, Schachter J, Barenholz Y, et al. Allogeneic human liposomal melanoma vaccine with or without IL-2 in metastatic melanoma patients: clinical and immunobiological effects. *Cancer Biother* 1995;10:293–306.

149. Oratz R, Shapiro R, Johnson D, et al. IL-2 liposomes markedly enhance the activity of a polyvalent melanoma vaccine. *Proc Annu Meet Am Soc Clin Oncol* 1996;15:Λ1356.

150. Kawakami Y, Eliejahu S, Jennings C, et al. Recognition of multiple epitopes in the human melanoma antigen gp100 by tumor infiltrating T-lymphocytes associated with in vivo tumor regression. *J Immunol* 1995;154:3461–3968.

151. van Pel A, van der Bruggen P, Coulie PG, et al. Genes coding for tumor antigens recognized by cytolytic T lymphocytes. *Immunol Rev* 1995;145:229–250.

152. Rosenberg SA. The immunotherapy of solid cancers based on cloning the genes encoding tumor-rejection antigens. *Annu Rev Med* 1996;47:481–491.

153. Cole DJ, Weil DP, Shilyansky J, et al. Characterization of the functional specificity of a cloned T-cell receptor heterodimer recognizing the MART-1 melanoma antigen. *Cancer Res* 1995;55:748–752.

154. Zhai Y, Yang JC, Kawakami Y, et al. Antigen-specific tumor vaccines: development and characterization or recombinant adenovirus encoding MART-1 or gp100 for cancer therapy. *J Immunol* 1996;156:700.

155. Parkhurst MR, Salgaller ML, Southwood S, et al. Improved induction of melanoma-reactive CTL with peptides from the melanoma antigen gp100 modified at HLA-A* 0201-binding residues. *J Immunol* 1996;157:2539–2548.

156. Rivoltini L, Kawakami Y, Sakaguchi K, et al. Induction of tumor-reactive CTLs from peripheral blood and tumor-infiltrating lymphocytes of melanoma patients by in vitro stimulation with an immuno-dominant peptide of the human melanoma antigen MART-1. *J Immunol* 1995;54:2257–2265.

157. Salgaller ML, Afshar A, Marencola FM, et al. Recognition of multiple epitopes in the human melanoma antigen gp100 by peripheral blood lymphocytes stimulated in vitro with synthetic peptides. *Cancer Res* 1995;55:4972–4979.

158. Marincola FM, Rivoltini L, Salgaller ML, et al. Differential anti-MART-1/Melan A CTL activity in peripheral blood of HLA-A2 melanoma patients in comparison to healthy donors: evidence for in vivo priming by tumor cells. *J Immunother* 1996;19:266–277.

159. Cormier JN, Salgaller ML, Prevette T, et al. Enhancement of cellular immunity in melanoma patients immunized with a peptide from MART-1Melan A. *Cancer J Sci Am* 1996;3:37–44.

160. Salgaller ML, Marincola FM, Comier JN, Rosenberg SA. Immunization against epitopes in the human melanoma antigen gp100 following patient immunization with synthetic peptides. *Cancer Res* 1996;56:4749–4757.

161. Rosenberg SA, Yang JC, Schwartzentruber DJ, et al. Immunologic and therapeutic evaluation of a synthetic peptide vaccine for the treatment of patients with metastatic melanoma. *Nat Med* 1998;4:321–327.

162. Stoter G, Aamdal S, Rodenhuis S, et al. Sequential administration of recombinant human interleukin-2 and dacarbazine in metastatic melanoma: a multicenter phase II study. *J Clin Oncol* 1991;9:1687–1691.

163. Dummer R, Gore ME, Hancock BW, et al. A multicenter phase II clinical trial using dacarbazine and continuous infusion interleukin-2 for metastatic melanoma. Clinical data and immunomonitoring. *Cancer* 1995;75:1038.

164. Richards JM, Gale D, Mehta N, Lestingi T. Combination of chemotherapy with interleukin-2 and interferon alfa for the treatment of metastatic melanoma. *J Clin Oncol* 1999;17:651–657.

165. Legha SS, Buzaid AC: Role of recombinant interleukin-2 in combination with interferon-alfa and chemotherapy in the treatment of advanced melanoma. *Semin Oncol* 1993;2[Suppl 9]:27–32.

166. Demchak PA, Mier JW, Robert NJ, et al. Interleukin-2 and high-dose cisplatin in patients with metastatic melanoma: a pilot study. *J Clin Oncol* 1991:9:1821–1830.

167. Atkins BM, O'Boyle KR, Sosman JA, et al. Multi-institutional phase II trial of intensive combination chemoimmunotherapy for metastatic melanoma. *J Clin Oncol* 1994;12:1553–1560.

168. Antoine EC, Benhammouda A, Bernard A, et al. Salpetiere Hospital Experience with biochemotherapy in metastatic melanoma. *Cancer J Sci Am* 1997;3:S16.

169. Legha SS, Sigrid R, Eton O, et al. Development and results of biochemotherapy in metastatic melanoma: the University of Texas M. D. Anderson Cancer Center Experience. *Cancer J Sci Am* 1997;3:S9–S15.

170. Mousseau M, Khayat D, Benhammouda A, et al. Feasibility study of chemo-immunotherapy (Ch-IM) with cisplatin (CDDP) interleukin-2 (IL-2) and interferon alpha 2a (IFNa) on 14 melanoma brain metastases patients (pts). *Proc ASCO* 1997;16:492a.

171. Keilholz U, Conradt C, Legha SS, et al. Results of interleukin-2-based treatment in advanced melanoma: a case record-based analysis of 631 patients. *J Clin Oncol* 1998;16:2921–2929.

172. Allen IE, Kupelnick B, Kumashiro M, et al. Efficacy of interleukin-2 in the treatment of metastatic melanoma: systematic review and meta-analysis. *Cancer Therapeutics* 1998;1:168.

173. Legha SA, Ring S, Eton O, et al. Development of a biochemotherapy regimen with concurrent administration of cisplatin, vinblastine, dacarbazine, interferon alfa and interleukin-2 for patients with metastatic melanoma. *J Clin Oncol* 1998;16:1752–1759.

174. McDermott DF, Mier JW, Lawrence DP, et al. A phase I pilot trial of concurrent biochemotherapy with cisplatin, vinblastine, dacarbazine (CVD), interleukin-2 (IL-2) and interferon alpha-2b (IFN) in patients with metastatic melanoma. *Proc ASCO* 1998;17:507.

175. O'Day SJ, Boasberg P, Guo M, et al. Phase II trial of concurrent biochemotherapy (c-BC) with decrescendo interleukin-2 (d-IL-2), tamoxifen (T), and G-CSF support in patients with metastatic melanoma (MM). *Proc ASCO* 1997;16:490.

176. Keilholz U, Scheibenbogen C, Brossart P, et al. Interleukin-2 based immunotherapy and chemoimmunotherapy in metastatic melanoma. *Recent Results Cancer Res* 1995:139:383–390.

177. O'Day SJ, Martin M, Boasberg P, et al. Escalating doses of tamoxifen in a phase I/II trial of concurrent biochemotherapy with decrescendo interleukin-2, and filgrastim (G-CSF) support in patients with metastatic melanoma. *Proc ASCO* 1998;17:1957.

178. Flaherty LE, Robinson W, Redman BG, et al. A phase II study of dacarbazine and cisplatin in combination with outpatient administered interleukin-2 in metastatic malignant melanoma. *Cancer* 1993;71:3520–3525.

179. Flaherty LE, Atkins M, Sosman J, et al. Randomized Phase II Trial of Chemotherapy and outpatient biotherapy with interleukin-2 and interferon alpha (IFN) in metastatic melanoma. *Proc Ann Meet Am Soc Clin Oncol* 18:1999; 536a.

180. Thompson JA, Gold PJ, Markowitz DR, et al. Updated analysis of an outpatient chemoimmunotherapy regimen for treating metastatic melanoma. *Cancer J Sci Am* 1997;3:S29–S34.

181. Atzpodien J, Lopez Hánninen E, Kirchner H, et al. Chemoimmunotherapy of advanced malignant melanoma: sequential administration of subcutaneous interleukin-2 and interferon- after intravenous dacarbazine and carboplatin or intravenous dacarbazine, cisplatin, carmustine and tamoxifen. *Eur J Cancer* 1995;31A:876–881.

182. Johnston SRD, Constenla DO, Moore J, et al. Randomized phase II trial of BCDT (BCNU, cisplatin, dacarbazine and tamoxifen) with or without interferon alpha and interleukin-2 (IL-2) in patients with metastatic melanoma. *Proc ASCO* 1997;16:490.

183. Rosenberg SA, Yang JC, Schwartzentruber DJ, et al. Prospective randomized trial of the treatment of patients with metastatic melanoma using chemotherapy with cisplatin, dacarbazine, and tamoxifen alone or in combination with interleukin-2 and interferon alfa-2b. *J Clin Oncol* 1999;17:968–975.

184. Keilholz U, Stoter G, Punt CJA, et al. Recombinant interleukin-2 based treatments for advanced melanoma: the experience of the European organization for research and treatment of cancer melanoma cooperative group. *Cancer J Sci Am* 1997;3:S22–S28.

185. Atkins MB. Biochemotherapy for Metastatic Melanoma: The Rationale for the Intergroup Phase III Trial, *Biotherapy Consideration for Oncology Nurses* 1997;3:1–4.

186. Schmittel A, Keilholz U, Max R, Thiel E, Scheibenbogen C. Induction of tyrosinase-reactive T cells by treatment with dacarbazine, cisplatin, interferon-alpha ± interleukin-2 in patients with metastatic melanoma. *Int J Cancer* 1999;80:39–43.

187. Scheibenbogen C, Goey SH, Proebstle T, Eggermont A, Keilholz U. Association of increased neopterin levels with response to therapy with CDDP and IFN alpha/IL-2 but not with IFN alpha/IL-2 alone in melanoma. *Anti-Cancer Treatment Sixth International Congress* 1996:109.

188. Anderson C, Buzaid A, Sussman J, et al. Nitric oxide (NO) and neopterin levels and clinical response in stage III melanoma patients receiving concurrent biochemotherapy. *Melanoma Res* 1998;8:149–155.

189. Buzaid AC, Ali-Osman F, Akande N, et al. DNA damage in peripheral blood mononuclear cells correlates with response to biochemotherapy in melanoma. *Melanoma Res* 1998;8:145–148.

190. Bleehan NM, Newlands ES, Lee SM, et al. Cancer research campaign Phase II trial of temozolomide in metastatic melanoma. *J Clin Oncol* 1995;13:910–913.

191. Buzaid AC, Ross M, Legha S, et al. Histologic response to preoperative concurrent biochemotherapy with cisplatin (C), vinblastine (V), DTIC (D), IL-2 and interferon-alfa-2a (IFN) in melanoma patients (pts) with local-regional disease. Anti-Cancer Treatment, Sixth International Congress, 1997:106.

192. Buzaid AC, Bedikian A, Eton O, et al. Importance of major histologic response in melanoma patients (pts) with local regional metastases (LRM) receiving neoadjuvant biochemotherapy. *Proc ASCO* 1997;16:A1808.

193. Miller DM, Jones D, Partin ML, et al. Effective interleukin-2 based adjuvant therapy for high risk malignant melanoma patients. *Proc ASCO* 1998;17:A1954.

194. Richards JM, Barker E, Latta J, et al. Phase I study of weekly 24-hour infusions of recombinant human IL-2. *J Natl Cancer Inst* 1998;80:1325–1328.

195. Atzpodien J, Korfer A, Evers P, et al. Low dose subcutaneous IL-2 in advanced human malignancy. A phase II outpatient study. *Mol Biother* 1990;2:18–26.

196. Hanninen EL, Korfer A, Hadam M, et al. Biological monitoring of low-dose IL-2 in humans: soluble IL-2 receptors, cytokines and cell surface phenotypes. *Cancer Res* 1991;51:6312–6316.

197. Tagliaferri P, Barile C, Caraglia M, et al. Daily low-dose subcutaneous recombinant interleukin-2 by alternate weekly administration: anti-tumor activity and immunomodulatory effects. *Am J Clin Oncol* 1998;21:48–53.

198. Budd GT, Murthy S, Finke J, et al. Phase I trial of high-dose bolus interleukin-2 and interferon-alpha-2a in patients with metastatic malignancy. *J Clin Oncol* 1992;10:804–809.

199. Lee KH, Talpaz M, Legha S, et al. Combination treatment of IL-2 and alfa2 a in patients with advanced melanoma. *Proc Am Soc Clin Oncol* 1989;8:290.

200. Mittelman A, Hubuman M, Puccio C, et al. A phase I study of recombinant IL-2 and alpha-interferon-2 A in patients with renal cell cancer, colorectal cancer and malignant melanoma. *Cancer* 1990;66:664.

201. Oldham RK, Blumenschein G, Schwartzberg L, et al. Combination biotherapy utilizing IL-2 and alfa interferon in patients with advanced cancer: a National Biotherapy Study Group trial. *Mol Biother* 1992;4:4–9.

202. Hidalgo OF, Aramendia JM, Alonso G, et al. Results of two sequential phase II studies of interleukin-2 (IL-2) in metastatic renal cell carcinoma and melanoma: high-dose continuous intravenous IL-2 infusion and subcutaneous IL-2 administration in combination with alpha interferon. *Rev Med Univ Navarra* 1996;40:6–12.

203. Gause BL, Snozl M, Kopp WC, et al. Phase I study of SC administered IL-2 in combination with IFN Alfa-2a in patients with advanced cancer. *J Clin Oncol* 1996;4:2234–2241.

204. Nasi ML, Frank SJ, Myers M, et al. Treatment with daily low dose subcutaneous IL-2 followed by monoclonal antibody R-24 against GD3 ganglioside in patients with metastatic melanoma. *Proc Annu Meet Am Soc Clin Oncol* 1997;16:A1770.

205. Richards JM, Gale D, Costello M, Smernoff N, Michel J. Ultra-low dose interleukin-2 following chemotherapy for metastatic melanoma. *Proc ASCO* 1996;15:1576A.

206. Andreas P, Cupissol D, Guillot B, Avril MF, Dreno B. Subcutaneous interleukin-2 and interferon-alpha therapy associated with cisplatin monotherapy in the treatment of metastatic melanoma. *Eur J Dermatol* 1998;8:235–239.

207. Hoffman R, Muller I, Neuber K, et al. Risk and outcome of meta-

static malignant melanoma patients receiving DTIC, cisplatin, BCNU and tamoxifen followed by immunotherapy with interleukin 2 and interferon alpha 2a. *Br J Cancer* 1998;78:1076–1080.

208. Honeycutt P, Wiemann M, Bury M, et al. Phase II trial of BCNU, DTIC, cisplatin, tamoxifen and outpatient interleukin-2 and interferon-alpha in the treatment of metastatic melanoma. *Proc ASCO* 1997;16:A1819.

209. Romanini A, Vezzani S, Zucchi V, et al. Recmombinant interleukin-2 and chemo-hormonotherapy in metastatic melanoma (MM): a phase II study. *Proc AACR* 1996;37:A1184.

210. Guida M, Latorre A, Mastria A, et al. Subcutaneous recombinant interleukin-2 plus chemotherapy with cisplatin and dacarbazine in metastatic melanoma. *Eur J Cancer* 1996;32A:730–733.

211. Bernengo MG, Doveil GC, Bertero M, et al. Low-dose integrated chemoimmuno-hormonotherapy with cisplatin, subcutaneous interleukin-2, alpha-interferon, and tamoxifen for advanced metastatic melanoma. *Melanoma Res* 1996;6:257.

212. Atkins MB, Gollob JA. Chemotherapy and cytokine-based immunotherapy for high-risk and metastatic melanoma. *Adv Oncol* 1999;15:22–29.

3.3

INTERLEUKIN-2: CLINICAL APPLICATIONS

Renal Cell Carcinoma

JAMES CHUNG-YIN YANG

Renal cell carcinoma (RCC) was diagnosed in approximately 25,000 patients in the United States in 1999, and its incidence has been increasing since 1994 (1). Metastatic disease develops in approximately 50% of patients (2). Metastatic RCC is a clinical entity that has been notoriously difficult to treat with cytotoxic chemotherapy or hormonal manipulation. In a review by Elson of 610 patients enrolled in Eastern Cooperative Oncology Group (ECOG) trials of therapeutic agents for advanced RCC (3), five prognostic factors that influenced overall patient survival were identified. These factors included number of metastatic sites, previous chemotherapy, performance status, weight loss, and time from diagnosis to study entry. The median survival of these patients was less than 7 months; a subset of 113 patients who possessed a combination of the most favorable prognostic factors had a 2-year survival rate of only 24%. Similar prognostic factors and overall results were described by Maldazys and deKernion (4). In a review of chemotherapy trials by Yagoda in 1989, initial response rates (RRs) [partial responses (PRs) and complete responses (CRs)] for 39 agents studied in more than 70 publications ranged from 0% to 19%, with a median RR of 2% (5). A study of patients treated with paclitaxel (Taxol) who had longer-term follow-ups available demonstrated that the survival of patients at 2 years was 8% (6). Despite these data, which document the poor prognoses of patients with metastatic RCC, this malignancy possesses a highly emphasized reputation for showing spontaneous regression (7). These anecdotes are often associated with major surgery (such as nephrectomy), sepsis, or other possible triggering events. Several series of patients undergoing nephrectomy indicate a spontaneous regression rate of approximately 1% exists. In one series, patients with excellent performance statuses underwent nephrectomy and maintained meticulous and frequent follow-ups; a 4% postnephrectomy rate of tumor regression was observed in the absence of therapy (8). Of the four regressing patients, only two experienced regressions of substantial durations, and the sole patient with an ongoing regression experienced life-threatening postoperative sepsis. The transient nature of these spontaneous regressions was also described in a randomized, placebo-controlled study on the efficacy of interferon-γ (IFN-γ) in RCC (9). Although the 6% response rate of the placebo arm is often cited as evidence of the frequency of spontaneous regression of RCC, this value represents a singularly high frequency for this phenomenon; five of the six regressing patients went on to relapse within 13 months. Thus, although spontaneous regression of RCC undoubtedly occurs, its true incidence is estimated to be between 1% and 4%, and regressions are rarely durable or of real clinical benefit. The fact that such occurrences are observed has led to the presumptions that the immune system is responsible and that RCC is a tumor of high immunogenicity. This idea was supported by early evidence that IFN-α could induce regression of RCC in some patients. However, responses to this agent are often of low frequency and modest duration (10).

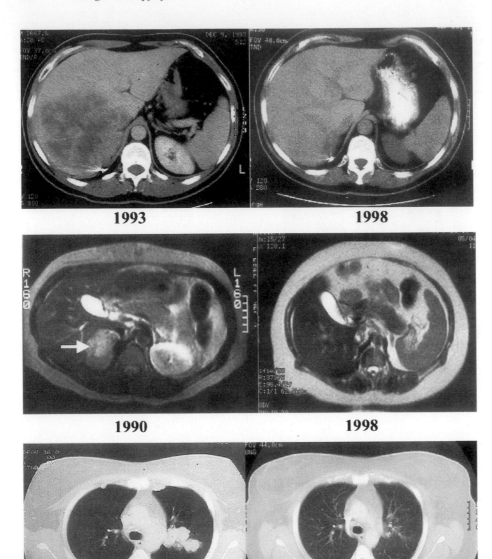

1993   1998

1990   1998

1992   1998

FIGURE 1. Durable complete responses to interleukin-2 in three patients with metastatic renal carcinoma at various sites. Left figures are pretreatment and right-sided figures are the last follow-up evaluation. Patients have responded with lung metastases, liver metastases, and a local recurrence site, as well as at all sites not shown, and remain in ongoing complete response at last evaluation.

In 1976, a glycoprotein with multiple immunostimulatory activities was identified (11). This product of lymphocytes, interleukin-2 (IL-2), included among its actions the generation of nonspecific tumoricidal activity in lymphoid cells [lymphokine-activated killer (LAK) cell activity] and T-cell growth-promoting activity (12,13). In preclinical animal models, this glycoprotein was able to cause the regression of a wide array of established tumors when given alone or with *in vitro*–generated antitumor cells (14–16). Clinical trials begun in 1983 with purified IL-2 derived from stimulated peripheral blood lymphocytes were restricted by drug supply (17). With the advent of recombinant IL-2 in 1984, clinical trials proceeded to higher doses and more prolonged administration schedules, which animal studies indicated would be more effective. The initial regimen used repeated bolus therapy every 8 hours. Animal experiments also predicted that IL-2 would be most effective when administered with LAK cells generated *in vitro* (18);

therefore, after a rapid escalation of IL-2 to maximum-tolerated dose, LAK cells were added to bolus IL-2 therapy. After treating patients with tumors of many different histologic types, those with RCC and melanoma showed more striking and frequent tumor regressions (19). Later, more extensive studies with IL-2 alone indicated that patients with RCC had significant RRs without LAK cells (20). Since then, many confirmatory studies support the conclusions that patients with RCC can attain complete and (what appear to be) permanent regressions of metastatic disease and that RCC is one of the most responsive tumors to IL-2–based immunotherapy (Fig. 1).

BOLUS INTRAVENOUS INTERLEUKIN-2

Initial experiences with IL-2 involved rapidly infused boluses of IL-2 administered every 8 hours to the maximum-tolerated

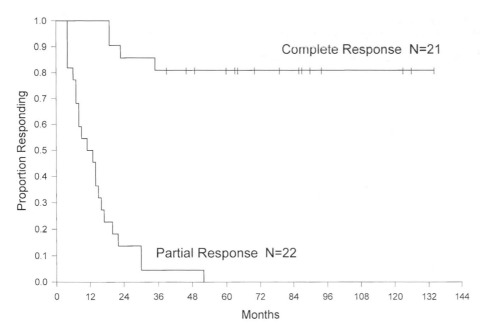

FIGURE 2. Actuarial curve of renal cancer patients completely responding to high-dose interleukin-2. Durations of response are measured from the start of therapy. The majority of completely responding patients have not relapsed (median follow-up is 7 years) and no patients have relapsed after 3 years. (From Rosenberg SA et al. Durability of complete responses in patients with metastatic cancer treated with high-dose interleukin-2. *Ann Surg* 1998;228:307–319, with permission.)

number of doses. This schedule and route resulted in high peak levels of IL-2 that fell to undetectable levels just before they were replenished by subsequent doses (17,21). Phase I dose-escalation studies showed that although large single doses of IL-2 (up to 6,000,000 IU per kg) could be administered once a week, when they were administered every 8 hours, the maximum tolerated dose was 600,000–720,000 IU per kg (with the number of consecutive doses tolerated ranging from seven to ten). This cycle was designated as a cycle of therapy and was repeated after 7–10 days of rest, with a pair of such cycles constituting a course of therapy. Treatment was limited by a host of toxic manifestations. In the initial National Cancer Institute (NCI) Surgery Branch experience (20), 1 of 21 patients with RCC exhibited a CR to treatment (that patient remained an ongoing complete responder 14 years later). An update of this experience (including 149 patients with RCC) shows an RR of 20%, with 7% CRs and 13% PRs (22). A larger experience derived from NCI and the IL-2 Cooperative Study Group reported a 7% CR and 8% PR rate for 255 patients with RCC who were given high-dose bolus IL 2 (23,24). The other striking factor in these studies is durability of the CRs. In the cooperative group study, the median response duration was 54 months for all responders. Patients who achieved CRs exhibited response durations of 7 to 107 or more months with few relapses that occurred doing so within the first 19 months. The NCI Surgery Branch reported that 81% of completely responding patients remained in ongoing CR (with no interval therapy or maintenance therapy) with a median follow-up of 7 years (range, 3 to 11 years) (Fig. 2) (25). A summary of literature on the treatment of RCC with bolus IL-2 alone is presented in Table 1.

Patients in these studies generally had an ECOG performance status of 0 or 1, were free of central nervous system (CNS) involvement, and were screened for normal hepatic, cardiac, pulmonary, and renal function. During therapy, approximately one-half of these patients required either low-dose dopamine or phenylephrine pressor support for oliguria or

hypotension. Although initial reports of high-dose bolus IL-2 described treatment-related mortalities of up to 4%, increasing experience has lowered mortality rates to less than 1%, with one series reporting up to 809 consecutive patients who were treated with high-dose IL-2 with no mortality (27). Only one randomized prospective study has been undertaken to determine whether toxicity incurred during high-dose bolus therapy is necessary to achieve optimal responses (28,29). This study compared 720,000 IU per kg of IL-2 administered every 8 hours by intravenous (i.v.) bolus to 72,000 IU per kg administered by the same route and schedule. The dose of 72,000 IU per kg was chosen as the highest dose that could be administered without inducing the same precipitous toxicities as high-dose IL-2 and avoiding intensive care unit support and use of vasopressors. Intermediate doses allowed the administration of a few more consecutive doses but induced exactly the same range of physiologic changes and side effects as high-dose IL-2. Although this study is scheduled to reach full accrual in 1999, an interim report in 1998 noted that 116 patients given 720,000 IU per kg of IL-2 tolerated a median of 12 total doses of IL-2 per course (compared with 27 total doses for the 112 patients receiving the lower dose). Patients who received low-dose IL-2 also showed significantly less thrombocytopenia, pulmonary toxicity, malaise, disorientation, and hypotension than patients who received high-dose IL-2. Vasopressor support was required in 43% of high-dose courses, compared with 4% of low-dose courses (although no treatment-related mortality was encountered in either arm). With a median follow-up of longer than 4 years, interim analysis shows nine CRs and 13 PRs (19% RR) among patients given high-dose bolus IL-2; five CRs and six PRs (10% RR) occurred among patients given low-dose IL-2 (p = .06). Overall survival and response duration data are not mature and are crucial to the final interpretation of this study.

A simple RR of 20% in patients with RCC treated with bolus IL-2 therapy is not significantly different from RRs of patients treated with various chemotherapeutic agents consid-

TABLE 1. THERAPY WITH INTERLEUKIN-2 (IL-2) ALONE

Author (Reference)	IL-2 Dose ($\times 10^{-6}$ IU/m^2)	Route	n	RR (%)	CR (%)	Comments
Rosenberg (25)	25.2 q8h[a]	Bolus i.v.	227	19	9	81% of CR ongoing at median follow-up of 7 yr
Cytokine Working Group (23,24)	21.0 q8h[a]	Bolus i.v.	71	17	7	Median response duration of 53 mo
Yang (29)	2.5 q8h × 5 days	Bolus i.v.	112	10	4	Randomized trial
Bukowski (26)	60.0 t.i.w.[a]	Bolus i.v.	41	12	2	—
Gold (32)	18–22 qd × 5 d, then 6–8 qd × 10 d	c.i.v.	47	13	6	—
von der Maase (33)	18.0 qd[a]	c.i.v.	51	16	4	—
Escudier (34)	24.0 qd × 2 d/wk	c.i.v.	104	19	4	—
Negrier (35)	18.0 qd[a]	c.i.v.	138	7	1	Randomized study vs. IL-2 + IFN or IFN alone
Lissoni (40)	3.0 b.i.d. 5 d/wk[b]	s.c.	91	23	2	
Buter (42)	9.0 qd × 5 d/wk, then 4.5 qd 5 d/wk[b]	s.c.	47	19	4	Many patients with cardiovascular disease
Tourani (43)	4.5 b.i.d. × 5 days/wk, then 4.5 b.i.d. × 2 and qd × 3/wk[b]	s.c.	39	18	3	—
Yang (29)	8.8 qd × 5 d/wk, then 4.4 qd × 5 d/wk	s.c.	53	11	6	Randomized trial

c.i.v., continuous intravenous infusion; CR, complete response; IFN, interferon; RR, response rate.
[a]Administered to patient tolerance.
[b]Fixed dose not adjusted for patient size. For comparison, dose here calculated for 2.0 m^2 pt.

ered to be of no benefit in RCC. The value of bolus IL-2 in RCC lies in the quality of some responses. One-third to one-half of patients responding to IL-2 achieve CRs and the majority of these patients have never relapsed. Rosenberg et al. noted that none of their 21 completely responding patients experienced a relapse after 3 years(with 3- to 11-year follow-up). Despite a modest overall RR of IL-2, the long-term CR rate of RCC to bolus IL-2 compares favorably with that of metastatic breast cancer and multiagent chemotherapy (30). PRs to IL-2 can last as long as several years, but nearly all eventually relapse (25). Therefore, efforts to improve the efficacy of IL-2 therapy in RCC must preserve and improve on this durable CR rate that, in the absence of randomized, controlled survival studies, represents the predominant evidence supporting the efficacy of this drug.

INTERLEUKIN-2 ADMINISTERED BY CONTINUOUS INTRAVENOUS INFUSION

In 1987, a report by West et al. indicated that IL-2 administered by continuous i.v. infusion (c.i.v.) over 3 to 5 days in conjunction with LAK cells, had antitumor activity comparable to high-dose bolus IL-2 and LAK cells but was associated with less toxicity (31). Although only six patients with RCC were included in this initial study, three of them experienced clinical responses. At IL-2 doses ranging from 6 to 42×10^6 IU per m^2 per day (7,000–50,000 IU/kg/h), universal fever, fatigue, a 35.0% incidence of hypotension, and 2.5% treatment-related mortality occurred. These results are well within the range of toxicities reported in studies of high-dose bolus IL-2, yet c.i.v. IL-2 has been widely pursued as a means of decreasing IL-2 toxicity. Results of subsequent studies of c.i.v. IL-2 are shown in Table 1. These studies indicate that the cumulative maximum tolerated dose (MTD) of IL-2 administered is less when

it is delivered by c.i.v. instead of bolus infusion. In addition, despite this difference in MTDs, the array and severity of toxicities seen with c.i.v. were not different from those observed with high-dose bolus IL-2. Therefore, only the relative efficacies of these two regimens (at MTD) have bearing on their clinical utility. Weiss et al. conducted a randomized trial comparing these two regimens in patients receiving LAK cells (36). The 46 patients randomized to LAK cells and c.i.v. IL-2 received 18.0 to 22.5×10^6 IU per m^2 per day; those randomized to LAK cells and bolus IL-2 received 600,000 IU per kg per dose every 8 hours (approximately 60×10^6 IU/m^2/day). The only significant differences in major toxicities were that more infections occurred in patients receiving c.i.v. IL-2, whereas more thrombocytopenia occurred in patients receiving bolus IL-2. Fifteen percent of patients receiving c.i.v. IL-2 and LAK cells responded (two CRs, five PRs), versus 20% of patients given bolus IL-2 and LAK cells (three CRs, six PRs; difference not significant). If the contribution of LAK cells to clinical response is small, insignificant, or equivalent in the two arm, this study suggests that at their respective MTDs, c.i.v. and bolus IL-2 are similar in toxicity and efficacy. What is unclear is whether the lower doses of c.i.v. IL-2 used in other studies to reduce toxicity preserve the efficacy of higher doses of c.i.v. IL-2. The nonrandomized data in Table 1 suggest that some of these regimens using low-dose IL-2 may be of inferior therapeutic efficacy.

SUBCUTANEOUS INTERLEUKIN-2

The need for frequent dosing when IL-2 is administered by i.v. delivery route led many investigators to try daily subcutaneous administration to maintain low levels of IL-2 and allow therapy to be administered in outpatient settings. Early dose escalation studies by Atzpodien et al. (37) and Whitehead et al. (38)

TABLE 2. THERAPY WITH INTERLEUKIN-2 (IL-2) AND LYMPHOKINE-ACTIVATED KILLER (LAK) CELLS

Author (Reference)	IL-2 Dose (x 10⁻⁶ IU/m²)	Route	Median LAK Cells Administered (x 10⁻¹⁰)	n	RR (%)	CR (%)	Comments
Rosenberg (45)	25.2 q8h	Bolus i.v.	10	72	35	11	—
Fisher (46)	21.0 q8h	Bolus i.v.	7	35	14	6	—
Weiss (36)	21.0 q8h	Bolus i.v.	14	46	20	7	Randomized for c.i.v. vs. bolus IL-2
Parkinson (47)	18.0 qd	c.i.v.	9	47	9	4	Prepheresis IL-2 administered by bolus i.v.
Negrier (48)	18.0 qd	c.i.v.	1	51	27	10	—
Dillman (49,50)	18.0 qd	c.i.v.	6–30	46	15	N/A	Data from five protocols
Thompson (51)	5.2–15.6 qd	c.i.v.	18	76	22	8	—
Weiss (36)	18–23 qd	c.i.v.	14	48	15	4	Randomized for c.i.v. vs. bolus IL-2

c.i.v., continuous intravenous infusion; CR, complete response; N/A, not applicable; RR, response rate.
Note: All IL-2 units converted to IU (1.0 Hoffman-LaRoche/Biologic Response Modifier Program unit = 2.6 IU and 1 Cetus unit = 6 IU).

described modest toxicity that usually consisted of local injection site inflammation and constitutional symptoms. Mild renal dysfunction and thyroid abnormalities were also observed, as well as the development of anti–IL-2 antibodies of unknown clinical significance (37,38). As doses were escalated between 2 and 30 million IU per m² per day in one or two divided doses administered subcutaneously for 5 or 6 days a week, appropriate alterations in peripheral blood phenotypes and natural killer cell activity were seen. The once-a-day, 5-days-per-week dosing used by Whitehead appeared to permit a higher MTD but resulted in no major tumor regressions in the 14 evaluable patients reported. Adzpodien's twice-a-day, 6-days-per-week dose schedule administered over 4 weeks could not deliver as much IL-2 per day or per week as the alternative regimen, but one of the six patients with RCC experienced a PR. Stein et al. (39) used approximately 1.8 million IU once a day for 5 days per week and reported two of nine patients achieving PRs. Lissoni et al. (40) administered IL-2 for 2 days at 9 million IU per m² per day followed by one-fifth of that dose 5 days per week for 6 weeks, obtaining four PRs in 14 patients. One regimen adopted by other investigators was first reported by Sleijfer et al. (41) and consisted of once-a-day dosing for 5 days per week (initially at 18 million IU per dose for the first week, followed by 9 million IU per dose for the next 5 weeks, without adjustment for body weight). Toxicity was typically modest, with elderly patients and patients with major cardiovascular disease receiving this regimen. Of 27 patients reported, one 76-year-old patient died of a myocardial infarction and cerebral ischemia. Six of 26 evaluable patients (23%) experienced major tumor regression (two CRs, four PRs) lasting from 2 to 19+ months. An update of this experience abbreviated the regimen to 4 weeks and reported a 19% RR (42) with two CRs and seven PRs among 47 patients. Pharmacokinetic studies of a subcutaneous regimen such as this one demonstrate that detectable levels of IL-2 are maintained throughout most of the day, but peak serum levels of IL-2 rarely exceed 5 ng per mL (in marked contrast to the peak serum levels greater than 300 ng per mL observed with high-dose bolus IL-2) (29). The relative efficacy of this subcutaneous regimen is currently being tested in a randomized prospective comparison to high-dose bolus IL-2, as well as against the low-dose i.v. regimen. Yang and Rosenberg (29) reported that the toxicity of the subcutaneous regimen was substantially less than that of high-dose i.v. IL-2,

especially with respect to hypotension, thrombocytopenia, pulmonary toxicity, and disorientation. High-dose IL-2 achieved four CRs and five PRs in 56 patients (16% RR), whereas three CRs and three PRs were observed in 53 patients given subcutaneous IL-2 (11% RR). This difference is not statistically significant, and no difference in survival rates occurred, but this study is ongoing.

Clinical studies of subcutaneous IL-2 show that it can achieve partial and complete regressions of tumors in patients with advanced RCC; for patients with major medical problems, such as cardiovascular disease, it may represent the only option for trying IL-2. Nevertheless, a major condition for using low-dose IL-2 in healthy patients with good performance statuses should be that its efficacy is equal or superior to that of high-dose IL-2. Such assessments should also carefully evaluate completeness and durability of responses, because such responses represent the major reason why IL-2 benefits patients with RCC.

INTERLEUKIN-2 ADMINISTERED WITH ADOPTIVE CELLULAR TRANSFER

Preclinical animal studies indicated that the addition of LAK cells to IL-2 markedly improved the antitumor activity over a range of IL-2 doses and against a variety of murine tumors (15,18). *In vitro* studies of human LAK cells indicated that tumors of virtually all histologic types (including RCC) were susceptible to LAK cell lysis (44). Based on these findings, many early clinical protocols included LAK cells administered with IL-2. Although several phase 2 trials suggested a higher RR exists for LAK cells and IL-2 compared with historical controls receiving IL-2 alone, other studies could not confirm this (Table 2) (45–50). The largest prospective randomized study involved 87 evaluable patients randomized to receive high-dose bolus IL-2 alone or the same IL-2 dose with LAK cells (45). Despite receiving a median of 10¹¹ LAK cells per course, no statistically significant improvement in the RR of patients randomized to receive LAK cells occurred; survival after a median follow-up of 63 months was not different (*p* >.5). An independent smaller study by Law et al. also failed to demonstrate a benefit in RR or overall survival with LAK cell administration (52). No evidence exists to demonstrate that patients with advanced RCC receive significant benefit from the administration of LAK cells; therefore, due to the expense and complexity of generating LAK cells, their use cannot be recommended.

In the treatment of melanoma, nonrandomized studies on the use of adoptive transfer of tumor infiltrating lymphocytes (TILs) expanded from patients' autologous tumors suggest they have benefits over using IL-2 alone (53). That the overall RR when TILs are added to IL-2 is nearly double that of historical RRs to IL-2 alone supports this contention; perhaps more compelling, some responders include patients who had recently received IL-2 alone and failed to respond. Furthermore, T cells with specific reactivity to autologous tumors can be found in the majority of TIL cultures from melanoma. Such data have led to exploration of TILs from RCC in combination therapy with IL-2. However, T cells with specific reactivity to autologous tumors are rare in RCC TIL (54). Figlin and Belldegrun have used RCC TIL in combination with IL-2 (and, in many cases, IFN-α) and report overall RRs that appear higher than IL-2 alone (55). This result has not yet been reproduced, however, and it is not clear if the improvement in RR is attributable to the administration of TIL. These questions should be investigated in randomized clinical trials, which have been undertaken.

COMBINATION THERAPY WITH INTERLEUKIN-2 AND INTERFERON-α

IL-2 and IFN-α represent the two biologic agents with reproducible activity in the treatment of RCC. Although the response frequency of either agent alone is low, preclinical animal models have suggested that combining these agents could result in synergistic therapeutic effects (56). Early patient studies included several combination regimens that seemed to have impressive RRs in the uncontrolled phase 2 setting. In different studies, IL-2 has been administered by i.v. bolus, continuous infusion, or subcutaneous injection, whereas IFN-α has been administered intravenously, subcutaneously, or intramuscularly. The IFNs

selected have included primarily IFN-α-2a and -2b, which are considered together and do not result in significant differences in efficacy or toxicity. The studies cited in Table 3 include a number of widely differing regimens and display RRs that vary greatly and overlap those reported for similar regimens using only IL-2. The i.v. regimens have been exemplified by a study from the NCI Surgery Branch in which escalating doses of IL-2 and IFN-α were given by periodic bolus dosing to the maximum-tolerated amount. The initial short-term RR for the combination of cytokines was 31% (57); a later report showed that this rate was 28% for a larger group of patients. The combination therapy seemed associated with increased CNS toxicity and myocarditis, and survival was not improved compared with an historical NCI Surgery Branch experience with IL-2 alone (58). Several randomized studies are included in Table 3. A large three-arm multiinstitutional trial in France reported by Negrier randomized patients to receive high-dose continuous infusion IL-2, with or without a modest dose of IFN or a greater dose of IFN alone (35). With 425 patients randomized and a median follow-up of 39 months, overall RRs for IL-2, IFN, or both agents were 7%, 7%, and 19%, respectively (p = .01, favoring both agents). Event-free survival at 1 year also significantly favored the combination, but an analysis of overall survival revealed no differences existed between any of the groups (p = .55). A smaller trial by Jayson using low-dose subcutaneous IL-2 and subcutaneous IFN also failed to demonstrate benefits for the combination by any parameters (63). These studies are notable for RRs for IL-2 alone that appear lower than those described for higher-dose regimens of IL-2. A third randomized study by Henriksson (which included tamoxifen in one arm and IL-2, IFN, and tamoxifen in the other), showed no difference in survival between these two regimens; it did not report overall RRs (64). A fourth randomized trial by Boccardo et al. (68) administered either high-dose, c.i.v. IL-2 for 4 days or low-dose IFN three times per week, or both regimens combined. In 66 randomized patients, the response to IL-2 alone was 23%, the response to IFN alone was 9%, and the RR for the combination

TABLE 3. THERAPY WITH INTERLEUKIN-2 (IL-2) AND INTERFERON-α (IFN-α)

Author (Reference)	IL-2 Dose (x 10⁻⁶ IU/m²)	Route	IFN-α (x 10⁻⁶ U/m²)	n	RR (%)	CR (%)	Comments
Marincola (58)	2.6–15.6 q8h	Bolus i.v.	3–6 qd or q8h i.v.	75	28	16	Increased toxicity vs. IL-2 alone
Taneja (59)	6 qd × 4 d	c.i.v.	6 b.i.w., s.c.	52	25	8	—
Kruit (60)	18 qd × 5 d	c.i.v.	5 q.d. × 5 d i.m.	68	34	13	Patients also received LAK cells
Negrier (48)	18 qd × 5 d	c.i.v.	6 t.i.w., s.c.	140	19	4	Randomized study vs. IL-2 and IFN alone
Bukowski (61)	9 qd × 5 d	c.i.v.	10 t.i.w., s.c.	36	17	8	—
Ravaud (62)	3.6 qd × 5 d	s.c.	5 t.i.w., s.c.	38	18	3	—
Jayson (63)	9 qd × 5 dᵃ	s.c.	9 t.i.w., s.c.	30	0	0	Randomized vs. IL-2
Henriksson (64)	14.4–4.8/d	s.c.	3–6 t.i.w., s.c.	65	N/A	8	Randomized study—all patients also received tamoxifen
Dutcher (65)	5 q8h × 3, then qd	s.c.	5 t.i.w., s.c.	47	17	4	Poor response duration
Atzpodien (66)	20 t.i.w. × 1 wk, then 5 t.i.w. × 2 wk	s.c.	6 q.w. or t.i.w., s.c.	152	25	6	—
Vogelzang (67)	6 qd × 4 d/wkᵃ	s.c.	9 b.i.w., s.c.	42	12	0	—

c.i.v., continuous intravenous infusion; CR, complete response; LAK, lymphokine-activated killer cell; N/A, not applicable; RR, response rate.
ᵃFixed dose not adjusted for patient size. For comparison, dose calculated for 2.0 m² pt.

of both was 9% (difference was not significant). For any randomized study of IL-2, large numbers of patients and long-term follow-up are needed because only a minority of patients substantially benefit from the therapy, and benefits consist of long-term durable responses. Unlike chemotherapy, no evidence exists that the agent markedly benefitting these few patients is having a lesser benefit on other patients treated. Therefore, one would not expect a change in median survival to occur; furthermore, analyses performed with less than 3-year median follow-ups may not identify that minority of patients who are potentially cured by IL-2–based therapy. This problem has significantly affected interpretations of every randomized trial of IL-2–based therapy performed. Even in the absence of such long-term data, experience with IL-2 and IFN combinations has varied, and results overlap extensively with results attained with IL-2 alone. With a few exceptions, the percentage of completely responding patients attained with this combination does not seem to be increased, and significant uncertainty as to the durability of these responses remains. Therefore, little conclusive data exists documenting synergistic benefits from the use of IL-2 and IFN in patients with advanced RCC; because the potential for increased toxicity exists, more compelling randomized studies are needed to recommend its use.

INTERLEUKIN-2, INTERFERON, AND CHEMOTHERAPY

In vivo animal data with a variety of chemotherapy agents and IL-2 demonstrated that, rather than antagonizing the activity of IL-2 by immunosuppressing the tumor-bearing host, many of these chemotherapy regimens exhibited (at least) additive or (at best) synergistic therapeutic results (69) when added to IL-2. Chemotherapy agents often had to show direct antitumor activity to be most effective, and candidates for such agents in RCC included 5-fluorouracil (5-FU) and vinblastine. In treatment of colon cancer, the addition of IFN to 5-FU was reported to augment therapeutic results, primarily through effects on the pharmacokinetics of 5-FU; therefore, many investigators combined IL-2, IFN, and 5-FU in exploring chemoimmunotherapeutic strategies in patients with metastatic RCC. Table 4 illustrates a number of such studies, using many different doses and schedules for all three agents. IL-2 was administered at high and low doses by i.v. bolus, continuous infusion, or subcutaneous injection, and IFN was administered intravenously, subcutaneously, and intramuscularly. Most investigators used 5-FU as a 750 mg per m^2 infusion once every week or as a 600 mg per m^2 per day continuous infusion for 5 days every 3 to 4 weeks. The variation in the RRs shown in Table 4 is quite evident, ranging from overall RRs of 0% to 39% and complete RRs of 0% to 13%. For the 434 patients in Table 4 who received IL-2, IFN, and 5-FU, the overall RR is 23% and the complete RR is 5%. Even more striking is that the protocols of Joffe (70), Dutcher (65), and Hanninen (75) are similar, patterned after the regimen developed and reported by Atzpodien; however, they exhibit disparate overall RRs of 16%, 16%, and 39% and complete RRs of 0%, 4%, and 11%. That significant toxicities are experienced when these agents are combined (despite the universal utilization of lower doses of IL-2) is evident. Several of the studies cited had treatment-related mortalities of 2% (70–72). As with the combination of IL-2 and IFN, some concern remains as to whether such combinations are able to achieve the same longevity of response initially reported with high-dose IL-2 alone (65). Again, large, long-term randomized studies are needed to investigate these critical issues. One study with vinblastine showed results similar to the more favorable results of studies with 5-FU, but these results have not been confirmed by others. In the end, it is important to determine whether responses observed are indeed durable and if concurrent administration of IL-2, IFN, and chemotherapy is superior to the sequential administration of these agents.

OTHER COMBINATIONS WITH INTERLEUKIN-2

A multitude of other agents have been combined with IL-2 in the treatment of advanced RCC, largely due to dissatisfaction with low RRs to IL-2 alone. Some combinations were identified as promising by preclinical animal data, others were proposed based on improving awareness of mechanisms of antitumor immune response. IL-4 was discovered to activate NK cells and generate LAK cells in murine systems and had some antitumor activity. Sosman et al. infused IL-4 by continuous infusion in a phase 1 setting and then infused it after IL-2 administration

TABLE 4. INTERLEUKIN-2 (IL-2) WITH INTERFERON-α (IFN-α) AND CHEMOTHERAPY

Author (Reference)	IL-2 Dose (x 10^{-6} IU/m^2)	IFN-α Dose (x 10^{-6} U/m^2)	Chemotherapy (mg/m^2)	n	RR (%)	CR (%)
Joffe (71)	10 b.i.d. × 3 d/wk, then 5 t.i.w., s.c.	6 qwk, then 6–9 t.i.w., s.c.	5-FU, 750 qwk	55	16	0
Ellerhorst (72)	5.2. qd × 5 d, c i v	4 qd, s.c.	5-FU, 600 qd × 5 d	52	31	8
Ravaud (73)	4.5 qd × 6 d, s.c.[a]	3 t.i.w.[a]	5-FU, 600 qd × 5 d	111	2	0
Tourani (74)	9 t.i.w., s.c.	4.5 t.i.w., s.c.[a]	5-FU, 750 qwk	62	19	2
Hofmockel (75)	20 t.i.w. × 1 wk, then 5 t.i.w., s.c.	6 qwk, then 6–9 t.i.w., s.c.	5-FU, 750 qwk	34	38	9
Hanninen (76)	20 t.i.w., × 1 wk, then 5 t.i.w., s.c.	6 qwk, then 6–9 t.i.w., s.c.	5-FU, 750 qwk	120	39	11
Dutcher (66)	10 b.i.d. × 3 d/wk, then 5 t.i.w., s.c.	6 qwk, then 6–9 t.i.w., s.c.	5-FU, 750 qwk	50	16	4
Pectasides (77)	4.5 t.i.w., s.c.[a]	1.5 t.i.w.[a]	Vinblastine, 4 q3wk	31	39	13

c.i.v., continuous intravenous infusion; CR, complete response; 5-FU, 5-fluorouracil; LAK, lymphokine-activated killer cell; N/A, not applicable; RR, response rate.
[a]Fixed dose not adjusted for patient size. For comparison, dose calculated for 2.0 m^2 pt.

(77). In the 14 patients who received both components of therapy, only one minor response occurred. Whitehead administered IL-2 and IL-4 by concurrent subcutaneous injections in the phase 1 setting to a group of patients with mixed tumor histologies; one of six patients with RCC appeared to have a transient PR (78). A larger unpublished study conducted by Lotze et al. in the NCI Surgery Branch demonstrated that IL-4 had no significant antitumor activity alone and, when it was combined with high-dose bolus IL-2, did not appear to enhance the RR seen with IL-2 alone (*personal communication*).

Stadler (79) reported a phase 2 study using IL-2 at modest doses via subcutaneous route combined with IFN and *cis*-retinoic acid (reported to potentiate the antiproliferative activities of IFN). He described a 17% overall RR with one completely responding patient. Levamisole, a veterinary antihelminthic reported to have immunostimulatory activity, has also been combined with IL-2 (80), but has only resulted in one partial regression among 22 evaluable patients. Despite the possible role of cyclophosphamide as an immunomodulator, Mitchell reported the use of cyclophosphamide with low-dose bolus IL-2 (without IFN) in 15 patients without observing any clinical responses (81). Other early phase efforts to combine IL-2 with IL-1β (82) or IFN-γ (83–85) are of insufficient size or design to determine efficacy against RCC.

These isolated efforts have not identified compounds that enhance responses of patients with RCC to IL-2; in general, reliable preclinical models for predicting effective combinations have not been identified.

THERAPY OF DISEASE RELAPSES AFTER IMMUNOTHERAPY

Patients who experience PRs to immunotherapy with IL-2–based regimens are likely to relapse and develop progressive disease within 2 years. Basic immunologic precepts suggest that an immune response against tumor-associated antigens could induce long-term memory T cells; therefore, the likelihood exists that repeat therapy with IL-2 could reinduce tumor remission. A review by Lee et al. (86) of patients with metastatic RCC who responded to a variety of IL-2–based therapies in the NCI Surgery Branch evaluated the chance that such a population may respond to further IL-2 therapy after disease relapse. These investigators found that this was not the case, however. Of 29 patients who received some form of IL-2 retreatment after relapse, the only one exhibiting a (brief) second response was a patient who had received TIL and IL-2 initially, responded and relapsed, then received only IL-2 afterwards (due to a lack of TIL availability). This experience supports the recommendation that patients who relapse after maximal IL-2 therapy should not be retreated with IL-2, but should instead move on to other modalities (or at least receive other modalities along with further IL-2). One area not adequately investigated is whether patients who respond to low-dose IL-2 and relapse could subsequently respond to a maximal dose of IL-2.

If these post–IL-2 relapses are caused by simple inadequate log-kill of tumor cells by activated immune cells, relapsing sites should be harbingers of multisite failures, and nonsystemic modalities, such as surgical resection, should be inadequate for maintaining a patient's tumor-free status for extended periods. However, Lee et al. found that surgical resections of isolated relapses in selected patients who had responded previously to immunotherapy maintained 30% of them free of progressive disease for 3 years or longer from time of resection. Therefore, surgical resection is recommended for patients who respond to IL-2 but suffer limited relapse. Studies on these resected tumor relapses may provide insights about mechanisms by which tumors escape immunotherapy.

SUMMARY

High-dose IL-2 by bolus administration or continuous infusion has endured as a therapy for metastatic RCC. Although RRs are consistently 15% to 20%, nearly one-half of these responses are complete and durable. Although lower doses of IL-2 have demonstrated comparable initial RRs in many series, duration and completeness of these responses remain to be evaluated. Once a caregiver departs from therapy with IL-2 alone, the benefits of regimens combining IL-2 with other agents are much less clear. Besides considering whether initial RRs are actually increased when other agents are added to IL-2, a more significant consideration is whether durability of responses is impaired when these agents are added. Long-term, randomized studies are necessary to address this important issue.

REFERENCES

1. Linehan WM, Shipley WU, Parkinson DR. Cancer of the kidney and ureter. In: DeVita VT Jr, Hellman S, Rosenberg SA, eds. *Cancer: principles and practice of oncology.* Philadelphia: JB Lippincott Co, 1993:1023.
2. Ritchie AWS, deKernion JB. The natural history and clinical features of renal carcinoma. *Semin Nephrol* 1987;7:131–139.
3. Elson PJ, Witte RS, Trump DL. Prognostic factors for survival in patients with recurrent or metastatic renal cell carcinoma. *Cancer Res* 1988;48:7310–7313.
4. Maldazys JD, deKernion JB. Prognostic factors in metastatic renal carcinoma. *J Urol* 1986;136:376–379.
5. Yagoda A. Chemotherapy of renal cell carcinoma: 1983–1989. *Semin Urol* 1989;7:199–206.
6. Walpole ET, Dutcher JP, Sparano J, et al. Survival after phase II treatment of advanced renal cell carcinoma with taxol or high-dose interleukin-2. *J Immunother* 1993;13:275–281.
7. Fairlarnb DJ. Spontaneous regression of retastases of renal cancer. *Cancer* 1981;47:2102–2106.
8. Marcus SG, Choyke PL, Reiter R, et al. Regression of metastatic renal cell carcinoma after cytoreductive nephrectomy. *J Urol* 1993; 150:463–466.
9. Gleave ME, Elhilali M, Fradet Y, et al. Interferon gamma-1b compared to placebo in metastatic renal-cell carcinoma. *N Engl J Med* 1998;338:1265–1271.
10. Quesada JR, Rios A, Swanson D, et al. Antitumor activity of recombinant-derived interferon alpha in metastatic renal cell carcinoma. *J Clin Oncol* 1985;3:1522–1528.
11. Morgan DA, Ruscetti FW, Gallo R. Selective in vitro growth of T lymphocytes from normal human bone marrows. *Science* 1976;193:1007–1008.
12. Mulé JJ, Shu S, Rosenberg SA. The antitumor efficacy of lymphokine-activated killer cells and recombinant interleukin-2 in vivo. *J Immunol* 1985;135:646–652.

13. Cantrell DA, Smith KA. The interleukin-2 T-cell system: a new cell growth model. *Science* 1984;224:1312–1316.
14. Rosenberg SA, Mulé JJ, Spiess PJ, et al. Regression of established pulmonary retastases and subcutaneous tumor mediated by the systemic administration of high-dose recombinant interleukin-2. *J Exp Med* 1985;161:1169–1188.
15. Mulé JJ, Shu S, Schwarz SL, Rosenberg SA. Adoptive immunotherapy of established pulmonary metastases with LAK cells and recombinant interleukin-2. *Science* 1984;225:1487–1489.
16. Lafreniere R, Rosenberg SA. Successful immunotherapy of experimental hepatic metastases with lymphokine activated killer cells and recombinant interleukin-2. *Cancer Res* 1985;45:3735–3741.
17. Lotze MT, Frana LW, Sharrow SO, Robb RJ, Rosenberg SA. In vivo administration of purified human interleukin-2. I. Half-life and immunologic effects of the Jurkat cell line-derived interleukin-2. *J Immunol* 1985;134:157–166.
18. Papa MZ, Mulé JJ, Rosenberg SA. Antitumor efficacy of lymphokine-activated killer cells and recombinant interleukin-2 in vivo: successful immunotherapy of established pulmonary metastases from weakly immunogenic and nonimmunogenic murine tumors of three distinct histological types. *Cancer Res* 1986; 46:4973–4978.
19. Rosenberg SA, Lotze MT, Muul LM, et al. Observations on the systemic administration of autologous lymphokine-activated killer cells and recombinant interleukin-2 to patients with metastatic cancer. *N Engl J Med* 1985;313:1485–1492.
20. Rosenberg SA, Lotze MT, Muul LM, et al. A progress report on the treatment of 157 patients with advanced cancer using lymphokine-activated killer cells and interleukin-2 or high-dose interleukin-2 alone. *N Engl J Med* 1987;316:889–897.
21. Konrad MW, Hemstreet G, Hersh EM, et al. Pharmacokinetics of recombinant interleukin-2 in humans. *Cancer Res* 1990;50:2009–2017.
22. Rosenberg SA, Yang JC, Topalian SL, et al. Treatment of 283 consecutive patients with metastatic melanoma or renal cell cancer using high-dose bolus interleukin-2. *JAMA* 1994;271:907–913.
23. Atkins MB, Sparano J, Fisher RI, et al. Randomized phase II trial of high-dose interleukin-2 either alone or in combination with interferon alpha-2b in advanced renal cell carcinoma. *J Clin Oncol* 1993;11:661–670.
24. Fisher RI, Rosenberg SA, Sznol M, Parkinson DR, Fyfe G. High-dose aldesleukin in renal cell carcinoma: long-term survival update. *Cancer J Sci Amer* 1997;[Suppl 1]:S70–S72.
25. Rosenberg SA, Yang JC, White DE, Steinberg SM. Durability of complete responses in patients with metastatic cancer treated with high-dose interleukin-2. *Ann Surg* 1998;228:307–319.
26. Bukowski RM, Goodman P, Crawford D, Sergi JS, Redman BG, Whitehead RP. Phase II trial of high-dose intermittent interleukin-2 in metastatic renal cell carcinoma: a Southwest Oncology Group Study. *J Natl Cancer Inst* 1990;82:143–146.
27. Kammula US, White DE, Rosenberg SA. Trends in the safety of high dose bolus interleukin-2 administration in patients with metastatic cancer. *Cancer* 1998;83:797–805.
28. Yang JC, Topalian SL, Parkinson D, et al. Randomized comparison of high-dose and low-dose intravenous interleukin-2 for the therapy of metastatic renal cell carcinoma; an interim report. *J Clin Oncol* 1994;12:1572–1576.
29. Yang JC, Rosenberg SA. An ongoing prospective randomized comparison of interleukin-2 regimens for the treatment of metastatic renal cell cancer. *Cancer J Sci Amer* 1997;3:S79–S84.
30. Greenberg PAC, Hortobagyi GN, Smith TL, Ziegler LD, Frye DK, Buzdar AU. Long-term follow-up of patients with complete remission following combination chemotherapy for metastatic breast cancer. *J Clin Oncol* 1996;14:2197–2205.
31. West WH, Tayer KW, Yannelli JR, et al. Constant-infusion recombinant interleukin-2 plus lymphokine-activated killer cells in metastatic renal cancer. *N Engl J Med* 1987;316:898–905.
32. Gold PJ, Thompson JA, Markowitz DR, Neumann S, Fefer A. Metastatic renal cell carcinoma: long-term survival after therapy with high-dose continuous-infusion interleukin-2. *Cancer J Sci Amer* 1997;3:S85–S91.
33. von der Maase H, Geertsen P, Thatcher N, et al. Recombinant interleukin-2 in metastatic renal cell carcinoma—a European multicentre phase II study. *Eur J Cancer* 1991;27:1583–1589.
34. Escudier B, Ravaud A, Fabbro M, et al. High-dose interleukin-2 two days a week for metastatic renal cell carcinoma: a FNCLCC multicenter study. *J Immunother* 1994;16:306–312.
35. Negrier S, Escudier B, Lasset C, et al. Recombinant human interleukin-2, recombinant human interferon alfa-2a or both in metastatic renal-cell carcinoma. *N Engl J Med* 1998;338:1272–1278.
36. Weiss GR, Margolin KA, Aronson FR, et al. A randomized phase II trial of continuous infusion interleukin-2 or bolus injection interleukin-2 plus lymphokine-activated killer cells for advanced renal cell carcinoma. *J Clin Oncol* 1992;10:275–281.
37. Atzpodien J, Korfer A, Evers P, et al. Low dose subcutaneous recombinant interleukin-2 in advanced human malignancy: a phase II outpatient study. *Mol Biother* 1990;2:18–26.
38. Whitehead RP, Ward D, Hemingway L, et al. Subcutaneous recombinant interleukin-2 in a dose escalating regimen in patients with metastatic renal cell adenocarcinoma. *Cancer Res* 1990;50:6708–6714.
39. Stein RC, Malkovska V, Morgan S, et al. The clinical effects of prolonged treatment of patients with advanced cancer with low-dose subcutaneous interleukin-2. *Br J Cancer* 1991;63:275–278.
40. Lissoni P, Barni S, Tancini G, et al. Clinical response and survival in metastatic renal carcinoma during subcutaneous administration of interleukin-2 alone. *Arch Ital Urol Androl* 1997;69:41–47.
41. Sleijfer DT, Janssen RA, Buter J, et al. Phase II study of subcutaneous interleukin-2 in unselected patients with advanced renal cell cancer on an outpatient basis. *J Clin Oncol* 1992;10:1119–1123.
42. Buter J, Sleijfer DT, Winette TA, et al. A progress report on the outpatient treatment of patients with advanced renal cell carcinoma using subcutaneous recombinant interleukin-2. *Semin Oncol* 1993;20: 16–21.
43. Tourani JM, Lucas V, Mayeur D, et al. Subcutaneous recombinant interleukin-2 (rIL-2) in out-patients with metastatic renal cell carcinoma. *Ann Oncol* 1996;7:525–528.
44. Grimm EA, Mazumder A, Zhang HZ, et al. Lymphokine-activated killer cell phenomenon: lysis of natural killer-resistant fresh solid tumor cells by interleukin-2 activated autologous human peripheral blood lymphocytes. *J Exp Med* 1982;155:1832–1841.
45. Rosenberg SA, Lotze MT, Yang JC, et al. Experience with the use of high-dose interleukin-2 in the treatment of 652 cancer patients. *Ann Surg* 1989;210:474–484.
46. Fisher RI, Coltman CA, Doroshow JH, et al. Metastatic renal cancer treated with interleukin-2 and lymphokine-activated killer cells. *Ann Intern Med* 1988;108:518–523.
47. Parkinson DR, Fisher RI, Rayner AA, et al. Therapy of renal cell carcinoma with interleukin-2 and lymphokine-activated killer cells. Phase II experience with a hybrid bolus and continuous infusion interleukin-2 regimen. *J Clin Oncol* 1990;8:1630–1636.
48. Negrier S, Philip T, Stoter G, et al. Interleukin-2 with or without lymphokine-activated killer cells in metastatic renal cell cancer: a report of the European multi-centre study. *J Clin Oncol* 1989; 25:21–28.
49. Dillman RO, Oldham RK, Tauer KW, et al. Continuous interleukin-2 and lymphokine-activated killer cells for advanced cancer: a national biotherapy study group. *J Clin Oncol* 1991;9:1233–1240.
50. Dillman RO, Church C, Oldham RK, West WH, Schwartzberg L, Birch R. Inpatient continuous-infusion interleukin-2 in 788 patients with cancer. *Cancer* 1993;71:2358–2370.
51. Thompson JA, Shulman KL, Benyunes MC, et al. Prolonged continuous intravenous infusion interleukin-2 and lymphokine-activated killer-cell therapy for metastatic renal cell carcinoma. *J Clin Oncol* 1992;10:960–968.
52. Law TM, Motzer R, Mazumdar M, et al. Phase III randomized trial of interleukin-2 with or without lymphokine activated killer cells in the treatment of patients with advanced renal cell carcinoma. *Cancer* 1995;76:824–832.
53. Rosenberg SA, Yanelli JR, Yang JC, et al. Treatment of patients with metastatic melanoma with autologous tumor-infiltrating lymphocytes and interleukin-2. *J Natl Cancer Inst* 1994;86:1159–1166.

54. Morita T, Salmeron MA, Hayakawa K, Swanson DA, von Eschenbach AC, Itoh K. T cell functions of IL-2-activated tumor-infiltrating lymphocytes from renal cell carcinoma. *Reg Immunol* 1993;4: 225–235.

55. Figlin RA, Pierce WC, Kaboo R, et al. Treatment of metastatic renal cell carcinoma with nephrectomy, interleukin-2 and cytokine-primed or CD8(+) selected tumor infiltrating lymphocytes from primary tumor. *J Urol* 1997;158:740–745.

56. Cameron RB, McIntosh JK, Rosenberg SA. Synergistic antitumor effects of combination immunotherapy with recombinant interleukin-2 and a recombinant hybrid alpha-interferon in the treatment of established murine hepatic metastases. *Cancer Res* 1988;48: 5810–5817.

57. Rosenberg SA, Lotze MT, Yang JC, et al. Combination therapy with interleukin-2 and alpha-interferon for the treatment of patients with advanced cancer. *J Clin Oncol* 1989;7:1863–1874.

58. Marincola FM, White DE, Wise AP, Rosenberg SA. Combination therapy with interferon alfa-2a and interleukin-2 for the treatment of metastatic cancer. *J Clin Oncol* 1995;13:1110–1122.

59. Taneja SS, Pierce W, Figlin R, Belldegrun A. Immunotherapy for renal cell carcinoma: the era of interleukin-2-based treatment. *Urology* 1994;45:911–924.

60. Kruit WHJ, Lamers CHJ, Gratama JW, et al. High-dose regimen of interleukin-2 and interferon-alpha in combination with lymphokine-activated killer cells in patients with metastatic renal cell cancer. *J Immunother* 1997;20:312–320.

61. Bukowski RM, Olencki T, Wang Q, et al. Phase II trial of interleukin-2 and interferon-α in patients with renal cell carcinoma: clinical results and immunologic correlates of response. *J Immunother* 1997;20:301–311.

62. Ravaud A, Negrier S, Cany L, et al. Subcutaneous low-dose recombinant interleukin-2 and alpha-interferon in patients with metastatic renal cell carcinoma. *Br J Cancer* 1994;69:1111–1114.

63. Jayson GC, Middleton M, Lee SM, Ashcroft L, Thatcher N. A randomized phase II trial of interleukin-2 and interleukin-2-interferon alpha in advanced renal cancer. *Br J Cancer* 1998;78:366–369.

64. Henriksson R, Nilsson S, Colleen S, et al. Survival in renal cell carcinoma: a randomized evaluation of tamoxifen vs. interleukin-2, α-interferon (leucocyte) and tamoxifen. *Br J Cancer* 1998;77: 1311–1317.

65. Dutcher JP, Fisher RI, Weiss G, et al. Outpatient subcutaneous interleukin-2 and interferon-α for metastatic renal cell cancer: five-year follow-up of the cytokine working group study. *Cancer J Sci Amer* 1997;3:157–162.

66. Atzpodien J, Hanninen EL, Kirchner H, et al. Multiinstitutional home-therapy trial of recombinant human interleukin-2 and interferon α-2 in progressive metastatic renal cell carcinoma. *J Clin Oncol* 1995;13:497–501.

67. Vogelzang NJ, Lipton A, Figlin RA. Subcutaneous interleukin-2 plus interferon alfa-2a in metastatic renal cancer: an outpatient multicenter trial. *J Clin Oncol* 1993;9:1809–1816.

68. Boccardo F, Rubagotti A, Canobbio L, et al. Interleukin-2, interferon-α and interleukin-2 plus interferon-α in renal cell carcinoma. A randomized phase II trial. *Tumori* 1998;84:534–539.

69. Papa MZ, Yang JC, Vetto JT, Shiloni E, Eisenthal A, Rosenberg SA. Combined effects of chemotherapy and interleukin-2 in the therapy of mice with advanced pulmonary tumors. *Cancer Res* 1988;48: 122–129.

70. Joffe JK, Banks RE, Forbes MA, et al. A phase II study of interferon-α, interleukin and 5-fluorouracil in advanced renal carcinoma: clinical data and laboratory evidence of protease activation. *Br J Urol* 1996;77:638–649.

71. Ellerhorst JA, Sella A, Amato RJ, et al. Phase II trial of 5-fluorouracil, interferon-α and continuous infusion interleukin-2 for patients with metastatic renal cell carcinoma. *Cancer* 1997;80:2128–2132.

72. Ravaud A, Audhuy B, Gomez F, et al. Subcutaneous interleukin-2, interferon alfa-2a, and continuous infusion of fluorouracil in metastatic renal cell carcinoma: a multicenter phase II trial. *J Clin Oncol* 1998;16:2728–2732.

73. Tourani JM, Pfister C, Berdah JF, et al. Outpatient treatment with subcutaneous interleukin-2 and interferon alfa administration in combination with fluorouracil in patients with metastatic renal cell carcinoma: results of a sequential nonrandomized phase II study. *J Clin Oncol* 1998;16:2505–2513.

74. Hofmockel G, Langer W, Theiss M, Gruss A, Frohmuller HGW. Immunochemotherapy for metastatic renal cell carcinoma using a regimen of interleukin-2, interferon-α and 5-fluorouracil. *J Urol* 1996;156:18–21.

75. Hanninen EL, Kirchner H, Atzpodien J. Interleukin-2 based home therapy of metastatic renal cell carcinoma: risks and benefits in 215 consecutive single institution patients. *J Urol* 1996;155:19–25.

76. Pectasides D, Varthalitis J, Kostopoulou M, et al. An outpatient phase II study of subcutaneous interleukin-2 and interferon-alpha-2b in combination with intravenous vinblastine in metastatic renal cell cancer. *Oncology* 1998;55:10–15.

77. Sosman JA, Fisher SG, Kefer C, Fisher RI, Ellis TM. A phase I trial of continuous infusion interleukin-4 (IL-4) alone and following interleukin-2 (IL-2) in cancer patients. *Ann Oncol* 1994;5:447–452.

78. Whitehead RP, Friedman KD, Clark DA, Pagani K, Rapp L. Phase I trial of simultaneous administration of interleukin-2 and interleukin-4 subcutaneously. *Clin Cancer Res* 1995;1:1145–1152.

79. Stadler WM, Kuzel T, Dumas M, Vogelzang NJ. Multicenter phase II trial of interleukin-2, interferon-α and 13-cis-retinoic acid in patients with metastatic renal-cell carcinoma. *J Clin Oncol* 1998;16:1820–1825.

80. Creagan ET, Hestorff RD, Suman VJ, et al. Combined levamisole with recombinant interleukin-2 (IL-2) in patients with advanced renal cell carcinoma. *Am J Clin Oncol* 1998;21:139–141.

81. Mitchell MS. Chemotherapy in combination with biomodulation: a 5-year experience with cyclophosphamide and interleukin-2. *Semin Oncol* 1992;19[Suppl 4]:80–87.

82. Triozzi PL, Kim JA, Martin EW, Young DC, Benzies T, Villasmil PM. Phase I trial of escalating doses of interleukin-1β in combination with a fixed dose of interleukin-2. *J Clin Oncol* 1995;13:482–489.

83. Baars JW, Wagstaff J, van Groeningen CJ, et al. Phase II study of interferon-γ and interleukin-2: tachyphylaxis of toxicity to the liver during increasing immune enhancement. *J Natl Cancer Inst* 1993;85:410–411.

84. Farace F, Pallardy M, Angevin E, Hercend T, Escudier B, Triebel F. Metastatic renal cell carcinoma patients treated with interleukin-2 or interleukin-2 plus interferon-α: immunological monitoring. *Int J Cancer* 1994;57:814–821.

85. Reddy SP, Harwood RM, Moore DF, Grimm EA, Murray JL, Vadhan-Raj S. Recombinant interleukin-2 in combination with recombinant interferon-gamma in patients with advanced malignancy: a phase I study. *J Immunother* 1997;20:79–87.

86. Lee DS, White DE, Hurst R, Rosenberg SA, Yang JC. Patterns of relapse and response to retreatment in patients with metastatic melanoma or renal cell carcinoma who responded to interleukin-2-based immunotherapy. *Cancer J Sci Am* 1998;4:86–93.

3.4

INTERLEUKIN-2: CLINICAL APPLICATIONS

Hematologic Malignancies

ALEXANDER FEFER

Several lines of preclinical evidence suggest a potential role for interleukin-2 (IL-2) in the treatment of hematologic malignancies:

1. In animal models, IL-2 eradicated widely disseminated hematologic malignancies (1) and augmented the therapeutic efficacy of adoptively transferred T lymphocytes sensitized to tumor-associated antigens (2).

2. Cells from patients with hematologic malignancies, such as acute myelogenous leukemia (AML), acute lymphoblastic leukemia (ALL), chronic myelogenous leukemia, malignant lymphoma, and multiple myeloma, are susceptible to lysis *in vitro* by human lymphocytes stimulated by IL-2 [i.e., lymphokine-activated killer (LAK) cells] (3–8).

3. Susceptibility to such lysis is non–cell cycle specific and maintained even in cell lines that demonstrate pleiotropic drug resistance markers, suggesting no cross-resistance between IL-2 and chemotherapy (9).

4. IL-2–activated natural killer (NK) cells can inhibit malignant colony proliferation by clonogenic human leukemic stem cells in colony-forming assays (10).

5. IL-2 can block the *in vivo* growth of human leukemic cells in immunosuppressed nude mice (11).

6. Peripheral blood lymphocytes from patients with acute leukemia at diagnosis or in relapse are defective in their ability to generate LAK activity against autologous leukemic cells in response to IL-2 *in vitro*—a defect that is reversed when the patient enters a complete remission (CR) (12).

7. An apparent correlation has been reported between the ability to respond with LAK cell generation and the clinical course of AML (13).

8. Because T-cell responses can be generated specifically directed against tumor-associated antigens (e.g., the immunoglobulin idiotype of B-cell lymphomas and multiple myeloma, the product of BCR-ABL in chronic myelogenous leukemia and antigens on AML, IL-2 might be clinically useful by augmenting such responses.

9. IL-2 might stimulate or augment an antitumor effect by NK cells, especially against tumors that do not express adequate class I major histocompatibility complex (MHC) antigens.

10. A state of minimal residual disease (MRD)—a setting in which immunotherapy is more likely to be effective—can be readily induced because hematologic malignancies are among the most sensitive to chemotherapy, radiation, or both.

Accordingly, IL-2 is being explored in the treatment of hematologic malignancies. Although the trials conducted involved heterogeneous patient populations and IL-2 regimens, some of the preliminary results are encouraging. Most trials targeted patients with AML or non-Hodgkin's lymphoma (NHL). This chapter briefly reviews the positive, negative, and inconclusive results and current status of such IL-2–based therapy trials.

CLINICAL TRIALS OF INTERLEUKIN-2 FOR REFRACTORY HEMATOLOGIC MALIGNANCIES

Several phase 1 and 2 trials were performed in patients with hematologic malignancies heavily pretreated with chemotherapy, radiation, or both. The prior exposure to aggressive therapy may influence the toxicity of IL-2 therapy. For example, such patients may be more susceptible than solid tumor patients to IL-2–associated toxicity, such as capillary leak syndrome and thrombocytopenia, a problem that may be exacerbated by marrow involvement in hematologic malignancies. Moreover, heavily pretreated patients may be less able to respond immunologically to IL-2.

Malignant Lymphoma

The patients treated were clinically heterogeneous with respect to disease, grade, stage, prior therapy, and so forth. The IL-2 regimens were empiric and varied in terms of source, dose, route, and schedule. Some of the trials involved infusion of autologous LAK cells.

Table 1 summarizes the results of eight trials of IL-2 with or without LAK cells in patients with NHL who relapsed after chemotherapy or autologous bone marrow transplantation (ABMT) (14–20). Most patients received high-dose IL-2 by continuous

TABLE 1. INTERLEUKIN-2 WITH OR WITHOUT LYMPHOKINE-ACTIVATED KILLER CELLS THERAPY FOR NON-HODGKIN'S LYMPHOMA

Regimen	Total No. Patients Evaluable	No. CR	No. PR	Overall Response Rate CR + PR (Total %)
IL-2	82	5	9	14/82 (17)
IL-2 + LAK	39	2	5	7/39 (17)
Total	**121**	**7**	**14**	**21/121 (17)**

CR, complete remission; IL-2, interleukin-2; LAK, lymphokine-activated cells; PR, partial response.
From West WH et al. Constant-infusion recombinant interleukin-2 in adoptive immunotherapy of advanced cancer. *N Engl J Med* 1987;316:898–905; Schoof DD et al. Adoptive immunotherapy of human cancer using low-dose recombinant interleukin-2 and lymphokine-activated killer cells. *Cancer Res* 1988;48:5007–5010; Margolin KA et al. Phase II trial of high-dose interleukin-2 and lymphokine-activated killer cells in Hodgkin's disease and non-Hodgkin's lymphoma. *J Immunother* 1991;10:214–220; Bernstein ZP et al. Interleukin-2 lymphokine-activated killer cell therapy of non-Hodgkin's lymphoma and Hodgkin's disease. *J Immunother* 1991;10:141–146; Tourani JM et al. Interleukin-2 therapy for refractory and relapsing lymphomas. *Eur J Cancer* 1991;27:1676–1680; Weber JS et al. The use of interleukin-2 and lymphokine-activated killer cells for the treatment of patients with non-Hodgkin's lymphoma [see comments]. *J Clin Oncol* 1992;10:33–40; Gisselbrecht C et al. Interleukin-2 treatment in lymphoma: a phase II multicenter study. *Blood* 1994;83:2081–2085, with permission.

intravenous infusion (c.i.v.), bolus infusion, or both and often required hospitalization. Overall, 6% of patients had a CR and 11% had a partial response (PR) with an overall response rate of 17%. Although most responses were short, a CR or PR occasionally persisted for longer than 2 or 3 years. Histology was reported for only 79 of the NHL patients. Of the 45 patients with diffuse NHL, three patients had a CR and four patients had a PR with an overall response rate of 16%. Of the 46 patients with follicular histologies, three patients had a CR and nine patients had a PR with an overall response rate of 26%.

Concern existed that IL-2 might serve as a growth factor *in vivo* for lymphoid malignancies expressing the IL-2 receptor. *In vitro* studies have been contradictory (11,21). In one trial, neither of the two patients with cutaneous T-cell lymphoma responded to IL-2 and LAK cells (17). In the largest reported series of IL-2–treated NHL patients, however, 8 of the 11 responders had T-cell lymphomas (20). The same series included seven patients with refractory mycosis fungoides or Sézary syndrome, five of whom responded to IL-2 (one CR, four PR). Although sparse, these results show that IL-2 can induce clinical regression of T-cell lymphomas in some patients and does not promote tumor growth.

Six reported clinical trials of IL-2 with or without LAK cells included 31 patients with Hodgkin's disease (HD) (16–18,20,22). All patients were extensively treated and eight had relapsed after ABMT. Of 16 patients who received IL-2 alone, one patient had a PR that lasted 11 months. Of 15 patients who received IL-2 plus LAK cells, three patients had short PRs (all <3 months).

Thus, some regimens of IL-2 with or without LAK cells can induce a PR or even a CR in some patients with malignant lymphoma. The therapies and patients, however, have been extremely heterogeneous. No trials have compared one IL-2

regimen with another, or one IL-2 regimen with and without LAK cells, in comparable patients so as to identify the subset of patients who are more or less likely to benefit from IL-2 therapy and to identify the most effective IL-2 regimen.

Acute Leukemia

Clinical trials of IL-2 for acute leukemia have focused on patients with AML who did not respond to chemotherapy or ABMT or who relapsed after such treatment. The most impressive clinical results were reported (23) and updated (24) by Meloni et al. Patients with AML [refractory, or in the first to fourth relapse (Rel 1–4)], whose marrow had less than 30% blasts (median, 15%) were treated with IL-2.

IL-2 was administered by c.i.v. for 5 days using a daily dose–escalating protocol. After 3 days of rest, IL-2 therapy was repeated at the maximum tolerated dose (MTD) for a total of 4 cycles. The first five patients received IL-2 from Glaxo; all subsequent patients received IL-2 from Chiron at a dose of $8–18 \times 10^6$ IU per m^2 per day. Responders to IL-2 received maintenance IL-2 as monthly 5-day courses at $4–8 \times 10^6$ IU per m^2 per day. After the first year, a lower dose of IL-2 was administered every other month.

Of 24 patients treated, 13 entered a CR. Although five of the CRs were of short duration and two were too early for evaluation, six patients remain in CR at 3+ to 9+ (median, 6+ years) years. The long-term disease-free survivors included patients who received IL-2 in Rel 2–4 with M1-, M2-, or M4-type AML. The results are quite encouraging and require confirmation and extension.

In another series (25), ten patients with AML in relapse with more than 30% blasts in their marrow were treated with high-dose IL-2 by i.v. bolus (8×10^6 IU per m^2 per 8 hours $\times$ 5 days per cycle for 3 cycles, each cycle separated by 9 days of rest). Two patients with 30% and 81% blasts in the marrow had a CR, but of only 3- to 4-months' duration. Finally, a CR of 6 months' duration was induced in one out of six AML patients treated with IL-2 while in "early relapse—partial remission" (26). The dose was largely 3×10^6 Cetus U per m^2 per day $\times$ 5 days by c.i.v. every other week, after which the dose was administered every month.

Nineteen patients with ALL treated with IL-2 were reported to have no response (27).

Thus, IL-2 induced clinical responses in some patients with refractory AML. Although most responses were of relatively short duration, some responses were quite durable. In patients with refractory disease, however, such clinical activity is significant and warrants further investigation in more favorable clinical settings, namely, in patients with MRD.

CLINICAL TRIALS OF INTERLEUKIN-2 AS AN ADJUNCT TO CHEMOTHERAPY

Theoretically, therapy with IL-2 is more likely to be effective in a setting of MRD [i.e., after chemotherapy or the more aggressive chemotherapy and radiotherapy used for bone marrow transplantation (BMT)]. Therefore, IL-2 has been administered to patients who were in CR after chemotherapy but at high risk for relapse in the hope of decreasing the relapse rate and prolonging disease-free survival.

Virtually all such trials have been performed in patients with AML in chemotherapy-induced CR1 or CR2. The trials involved small groups of heterogeneous patients and a variety of IL-2 regimens and yielded variable, inconsistent, and inconclusive results. The effects of IL-2 in patients with AML in CR1 can be evaluated retrospectively only by comparing their results with those expected with chemotherapy alone, which, in turn, vary greatly depending on clinical and cytogenetic prognostic indicators. Therefore, large numbers of well-characterized patients must be studied. This has not been done.

In one trial (28), patients with AML in CR1 at high risk for relapse were randomized to receive 4 cycles of IL-2 by c.i.v. at 9 $\times$ 10^6 IU per m^2 per day (n = 10) or 0.9 $\times$ 10^6 IU per m^2 per day (n = 8) for two 5-day cycles. The median CR duration for both groups was approximately 1 year. Another group of nine patients with AML in CR1 received a low dose of IL-2. Six patients in this group relapsed early (29). No benefit from IL-2 therapy was detectable in these small groups.

Several low-dose IL-2 regimens have been used in patients with AML in CR1. Cortes et al. (30) treated 18 consecutive patients with AML in CR1 with IL-2 by c.i.v. (4.5 $\times$ 10^5 IU per m^2 per day) and i.v. bolus (1 $\times$ 10^6 IU per m^2 once a week). For comparison, two historical control groups with similar prognostic factors, including cytogenetics, were selected. These control groups met the eligibility criteria for IL-2 therapy but had not received it. The median CR duration of the IL-2–treated group was 53 weeks. At 4 years, 6 out of 18 (33%) patients in the IL-2 group and 5 out of 36 (14%) patients in the control group (*p* = .09) were in CR. The results suggest that postremission IL-2 therapy might have reduced the relapse rate.

In a small, multicenter randomized trial (31), 14 patients with AML in CR1 received IL-2 and ten did not. The low-dose IL-2 regimen consisted of 0.2 $\times$ 10^6 IU per m^2 subcutaneously twice a day for 3 months. Eight of the 16 patients who received IL-2 and six of the ten patients who did not relapsed with a median disease-free survival of 52 and 40 weeks. Thus, no significant effect was noted.

A low-dose IL-2 regimen with minor variations developed at Dana Farber/Roswell Park is being studied in a number of clinical settings. In one study (32), patients with AML in CR1 received IL-2 at 4.5 $\times$ 10^5 IU per m^2 per day by c.i.v. (18 patients) or 1.2 $\times$ 10^6 IU per m^2 per day subcutaneously (5 patients) for 90 to 160 days with i.v. boluses of higher doses (i.e., 1, 2, and 3 $\times$ 10^6 IU per m^2 administered on 3 successive days every 14 days). The regimen was well tolerated. Of 23 patients treated, 13 did not complete therapy because of early relapse. The median CR duration for the ten patients who completed IL-2 therapy was 22 months (range, 8+ to 77+ months). No conclusions can be drawn about the clinical benefit of IL-2 therapy.

A phase 2 trial with a similar low-dose IL-2 regimen is in progress by CALGB (protocol 9,621) for AML patients younger than 60 years in CR1 with favorable cytogenetics. The IL-2 regimen consists of 1 $\times$ 10^6 IU per m^2 per day subcutaneously on

TABLE 2. SEATTLE INTERLEUKIN-2 REGIMEN

	IL-2 Dose by c.i.v.
Induction	9 $\times$ 10^6 IU/m^2/d $\times$ 4 d
Rest	4 d
Maintenance	1.6 $\times$ 10^6 IU/m^2/d $\times$ 10 d

c.i.v., continuous i.v. infusion; IL-2, interleukin-2.
From Robinson N et al. Interleukin-2 after autologous stem cell transplantation for hematologic malignancy: a phase I/II study. *Bone Marrow Transplant* 1997;19:425–442, with permission.

days 1 to 14, 19 to 28, 33 to 42, 47 to 56, 61 to 70, and 75 to 90 with a high-dose s.c. bolus of 12 $\times$ 10^6 IU per m^2 on days 15 to 17, 29 to 31, 43 to 45, 57 to 59, and 71 to 73. A phase 3 trial is planned. The same IL-2 regimen is being tested in the phase 3 trial of IL-2 versus no IL-2 (CALGB, protocol 9,720) in patients older than 60 years with AML in CR1.

A combination of histamine and low-dose IL-2 is also being explored in patients with AML in CR1. This is based on studies that suggest that IL-2–induced NK-mediated lysis of AML cells is inhibited by a monocyte-derived inhibitory signal that, in turn, is inhibited by histamine. In one reported (33) and updated (34) trial, 26 patients received histamine plus IL-2 (18,000 IU per kg s.c. twice a day) in 21-day cycles with 3- to 6-week rest periods until relapse or 24 months of CR. Fifteen of 26 patients remain in CR with a median follow-up of 26 months. A randomized phase 3 trial of IL-2 and histamine versus no IL-2 or histamine is in progress.

One trial (35) involved a higher dose of IL-2 administered for a shorter period of time. In a trial to assess the feasibility, toxicity, and biologic response of IL-2 administered after consolidation chemotherapy for AML in CR1, the Children's Cancer Group treated 21 patients with an IL-2 regimen that had been identified as an MTD in a phase 1 trial in patients who had undergone ABMT for hematologic malignancies. The regimen, designated as *Seattle Regimen*, is highlighted in Table 2 because it is being extensively tested in large phase 2 and 3 trials.

This IL-2 regimen was more toxic than the low-dose regimens because of the occurrence of fever (57%), vascular leak (48%), hypotension (38%), rash (29%), septicemia (5%), and thrombocytopenia (29%). The IL-2 regimen was considered tolerable. With a median follow-up of 7 months, seven patients had relapsed. A randomized prospective trial to determine whether this IL-2 regimen will prevent relapses and prolong disease-free survival in such children is in progress (Children's Cancer Group, protocol 2,961).

Because patients with AML in CR2 have a poor prognosis, they, too, have been subjects for IL-2 trials. Shepherd et al. (36) treated patients in CR2 or PR with IL-2 (3 $\times$ 10 IU or 9 $\times$ 10^6 IU per day, 5 days per week for 3 weeks s.c.) with cycles repeated with 1-week rest periods until relapse. Of 29 CR2 patients, two had a CR that was longer than the duration of their CR1 (19 and 20+ months). Three of 21 patients treated in PR achieved a CR2, two of which lasted longer than 2 years. Similarly, of seven patients in CR2 treated with polyethylene glycolated IL-2, three had a CR2 duration substantially longer than their CR1 (37).

Finally, 21 patients with AML were treated in CR2 with 4 cycles of IL-2 at 9×10^6 IU per m² per day on days 1 to 5 and 8 to 12 per cycle by a 1-hour infusion every 6 weeks (38). The duration of the CR2 in five patients exceeded that of their CR1. The authors concluded that the IL-2 regimen was feasible and the data sufficiently encouraging to justify a phase 3 trial. Such a trial, however, was never performed. Cumulatively, results of all these studies are inconclusive or, at best, slightly encouraging.

CLINICAL TRIALS OF INTERLEUKIN-2 AFTER BONE MARROW AND STEM CELL TRANSPLANTATION

Autologous

If MRD is truly the setting in which IL-2 therapy is most likely to be effective, then the most suitable patients may be those who have undergone BMT after otherwise lethal doses of chemoradiotherapy but who are at high risk for post-transplant relapse. For example, patients who undergo ABMT for advanced hematologic malignancies (i.e., AML or malignant lymphoma beyond CR1) have more than a 50% probability of relapse, most often within a few months.

BMT as a setting for IL-2 therapy is based on the following rationale, in addition to its setting as an MRD:

1. After BMT, a greater increase in circulating IL-2–responsive lytic CD56⁺ cells occurs than after conventional chemotherapy (39).
2. IL-2 might induce or augment a graft-versus-leukemia (GVL) or a graft-versus- tumor effect after allogeneic bone marrow transplantation (AlloBMT) or perhaps even after ABMT.
3. IL-2 after ABMT might destroy whatever clonogenic tumor cells might be transplanted with the marrow/stem cells, and, thus, might represent a form of purging tumor cells *in vivo*.

A number of clinical trials have been performed using IL-2 as consolidative immunotherapy after ABMT in the hope of reducing the relapse rate and prolonging disease-free survival. IL-2 has been used in the following ways:

1. In a few trials, IL-2 was administered immediately after marrow infusion.
2. In most trials, IL-2 was administered after some degree of documented hematologic recovery.
3. In some trials based on preclinical data, the marrow or stem cells were incubated with IL-2 before infusion, after which systemic IL-2 was administered.
4. IL-2 is being explored as part of a cocktail of growth factors to mobilize autologous stem cells with potential antitumor killer activity.

The chemoradiotherapy used for BMT is often associated with toxicity, which makes recipients less able to tolerate IL-2 than nontransplant patients with solid tumors. Therefore, several trials have been performed to determine the toxicity and immunomodulatory effects of different sources, schedules, and regimens of IL-2 administered after ABMT. Peripheral blood is increasingly replacing marrow as a source of stem cells for autologous transplantation. Accordingly, ABMT should be used when the source is known to be marrow, and autologous stem-cell transplantation (ASCT) should be used when the source is blood, a combination of blood and marrow, or unknown.

Timing and dosage are important. For example (40), when children with ALL were treated with Roche IL-2 (0.5 to 2.0 $\times$ 10^6 IU per m² per day $\times$ 4 days per week) beginning 1 day after ABMT, unacceptably serious nonhematologic toxicity was observed without any immunomodulatory effects. Severe toxicity was also reported in two patients with AML given high-dose IL-2 beginning 2 days after ABMT; a lower dose of IL-2 administered at a later time was far less toxic (41).

Theoretically, IL-2 should be administered sufficiently early after ABMT before relapses are likely to occur but after the reconstitution of IL-2–responsive lymphocytes in the circulation. Such cells capable of lysing tumor targets *in vitro* with or without incubation with IL-2 have been detected within 2 to 3 weeks after ABMT and ASCT (39,42,43).

A variety of empirically derived IL-2 regimens have been used after ASCT. Although a variety of immunologic changes are induced, none of these changes can serve as proxies or predictors of clinical benefit because none of the regimens has been documented definitively as clinically beneficial. Therefore, the optimal regimen of IL-2 in terms of dose, route, schedule, and duration remains unknown. Although some trials identified and used the MTD for IL-2, it is unknown if the MTD is the optimal dose.

The following three broadly defined types of IL-2 regimens have been used after ASCT:

1. The French-type regimen (44)—This regimen involves a high dose of IL-2 administered for 5 cycles. The first cycle lasts 5 days and the subsequent cycles last 2 days each every other week.
2. The Seattle-type regimen (45,46)—This regimen is a single cycle consisting of a short course of a moderate induction dose of IL-2 for 4 to 5 days, 4 to 6 days of rest, and a low-maintenance dose for 10 days. All doses are administered by c.i.v.
3. The Dana Farber/Roswell Park–type regimen (47)—This regimen involves a low dose of IL-2 chronically administered by c.i.v. or subcutaneously for 3 months or longer. Low-dose regimens are better tolerated than moderate- or high-dose regimens and require no hospitalization.

The immunomodulatory effects induced by the low-dose and moderate- to high-dose regimens differ. Although both types of regimens induce NK expansion with an increase in circulating lymphocytes expressing CD16 and CD56, the moderate- to high-dose regimens also induce increases in circulating CD3⁺ and CD8⁺ T cells, as well as increases in cytotoxic reactivity by circulating cells with and without exposure to IL-2 *in vitro* whereas low-dose regimens do not (41,48–50). For this reason, low-dose regimens have incorporated intermittent administration of moderate- to high-dose IL-2 to enhance cytotoxicity. New regimens are also being studied that involve low-dose IL-2 immediately after ASCT and higher doses thereafter (51).

Lymphomas

Patients with NHL have been included in a few phase 1 and 2 trials of IL-2 after ASCT. One of the trials was designed to identify the MTD of IL-2 (Roche) and its immunomodulatory effects (48) when administered to 16 patients with advanced hematologic malignancies beginning 33 days (median) after ABMT. Patients were sequentially assigned to escalating IL-2 "induction" doses on days 1 to 5 of the IL-2 protocol and a nonescalating, low IL-2 "maintenance" dose on days 12 to 21. The dose-limiting side effects of induction IL-2 were reversible hypotension and thrombocytopenia. Its MTD was 3×10^6 RU per m^2 per day (equivalent to 9×10^6 IU). The IL-2 regimen induced marked, rebound lymphocytosis with an increase in CD3$^+$ and CD8$^+$ cells, as well as an increase in NK cells expressing CD16 and CD56. This IL-2 regimen was associated with an increased ability of cells to lyse NK-resistant tumors with and without IL-2 *in vitro*.

In animal models, the combination of IL-2 plus LAK cells has been therapeutically more effective than IL-2 alone (52,53). Therefore, a trial was performed to determine whether LAK cells could be generated, characterized, and infused with IL-2 in patients after ABMT for advanced hematologic malignancies (54–56). Beginning 35 days (median) after ABMT, patients received the MTD IL-2 induction course identified above. Patients underwent leukaphereses during the period of maximal lymphocytosis (days 7 to 9 of the IL-2 protocol). The cells were cultured for 5 days in IL-2 (1,000 U per mL) and reinfused on days 12 to 14. Low-dose "maintenance" IL-2 was administered on days 12 to 21. A total of 0.4 to 3.8×10^{11} (median, 1.7×10^{11}) cells were infused per patient.

The LAK cells infused were quite lytic against the Daudi tumor target. The infused cells expressed CD3 (65%), CD8 (61%), and CD56 (43%). The most common toxicities associated with LAK cell infusions were fever, chills, and dyspnea. These toxicities usually resolved within 2 to 4 hours (56). LAK cell infusions induced a thrombocytopenia more severe than that observed with IL-2 alone, however, especially in patients with AML (56). The use of LAK cells was abandoned by the Seattle group primarily for financial reasons.

The clinical end-results of IL-2 with or without LAK cell therapy after ABMT in patients with NHL were encouraging. Of 22 patients at a high risk for relapse thus treated with IL-2 plus LAK cells (16 patients) or IL-2 alone (6 patients), 11 relapsed, two died in CR, and nine remained in CR 27 to 51 (median, 37+) months after BMT (56).

When IL-2 could no longer be obtained from Hoffman LaRoche, a phase 1/2 trial was performed with IL-2 from Chiron Therapeutics, Inc. Patients with advanced hematologic malignancies received IL-2 beginning a median of 46 days after ASCT. The MTD of induction IL-2 administered in the hospital was identified and maintenance IL-2 was administered in the outpatient clinic. The resultant "Seattle regimen" (see Table 2) was then tested in a phase 2 trial in 52 patients after ASCT for hematologic malignancies (57). Eighty percent of patients completed the induction IL-2. Most patients exhibited some degree

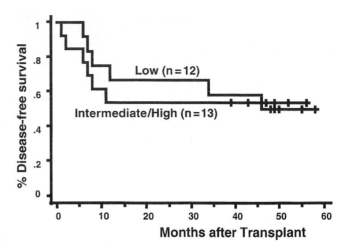

FIGURE 1. Interleukin-2 therapy after autologous bone marrow and stem cell transplantation for patients with non-Hodgkin's lymphoma (low or intermediate/high grade) at high risk for relapse. (From Robinson N et al. Interleukin-2 after autologous stem cell transplantation for hematologic malignancy: a phase I/II study. *Bone Marrow Transplant* 1997;19:425–442, with permission.)

of capillary leak. One patient died of cytomegalovirus pneumonia and one patient died of adult respiratory distress syndrome. Maintenance IL-2 was well tolerated. The regimen was well tolerated in the majority of patients.

Lymphocytosis was observed after induction IL-2. It reflected a rise in the number of cells expressing CD3, CD8, CD56, and P75 and was associated with significant cytotoxic activity. The results in the 25 patients thus treated for high-risk NHL, updated since the report (57) are shown in Figure 1. Patients with low-grade NHL numbered three in relapse 1 (Rel 1) or CR2 and nine beyond CR2. Those patients with intermediate or high-grade NHL represented nine in Rel1 or CR2 and four beyond CR2. The results compare favorably with historical controls at our institution. A phase 3 trial of this Seattle IL-2 regimen versus observation after ASCT for NHL in relapse is in progress at Southwest Oncology Group (protocol 9,438) to determine whether IL-2 will decrease the relapse rate and prolong disease-free survival. To date, approximately 230 patients have been entered in the trial.

A different approach evolved from studies in murine models in which marrow incubated with IL-2 *in vitro* before transplantation and combined with systemic IL-2 was injected into tumor-bearing mice. This approach was reported as more effective against tumors than marrow not incubated with IL-2 (58). Accordingly (59), in the largest trial of NHL patients, marrow or stem cells were incubated with IL-2 for 24 hours and then infused into patients conditioned for ASCT. These patients then received systemic IL-2 at a dose of 1 to 2×10^6 IU per m^2 per day by c.i.v. beginning on day 1 for at least 21 days. Subsequently, all patients received 6 cycles of maintenance IL-2 at a dose of 6×10^6 IU per m^2 per day × 5 days per week in weeks 1 and 2 every 28 days. Hematologic engraftment occurred. Clinically, of 19 patients treated for recurrent or refractory NHL, two died as a result of treatment, eight relapsed a median of 4 months after ASCT, and nine remain disease free with a median follow-up of 8 months. The results show that this approach is feasible and clinically tolerable but more cumbersome than the use of IL-2 alone. The clinical outcome cannot be evaluated in this group of patients because only a small number of individuals were studied for a short period.

IL-2 administered after ABMT for lymphoma has also been used in combination with interferon-α (IFN-α) (60) in a trial of 32 patients with NHL and 24 patients with HD. Sixty-one patients (NHL, 36; HD, 25) served as historical controls. IL-2 and IFN-α were self-administered in 2 cycles beginning a median of 4 months post-transplant and separated by a 4-week period. Each cycle consisted of IFN-α combined with IL-2 at 3 to 6 × 106 IU per m^2 per day × 5 days per week for 4 weeks administered subcutaneously. After a median follow-up of 34 months, 45 out of 56 (80%) patients treated with IFN-α plus IL-2 are disease free compared with only 32 out of 61 (53%) historical controls. The disease-free survival benefit applied to NHL and HD. The relative contributions of IFN-α or IL-2 are unknown. A phase 3 trial of IFN-α and IL-2 versus no cytokines is in progress.

Acute Lymphoblastic Leukemia

Although patients with ALL have been included in some of the phase 1 and 2 trials after ABMT, only two trials specifically dealt with patients with ALL. In Weisdorf et al.'s study (61), in which IL-2 was administered immediately after ABMT, ALL recurred in nine of ten patients in a median of 3 months. One randomized trial was reported (62) in which adult patients with ALL in CR1 were randomized to receive (n = 30) or not receive (n = 30) IL-2 (the French regimen) after ABMT. The 3-year post-BMT probability of CR was similarly low in both groups (29% and 27%). Thus, no clinical benefit of IL-2 therapy was observed.

Acute Myelogenous Leukemia

AML has been the major target of clinical trials of IL-2 after ASCT. Patients who undergo ASCT while in relapse have a 75% probability of post-transplant relapse and a 20% probability of long-term disease-free survival. The corresponding figures for patients treated in CR2 are 50% to 60% and 30%. The results for patients transplanted for AML in CR1 are far more variable, depending on a number of prognostic indicators, including cytogenetics, but, overall, the probability of post-transplant relapse and disease-free survival is approximately 40% to 50%.

For IL-2 trials, AML patients with a poor prognosis (i.e., beyond CR1) have an advantage because the beneficial effects of IL-2, if any, can be more quickly assessed because the controls are likely to relapse and to do so early. Such studies, however, are logistically difficult to assess because the patients become ill too quickly and require rapid initiation of therapy. Furthermore, only a fraction of the patients who relapse enter a CR2.

The phase 1 trial with Roche IL-2 by Higuchi et al. (48) and the feasibility trial of IL-2 plus LAK cells by Benyunes et al. (55) included 17 such AML patients who were treated with IL-2 alone (12 patients) or IL-2 plus LAK cells (5 patients) beginning a median of 54 days after ABMT. At the time of BMT, 11 patients were in Rel1, three were in CR2, and three were beyond CR2—all associated with poor post-transplant prognosis.

The clinical details of the patients treated have been published (55). The updated results (63) are shown in Figure 2. Of

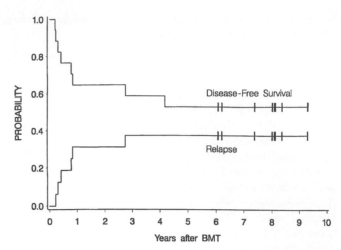

FIGURE 2. Kaplan-Meier product limit estimates of relapse and disease-free survival of patients treated with autologous bone marrow transplantation (BMT) plus IL-2 ± lymphokine-activated killer cells for acute myelogenous leukemia in first relapse or later (n = 17). (From Benyunes MC et al. Interleukin-2 with or without lymphokine-activated killer cells as consolidative immunotherapy after autologous bone marrow transplantation for acute myelogenous leukemia. *Bone Marrow Transplant* 1993;12:159–163; and Fefer A. Graft-versus-tumor responses. In: Thomas ED, Blume KG, Forman S, eds. *Hematopoietic cell transplantation*. Cambridge, MA: Blackwell, 1999:316–326, with permission.)

17 patients treated, one died of infection, six relapsed, one died in CR with a secondary malignancy at 5 years, and nine remain in continuous CR beyond 6 years. For comparison, a historical control group was identified that consisted of all patients with comparable clinical characteristics who underwent ABMT at our institution for AML beyond CR1 during the same period. The patients received the same preparative and purging regimens and met the eligibility criteria for IL-2 therapy. These patients did not receive IL-2, however, because they refused treatment or had financial problems, or because IL-2 was temporarily unavailable (54). Of the 15 control patients thus identified, one died of infection, ten relapsed at a median of 4 months, and four (27%) remain in CR beyond 6 years—consistent with results that are expected with ABMT for such patients.

A subsequent phase 1 and 2 trial with the Seattle IL-2 regimen (Chiron) after ASCT included 16 patients with AML beyond CR1, some with secondary AML. The published, updated results (57) reveal that one patient with a history of mantle radiation for prior HD died early of adult respiratory distress syndrome, two patients died in CR as a result of cytomegalovirus pneumonia or cardiac fibrosis, nine relapsed at a median of 8 months, and only four remain in CR beyond 6 years. The somewhat discrepant results between two different Seattle trials involving small groups of heterogeneous AML patients highlight the need for a prospective randomized phase 3 trial.

Virtually all other trials reported with IL-2 after ASCT for AML have involved patients in CR1. In the smallest series (64), six patients received high-dose IL-2 after ABMT. Five of these patients were still in CR at 1.5 to 5 years.

The effectiveness of the Seattle IL-2 regimen is being tested after ASCT for AML in CR1 at the City of Hope. To date (65), 46 such patients underwent ASCT after conditioning with total body irradiation, VP16, and cyclophosphamide (Cytoxan). At a median of 36 days after ASCT, 35 of these patients received IL-2. At 2 years, the disease-free survival for all 46 patients is 82%. The results are sufficiently encouraging to justify a phase 2 trial by SWOG with a view to a subsequent phase 3 trial to determine whether IL-2 will reduce the relapse rate and prolongs disease-free survival.

A small French trial, however, yielded no evidence of benefit (27). Twenty-two patients with AML in CR1 received IL-2 (from Roussel-Uclaf) beginning an average of 72 days after ABMT. Two patients died from toxicity. At 3 years, the probability of relapse was 59%, and leukemia-free survival was only 41%. These results are consistent with those expected without IL-2 therapy. IL-2 was administered later than other trials, and the IL-2 regimen delivered was somewhat unusual. Although a median of 69% of the scheduled dose of IL-2 was administered, the doses that were not tolerated and, therefore, not administered, were probably during the last 2 or 3 days of the first cycle because patients tend to tolerate the first 2 days of most IL-2 doses. If so, then these patients most likely received 2 days of IL-2 every other week for 5 weeks—a regimen not consistent with any of the short-term high-dose or chronic low-dose IL-2 regimens in any murine models.

The low-dose IL-2 regimen of Dana Farber/Roswell Park is being evaluated in a large phase 2 trial (CALGB, protocol 9,621) in patients who undergo ASCT for AML in CR1 with average to poor cytogenetic prognostic features. The IL-2 regimen consists of low-dose chronic s.c. IL-2 with intermittent 3-day periods of intermediate-dose bolus IL-2.

The use of stem cells incubated *in vitro* with IL-2 followed by systemic IL-2 is also being explored (66). Thirty-one patients with AML in CR1 at high risk for relapse underwent ASCT with marrow or stem cells cultured with IL-2 for 8 to 9 days. Beginning right after the infusion, the patients received IL-2 at a s.c. dose of 2 to 10×10^5 IU per m^2 per day for 7 days. Six patients died as a result of complications of ASCT, 12 relapsed, and 13 remain in CR at a median of 4 years. The results demonstrate that this approach is feasible, although probably rather cumbersome, and that incubated cells can reconstitute the patient hematologically. No conclusion can be drawn, however, about clinical benefit. Large phase 2 and 3 trials would have to be performed to determine if this approach is beneficial and to identify the treatment component required (i.e., IL-2, activated cells, or both).

Finally, IL-2 is being studied as part of a cocktail of cytokines and chemotherapy to mobilize stem cells for ASCT for patients with AML in CR1. In one such study (67), the actual leukemia-free survival for the 23 patients who received a systemic s.c. IL-2 dose of 3×10^6 IU per m^2 twice a day $\times$ 10 days was 63%. The median follow-up from CR, however, was less than a year. This approach seems feasible, but assessment of its clinical efficacy must await more trials and longer follow-up.

Interleukin-2 after Allogeneic Bone Marrow Transplant

AlloBMT for advanced hematologic malignancies is associated with a high relapse rate (e.g., >50%). The major rationale for using IL-2 as an adjunct to AlloBMT is to induce or augment a GVL effect, because the potential effector mechanisms of GVL (i.e., cytotoxic and noncytotoxic T cells, NK cells, and the secreted cytokines) may be enhanced by IL-2. The major concern, however, is that GVL and graft-versus-host disease (GVHD) share at least some effector mechanisms and targets. Thus, IL-2 therapy might increase the incidence or severity of GVHD.

Rare case reports exist of IL-2, alone or in combination with chemotherapy or IFN-α, inducing clinical antileukemic effects when given to patients whose leukemia relapsed after AlloBMT (68–71). Attempts to use IL-2 after AlloBMT to prevent relapses, however, have been limited by concern that it might induce fatal GVHD. To reduce this possibility, IL-2 was first used only in recipients of marrow depleted of T cells who were less likely to develop GVHD (72). Beginning a median of 67 days after BMT for a variety of hematologic malignancies, low-dose IL-2 was administered by c.i.v. at 2 to 4×10^5 IU per m^2 per day for 3 months. The number of circulating NK cells increased without a significant change in T-cell number. Only one patient developed GVHD. The relapse rate in the 25 patients who completed more than 4 weeks of IL-2 was significantly lower than that of historical controls who were transplanted for the same conditions in the same way without IL-2 and survived disease-free beyond 100 days. The results are interesting and encouraging and call for follow-up trials.

IL-2 therapy after unmodified AlloBMT could theoretically exert a greater GVL effect than after T cell–depleted BMT, but could also present a greater risk for GVHD. The relevant clinical data reported are sparse. Based on a report (73) that IL-2 protected against fatal GVHD in a murine model, seven leukemic patients received IL-2 at 3×10^6 IU per m^2 per day for 5 days by c.i.v. beginning 4 hours after BMT from a 2- to 3-antigen mismatched donor (74). All patients developed severe GVHD. Six patients died; three died as a result of GVHD. Clearly, this regimen of IL-2 administered early to mismatched recipients had unacceptable toxicity and no benefit.

The only reported trial of IL-2 in recipients of non–T cell–depleted allogeneic marrow was a phase 1 trial (75) conducted among 17 children who underwent matched sibling AlloBMT for acute leukemia beyond CR1. They began receiving IL-2 (Roche) by c.i.v. a median of 68 days after BMT. Cohorts of patients received escalating doses of induction IL-2 (0.9, 3.0, or 6.0×10^6 IU per m^2 per day for 5 days, representing levels 1, 2, and 3) as inpatients and were then discharged. After 6 days of rest, they received maintenance IL-2 (0.9×10^6 IU per m^2 per day for 10 days) as outpatients.

Because IL-2 could potentially exacerbate GVHD, and because the immunosuppressive agents used for GVHD prophylaxis could interfere with an immunologically mediated antileukemic effect of IL-2, the IL-2 was administered only to children whose GVHD prophylaxis was withdrawn and who developed no GVHD during the susequent 2 weeks. Three patients received level 1, eight patients received level 2, and six patients received level 3. The MTD of induction IL-2 was determined to be level 2.

All induction doses of IL-2 at levels 1 and 2 were received by all patients. Fever, nausea, vomiting, diarrhea, weight gain, and mild rash were common, reversible, and not dose limiting. Levels 1 and 2 were not associated with any toxicities greater than

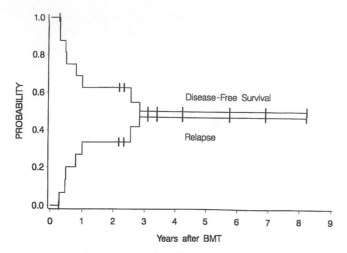

FIGURE 3. Kaplan-Meier product limit estimates of relapse and disease-free survival of children treated with allogeneic HLA-identical matched-sibling bone marrow transplantation (BMT) plus interleukin-2 for acute leukemia in first relapse (n = 17) or later. (From Fefer A. Graft-versus-tumor responses. In: Thomas ED, Blume KG, Forman S, eds. *Hematopoietic cell transplantation.* Cambridge, MA: Blackwell, 1999:316–326; and Robinson N et al. Phase 1 trial of interleukin-2 after unmodified HLA-matched sibling bone marrow transplantation for children with acute leukemia. *Blood* 1996;87:1249–1254, with permission.)

grade 2. Most patients exhibited a mild, reversible thrombocytopenia with a nadir during the rest period and a return to baseline during maintenance. Neutropenia did not occur.

Acute GVHD during IL-2 therapy was observed in only two patients—one after completing level 1 and one at level 3. In both patients, GVHD resolved within a week of discontinuing IL-2 without additional therapy. Extensive, chronic GVHD of variable severity occurred in five patients (one out of three patients at level 1, zero out of eight patients at level 2, and four out of five patients at level 3). The immunologic changes induced were comparable to those observed with IL-2 after ABMT with lymphocytosis and increases in cells expressing CD8 and CD56. Thus, level 2 (MTD) induction IL-2 induced immunomodulatory effects, was relatively well tolerated, and was not associated with a high incidence or great severity of acute or chronic GVHD.

The clinical outcomes for the 17 patients reported (75) are updated (63) in Figure 3. One patient died early of infection, seven relapsed, and nine remain in CR at 3 to 8 years. These long-term disease-free survivors include four out of six patients with AML and 5 out of 11 patients with ALL—all at high risk for relapse. The results are better than expected for such patients with AlloBMT alone. A multisite phase 2 trial has been initiated.

SUMMARY AND CONCLUSIONS

The role of IL-2 in the treatment of hematologic malignancies has yet to be defined. The most cogent and relevant observation is that some patients with some refractory hematologic malignancies, especially AML and NHL, have responded to some regimen of IL-2 with or without LAK cells, usually with PRs, but occasionally with durable CRs. These results need to be

confirmed, and anecdotal responses in other hematologic malignancies need to be validated. The optimal regimen remains unknown and can be identified only by comparative trials in more homogeneous patients because the trials involved small numbers of clinically heterogeneous patients and different IL-2 regimens.

Theoretically, IL-2 therapy should be more effective in a setting of MRD (e.g., after conventional chemotherapy or high-dose therapy plus blood or marrow stem-cell rescue). Several small phase 2 trials have been performed with IL-2 for AML patients in chemotherapy-induced CR1 with inconclusive results. One randomized phase 3 trial of one regimen of IL-2 for AML in CR1 has been initiated by the Children's Cancer Group. Similar trials are anticipated by other groups with other regimens. Two phase 2 trials are in progress by CALGB and are likely to lead to phase 3 trials.

The post-transplant setting may be preferable to the post-chemotherapy setting for IL-2 therapy. In the post-transplant setting, fewer residual tumor cells exist and more CD56+ cells are present with MHC-unrestricted lytic activity against tumors, particularly those hematologic malignancies that express few MHC molecules. Pilot or phase 1 and 2 trials of various IL-2 regimens administered after ABMT yielded some encouraging but inconsistent and inconclusive results. Based on encouraging results of one phase 2 trial, a phase 3 trial of IL-2 versus observation after ASCT for relapsed NHL is in progress by SWOG. Moreover, rigorous phase 2 trials of IL-2 for patients who have undergone ABMT or ASCT for AML in CR1 are in progress or about to be initiated by SWOG and CALGB.

The use of IL-2 after allogeneic transplantation is based on the hope that a donor lymphocyte-mediated GVL effect can be induced or augmented without concomitant exacerbation of GVHD. Trials have been limited by concern that IL-2 might induce severe or fatal GVHD. The encouraging clinical results of two phase 1 and 2 trials of IL-2 administered to recipients of allogeneic T cell–depleted or non–T cell–depleted marrow for leukemia, however, warrant larger phase 2 and, ultimately, phase 3 trials.

The MRD setting is one in which the efficacy of IL-2, or any other immunotherapy, is most difficult to evaluate because it ultimately requires randomized phase 3 trials with large numbers of patients and a long follow-up time. The lower the amount of MRD at initiation of IL-2 therapy (e.g., AML in CR1), the more patients and longer follow-up time is required. Moreover, it is extraordinarily difficult to identify the optimal regimen of IL-2 without measurable disease to follow and without surrogate markers or proxy laboratory assays predictive of clinical efficacy. Thus, the optimal therapeutic dose of IL-2 may or may not be the MTD.

The impact of any additional therapeutic variable, such as exogenously generated LAK cells obtained after chemotherapy, after recovery from BMT, or as part of the infused marrow and stem cells, is even more difficult to assess in an adjuvant clinical setting. It requires phase 2 and 3 trials to determine not only the therapeutic efficacy of the entire combination of IL-2–activated cells and systemic IL-2, but also whether all components are required.

In summary, the role of IL-2 in the treatment of hematologic malignancies remains unknown but deserves continued investigation. The encouraging clinical results reported, however sparse, suggest that its role will be clarified with additional basic research and clinical trials that are in progress or soon to be initiated. Until then, IL-2 should be used for hematologic malignancies only in the investigative setting of a clinical trial.

REFERENCES

1. Thompson JA, Peace DJ, Klarnet JP, Kem DE, Greenberg PD, Cheever MA. Eradication of disseminated murine leukemia by treatment with high-dose interleukin 2. *J Immunol* 1986;137:3675–3680.
2. Cheever M, Greenberg P, Fefer A, Gillis S. Augmentation of the antitumor therapeutic efficacy of long-term cultured T lymphocytes by *in vivo* administration of purified interleukin-2. *J Exp Med* 1982;155:968–980.
3. Lotzova E, Savary CA, Herberman RB. Induction of NK cell activity against fresh human leukemia in culture with interleukin 2. *J Immunol* 1987;138:2718–2727.
4. Mackinnon S, Hows JM, Goldman JM. Induction of in vitro graft-versus-leukemia activity following bone marrow transplantation for chronic myeloid leukemia. *Blood* 1990;76:2037–2045.
5. Oshimi K, Oshimi Y, Akutsu M, et al. Cytotoxicity of interleukin 2-activated lymphocytes for leukemia and lymphoma cells. *Blood* 1986;68:938–948.
6. Dawson MM, Johnston D, Taylor GM, Moore M. Lymphokine activated killing of fresh human leukaemias. *Leuk Res* 1986;10:683–688.
7. Allavena P, Damia G, Colombo T, Maggioni D, D'Incalci M, Mantovani A. Lymphokine-activated killer (LAK) and monocyte-mediated cytotoxicity on tumor cell lines resistant to antitumor agents. *Cell Immunol* 1989;120:250–258.
8. Shimazaki C, Atzpodien J, Wisniewski D, et al. Cell-mediated toxicity of interleukin-2-activated lymphocytes against autologous and allogeneic human myeloma cells. *Acta Haematol* 1988;80:203–209.
9. Landay AL, Zarcone D, Grossi CE, Bauer K. Relationship between target cell cycle and susceptibility to natural killer lysis. *Cancer Res* 1987;47:2767–2770.
10. Lista P, Fierro MT, Liao XS, et al. Lymphokine-activated killer (LAK) cells inhibit the clonogenic growth of human leukemic stem cells. *Eur J Haematol* 1989;42:425–430.
11. Foa R, Caretto P, Fierro MT, et al. Interleukin-2 does not promote the in vitro and in vivo proliferation and growth of human acute leukaemia cells of myeloid and lymphoid origin. *Br J Haematol* 1990;75:34–40.
12. Foa R. Interleukin-2 in the management of acute leukaemia. *Br J Haematol* 1996;92:1–8.
13. Archimbaud E, Bailly M, Dore JF. Inducibility of lymphokine activated killer (LAK) cells in patients with acute myelogenous leukaemia in complete remission and its clinical relevance. *Br J Haematol* 1991;77:328–334.
14. West WH, Tauer KW, Yannelli JR, et al. Constant-infusion recombinant interleukin-2 in adoptive immunotherapy of advanced cancer. *N Engl J Med* 1987;316:898–905.
15. Schoof DD, Gramolini BA, Davidson DL, Massaro AF, Wilson RE, Eberlein TJ. Adoptive immunotherapy of human cancer using low-dose recombinant interleukin-2 and lymphokine-activated killer cells. *Cancer Res* 1988;48:5007–5010.
16. Margolin KA, Aronson FR, Sznol M, et al. Phase II trial of high-dose interleukin-2 and lymphokine-activated killer cells in Hodgkin's disease and non-Hodgkin's lymphoma. *J Immunother* 1991;10:214–220.
17. Bernstein ZP, Vaickus L, Friedman N, et al. Interleukin-2 lymphokine-activated killer cell therapy of non-Hodgkin's lymphoma and Hodgkin's disease. *J Immunother* 1991;10:141–146.
18. Tourani JM, Levy V, Briere J, Levy R, Franks C, Andrieu JM. Interleukin-2 therapy for refractory and relapsing lymphomas. *Eur J Cancer* 1991;27:1676–1680.
19. Weber JS, Yang JC, Topalian SL, Schwartzentruber DJ, White DE, Rosenberg SA. The use of interleukin-2 and lymphokine-activated killer cells for the treatment of patients with non-Hodgkin's lymphoma [see comments]. *J Clin Oncol* 1992;10:33–40.
20. Gisselbrecht C, Maraninchi D, Pico JL, et al. Interleukin-2 treatment in lymphoma: a phase II multicenter study. *Blood* 1994;83:2081–2085.
21. Rosolen A, Nakanishi M, Poplack DG, et al. Expression of interleukin-2 receptor beta subunit in hematopoietic malignancies. *Blood* 1989;73:1968–1972.
22. Paciucci PA, Holland JF, Glidewell O, Odchimar R. Recombinant interleukin-2 by continuous infusion and adoptive transfer of recombinant interleukin-2 activated cells in patients with advanced cancer. *J Clin Oncol* 1989;7:869–878.
23. Meloni G, Foa R, Vignetti M, et al. Interleukin-2 may induce prolonged remissions in advanced acute myelogenous leukemia. *Blood* 1994;84:2158–2163.
24. Meloni G, Vignetti M, Pogliani E, et al. Interleukin-2 therapy in relapsed acute myelogenous leukemia. *Cancer J Sci Am* 1997;3[Suppl 1]:S43–S47.
25. Maraninchi D, Blaise D, Viens P, et al. High-dose recombinant interleukin-2 and acute myeloid leukemias in relapse. *Blood* 1991;78:2182–2187.
26. Lim SH, Newland AC, Kelsey S, et al. Continuous intravenous infusion of high-dose recombinant interleukin-2 for acute myeloid leukaemia—a phase II study. *Cancer Immunol Immunother* 1992;34:337–342.
27. Blaise D, Maraninchi D. Interleukin 2 in the treatment of acute leukemia. *Leuk Res* 1998;22:1165–1170.
28. Ganser A, Heil G, Hofmann WK, et al. Aggressive chemotherapy with idarubicin, ARA-C, VP-16, amsacrine, followed by G-CSF and maintenance immunotherapy with interleukin-2 for advanced myelodysplastic syndromes and high-risk ANLL. *Blood* 1995;86:434A.
29. Macdonald D, Jiang YZ, Gordon AA, et al. Recombinant interleukin-2 for acute myeloid leukaemia in first complete remission: a pilot study. *Leuk Res* 1990;14:967–973.
30. Cortes JKH, O'Brien S, Keating M, Estey E. Interleukin-2 (IL-2) therapy for adult patients (PTS) with acute myelogenous leukemia (AML) in first complete remission (CR). *Blood* 1997;90[Suppl 1]:505A.
31. Faber ELK, Mocikova K, Kuvikova A, et al Low-dose interleukin-2 in AML in first remission—a multicentre randomized study. *Blood* 1997;92[Suppl 1]:240B.
32. Baer MR, Pixley LA, Schriber JR, et al. Prolonged administration of low-dose interleukin-2 (IL-2) to patients (pts) with acute myeloid leukemia (AML) in remission (CR) expands natural killer (NK) cells without significant clinical toxicity. *Blood* 1998;92[Suppl 1]:614A.
33. Hellstrand K, Meliqvist UH, Walihult E, et al. Histamine and interleukin-2 in acute myelogenous leukemia. *Leuk Lymphoma* 1997;27:429–438.
34. Walihult E, Meliqvist UH, Celsing F, et al. Safety and feasibility of IL-2 + histamine dihydrochloride (Maxamine) in AML patients in first or subsequent complete remission. *Blood* 1998;92:614A.
35. Sievers EL, Lange BJ, Sondel PM, et al. Feasibility, toxicity and biologic response of interleukin-2 after consolidation chemotherapy for acute myelogenous leukemia: a report from the Children's Cancer Group. *J Clin Oncol* 1998;16:1914–1919.
36. Shepherd JDJE, Gratwohl A, Helbig W, et al. Phase II study of subcutaneous rHu interleukin-2 in patients with acute myelogenous leukemia in partial or complete second remission and partial relapse. *Br J Hematol* 1994;87[Suppl 1].
37. Wiernik PH, Dutcher JP, Todd M, Caliendo G, Benson L. Polyethylene glycolated interleukin-2 as maintenance therapy for acute myelogenous leukemia in second remission. *Am J Hematol* 1994;47:41–44.
38. Bergmann L, Heil G, Kolbe K, et al. Interleukin-2 bolus infusion as late consolidation therapy in 2nd remission of acute myeloblastic leukemia. *Leuk Lymphoma* 1995;16:271–279.

39. Reittie JE, Gottlieb D, Heslop HE, et al. Endogenously generated activated killer cells circulate after autologous and allogeneic marrow transplantation but not after chemotherapy. *Blood* 1989;73:1351–1358.

40. Weisdorf DJ, Nesbit ME, Ramsay NK, et al. Allogeneic bone marrow transplantation for acute lymphoblastic leukemia in remission: prolonged survival associated with acute graft-versus-host disease. *J Clin Oncol* 1987;5:1348–1355.

41. Gottlieb DJ, Brenner MK, Heslop HE, et al. A phase I clinical trial of recombinant interleukin-2 following high dose chemo-radiotherapy for haematological malignancy: applicability to the elimination of minimal residual disease. *Br J Cancer* 1989;60:610–615.

42. Higuchi C, Thompson J, Cox T, Lindgren C, Buckner C, Fefer A. Lymphokine-activated killer function following autologous bone marrow transplantation for refractory hematologic malignancies. *Cancer Res* 1989;49:5509–5513.

43. Neubauer M, Benyunes M, Thompson J, et al. Lymphokine-activated killer (LAK) precursor cell activity is present in infused peripheral blood stem cells and in the blood after autologous peripheral blood stem cell transplantation. *Bone Marrow Transplant* 1994;13: 311–316.

44. Butturini A, Bortin MM, Gale RP. Graft-versus-leukemia following bone marrow transplantation. *Bone Marrow Transplant* 1987;2: 233–242.

45. Brunda MJ, Luistro L, Warrier RR, et al. Antitumor and antimetastatic activity of interleukin 12 against murine tumors. *J Exp Med* 1993;178:1223–1230.

46. Cheever M, Greenberg P, Fefer A. Potential for specific cancer therapy with immune T lymphocytes. *J Biol Resp Mod* 1984;3:113–127.

47. Brunvand MW, Bensinger WI, Soll E, et al. High-dose fractionated total-body irradiation, etoposide and cyclophosphamide for treatment of malignant lymphoma: comparison of autologous bone marrow and peripheral blood stem cells. *Bone Marrow Transplant* 1996;18:131–141.

48. Higuchi C, Thompson J, Petersen F, Buckner C, Fefer A. Toxicity and immunomodulatory effects of interleukin-2 after autologous bone marrow transplantation for hematologic malignancies. *Blood* 1991;77:2561–2568.

49. Soiffer RJ, Murray C, Cochran K, et al. Clinical and immunologic effects of prolonged infusion of low-dose recombinant interleukin-2 after autologous and T-cell-depleted allogeneic bone marrow transplantation. *Blood* 1992;79:517–526.

50. Blaise D, Viens P, Olive D, et al. Recombinant interleukin-2 (rIL-2) after autologous bone marrow transplantation (BMT): a pilot study in 19 patients. *Eur Cytokine Netw* 1991;2:121–129.

51. Stoppa AM, Vey N, Viret F, et al. Early and prolonged D1-86 administration of low dose interleukin-2 (IL-2) after autologous stem cell transplantation (ASCT) for haematologic malignancies. *Blood* 1998;92(Suppl 1):295a

52. Mulé JJ, Shu S, Schwarz SL, Rosenberg SA. Adoptive immunotherapy of established pulmonary metastases with LAK cells and recombinant interleukin-2. *Science* 1984;225:1487–1489.

53. Mulé JJ, Shu S, Rosenberg SA. The anti-tumor efficacy of lymphokine-activated killer cells and recombinant interleukin 2 *in vivo*. *J Immunol* 1985;135:646–652.

54. Fefer A, Benyunes MC, Massumoto C, et al. Interleukin-2 therapy after autologous bone marrow transplantation for hematologic malignancies. *Semin Oncol* 1993;20:41–45.

55. Benyunes MC, Massumoto C, York A, et al. Interleukin-2 with or without lymphokine-activated killer cells as consolidative immunotherapy after autologous bone marrow transplantation for acute myelogenous leukemia. *Bone Marrow Transplant* 1993;12:159–163.

56. Benyunes MC, Higuchi C, York A, et al. Immunotherapy with interleukin 2 with or without lymphokine-activated killer cells after autologous bone marrow transplantation for malignant lymphoma: a feasibility trial. *Bone Marrow Transplant* 1995;16:283–288.

57. Robinson N, Benyunes MC, Thompson JA, et al. Interleukin-2 after autologous stem cell transplantation for hematologic malignancy: a phase I/II study. *Bone Marrow Transplant* 1997;19:425–442.

58. Again R, Malloy B, Kemer M, et al. Potent graft antitumor effect in natural killer-resistant disseminated tumors by transplantation of interleukin-2-activated syngeneic bone marrow in mice. *Cancer Res* 1989;49:5959–5963.

59. van Besien K, Champlin R. Activity of interleukin-2 in non-Hodgkin's lymphoma following transplantation of interleukin-2-activated autologous bone marrow or stem cells. Cancer J Sci Am 1997;3:S54.

60. Nagler A, Ackerstein A, Or R, Naparstek E, Slavin S. Immunotherapy with recombinant human interleukin-2 and recombinant interferon-alpha in lymphoma patients postautologous marrow or stem cell transplantation. *Blood* 1997;89:3951–3959.

61. Weisdorf DJ, Anderson PM, Blazar BR, Uckun FM, Kersey JH, Ramsay NK. Interleukin-2 immediately after autologous bone marrow transplantation for acute lymphoblastic leukemia—a phase 1 study. *Transplantation* 1993;55:61–66.

62. Attal M, Blaise D, Marit G, et al. Consolidation treatment of adult acute lymphoblastic leukemia: a prospective, randomized trial comparing allogeneic versus autologous bone marrow transplantation and testing the impact of recombinant interleukin-2 after autologous bone marrow transplantation. BGMT Group. *Blood* 1995; 86:1619–1628.

63. Fefer A. Graft-versus-tumor responses. In: Thomas ED, Blume KG, Forman S, eds. *Hematopoietic cell transplantation*. Cambridge, MA: Blackwell Science, 1999:316–326.

64. Hamon MD, Prentice HG, Gottlieb DJ, et al. Immunotherapy with interleukin-2 after ABMT in AML. Bone Marrow Transplant 1993;11:399–401.

65. Stein AODMR, Parker P, Snyder DS, et al. Interleukin 2(IL-2) post high dose cytarabine mobilized autologous stem cell transplant (ASCT) for adult patients with acute myelogenous leukemia (AML) in first complete remission (CR). *Blood* 1998;92[Suppl 1]:292A.

66. Hogge D, Eaves C, Barnett M, et al. Autologous stem cell transplants (ASCT) cultured in interleukin-2 (IL-2) for high risk acute myelogenous leukemia (AML) in first complete remission (CR). *Blood* 1998;92:292A.

67. Schiller GM, Sawyers C, Paquette R, Wolin M, Kunkel L, Territo M. Transplantation of interleukin-2-mobilized autologous peripheral blood progenitor cells procured after high-dose cytarabine/G-CSF-based consolidation for adults with acute myelogenous leukemia in first complete remission. *Blood* 1998;92[Suppl 1]:293A.

68. O'Brien D, Boughton B. High and low affinity IL-2 receptors on human leukaemic blast cells [letter]. *Br J Haematol* 1990;76: 315–317.

69. Butturini A, Bonilauri E, Izzi G, et al. Therapy of advanced acute myeloblastic leukemia with cytarabine and interleukin-2. *Leuk Res* 1991;15:759–763.

70. Mehta J, Powles R, Singhal S, Tait D, Swansbury J, Treleaven J. Cytokine-mediated immunotherapy with or without donor leukocytes for poor-risk acute myeloid leukemia relapsing after allogeneic bone marrow transplantation. *Bone Marrow Transplant* 1995;16: 133–137.

71. Verdonck LFVH, Hans G, Giltay J, Franks CR. Amplification of the graft-versus-leukemia effect in man by interleukin-2. *Transplantation* 1991;51:1120–1124.

72. Soiffer RJ, Murray C, Gonin R, Ritz J. Effect of low-dose interleukin-2 on disease relapse after T-cell-depleted allogeneic bone marrow transplantation. *Blood* 1994;84:964–971.

73. Sykes M, Romick ML, Sachs DH. Interleukin-2 prevents graft-versus-host disease while preserving the graft-versus-leukemia effect of allogeneic T cells. *Proc Natl Acad Sci USA* 1990;87:5633–5637.

74. Przepiorka D, Ippoliti C, Koberda J, et al. Interleukin-2 for prevention of graft-versus-host disease after haploidentical marrow transplantation. *Transplantation* 1994;58:858–860.

75. Robinson N, Sanders JE, Benyunes MC, et al. Phase I trial of interleukin-2 after unmodified HLA-matched sibling bone marrow transplantation for children with acute leukemia. *Blood* 1996;87: 1249–1254.

4

INTERLEUKIN-4: CLINICAL APPLICATIONS

HIDEHO OKADA
MICHAEL T. LOTZE

BIOLOGY OF INTERLEUKIN-4

Molecular Aspects

Interleukin-4 (IL-4) is a glycoprotein with an approximate molecular mass of 15 to 19 kd. A mouse IL-4 complementary DNA (cDNA) was first isolated from a mouse T helper 2 (Th2) cell library as a cDNA encoding for a unique mouse interleukin that expressed B-cell, T-cell, and mast-cell stimulating activities (1). Subsequently, a human IL-4 cDNA was isolated by cross-hybridization from an activated human T-cell clone cDNA library (2). Mouse chromosomal DNA segments for IL-4 were isolated based on homology with the IL-4 cDNA and mapped to chromosome 11 (3). The gene for human IL-4 consists of four exons and three introns located on chromosome 5 at position q23.3–31.2 (4). It is produced mostly by activated Th2 cells (5) and mast cells (6). Multiple stimulatory and regulatory effects on the immune system can be demonstrated (Table 1). IL-4 mediates its biologic activity by binding to a high-affinity receptor expressed on B and T lymphocytes, myeloid cells, monocytes, macrophages, mast cells, fibroblasts, endothelial cells, and some cancer cells (7–9). Initially, it was shown that IL-4 binds to three molecular species of 140-, 70- to 75-, and 65-kd molecular weight (10,11). The 140-kd protein is termed *IL-4 receptor α* (IL-4Rα) (12) and the 65-kd form is termed the γ *common chain* (γ_c), which is shared with other cytokine receptors, including IL-2, IL-7, IL-9, and IL-15. The γ_c chain increases by two- to threefold the affinity of IL-4 for gp140 and IL-4Rα in lymphoid cells (13,14). Binding of IL-4 to the IL-4Rα chain induces dimerization of the IL-4Rα chain with the γ_c chain in these cells. It has been demonstrated that two different forms of IL-4R exist: the classical and alternative forms (15) (Fig. 1). The classical IL-4Rα form is predominantly expressed in hematopoietic cells and consists of IL-4Rα and γ_c chains. The alternative form of IL-4R is predominantly expressed in nonhematopoietic cells and consists of IL-4Rα and IL-13Rα' chains. Moreover, the alternative form of IL-4R is used as a functional component of the IL-13R complex (15,16). Sanafelt et al. created a mutant form of IL-4 that was substituted in the region of IL-4 implicated in interactions with the γ_c chain. The mutant containing the mutation Arg-121 to Glu (IL-4/R121E) exhibited complete functional and binding selectivity for T cells, B cells, and monocytes. The mutant showed no activity on endothelial cells, which express only alternative forms of IL-4R, suggesting its use in the treatment of certain autoimmune diseases (17). It has been shown that the phosphorylation and acti-

vation of Janus tyrosine kinase (Jak)3 is crucial for IL-4–induced activation of signal transducer and activator of transcription (STAT) 6 in hematopoietic cells. It has been demonstrated that nonhematopoietic cells, however, lack Jak3 expression. In these cells, Jak1 and Jak2 mediate activation of STAT6 instead (16). Furthermore, IL-4 and IL-13 signals are transmitted through the alternative form of IL-4R in these cells (18). The structure and signal transduction through IL-4R and IL-13R appear to be different in hematopoietic versus nonhematopoietic cells. The crystal structural analysis of the complex between the human IL-4 and IL-4Rα chain revealed a novel spatial orientation of the two proteins; a small, but unexpected, conformational change in the receptor-bound IL-4 and an interface with separate clusters of transinteracting residues (19). Downstream events involve insulin receptor substrate–2, phosphoinositol-3 kinase activation, and STAT6 translocation (20) to the nucleus.

Immunology

IL-4 promotes growth and differentiation of B cells (21,22), T cells, and mast cells and mediates profound regulatory effects on macrophages (23). IL-4 increases surface class II major histocompatibility complex (MHC) antigens in B cells (24), low-affinity Fc receptors (CD23), surface immunoglobulin (Ig) M, CD40, and cell adhesion molecules (i.e., leukocyte function–associated antigens 1 and 3) (25). IL-4 induces Ig isotype switching for IgG1 and IgE production (26,27); stimulates the growth of normal helper and cytotoxic T cells (28), including tumor-infiltrating lymphocytes (29); and acts synergistically with IL-2 to enhance proliferation of precursor cytotoxic T lymphocytes, inducing their differentiation into active cytotoxic T lymphocytes (30). IL-4 also upregulates the expression of vascular cell adhesion molecule 1 on activated endothelia (31). IL-4 in combination with granulocyte-macrophage colony-stimulating factor, promotes the differentiation of bone marrow precursor cells to dendritic cells (DC), as described in the section Interleukin-4 in Dendritic Cell Biology and Its Use in Dendritic Cell–Based Therapy (32–36).

Interleukin-4 in T-Helper Cell Responses

IL-4 is a Th2-type response mediator. Naïve helper T cells differentiate preferentially to Th2-type cells, which produce predominantly IL-4, IL-5, IL-6, and IL-10; drive isotype switching in the

TABLE 1. BIOLOGIC PROPERTIES OF INTERLEUKIN-4

Human IL-4: Glycoprotein with molecular weight of 15–19 kd encoded on chromosome 5 at q23.3–31.2

Mouse IL-4: Molecular weight: 19 kd (EL-4 cells) and 24 kd (COS7-derived recombinant) encoded on chromosome 11

Produced by CD4$^+$ T cells (Th2 subset), basophils, and mast cells

Other names: B-cell growth factor–1, B-cell stimulating factor, mast-cell growth factor, and T-cell growth factor–2

Effects on B Cells

    Increases surface class II major histocompatibility complex antigens in B cells

    Induces Ig isotype switching for IgG1 and IgE production

    Enhances Ig production and expression of CD23 on B cells

Effects on T Cells

    Stimulates the growth of normal helper and cytotoxic T cells, including tumor-infiltrating lymphocytes

    Promotes Th2 cell growth

    Stimulates the growth of normal helper and cytotoxic T cells, including tumor-infiltrating lymphocytes; acts synergistically with IL-2 to enhance proliferation of precursor cytotoxic T lymphocytes and induce their differentiation into active cytotoxic T lymphocytes

    In concert with TGF-β, promotes the differentiation of naïve CD4$^+$ T cells into Th1-type cells

    Roles in induction of Th1-type response and antitumor-immune response shown in experiments using IL-4 gene knockout mice

Effects on Myeloid Cells

    In combination with GM-CSF, promotes the differentiation of bone marrow precursor cells to DCs

    Drives Th1 response by inducing apoptotic death of lymphoid DCs and mature myeloid DCs

    Decreases macrophage production of IL-1β, IL-6, and TNF-α

Effects on Other Cells

    Direct growth-inhibitory effect on human cancer cells, including induction of apoptotic cell death

    Inhibits angiogenesis

    Upregulates the expression of vascular cell adhesion molecule 1 on endothelia, allowing enhanced recruitment of VLA-4$^+$ cells (i.e., memory T cells, eosinophils, and DCs)

DCs, dendritic cells; GM-CSF, granulocyte-macrophage colony-stimulating factor; Ig, immunoglobulin; IL, interleukin; TGF-β, tumor growth factor–β; Th1, T helper 1; Th2, T helper 2; TNF-α, tumor necrosis factor–α; VLA, very late antigen.

differentiation of B cells; and enhance CD8$^+$ T-cell production of IL-4 (i.e., Tc2). The view of IL-4 as solely a Th2 inducer, however, oversimplifies its biology. In the presence of IL-4 and tumor growth factor–β, both of which are known as Th2 differentiation factors, naïve CD4$^+$ T cells can differentiate into Th1-type cells, at least *in vitro* (37). Critical roles of IL-4 in the induction of Th1-type responses and antitumor immune responses have been demonstrated in experiments using IL-4 gene knockout mice (38). Initiation of the immune response to otherwise immunogenic tumors is markedly suppressed in these animals. Peritumoral IL-4 expression after transfection with the IL-4 gene, however, restores the Th1-mediated antitumor immune response in these IL-4–deficient mice, suggesting the potent ability of IL-4 to induce a response even in immunologically compromised hosts.

Interleukin-4 in Dendritic Cell Biology and Its Use in Dendritic Cell–Based Therapy

Figdor et al. noted that IL-4 is capable of enhancing the antigen-presenting capacity of human monocytes accompanied by upregu-

lation of MHC class II and reduced secretion of IL-1β, IL-6, and tumor necrosis factor–α (TNF-α) (39). Later, it was found that IL-4 in combination with granulocyte-macrophage colony-stimulating factor also promotes the acquisition of a DC phenotype and function in mouse bone marrow (34) and human monocyte precursors or CD34$^+$ cell (32–36) cultures. Thus, IL-4 is widely used *ex vivo* in clinical trials of DC-based cancer therapy (40–42). It has been demonstrated that myeloid DCs produce large amounts of IL-12 and induce Th1 differentiation; in contrast, lymphoid DCs derived from CD4$^+$, CD3$^-$, and CD11$^-$ plasmacytoid cells cause Th2 differentiation. Furthermore, IL-4 has been demonstrated to drive Th1 responses by inducing apoptotic death of lymphoid DCs and maturing myeloid DCs (44). These findings suggest a possible mechanism by which local exogenous IL-4 mediates immune modulation at the level of the antigen-presenting cell.

Other Biologic Functions

Human IL-4 has a direct growth-inhibitory effect on human renal cell carcinoma and malignant melanoma cells (44–48). These cells express the high-affinity receptor for IL-4. Lahm et al. examined the effect of IL-4 on the growth of seven human colorectal carcinoma cell lines. In five of seven cell lines, a dose-dependent reduction of proliferation was observed, and those cells expressed functional IL-4R (49). The growth inhibition mediated by IL-4 involves suppression of insulinlike growth factor 2 (50). Similar observations were found in human astrocytes and astrocytic tumors (51). Growth inhibition of glioma cells by IL-4 appears to involve upregulation of p27Kip1, a cyclin-dependent kinase inhibitor (52). One report (53) demonstrated an IL-4R–dependent growth inhibition by IL-4, as well as human breast cancer cell lines. Apoptotic cell death was detected as a mechanism of IL-4–induced growth inhibition. Taken together, the antitumor effect of IL-4 on human cancer cells appears to be mediated, at least in part, by the direct inhibition of tumor growth via IL-4R–mediated signaling. IL-4 may promote the growth of some types of human cancer cells, however, such as squamous cell carcinoma of the head and neck cell lines (54).

Antiangiogenesis is an important strategy to control tumor growth *in vivo*. Murine IL-4 downregulates the expression of vascular endothelial growth factor receptor 2, one of the receptors for vascular endothelial growth factor on endothelial cells *in vitro* (55). The inhibited growth of C6 rat glioma cells engineered to express murine IL-4 in athymic mice is accompanied by reduced levels of vascularization. Volpert et al. (56) demonstrated that IL-4 blocks the basic fibroblast growth factor–mediated neovascularization in rat cornea. No species specificity was observed in the effect. IL-13 inhibited the migration of human or bovine microvascular cells, as well as IL-4.

RECOMBINANT INTERLEUKIN-4 IN CANCER THERAPY

Animal Models

The availability of recombinant IL-4 led investigators to test its antitumor effect *in vivo*. Hillman et al. demonstrated the therapeutic potential of systemic IL-4 administration for the treatment

Classical IL-4R

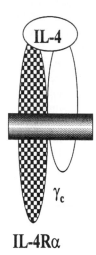

IL-4Rα

Hematopoietic Cells

Alternative IL-4R

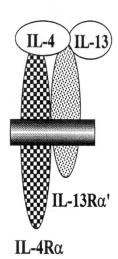

IL-13Rα'

IL-4Rα

Nonhematopoietic Cells
Including Cancer Cells

Type I IL-13R

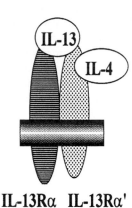

IL-13Rα IL-13Rα'

Renal Cell Carcinoma
Glioblastoma
Ovarian Carcinoma

FIGURE 1. Interleukin-4 receptor (IL-4R) structure model. The classical IL-4R is predominantly expressed in hematopoietic cells and consists of the 140-kd protein, IL-4Rα, and the 65-kd form of the γ common chain (γ_c), which is shared with other cytokine receptors, including IL-2, IL-7, IL-9, and IL-15. An alternative form of IL-4R is predominantly expressed in nonhematopoietic cells, including endothelia, and consists of IL-4Rα and IL-13Rα' chains. IL-4 and IL-13 signal through the alternative IL-4R in nonhematopoietic cells. Thus, the structure and signal transduction through IL-4R and IL-13R appear to be different between hematopoietic and nonhematopoietic cells. IL-4Rα chain is also required in functional type 1 IL-13R. This chain binds to both IL-4 and IL-13 in type I IL-13R system. In this complex, IL-13 binds to all three chains, whereas IL-4 binds to only two chains. (Modified from Murata T, Obiri NI, Debinski W, Puri RK. Structure of IL-13 receptor: analysis of subunit composition in cancer and immune cells. *Biochem Biophys Res Commun* 1997;238:90–94; and Obiri NI, Leland P, Murata T, Debinski W, Puri RK. The IL-13 receptor structure differs on various cell types and may share more than one component with IL-4 receptor. *J Immunol* 1997;158:756–764, with permission.)

of pulmonary metastases in a murine RenCa renal adenocarcinoma model (57). A dose-dependent (up to 2 µg per animal per day for 5 consecutive days since day 5) reduction in the number of metastasis and augmented survival was observed. *In vivo* depletion of lymphocyte subpopulations indicated that CD8$^+$ T cells and asialo GM1$^+$ cells were involved in the rejection of tumors. When IL-4 was intralesionally administered to the same RenCa tumors implanted below the renal capsule (6 µg per animal, single injection), marked inhibition of primary tumor growth was observed. Little effect on the progression of distant metastatic sites was detected (58). A unique route of IL-4 administration was tested by Bosco et al. (59). Using BALB/c mice bearing a chemically induced fibrosarcoma or a spontaneous adenocarcinoma (TS/A), IL-4 was administered by daily, local subcutaneous injection at the site of tumor-draining lymph nodes. Small amounts (0.00001 to 1,000 µg per day) of recombinant IL-4 inhibited tumor growth and led to induction of immunologic memory specific for the tumor. Delivery of 0.1 µg per day of IL-4 led to the best survival among the dosages tested, suggesting a dichotomous response to IL-4. IL-4 inhibited tumor growth far better than the direct injection of the most effective doses of IL-2, IL-1, or interferon-γ. Tumor-draining lymph nodes from animals treated in these studies displayed numerous macrophages, activated lymphocytes, and eosinophils. Combination therapy was also tested. Coadministration of IL-1 with IL-4 was much better at eliciting tumor rejection and long-term memory superior to that observed with other cytokines used singly or in combination.

Other trials demonstrated a compromised tumor-rejection response after systemic administration of IL-4. Terres et al. (60) examined the effect of systemic administration of recombinant IL-4, IL-10, or both in mice harboring a syngeneic p815 tumor line transfected with B7.1. In nontreated animals, these tumors were rejected by T cell–mediated responses. Treatment of animals

with IL-4 particularly at higher doses when compared with other studies (10 µg per mouse begun on day 7 and ended on day 22 every 3 days) resulted in a compromised rejection response accompanied with splenomegaly characterized by a marked increase in neutrophils and natural killer cell activity. IL-10, in contrast, was not immunosuppressive. When given in combination with IL-4, IL-10 countered the IL-4–suppressive effect. Suppressive effects of systemic IL-4 administration in antitumor immunity were demonstrated in another trial (61). A higher number of pulmonary metastases in the murine melanoma cell line B16F10 was associated with enhanced production of IL-4 and IL-10 by CD4$^+$ T cells in the spleen. Such cells were not detected in animals inoculated with the same number of B16F1, a less metastatic B16 subclone compared with B16F10. When animals were treated with anti–IL-4 antibody, the number of metastases decreased. Animals with B16F1 cells had an increased number of metastases after treatment with 10 µg per kg of recombinant IL-4. This study suggested that IL-4 secreted from tumor-associated Th2 cells enhanced the metastatic ability of tumors *in vivo*, perhaps by activating the endothelium (IL-4 enhances expression of vascular cell adhesion molecule 1 on endothelial cells, enhancing recruitment of memory T cells and DCs). The impact of systemic IL-4 administration in tumor-bearing animals may differ depending on cell line, animal strains, and so forth, as well as timing, dosage, and the duration of administration. IL-4 mimics the immunobiology of other cytokines in which issues such as timing and location are important to function.

Clinical Trials of Recombinant Interleukin-4

Recombinant human IL-4 (rhIL-4) has been tested on various types of human tumors. Possible mechanisms that propagate trafficking of the antitumor effects of IL-4 include induction of immune responses, antiangiogenic effects, and induction of apoptotic death or direct growth inhibition of tumor cells or both. Phase 1 clinical trials with rhIL-4 as a single antitumor agent began in 1988. In general, rhIL-4 has been relatively well tolerated at lower doses, but dose-limiting toxicities have been reached with the glycosylated and nonglycosylated forms (61–65). Side effects include fatigue, diarrhea, gastric ulceration, arthralgia, dyspnea, headache, sinus congestion, and hyponatremia. The more common side effects are headache, nasal congestion, fever, fluid retention, anorexia, fatigue, nausea and vomiting, and diarrhea. With the exception of some inflammatory reactions at subcutaneous injection sites, no allergic reactions have been reported and no antibodies to rhIL-4 have been described. Pharmacokinetic studies indicate that IL-4 can be detected in the serum 8 to 12 hours after subcutaneous administration but is rapidly cleared after intravenous administration with a half-life of less than 1 hour (65). Elevated liver enzymes (i.e., alkaline phosphatase and transaminase) are frequently reported, especially in patients with hepatic disease. Following are some of the published results from single-agent phase 1 and 2 clinical trials with rhIL-4.

Atkins et al. tested relatively high doses (10 or 15 μg per kg, thrice-daily intravenous bolus injection) in ten patients (63). A dose of 10 μg per kg of IL-4 was found to be the maximum tolerated dose for this schedule. No clinical benefit, however, was observed. Vokes et al. (66) reported our clinical study with 62 patients with advanced non–small-cell lung cancer. A dose of 0.25 μg per kg or 1.0 μg per kg of rIL-4 was administered subcutaneously three times per week. Therapy was well tolerated with no myelosuppression or elevation of liver enzymes, bilirubin, or blood glucose. Symptoms encountered in patients with 1.0 μg per kg included fatigue (18 of 41 patients), fever (14 of 41 patients), and anorexia (12 of 41 patients). Among 55 evaluable patients, one partial response occurred that lasted longer than 5 years. Eight patients had stable disease lasting 106 to 350 days. Leach et al. (67,68) summarized the results of preclinical safety evaluation and found that *Escherichia coli*–derived rhIL-4 is safe and well tolerated in doses up to 5 μg per kg per day and 10 μg per kg when administered three times a week. Diverse effects observed in primates have not been generally observed in human patients.

We initially began phase 1 studies in the fall of 1988 with recombinant IL-4 provided by Sterling Pharmaceuticals (Malvern, PA). Patients were started at 1 μg per kg given as a rapid intravenous infusion once a day for 2 cycles of 7 days separated by a week of rest. This dose was escalated in 12 patients to a final dose of 30 μg per kg administered on the same schedule (61). Toxicities were minimal but included symptoms described previously in this section. Using a biologic assay with the induction of CD23 on a malignant B-cell line (69), we defined an α *phase* as approximately 8 minutes and a β *clearance* as approximately 48 minutes. Ultimately, a total of 100 patients were treated, 99 eligible for analysis. A review of this experience is being prepared for publication. Three patients per cohort were treated with rIL-4 at 1, 3, 10, or 30 μg per kg per day as a single intravenous bolus. Subsequent patients in group 1 (IL-4 alone) were administered IL-4 three times daily for a total of 15 doses at 3, 10, or 20 μg per kg per dose. In group 2, patients received a combination of IL-4 and IL-2 intravenous bolus at low doses of IL-2 (216,000 U per kg) with 2, 6, or 20 μg per kg IL-4 every 8 hours or at high doses of IL-2 (720,000 U per kg) with 2, 6, 10, or 20 μg per kg IL-4 in cohorts of three patients. Twenty-seven and ten patients, respectively, were treated with 20 μg of IL-4 every 8 hours and either 216,000 or 720,000 U per kg of IL-2, respectively. Toxicity of IL-4 was associated with mild hypotension, peripheral swelling, nasal congestion, and headache and was observed in a dose-dependent fashion. No responses were observed in the 48 patients who received IL-4 alone. Partial responses were observed in patients who received the combination therapies, including 51 evaluable patients. Two of 19 patients treated with melanoma who received the 720,000 U per kg per dose IL-2 with IL-4 had partial responses. Three out of 18 patients with renal cell carcinoma who received 216,000 or 720,000 U per kg per dose IL-2 with IL-4 had partial responses (2) or complete remissions (1). No patient (zero out of eight) with colon cancer responded. One of two patients with breast cancer responded to this therapy. In conclusion, no increases in survival were observed with IL-4 alone. Although responses were observed in combination with IL-2 treatment, the enhanced toxicity precluded effective application, suggesting the need for locoregional therapy with delivery by gene transfer approaches.

INTERLEUKIN-4 AND ITS USE IN GENE THERAPY

Animal Models

As is true for other cytokines, intrinsic potency and toxicity have complicated application of IL-4 as a therapeutic agent when applied systemically. Many cytokines mediate a variety of antagonistic and synergistic immunologic effects when encountered by immune cells, which are activated during the process of ongoing immune responses, at various stages subsequent to hematopoiesis and lineage commitment. Indeed, one of the major characteristics of most cytokines is their ability to regulate immunity at a local or regional level. Systemic levels provided by most conventional schema fail to mimic the induction of an effective immune response, particularly in the context of an established tumor. Introduction of genetic engineering of cells made it possible to assess the effects of sustained IL-4 production at local tumor sites (Table 2). The initial reports of Tepper et al. (70) demonstrated that tumor rejection could be initiated with IL-4 transfection of murine tumors. Tumor rejection was initially thought to be solely mediated by eosinophils and macrophage infiltration. In retrospect, it was almost certainly caused in part by endothelial activation and antiangiogenic effects mediated directly by IL-4 or through recruitment and activation of innate immune effectors, which can regulate the local angiogenic response alone. Transfecting the IL-4–dependent T-cell line with IL-4 led to autocrine growth *in vitro* (71,72). These cells could not grow *in vivo*, however, even in nude mice, presumably because of the local biologic activity of IL-4. Introducing the IL-4 gene into a murine renal cell carcinoma (RenCa) or a colorectal carcinoma (CT26) caused rejection, systemic immunity mediated predominantly by CD8+ T cells, and therapeutic effects, even when administered as late as 9 days after establishment of the primary tumor. Macrophages and eosinophils were observed to infiltrate the tumors early. T cells were observed to enter the tumor site mostly during the second week (73).

TABLE 2. GENE THERAPY APPROACHES USING INTERLEUKIN-4

Murine Models

Authors	Year	Tumor Type	Effector Type or Mechanisms
Tepper	1989	Plasmacytomas and mammary adenoca	Eosinophils and macrophages
Blankenstein	1990	IL-4–dependent T cell CT4S	Loss of tumorigenicity even in nu/nu mice
Golumbeck	1991	Renal cell carcinoma (RenCa)	CD8$^+$ T-cell mediated specific immunity
Pippin	1994	Colorectal (MC-38) and fibrosarcoma (MC-105)	Synergy with IL-2
Pericle	1994	Mammary adenoca (TS/A)	Cellular and humoral immunity
Stoppacciaro	1997	Colon cancer	Influx of dendritic cells
Cayeux	1997	β-galactosidase–expressing MCA-205 and TS/A	Enhancement of cross-printing
Okada	1999	Gliosarcoma (9L)	Effective peripheral vaccine against intracranial tumors
Schüler	1999	Colorectal (CT-26)	Required for antitumor T-cell priming in IL-4 knockout mice

Human Trials

Authors	Year	Tumor Type	Vaccine Formulation	Efficacy and Toxicity
Belli	1998	Melanoma	Transduced allogeneic melanoma cell line	Three out of seven patients with local response
Lotze	1999	Melanoma, etc. (see Table 3)	Transduced autologous fibroblasts	Three out of six melanoma patients and three out of 18 patients with local response

IL, interleukin.

We confirmed such studies in murine models and demonstrated synergy with systemic administration of IL-2 (74). Pericle et al. highlighted an aspect of IL-4 biology as the Th2-type response-inducing factor (75). Although morphologic observation suggested that the rejection of IL-4–transfected TS/A tumors depended on eosinophil cytolysis, lymphocyte depletion experiments showed that this rejection also required CD8$^+$ lymphocytes. The memory response induced by this initial rejection appears to be mediated partially by Th2-type humoral response, as well as antibody-dependent cellular cytotoxicity and other cellular-effector mechanisms. Comparison of these mechanisms mediating memory with those elicited by IL-2 gene-transduced TS/A cells shows that Th2 memory is more efficient in protecting against a subsequent challenge of TS/A-pc than the Th1-type memory elicited by IL-2 gene-transduced TS/A cells. As described in the Interleukin-4 in Dendritic Cell Biology and Its Use in Dendritic Cell–Based Therapy section, IL-4 plays an important role in DC maturation. IL-4–transduced cancer cells increased the influx of DCs to the tumor site relative to other cytokines (76), suggesting that local IL-4 expression at the vaccine site may enhance leukocyte recruitment, including DCs, thereby enhancing tumor-antigen presentation.

Cytokine gene-transfected tumor cells conferred protection against a subsequent lethal tumor challenge that was comparable with a tumor cell/adjuvant vaccine (77). Cayeux et al. (78) reported that IL-4/B7.1 cotransfected cells are clearly superior to a tumor cell/adjuvant vaccine. The mechanism responsible for enhanced antitumor immunity was addressed using the TS/A (H-2d) and MCA 205 (H-2b) tumors transfected with the individual cytokine gene or B7.1, or both (79). β-galactosidase (β-gal) was chosen as a surrogate tumor Ag. β-gal has well-defined MHC class I epitopes in H-2b and H-2d mice. Immunization of (H-2b × d) F1 mice with MCA-205/β-gal CD80 or IL-4 transfectants enhanced cross-priming and rejection of an otherwise lethal challenge with TS/A/β-gal. On the other hand, direct antigen presentation was examined using H-2b nu/nu mice reconstituted with F1 lymphocytes in which antigen-presenting cells expressed only the H-2b haplotype. These animals were immunized with H-2d TS/A/β-gal transfectants and challenged with TS/A/β-gal. CD80 enhanced direct antigen presentation by tumor cells. Cytokine gene transfection did not. This elegant set of studies demonstrated that combinations of cytokine (e.g., IL-4) and costimulatory molecule (CD80) gene therapy enhanced antitumor immunity by enhancing antigen-presenting cell function and defining effector pathways.

Interleukin-4 Gene Therapy in Central Nervous System Tumors

The central nervous system (CNS) has been regarded as a partly immune-privileged site. CNS tumors are indeed challenging targets for immunotherapy (80). Although cytokine gene therapy for CNS tumors is an attractive approach, inducing considerable inflammation after cytokine gene expression in the CNS may cause life-threatening brain edema or elevation of intracranial pressure (81). In murine brain tumor models, however, accumulating findings demonstrate that IL-4 can be expressed in the CNS as an effective treatment for brain tumors. For example, investigation of a spontaneously generated mouse glioma cell line transduced with a panel of cytokines demonstrated that IL-4–transduced glioma cells conferred antitumor immunity with the least toxic response to surrounding normal brain among the cytokines tested (82). Prolonged survival was observed in animals who received IL-2, TNF-α, or IL-4–secreting tumors. IL-2 and TNF-α, however, seemed to have a detrimental effect on survival in some animals when expressed intracerebrally. IL-4–encoding retroviral vector (83) or its combination with the herpes simplex thymidine kinase (HSV-TK) gene (84) or herpes simplex viruses (85) produces safe and effective antibrain tumor responses in murine brain tumor models.

We explored the potential of IL-4–transduced glioma peripheral vaccine to induce immunoreactivity to CNS tumors (86). As a mechanism for enhancing the safety of vaccine administration, we introduced the HSV-TK gene, a so-called suicide gene, into a

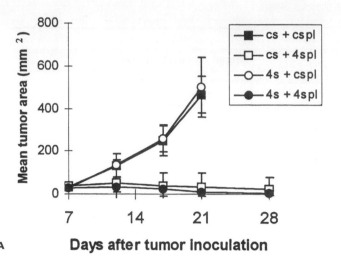

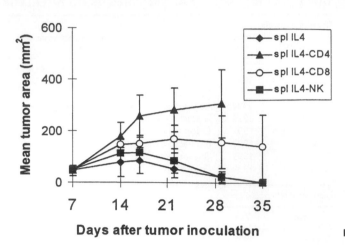

FIGURE 2. CD4$^+$ and CD8$^+$ cells play major roles in memory immune response against 9L gliosarcoma. **A:** Adoptive transfer of serum, splenocytes, or both, from 9L–IL-4–immunized rats. Four weeks after a single injection of 9L–IL-4, serum and splenocytes were harvested and transferred to irradiated recipient rats. Recipient rats were injected with 9L cells after 1 day. (cs, serum from control rats; cspl, splenocytes from control rats; 4s, serum from 9L–IL-4 immunized rats; 4spl, splenocytes from 9L–IL-4 immunized rats.) **B:** Depletion of subpopulations of splenocytes (spl) from 9L–IL-4 abrogates anti-9L immunity. Four weeks after a single injection of 9L–IL-4, splenocytes were harvested and depleted for CD4$^+$, CD8$^+$, and natural killer cells before being transferred to irradiated recipient rats. Recipient rats were injected with 9L cells after 1 day.

retroviral vector encoding the murine IL-4 and neomycin phosphotransferase genes. By incorporating the HSV-TK gene into IL-4–transduced glioma vaccines and subsequently treating vaccinated patients with ganciclovir, we hope to eliminate the small potential for local tumor growth at the site of vaccination and enhance the delivery of tumor antigens to antigen-presenting cells. Subcutaneous immunization of rats with nonirradiated IL-4 plus HSV-TK–transduced syngeneic rat gliosarcoma 9L (9L–IL-4-Tk) cells followed by treatment with ganciclovir completely protected animals from a subsequent intracranial challenge with wild-type 9L cells. More important, treatment of established (day 3) intracranial 9L tumors with genetically engineered tumor cells resulted in long-term survival (>100 days) for 25% to 43% of 9L–IL-4-Tk–immunized animals using various concentrations of ganciclovir and for 27% of nonirradiated IL-4–transfected 9L (9L–IL-4) immunized animals. These findings support the potential use of tumor cell vaccines expressing the IL-4 and HSV-TK genes for the treatment of malignant gliomas.

The mechanisms by which IL-4 induces anti-9L immune responses have been evaluated. 9L–IL-4 grew at a rate comparable to sham-transduced 9L (9L-neo) for a period of 10 to 14 days and then regressed. This occurred only in immunocompetent rats. Regression of 9L–IL-4 was not observed in nude athymic rats. These data clearly suggest a role for T cells in the regression of 9L–IL-4 tumors. In addition to evidence supporting T-cell involvement, we also determined that serum concentrations of Ig of the IgG1 isotype were markedly elevated in the sera of rats bearing 9L–IL-4. We were able to take advantage of this enhanced humoral-immune response to isolate tumor-associated antigens by combining IL-4 tumor vaccine and serologic identification of antigens by recombinant expression cloning (87). A series of adoptive transfer experiments were performed to determine whether transfer of humoral or cellular elements from immune to naïve rats were able to mediate protection against 9L because immunization with 9L–IL-4 apparently affects the cellular and

humoral immune response (88). Rats were immunized by implanting 2×10^6 9L–IL-4 cells subcutaneously; after 4 weeks, sera and splenocytes were harvested from rats in which 9L–IL-4 regressed. Sera or nylon wool nonadherent splenocytes or both were transferred to naïve, irradiated (1,000 rad) recipient rats. One day after transfer, recipient rats were implanted subcutaneously with 2×10^6 parental 9L cells. As shown in Figure 2A, tumor growth was observed in groups where nonimmunized splenocytes or serum from 9L–IL-4–immunized rats were transferred. Only transfer of splenocytes from 9L–IL-4–immunized rats with or without immune serum eradicated tumor growth in recipient rats. Further analysis using specific antibodies to deplete lymphocyte subsets from splenocytes revealed that CD4$^+$ and CD8$^+$ T cells play important roles in rejection (Fig. 2B). Natural killer cells do not. We are initiating clinical trials of IL-4$^+$ HSV-TK gene-transduced tumor vaccines for patients with malignant gliomas (89) based on these studies.

Clinical Trials of Interleukin-4 Gene Therapy

We demonstrated in clinical trials (90,91) that IL-4 expressed from genetically modified fibroblasts could indeed cause local endothelial activation and recruitment of immune effectors. We treated 18 patients in the context of phase 1 and 2 (immunologic end points) trials designed to determine whether IL-4 gene therapy could be administered safely and effectively to patients with cancer. This study was terminated prematurely because of a shortage of the initial vector. The results in the original study still are of considerable interest, revealing antitumor responses in three patients with melanoma (all partial), including extensive vitiligo in one patient with a partial response. A surgical complete remission was realized in one patient who remains disease free 5 years later in spite of pretreatment crescendo recurrences in the skin, small bowel, and brain metastases. Table 3 demonstrates IL-4 production in vac-

TABLE 3. INTERLEUKIN-4 GENE THERAPY AT THE UNIVERSITY OF PITTSBURGH

| Disease | Primary Vaccine | | Secondary Vaccine | | |
	Maximum Dose of IL-4[a]	No. of IL-4–Producing Fibroblasts	No. of Tumor Cells	Maximum Dose of IL-4[a]	No. of IL-4–Producing Fibroblasts
Mel	2,073	9.0×10^6	5.0×10^6	—	—
Mel[b]	2,482	1.0×10^7	4.0×10^6	2,472	4.0×10^6
Renal cell	3,440	1.0×10^7	3.6×10^6	4,181	5.8×10^6
Mel[b]	25,900	1.0×10^7	2.9×10^6	31,500	1.0×10^7
Mel	27,650	7.0×10^6	5.0×10^6	—	—
Mel[b]	51,830	1.0×10^7	5.0×10^6	21,950	3.0×10^6
Colon	85,328	1.0×10^7	2.2×10^6	23,890	5.8×10^6
Colon	28,663	8.6×10^6	3.0×10^6	13,368	2.8×10^6
Colon	5,598	4.3×10^6	3.9×10^6	—	—
Colon	86,661	4.6×10^6	5.0×10^6	—	—
Renal cell	97,353	9.0×10^6	5.0×10^6	6,606	3.0×10^6
Breast	825	1.2×10^6	4.0×10^6	—	—
Colon	11,724	1.8×10^6	3.0×10^6	—	—
Breast	73,460	1.0×10^6	5.0×10^6	7,181	1.0×10^6

IL-4, interleukin-4; mel, melanoma.
[a]U/24 h.
[b]Patients with partial response.

cination in 14 patients. Tissue biopsies of multiple vaccination sites were obtained from the patients to determine the level of gene expression *in situ* for IL-4 and neomycin-resistance gene (91). Two weeks after the first vaccination, both IL-4 and neomycin-resistance transgene transcripts were still detectable. After the second vaccination, expression of the individual transgenes peaked on day 1 after the vaccination but were still detectable on day 14. Immunohistochemical analysis of the injection sites of IL-4–transfected fibroblasts and tumors revealed endothelial activation and recruitment of DC and T cells to the injected site. With vector TFG human IL-4–neo-TK, we will be able to launch our next phase of protocols in the combination with IL-2 administration (melanoma) and alone in the setting of glioma (92). It is likely that the complexity of immune reactivity will preclude the use of a single cytokine to elicit or maintain long-term effective immune reactivity to human tumors.

Belli et al. reported the application of a melanoma vaccine using a HLA A2+ allogeneic cell line transduced with IL-2 or IL-4 (93). Seven patients were given 5×10^7 irradiated IL-4–transduced cells per vaccination, and each patient received at least three vaccinations subcutaneously. Although some patients demonstrated regression of skin nodules, no changes were observed in other lesions. The side effects, including transient fever and erythema, were mild at the site of injection.

INTERLEUKIN-4 TOXIN THERAPY

Debinski et al. and Puri et al. (94,95) investigated the possibility of targeting IL-4R with chimeric proteins composed of human IL-4 and mutant forms of *Pseudomonas* exotoxin A because IL-4Rs are present on a variety of human cancer cells. Administration of chimeric toxin to animals caused regression of established xenografts. To improve the efficacy, the researchers constructed circularly permuted forms of IL-4 that retain proliferative and binding activity (96). A toxin-fused circularly permuted IL-4 was

found to have several-fold higher affinity to IL-4R and to be at least several-fold more toxic to human renal cell carcinoma cells (97) and human malignant astrocytomas (98) compared with an original form of nonpermuted IL-4 toxin. Intratumoral administration of the IL-4 toxin into well-established human glioblastoma (99) and acquired immunodeficiency syndrome–associated Kaposis's sarcoma (100) xenografts demonstrated a complete remission of flank tumors in all animals. On the basis of this observation, Debinski et al. have begun a phase 1 trial for glioblastoma patients (101).

FUTURE DIRECTIONS WITH INTERLEUKIN-4 IN CANCER THERAPY

Systemic administration of recombinant IL-4 administered alone to cancer patients did not produce apparent benefit. It is clear from the clinical trials performed with rhIL-4 that IL-4 can be repeatedly administered without life-threatening toxicity. The complex regulatory responses after systemic IL-4 administration have been quite apparent in animal models. The results with local IL-4 produced at the tumor site by cells transduced with IL-4 gene, in contrast, are encouraging. IL-4 is capable of inducing Th1-type responses in combination with tumor growth factor–β (37) or by eliminating lymphoid DCs (43). Thus, future applications of the use of IL-4 in cancer therapy should include gene transfection and combination approaches. With regard to gene therapy strategies, we generated substantial evidence demonstrating the efficacy of local delivery of IL-4 by retroviral-transduced fibroblasts when admixed with tumor cells and injected as a tumor vaccine. We (102) demonstrated that IL-12 gene-transduced DCs, however, elicit a more effective immune response against tumors than gene-transduced fibroblasts expressing a comparable amount of cytokine when these cells are injected directly into tumor nodules. Cytokine-transduced DCs are significantly more effective than nontransduced DCs, suggesting a possible role for

IL-12 in the protection of DCs from tumor cell suppressive signals, death signals, or both (103). When considering the efficacy of local cytokine expression delivered at the tumor site, responses induced by other methods of cytokine delivery should be evaluated. Adenoviral vectors, for example, have emerged as effective vehicles for *in vivo* gene delivery for various purposes. Effective local expression of IL-4 mediated by adenoviral vectors may also serve as a signal for migration of DCs into inflammatory sites via upregulation of vascular cell adhesion molecule 1. Gene transfer approaches should be evaluated to determine various strategies of gene delivery. The use of IL-4 in DC-based therapy in combination with granulocyte-macrophage colony-stimulating factor and other cytokines should be pursued extensively. Adding other cytokine genes to DC-based subcutaneous or intradermal vaccines may optimize recruitment of immune cells to the DC-vaccine site by creating a local inflammatory environment. In addition, combination with other antiangiogenic factors may be an attractive strategy for the use of IL-4.

REFERENCES

1. Lee F, Yokota T, Otsuka T, et al. Isolation and characterization of a mouse interleukin cDNA clone that expresses B-cell stimulatory factor 1 activities and T-cell- and mast-cell-stimulating activities. *Proc Natl Acad Sci U S A* 1986;83:2061–2065.
2. Yokota T, Otsuka T, Mosmann T, et al. Isolation and characterization of a human interleukin cDNA clone, homologous to mouse B-cell stimulatory factor 1, that expresses B-cell- and T-cell-stimulating activities. *Proc Natl Acad Sci U S A* 1986;83:5894–5898.
3. Otsuka T, Villaret D, Yokota T, et al. Structural analysis of the mouse chromosomal gene encoding interleukin 4 which expresses B cell, T cell and mast-cell-stimulating activities. *Nucleic Acids Res* 1987;15:333–344.
4. Le BM, Lemons RS, Espinosa R, Larson RA, Arai N, Rowley JD. Interleukin-4 and interleukin-5 map to human chromosome 5 in a region encoding growth factors and receptors and are deleted in myeloid leukemias with a del(5q). *Blood* 1989;73:647–650.
5. Mosmann TR, Cherwinski H, Bond MW, Giedlin MA, Coffman RL. Two types of murine helper T cell clone. I. Definition according to profiles of lymphokine activities and secreted proteins. *J Immunol* 1986;136:2348–2357.
6. Plaut M, Pierce JH, Watson CJ, Hanley-Hyde J, Nordan RP, Paul WE. Mast cell lines produce lymphokines in response to cross-linkage of Fc epsilon RI or to calcium ionophores. *Nature* 1989;339:64–67.
7. Boulay JL, Paul WE. The interleukin-4-related lymphokines and their binding to hematopoietin receptors. *J Biol Chem* 1992;267: 20525–20528.
8. Cabrillat H, Galizzi JP, Djossou O, et al. High affinity binding of human interleukin 4 to cell lines. *Biochem Biophys Res Commun* 1987;149:995–1001.
9. Park LS, Friend D, Sassenfeld HM, Urdal DL. Characterization of the human B cell-stimulatory factor 1 receptor. *J Exp Med* 1987;166: 476–488.
10. Foxwell BM, Woerly G, Ryffel B. Identification of interleukin-4 receptor-associated proteins and expression of both high- and low-affinity binding on human lymphoid cells. *Eur J Immunol* 1989; 19:1637–1641.
11. Galizzi JP, Zuber CE, Cabrillat H, Djossou O, Bancherau J. Internalization of human interleukin-4 and transient down-regulation of its receptor in the CD23-inducible Jijoye cells. *J Biol Chem* 1989;264: 6984–6989.
12. Galizzi JP, Zuber CE, Harada N, et al. Molecular cloning of a cDNA encoding the human interleukin-4 receptor. *Int Immunol* 1990;2: 669–675.
13. Noguchi M, Nakamura Y, Russell SM, et al. Interleukin-2 receptor gamma chain: a functional component of the interleukin-7 receptor [see comments]. *Science* 1993;262:1877–1880.
14. Russell SM, Keegan AD, Harada N, et al. Interleukin-2 receptor gamma chain: a functional component of the interleukin-4 receptor [see comments]. *Science* 1993;262:1880–1883.
15. Murata T, Obiri NI, Puri RK. Structure of and signal transduction through interleukin-4 and interleukin-13 receptors. *Int J Mol Med* 1998;1:551–557.
16. Murata T, Noguchi PD, Puri RK. Receptors for IL-4 do not associate with the common K chain and IL-4 induces the phosphorylation of JAK2 tyrosine kinase in human colon carcinoma cells. *J Biol Chem* 1995;270:30829–30836.
17. Shanafelt AB, Forte CP, Kasper JJ, et al. An immune cell-selective interleukin-4 agonist. *Proc Natl Acad Sci U S A* 1998;95:9454–9458.
18. Murata T, Noguchi PD, Puri RK. Interleukin-13 induces phosphorylation and activation of JAK2 Janus kinase in human colon carcinoma cell lines: Similarities between interleukin-4 and 13 signalling. *J Immunol* 1996;156:2972–2978.
19. Hage T, Sebald W, Reinemer P. Crystal structure of the interleukin-4/receptor alpha chain complex reveals a mosaic binding interface. *Cell* 1999;97:271–281.
20. Chomarat P, Rybak ME, Bancherau J. Interleukin-4 In: Thomson A, ed. *The cytokine handbook*. San Diego: Academic Press, 1998; 6,133–174.
21. Howard M, Farrar J, Hilfiker M, et al. Identification of a T cell-derived B cell growth factor distinct from interleukin-2. *J Exp Med* 1982;155:914–923.
22. Rabin EM, Ohara J, Paul WE. B-cell stimulatory factor 1 activates resting B cells. *Proc Nat Acad Sci U S A* 1985;82:2935–2939.
23. Puri RK, Siegel JP. Interleukin-4 and cancer therapy. *Cancer Invest* 1993;11:473–486.
24. Noelle R, Kramer PH, Ohara J, Uhr JW, Vitetta ES. Increased expression of Ia antigens on resting B cells. *Proc Natl Acad Sci U S A* 1984;81:6149–6153.
25. Bancherau J, Defrance T, Galizzi JP, Miossec P, Rousset F. Human interleukin-4. *Bull Cancer* 1991;78:299–306.
26. Snapper CM, Finkelman FD, Paul WE. Differential regulation of IgG1 and IgE synthesis by interleukin 4. *J Exp Med* 1988;167:183–196.
27. Snapper CM, Finkelman FD, Paul WE. Regulation of IgG1 and IgE production by interleukin-4. *Immunol Rev* 1988;102:51–75.
28. Hu-Li J, Shevach EM, Mizuguchi J, Ohara J, Mostmann T, Pawl WE. B cell stimulatory factor I (interleukin-4) is a potent co-stimulant for normal resting T lymphocytes. *J Exp Med* 1987;165:157–161.
29. Kawakami Y, Rosenberg SA, Lotze MT. Interleukin-4 promotes the growth of tumor-infiltrating lymphocytes cytotoxic for human autologous melanoma. *J Exp Med* 1988;168:2183–2191.
30. Nagler A, Lanier LL, Phillips JH. The effects of IL-4 on human natural killer cells. A potent regulator of IL-2 activation and proliferation. *J Immunol* 1988;141:2349–2351.
31. Barks JL, McQuillan JJ, Iademarco MF. TNF-alpha and IL-4 synergistically increase vascular cell adhesion molecule-1 expression in cultured vascular smooth muscle cells. *J Immunol* 1997;159:4532–4538.
32. Sallusto F, Lanzavecchia A. Efficient presentation of soluble antigen by cultured human dendritic cells is maintained by granulocyte/macrophage colony-stimulating factor plus interleukin-4 and down-regulated by tumor necrosis factor alpha. *J Exp Med* 1994;179:1109–1118.
33. Romani N, Gruner S, Brang D, et al. Proliferating dendritic cell progenitors in human blood. *J Exp Med* 1994;180:83–93.
34. Mayordomo JI, Zorina T, Storkus WJ, et al. Bone marrow-derived dendritic cells pulsed with synthetic tumour peptides elicit protective and therapeutic antitumor immunity. *Nat Med* 1995;1:1297–1302.
35. Romani N, Reider D, Heuer M, et al. Generation of mature dendritic cells from human blood. An improved method with special regard to clinical applicability. *J Immunol Methods* 1996;196: 137–151.
36. Rosenzwajg M, Camus S, Guigon M, Gluckman JC. The influence of interleukin (IL)-4, IL-13, and Flt3 ligand on human dendritic cell differentiation from cord blood CD34+ progenitor cells. *Exp Hematol* 1998;26:63–72.
37. Lingnau K, Hoehn P, Kerdine S, et al. IL-4 in combination with

TGF-beta favors an alternative pathway of Th1 development independent of IL-12. *J Immunol* 1998;161:4709–4718.

38. Schüler T, Qin Z, Ibe S, et al. TH1-associated and cytotoxic T lymphocyte-mediated tumor immunity is impaired in IL-4-deficient mice. *J Exp Med* 1999 (*in press*).

39. Figdor CG, te Velde AA. Regulation of human monocyte phenotype and function by interleukin-4. In: Spits H, ed. *IL-4: structure and function.* Boca Raton: CRC Press, 1992;12,187–202.

40. Lotze MT. Getting to the source: Dendritic cells as therapeutic reagents for the treatment of cancer patients [Editorial]. *Ann Surg* 1997;226:1–5.

41. Morse MA, Zhou LJ, Tedder TF, Lyerly HK, Smith C. Generation of dendritic cells in vitro from peripheral blood mononuclear cells with granulocyte-macrophage-colony-stimulating factor, interleukin-4, and tumor necrosis factor-alpha for use in cancer immunotherapy [see comments]. *Ann Surg* 1997;226:6–16.

42. Nestle FO, Alijagic S, Gilliet M, et al. Vaccination of melanoma patients with peptide- or tumor lysate-pulsed dendritic cells. *Nat Med* 1998;4:328–332.

43. Rissoan MC, Soumelis V, Kadowaki N, et al. Reciprocal control of T helper cell and dendritic cell differentiation. *Science* 1999;36:(8075)1183–1186.

44. Obiri NI, Hillman GG, Haas GP, Sud S, Puri RK. Expression of high affinity interleukin-4 receptors on human renal cell carcinoma cells and inhibition of tumor cell growth in vitro by interleukin-4. *J Clin Invest* 1993;91:88–93.

45. Topp MS, Papadimitriou CA, Eitelbach F, et al. Antiproliferative effect of human interleukin-4 in human cancer cell lines: studies on the mechanism. *Leuk Lymphoma* 1995;19:319–328.

46. Topp MS, Papadimitriou CA, Eitelbach F, et al. Recombinant human interleukin 4 has antiproliferative activity on human tumor cell lines derived from epithelial and nonepithelial histologies. *Cancer Res* 1995;55:2173–2176.

47. Topp MS, Koenigsmann M, Mire-Sluis A, et al. Recombinant human interleukin-4 inhibits growth of some human lung tumor cell lines in vitro and *in vivo. Blood* 1993;82:2837–2844.

48. Obiri NI, Siegel JP, Varricchio F, Puri RK. Expression and function of high affinity interleukin-4 receptors on human melanoma, ovarian and breast carcinoma cells. *Clin Exp Immunol* 1994;95:148–155.

49. Lahm H, Schnyder B, Wyniger J, et al. Growth inhibition of human colorectal-carcinoma cells by interleukin-4 and expression of functional interleukin-4 receptors. *Int J Cancer* 1994;59:440–447.

50. Lahm H, Amstad P, Yilmaz A, Fischer JR, Givel JC, Odartchenko N, Sordat B. Differential effect of interleukin-4 and transforming growth factor beta 1 on expression of proto-oncogenes and autocrine insulin-like growth factor II in colorectal carcinoma cells. *Biochem Biophys Res Commun* 1996;220:334–340.

51. Barna BP, Estes ML, Pettay J, Iwasaki K, Zhou P, Barnett GH. Human astrocyte growth regulation: interleukin-4 sensitivity and receptor expression. *J Neuroimmunol* 1995;60:75–81.

52. Liu J, Flanagan WM, Drazba JA, et al. The CDK inhibitor, p27Kip1, is required for IL-4 regulation of astrocyte proliferation. *J Immunol* 1997;159:812–819.

53. Gooch JL, Lee A, Yee D, et al. Interleukin 4 inhibits growth and induces apoptosis in human breast cancer cells. *Cancer Res* 1998;58:(18)4199–4205.

54. Myers JN, Yasumura S, Suminami Y, et al. Growth stimulation of human head and neck squamous cell carcinoma cell lines by interleukin 4. *Clin Cancer Res* 1996;2:127–135.

55. Saleh M, Davis ID, Wilks AF. The paracrine role of tumour-derived mIL-4 on tumour-associated endothelium. *Int J Cancer* 1997;72:664–672.

56. Volpert OV, Fong T, Koch AE, et al. Inhibition of angiogenesis by interleukin 4. *J Exp Med* 1998;188:1039–1046.

57. Hillman GG, Younes E, Visscher D, et al. Systemic treatment with interleukin-4 induces regression of pulmonary metastases in a murine renal cell carcinoma model. *Cell Immunol* 1995;160:(2)257–263.

58. Younes E, Haas GP, Visscher D, et al. Intralesional treatment of established murine primary renal tumor with interleukin-4: localized effect on primary tumor with no impact on metastases. *J Urol*

59. 1995;153:490–493.

Bosco M, Riovarelli M, Forni M, et al. Low doses of IL-4 injected perilymphatically in tumor-bearing mice inhibit the growth of poorly and apparently nonimmunogenic tumors and induce a tumor-specific immune memory. *J Immunol* 1990;145:3136–3143.

60. Terres G, Coffman RL. The role of IL-4 and IL-10 cytokines in controlling an anti-tumor response *in vivo. Int Immunol* 1998;10:823–832.

61. Kobayashi M, Kobayashi H, Pollard RB, Suzuki F. A pathogenic role of Th2 cells and their cytokine products on the pulmonary metastasis of murine B16 melanoma. *J Immunol* 1998;160:5869–5873.

62. Lotze MT, Custer MC, Bolton ES, Wiebke EA, Kawakami Y, Rosenberg SA. Mechanisms of immunologic antitumor therapy: lessons from the laboratory and clinical applications. *Hum Immunol* 1990;28:198–207.

63. Atkins MB, Vachino G, Tilg HJ, et al. Phase I evaluation of thrice-daily intravenous bolus interleukin-4 in patients with refractory malignancy. *J Clin Oncol* 1992;10:1802–1809.

64. Gilleece MH, Scarffe JH, Ghosh A, et al. Recombinant human interleukin 4 (IL-4) given as daily subcutaneous injections—a phase I dose toxicity trial. *Br J Cancer* 1992;66:204–210.

65. Prendiville J, Thatcher N, Lind M, et al. Recombinant human interleukin-4 (rHu IL-4) administered by the intravenous and subcutaneous routes in patients with advanced cancer—a phase I toxicity study and pharmacokinetic analysis. *Eur J Cancer* 1993;29A:1700–1707.

66. Vokes EE, Figlin R, Hochster H, Lotze M, Rybak ME. A phase II study of recombinant human interleukin-4 for advanced or recurrent non-small cell lung cancer. *Cancer J* 1998;4:46–51.

67. Leach MW, Rybak ME, Rosenblum IY. Safety evaluation of recombinant human interleukin-4. II. Clinical studies. *Clin Immunol Immunopathol* 1997;83:12–14.

68. Leach MW, Snyder EA, Sinha DP, et al. Safety evaluation of recombinant human interleukin-4. I. Preclinical studies. *Clin Immunol Immunopathol* 1997;83:(1)8–11(abst).

69. Custer MC, Lotze MT. Rapid fluorescence assay for IL-4 detection in supernatants and serum. *J Immunol Methods* 1990;128:109–117.

70. Tepper RI, Pattengale PK, Leder P. Murine interleukin-4 displays potent anti-tumor activity *in vivo. Cell* 1989;57:503–512.

71. Li WQ, Diamantstein T, Blankenstein T. Lack of tumorigenicity of interleukin 4 autocrine growing cells seems related to the anti-tumor function of interleukin 4. *Mol Immunol* 1990;27:1331–1337.

72. Blankenstein T, Li WQ, Muller W, Diamantstein T. Retroviral interleukin 4 gene transfer into an interleukin 4-dependent cell line results in autocrine growth but not in tumorigenicity. *Eur J Immunol* 1990;20:935–938.

73. Golumbek PT, Lazenby AJ, Levitsky HI, et al. Treatment of established renal cancer by tumor cells engineered to secrete interleukin-4. *Science* 1991;254:713–716.

74. Pippin BA, Rosenstein M, Jacob WF, Chiang Y, Lotze MT. Local IL-4 delivery enhances immune reactivity to murine tumors: gene therapy in combination with IL-2. *Cancer Gene Ther* 1994;1:35–42.

75. Pericle F, Giovarelli M, Colombo MP, et al. An efficient Th2-type memory follows CD8+ lymphocyte-driven and eosinophil-mediated rejection of a spontaneous mouse mammary adenocarcinoma engineered to release IL-4. *J Immunol* 1994;153:5659–5673.

76. Stoppacciaro A, Paglia P, Lombardi L, Parmiani G, Baroni C, Colombo MP. Genetic modification of a carcinoma with the IL-4 gene increases the influx of dendritic cells relative to other cytokines. *Eur J Immunol* 1997;27:2375–2382.

77. Hock H, Dorsch M, Kunzendorf U, et al. Vaccinations with tumor cells genetically engineered to produce different cytokines: effectively not superior to a classical adjuvant. *Cancer Res* 1993;53:714–716.

78. Cayeux S, Beck C, Dorken B, Blankenstein T. Co-expression of interleukin-4 and B7.1 in murine tumor cells leads to improved tumor rejection and vaccine effect compared to single gene transductants and a classical adjuvant. *Human Gene Ther* 1996;7:525–529.

79. Cayeux S, Richter G, Noffz G, Dorken B, Blankenstein T. Influence of gene-modified (IL-7, IL-4, and B7) tumor cell vaccines on tumor antigen presentation. *J Immunol* 1997;158:2834–2841.

80. Mitchell MS. Relapse in the central nervous system in melanoma

patients successfully treated with biomodulators. *J Clin Oncol* 1989;7:1701–1709.

81. Tjuvajev J, Gansbacher B, Desai R, et al. RG-2 glioma growth attenuation and severe brain edema caused by local production of interleukin-2 and interferon-gamma. *Cancer Res* 1995;55:1902–1910.

82. Sampson JH, Ashley DM, Archer GE, et al. Characterization of a spontaneous murine astrocytoma and abrogation of its tumorigenicity by cytokine secretion. *Neurosurg* 1997;41(6):1365–1373.

83. Benedetti S, Bruzzone MG, Pollo B, et al. Eradication of rat malignant gliomas by retroviral-mediated, *in vivo* delivery of the interleukin 4 gene. *Cancer Res* 1999;59:645–652.

84. Benedetti S, Dimeco F, Pollo B, et al. Limited efficacy of the HSV-TK/GCV system for gene therapy of malignant gliomas and perspectives for the combined transduction of the interleukin-4 gene. *Human Gene Ther* 1997;8:1345–1353.

85. Andreansky S, He B, van Cott J, et al. Treatment of intracranial gliomas in immunocompetent mice using herpes simplex viruses that express murine interleukins. *Gene Ther* 1998;5:121–130.

86. Okada H, Giezeman-Smits KM, Tahara H, et al. Effective cytokine gene therapy against an intracranial glioma using a retrovirally transduced IL-4 plus HSV-TK tumor vaccine. *Gene Ther* 1999;6: 219–226.

87. Okada H, Attanucci J, Katinka M, et al. Identification of a rat glioma rejection antigen by cytokine tumor vaccine-assisted SEREX (CAS). *Cancer Res* 1999 (submitted).

88. Giezeman-Smits KM, Okada H, Brissette-Storkus CS, et al. CD4+ T cells mediate the tumor specific immune response, generated from vaccination with interleukin-4-producing glioma cells. *Cancer Res* 1999 (submitted).

89. Okada H, Attanucci J, Tahara H, et al. Characterization and transduction of a retroviral vector encoding human interleukin-4 and the herpes simplex-thymidine kinase for glioma tumor vaccine therapy. *Cancer Gene Ther* 1999 (in press).

90. Lotze MT. Transplantation and adoptive cellular therapy of cancer: the role of T cell growth factors. *Transplantation* 1993;2:33–47.

91. Suminami Y, Elder EM, Lotze MT, Whiteside TL. In situ interleukin-4 gene expression in cancer patients treated with genetically modified tumor vaccine. *J Immunother* 1995;17:238–248.

92. Okada H, Pollack IF, Lotze MT, et al. Gene therapy of malignant gliomas: a phase I study of IL-4 HSV-TK gene-modified autologous tumor to elicit an immune response. *Hum Gene Ther* 1999 (in press).

93. Belli F, Mascheroni L, Gallino G, et al. Active immunization of metastatic melanoma patients with IL-2 or IL-4 gene transfected, allogeneic melanoma cells. *Adv Exp Med Biol* 1998;451:543–545.

94. Debinski W, Puri RK, Pastan I. Interleukin-4 receptors expressed on tumor cells may serve as a target for anticancer therapy using chimeric *Pseudomonas* exotoxin. *Int J Cancer* 1994;58:744–748.

95. Puri RK, Debinski W, Obiri N, Kreitman R, Pastan I. Human renal cell carcinoma cells are sensitive to the cytotoxic effect of a chimeric protein comprised of human interleukin-4 and Pseudomonas exotoxin. *Cell Immunol* 1994;154:369–379.

96. Kreitman RJ, Puri RK, McPhie P, Pastan I. Circularly permuted interleukin 4 retains proliferative and binding activity. *Cytokine* 1995;7:311–318.

97. Puri RK, Leland P, Obiri NI, et al. An improved circularly permuted interleukin 4-toxin is highly cytotoxic to human renal cell carcinoma cells. Introduction of gamma c chain in RCC cells does not improve sensitivity. *Cell Immunol* 1996;171:80–86.

98. Puri RK, Hoon DS, Leland P, et al. Preclinical development of a recombinant toxin containing circularly permuted interleukin-4 and truncated *Pseudomonas* exotoxin for therapy of malignant astrocytoma. *Cancer Res* 1996;56:5631–5637.

99. Husain SR, Behari N, Kreitman RJ, Pastan I, Puri RK. Complete regression of established human glioblastoma tumor xenograft by interleukin-4 toxin therapy. *Cancer Res* 1998;58:3649–3653.

100. Husain SR, Kreitman RJ, Pastan I, Puri RK. Interleukin-4 receptor directed cytotoxin therapy of AIDS-associated Kaposi's sarcoma tumors in xenograft model. *Nat Med* 1999;5:817–822. (Accompanying News and Views, pages 738–739).

101. Rand RW, Kreitman RJ, Pastan I, Puri RK. A circularly permuted interleukin-4-Pseudomonas exotoxin for treatment of malignant gliomas. Phase I trial for glioblastoma patients. 44th Annual Meeting of Western Neurological Society; September 12-15, 1998; Silverado, Napa, CA.

102. Nishioka Y, Hirao M, Robbins PD, Lotze MT, Tahara H. Delivering antigen presenting cells to the site of tumor antigen: Induction of systemic and therapeutic antitumor immunity using intratumoral injection of dendritic cells genetically engineered to express Interleukin-12 (IL-12). *Cancer Res* 1999; 59:4035–4041.

103. Grohmann U, Belladonna ML, Bianchi R, et al. IL-12 acts directly on DC to promote nuclear localization of NF-kappaB and primes DC for IL-12 production. *Immunity* 1998;9:315–323.

5

INTERLEUKIN-12: CLINICAL APPLICATIONS

HIDEAKI TAHARA
MICHAEL T. LOTZE

INITIAL FINDINGS IN INTERLEUKIN-12 BIOLOGY

Interleukin-12 (IL-12) was initially identified as a natural killer (NK) cell stimulatory factor (1) and a cytotoxic-lymphocyte maturation factor (2). IL-12 is a disulfide-linked heterodimeric cytokine composed of a 35-kd light chain (p35) and a 40-kd heavy chain (p40) (1,2). The complementary DNA encoding the p35 and p40 chains of IL-12 from the mouse and human have been cloned. Unlike most other cytokines, simultaneous transfection of mammalian cells with two different genes is necessary for production of biologically active IL-12 (3,4). This cytokine exerts a variety of biologic effects *in vitro* and *in vivo* (Table 1). These include the ability to synergize with IL-2 in augmenting allogeneic, cytotoxic T-lymphocyte responses (5), lymphokine-activated killer cell activity (2), and interferon-γ (IFN-γ) production from NK and T cells (1,6). IL-12 also directly stimulates the production of IFN-γ and other cytokines from these cells (1,2), enhances the lytic activity of T and NK cells (1,7), and promotes their expansion (8). Under most circumstances, IL-12 induces primarily a T helper 1 (Th1) (cellular immune) response *in vitro* (9). Under conditions of limited IFN-γ production, as seen in IFN-γ gene-disrupted animals or neonates, IL-12 induces and promotes a Th2 (T helper 2) response. Studies of administration of recombinant murine IL-12 (rIL-12) to normal mice revealed that rIL-12 also enhances NK and cytotoxic T-lymphocyte activity and induces IFN-γ production *in vivo* (10). IL-12 is a potent adjuvant in a murine Leishmania model (11). These findings suggest that IL-12 might be an appropriate cytokine for enhancing antitumor immunity.

Production of Interleukin-12

Although IL-12 was originally isolated from B-cell lines, normal B cells do not secrete IL-12 heterodimer (12). Macrophages and dendritic cells appear to be the principal producers of IL-12 (Table 2). Macatonia et al. (13) demonstrated that monocytes treated with heat-inactivated *Listeria monocytogenes* produce IL-12 and direct the promotion of cellular immunity of the Th1 type *in vitro* and *in vivo*. Similarly, murine macrophages expressing the CD40 costimulatory molecule and interacting with anti-CD3–activated CD40L⁺ splenic T cells or

CD40L⁺ T-cell clones are induced to secrete IL-12 (14). The IL-12 production by antigen-presenting cells (APCs) is believed to be dependent of CD40/CD40L interaction by APCs based on the findings using anti-CD40L antibodies and CD40L gene-disrupted mice. Administration of anti-CD40L antibodies has the ability to block IL-12 production. Activated T cells derived from CD40L gene-disrupted mice are incapable of eliciting IL-12 secretion from splenic monocytes. Activated T cells cannot mount Th1-type immunity (15,16). In addition, soluble trimeric CD40L promotes the secretion of IL-12 from macrophages at levels lower than those observed in macrophage-activated T-cell cultures (14). Additional stimuli that enhance APC production include microparticulate ingestion (17), IFN-γ plus lipopolysaccharide (18), *Mycobacterium tuberculosis* (19), *Listeria* (9), *Neisseria meningitidis*-derived lipopolysaccharide (20), polyinosinic acid (21), phagocytosis of *Borrelia burgdorferi* (22), lipoteichoic acid preparations of gram-positive bacteria (23), recombinant human immunodeficiency virus gp120 protein (24), and nitric oxide–generating compounds (25). CpG motifs present in hypomethylated oligodeoxynucleotides or bacterial DNA also elicit IL-12 production from human and murine responder APC cells (26,27). The production of IL-12 by activated APC appears to represent a critical early physiologic event in cellular immunity because dendritic cells appear to represent the principal producers of IL-12 *in situ* in draining lymphoid organs (28).

Receptor and Signaling of Interleukin-12

Initial studies using radiolabeled Scatchard binding assays implementing Iodine-125–labeled IL-12 showed that IL-12 receptors (IL-12R) are expressed on only the cell surface of NK cells and T cells activated with IL-2 or phytohemagglutinin (29). This result confirmed in principle that IL-12 has the ability to promote the secretion of IFN-γ from these two cell types. IFN-γ induced by IL-12 enhances APC functions by increasing the expression of major histocompatibility antigen gene products and antigen-processing functions required for the promotion of primary T-cell immune responsiveness (30). When stimulated for 4 days with phytohemagglutinin, T lymphocytes were found to express approximately 1,000 to 10,000 binding sites per cell with three classes of binding affinities.

TABLE 1. BIOLOGIC CHARACTERISTICS OF INTERLEUKIN-12

Identified as "cytotoxic lymphocyte maturation factor" (CLMF) or "natural killer cell stimulatory factor" (NKSF)

A disulfide-linked heterodimeric cytokine

Simultaneous expression of p35 and p40 subunits required for biologic activity

Produced by professional antigen-presenting cells (macrophages and dendritic cells), lesser amounts by keratinocytes and polymorphonuclear leukocytes

Promotes the expansion of activated T, natural killer, and natural killer–T cells

Enhances natural killer cell and T-cell cytotoxicity

Strongly induces interferon-γ production from T and natural killer cells synergistically with interleukin-2 or interleukin-18

Promotes T helper 1 (Th1)-type response (directly stimulates the production of Th1-type cytokines, including interferon-γ and interleukin-2)

Strongly inhibits angiogenesis (through secondary elaboration of chemokines, including IP-10 induced by interferon-γ)

They were consistent with low-, intermediate-, and high-affinity IL-12 receptors displaying Kd in the range of 2 to 6, 50 to 200, and 5 to 20 pm, respectively (29). The low-affinity IL-12R was characterized as a multichain complex with an approximate molecular weight of 135 to 210 kd. The low-affinity IL-12R was expressed optimally 2 to 4 days after phytohemagglutinin stimulation on T cells or 7 to 8 days after IL-2 activation of T cells or NK cells.

Expression cloning studies performed by Presky et al. (31) and Wu et al. (32) subsequently showed that the IL-12R is composed of a dimeric complex ($\beta1\beta2$) in which the $\beta1$ and $\beta2$ chains confer low to intermediate binding affinity of the complex for IL-12 (Table 3, Fig. 1). Each subunit was designated as a *β chain* because of its homology to gp120 molecule, serving as a common β chain for a number of alternate cytokines (33).

TABLE 2. INTERLEUKIN-12 PRODUCERS AND STIMULI

IL-12 Producer	Stimuli
DC	Anti-CD40 antibody
	T cells with antigen particulates
	Bacteria
	Bacterial products
Macrophages	Anti-CD40
	LPS
	IFN-γ
	Polyinosidic acid
	Human immunodeficiency virus gp120
	Bacteria
	Bacterial products
Langerhans' cells	Culture (*in vitro*)
B cells	LPS + IFN-γ
	Phorbol esters
	SAC
Neutrophils	LPS
Keratinocytes	UV irradiation
	Phorbol esters
	Culture (*in vitro*)
Microglia	LPS
Astrocytes	LPS

DC, dendritic cell; IFN-γ, interferon-γ; LPS, bacterial lipopolysaccharide; SAC, *Staphylococcus aureus* Cowan A strain.

TABLE 3. CHARACTERISTICS OF INTERLEUKIN-12 RECEPTOR SUBUNITS

Subunit	Kd for IL-12	Distribution	Author (Reference)
$\beta1$	2–5 nM	T (Th1, Th2, CD8$^+$), NK, B	Wu et al. (32) Rogge et al. (45)
$\beta2$	3–5 nM	Th1 CD4$^+$ T cells	Rogge et al. (45)
$\beta1 + \beta2$ (COS)	50 pM	Th1 CD4$^+$ T cells	Presky et al. (31)

IL-12, interleukin-12; NK, natural killer; Th1, T helper 1; Th2, T helper 2.

The β chains of murine IL-12R DNA have been isolated and cloned using cross-hybridization techniques (34). In the mouse system, the $\beta1$ chain of IL-12R appears to play the dominant role in binding the IL-12 ligand. The $\beta1$ and $\beta2$ chains appear to play significant roles in binding IL-12 in human cells expressing the high-affinity IL-12R (33,35). The $\beta1$ chain appears to be principally occupied with binding to the IL-12 p40 chain, whereas the β chain of IL-12R appears to associate with the p35 chain of IL-12 (35,36). This mechanism explains the capacity to bind to the IL-12–p40 homodimer, which has the capability to bind to IL-12R$\beta1$, but not to IL-12R$\beta2$, to effectively antagonize the binding of the IL-12 heterodimer to IL-12R. Antibodies directed against the IL-12β chains efficiently inhibit IL-12–induced IFN-γ production and activated T-cell proliferation. Antibodies have no effect, however, on the ability of other T-cell growth factors, including IL-2, IL-4, or IL-7, to promote T-cell expansion (32).

The IL-12R appears to use intracellular signaling apparatus that distinguish IL-12 from most of the other cytokines. Specifically, functional signaling through the IL-12R results in the phosphorylation of p56^{lck}, the Janus kinases tyk2 and Jak2, and the signal transducer and activator of transcription (STAT) kinases 3 and 4 (37–42). STAT 4 is also similarly used in the signaling mediated by IFN-αR (43). To evaluate the individual and combined signaling capacity mediated by each of the IL-12R subunits, the transmembrane and intracellular domains of

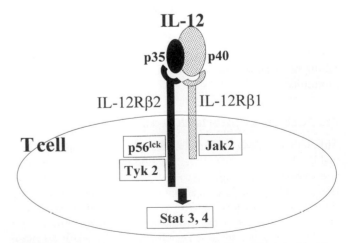

FIGURE 1. Schematic of the high-affinity receptor of interleukin-12.

the IL-12Rβ1 and IL-12Rβ2 subunits were fused to the extracellular domain of the receptor of epidermal growth factor–R, resulting in the production of chimeric molecules (44). Only cells transfected with the fusion protein containing the intracellular domain of the IL-12Rβ2 subunit were able to mediate signals on epidermal growth factor–R stimulation, resulting in proliferation and phosphorylation of Jak2 kinase. Although unable to promote proliferation by themselves, cells transfected with IL-12Rβ1 alone or with IL-12Rβ2 (but not IL-12Rβ2 alone) demonstrated association with tyks. Overall, activation through these chimeric receptors resulted in the phosphorylation of Jak2, tyk2, and STAT3 (in STAT4–deficient BaF3 cells). In addition to IL-12 to Th1, CD4⁺ T cells lead to the rapid phosphorylation of STAT4 kinase (45). Th2 CD4⁺ T-cell clones do not phosphorylate STAT4 in response to IL-12, despite expressing the low-affinity IL-12R (46). Studies performed in STAT4 gene–disrupted mice support a similar biology to that observed in IL-12–p40 gene–disrupted animals. Th2 immune responses (and IL-4, IL-5, and IL-10 production) were predominant in the absence of functional STAT4 kinase activity (47). Although Th1-associated immune responses do occur, they are generally far weaker that those observed in heterozygous or wild-type control animals in response to IL-12 or pathogenic organisms, such as *L. monocytogenes* (47,48). IL-12 activation of NK cells does not occur in STAT4 gene–disrupted mice (48). IFN-γ produced as a consequence of IL-12 administration is minimized, and long-term antigen-specific cellular immunity is lessened in these gene-disrupted animals.

PRECLINICAL TUMOR MODELS

Antitumor Effects of Systemic Administration of Recombinant Interleukin-12 Protein

We initiated murine therapeutic studies to investigate the possible antitumor effect of IL-12 (49). These experiments demonstrated that systemic application of IL-12 suppressed tumor growth and prolonged survival of tumor-bearing mice, even when IL-12 treatment was started as late as 14 days after tumor inoculation. Such therapeutic effects were also reported in similar models by Brunda et al. (50). In these studies, therapeutic intervention with systemic administration of IL-12 could be initiated as late as day 28 after injection of tumor cells (M5076 reticulum cell sarcoma), resulting in inhibition of tumor growth, reduction in the number of metastases, and an increase in survival time. Similar findings related to the potent antitumor effects have been reported by other investigators using diverse tumor models (41,51–53). Virtually every murine tumor model carefully studied has demonstrated significant antitumor effects.

Antitumor Effects of Paracrine Administration of Interleukin-12 Using Gene Transfer Technique

Although IL-12 has potent antitumor effects when injected systemically, induction of long-term immunity is less frequent and variable from experiment to experiment (49,50). Brunda et al. observed that the best results with systemic IL-12 administra-

tion (complete regression of the tumor and induction of protective immunity against tumor rechallenge) was observed after peritumoral injections of IL-12 in a subcutaneous (s.c.) renal cell carcinoma (RenCa) tumor model (50). Local administration of IL-12 at the site of tumor may more closely mimic an endogenous immune response because IL-12 is secreted primarily by "professional" antigen-presenting cells (i.e., macrophages and dendritic cells). IL-12 plays a critical costimulatory role with CD80 (B7) on APC in inducing proliferation and IFN-γ production from Th1 clones (54). Thus, IL-12 may be the proximal cytokine for inducing tumor-specific immunity when administered at the tumor site.

Using plasmid or retroviral expression systems, we studied the effects of IL-12 gene therapy in murine tumor models (55,56). Paracrine secretion of IL-12 using genetic engineering was highly effective in preventing tumor establishment and the induction of protective antitumor immunity. Furthermore, intradermal inoculation of genetically modified tumor cells or intratumoral injection of genetically modified fibroblasts can lead to regression of a nontransfected tumor inoculated at a distant site before therapy (56,57). Other investigators reported the usefulness of *in vivo* transduction using IL-12 adenoviral vectors (58,59) in the treatment of established tumors. Such strategies may be appropriate for clinical application and are in the process of being tested.

Combination Therapy with Interleukin-12

Synergy of IL-12 and CD28/CD80 signaling in promoting T-cell responses (54) supported the evaluation of this approach in murine tumor models (60). Zitvogel et al. (61) evaluated the antitumor benefit associated with combined IL-12 and CD80 gene delivery in two poorly immunogenic tumor models (MCA-207 sarcoma and TS/A mammary adenocarcinoma). Coinoculation of tumor cells infected with retroviruses encoding IL-12 induced specific immunity at a significantly higher rate when compared with animals injected with tumor cells transduced to express IL-12 or CD80 alone. The therapeutic efficacy of these vaccines was dependent on the dose of IL-12 delivered by the transduced tumor cells and blocked by the administration of CTLA4-immunoglobulin fusion protein or neutralizing antibodies against murine IFN-γ or murine tumor necrosis factor–α. Similar synergistic effects of IL-12 and CD80 have been noted in C3H mice bearing mCD80-transfected K1735 melanoma, as well as serum creatine kinase mammary carcinomas (62).

Other molecules reported for synergistic effect with IL-12 include IL-2 and IL-18. As initial studies suggested using transfected fibroblasts (63), treatment using IL-2 in combination with IL-12 appears to be associated with potent antitumor effects (64) possibly related to nitric oxide production (65). This combination could be applied in humans if reduction in side effects could be accomplished (66). IL-18 has also been suggested as useful in combination with IL-12. Combination therapy using systemic administration of rIL-12 and rIL-18 induced serious side effects in our mouse models primarily because of the markedly enhanced induction of high levels of IFN-γ (67). Treatment strategies using local expression of IL-12, IL-18, or both have been actively pursued (68,69).

TABLE 4. CLINICAL TRIALS USING SYSTEMIC ADMINISTRATION OF RECOMBINANT INTERLEUKIN-12 IN CANCER PATIENTS

Author (Reference)	Route	Tumor types	Dose	Schedule	Total no. of pts.	MTD
Atkins et al. (74)	i.v.	Multiple	Dose escalation (0.03–1.0 mg/kg)	Test dose + 5 d injections (1 to 6 cycles)	40	0.5 mg/kg
Motzer et al. (77)	s.c.	Renal cell	Dose escalation[a] (0.1–1.5 mg/kg)	D 1, 8, and 15 (multiple cycles allowed)	51	Fixed dose: 1.0 mg/kg Up-titration: 1.5 mg/kg

MTD, maximum tolerated dose.
[a]Fixed dose schedule: 24 patients; up-titration schedule: 27 patients.

Mechanism of the Antitumor Effects of Interleukin-12 Administration

Although the precise mechanism of the IL-12–induced antitumor effects are still under investigation, substantial information is already available. IL-12 is an effective antitumor reagent in NK cell–deficient beige mice and in mice depleted of NK cell activity by pretreatment with antiasialo GM1. IL-12 is less effective in nude mice (50). These results suggested that T cells, rather than NK cells, were primarily involved in mediating the antitumor effects of this cytokine. Depletion of CD8$^+$, not CD4$^+$, T cells appears to significantly reduce the efficacy of IL-12 as well. In our mouse models (49), only the coordinate depletion of CD4$^+$ and CD8$^+$ T cells resulted in significant abrogation of the IL-12 antitumor effect. Although some differences in the results of T-cell depletion studies exist between the various tumor models used, these studies clearly demonstrate the critical involvement of T cells in IL-12 antitumor effects. After systemic administration of rIL-12, INF–γ depletion only partially abrogated the antitumor effects of IL-12, suggesting the importance of additional antitumor mechanisms induced by IL-12.

NK T cells are also involved in the antitumor effects of IL-12 (70,71). NK T cells, the Vα14-expressing murine NK T cells (homologous to the Vα24 human NK T cells), express NK1.1 and a single invariant T-cell receptor encoded by the Vα14 and Jα281 gene segments. Cui et al. (72) have shown that Vα14 NK T cell–deficient mice no longer mediate the IL-12–induced rejection of tumors. These results suggest that Vα14 NK T cells are essential targets of IL-12, especially in the metastatic tumor models. Furthermore, NK T cells mediate their cytotoxicity by an NK-like effector mechanism after activation with IL-12.

These results collectively suggest that IL-12 affects multiple cell populations within immunity to mediate its antitumor effects. Furthermore, IL-12 may affect additional nonimmune events associated with tumor progression. IL-12–induced IFN-γ triggers the subsequent production of a variety of other cytokines and chemokines from a variety of cells, including tumor cells (68). These include the CXC chemokines, IP-10 and Mig, which inhibit angiogenesis. Kanegane et al. (73) showed that local and systemic treatment with IL-12 was associated with expression of IFN-γ, IP-10, and Mig genes and proteins within the tumor. Levels of IP-10 and Mig expression in the tumor, liver, and kidney were inversely correlated with tumor size. Furthermore, administration *in vivo* of neutralizing antibodies to IP-10 and Mig substantially reduced the antitumor effects of IL-12 inoculated locally into the tumors. These results support the notion that IP-10 and Mig contribute to the antitumor effects of IL-12 through their inhibitory effects on tumor angiogenesis.

CLINICAL STUDIES OF INTERLEUKIN-12

Clinical studies to treat cancer patients using IL-12 have been initiated using systemic administration (intravenous or s.c.) or gene therapy strategy. Although it is still in the early stage of clinical development, some information is available from the phase 1 and 2 studies.

Systemic Administration of Recombinant Interleukin-12

We began the first clinical evaluation of rIL-12 in the spring of 1994 (Table 4). This phase 1 dose-escalation trial (74) was designed to determine the toxicity, maximum tolerated dose (MTD), pharmacokinetics, and biologic and potential antineoplastic effects of IL-12. Cohorts of four to six patients in sequential doses escalating from 3 ng per kg per day to 1,000 ng per kg per day were treated. Patients with advanced cancer and a performance status of more than 70% received escalating doses of recombinant human IL-12 (rhIL-12) by bolus intravenous injection once as an inpatient and once daily for 5 days every 3 weeks as an outpatient, after a 2-week rest period. After establishment of the MTD as less than 1,000 ng per kg per day (because of stomatitis and liver function test abnormalities), eight more patients were enrolled to further assess the safety, pharmacokinetics, and immunobiology at a dose of 500 ng per kg per day. Forty patients were enrolled, including 20 with renal cancer, 12 with melanoma, and five with colon cancer.

Mild anemia, leucopenia, thrombocytopenia, lymphopenia, hyperglycemia, and hypoalbuminemia were noted in some patients but were rapidly reversed after discontinuation of therapy. Fever was observed at doses as low as 3 ng per kg and was largely preventable with acetaminophen and nonsteroidal anti-inflammatory agents. Other symptoms included fatigue, myalgia, mild nausea and rare emesis, and headache. Oral stomatitis of undetermined etiology was a frequent complaint and limited therapy in some patients at higher doses. Mild elevation of transaminases was observed with 1,000 ng per kg rhIL-2 in three-fourths of patients, causing this dose to be declared as an intolerable daily dose on this schedule. The half-life elimination was 5.3 to 9.6 hours. Biologic effects included dose-dependent increases in circulating IFN-γ, which decreased with subsequent cycles (Fig. 2). Serum neopterin rose in a reproducible fashion regardless of dose or cycle. Tumor necrosis factor–α was not detected by enzyme-linked immunosorbent assay. One of 40 patients developed a low titer antibody to rhIL-12. Lymphopenia was observed at all dose levels with recovery occurring within several days of completing treatment without rebound lymphocytosis. In this phase 1 study, rhIL-12 administered according to this schedule is biologically active at doses tolerable by most patients in an outpatient setting.

This phase 1 study allowed initiation of treatment in a subsequent phase 2 trial in patients with renal cancer at a dose of 500 ng per kg. The phase 2 study was abbreviated after 17 patients entered the trial because profound neurasthenia required admission in over one-half of the patients. Neurasthenia was associated with two treatment-related deaths, one in a patient with advanced atherosclerotic disease who developed renal failure and subsequent complications of dialysis and one in a patient with a gastrointestinal bleed who did not undergo autopsy evaluation.

A thorough scientific investigation was subsequently initiated to determine the cause of the striking difference between the phase 1 and 2 studies. It failed to identify, however, any difference in the drug products used or the patient populations enrolled, which could have illuminated the difference between the two trials. The difference was attributed to the modification of the administration schedule in the subsequent trial. The phase 2 trial used an administration schedule omitting the initial test dose of IL-12, which was received 2 weeks before the daily dosing schedule applied in the phase 1 study. This suggested that IL-12 "protected" against subsequent IL-12 toxicity. This theory has been lent credence by mouse studies, as described below.

A single injection of rIL-12 administered 2 weeks before subsequent dosing included in the phase 1 study had a profound effect on IL-12–induced IFN-γ, diminishing its production and associated toxicity (75). The schedule-dependent toxicity of IL-12 has been confirmed in primates and mice. Coughlin et al. (76) examined the influence of giving a single dose of rIL-12 a week before (predosing) subsequent, daily, consecutive rIL-12 administration. In C3H/HeN mice, treatment without predosing induced rejection of syngeneic K1735 melanomas in 33% of mice. In A/J mice, treatment induced rejection of syngeneic B8–11+SCK (SCK.B7-1) mammary carcinomas in 63% of mice. Administration of a predose of rIL-12 markedly reduced cytokine toxicity in a dose-dependent manner and allowed safe administration of up to eightfold higher doses of daily rIL-12 in C3H mice and fourfold higher doses of rIL-12 in A/J mice. Predosing followed by either standard or high daily doses of rIL-12, however, did not significantly alter the response to rIL-12 treatment in either tumor type. Predosing desensitizes mice to the toxic effects of rIL-12 and allows much higher doses to be given. Predosing does not improve treatment and, by some criteria, attenuates rIL-12 therapeutic outcome. The use of predosing alone does not enhance the effectiveness of rIL-12 in cancer clinical trials.

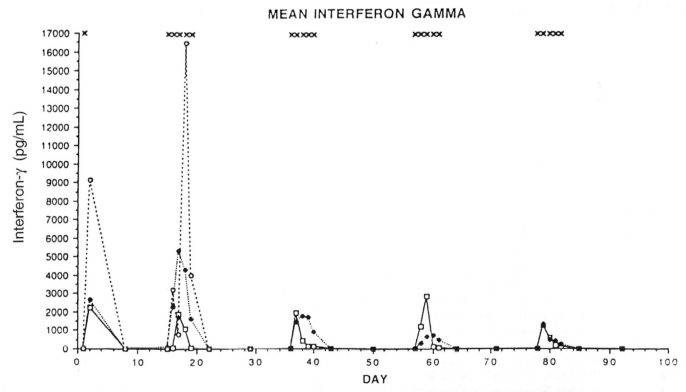

MEAN INTERFERON GAMMA

FIGURE 2. Serial mean serum interferon-γ (IFN-γ) levels for patients treated at the top three recombinant human interleukin-12 dose levels. (☐, 250 ng/kg; ◆, 500 ng/kg; ○, 1,000ng/kg.) (From Atkins BA et al. Phase I evaluation of intravenous recombinant human interleukin-12 (rhIL-12) in patients with advanced malignancies. *Clin Cancer Res* 1997;3:409–417, with permission.)

A phase 1 trial of escalating doses of s.c. rIL-12 given on days 1, 8, and 15 of each 28-day cycle in patients with advanced renal cell carcinoma was carried out (77). Treatment in the initial dosage scheme consisted of a fixed dose level of 0.1, 0.5, or 1.0 mg per kg given in cohorts of three or six patients. On the basis of the toxicity profile, a second scheme ("up-titration") was undertaken, wherein rhIL-12 was escalated sequentially for each patient from week 1 to week 2, to a target maximum dose given week 3 and thereafter; cohort target dose levels were 0.5, 0.75, 1.0, 1.25, and 1.5 mg per kg. Fifty-one patients were treated. The MTD for the fixed dose scheme was 1.0 mg per kg. Dose-limiting toxicities included increase in transaminase concentration, pulmonary toxicity, and leukopenia. The most severe toxicities occurred with the first injection and were milder during further treatment. With the escalation dose scheme (up-titration), the MTD was reached at 1.5 mg per kg and dose-limiting toxicity consisted of an increase in serum transaminase levels. At the MTD of 1.5 mg per kg, serum IL-12 levels increased to a mean peak level of 706 pg per mL. Serum levels of IFN-γ increased to a mean peak level of approximately 200 pg per mL at 24 hours after achieving a maintenance dose of 1.5 mg per kg. The rIL-12 was relatively well tolerated when administered by s.c. injection. Phase 2 trials of rIL-12 were initiated in previously untreated patients with renal cell carcinoma and in patients with melanoma using the up-titration schedule of rhIL-12 (mg per kg) for phase 2 trials as follows: cycle 1–0.1 (day 1), 0.5 (day 8), 1.25 (day 15); cycle 2–1.25 (fixed).

Antitumor Activity and Immunologic Modulation After Systemic Administration of Recombinant Interleukin-12

In our initial phase 1 study using intravenous administration of rIL-12, four patients were noted to have stable disease, one patient with melanoma had a complete response that was transient, and one patient with renal cell cancer has continued a partial response without progression for almost 2 years (74). In a phase 1 study using s.c. delivery of rIL-12, one patient had a complete response, 34 patients had stable disease, 14 patients progressed, and one patient was not evaluable (77). Although it is premature to draw any conclusions from these phase 1 studies, initiation of succeeding phase 2 studies are warranted to define the antitumor effects of rIL-12.

Limited but interesting results are available on the immunomodulatory effects of rIL-12 in humans as well. Robertson et al. (78) reported the immunologic effects of intravenous rIL-12 during the conduct of a phase 1 clinical trial. Forty patients with advanced cancer received bolus intravenous injections of rIL-12 at doses ranging between 3 and 1,000 ng per kg. Dose-dependent increases in serum IFN-γ levels were observed during rIL-12 therapy. rIL-12–induced lymphopenia involved all major lymphocyte subsets. NK cell numbers were the most profoundly affected and CD4 T-cell numbers were the least affected. CD2, LFA-1, and CD56 were transiently upregulated on the surface of NK cells obtained during rIL-12 treatment. Peripheral blood mononuclear cells obtained from cancer patients before rIL-12 therapy exhibited defective NK–cell cytotoxicity and T-cell proliferative responses. Peripheral blood mononuclear cells obtained after lymphocyte recovery after the administration of a single 500 ng per kg dose of rhIL-12 displayed augmented NK-cell cytolytic activity in four out of four patients tested and enhanced T-cell proliferation in three-fourths of patients tested. These studies confirm that doses of rIL-12 resulting in significant immunologic activity can be administered with acceptable toxicity to cancer patients. Furthermore, rhIL-12 therapy reverses defects in NK and T-cell function that are associated with advanced cancer.

Gollob et al. (79) showed that repeated s.c. injections of IL-12 in patients with cancer resulted in the selective expansion of a subset of peripheral blood CD8$^+$ T cells. This T-cell subset expressed high levels of CD18 and further upregulated IL-12 receptor expression after systemic rIL-12 treatment. These CD3$^+$CD8$^+$CD18^{++} T cells have been identified as well in normal subjects and express IL-12, IL-2R, and other adhesion or costimulatory molecules, or both to a greater degree than other CD8$^+$ and CD4$^+$ T cells. They appeared morphologically as large granular lymphocytes although they did not express NK cell markers, such as CD56. In addition, CD8$^+$CD18^{++} T cells were almost exclusively T-cell receptor $\alpha\beta$+ and exhibited a T-cell receptor Vβ repertoire that was strikingly oligoclonal, whereas the Vβ repertoire of CD18 with or without T cells was polyclonal. Although CD8$^+$CD18(bright) T cells demonstrated little functional responsiveness to IL-12 or IL-2 alone *in vitro*, they responded to the combination of IL-2 plus IL-12 with enhanced IFN-γ production and proliferation, as well as non–MHC-restricted cytolytic activity. These CD8$^+$CD18^{++} T cells appear to be a unique population of peripheral blood lymphocytes with features of memory or effector cells, or both, which are capable of T-cell receptor–independent activation after combined stimulation with IL-2 plus IL-12. As this activation results in IFN-γ production and enhanced cytolytic activity, these T cells may play a role in innate, as well as acquired, immunity to tumors and infectious pathogens. Additional studies will be necessary to determine whether CD8$^+$CD18^{++} T cells mediate some of the antitumor effects of IL-12 or IL-2 administered to cancer patients or whether they have additional biologic roles. IL-12 has been used also at lesser doses as a vaccine adjuvant. We treated 25 melanoma patients of doses up to 300 ng per kg in conjunction with immunization using synthetic peptides (i.e., MART1/MelanA, gp100, tyrosinase) without a single objective response (Lotze et al., *unpublished observation*). Similar studies performed by Rosenberg's group have reported at best a minimal response. IL-12 as an adjuvant seems to have little use based on these findings.

Feasibility and Safety of Phase 1 and 2 Studies of Interleukin-12 Gene Therapy

Clinical studies showed that systemic administration of rIL-12 has significant side effects that were not predicted from the animal models. The MTD of the systemic administration of rIL-12 in humans, 500 ng per kg, was found to be significantly lower by 2 to 3 orders of magnitude than that in the mouse (100 μg per kg in C57BL/6 mice) because of significant dose-dependent toxicities. Although phase 2 studies have not been completely reported, the antitumor effects of systemic administration of

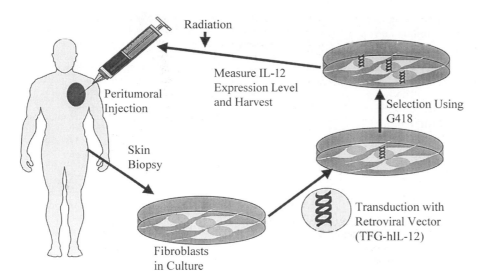

FIGURE 3. Clinical protocol of interleukin-12 (IL-12) gene therapy.

rIL-12 at reported tolerable outpatient doses administered in humans appear to be less potent than those in mice. In contrast, gene therapy strategies can provide high local concentration of IL-12 at the tumor site without the need for attaining high systemic levels of IL-12. In murine tumor models (55–57), eradication of locally treated tumors leads to induction of systemic immune responses that are tumor specific.

Phase 2 clinical trials of IL-12 gene therapy were initiated in the summer of 1995 using direct injection of tumors with genetically engineered autologous fibroblasts (Fig. 3) (80). Patients with advanced malignancies of any histologic type with tumor lesions accessible from the body surface were eligible for this dose-escalating (10 to 3,000 ng per 24 hours) protocol. Primary fibroblast cultures from the patients were transduced using the retroviral vector carrying human IL-12 genes, p35 and p40, as well as the gene encoding neomycin phosphotransferase (TFG-hIL-12-neo). We used transduced autologous fibroblasts because they are readily available from the patients' dermal skin, can be induced to proliferate in cultures, and be retrovirally transduced. Furthermore, autologous fibroblasts can express cytokines at high levels. Minimal immune response to cultured autologous fibroblasts from individual patients was thought to enable repeated administration, which is not possible with immunogenic viral vectors, including adenoviral vectors or allogeneic cell lines. The results of such clinical studies revealed that these advantages are also present in the clinical setting (Tahara et al., *unpublished observation*). Fibroblast cultures were obtained and retrovirally transduced with a success rate of greater than 90%. The average IL-12 transgene expression after selection was approximately 150 ng per 10^6 per 24 hours, which is higher than what we observed in the mouse. The lack of RCR in the fibroblast preparation and patients' serum also supports the feasibility of this approach. Even though retroviral vector systems generally have modest transgene expression, we achieved 9,000 ng per 24 hours dose level (per injection) and *in vivo* expression of p40 transgene in 57% of the patients examined 7 days after the fourth injection. Thus, local and presumably continuous expression of IL-12 can be maintained for at least 4 weeks with 4 weekly injections.

This therapy was associated with minimal side effects in patients treated at dose levels at or below 5,000 ng per 24 hours. Dose-limiting side effects (Shwartzmanlike skin reaction) were observed in some patients who were treated at 7,000 and 9,000 ng per 24-hour dose levels. No systemic toxicities, however, were observed in these patients. The mechanism of inducing this skin reaction is not clear. With rare exception, IL-12 was not detectable in the serum and only marginally increased after treatment, suggesting that high local concentrations of IL-12 can be achieved without detectable systemic levels.

Preliminary Information on the Antitumor Activity of Interleukin-12 Gene Therapy

In several patients with breast cancer, head and neck cancer, and melanoma, objective antitumor effects were observed. Antitumor effects were not limited to the injected tumor. IL-12 alone or other induced cytokines, such as IFN-γ and IL-10, were not detected in these patients. Although the therapeutic effects were transient in most of the patients, sustained systemic antitumor responses were observed in two patients with melanoma. These results suggest that such a local therapy could induce sustained systemic immune responses against tumors in some patients.

Based on these results, phase 2 studies have been initiated in patients with melanoma or head and neck cancer at a dose level of 5,000 ng per 24 hours. Six and three patients have been treated so far on these protocols, respectively. These studies at a fixed dose may confirm some of the favorable findings observed with phase 1 study and provide an opportunity for a more detailed analysis regarding modulation of the local tumor environment.

CONCLUSIONS

Clinical application of IL-12 using systemic administration of rIL-12 has been of limited use in part because of the demise to limit systemic toxicity and development as an outpatient regimen. Gene therapy strategies appear to be more promising at this time. Both strategies have revealed additional unique and unpredicted biologic effects of IL-12. The results obtained in phase 1 studies warrant further investigation of this very interesting molecule in the clinic. Additional efforts to optimize the methods of application in association with optimal antitumor effects and tolerable toxicity are necessary. A more complete understanding of the role of IL-12 in human tumor immunity, especially with dendritic cells or adaptive T-cell responses, will likely lead to successful application of this molecule to cancer and antiviral therapies.

REFERENCES

1. Kobayashi M, Fitz L, Ryan M, et al. Identification and purification of natural killer cell stimulatory factor (NKSF), a cytokine with multiple biologic effects on human lymphocytes. *J Exp Med* 1989;170: 827–845.
2. Stern AS, Podlaski FJ, Hulmes JD, et al. Purification to homogeneity and partial characterization of cytotoxic lymphocyte maturation factor from human B-lymphoblastoid cells. *Proc Natl Acad Sci U S A* 1990;87:6808–6812.
3. Wolf SF, Temple PA, Kobayashi M, et al. Cloning of cDNA for natural killer cell stimulatory factor, a heterodimeric cytokine with multiple biologic effect on T and natural killer cells. *J Immunol* 1991;146:3074–3081.
4. Gubler U, Chua AO, Schoenhout DS, et al. Coexpression of two distinct genes is required to generate secreted bioactive cytotoxic lymphocyte maturation factor. *Proc Natl Acad Sci U S A* 1991;88: 4143–4147.
5. Wong HL, Wilson DE, Jenson JC, Familletti PC, Stremlo DL, Gately MK. Characterization of a factor(s) which synergizes with recombinant interleukin 2 in promoting allogeneic human cytolytic T-lymphocyte responses in vitro. *Cell Immunol* 1988;111:39–54.
6. Chan SH, Perussia B, Gupta JW, et al. Induction of interferon-γ production by natural killer cell stimulatory factor: characterization of the responder cells and synergy with other inducers. *J Exp Med* 1991;173:869–879.
7. Naume B, Gately M, Espevik T. A comparative study of IL-12 (cytotoxic lymphocyte maturation factor)-, IL-12- and IL-7 induced effects on immunomagnetically purified CD56+ NK cells. *J Immunol* 1992;148:2429–2436.
8. Gately MK, Desai BB, Wolitzky AG, et al. Regulation of human lymphocyte proliferation by a heterodimeric cytokine, IL-12 (cytotoxic lymphocyte maturation factor). *J Immunol* 1991;147:874–882.
9. Hsieh C-S, Macatonia S, Tripp C, Wolf S, O'Garra A, Murphy K. Development of Th1 CD4+ T cells through IL-12. Produced by *Listeria*-induced macrophages. *Science* 1993;260:547–549.
10. Gately MK, Warrier RR, Honasoge S, et al. Administration of recombinant IL-12 to normal mice enhances cytolytic lymphocyte activity and induces production of IFN-γ in vivo. *Int Immunol* 1994;6:157–166.
11. Afonso LCC, Scharton TM, Vieira LQ, Wysocka M, Trinchieri G, Scott P. The adjuvant effect of interleukin-12 in a vaccine against Leishmania major. *Science* 1994;263:235–237.
12. Guery J-C, Ria F, Galbaiati F, Adorini L. Normal B cells fail to secrete interleukin-12. *Eur J Immunol* 1997;27:1632–1639.
13. Macatonia SE, Hsieh CS, Murphy KM, O'Garra A. Dendritic cells and macrophages are required for Th1 development of CD4+ T cells from TCRα/β transgenic mice: IL-12 substitution for macrophages to stimulate IFN-γ production is IFN-gamma-γ. *Int Immunol* 1993;5:1119–1128.
14. Kennedy MK, Picha KS, Fanslow WC, et al. CD40/Cd40 ligand interactions are required for T cell-dependent production of interleukin-12 by mouse macrophages. *Eur J Immunol* 1996;26:370–378.
15. Koch F, Stanbl U, Jennewein P, et al. High level IL-12 production by murine dendritic cells: upregulation via MHC class II and CD40 molecules and downregulation by IL-4 and IL-10. *J Exp Med* 1996;184:741–746.
16. Stuber E, Strober W, Neurath M. Blocking the CD40L-CD40 interaction in vivo specifically prevents priming of T helper 1 cells through the inhibition of interleukin 12 secretion. *J Exp Med* 1996;183:693–698.
17. Scheicher C, Mehlig M, Dienes H-P, Reske K. Uptake of microparticulate-absorbed protein antigen by bone-marrow derived dendritic cells results in up-regulation of interleukin-1α and interleukin-12 p40/p35 and triggers prolonged efficient antigen presentation. *Eur J Immunol* 1995;24:1566–1572.
18. Hayes MP, Wang J, Norcross MA. Regulation of interleukin-12 expression in human monocytes: selective priming by interferon-gamma of lipopolysaccharide-inducible p35 and p40 genes. *Blood* 1995;86:646–650.
19. Cooper AM, Roberts AD, Rhoades ER, Callahan JE, Getzy DM, Orme IM. The role of interleukin-12 in acquired immunity to *Mycobacterium tuberculosis* infection. *Immunology* 1995; 84:423–432.
20. Van der Pouw Kraan TC, Boeije LC, Smeek RJ, Wijdened J, Aarden LA. Prostaglandin-E2 is a potent inhibitor of human interleukin 12 production. *J Exp Med* 1995;181:775–779.
21. Manetti R, Annunziato F, Tomasevic L, et al. Polyinosinic acid: polysytidylic acid promotes T helper type 1-specific immune responses by stimulating macrophage production of interferon-alpha and IL-12. *Eur J Immunol* 1995;25:2656–2660.
22. Filgueira L, Nestle FO, Rittig M, Juller HI, Groscurth P. Human dendritic cells phagocytose and process Borrelia burgdorferi. *J Immunol* 1996;157:2998–3005.
23. Cleveland MG, Gorham JD, Murphy TL, Tuomanen E, Murphy KM. Lipoteichoic acid preparations of gram-positive bacteria induce interleukin-12 through a CD14-dependent pathway. *Int Immunol* 1996;64:1906–1912.
24. Fantuzzi L, Gessani S, Birghi P, et al. Induction of interleukin-12 (IL-12) by recombinant glycoprotein gp120 of human immunodeficiency virus type I in human monocytes/macrophages: requirement of gamma interferon for IL-12 secretion. *J Virol* 1996;70: 4121–4124.
25. Rothe H, Hartmann B, Geerlings P, Kolb H. Interleukin-12 gene-expression of macrophages is regulated by nitric oxide. *Biochem Biophys Res Commun* 1996;224:159–163.
26. Ballas ZK, Rasmussen WL, Kreig AM. Induction of NKI activity in murine and human cells by CpG motifs in oligodeoxynucleotides and bacterial DNA. *J Immunol* 1996;157:1840–1845.
27. Klinman DM, Yi AK, Beaucage SL, Conover J, Kreig AM. CpG motifs present in bacterial DNA rapidly induce lymphocytes to secrete interleukin-6, interleukin-12, and interferon gamma. *Proc Natl Acad Sci U S A* 1996;93:2879–2883.
28. Muller G, Salga J, Germann T, Schuler G, Knop J, Enk AH. IL-12 as mediator and adjuvant for the induction of contact sensitivity in vitro. *J Immunol* 1995;155:4661–4668.
29. Chizzonite R, Truitt T, Desai B, et al. IL-12 receptor I. Characterization of the receptor on phytohemagglutinin-activated human lymphoblasts. *J Immunol* 1992;148:3117–3124.
30. Robertson M. Antigen processing: proteasomes in the pathway. *Nature* 1991;353:300–309.
31. Presky DH, Yang H, Minetti LJ, et al. A functional interleukin-12 receptor complex is composed of two beta-type cytokine receptor subunits. *Proc Natl Acad Sci U S A* 1996;93:14002–14007.
32. Wu CY, Warrier RR, Carvajal DM, et al. Biological function and distribution of human interleukin-12 receptor beta chain. *Eur J Immunol* 1996;26:345–350.
33. Gubler U, Presky DH. Molecular biology of interleukin-12 receptors. *Ann N Y Acad Sci* 1996;795:36–40.
34. Chua AO, Wilkinson VL, Presky DH, Gubler U. Cloning and characterization of a mouse IL-12 receptor-beta component. *J Immunol* 1995;155:4286–4294.

35. Presky DH, Minetti LJ, Gillessen S, et al. Evidence for multiple sites of interaction between IL-12 and its receptor. *Ann N Y Acad Sci* 1996;795:390–393.

36. Gillessen S, Carvehal D, Ling P, et al. Mouse interleukin-12 (IL-12) p40 homodimer: a potent IL-12 antagonist. *Eur J Immunol* 1995;25:200–206.

37. Bacon CM, McVicar DW, Ortaldo JR, Rees RC, O'Shea JJ, Johnson JA. Interleukin 12 (IL-12) induces tyrosine phosphorylation of JAK2 and TYK2: differential use of Janus family tyrosine kinases by IL-2 and IL-12. *J Exp Med* 1995;181:399–404.

38. Bacon CM, Petricoin EF III, Ortaldo JR, et al. Interleukin 12 induces tyrosine phosphorylation and activation of STAT4 in human lymphocytes. *Proc Natl Acad Sci U S A* 1995;92:7307–7311.

39. Pignata C, Prasad KV, Haliek M, et al. Phosphorylation of src family lck tyrosine kinase following interleukin-12 activation of human natural killer cells *Cell Immunol* 1995;65:211–216.

40. Klein JL, Fichenscher H, Holliday JE, Biesinger B, Fleckenstein B. Herpesvirus saimiri immortalized gamma delta T cell line activated by IL-12. *J Immunol* 1996;56:2754–2760.

41. Yu WG, Yamamoto N, Takeeenaka H, et al. T. Molecular mechanisms underlying IFN-γ mediated tumor growth inhibition induced during tumor immunotherapy with rIL-12. *Int Immunol* 1996;8:855–865.

42. Yu CR, Kin JK, Fink DW, Akira S, Bloom ET, Yamauchi A. Differential utilization of Janus kinase-signal transducer activator of transcription signaling pathways in the stimulation of human natural killer cells by IL-2, IL-12 and interferon-gamma. *J Immunol* 1996;157:126–137.

43. Cho SS, Bacon CM, Sudarshan C, et al. Activation of STAT4 by IL-12 and IFN-α: evidence for the involvement of ligand-induced tyrosine and serine phosphorylation. *J Immunol* 1996;157:4781–4789.

44. Zou J, Presly DH, Wu CY, Gubler U. Differential associations between the cytoplasmic regions of the interleukin-12 receptor subunits β1 and β2 and JAK kinases. *J Biol Chem* 1997;272:6073–6077.

45. Rogge L, Barberis-Maino L, Biffi M, et al. Selective expression of an interleukin-12 receptor component by human T helper 1 cells. *J Exp Med* 1997;185:825–831.

46. Hilkens CM, Messer G, Tesselaar K, van Rietshoten AG, Kapsenberg ML, Wierenga EA. Lack of IL-12 signaling in human allergen-specific Th2 cells. *J Immunol* 1996;157:4316–4321.

47. Kaplan MH, Sun YL, Hoey T, Grusby MJ. Impaired IL-12 responses and enhanced development of Th2 cells in Stat4-deficient mice. *Nature* 1996;382;174–177.

48. Thierfelder WE, van Deursen JM, Yamamoto K, et al. Requirement for Stat4 in interleukin-12-mediated responses of natural killer cells and T-cells. *Nature* 1996;82:171–174.

49. Nastala CL, Edington H, Storkus W, et al. Recombinant interleukin-12 administration induces tumor regression in association with interferon-gamma and nitric oxide production. *J Immunol* 1994;153:169–178.

50. Brunda MJ, Luistro L, Warrier RR, et al. Antitumor and antimetastatic activity of interleukin-12 against murine tumors. *J Exp Med* 1993;178:1223–1230.

51. Nishimura T, Watanabe K, Lee U, et al. Systemic *in vivo* antitumor activity of interleukin-12 against both transplantable and primary tumor. *Immunol Lett* 1995;48:149–152.

52. Nishimura T, Watanabe K, Yahata T, et al. Application of interleukin-12 to antitumor and gene therapy. *Cancer Chemother Pharmacol* 1996;38:S27–S34.

53. Verbik LA, Showe LC, Lester TL, McNutt RM, Van Cleave VH, Metzger DW. Direct binding of IL-12 to human and murine B lymphocytes. *Int Immunol* 1996;8:1955–1962.

54. Kubin M, Kamoun M, Trinchieri G. Interleukin-12 synergizes with B7/CD28 interaction in inducing efficient proliferation and cytokine production of human T cells. *J Exp Med* 1994;180(1): 211–222.

55. Tahara H, Zeh HJZ III, Storkus WJ, et al. Fibroblasts genetically engineered to secrete interleukin-12 can suppress tumor growth and induce anti-tumor immunity to a murine melanoma *in vivo*. *Cancer Res* 1994;54:182–189.

56. Tahara H, Zitvogel L, Storkus WJ, et al. Effective eradication of established murine tumors with interleukin 12 (IL-12) gene therapy using a polycistronic retroviral vector. *J Immunol* 1995;154: 6466–6474.

57. Zitvogel L, Tahara H, Robbins PD, et al. Cancer immunotherapy of established tumors with interleukin-12: effective delivery by genetically engineered fibroblasts. *J Immunol* 1995;155:1393–1403.

58. Addison CL, Bramson JL, Hitt MM, Muller WJ, Gauldie J, Graham FL. Intratumoral coinjection of adenoviral vectors expressing IL-2 and IL-12 results in enhanced frequency of regression of injected and untreated distal tumors. *Gene Ther* 1998;5:1400–1409.

59. Gambotto A, Tuting T, McVey DL, et al. Induction of antitumor immunity by direct intratumoral injection of a recombinant adenovirus vector expressing interleukin-12. *Cancer Gene Ther* 1999;6: 45–53.

60. Zitvogel L, Lotze MT. Role of interleukin-12 as an anti-tumor agent: experimental biology and clinical application. *Res Immunol* 1995;46:628–638.

61. Zitvogel L, Robbins PD, Storkus WJ, et al. B7.1 costimulation markedly enhances IL-12-mediated antitumor immunity *in vivo*. *Eur J Immunol* 1996;26:1335–1341.

62. Coughlin CM, Wysocka M, Kurzawa HL, Lee WM, Trinchieri G, Eck SL. B7-1 and interleukin 12 synergistically induce effective antitumor immunity. *Cancer Res* 1995;55:4980–4987.

63. Pappo I, Tahara H, Robbins PD, Wolf SF, Lotze MT. Administration of systemic or local interleukin-2 enhances the anti-tumor effects of interleukin-12 gene therapy. *J Surg Res* 1995;58:218–226.

64. Vagliani M, Rodolfo M, Cavallo F, et al. Interleukin 12 potentiates the curative effect of a vaccine based on interleukin-2-transduced tumor cells. *Cancer Res* 1996;56:467–470.

65. Wigginton JM, Kuhns DB, Back TC, Brunda MJ, Wiltrout RH, Cox GW. Interleukin 12 primes macrophages for nitric oxide production *in vivo* and restores depressed nitric oxide production by macrophages from tumor-bearing mice: implications for the antitumor activity of interleukin-12 and/or interleukin-2. *Cancer Res* 1996;56:1131–1136.

66. Wigginton JM, Komschlies KL, Back TC, Franco JL, Brunda MJ, Wiltrout RH. Administration of interleukin-12 with pulse interleukin-2 and the rapid and complete eradication of murine renal carcinoma. *J Natl Cancer Inst* 1996;88:38–43.

67. Osaki T, Péron J-M, Cai Q, et al. IFN-γ-inducing factor/IL-18 administration mediates IFN-γ and IL-12 independent anti-tumor effects. *J Immunol* 1998;160:1742–1749.

68. Coughlin CM, Salhany KE, Gee MS, et al. Tumor cell responses to IFN-gamma affect tumorigenicity and response to IL-12 therapy and antiangiogenesis. *Immunity* 1998;9:25–34.

69. Osaki T, Hashimoto W, Gambotto A, et al. Potent anti-tumor effects mediated by local expression of the mature form of the IFN-gamma inducing factor, IL-18. *Gene Therapy* 1999;6:808–815.

70. Hashimoto W, Takeda K, Anzai R, et al. Cytotoxic NK1.1 Ag+ T cells with intermediate TCR induced in the liver of mice by IL-12. *J Immunol* 1995;154:4333–4340.

71. Takeda K, Seki S, Ogasawara K, et al. Liver NK1.1 CD4+ T cells activated by IL-12 as a major effect in inhibition of experimental tumor metastases. *J Immunol* 1996;156:3366–3373.

72. Cui J, Shin T, Kawano T, et al. Requirement for Valpha14 NKT cells in IL-12-mediated rejection of tumors. *Science* 1997;278: 1623–1626.

73. Kanegane C, Sgadari C, Kanegane H, et al. Contribution of the CXC chemokines IP-10 and Mig to the antitumor effects of IL-12. *J Leukoc Biol* 1998;64:384–392.

74. Atkins BA, Robertson MJ, Gordon M, et al. Phase 1 evaluation of intravenous recombinant human interleukin-12 (rhIL-12) in patients with advanced malignancies. *Clin Cancer Res* 1997;3:409–417.

75. Leonard JP, Sherman ML, Fisher GL, et al. Effects of single-dose interleukin-12 exposure on interleukin-12-associated toxicity and interferon-gamma production. *Blood* 1997;90:2541–2548.

76. Coughlin CM, Wysocka M, Trinchieri G, Lee WM. The effect of interleukin-12 desensitization on the antitumor efficacy of recombinant interleukin-12. *Cancer Res* 1997;57:2460–2467.

77. Motzer RJ, Rakhitt A, Schwartz LH, et al. Phase I trial of subcutaneous recombinant human interleukin-12 in patients with advanced renal cell carcinoma. *Clin Cancer Res* 1998;4:1183–1191.

78. Robertson MJ, Cameron C, Atkins MB, et al. Immunological effects of interleukin 12 administered by bolus intravenous injection to patients with cancer. *Clin Cancer Res* 1999;5:9–16.

79. Gollob JA, Schnipper CP, Orsini E, et al. Characterization of a novel subset of CD8(+) T cells that expands in patients receiving interleukin-12. *J Clin Invest* 1998;102:561–575.

80. Tahara H, Lotze MT. IL-12 gene therapy using direct injection of tumors with genetically engineered autologous fibroblasts. *Hum Gene Ther* 1995;6:1607–1624.

6

COLONY-STIMULATING FACTORS: BASIC PRINCIPLES AND PRECLINICAL STUDIES

MALCOLM A. S. MOORE

Colony-stimulating factors (CSFs) belong to a large family of cytokines with pleiotropic and frequently overlapping activities that orchestrate steady-state lymphohematopoiesis, as well as mediate acute responses involving specific cell lineages. For historic reasons, hematopoietic growth factors have been named after the lineages they regulate [e.g., erythropoietin (Epo), thrombopoietin (Tpo)] or after the assays that permitted their detection [e.g., CSF, granulocyte colony-stimulating factor (G-CSF), macrophage colony-stimulating factor (M-CSF), and granulocyte-macrophage colony-stimulating factor (GM-CSF)]. Others are termed *interleukins*, numbered consecutively in order of discovery, indicating cytokines produced by and acting on leukocytes. Eighteen interleukins exist, many of which can be produced by nonleukocytic populations. These have actions on cells outside the hematopoietic system, as well as on leukocytes and their progenitors. Interleukin-3 (IL-3) was independently identified as a multilineage CSF and has been termed *multi-CSF*. Due to its close relationship with other members of the CSF family, it is included in this review. Other cytokines are identified by their receptors (c-kit and Flk-2/Flt-3 ligands).

Early attempts to functionally classify hematopoietic growth factors as early-acting, late-acting, or lineage-specific (versus multilineage-stimulating) have not held up to detailed analysis. Apparently, for example, lineage-specific, late-acting factors, such as G-CSF and Tpo, exhibit potent synergistic interactions influencing pluripotential stem-cell proliferation and differentiation. Early-acting, multilineage factors, such as c-kit and Flk-2/Flt-3 ligands, can affect early stem-cell proliferation and differentiation, as well as highly differentiated cells such as mast cells (c-kit ligand–stimulated) or dendritic cells (DCs) (Flk-2/Flt-3 ligand–stimulated).

MACROPHAGE COLONY-STIMULATING FACTOR
Molecular Characterization

In the early 1970s, a CSF that had a restricted ability to stimulate the development of colonies containing only macrophages was identified in serum, urine, and fibroblast cell-line–conditioned media (1,2). One unit of this M-CSF was defined as the amount of factors required to stimulate a single macrophage colony in a 7-day agar or methylcellulose culture of mouse bone marrow cells in the linear part of the dose-response curve (representing 0.44 fmol of murine M-CSF). This sensitive bioassay permitted detection of activity in human serum, urine, or cell-line conditioned media at concentrations as low as 1 pm and facilitated purification of the factor. Murine M-CSF was isolated from mouse L-cell conditioned medium as a glycoprotein of 70 kd, composed of two 35-kd polypeptide chains with disulfide bonds (3). M-CSF purified from human urine or tumor cell lines is a 44-kd to 86-kd homodimeric glycoprotein (Table 1) (3,4). Oligonucleotide probes predicted from the N-terminal sequence were used to isolate human M-CSF genomic clones. Messenger ribonucleoproteins (mRNAs) of different sizes are produced by alternative splicing of exon 6 (5,6). Three spliced variants of biologically active M-CSF are produced: a short, or alpha form (α-form), with a leader sequence of 32 amino acids followed by 256 amino acids; a long, or beta form (β-form) of 554 amino acids; and a gamma form (γ-form) of 438 amino acids. The COOH-terminus anchors some forms of M-CSF in an active cell-associated form, with the native secreted form of macrophage colony-stimulating factor-alpha (M-CSF-α) being generated by cotranslational N-linked glycosylation and proteolytic cleavage at or near amino acid 158. The 18 cysteines in the homodimeric species form three intermolecular and three intramolecular disulfide bonds, rendering the protein resistant to proteolytic cleavage. The 64-kd homodimer consists of two bundles of four alpha helices laid end-to-end with an interchain disulfide bond, together with mannose-rich asparagine-(N)-linked oligosaccharide chains (7). A portion of this molecule is released by proteolysis as a 44-kd extracellular protein. A second soluble form of 86-kd is composed of two identical subunits of 223 amino acids with O- and N-linked sugar residues. This form is cleared from the membrane within the intracellular secretory compartment before its release from the cell, and does not appear as a surface membrane–bound molecule. A high-molecular-weight proteoglycan form of M-CSF (> 200 kd) with a core protein of 45 kd and a chondroitin sulfate glycosaminoglycan chain has been reported (8). The proteoglycan

TABLE 1. CHARACTERISTICS OF COLONY-STIMULATING FACTORS

	M-CSF	G-CSF	GM-CSF	IL-3
Mature molecular weight (kd)	44–86	19.6	14–32	14–28
Amino acids	223/438/554	174/177	127	133
Carbohydrate	2–4 N–O[a]	1-O	2-N	2-N
Cysteines (half)	9	4	4	2
Messenger RNA (kb)	1.6–4.2	1.6	0.7	1.0
Gene size (kb)	~21	2.5	0.7	~3.2
Number of exons	10	5	4	5
Chromosome	1p13-21	17q11-21	5q33	5q31

G-CSF, granulocyte colony-stimulating factor; GM-CSF, granulocyte-macrophage colony-stimulating factor; IL-3, interleukin-3; kb, kilobase; M-CSF, macrophage colony-stimulating factor.
[a]Number of *N*- or *O*-linked glycosylation sites.

form is not a latent form or precursor of the 85-kd M-CSF because it rapidly phosphorylates tyrosine residues of the M-CSF receptor (9). This form is found in bone matrix, suggesting it plays a role in bone metabolism, and because it can bind and neutralize the biologic activity of basic fibroblast growth factor (bFGF), it may regulate fibroblast proliferation (10). The membrane-anchored form of M-CSF expressed by marrow stromal cells has been shown to mediate intercellular adhesion of M-CSF-receptor–expressing hematopoietic cells (11). The soluble, matrix-associated, membrane-bound cell-associated forms of M-CSF play different specific roles on receptor-bearing target cells, with ligand-receptor interactions involving endocrine, paracrine, juxtacrine, or autocrine pathways (12).

The human M-CSF gene maps to the short arm of chromosome 1, bands p13–21 (see Table 1) (13).

Macrophage Colony-Stimulating Factor Receptor

High-affinity (kd = 10^{-13} m) M-CSF binding sites are expressed at levels of 1×10^4 to 1×10^5 per cell on mature monocytes, macrophages, and osteoclasts (Table 2) (4). During differentiation within the macrophage lineage, the number of receptors increases while proliferative response to M-CSF declines. The M-CSF receptor is encoded by the c-fms oncogene and is a member of the growth-factor receptor family that

exhibits ligand-induced tyrosine-specific protein kinase activity (14,15). C-fms maps on chromosome 5 at band 5q 33.3 in relative proximity to other growth-factor receptors and genes (see Table 2) (4). The receptor is an integral membrane glycoprotein of 972 amino acids that include a signal peptide. The extracellular ligand-binding domain has 512 amino acids, with five immunoglobulin-like domains joined to a 435 amino-acid cytoplasmic-protein kinase domain through a single membrane-spanning helix. On ligand binding, the receptor undergoes noncovalent dimerization, rapid autophosphorylation (30 seconds), and signaling, followed by covalent dimerization via disulfide bonds, leading to further modification, tyrosine dephosphorylation, and internalization (15). Specific autophosphorylation sites determine whether the receptor mediates proliferation versus differentiation signals, and whether mutations of mouse fms at Tyr807 totally abrogate differentiation but increase the rate of M-CSF–dependent proliferation and provide a paradigm for fms involvement in leukemogenesis (16). Phosphorylated receptor tyrosine residues are sites of interaction for a number of proteins containing src homology type 2 (SH2) domains. In c-fms, Grb2 interacts with Tyr-697, whereas the p85 subunit of phosphatidylinositol 3′ (PI3)-kinase interacts with Tyr-721. Tyr-809 is the site of interaction for members of the src kinase family. Signaling involves phosphorylation of many cytosolic proteins, including tyrosine phosphorylation of Tyk2, a protein kinase of the Janus protein tyrosine kinase (Jak) family, and the signal transducers and activators of transcription [STAT (STAT1, STAT3, and STAT5)] proteins (see Table 2) (15,17). Multimeric cytosolic complexes of signaling proteins and cytoskeletal components form in macrophages on M-CSF stimulation; these incorporate the STATs, Cb1, SHP-1, Shc, cytoskeletal, and contractile proteins (e.g., vimentin, actin, myosin regulatory light chain, tropomyosin, and paxillin), Ras family signaling proteins, NnaJ-like proteins, and glyceraldehyde-3-phosphate dehydrogenase (18). STAT5 homodimer or STAT5-α/STAT5-β heterodimers formed in response to M-CSF signaling bind to the prolactin-inducible element (PIE) forming novel PIE-binding complexes (19). Mitogen-activated protein (MAP) kinases p42 and p44 are phosphorylated and constitutively activated by raf kinase in response to M-CSF binding to fms (20). Persistent activation of the raf-MAP kinase pathway by M-CSF is necessary for Ets-2 expression

TABLE 2. CHARACTERISTICS OF THE COLONY STIMULATING-FACTOR RECEPTORS

	M-CSFR	G-CSFR	IL-3Rα	GM-CSFR-α	GM-CSFR-βc	GM-CSFR-αβ
Affinity (kd/nm)	0.002	0.1	0.1–10.0	0.9–20.0	—	0.01–0.10
Number/cell	2×10^3–10^5	50–500	< 1,000	300–2,400	881	< 10,000
Amino acids	972	813	360	378	881	—
Messenger RNA (kb)	~3.0	3.7	2.0	2.1	~3.0	—
Chromosome	5q33.3	1p32-34	PA–XY	PA–XY	22q31	—
Signals via	Tyk2, Grb, p13 kinase	Jak1, 2, Tyk2	Jak1, 2	Jak1, 2	Jak1, 2	Jak1, 2
Signals via	STAT1, 3, 5	STAT1, 3, 5	STAT1, 3, 5	STAT1, 3, 5	STAT1, 3, 5	STAT1, 3, 5

βc, beta common; G-CSF, granulocyte colony-stimulating factor receptor; GM-CSF, granulocyte-macrophage colony-stimulating factor; IL-3, interleukin-3; kb, kilobase; M-CSF, macrophage colony-stimulating factor; PA, pseudoautosomal region of X and Y chromosomes; p13, phosphatidylinositol 3′ kinase; STAT, signal transducers and activators of transcription proteins.

TABLE 3. CELLULAR SOURCES OF COLONY-STIMULATING FACTORS

Cell Type	Stimuli	M-CSF	G-CSF	GM-CSF	IL-3
T lymphocyte	Ag, lectin, IL-2	+	–	++	++
B lymphocyte	Ag, LPS, IL-1	–	–	++	–
Monocyte/Macrophage	LPS, adh, phag	++	++	++	–
Mesothelium	LPS,	+	+	+	–
Keratinocytes	+	+	+	–	
Osteoblasts	PH, LPS	+	+	+	–
Synoviocytes	RA	+	+	+	–
Mast cells	IgE	–	–	+	+
Fibroblasts	IL-1, TNF, IL-17	+	+	+	–
Marrow stroma	IL-1, TNF, IL-17	+	++	++	–
Endothelium	IL-1, TNF, LPS, shear	+	+	+	–
Astrocytes	IL-1, TNF	+	?	+	–
Microglia	IL-1, TNF	+	+	+	–
Placenta	None or IL-1	+	+	+	–
Trophoblast	None or IL-1	+	+	+	–

adh, stimulus of adherence; ag, antigen; G-CSF, granulocyte colony-stimulating factor; GM-CSF, granulocyte-macrophage colony-stimulating factor; IgE, immunoglobulin E; IL-1, interleukin-1; IL-2, interleukin-2; IL-3, interleukin-3; IL-17, interleukin-17; LPS, lipopolysaccharide; M-CSF, macrophage colony-stimulating factor; phag, phagocytosis; PH, parathyroid hormone; RA, rheumatoid arthritis; shear, hydrodynamic shear forces; TNF, tumor necrosis factor; –, no factor produced; +, low level factor production; ++, high level factor production.

and posttranslational activation in macrophages. A novel non-receptor protein kinase, RAFTK, associates with c-fms in response to M-CSF and participates in signal-transduction pathway (21). RAFTK is involved in focal-adhesion signal-transduction pathways in many cell types; focal adhesions may modulate cytoskeletal functions and thereby alter phagocytosis, cell migration, and adhesion of macrophages.

Origin of Macrophage Colony-Stimulating Factor and Regulation of Production

M-CSF is present in normal plasma at levels of 100 to 200 units per mL, and most tissues produce M-CSF transcripts of several sizes. This ubiquitous expression may reflect production by cells common to many organs (e.g., macrophages, endothelial cells, fibroblasts, or mesothelial cells) (Table 3) (4). Fluctuations in levels of circulating M-CSF reflect a balance between production and excretion, with M-CSF receptors on Kupffer's cells in the liver and on splenic macrophages responsible for significant clearance by specific binding of M-CSF with subsequent endocytosis and intracellular destruction (22). Adherence and bacterial lipopolysaccharides are potent inducing stimuli for monocyte and macrophage M-CSF production, with further enhancement by cyclooxygenase inhibitors and inhibition by prostaglandin-E (PGE), which participates in a negative feed-back loop (4,12,23). GM-CSF is a strong inducer of M-CSF mRNA in monocytes, and tumor necrosis factor–α (TNF-α) synergizes with it to induce M-CSF secretion. IL-2 is also an inducer of monocyte M-CSF production and IL-1 strongly augments M-CSF secretion. IL-4 and IL-10 strongly inhibit M-CSF production by repressing M-CSF gene transcription. Constitutive production of M-CSF is found in alveolar macrophages; production is increased after endotoxin treatment of macrophages from individuals who have smoked (but not from nonsmokers). Activated T cells produce M-CSF, as can keratinocytes, endothelial cells

and IL-1, IL-6, or TNF-stimulated fibroblasts, and marrow stromal cells (see Table 3) (4).

Biologic Activities of Macrophage Colony-Stimulating Factor

Action on Progenitor Cells

Whereas the pathway of differentiation stimulated by M-CSF is restricted to cells of the phagocytic mononuclear lineage, its action is not limited to progenitors restricted to this lineage. At the progenitor level, highly purified populations are stimulated by M-CSF alone, as well as by GM-CSF and IL-3, with a frequency indicating that many oligopotential progenitors have receptors for all three growth factors. Furthermore, cultures of marrow cell initiated with M-CSF, followed by delayed addition of GM-CSF, form colonies of granulocytes and macrophages indistinguishable from those initiated with GM-CSF (24). This indicates that M-CSF sustains a progenitor population with the potential to form granulocytes, although it is responsible only for macrophage-lineage terminal differentiation. In the murine system, M-CSF can act on multipotent high proliferative potential cells, including pluripotent stem cells, but only in synergistic interaction with IL-1, IL-6, IL-3, or KL (25).

Action on Monocytes and Macrophages

Insight into the physiologic importance of M-CSF has come from studies of the osteopetrotic (op/op) mouse characterized by an autosomal recessive inactivating mutation of the M-CSF gene, resulting in absence of M-CSF (26). Quantitative defects in macrophage populations characterize op/op mice with marrow macrophages 1% of numbers in normal mice and with no splenic marginal zone macrophages. Strong evidence exists that M-CSF is involved in survival, proliferation, and differentiation on at least some monocyte-macrophage populations; evidence that the factor functions as a macrophage activator as part of an inflammatory host defense response also exists. Acute events after M-CSF interaction with monocytes include increased cell spreading, membrane ruffling, and receptor turnover, as well as induction of a variety of cytokines (IL-1, G-CSF, TNF, IL-6). The latter response may be observed only with adherent cells. M-CSF activation enhances macrophage phagocytosis, bacteriocidal and amebicidal capacity, and upregulates Fc receptor gamma (FcR-γ) and antibody-dependent cell-mediated cytotoxicity (ADCC) (4). Nitric oxide is also produced by macrophages after synergistic stimulation by M-CSF and endotoxin or interferon-gamma (IFN-γ). M-CSF induces the transcriptional activation of heat shock genes (*HSP60*, *HSP70*, and *HSP90*); these may play important roles in macrophage activation by functioning as molecular chaperones and protecting cells against autooxidative damage associated with respiratory burst (27). M-CSF activation of monocytes and macrophages enhances their capacity to kill or inactivate a wide range of pathogens, including *Mycobacterium*, *Leishmania*, *Candida albicans*, *Histoplasma* and *Entamoeba histolytica*, *Staphylococcus aureus*, and *Cryptococcus neoformans* (4,28,29). M-CSF inhibits macrophage metalloelastase production, whereas GM-CSF induces it, suggesting that these molecules may control degradation of elastin fibers in lung or blood vessels (30). Differences in functional states of macrophages mediated by M-CSF include downregulation (perhaps irreversibly) of IL-12 production (31); upregulation of CD14 (a receptor for endotoxin, rendering monocytes more sensitive to this agent) (32), and release of immunoglobulin E (IgE)–dependent histamine, releasing M-CSF primes elicited–peritoneal macrophages for differential expression of adhesion molecules, enhancing very late antigens-5 (VLA-5) expression, adhesion to extracellular matrix components, and subsequent secretion of IL-6 (34). Transwell migration studies have shown that M-CSF is a chemotactic and chemokinetic agent for macrophages (35). Human macrophages express chemokine receptors (CCR5, CXCR4) that act as coreceptors for human immunodeficiency virus type 1 (HIV-1) and are major targets for HIV-1 infection *in vivo*. M-CSF and GM-CSF markedly increase the extent of HIV-1 entry and replication, as well as expression of CCR5 on macrophages (36).

M-CSF activates antibody-dependent (ADCC) and -independent tumor cell cytolysis. Human macrophages cultured with IL-2 and M-CSF show high tumoricidal activity against human and murine leukemic cell lines; the effector mechanism involves production of cytotoxic molecules (37). Synergy between M-CSF and IFN-γ also induces tumoricidal macrophages (38). Monocytes and macrophages exposed to M-CSF for 48 hours exhibit enhanced FcR-γ expression and mediate ADCC killing of tumor cells with phagocytosis of intact cells as the principal mechanism of antitumor cytotoxicity (37,38).

Action on Osteoclasts

M-CSF–deficient op/op mice are toothless, and marrow cavities are occluded by bone overgrowth owing to an osteoclast deficit (26). This defect in osteoclastogenesis can be cured by M-CSF treatment (39). Whereas a specific osteoclast CSF supports the proliferation of osteoclast progenitors and formation of colonies of tartrate-resistant acid phosphatase–positive osteoclasts, M-CSF plays a role in later development of osteoclasts, inducing osteoclast fusion and stimulating their motility (chemotaxis), spread, and survival (40,41). Bone stromal cells produce M-CSF in response to IL-1 and TNF, cytokines produced locally by bone marrow mononuclear cells that are recognized for their ability to promote osteoclast formation and bone resorption (41).

Role of Macrophage Colony-Stimulating Factor in Pregnancy

Impaired fertility is observed in op/op mice and a marked pregnancy-associated increase in serum levels of M-CSF suggests a role exists for M-CSF in blastocyst attachment, trophoblast outgrowth, implantation, and proliferation of placental tissue (42). The major effect of M-CSF on female reproductive function is on frequency and rate of ovulation, indicating a major role for the factor in regulating follicular development and ovulation (43). In male op/op mice, a greatly reduced serum testosterone level owing to reduced testicular Leydig cell steroidogenesis exists, indicating M-CSF plays a novel role in the development or regulation, or both, of male hypothalamic-pituitary-gonadal axis (44). The expression of c-fms and M-CSF by normal human first trimester–invasive extravillous trophoblast cells, and evidence of the role of M-CSF in stimulation of proliferation of this tissue, suggests an autocrine and possibly paracrine role exists for M-CSF in invasive trophoblast *in situ* (see Table 3) (45). M-CSF may also have a role in mammary gland development during pregnancy; in mid-gestation op/op mice, ductal branching is impaired, and after parturition, a failure to switch to lactation occurs (46).

Role of Macrophage Colony-Stimulating Factor in the Central Nervous System

The numeric density of microglia, resident brain macrophages, is significantly reduced in op/op mice; cells are smaller and have shorter cytoplasmic processes (47). The relative failure of op/op mice to respond to external stimuli also suggests a role for M-CSF in the brain. M-CSF mRNA is expressed in a regional-specific manner in the brain throughout development, whereas *c-fms* is expressed throughout the brain in the microglia (46,48). M-CSF is neurotrophic in embryonal neuronal cultures; its absence in op/op mice results in severe electrophysiologic abnormalities in the cortex that can be corrected by M-CSF therapy (48). M-CSF is a neurotrophic factor that acts through microglia. M-CSF dramatically augmented β-amyloid peptide-induced microglial production of inflammatory cytokines (IL-1 and IL-6) and nitric oxide (NO) (49). These mediators, in turn, could intensify cerebral inflammatory states by activating astrocytes and additional microglia, as well as by directly injuring neurones. These pathways may be involved in Alzheimer's disease, a chronic cerebral inflammatory state that leads to neuronal injury. Intraparenchymal migration of macrophages occurs in the central nervous system (CNS) during development or as a consequence of tissue injury. Astrocytes, through their ability to secrete M-CSF, can trigger polarized migration of brain macrophages (see Table 3) (50).

Role of Macrophage Colony-Stimulating Factor in Atherosclerosis

Macrophages serve as the principal inflammatory cell in the atheromatous plaque microenvironment. Their localization within the artery wall is probably determined by M-CSF produced locally by endothelial and smooth muscle cells after activation by inflammatory cytokines or modified low-density lipoprotein (LDL) (4,51,52). Lipid-laden "foamy" macrophages that develop in plaques produce M-CSF and express acetyl–LDL receptors. These scavenger receptors mediate uptake of modified lipoprotein-cholesterol with subsequent cholesterol ester accumulation and foam cell formation (4,51,52). The influence of M-CSF on atherogenesis was studied in an atherogenesis-induction model involving feeding op/op or control mice a high-fat, high-cholesterol diet, or crossing op/op mice with apolipoprotein-E knockout mice (53). Crossing of op/op mice with LDL receptor-deficient mice (an animal model of familial hypercholesterolemia) significantly reduced atherosclerosis, producing a 100-fold decrease in lesion size (54). Absence of M-CSF was associated with complete protection from atherosclerosis, an effect that may have resulted due to decreased circulating monocytes, reduced tissue macrophages, or diminished arterial M-CSF.

Role of Macrophage Colony-Stimulating Factor in Adipose Tissue Growth

Adipose tissue growth results from *de novo* adipocyte recruitment (hyperplasias) and increased size of preexisting adipocytes. M-CSF mRNA and protein are expressed in human adipocytes, and expression is upregulated in rapidly growing adipose tissue. Localized overexpression of M-CSF resulting from an adenovector gene transfer was associated with a 16-fold increase in adipose tissue growth owing to proliferation rather than hypertrophy (55). The proximity of the chromosomal locus for M-CSF (1p21) to sites linked with obesity and insulin action heightens the potential importance of M-CSF in the biology of adipose tissue growth and pathogenesis of obesity.

Preclinical *in Vivo* Studies of Macrophage Colony-Stimulating Factor

Treatment of mice, rats, rabbits, and primates with recombinant human M-CSF for 7 to 14 days at doses of 10 to 300 μg per kg per day leads to an increase in circulating monocytes (up to tenfold), promonocytes, and macrophagelike cells that can comprise up to 30% to 70% of circulating nucleated cells (4,56–58). The FcR-γ III (CD16 receptor) is found on tissue macrophages, but its expression is restricted to a small subset of circulating monocytes. This CD16+ monocyte population is selectively expanded by administration of recombinant human (rh) M-CSF in primates, with a 50-fold increase in numbers (58). This increase was paralleled by the emergence of a population of circulating CD16+ cells morphologically resembling

large granular lymphocytes. The number of natural killer (NK) cells is increased in mouse spleen and blood after M-CSF treatment; the cells are activated as indicated by their higher cytotoxic activity against NK-sensitive tumor targets, enhanced proliferative response to IL-2, and a greater production of IFN-γ in response to IL-2 and IL-12 (59). M-CSF treatment of mice also produces a redistribution of myeloid progenitors with an initial decrease in marrow colony forming unit M, -GM, and -G, with a progressive increase in these populations occurring in the spleen, peaking at levels of four- to 15-fold of baseline by day 3 or 4 (60). Splenic macrophages are also increased in number and activation state in M-CSF–treated mice, being primed for heightened response to endotoxin, as indicated by a tenfold higher level of serum IL-6 (61). Dose-dependent delayed thrombocytopenia, seen in all species after M-CSF treatment, is usually transient and resolves rapidly on cessation of treatment; it resolves on prolonged treatment in mice (62). This thrombocytopenia is not caused by suppressed thrombopoiesis, but by increased activity of the monocyte/macrophage system, which causes hemophagocytosis and shortened platelet survival with increased platelet production, compensating for ongoing platelet destruction with restoration of normal platelet levels (62). M-CSF and IL-1 interact synergistically to enhance restoration of stem and progenitor populations in murine marrow and accelerate hematopoietic recovery in 5-fluorouracil (5-FU) myelosuppressed mice (63). Monocyte ADCC and tumoricidal capacity are enhanced by *in vivo* M-CSF therapy; this is correlated with a significant reduction in metastasis in an experimental melanoma tumor system (64,65). Treatment of mice bearing melanoma or lung carcinoma with fractionated radiation therapy and M-CSF resulted in an M-CSF dose–dependent increase in tumor killing (65). The combination of IL-12 and M-CSF was most effective with radiation therapy in the clinically relevant dosage of 2 and 2 Gy per fraction with a synergistic antitumor action.

In normal rabbits and young Watanabe hyperlipidemic rabbits deficient in LDL receptors, M-CSF reduced cholesterol levels by one-third (66).

The cholesterol-lowering effect may be attributed to enhanced macrophage activities of neutral and acidic cholesteryl ester hydrolases, enhancing net hydrolysis of acidic cholesterol ester (67).

GRANULOCYTE COLONY-STIMULATING FACTOR

Isolation of Granulocyte Colony-Stimulating Factor Gene and Protein Structure

G-CSF was first identified in the serum of endotoxin-treated mice as a neutrophil G-CSF with the capacity to induce granulocyte differentiation of a murine myelomonocytic leukemic cell line (68,69). The purification and molecular cloning of human G-CSF was performed between 1984 and 1986 (70,71), and clinical development commenced in 1986 with approval for clinical use in cancer patients treated with chemotherapy (72). Human G-CSF is glycoprotein of 19,600 d with threonine at amino-acid position 133 being O-glycosylated; structurally, it has four antiparallel α helices arranged to form a helic bundle (see Table 1) (73). G-CSF is encoded by a single gene on chromosome 17q21-22 that is comprised of five exons and four introns (see Table 1) (74). Alternative use of the two donor splice sites nine nucleotides apart at the 5' end of intron 2 leads to production of two different mRNAs, encoding one G-CSF of 174 amino acids (71) and one of 177 amino acids (75), which is less active in stimulating granulocyte colony formation. Murine G-CSF has a nucleotide sequence that is 69% homologous, and a deduced amino acid sequence that is 73% homologous to the corresponding sequence of human factor (76). This close homology accounts for species cross-reactivity of the molecules.

Granulocyte Colony-Stimulating Factor Receptor

The expression of the specific transmembrane receptor for G-CSF is largely confined to the hematopoietic system—predominantly, it is confined to mature neutrophils and their morphologically recognizable precursors, with some expression on monocytes. Mature human neutrophils possess 500 to 3,000 high-affinity receptors that bind G-CSF with an affinity of 60 to 300 pm (see Table 2) (77). Intermediate myeloid precursors in the marrow express 300 to 500 receptors; receptor expression is found on purified stem-cell populations (78). Receptors are also found on endothelial cells and placenta and trophoblastic cells (77). Receptors are rapidly internalized after ligand binding, and are also rapidly "trans–down-modulated" after exposure of receptor-bearing neutrophils to GM-CSF, TNF-α, lipopolysaccharide (LPS), and chemotactic peptide f-Met-leu-phe (fMLP-$t_{1/2}$ 15 minutes) (79).

The murine G-CSF receptor (G-CSFR) is an 812 amino-acid polypeptide (Mr 90, 814) with a single transmembrane domain. The extracellular domain consists of 601 amino acids with a region of 220 amino acids that shows remarkable similarity to the rat prolactin receptor (80). The cytoplasmic domain shows significant homology with the murine IL-4 receptor. Two human complementary deoxyribonucleic acids (cDNAs) have been identified that encode integral membrane proteins of 759 and 812 amino acids with identical extracellular and membrane spanning sequences, but which differ at the COOH termini (with one alternative spliced form with 24 residues and the other with 87) (81). The predicted molecular masses of these G-CSFRs, 86 and 92 kd, are substantially less than the 150 kd demonstrated by cross-linking, suggesting that some (or all) of the nine potential glycosylation sites contain carbohydrate. The long form of the receptor is predominantly expressed on hematopoietic cells, whereas the short form is expressed in tissues such as placenta (81,82). The alternative cytoplasmic domains may confer functional differences, with the smaller form possibly functioning in ligand transport or sequestration in the placenta. Alternatively, the two forms may differ in signal transduction properties because the long form contains one potential C–kinase phosphorylation site.

The extracellular region of the G-CSFR is composed of four distinct types of structural domain. Two domains are identified by the presence of highly conserved cysteine residues and a WSXWS motif with a less well-conserved 100 amino-acid stretch that char-acterizes a hematopoietin receptor superfamily (17). The receptor also incorporates one amino terminal immunoglobulinlike domain characteristic of the Ig superfamily of receptors. Three additional repeats of fibronectin type III domains are present and are also found in the leukemia inhibitory factor (LIF) receptor, gp130 (the common subunit of IL-6, LIF, ciliary neutropic factor, oncostatin-M, and IL-11 receptors), and the alpha chain of IL-3, IL-5, and GM-CSF. Two G-CSF-R domains make direct contact with one G-CSF molecule, leading to dimerization of the receptor (so that the two C-terminal receptor domains interact with each other, probably extending to the transmembrane and cytoplasmic domains, leading to signal transduction).

The gene for G-CSFR is localized on the p32-34 region of human chromosome 1 (see Table 2) (82). It consists of 17 exons, is 165 kilobase (kb) in length, and is present as a single copy per haploid human genome. Exons 3-17 code for G-CSFR protein; each subdomain of the receptor is encoded by a set of exons. Approximately 110 nucleotides upstream of the transcription initiation site of the gene an element of 18 nucleotides homologous to the sequences found in the promoter of human myeloperoxidase and neutrophil elastase genes exist (83).

The G-CSFR does not have a catalytic domain; nevertheless, it induces tyrosine phosphorylation of multiple cellular substrates (77). Structure-function studies have demonstrated that different regions of the cytoplasmic domain of the G-CSFR are responsible for distinct signals driving proliferation versus differentiation. Using murine cell lines transfected with deletion-mutant and chimeric-mutant receptors showed that the region responsible for transduction of growth signals lies within the cytoplasmic region of 100 amino acids proximal to the cell membrane. Indeed, the region homologous to the conserved box-domains of other receptors, lying within the first 57 residues, is absolutely required and sufficient to deliver the proliferative signal (84,85). Additional sequences in the first 96 amino acids are required for a maximal proliferative response. The membrane proximal and the COOH-terminal region are required to transduce a differentiation signal, as measured by induction of expression of the myeloperoxidase gene (85). Because multiple hematopoietic cytokines can stimulate granulopoiesis, the relative importance of the G-CSFR to the process was evaluated in receptor-deficient mice. These mice have severe quantitative defects in granulopoiesis but phenotypically normal neutrophils are still detectable (86). In IL-6 × G-CSFR doubly deficient mice, the additional loss of IL-6 worsened the neutropenia; near normal numbers of myeloid progenitors were detected in the marrow, however, and could terminally differentiate into mature neutrophils (86). Thus, neither G-CSFR nor IL-6 signaling is required for the commitment of multipotent progenitors to the myeloid lineage or their terminal differentiation. In further studies, retroviral transduction of wild-type G-CSFR allowed ectopic expression in hematopoietic progenitors of G-CSFR–deficient mice, resulting in their G-CSF–dependent differentiation into mature granulocytes, macrophages, megakaryocytes, and erythroid cells. Furthermore, two mutant G-CSFR proteins, a truncated mutant that deletes the carboxy-terminal 96 amino acids and a chimeric receptor containing the extracellular and transmembrane domain of G-CSFR fused to the cytoplasmic domain of the erythropoietin receptor, are able to support the production of morphologically mature, chloracetate esterase and Gr-/Mac-1–positive neutrophils in response to G-CSF (87). This indicates that unique signals generated by the cytoplasmic domain of the G-CSFR are not required for G-CSF–dependent granulocytic differentiation.

Possible defects in the G-CSF receptor or its downstream signaling pathway, or both, have been proposed to explain the pathophysiology of severe congenital neutropenia (SCN) or Kostmann's syndrome. SCN is a rare autosomal recessive disorder characterized by severe neutropenia present from birth with maturation arrest of the myeloid series in marrow at the promyelocyte/myelocyte stage. G-CSF levels are normal to elevated in these patients, but treatment with G-CSF leads to an increase in neutrophils to greater than 1,000 cells per mm^3 in 90% of patients, resulting in significant improvement in survival and quality of life (88,89). G-CSFR is present at normal or increased levels on patient cells; these receptors bind and internalize G-CSF normally. In approximately 25% of patients with SCN, mutations in one allele of the G-CSFR have been detected (89,90). These mutations are invariably single nucleotide substitutions that introduce premature stop codons, leading to truncation of the distal cytoplasmic portion of the G-CSFR, the region implicated in generating maturation signals. Patients with G-CSFR mutations appear at greatest risk of developing acute myeloid leukemia (AML) or myelodysplastic syndrome, with one-half of patients with receptor mutations developing leukemia (88–90). Conversely, no SCN patient has developed leukemia without this receptor mutation. Mice have been generated that carry a targeted mutation of G-CSFR that reproduces the mutation found in patients with SCN and AML (91). These mice have normal levels of neutrophils and no evidence of a block in neutrophil maturation. In response to G-CSF, however, they show an enhanced neutrophil leukocytosis indicative of an enhanced proliferative response (91). To date, no case of AML or myelodysplastic syndrome has been found in these mice.

Signal Transduction

In common with all members of the cytokine receptor superfamily, ligand binding to G-CSFR induces tyrosine phosphorylation and activation of members of the Jak family. G-CSF induces tyrosine phosphorylation and activation of Jak1, Jak2, and Tyk2 (89,92,93). In addition, G-CSF induces the tyrosine phosphorylation of the receptor and members of the STAT family, including STAT3, as well as STAT1 and STAT5, depending on the cells involved. Jak1 is critical for G-CSF–mediated STAT activation, whereas Jak2 or Tyk2 are either not required or play redundant or ancillary roles (see Table 2) (93). Because the requirement for Jak1 is similar to that previously shown for IL-6 signaling, data supports the concept that G-CSFR and gp130 are structurally and functionally similar. Activation of the Jak/STAT pathway correlates with proliferative signals by the G-CSFR and requires the membrane-proximal box 1 and box 2 proline X proline motifs for STAT1 and STAT5 phosphorylation, whereas STAT3 phosphorylation requires a region distal to box 2 that contains four tyrosines (93–95). Although the membrane-proximal 55 amino acids of the G-CSF receptor are sufficient for activation of STAT5, the maximal rate of STAT5 activation requires an additional 30 amino acids of the cytoplasmic domain. In contrast, the distal carboxyl-terminal region of the receptor appears to downregulate STAT5 activation, in that deletion of this region results in increased amplitude and prolonged duration of STAT5 activation by G-CSF (93,94). The role of tyrosines in the cytoplasmic region of G-CSFR in STAT3 activation has been evaluated using mutant receptors either completely lacking tyrosines or retaining just one of the four cytoplasmic tyrosines (95). At saturating G-CSF concentrations, STAT3 activation occurred in the absence of tyrosines. In contrast, at low G-CSF concentrations, Tyr704 and Tyr744 of G-CSFR play major roles in STAT3 activation (95). This suggests that G-CSF–induced STAT3 activation during basal granulopoiesis (low G-CSF) and "emergency" granulopoiesis (high G-CSF) are controlled differentially. Furthermore, this establishes the importance of the G-CSFR C-terminus for STAT3 in activation, with implications for understanding of the defective signaling seen with the truncated G-CSFR observed in some SCN patients. Three isoforms of STAT3 have been identified, -α (p92), -β (p83), and -γ (p72), each derived from a single gene. STAT3-α is the predominant isoform expressed in most cells. STAT3-β is derived from STAT3-α by alternative splicing, whereas STAT3-γ is derived from STAT3-α by limited proteolysis (96). Mapping of STAT3-α and STAT3-β activation in murine myeloid cells shows that their optimal activation requires G-CSFR constructs containing Tyr704 and Tyr744. Tyr744 is followed at the +3 position by Cys; the sequence YXXC represents a novel motif implicated in the recruitment and activation of STAT3-α, -β, and -γ (95,96). In immature myeloid cells, G-CSF activates STAT3-β but not STAT3α, suggesting the β form may be more critical for G-CSF–mediated differentiation. In mature, nondividing neutrophils, no activation of Jak1, Jak2, Tyk2, STAT3, or Jak3 kinase was observed after G-CSF stimulation (92). This suggests utilization in mature neutrophils of alternative signal transduction pathways is distinct from those in proliferating cells. In other studies, however, activation of STAT3-γ has been shown to occur predominantly in terminally differentiated neutrophils, suggesting that it may be part of a controlled proteolytic mechanism modulating pro-proliferative proteins in mature myeloid cells (96,97). Hematopoietic cell kinase (Hck) is a member of the Src-family of kinases and is known to be expressed in cells of granulocytic lineages. It interacts with the gp130 subunit of the LIF/IL-6 receptor, directly binding via its SH2 domain to multiple phosphotyrosines of G-CSFR (98). Hck becomes activated on G-CSF treatment and is, in turn, able to phosphorylate G-CSFR, indicating a clear functional and physical involvement in G-CSF signaling. The G-CSFR proliferative stimulus also leads to rapid activation of the p21 ras and p42, p44 MAP kinase signaling pathway (99). G-CSF–induced differentiation can occur in the absence of p42 MAP kinase activation, however (52).

Role of Myeloid Transcription Factors in Development of Granulocyte Colony-Stimulating Factor Responsiveness

The Ets factor PU-1, and the CCAAT/enhancer binding protein-alpha (C/EBPα) are master transcription factors that regulate myeloid development (101–103). C/EBPα is a basic leucine zipper transcription factor that regulates a number of myeloid-specific genes and acts as a myeloid differentiation switch on bipotent granulocyte-macrophage (GM) progenitors and directing them to mature to granulocytes (100,101). Analysis of C/EBPα knockout mice has shown these animals to be absolutely deficient in granulopoiesis (102), a phenotype different from that of G-CSFR –/– mice, which have quantitative defects in granulopoiesis but mature granulocytes detected at reduced levels (approximately 12% of wild type) (86). C/EBPα –/– mice have greatly reduced mRNA levels and no detectable G-CSFR or IL-6 receptor (IL-6R) proteins. Restoration of either receptor in C/EBPα –/– hematopoietic cells by retroviral transduction restores cytokine response and granulocytic differentiation (103).

Hematopoiesis in Granulocyte Colony-Stimulating Factor and Granulocyte Colony-Stimulating Factor Receptor Knockout Mice

Homozygous inactivation of G-CSF (104) or G-CSFR (86) genes leads to a quantitative impairment of granulopoiesis with an approximately 80% to 90% reduction in neutrophils and a 50% reduction in granulocyte-macrophage progenitor cells, maturing granulocytes, and macrophages in marrow. These mice have reduced ability to mobilize neutrophils on challenge, and impaired resistance to challenge infections with *Listeria monocytogenes* (105). Peritoneal macrophage tumoricidal activity and phagocytosis of *Listeria*, together with bactericidal NO production, were reduced in –/– mice; these reductions were associated with expansion of a poorly differentiated population of cells, morphologically intermediate between typical macrophages and typical lymphocytes (105). G-CSF–deficient animals have marked predispositions to spontaneous infection, reduced long-term survival, and high incidences of reactive type-AA amyloidosis. Mice lacking G-CSF and GM-CSF are more severely neutropenic (up to 2 weeks of age) than those with additive features of the constituent genotypes lacking G-CSF alone. In addition, three novel features are present: greater degrees of neutropenia in neonates, increased neonatal mortality, and a dominant influence of lack of G-CSF on splenic hematopoiesis, resulting in significantly reduced numbers of splenic progenitors (106).

Production of Granulocyte Colony-Stimulating Factor: Cell Sources and Regulation of Production

G-CSF can be produced by a variety of organs and tissues on stimulation; constitutive production is normally low or absent (see Table 1). G-CSF production is highly inducible and can be elicited by exposure of cells to bacterial cell wall products (e.g., LPS) and proinflammatory cytokines (e.g., IL-1, TNF, or IL-17). Specific cellular sources of G-CSF include monocytes and macrophages, endothelial cells, fibroblasts and related mesenchymal cells, and bone marrow stromal cells (77). With the latter, a 6-hour *in vitro* pulse exposure to IL-1 was necessary to induce G-CSF production, which continued for 48 hours;

thereafter, stromal cells could not be restimulated by IL-1, although IL-4 was able to promote further production (107). Primitive CD34$^+$ hematopoietic cells may be capable of conditioning their own hematopoietic microenvironments because they can induce four- to fivefold increases in marrow stromal cell production of G-CSF and IL-6 on coculture (108). IL-1 beta (IL-1β) serves as a potent primary stimulus for endothelial cell release of G-CSF, IL-6, and IL-8; a further increase in G-CSF was observed when IL-1–primed cells were exposed to *Staphylococcus aureus* and *Staphylococcus* exotoxins (109). IL-17, a cytokine produced by activated memory CD4$^+$ T cells, stimulates epithelial, endothelial, and fibroblastic cells to secret G-CSF, IL-6, IL-8, and PGE (110,111). The action on fibroblasts results in increased steady-state G-CSF mRNA levels within 2 to 4 hours, due to message stabilization with augmented protein production (110). An additive effect on G-CSF production was observed when IL-17 and LPS were combined. When stimulated with IL-17, fibroblasts can sustain proliferation of CD34$^+$ progenitor cells and their preferential maturation to neutrophils (111). Serum levels of G-CSF are low to undetectable in normal mice or humans; in response to LPS treatment or significant infection, however, serum levels are rapidly and markedly elevated (77). A number of studies have demonstrated that the plasma half-life of G-CSF is inversely related to absolute neutrophil count (112). Mature neutrophils and immature myeloid cells in marrow negatively regulate neutropoiesis—at least in part—by decreasing G-CSF levels through receptor-mediated continual absorption, internalization, and destruction. Inhibitors of exocytosis of ligand receptor complexes abrogated the ability of neutrophils to reduce G-CSF levels (113).

Granulocyte Colony-Stimulating Factor Action on Progenitor Cells

The functional characterization of murine and human G-CSF was undertaken in clonogenic assays in semisolid medium, using either normal bone marrow colony-forming unit (CFU)–granulocyte assay, or murine myeloid leukemic cells inducible to differentiate (WEHI-3 colony differentiation assay). Murine marrow progenitors form small colonies of up to 200 cells within 5 to 6 days in the presence of G-CSF in mice or humans. These colonies contain mature neutrophils; with higher concentrations of G-CSF in serum-containing cultures, however, monocyte-macrophage populations develop. The frequency of G-CSF–stimulated colonies in murine marrow is always two- to tenfold lower than the frequency of colonies stimulated by IL-3, GM-CSF, and M-CSF. In human marrow cultures, G-CSF–stimulated colonies outnumber GM-CSF or IL-3 colonies by day 7 (although the reverse is the case by day 14, when human cultures are normally scored). Pluripotent stem cells express G-CSFR (78) but are not stimulated by G-CSF alone. The factor does, however, synergize in the murine system with IL-3, GM-CSF, M-CSF, and KL in accelerating cell-cycle entry of primitive cells detected in the CFU-blast assay and stimulating subsequent proliferation (114). Synergy is also seen with IL-1, IL-3, GM-CSF, and KL in the murine high proliferative potential (HPP) assay, and in *ex vivo* expansion cultures of primitive progenitors (Delta assay) (115,116). In suspension cultures of human CD34$^+$ cells, or of more purified primitive progenitors in the CD38-ve fraction, G-CSF synergizes with multiple other cytokines [e.g., GM-CSF, IL-3, IL-1, IL-6, KL, Flk-2 ligand, Epo, and Tpo], resulting in extensive expansion of total cells, progenitors, and, to a much lesser degree, stem cells (116–119). Such expanded populations have been used for autologous transplantation (119).

Action of Granulocyte Colony-Stimulating Factor on Neutrophils

G-CSF is a potent activator of neutrophils (PMN), mobilizing secretory vesicles (leukocyte alkaline phosphatase, CD11b) and inducing the release of specific granules (lactoferrin, CD11b, and CD66b) and azurophil granules (elastase, alpha$_1$-antitrypsin complexes) (77,120). G-CSF enhances PMN–superoxide anion release, enhancing respiratory burst metabolism (120). Amounts as small as 0.1 ng per mL of G-CSF increase binding of the chemotactic peptide fMLP to neutrophils; increase *in vitro* response to this agent, with enhanced superoxide release and upregulation of C3b receptors; and enhance phagocytosis of opsonized microspheres (77,121). G-CSF enhances neutrophil antibody–dependent cell-mediated cytotoxicity against antibody-coated leukemic cells. Immunoglobulin A (IgA)–mediated phagocytosis is upregulated by G-CSF induction of increased FcR affinity for IgA (77). Anti-*Candida albicans* activity of human PMN *in vitro* is also shown to be stimulated by G-CSF *in vitro* (122). IL-6 mRNA and protein are upregulated in neutrophils after G-CSF treatment *in vivo* or *in vitro* and may contribute to a clinical engraftment syndrome occurring during periods of rapid increase in PMN numbers in patients receiving G-CSF (123). G-CSF has been reported to stimulate PMN production of IFN-α, is chemotactic for neutrophils and monocytes, and induces neutrophil adhesion (124,125). The leukocyte adhesion molecule-1, which plays a central role in neutrophil localization at inflammatory sites, is rapidly downregulated on neutrophils by G-CSF (77). G-CSF enhances vitamin C uptake in neutrophils by promoting the conversion of ascorbic acid to dehydroascorbic acid as a result of enhanced oxidation in the pericellular milieu and increasing transport of dehydroascorbic acid through facilitative glucose transporters at the cell membrane (126).

In Vivo Preclinical Studies of Granulocyte Colony-Stimulating Factor

Because G-CSF has been in extensive clinical use since 1988, a review of preclinical studies for other than historic reasons may seem redundant. Nevertheless, a number of lessons learned from animal model systems have yet to be applied in clinical practice. The first *in vivo* studies of rhG-CSF were carried out by Moore in 1986. Species cross-reactivity and relatively low immunogenicity of rhG-CSF permitted extensive studies in mice, primates, and dogs. In various mouse strains, 50 μg to 100 μg rhG-CSF per kg per day induced a rapid neutrophil leukocytosis with PMN counts elevated approximately 50-fold, remaining elevated up to 5 weeks with daily G-CSF treatment (127). This is associated with mild monocytosis and lymphocytosis. Although mar-

row cellularity does not change, a marked transition to myelopoiesis exists to the exclusion of erythropoiesis; spleen cellularity increases three- to fivefold within 2 weeks, with extensive extramedullary granulopoiesis and compensatory erythropoiesis and megakaryopoiesis. Myeloid, erythroid, megakaryocyte, and pluripotent progenitors increase markedly in the spleen, with total numbers per mouse increasing three- to sixfold. G-CSF also increases numbers of circulating progenitors in a dose-dependent manner, increasing levels of CFU–spleen (CFU-s) four- to 32-fold but not altering their self-renewal capacities (128). Genetic marking studies have shown that mobilization includes cells with long-term lymphomyeloid reconstituting capacity (129). A tenfold range in progenitor mobilization response to G-CSF that does not correlate with white blood cell count (WBC) increase is reported among different mouse strains, and F2 intercrosses of low-responding C57BL/6 and intermediate-responding SJL mice indicate that regulation of progenitor mobilization is a complex genetic trait (130). The mechanism by which G-CSF mobilizes stem and progenitors into the peripheral blood may be related in part to its ability to downmodulate endothelial intercellular adhesion molecule 1 (ICAM-1), induced by IL-1, and upmodulate vascular cell adhesion molecule-1 on IL-1–treated endothelium (131). Transendothelial migration of granulocytes (lacking vascular cell adhesion molecule-1 receptor VLA-4) through IL-1–activated endothelium is inhibited by G-CSF in a concentration-dependent manner (131). Additive or synergistic elevation of progenitors and stem cells in mouse peripheral blood is reported when G-CSF is combined with other cytokines, including IL-6, KL, and FL (132–134). A population of cells that facilitate engraftment of highly purified stem cells across major histocompatibility complex barriers without causing graft-versus-host disease is mobilized after treatment of mice with G-CSF and FL (136). Comparison of allogeneic engraftment potential of mobilized cells indicates that day 10 of treatment coincides with maximum mobilization of repopulating stem cells and facilitator cells.

Transgenic mice expressing hG-CSF produced approximately 1,000 pg per mL of G-CSF in sera, associated with an expected granulocytosis, elevation of hematopoietic progenitor numbers, and mobilized stem cells; unexpectedly, however, a lymphocytosis occurred, as well as a fivefold increase in peripheral blood and a twofold increase in spleen cellularity (137). Transgenic mice developed osteoporosis due to increased osteoclastic activity. Retroviral gene transfer of the G-CSF gene into vascular smooth muscle or primary myoblasts in rat models resulted in prolonged granulocytosis (7 to 26 weeks, two- to 15-fold increase), suggesting this strategy has potential for treating congenital and cyclic neutropenic disorders in humans (138,139). Chronic exposure of mice to G-CSF resulting from transplantation of bone marrow infected with a retroviral vector bearing a G-CSF cDNA produced a nonneoplastic granulocytic and progenitor cell hyperplasia (140). Most animals remained healthy despite dramatic neutrophil leukocytosis with neutrophil infiltration of many organs. Progenitors of all lineages were raised ten- to 100-fold in the spleen, blood, and peritoneal cavity but remained unaffected, or slightly depressed, in the marrow. No tumors developed, and no evidence of tissue damage over a 30-week period was observed.

G-CSF protected a significant number of mice from lethal effects of lethal-dose 100/30 total body irradiation, and a single intraperitoneal injection of 1 mg per kg 2 hours after a dose of lethal-dose 95/30 irradiation significantly improved survival (141,142). G-CSF was effective in reducing chemotherapy-induced myelosuppression in mice treated with single or multiple doses of cyclophosphamide, doxorubicin, vinblastine, mitomycin-c, busulphan, or 5-FU (115,143). Repeated treatment with cyclophosphamide, followed by G-CSF treatment to accelerate neutrophil recovery, induced stem cell damage as measured by serial bone marrow transplantation (144). Mice treated with etoposide plus chlorambucil, bischloroethyl-nitrosourea, or total body irradiation (80c Gy) also experienced greater long-term damage to primitive stem cell populations when chemotherapy was combined with G-CSF (145). This toxicity can be abrogated using a suitable delay between the end of G-CSF treatment and the beginning of the next cycle of chemotherapy, to ensure rebound quiescence occurs in the stem-cell pool. Other protective strategies include administration of IL-1 24 hours before each chemotherapy cycle (145) or treatment with negative regulators, such as transforming growth factor-β or macrophage inflammatory protein-1α, to actively place stem cells into a noncycling state (146). In primates, G-CSF shortened the time to recovery of WBCs after cyclophosphamide treatment to 1 week, compared to greater than 4 weeks in controls (147).

In murine and primate models of bone marrow transplantation, G-CSF has been shown to markedly accelerate recovery of neutrophils, marrow, and spleen hematopoietic progenitor cells and stem cells (77). Autologous bone marrow transplantation in monkeys after myeloablative TBI (100 Gy) was enhanced by G-CSF treatment with neutrophil counts of control animals taking 3 weeks to reach 1,000 per mm³, whereas animals receiving 100 μg per kg per day of rhG-CSF achieved an equivalent neutrophil count 9 days earlier (77).

G-CSF has been shown to prevent progression of systemic nonresponsiveness in various animal models of systemic inflammatory response syndrome (SIRS) and sepsis (148). SIRS constitutes the primary host response to a variety of severe insults such as trauma, burns, pancreatitis, or major surgical intervention. Distinct from SIRS, the term *sepsis* is applied to the state when bacterial infections cause a systemic hyperinflammatory immune response. Rodent models in which G-CSF has been shown efficacious include rodent LPS or fecal septic shock (149,150) or cecal perforation models (151), dog intraperitoneal *Escherichia coli* infection (152), and a porcine *Pseudomonas* sepsis (153). In all cases, G-CSF improved survival and reduced endotoxemia, bacterial count, and TNF release. G-CSF attenuated the proinflammatory cytokines that would otherwise predominate. Upregulation of the endotoxin-binding protein CD14 on neutrophils may be responsible for enhanced endotoxin binding and accelerated clearance. In a rat intraabdominal sepsis model, G-CSF increased microvascular flow and prevented neutrophil-mediated damage by downmodulating the potent vasoconstrictor endothelin-1 (151). Hemoconcentration and lactic acidosis were also attenuated, which is consistent with reduced endothelial damage and plasma leakage. In a rat pneumonia model (154), all control animals died but more than 90% of G-CSF treated animals survived. Exogenous G-CSF has improved survival in a number of models of pneumonia induced by *Klebsiella pneumoniae*, *Streptococcus pneumoniae*, and *Pseudomonas aeruginosa* (148). It has also protected mice against T-cell–mediated lethal shock triggered by superantigen, decreasing LPS-induced pulmonary edema and alveolar capillary leakage (155). G-CSF treatment of rats with visceral ischemia or reperfusion injury, or both, resulted in increased survival and reduced TNF release (156). G-CSF stimulates hemoxygenase-1 expression in microvascular endothelial cells *in vitro*; this may be an important response against oxidative damage (148). In a rabbit model of immune complex colitis, treatment with G-CSF markedly decreased production of proinflammatory mediators such as LTB4 and thromboxane B₂; mucosal generation of protective PGE, however, was preserved (157). Inflammatory bowel disease is associated with mucosal neutrophil recruitment and activation mediated in part by arachidonic acid metabolites. The potential of G-CSF for treatment of SIRS and sepsis is suggested by these animal models, in which improved survival is observed with evidence of functional activation (CD64 expression, phagocytic activity, decreased apoptosis), decreased neutrophil L-selectin expression, increased serum IL-1 receptor antagonist (IL-1ra), and decreased serum proinflammatory cytokine concentrations (IL-1, TNF, IL-8) (148).

GRANULOCYTE-MACROPHAGE COLONY-STIMULATING FACTOR

Molecular Characterization

Murine GM-CSF was first purified from lung-conditioned medium and shown to be a heavily *N*-glycosylated polypeptide of 124 amino acids and a molecular weight of 23,000 to 29,000 d (see Table 1) (158). Subsequent cloning of the murine gene revealed a polypeptide of 142 amino acids with an 18 amino-acid leader sequence (159,160). Human GM-CSF was first purified from a T-lymphoblastoid cell line as a glycoprotein of 22,000 Da (161). Human GM-CSF cDNA encodes a polypeptide of 144 amino acids with a 17 amino-acid leader sequence (162). The primary GM-CSF transcript expressed from four exons in mouse and humans is processed to a mature mRNA of approximately 780 nucleotides (160). Despite a 60% homology at the nucleotide level and 54% identity at the amino acid level, murine and human GM-CSFs are species restricted in their actions. The crystal structure has been determined at 2.8 A (163). The main structural feature is a four-alpha-helix bundle that represents approximately 42% of the structure. The helices are arranged in a left-handed, antiparallel bundle with two overhead connections. Within these connections is a two-stranded antiparallel beta-sheet. Most of the critical regions for receptor binding are located on a continuous surface at one end of the molecule that includes the C-terminus. Structure-function analysis using monoclonal antibodies (164,165) or scanning deletion (166) has shown four critical regions, residues 18 to 21, 34 to 41, 52 to 56, and 94 to 115. The disulfide bridge between cysteines 51 and 93 (but not that between cysteines 85 and 118) is essential for activity. Two N-glycosylation sites are present, and mature GM-CSF is also modified by O-glycosylation. Variations in the molecular weight of mature GM-CSF from 14 kd to 30 kd result from variable glycosylation; up to 50% of the molecule is carbohydrate (see Table 1). rhGM-CSF produced commercially from yeast (sargramostim) or baculovirus is glycosylated, although differently from the native molecule; in the former, proline at position 23 is replaced by valine. In contrast, *E. coli*–derived rhGM-CSF (molgramostim) is not glycosylated and contains six fewer residues and an extra initial methionine (167,168). *E. coli*–derived rhGM-CSF has a significantly faster elimination phase *in vivo* compared to mammalian Chinese hamster ovary cell–derived rhGM-CSF (regramostim), yet it retains high biologic activity and is tenfold more active in stimulating myeloid proliferation and binding to the GM-CSFR than the fully glycosylated form (169).

The GM-CSF gene is located on chromosome 5q23-31 in close proximity to the IL-3 gene (9 kbp downstream) (see Table 1) (170). The long arm of chromosome 5 contains a clustering of hematopoietic regulatory genes that include GM-CSF, IL-3, IL-4, IL-5, IL-9, IL-13, and M-CSF and the receptors for platelet-derived growth factor and M-CSFR (*c-fms*) (171). Deletion of the long arm of chromosome 5 from 5q11-21 to 5q22-34 is associated with primary and familial myelodysplastic syndrome and therapy-related leukemia, but it is more likely that the candidate for pathogenesis of 5q is the interferon regulatory factor-1 gene mapping to 5q31.1 (172).

Granulocyte-Macrophage Colony-Stimulating Receptor

The GM-CSFR is a member of the hematopoietin receptor superfamily and is comprised of an 85-kd α-chain that binds GM-CSF with a low affinity (kd = 1 to 10 nm) and a 130-kd β-chain with no intrinsic binding affinity for GM-CSF alone, but converts the GM-CSF α-chain complex to a high affinity state (kd = 30 pm to 100 pm) (see Table 2) (167,173). The α-chain exhibits rapid dissociation kinetics, whereas the α/β GM-CSFR displays slow dissociation kinetics. Both chains share a common conserved ~200–amino-acid hematopoietin extracellular domain common to members of the superfamily (167,173). This domain has four conserved cysteine residues that form two internal disulfide loops: a Pro-Pro pair that divides the domain into two subdomains, each of which adopt a seven-stranded beta-barrel structure similar to the immunoglobulin constant chain; and a largely conserved membrane proximal WSXWS motif. The β chain is shared by the IL-3 and IL-5 receptor α-chains (174). GM-CSF, IL-3, and IL-5 bind to their specific α-chains with absolute specificity, followed by signaling in association with the common compatible β-chain. This cross-competition accounts for much of the redundancy of these cytokines and their homologous actions (observed, for example, in eosinophil development and effector function). It is distinct from receptor trans-down-modulation of GM-CSFR, observed under conditions permitting receptor internalization when cells are exposed to IL-3 or TNF (175). Three isoforms of the GM-CSFR-α chain have been described and are generated by alternative splicing (167). Two forms of 400 and 401 amino acids are identical except for the terminal 54 and 64 amino acids of the cytoplasmic domain. The third form has a transmembrane deletion and can occur as a sol-

uble form. The GM-CSF receptor α-chain is encoded by a gene situated within the pseudoautonomous region, an area of homology between the ends of the human sex chromosomes that undergo obligatory exchange during meiosis, thereby behaving "pseudo-autosomally" (176). The common β-subunit of GM-CSF is encoded by a gene located on chromosome 22q12-13 (177).

GM-CSF receptors are expressed on neutrophils as a single class of high-affinity receptor (kd of 99 pm, 300 to 2,800 receptors per cell) (see Table 2). This receptor is expressed at levels of 50 to 500 receptors per cell on myeloid progenitors, monocytes, eosinophils, and DCs (but not on lymphoid or erythroid populations) (167). On monocytes and myeloid leukemic cells, a high-affinity (kd 10 to 40 pm) and more frequent low-affinity (kd less than 2 pm) class of receptor is expressed (178). Primitive progenitor/stem-cell populations (CD34$^+$, CD38$^-$) express receptors for GM-CSF at levels 20% to 30% of more committed granulomonocytic progenitors (179).

Granulocyte-Macrophage Colony-Stimulating Receptor Signal Transduction

The GM-CSFR exists as an inducible and preformed complex, unlike the IL-3 receptor (or any other member of the cytokine receptor superfamily) (180). This complex of the GM-CSFR-α and -β common chains required only the extracellular domains, and the β common component of the complex was phosphorylated by GM-CSF binding and IL-3 and IL-5. Analysis of cytoplasmic truncation mutants of β common showed that the residues to amino acid 783 (numbering from the first amino acid of the leader sequence) were sufficient for GM-CSF–dependent induction of all aspects of myeloid differentiation (181). Shorter truncations selectively lost (in a cell-specific manner) the capacity to induce macrophage migration and cell-surface differentiation antigens and clonal suppression of proliferative potential, however (181). This suggests that different aspects of the differentiation phenotype require signaling pathways that originate from distinct regions of the receptor cytoplasmic domain. The GM-CSFR-α subunit is essential for GM-CSF–mediated growth and differentiation. The membrane proximal proline-rich domain and adjacent 16 residues are necessary for cell proliferation and differentiation and Jak2 activation (182). In contrast, the C-terminal region was not necessary for differentiation, but removal of this region severely impaired the ability of GM-CSF to support cell survival.

Jak2 is the primary kinase regulating GM-CSF activities and inducing c-fos activation through receptor phosphorylation (183). The importance of c-fos and related AP-1 activity in GM-CSF signaling is suggested by the tight correlation between GM-CSF–dependent activation of the c-fos promoter and cell proliferation, and by the inhibitory effect of a trans-dominant c-fos mutation on the growth of GM-CSF–dependent cells (184). Activation of Jak2, Shc, Erk, and STAT5 proteins correlates with GM-CSF–mediated cell growth. In myeloid leukemic cells, GM-CSF enhances DNA binding and tyrosine phosphorylation of STAT3, which is directly activated by c-fes tyrosine kinase (185). In early stages of GM-CSF–induced proliferation of CD34$^+$ cells, the 94 kd STAT5-β protein is activated at later stages of differentiation and increased expression of the 80 kd STAT5 isoform is observed, resulting in heterodimeric DNA binding (186). CrkL, an adaptor protein comprising Src homology (SH)2 and SH3 domains participates in the GM-CSF activated Jak-STAT pathway by directly associating with STAT5 (187). In mature neutrophils, GM-CSF activation is reported to result solely in Jak2, STAT3, and STAT5-β phosphorylation (not involving other members of the Jak/STAT family) (188). However, earlier reports indicate that STAT1, STAT3, and the product of the c-fps/fes protooncogene become tyrosine phosphorylated and physically associate with the GM-CSFR-β common chain and Jak2 (189). Jak2 phosphorylation of the p85 subunit of p13-kinase in neutrophils is mediated by an as-yet-unidentified adaptor protein (190). In neutrophils, GM-CSF stimulation leads to phosphorylation of MKK3/MKK6 (upstream kinases of p38 MAPK), and the upstream kinase of Erk. Phosphorylation of MAPK and Erk occur within 1 to 5 minutes after stimulation; inhibitors of p35 MAPK inhibit GM-CSF–induced neutrophil superoxide release (191). In monocytes and macrophages activated directly by GM-CSF—or indirectly by LPS-inducing autocrine GM-CSF production—Cox-2 gene activation occurs after STAT5 is activated (192,193). In DCs, GM-CSF induces a broad complex of STAT isoforms (STAT1, STAT3, STAT5-α, STAT5-β, and STAT6) not seen in any other type of GM-CSF–responsive cell (193). Other known intermediates that are phosphorylated and activated as a consequence of GM-CSF include SH collagen (SCH) protein, GRB2, Ras, p21, pp100, pim-1 kinase, raf-1 kinase, p92c-fps/fes kinase, p53/p56 lyn kinase, and p62 yes kinase (167). The signaling pathway ultimately involves transcriptional activation of nuclear factors, such as c-fos, c-jun, c-myc and, possibly, p53, important in the cell cycle. GM-CSF has been shown to abrogate transforming growth factor-β1–mediated cell-cycle arrest of a myeloid cell line by constitutively overexpressing cdk4 and cyclin D2, which had been downregulated by TGF-β1 (194).

Origin of Granulocyte-Macrophage Colony-Stimulating Factor and Regulation of Production

GM-CSF is an inducible product of a variety of cell types (see Table 3). GM-CSF is not detectable in normal resting cells, although transcription of the GM-CSF gene can be detected using sensitive nuclear run-on assays (195). It is produced by antigen or lectin; or IL-2–stimulated T lymphocytes, antigen, or LPS; or IL-1–stimulated B lymphocytes and macrophages activated by LPS, phagocytosis, or adherence. In these various inducible cells, the accumulation of GM-CSF mRNA is due to increased transcription rate and posttranscriptional stabilization of mRNA. IL-1 or TNF stimulates fibroblast and endothelial cell GM-CSF expression by predominantly posttranscriptional mechanisms. The A/T-rich region at the 3' end of GM-CSF is important in determining mRNA stability, and similar AT-rich sequences are located at the 3' end of a variety of genes that must be turned on and off quickly (195). A variety of transcriptional regulatory elements in the 5' flanking

region of the GM-CSF gene control its expression. Contained within the GM-CSF promoter region is the repeated sequence CATT (A/T) located in the region bp -48 to -37 relative to the GM-CSF mRNA initiation site, which is a recognition site for cellular transcription factors. Other regulatory elements, including negative regulatory elements located at 5' in these sequences, modulate transcription of GM-CSF (195). *Cis*-acting elements with NF-kappa-beta (NFκβ), AP1, and ETS-like binding motifs in the promoter region of the GM-CSF gene are important for transcriptional activity after T–helper-cell activation. ETS1 can transactivate GM-CSF in T cells, but only after these cells have been stimulated by phorbol esters or ionomycin, agents that mimic T-cell activation (196). ETS1, NFκB and Ap1 synergistically transactivate the human GM-CSF promoter. IL-1–induced GM-CSF production in endothelium was associated with increased GM-CSF mRNA levels (which, in turn, are linked to nuclear-protein kinase-C and low-molecular-weight G-protein activation) (197). Neither activity alone was sufficient to increase levels of mRNA (197). Production of GM-CSF by vascular endothelium may be regulated by hemodynamic force because elevated GM-CSF mRNA and protein production are observed when vascular endothelium is exposed to a shear stress of 15 to 25 dyne per cm^2. This response depends on protein synthesis and results from mRNA stabilization (198). GM-CSF is released from lung mast cells after cross-linkage of their high-affinity Fc epsilon receptors by IgE (199). In turn, GM-CSF in mast cell supernatant can release eosinophil cationic protein from eosinophils, contributing to chronic eosinophil-mediated inflammation (199). In the brain, GM-CSF may be released by infiltrating cells of the immune system or by resident cells, such as microglia and astrocytes (200). Astrocyte-secreted GM-CSF may play an important role in enhancing local inflammatory response to CNS injury and recruiting microglia and activated macrophages. Astrocytes express the α-subunit of the GM-CSF receptor and proliferate in response to GM-CSF (200). Autocrine astrocyte production of and response to GM-CSF may be involved in astrocytosis, a hallmark of various neurologic injuries, and in inflammatory processes.

Granulocyte-Macrophage Colony-Stimulating Factor Action at the Progenitor Level

The biologic effects of GM-CSF were initially related to its ability to stimulate proliferation and differentiation of myeloid-committed progenitors (CFU-GM) at concentrations of 2 to 80 pg per mL. In the murine system, higher concentrations of GM-CSF can stimulate eosinophil colony formation, and tenfold higher concentrations stimulate CFU, megakaryocyte (CFU-Meg); burst-forming unit, erythroid (BFU-E); and mixed (CFU-granulocyte, erythroid, megakaryocyte, macrophage) progenitor colony formation (200). Dose-dependency is less evident in human colony assays, and synergy is observed with a variety of other hematopoietic growth factors (IL-3, M-CSF, KL, and Epo). Although GM-CSF has minimal effects on survival or proliferation of primitive progenitor/stem-cell populations when added alone, cytokine-enhanced

KL induced cell-cycle entry, an effect not observed when cells were incubated sequentially with KL and GM-CSF (179).

Action of Granulocyte-Macrophage Colony-Stimulating Factor on Mature Leukocytes

GM-CSF has a direct action on random migration of neutrophils; a 1-minute exposure is sufficient (201). *In vitro*, GM-CSF increases PMN half-life threefold and protects the cells from ultraviolet or x-irradiation–induced apoptosis (202,203). Increased viability and longevity of neutrophils is achieved with approximately $1/100$ the concentration of GM-CSF required to stimulate cell proliferation. The Erk-signaling pathway plays an important role in protection and rescue of PMN from apoptosis but appears to be a proximal event in the process (202). GM-CSF also suppresses anti-Fas antibody–induced neutrophil apoptosis with retention of superoxide production and enzyme release (204). GM-CSF induces neutrophil degranulation with release of primary and secondary granules (205). Neutrophils exposed to fMLP or its complement (C5a) produce much higher levels (sixfold) of reactive oxygen products when primed by GM-CSF (206). One mechanism of GM-CSF priming of the fMLP-induced respiratory burst is the synergistic activation of PI3 kinase by heterotrimeric Gi proteins in the presence of tyrosine-phosphorylated proteins, and phosphorylation of p47 phox (207). GM-CSF also rapidly upregulates fMLP receptors on neutrophils (208). GM-CSF primes neutrophils for arachidonic acid release and leukotriene B4 synthesis elicited by fMLP, IL-8, or platelet-activating factor (PAF) (209) by a mechanism involving rapid upregulation of 5-lipoxygenase, a key enzyme in the leukotriene synthetic pathway (210). GM-CSF and IL-8 synergistically interact to enhance PMN synthesis of PAF and LTB4 (211).

Antimicrobial effects of GM-CSF include enhanced bactericidal activity of neutrophils against *S. aureus* (120) and enhanced phagocytosis and intracellular killing of *C. albicans* (212,213). GM-CSF enhances killing of *Trypanosoma cruzi* (214) and opsonized *Torulopsis glabrata* (215). IgA FcR is induced by GM-CSF (216) and enhanced ADCC toward tumor cells involves upregulation of FcR II (217). This tumor lysis involves an increased release of lytic granular molecules, including defensins and cathepsin-G, a neutrophil protease that mediates tumor lysis (218). GM-CSF increases the expression of class I heavy and light chains and beta$_2$-microglobulin (219) and class II mixed leukocyte culture antigens (220). GM-CSF increases neutrophils' vitamin C uptake by enhancing oxidation in the pericellular milieu and increasing transport through facilitative glucose transporters in the cell membrane (126).

The leukocyte adhesion molecule, which plays a crucial role in neutrophil localization at inflammatory sites and endothelial interaction, is rapidly downregulated by GM-CSF (221), whereas the beta$_2$-integrin molecules CD11b/CD18 and CD11c/CD18 are upregulated (208). Integrins mediate PMN adhesion to endothelium, homeotypic adhesion, chemotaxis and phagocytosis, and respiratory burst. GM-CSF–enhanced neutrophil migration across a nonactivated endothelium independent of concentration gradients, but inhibited migration across IL-1–activated endothelium (i.e., inflamed endothelium) (222).

Eosinophils are potent inflammatory cells involved in allergic reactions, and GM-CSF (and IL-3 and IL-5) can prolong eosinophil survival *in vitro* and *in vivo*, providing an important mechanism for causing tissue eosinophilia (223,224). Spontaneous eosinophil apoptosis is associated with a decrease in Bcl-xL mRNA and protein levels, and the antiapoptotic action of GM-CSF involves maintenance or upregulation of Bcl-xL (but not Bcl-2) (225). Glucocorticoids inhibit this survival-promoting effect, suggesting a mechanism for their efficiency exists in the treatment of eosinophilia-associated disorders (224). GM-CSF enhances the eosinophil respiratory burst induced by opsonized particles (226). Eosinophil degranulation and release of toxic granular proteins is induced by IgA cross-linking of Ig receptors; this is enhanced by GM-CSF (227), which also upregulates FcR-γ II and CR3 (228). GM-CSF upregulates CD11b adhesion molecules on eosinophils after fMLP or PAF treatment (229), which may facilitate their adherence to endothelium and subsequent migration to inflammatory sites. Enhancement of eosinophil ADCC (230) and enhanced phagocytosis of *C. albicans* and *Staphylococcus* killing is observed after GM-CSF treatment (231). GM-CSF enhances the generation of leukotriene C4 induced by calcium ionophore and the release of arylsulfatase and beta-glucuronidase from specific and small granules of eosinophils (231). Release of eosinophil cationic protein after GM-CSF treatment may contribute to chronic eosinophil inflammation (199).

GM-CSF prevents the apoptotic death of macrophages and enhances their differentiation into macrophages (232). It is chemotactic for monocytes and macrophages (233), and induces M-CSF (234) and TNF-α (235) production by these cells. Synergy between GM-CSF and IFN-γ increases TNF-α release from the surface of monocytic cells by a protease cleavage mechanism (236). IL-1β and IL-receptor (IL-R) antagonist protein are induced in macrophages by GM-CSF; this factor primes monocytes for enhanced reactive oxygen release after fMLP or C5a treatment (237–239) and plasminogen activator secretion (340). Activation of monocytes and macrophages by GM-CSF is associated with upregulation of CR3 and IFN-γ receptors (42), the fMLP receptor (241) and the FcR-γ II, which are largely responsible for immune clearance of IgG–sensitized cells (242). The delta integrin Vβ3 is induced on monocytes by GM-CSF (243), as are CD1 (a, b, and c) molecules, thereby enhancing macrophages' roles as accessories to T cells (244). GM-CSF, in synergy with glucocorticoids, upregulates class I and II antigens on monocytes, and enhances macrophage ADCC (245,246). Significant growth inhibition of *Mycobacterium avium* was observed in human macrophages treated with GM-CSF (247,248). GM-CSF –activated monocytes and macrophages inhibit replication of *Leishmania* (249), *L. monocytogenes* (247), *C. albicans* (250), *Histoplasma capsulatum* (251), and *T. cruzi* (252) by mechanisms involving augmented superoxide, NO production, and elevation of mannose receptors. Monocytes from septic patients had depressed membrane expression of CD71 and HLA-DR, enhanced apoptosis and priming of such cells with GM-CSF–abrogated apoptosis, and restored LPS responsiveness and cytokine secretion (253). GM-CSF–enhanced LPS or IFN-γ–induced monocyte production of endothelin, a potent vasoconstrictor molecule with immune modulating properties (254).

Human macrophages express chemokine receptors (CCR5, CXCR4) that act as coreceptors for HIV-1. CCR5 is virtually undetectable on freshly isolated monocytes; on exposure to GM-CSF (or M-CSF), however, CCR5 is upregulated, and entry and replication of HIV-1 is markedly increased (35).

Morphogenesis and remodeling of bone involves the synthesis of bone matrix by osteoblasts and coordinated resorption of bone by osteoclasts. Osteoblasts arise from mesenchymal stem cells; osteoclasts differentiate from hematopoietic monocyte and macrophage precursors. CD14$^+$ adherent human monocytes differentiate into tartrate-resistant acid phosphatase (TRAP)–positive osteoclast-like multinucleate giant cells in the presence of GM-CSF and IL-4 (255). Endogenous GM-CSF is an autocrine growth factor for human osteoblastic cells; such cells express GM-CSF and the α and β chains of GM-CSFR (256). Exogenous GM-CSF induced a dose-dependent proliferation of osteoblasts. Antibody or antisense to GM-CSF inhibited proliferation (256).

The tumoricidal capacity of monocytes is enhanced by GM-CSF, and ADCC activity with tumor-specific antibody has been demonstrated *in vitro* (257) and *in vivo* on transfer of activated human cells to nude mice bearing human tumors (246). GM-CSF also enhances IL-2–mediated LAK cell function (258). In tumor-infiltrating macrophages, it also increases secretion of matrix metalloelastase with subsequent production of angiotensin, inhibiting angiogenesis and suppressing growth of lung metastases (259). GM-CSF may also facilitate tumor antigen presentation and enhance immunogenicity of tumor cells (168).

Granulocyte-Macrophage Colony-Stimulating Factor and Dendritic Cells

DCs are irregularly shaped with numerous cell membrane processes, including spiny dendrites, bulbous pseudopods, and lamellipodia or veils. Mature DCs lack phagocytic capacity and are nonadherent. They express high levels of class II major histocompatibility complex, CD40, CD83, and CD1a, lacking the monocyte/macrophage marker CD14 (260). These cells are professional antigen presenters, stimulating primary T-cell responses and autologous mixed lymphocyte response, which probably relates to the primary response to exogenous antigen. DCs are heterogeneous in lineage, and origin can arise from lymphoid or myeloid precursors. CD34$^+$ precursors in normal marrow generate dendritic colonies when stimulated with GM-CSF and TNF (260,261). Large numbers of functionally mature DCs can also be generated over 12 to 14 days in suspension cultures of CD34$^+$ cells with the same cytokines; absolute recovery is enhanced by addition of c-kit or flt3 ligands (probably by expanding production of CFU-GM progenitors) (262). Development of DCs in this system occurs via development of an intermediate CD14$^+$, HLA-DR$^+$, or c-fms$^+$ cell that lacks myeloperoxidase and nonspecific esterase. These cells possess substantial phagocytic capacities and are bipotential, generating typical adherent CD14$^+$ phagocytic macrophages in the presence of M-CSF, and CD14-ve, c-fms-ve, CD1a$^+$, CD83$^+$, HLA-DR^{+++} DC in the presence of GM-CSF and TNF (263). Blood monocytes also differentiate into DC without proliferation; in the presence of GM-CSF, this pathway is reversible. Exposure to proinflammatory cytokines, such as TNF, however, induces an apparently irreversible maturation to DC with downmodulation of *c-fms* (255,260). GM-CSF, TNF, and IL-4 are widely used to induce DC development from blood monocytes (264). CD40 to CD40 ligand interactions play central roles in antigen presentation and T-cell–dependent effector function; CD40 is upregulated by GM-CSF (264). Physiologic conditions inducing monocyte differentiation to DC include a combination of phagocytosis and transendothelial migration. In one *in vitro* model, monocytes first cross a layer of endothelial cells and lodge in an underlying collagen matrix, mimicking entry of monocytes into tissues from circulation (265). A proportion of these cells then "reverse transmigrate" and become DCs, mimicking the migration of DCs out of tissues into lymphatics. Those cells that remain in the collagen "tissue" become macrophages. The phagocytosis process provides a strong stimulus for DC maturation, and the endothelium may be a source of GM-CSF and proinflammatory cytokines (265).

Action of Granulocyte-Macrophage Colony-Stimulating Factor on Leukemic Cells

In vitro analysis of most human leukemias at diagnosis reveals their dependences on exogenous CSFs for *in vitro* proliferation when cultured at low cell densities. At high cell densities, however, autonomous proliferation is seen (266). Genuine cases of autocrine GM-CSF production have been documented in B-lineage acute lymphoblastic leukemia (267) and acute myeloid leukemia, some cases expressing large transcripts from rearranged GM-CSF loci (167). The nontumorigenic FDC-P1 factor-dependent hematopoietic cell line becomes leukemogenic when transplanted into irradiated recipients; in many cases, factor-independent lines that were producing GM-CSF or IL-3 due to rearrangements associated with transposition of intracisternal A-particles can be isolated (268). Enforced expression of GM-CSF by FDC-P1 cells gave rise to autocrine leukemogenic variants (167). The *bcr-abl* oncogene plays a critical role in chronic myeloid leukemia (CML). Retroviral transduction of human Bcr-Abl/p210 into mouse bone marrow cells induced a transplantable myeloproliferative CML-like disease in 100% of mice in approximately 3 weeks; this was associated with excess production of IL-3 and GM-CSF, suggesting that autocrine cytokine production is a component of the pathophysiology of CML (269). The recruitment of chemoresistant leukemic cells into sensitive phases of the cell cycle by GM-CSF may enhance the antileukemic effect of chemotherapy. GM-CSF–induced increases in leukemic cells in S-phase and intracellular phosphorylation of cytarabine have been shown to promote drug-induced cell kill (270).

Mice with Targeted Deletions of Granulocyte-Macrophage Colony-Stimulating Factor, Granulocyte-Macrophage Colony-Stimulating Factor Receptor-Alpha, or Granulocyte-Macrophage Colony-Stimulating Factor Receptor-Beta Common Chains

Mice in which the GM-CSF gene is knocked-out exhibit normal steady-state hematopoiesis, suggesting either functional redundancy of the myeloid regulatory factors or lack of a role for the factor in normal hematopoiesis (271). A universal abnormality in these mice is a pulmonary pathology with similarities to human alveolar proteinosis that involves accumulation of pulmonary surfactant protein and associated opportunistic infection. After *L. monocytogenes* infection, these mice showed 50-fold more organisms in spleen and liver than similarly infected wild-type mice, accompanied by severe depletion of bone marrow hematopoietic cells and defective inflammatory response (106). Mice lacking GM-CSF and G-CSF have greater degrees of neutropenia at birth and higher mortality than those lacking G-CSF only; in adult mice, however, neutrophil levels are comparable (107). The cellular delayed hypersensitivity response to type II chick collagen was significantly reduced in GM-CSF–deficient mice, supporting the view that GM-CSF is required for the development of collagen-induced arthritis (272). Defects in T-cell function involving generation of cytotoxic CD8 T cells, impaired CD4$^+$ T-cell proliferation, and cytokine production has been reported in GM-CSF –/– mice (273). In GM-CSF –/– and GM-CSFRβc –/– mice, DCs of all surface phenotypes were still present in all lymphoid organs (only small decreases occurred in most sites, but a threefold decrease occurred in the lymph nodes of receptor-null mice) (274). In GM-CSF transgenic mice, a threefold increase in lymph node DCs occurred (274). More surprising is the normality of hematopoiesis in GM-CSFRβc/IL-3 double-mutant mice lacking entire GM-CSF, IL-3, and IL-5 functions (275). These mice showed normal hematopoietic parameters except for reduced numbers of eosinophils and lack of an eosinophil response to *L. monocytogenes*. Hematopoietic recovery after administration of the myelosuppressive drug 5-FU was unimpaired, indicating that these three cytokines were dispensable for hematopoiesis in an emergency, as well as in steady state. On injection of endotoxin or casein, βc –/– mice showed much greater elevations of serum GM-CSF than wild-type mice, indicating that receptor-mediated clearance for normal regulation of local and systemic levels of the cytokine is important (276).

Preclinical *in Vivo* Studies of Granulocyte-Macrophage Colony-Stimulating Factor

In mice, chronic intraperitoneal administration of murine GM-CSF caused a local peritoneal accumulation of macrophages, eosinophils, and neutrophils, with little systemic changes in hematopoiesis occurring elsewhere (227,228). Transgenic mice expressing GM-CSF under control of a retroviral promoter exhibited chronic elevation of GM-CSF associated with an abnormal accumulation of macrophages in pleural, peritoneal, and ocular cavities (279). The transgenic mice exhibited a frequently fatal syndrome involving blindness, muscle wasting, and tissue destruction, probably related to GM-CSF induction of various inflammatory mediators. A similar lethal myeloproliferative syndrome was associated with introduction of the GM-CSF gene via retrovirally transduced bone marrow stem-cell transplantation (280).

Continuous infusion, or multiple injections of GM-CSF in mice before sublethal irradiation or chemotherapy, led to accelerated reconstitution of hematopoiesis (167,168). It is also effective in accelerating hematopoietic recovery after chemotherapy, although greater long-term damage to the stem-cell population is found to occur with repeated cycles of cyclophosphamide plus GM-CSF than with the drug alone (144).

GM-CSF protected neonatal rats from morbidity and death produced by *Streptococcus* infection and *Salmonella typhimurium*–sensitive mouse strains from infectious challenge (315,316). Protection of rodents from mortality was also observed in otherwise lethal infections with *P. aeruginosa, M. avium, C. albicans*, and aspergillosis (167,168).

In primates, continuous GM-CSF administration induces a dose-dependent leukocytosis, which can be maintained at 50,000 WBCs per mm^3 for up to 1 month (283). The leukocytosis involved neutrophils, band forms, eosinophils, monocytes, lymphocytes, and reticulocytes. WBCs fell to near pretreatment levels within a few days of discontinuation of therapy. GM-CSF also stimulated recovery of neutrophils in monkeys receiving autologous bone marrow transplantation with recovery of neutrophils at least 1 week earlier than in nontreated controls (284). Coadministration of GM-CSF and thrombopoietin in sublethally irradiated primates augmented platelet, red blood cell, and neutrophil recovery to a greater degree than either cytokine alone (285).

In vivo preclinical studies have shown that GM-CSF has an antitumor effect owing to enhancement of LAK and monocyte/neutrophil ADCC (168). Based on its enhancement of functional effects on macrophages and DCs, GM-CSF has been studied for its potential to enhance immune responses to antitumor immunotherapies. GM-CSF in rats elicited a delayed hypersensitivity response to tetanus toxoid similar to that seen with standard Freund's adjuvant (286). Retroviral (287) and adenoviral (288) gene delivery systems have been used to transduce GM-CSF into tumor cells and demonstrate, in syngeneic mouse transplantation models, protective antitumor immunity.

An interesting cholesterol-lowering effect of GM-CSF has been reported in rabbits and may be mediated by enhancement of macrophage functions in lipid metabolism and an increase in very-low-density lipoprotein receptor expression (289).

INTERLEUKIN-3

Molecular Characterization

In the early 1980s, a murine factor purified from a conditioned medium of a murine myelomonocytic leukemic cell line (WEHI-3) was shown to stimulate multiple different murine hematopoietic lineages. The factor, an extensively glycosylated molecule of 28,000 d, was initially termed *multi-CSF* but subsequently renamed *IL-3* (290). A cDNA clone from this cell line encoded a molecule of 266 amino acids with a 27 amino acid signal peptide (see Table 1) (291). Mature processed IL-3 has a molecular weight of 15,102, with four potential glycosylation sites. Human IL-3, which is species-restricted in its activity, is a glycoprotein of 25 to 30 kd, with a core protein of 14.6 kd consisting of 152 amino acids with a 19 amino-acid signal peptide (292). Murine and human IL-3 coding sequences show 45% identity at the nucleotide level and 29% at the amino acid level. The protein consists of four α-helix bundles and two β-sheets.

Structure–function relation studies have shown that two non-contiguous helic domains located near the NH_2 terminus and the COOH-terminus of the molecule are responsible for receptor binding (293). Two contiguous residues (Asp-21 and Glu-22) in the NH_2-terminal region of human IL-3 mediate binding to the two different chains of the IL-3 receptor; this emphasizes the functional significance of the conserved glutamic acid residue in the first helix of the IL-3, GM-CSF, IL-5 subfamily (294). The gene encoding IL-3 is located on the long arm of chromosome 5 (5q23-32), only 9 kb from the gene for GM-CSF (see Table 1) (17).

Interleukin-3 Receptor Complex and Signal Transduction

The receptor for IL-3 consists of two subunits, a 70-kd ligand-binding subunit [IL-3 receptor alpha (IL-3Rα)], which binds IL-3 with low affinity, and a 120-kd signal transducing chain (βc), which is shared by GM-CSF and IL-3 (see Table 2) (293,295). The cytoplasmic portion of βc is believed to contain most of the domains responsible for ligand-induced proliferation. Additionally, in murine cells, a highly related protein [beta IL-3 (β-IL-3)] can form a functional subunit with IL-3Rα (296). Ligand binding is believed to activate the receptor by inducing the formation of heterodimers. Synergy occurs between IL-3 and Epo in stimulation of erythropoiesis. A molecular explanation for this synergy is provided by the observation that the βc chain functionally and physically associates with the Epo receptor, and these receptors exist as a large super-complex in erythroid progenitor cells (297). The IL-3α chain gene has been mapped to the pseudoautosomal region of the sex chromosomes (298); the common β chain gene has been mapped to chromosome 22q31 (see Table 2) (177).

Signal Transduction by the Interleukin-3 Receptor Complex

Because the 120-kd signal transducer βc is a common signaling pathway for IL-3 and GM-CSF, then the Jak/STAT pathways activated by cytokines are common and have been reviewed in the section Granulocyte-Macrophage Colony-Stimulating Factor. The Src family of tyrosine kinases participate in the signal transduction pathway of many cytokines. On binding to its receptor, IL-3 activates c-Src kinase activity, which, in turn, facilitates binding of c-Src to STAT3, activated via phosphorylation of Tyr701 (translocated to the nucleus and signaling myeloid cell proliferation) (299). IL-3 stimulates rapid and transient phosphorylation of SHC protein, Jak2 and MAPK kinase, and isoforms Erk1 and Erk2, which provide antiapoptotic signals (299,300). In multipotent hematopoietic progenitor cells, synergy is observed between c-kit ligand and IL-3 in the activation of Erk1, possibly representing a point where the two cytokine signaling pathways interact to generate synergistic enhancement of proliferation (300). It has been proposed that IL-3 inhibits G-CSF–induced neutrophil differentiation of the 32D IL-3–dependent murine myeloblast cell line by blocking G-CSF–induced activation of STAT3–DNA binding (301). Such cross-modulation of STAT pathway signaling could be a physiologic

mechanism for establishing a hierarchy of growth factor effects on cells exposed to multiple cytokines. The addition of proteosome inhibitors to IL-3–stimulated cells leads to a prolongation of activation of Jak1 and Jak2, and SHC and MAPK kinase phosphorylation (consistent with the hypothesis that proteosome-mediated protein degradation can modulate the activity of the Jak/STAT pathway by regulating the deactivation of Jak) (302). IL-3 activates PI3-kinase, leading to phosphorylation of BAD, a distant member of the Bcl-2 family that promotes cell death (at least in part) through heterodimerization with the survival proteins Bcl-2 and Bcl-x (303). Akt, a survival-promoting serine–threonine protein kinase, is activated by IL-3 in a PI3-kinase–dependent manner; in its active form, it is able to phosphorylate BAD, thus mediating antiapoptosis signaling (304). Bcl-2 and related protein Bax regulate the effector stage of apoptosis and can modulate the entry of quiescent cells into cell cycle. In the presence of IL-3, constitutively expressed Bcl-2 is phosphorylated on serine, losing its capacity to heteodimerize with Bax; therefore, IL-3–induced phosphorylation of a distinct pool of Bcl-2 may contribute to the inactivation of its antiproliferative function (305). The activation of Ras, followed by the activation of the kinase cascade of Raf-1, MAPK kinase, and MAPK that leads to induction of c-fos and c-jun, has been well documented in the human IL-3 system (293). Many adaptor proteins, such as SHC, Grb2 and the c-vav oncogene, have been linked to this pathway and phosphorylated after IL-3 stimulation (293). The Ras–guanine nucleotide exchange factor mSos is indispensable for activation of the Ras pathway and downstream enhancement of kinase activity of cRaf-1, Erk2, and Jnk1 in IL-3 treated cells (306).

NFκβ plays an important role in maintaining cell survival in response to IL-3; c-Myc may be a downstream effector mediating this effect (307). Activation of p38 MAP kinase and amino terminal kinase Jnk stress-activated protein kinase has been described as being induced by a variety of environmental stresses, such as ultraviolet radiation, heat shock, or proinflammatory cytokines; IL-3 and Epo activate these cascades in murine hematopoietic progenitors, however (308). IL-3 stimulation results in the induction of c-myc, c-fos, c-jun, and pim-1 (293).

Origin of Interleukin-3 and Regulation of Production

IL-3 mRNA is not detectable in unstimulated T cells but is produced by activated T cells, NK cells, and mast cells after transient increase in gene transcription and mRNA stabilization (see Table 3) (293). It is probably a local-acting factor because it does not normally circulate at detectable levels in blood. Measurable amounts of IL-3 are produced in a subgroup of patients experiencing extensive graft-versus-host disease (293). In activated T lymphocytes, positive and negative elements control expression of the IL-3 gene. Two positive control sequences and an interposed repressor sequence reside within 315 nucleotides upstream from the transcriptional start site (309–311). The proximal regulatory region is specific to IL-3, binds an inducible T-cell–specific factor and Oct-1, and is essential for its efficient transcription. Transcriptional activation of this region can be enhanced by a second, more distal activating site consisting of AP-1 and Ef1-binding sites, conferring some specificity (310). A transcription silencer that represses in the absence of the AP-1 site lies between the two activator sites (309).

Action on Progenitor Cells

IL-3 stimulates colony formation by a spectrum of progenitors, including CFU-GEMM, CFU-GM, neutrophil-, eosinophil-, and basophil-restricted progenitors, and, in synergy with other factors, CFU-Meg and BFU-E (293). In marrow culture, approximately one-third of colonies stimulated are granulocyte-macrophage; the remainder is approximately equal numbers of pure neutrophil or macrophage colonies with low numbers (5%) of eosinophil colonies in mice and significantly more (30%) in humans (130). In cultures of highly enriched progenitors, or after serum or monocyte depletion, neutrophil and macrophage colonies are greatly reduced in number (312). Although IL-3 supports the survival and initial proliferation of unipotent neutrophil progenitors, G-CSF is necessary for terminal neutrophil proliferation and differentiation (312). IL-3 acts optimally in a concatenate manner with IL-5 to stimulate eosinophil development (313). Erythroid progenitors (BFU-E and CFU-GEMM) are stimulated by IL-3, with erythropoietin necessary for terminal differentiation and synergistic enhancement seen with c-kit ligand. IL-3 increases the numbers of subcolonies in each erythroid burst, whereas KL increases the size of the subcolonies themselves (314). Experiments involving combinations of IL-3, KL, and Epo (with delayed addition of one or more factors) indicated that the actions of IL-3 and KL were largely independent of one another in the BFU-E assay, and IL-3 acted at an earlier stage of erythroid differentiation than KL (314). Human and murine megakaryocyte progenitors (CFU-Meg) can be stimulated by IL-3 or Tpo alone, but number and size of colonies is greatly augmented by the combination of IL-3, Tpo, and KL (315). In CD34$^+$ suspension cultures, although IL-3 and Tpo stimulate CD41$^+$ megakaryocyte-lineage cells and IL-3 plays an important role early in megakaryocyte development *in vitro*, it appears to inhibit further maturation after endoreduplication begins (315). In assays of more primitive blast-cell colonies and HPP-CFU, IL-3 stimulates in synergy with factors like IL-1, IL-6, IL-11, G-CSF, KL, and FL (25). In addition to growth stimulation, shortening the "go" period, and doubling time of early hematopoietic cells, IL-3 also has an antiapoptotic action on progenitor populations at concentrations lower than necessary to initiate proliferation.

IL-3 can induce integrin expression in a dose-dependent manner, upregulating VLA-4 and VLA-5 on the murine Baf3 murine precursor B-cell line by an inside-out pathway involving H-Ras (316). Conflicting reports on the effects of brief cytokine exposure on marrow-repopulating ability exist. Brief 2- to 3-hour preincubations of mouse bone marrow with IL-3 have been reported to enhance repopulating ability, possibly due to upregulation of homing receptors (317). In contrast, other studies have found that a similar preincubation with IL-3 alone or IL-3, IL-12, and KL led to sustained decreases in marrow and spleen seeding of early and late CAFC, cobblestone area–forming cell and an 11.4% to 7.3% reduction in day 12 CFU-s seeding, together with a decrease in long-term repopulation, occurred (318). IL-3 reduced the $\alpha4\beta1$ integrin-mediated adhesion of human CD34$^+$ cells to fibronectin-coated surfaces in a 30-minute adhesion assay while enhancing migration of progenitor cells through fibronectin-coated transwell filters (318). IL-3 addition can lead to reduction in long-term repopulating ability of cultured marrow (320–322). Its addition to combinations of FL and Tpo inhibited long-term generation of long-term culture–initiating cells in cord blood cultures (323). This negative regulation by IL-3 acts at the level of stem-cell self-renewal versus differentiation-decision; it appears to be mediated by the common receptor-signaling subunit βc and the additional IL-3 signaling protein β-IL-3, which is specific to IL-3 and is found in mice but not in humans (322). In apparent contradiction to the inhibitory effects of IL-3 on stem cells *in vitro*, *in vivo* treatment of nonobese diabetic/severe combined immunodeficiency disease mice engrafted with human CD34$^+$ cells with human IL-3 resulted in substantial expansion of the most primitive stem-cell population (323).

Action of Interleukin-3 on Leukocyte Subpopulations

In addition to being an eosinopoietic factor, IL-3 has effects on mature eosinophil functions, many of which are also mediated by GM-CSF. These effects include prolongation of survival (325–327), enhanced respiratory burst activity induced by opsonized particles (328), and enhanced FcR-γ II- and CR3-binding activity (329,330). Eosinophil degranulation induced by cross-linking of IgA receptors is enhanced by IL-3 (331). The intracellular cytoadhesion molecule ICAM-1 is expressed on eosinophils after IL-3 exposure; synergistic upregulation is observed with TNF-α, resulting in enhanced eosinophil capacity for interaction with leukotactic factor activity-1–expressing inflammatory leukocytes (332). IL-3 enhances leukotriene C4 production induced by calcium ionophore and the release of arylsulfatase and beta-glucuronidase from specific and small granules of eosinophils (327,333).

IL-3 was originally identified as a murine mast cell growth factor, allowing long-term proliferation of mast cells from bone marrow (334). IL-3 enhances the viability of human basophils *in vitro* and may modulate delayed-type hypersensitivity *in vivo* by prolonging basophil survival (335). IL-3 induces basophil chemotaxis (336,337) and homotypic aggregation of basophils mediated by $\beta2$ integrins (338), features associated with basophil accumulation in late-phase allergic responses. IL-3 induces basophil adhesion to endothelium (339); local production of IL-3 during allergic reactions may selectively promote basophil CD11b upregulation, with recruitment of these cells to extravascular sites of inflammation. IL-3 induces histamine release from basophils and mast cells (340). Pretreatment with the cytokine causes a modest release of histamine; subsequent stimulation with IgE or fMLP, however, causes marked increase (341). IL-3 induces the release of an IgE–dependent histamine-releasing factor, which stimulates histamine release from other basophils, in a dose-dependent manner (342). Secretory IgA mediates basophil granulation and histamine release that is totally dependent on IL-3 pretreatment (343). IL-3 induces secretion of several mediators from basophils. The combination of C5a with IL-3 induces basophil leukotriene release (344). IL-4, normally a T-cell product, is produced by human basophils on IgE–receptor activation in the presence of IL-3 (345).

IL-3 directly induces the expression of class II antigens and members of the $\beta 2$ integrin family (e.g., leukotactic factor activity-1) on macrophages, thereby altering the function of mature phagocytes (345,346). IL-3 acts as a survival factor for monocytes and induces macrophage secretion of TNF-α, IL-1β, and IL-6 (347,348). CD40, a member of the TNF-receptor family and a facilitator of T-cell stimulation and antigen presentation, is upregulated on monocytes by IL-3 (349). IL-3 stimulates phagocytic activity, DNA synthesis, and endotoxin uptake by alveolar macrophages, facilitating their roles in host defense (350). IL-3 can prime monocytes for enhanced respiratory burst activity to a greater extent than either IFN-γ or TNF-α, and stimulates TNF-α release from macrophages; it may decrease IL-2–induced macrophage activation, however (351). As members of the phagocytic mononuclear phagocyte family, osteoclasts are responsive to IL-3. IL-3 administration to op mutant mice significantly increased numbers of macrophages and osteoclasts in these M-CSF–deficient mice (352).

Interleukin-3 and Leukemic Cells

Murine IL-3 was first identified as an autocrine product of a murine myeloid leukemia (293), and the initial identification and cloning of human IL-3 was based on its ability to stimulate proliferation of human CML cells. Extensive subsequent studies have shown the responsiveness of primary blast cells from patients with AML (293,353). Pretreatment of leukemic cells with IL-3 increases their sensitivity to cycle-specific chemotherapeutic agents (e.g., cytarabine) (354), nonspecific drugs (e.g., daunorubicin), or alkylating agents (e.g., 4-hydroxyperoxycyclophosphamide) (293). Pretreatment also increases AML cell susceptibility to lymphokine-activated killer (LAK) cells, possibly mediated through expression of the cell adhesion molecule LFA-3 (355). Oncogene-transformed murine hematopoietic cells and factor-dependent cell lines show enhanced glucose uptake on IL-3 stimulation due to increased glucose transporter expression (356); in Ras transformed cells, this was associated with an increased affinity of the glucose transporter. Autocrine production of IL-3 and GM-CSF is associated with expression of the bcr-abl oncogene in hematopoietic stem cells, and raises the possibility that excess production of these hematopoietic growth factors may contribute to the clinical phenotype of CML (262).

Interleukin-3 Action on Nonhematopoietic Cells

IL-3 receptors are expressed on certain nonhematopoietic cells (e.g., umbilical vein endothelium constitutively expresses functional high-affinity receptors) (293). Functional activation of endothelium by IL-3 induced endothelial-leukocyte adhesion molecule-1 and enhanced endothelial adhesion of neutrophils and CD4$^+$ T cells (357). TNF-α– or IL-1–induced expression of IL-3 receptors on endothelium primes cells for enhanced IL-8 production, E-selectin expression, and neutrophil transmigration in response to IL-3 (358). Cholinergic neurons in the CNS express the IL-3Rα and βc subunits; choline acetyltransferase and vesicular acetylcholine transporter mRNA were significantly increased in a central cholinergic neuronal cell line, indicating a potential role of IL-3 exists in differentiating and maintaining these neurons (359).

Preclinical *in Vivo* Studies of Interleukin-3

Mice lacking IL-3 (IL-3 –/–) mice produced by gene targeting are healthy and fertile (360), as are mice that carry an inactivating mutant in heterodimeric IL-3Rα (361) or lack IL-3 and the βc-subunit of receptors for IL-3, IL-5, and GM-CSF (275), with no detectable abnormalities in multiple aspects of hematopoiesis *in vivo* and *in vitro* (360). Studies in these mice indicated that IL-3 is not necessary for the generation of mast cells or basophils under physiologic conditions, but it does contribute to increased numbers of tissue mast cells, enhanced basophil production, and immunity in mice infected with nematodes, indicating a role for IL-3 exists in host defense against infection (360). In IL-3 –/– mice, contact hypersensitivity reactions were compromised; IL-3 was shown to be required for efficient priming of hapten-specific contact hypersensitivity responses but was dispensable for T-cell–dependent sensitization to tumor cells (362).

In mice, recombinant murine IL-3 produced a modest elevation in circulating neutrophils, eosinophils, and monocytes, with increased splenic myelopoiesis, mast cell content, and CFU-S, CFU-GM, and a greater than tenfold increase in BFU-E incidence (363,364). Chronic elevation of IL-3 levels after transplantation of marrow cells transduced with an IL-3–expressing vector was associated with 80% mortality in mice within 5 weeks (365). This was associated with a nonneoplastic, myeloproliferative syndrome involving multiorgan neutrophil and eosinophil infiltration.

In preclinical studies in cynomolgus monkeys, IL-3 administration produced a modest leukocytosis, with increases in neutrophils, eosinophils, basophils, and lymphocytes (366). In rhesus monkeys, IL-3 slightly raised leukocyte counts and substantially expanded (nine- to 13-fold) numbers of circulating progenitors (367). Synergistic increases in numbers of circulating progenitors were observed when IL-3 was administered sequentially with either GM-CSF or IL-1.

In sublethally irradiated primates, IL-3 administered for 7 days, followed by GM-CSF administered for 7 to 21 days, was optimally effective in promoting neutrophil and platelet recovery (368). A GM-CSF/IL-3 fusion protein (PIXY) produced enhanced rates of platelet and neutrophil recovery in irradiated monkeys (369). IL-3 treatment of primates after intensive myelosuppressive chemotherapy with 5-FU or cyclophosphamide dramatically enhanced myeloid recovery and reduced duration of neutropenia (370). Enhanced recovery of thymocytes and splenic T and B cells were observed after IL-3 treatment of sublethally irradiated mice; synergy was observed with IL-11 enhancing immune reconstitution (371). IL-3 *in vivo* appears to be capable of regulating extrathymic T-cell development and augments alloreactive bone marrow-derived suppressor activity *in vitro* and *in vivo*. Administration of IL-3 to autoimmune diabetic NOD mice delayed the onset and overall incidence of diabetes via enhanced generation of T cells capable of suppressing cyclophosphamide-induced diabetes (372).

CONCLUSIONS

Hematopoiesis is a complex process encompassing the continuous generation of a spectrum of highly specialized, differentiated cell types whose life spans can be measured in hours or years. What is particularly remarkable is the continual generation of these multiple lineages from a population of rare pluripotent, self-renewing stem cells under steady-state conditions and conditions of increased demand for one or a number of lineages. In adult humans, for example, bone marrow produces approximately 10^{10} erythrocytes and 4×10^8 leukocytes every hour. In the 1990s, a remarkable revolution occurred in the understanding of hematopoiesis at molecular levels. Indeed, hematopoiesis is close to being defined as the consequence of a pattern of expression of more than 50 gene products variously defined as hematopoietic growth factors, cytokines, and chemokines, produced within hematopoietic tissues and orchestrating a complex process of multilineage proliferation and differentiation. Furthermore, dysregulation of the complex pattern of autocrine, paracrine, and endocrine regulation provides a molecular basis for understanding malignant hematopoiesis.

The four hematopoietic growth factors reviewed have many overlapping functional activities in hematopoiesis, and considerable redundancy is seen in knockout models. In the cases of GM-CSF and IL-3, this can be explained in part by their sharing of a common receptor signaling chain, whereas sharing common downstream signaling pathways (such as Jak/STAT) can explain much additional functional overlap. The Jak/STAT signaling cascade that ultimately results in the appropriate cellular response to an initial stimulus is under strict regulatory control. A growing family of cytokine-inducible SH2 proteins (CISs), also termed *suppressors of cytokine signaling* (SOCS) have been identified (373,374). These molecules are negative regulators of Jak/STAT signaling. CIS1 is induced by EpoR, IL-3R, or IL-2R signaling via STAT5, binding to receptors and thereby inhibiting further activation of STAT5 (375). SOCS1 is an inhibitor of IL-6 signaling induced via gp130 and STAT3 that inhibits Jak–tyrosine kinase activity (376). CIS3 is strongly induced by IFN-γ, probably via STAT1, and inhibits signaling via binding to Jaks (373). Growing awareness exists that these negative regulators are critical in self-limiting the signaling mediated by most, if not all, members of the hematopoietin receptor superfamily. Potential dysregulation of these negative regulators of signaling may be expected to lead or predispose subjects to leukemic transformation.

An increased understanding of the role of certain key regulatory proteins in regulation of myelopoiesis exists. The Ets factor PU-1, and the C/EBPα are master transcription factors that regulate myeloid development (102). PU-1 is a unique protein that functions exclusively in a cell-intrinsic matter to control development of granulocytes, macrophages, and B and T lymphocytes. PU-1 –/– progenitors can proliferate in response to IL-3 but not G-CSF, GM-CSF, or M-CSF (377). The failure of PU –/– progenitors to respond to G-CSF is bypassed by transient signaling with IL-3 because, in the presence of factors, progenitors differentiate to myeloperoxidase-positive cells, indicating that PU-1 is not essential for specification of granulocyte precursors (although it is required for further differentiation) (377). The defect in M-CSF proliferative response is due to lack of expression of the M-CSF receptor *c-fms*; even if this is bypassed by fms transduction, however, a persisting defect in macrophage differentiation in PU-1 –/– cells exists. Another important myeloid regulatory gene is C/EBPα, a basic leucine zipper transcription factor that regulates a number of myeloid-specific genes and acts as a myeloid differentiation switch on bipotent GM progenitors, directing them to mature to granulocytes (102). C/EBPα knockout mice have no detectable G-CSFRs and are absolutely deficient in granulopoiesis (103). Increased understanding of the control of myelopoiesis at this level may also provide insight into the nature of lineage commitment and permissive role of CSFs on the expression of the differentiated phenotype in normal and malignant hematopoiesis.

REFERENCES

1. Robinson W, Metcalf D, Bradley TR. Stimulation by normal and leukemic mouse sera of colony formation in vitro by mouse bone marrow cells. *J Cell Physiol* 1967;69:83–92.
2. Stanley ER, Metcalf D. Partial purification and some properties of the factor in normal and leukaemic human urine stimulating mouse bone marrow colony growth in vitro. *Aust J Exp Biol Med Sci* 1969;47:467–483.
3. Stanley ER, Heard PM. Factors regulating macrophage production and growth. Purification and some properties of the colony-stimulating factor from medium conditioned by mouse L cells. *J Biol Chem* 1977;252:4305–4312.
4. Moore MAS. Macrophage colony-stimulating factor. In: Garland JM, Quesenberry PJ, Hilton DJ, eds. *Colony-stimulating factors: molecular and cellular biology*, 2nd ed. New York: Marcel Dekker, 1997:255–289.
5. Kawasaki ES, Ladner MB, Wang AM, et al. Molecular cloning of a complementary DNA encoding human macrophage-specific colony-stimulating factor (CSF-1). *Science* 1985;230:291–296.
6. Wong GG, Temple PA, Leary AC, et al. Human CSF-1: molecular cloning and expression of 4 kb cDNA encoding the human urinary protein. *Science* 1987;235:1504–1508.
7. Glocker MO, Arbogast B, Schreurs J, Deinzer ML. Assignment of the inter- and intramolecular disulfide linkages in recombinant human macrophage colony-stimulating factor using fast atom bombardment mass spectrometry. *Biochemistry* 1993;32:482–488.
8. Teicher BA, Ara G, Menon K, Schaub RG. In vivo studies with interleukin-12 alone and in combination with monocyte colony-stimulating factor and/or fractionated radiation treatment. *Int J Cancer* 1996;65:80–84.
9. Suzu S, Kimura F, Ota J, et al. Biologic activity of proteoglycan macrophage colony-stimulating factor. *J Immunol* 1997;159:1860–1867.
10. Suzu S, Kimura F, Matsumoto H, et al. Identification of binding domains for basic fibroblast growth factor in proteoglycan macrophage colony-stimulating factor. *Biochem Biophys Res Commun* 1997;230:392–397.
11. Uemura N, Ozawa K, Takahashi K, et al. Binding of membrane-anchored macrophage colony stimulating factor (M-CSF) to its receptor mediates specific adhesion between stromal cells and M-CSF receptor-bearing hematopoietic cells. *Blood* 1993;82:2634–2640.
12. Fixe P, Praloran V. M-CSF haematopoietic growth factor or inflammatory cytokine? *Cytokine* 1998;10:32–37.
13. Morris SW, Valentine MB, Shapiro DN, et al. Reassignment of the human CSF-1 gene to chromosome 1p13-p21. *Blood* 1991;78:2013–2020.

14. Sherr CJ. Colony-stimulating factor-1 receptor. *Blood* 1990;75:1–12.
15. Hamilton JA. CSF-1 signal transduction. *J Leukoc Biol* 1997;62: 145–155.
16. Rohrschneider LR, Bourette RP, Lioubin MN, Algate PA, Myles GM, Carlberg K. Growth and differentiation signals regulated by the M-CSF receptor. *Mol Reprod Dev* 1997;46:96–103.
17. Hilton DJ. Receptors for hematopoietic regulators. In: Garland JM, Quesenberry PJ, Hilton DJ, eds. *Colony-stimulating factors: molecular and cellular biology,* 2nd ed. New York: Marcel Dekker, 1997:49–70.
18. Yeung YG, Wang Y, Einstein DB, Lee PS, Stanley ER. Colony-stimulating factor-1 stimulates the formation of multimeric cytosolic complexes of signaling proteins and cytoskeletal components in macrophages. *J Biol Chem* 1998;273:17128–17137.
19. Novak U, Mui A, Miyajima A, Paradiso L. Formation of STAT5-containing DNA binding complexes in response to colony-stimulating factor-1 and platelet-derived growth factor. *J Biol Chem* 1996;271:18350–18354.
20. Fowles LF, Martin ML, Nelsen L, et al. Persistent activation of mitogen-activated protein kinases p42 and p44 and ets-2 phosphorylation in response to colony-stimulating factor 1/c-fms signaling. *Mol Cell Biol* 1998;18:5148–5156.
21. Hatch WC, Ganju RK, Hiregowdawa D, Avraham S, Groopman JE. The related adhesion focal tyrosine kinase (RAFTK) is tyrosine phosphorylated and participates in colony-stimulating factor-1/macrophage colony-stimulating factor signaling in monocyte-macrophages. *Blood* 1998;91:3967–3973.
22. Bartocci A, Mastrogiannis DS, Migliorati G, et al. Macrophages specifically regulate the concentration of their own growth factor in the circulation. *Proc Natl Acad Sci U S A* 1987;84:6179–6183.
23. Hamilton JA. Coordinate and noncoordinate colony-stimulating factor formation by human monocytes. *J Leukoc Biol* 1994;55:355–361.
24. Rothstein G, Rhondeau SM, Peters CA, et al. Stimulation of neutrophil production in CSF-1 responsive clones. *Blood* 1988;72:898–902.
25. Muench MO, Schneider JG, Moore MAS. Interactions among colony stimulating factors, IL-1ß, IL-6 and Kit-Ligand (KL) in the regulation of primitive murine hematopoietic cells. *Exp Hematol* 1992;20:339–349.
26. Wiktor-Jedrezjczak W, Bartocci A, et al. Total absence of colony-stimulating factor 1 in the macrophage-deficient osteopetrotic (op/op) mouse. *Proc Natl Acad Sci U S A* 1990;87:4828–4832.
27. Teshima S, Rokutan K, Takahashi M, Nikawa T, Kishi K. Induction of heat shock proteins and their possible roles in macrophages during activation by macrophage colony-stimulating factor. *Biochem J* 1996;315:497–504.
28. Roilides E, Lyman CA, Mertins SD, et al. Ex vivo effects on macrophage colony-stimulating factor on human monocyte activity against fungal and bacterial pathogens. *Cytokine* 1996;8:42–48.
29. Brummer E, Gilmore GL, Shadduck RK, Stevens DA. Development of macrophage anticryptococcal activity in vitro is dependent on endogenous M-CSF. *Cell Immunol* 1998;189:144–148.
30. Kumar R, Dong Z, Fidler IJ. Differential regulation of metalloelastase activity in murine peritoneal macrophages by granulocyte-macrophage colony-stimulating factor and macrophage colony-stimulating factor. *J Immunol* 1996;157:5104–5111.
31. Smith W, Feldmann M, Londei M. Human macrophages induced in vitro by macrophage colony-stimulating factor are deficient in IL-12 production. *Eur J Immunol* 1998;28:2498–2507.
32. Asakura E, Hanamura T, Umemura A, Yada K, Yamauchi T, Tanabe T. Effects of macrophage colony-stimulating factor (M-CSF) on lipopolysaccharide (LPS)-induced mediator production from monocytes in vitro. *Immunobiology* 1996;195:300–313.
33. Teshima S, Rokutan K, Nikawa T, Kishi K. Macrophage colony-stimulating factor stimulates synthesis and secretion of a mouse homolog of a human IgE-dependent histamine-releasing factor by macrophages in vitro and in vivo. *J Immunol* 1998;161:6356–6366.
34. Kemley SG, Chapoval AI, Evans R. Cytokine release by macrophages after interacting with CSF-1 and extracellular matrix proteins: Characteristics of a mouse model of inflammatory responses in vitro. *Cell Immunol* 1998;185:59–64.
35. Webb SE, Pollard JW, Jones GE. Direct observation and quantification of macrophage chemoattraction of the growth factor CSF-1. *J Cell Sci* 1996;109:793–803.
36. Wang J, Roderiquez G, Oravecz T, Norcross MA. Cytokine regulation of human immunodeficiency virus type 1 entry and replication in human monocytes/macrophages through modulation of CCR5 expression. *J Virol* 1998;72:7642–7647.
37. Grabstein KH, Urdal DL, Tushinski RJ, et al. Induction of macrophage tumoricidal activity by granulocyte-macrophage colony-stimulating factor. *Science* 1986;232:506–508.
38. Charak BS, Agah R, Mazumder A. Granulocyte macrophage colony-stimulating factor-induced antibody-dependent cellular cytotoxicity in bone marrow macrophages: application in bone marrow transplantation. *Blood* 1993;81:3474–3479.
39. Marks SC Jr, Iizuka T, MacKay CA, Mason-Savas A, Cielinski MJ. The effects of colony-stimulating factor-1 on the number and ultrastructure of osteoclasts in toothless (tl) rats and osteopetrotic (op) mice. *Tissue Cell* 1997;29:589–595.
40. Cecchini MG, Hofstetter W, Halasy J, Wetterwald A, Felix R. Role of CSF-1 in bone and bone marrow development. *Mol Reprod Dev* 1997;46:75–83 [discussion 83–84].
41. Amano H, Yamada S, Felix R. Colony-stimulating factor-1 stimulates the fusion process in osteoclasts. *J Bone Miner Res* 1998;13:846–853.
42. Finbloom DS, Larner AC, Nakagawa Y, et al. Culture of human monocytes with granulocyte-macrophage colony-stimulating factor results in enhancement of IFN-gamma receptors but suppression of IFN-gamma-induced expression of the gene IP-10. *J Immunol* 1993;150:2382–2390.
43. Cohen PE, Zhu L, Pollard JW. Absence of colony-stimulating factor-1 in osteopetrotic (csfmop/csfmop) mice disrupts estrous cycles and ovulation. *Biol Reprod* 1997;56:110–118.
44. Cohen PE, Hardy MP, Pollard JW. Colony-stimulating factor-1 plays a major role in the development of reproductive function in male mice. *Mol Endocrinol* 1997;11:1636–1650.
45. Hamilton GS, Lysiak JJ, Watson AJ, Lala PK. Effects of colony-stimulating factor-1 on human extravillous trophoblast growth and invasion. *J Endocrinol* 1998;159:69–77.
46. Pollard JW. Role of colony-stimulating factor-1 in reproduction and development. *Mol Reprod Dev* 1997;46:54–60 [discussion 60–61].
47. Wegiel J, Wisniewski HM, Dziewiatkowski J, et al. Reduced number and altered morphology of microglial cells in colon stimulating factor-1-deficient osteopetrotic op/op mice. *Brain Res* 1998;804:135–139.
48. Michaelson MD, Bieri PL, Mehler MF, et al. CSF-1 deficiency in mice results in abnormal brain development. *Development* 1996;122:2661–2672.
49. Murphy GM Jr, Yang L, Cordell B. Macrophage colony-stimulating factor augments beta-amyloid-induced interleukin-1, interleukin-6, and nitric oxide production by microglial cells. *J Biol Chem* 1998;273:20967–20971.
50. Calvo CF, Dobbertin A, Gelman M, Glowinski J, Mallat M. Identification of CSF-1 as a brain macrophage migratory activity produced by astrocytes. *Glia* 1998;24:180–186.
51. Yuo A, Kitagawa S, Azuma E, et al. Tyrosine phosphorylation and intracellular alkalinization are early events in human neutrophils stimulated by tumor necrosis factor-alpha, granulocyte-macrophage colony-stimulating factor and granulocyte colony stimulating factor. *Biochim Biophys Acta* 1993;1156:197–203.
52. Bashey A, Healy L, Marshall CJ. Proliferative but not nonproliferative responses to granulocyte colony stimulating factor are associated with rapid activation of the p21ras/MAP kinase signalling pathway. *Blood* 1994;83:949–957.
53. Qiao JH, Tripathi J, Mishra NK, et al. Role of macrophage colony-stimulating factor in atherosclerosis: studies of osteopetrotic mice. *Am J Pathol* 1997;150:1687–1699.
54. Rajavashisth T, Qiao J-H, Tripathi S, et al. Heterozygous osteopetrotic (op) mutation reduces atherosclerosis in LDL receptor-deficient mice. *J Clin Invest* 1998;101:2702–2710.
55. Levine JA, Jensen MD, Eberhardt NL, O'Brien T. Adipocyte macrophage colony-stimulating factor is a mediator of adipose tissue growth. *J Clin Invest* 1998;101:1557–1564.

56. Hume DA, Pavli P, Donahue RE, et al. The effect of human recombinant macrophage colony-stimulating factor (CSF-1) on the murine mononuclear phagocyte system in vivo. *J Immunol* 1988; 141:3405–3409.

57. Chikkappa G, Broxmeyer HE, Cooper S, et al. Effect in vivo of multiple injections of purified murine and recombinant human macrophage colony-stimulating factor to mice. *Cancer Res* 1989;49:3558–3561.

58. Munn DH, Bree AG, Beall AC, et al. Recombinant human macrophage colony-stimulating factor in nonhuman primates: selective expansion of a CD16$^+$ monocyte subset with phenotypic similarity to primate natural killer cells. *Blood* 1996;88:1215–1224. [Erratum in *Blood* 1996;88:4083.]

59. Sakurai T, Wakimoto N, Yamada M, Shimamura S, Motoyoshi K. Effect of macrophage colony-stimulating factor on mouse NK 1.1$^+$ cell activity in vivo. *Int J Immunopharmacol* 1998;20:401–413.

60. Yamauchi T, Yada K, Umemura A, Asakura E, Hanamura T, Tababe T. Effect of recombinant human macrophage colony-stimulating factor on marrow, splenic, and peripheral hematopoietic progenitor cells in mice. *J Leukoc Biol* 1996;59:296–301.

61. Asakura E, Yamauchi T, Umemura A, Hanamura T, Tanabe T. Intravenously administered macrophage colony-stimulating factor (M-CSF) specifically acts on the spleen, resulting in the increasing and activating spleen macrophages for cytokine production in mice. *Immunopharmacology* 1997;37:7–14.

62. Baker GR, Levin J. Transient thrombocytopenia produced by administration of macrophage colony-stimulating factor: investigations of the mechanism. *Blood* 1998;91:89–99.

63. Kovacs CJ, Kerr JA, Daly BM, Evans MJ, Johnke RM. Interleukin 1 alpha (IL-1) and macrophage colony-stimulating factor (M-CSF). *Anticancer Res* 1998;18:1805–1812.

64. Orchard PJ, Dahl N, Aukerman SL, et al. Circulating macrophage colony-stimulating factor is not reduced in malignant osteopetrosis. *Exp Hematol* 1992;20:103–105.

65. Hume DA, Donahue RE, Fidler IJ: The therapeutic effect on human recombinant macrophage colony-stimulating factor (CSF-1) in experimental murine metastatic melanoma. *Lymphokine Res* 1989; 8:69–77.

66. Perkins RC, Vadhan-Raj S, Scheule RK, et al. Effects of continuous high-dose rhGM-CSF infusion on human monocyte activity. *Am J Hematol* 1993;43:279–285.

67. Inaba T, Shimano H, Gotoda T, et al. Macrophage colony-stimulating factor regulates both activities of neutral and acidic cholesteryl ester hydrolases in human monocyte-derived macrophages. *J Clin Invest* 1993;92:750–757.

68. Burgess A, Metcalf D. Characterization of a serum factor stimulating the differentiation of myelomonocytic leukemia cells. *Int J Cancer* 1980:6:254–264.

69. Moore MAS. G-CSF: its relationship to leukemia differentiation-inducing activity and other hematopoietic regulators. *J Cell Physiol Suppl* 1982;1:53–64.

70. Welte K, Platzer E, Lu L, et al. Purification and biochemical characterization of human pluripotent hematopoietic colony-stimulating factor. *Proc Natl Acad Sci U S A* 1985;82:1526–1530.

71. Souza LM, Boone TC, Gabrilove JL, et al. Recombinant human granulocyte colony-stimulating factor: Effects on normal and leukemic myeloid cells. *Science* 1986;232:61–65.

72. Gabrilove JL, Jakubowski A, Scher H, et al. Effect of granulocyte colony-stimulating factor on neutropenia and associated morbidity due to chemotherapy for transitional-cell carcinoma of the urothelium. *N Engl J Med* 1988;318:1414–1422.

73. Hill CP, Osslund TD, Eisenberg D. The structure of granulocyte colony-stimulating factor and its relationship to other growth factors. *Proc Natl Acad Sci U S A* 1993;90:5167–5171.

74. LeBeau MM, Lemons RS, Carrino JJ, et al. Chromosomal localization of the human G-CSF gene to 17q11 proximal to the breakpoint of the t(15;17) in acute promyelocytic leukemia. *Leukemia* 1987;1:795–799.

75. Nagata S, Tsuchiya M, Asano S, et al. Molecular cloning and expression of cDNA for murine granulocyte colony-stimulating factor. *Nature* 1986;319:415–418.

76. Tsuchiya M, Asano S, Kaziro Y. Isolation and characterization of the cDNA for murine granulocyte colony-stimulating factor. *Proc Natl Acad Sci U S A* 1986;83:7633–7637.

77. Roberts AW, Nicola NA. Granulocyte colony-stimulating factor. In: Garland JM, Quesenberry PJ, Hilton DJ, eds. *Colony-stimulating factors: molecular and cellular biology*, 2nd ed. New York: Marcel Dekker, 1997:203–225.

78. McKinstry WJ, Chung-Leung L, Rasko JEJ, et al. Cytokine receptor expression on hematopoietic stem and progenitor cells. *Blood* 1997;89:65–71.

79. Shieh J-H, Moore MAS. Hematopoietic growth factor receptors. *Cytotechnology* 1989;2:269–286.

80. Fukanaga R, Ishizaka-Ikeda E, Seto Y, et al. Expression cloning of human granulocyte macrophage colony stimulating factor. *Cell* 1990;61:341–350.

81. Larsen A, Davis T, Curtis BM, et al. Expression cloning of human granulocyte macrophage colony stimulating factor receptor. A structural mosaic of hematopoietin receptor, immunoglobulin, and fibronectin domains. *J Exp Med* 1990;172:1559–1603.

82. Tweardy DJ, Anderson K, Cannizzaro LA, et al. Molecular cloning of the cDNA's for the human granulocyte macrophage colony stimulating factor receptor from HL-60 and mapping of the gene to chromosome region 1p32-34. *Blood* 1992;79:1148–1160.

83. Seto Y, Fukunaga R, Nagata S. Chromosomal gene organization of the human granulocyte macrophage colony stimulating factor receptor. *J Immunol* 1992;148:259–266.

84. Fukunga R, Ishizaka-Ikeda E, Nagata S. Growth and differentiation signals mediated by different regions in the cytoplasmic domain of granulocyte colony-stimulating factor receptor. *Cell* 1993;74:1079–1087.

85. Ziegler SF, Bird TA, Morella KK, Mosely B, Gearing DB, Baumannn H. Distinct regions of the human granulocyte colony-stimulating factor receptor cytoplasmic domain are required for proliferation and gene induction. *Mol Cell Biol* 1993;13:2384–2390.

86. Liu F, Poursine-Laurent J, Wu HY, Link DC. Interleukin-6 and the granulocyte colony-stimulating factor are major independent regulators of granulopoiesis in vivo but are not required for lineage commitment or terminal differentiation. *Blood* 1997;90:2583–2590.

87. Jacob J, Haug JS, Raptis S, Link DC. Specific signals generated by the cytoplasmic domain of the granulocyte colony-stimulating factor (G-CSF) receptor are not required for G-CSF-dependent granulocytic differentiation. *Blood* 1998;92:353–361.

88. Welte K, Gabrilove J, Bronchud MH, Platzer E, Morstyn G. Filgrastim (r-metHuG-CSF): the first 10 years. *Blood* 1996;88: 1907–1929.

89. Tidow N, Welte K. Advances in understanding postreceptor signaling in response to granulocyte colony-stimulating factor. *Curr Opin Hematol* 1997;4:171–175.

90. Tidow N, Kasper B, Welte K. Clinical implications of G-CSF receptor mutations. *Crit Rev Oncol Hematol* 1998;28:1–6.

91. McLemore ML, Poursine-Laurent J, Link DC. Increased granulocyte colony-stimulating factor responsiveness but normal resting granulopoiesis in mice carrying a targeted granulocyte colony-stimulating factor receptor mutation derived from a patient with severe congenital neutropenia. *J Clin Invest* 1998;102:483–492.

92. Avalos BR, Parker JM, Ware DA, Hunter MG, Sibert KA, Druker BJ. Dissociation of the Jak kinase pathway from G-CSF receptor signaling in neutrophils. *Exp Hematol* 1997;25:160–168.

93. Shimoda K, Feng J, Murakami H, et al. Jak 1 plays an essential role for receptor phosphorylation and Stat activation in response to granulocyte colony-stimulating factor. *Blood* 1997;90:597–604.

94. Dong F, Liu X, de Koning JP, et al. Stimulation of Stat5 by granulocyte colony-stimulating factor (G-CSF) is modulated by two distinct cytoplasmic regions of the G-CSF receptor. *J Immunol* 1998;161: 6503–6509.

95. Ward AC, Hermans MH, Smith L, et al. Tyrosine-dependent and independent mechanisms of STAT3 activation by the human granulocyte colony-stimulating factor (G-CSF) receptor are differentially utilized depending on G-CSF concentration. *Blood* 1999;93: 113–124.

96. Chakraborty A, Tweardy DJ. Stat3 and G-CSF-induced myeloid differentiation. *Leuk Lymphoma* 1998;30:433–442.

97. Chakraborty A, Tweardy DJ. Granulocyte colony-stimulating factor activates a 72-kDA isoform of STAT3 in human neutrophils. *J Leukoc Biol* 1998;64:675–680.

98. Ward AC, Monkhouse JL, Csar XF, Touw IP, Bello PA. The Src-like tyrosine kinase Hck is activated by granulocyte colony-stimulating factor (G-CSF) and docks to the activated G-CSF receptor. *Biochem Biophys Res Commun* 1998;251:117–123.

99. Nicholson SE, Novak U, Ziegler SF, Layton JE. Distinct regions of the granulocyte colony-stimulating factor receptor are required for tyrosine phosphorylation of the signaling molecules JAK2, Stat3, and p42, p44MAPK. *Blood* 1995;86:3698–3703.

100. Radomska HS, Huettner CS, Zhang P, Cheng T, Scadden DT, Tenen DG. CCAAT/Enhancer binding protein α is a regulatory switch sufficient for induction of granulocytic development from bipotential myeloid progenitors. *Mol Cell Biol* 1998;18:4301–4314.

101. Tenen DG, Hromas R, Licht J, Zhang D-E. Transcription factors, normal myeloid development and leukemia. *Blood* 1997:90: 489–519.

102. Zhang DE, Zhang P, Wang ND, Hetherington CJ, Durlington GJ, Tenen DG. Absence of granulocyte colony-stimulating factor signaling and neutrophil development in CCAAT enhancer binding protein alpha-deficient mice. *Proc Natl Acad Sci U S A* 1997;94:569–574.

103. Zhang P, Iwama A, Datta MW, Darlington GJ, Link DC, Tenen DG. Upregulation of interleukin 6 and granulocyte colony-stimulating factor receptors by transcription factor CCAAT enhancer binding protein alpha (C/EBP alpha) is critical for granulopoiesis. *J Exp Med* 1998;188:1173–1184.

104. Lieschke GJ, Grail D, Hodgson G, et al. Mice lacking granulocyte colony-stimulating factor have chronic neutropenia, granulocyte and macrophage progenitor cell deficiency, and impaired neutrophil mobilization. *Blood* 1994;84:1737–1746.

105. Zhan Y, Basu S, Lieschke GJ, Grail D, Dunn AR, Cheers C. Functional deficiencies of peritoneal cells from gene-targeted mice lacking G-CSF or GM-CSF. *J Leukoc Biol* 1999;65:256–264.

106. Seymour JF, Lieschke GJ, Grail D, Quilici C, Hodgson G, Dunn AR. Mice lacking both granulocyte colony-stimulating factor (CSF) and granulocyte-macrophage CSF have impaired reproductive capacity, perturbed neonatal granulopoiesis, lung disease, amyloidosis, and reduced long-term survival. *Blood* 1997;90:3037–3049.

107. Ogawa Y, Yonekura S, Nagao T. Granulocyte colony-stimulating factor production by human bone marrow fibroblasts stimulated with interleukins. *Am J Hemat* 1996;52:71–76.

108. Gupta P, Blazar BR, Gupta K, Verfaillie CM. Human CD34(+) bone marrow cells regulate stromal production of interleukin-6 and granulocyte colony-stimulating factor and increase the colony-stimulating activity of stroma. *Blood* 1998;91:3724–3733.

109. Soderquist B, Kallman J, Holmbefg H, Vikerfors T, Kihlstrom E. Secretion of IL-6, IL-8, and G-CSF by human endothelial cells in vitro in response to *Staphylococcus aureus* and staphylococcal exotoxins. *APMIS* 1998;106:1157–1164.

110. Cai XY, Gommoll CP Jr, Justice L, Narula SK, Fine JS. Regulation of granulocyte colony-stimulating factor gene expression by interleukin-17. *Immunology Lett* 1998;62:51–58.

111. Fossiez F, Djossou O, Chomarat P, et al. T cell interleukin-17 induces stromal cells to produce proinflammatory and hematopoietic cytokines. *J Exp Med* 1996;183:1593–2603.

112. Ericson SG, Gao H, Gericke GH, Lewis LD. The role of polymorphonuclear neutrophils (PMNs) in clearance of granulocyte colony-stimulating factor (G-CSF) in vivo and in vitro. *Exp Hematol* 1997;25:1313–1325.

113. Siato K, Nakamura Y, Waga K, et al. Mature and immature myeloid cells decrease the granulocyte colony-stimulating factor level by absorption of granulocyte colony-stimulating factor. *Int J Hemat* 1998;67:145–151.

114. Ikebuchi K, Ihle JN, Hirai Y, et al. Synergistic factors for stem cell proliferation: further studies of the target stem cells and the mechanism of stimulation by interleukin-1, interleukin-6, and granulocyte colony-stimulating factor. *Blood* 1988;72:2007–2014.

115. Moore MAS, Warren DJ. Synergy of interleukin 1 and granulocyte colony-stimulating factor: in vivo stimulation of stem-cell recovery and hematopoietic regeneration following 5-fluorouracil treatment of mice. *Proc Natl Acad Sci U S A* 1987;84:7134–7138.

116. Moore MAS. The use of colony-stimulating factors in combinations. *Curr Opin Biotechnol* 1991;2:854–874.

117. Shapiro F, Yao T-J, Raptis G, Reich L, Norton L, Moore MAS. Optimization of conditions for ex vivo expansion of CD34⁺ cells from patients with stage IV breast cancer. *Blood* 1994;84:3567–3574.

118. Shapiro F, Pytowski B, Rafii S, et al. The effects of Flk-2/flt3 ligand as compared with c-kit ligand on short-term and long-term proliferation of CD34⁺ hematopoietic progenitors elicited from human fetal liver, umbilical cord blood, bone marrow, and mobilized peripheral blood. *J Hematother* 1996;5:655–662.

119. Brugger W, Heimfeld S, Berenson RJ, et al. Reconstitution of hematopoiesis after high-dose chemotherapy by autologous progenitor cells generated ex vivo. *N Engl J Med* 1995;333:283–287.

120. Pitrak DL. Effects of granulocyte colony-stimulating factor and granulocyte-macrophage colony-stimulating factor on the bactericidal functions of neutrophils. *Curr Opin Hematol* 1997;4:183–190.

121. Stevens P, Shatzer EM, Hanson ES, Allen RC. Phamacodynamics of recombinant human G-CSF with respect to an increase of neutrophil oxidative metabolism. *J Leukoc Biol* 1991;2:40(abst).

122. Yamamoto Y, Klein TW, Friedman H, Kimura S, Yamaguchi H. Granulocyte colony-stimulating factor potentiates anti-*Candida albicans* growth inhibitory activity of polymorphonuclear cells. *FEMS Immunol Med Microbiol* 1993;7:15–22.

123. Ericson SG, Zhao Y, Gao H, et al. Interleukin-6 production by human neutrophils after Fc-receptor cross-linking or exposure to granulocyte colony-stimulating factor. *Blood* 1998;91:2099–2107.

124. Shirafuji N, Matsuda S, Ogura H, et al. Granulocyte colony-stimulating factor stimulates human mature neutrophilic granulocytes to produce interferon-α. *Blood* 1990;75:17–19.

125. Wang JM, Chen ZG, Colella S, et al. Chemotactic activity of recombinant human granulocyte colony-stimulating factor. *Blood* 1988;72:1456–1460.

126. Vera JC, Rivas CI, Shang RH, Golde DW. Colony-stimulating factors signal for increased transport of vitamin C in human host defense cells. *Blood* 1998;91:2536–2546.

127. Moore MAS. Coordinate actions of hematopoietic growth factors in stimulation of bone marrow function. In: Sporn MB, Roberts AB, eds. *Handbook of experimental pharmacology-peptide growth factors and their receptors.* Vol 95/II. New York: Springer-Verlag, 1990:299–344.

128. Drize N, Gan O, Zander A. Effect of recombinant granulocyte colony stimulating factor treatment of mice on spleen colony-forming unit number and self-renewal capacity. *Exp Hematol* 1993;21:1289–1293.

129. Molineux G, Pojda Z, Hampson IN, et al. Transplantation potential of peripheral blood stem cells induced by granulocyte colony-stimulating factor. *Blood* 1990;76:2153–2158.

130. Roberts AW, Foote S, Alexander WS, Scott C, Robb L, Metcalf D. Genetic influences determining progenitor cell mobilization and leukocytosis induced by granulocyte colony-stimulating factor. *Blood* 1997;98:2736–2744.

131. Eissner G, Lindner H, Reisbach G, Kaluke J, Holler E. Differential modulation of IL-1-induced endothelial adhesion molecules and transendothelial migration of granulocytes by G-CSF. *Br J Haematol* 1997;97:726–733.

132. Suzuki H, Ikebuchi K, Wada Y, et al. An increase in peripheral blood progenitor cells in primates by coadministration of recombinant human interleukin-6 and recombinant human granulocyte colony-stimulating factor. *Transplantation* 1997;64:1468–1473.

133. Briddell RA, Hartley CA, Smith KA, et al. Recombinant rat stem cell factor synergises with recombinant human granulocyte colony-stimulating factor in vivo in mice to mobilize peripheral blood progenitor cells that have enhanced repopulation potential. *Blood* 1993;82:1720–1723.

134. Sudo Y, Shimazaki C, Ashihara E, et al. Synergistic effect of FLT-3 ligand on the granulocyte colony-stimulating factor-induced mobilization of hematopoietic stem cells and progenitor cells into blood in mice. *Blood* 1997;89:3186–3191.

135. Pless M, Wodnar-Filipowicz A, John L, et al. Synergy of growth factors during mobilization of peripheral blood precursor cells with recombinant human Flt-3-ligand and granulocyte colony-stimulating factor in rabbits. *Exp Hematol* 1999;27:155–161.

136. Neipp M, Zorina T, Domenick MA, Exner BG, Ildstad ST. Effect of FLT3 ligand and granulocyte colony-stimulating factor on expansion and mobilization of facilitating cells and hematopoietic stem cells in mice kinetics and repopulating potential. *Blood* 1998; 92:3177–3188.

137. Yamada T, Kaneko H, Iizuka K, Matsubayashi Y, Kokai Y, Fujimoto J. Elevation of lymphocyte and hematopoietic stem cell numbers in mice transgenic for human granulocyte CSF. *Lab Invest* 1996;74:384–394.

138. Lejnieks DV, Hans SW, Ramesh N, Lau S, Osborne WR. Granulocyte colony-stimulating factor expression from transduced vascular smooth muscle cells provides sustained neutrophil increases in rats. *Hum Gene Ther* 1996;7:1431–1436.

139. Bonham L, Palmer T, Miller AD. Prolonged expression of therapeutic levels of human granulocyte colony-stimulating factor in rats following gene transfer to skeletal muscle. *Hum Gene Ther* 1996;7: 1423–1429.

140. Chang JM, Metcalf KD, Gonda TJ, et al. Long-term exposure to retrovirally expressed granulocyte-colony-stimulating factor induces a nonneoplastic granulocytic and progenitor cell hyperplasia without tissue damage in mice. *J Clin Invest* 1989;84:1488–1496.

141. Waddick KG, Song CW, Zouza L, et al. Comparative analysis of the in vivo radioprotective effects of recombinant granulocyte colony-stimulating factor (G-CSF), recombinant granulocyte-macrophage CSF, and their combination. *Blood* 1991;77:2364–2371.

142. Sureda A, Kadar E, Valls A, Garcia-Lopez J. Granulocyte colony-stimulating factor administered as a single intraperitoneal injection modifies the lethal dose 95/30 in irradiated B6D2F1 mice. *Haematologica* 1998;83:863–864.

143. Shimamura M, Takigawa T, Urabe A, et al. Synergistic effect of dolichyl phosphate and human recombinant granulocyte colony-stimulating factor on recovery from neutropenia in mice treated with anticancer drugs. *Exp Hematol* 1988;16:681–685.

144. Hornung RL, Longo DL. Hematopoietic stem cell depletion by restorative growth factor regimens during repeated high-dose cyclophosphamide therapy. *Blood* 1992;80:77–83.

145. van Os R, Robinson S, Sheridan T, Mislow JM, Dawes D, Mauch PM. Granulocyte colony-stimulating factor enhances bone marrow stem cell damage caused by repeated administration of cytotoxic agents. *Blood* 1998;92:1950–1956.

146. Moore MAS. Does stem cell exhaustion result from combining hematopoietic growth factors with chemotherapy? If so, how do we prevent it? *Blood* 1992;80:3–7.

147. O'Reilly J, Souza LM. Recombinant human granulocyte colony-stimulating factor: effects on hematopoiesis in normal and cyclophosphamide-treated primates. *J Exp Med* 1987;164:941–948.

148. Weiss M, Moldawer LL, Schneider EM. Granulocyte colony-stimulating factor to prevent the progression of systemic nonresponsiveness in systemic inflammatory response syndrome and sepsis. *Blood* 1999;93:425–439.

149. Gorgen I, Hartung T, Leist M, et al. Granulocyte colony-stimulating factor treatment protects rodents against lipopolysaccharide-induced toxicity via suppression of systemic tumor necrosis factor-alpha. *J Immunol* 1992;149:918–924.

150. Lorenz W, Reimund KP, Weitzel F, et al. Granulocyte colony-stimulating factor prophylaxis before operation protects against lethal consequences of postoperative peritonitis. *Surgery* 1994;116:925–934.

151. Lundblad R, Nesland JM, Giercksky KE. Granulocyte colony-stimulating factor improves survival rate and reduces concentrations of bacteria, endotoxin, tumor necrosis factor, and endothelin-1 in fulminant intra-abdominal sepsis in rats. *Crit Care Med* 1996;24:820–826.

152. Eichacker PQ, Waisman Y, Natanson C, et al. The cardiopulmonary effect of granulocyte colony-stimulating factor in a canine model of bacterial sepsis. *J Appl Physiol* 1994;77:2366–2373.

153. Haberstroh J, Breuer H, Lucke I, et al. Effect of recombinant human granulocyte colony-stimulating factor on hemodynamic and cytokine response in a porcine model of pseudomonas sepsis. *Shock* 1995;4:216–224.

154. Nelson S, Summer W, Bagby G, et al. Granulocyte colony-stimulating factor enhances pulmonary host defenses in normal and ethanol-treated rats. *J Infect Dis* 1991;164:901–906.

155. Aoki Y, Hiromatsu K, Kobayashi N, et al. Protective effect of granulocyte colony-stimulating factor against T-cell-mediated lethal shock triggered by superantigens. *Blood* 1995;86:1420–1427.

156. Squadrito F, Altavilla D, Squadrito G, et al. The effects of recombinant human granulocyte colony-stimulating factor on vascular dysfunction and splanchnic ischemia-reperfusion injury. *Br J Pharmacol* 1997;120:333–339.

157. Hommes DW, Meenan J, Dijkhuizen S, et al. Efficacy of recombinant granulocyte colony-stimulating factor (rhG-CSF) in experimental colitis. *Clin Exp Immunol* 1996;106:529–530.

158. Burgess AW, Camakaris J, Metcalf D. Purification and properties of colony-stimulating factor from mouse lung-conditioned medium. *J Biol Chem* 1977;252:1998–2003.

159. Gough NM, Gough J, Metcalf D, et al. Molecular cloning of cDNA encoding a murine haematopoietic growth regulator, granulocyte-macrophage colony-stimulating factor. *Nature* 1985;309:763–767.

160. Miyatake S, Otsuka T, Yokota T, et al. Structure of the chromosomal gene for granulocyte macrophage colony-stimulating factor. Comparison of the mouse and human genes. *EMBO J* 1985;4: 2561–2565.

161. Gasson JC, Weisbart RH, Kaufman SE, et al. Purified human granulocyte-macrophage colony-stimulating factor: direct action on neutrophils. *Science* 1984;226:1339–1342.

162. Wong GG, Witek JS, Temple PA, et al. Molecular cloning of human and gibbon GM-CSF cDNA's and purification of the natural and recombinant human proteins. *Cancer Cells* 1985;3:235–242.

163. Walter MR, Cook WH, Ealick SE, et al. Three-dimensional structure of recombinant human granulocyte macrophage colony-stimulating factor. *J Mol Biol* 1992;224:1075–1085.

164. Kaushansky K, Shoemaker SG, Alfar S, et al. Hematopoietic activity of granulocyte macrophage colony-stimulating factor is dependent upon two distinct regions of the molecule: functional analysis based upon the activities of interspecies hybrid growth factors. *Proc Natl Acad Sci U S A* 1989;86:1213–1217.

165. Greenfield RS, Braslawsky GR, Kadow KF, et al. Identification of functional domains in murine granulocyte macrophage colony-stimulating factor using monoclonal antibodies to synthetic peptides. *J Immunol* 1993;150:5241–5251.

166. Shanafelt AB, Kastelein RA. Identification of critical regions in mouse granulocyte macrophage colony-stimulating factor by scanning-deletion analysis. *Proc Natl Acad Sci U S A* 1989;86:4872–4876.

167. Rasko JEJ. Granulocyte-macrophage colony-stimulating factor and its receptor. In: Garland JM, Quesenberry PJ, Hilton DJ, eds. *Colony-stimulating factors: molecular and cellular biology*, 2nd ed. New York: Marcel Dekker, 1997:163–202.

168. Armitage JO. Emerging applications of recombinant human granulocyte-macrophage colony-stimulating factor. *Blood* 1998;92; 4491–4508.

169. Kelleher CA, Wong GG, Clark SC, et al. Binding of iodinated recombinant human GM-CSF to the blast cells of acute myeloblastic leukemia. *Leukemia* 1988;2:211–215.

170. Huebner K, Isobe M, Croce CM, et al. The human gene encoding GM-CSF is at 5q21-q32, the chromosome region deleted in the 5q-anomaly. *Science* 1985;230:1282–1285.

171. Kluck PM, Weigant J, Raap AK, et al. Order of human hematopoietic growth factor and receptor genes on the long arm of chromosome 5, as determined by fluorescence in situ hybridization. *Ann Hematol* 1993;66:15–20.

172. Willman CL, Sever CE, Pallavicini MG, et al. Deletion of IRF-1 mapping to chromosome 5q31.1, in human leukemia and preleukemic myelodysplasia. *Science* 1993;259:968–971.

173. Hilton DJ. Receptors for hematopoietic regulators. In: Garland JM, Quesenberry PJ, Hilton DJ, eds. *Colony-stimulating factors: molecular and cellular biology*, 2nd ed. New York: Marcel Dekker, 1997:49–70.

174. Lopez AF, Shannon MF, Barry S, et al. A human interleukin 3 analog with increased biological and binding activities. *Proc Natl Acad Sci U S A* 1992;89:11842–11846.

175. Shieh J-H, Moore MAS. Hematopoietic growth factor receptors. *Cytotechnology* 1989;2:269–286.

176. Gough NM, Gearing DP, Nicola NA, et al. Localization of the human GM-CSF receptor gene to the X-Y pseudoautosomal region. *Nature* 1990;345:734–736.

177. Shen Y, Baker E, Callen DF, et al. Localization of the human GM-CSF receptor beta chain gene (CSF2RB) to chromosome 22q12. 2→q13.1. *Cytogenet Cell Genet* 1992;61:175–177.

178. Budel LM, Elbaz O, Hoogerbrugge H, et al. Common binding structure for granulocyte macrophage colony-stimulating factor and interleukin-3 on human acute myeloid leukemia cells and monocytes. *Blood* 1990;75:1439.

179. Lund-Johansen F, Houck D, Hoffman R, Davis K, Olweus J. Primitive human hematopoietic progenitor cells express receptors for granulocyte-macrophage colony-stimulating factor. *Exp Hematol* 1999;27:762–772.

180. Woodcock JM, McClure BJ, Stomski FC, Elliott MJ, Bagley CJ, Lopez AF. The human granulocyte-macrophage colony-stimulating factor (GM-CSF) receptor exists as a preformed receptor complex that can be activated by GM-CSF, interleukin-3, or interleukin-5. *Blood* 1997;90:3005–3017.

181. Smith A, Metcalf D, Nicola NA. Cytoplasmic domains of the common beta-chain of the GM-CSF/IL-3/IL-5 receptors that are required for inducing differentiation or clonal suppression in myeloid leukaemic cell lines. *EMBO J* 1997;16:451–464.

182. Matsuguchi T, Lilly MB, Kraft AS. Cytoplasmic domains of the human granulocyte-macrophage colony-stimulating factor (GM-CSF) receptor beta chain (hbetac) responsible for human GM-CSF-induced myeloid cell differentiation. *J Biol Chem* 1998;273:19411–19418.

183. Watanabe S, Itoh T, Arai K. Roles of JAK kinase in human GM-CSF receptor signals. *Leukemia* 1997;11[Suppl 3]:76–78.

184. Rajotte D, Sadowski HB, Haman A, et al. Contribution of both STAT and SRF/TCF to c-fos promoter activation by granulocyte-macrophage colony-stimulating factor. *Blood* 1996;88:2906–2916.

185. Park WY, Ahn JH, Feldman RA, Seo JS. c-Fes tyrosine kinase binds to and activates STAT3 after granulocyte-macrophage colony-stimulating factor stimulation. *Cancer Lett* 1998;129:29–37.

186. Caldenhoven E, van Dijk TB, Tijmensen A, et al. Differential activation of functionally distinct STAT5 proteins by IL-5 and GM-CSF during eosinophil and neutrophil differentiation from human CD34⁺ hematopoietic stem cells. *Stem Cells* 1998;16:397–403.

187. Ota J, Kimura F, Sato K, et al. Association of CrkL with STAT5 in hematopoietic cells stimulated by granulocyte-macrophage colony-stimulating factor or erythropoietin. *Biochem Biophys Res Commun* 1998;252:779–786.

188. Al-Shami A, Mahanna W, Naccache PH. Granulocyte-macrophage colony-stimulating factor-activated signaling pathways in human neutrophils. Selective activation of Jak2, STAT3, and STAT5b. *J Biol Chem* 1998;273:1058–1063.

189. Brizzi MF, Aronica MG, Rosso A, Bagnara GP, Yarden Y, Pegoraro L. Granulocyte-macrophage colony-stimulating factor stimulates Jak2 signaling pathway and rapidly activates p93fes, STAT1 p91, and STAT3 p92 in polymorphonuclear leukocytes. *J Biol Chem* 1996;271:3562–3567.

190. Al-Shami A, Naccache PH. Granulocyte-macrophage colony-stimulating factor-activated signaling pathways in human neutrophils. Involvement of Jak2 in the stimulation of phosphatidylinositol 3-kinase. *J Biol Chem* 1999;274:5333–5338.

191. Suzuki K, Hino M, Hato F, Tatsumi N, Kitagawa S. Cytokine-specific activation of distinct mitogen-activated protein kinase subtype cascades in human neutrophils stimulated by granulocyte colony-stimulating factor, granulocyte-macrophage colony-stimulating factor, and tumor necrosis factor-alpha. *Blood* 1999;93:341–349.

192. Yamaoko K, Otsuka T, Niiro H, et al. Activation of STAT5 by lipopolysaccharide through granulocyte-macrophage colony-stimulating factor production in human monocytes. *J Immunol* 1998;160: 838–845.

193. Welte T, Koch F, Schuler G, Lechner J, Doppler W, Heufler C. Granulocyte-macrophage colony-stimulating factor induces a unique set of STAT factors in murine dendritic cells. *Eur J Immunol* 1997;27:2737–2740.

194. Ohtsuki F, Yamamoto M, Nakagawa T, Tanizawa T, Wada H. Granulocyte-macrophage colony-stimulating factor abrogates transforming growth factor-beta 1-mediated cell cycle arrest by upregulating cyclin D2/Cdk6. *Br J Haematol* 1997;98:520–527.

195. Nimer SD, Uchida H. Regulation of granulocyte-macrophage colony-stimulating factor and interleukin-3 expression. *Stem Cells* 1995;13:324–335.

196. Thomas RS, Tymms MJ, McKinlay LH, Shannon MF, Seth A, Kola I. ETS1, NfkappaB, and AP1 synergistically transactivate the human GM-CSF promoter. *Oncogene* 1997;14:2845–2855.

197. Patterson CE, Stasek JE, Bahler C, Verin AD, Harrington MA, Garcia JG. Regulation of interleukin-1 stimulated GMCSF mRNA levels in human endothelium. *Endothelium* 1998;6:45–59.

198. Kosaki K, Ando J, Korenaga R, Kurokawa T, Kamiya A. Fluid shear stress increases the production of granulocyte-macrophage colony-stimulating factor by endothelial cells via mRNA stabilization. *Circ Res* 1998;82:794–802.

199. Okayama Y, Kobayashi H, Ashman LK. Human lung mast cells are enriched in the capacity to produce granulocyte-macrophage colony-stimulating factor in response to IgE-dependent stimulation. *Eur J Immunol* 1998;28:708–715.

200. Guillemin G, Boussin FD, Le Grand B, Croitoru J, Coffigny H, Dormont D. Granulocyte macrophage colony-stimulating factor stimulates in vitro proliferation of astrocytes derived from simian mature brains. *Glia* 1996;16:71–80.

201. Harakawa N, Sasada M, Maeda A, et al. Random migration of polymorphonuclear leukocytes induced by GM-CSF involving a signal transduction pathway different from that of fMLP. *J Leukoc Biol* 1997;61:500–506.

202. Sweeney JF, Nguyen PK, Omann G, Hinshaw DB. Granulocyte-macrophage colony-stimulating factor rescues human polymorphonuclear leukocytes from ultraviolet irradiation-accelerated apoptosis. *J Surg Res* 1999;81:108–112.

203. Escribano S, Cuenllas E, Gaitan S, Tejero C. Delayed neutrophil apoptosis after total body irradiation in mice. The role of granulocyte-macrophage colony-stimulating factor in neutrophil function. *Exp Hematol* 1998;26:942–949.

204. Hu B, Yasui K. Effects of colony-stimulating factor (Csfs) on neutrophil apoptosis: possible roles at inflammation site. *Int J Hematol* 1997;66:179–188.

205. Smith RJ, Justen JM, Sam LM. Recombinant human granulocyte-macrophage colony-stimulating factor induces granule exocytosis from human polymorphonuclear neutrophils. *Inflammation* 1990;14:83–92.

206. Khwaja A, Carver JE, Linch DC. Interactions of granulocyte-macrophage colony-stimulating factor (CSF), granulocyte CSF, and tumor necrosis factor alpha in the priming of the neutrophil respiratory burst. *Blood* 1992;79:745–753.

207. Kodama T, Hazeki K, Hazeki O, Okada T, Ui M. Enhancement of chemotactic peptide-induced activation of phosphoinositide 3-kinase by granulocyte-macrophage colony-stimulating factor and its relation to the cytokine-mediated priming of neutrophil superoxide-anion production. *Biochem J* 1999;337:201–209.

208. Novella A, Bergamaschi G, Canale C, et al. Expression of adhesion molecules and functional stimulation in human neutrophils: modulation by GM-CSF and role of the Bcr gene. *Br J Haematol* 1997; 98:621–626.

209. Poubelle PE, Bourgoins, Naccache PH, et al. Granulocyte-macrophage colony-stimulating factor (GM-CSF) and opsonization synergistically enhance leukotriene B₄ (LTB₄) synthesis induced by phagocytosis in human neutrophils. *Agents Actions Suppl* 1989;27: 388–390.

210. Pouliot M, McDonald PP, Khamzina L, et al. Granulocyte-macrophage colony-stimulating factor enhances 5-lipoxygenase levels in human polymorphonuclear leukocytes. *J Immunol* 1994;152:851.

211. McDonald PP, Pouliot M, Borgeat P, et al. Induction by chemokines of lipid mediator synthesis in granulocyte-macrophage colony-

stimulating factor-treated human neutrophils. *J Immunol* 1993; 151:6399–6409.

212. Moore MAS. Coordinate actions of hematopoietic growth factors in stimulation of bone marrow function. In Sporn MB, Roberts AB, eds. *Handbook of experimental pharmacology–peptide growth factors and their receptors*, Vol 95/II. New York, Springer-Verlag, 1990:299–344.

213. Richardson MD, Brownlie CE, Shankland GS. Enhanced phagocytosis and intracellular killing of *Candida albicans* by GM-CSF-activated human neutrophils. *J Med Vet Mycol* 1992;30:433–441.

214. Villalta F, Kierszenbaum F. Effects of human colony-stimulating factor on the uptake and destruction of a pathogenic parasite (trypanosoma cruzi) by human neutrophils. *J Immunol* 1986;137:1703–1707.

215. Kowanko IC, Ferrante A, Harvey DP, et al. Granulocyte-macrophage colony-stimulating factor augments neutrophil killing of Torulopsis glabrata and stimulates neutrophil respiratory burst and degranulation. *Clin Exp Immunol* 1991;83:225–230.

216. Weisbart RH, Kacena A, Schuh A, et al. GM-CSF induces human neutrophil IgA-mediated phagocytosis by an IgA Fc receptor activation mechanism. *Nature* 1988;332:647–648.

217. Baldwin GC, Chung GY, Kaslander C, et al. Colony-stimulating factor enhancement of myeloid effector cell cytotoxicity towards neuroectodermal tumour cells. *Br J Haematol* 1993;83:545–553.

218. Barker E, Reisfeld RA. A mechanism for neutrophil-mediated lysis of human neuroblastoma cells. *Cancer Res* 1993;53:362–367.

219. Neuman E, Huleatt JW, Vargas H, et al. Regulation of MHC class I synthesis and expression by human neutrophils. *J Immunol* 1992;148:3520–3527.

220. Gosselin EJ, Wardwell K, Rigby WF, et al. Induction of MHC class II on human polymorphonuclear neutrophils by granulocyte-macrophage colony-stimulating factor, IFN-gamma, and IL-3. *J Immunol* 1993;151:1482–1490.

221. Griffin JD, Spertini O, Ernst TJ, et al. Granulocyte-macrophage colony-stimulating factor and other cytokines regulate surface expression of the leukocyte adhesion molecule-1 on human neutrophils, monocytes, and their precursors. *J Immunol* 1990;145:576–584.

222. Yong KL. Granulocyte colony-stimulating factor (G-CSF) increases neutrophil migration across vascular endothelium independent of an effect on adhesion: comparison with granulocyte-macrophage colony-stimulating factor (GM-CSF). *Br J Haematol* 1996;94:40–47.

223. Masuda T, Suda Y, Shimura S, et al. Airway epithelial cells enhance eosinophil survival. *Respiration* 1992;59:238–242.

224. Hallsworth MP, Litchfield TM, Lee TH. Glucocorticoids inhibit granulocyte-macrophage colony-stimulating factor-1 and interleukin-5 enhanced in vitro survival of human eosinophils. *Immunology* 1992;75:382–385.

225. Dibbert B, Daigle J, Braun D, et al. Role for Bcl-xL in delayed eosinophil apoptosis mediated by granulocyte-macrophage colony-stimulating factor and interleukin-5. *Blood* 1998;92:778–783.

226. Van der Bruggen T, Kok PT, Raaijmakers JA, et al. Cytokine priming of the respiratory burst in human eosinophils in Ca2+ independent and accompanied by induction of tyrosine kinase activity. *J Leukoc Biol* 1993;53:347–353.

227. Abu-Ghazalch RI, Kita H, Gleich GJ. Eosinophil activation and function in health and disease. *Immunol Ser* 1992;57:137–167.

228. Koenderman L, Hermans SW, Capel PJ, et al. Granulocyte-macrophage colony-stimulating factor induces sequential activation and deactivation of binding via a low-affinity IgG Fc receptor, hFc gamma R11, on human eosinophils. *Blood* 1993;81:2413–2419.

229. Tomioka K, MacGlashan DW Jr, Lichtenstein LM, et al. GM-CSF regulates human eosinophil responses to F-Met peptide and platelet activating factor. *J Immunol* 1993;151:4989–4997.

230. Lopez AF, Williamson DJ, Gamble JR, et al. Recombinant human granulocyte-macrophage colony-stimulating factor stimulates in vitro mature human neutrophil and eosinophil function, surface receptor expression and survival. *J Clin Invest* 1986;78:1220–1228.

231. Fabian I, Kletter Y, Mor S, et al. Activation of human eosinophil and neutrophil functions by haematopoietic growth factors: comparisons of IL-1, IL-3, IL-5 and GM-CSF. *Br J Haematol* 1992;80:137–143.

232. Lopez M, Martinache C, Canepa S, et al. Autologous lymphocytes prevent the death of monocytes in culture and promote, as do GM-CSF, IL-3, and M-CSF, their differentiation into macrophages. *J Immunol Methods* 1993;159:29–38.

233. Wang JM, Colella S, Allavena P, et al. Chemotactic activity of human recombinant granulocyte-macrophage colony-stimulating factor. *Immunology* 1987;60:439–444.

234. Horiguchi J, Warren MK, Kufe D. Expression of the macrophage-specific colony-stimulating factor in human monocytes treated with granulocyte-macrophage colony-stimulating factor. *Blood* 1987;69: 1259–1261.

235. Cannistra SA, Rambaldo A, Spriggs DR, et al. Human granulocyte-macrophage colony-stimulating factor induces expression of the tumor necrosis factor gene by the U937 cell line and by normal human monocytes. *J Clin Invest* 1987;79:1720–1728.

236. Kelsey SM, Allen PD, Razak K, et al. Induction of surface tumor necrosis factor (TNF) expression and possible facilitation of surface TNF release from human monocytic cells by granulocyte-macrophage colony-stimulating factor or gamma interferon in combination with 1,25-dihydroxyvitamin D3. *Exp Hematol* 1993;21:864–869.

237. Oster W, Brach MA, Gruss HJ, et al. Interleukin-1 beta (IL-1 beta) expression in human blood mononuclear phagocytes is differentially regulated by granulocyte-macrophage colony-stimulating factor (GM-CSF), M-CSF, and IL-3. *Blood* 1992;79:1260–1265.

238. Berger AE, Carter DB, Hankey SO, et al. Cytokine regulation of the interleukin-1 receptor antagonist protein in U937 cells. *Eur J Immunol* 1993;23:39–45.

239. Yuo A, Kitagawa S, Motoyoshi K, et al. Rapid priming of human monocytes by human hematopoietic growth factors: granulocyte-macrophage colony-stimulating factor (CSF), macrophage-CSF, and interleukin-3 selectively enhance superoxide release triggered by receptor-mediated agonists. *Blood* 1992;79:1553–1557.

240. Hamilton JA, Whitty GA, Stanton H, et al. Effects of macrophage-colony-stimulating factor on human monocytes: induction of expression of urokinase-type plasminogen activator, but not of secreted prostaglandin E2, interleukin-6, interleukin-1, or tumor necrosis factor-alpha. *J Leukoc Biol* 1993;53:707–714.

241. Gabrilove JL, Welte K, Harris P, et al. Pluripoietin alpha: a second human hematopoietic colony-stimulating factor produced by the human bladder carcinoma cell line 5637. *Proc Natl Acad Sci U S A* 1986;83:2478–2482.

242. Rossman MD, Ruiz P, Comber P, et al. Modulation of macrophage Fc gamma receptors by rGM-CSF. *Exp Hematol* 1993;21:177–183.

243. De Nichilo MO, Burns GF. Granulocyte macrophage and macrophage colony-stimulating factors differentially regulate alpha v integrin expression on cultured human macrophages. *Proc Natl Acad Sci U S A* 1993;90:2517–2521.

244. Kasinrerk W, Baumruker T, Majdic O, et al. CD1 molecule expression on human monocytes induced by granulocyte-macrophage colony-stimulating factor. *J Immunol* 1993;150:579–584.

245. Sadhegi R, Feldmann M, Hawrylowicz C. Upregulation of HLA class II, but not intercellular adhesion molecule 1 (ICAM-1) by granulocyte-macrophage colony-stimulating factor (GM-CSF) or interleukin-3 (IL-3) in synergy with dexamethasone. *Eur Cytokine Netw* 1992;3:373–380.

246. Charak BS, Agah R, Mazumder A. Granulocyte macrophage colony-stimulating factor-induced antibody-dependent cellular cytotoxicity in bone marrow macrophages: application in bone marrow transplantation. *Blood* 1993;81:3474–3479.

247. Ho JL, He SH, Rios MJ, et al. Interleukin-4 inhibits human macrophage activation by tumor necrosis factor, granulocyte-macrophage colony-stimulating factor, and interleukin-3 for anti-leishmanial activity and oxidative burst capacity. *J Infect Dis* 1992;165:344–351.

248. Bermudez LE. Differential mechanisms of intracellular killing of mycobacterium avium and listeria monocytogenes by activated human and murine macrophages. The role of nitric-oxide. *Clin Exp Immunol* 1993;91:277–281.

249. Weiser SY, van Niel A, Clark SC, et al. Recombinant human granulocyte-macrophage colony-stimulating factor activates intracellular killing of Leishmania donovanii by human monocyte-derived macrophages. *J Exp Med* 1987;166:1436–1446.

250. Calderone R, Sturtevant J. Macrophage interactions with Candida. [Review] *Immunol Ser* 1994;60:505–515.

251. Newman SL, Gootee L. Colony-stimulating factors activate human

macrophages to inhibit intracellular growth of Histoplasma capsulatum yeasts. *Infect Immun* 1992;60:4593–4597.

252. Fontt FO, De Baetselier P, Heirman C, Thielemans K, Lucas R, Vray B. Effects of granulocyte-macrophage colony-stimulating factor and tumor necrosis factor alpha on Trypanosoma cruzi trypomastigotes. *Infect Immun* 1998;66:2722–2727.

253. Williams MA, Withington S, Newland AC, Kelsey SM. Monocyte anergy in septic shock is associated with a predilection to apoptosis and is reversed by granulocyte-macrophage colony-stimulating factor ex vivo. *J Infect Dis* 1998;178:1421–1433.

254. Salh B, Hoeflick K, Kwan W, Pelech S. Granulocyte-macrophage colony-stimulating factor and interleukin-3 potentiate interferon-gamma-mediated endothelin production by human monocytes: Role of protein kinase C. *Immunology* 1998;95:473–479.

255. Akagawa KS, Takasuka N, Nozaki Y, et al. Generation of CD1⁺ReIB⁺ dendritic cells and tartrate-resistant acid phosphatase-positive osteoclast-like multinucleate giant cells from human monocytes. *Blood* 1996;88:4029–4039.

256. Modrowski D, Lomri A, Marie PJ. Endogenous GM-CSF is involved as an autocrine growth factor for human osteoblastic cells. *J Cell Phys* 1997;170:35–46.

257. Ragnahammar P, Frodin J-E, Trotta PP, Mellstedt H. Cytotoxicity of white blood cells activated by granulocyte-colony stimulating factor, granulocyte-macrophage colony stimulating factor and macrophage-colony stimulating factor against tumor cells in the presence of various monoclonal antibodies. *Cancer Immunol Immunother* 1994;39:254–260.

258. Baxevanis CN, Dedoussis GVZ, Papadopoulos NG, et al. Enhanced human lymphokine-activated killer cell function after brief exposure to granulocyte-macrophage colony stimulating factor. *Cancer* 1995; 76:1253–1260.

259. Dong Z, Kumar R, Yang X, Fiedler IJ. Macrophage metalloelastase is responsible for the generation of angiostatin in Lewis lung carcinoma. *Cell* 1997;88:801–805.

260. Banchereau J, Steinman RM. Dendritic cells and the control of immunity. *Nature* 1998;392:245–252.

261. Young JW, Szabolcs P, Moore MAS. Identification of dendritic cell colony-forming units among normal human CD34⁺ bone marrow progenitors that are expanded by c-kit-ligand and yield pure dendritic cell colonies in the presence of granulocyte/macrophage colony-stimulating factor and tumor necrosis factor a. *J Exp Med* 1995;182:1111–1120.

262. Zhang X, Ren R. Bcr-Abl efficiently induces a myeloproliferative disease and production of excess interleukin-3 and granulocyte-macrophage colony-stimulating factor in mice: A novel model for chronic myelogenous leukemia. *Blood* 1998;92:3829–3840.

263. Szabolcs P, Avigan D, Gezelter S, et al. Dendritic cells and macrophages can mature independently from a human bone marrow-derived, post-colony-forming unit intermediate. *Blood* 1996;87:4520–4530.

264. Tarte R, Klein B. Dendritic cell-based vaccine: a promising approach for cancer immunotherapy. *Leukemia* 1999;13:653–663.

265. Randolph GJ, Beaulieu S, Lebecque S, Steinman RM, Muller WA. Differentiation of monocytes into dendritic cells in a model of transendothelial trafficking. *Science* 1998;282:480–483.

266. Moore MAS, Spitzer G, Williams N, Metcalf D, Buckley J. Agar culture studies in 127 cases of untreated acute leukemia. The prognostic value of reclassification of leukemia according to in vitro growth characteristics. *Blood* 1974;44:1–6.

267. Freedman MH, Grunberger T, Correra P, Axelrad AA, Dube ID, Cohen A. Autocrine and paracrine growth control by granulocyte-macrophage colony-stimulating factor of acute lymphoblastic leukemia cells. *Blood* 1993;81:3068–3075.

268. Duhrsen U, Stahl J, Gough NM. In vivo transformation of factor-dependent hemopoietic cells: role of intracisternal A-particle transposition for growth factor gene activation. *EMBO J* 1990;9:1087–1096.

269. Zhang X, Ren R. Bcr-Abl efficiently induces a myeloproliferative disease and production of excess interleukin-3 and granulocyte-macrophage colony-stimulating factor in mice: a novel model for chronic myelogenous leukemia. *Blood* 1998;92:3829–3840.

270. Cannistra SA, Groshek P, Griffin JD. Granulocyte-macrophage colony-stimulating factor enhances the cytotoxic effect of cytosine arabinoside in acute myeloblastic leukemia and in the myeloid blast crisis phase of chronic myeloid leukemia. *Leukemia* 1989;3: 328–334.

271. Stanley E, Lieschke GJ, Grail D, et al. Granulocyte-macrophage colony-stimulating factor-deficient mice show no major perturbation of hematopoiesis but develop a characteristic pulmonary pathology. *Proc Natl Acad Sci U S A* 1994;91:5592–5596.

272. Campbell JK, Rich MJ, Bischof RJ, Dunn AR, Grail D, Hamilton JA. Protection from collagen-induced arthritis in granulocyte-macrophage colony-stimulating factor-deficient mice. *J Immunol* 1998;161:3639–3644.

273. Wada H, Noguchi Y, Marino MW, Dunn AR, Old LJ. T cell functions in granulocyte/macrophage colony-stimulating factor deficient mice. *Proc Natl Acad Sci U S A* 1997;94:12557–12561.

274. Vremec D, Lieschke GJ, Dunn AR, Robb L, Metcalf D, Shortman K. The influence of granulocyte/macrophage colony-stimulating factor on dendritic cell levels in mouse lymphoid organs. *Eur J Immunol* 1997;27:40–44.

275. Nishinakamura R, Miyajima A, Mee PJ, Tybulewicz VLJ, Murray R. Hematopoiesis in mice lacking the entire granulocyte-macrophage colony-stimulating factor/Interleukin-3/Interleukin-5 functions. *Blood* 1996;88:2458–2464.

276. Metcalf D, Nicola NA, Mifsud S, Di Rago L. Receptor clearance obscures the magnitude of granulocyte-macrophage colony-stimulating factor responses in mice to endotoxin or local infections. *Blood* 1999;93:1579–1585.

277. Metcalf D, Begley CG, Williamson DJ, et al. Hemopoietic responses in mice injected with purified recombinant murine GM-CSF. *Exp Hematol* 1987;15:1–10.

278. Pojda Z, Molineux G, Dexter TM. Effects of long-term in vivo treatment of mice with purified murine recombinant GM-CSF. *Exp Hematol* 1989;17:1100–1104.

279. Lang RA, Metcalf D, Cuthbertson RA, et al. Transgenic mice expressing a hemopoietic growth factor gene (GM-CSF) develop accumulations of macrophages, blindness, and a fatal syndrome of tissue damage. *Cell* 1987:51:675–686.

280. Johnson JR, Gonda TJ, Metcalf D, et al. A lethal myeloproliferative syndrome in mice transplanted with bone marrow. cells infected with a retrovirus expressing granulocyte-macrophage colony-stimulating factor. *EMBO J* 1989;8:441–448.

281. Givner LB, Nagaraj SK, Hyperimmune human IgG or recombinant human granulocyte-macrophage colony-stimulating factor as adjunctive therapy for group B streptococcal sepsis in newborn rats. *J Pediatr* 1993;122:774–779.

282. Morrissey PJ, Charrier K. GM-CSF administration augments the survival of ITY-resistant A/J mice. but not ITY-susceptible C57BL/6 mice to a lethal challenge with salmonella typhimurium. *J Immunol* 1990;144:557–561.

283. Donohue RE, Schra J, Metzger M, et al. Human IL-3 and GM-CSF act synergistically in stimulating hematopoiesis in primates. *Science* 1989;241:1820–1823.

284. Nienhuis AW, Donahue RE, Karlsson S, et al. Recombinant human granulocyte-macrophage colony-stimulating factor shortens the period of neutropenia after autologous bone marrow transplantation in a primate model. *J Clin Invest* 1987;80:573–577.

285. Neelis KJ, Hartong SCC, Egeland T, Thomas GR, Elton DL, Wagemaker G. The efficacy of single-dose administration of thrombopoietin with coadministration of either granulocyte/macrophage or granulocyte colony-stimulating factor in myelosuppressed rhesus monkeys. *Blood* 1997;90:2565–2568.

286. Disis ML, Bernhard H, Shiota FM, et al. Granulocyte-macrophage colony-stimulating factor: an effective adjuvant for protein and peptide-based vaccines. *Blood* 1996;88:202–210.

287. Nakazaki Y, Tani K, Lin ZT, et al. Vaccine effect of granulocyte-macrophage colony-stimulating factor or CD80 gene-transduced murine hematopoietic tumor cells and their cooperative enhancement of antitumor immunity. *Gene Ther* 1998;5:1355–1362.

288. Nagai E, Ogawa T, Kielian T, Ikubo A. Suzuki T. Irradiated tumor cells adenovirally engineered to secrete granulocyte/macrophage colony-stimulating factor establish antitumor immunity and eliminate pre-existing tumors in syngeneic mice. *Cancer Immunol Immunother* 1998;47:72–80.

289. Ishibashi T, Yokoyama K, Shindo J, et al. Potent cholesterol-lowering effect by human granulocyte-macrophage colony-stimulating factor

in rabbits. Possible implication of enhancement of macrophage functions and an increase in mRNA for VLDL receptor. *Arterioscler Thromb* 1994;14:1534–1541.

290. Ihle JN, Keller J, Oroszlan S, et al. Biological properties of homogeneous interleukin-3. I. Demonstration of WEHI-3 growth factor activity, mast cell growth factor activity, P-cell stimulating factor activity, colony-stimulating factor activity, and histamine-producing factor activity. *J Immunol* 1983;131:282–287.

291. Fung MC, Hapel AJ, Ymer S, et al. Molecular cloning of cDNA for mouse interleukin-3. *Nature* 1984;307:233–236.

292. Yang YC, Ciarletta AB, Temple PA, et al. Human IL-3 (multi-CSF): identification by expression cloning of a novel hematopoietic growth factor related to murine IL-3. *Cell* 1986;47:3–10.

293. Yang Y-C. Human interleukin-3: an overview. In: Garland JM, Quesenberry PJ, Hilton DJ, eds. *Colony-stimulating factors: molecular and cellular biology*, 2nd ed. New York: Marcel Dekker, 1997:227–254.

294. Barry SC, Bagley CJ, Phillips J, et al. Two contiguous residues in human interleukin-3, Asp21 and Glu22 selectively interact with the alpha- and beta-chains of its receptor and participate in function. *J Biol Chem* 1994;269:8488–8492.

295. Sato N, Miyajima A. A multimeric cytokine receptor: common versus specific functions. *Curr Opin Cell Biol* 1994;6:174–179.

296. Hara T, Miyajima A. Two distinct functional high affinity receptors for mouse interleukin-3 (IL-3). *EMBO J* 1993;11:1875–1880.

297. Jubinsky PT, Krijanovski OI, Nathan DG, Tavernier J, Sieff CA. The beta chain of the interleukin-3 receptor functionally associates with the erythropoietic receptor. *Blood* 1997;90:1867–1873.

298. Itoh N, Yonehara S, Schreurs J, et al. Cloning of an interleukin-3 receptor: a member of a distinct receptor gene family. *Science* 1990;247:324–327.

299. Chaturvedi P, Reddy MV, Reddy EP. Src kinases and not JAKs activate STATs during IL-3 induced myeloid cell proliferation. *Oncogene* 1998;16:1749–1758.

300. Pearson MA, O'Farrell AM, Dexter TM, Whetton AD, Owen-Lynch PJ, Heyworth CM. Investigation of the molecular mechanism underlying growth factor synergy: the role of ERK 2 activation in synergy. *Growth Factors* 1998;15:293–306.

301. Steinman RA, Iro A. Suppression of G-CSF-mediated Stat signaling by IL-3. *Leukemia* 1999;13:54–61.

302. Callus BA, Mathey-Prevot B. Interleukin-3-induced activation of the JAK/STAT pathway is prolonged by proteasome inhibitors. *Blood* 1998;91:3182–3192.

303. del Peso L, Gonzalez-Garcia M, Page C, Herrera R, Nunez G. Interleukin-3-induced phosphorylation of BAD through the protein kinase Akt. *Science* 1997;278:687–689.

304. Songyang Z, Baltimore D, Cantley LC, Kaplan DR, Franke TF. Interleukin-3-dependent survival by the Akt protein kinase. *Proc Natl Acad Sci U S A* 1997;94:11345–11350.

305. Poommopanit PB, Chen B, Oltvai ZN. Interleukin-3 induces the phosphorylation of a distinct fraction of bcl-2. *J Biol Chem* 1999;274:1033–1039.

306. Tago K, Kaziro Y, Satoh T. Functional involvement of mSos in interleukin-3 and thrombin stimulation of the Ras, mitogen-activated protein kinase pathway in BaF3 murine hematopoietic cells. *J Biochem* 1998;123:659–667.

307. Besancon F, Atfi A, Gespach C, Cayre YE, Bourgeade MF. Evidence for a role of NF-kappaB in the survival of hematopoietic cells mediated by interleukin 3 and the oncogenic TEL/platelet-derived growth factor receptor beta fusion protein. *Proc Natl Acad Sci U S A* 1998;95:8081–8086.

308. Nagata Y, Moriguchi T, Nishida E, Todokoro K. Activation of p38 MAP kinase pathway by erythropoietin and interleukin-3. *Blood* 1997;90:929–934.

309. Mathey-Prevot B, Andrews NC, Murphy HS, Kreissman SG, Nathan DG. Positive and negative elements regulate human interleukin-3 expression. *Proc Natl Acad Sci U S A* 1990;87:5046–5050.

310. Davies K, TePas EC, Nathan DG, Mathey-Prevot B. Interleukin-3 expression in activated T-cells involves an inducible T-cell specific factor and an octamer binding protein. *Blood* 1993;81:928–934.

311. Gottschalk LR, Giannoa DM, Emerson SG. Molecular regulation of the human IL-3 gene: inducible T-cell-restricted expression requires

312. Sonoda Y, Yang YC, Wong GG, et al. Analysis in serum-free culture of the targets of recombinant human hemopoietic growth factors: interleukin-3 and granulocyte-macrophage colony-stimulating factor are specific for early developmental stages. *Proc Natl Acad Sci U S A* 1988;85:4360–4364.

313. Warren DJ, Moore MAS. Synergism among interleukin-1, interleukin-3, and interleukin-5 in the production of eosinophils from primitive hemopoietic stem cells. *J Immunol* 1988;140:94–99.

314. Lewis JL, Marley SB, Blackett NM, Szydlo R, Goldman JM, Gordon MY. Interleukin-3 (IL-3), but not stem cell factor (SCF), increases self-renewal by human erythroid burst-forming units (BFU-E) in vitro. *Cytokine* 1998;10:49–54.

315. Dolzhanskiy A, Hirst J, Basch RS, Karpatkin S. Complementary and antagonistic effects of IL-3 in the early development of human megakaryocytes in culture. *Br J Haematol* 1998;100:415–426.

316. Shibayama H, Anzai N, Braun SE, Fukuda S, Mantel C, Broxmeyer HE. H-Ras is involved in the inside-out signaling pathway of interleukin-3-induced integrin activation. *Blood* 1999;93:1540–1548.

317. Tavassoli M, Konno M, Shiota Y, et al. Enhancement of the grafting efficiency of transplanted marrow cells by preincubation with interleukin-3 and granulocyte-macrophage colony-stimulating factor. *Blood* 1991;77:1599–1606.

318. Van der Loo NCM, Ploemacher RE. Marrow- and spleen-seeding efficiencies of all murine hematopoietic stem cell subsets are decreased by preincubation with hematopoietic growth factors. *Blood* 1995;85:2598–2606.

319. Schofield KP, Rushton G, Humphries MJ, Dexter TM, Gallagher JT. Influence of interleukin-3 and other growth factors on alpha4 beta1 integrin-mediated adhesion and migration of human hematopoietic progenitor cells. *Blood* 1997;90:1858–1866.

320. Peters SO, Kittler ELW, Ramshaw HS, Quesenberry PJ. Ex vivo expansion of murine marrow cells with interleukin-3 (IL-3), IL-6, IL-11, and stem cell factor leads to impaired engraftment in irradiated hosts. *Blood* 1996;87:30–37.

321. Ogawa M, Yonemura Y, Ku H. In vitro expansion of hematopoietic stem cells. *Stem Cells* 1997;15[Suppl 1]:7–11.

322. Matsunaga T, Hirayama F, Yonemura Y, Murray R, Ogawa M. Negative regulation by interleukin-3 (IL-3) of mouse early B-cell progenitors and stem cells in culture: transduction of negative signals by βc and βIL-3 proteins of IL-3 receptor and absence of negative regulation by granulocyte-macrophage colony-stimulating factor. *Blood* 1998;92:901–907.

323. Piacibello W, Sanavio F, Garetto L, et al. Extensive amplification and self-renewal of human primitive hematopoietic stem cells from cord blood. *Blood* 1997;89:2644–2653.

324. Cashman JD, Eaves CJ. Human growth factor-enhanced regeneration of transplantable human hematopoietic stem cells in nonobese diabetic/severe combined immunodeficient mice. *Blood* 1999;93:481–487.

325. Begely CG, Lopez AF, Metcalf D, et al Purified colony-stimulating factor enhances the survival of human neutrophils and eosinophils in vitro: a rapid and sensitive microassay for colony-stimulating factors. *Blood* 1986;68:162–166.

326. Hallsworth MP, Litchfield TM, Lee TH. Glucocorticoids inhibit granulocyte-macrophage colony-stimulating factor-1 and interleukin-5 enhanced in vitro survival of human eosinophils. *Immunology* 1991;75:382–385.

327. Owen WF Jr, Rothenberg ME, Silberstein DS, et al. Regulation of human eosinophil viability, density, and function by granulocyte-macrophage colony stimulating factor in the presence of 3T3 fibroblasts. *J Exp Med* 1987;166:129–141.

328. van der Bruggen T, Kok PT, Raaijmakers A, et al. Cytokine priming of the respiratory burst in human eosinophils is Ca2+ independent and accompanied by induction of tyrosine kinase activity. *J Leukoc Biol* 1993;53:347–353.

329. Koenderman L, Hermans SW, Capel PI, et al. Granulocyte-macrophage colony stimulating factor induces sequential activation and deactivation of binding via a low-affinity IgG Fc receptor, hFc gamma RII, on human eosinophils. *Blood* 1993;81:2413–2419.

330. Hartnell A, Kay AB, Wardlaw AJ. Interleukin-3-induced up-regulation of CR3 expression on human eosinophils is inhibited by dexamethasone. *Immunology* 1992;77:488–493.

intact AP-1 and Elf-1 nuclear protein binding sites. *J Exp Med* 1993;178:1681–1692.

331. Abu-Ghazaleh RI, Kita H, Gleich GJ. Eosinophil activation and function in health and disease. *Immunol Ser* 1992;57:137–167.

332. Czech W, Krutmann J, Budnik A, et al. Induction of intercellular adhesion molecule 1 (ICAM-]) expression in normal human eosinophils by inflammatory cytokines. *Invest Derm* 1993;100:417–423.

333. Fabian I, Kletter Y, Mor S, et al. Activation of human eosinophil and neutrophil functions hy haematopoietic growth factors: comparisons of IL-1, IL-3, IL-5 and GM-CSF. *Br J Haematol* 1992;80:137–143.

334. Yung YP, Eger R, Tertian G, et al. Long term in vitro culture of murine mast cells. II. Purification of a mast cell growth factor and its dissociation from TCGF. *J Immunol* 1981;12:794–799.

335. Yamaguchi M, Hirai K, Morita Y, et al. Hemopoietic growth factors regulate the survival of human basophils in vitro. *Int Arch Allergy Immunol* 1992;97:322–329.

336. Tanimoto Y, Takahashi K, Kimura I. Effects of cytokines on human basophil chemotaxis. *Clin Exp Allergy* 1992;27:1020–1025.

337. Yamaguchi M, Hirai K, Shoji S, et al. Haemopoietic growth factors induce human basophil migration in vitro. *Clin Exp Allergy* 1992;22:379–383.

338. Knol EF, Kuijpers TW, Mul FP, et al. Stimulation of human basophils results in homotypic aggregation. A response independent of degranulation. *J Immunol* 1993;151:4926 4933.

339. Bochner BS, McKelvey AA, Strebinsky SA, et al. IL-3 augments adhesiveness for endothelium and CD 11b expression in human basophils but not neutrophils. *J Immunol* 1990;145:1832–1837.

340. Liao TN, Hsieh KH. Characterization of histamine-releasing activity: role of cytokines and IgE heterogeneity. *J Clin Immunol* 1992:12: 248–258.

341. Miadonna A, Salmaso C, Macro MP, et al. Priming and inducing effects of interleukin-3 on histamine release from cord-blood basophils. *Allergy* 1997;52:992–998.

342. Nielsen HV, Johnsen AH, Sanchez JC, Hochstrasser DF, Schiotz PO. Identification of a basophil leukocyte interleukin-3-regulated protein that is identical to IgE-dependent histamine-releasing factor. *Allergy* 1998;53:642–652.

343. Iikura M, Yamaguchi M, Fujisawa T, et al. Secretory IgA induces degranulation of IL-3-primed basophils. *J Immunol* 1998;16:1510–1515.

344. MacGlashan DW Jr, Hubbard WC. IL-3 alters free arachidonic acid generation in C5a-stimulated human basophils. *J Immunol* 1993; 151:6358–6369.

345. Brunner T, Heusser CH, Dahinden CA. Human peripheral blood basophils primed by interleukin 3 (IL-3) produce IL-4 in response to immunoglobulin E receptor stimulation. *J Exp Med* 1993:177:605–611.

346. Sadhegi R, Feldmann M, Hawrylowicz C. Upregulation of HLA class II, but not intercellular adhesion molecule 1 (ICAM-l) by granulocyte-macrophage colony-stimulating factor (GM-CSF) or interleukin-3 (IL-3) in synergy with dexamethasone. *Eur Cytokine Netw* 1992;3:373–380.

347. Frendl G. Interleukin 3: from colony-stimulating factor to pluripotent immunoregulatory cytokine. *Int J Immunopharmacol* 1992;14:421–430.

348. Thomassen MJ, Antal JM, Connors MJ, et al. Immunomodulatory effects of recombinant interleukin-3 treatment on human alveolar macrophages and monocytes. *J Immunother* 1993;14:43–50.

349. Alderson MR, Armitage RJ, Tough TW. CD40 expression by human monocytes: regulation by cytokines and activation of monocytes by the ligand for CD40. *J Exp Med* 1993;178:669–674.

350. Thomassen MJ, Antal JM, Connors MJ, et al. Immunomodulatory effects of recombinant interleukin-3 treatment on human alveolar macrophages and monocytes. *J Immunother* 1993;14:43–50.

351. Lissoni P, Pittalis S, Brivio F, et al. In vitro modulatory effects of interleukin-3 on macrophage activation induced by interleukin-2. *Cancer* 1993;71:2076–2081.

352. Myint YY, Miyakawa K, Naito M, et al. Granulocyte/macrophage colony-stimulating factor and interleukin-3 correct osteopetrosis in mice with osteopetrosis mutation. *Am J Pathol* 1999;154:553–566.

353. Saeland S, Caux C, Favre C, et al. Effects of recombinant human interleukin-3 on CD34-enriched normal hematopoietic progenitors and on myeloblastic leukemic cells. *Blood* 1988;72:1580–1588.

354. Asano Y, Shibata S, Kobayashi S, Okamura S, Akazawa K, Niho Y. Action of interleukin-3 on the proliferation of leukaemic progenitor cell from patients with acute myeloblastic leukaemia. *Clin Lab Haematol* 1998;20:225–229.

355. Cesano A, Lista P, Bellone G, et al. Effect of human interleukin 3 on the susceptibility of fresh leukemic cells to interleukin-2 induced lymphokine activated killing activity. *Leukemia* 1992;6:567–573.

356. Ahmed N, Berridge MV. Regulation of glucose transport by interleukin-3 in growth factor-dependent and oncogene-transformed bone marrow-derived cell lines. *Leukemia Res* 1997;21:609–618.

357. Brizzi MF, Garbarini G, Rossi PR, et al. Interleukin 3 stimulates proliferation and triggers endothelial-leukocyte adhesion molecule-1 gene activation of human endothelial cells. *J Clin Invest* 1993;91: 2887–2892.

358. Korpelainen EI, Gamble JR, Smith WB, et al. The receptor for interleukin-3 is selectively induced in human endothelial cells by tumor necrosis factor alpha and potentiates IL-8 secretion and neutrophil transmigration. *Proc Natl Acad Sci U S A* 1993;90:11137–11141.

359. Tabira T, Chui DH, Fan JP, Shirabe T, Konishi Y. Interleukin-3 and interleukin-3 receptors in the brain. *Ann N Y Acad Sci* 1998;840: 107–116.

360. Lantz CS, Boesiger J, Song CH, et al. Role for interleukin-3 in mast-cell and basophil development and in immunity to parasites. *Nature* 1998;392:90–93.

361. Ichihara M, Hara T, Takagi M, et al. Impaired interleukin-3 (IL-3) response of the A/J mouse is caused by a branch point deletion in the IL-3 receptor alpha subunit gene. *EMBO J* 1995;14:939–950.

362. Mach N, Lantz CS, Galli SJ, et al. Involvement of interleukin-3 in delayed-type hypersensitivity. *Blood* 1998;91:778–783.

363. Lord BI, Molineux G, Testa NG. The kinetic response of haemopoietic precursor cells, in vivo, to highly purified, recombinant interleukin-3. *Lymphokine Res* 1986;5:97–104.

364. Kimoto M, Kindler V, Higaki M, et al. Recombinant murine IL3 fails to stimulate T or B lymphopoiesis in vivo, but enhances immune responses to T cell-dependent antigens. *J Immunol* 1988; 140:1889–1894.

365. Chang JM, Metcalf D, Lang RA, et al. Nonneoplastic hematopoietic myeloproliferative syndrome induced by dysregulated multi-CSF (IL-3) expression. *Blood* 1989;73:1487–1497.

366. Donahue RE, Sechra I, Metzger M, et al. Human IL-3 and GM-CSF act synergistically in stimulating hematopoiesis in primates. *Science* 1989;241:1820–1823.

367. Geissler K, Valent P, Mayer P, et al. Recombinant human interleukin-3 expands the pool of circulating hematopoietic progenitor cells in primates—synergism, with recombinant human granulocyte-macrophage colony-stimulating factor. *Blood* 1990;75:2305–2310.

368. Farese AM, Douglas EW, Seiler FR, et al. Combination protocols of cytokine therapy with interleukin-3 and granulocyte-macrophage colony-stimulating-factor in a primate model of radiation-induced marrow aplasia. *Blood* 1993;82:3012–3018.

369. Williams DE, Dunn JT, Park LS, et al. A GM-CSF/IL-3 fusion protein promotes neutrophil and platelet recovery in sublethally irradiated rhesus monkeys. *Biotechnol Ther* 1993;4:17–29.

370. Gillio AP, Gasparetto C, Laver J, et al. Effects of Interleukin-3 on hematopoietic recovery after 5-fluorouracil or cyclophosphamide treatment of cynomolgus primates. *J Clin Invest* 1990;85:1560–1565.

371. Frasca D, Guidi F, Arbitrio M, et al. Use of hematopoietic cytokines to accelerate the recovery of the immune system in irradiated mice. *Exp Hematol* 1997;25:1167–1171.

372. Ito A, Aoyanagi N, Maki T. Regulation of autoimmune diabetes by interleukin-3-dependent bone marrow-derived cells in NOD mice. *J Autoimmun* 1997;10:331–338.

373. Yoshimura A. The CIS family: Negative regulators of Jak-STAT signaling. *Cytokine Growth Factor Rev* 1998;9:197–204.

374. Nicholson SE, Hilton DJ. The SOCS proteins: A new family of negative regulators of signal transduction. *J Leukoc Biol* 1998;63:665–668.

375. Yoshimura A, Ohkubo T, Kiguchi T, et al. A novel cytokine-inducible gene CIS encodes an SH2-containing protein that binds to tyrosine-phosphorylated interleukin-3 and erythropoietin receptors. *EMBO J* 1995;14:2816–2826.

376. Starr R, Willson TA, Viney EM, et al. A family of cytokine-inducible inhibitors of signalling. *Nature* 1997;387:917–920.

377. DeKoter RP, Walsh JC, Singh H. PU.1 regulates both cytokine-dependent proliferation and differentiation of granulocyte/macrophage progenitors. *EMBO J* 1998;17:4456–4468.

COLONY-STIMULATING FACTORS: CLINICAL APPLICATIONS

Colony-Stimulating Factors in Oncology

JOHN A. GLASPY

The purification and cloning of several cytokines involved in the regulation of neutrophil production or function in the 1980s was a watershed event in experimental hematology and cancer medicine. These cytokines included granulocyte-macrophage colony-stimulating factor (GM-CSF), granulocyte colony-stimulating factor (G-CSF), macrophage colony-stimulating factor, and inter-leukin-3. The availability of recombinant preparations of these molecules facilitated rapid advances in the understanding of basal hematopoiesis and the systemic and local responses to infection. Later, their clinical application led to new approaches for the supportive care of patients undergoing myelosuppressive chemotherapy and chemotherapy dose intensification. The availability of these factors also transformed the practice of bone marrow transplantation. More than a decade after the first patients were treated with recombinant myeloid growth factors, the refinement of these applications continues and new applications are being explored in the fields of cancer immunotherapy and gene therapy.

BIOLOGY OF GRANULOCYTE-MACROPHAGE COLONY-STIMULATING FACTOR AND GRANULOCYTE COLONY-STIMULATING FACTOR

Although several other cytokines influence neutrophil production, survival, and function, two of these molecules, GM-CSF and G-CSF, have been shown to have clear clinical value and are used in most countries in the management of cancer patients. These two cytokines have been the subject of previous review (1,2) and are the focus of this chapter. Although G-CSF and GM-CSF were originally discovered, purified, and cloned based on the ability of conditioned media containing them to support myeloid differentiation and development *in vitro*, the roles played by these factors in the regulation of *in vivo* hematopoiesis and inflammation are distinct. Preclinical and clinical data are reviewed separately because GM-CSF and G-CSF differ in biology and clinical effects.

Human GM-CSF is a 127–amino acid glycoprotein product of a gene located on chromosome 5. GM-CSF acts on a specific receptor complex present on hematopoietic progenitor cells, as well as mature neutrophils, macrophages, and eosinophils. When exposed to GM-CSF *in vitro*, mature macrophages are activated and release secondary cytokines, including G-CSF and inter-feron-α (3). *In vitro*, GM-CSF acts on mature neutrophils to prime them to enhance activity in a variety of neutrophil function assays, including bacterial killing and antibody-dependent cellular cytotoxicity. When recombinant GM-CSF is administered *in vivo*, a transient decrease in neutrophil, eosinophil, and monocyte counts is observed, followed by an increase in the number of these cells circulating (4–6). Neutrophil adhesion to vascular endothelium is enhanced (7), and migration to sites of injury may be inhibited (8). Therapy with GM-CSF results in a prolongation of the circulating half-life of neutrophils and a modest increase in the neutrophil production rate in the marrow (9).

The constitutive role, if any, of GM-CSF in basal hematopoiesis or in the increased neutrophil production rate observed in response to infection ("emergency hematopoiesis") is unclear. Gene knockout studies have shown that mice deficient in GM-CSF have normal numbers of hematopoietic progenitor cells and mature circulating leukocytes but develop alveolar proteinosis and infections in the lung (10). GM-CSF is usually not detectable in the serum of animals or humans, even during neutropenia, active infection, or both. These observations suggest that natural GM-CSF may be produced locally in the tissues as part of the regulation of the inflammatory response and acts in part to immobilize and prime local neutrophils.

Human G-CSF is a 174–amino acid glycoprotein product of a gene located on chromosome 17. G-CSF acts on a specific receptor complex present on hematopoietic progenitor cells, as well as mature neutrophils. G-CSF acts on mature neutrophils to prime them to enhanced activity in a variety of neutrophil function assays, including bacterial killing and antibody-dependent cellular cytotoxicity. The administration of G-CSF results in a

TABLE 1. GOALS OF MYELOID GROWTH FACTOR USE DURING MYELOSUPPRESSIVE CHEMOTHERAPY AND APPROPRIATE CLINICAL EFFICACY AND COST EVALUATIONS

	Goal		
	Decrease Infection Risk during Chemotherapy	Increased Dose Intensity of Chemotherapy	Treatment of Infection with Neutropenia
Appropriate randomized clinical trial	Same chemotherapy regimen in both groups, one group treated with CSF	"Standard" dose chemotherapy vs. higher dose intensity regimen with CSF	Patients with established febrile neutropenia treated with antibiotics with or without CSF
Appropriate clinical end point	Incidence of infection in the treated and untreated groups	Response rate, time to progression, and survival in the two groups	Duration of antibiotic use and hospitalization in the two groups
Appropriate cost-benefit analysis	Cost of CSF treatment balanced against cost of prevented infections and impact of infections on quality of life	Cost of higher chemotherapy doses, toxicity, and CSF balanced against improvement in survival outcomes	Cost of CSF treatment balanced against cost savings in resource use and any quality of life improvements

CSF, colony-stimulating factor.

rapid increase in circulating neutrophils without increases in the numbers of monocytes or eosinophils (11). This increase in neutrophil counts is caused by a significant increase in neutrophil release and production by the marrow and not an increase in the survival of neutrophils in the circulation.

G-CSF appears to be central to basal and emergency hematopoiesis. A nonsense mutation of the G-CSF receptor has been identified in a patient with severe congenital neutropenia. Serum levels of G-CSF are measurable and increase with infection in neutropenic individuals, normal adults, and neonates (12–14), suggesting a systemic role for G-CSF in the regulation of neutrophil numbers and function.

RECOMBINANT MOLECULES

Recombinant human G-CSF (rhG-CSF) is produced in bacteria. Worldwide, two preparations are available: filgrastim and lenograstim. The clinical data regarding their effects are pooled for presentation in this chapter as rhG-CSF because no comparative studies have demonstrated a difference between the biologic or clinical qualities of these two preparations. Three preparations of rhGM-CSF have been introduced into clinical trials, one produced in bacteria, one produced in Chinese hamster ovary cells, and one produced in yeast. Results are pooled for presentation in this chapter as rhGM-CSF because no comparative studies exist that demonstrate a significant difference between these preparations in terms of biology, efficacy, or toxicity. Most of the data available was obtained with the glycosylated proteins (Chinese hamster ovary and yeast–derived) (15,16).

CLINICAL APPLICATIONS OF RECOMBINANT HUMAN GRANULOCYTE-MACROPHAGE COLONY-STIMULATING FACTOR AND RECOMBINANT HUMAN GRANULOCYTE COLONY-STIMULATING FACTOR

The risk of infection during myelosuppressive cancer chemotherapy is directly related to the duration and severity of neutropenia. When the myeloid growth factors were introduced into clinical practice in the early 1990s, the chemotherapy regimens

in use for the treatment of most common cancers used doses and intertreatment intervals chosen to provide the maximum dose intensity with acceptable risks of complicating myelosuppression. Therefore, three distinct possible goals for the integration of myeloid growth factors into clinical practice were developed:

1. Decrease the infection risk associated with chemotherapy.
2. Increase the dose intensity of chemotherapy.
3. Decrease the severity of the established infections in neutropenic patients.

Each approach implies an appropriate design for controlled clinical trials of efficacy and a logical perspective for cost-benefit analysis (Table 1).

Prevention of Infection during Chemotherapy for Nonmyeloid Malignancies

The best-studied application of the myeloid growth factors is their use to decrease the risk of infection associated with a given regimen of myelosuppressive chemotherapy. In evaluating these studies, it is important to recognize that the duration of neutropenia is only an adequate surrogate end point for infection risk to patients if the neutrophils produced during growth factor therapy function normally and the growth factor has no other effects that increase infection risk, such as impairment of migration of otherwise normally functioning neutrophils to sites of tissue injury. This is the rationale underlying the emphasis on randomized trials with a measure of infection rather than the duration or severity of neutropenia as the end point for definitive demonstration of efficacy.

In nonrandomized clinical trials in patients receiving myelosuppressive chemotherapy, treatment with rhG-CSF in doses of 5 to 60 µg per kg per day beginning 24 hours after the chemotherapy was given was associated with a significant shortening of the duration of neutropenia (17–20). In these studies, patients received rhG-CSF during one of two chemotherapy cycles. The duration of neutropenia and incidence of infections observed during treated cycles were compared with earlier or subsequent cycles of the same chemotherapy given without growth factor support. The neutrophils produced during rhG-CSF therapy

TABLE 2. RANDOMIZED CLINICAL TRIALS OF RECOMBINANT HUMAN GRANULOCYTE COLONY-STIMULATING FACTOR FOR THE PREVENTION OF INFECTION DURING MYELOSUPPRESSIVE CHEMOTHERAPY

Clinical Setting (Reference)	Design Features	FN Incidence	Other Observations
Small-cell lung cancer in adults (23)	n = 199 Dose = 230 µg/m²/d Off study if FN event occurred Crossover	77% vs. 40% over six cycles of chemotherapy[a]	Decreased hospitalization,[a] antibiotic use,[a] and confirmed infections[a] in treated group
Small-cell lung cancer in adults (24)	n = 130 Dose = 230 µg/m²/d Dose reduction if FN event occurred No crossover	53% vs. 26% over all cycles[a]	Decreased hospitalization,[a] antibiotic use,[a] dose reduction, and dose delay[a] in the treated group
Advanced cancer in adults (25)	n = 100 Dose = 5 µg/kg/d rhG-CSF ± thymopentin vs. thymopentin vs. placebo	64% vs. 22%[a] No rhG-CSF vs. rhG-CSF groups[a]	—
Inflammatory breast cancer, neoadjuvant (26)	n = 120 Dose = 5 µg/kg/d	Decreased need for hospitalization[a]	Decreased culture-confirmed infections[a] and antibiotic use[a] in the treated group
Acute lymphoblastic leukemia in children, up to nine cycles (27)	n = 34 Dose = 5 µg/kg/d	40% vs. 17% over all cycles[a]	Decreased duration of FN,[a] antibiotic use,[a] and culture-confirmed infections[a] in the treated group
Acute lymphoblastic leukemia in children, induction cycle only (28)	n = 148 Dose = 10 µg/kg/d	Not significantly different	Shorter hospital stays,[a] fewer culture-confirmed infections[a] in the treated group
Acute lymphoblastic leukemia in adults, induction, and consolidation (29)	n = 198 Dose = 5 µg/kg/d		Fewer days in hospital during induction only,[a] fewer deaths during induction[a] in the treated group
Neuroblastoma in children, four cycles of therapy (30)	n = 59 Dose = 5 µg/kg/d No placebo	Not significantly different	Shorter duration of neutropenia,[a] decreased antibiotic use,[a] higher dose intensity,[a] and improved event-free survival[a] in the treated group

FN, febrile neutropenia; rhG-CSF, recombinant human granulocyte colony-stimulating factor.
[a] $p < .05$.

functioned normally in *in vitro* testing (11,21,22). Fewer febrile episodes were observed during rhG-CSF–protected chemotherapy cycles. Although these studies demonstrated that rhG-CSF therapy was associated with a shorter duration of neutropenia after chemotherapy and that the neutrophils produced in response to rhG-CSF appeared to function normally, they did not demonstrate conclusively that rhG-CSF was associated with a reduction in the incidence of infection.

In randomized clinical trials of rhG-CSF for the prevention of infection during chemotherapy, the incidence of febrile neutropenia has been the most commonly used end point for estimating overall infection risk. Eight randomized, placebo-controlled clinical trials of rhG-CSF for the prevention of infection during myelosuppressive chemotherapy have been conducted (23–30). These trials are summarized in Table 2. In these studies, rhG-CSF therapy was initiated 24 hours after the completion of chemotherapy and continued until the nadir in the absolute neutrophil count had resolved. In all instances, rhG-CSF therapy was associated with a decrease in the duration of severe neutropenia. In all but one study (28), the incidence of infectious complications of chemotherapy as measured by the incidence of febrile neutropenia (23–25,27) or hospitalization for infectious complications (26,29) was reduced in patients receiving rhG-CSF. The two small-cell lung cancer studies used the same chemotherapy regimen and were designed in a complementary fashion (23,24). In the Crawford study, patients in the two comparison

groups received the same chemotherapy throughout the study; if a patient developed febrile neutropenia, he or she was withdrawn from blinded study medication and offered open-label rhG-CSF if he or she received placebo. This design permitted insight into the impact of therapy with rhG-CSF on the risk of infection without the complicating factor of differences between study groups in chemotherapy dose intensity. The open-label data also demonstrated the efficacy of rhG-CSF when used as secondary prophylaxis. In the Trillet-Lenoir study, chemotherapy doses were reduced in patients experiencing febrile neutropenia, and patients were removed from study medication. This design facilitated understanding of the impact of rhG-CSF on overall chemotherapy dose intensity and of this dose intensity on other hematologic toxicities and survival outcomes. In the study of children undergoing induction chemotherapy for acute lymphoblastic leukemia, which reported no statistically significant reduction in the incidence of febrile neutropenia associated with rhG-CSF therapy, significant reductions in days of hospitalization and culture-confirmed infections in the treated patients (28) were found. One small randomized, but not placebo-controlled, study of rhG-CSF administered during chemotherapy for Hodgkin's disease did not show a difference in infection outcomes but was substantially underpowered (31). Overall, the large randomized trials of rhG-CSF demonstrated that the use of this agent at doses of 5 to 10 µg per kg per day beginning 24 hours after the last dose of chemother-

TABLE 3. RANDOMIZED CONTROLLED CLINICAL TRIALS OF RECOMBINANT HUMAN GRANULOCYTE-MACROPHAGE COLONY-STIMULATING FACTOR FOR THE PREVENTION OF INFECTION DURING MYELOSUPPRESSIVE CHEMOTHERAPY

Clinical Setting (Reference)	Design Features	Infection Incidence	Other Observations
Lymphoma in adults (35,36)	n = 125 Dose = 400 µg/d for 7 d	Fewer clinically relevant infections 70% vs. 48%[a]	Fewer patients with infection[a] and days of hospitalization for infection[a]
Small-cell lung cancer in adults (38)	n = 290 No placebo Dose = 5, 10, or 20 µg/kg/d for 9 d Chemotherapy dose intensity higher in the rhGM-CSF after cycle 1	Fewer patients receiving 10 µg/kg/d required i.v. antibiotics in cycle 1 (29% vs. 11%)[a]	Fever more common in 10- and 20-µg/kg cohorts than observation arm
Acute lymphoblastic leukemia in children, induction and intensification cycles (37)	n = 40 Dose = 5.5 µg/kg/d for 6 d	Not significantly different	No difference in number of days of fever, days of neutropenia, days in hospital or infections
Germ cell tumors in adults (39)	n = 104 No placebo Dose = 10 µg/kg/d for 9 d Randomized to rhGM-CSF on cycles 1 and 2 vs. 3 and 4	Fewer clinically relevant infections in cycle 1, 45% vs. 24%[a] No difference in cycle 2	Fewer infections during neutropenia,[a] infections requiring antibiotics[a] and infections[a] in cycle 1 14% of cycles of rhGM-CSF discontinued for toxicity
Non–small-cell lung cancer in adults (40)	n = 230 No placebo Patients received concurrent radiotherapy and chemotherapy	Higher incidence of intravenous antibiotic use with rhGM-CSF	Increased thrombocytopenia[a] and days in hospital[a] with rhGM-CSF[a]
Lymphoma or breast cancer in adults (41)	n = 56 Dose = 500 µg/m²/d	Not significantly different	Shorter duration of FN in cycle 1[a] not subsequent cycles, possible worsening of thrombocytopenia in the rhGM-CSF group
Sarcoma in children and young adults (42)	n = 37 No placebo Dose = 5–15 µg/kg/d, begun in cycle 3	Not significantly different	More severe thrombocytopenia with rhGM-CSF
Breast cancer, adjuvant treatment (43)	n = 142 Dose = 250 µg/m²/d for 12 days All patients received ciprofloxacin	Not significantly different	Higher dose intensity and more thrombocytopenia in the rhGM-CSF group

FN, febrile neutropenia; rhGM-CSF, recombinant human granulocyte-macrophage colony-stimulating factor.
[a]$p <.05$.

apy and continuing until hematologic recovery has occurred is associated with a reduction in infectious complications.

In nonrandomized trials in patients undergoing myelosuppressive chemotherapy, therapy with rhGM-CSF was associated with reduction in the duration of neutropenia (32). In these studies, the duration of neutropenia after a first cycle of chemotherapy during which patients received rhGM-CSF was compared with the duration during a subsequent untreated cycle. Although the neutrophils produced in response to rhGM-CSF functioned normally in *ex vivo* functional assays, some data suggested that rhGM-CSF therapy may inhibit neutrophil migration to sites of tissue injury (33,34).

Eight randomized controlled trials of rhGM-CSF during myelosuppressive chemotherapy have been published (35–43). They are summarized in Table 3. In addition to these studies, a randomized clinical trial of rhGM-CSF administered at a dose of 5 mcg per kg per day compared with observation during chemotherapy for breast cancer showed no difference in the rate of febrile neutropenia but was underpowered (n = 20) to detect a difference if present (44). Another small but nonrandomized, historically controlled trial of rhGM-CSF during intensive chemotherapy for solid tumors in children showed no impact of the factor on the incidence of febrile neutropenia (45).

The results of these studies are less consistent than those observed with rhG-CSF, and their interpretation is more prob-

lematic. None of the studies were designed in the same fashion as the Crawford rhG-CSF study with patients meeting the primary infection end point removed from the study drug (23). Hence, an imbalance in chemotherapy dose intensity over multiple chemotherapy cycles between the study arms in some studies complicates the analysis of the impact of rhGM-CSF on infection risk. The lack of double-blinding in several of the studies complicates the analysis of efficacy and toxicity (38–40,42). The analysis and reporting of alpha error estimates for multiple secondary end points for measuring infection incidence in several of the studies introduced statistical issues that were not addressed in study design or compensated for in the reported analyses. The intensity of surveillance for infection end points, coadministration of prophylactic antibiotics, and incidence of infection in the control group were too low in one study for it to have the power to detect an impact of rhGM-CSF on infection risk because of the choice of chemotherapy regimen (43). The use of fixed durations of rhGM-CSF therapy rather than treatment until neutropenia had resolved may have resulted in underestimates of the efficacy and toxicity of rhGM-CSF in several studies (35,37,39,43,46).

Three potential explanations exist for the differences observed in these randomized trials of rhG-CSF and rhGM-CSF, each of which is consistent with the data available to date. First, it is possible that rhGM-CSF does not decrease the risk of infection in patients undergoing myelosuppressive chemotherapy. This may be because of its relatively modest impact on neutrophil production rate or a deleterious effect on neutrophil migration into tissues. Second, it is possible that rhGM-CSF does lower infection risk, but fevers induced by the drug have obscured the benefit in randomized trials. Finally, rhGM-CSF given at doses of 5 to 10 μg per kg per day may reduce the risk of infection in this setting, and one or all of the available preparations may not produce fever in a proportion of patients large enough to obscure this effect (35,43). It is possible that some of the randomized trials have failed to detect this benefit because of design and power issues. It will be possible to design future clinical trials to further clarify the efficacy of rhGM-CSF.

The efficacy of rhGM-CSF therapy for decreasing infection risks in patients undergoing myelosuppressive chemotherapy remains controversial. The American Society of Clinical Oncology guidelines for myeloid growth factor use do not distinguish between rhGM-CSF and rhG-CSF (47,48); rhG-CSF, not rhGM-CSF, is approved for this indication by the U.S. Food and Drug Administration. No adequate randomized trials comparing the efficacy of the two factors for the prevention of infection during chemotherapy have been conducted. One randomized study compared rhG-CSF and rhGM-CSF for the treatment of patients who were afebrile but neutropenic after myelosuppressive chemotherapy, a setting in which neither factor has been clearly shown to alter infection risk (49). This study showed no difference in infection end points between the two groups. It was substantially underpowered to demonstrate equivalence and did not include a placebo group.

In randomized trials, therapy with a myeloid growth factor has not been shown to increase survival in any group of patients undergoing myelosuppressive chemotherapy. Indirect evidence exists, particularly in studies of patients receiving chemotherapy for Hodgkin's disease or early stage breast cancer, that chemotherapy dose reductions or delays may compromise survival outcomes. These observations may be relevant to secondary prophylaxis with myeloid growth factors after an episode of febrile neutropenia during a prior cycle of chemotherapy in patients undergoing chemotherapy with curative intent. Similarly, randomized trials have not demonstrated that myeloid growth factor therapy is associated with an improvement in quality of life, although evidence exists that a reduction in mucositis may occur (43,50). It seems plausible that a serious infection would, if measured, be shown to compromise quality of life more than daily growth factor injections.

The lack of definitive demonstration in randomized trials of a survival or quality of life advantage of myeloid growth factors given to patients during myelosuppressive chemotherapy has resulted in an intense focus on the costs associated with their use. The cost impact of the myeloid factors used in this setting depends on the cost of treating the patients with myeloid growth factors and the cost savings realized through prevented infections. Using the clinical data from the randomized trial of rhG-CSF, which served as the registration trial in the United States (23), coupled with additional cost data, two studies examined these cost offsets (51,52). In both analyses, the cost offsets were found to depend on several variables but were most sensitive to the risk of febrile neutropenia if the growth factor was not given (53). Both studies estimated that, in most situations, the cost of administering the growth factor to all patients would be completely offset by the cost savings in prevented infections if the risk of febrile neutropenia without growth factor was approximately 40% or greater. These models predicted that at lower risks of febrile neutropenia, myeloid growth factor use is associated with an increase in overall cost, the magnitude of this increase dependent on the magnitude of the risk. These increased costs must be justified by an improvement in survival or quality of life outcomes (54–56).

It is hoped that additional data clarifying the survival or quality of life benefits of myeloid growth factors will be forthcoming. It is reasonable to use myeloid growth factors as primary prophylaxis in patients in whom the risk of serious infection approaches 40% and as secondary prophylaxis in patients in whom the goal of therapy is cure or prolonged survival. Evidence exists that dose delay or dose reduction compromises that outcome (57).

Treatment of Febrile Neutropenia

Although patients with febrile neutropenia usually have increased serum levels of endogenous G-CSF by the time they present clinically, pharmacologic doses of myeloid growth factors might increase the rate of their recovery and benefit these patients. The myeloid growth factors have been used in the treatment of patients in whom febrile neutropenia has developed in the absence of prophylactic growth factor use. In this setting, the evaluation of efficacy can only be made in randomized trials comparing antibiotic therapy alone with antibiotics with growth factor. Such trials have been published using rhGM-CSF in adults (58–60) and children (61) or rhG-CSF in adults (58,62). They are summarized in Table 4. For adults with established febrile neutropenia, the routine use of myeloid growth factor therapy is not supported by this group of studies and is probably not cost effective, although some evidence to the contrary exists (58). It is reasonable to use myeloid growth factor therapy in the occasional ill patient in whom a 1- to 3-day reduction in the duration of neutropenia may favorably impact outcome, because both growth factors have been shown to increase the rate of neutrophil recovery. This approach is consistent with the American Society of Clinical Oncology guidelines. The duration of neutropenia is longer after many pediatric chemotherapy regimens, and this may explain the efficacy of myeloid growth factor therapy for febrile neutropenia in these patients. In this setting, the use of rhGM-CSF is supported by the current data, although confirmatory studies and cost analyses are desirable.

Use in Patients with Acute Nonlymphocytic Leukemia

Early concerns existed regarding the safety of myeloid growth factor therapy for patients with acute nonlymphocytic leukemia (ANL) because ANL cells frequently bear receptors for G-CSF and GM-CSF. Four randomized trials have been published (63–66). These trials are summarized in Table 5. These data indicate that

TABLE 4. RANDOMIZED CLINICAL TRIALS OF RECOMBINANT HUMAN GRANULOCYTE-MACROPHAGE COLONY-STIMULATING FACTOR OR RECOMBINANT HUMAN COLONY-STIMULATING FACTOR FOR THE TREATMENT OF FEBRILE NEUTROPENIA

Growth Factor and Dose (Reference)	Design Features	Impact on Hospital or Antibiotic Days	Other Observations
rhGM-CSF 5 μg/kg/d (61)	n = 58 children Double-blind Placebo-controlled	Decreased days of hospitalization[a] and of antibiotics[a] in the treated patients	Decreased number of patients requiring antibiotics for 10 d or more[a]
rhGM-CSF, 5 μg/kg/d (59)	n = 134 adults Placebo-controlled	No significant difference	Decreased duration of neutropenia[a] and quality of life[a] in treated group
rhGM-CSF, 5 μg/kg/d (60)	n = 68 adults Randomized No placebo control	Decreased days of hospitalization[a] and antibiotics[a] (only in "low risk" chemotherapy cycles)	Decreased duration of neutropenia,[a] No effect with "high risk" chemotherapy
rhG-CSF, 12 μg/kg/d (126)	n = 218 adults Randomized Double-blind Placebo-controlled	No significant difference	Decreased duration of neutropenia[a] and risk of prolonged hospitalization[a] in treated group
rhG-CSF, or rhGM-CSF, both at 5 μg/kg/d (58)	n = 121 Randomized (rhG-CSF vs. rhGM-CSF vs. placebo)	Decreased days of hospitalization[a] (5 vs. 7 days) for the rhG-CSF or rhGM-CSF groups compared with placebo	Decreased duration of neutropenia in the treated groups[a]

rhG-CSF, recombinant human granulocyte colony-stimulating factor; rhGM-CSF, recombinant human granulocyte-macrophage colony-stimulating factor.
[a]$p <.05$.

myeloid growth factor therapy is probably safe during induction chemotherapy for ANL, but the benefit in this setting is unclear. Issues that require clarification include the identification of a subset of patients who benefit consistently, the best schedule for their use during induction therapy, the safety of these factors during consolidation therapy, and the cost impacts of myeloid growth factors during therapy for ANL.

A second strategy for treating patients with ANL is the use of myeloid growth factors for priming before or during induction chemotherapy. The goal of this approach is to recruit leukemic cells into more chemotherapy-sensitive phases of the cell cycle by appropriately timed administration of growth factor. This approach has been explored and has not been shown to benefit patients (67–71).

TABLE 5. RANDOMIZED CLINICAL TRIALS OF RECOMBINANT HUMAN GRANULOCYTE-MACROPHAGE COLONY-STIMULATING FACTOR OR RECOMBINANT HUMAN GRANULOCYTE COLONY-STIMULATING FACTOR PATIENTS WITH ACUTE NONLYMPHOCYTIC LEUKEMIA

Growth Factor and Dose (Reference)	Design Features	Impact on Remission or Survival	Other Observations
rhG-CSF, 200 μg/m^2/d beginning on d 2 (63)	n = 67 Refractory or relapsed ANL Induction chemotherapy Randomized	No significant difference in remission frequency or duration	Fewer documented infections[a] in treated patients
rhG-CSF, 5 μg/kg/d beginning on d 9 of induction Adults, 65 yr and older (64)	n = 173 Newly diagnosed ANL undergoing induction Randomized, placebo-controlled	Higher remission rate[a] (70% vs. 47%) in the treated group No difference in survival	Shorter duration of neutropenia[a] in treated patients No difference in leukemic regrowth
rhGM-CSF, 5 μg/kg/d beginning on d 8 of induction Adults 60 yr and older (65)	n = 388 Newly diagnosed ANL undergoing induction Randomized, placebo-controlled	No difference in remission or survival in the treated group	Shorter duration of neutropenia[a] in treated patients No difference in leukemic regrowth
rhGM-CSF, 5 μg/kg/d beginning on d 10 of induction if marrow hypoplastic Adults 55–70 yr old (66)	n = 124 Newly diagnosed ANL undergoing induction Randomized, placebo-controlled	No significant difference in remission rate in the treated group Median survival longer[a] in the treated group (10.6 vs. 4.8 months)	Shorter duration of neutropenia[a] and decreased infectious toxicity[a] in treated patients No difference in leukemic regrowth

ANL, acute nonlymphocytic leukemia; rhG-CSF, recombinant human granulocyte colony-stimulating factor, rhGM-CSF, recombinant human granulocyte-macrophage colony-stimulating factor.
[a]$p <.05$.

Chemotherapy Dose Intensification without Progenitor Cell Support

In this approach, the myeloid growth factors are used to enhance anticancer therapy by increasing the dose intensity of the chemotherapy that can be administered with acceptable toxicity. In randomized clinical trials, the appropriate control group would receive the same chemotherapy drugs without growth factor support and both groups would receive maximal dose intensity within established safety guidelines. The appropriate measure of a successful outcome would be increased dose intensity coupled with an increased complete response rate, time to tumor progression, survival, or quality of life. No randomized studies meeting these criteria have been reported, and the use of mycloid growth factors to support routine chemotherapy dose escalation cannot be supported.

Studies demonstrate that therapy with rhG-CSF or rhGM-CSF is associated with a more rapid recovery of neutrophil counts after dose-intensive chemotherapy. These studies suggest that patients receiving rhG-CSF or rhGM-CSF during chemotherapy adjusted for each cycle based on neutrophil counts can receive 1.3- to twofold greater dose intensity compared with patients who are not receiving a cytokine (72–77). At higher dose intensities, thrombocytopenia and nonmyeloid toxicities occur. The clinical benefit of this degree of dose intensification remains unclear. In one randomized trial in patients with myeloid growth factor–facilitated dose intensification of chemotherapy for germ cell tumors, the increased dose intensity was not associated with improvement in survival outcomes (77).

A closely related but distinct approach is the use of myeloid growth factors to maintain full-planned chemotherapy dose intensity in as many patients as possible over all cycles of chemotherapy. Retrospective analyses of survival outcomes in several studies of chemotherapy given with curative intent have suggested that patients who received lower dose intensity caused by dose delays or reductions have a significantly lower rate of survival. It is not clear whether this observed inferior survival is caused by the lower chemotherapy dose intensity received or whether the decreased tolerance of chemotherapy and the inferior survival are caused by more aggressive cancer or comorbidities. These issues can only be addressed in randomized clinical trials that are difficult to carry out. It is encouraging that in a randomized study in patients with neuroblastoma, the higher chemotherapy doses achieved in conjunction with growth factor therapy were associated with improved cancer outcomes (30).

Hematopoietic Recovery after Hematopoietic Progenitor Cell Transplantation

One of the first applications of the myeloid growth factors was their administration after autologous bone marrow transplantation (78). Subsequently, controlled trials of rhGM-CSF (79–81) and rhG-CSF (82,83) demonstrated that therapy with these factors is associated with an acceleration of neutrophil engraftment. The myeloid growth factors have been administered to patients after allogeneic marrow transplant. This therapy has been associated with accelerated neutrophil recovery without a change in the incidence of graft rejection or graft-versus-host disease (84–86). The results of myeloid growth factor therapy for patients with graft failure after marrow transplantation have been disappointing (87). Some indication exists that therapy with rhG-CSF may be efficacious in the management of patients with myeloid malignancies who relapse after allogeneic transplantation (88). It is unclear what role G-CSF plays in these patients who are also undergoing cyclosporin withdrawal, which may contribute to the remissions observed.

Mobilization of Peripheral Blood Progenitor Cells

The most significant impact of myeloid growth factors in the field of marrow transplantation followed the observation that, during therapy with these factors, particularly when patients are recovering from myelosuppressive chemotherapy, hematopoietic progenitor cells circulate in increased numbers. These peripheral blood progenitor cells (PBPC) can be harvested and used as an alternative to marrow in the support of myeloablative chemotherapy. The use of autologous PBPC mobilized during therapy with rhG-CSF or rhGM-CSF has been associated with durable engraftment and a more rapid recovery of platelet production compared with traditional bone marrow (89,90). PBPC are a superior and more flexible source of progenitor cells and multiple cycles of high-dose therapy are feasible and under study (91,92). Despite concerns about graft failure or graft-versus-host disease, PBPC appear to be safe and effective in allogeneic transplantation (93,94).

Although they are usually used, the benefit of therapy with myeloid growth factors after the infusion of cytokine-mobilized PBPC has not been fully established. In one study, the combination of rhG-CSF and rhGM-CSF after PBPC infusion was associated with accelerated neutrophil engraftment and shorter hospital stay (95). In another study, rhG-CSF administered after PBPC was not associated with more rapid engraftment (96).

The optimal approach to the mobilization of PBPC is a subject of current investigation. While doses of rhG-CSF or rhGM-CSF of 5 to 10 μg per kg per day given alone or after a mobilizing dose of chemotherapy are effective in mobilizing PBPC, one comparative study has been published that suggests that rhG-CSF is a superior mobilizing agent (97). Further comparative studies are warranted. Moreover, better quality grafts may be obtainable with higher doses of mycloid growth factors or with newer cytokine combinations (98–100).

Myelodysplasia

In early nonrandomized studies, therapy with rhGM-CSF or rhG-CSF was shown to produce transient increases in circulating neutrophil counts in neutropenic patients with myelodysplastic syndromes (101–104). No randomized clinical trials have been published establishing the safety or efficacy of chronic myeloid growth factor therapy. Outside the setting of a clinical trial, these agents are best used for short-term therapy of the neutropenic-infected patient (105). Some evidence exists that combinations of cytokines may have synergy in patients with myelodysplastic syndromes (106,107).

FUTURE APPLICATIONS IN CANCER THERAPY

Interest is growing in the application of the myeloid growth factors, particularly rhGM-CSF, to cancer immunotherapy because of their effect on mature effector cell function. In early phase 1 and 2 studies in patients with cancer, therapy with these factors alone was not associated with tumor regression (108–121). Studies have explored the potential of rhGM-CSF administered to the patient or produced by transfected vaccine cells to enhance the effects of monoclonal antibody or tumor vaccines strategies. PBPC mobilized by myeloid growth factors can be used to generate dendritic cells used in immunotherapy (122–125). *Ex vivo* application of the myeloid growth factors enhances transduction efficiency in gene therapy strategies in which PBPC or dendritic cells are the target (122).

CONCLUSION

Since the early 1990s, the myeloid growth factors have become established tools in the treatment of cancer patients. The availability of rhGM-CSF and rhG-CSF have improved the supportive care of cancer patients and transformed the field of bone marrow transplantation. Although these advances are important, therapy with the myeloid factors has not been shown to improve survival and the effects of the supportive care advances on the quality of life for patients remains largely unstudied. The next generation of myeloid growth factor studies should focus on the following goals:

1. Characterize the patient benefits associated with the use of myeloid growth factor in supportive care. Focus their use on patients in whom a benefit is demonstrable.
2. Explore the effect of maintaining chemotherapy dose intensity and chemotherapy dose escalation on cancer outcomes.
3. Refine PBPC technology and its clinical applications.
4. Pursue the potential of the mature effector cell activation effects of rhGM-CSF in cancer immunotherapy.

REFERENCES

1. Lieschke GJ, Burgess AW. Granulocyte colony-stimulating factor and granulocyte-macrophage colony-stimulating factor (1). *N Engl J Med* 1992;327:28–35.
2. Lieschke GJ, Burgess AW. Granulocyte colony-stimulating factor and granulocyte-macrophage colony-stimulating factor (2). *N Engl J Med* 1992;327:99–106.
3. Coleman DL, Chodakewitz JA, Bartiss AH, Mellors JW. Granulocyte-macrophage colony-stimulating factor enhances selective effector functions of tissue-derived macrophages. *Blood* 1988;72:573–578.
4. Lieschke GJ, Maher D, Cebon J, et al. Effects of bacterially synthesized recombinant human granulocyte-macrophage colony-stimulating factor in patients with advanced malignancy. *Ann Intern Med* 1989;110:357–364.
5. Lord BI, Molineux G, Chang J, Bronchud MH, Gurney H, Dexter TM. Hemopoietic cell kinetics in mice and humans during treatment *in vivo* with hemopoietic growth factors [Meeting Abstract]. *Exp Hematol* 1990;18:598.
6. Lord BI, Gurney H, Chang J, Thatcher N, Crowther D, Dexter TM. Haemopoietic cell kinetics in humans treated with rGM-CSF. *Int J*

7. *Cancer* 1992;50:26–31.
7. Yong KL, Rowles PM, Patterson KG, Linch DC. Granulocyte-macrophage colony-stimulating factor induces neutrophil adhesion to pulmonary vascular endothelium *in vivo*: role of beta 2 integrins. *Blood* 1992;80:1565–1575.
8. Peters WP, Stuart A, Affronti ML, Kim CS, Coleman RE. Neutrophil migration is defective during recombinant human granulocyte-macrophage colony-stimulating factor infusion after autologous bone marrow transplantation in humans. *Blood* 1988;72:1310–1315.
9. van Pelt LJ, Huisman MV, Weening RS, von dem Borne AK, Roos D, van Oers RH. A single dose of granulocyte-macrophage colony-stimulating factor induces systemic interleukin-8 release and neutrophil activation in healthy volunteers. *Blood* 1996;87:5305–5313.
10. Stanley E, Lieschke GJ, Grail D, et al. Granulocyte-macrophage colony-stimulating factor-deficient mice show no major perturbation of hematopoiesis but develop a characteristic pulmonary pathology. *Proc Natl Acad Sci U S A* 1994;91:5592–5596.
11. Bronchud MH, Potter MR, Morgenstern G, et al. *In vitro* and *in vivo* analysis of the effects of recombinant human granulocyte colony-stimulating factor in patients. *Br J Cancer* 1988;58:64–69.
12. Watari K, Asano S, Shirafuji N, et al. Serum granulocyte colony-stimulating factor levels in healthy volunteers and patients with various disorders as estimated by enzyme immunoassay. *Blood* 1989;73:117–122.
13. Kawakami M, Tsutsumi H, Kumakawa T, et al. Levels of serum granulocyte colony-stimulating factor in patients with infections. *Blood* 1990;76:1962–1964.
14. Gessler P, Kirchmann N, Kientsch-Engel R, Haas N, Lasch P, Kachel W. Serum concentrations of granulocyte colony-stimulating factor in healthy term and preterm neonates and in those with various diseases including bacterial infections. *Blood* 1993;82:3177–3182.
15. Lindemann A, Herrmann F, Oster W, et al. Hematologic effects of recombinant human granulocyte colony-stimulating factor in patients with malignancy. *Blood* 1989;74:2644–2651.
16. Duhrsen U, Villeval JL, Boyd J, Kannourakis G, Morstyn G, Metcalf D. Effects of recombinant human granulocyte colony-stimulating factor on hematopoietic progenitor cells in cancer patients. *Blood* 1988;72:2074–2081.
17. Bronchud MH, Scarffe JH, Thatcher N, et al. Phase I/II study of recombinant human granulocyte colony-stimulating factor in patients receiving intensive chemotherapy for small cell lung cancer. *Br J Cancer* 1987;56:809–813.
18. Morstyn G, Campbell L, Souza LM, et al. Effect of granulocyte colony-stimulating factor on neutropenia induced by cytotoxic chemotherapy. *Lancet* 1988;1:667–672.
19. Gabrilove JL, Jakubowski A, Scher H, et al. Effect of granulocyte colony stimulating factor on neutropenia and associated morbidity due to chemotherapy for transitional-cell carcinoma of the urothelium. *N Engl J Med* 1988;318:1414–1422.
20. Riikonen P, Rahiala J, Salonvaara M, Perkkio M. Prophylactic administration of granulocyte colony-stimulating factor (filgrastim) after conventional chemotherapy in children with cancer. *Stem Cells* 1995;13:289–294.
21. Gabrilove JL, Jakubowski A, Fain K, et al. Phase I study of granulocyte colony-stimulating factor in patients with transitional cell carcinoma of the urothelium. *J Clin Invest* 1988;82:1454–1461.
22. Glaspy JA, Baldwin GC, Robertson PA, et al. Therapy for neutropenia in hairy cell leukemia with recombinant human granulocyte colony-stimulating factor. *Ann Intern Med* 1988;109:789–795.
23. Crawford J, Ozer H, Stoller R, et al. Reduction by granulocyte colony-stimulating factor of fever and neutropenia induced by chemotherapy in patients with small cell lung cancer. *N Engl J Med* 1991;325:164–170.
24. Trillet-Lenoir V, Green J, Manegold C, et al. Recombinant granulocyte colony-stimulating factor reduces the infectious complications of cytotoxic chemotherapy. *Eur J Cancer* 1993;29A:319–324.
25. Gebbia V, Valenza R, Testa A, Cannata G, Borsellino N, Gebbia N. A prospective randomized trial of thymopentin versus granulocyte colony-stimulating factor with or without thymopentin in the pre-

vention of febrile episodes in cancer patients undergoing highly cyto-toxic chemotherapy. *Anticancer Res* 1994;14:731–734.

26. Chevallier B, Chollet P, Merrouche Y, et al. Lenograstim prevents morbidity from intensive induction chemotherapy in the treatment of inflammatory breast cancer. *J Clin Oncol* 1995;13:1564–1571.

27. Welte K, Reiter A, Mempel K, et al. A randomized phase-III study of the efficacy of granulocyte colony-stimulating factor in children with high-risk acute lymphoblastic leukemia. Berlin-Frankfurt-Munster Study Group. *Blood* 1996;87:3143–3150.

28. Pui CH, Boyett JM, Hughes WT, et al. Human granulocyte colony-stimulating factor after induction chemotherapy in children with acute lymphoblastic leukemia. *N Engl J Med* 1997;336:1781–1787.

29. Larson RA, Dodge RK, Linker CA, et al. A randomized controlled trial of filgrastim during remission induction and consolidation chemotherapy for adults with acute lymphoblastic leukemia: CALGB study 9111. *Blood* 1998;92:1556–1564.

30. Michon JM, Hartmann O, Bouffet E, et al. An open-label, multi-centre, randomised phase 2 study of recombinant human granulo-cyte colony-stimulating factor (filgrastim) as an adjunct to combination chemotherapy in paediatric patients with metastatic neuroblastoma. *Eur J Cancer* 1998;34:1063–1069.

31. Dunlop DJ, Eatock MM, Paul J, et al. Randomized multicentre trial of filgrastim as an adjunct to combination chemotherapy for Hodgkin's disease. West of Scotland Lymphoma Group. *Clin Oncol (R Coll Radiol)* 1998;10:107–114.

32. Antman KS, Griffin JD, Elias A, et al. Effect of recombinant human granulocyte-macrophage colony-stimulating factor on chemother-apy-induced myelosuppression. *N Engl J Med* 1988;319:593–598.

33. Addison IE, Johnson B, Devereux S, Goldstone AH, Linch DC. Granulocyte-macrophage colony-stimulating factor may inhibit neu-trophil migration *in vivo*. *Clin Exp Immunol* 1989;76:149–153.

34. Rapoport AP, Abboud CN, DiPersio JF. Granulocyte-macrophage colony-stimulating factor (GM-CSF) and granulocyte colony-stimu-lating factor (G-CSF): receptor biology, signal transduction, and neutrophil activation. *Blood Rev* 1992;6:43–57.

35. Gerhartz HH, Engelhard M, Meusers P, et al. Randomized, double-blind, placebo controlled, phase III study of recombinant human granulocyte-macrophage colony-stimulating factor as adjunct to induction treatment of high-grade malignant non-Hodgkin's lym-phomas [see comments]. *Blood* 1993;82:2329–2339.

36. Engelhard M, Gerhartz H, Brittinger G, et al. Cytokine efficiency in the treatment of high-grade malignant non-Hodgkin's lymphomas: results of a randomized double-blind placebo-controlled study with intensified COP-BLAM +/-rhGM-CSF. *Ann Oncol* 1994;5[Suppl 2]:123–125.

37. Calderwood S, Romeyer F, Blanchette V, et al. Concurrent RhGM-CSF does not offset myelosuppression from intensive chemotherapy: randomized placebo-controlled study in childhood acute lympho-blastic leukemia. *Am J Hematol* 1994;47:27–32.

38. Hamm J, Schiller JH, Cuffie C, et al. Dose-ranging study of recom-binant human granulocyte-macrophage colony-stimulating factor in small-cell lung carcinoma. *J Clin Oncol* 1994;12:2667–2676.

39. Bajorin DF, Nichols CR, Schmoll HJ, et al. Recombinant human granulocyte-macrophage colony-stimulating factor as an adjunct to conventional-dose ifosfamide-based chemotherapy for patients with advanced or relapsed germ cell tumors: a randomized trial. *J Clin Oncol* 1995;13:79–86.

40. Bunn PA Jr, Crowley J, Kelly K, et al. Chemoradiotherapy with or without granulocyte-macrophage colony-stimulating factor in the treatment of limited-stage small cell lung cancer: a prospective phase III randomized study of the Southwest Oncology Group. *J Clin Oncol* 1995;13:1632–1641.

41. Yau JC, Neidhart JA, Triozzi P, et al. Randomized placebo-controlled trial of granulocyte-macrophage colony-stimulating-factor support for dose-intensive cyclophosphamide, etoposide, and cisplatin. *Am J Hematol* 1996;51:289–295.

42. Wexler LH, Weaver-McClure L, Steinberg SM, et al. Randomized trial of recombinant human granulocyte-macrophage colony-stimu-lating factor in pediatric patients receiving intensive myelosuppres-sive chemotherapy. *J Clin Oncol* 1996;14:901–910.

43. Jones SE, Schottstaedt MW, Duncan LA, et al. Randomized double-blind prospective trial to evaluate the effects of sargramostim versus placebo in a moderate-dose fluorouracil, doxorubicin, and cyclo-phosphamide adjuvant chemotherapy program for stage II and III breast cancer. *J Clin Oncol* 1996;14:2976–2983.

44. Hansen F, Stenbygaard L, Skovsgaard T. Effect of granulocyte-mac-rophage colony-stimulating factor (GM-CSF) on hematologic toxic-ity induced by high-dose chemotherapy in patients with metastatic breast cancer. *Acta Oncol* 1995;34:919–924.

45. Marina NM, Shema SJ, Bowman LC, et al. Failure of granulocyte-macrophage colony-stimulating factor to reduce febrile neutropenia in children with recurrent solid tumors treated with ifosfamide, car-boplatin, and etoposide chemotherapy. *Med Pediatr Oncol* 1994;23:328–334.

46. Hamm J, Crawford J, Figlin R, et al. A phase I/II study of the simultaneous administration of recombinant human interleukin-6 (rhIL-6, *E. coli*) and Neupogen (rhG-CSF, *E. coli*) following ICE chemotherapy in pts with advanced non small cell lung carcinoma [Meeting Abstract]. *Proc Annu Meet Am Soc Clin Oncol* 1994;13: 1100–1994.

47. Anonymous. American Society of Clinical Oncology. Recommenda-tions for the use of hematopoietic colony-stimulating factors: evi-dence-based, clinical practice guidelines. *J Clin Oncol* 1994;12: 2471–2508.

48. Ozer H. American Society of Clinical Oncology guidelines for the use of hematopoietic colony-stimulating factors. *Curr Opin Hematol* 1996;3:3–10.

49. Beveridge RA, Miller JA, Kales AN, et al. A comparison of efficacy of 1 sargramostim (yeast-derived RhuGM-CSF) and filgrastim (bacte-ria-derived RhuG-CSF) in the therapeutic setting of chemotherapy-induced myelosuppression. *Cancer Invest* 1998;16:366–373.

50. Crawford J, Glaspy J, Vincent M, Tomita D, Mazanet R. Effect of filgrastim (r-metHug-CSF) on oral mucositis in patients with small cell lung cancer (SCLC) receiving chemotherapy (cyclophospha-mide, doxorubicin and etoposide, CAE) [Meeting abstract]. *Proc Annu Meet Am Soc Clin Oncol* 1994;13:A15–A23.

51. Lyman GH, Lyman CG, Sanderson RA, Balducci L. Decision analy-sis of hematopoietic growth factor use in patients receiving cancer chemotherapy [see comments]. *J Natl Cancer Inst* 1993;85:488–493.

52. Glaspy JA, Bleecker G, Crawford J, Stoller R, Strauss M. The impact of therapy with filgrastim (recombinant granulocyte colony-stimu-lating factor) on the health care costs associated with cancer chemo-therapy. *Eur J Cancer* 1993;29A[Suppl 7]:S23–S30.

53. Glaspy J. Economic effect of myeloid growth factors on cancer treat-ment. *Clin Immunother* 1994;2:192–205.

54. Glaspy JA. Economic outcomes associated with the use of hemato-poietic growth factors. *Oncology* (Huntingt) 1995;9:93–105.

55. Smith TJ. Economic analysis of the clinical uses of the colony-stimu-lating factors. *Curr Opin Hematol* 1996;3:175–179.

56. Lyman GH, Kuderer NM, Balducci L. Economic impact of granu-lopoiesis stimulating agents on the management of febrile neutrope-nia. *Curr Opin Oncol* 1998;10:291–296.

57. Aglietta M, Monzeglio C, Pasquino P, Carnino F, Stern AC, Gavosto F. Short-term administration of granulocyte-macrophage colony-stimulating factor decreases hematopoietic toxicity of cytostatic drugs. *Cancer* 1993;72:2970–2973.

58. Mayordomo JI, Rivera F, Diaz-Puente MT, et al. Improving treat-ment of chemotherapy-induced neutropenic fever by administration of colony-stimulating factors [see comments]. *J Natl Cancer Inst* 1995;87:803–808.

59. Vellenga E, Uyl-de Groot CA, de Wit R, et al. Randomized placebo-controlled trial of granulocyte-macrophage colony-stimulating factor in patients with chemotherapy-related febrile neutropenia. *J Clin Oncol* 1996;14:619–627.

60. Ravaud A, Chevreau C, Cany L, et al. Granulocyte-macrophage col-ony-stimulating factor in patients with neutropenic fever is potent after low-risk but not after high-risk neutropenic chemotherapy regi-mens: results of a randomized phase III trial. *J Clin Oncol* 1998;16: 2930–2936.

61. Riikonen P, Saarinen UM, Makipernaa A, et al. Recombinant

human granulocyte-macrophage colony-stimulating factor in the treatment of febrile neutropenia: a double blind placebo-controlled study in children. *Pediatr Infect Dis J* 1994;13:197–202.

62. Maher DW, Lieschke GJ, Green M, et al. Filgrastim in patients with chemotherapy-induced febrile neutropenia: a double-blind, placebo-controlled trial. *Ann Intern Med* 1994;121:492–501.

63. Ohno R, Tomonaga M, Kobayashi T, et al. Effect of granulocyte colony-stimulating factor after intensive induction therapy in relapsed or refractory acute leukemia. *N Engl J Med* 1990;323:871–877.

64. Dombret H, Chastang C, Fenaux P, et al. A controlled study of recombinant human granulocyte colony-stimulating factor in elderly patients after treatment for acute myelogenous leukemia. AML Cooperative Study Group. *N Engl J Med* 1995;332:1678–1683.

65. Stone RM, Berg DT, George SL, et al. Granulocyte-macrophage colony-stimulating factor after initial chemotherapy for elderly patients with primary acute myelogenous leukemia. Cancer and Leukemia Group B. *N Engl J Med* 1995;332:1671–1677.

66. Rowe JM, Andersen JW, Mazza JJ, et al. A randomized placebo-controlled phase III study of granulocyte-macrophage colony-stimulating factor in adult patients (>55 to 70 years of age) with acute myelogenous leukemia: a study of the Eastern Cooperative Oncology Group (E1490). *Blood* 1995;86:457–462.

67. Hansen PB, Johnsen HE, Jensen L, Gaarsdal E, Simonsen K, Ralfkiaer E. Priming and treatment with molgramostim (rhGM-CSF) in adult high-risk acute myeloid leukemia during induction chemotherapy: a prospective, randomized pilot study. *Eur J Haematol* 1995;54:296–303.

68. Hansen PB, Johnsen HE, Lund JO, Hansen MS, Hansen NE. Unexpected hepatotoxicity after priming and treatment with molgramostim (rhGM-CSF) in acute myeloid leukemia during induction chemotherapy. *Am J Hematol* 1995;48:48–51.

69. Hansen PB, Knudsen H, Gaarsdal E, Jensen L, Ralfkiaer E, Johnsen HE. Short-term *in vivo* priming of bone marrow haematopoiesis with rhG-CSF, rhGM-CSF or rhIL-3 before marrow harvest expands myelopoiesis but does not improve engraftment capability. *Bone Marrow Transplant* 1995;16:373–379.

70. Ganser A, Heil G. Use of hematopoietic growth factors in the treatment of acute myelogenous leukemia. *Curr Opin Hematol* 1997;4: 191–195.

71. Rowe JM, Liesveld JL. Hematopoietic growth factors and acute leukemia. *Cancer Treat Res* 1999;99:195–226.

72. Crawford J, O'Rourke MA. Vinorelbine (Navelbine)/carboplatin combination therapy: dose intensification with granulocyte colony-stimulating factor. *Semin Oncol* 1994;21:73–78.

73. Gisselbrecht C. Chemotherapy dose intensity facilitated by use of lenograstim—implications for quality of life and survival. *Eur J Cancer* 1994;30A[Suppl 3]:S30–S33.

74. Piccart MJ, Bruning P, Wildiers J, et al. An EORTC pilot study of filgrastim (recombinant human granulocyte colony stimulating factor) as support to a high dose-intensive epiadriamycin-cyclophosphamide regimen in chemotherapy-naive patients with locally advanced or metastatic breast cancer. *Ann Oncol* 1995;6:673–677.

75. Bergmann L, Karakas T, Knuth A, Lautenschlager G, Mitrou PS, Hoelzer D. Recombinant human granulocyte-macrophage colony-stimulating factor after combined chemotherapy in high-grade non-Hodgkin's lymphoma—a randomised pilot study. *Eur J Cancer* 1995;31A:2164–2168.

76. Woll PJ, Hodgetts J, Lomax L, Bildet F, Cour-Chabernaud V, Thatcher N. Can cytotoxic dose-intensity be increased by using granulocyte colony-stimulating factor? A randomized controlled trial of lenograstim in small cell lung cancer. *J Clin Oncol* 1995;13:652–659.

77. Fossa SD, Kaye SB, Mead GM, et al. Filgrastim during combination chemotherapy of patients with poor-prognosis metastatic germ cell malignancy. European Organization for Research and Treatment of Cancer, Genito-Urinary Group, and the Medical Research Council Testicular Cancer Working Party, Cambridge, United Kingdom. *J Clin Oncol* 1998;16:716–724.

78. Brandt SJ, Peters WP, Atwater SK, et al. Effect of recombinant human granulocyte-macrophage colony-stimulating factor on hematopoietic reconstitution after high-dose chemotherapy and autologous bone marrow transplantation. *N Engl J Med* 1988;318: 869–876.

79. Nemunaitis J, Rabinowe SN, Singer JW, et al. Recombinant granulocyte-macrophage colony-stimulating factor after autologous bone marrow transplantation for lymphoid cancer. *N Engl J Med* 1991; 324:1773–1778.

80. Gulati SC, Bennett CL. Granulocyte-macrophage colony-stimulating factor (GM-CSF) as adjunct therapy in relapsed Hodgkin disease. *Ann Intern Med* 1992;116:177–182.

81. Rabinowe SN, Neuberg D, Bierman PJ, et al. Long-term follow-up of a phase III study of recombinant human granulocyte-macrophage colony-stimulating factor after autologous bone marrow transplantation for lymphoid malignancies. *Blood* 1993;81:1903–1908.

82. Sheridan WP, Morstyn G, Wolf M, et al. Granulocyte colony-stimulating factor and neutrophil recovery after high-dose chemotherapy and autologous bone marrow transplantation. *Lancet* 1989;2:891–895.

83. Stahel RA, Jost LM, Cerny T, et al. Randomized study of recombinant human granulocyte colony-stimulating factor after high-dose chemotherapy and autologous bone marrow transplantation for high-risk lymphoid malignancies. *J Clin Oncol* 1994;12:1931–1938.

84. Nemunaitis J, Anasetti C, Storb R, et al. Phase II trial of recombinant human granulocyte-macrophage colony-stimulating factor in patients undergoing allogeneic bone marrow transplantation from unrelated donors. *Blood* 1992;79:2572–2577.

85. Hiraoka A, Masaoka T, Mizoguchi H, et al. Recombinant human non-glycosylated granulocyte-macrophage colony-stimulating factor in allogeneic bone marrow transplantation: double-blind placebo-controlled phase III clinical trial. *Jpn J Clin Oncol* 1994;24:205–211.

86. Schriber JR, Chao NJ, Long GD, et al. Granulocyte colony-stimulating factor after allogeneic bone marrow transplantation. *Blood* 1994;84:1680–1684.

87. Weisdorf DJ, Verfaillie CM, Davies SM, et al. Hematopoietic growth factors for graft failure after bone marrow transplantation: a randomized trial of granulocyte-macrophage colony-stimulating factor (GM-CSF) versus sequential GM-CSF plus granulocyte-CSF. *Blood* 1995;85:3452–3456.

88. Giralt S, Escudier S, Kantarjian H, et al. Preliminary results of treatment with filgrastim for relapse of leukemia and myelodysplasia after allogeneic bone marrow transplantation. *N Engl J Med* 1993;329: 757–761.

89. Sheridan WP, Begley CG, Juttner CA, et al. Effect of peripheral-blood progenitor cells mobilised by filgrastim (G-CSF) on platelet recovery after high-dose chemotherapy [see comments]. *Lancet* 1992;339:640–644.

90. Bishop MR, Anderson JR, Jackson JD, et al. High-dose therapy and peripheral blood progenitor cell transplantation: effects of recombinant human granulocyte-macrophage colony-stimulating factor on the autograft. *Blood* 1994;83:610–616.

91. Shea TC, Mason JR, Storniolo AM, et al. Sequential cycles of high-dose carboplatin administered with recombinant human granulocyte-macrophage colony-stimulating factor and repeated infusions of autologous peripheral-blood progenitor cells: a novel and effective method for delivering multiple courses of dose-intensive therapy. *J Clin Oncol* 1992;10:464–473.

92. Tepler I, Cannistra SA, Frei ED, et al. Use of peripheral-blood progenitor cells abrogates the myelotoxicity of repetitive outpatient high-dose carboplatin and cyclophosphamide chemotherapy. *J Clin Oncol* 1993;11:1583–1591.

93. Dreger P, Haferlach T, Eckstein V, et al. G-CSF-mobilized peripheral blood progenitor cells for allogeneic transplantation: safety, kinetics of mobilization, and composition of the graft. *Br J Haematol* 1994;87:609–613.

94. Pan L, Bressler S, Cooke KR, Krenger W, Karandikar M, Ferrara JL. Long-term engraftment, graft-versus-host disease, and immunologic reconstitution after experimental transplantation of allogeneic peripheral blood cells from G-CSF-treated donors [see comments]. *Biol Blood Marrow Transplant* 1996;2:126–133.

95. Spitzer G, Adkins DR, Spencer V, et al. Randomized study of growth factors post-peripheral-blood stem-cell transplant: neutrophil recovery is improved with modest clinical benefit. *J Clin Oncol*

1994;12:661–670.

96. Dunlop DJ, Fitzsimons EJ, McMurray A, et al. Filgrastim fails to improve haemopoietic reconstitution following myeloablative chemotherapy and peripheral blood stem cell rescue. *Br J Cancer* 1994;70:943–945.

97. Peters WP, Rosner G, Ross M, et al. Comparative effects of granulocyte-macrophage colony-stimulating factor (GM-CSF) and granulocyte colony-stimulating factor (G-CSF) on priming peripheral blood progenitor cells for use with autologous bone marrow after high-dose chemotherapy. *Blood* 1993;81:1709–1719.

98. Lee ME, Crawford J, Issaacs R, Manfreda S, Kurtzberg J. Mobilization of peripheral blood progenitor cells with interleukin 6+ granulocyte-colony stimulating factor [Meeting Abstract]. *Proc Annu Meet Am Assoc Cancer Res* 1994;35:A3108.

99. Glaspy JA, Shpall EJ, LeMaistre CF, et al. Peripheral blood progenitor cell mobilization using stem cell factor in combination with filgrastim in breast cancer patients. *Blood* 1997;90:2939–2951.

100. Shpall EJ, Wheeler CA, Turner SA, et al. A randomized phase 3 study of peripheral blood progenitor cell mobilization with stem cell factor and filgrastim in high-risk breast cancer patients. *Blood* 1999;93:2491–2501.

101. Vadhan-Raj S, Keating M, LeMaistre A, et al. Effects of recombinant human granulocyte-macrophage colony-stimulating factor in patients with myelodysplastic syndromes. *N Engl J Med* 1987;317:1545–1552.

102. Ganser A, Volkers B, Greher J, et al. Recombinant human granulocyte-macrophage colony-stimulating factor in patients with myelodysplastic syndromes—a phase I/II trial. *Blood* 1989;73:31–37.

103. Thompson JA, Lee DJ, Kidd P, et al. Subcutaneous granulocyte-macrophage colony-stimulating factor in patients with myelodysplastic syndrome: toxicity, pharmacokinetics, and hematological effects. *J Clin Oncol* 1989;7:629–637.

104. Negrin RS, Haeuber DH, Nagler A, et al. Treatment of myelodysplastic syndromes with recombinant human granulocyte colony-stimulating factor. A phase I-II trial. *Ann Intern Med* 1989;110:976–984.

105. Greenberg PL. Treatment of myelodysplastic syndromes with hemopoietic growth factors. *Semin Oncol* 1992;19:106–114.

106. Negrin RS, Stein R, Doherty K, et al. Maintenance treatment of the anemia of myelodysplastic syndromes with recombinant human granulocyte colony-stimulating factor and erythropoietin: evidence for *in vivo* synergy. *Blood* 1996;87:4076–4081.

107. Hansen PB, Penkowa M, Johnsen HE. Hematopoietic growth factors for the treatment of myelodysplastic syndromes. *Leuk Lymphoma* 1998;28:491–500.

108. Dranoff G, Jaffee E, Lazenby A, et al. Vaccination with irradiated tumor cells engineered to secrete murine granulocyte-macrophage colony-stimulating factor stimulates potent, specific, and long-lasting anti-tumor immunity. *Proc Natl Acad Sci U S A* 1993;90:3539–3543.

109. Tao MH, Levy R. Idiotype/granulocyte-macrophage colony-stimulating factor fusion protein as a vaccine for B-cell lymphoma [see comments]. *Nature* 1993;362:755–758.

110. Ragnhammar P, Frodin JE, Trotta PP, Mellstedt H. Cytotoxicity of white blood cells activated by granulocyte-colony stimulating factor, granulocyte/macrophage-colony-stimulating factor and macrophage-colony-stimulating factor against tumor cells in the presence of various monoclonal antibodies. *Cancer Immunol Immunother* 1994;39:254–262.

111. Jones T, Stern A, Lin R. Potential role of granulocyte-macrophage colony-stimulating factor as vaccine adjuvant. *Eur J Clin Microbiol Infect Dis* 1994;13[Suppl 2]:S47–S53.

112. Jaffee EM, Lazenby A, Pardoll DM. Murine tumor vaccines: models for designing human vaccine trials [Meeting Abstract]. *Proc Annu Meet Am Assoc Cancer Res* 1995;36:A29–47.

113. Pardoll DM. Immunotherapy with tumor vaccines in renal cancer [Meeting Abstract]. *Ann Oncol* 1996;7:18.

114. Kwak LW, Young HA, Pennington RW, Weeks SD. Vaccination with syngeneic, lymphoma-derived immunoglobulin idiotype combined with granulocyte/macrophage colony-stimulating factor primes mice for a protective T-cell response. *Proc Natl Acad Sci U S A* 1996;93:10972–10977.

115. Armstrong CA, Botella R, Galloway TH, et al. Antitumor effects of granulocyte-macrophage colony-stimulating factor production by melanoma cells. *Cancer Res* 1996;56:2191–2198.

116. Cole DJ, Gattoni-Celli S, McClay EF, et al. Characterization of a sustained release delivery system for combined cytokine/peptide based vaccination using a fully-acetylated poly-*N*-acetyl glucosamine matrix [Meeting Abstract]. *Proc Annu Meet Am Assoc Cancer Res* 1996;37:A32–62.

117. Hornick JL, Khawli LA, Hu P, Anderson PM, Gasson JC, Epstein AL. Antibody fusion proteins containing GM-CSF or IL-2 with specificity for B-cell malignancies exhibit enhanced effector functions while retaining tumor targeting properties [Meeting Abstract]. *Proc Annu Meet Am Assoc Cancer Res* 1997;38:A555.

118. Hogge G, Burkholder J, Culp J, et al. Phase I clinical trial of hGM-CSF transfected autologous tumor cell vaccines in canines [Meeting Abstract]. *Proc Annu Meet Am Assoc Cancer Res* 1997;38:A26–A66.

119. Botella R, Sarradet MD, Potter LE, et al. Inhibition of murine melanoma growth by granulocyte-macrophage colony stimulating factor gene transfection is not haplotype specific. *Melanoma Res* 1998;8:245–254.

120. Hurwitz AA, Yu TF, Leach DR, Allison JP. CTLA-4 blockade synergizes with tumor-derived granulocyte-macrophage colony-stimulating factor for treatment of an experimental mammary carcinoma. *Proc Natl Acad Sci U S A* 1998;95:10067–10071.

121. Thomas MC, Greten TF, Pardoll DM, Jaffee EM. Enhanced tumor protection by granulocyte-macrophage colony-stimulating factor expression at the site of an allogeneic vaccine. *Hum Gene Ther* 1998;9:835–843.

122. Bernhard H, Disis ML, Heimfeld S, Hand S, Gralow JR, Cheever MA. Generation of immunostimulatory dendritic cells from human CD34+ hematopoietic progenitor cells of the bone marrow and peripheral blood. *Cancer Res* 1995;55:1099–1104.

123. Bui LA, Butterfield LH, Roth MD, et al. A direct comparison of DC propagated from different progenitor cell populations from one donor [Meeting Abstract]. *Proc Annu Meet Am Assoc Cancer Res* 1997;38:A208.

124. Paquette RL, Hsu NC, Kiertscher SM, et al. Interferon-alpha and granulocyte-macrophage colony-stimulating factor differentiate peripheral blood monocytes into potent antigen-presenting cells. *J Leukoc Biol* 1998;64:358–367.

125. Soiffer R, Lynch T, Mihm M, et al. Vaccination with irradiated autologous melanoma cells engineered to secrete human granulocyte-macrophage colony-stimulating factor generates potent antitumor immunity in patients with metastatic melanoma. *Proc Natl Acad Sci U S A* 1998;95:13141–13146.

126. Maher DW, Lieschke GJ, Green M, et al. Filgrastim in patients with chemotherapy-induced febrile neutropenia: a double-blind, placebo-controlled trial [see comments]. *Ann Intern Med* 1994;121:492–501.

COLONY-STIMULATING FACTORS: CLINICAL APPLICATIONS

Platelet-Stimulating Factors

KENNETH KAUSHANSKY

Thrombocytopenia is a major problem facing clinicians. In the United States, approximately 8,000,000 units of platelets are transfused yearly into patients to reduce their risks of severe bleeding (1). Platelet transfusion therapy is less than ideal, however. At least 30% are complicated (2), usually by cytokine-mediated febrile reactions but occasionally by bacteremia, graft-versus-host disease, or acute pulmonary injury. Moreover, an inadequate platelet response due to HLA alloimmunization occurs in a number of patients who require repeated platelet transfusions, the frequency ranging from 10% to 30% of individuals, depending on a patient's underlying disease (3,4). Platelet transfusions are expensive; the approximate cost of a standard six units of platelets (usually sufficient to raise the platelet count 30,000 to 50,000 per mm^3) is $300, rising substantially if a single donor pheresis, removal of leukocytes, or HLA matching is required. The distinguished physician and teacher Dr. William Osler stated, "We are still without a trustworthy medicine which can always be relied upon to control purpura." In many ways, Osler's dilemma is as true today as it was when it was first penned in 1892 (5). Clearly, stimulation of marrow platelet production will prove superior to transfusion of allogeneic platelets. The understanding of thrombopoiesis, however, was for a long time inadequate to allow therapeutic intervention.

Generation of platelets from their marrow progenitors is an enormous and complex process. Each day, an adult produces 1 $\times$ 10^{11} platelets, a number that can easily increase tenfold in times of increased demand for platelet production. Megakaryocyte (MK) and platelet formation are dependent on the productive interaction of hematopoietic stem and progenitor cells, marrow stromal elements, and multiple protein growth and survival factors. The evolving understanding of the humoral regulation of MK development—and how this process may be manipulated (and already has been manipulated) for therapeutic benefit—forms the basis of this chapter.

Several cytokines and hormones have been reported to influence the development of the megakaryocytic lineage. Classically, these have been divided into MK colony-stimulating factors

(MK-CSFs) and potentiators of MK differentiation (6). Several investigators have shown that interleukin-3 (IL-3), granulocyte-macrophage CSF (GM-CSF), and stem-cell factor (SCF) all display colony-stimulating activity for MKs (7–11). MK potentiators, initially defined by their capacity to augment colony numbers when added to marrow cultures containing MK-CSFs and to induce terminal maturation of developing cells, include IL-6, IL-11, and leukocyte inhibitory factor (12,13). None of these cytokines can support MK colony growth when added to marrow cells alone. In contrast, thrombopoietin (Tpo) was initially defined as the substance in blood responsible for platelet recovery after thrombocytopenic insults (14,15); with the recent cloning of the molecule, however, it was found to stimulate all aspects of MK development (16).

MOLECULAR AND CELLULAR BIOLOGY OF THE MEGAKARYOPOIETIC AND THROMBOPOIETIC CYTOKINES AND HORMONES

Interleukin-3

The human IL-3 gene was cloned in 1986 and encodes a 152–amino acid polypeptide processed to a mature 133-residue cytokine (17). The 25- to 30-kd monomeric polypeptide is produced almost exclusively by stimulated T lymphocytes, natural killer cells, and mast cells. Like many of the other hematopoietic cytokines, significant amounts of N-linked carbohydrate modification account for approximately 40% of its apparent molecular weight (M$_r$).

Although initially defined as an activity that stimulates lymphocyte-20 α-steroid dehydrogenase (18), IL-3 has been shown to possess a number of hematopoietic activities. Cultures of marrow cells containing IL-3 develop colonies composed of basophils, eosinophils, neutrophils, monocytes, and MKs, alone and in combination; if erythropoietin (Epo) is added, large erythroid bursts and small erythroid colonies also develop

(12,19–23). Colony formation is significantly enhanced when other cytokines and hormones are added to IL-3. This appears to be particularly important for MK development, because although the cytokine alone can promote the expansion of immature MKs (i.e., diploid CD41$^+$ cells), blockade of thrombopoietin action in IL-3–containing cultures prevents the development of mature polyploid cells (16). Like many other hematopoietic cytokines, IL-3 primes the mature cells it helps produce to become functionally activated (24). These findings have clinical repercussions. The administration of IL-3 to humans has been associated with toxicities related to its activation of multiple types of mature leukocytes.

Although one of the most pleiotropic and potent of CSFs *in vitro*, the physiologic role of IL-3 has been called into question. For example, minimal hematopoietic effects are noted in animals in which the IL-3 gene has been genetically eliminated (25); the sole phenotype is a loss in delayed-type hypersensitivity reaction (26). Moreover, other than a mild eosinophilia, administration of large amounts of the cytokine (in animals and in patients) fails to substantially alter steady-state or stimulated hematopoiesis (27–29). As such, further discussion of IL-3 is limited to a brief review of the clinical trials that have been conducted.

Granulocyte-Macrophage Colony-Stimulating Factor

GM-CSF, an 18- to 30-kd monomeric protein, is produced by activated T lymphocytes, endothelial cells, monocytes, and fibroblasts; like IL-3, it is highly modified with *N*- and *O*-linked carbohydrates. The human GM-CSF gene predicts a polypeptide of 144 amino acids, including a 17-residue secretory leader (30). As its name implies, GM-CSF can support the growth of colonies containing all types of granulocytes and monocytes, alone and in combination. This polypeptide can also act in synergy with Epo to support the development of erythroid bursts or with serum or plasma (presumably with the Tpo in these sources) to stimulate the production of MK-containing colonies (7,31). It is often commented that IL-3 and GM-CSF are not physiologically relevant, as plasma levels of the cytokines are almost never detectable. When examined in mice made deficient in the β-subunit of its receptor, however, GM-CSF becomes detectable in plasma, suggesting the receptor plays an important role in GM-CSF clearance. GM-CSF has been shown to prime neutrophils, eosinophils, and monocytes for functional activity (32). This role appears to be its most important—or at least its only unique—physiologic function. Although genetic elimination of the GM-CSF gene in mice fails to affect granulocyte or monocyte production, it is associated with pulmonary alvcolar proteinosis (33), thought to be related to inadequate pulmonary alveolar number or function. In addition, approximately one-half of humans with this disease harbor a mutation in the β$_C$ subunit of the GM-CSF receptor (34). Neither deficiency of GM-CSF nor of its receptor, however, led to any defects in platelet numbers or function.

As preclinical trials of IL-3 and GM-CSF were beginning, a novel fusion protein was designed and constructed in an attempt to capitalize on the beneficial effects of cytokines, including their effects on MK development. PIXI321, as it was termed, joined full-length IL-3 and GM-CSF proteins, together with a flexible polyglycine linker. The recombinant protein was produced in yeast and has shown pronounced effects on hematopoiesis *in vitro* (35) and *in vivo* in preclinical trials (36).

Interleukin-6

IL-6, cloned using several different end points (assays for IL-6 include antiviral activity, myeloma cell growth, hepatocyte growth, and immunoglobulin secretion), was found to affect primitive hematopoietic cells and megakaryocytic development (37). The IL-6 gene encodes a 26-kd polypeptide produced in almost all tissues from activated T cells, fibroblasts, macrophages, and stromal cells (37). The mature protein is composed of 184 amino acids and displays *N*- and *O*-linked carbohydrate modification. IL-6 is normally produced in response to inflammatory stimuli, including IL-1 and tumor necrosis factor. The production of these inflammatory cytokines is induced by IL-6, contributing to a positive feedback loop designed to maintain or amplify inflammatory responses. As such, the administration of IL-6 has met with considerable toxicity.

Alone, IL-6 does not exert any significant hematopoietic effects *in vitro*. However, it acts in synergy with SCF or IL-3 to induce primitive hematopoietic cells into the cell cycle (12,38), to augment myelopoiesis (39,40), and to modestly enhance MK development (22,41,42). The role of IL-6 in steady-state hematopoiesis is uncertain. The predominant phenotype of IL-6–deficient mice is liver failure and defective hepatic regeneration (43), but these animals also display modest reductions in number of T lymphocytes. In contrast, myeloid cell numbers are normal (44). The combined genetic elimination of G-CSF and IL-6, however, was shown to produce a more severe neutropenia than was found in the absence of G-CSF alone (45). Combined elimination of the IL-6– and Tpo-receptor genes has not been found to reduce platelet production below that found in Tpo receptor–deficient animals alone (W. Alexander and C. G. Begley, *personal communication*, January 1999). Combined genetic elimination of IL-6 and the signaling subunit of the IL-6 receptor leads to modest thrombocytopenia, however, suggesting the cytokine and its receptor play some role in normal MK production.

Interleukin-11

IL-11 was cloned as a marrow stromal cell-derived activity that induces differentiation of an IL-6–responsive myeloma cell line (46). IL-11 was also shown to act in synergy with IL-3 to stimulate MK colony formation (23,46,47), however, enlisting it in the ranks of hematopoietic cytokines.

The human IL-11 gene encodes a mature protein containing 199 amino acids. The cytokine is produced constitutively from cells of the marrow stroma, especially fibroblasts, and production increases when these cells are exposed to inflammatory stimuli (48). This appears to occur *in vivo*, as high levels of this cytokine have been found in rheumatoid synovial fluid (49). Blood levels of IL-11 are thought to react to other stimuli; some (50,51) but not all investigators (52) have found increased IL-11 blood levels in thrombocytopenic patients, suggesting IL-11 possibly plays a role in steady-state thrombopoiesis. Studies conducted on mice that are genetically deficient in the IL-11 receptor, however, have failed to demonstrate any role for the cytokine in baseline or in stimulated platelet production (53).

IL-11 is a pleiotropic cytokine that exerts a multitude of growth stimulatory effects on hepatic, osteoclastic, intestinal, neural and adipocytic cells (54). However, hematopoietic effects of this cytokine have been the most well studied. Like IL-6, IL-11 acts in synergy with IL-3, SCF, or Flt-3 ligand to induce primitive hematopoietic cells into the cell cycle (55) resulting in expansion in the subsequent numbers of committed progenitor cells (38,56,57). IL-11 acts together with IL-3 or SCF to enhance erythropoiesis (58), with SCF and G-CSF to augment myelopoiesis (54) and with IL-3, SCF, or Tpo to promote MK development (13,16,23,46,47,59,60). The hematopoietic effects of combining IL-3 and IL-11 are similar to that reported for IL-3 and IL-6 (55), a finding that can be readily explained by the common receptor signaling components of the complete IL-6 and IL-11 receptors (61). One exception to this general rule may be the differential effects of IL-6 and IL-11 on platelet function; when administered to animals, IL-6 activates platelets and enhances their sensitivity to aggregation in the presence of several platelet agonists (62), effects not reported for IL-11. The explanation for this apparent discrepancy may be the differential expression of the two receptors; IL-11 receptors are not found on platelets (63).

Thrombopoietin

The human Tpo gene encodes a mature polypeptide of 332 amino acids (64–67), considerably longer than any other member of the hematopoietic growth factor family. This polypeptide can be conveniently divided into two domains. The amino-terminal-154 residues of the mature polypeptide bears striking primary sequence homology with Epo and secondary sequence homology with all the other hematopoietic cytokines, and acts by binding to the MPL receptor (66). In contrast, the carboxyl-terminal domain of Tpo bears no resemblance to any known proteins and contains multiple sites of N- and O-linked carbohydrates, accounting for the large discrepancy between predicted and actual M_r of the protein. Nearly 50% of the 70-kd thrombopoietin molecule is carbohydrate. Functions for the carbohydrate-containing carboxyl-terminal domain include increased circulatory survival and improved secretory efficiency in cells that produce the hormone (68).

The biologic activities of Tpo have been rapidly identified in the short time since its cloning; the hormone is the major regulator of MK maturation (16). In suspension cultures of murine or human marrow cells, Tpo increases size and number of MKs, leads to their expression of platelet-specific markers, such as CD41 and CD61, and is a potent stimulus of MK endomitosis and polyploidy (64,66,69). Tpo is a potent MK-CSF, capable of inducing colony formation from up to two-thirds of all megakaryocytic progenitors (60,69); it acts in synergy with other molecules that influence MK growth (IL-3, IL-11, SCF, and Epo) (60), with Epo to stimulate the growth of primitive erythroid progenitor cells (70,71), and with IL-3 or SCF to support survival and stimulate proliferation of hematopoietic stem cells and primitive progenitors (72,73).

Like many of the hematopoietic cytokines that affect cellular production and the state of activation of corresponding mature cells, Tpo was predicted to activate, or at least enhance, platelet response to activating substances. Initial reports suggested that although Tpo does not cause platelets to aggregate in the absence of well-established agonists (e.g., thrombin, adenosine 5'-diphosphate, collagen), it does sensitize the cells to the aggregatory effects of these agents (74). Such "priming" has also been documented *in vivo*; platelets derived from Tpo-treated animals have heightened sensitivity to standard platelet agonists (75). Thus, the potential to aggravate thrombogenic conditions in Tpo recipients exists, and should be carefully evaluated when it is administered to patients.

Finally, additional attempts have been made to combine two megakaryopoietic cytokines to provide a more effective stimulus of MK growth than that seen with either single agent alone. Investigators have combined optimized versions of IL-3 and Tpo (initial studies identified several amino acid substitutions that increased their individual biologic activities) to produce a protein termed *promegapoietin*. Although no published reports of its effects have appeared, several presented abstracts have indicated its capacity to expand immature CD41+ cells from marrow or peripheral blood progenitor cells (76,77) and to prevent thrombocytopenia in a nonhuman primate model of radiation-induced myelosuppression (78). In most of these studies, promegapoietin was compared to the combination of IL-3 plus Tpo; it has been claimed by the same investigators that the combination molecule is more active than the combination of the two native sequence recombinant cytokines. Data should be evaluated in a peer-reviewed setting, however, and the potential for immunogenicity of the combination molecule must be carefully monitored.

PHARMACOLOGY OF PLATELET-PRODUCING AGENTS

Unlike most polypeptide endocrine hormones, such as insulin or growth hormone, a major route of elimination of exogenously administered hematopoietic growth factors is specific receptor-mediated clearance. Although postulated to account for the metabolism of Epo in the 1950s, Stanley and colleagues were the first to show that this mechanism plays a major role in the removal of CSFs, demonstrating that macrophages account for much of the M-CSF clearance from circulation (79).

IL-3 is rapidly cleared from blood after an intravenous (i.v.) bolus infusion, with an equilibration phase of 17 minutes and a 59-minute β-phase elimination (80). As a result, the cytokine is usually administered as an extended i.v. infusion (i.e., greater than or equal to 2 hours per day) or by subcutaneous injection. The elimination of GM-CSF follows similar kinetics; an α-phase of 7 to 20 minutes and a β-phase of 68 to 75 minutes (bacterial versus mammalian cell–derived material, respectively) (81). Although it has not been extensively studied, reports suggest that specific receptor-mediated uptake by leukocytes is responsible for this finding.

IL-6 has been tested in a number of patients with cancer. Half-life of elimination is approximately 4.2 hours after a single

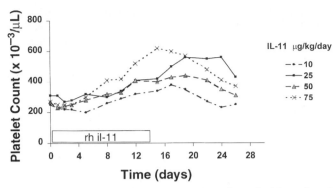

FIGURE 1. Platelet response to graded doses of interleukin-11 (IL-11). Cancer patients just before chemotherapy were administered from 10 to 75 mg per kg recombinant human IL-11 (rhIL-11) subcutaneously for 14 consecutive days. The data represent the mean platelet counts of three patients at each dose level. [From Gordon MS et al. A phase I trial of recombinant interleukin-11 (Neumega rhIL-11 growth factor) in women with breast cancer receiving chemotherapy. *Blood* 1996;87:3615–3624, with permission.]

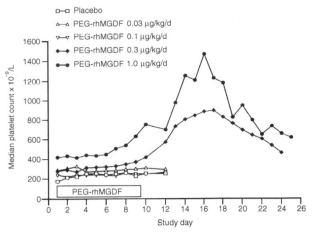

FIGURE 2. Platelet response to graded doses of thrombopoietin. Just before chemotherapy, cancer patients were administered 0.03–1.00 mg/kg of polyethylene-glycol–modified recombinant human MK growth and differentiation factor (PEG-rhMGDF) daily for 10 consecutive days. The data represent the mean platelet counts of three to four patients and four control patients. [From Basser RL et al. Thrombopoietic effects of pegylated recombinant human MK growth and development factor (PEG-rHuMGDF) in patients with advanced cancer. *Lancet* 1996;348:1279–1281, with permission.]

subcutaneous dose (82). The pharmacokinetics of IL-11 are similar, with a half-life of 1.8 to 2.4 hours after a single i.v. infusion (83). Subcutaneous administration results in a slightly longer circulatory life of 8 hours (84). However, unlike the cases of M-CSF, G-CSF, or Tpo, radiolabeled IL-11 localized primarily to the liver and kidneys after injection into mice, suggesting that hematopoietic cells are not the most common sites of cytokine metabolism (85). Thrombopoietic effects of IL-11 administration begin 5 to 9 days after initiation of therapy (Fig. 1), and are maximal for approximately 1 week after discontinuation of the drug (84).

The survival of Tpo in circulation is longer than any other hematopoietic growth factor, with an elimination half-life approaching 30 hours (86). The molecule's carboxyl-terminal region appears responsible for this property. Although a truncated form of Tpo that contains only the amino-terminal region retains full activity *in vitro*, it has little *in vivo* thrombopoietic action. The addition of a single polyethylene glycol moiety (which increases its plasma half-life tenfold) increases its biologic activity in animals substantially, however (87,88). The long half-life of elimination also makes it possible to administer the drug less frequently than other thrombopoietic agents and to provide full efficacy.

The effects of exogenous cytokines on the kinetics of platelet production have been studied extensively (Fig. 2). Unlike the immediate release of reticulocytes prompted by Epo and the immediate release of marrow storage pool neutrophils prompted by G-CSF, none of the thrombopoietic cytokines trigger a rapid release of platelets. Instead, the rise in platelets appears on average 3 to 4 days after the onset of cytokine administration (86,89), strongly suggesting that all platelet-producing effects of these proteins are due to enhanced MK production. This conclusion is consistent with the failure of Tpo or other cytokines to accelerate fragmentation of proplatelet processes, long evaginations of MK cytoplasm considered to represent the most immediate platelet precursor *in vitro* (90). Once size and numbers of MKs increase, platelet count begins to rise until a new steady-state level is reached, the height of which depends on a log-linear relationship

with administered dose, at least for Tpo (88). For IL-6 and IL-11, peak platelet count occurs within several days after administration of the cytokine is begun (91,92). Due to a prolonged biologic effect (the result of its action on primitive and mature hematopoietic cells) and slow plasma clearance, however, enhanced platelet production resulting from parenteral administration of Tpo for 7 to 10 days occurs 6 to 16 days later (86,89). Thus, careful attention to the pharmacokinetics of Tpo administration is necessary to ensure that excessive thrombocytosis is avoided.

PRECLINICAL TRIALS OF THROMBOPOIETIC AGENTS IN STATES OF MARROW FAILURE

IL-3 effectively promotes MK colony growth *in vitro* (9,46), leading to testing of its capacity to accelerate platelet recovery after chemotherapy-induced myelosuppression. Results from preclinical trials have been mixed, however. Gillio and coworkers administered IL-3 to primates after 5-fluorouracil treatment, finding earlier recovery of neutrophils and platelets (93). In contrast, the same group reported that IL-3 failed to affect recovery from cyclophosphamide-induced marrow suppression (94).

Although GM-CSF was initially found to promote MK colony growth *in vitro* (7,8), most animal studies failed to demonstrate any significant effect on cells other than leukocytes. In contrast, human IL-6 has been administered to normal mice in a number of preclinical trials designed to test its thrombopoietic potential. Most studies report a 30% to 60% rise in platelet counts of normal mice owing to enhanced MK maturation (41,42,95). Although not found by all investigators (96), the administration of IL-6 to irradiated mice hastened the recovery of all types of hematopoietic progenitors and was associated with a modest improvement in erythrocyte, leukocyte, and platelet levels (97). Irradiated and control dogs were treated with graded doses of human IL-6. Platelet counts rose in a dose-dependent fashion to 220% of baseline values in the control animals; platelet recovery was enhanced in irradiated dogs receiving the cytokine (98). Low doses of IL-6 increased platelet production two- to threefold in normal cynomolgus macaques, and although much higher doses were required, administration of the cytokine improved platelet recoveries in irradiated animals (91,99).

The preclinical effects of IL-11 have been evaluated in mice, rats, and subhuman primates. In normal rodents, administration of human IL-11 leads to a modest rise in marrow progenitor cells and peripheral blood platelet levels (92,100,101). Moreover, administration of IL-11 accelerates recovery of progenitors and mature cells after myelosuppressive therapies. For example, platelet recovery to 50% of baseline values occurred 5 days earlier in mice that were administered IL-11 after combined radiation and chemotherapy than it did in control animals (102). Favorable effects were also noted on red cell recovery, owing, at least in part, to accelerated red cell production. IL-11 appears to accelerate platelet recovery after stem-cell transplantation (54).

More pronounced effects on thrombopoiesis have been noted in primates administered IL-11, likely due to incomplete cross-reactivity of the human cytokine in rodents. For example, its administration to cynomolgus monkeys doubled platelet counts (compared to 17% to 38% in rodents) and prevented severe thrombocytopenia when administered after carboplatinum-induced myelosuppression (103).

Toxicity and therapeutic efficacy of Tpo have been tested in mice, rats, dogs, and nonhuman primates. In all studies, administration of Tpo has been safe; no signs of hepatic, renal, or pulmonary toxicity, capillary leak, coagulopathy, or hematopoietic toxicity have appeared. As would be expected from its profound megakaryopoietic effects *in vitro*, the administration of Tpo to mice or nonhuman primates increases marrow MK numbers up to tenfold, and peripheral blood platelet counts by an equal degree (64–66,75). Moreover, the panhematopoietic *in vitro* effects of Tpo were also found to correlate with its *in vivo* properties; administration of Tpo to control or myelosuppressed animals increased numbers of all types of hematopoietic progenitor cells (104). Genetic elimination of Tpo or its receptor resulted in a 65% to 95% reduction in numbers of transplantable stem cells and hematopoietic precursors of multiple lineages (105–107).

When administered to animals treated with nonablative myelosuppressive regimens, the use of Tpo has resulted in higher nadir platelet counts and 7- to 14-day accelerations of platelet recovery (104,108–112). It also has favorable effects on erythrocyte and granulocyte recovery in these animals, consistent with its *in vitro* stimulatory effects on cells of these hematopoietic lineages (72,73,104). In one study of nonhuman primates, administration of Tpo after sublethal irradiation resulted in functional iron deficiency (112), confirming its profound effect on erythropoiesis, and arguing for prophylactic use of iron supplementation in patients receiving Tpo.

In contrast to the near-universal preclinical success of Tpo in ameliorating thrombocytopenia (and often pancytopenia) associated with myelosuppressive therapy, its effectiveness after stem-cell transplantation has been less impressive. The administration of Tpo to lethally irradiated mice receiving bone marrow cells

accelerated platelet recovery by 2 to 4 days in two studies (113,114) but did not augment hematopoietic recovery when fewer bone marrow cells were administered (115). In mice receiving peripheral blood stem-cell transplants compared with mice receiving transplants but no Tpo, the hormone accelerated platelet recovery by only 1 or 2 days (113). Tpo also did not facilitate hematopoietic reconstitution in nonhuman primates undergoing autologous bone marrow or peripheral blood stem-cell transplantations (116). Two studies suggest its use in stem-cell donors might improve the quality of the transplantation product, however, leading to enhanced hematopoietic recovery (113,115).

CLINICAL TRIALS OF THROMBOPOIETIC AGENTS

Before discussing results of studies testing therapeutic efficacy of thrombopoietic agents, the goals of such therapy should be considered. In clinical practice, even severe treatment-related thrombocytopenia only rarely induces life-threatening morbidity or mortality; the availability of platelet transfusions has ensured that few thrombocytopenic patients die due to hemorrhage. Most of the adverse effects of thrombocytopenia are mucosal or petechial bleeding, which are not easily quantified, and are thus unlikely to serve as convenient markers of therapeutic efficacy. Rather, as platelet transfusions are associated with multiple adverse reactions, refractoriness to repeated therapy and high cost, a more suitable end point for judging the efficacy of any thrombopoietic agent is reduction in the need for platelet transfusions or earlier release from hospital after episodes of iatrogenic or naturally occurring thrombocytopenia. Alternately, because dose intensities of many forms of chemotherapy are important determinants of success, the ability to administer repeated cycles of chemotherapy on schedule might also serve as an important marker of therapeutic advance.

Recombinant human IL-3 was approved for use in human clinical trials in the late 1980s. Initial reports in individuals with normal hematopoiesis were modestly encouraging (117,118). In general, its use was well tolerated, with toxicity limited to mild fever, flulike symptoms, myalgias, malaise, and headache. In some patients undergoing autologous marrow transplantation, however, its use leads to intolerable side effects (119).

A number of clinical trials using IL-3 to attempt to accelerate platelet recovery from combination chemotherapy have been reported. Four studies in patients being treated for small cell lung or ovarian cancers have suggested that its use accelerates platelet recovery (120–123). In contrast, its use in patients undergoing chemotherapy for non–small-cell lung cancers, relapsed non-Hodgkin's lymphoma, or those undergoing autologous bone marrow transplantation for lymphoma did not significantly affect platelet recovery (119,124,125). Similar results were reported for the use of IL-3 in various states of naturally occurring thrombocytopenia (28,126) with one exception (127). Overall, these studies demonstrate that in selected clinical settings, IL-3 can modestly accelerate platelet recovery and may reduce some of the complications and costs of prolonged thrombocytopenia. As most of the beneficial effects on platelet recovery have been noted at higher doses and are associated with more profound side effects, however, its clinical utility as a single agent appears to be limited.

Although GM-CSF has proven useful in alleviating neutropenia after moderately aggressive myelosuppressive therapy (128) the weight of available evidence suggests that this cytokine fails to significantly impact thrombocytopenia in the same patients (129–131). Similar results have been reported in naturally occurring states of thrombocytopenia (132,133). One of the few exceptions has occurred in patients undergoing autologous transplantation for Hodgkin's disease, in which patients receiving GM-CSF became platelet transfusion–independent approximately 8 days sooner than a control group (134). Altogether, however, these data suggest that if GM-CSF has an effect on platelet recovery, it is not striking; studies to investigate the efficacy of the cytokine in patients with thrombocytopenia have been abandoned.

When administered to cancer patients before chemotherapy, PIXY321 induced a modest increase in neutrophil and platelet levels (135). In general, toxicity has been tolerable in the majority of the trials of this fusion protein; most patients experience fever, rash, and injection-site erythema. The vast majority of studies have failed to reveal any beneficial effects of the drug on platelet recovery, however (136,137). On the basis of these and other negative studies, clinical development of PIXY321 for thrombocytopenia has been abandoned.

In contrast to the minimal effects of IL-3, GM-CSF, and PIXY321 on platelet production in individuals with normal hematopoiesis, IL-6 appears to increase platelet counts by 80 to 100% when administered before chemotherapy to cancer patients (138–140). This level of thrombocytosis is remarkably similar to that observed in patients with inflammation, in whom the overwhelming majority display elevated endogenous levels of IL-6 (141). Its therapeutic efficacy in patients undergoing chemotherapy for malignancy has been mixed, however, even within seemingly homogeneous patient groups. In studies using apparently identical patient populations undergoing identical chemotherapeutic regimens, for example, the drug showed a promising elevation in mean platelet nadirs in one study (55,000 versus 30,000 in IL-6 and control patients, respectively) (142) but no apparent effect in another report (143). Adding further complexity to the interpretation of effects of IL-6 on platelet recovery, D'Hondt reported favorable effects of IL-6 administration only 17 days after the start of chemotherapy (140). As a result, patients were able to receive subsequent cycles of chemotherapy on schedule more often than only after control chemotherapy cycles. Despite the modest therapeutic efficacy in some of these early clinical trials, however, toxicity of IL-6 has been substantial. In all reported studies, patients receiving IL-6 (compared to control patients) developed modest to significant levels of anemia and mild to modest constitutional symptoms; some studies have been marked by severe complications, such as venoocclusive liver disease. As such, the usefulness of IL-6 in alleviating thrombocytopenia is limited.

Unlike IL-3, IL-6, GM-CSF, and PIXY321, recombinant IL-11 has proven effective and relatively safe in clinical trials. The major side effects of IL-11 are related to sodium and fluid retention, causing generalized edema, dilutional anemia, dyspnea, and secondary atrial tachyarrhythmias (144,145). Use of diuret-

TABLE 1. EFFECTS OF INTERLEUKIN-11 AFTER CHEMOTHERAPY IN TWO CLINICAL TRIALS

Reference	n	Percent of patients requiring platelet transfusion
Tepler et al. (146)		
Placebo	27	96
rhIL-11; 25 μg/kg/d	28	82[b]
rhIL-11; 50 μg/kg/d	27	70[c]
Isaacs et al. (147)[a]		
Placebo	37	60
rhIL-11; 50 μg/kg/d	40	33[d]

n, number of evaluable patients.
[a]Intent-to-treat analysis.
[b]$p = .23$.
[c]$p < .05$.
[d]$p = .02$.
Note: Patients received many different chemotherapeutic regimens in the study of Tepler et al. and cyclophosphamide/doxorubicin in the Isaacs et al. study.

ics with IL-11 has been recommended, but dangerous degrees of hypokalemia have also been noted even without diuretic use. Approximately 1% of patients develops antibodies to the cytokine that appear to be of no clinical importance. Two major clinical trials of IL-11 have been published, the results of which are shown in Table 1. In a phase 1/2 randomized trial of 93 cancer patients who required at least one platelet transfusion during their previous cycle of chemotherapy, administration of IL-11 reduced the need for platelet transfusions during a subsequent cycle of the same chemotherapy (146). In a second intent to treat study of 77 patients with breast cancer who needed one or more platelet transfusions during their first cycle of intensive chemotherapy, the use of IL-11 reduced the need for a platelet transfusion from 68% to 41% in the subsequent treatment cycle, a statistically significant difference if based on intent-to-treat analysis (147). Most of the reduction in transfusional needs occurred during the second cycle of chemotherapy. These studies led to recent FDA approval of the drug for the secondary prophylaxis of thrombocytopenia after chemotherapy.

Results of several clinical trials of Tpo therapy are summarized in Table 2. In all studies, the administration of either of two forms of recombinant human Tpo was safe and, when administered before chemotherapy, resulted in profound stimulation of platelet production (86,89,148). Specifically, no significant changes in vital signs or weight occurred, and the frequency of symptoms or signs of bone pain, organ dysfunction, superficial or deep venous thrombosis, and platelet activation were similar in treatment and placebo groups. It must be noted, however, that patients with histories of cardiac, pulmonary, vascular, or thrombotic disease were excluded from all studies. Only a rare patient in any of the reported trials developed antibodies to Tpo (85,148). Few patients have been given more than a single course of treatment in these trials, however, making any conclusions on the immunogenicity of the two products premature.

Results from several clinical trials of Tpo in patients with cancer treated with carboplatin-based chemotherapeutic regimens have been reported (148–152). In all studies, platelet counts returned to baseline significantly faster; in four studies, nadir platelet counts were higher in the patients receiving Tpo (com-

TABLE 2. EFFECTS OF THROMBOPOIETIN AFTER CHEMOTHERAPY IN FIVE CLINICAL TRIALS

Reference	n	Nadir plt count (x 10^{-3}/mm^3) (range)	Days for plt recovery to baseline	Percent plt >50,000/mm^3	Percent requiring platelet transfusion
Fanucchi et al. (148)					
Placebo	12	111 (21–307)	>21	N.S.	8
MGDF	38	188 (68–373)	14	N.S.	0
Crawford et al. (149)					
Placebo	10	27	N.S.	N.S.	64
MGDF, 2.5 µg/kg/d	12	21	N.S.	N.S.	50
MGDF, 5 µg/kg/d	18	89	N.S.	N.S.	17
Basser et al. (150)					
Placebo	10	50	22	N.S.	20
MGDF[a]	41	55	17[c]	N.S.	23[d]
Vadhan-Raj et al. (151)[b]					
First cycle without rhTpo	22	N.S.	N.S.	N.S.	50
Second cycle with rhTpo	22	N.S.	N.S.	N.S.	23
Moskowitz et al. (152)					
Placebo	15	36 (8–118)	N.S.	47	20
MGDF, 2.5 µg/kg/d	15	105 (11–438)	N.S.	87	0
MGDF, 5 µg/kg/d	21	147 (31–491)	N.S.	95	0

MGDF, pegylated recombinant human megakaryocyte growth and development factor; N.S., not stated; plt, platelet; rhTpo, recombinant human thrombopoietin.
[a]All doses from 0.03 to 5.00 µg/kg/d are included.
[b]Study designed to hold thrombopoietin during first cycle, and administer thrombopoietin after the second cycle of therapy.
[c]$p = .014$.
[d]$p = .7$.
Note: Patients received carboplatin/paclitaxel (148,149), carboplatin/cyclophosphamide (150), high-dose carboplatin alone (151), or ifosfamide/carboplatin/etoposide (152) for their malignancies.

pared with either those patients receiving placebos or the same patients during their first cycles of chemotherapy). Chemotherapy regimens administered in the first two of these trials induced only modest thrombocytopenia (mean nadir platelet counts in the placebo groups of 60,000 per mm^3 to 111,000 per mm^3); in neither study was hospital discharge delayed due to thrombocytopenia, nor were significant numbers of platelet transfusions required. In the other three studies (149,151,152), nadir platelet values (the number of days with less than or equal to 20,000 or 50,000 platelets per µl) and the number of patients requiring platelet transfusions were all improved compared to cycles of therapy without Tpo. As these studies had accrued small numbers of patients at the time of writing, additional results from these and additional trials enrolling greater numbers of patients is required to confirm the beneficial effects of the use of Tpo to alleviate chemotherapy-induced thrombocytopenia, the need to use platelet transfusions, and to ensure the timely return of platelet counts to safe levels to allow the on-time administration of subsequent cycles of chemotherapy.

Tpo increases the number of megakaryocytic and other hematopoietic progenitors *in vitro* and *in vivo* (72,73,104), properties that may benefit patients receiving stem-cell transplants. Although the hormone was of only marginal benefit in several preclinical trials, Tpo has now been tested in several clinical trials of bone marrow or peripheral blood stem-cell transplantation. In 40 patients with breast cancer undergoing autologous bone marrow transplantation, administration of pegylated (MGDF) recombinant human MK growth and development factor led to a 5 to 6 day earlier rise in platelet count (20,000 per mm^3) and a 48% reduction in use of platelet transfusions (as compared with placebo) (152). It has not been effective in

patients undergoing autologous peripheral blood stem-cell transplants, however. In a total of 75 patients with breast cancer undergoing autologous peripheral blood stem-cell transplantation, the use of Tpo (either before conditioning chemotherapy or after stem-cell infusion) did not alter platelet recovery or need for platelet transfusion (153–155). In a study of 38 patients with delayed platelet recovery after peripheral blood stem-cell or bone marrow transplantation, the use of recombinant human Tpo led to platelet transfusion independence in only two individuals (156).

Because of the dynamics of modern platelet pheresis technology, relatively small increments in peripheral blood platelet counts result in large increases in the numbers of platelets that can be recovered. A single dose of Tpo administered to subjects with normal hematopoietic functions increased yield of platelets threefold and was associated with a fourfold improvement in platelet counts in recipients of the pheresed platelets (157). When this study was expanded to include more than 1,000 normal platelet donors, however, approximately 1% developed antirecombinant Tpo antibodies that cross-reacted with endogenous hormones, leading to donor thrombocytopenia. Although most of these individual platelet donors have recovered, the form of recombinant Tpo used in this study has been withdrawn from further clinical testing in this setting.

CONCLUSION

Erythropoietin, GM-CSF, and G-CSF have proven effective in many—but not all—patients with anemia and neutropenia. These successes provide the bases for optimism that thrombopoietic agents can be similarly identified. Although many cytokines and hormones affect MK development *in vivo*, only two, IL-11 and Tpo, and an engineered molecule that combines sequences from IL-3 and Tpo, continue to be tested for efficacy in clinical trials. Initial trials suggest that one or more of these agents prove effective in ameliorating thrombocytopenia in some—but not all—clinical settings. On the basis of its ability to reduce need for platelet transfusions in secondary prophylaxis settings, IL-11 has been approved by the U.S. Food and Drug Administration for use, and it is likely that one or more forms of Tpo will also be approved for use. Promegapoietin, the combination molecule, has been effective in preclinical trials; its toxicity and immunogenicity profile will determine its usefulness. Clearly, applying physiology-based biotechnologic strategies to Osler's dilemma is yielding therapeutic dividends.

REFERENCES

1. Wallace EL, Churchill WH, Surgenor DM, Cho G, McGurk S. Collection and transfusion of blood and blood components in the United States, 1994. *Transfusion* 1998;38:622–624.
2. Heddle NM, Klama L, Singer J, et al. The role of the plasma from platelet concentrates in transfusion reactions. *N Engl J Med* 1994;331:625–628.
3. Sniecinski I, O'Donnell MR, Nowicki B, Hill LR. Prevention of refractoriness and HLA-alloimmunization using filtered blood products. *Blood* 1988;71:1402–1407.
4. Slichter SJ. Platelet refractoriness and alloimmunization. *Leukemia* 1998;12[Suppl 1]:S51–S53.
5. Osler W. *The principles and practice of medicine*. Purpura: D. Appleton and Co. 1892:320–322.
6. Williams N, Eger RR, Jackson HM, Nelson DJ. Two-factor requirement for murine megakaryocyte colony formation. *J Cell Physiol* 1982;110:101–104.
7. Kaushansky K, O'Hara PJ, Berkner K, Segal GM, Hagen FS, Adamson JW. Genomic cloning, characterization, and multilineage expression of human granulocyte-macrophage colony-stimulating factor. *Proc Natl Acad Sci U S A* 1986;83:3101–3105.
8. Robinson BE, McGrath HE, Quesenberry PJ. Recombinant murine granulocyte macrophage colony stimulating factor has megakaryocyte colony stimulating activity and augments megakaryocyte colony stimulation by interleukin-3. *J Clin Invest* 1987;79:1648–1652.
9. Segal GM, Stueve T, Adamson JW. Analysis of murine megakaryocyte colony size and ploidy. Effects of interleukin-3. *J Cell Physiol* 1988;137:537–544.
10. Briddell RA, Bruno E, Cooper RJ, Brandt JE, Hoffman R. Effect of *c-kit* ligand on *in vitro* human megakaryocytopoiesis. *Blood* 1991;78:2854–2859.
11. Avraham H, Vannier E, Cowley S, et al. Effects of the stem cell factor, *c-kit* ligand, on human megakaryocytic cells. *Blood* 1992;79:365–371.
12. Ikebuchi K, Wong GG, Clark SC, Ihle JN, Hirai Y, Ogawa M. Interleukin-6 enhancement of interleukin-3-dependent proliferation of multipotential hemopoietic progenitors. *Proc Natl Acad Sci U S A* 1987;84:9035–9039.
13. Burstein SA, Mei R-L, Henthorn J, Friese P, Turner K. Leukemia inhibitory factor and interleukin-11 promote maturation of murine and human megakaryocytes *in vitro*. *J Cell Physiol* 1992;153:305–312.
14. McDonald TP. Thrombopoietin: its biology, purification, and characterization. *Exp Hematol* 1988;16:201–205.
15. Hill RJ, Levin J. Regulators of thrombopoiesis. Their biochemistry and physiology. *Blood Cells* 1989;15:141–166.
16. Kaushansky K. Thrombopoietin. The primary regulator of platelet production. *Blood* 1995;86:419–431.
17. Yang YC, Ciarletta AB, Temple PA, et al. Human IL-3 (mutli-CSF). Identification by expression cloning of a novel hematopoietic growth factor related to murine IL-3. *Cell* 1986;47:3–10.
18. Ihle JN, Peppersack L, Rebar L. Regulation of T cell differentiation. *In vitro* induction of 20 α-hydroxysteroid dehydrogenase in splenic lymphocytes from thymic mice by a unique lymphokine. *J Immunol* 1981;126:2184.
19. Kindler V, Thorens B, de Kossodo S, et al. Stimulation of hematopoiesis *in vivo* by recombinant bacterial murine interleukin-3. *Proc Natl Acad Sci U S A* 1986;83:1001–1005.
20. Emerson SG, Yang YC, Clark SC, Long MW. Human recombinant granulocyte-macrophage colony stimulating factor and interleukin-3 have overlapping but distinct hematopoietic activity. *J Clin Invest* 1988;82:1282–1287.
21. Clutterbuck EJ, Hirst EMA, Sanderson CJ. Human interleukin-5 (IL-5) regulates the production of eosinophils in human bone marrow cultures. Comparison and interaction with IL-1, IL-3, IL-6, and GM-CSF. *Blood* 1989;73:1504–1512.
22. Carrington PA, Hill RJ, Stenberg PE, et al. Multiple *in vivo* effects of interleukin-3 and interleukin-6 on mouse megakaryocytopoiesis. *Blood* 1991;77:34–41.
23. Yonemura Y, Kawakita M, Masuda T, Fujimoto K, Kato K, Takatsuki K. Synergistic effects of interleukin-3 and interleukin-11 on murine megakaryopoiesis in serum-free culture. *Exp Hematol* 1992;20:1011.
24. Valent P, Besemer J, Muhm M, Majdic O, Lechner K, Bettelheim P. Interleukin-3 activates human blood basophils via high-affinity binding sites. *Proc Natl Acad Sci U S A* 1989;86:5542–5546.
25. Nishinakamura R, Miyajima A, Mee PJ, Tybulewicz VLJ, Murray R. Hematopoiesis in mice lacking the entire granulocyte-macrophage colony-stimulating factor/interleukin-3/interleukin-5 functions. *Blood* 1996;88:2458–2464.
26. Mach N, Lantz CS, Galli SJ, et al. Involvement of interleukin-3 in delayed-type hypersensitivity. *Blood* 1998;91:778–783.
27. Metcalf D, Begley CG, Johnson GR, Nicola NA, Lopez AF, Williamson DJ. Effects of purified bacterially synthesized murine multi-CSF (IL-3) on hematopoiesis in normal adult mice. *Blood* 1986;68:46.
28. Nimer SD, Paquette RL, Ireland P, Resta D, Young D, Golde DW. A phase I/II study of interleukin-3 in patients with aplastic anemia and myelodysplasia. *Exp Hematol* 1994;22:875–880.
29. Kaushansky K. The thrombopoietin of cancer. Prospects for effective cytokine therapy. *Hematol Oncol Clin North Am* 1996;10:431–455.
30. Wong GG, Witek JS, Temple PA, et al. Human GM-CSF. Molecular cloning of the complementary DNA and purification of the natural and recombinant proteins. *Science* 1985;228:810–815.
31. Emerson SG, Sieff CA, Wang EA, Wong GG, Clark SC, Nathan DG. Purification of fetal hematopoietic progenitors and demonstration of recombinant multipotential colony stimulating activity. *J Clin Invest* 1985;76:1286–1290.
32. Weisbart RH, Kwan L, Golde DW, Gasson JC. Human GM-CSF primes neutrophils for enhanced oxidative metabolism in response to the major physiological chemoattractants. *Blood* 1987;69:18–21.
33. Dranoff G, Crawford AD, Sadelain M, et al. Involvement of granulocyte-macrophage colony-stimulating factor in pulmonary homeostasis. *Science* 1994;264:713–716.
34. Dirksen U, Nishinakamura R, Groneck P, et al. Human pulmonary alveolar proteinosis associated with a defect in GM-CSF/IL-3/IL-5 receptor common β chain expression. *J Clin Invest* 1997;100:2211–2217.
35. Curtis BM, Williams DE, Broxmeyer HE, et al. Enhanced hematopoietic activity of a human granulocyte/macrophage colony-stimulating factor-interleukin 3 fusion protein. *Proc Natl Acad Sci U S A* 1991;88:5809.
36. Williams DE, Dunn JT, Park LS, et al. A GM-CSF/IL-3 fusion protein promotes neutrophil and platelet recovery in sublethally irradiated rhesus monkeys. *Biotechnol Ther* 1993;4:17–29.
37. Kishimoto T. The biology of interleukin-6. *Blood* 1989;74:1–10.
38. Ariyama Y, Misawa S, Sonoda Y. Synergistic effects of stem cell factor and interleukin-6 or interleukin-11 on the expansion of murine

hematopoietic progenitors in liquid suspension culture. *Stem Cells* 1995;13(4):404–413.

39. Ulich TR, del Castillo J, Guo KZ. *In vivo* hematologic effects of recombinant interleukin 6 on hematopoiesis and circulating numbers of RBCs and WBCs. *Blood* 1989;73:108–110.

40. Hudak S, Thompson-Snipes L, Rocco C, Jackson J, Pearce M, Rennick D. Anti-IL-6 antibodies suppress myeloid cell production and the generation of CFU-c in long term bone marrow cultures. *Exp Hematol* 1992;20;412–417.

41. Ishibashi T, Kimura H, Uchida T, Kariyone S, Friese P, Burstein SA. Human interleukin-6 is a direct promoter of maturation of megakaryocytes in vitro. *Proc Natl Acad Sci U S A* 1989;86:5953–5957.

42. Hill RJ, Warren MK, Levin J. Stimulation of thrombopoiesis in mice by human recombinant interleukin-6. *J Clin Invest* 1990;85:1242–1247.

43. Cressman DE, Greenbaum LE, DeAngelis A, et al. Liver failure and defective hepatocyte regeneration in interleukin-6-deficient mice. *Science* 1996;274:1379–1383.

44. Bluethmann H, Rothe J, Schultze N, Tkachuk M, Koebel P. Establishment of the role of IL-6 and TNF receptor 1 using gene knock-out mice. *J Leukoc Biol* 1994;56:565–570.

45. Liu F, Poursine-Laurent J, Wu HY, Link DC. Interleukin-6 and the granulocyte colony-stimulating factor receptor are major independent regulators of granulopoiesis *in vivo* but are not required for lineage commitment or terminal differentiation. *Blood* 1997;90:2583–2590.

46. Paul SR, Bennett F, Calvetti JA, et al. Molecular cloning of a cDNA encoding interleukin 11, a stromal cell-derived lymphopoietic and hematopoietic cytokine. *Proc Natl Acad Sci U S A* 1990;87:7512–7516.

47. Bruno E, Briddell RA, Cooper RJ, Hoffman R. Effects of recombinant interleukin-11 on human megakaryocyte progenitor cells. *Exp Hematol* 1991;19:378–381.

48. Elias JA, Zheng T, Whiting NL, Trow TK, Merrill WW, Zitnik R, Ray P, Alderman EM. IL-1 and transforming growth factor beta regulation of fibroblast derived IL-11. *J Immunol* 1994;152:2421–2429.

49. Okamoto H, Yamamura M, Morita Y, Harada S, Makino H, Ota Z. The synovial expression and serum levels of interleukin-6, interleukin-11, leukemia inhibitory factor, and oncostatin M in rheumatoid arthritis. *Arthritis Rheum* 1997;40:1096–1105.

50. Chang M, Suen Y, Meng G, et al. Differential mechanisms in the regulation of endogenous levels of thrombopoietin and interleukin-11 during thrombocytopenia. Insight into the regulation of platelet production. *Blood* 1996;88:3354–3362.

51. Endo S, Inada K, Arakawa N, et al. Interleukin-11 levels in patients with disseminated intravascular coagulation. *Res Commun Mol Pathol Pharmacol* 1996;91(2):253–256.

52. Heits F, Katschinski DM, Wilmsen U, Wiedemann GJ, Jelkmann W. Serum thrombopoietin and interleukin-6 concentrations in tumour patients and response to chemotherapy-induced thrombocytopenia. *Eur J Haematol* 1997;59:53–58.

53. Nandurkar HH, Robb L, Tarlinton D, Barnett L, Köntgen F, Begley CG. Adult mice with targeted mutation of the interleukin-11 receptor (IL11Ra) display normal hematopoiesis. *Blood* 1997;90:2148–2159.

54. Du X, Williams DA. Interleukin-11. Review of molecular, cell biology and clinical use. *Blood* 1997;89:3897–3908.

55. Musashi M, Yang YC, Paul SR, Clark SC, Sudo T, Ogawa M. Direct and synergistic effects of interleukin-11 on murine hemopoiesis in culture. *Proc Natl Acad Sci U S A* 1991;88:765–769.

56. Neben S, Donaldson D, Sieff C, et al. Synergistic effects of interleukin-11 with other growth factors on the expansion of murine hematopoietic progenitors and maintenance of stem cells in liquid culture. *Exp Hematol* 1994;22:353–359.

57. Du XX, Scott D, Yang ZX, Cooper R, Xiao XL, Williams DA. Interleukin-11 stimulates multilineage progenitors, but not stem cells, in murine and human long-term marrow cultures. *Blood* 1995;86:128–134.

58. Quesniaux VFJ, Clark SC, Turner K, Fagg B. Interleukin-11 stimulates multiple phases of erythropoiesis *in vitro*. *Blood* 1992;80:1218–1223.

59. Teramura M, Kobayashi S, Hoshino S, et al. Interleukin-II enhances human megakaryocytopoiesis in vitro. *Blood* 1992;79:327–331.

60. Broudy VC, Lin NL, Kaushansky K. Thrombopoietin (c-*mpl* ligand) acts synergistically with erythropoietin, stem cell factor, and IL-11 to enhance murine megakaryocyte colony growth and increases megakaryocyte ploidy *in vitro*. *Blood* 1995;85:1719–1726.

61. Taga T, Kishimoto T. gp130 and the interleukin-6 family of cytokines. *Annu Rev Immunol* 1997;15:797–819.

62. Peng J, Friese P, Wolf RF, et al. Relative reactivity of platelets from thrombopoietin and interleukin-6 treated dogs. *Blood* 1996;87:4158–4163.

63. Weich NS, Wang A, Fitzgerald M, et al. Recombinant human interleukin-11 directly promotes megakaryocytopoiesis in vitro. *Blood* 1997;90:3893–3902.

64. de Sauvage FJ, Hass PE, Spencer SD, et al. Stimulation of megakaryocytopoiesis and thrombopoiesis by the c-Mpl ligand. *Nature* 1994;369:533–538.

65. Lok S, Kaushansky K, Holly RD, et al. Cloning and expression of murine thrombopoietin cDNA and stimulation of platelet production *in vivo*. *Nature* 1994;369:565–568.

66. Bartley TD, Bogenberger J, Hunt P, et al. Identification and cloning of a megakaryocyte growth and development factor that is a ligand for the cytokine receptor Mpl. *Cell* 1994;77:1117–1124.

67. Sohma Y, Akahori H, Seki N, et al. Molecular cloning and chromosomal localization of the human thrombopoietin gene. *FEBS Lett* 1994;353:57–61.

68. Linden H, Kaushansky K. The glycan domain of thrombopoietin (TPO) functions alone in trans to enhance secretion of the receptor binding domain of TPO and other cytokines. *Blood* 1998;92[Suppl 1]:674a(abst).

69. Kaushansky K, Lok S, Holly RD, et al. Promotion of megakaryocyte progenitor expansion and differentiation by the c-Mpl ligand thrombopoietin. *Nature* 1994;369:568–571.

70. Kaushansky K, Broudy VC, Grossmann A, et al. Thrombopoietin expands erythroid progenitors, increases red cell production, and enhances erythroid recovery after myelosuppressive therapy. *J Clin Invest* 1995;96:1683–1687.

71. Kobayashi M, Laver JH, Kato T, Miyazaki H, Ogawa M. Recombinant human thrombopoietin (Mpl ligand) enhances proliferation of erythroid progenitors. *Blood* 1995;86:2494–2999.

72. Ku H, Yonemura Y, Kaushansky K, Ogawa M. Thrombopoietin, the ligand for the Mpl receptor, synergizes with steel factor and other early-acting cytokines in supporting proliferation of primitive hematopoietic progenitors of mice. *Blood* 1996;87:4544–4551.

73. Sitnicka E, Lin N, Priestley GV, et al. The effect of thrombopoietin on the proliferation and differentiation of murine hematopoietic stem cells. *Blood* 1996;87:4998–5005.

74. Chen J, Herceg-Harjacek L, Groopman JE, Grabarek J. Regulation of platelet activation in vitro by the c-Mpl ligand, thrombopoietin. *Blood* 1995;86:4054–4062.

75. Harker LA, Marzec UM, Hunt P, et al. Dose response effects of pegylated human megakaryocyte growth and development factor on platelet production and function in nonhuman primates. *Blood* 1996;88:511–521.

76. Giri JG, Kahn LE, Doshi PD, et al. Promegapoietin, an engineered chimeric growth factor for platelet producing cells. *Blood* 1996;88[Suppl 1]:351a(abst).

77. Lin J, Nachtrieb E, Bensinger W, et al. Ex vivo expansion of myeloid and megakaryocytic progenitors using HS-5 stromal cell conditioned medium plus promegapoietin. *Blood* 1997;90[Suppl 1]:538a(abst).

78. Giri JG, Smith WG, Kahn LE, et al. Promegapoietin, a chimeric growth factor for megakaryocyte and platelet restoration. *Blood* 1997;90[Suppl 1]:580a(abst).

79. Bartocci A, Mastrogiannis DS, Migliorati G, Stockert RJ, Wolkoff AW, Stanley ER. Macrophages specifically regulate the concentration of their own growth factor in the circulation. *Proc Natl Acad Sci U S A* 1987;84:6179–6183.

80. Hovgaard DJ, Folke M, Mortensen BT, Nissen NI. Recombinant human interleukin-3. Pharmacokinetics after intravenous and subcutaneous bolus injection and effects on granulocyte kinetics. *Br J Haematol* 1994;87:700–707.

81. Hovgaard DJ, Mortensen BT, Schifter S, Nissen NI. Comparative pharmacokinetics of single-dose administration of mammalian and bacterially derived recombinant human granulocyte-macrophage colony-stimulating factor. *Eur J Haematol* 1993;50:32–36.

82. Weber J, Yang JC, Topalian SL, et al. Phase I trial of subcutaneous interleukin-6 in patients with advanced malignancies. *J Clin Oncol* 1993;11:499–506.

83. Aoyama K, Uchida T, Takanuki F, Usui T, Watanabe T, Higuchi S, Toyoki T, Mizoguchi H. Pharmacokinetics of recombinant human interleukin-11 in healthy male subjects. *Br J Clin Pharm* 1997;43:571–578.

84. Gordon MS, McCaskill-Stevens WJ, Battiato LA, et al. A phase I trial of recombinant intereleuikin-11 (Neumega rhIL-11 growth factor) in women with breast cancer receiving chemotherapy. *Blood* 1996;87:3615–3624.

85. Takagi A, Masuda H, Takakura Y, Hashida M. Disposition characteristics of recombinant human interleukin-11 after a bolus intravenous administration in mice. *J Pharm Exp Ther* 1995;275:537–543.

86. Vadhan-Raj S, Murray LJ, Bueso-Ramos C, et al. Stimulation of megakaryocyte and platelet production by a single dose of recombinant human thrombopoietin in cancer patients. *Ann Intern Med* 1997;126:673–681.

87. Hokum MM, Lacey D, Kintsler OB, et al. Pegylated megakaryocyte growth and development factor abrogates the lethal thrombocytopenia associated with carboplatin and irradiation in mice. *Blood* 1995;86:4486–4492.

88. Harker LA, Hunt P, Marzek UM, et al. Regulation of platelet production and function by megakaryocyte growth and development factor in nonhuman primates. *Blood* 1996;87:1833–1844.

89. Basser RL, Rasko JEJ, Clarke K, et al. Thrombopoietic effects of pegylated recombinant human megakaryocyte growth and development factor (PEG-rHuMGDF) in patients with advanced cancer. *Lancet* 1996;348:1279–1281.

90. Choi ES, Nichol JL, Hokom MM, Hornkohl AC, Hunt P. Platelets generated *in vitro* from proplatelet-displaying human megakaryocytes are functional. *Blood* 1995;85:402–413.

91. Asano S, Okano A, Ozawa K, et al. *In vivo* effects of recombinant human interleukin-6 in primates. Stimulated production of platelets. *Blood* 1990;75:1602–1605.

92. Neben TY, Loebelenz J, Hayes L, McCarthy K, Stoudemire J, Schaub R, Goldman SJ. Recombinant human interleukin-11 stimulates megakaryocytopoiesis and increases peripheral platelets in normal and splenectomized mice. *Blood* 1993;81:901–908.

93. Gillio AP, Gasparetto C, Laver J, et al. Effects of interleukin-3 on hematopoietic recovery after 5-fluorouracil or cyclophosphamide treatment of cynomolgus primates. *J Clin Invest* 1990;85:1560.

94. Garnick MB, O'Reilly RJ. Clinical promise of new hematopoietic growth factors. M-CSF, IL-3, IL-6. *Hematol Oncol Clin North Am* 1989;3:495.

95. Ishibashi T, Shikama Y, Kimura H, et al. Thrombopoietic effects of interleukin-6 in long-term administration in mice. *Exp Hematol* 1993;21:640–646.

96. Pojda Z, Aoki Y, Sobiczewska E, et al. *In vivo* administration of interleukin-6 delays hematopoietic regeneration in sublethally irradiated mice. *Exp Hematol* 1992;20:862.

97. Patchen ML, MacVittie TJ, Williams JL, et al. Administration of interleukin-6 stimulates multilineage hematopoiesis and accelerates recovery from radiation-induced hematopoietic depression. *Blood* 1991;77:472.

98. Burstein SA, Downs T, Friese P, et al. Thrombocytosis in normal and sublethally irradiated dogs. Response to human interleukin-6. *Blood* 1992;80:420–428.

99. Zeidler C, Kanz L, Hurkuck F, et al. *In vivo* effects of interleukin-6 on thrombopoiesis in healthy and irradiated primates. *Blood* 1992;80:2740–2745.

100. Hangoc G, Yin T, Cooper S, Schendel P, Yang Y-C, Broxmeyer HE. *In vivo* effects of recombinant interleukin-11 on myelopoiesis in mice. *Blood* 1993;81:965–972.

101. Yonemura Y, Kawakita M, Masuda T, Fujimoto K, Takatsuki K. Effect of recombinant human interleukin-11 on rat megakaryopoie-

sis and thrombopoiesis *in vivo*. Comparative study with interleukin-6. *Br J Haematol* 1993;84:16–23.

102. Leonard JP, Quinto CM, Kozitza MK, Neben TY, Goldman, SJ. Recombinant human interleukin-11 stimulates multilineage hematopoietic recovery in mice after a myelosuppressive regimen of sublethal irradiation and carboplatin. *Blood* 1994;83:1499–1506.

103. Schlerman E, Bree AG, Kaviani MD, et al. Thrombopoietic activity of recombinant human interleukin-11 (rhIL-11) in normal and myelosuppressed nonhuman primates. *Stem Cells* 1996;4:517–532.

104. Kaushansky K, Lin N, Grossmann A, Humes J, Sprugel KH, Broudy VC. Thrombopoietin expands erythroid, granulocyte-macrophage and megakaryocytic progenitor cells in normal and myelosuppressed mice. *Exp Hematol* 1996;23:265–269.

105. Alexander WS, Roberts AW, Nicola NA, Li R, Metcalf D. Deficiencies in progenitor cells of multiple hematopoietic lineages and defective megakaryocytopoiesis in mice lacking the thrombopoietin receptor c-Mpl. *Blood* 1996;87:2162–2170.

106. Kimura S, Roberts AW, Metcalf D, Alexander WS. Hematopoietic stem cell deficiencies in mice lacking c-Mpl, the receptor for thrombopoietin. *Proc Natl Acad Sci U S A* 1998;95:1195–1200.

107. Solar GP, Kerr WG, Zeigler FC, et al. Role of c-mpl in early hematopoiesis. *Blood* 1998;92:4–10.

108. Ulich TR, del Catillo J, Senaldi G, et al. Systemic hematologic effects of PEG-rHuMGDF-induced megakaryocyte hyperplasia in mice. *Blood* 1996;87:5006–5015.

109. Grossmann A, Lenox J, Deisher T, et al. Synergistic effects of thrombopoietin and G-CSF on neutrophil recovery in myelosuppressed mice. *Blood* 1996;88:3363–3370.

110. Akahori H, Shibuya K, Obuchi M, et al. Effect of recombinant human thrombopoietin in nonhuman primates with chemotherapy-induced thrombocytopenia. *Br J Haematol* 1996;94:722–728.

111. Harker LA, Marzec UM, Kelly AB, et al. Prevention of thrombocytopenia and neutropenia in a nonhuman primate model of marrow suppressive chemotherapy by combining pegylated recombinant human megakaryocyte growth and development factor and recombinant human granulocyte colony-stimulating factor. *Blood* 1997;89:155–165.

112. Neelis KJ, Qingliang L, Thomas GR, Cohen BL, Eaton DL, Wagemaker G. Prevention of thrombocytopenia by thrombopoietin in myelosuppressed rhesus monkeys accompanied by prominent erythropoietic stimulation and iron depletion. *Blood* 1997;90:58–63.

113. Molineaux G, Hartley C, McElroy P, McCrea C, McNiece IK. Megakaryocyte growth and development factor accelerates platelet recovery in peripheral blood progenitor cell transplant recipients. *Blood* 1996;88:366–376.

114. Kabaya K, Shibuya K, Torii Y, et al. Improvement of thrombocytopenia following bone marrow transplantation by pegylated recombinant human megakaryocyte growth and development factor in mice. *Bone Marrow Transplant* 1996;18:1035–1041.

115. Fibbe WE, Heemskerk DPM, Laterveer L, Pruijt JFM, Foster D, Kaushansky K, Willemze R. Accelerated reconstitution of platelets and erythrocytes following syngeneic transplantation of bone marrow cells derived from thrombopoietin pretreated donor mice. *Blood* 1995;86:3308–3313.

116. Neelis KJ, Dubbelman YD, Wognum AW, et al. Lack of efficacy of thrombopoietin and granulocyte colony-stimulating factor after high dose total body irradiation and autologous stem cell or bone marrow transplantation in rhesus monkeys. *Exp Hematol* 1997;25:1094–1103.

117. Ganser A, Lindemann A, Seipelt G, et al. Effects of recombinant human interleukin-3 in patients with normal hematopoiesis and in patients with bone marrow failure. *Blood* 1990;76:666.

118. Lindemann A, Ganser A, Herrmann F, et al. Biologic effects of recombinant human interleukin-3 *in vivo*. *J Clin Oncol* 1991;9:2120.

119. Nemunaitis J, Appelbaum FR, Singer JW, et al. Phase I trial with recombinant human interleukin-3 in patients with lymphoma undergoing autologous bone marrow transplantation. *Blood* 1993;82:3273–3278.

120. Postmus PE, Gietema JA, Damsma O, et al. Effects of recombinant human interleukin-3 in patients with relapsed small-cell lung cancer

treated with chemotherapy. A dose-finding study. *J Clin Oncol* 1992;10:1131.

121. Biesma B, Willemse PHB, Mulder NH, et al. Effects of interleukin-3 after chemotherapy for advanced ovarian cancer. *Blood* 1992;80:1141.

122. D'Hondt V, Weynants P, Humblet Y, et al. Dose-dependent interleukin-3 stimulation of thrombopoiesis and neutropoiesis in patients with small-cell lung carcinoma before and following chemotherapy. A placebo-controlled randomized phase Ib study. *J Clin Oncol* 1993;11:2063.

123. Speyer J, Mandeli J, Hochster H, et al. A phase I trial of cyclophosphamide and carboplatinum combined with interleukin-3 in women with advanced stage ovarian cancer. *Gynecol Oncol* 1995;56:387–394.

124. Raemaekers J, Imhoff GW, Verdonck MF, Hessels JA, Fibbe W. The tolerability of continuous intravenous infusion of interleukin-3 after DHAP chemotherapy in patients with relapsed malignant lymphoma. A phase I study. *Ann Hematol* 1993;67:175–181.

125. Tepler I, Elias A, Kalish L, et al. Effect of recombinant human interleukin-3 on haematological recovery from chemotherapy-induced myelosuppression. *Br J Haematol* 1994;87:678.

126. Kurzrock R, Talpaz M, Estrov Z, et al. Phase I study of recombinant human interleukin-3 in patients with bone marrow failure. *J Clin Oncol* 1991;9:1241.

127. Guinan EC, Lee YS, Lopez KD, et al. Effects of interleukin-3 and granulocyte-macrophage colony-stimulating factor on thrombopoiesis in congenital amegakaryocytic thrombocytopenia. *Blood* 1993;81:1691.

128. Armitage JO. Emerging applications of recombinant human granulocyte-macrophage colony-stimulating factor. *Blood* 1999;92:4491–4508.

129. Antman KS, Griffin JD, Elias A, et al. Effect of recombinant human granulocyte-macrophage colony-stimulating factor on chemotherapy-induced myelosuppression. *N Engl J Med* 1988;319:593.

130. Nemunaitis J, Robinowe SN, Singer JW, et al. Recombinant granulocyte-macrophage colony-stimulating factor after autologous bone marrow transplantation for lymphoid cancer. *N Engl J Med* 1991;324:1773.

131. Brandt SJ, Peters WP, Atwater SK, et al. Effect of recombinant human granulocyte-macrophage colony-stimulating factor on hematopoietic reconstitution after high-dose chemotherapy and autologous bone marrow transplantation. *N Engl J Med* 1988;318:869.

132. Vadhan-Raj S, Buescher S, Broxmeyer HE, et al. Stimulation of myelopoiesis in patients with aplastic anemia by recombinant human granulocyte-macrophage colony-stimulating factor. *N Engl J Med* 1988;319:1628.

133. Thompson JA, Lee DJ, Kidd P, et al. Subcutaneous granulocyte-macrophage colony-stimulating factor in patients with myelodysplastic syndrome. Toxicity, pharmacokinetics, and hematological effects. *J Clin Oncol* 1989;7:629.

134. Gulati SC, Bennett CL. Granulocyte-macrophage colony-stimulating factor (GM-CSF) as adjunct therapy in relapsed Hodgkin disease. *Ann Intern Med* 1992;116:177–182.

135. Vadhan-Raj S, Papadopoulos NE, Burgess MA, et al. Effects of PIXY321, a granulocyte-macrophage colony-stimulating factor/interleukin-3 fusion protein, on chemotherapy-induced multilineage myelosuppression in patients with sarcoma. *J Clin Oncol* 1994;12:715.

136. Vose JM, Pandite AN, Beveridge RA, et al. Granulocyte-macrophage colony-stimulating factor/interleukin-3 fusion protein versus granulocyte macrophage colony stimulating factor after autologous bone marrow transplantation for non-Hodgkin's lymphoma. Results of a randomized double-blind trial. *J Clin Oncol* 1997;15:1617–1623.

137. Furman WL, Rodman JH, Tonda ME, et al. Clinical effects and pharmacokinetics of the fusion protein PIXY321 in children receiving myelosuppressive chemotherapy. *Cancer Chemother Pharmacol* 1998;41:229–236.

138. Demetri GD, Samuels B, Gordon M, et al. Recombinant human interleukin-6 (IL-6) increases circulating platelet counts and C-reactive protein levels *in vivo*. Initial results of a phase I trial in sarcoma

patients with normal hemopoiesis. *Blood* 1992;80[Suppl 1]:88a(abst).

139. Samuels B, Bukowski R, Gordon M, et al. Phase I study of rhIL-6 with chemotherapy in advanced sarcoma. *Proc ASCO* 1993;12:291(abst).

140. D'Hondt V, Humblet Y, Guillaume TH, et al. Thrombopoietic effects and toxicity of interleukin-6 in patients with ovarian cancer before and after chemotherapy. A multicentric placebo-controlled, randomized phase Ib study. *Blood* 1995;85:2347.

141. Uppenkamp M, Makarova E, Petrasch S, Brittinger G. Thrombopoietin serum concentrations in patients with reactive and myeloproliferative thrombocytosis. *Ann Hematol* 1998;77:217–223.

142. Demetri GD, Bukowski RM, Samuels B, et al. Stimulation of thrombopoiesis by recombinant human interleukin-6 (IL-6) pre- and post-chemotherapy in previously untreated sarcoma patients with normal hematopoiesis. *Blood* 1993;82[Suppl 1]:367a(abst).

143. Budd GT, Pelley R, Samuels B, et al. Phase II randomized trial of simultaneous rhIL-6 and G-CSF following MAID chemotherapy in patients with sarcomas. Preliminary results. *Proc ASCO* 1995;14:256.

144. Ault A, Mitchell J, Knowles C, et al. Recombinant human interleukin-11 increases plasma volume and decreases urine sodium excretion in normal human subjects. *Blood* 1994;84[Suppl 1]:276a(abst).

145. Dykstra K, Rogge H, Stone A, Loewy J, Schwertschlag U. Effect of diuretic treatment on rhIL-11 induced salt and water retention. *Blood* 1996;88[Suppl 1]:346a(abst).

146. Tepler I, Elias L, Smith W, et al. A randomized placebo-controlled trial of recombinant IL-11 in cancer patients with severe thrombocytopenia due to cancer. *Blood* 1996;87:3607–3614.

147. Isaacs C, Robert NJ, Bailey FA, et al. Randomized placebo-controlled study of recombinant interleukin-11 to prevent chemotherapy-induced thrombocytopenia in patients with breast cancer receiving dose-intensive cyclophosphamide and doxorubicin. *J Clin Oncol* 1997;15:3368–3377.

148. Fanucchi M, Glaspy J, Crawford J, et al. Effects of polyethylene glycol-conjugated recombinant human megakaryocyte growth and development factor on platelet counts after chemotherapy for lung cancer. *N Engl J Med* 1997;336:404–409.

149. Crawford J, Glaspy J, Belani C, et al. A randomized, placebo-controlled, blinded, dose scheduling trial of pegylated recombinant human megakaryocyte growth and development factor with filgrastim support in non-small cell lung cancer patients treated with paclitaxel and carboplatin during multiple cycles of chemotherapy. *Proc ASCO* 1998;17:73a(abst).

150. Basser RL, Rasko J, Clarke K, et al. Randomized, blinded, placebo-controlled phase I trial of pegylated recombinant human megakaryocyte growth and development factor with filgrastim after dose-intensive chemotherapy in patients with advanced cancer. *Blood* 1997;89:3118–3128.

151. Vadhan-Raj S, Verschraegen C, McGarry L, et al. Recombinant human thrombopoietin (rhTPO) attenuates high-dose carboplatin (C)-induced thrombocytopenia in patients with gynecologic malignancy. *Blood* 1997;90[Suppl 1]:580a(abst).

152. Moskowitz C, Nimer S, Gabrilove J, et al. A randomized, double-blind, placebo-controlled, dose finding, efficacy and safety study of PEG-rHuMGDF in non-Hodgkin's lymphoma patients treated with ICE. *Proc ASCO* 1998;17:76a(abst).

153. Beveridge R, Schuster M, Waller E, et al. Randomized, double-blind, placebo-controlled trial of pegylated recombinant human megakaryocyte growth and development factor (PEG-rHuMGDF) in breast cancer patients following autologous bone marrow transplantation (ABMT). *Blood* 1997;90[Suppl 1]:580a(abst).

154. Glaspy J, Vredenburgh J, Demetri GD, et al. Effects of PEGylated recombinant human megakaryocyte growth and development factor (PEG-rHuMGDF) before high dose chemotherapy (HDC) with peripheral blood progenitor cell (PBPC) support. *Blood* 1997;90[Suppl 1]:580a(abst).

155. Bolwell B, Vredenburgh J, Overmoyer B, et al. Safety and biologic effect of pegylated recombinant human megakaryocyte growth and development factor (PEG-rHuMGDF) in breast cancer patients fol-

lowing autologous peripheral blood progenitor cell transplantation (PBPC). *Blood* 1997;90[Suppl 1]:171a(abst).

156. Nash R, Kurzrock R, DiPersio J, et al. Safety and activity of recombinant human thrombopoietin (rhTPO) in patients with delayed platelet recovery. *Blood* 1997;90[Suppl 1]:262a(abst).

157. Kuter D, McCullough J, Romo J, et al. Treatment of platelet donors with pegylated recombinant human megakaryocyte growth and development factor (PEGrHuMGDF) increases circulating platelet counts and apheresis yields and increases platelet increments in recipients of platelet transfusions. *Blood* 1997;90[Suppl 1]:579a(abst).

7.3

COLONY-STIMULATING FACTORS: CLINICAL APPLICATIONS

Erythropoietin Therapy for the Cancer Patient

JOHN A. GLASPY

Patients with cancer are frequently anemic (1). In some clinical settings, this anemia is attributable to specific complications of a particular malignancy, including hemolytic anemias associated with B-cell malignancies; blood loss or iron deficiency associated with cancers of the gastrointestinal tract, uterus, uterine cervix, or urothelium; bone marrow infiltration by breast cancer, prostate cancer, or hematologic malignancies; and red blood cell aplasia associated with thymoma. In addition, some patients with cancer develop anemia related to nutritional deficiencies or the cytotoxic effects of cancer chemotherapy. It is important to recognize and, when possible, treat these causes of the anemia of cancer.

A frequent and often dominant pathophysiologic factor in the anemia associated with cancers of all sites is the anemia of chronic disease. This entity was first described in association with chronic inflammatory disorders and was attributed to demonstrable alterations in iron metabolism with increased reticuloendothelial retention of recycled iron, coupled with decreased survival of endogenous and transfused red blood cells (2,3). This anemia is usually characterized by normocytic or microcytic and normochromic or hyperchromic red blood cell indices and an inappropriately low reticulocyte count. Iron studies, particularly serum ferritin levels, frequently suggest normal or increased iron stores. The anemia of chronic disease is usually mild to moderate in severity with hemoglobin concentrations of 7.5 to 11.0 g per dL. It has been recognized that the anemia of chronic disease is characterized by a diminished erythropoietin response to the decreased hemoglobin levels.

This blunting of the erythropoietin response axis has been specifically demonstrated in patients with cancer (4). These studies have also shown that endogenous erythropoietin levels are further diminished when cancer patients are treated with cytotoxic chemotherapy.

Erythropoietin is the major regulator of red blood cell production in mammalian species and is produced in the kidney with the quantity of erythropoietin released related to the tissue partial pressure of oxygen in the oxygen sensor. A high degree of species-to-species homology exists in the sequence and structure of erythropoietin. Human erythropoietin is a 193–amino acid protein with two disulfide bonds and four sites of glycosylation. Recombinant human erythropoietin for clinical use is produced in Chinese hamster ovary cells and bears four linked oligosaccharide chains because removal of the linked oligosaccharide moieties results in decreased biologic activity and complete deglycosylation in a biologically inactive molecule. Glycosylated erythropoietin binds to a specific receptor complex that lacks a tyrosine kinase domain and has sequence homology to receptors for other hematopoietic cytokines, including granulocyte-macrophage colony-stimulating factor, interleukin-3, interleukin-6, and thrombopoietin. The erythropoietin-receptor complex is internalized after binding, inducing proliferation, differentiation, and enhanced survival of erythroid progenitors in the bone marrow. Two recombinant human erythropoietin (rhEpo) preparations are available for clinical application—epoetin-α and epoetin-β. In the United States, only epoetin-α is marketed; in other parts of the world, both preparations are available. The biologic properties and clinical effects of epoetin-α and epoetin-β are similar, although some differences may exist in isoform composition, glycosylation, and pharmacokinetics (5,6). Their clinical data are pooled for discussion as rhEpo in this chapter because a comparative clinical trial demonstrating a significant difference in potency per unit or in safety or efficacy between the two preparations has not been conducted.

rhEpo became available for clinical testing in 1985. The first clinical trials were in patients with chronic renal failure. Chronic renal failure is the clinical setting in which the erythropoietin response to anemia is the most deficient. In these studies, therapy with rhEpo was shown to be effective in increasing hemoglobin levels and decreasing red blood cell transfusion requirements and iron overload. The initial studies were carried out with intravenously administered rhEpo; subsequent studies demonstrated that subcutaneous dosing was more efficient and permitted a one-third reduction in the intravenous dose. The toxicities observed included local injection-site pain when the drug was administered subcutaneously, an increase in diastolic blood pressure in as many as one-third of patients treated with rhEpo, and seizures in 4% of patients, the latter attributable to rapid increases in blood pressure. Iron deficiency developed in the majority of patients because of an increase in iron use, decrease in transfusions, and the chronic blood loss of hemodialysis. An increased frequency of thromboembolic events were not observed in patients receiving rhEpo, and neutralizing antibodies were not detected. The clinical benefits and safety profile of rhEpo therapy observed in hemodialysis patients were subsequently observed in predialysis patients with chronic renal insufficiency and those undergoing chronic ambulatory peritoneal dialysis.

One aspect of these studies was particularly relevant to the current evolution of thought regarding the role of rhEpo in the management of the cancer patient. In these clinical trials, rhEpo therapy was associated with an increased hemoglobin level despite a decrease in red blood cell transfusion requirement, the primary study end point. It was therefore logical to ask whether this increase in hemoglobin level was associated with any benefit to the patients in terms of symptom status. In the hemodialysis patient population, rhEpo therapy was associated with significant improvements in functional ability, health status, life satisfaction, social and sexual functioning, appetite, affect, and happiness (7–18). These quality of life (QOL) questionnaire–based observations were supported by studies documenting objective improvements in peak oxygen consumption and ventilatory anaerobic threshold in rhEpo–treated patients (19). Similar effects on QOL outcomes were reported in predialysis patients (20–23) and in patients undergoing peritoneal dialysis (24). These improvements were observed in pediatric (25) and elderly (26) subsets of renal failure patients. Analogous findings were reported in patients with acquired immunodeficiency syndrome treated with rhEpo (27,28). The demonstrations of increased energy level, functional capacity, and QOL associated with rhEpo therapy were consistent across different clinical settings, age groups, and countries. This had important implications for the palliative management of anemic cancer patients (29).

The insights into the frequency and pathophysiology of anemia in cancer patients summarized above, coupled with the clinical experience with rhEpo in chronic renal failure and, later, in patients with acquired immunodeficiency syndrome provided the rationale for the initiation and design of clinical trials of rhEpo in patients with cancer.

EFFECTS OF RECOMBINANT HUMAN ERYTHROPOIETIN ON THE ANEMIA OF CANCER

For obvious reasons, cancer patients with anemia caused by bleeding, nutritional deficiencies, or hemolysis have been excluded from clinical trials of rhEpo. rhEpo therapy may be associated with enhanced proliferation or survival of immature myeloid cells because these cells bear erythropoietin receptors. Patients with myeloid malignancies have therefore been excluded, and safety in these patients has not been established. Treatment of patients with myelodysplastic syndromes, however, has not been associated with a higher risk of progression to acute leukemia.

Some aspects of rhEpo clinical trials have made a full understanding of this agent's potential in cancer treatment more elusive. In many clinical trials, rhEpo has been given to all patients at a predefined dose with one or two dose escalations permitted in unresponsive patients. These studies have reported a "response rate" for the dose and schedule used, usually indicating the proportion of patients in whom an increase of hemoglobin concentration by 2 g per dL or an increase in hematocrit of 6% was observed during a defined period of rhEpo therapy. Although this approach is frequently taken in the development of cytotoxic chemotherapeutic agents, it may not be the most biologically sound design for clinical trials of a protein hormone, such as rhEpo. This approach in rhEpo development has not fully elucidated the dose-response relationship in patients with cancer and has left the impression, perhaps mistakenly, that 25% to 50% of patients with cancer will be biologically unresponsive to the drug. The results of rhEpo therapy for patients with cancer-associated anemia and patients with anemia associated with cancer during chemotherapy have been analyzed separately because of differences in the degree of relative erythropoietin deficiency and pathophysiology of the anemia. Studies in cancer patients not receiving chemotherapy have included fewer patients treated with lower rhEpo doses or for shorter durations of time before response assessment. Moreover, fewer patients requiring red blood cell transfusions have been included in these studies. This has made the determination of the clinical benefits to this group of patients more problematic.

Clinical Trials of Recombinant Human Erythropoietin for the Anemia of Cancer

Until recently, most rhEpo clinical trials used at least thrice-weekly dosing. In phase 2 studies, therapy with rhEpo with divided weekly doses of 66 to 450 U per kg was associated with an increase in hemoglobin concentration in some patients with cancer-associated anemia (30–32). The proportion of patients identified as hematologic responders in these small studies varied from 33% to 83% with the higher response rates generally observed with higher weekly rhEpo doses. In one study, which also included patients receiving chemotherapy, the results suggested that patients not receiving chemotherapy were more responsive to rhEpo; slightly higher response rates were achieved with somewhat lower weekly doses (32).

Osterborg studied the relationship of rhEpo dose and schedule to hematologic response in transfusion-dependent patients with multiple myeloma or low-grade lymphoma (33). In this study, 126 patients were randomized to receive subcutaneous rhEpo at a fixed dose of 10,000 U per day, 7 days a week, or at an initial dose of 2,000 U per day for 8 weeks followed by stepwise titration of dose or no rhEpo therapy at all. The response rate, defined as transfusion independence and a 2 g per dL increase in hemoglobin concentration, was 60% in the two rhEpo groups and 24% in the untreated patients. Maximal rhEpo efficacy was observed more rapidly in the high fixed-dose group; only 14% of patients responded to the initial dose in the titration group. The authors suggested a starting dose of 5,000 U per day (35,000 U per week, approximately 500 U per kg per week). In a second dose study, similar findings were reported, and 5,000 U per day was also the suggested dose (34). In a small study, 16 patients with gastrointestinal malignancies were randomized to receive subcutaneous rhEpo at 2,000 or 10,000 U three times weekly (35). Five of eight patients receiving 30,000 U per week met the criteria for a hematologic response; one of eight patients in the low-dose group responded.

In the phase 3 registration trial of rhEpo in the United States, 124 patients with the anemia of cancer were randomized to placebo or rhEpo, 100 U per kg subcutaneously thrice weekly, a somewhat lower dose than that suggested in the later dose-finding studies (36,37). Although transfusion dependence was not an entry criteria, the clinical end point was a decrease in the proportion of patients requiring transfusion or in the number of transfusions administered to the treated population compared with control. The response assessment was made after only 8 weeks of therapy. Although a significant increase occurred in the hematocrit level in the rhEpo–treated group compared with placebo, the response rate in the treated group was only 40%, and a statistically significant reduction in transfusions was not observed. This failure to achieve the clinical end point was probably related to the relatively low dose and short duration of rhEpo therapy and to the study being statistically underpowered to identify a true difference in transfusions between the two groups. Nevertheless, rhEpo is not registered for this indication in the United States. In contrast to the experience in patients with renal failure, serious adverse events were not observed with increased frequency in the rhEpo group.

Therapy with rhEpo has been shown to decrease perioperative transfusion requirements in patients undergoing abdominal surgery for cancer (38). Twenty patients were randomized to receive rhEpo, 300 U per kg 12 days before surgery, then 100 U per kg 4 and 8 days later, or no preoperative rhEpo therapy. Significantly fewer patients in the rhEpo group required allogeneic red blood cell transfusion. In two randomized studies, rhEpo was shown to facilitate preoperative autologous blood donation in cancer patients (39,40).

Clinical Trials of Recombinant Human Erythropoietin for the Anemia Occurring during Cancer Chemotherapy

The first clinical trials of rhEpo in cancer treatment were carried out in patients undergoing chemotherapy. In phase 1 and 2 clinical trials, intravenous rhEpo doses of 25, 50, 100, 200, or 300 U per kg per day, all 5 times weekly for 5 weeks, were given to patients undergoing cancer chemotherapy (41,42). No dose-related toxicities were encountered. An apparent dose-response effect occurred with the majority of hematologic responses noted in patients receiving 100 U per kg per day (500 U per kg per week) or higher doses and response rates of 83% in patients receiving 200 or 300 U per kg per day (1,000 or 1,500 U per kg per week). Several series have been published confirming the safety and efficacy of rhEpo in the setting of cancer chemotherapy, usually using subcutaneous doses of 450 U per kg per week given in three divided doses (43–47). The efficacy and safety of rhEpo therapy given during chemotherapy also has been confirmed in studies of elderly patients. Therapy with rhEpo has been safe in pediatric chemotherapy patients, but efficacy studies have yielded mixed results (49–51).

After the initial dose-ranging studies, several trials explored the effects of rhEpo dose on its hematologic efficacy. Tsuda et al. compared the hematologic effects of rhEpo in 12 patients treated with 3,000 U three times weekly with those in 14 patients treated with twice that dose, concluding that the 6,000 U dose (approximately 250 U per kg per week) was superior in terms of hemoglobin response (52). Glimelius et al. randomized 84 patients with gastrointestinal cancers to receive subcutaneous rhEpo at 2,000 U or 10,000 U given thrice weekly (35). Responses, defined as an increase of 1 g per dL in hemoglobin concentration, occurred more rapidly and in a significantly greater proportion of patients in the higher dose group with a 73% response rate at 4 weeks compared with 30% of responders at 10 weeks in the lower dose group. Mantovani et al. randomized 20 patients receiving cisplatin-based chemotherapy to receive subcutaneous rhEpo at a dose of 150 U per kg thrice weekly (nine evaluable patients) or 50 U per kg daily (eight evaluable patients). Both groups were treated for 12 weeks (53). This small study was relatively underpowered to detect a difference between the 350 and 450 U per kg per week groups; no significant difference between the groups in hematologic response or transfusion requirements was observed.

Cisplatin therapy results in erythropoietin deficiency and is frequently complicated by anemia because of its direct renal effects (54). Some studies have therefore focused on the use of rhEpo therapy for patients receiving cisplatin (42,47,53,55). Others have randomized or analyzed patients receiving cisplatin-based chemotherapy separately from those treated with other regimens (36,37,44,46,52,56). In some studies, the data have suggested that patients receiving cisplatin are most likely to respond or respond more rapidly to rhEpo therapy than patients receiving non–cisplatin-containing regimens. Anemic patients receiving non–cisplatin-containing chemotherapy, however, have also responded to rhEpo. Taken in aggregate, the studies do not demonstrate that rhEpo is more effective or requires a different dosing regimen in either group.

Two randomized, placebo-controlled clinical trials of rhEpo for patients undergoing cytotoxic chemotherapy have been reported. Cassinu et al. randomized 100 anemic patients receiving cisplatin-based chemotherapy to receive subcutaneous rhEpo, 100 U per kg thrice weekly, or placebo (55). Significantly higher hemoglobin concentrations were observed in the rhEpo arm within 3 weeks of beginning the study drug. A significantly smaller proportion of patients in the rhEpo group required red blood cell transfusions (20% vs. 56%) and significantly fewer red blood cell transfusions were given per patient in the rhEpo group over the 9 weeks of the trial. In a large, multicenter, randomized, placebo-controlled study that served as the U.S. registration trial for rhEpo, 289 patients receiving chemotherapy, 132 patients receiving cisplatin, and 157 patients receiving non–cisplatin-based regimens were randomized separately to receive rhEpo 150 U per kg subcutaneously thrice weekly or placebo for 12 weeks (37,57,58). The clinical end point of the study was the number of red blood cell transfusions received by the two groups. The data from these two groups were pooled for the final efficacy analysis because no significant differences existed between the cisplatin and noncisplatin subsets in terms of hematologic response (58% vs. 56%, response defined as at least a 6% increase in hematocrit). In the second and third months of study drug treatment, a statistically significant smaller proportion of transfused patients and a significantly lower number of transfused red blood cell units in rhEpo–treated group existed. After the blinded portion of the study, patients receiving placebo were permitted to cross over and receive rhEpo; these patients responded similarly to those initially randomized to rhEpo. Patients who had been receiving rhEpo but had not responded were permitted dose increases to 300 U per kg thrice weekly. Some patients did not respond to 150 U per kg but responded to a higher dose, demonstrating a link between dose and the proportion of patients with a hematologic response. This observation was supported by the study of Ludwig et al. in which patients receiving chemotherapy were treated initially with rhEpo 150 U per kg thrice weekly for 6 weeks, at which point the dose was increased to 300 U per kg in patients in whom the hemoglobin concentration did not increase by at least 2 g per dL (43). In this study, 52% of patients ultimately responded to rhEpo, and the mean dose required was 570 U per kg per week.

Therapy with rhEpo has been studied as a strategy to prevent rather than treat anemia and red blood cell transfusion dependence in patients receiving chemotherapy. In a study of small-cell lung cancer patients receiving intensive non–cisplatin-containing chemotherapy, de Campos et al. randomized 36 patients to receive either rhEpo 150 U per kg thrice weekly, rhEpo 300 U per kg thrice weekly, or no rhEpo for the duration of chemotherapy (59). Hemoglobin levels decreased in all patients, but significantly fewer red blood cell transfusions were administered to the rhEpo–treated groups. No differences were observed between the two dose cohorts. In another study, 62 patients with breast cancer undergoing intensive adjuvant chemotherapy were randomized to receive rhEpo 150 U per kg thrice weekly or no rhEpo treatment (60). In the rhEpo–treated patients, hemoglobin levels were maintained over 6 cycles of chemotherapy; a progressive decrease in hemoglobin was observed in the control group.

The results of phase 2 and 3 studies of rhEpo demonstrate that, when administered to anemic cancer patients receiving cytotoxic chemotherapy, rhEpo therapy is associated with an increase in hemoglobin level and a decrease in the proportion of patients who require red blood cell transfusion. The data available strongly suggest that the proportion of patients who benefit and, perhaps, the rapidity with which they realize that benefit are

related to the dose of rhEpo administered, at least up to doses of 500 to 900 U per week when the drug is administered subcutaneously and three times weekly. At these higher doses, 50% to 75% of these patients respond to rhEpo with an increase in hemoglobin levels and a 50% or greater decrease in transfusion risk. Relatively little is known about the benefits of rhEpo doses higher than 1,000 U per week; doses of 1,500 U per week have been administered without encountering dose-limiting toxicities. The proportion of cancer patients who are unresponsive to rhEpo at any dose is unknown. When administered at doses of 450 U per kg per week, rhEpo therapy can prevent the progressive decline in hemoglobin levels observed during chemotherapy. When rhEpo is used to prevent anemia, a significant decrease in transfusion risk has been demonstrated only for patients at high risk for transfusion, such as those receiving carboplatin and ifosfamide chemotherapy. In the setting of cancer chemotherapy, rhEpo therapy is safe. Acute, serious, adverse events and longer-range toxicities, such as stem-cell exhaustion, lineage steal, and increased rates of acute leukemia have not been reported with increased frequency in rhEpo–treated patients.

Clinical Trials in Myelodysplasia

Patients with myelodysplastic syndromes most frequently present with anemia and often become red blood cell transfusion–dependent and alloimmunized. Several uncontrolled clinical trials of rhEpo intravenously at doses of 210 to 3,200 U per kg per week (61–67) or subcutaneously at doses of 150 to 2,100 U per kg per week (68–76) have been reported with improvement in anemia, decrease in transfusion requirements, or both, observed in zero to 50% of treated patients with an average response rate of approximately 30% in pooled data. Clinical trials of cytokine combinations have suggested that erythropoietic synergy may exist between granulocyte-macrophage colony-stimulating factor (77) or granulocyte colony-stimulating factor (78) and rhEpo in some patients with myelodysplasia, although these findings have not been consistent (79,80), and the safety of routine use of myeloid growth factors in these patients has not been established.

In a randomized, placebo-controlled clinical trial, rhEpo given subcutaneously at a dose of 150 U per kg per day for 8 weeks was compared with placebo in 87 patients with myelodysplasia (81). The overall hematologic response rate was 37% with a higher frequency of response in patients in the refractory anemia group compared with refractory anemia with excess blasts subset. Serious toxicities or progression to leukemia were not observed with increased frequency in the rhEpo group. Small studies in patients selected for refractory anemia, normal platelet counts and lactate dehydrogenase levels, and a short duration of disease have suggested that, in this subset of patients with myelodysplasia, rhEpo may have hematologic responses and dose requirements similar to patients with cancer-receiving chemotherapy (82,83).

The available data support the conclusion that rhEpo is safe in patients with myelodysplasia. For the whole population of patients, however, doses of at least 450 U per kg per week or greater are required to achieve hematologic improvement in one-third of patients. Some studies have reported that baseline serum erythropoietin or other cytokine levels can be used to select patients more likely to respond but this has not been a consistent finding. Data suggest that it may be possible to select a subset of patients, such as those with refractory anemia without excess blasts, in whom lower doses will be required and higher response rates observed.

PRACTICAL ASPECTS OF RECOMBINANT HUMAN ERYTHROPOIETIN THERAPY IN CANCER

Iron

Some patients with cancer are iron deficient before the initiation of rhEpo therapy. Any patient with a low serum ferritin or a transferrin iron saturation of less than 20% should be treated with iron during the first 1 to 2 months after the initiation of rhEpo therapy. Many more patients develop iron deficiency during rhEpo therapy. Any patient in whom a response to rhEpo is observed initially but who later begins to become anemic despite continued treatment should be evaluated for iron deficiency and treated. Interest is increasing in the use of intravenous iron repletion in conjunction with rhEpo to prevent and treat iron deficiency. This is a result of the small quantities of orally administered iron that can be absorbed daily, the gastrointestinal toxicity and resultant noncompliance associated with oral iron supplementation, and the improved safety profile of currently available paternal iron preparations.

Recognition is emerging that patients treated with rhEpo frequently develop functional iron deficiency (84,85). In this syndrome, total body stores of iron, as assessed by iron studies, serum ferritin, or bone marrow–stainable iron, may be normal or increased while erythropoiesis is iron deficient, because demand by the stimulated erythron exceeds supply from body iron stores and oral absorption. Functional iron deficiency has been described in patients treated with rhEpo undergoing hemodialysis, as well as in normal autologous blood donors (86). Given the abnormalities of iron metabolism that accompany chronic diseases with avid retention of body iron stores in the reticuloendothelial system, it is likely that functional iron deficiency is more common in the setting of cancer than in healthy individuals or hemodialysis patients (87). Physicians are learning that parenteral iron administered during rhEpo therapy in patients with renal failure frequently improves the efficacy of a given rhEpo dose. Clinical trials of cotherapy with parenteral iron and rhEpo in cancer patients with normal or increased iron body stores are in progress. The goal of these studies is to determine whether cotherapy with iron improves rhEpo response rates or decreases the dose required to obtain a hematologic response.

Dose and Schedule of rhEpo

As discussed previously, the dose-response relationship for rhEpo in cancer patients is incompletely understood with respect to the overall hematologic response and the rapidity of response. It is reasonable to begin therapy with 10,000 U subcutaneously three times weekly with the dose doubled if an increase in hemoglobin concentration is not observed within 4 weeks in an iron-replete patient.

Studies of less frequent dosing have been carried out because thrice-weekly dosing is inconvenient, particularly for patients who must be treated in a physician's office. It appears that once-weekly subcutaneous dosing with 40,000 U is equivalent to 10,000 U thrice weekly in terms of hematologic response in patients receiving cancer chemotherapy.

Prediction of Response to rhEpo

Interest is growing in identifying patients who will not respond to a given dose of rhEpo. Because rhEpo is expensive, inefficient use of the drug should be minimized. Although some studies have suggested that higher baseline serum erythropoietin levels are predictive of a failure to respond, this has not been a consistent observation. Moreover, most patients with cancer and many patients with myelodysplastic syndromes have low erythropoietin; some of these patients do not respond to the customarily used doses of rhEpo. One approach has been to calculate the erythropoietin level that would be predicted in the absence of chronic disease (log Epo = 3.420–0.056 × hematocrit) and divide this figure into the observed level to generate the observed:predicted ratio (88). Ratios of less than .83 are associated with an increased proportion of responders to rhEpo, although some patients with higher ratios respond.

No pretreatment response–prediction strategy has emerged that can be used to consistently predict a less than 30% chance of nonresponse or a greater than 75% chance of response to the usual starting doses of rhEpo. Newer approaches have focused on evaluating patients after 4 weeks of rhEpo therapy and coupling the hematologic response observed with pretreatment assessments to generate a prediction of response (88–90). Patients in whom an increase of 1 g per dL in hemoglobin concentration is observed after 4 weeks of rhEpo therapy who also have an observed:predicted ratio of less than .82 have approximately an 85% chance of responding satisfactorily to that dose of rhEpo. Future work on prediction of rhEpo response and early identification of nonresponders will be important to maximize the cost-effectiveness of this drug in cancer patients.

Cost-Effectiveness

Several studies have examined the cost-effectiveness of rhEpo in the treatment of anemia in cancer patients (91–94). In general, these studies have compared the cost of rhEpo therapy for the whole population of treated patients with the cost of the prevented transfusions. These studies have concluded that routine rhEpo therapy adds to overall health care costs. If the only benefit derived from rhEpo therapy is the prevention of some red blood cell transfusions, the prevented transfusions may be less expensive than the rhEpo. As more is learned about the most efficient uses of rhEpo, the balance of costs in these analyses will change to some extent. More important, these analyses have focused on the prevention of red blood cell transfusion effects of rhEpo therapy and have not included the increase in hemoglobin level seen in treated patients compared with controls. These increased hemoglobin levels have been associated with improvements in QOL (see Relationship of Anemia to Quality of Life) and these benefits, if confirmed in randomized trials, should be incorporated into future cost-utility studies.

RELATIONSHIP OF ANEMIA TO OUTCOMES IN CANCER TREATMENT

Fatigue in Cancer Patients

Fatigue is the most frequent symptom of cancer patients. In a study of 419 cancer patients, 78% stated that they had fatigue, defined as debilitating tiredness, and 32% reported this symptom to be present and affecting their lives on a daily basis (95). Although the oncologists questioned believed that pain was more important than fatigue to cancer patients, 61% of the patients in this study reported that fatigue affected their lives more than pain. Fatigue is prevalent and important to patients and their caregivers; its importance may be underappreciated by physicians.

Several causes of fatigue exist in cancer patients. It is likely that alterations in endogenous cytokine levels, depression, the effects of therapy, poor nutritional status, and the direct effects of the cancer all play a role. Although the earlier experience in patients with renal failure indicated that anemia not believed to be severe enough to warrant transfusion still impacts functional status and QOL, the anemia of chronic disease associated with cancer has not been recognized as a factor in the debilitating tiredness reported by these patients.

Relationship of Anemia to Quality of Life

Most physicians have been trained to refrain from treating mild and moderate degrees of anemia with red blood cell transfusions unless potentially life-threatening complications exist. This mindset has resulted in an assumption on the part of many physicians that mild and moderate degrees of anemia are asymptotic and unimportant. In most practices, patients with mild and moderate anemias have been left untreated, and patients with severe anemia (hemoglobin concentration <7.5 g per dL) have been transfused and maintained in a state of mild or moderate anemia. In the early studies of rhEpo therapy for cancer patients, some investigators reported improvements in functional status, energy level, or overall QOL in responding patients (36,43,96,97). These studies were not designed or statistically powered to define the QOL benefits of increasing hemoglobin levels above that usually achieved with current red blood cell transfusion practices. Nevertheless, they indicated that a palliative benefit to cancer patients associated with increased hemoglobin levels may exist.

The results of two large, open-label phase 4 studies of rhEpo therapy in cancer patients undergoing chemotherapy in community oncology practices in the United States, each including more than 2,000 patients, have been reported (98,99). In both studies, therapy with rhEpo was effective in increasing hemoglobin levels and decreasing red blood cell transfusion requirements without severe adverse events. In these studies, physicians remained at liberty to transfuse patients whenever it was deemed appropriate. In neither study was the anemia before rhEpo therapy severe; mean baseline hemoglobin levels were 9.2 and 9.3 g per dL. The rhEpo was administered subcutaneously three times weekly for 4 months in one study at a dose of 150 U per kg per dose and in the other study at a fixed 10,000 U per dose.

In the first study, rhEpo therapy was associated with an increase in mean hemoglobin level to 11.2 g per dL (98).

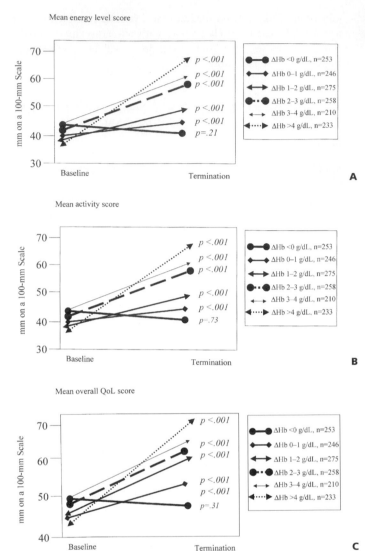

FIGURE 1. Changes in mean linear analog scale score for patients at the beginning and termination of recombinant human erythropoietin therapy. The results for different hemoglobin (Hb) response cohorts are shown. The p values shown for each cohort were by paired tests. The mean energy level scores **(A)**, mean activity level scores **(B)**, and mean overall quality of life scores **(C)** are shown. (Adapted from Glaspy J et al. Impact of therapy with epoetin-α on clinical outcomes in patients with nonmyeloid malignancies during cancer chemotherapy in community oncology practice. *J Clin Oncol* 1997;15:1218–1234, with permission.)

QOL was assessed at the initiation of rhEpo therapy and when the drug was discontinued. The QOL tool used was a three-question linear analog scale that provided a self-assessment, on a scale of 0 to 100, of the patient's energy level, activity level, and overall QOL over the previous week. Statistically significant increases in mean scores for all three questions were found (p <.001). The magnitude of the effective size of each of these changes was similar to those reported in other studies of cancer pain control. The increases in scores for each patient correlated with the magnitude of the increase in hemoglobin level (p <.001) (Fig. 1). Tumor response data was collected retrospectively for more than 600 patients. The correlation between

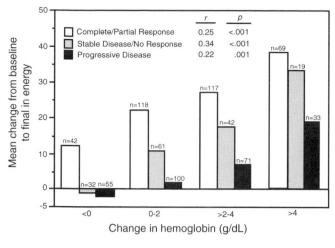

A

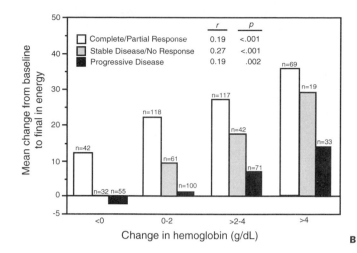

B

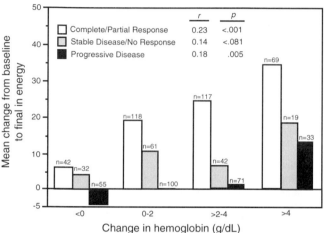

C

FIGURE 2. The relationship of changes in mean linear analog scale score during recombinant human erythropoietin therapy to the increase in hemoglobin level for patients with cancer undergoing chemotherapy. Patients were segregated into three chemotherapy response groups, based on the physician's assessment of their tumor response. The correlation between increase in hemoglobin and the increase in score was assessed using a simple linear regression model and the corresponding *p* values shown. The results for questions regarding energy level **(A)**, ability to carry out daily activities **(B)**, and overall quality of life **(C)** are shown. (Adapted from Glaspy J. The impact of epoetin alfa on quality of life during cancer chemotherapy. A fresh look at an old problem. *Semin Hematol* 1998;34:20–26, with permission.)

hemoglobin increase and QOL scores were seen within each tumor response category (Fig. 2).

In the second study, the mean hemoglobin level increased to 11.3 g per dL (99). In this study, tumor response data were collected prospectively, and the Functional Assessment of Cancer Therapies anemia QOL tool was added to the linear analog scale as a more validated measure of the impact of rhEpo. In this study, significant increases in QOL as assessed by the linear analog scale were observed. In addition, for each tumor response category, an increase in QOL as measured by the Functional Assessment of Cancer Therapies anemia scale was observed with the magnitude of the increase related to the magnitude of the hemoglobin rise (Fig. 3). Taken together, these two phase 4 studies strongly suggest that mild and moderate anemia in cancer patients negatively impacts functional status and overall QOL. The negative effects of anemia on QOL were observed despite continued red blood cell transfusion administered whenever clinically indicated. Similar findings have been observed in a third phase 4 study that used weekly rhEpo dosing (100) and in a randomized, placebo-controlled trial in Europe (101).

This raises the question as to what is the minimum hemoglobin level requisite for optimal palliation in cancer patients. The data from the two phase 4 studies have been pooled in an incremental analysis (102). The results suggest a nonlinear relation-

ship of hemoglobin level to QOL with QOL improving with each hemoglobin increase of 1 g per dL between 8 and 14 g per dL. The greatest improvement was observed between 11 and 12 g per dL. These data are provocative and have important implications for the palliation of cancer patients. Nevertheless, it is still possible that these results reflect a placebo effect of the rhEpo and not a true biologic effect of increased hemoglobin level. The results of one randomized placebo controlled trial have been reported in abstract form and suggest that the improved QOL observed in the rhEpo-treated patients is not a placebo effect (101). Moreover, rhEpo therapy in advanced cancer patients has been shown to be associated with the objective improvements in measured metabolic efficiency and exercise capacity (103).

It is important to note that these data relate to the relationship of hemoglobin level to QOL. It is possible that similar improvements could be achieved by restructuring our approach to red blood cell transfusion treatment for cancer patients. No data exist regarding the effect of red blood cell transfusion for mild and moderate anemia on QOL. In addition to the risks associated with transfusions, some properties of transfused red blood cells, specifically decreased 2- and 3-diphosphoglycerate levels, may compromise tissue oxygen delivery and render them less effective than red blood cells produced in response to rhEpo (104).

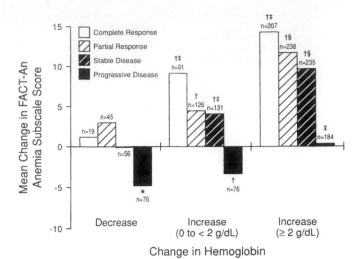

FIGURE 3. The relationship of change in quality of life (QOL) score during recombinant human erythropoietin therapy, as measured by the Functional Assessment of Cancer Therapies tool to the observed change in hemoglobin level. Patients are divided into cohorts based on tumor chemotherapy response. (Adapted from Demetri GD et al. Quality-of-life benefit in chemotherapy patients treated with epoetin-α is independent of disease response or tumor type. Results from a prospective community oncology study. Procrit Study Group. *J Clin Oncol* 1998;16:3412–3425, with permission.)

Potential Effects of Anemia on Survival Outcomes

It has long been recognized that anemia or red blood cell transfusion dependence, or both, correlated with a poor prognosis for a variety of solid tumors. This has been attributed to the anemia being a reflection of the advanced stage of the malignancy, although the immunosuppressive effects of red blood cell transfusions or radioresistance conferred by decreased tissue oxygen levels have also been postulated. It is possible that clinical settings will be identified in which rhEpo therapy is associated with improved survival outcomes. The focus of this research has been on the use of rhEpo to increase hemoglobin levels in patients scheduled to undergo or undergoing radiotherapy, with the goal of increasing the efficacy of radiation. Several studies have demonstrated the safety and hematologic efficacy of rhEpo in patients undergoing radiotherapy (52,105–108). Randomized clinical trials designed to study the survival impact of rhEpo administered to correct anemia and maintain hemoglobin levels in cervical cancer patients undergoing radiotherapy are under way.

CONCLUSION

Therapy with rhEpo is well established as an adjunct to cancer treatment; however, the role of this factor continues to evolve. The focus of rhEpo treatment is moving from the prevention of red blood cell transfusions to the maintenance of maximal performance status, comfort level, and QOL in patients with cancer. The importance of iron supplementation, including its potential role in rhEpo–treated patients with normal body iron stores, is being recognized. Future developments in the field are likely to include the following:

1. Further refinements in rhEpo iron supplementation, dosing and response prediction, and improvements in the efficiency of its use
2. Better definition of the cost-utility of rhEpo in cancer patients, including its effects on functional status and QOL
3. Exploration of the potential of rhEpo to improve survival outcomes
4. The introduction of additional erythropoietic agents into clinical trials

REFERENCES

1. Skillings JR, Sridhar FG, Wong C, et al. The frequency of red cell transfusion for anemia in patients receiving chemotherapy. A retrospective cohort study. *Am J Clin Oncol* 1993;16:22–25.
2. Haurani F, Young K, Tocantins L. Reutilization of iron in anemia complicating malignant neoplasms. *Blood* 1963;22:73.
3. Cartwright GE. The anemia of chronic disorders. *Semin Hematol* 1966;3:351.
4. Miller CB, Jones RJ, Piantadosi S, et al. Decreased erythropoietin response in patients with the anemia of cancer. *N Engl J Med* 1990;322;1689–1692.
5. Halstenson CE, Macres M, Katz SA, et al. Comparative pharmacokinetics and pharmacodynamics of epoetin alfa and epoetin beta. *Clin Pharmacol Ther* 1991;50:702–712.
6. Storring PL, Tiplady RJ, Gaines Das RE, et al. Epoetin alfa and beta differ in their erythropoietin isoform compositions and biological properties. *Br J Haematol* 1998;100:79–89.
7. Eschbach JW, Abdulhadi MH, Browne JK, et al. Recombinant human erythropoietin in anemic patients with end-stage renal disease. Results of a phase III multicenter clinical trial. *Ann Intern Med* 1989;111:992–1000.
8. Wolcott DL, Marsh JT, La Rue A, et al. Recombinant human erythropoietin treatment may improve quality of life and cognitive function in chronic hemodialysis patients. *Am J Kidney Dis* 1989;14:478–485.
9. Delano BG. Improvements in quality of life following treatment with r–HuEPO in anemic hemodialysis patients. *Am J Kidney Dis* 1989;14:14–18.
10. Barany P, Pettersson E, Bergstrom J. Erythropoietin treatment improves quality of life in hemodialysis patients. *Scand J Urol Nephrol Suppl* 1990;131:55–60.
11. Evans RW. Recombinant human erythropoietin and the quality of life of endstage renal disease patients: a comparative analysis. *Am J Kidney Dis* 1991;18:62–70.
12. Laupacis A, Wong C, Churchill D. The use of generic and specific quality-of-life measures in hemodialysis patients treated with erythropoietin. The Canadian Erythropoietin Study Group. *Control Clin Trials* 1991;12:S168–S179.
13. Deniston OL, Luscombe FA, Buesching DP, et al. Effect of long-term epoetin beta therapy on the quality of life of hemodialysis patients. *ASAIO Trans* 1990;36:M157–160.
14. Association between recombinant human erythropoietin and quality of life and exercise capacity of patients receiving haemodialysis. Canadian Erythropoietin Study Group. *BMJ* 1990;300:573–578.
15. Levin NW, Lazarus JM, Nissenson AR. National Cooperative rHu Erythropoietin Study in patients with chronic renal failure—an interim report. The National Cooperative rHu Erythropoietin Study Group. *Am J Kidney Dis* 1993;22:3–12.
16. Barany P, Pettersson E, Konarski-Svensson JK. Long-term effects on quality of life in haemodialysis patients of correction of anaemia with erythropoietin. *Nephrol Dial Transplant* 1993;8:426–432.

17. Hosokawa S, Yoshida O. Effect of erythropoietin (rHuEPO) on trace elements and quality of life (Qol) in chronic hemodialysis patients. *Int J Clin Pharmacol Ther* 1994;32:415–421.

18. Beusterien KM, Mssenson AR, Port FK, et al. The effects of recombinant human erythropoietin on functional health and well-being in chronic dialysis patients. *J Am Soc Nephrol* 1996;7:763–773.

19. Levin NW. Quality of life and hematocrit level. *Am J Kidney Dis* 1992;20;16–20.

20. Kleinman KS, Schweitzer SU, Perdue ST, et al. The use of recombinant human erythropoietin in the correction of anemia in predialysis patients and its effect on renal function: a double-blind, placebo-controlled trial. *Am J Kidney Dis* 1989;14:486–495.

21. Double-blind, placebo-controlled study of the therapeutic use of recombinant human erythropoietin for anemia associated with chronic renal failure in predialysis patients. The US Recombinant Human Erythropoietin Predialysis Study Group. Published erratum appears in *Am J Kidney Dis* 1991;18:50–59.

22. Lim VS. Recombinant human erythropoietin in predialysis patients. *Am J Kidney Dis* 1991;18:34–37.

23. Revicki DA, Brown RE, Feeny DH, et al. Health-related quality of life associated with recombinant human erythropoietin therapy for predialysis chronic renal disease patients. *Am J Kidney Dis* 1995;25:548–554.

24. Auer J, Simon G, Stevens J, et al. Quality of life improvements in CAPD patients treated with subcutaneously administered erythropoietin for anemia. *Perit Dial Int* 1992;12:40–42.

25. Morris KP, Sharp J, Watson S, et al. Non-cardiac benefits of human recombinant erythropoietin in end stage renal failure and anaemia. *Arch Dis Child* 1993;69:580–586.

26. Moreno F, Aracil FJ, Perez R, et al. Controlled study on the improvement of quality of life in elderly hemodialysis patients after correcting end-stage renal disease-related anemia with erythropoietin. *Am J Kidney Dis* 1996;27:548–556.

27. Henry DH, Beall GN, Benson CA, et al. Recombinant human erythropoietin in the treatment of anemia associated with human immunodeficiency virus (HIV) infection and zidovudine therapy. Overview of four clinical trials. *Ann Intern Med* 1992;117:739–748.

28. Revicki DA, Brown RE, Henry DH, et al. Recombinant human erythropoietin and health-related quality of life of AIDS patients with anemia. *J Acquir Immune Defic Syndr* 1994;7:474–484.

29. Glaspy J. The impact of epoetin alpha on quality of life during cancer chemotherapy. A fresh look at an old problem. *Semin Hematol* 1998;34:20–26.

30. Ponchio L, Beguin Y, Farina G, et al. Evaluation of erythroid marrow response to recombinant human erythropoietin in patients with cancer anaemia. *Haematologica* 1992;77:494–501.

31. Falkson CI, Keren-Rosenberg S, Uys A, et al. Recombinant human erythropoietin in the treatment of cancer-related anaemia. *Oncology* 1994;51:497–501.

32. Ludwig H, Leitgeb C, Pecherstorfer J, et al. Epoetin alfa for the correction of anemia in various cancers [Meeting Abstract]. *Proc Annu Meet Am Soc Clin Oncol* 1995;14:A714.

33. Osterborg A, Boogaerts MA, Cimino R, et al. Recombinant human erythropoietin in transfusion-dependent anemic patients with multiple myeloma and non-Hodgkin's lymphoma—a randomized multicenter study. The European Study Group of Erythropoietin (Epoetin Beta) Treatment in Multiple Myeloma and Non-Hodgkin's Lymphoma. *Blood* 1996;87:2675–2682.

34. Kasper C, Terhaar A, Fossa A, et al. Recombinant human erythropoietin in the treatment of cancer-related anaemia: *Eur J Haematol* 1997;58:251–256.

35. Glimelius B, Linne T, Hoffman K, et al. Epoetin beta in the treatment of anemia in patients with advanced gastrointestinal cancer. *J Clin Oncol* 1998;16:434–440.

36. Abels RI. Recombinant human erythropoietin in the treatment of the anemia of cancer. *Acta Haematol* 1992;1:4–11.

37. Henry DH, Abels RI. Recombinant human erythropoietin in the treatment of cancer and chemotherapy-induced anemia: results of double-blind and open-label follow-up studies. *Semin Oncol* 1994;21:21–28.

38. Braga M, Gianotti L, Gentilini O, et al. Erythropoietic response induced by recombinant human erythropoietin in anemic cancer patients candidate to major abdominal surgery. *Hepatogastroenterology* 1997;44:685–690.

39. Braga M, Gianotti L, Vignali A, et al. Evaluation of recombinant human erythropoietin to facilitate autologous blood donation before surgery in anaemic patients with cancer of the gastrointestinal tract. *Br J Surg* 1995;82:1637–1640.

40. Rau B, Schlag PM, Willeke F, et al. Increased autologous blood donation in rectal cancer by recombinant human erythropoietin (rhEPO) [see comments]. *Eur J Cancer* 1998;34:992–998.

41. Platanias LC, Miller CB, Mick R, et al. Treatment of chemotherapy-induced anemia with recombinant human erythropoietin in cancer patients. *J Clin Oncol* 1991;9:2021–2026.

42. Miller CB, Platanias LC, Mills SR, et al. Phase I-II trial of erythropoietin in the treatment of cisplatin-associated anemia. *J Natl Cancer Inst* 1992;84:98–103.

43. Ludwig H, Sundal E, Pecherstorfer M, et al. Recombinant human erythropoietin for the correction of cancer associated anemia with and without concomitant cytotoxic chemotherapy. *Cancer* 1995;76:2319–2329.

44. Bosze P, Mayer A, Thurzo L, et al. Recombinant human erythropoietin in the treatment of anemic patients undergoing chemotherapy for cancer. *Orv Hetil* 1995;136:2567–2572.

45. Chiou TJ, Chim YS, Wei CH, et al. The effect of subcutaneous r-HuEPO in cancer patients receiving chemotherapy with anemia: a preliminary report. *Chung Hua I Hsueh Tsa Chih* (Taipei) 1997;60:229–235.

46. Pawlicki M, Jassem J, Bosze P, et al. A multicenter study of recombinant human erythropoietin (epoetin alpha) in the management of anemia in cancer patients receiving chemotherapy. *Anticancer Drugs* 1997;8:949–957.

47. Malik IA, Khan ZK, Hakimali A, et al. The effect of subcutaneous recombinant human erythropoietin (r-HuEPO) on anemia in cancer patients receiving platinum-based chemotherapy. *JPMA J Pak Med Assoc* 1998;48:127–131.

48. Cascinu S, Del Ferro E, Fedeli A, et al. Recombinant human erythropoietin treatment in elderly cancer patients with cisplatin-associated anemia. *Oncology* 1995;52:422–426.

49. Beck MN, Beck D. Recombinant erythropoietin in acute chemotherapy-induced anemia of children with cancer. *Med Pediatr Oncol* 1995;25:17–21.

50. Leon Molinari P, Jimenez Monteagudo M, Barona Zamora P, et al. [Recombinant human erythropoietin in anemia associated with pediatric cancer: study of the identification of predictors of response]. *An Esp Pediatr* 1998;49:17–22.

51. MacMillan ML, Freedman MH. Recombinant human erythropoietin in children with cancer. *J Pediatr Hematol Oncol* 1998;20:187–189.

52. Tsukuda M, Mochimatsu I, Nagahara T, et al. Clinical application of recombinant human erythropoietin for treatments in patients with head and neck cancer. *Cancer Immunol Immunother* 1993;36:52–56.

53. Mantovani G, Ghiani M, Curreli L, et al. Assessment of the efficacy of two dosages and schedules of human recombinant erythropoietin in the prevention and correction of cisplatin-induced anemia in cancer patients. *Oncol Rep* 1999;6:421–426.

54. Wood PA, Hrushesky WJ. Cisplatin-associated anemia. An erythropoietin deficiency syndrome. *J Clin Invest* 1995;95:1650.

55. Cascinu S, Fedeli A, Del Ferro E, et al. Recombinant human erythropoietin treatment in cisplatin-associated anemia: a randomized, double blind trial with placebo. *J Clin Oncol* 1994;12:1058–1062.

56. Case D Jr, Bukowski RM, Carey RW, et al. Recombinant human erythropoietin therapy for anemic cancer patients on combination chemotherapy. *J Natl Cancer Inst* 1993;85:801–806.

57. Abels RI. Use of recombinant human erythropoietin in the treatment of anemia in patients who have cancer. *Semin Oncol* 1992;19:29–35.

58. Case DC Jr, Bukowski RM, Carey RW, et al. Recombinant human erythropoietin therapy for anemic cancer patients on combination chemotherapy. *J Natl Cancer Inst* 1993;85:801–806.

59. de Campos E, Radford J, Steward W, et al. Clinical and *in vitro* effects of recombinant human erythropoietin in patients receiving intensive chemotherapy for small-cell lung cancer. *J Clin Oncol* 1995;13:1623–1631.

60. Del Mastro L, Venturini M, Lionetto R, et al. Randomized phase III trial evaluating the role of erythropoietin in the prevention of chemotherapy-induced anemia. *J Clin Oncol* 1997;15:2715–2721.

61. Stebler C, Tichelli A, Dazzi H, et al. High-dose recombinant human erythropoietin for treatment of anemia in myelodysplastic syndromes and paroxysmal nocturnal hemoglobinuria: a pilot study. *Exp Hematol* 1990;18:1204–1208.

62. Bessho M, Jinnai I, Matsuda A, et al. Improvement of anemia by recombinant erythropoietin in patients with myelodysplastic syndromes and aplastic anemia. *Int J Cell Cloning* 1990;8:445–458.

63. Stein RS, Abels RI, Krantz SB. Pharmacologic doses of recombinant human erythropoietin in the treatment of myelodysplastic syndromes [see comments]. *Blood* 1991;78:1658–1663.

64. Hellstrom E, Birgegard G, Lockner D, et al. Treatment of myelodysplastic syndromes with recombinant human erythropoietin. *Eur J Haematol* 1991;47:355–360.

65. Casadevall N, Belanger C, Goy A, et al. High-dose recombinant human erythropoietin administered intravenously for the treatment of anaemia in myelodysplastic syndromes. *Acta Haematol* 1992; 87[Suppl 1]:25–27.

66. Goy A, Belanger C, Casadevall N, et al. High doses of intravenous recombinant erythropoietin for the treatment of anaemia in myelodysplastic syndrome. *Br J Haematol* 1993;84:232–237.

67. Mohr B, Herrmann R, Huhn D. Recombinant human erythropoietin in patients with myelodysplastic syndrome and myelofibrosis [see comments]. *Acta Haematol* 1993;90:65–70.

68. van Kaam AH, Egeler RM. Recombinant human erythropoietin for the correction of cancer associated anemia with and without concomitant cytotoxic chemotherapy [letter; comment]. *Cancer* 1991; 78:1144–1145.

69. Bowen D, Culligan D, Jacobs A. The treatment of anaemia in the myelodysplastic syndromes with recombinant human erythropoietin. *Br J Haematol* 1991;77:419–423.

70. Adamson JW, Schuster M, Allen S, et al. Effectiveness of recombinant human erythropoietin therapy in myelodysplastic syndromes. *Acta Haematol* 1992;87[Suppl 1]:20–24.

71. Rafanelli D, Grossi A, Longo G, et al. Recombinant human erythropoietin for treatment of myelodysplastic syndromes. *Leukemia* 1992;6:323–327.

72. Ghio R, Balleari E, Ballestrero A, et al. Subcutaneous recombinant human erythropoietin for the treatment of anemia in myelodysplastic syndromes [see comments]. *Acta Haematol* 1993;90:58–64.

73. Aloe Spiriti MA, Petti MC, Latagliata R, et al. Recombinant human erythropoietin in the treatment of myelodysplastic syndromes. An interim report. *Haematologica* 1993;78:123–126.

74. Negrin RS, Stein R, Vardiman J, et al. Treatment of the anemia of myelodysplastic syndromes using recombinant human granulocyte colony-stimulating factor in combination with erythropoietin [see comments]. *Blood* 1994;82:737–743.

75. Stone RM, Bernstein SH, Demetri G, et al. Therapy with recombinant human erythropoietin in patients with myelodysplastic syndromes. *Leuk Res* 1994;18:769–776.

76. Stasi R, Brunetti M, Bussa S, et al. Response to recombinant human erythropoietin in patients with myelodysplastic syndromes. *Clin Cancer Res* 1997;3:733–739.

77. Hansen PB, Johnsen HE, Hippe E, et al. Recombinant human granulocyte-macrophage colony-stimulating factor plus recombinant human erythropoietin may improve anemia in selected patients with myelodysplastic syndromes. *Am J Hematol* 1993;44:229–236.

78. Negrin RS, Stein R, Doherty K, et al. Maintenance treatment of the anemia of myelodysplastic syndromes with recombinant human granulocyte colony-stimulating factor and erythropoietin. Evidence for *in vivo* synergy. *Blood* 1996;87:4076–4081.

79. Runde V, Aul C, Ebert A, et al. Sequential administration of recombinant human granulocyte-macrophage colony-stimulating factor and human erythropoietin for treatment of myelodysplastic syn-

80. Imamura M, Kobayashi M, Kobayashi S, et al. Failure of combination therapy with recombinant granulocyte colony-stimulating factor and erythropoietin in myelodysplastic syndromes. *Ann Hematol* 1994;68:163–166.

81. Anonymous. A randomized double-blind placebo-controlled study with subcutaneous recombinant human erythropoietin in patients with low-risk myelodysplastic syndromes. Italian Cooperative Study Group for rHuEpo in Myelodysplastic Syndromes. *Br J Haematol* 1998;103:1070–1074.

82. Isnard F, Najman A, Jaar B, et al. Efficacy of recombinant human erythropoietin in the treatment of refractory anemias without excess of blasts in myelodysplastic syndromes. *Leuk Lymphoma* 1994;12: 307–314.

83. Di Raimondo F, Longo G, Cacciola E Jr, et al. A good response rate to recombinant erythropoietin alone may be expected in selected myelodysplastic patients. A preliminary clinical study. *Eur J Haematol* 1996;56:7–11.

84. Skikne BS, Cook JD. Effect of enhanced erythropoiesis on iron absorption. *J Lab Clin Med* 1992;120:746–751.

85. Adamson JW. The relationship of erythropoietin and iron metabolism to red blood cell production in humans. *Semin Oncol* 1997;21: 9–15.

86. Brugnara C, Chambers LA, Malynn E, et al. Red blood cell regeneration induced by subcutaneous recombinant erythropoietin: iron-deficient erythropoiesis in iron-replete subjects [see comments]. *Blood* 1993;81:956–964.

87. Cazzola M, Ponchio L, Beguin Y, et al. Subcutaneous erythropoietin for treatment of refractory anemia in hematologic disorders. Results of a phase I/II clinical trial [see comments]. *Blood* 1992;79:29–37.

88. Henry D, Glaspy J. Predicting response to epoetin alfa in anemic cancer patients receiving chemotherapy [Meeting Abstract]. *Proc Annu Meet Am Soc Clin Oncol* 1996;16:A1971–1997.

89. Henry DH. Recombinant human erythropoietin treatment of anemic cancer patients. *Cancer Pract* 1996;4:180–184.

90. Adamson JW, Ludwig H. Predicting the hematopoietic response to recombinant human erythropoietin (Epoetin alfa) in the treatment of the anemia of cancer. *Oncology* 1999;56:46–53.

91. Meadowcroft AM, Gilbert CJ, Maravich-May D, et al. Cost of managing anemia with and without prophylactic epoetin alfa therapy in breast cancer patients receiving combination chemotherapy. *Am J Health Syst Pharm* 1997;55:1898–1902.

92. Finkelstein SN, Huber SL, Greenberg PE. Cost comparison of recombinant human erythropoietin and blood transfusion in cancer chemotherapy-induced anemia [letter; comment]. *Ann Pharmacother* 1997;31:1094–1095.

93. Sheffield R, Sullivan SD, Saltiel E, et al. Cost comparison of recombinant human erythropoietin and blood transfusion in cancer chemotherapy-induced anemia [see comments]. *Ann Pharmacother* 1997;31:15–22.

94. Ortega A, Dranitsaris G, Puodziunas A. What are cancer patients willing to pay for epoetin alfa? A cost-benefit analysis. *Annu Meet Int Soc Technol Assess Health Care* 1998;14:100(abst).

95. Vogelzang NJ, Breitbart W, Cella D, et al. Patient, caregiver, and oncologist perceptions of cancer-related fatigue: results of a tripart assessment survey. The Fatigue Coalition. *Semin Hematol* 1997;34: 4–12.

96. Leitgeb C, Pecherstorfer M, Fritz E, et al. Quality of life in chronic anemia of cancer during treatment with recombinant human erythropoietin. *Cancer* 1994;73:2535–2542.

97. Borsi JD, Ferencz T, Csaki C, et al. Transfusion requirements of children with cancer and the use of human recombinant erythropoietin for the prevention and treatment of cytostatics induced anemia in children [Meeting Abstract]. *Can J Infect Dis* 1995;6:235C.

98. Glaspy J, Bukowski R, Steinberg D, et al. Impact of therapy with epoetin alfa on clinical outcomes in patients with nonmyeloid malignancies during cancer chemotherapy in community oncology practice. *J Clin Oncol* 1997;15:1218–1234.

99. Demetri GD, Kris M, Wade J, et al. Quality-of-life benefit in chemotherapy patients treated with epoetin alfa is independent of dis-

ease response or tumor type. Results from a prospective community oncology study. Procrit Study Group. *J Clin Oncol* 1998;16:3412–3425.

100. Gabrilove JL, Einhorn LH, Livingston RB, et al. Once-weekly dosing of epoetin alfa is similar to three-times-weekly dosing in increasing hemoglobin and quality of life. *Proc Am Soc Clin Oncol* 1999;18:574a(abst).

101. Littlewood TJ, Bajetta E, Cella D. Efficacy and quality of life outcomes of epoetin alfa in a double-blind, placebo-controlled multicenter study of cancer patients receiving non-platinum containing chemotherapy. *Proc Am Soc Clin Oncol* 1999;18:574a(abst).

102. Cleeland CS, Demetri GD, Glaspy J, et al. Identifying hemoglobin level for optimal quality of life: results of an incremental analysis. *Proc Am Soc Clin Oncol* 1999;18:574a(#2215).

103. Daneryd P, Svanberg E, Korner U, et al. Protection of metabolic and exercise capacity in unselected weight-losing cancer patients following treatment with recombinant erythropoietin: a randomized pro-

spective study. *Cancer Res* 1998;58:5374–5379.

104. Sowade O, Gross J, Sowade B, et al. Evaluation of oxygen availability with oxygen status algorithm in patients undergoing open heart surgery treated with epoetin beta. *J Lab Clin Med* 1997;129:97–105.

105. Lavey RS, Dempsey WH. Erythropoietin increases hemoglobin in cancer patients during radiation therapy. *Int J Radiat Oncol Biol Phys* 1993;27:1147–1152.

106. Vijayakumar S, Roach MD, Wara W, et al. Effect of subcutaneous recombinant human erythropoietin in cancer patients receiving radiotherapy. Preliminary results of a randomized, open-labeled, phase II trial. *Int J Radiat Oncol Biol Phys* 1993;26:721–729.

107. Dusenbery KE, McGuire WA, Holt PJ, et al. Erythropoietin increases hemoglobin during radiation therapy for cervical cancer. *Int J Radiat Oncol Biol Phys* 1994;29:1079–1084.

108. Sweeney PJ, Nicolae D, Ignacio L, et al. Effect of subcutaneous recombinant human erythropoietin in cancer patients receiving radiotherapy. Final report of a randomized, open-labelled, phase II trial. *Br J Cancer* 1998;77:1996–2002.

8

TUMOR NECROSIS FACTOR: BASIC PRINCIPLES AND CLINICAL APPLICATIONS IN SYSTEMIC AND REGIONAL CANCER TREATMENT

H. RICHARD ALEXANDER, JR.
ANDREW L. FELDMAN

Tumor necrosis factor (TNF) has had a long and fascinating history as a potential antitumor agent (Table 1). TNF became available in recombinant form in the mid-1980s after dramatic antitumor effects were observed in experimental models. High expectations existed for its clinical use. It was found, however, that humans are sensitive to the toxic effects of systemically administered TNF. Therefore, its clinical use was largely abandoned until 1992, when the initial results of its remarkable efficacy when given via isolated limb perfusion (ILP) were reported. The words of Emil Frei hold true today, as they did in 1989: "Our task is to learn to use TNF . . . appropriately." (1)

William Coley, a surgeon practicing in New York City in the late 1800s, was the first to investigate the therapeutic potential of inducing tumor necrosis using a crude extract of bacteria (2). Although the phenomenon of tumor necrosis in the presence of an infection was well known at the time, Coley administered preparations of gram-positive and gram-negative bacteria or bacterial products to humans with inoperable cancer and claimed success in some patients (3,4). The side effects of *Coley's toxins*, as these preparations were called, were unacceptable. For this and other reasons, their use was largely abandoned.

In the 1940s, Shear et al. (5) sought to isolate an active agent from Coley's toxins and purified bacterial polysaccharide from *Serratia marcescens*, known as *lipopolysaccharide* (LPS). It was shown that LPS, like Coley's original preparations, induced hemorrhagic necrosis of transplantable tumors in mice, although its toxicity profile also was similar (6). In 1962, O'Malley et al. (7) reported identifying an endogenous factor present in the serum of LPS-treated animals that induced hemorrhagic necrosis of tumors in naïve animals. Further characterization of this factor and the name *tumor necrosis factor* awaited the reports of Carswell and Old in 1975 (8). These authors showed that TNF was produced in mice pretreated with bacillus Calmette-Guérin and then given LPS. This caused hemorrhagic necrosis of methylcholanthrene-induced tumors when adminis-

tered to naïve mice. In addition, TNF was recognized to cause lysis of various neoplastic cells *in vitro* (9).

It was not until 1984 that the TNF gene was cloned (10). Recombinant TNF became available in 1985 (11), spurring a large number of preclinical murine studies. Prominent antitumor activity at doses associated with minimal toxicity in mice prompted multiple phase 1 and 2 trials of systemic and regional TNF between 1987 and 1991. These trials produced disappointing results.

In 1992, however, Liénard and Lejeune (12) published their first report of the efficacy of ILP using melphalan and high-dose TNF, sparking renewed interest in clinical TNF application. Reports on the use of isolated perfusion to treat tumors in the lung, liver, and kidney soon followed. This chapter reviews the biologic properties of TNF, its use in early clinical trials, and, particularly, its current use in regional administration via isolation perfusion.

BIOLOGIC PROPERTIES OF TUMOR NECROSIS FACTOR

Tumor Necrosis Factor Gene, Protein, and Biosynthesis

The term *TNF*, as used in this chapter, refers to *TNF-α*, also known previously as *cachectin* (13). TNF-β or lymphotoxin bears sequence homology to TNF but differs functionally (14,15). The human TNF (hTNF) gene has been localized to the short arm of chromosome 6 (chromosome 17 in mice) in the middle of the major histocompatibility complex (16).

hTNF messenger RNA codes for a 76–amino acid presequence and a 157–amino acid mature protein (11). In addition to the 17-kd secreted form of the protein, TNF can exist as an uncleaved 26-kd cell surface protein, which is biologically active, as measured by *in vitro* cytotoxicity (17). The tertiary structure of TNF is maintained by a disulfide bridge and the

TABLE 1. HISTORY OF THE STUDY OF TUMOR NECROSIS FACTOR AS AN ANTICANCER AGENT

Date	Event
1891–1906	Coley reports use of bacterial toxins in patients with cancer
1936–1944	Shear and others purify LPS from *Serratia marcescens*
1962	O'Malley et al. discover factor in LPS–treated animal that causes tumor necrosis
1975	Carswell and Old coin the term *TNF* and show antitumor activity *in vitro* and *in vivo* in mice
1984	TNF gene cloned
1985	Recombinant TNF first available
1985–1987	Preclinical studies show impressive antitumor effect of recombinant TNF in mice
1987–1991	Phase 1 and 2 human trials of systemic TNF show unacceptable toxicity at therapeutic doses
1992	Liénard and Lejeune report success of TNF and melphalan in isolated limb perfusion
1993	Uses of high-dose TNF in liver and lung perfusions

LPS, lipopolysaccharide; TNF, tumor necrosis factor.

molecule has a tendency to form noncovalently linked trimers held together by hydrophobic forces (18).

TNF is a cytokine produced mainly by macrophages and monocytes but can be secreted by various other cell types, including natural killer cells and lymphocytes (19,20). Although LPS is the best-characterized inducer of TNF (21), many other agents increase TNF synthesis *in vivo*, including tumor promoters and mitogens; viruses; and cytokines, such as interleukin (IL)-1, interferon (IFN)-γ, and granulocyte-macrophage colony-stimulating factor (22). Multiple inhibitors of TNF synthesis also are known, including glucocorticoids (21); phosphodiesterase inhibitors; and cyclic adenosine monophosphate analogues, such as pentoxifylline (23), tumor growth factor–β (24), and IL-4 (25).

Tumor Necrosis Factor Receptors

Two TNF receptors (TNF-R) have been characterized (26,27) and are generally known as *TNF-R1* and *TNF-R2*. These receptors previously have been termed *TNF-R55* and *TNF-R75*, respectively, based on their molecular weights. TNF-Rs are present on the surfaces of almost all cell types with the exception of red blood cells and unstimulated lymphocytes (28,29). Preclinical studies showed that a marked cross-reactivity exists between murine and hTNF and the murine receptors and hTNF-Rs, except that hTNF does not bind to murine TNF-R2 (30,31).

Although TNF-R1 is present on nearly all nucleated cells, it is maintained in relatively low concentrations on cell surfaces and is relatively refractory to upregulation or downregulation (32). Several inducers of TNF-R1 expression, however, have been identified, including IL-1β and a newly described cytokine, endothelial-monocyte–activating polypeptide II, which is capable of rendering TNF-resistant tumors TNF-sensitive *in vivo* (33–35). IFN-γ also may induce TNF-R1 expression, but this effect appears less consistent (32,33). TNF-R2 expression is widely variable and is induced by IFN-γ, IL-2 activation of T-

cell lymphocytes, and increased intracellular levels of cyclic adenosine monophosphate and protein kinase A (36–38). Protein kinase C activation downregulates expression of TNF-R2 (38).

TNF-R1 and TNF-R2 are transmembrane glycoproteins with similar extracellular domains but markedly differing intracellular domains (39). TNF-R1 appears chiefly responsible for TNF-induced cytotoxicity, activation of nuclear factor (NF)-κB, and possibly induction of nitric oxide synthetase (40–42). The intracellular effects of TNF-R2 have been observed mainly in T-cell lymphocytes, where TNF-R2 can mediate TNF-induced cytotoxicity (43). An extracellular role of TNF-R2 in "ligand passing" of TNF from TNF-R2 to TNF-R1, however, also has been proposed (44).

Both TNF receptors are known to be shed from cell surfaces, resulting in circulating levels of soluble receptors (45–47). This phenomenon may have major clinical consequences and potential therapeutic applications because soluble TNF-R has been shown to block TNF bioactivity *in vitro* and *in vivo* (48). Low concentrations of soluble TNF-R, however, also appear to stabilize the structure of TNF, prolonging its bioactivity and, thus, potentially enhancing its effect (49).

Biologic Actions of Tumor Necrosis Factor

The major actions of TNF on cells *in vitro* are cytotoxicity (8,9,50) and induction of gene expression, including the release of soluble factors (51). Occasionally, TNF can induce cellular proliferation (i.e., fibroblasts) (52,53). Soluble mediators released in the presence of TNF include PGE_2, leukotrienes, platelet-activating factor, nitric oxide, and reactive oxygen intermediates. The list of proteins induced by TNF has become voluminous but includes (1) nuclear factors, such as c-fos and c-jun; (2) cytosolic proteins, including nitric oxide synthetase; (3) mitochondrial manganese superoxide dismutase; (4) cell surface molecules, including intercellular adhesion molecule–1, IL-2 receptor-α, and class I and II major histocompatibility complex molecules; and (5) secreted proteins, including IL-1, IL-6, IL-8, IFN-β, granulocyte-macrophage colony-stimulating factor, platelet-derived growth factor, u-PA, and TNF itself (54–59).

The *in vitro* cytotoxic activity of TNF has been best characterized using L929 fibrosarcoma cells, the cell line in which this effect was first documented by Carswell and Old (8). Since then, the TNF sensitivity of many cell lines has been studied. Although no single mechanism for cytotoxicity emerges as the predominant one, traditional apoptosis and directly induced cellular necrosis contribute to this process (60). After TNF binds to its receptors, these complexes are internalized and phospholipase A_2 is activated (61,62). This releases arachidonic acid, prostaglandins, or both, and other eicosanoids (63). The result is the formation of reactive oxygen intermediates by the mitochondria, leading to cellular damage, as well as a chain of intracellular events triggered by the activation of transcription factors, such as NF-κB (64–66). Cells subsequently develop increased permeability and undergo "cellular collapse" (67). Hyperthermia increases sensitivity to the cytotoxic effects of TNF (68).

In vivo, high concentrations of TNF produce a toxicity syndrome similar to septic shock (69). In various laboratory mammals, TNF causes hypotension, acidosis, transient hyperglycemia followed by hypoglycemia, oliguria and renal failure, hemorrhagic infarction of the gastrointestinal tract, disseminated intravascular coagulopathy, and death by respiratory arrest (70,71). In addition, chronic administration of TNF (cachectin) causes cachexia in mice, and TNF is at least partially responsible for cancer-associated cachexia (72,73). In smaller doses, human subjects experience fever, headache, and a broad range of constitutional symptoms (74). Most of these effects are attributed to the TNF-induced release of multiple cytokines and other mediators, including IL-1, prostaglandins, and nitric oxide (75–77).

Antitumor Activity of Tumor Necrosis Factor

In addition to the direct cytotoxicity on malignant cell lines *in vitro*, as described in the Biologic Actions of Tumor Necrosis Factor section, TNF clearly has other antitumor activity. This was well documented by Carswell and Old, who discovered that TNF causes hemorrhagic necrosis in methylcholanthrene-induced fibrosarcomas in mice, despite the fact that these cells are resistant to the cytotoxic action *in vitro* (8). Further study of this phenomenon led to the understanding that TNF induces effects of the tumor microvasculature, ultimately resulting in necrosis in the central portion of the tumor. Specifically, TNF induces tissue factor expression by endothelial cells, promoting fibrin deposition and clot formation (78,79). This induction is enhanced by tumor-derived factors, such as endothelial-monocyte activating polypeptide II, which upregulates endothelial cell expression of TNF-R1 (35,78). In addition, TNF increases vascular permeability and induces expression of various adhesion molecules by endothelial cells, contributing to neutrophil invasion (80,81). The importance of the vascular effects of TNF on tumors is supported by the normalization of the hypervascular angiographic findings after treatment of sarcomas by ILP with TNF and melphalan (82).

Evidence exists that T-cell lymphocytes play a role in the antitumor effects of TNF (83). Tumor regression also has been documented after treatment of nude mice bearing transplantable human tumors with TNF (84,85). Although the degree of necrosis was less in this model than in immune-competent models, necrosis was still present, implicating a complex antitumor mechanism with multiple effectors. Some of this antitumor activity may be caused by synergy between TNF and IFN-γ (84). A large number of conventional chemotherapeutic agents have been screened for potential synergy with TNF with some success (86,87). This research, along with the known synergy between TNF and hyperthermia, has yielded the current combination of melphalan and hyperthermia as the most common agents used in conjunction with TNF in isolated perfusion (12).

EARLY CLINICAL STUDIES USING TUMOR NECROSIS FACTOR

Preclinical studies demonstrated that single-bolus intravenous (i.v.) administration of recombinant TNF could induce antitumor activity in a variety of murine tumor models (88,89). These

findings led to a concerted effort to identify clinical applications of TNF to treat cancer in humans. The majority of phase 1 and phase 2 trials indicated that systemic administration of TNF yielded unacceptable toxicity at subtherapeutic doses. The pharmacokinetic data obtained in these trials, however, paved the way for the refinement of regional applications of TNF and the current use of TNF in isolation perfusion.

Phase 1 Studies of Systemic Tumor Necrosis Factor

Early phase 1 trials were instrumental in defining the pharmacokinetics of bolus i.v. TNF (90–95). The rate of clearance of TNF from the circulation is highly dose dependent. At doses up to 100 µg per m^2, peak serum levels ranged from undetectable to 8 ng per mL, a half-life ranging from 10 to 17 minutes, and a high volume of distribution and rapid clearance (90,92,94,95). At higher dose levels (150 to 727 µg per m^2), however, the half-life ranged from 27 to 80 minutes (91–95), and a single study reported a half-life of 144 minutes using a high dose of 1,667 µg per m^2 (93). In addition, the ratio of peak serum level to dose level was found to increase dramatically as higher doses were given. For example, in one study, a dose of 45 mg per m^2 yielded a peak serum level of 2.2 ng per mL, whereas a 16-fold dose escalation (727 µg per m^2) yielded a 185-fold increase in the peak serum level (407 ng per mL) (91).

Two mechanisms for the nonlinear pharmacokinetics of i.v. TNF have been proposed. First, clearance of circulating TNF appears to exhibit saturation kinetics with preclinical studies, demonstrating enhanced tissue distribution to the liver and kidney (96) and increased clearance time in nephrectomized mice (97). Second, the binding of circulating TNF to soluble TNF-Rs represents a saturable system with complex implications because levels of bioactive TNF and immunologically detectable TNF appear to be different (97).

Phase 1 trials using continuous infusion of TNF demonstrated a pattern of high early circulating levels with a subsequent decrease and failure to reach a steady serum level (98,99). For example, one study measured serum TNF levels ranging from 90 to 900 pg per mL up to 3 hours after initiating the infusion but reported subsequent undetectable serum levels despite continued infusion at the same dose (98). Again, the presence and possible increased production of soluble TNF-Rs receptors may contribute to this phenomenon (100).

Attempts to deliver systemic TNF via intramuscular or subcutaneous (s.c.) injection yielded measurable serum levels only at high-dose levels (>150 µg per m^2) with peak circulating levels occurring 4 to 12 hours after s.c. injection, and somewhat higher peak levels occurring 12 to 24 hours after intramuscular injection (101–104).

The majority of phase 1 trials of systemic recombinant TNF used single- or repetitive-dose i.v. bolus TNF or continuous i.v. TNF. Maximum tolerated doses achieved with repetitive-dose bolus TNF (150 to 300 µg per m^2) (94,105–110) were no higher than those achieved with single-dose treatment (218 to 410 µg per m^2), except for one trial that delivered 818 µg per m^2 (91,92,111,112). Preclinical rodent studies have demonstrated a tachyphylactic or tolerant effect to repetitive TNF dos-

TABLE 2. DOSE-LIMITING TOXICITIES IN PHASE 1 TRIALS OF INTRAVENOUS TUMOR NECROSIS FACTOR

Dose-Limiting Toxicity	Bolus i.v. (n = 12)	Continuous i.v. Infusion (n = 6)	Total (n = 18)
Hypotension	11 (92)	2 (33)	13 (72)
Hepatotoxicity	5 (42)	1 (17)	6 (33)
Malaise, myalgia, fatigue	2 (17)	2 (33)	4 (22)
Thrombocytopenia	1 (8)	3 (50)	4 (22)
CNS toxicity, confusion	1 (8)	2 (33)	3 (17)
Leukopenia	1 (8)	1 (17)	2 (11)
Headache	—	2 (33)	2 (11)
Nausea	1 (8)	—	1 (6)
Fever, chills	—	1 (17)	1 (6)

(Header: Number of Trials (%))

CNS, central nervous system.

ing, which may explain the findings of these phase 1 human trials (113,114).

All phase 1 trials produced single or multiple dose-limiting toxicities with hypotension being by far the most common toxicity (Table 2). Hypotension was the most prominent side effect in 11 of 12 bolus i.v. trials that defined a dose-limiting toxicity (91–95,106–112). The incidence and severity of hypotension was dose related and occurred in 30% to 60% of patients. Other common grade III and IV toxicities included hepatotoxicity (elevated hepatic transaminases, 10% to 50% of patients), constitutional symptoms, and thrombocytopenia or leukopenia (0% to 40% of patients). Between 15 and 30 minutes after bolus administration of TNF, most patients experienced rigors, followed by hypertension and tachycardia. Between 60 and 90 minutes after infusion, almost all patients developed fever. These sequelae did not appear to be dose related. Hypotension was seen 6 to 12 hours after administration and clearly was dose related, requiring vigorous resuscitation, including vasopressors, in all patients at the highest dose level (1,667 µg per m^2) (93). Nadir platelet counts generally occurred 1 to 2 days after infusion, but few patients had counts less than 100,000 per mm^3. Leukocyte counts generally decreased 30 to 60 minutes after infusion of TNF, after which a return to normal or mildly ele-

vated levels was followed by a gradual decrease; significant neutropenia was seen only rarely.

Constitutional and hematologic side effects were more frequently dose limiting in phase 1 trials of continuous i.v. TNF than in the bolus i.v. trials (see Table 2) (98,99,115–118). With maximum tolerated doses as low as 40 to 160 µg per m^2 per day, however (99, 115,118), it is likely that the doses necessary to cause the more severe side effect of hypotension never were reached. Phase 1 trials of s.c. or intramuscular TNF (101–104) yielded similar maximum tolerated doses and side-effect profiles as the i.v. trials, with the addition of severe inflammation at the site of injection as a dose-limiting toxicity in two studies (101,104). Most phase 1 studies reported no evidence of antitumor activity. The occasional responses in these trials are discussed in the following section.

Phase 2 Studies of Systemic Tumor Necrosis Factor

The results of nine phase 2 studies using intermittent bolus i.v. administration of TNF were reported between 1989 and 1992 (Table 3) (119–127). These studies represented treatment of 168 patients (156 evaluable) with tumors of various histologies. The majority of patients were part of a series of Southwest Oncology Group trials in which the TNF administration schedule was 150 µg per m^2 daily for 5 days given every other week for 8 weeks; experience with 127 of these patients was reported in 1991 (128). Seventeen percent of patients were removed from this study because of drug toxicity. Grade III toxicity consisted mostly of constitutional symptoms and was seen in 47% of patients. Grade IV toxicity was seen in 13% of patients and, in addition to the toxicities seen in phase 1 studies, included a subset of patients with disseminated intravascular coagulation, most of whom had pancreatic cancer.

The therapeutic outcome of the phase 2 trials was disappointing (see Table 3). Only 2 of the 156 patients summarized in Table 3, both with renal cell cancer, achieved an objective response (126). Similarly, among 410 patients in phase 1 trials whose responses were recorded, only 11 had an objective response (93,95,105–108,110). The only complete response within this group was in a patient with renal cell cancer (110).

TABLE 3. PHASE 2 TRIALS OF INTRAVENOUS TUMOR NECROSIS FACTOR

Authors (Reference)	Dose Schedule	Histology	Evaluable Patients (n)	CR	PR	MR/SD	PD
Lenk et al. (120)	683–956 µg/m^2 q8–12d	Mixed	18	—	—	4	14
Aboulafia et al. (121)	100 µg/m^2 qwk	Kaposi's sarcoma	5	—	—	—	5
Kemeny et al. (122)	100–150 µg/m^2 qd × 5 d	Colorectal	14	—	—	3	11
Whitehead et al. (123)	150 µg/m^2 qd × 5 d	Colorectal	20	—	—	2	18
Schaadt et al. (124)	217–652 µg/m^2 3 × wk	Colorectal	15	—	—	1	14
Budd et al. (125)	150 µg/m^2 qd × 5 d	Breast	19	—	—	—	19
Brown et al. (119)	150 µg/m^2 qd × 5 d	Pancreas	22	—	—	—	22
Skillings et al. (126)	150 µg/m^2 qd × 5 d	Renal cell	22	1	1	—	20
Feldman et al. (127)	150 µg/m^2 qd × 5 d	Melanoma	21	—	—	1	20
Total			**156**	**1**	**1**	**11**	**143**

(Header: Responses)

CR, complete response; MR, minimal or mixed response; PD, progressive disease; PR, partial response; SD, stable disease.

TABLE 4. TRIALS OF INTRATUMORAL OR INTRACAVITY ADMINISTRATION OF TUMOR NECROSIS FACTOR

Authors (Reference)	Dose		Histology	Patients (n)	Response Rate (%)
	μg	μg/m²			
Intratumoral					
Ijzermans et al. (143)	100–350	—	GI (liver metastases)	15	—
Taguchi (93)	33–667	—	Mixed	9	—
Kahn et al. (144)	—	5–100	Kaposi's sarcoma	28	50
Bartsch et al. (145)	25–300	—	Mixed	14	21
Pfreundschuh et al. (146)	—	87–522	Mixed	21	19
Tada et al. (147)	0.004–0.033	—	Glioma	6	Not reported
Intraperitoneal					
Markman et al. (149)	—	10–50	Mixed	11	—
Rath et al. (150)	—	40–350	Mixed	29	76
Hardy et al. (151)	—	89	Ovarian	4	—
Rath et al. (152)	—	80	Mixed	32	100
Intravesical					
Serretta et al. (153)	—	60–600	Bladder	24	23
Sternberg et al. (154)	—	400–1,800	Bladder	20	22

GI, gastrointestinal.

Duration of response likewise was disappointing, lasting no longer than 9 months in all but one patient (renal cell cancer, ongoing partial response at 2 years) (93,95,98,105–108, 110,126).

Systemic Tumor Necrosis Factor Combined with Other Agents

Several studies sought to demonstrate a synergistic effect between TNF and other biologic agents because of the disappointing results in the phase 1 and 2 trials using systemic TNF alone. Such synergism previously had been demonstrated in mice using IL-2 (129,130), IFN-γ and IFN-α (84), standard chemotherapeutic agents (131,87), and hyperthermia (132). A human phase 1 and 2 trial of TNF and IL-2 yielded four objective responses in 38 patients (10.5%), a response rate somewhat lower than that seen with IL-2 alone (133). Other studies with this therapeutic combination demonstrated low maximum tolerated doses of TNF and similarly low response rates (134,135). Several trials combined TNF with IFN-γ and also demonstrated enhanced TNF toxicity without therapeutic benefit (136–138). The combination of TNF and IFN-α has shown occasional objective responses in humans (94,139,140). At this time, however, too few patients have been treated to draw any definitive conclusions. No evidence exists to suggest that TNF enhances the effectiveness of systemic chemotherapy in humans. One phase 3 study randomized patients to bischloromethyl-nitrosourea or bischloromethyl-nitrosourea and TNF. The response rate for bischloromethyl-nitrosourea was almost double that for the combined therapy with less systemic toxicity (141). Finally, although anecdotal reports exist of systemic TNF-inducing responses when combined with regional hyperthermia (142), by far the most widely used application of TNF and hyperthermia is in isolated perfusion, which is discussed in the section on Application of Tumor Necrosis Factor in Isolation Perfusion.

Early Trials of Regional Administration of Tumor Necrosis Factor

Because of the promising results of TNF in preclinical studies but disappointing outcome of phase 1 and 2 studies resulting from unacceptable systemic toxicity, the strategy of regional administration of TNF became increasingly attractive. Isolated perfusion with TNF is discussed in the section on Application of Tumor Necrosis Factor in Isolation Perfusion. Several other techniques of regional administration of TNF have been investigated (Table 4).

Several phase 1 trials have been conducted using intratumoral injection (see Table 4) (93,143–147). Although the applicability of this technique to patients with metastatic cancer is limited, these studies did show that TNF has antitumor effects in humans when sufficiently high local concentrations can be achieved. Response rates ranged from 0% to 50%. Even in nonresponders, however, hemorrhagic necrosis has been noted (93), and growth arrest has been documented in injected lesions while noninjected lesions in the same patient progressed (143). In addition, these studies showed that TNF could be injected locally without systemic toxicity, even to the liver or brain under radiologic guidance (143,147).

Murine studies that suggested that TNF demonstrated less toxicity when delivered intraperitoneally rather than intravenously (148) prompted several human trials treating peritoneal carcinomatosis or malignant ascites with intraperitoneal TNF (see Table 4) (149–152). In two of these studies that used TNF prepared by Knoll AG, response rates of 76% and 100% were achieved in patients with malignant ascites (150,152). Despite mild constitutional and gastrointestinal symptoms, no dose-limiting toxicity was reached. In two other studies using other commercial preparations of TNF (Genentech and Asahi), however, no objective responses were achieved, and dose-limiting abdominal pain and infectious complications were observed (149,151). These studies suggest some pharmacokinetic advantage may exist to using intraperitoneal TNF, but poorly understood differences in commercial preparations warrant further investigation of this route of administration.

The use of intravesical TNF has been studied as an adjuvant and a therapeutic agent because of the high rate of local recurrence after transurethral resection of superficial bladder cancer (see Table 4) (153,154). Objective response rates of 22% and 23% have been reported. Even at high-dose levels (1,800 µg per m^2), neither systemic toxicity nor measurable TNF in the systemic circulation was observed. Although few patients achieved complete responses in these trials, the results emphasize the potential benefits of regional application of TNF.

Finally, direct intraarterial infusion has been attempted to deliver TNF regionally (155,156). Mavligit et al. have reported a 14% partial response rate in patients with hepatic metastases refractory to standard therapies using a continuous 5-day infusion of TNF into the hepatic artery (155). The maximum tolerated dose (150 µg per m^2) was similar to that achieved in trials using continuous i.v. infusion with grade IV hypophosphatemia as the dose-limiting toxicity and a notable absence of hypotensive episodes (155,157). Intraarterial TNF also has been used in patients with gliomas with objective responses in 20% of patients, symptomatic improvement in 47% of patients despite absence of tumor shrinkage, and radiographic evidence of necrosis in 70% of patients (156). Therefore, traditional radiographic follow-up may underestimate tumor response to TNF. These studies again support the concept of regional administration of TNF, which is discussed further in the section on Application of Tumor Necrosis Factor in Isolation Perfusion.

Gene Therapy with Tumor Necrosis Factor

The safe administration to patients with tumor-infiltrating lymphocytes retrovirally transduced with a marker gene by Rosenberg et al. established the feasibility of gene therapy in humans (158). The first potentially therapeutic gene investigated for use in cancer patients was TNF, based on the hypothesis that trafficking of transduced tumor-infiltrating lymphocytes to tumor would produce high local concentrations of TNF while avoiding systemic toxicity (159). Although some patients experienced tumor regression after such therapy (160), lymphocytes proved to have transcriptional and secretory limitations that precluded the widespread clinical use of this approach (161). These studies, however, encouraged the development of multiple strategies for the gene therapy of cancer with TNF and other cytokines.

Intratumoral injection of retroviral or adenoviral vectors carrying the TNF gene have demonstrated reliable TNF production and significant antitumor effects in mice (162,163), although systemic toxicity remains a significant concern (164). Studies using a membrane-bound mutant of TNF demonstrated greater safety (165). The use of conditional gene-expression systems may represent another means to control systemic toxicity (166). TNF gene therapy also may be synergistic with other forms of cancer therapy, including ionizing radiation (167,168), chemotherapy (169), and suicide gene therapy (170). Intraarterial injection of liposomes encapsulating the TNF gene has been shown to lead to an antitumor immune response and tumor regression in mice (171). These findings, along with the clinical use of TNF in the

isolation perfusion setting, raise the possibility of regional administration of TNF gene therapy in humans.

APPLICATION OF TUMOR NECROSIS FACTOR IN ISOLATION PERFUSION

Background

Interest in the use of TNF as an anticancer agent was rekindled in 1992 with the initial report of Liénard and Lejeune regarding 23 patients who were treated with a combination of IFN-γ, TNF, and melphalan administered as a hyperthermic ILP for intransit extremity melanoma or unresectable high-grade extremity sarcoma (12). In this initial report, the overall response rate was 100% in 23 assessable patients with a complete response rate of 89%. Subsequently, a number of institutions have been evaluating the use of TNF applied via isolation perfusion using ILP for the treatment of intransit melanoma or unresectable extremity sarcoma and isolated organ perfusion of the liver, lung, or kidney for primary or metastatic unresectable cancers confined to these organs.

Rationale for the Use of Tumor Necrosis Factor in Isolation Perfusion

Isolation perfusion is a specialized surgical technique in which the vascular supply to a cancer-bearing region (extremity) or organ (i.e., liver, lung) is isolated, cannulated, and connected to an extracorporeal bypass machine consisting of an oxygenator, reservoir, heat exchanger, and roller pump similar to that used in cardiac surgical procedures. The organ or region of the body can then be perfused with therapeutic agents added into a solution that is composed of 1 U of packed red blood cells diluted in 700 mL of a balanced salt solution containing heparin. At the completion of treatment, the perfused organ or region is flushed with saline and colloid solution to remove the residual therapeutic agents before reestablishing the native vascular blood flow.

One advantage of isolation perfusion is that complete or near complete separation of the regional and systemic circulation should be theoretically possible in virtually all circumstances, so that leak of perfusate into the systemic circulation can be eliminated or minimized, thereby reducing systemic exposure and toxicity. Another advantage is that dose escalation of the therapeutic agents is limited largely by the tissue tolerance of the perfused organ or limb. Finally, the use of isolation perfusion allows delivery of hyperthermia to the perfused tissues, which has known synergistic tumoricidal effect with TNF (172,173) and chemotherapeutic agents (174,175), as well as direct tumoricidal effects in experimental models (176).

When using TNF via isolation perfusion, continuous monitoring of potential perfusate leak into the systemic circulation is an essential component of treatment because the 3- to 4-mg dose of TNF that is typically used in ILP is approximately tenfold higher than the maximum systemic tolerated dose of TNF in previous phase 1 trials (90,91,94,106). Several leak monitoring techniques using radiolabeled iodine-131–radiolabeled albumin (177,178) or technetium-99–labeled red blood cells (179,180) have been used and have been shown to be sensitive and reliable methods of detecting leak rates less than 1%. Leak rates greater

TABLE 5. RATIONALE FOR TUMOR NECROSIS FACTOR USE IN ISOLATION PERFUSION

Can achieve high and sustained perfusate concentrations
Limited or no systemic exposure
Efficacy with single-dose administration
Synergy with chemotherapy and hyperthermia
Selective effects on tumor neovasculature

than 1% occur in 10% to 12% of patients undergoing ILP (177), due to the fact that, despite careful dissection of the iliac artery and vein and the use of a tourniquet at the root of the extremity, it is impossible to completely control small collateral blood vessels present in the pelvis. Control of perfusate leaks during ILP can be improved using various technical maneuvers, such as repositioning of the cannulae, tightening of the tourniquet, placing a partial occluding clamp on the venous outflow line to increase venous pressure within the perfusion circuit, or changing flow rates, which secondarily increases or decreases arterial pressures within the circuit (181). Thom and colleagues have shown that systemic perfusate leak during ILP with TNF, melphalan, and IFN as small as 1% result in significantly higher systemic levels of TNF and other inflammatory cytokines, such as IL-6 and IL-8, compared with patients with no leak (182). Leak of perfusate during liver perfusion does not typically occur because of the unique vascular anatomy of the liver.

TNF appears to be an ideally suited agent for isolation perfusion because sustained high perfusate concentrations of the protein can be routinely achieved during isolation organ or extremity perfusion (182,183). In fact, the perfusate doses of TNF initially measured at the beginning of treatment in the perfusate are approximately equal to the calculated concentration based on the dose of TNF administered into a fixed volume consisting of 1 L of perfusate and 300 to 400 mL of existing blood volume in the liver or extremity. Over the course of isolated limb or other perfusion, TNF concentrations stay largely stable, indicating little degradation or tissue absorption of the protein. Other factors that support the rationale for TNF applied via isolation perfusion are

shown in Table 5. Data from experimental models (78–80) and clinical reports (81,82) exist that support the notion that TNF exerts its antitumor effects primarily via actions on tumor-associated neovasculature and explain, in some part, the observation that TNF-based therapy administered via isolation perfusion is effective against a wide range of different tumor histologies.

Treatment of Intransit Melanoma with Tumor Necrosis Factor Administered via Isolated Limb Perfusion

The initial clinical results with TNF, IFN-γ, and melphalan administered as a 90-minute hyperthermic ILP for intransit melanoma was confirmed in a subsequent report by Liénard and Lejeune regarding 29 patients with intransit melanoma who underwent 31 ILPs (184). The combination and doses of TNF and IFN-γ initially used in ILP were derived mostly empirically based on the fact that chemotherapeutic doses used in ILP historically have been approximately tenfold higher than the maximally tolerated systemic i.v. dose. A tenfold higher dose of TNF than that tolerated intravenously (200 to 250 µg per m^2) would be approximately 4 mg. Because leak rates greater than 10% occur in less than 2% of patients undergoing ILP, and because treatment can be terminated if unacceptable leak rates (>10%) occur by using a continuous leak monitoring system, that dose of TNF should be considered safe. IFN-γ was included in the regimen because of its ability to upregulate TNF-Rs on tumor and endothelium (185) and its synergistic antitumor activity with TNF in experimental models (84,186). The sequence in which agents were administered was also largely empirical. IFN-γ was administered subcutaneously at a dose of 200 µg for 2 days before ILP and given at the beginning of treatment into the perfusion circuit with TNF. After 30 minutes, melphalan was added slowly to the circuit, and treatment continued for 60 additional minutes. This regimen was modified in subsequent clinical trials.

The overall response rate in 23 assessable patients reported by Liénard and Lejeune was 100% with 21 patients or 90% experiencing a complete response to treatment (Table 6). Of

TABLE 6. RESULTS OF CLINICAL TRIALS USING TUMOR NECROSIS FACTOR FOR ISOLATED LIMB PERFUSION TO TREAT EXTREMITY MELANOMA

Authors (Reference)	Trial Type (Phase)	Regimens	Assessable (n)	CR (%)	PR (%)	Overall (%)
				Response Rates		
Liénard et al. (184)	2	Melp/IFN/TNF	23	21 (90)	2 (10)	23 (100)
Posner et al. (193)	1	TNF alone (1–4 mg)	6	1 (17)	—	1 (17)
Fraker et al. (192)	1/2	Melp/IFN/TNF (4 mg)	26	20 (76)	4 (16)	24 (92)
		Melp/IFN/TNF (6 mg)	11	4 (36)	7 (64)	11 (100)
Fraker et al. (189)	3	Melp	23	14 (61)	9 (39)	23 (100)
		Melp/IFN/TNF	20	16 (80)	2 (10)	18 (90)
Liénard et al. (188)	3	Melp/TNF	33	23 (69)	7 (22)	30 (91)
		Melp/IFN/TNF	31	24 (78)	7 (22)	31 (100)
Vaglini et al. (190)	2	Melp/IFN/TNF (0.5–4.0 mg)	11	7 (64)	—	7 (64)

CR, complete remission; IFN, interferon; Melp, melphalan; PR, partial response; TNF, tumor necrosis factor.
Note: Melp/IFN/TNF: 90-minute perfusion described by Liénard et al. (184) with preoperative IFN-γ. Time 0 perfusate: IFN-γ, 0.2 mg; TNF, 4 mg; and melphalan, 10 mg per L (lower extremity), 13 mg per L (upper extremity) at time 30 minutes. Melp: Other regimens with standard melphalan dose as with the triple combination.

note, this cohort included 18 patients who failed a prior ILP. One-third of patients had more than ten intransit lesions present on extremity. The mean duration of response was 33 weeks, although median follow-up time was short (41 weeks) in this study (184).

Regional (extremity) toxicity was considered acceptable with most patients experiencing reversible grade II erythema, as defined by Wieberdink (187). All patients were treated with prophylactic dopamine during ILP and for 48 hours thereafter to prevent hypotension and tachycardia. With considerably more experience, most investigators would agree that regional toxicity from TNF and melphalan is more severe than that of the original report. The incidence of severe systemic toxicity, however, has been overestimated, and the routine use of perioperative dopamine has been abandoned.

A subsequent multicenter, randomized trial was conducted in Europe in which patients received the original three-agent regimen versus melphalan and TNF while eliminating the preoperative and perfusate doses of IFN-γ. Two interesting results were reported from this trial (188). The complete response rates in either arm of this study were less than the 89% complete response rates in the initial series of patients. In addition, no significant difference existed in the response rates observed with the two arms, with the complete response rates being 78% and 69% with and without IFN, respectively (see Table 6).

A phase 3 random assignment trial was initiated at the National Cancer Institute in Bethesda, Maryland, and expanded to a multicenter trial comparing the three-agent regimen with a standard treatment arm consisting of a melphalan (alone) ILP administered in an otherwise identical fashion to the experimental regimen. Although this trial was terminated early because of the loss of TNF for clinical trials in the United States, an interim analysis reported a complete response of 80% for the three-drug regimen and 61% for the melphalan alone group (189). The duration of complete responses were similar in both arms of the trial. In an unplanned subgroup analysis of a small number of patients, it appeared that the complete response rate was greater for patients who had bulky or numerous lesions when TNF was included in the regimen.

The question as to the optimal dose of TNF used in conjunction with melphalan administered via ILP has not been critically evaluated. A study was reported by Vaglini et al. from Milan in which 12 patients with extremity melanoma were treated with the three-agent regimen (190). Of interest, three patients were treated with a dose of 2 mg of TNF. Two of the three patients had a complete response to treatment. Of 11 evaluable patients, seven complete responses occurred with an overall response rate of 64%. One institutional report of ILP in patients with various types of extremity tumors using TNF in a relatively unusual dose-deescalation regimen was reported in 1993 by Hill and coworkers (191). Nine patients were treated with a regimen using a short 45-minute total perfusion time, which included melphalan given at time 0 at a dose of 1.5 mg per kg followed 15 minutes later by TNF at doses of 500, 250, and 125 μg in three patients at each level. Of the patients on this deescalating study, four had melanoma and all had complete responses to therapy. The extremely low doses used in the report by Hill and coworkers are approximately 10% of the

usual 4-mg dose. This dose was given for only 30 minutes compared with the usual 90-minute interval. The complete responses observed in the four patients treated using this strategy are remarkable and suggest that further work is necessary to determine the optimal dose of TNF.

A phase 1 study was reported in which the dose of TNF was escalated in the perfusion circuit from 4 to 6 mg (192). The peak perfusate levels of TNF were significantly higher when the higher dose of TNF was administered into the perfusion circuit. The complete response rate, however, was 76% in 26 patients treated in the 4-mg TNF group and only 36% in 12 patients in the 6-mg TNF group. This response rate was explained by differences in disease burden before therapy. Most notably, regional toxicity, including myopathy and neuropathy, was greater with the addition of higher doses of TNF. Taken together, these data suggest that lower, rather than higher, doses of TNF may be optimal in ILP.

Posner et al. have reported the only experience using TNF alone administered via ILP for intransit melanoma of the extremity (193). Six patients were treated with a 60- to 90-minute hyperthermic ILP in which three patients received either 1, 2, or 3 mg of TNF, and three patients received a total of 4 mg of TNF. Of these six patients, only one patient had a complete response of 7 months' duration and then relapsed. Three of the cohort underwent a second perfusion with the three-agent regimen, including melphalan, TNF, and IFN-γ, and all had a response to therapy. These data indicate that TNF alone applied via ILP for melanoma has essentially no meaningful antitumor activity. This raises many important questions with respect to the role of TNF in this setting. A prospective randomized trial is under way in Europe comparing melphalan alone with melphalan and TNF. A second similarly designed trial has been initiated in the United States.

Although the data do not definitively demonstrate any bonafide improvement in response rates when TNF is included in the regimen, some compelling data exist that indicate that TNF may be important in some patients. When TNF is included in the regimen with melphalan, the antitumor effects are rapid, and the mean time to response is 9 days (184), which is considerably different from the character and time course of responses in patients treated with melphalan alone (194). Secondly, a frequently rapid necrosis and eschar formation of cutaneous lesions are present that occurs with TNF reminiscent of the findings in preclinical murine models (195) (Fig. 1). Nevertheless, the complete response rate with ILP using melphalan alone for intransit melanoma has been reported to be between 50% and 65% (194). It is possible that the therapeutic benefit from the addition of TNF may be limited in patients with extensive or bulky disease. The duration of complete responses with melphalan alone or with melphalan combined with TNF was 320 and 495 days, respectively (188), illustrating the limitations of ILP with any regimen to provide durable disease control in the limb.

Isolated Limb Perfusion with Tumor Necrosis Factor for Unresectable Extremity Sarcoma

Despite significant improvement in limb-sparing techniques to control high-grade extremity sarcoma, approximately 10% to

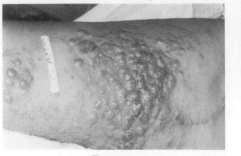

Pre-op

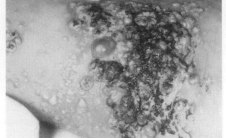

4 days post-op

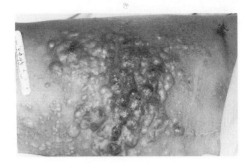

1 day post-op

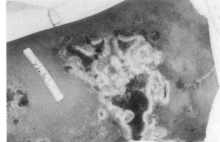

18 days post-op

FIGURE 1. Sequential photographs of extensive cutaneous and subcutaneous metastases from a primary eccrine gland adenocarcinoma. The patient did not respond to combination systemic chemotherapy and intraarterial doxorubicin hydrochloride (Adriamycin) and platinum. The patient was treated with an isolated limb perfusion using tumor necrosis factor, interferon-γ, and melphalan at the National Cancer Institute in Bethesda, Maryland. Note the rapid eschar formation apparent within days of treatment and the selective effects of treatment on the tumor with sparing of normal skin along the edge and within the tumor bed.

15% of patients present with primary or recurrent tumors that are not amenable to local therapy. Despite amputation in this group of patients, systemic metastases occur in more than 50% of patients. Therefore, strategies to preserve limb function translate into markedly improved quality of life for patients afflicted with this disease. Although ILP using various chemotherapeutics has been used in the past for extremity sarcoma, the data represent poorly controlled trials for which the benefit for limb perfusion has not been clearly established (196).

Most of the experience using TNF-based regimens administered via ILP for extremity sarcoma has come from a large multicenter trial. Results have been presented in several reports (197,198). The application of ILP in extremity sarcoma differs in several ways from ILP for intransit melanoma. For patients who have a large but potentially curable, locally unresectable extremity sarcoma as a result of its proximity or involvement with neurovascular or bony structures, ILP is administered as a neoadjuvant therapy with the goal of converting an unresectable lesion to a resectable one. Under these circumstances, after maximal tumor response to perfusion, an interval procedure is performed in which the tumor is excised usually between 4 to 12 weeks later. For patients who have multifocal sarcoma with no local resection option, ILP is administered primarily with curative intent. Lastly, in patients who have unresectable metastatic disease and a symptomatic primary tumor in place, limb perfusion is administered primarily as a palliative measure in which the success of therapy is gauged by its ability to provide sufficient tumor regression for relief of symptoms during the life of the patient. In the initial report from Liénard and Lejeune, four patients with extremity sarcoma were treated, all of whom had an objective response, including two patients who had a complete response at a follow-up of 12 and 23 months (12) (Table 7).

Eggermont et al. initially reported the results of ILP with TNF, IFN, and melphalan for unresectable extremity soft tissue sarcoma in which 55 patients were treated (197). This cohort represented a relatively heterogeneous population, including 30 patients with primary lesions, 25 with recurrent sarcomas, and seven patients with low-grade tumors. Limb perfusion was administered exactly as described in the setting of intransit melanoma, using IFN administered for 2 days subcutaneously before limb perfusion. Tumor response was graded according to radiographic and pathologic criteria. If the lesion showed more than 50% necrosis on careful histopathologic examination, this was scored as a partial response in patients who underwent tumor resection, although, radiographically or clinically, the lesion may have shown only minimal or no size regression. If no evidence of tumor viability existed on histopathologic evaluation, the final outcome was scored as a complete response, even if a residual lesion was present radiographically or clinically. The clinical complete response rate was 18% and increased to 36% after pathologic evaluation. The clinical partial response rate was 64% and decreased slighly after the pathologic evaluation because some lesions that had partially regressed radiographically or clinically were found to be 100% necrotic. The overall response rate was 87%. Limb salvage was achieved in 84% of patients with follow-up ranging from 20 to 50 months (see Table 7). Of note, one-third of the 39 patients who underwent tumor resection after ILP received adjuvant external beam radiation therapy (EBRT). Olieman et al. have reported results in 34 patients with high-grade unresectable extremity sarcoma treated with TNF, IFN-γ, and melphalan ILP (199). In 15 patients with close or positive margins after resection, EBRT was administered with a local control rate of 100%. EBRT has been shown to provide excellent local control, however, even for large high-

TABLE 7. SUMMARY OF ISOLATED LIMB PERFUSION TRIALS USING TUMOR NECROSIS FACTOR FOR EXTREMITY SOFT TISSUE SARCOMA

Authors (Reference)	n	Agents	Dose	Response Rate		Limb Salvage (%)	Comments
				CR (%)	PR (%)		
Liénard et al. (12)	4	TNF Melphalan	2–4 mg 10–13 mg/L	3 (75)	1 (25)	N/A	Initial pilot study, short F/U
Hill et al. (191)	9	TNF Melphalan	125–500 µg 10–13 mg/L	9 (100)	—	56	Short (45 min) ILP severe limb toxicity
Eggermont et al. (198)	186	TNF Melphalan	3–4 mg 10–13 mg/mL	54 (29)	99 (53)	82	Multicenter trial, regimen approved for STS in Europe, median F/U 2 yr
Gutman et al. (204)	35	TNF Melphalan	3–4 mg 1.0–1.5 mg/kg	13 (37)	19 (54)	85	Second ILP in five of six converted PR to CR
Olieman et al. (199)	34	TNF Melphalan	3–4 mg 10–13 mg/L	12 (33)	20 (40)	85	Median F/U 34 months, EBRT decreased local recurrences
Fraker et al. (203)	43[a]	TNF Melphalan	3–6 mg 10–13 mg/L	11 (26)	13 (30)	68	Entire U.S. experience

CR, complete remission; EBRT, external beam radiation therapy; F/U, follow-up; ILP, isolated limb perfusion; PR, partial response; STS, short-term storage; TNF, tumor necrosis factor.
[a]Two patients received TNF without melphalan.

grade, deep-seated lesions or in the presence of microscopically positive margins after resection without a prior ILP (200–202). Lastly, it is interesting that in the series reported by Olieman et al., 19 patients did not receive EBRT because of a possible adequate resection margin, or because a complete pathologic response to ILP occurred. In this cohort, the local recurrence rate was high at 26%.

The last update reported by Eggermont et al. included data on 186 patients with locally advanced soft tissue extremity sarcoma with results that largely confirmed the earlier experience (198) (see Table 7). At a median follow-up of almost 2 years with a range of 6 to 58 months, an 82% limb salvage rate occurred in the setting of an overall clinical and pathologic response rate of 82%. Of note, only the first 55 patients received IFN-γ, and the effectiveness of therapy did not appear to be compromised when it was omitted from the treatment regimen. Based on the considerable efforts of the European investigators to establish ILP as a reasonable treatment option for patients with unresectable extremity sarcoma, it has been approved and licensed in Europe for this indication.

The cumulative U.S. experience of ILP with TNF for unresectable extremity sarcoma has been presented in abstract form (203) and includes results of 43 patients treated with TNF and melphalan, 12 of whom received IFN-γ (see Table 7). Using standard radiographic size criteria to define outcome, 56% of patients were shown to have an objective response to therapy with 11 patients (26%) having a complete response. Of the 11 patients who had a complete response, eight had multifocal sarcoma, such as angiosarcoma or epithelioid sarcoma. Fourteen patients (32%) eventually underwent amputation, resulting in a limb salvage rate of 68%.

Some of the most compelling clinical data that TNF exerts selective and significant effects on tumor neovasculature comes from results observed after ILP for advanced extremity sarcoma. Gutman et al. reported an overall response rate of 91% and a limb salvage rate of 85% in 34 patients with advanced extremity soft tissue sarcoma (204) (see Table 7). Pre- and post-ILP arteriograms showed complete obliteration of tumor-associated neovasculature with sparing of normal vessels. This phenomenon has been reported by others (82,205) (Fig. 2). We have observed this effect in a patient with large, high-grade thigh sarcoma treated with TNF alone, however, who had clinical and radiographic evidence of progression 2 months after ILP. Because of the fact that TNF alone has minimal antitumor efficacy in any isolation perfusion setting, the significance, if any, of these vascular effects must be questioned.

Results of Tumor Necrosis Factor Administered via Isolated Hepatic Perfusion for Unresectable Liver Cancers

Regional treatment strategies for primary or metastatic cancers confined to the liver have been under clinical evaluation because of their common ability to apply dose-intensive therapy to a cancer-bearing region of the body with apparently improved efficacy over the best available systemic treatments for many patients with colorectal cancer, neuroendocrine tumors, ocular melanoma, or primary hepatocellular cancers (206). The first application of isolated hepatic perfusion (IHP) for unresectable cancers of the liver was performed in the late 1950s.

IHP has never gained widespread clinical application, however, because of its complexity, the risks associated with the major operative procedure necessary to deliver this therapy, and the overall lack of established efficacy using standard therapeutics. Based on the results using TNF and melphalan administered via ILP for bulky intransit melanoma metastasis or high-grade unresectable extremity sarcoma, a number of institutions evaluated this regime administered via IHP in the early 1990s.

The technique of IHP has been described in detail and conceptually is similar to ILP. During hepatic perfusion, however,

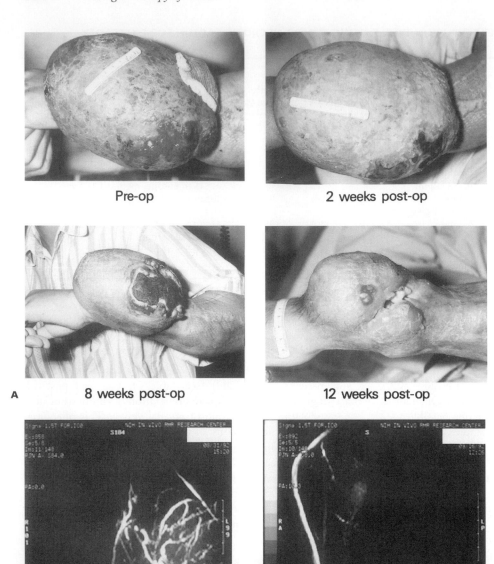

Pre-op

2 weeks post-op

8 weeks post-op

12 weeks post-op

A

B   **Pre- and Post-ILP MRA**

FIGURE 2. A large, multiple, recurrent symptomatic Ewing's sarcoma arising from the dorsum of the left forearm in a patient with small-volume metastatic disease. The patient was treated with an isolated limb perfusion (ILP) using tumor necrosis factor, interferon, and melphalan at the National Cancer Institute in Bethesda, Maryland. **A:** Photographs show a significant antitumor response observed after ILP. The patient had a stable response in the arm but died approximately 2 years later from progressive systemic metastases. **B:** Magnetic resonance angiogram (MRA) shows a pre- and post-ILP tumor neovasculature before therapy (*left*) and the complete obliteration of the neovasculature after ILP (*right*).

inferior vena caval and portal blood flow must be temporarily interrupted. To maintain hemodynamic stability during IHP, a second veno-veno bypass circuit is used to shunt venous return from these vessels to the heart. A schema of the hepatic perfusion setup is shown in Figure 3.

Because little information was available regarding liver tolerance to IHP with TNF alone or TNF and melphalan, a phase 1 trial was initiated by the Surgery Branch of the National Cancer Institute. This trial used a fixed low dose of IFN-γ administered in a schedule identical to the ILP schedule with escalating-dose TNF administered as a 60-minute IHP. A subsequent phase 1 trial of alternating dose escalation of TNF and melphalan was then conducted omitting IFN-γ from the treatment regimen. In the initial 16 patients treated with escalating-dose TNF alone, dose-limiting toxicity was observed at 2 mg of TNF, which was manifested by coagulopathy. In the subsequent phase 1 trial, the maximum safe, tolerated doses of TNF and melphalan when used in combination were 1 mg and 1.5 mg per kg, respectively, with dose-limiting toxicity manifested as veno-occlusive disease for melphalan and coagulopathy again for TNF (207). Using a dosing schedule of 1.5 mg per kg of melphalan, the mean dose administered in a subsequent phase 2 trial of TNF and melphalan was approximately 105 mg, which is similar to the total dose administered in isolated lower extremity perfusion for intransit melanoma or sarcoma. The dose of TNF that the liver can tolerate, however, is substan-

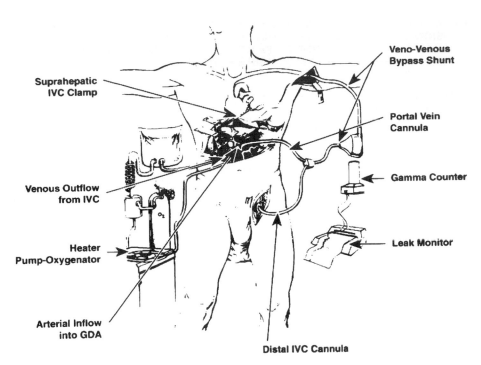

FIGURE 3. Isolated hepatic perfusion procedure shows the extracorporeal bypass circuit on the patient's right with inflow through the gastroduodenal artery (GDA) and outflow obtained from a cannula positioned in an isolated segment of retrohepatic inferior vena cava. Portal venous and inferior vena cava (IVC) flow are shunted externally to the axillary vein to maintain venous return to the heart during treatment. The bypass circuit is shown on the patient's left. Just below the bypass circuit is the gamma detection camera, which is used for continuous intraoperative leak monitoring.

tially lower than that administered into the extremity, which reflects the highly variable tissue tolerances to this protein.

The results of IHP using TNF and melphalan from several centers around the world are shown in Table 8. de Vries and coworkers reported results in eight patients treated with 1 mg per kg of melphalan and 0.4 mg of TNF administered as a 1-hour hyperthermic perfusion (208). The treatment mortality in this series was significant, with 33% of patients suffering fatal perioperative treatment–related complications. In five of six evaluable patients, however, evidence existed of significant antitumor effects from treatment. Hafström reported results in 11 patients treated with a combination of agents at doses somewhat lower than used in other centers. Treatment-related mortality in this series was 18% (209). The low efficacy of the treatment most likely reflects the fact that doses of melphalan and TNF were lower than those used at other centers. Oldhafer reported a series of 12 patients treated with IHP, of whom six patients received TNF and melphalan (210). In this group of six

patients, however, no treatment mortality was evident in the overall cohort of 12 patients. Two patients treated with mitomycin alone succumbed to hepatic veno-occlusive disease after treatment. In the six patients treated with TNF and melphalan, three patients had a response to treatment.

The largest institutional trial with IHP using TNF and melphalan has been reported from the National Cancer Institute and includes more than 50 patients treated with melphalan and TNF at doses derived from initial phase 1 dose-seeking studies (see Table 8). In a cohort of 50 patients, a treatment-related mortality of 4% was evident, of which one was secondary to hepatic veno-occlusive disease. The overall response rate in this trial was 75%. Responses were observed across all histologies treated (Table 9).

Response data in 34 patients who had been evaluated in detail (211) are shown in Table 10. Of note, responses were observed in patients regardless of tumor size, number of lesions, or percent of liver replaced by tumor. The duration of responses

TABLE 8. SUMMARY OF ISOLATED HEPATIC PERFUSION TRIAL USING TUMOR NECROSIS FACTOR

Authors (Reference)	n	Agent(s)	Dose	Duration	Temp (°C)	Results
de Vries et al. (208)	8	Melphalan TNF	1 mg/kg 0.4 mg	1 hr	>41	Mortality, 33% 5/6 PRs
	1	TNF Alone	0.8 mg			
Hafström and Naredi (209)	11	Melphalan TNF	0.5 mg/kg 30–200 µg	1 hr	39	Mortality, 18% Morbidity, 45% 3/11 PRs
Oldhafer et al. (210)	6	Melphalan TNF	60–140 mg 200–300 µg	1 hr	40–41	Mortality, 0% 1/6 CR, 2/6 PR
Alexander et al. (211)	50	Melphalan TNF	1.5 mg/kg 1.0 mg	1 hr	39.5–40	Mortality, 4% 1/48 CR, 36/48 PRs

CR, complete response; PR, partial response; TNF, tumor necrosis factor.

TABLE 9. RESPONSE TO TUMOR NECROSIS FACTOR AND MELPHALAN ISOLATED HEPATIC PERFUSION IN 50 PATIENTS

Histology	n	Assessable	CR	PR	Overall Response Rate (%)
Overall	50	48	1	35	75
Colorectal	37	35	—	25	71
Ocular melanoma	8	8	1	6	88
Other	5	5	—	4	80

CR, complete radiographic response; PR, partial radiographic response.

TABLE 10. RESPONSE TO ISOLATED HEPATIC PERFUSION BASED ON NUMBER OF LESIONS, DIAMETER OF LARGEST TUMOR, OR PERCENT HEPATIC REPLACEMENT IN 33 EVALUABLE PATIENTS

	n	PR or CR	%
Overall	33	25	25
Number[a]			
1–4	9	7	78
5–19	13	9	69
≥20	11	9	81
Diameter largest lesion (cm)			
<5	4	2	50
5.0–9.9	12	9	75
≥10	17	14	82
% Hepatic replacement			
<20	6	5	83
20–49	15	10	66
≥50	12	10	83

CR, complete response; PR, partial response.
[a]Radiographically imageable lesions.
(From Alexander HR Jr, Bartlett DL, Libutti SK, Fraker DL, Moser T, Rosenberg SA. Isolated hepatic perfusion with tumor necrosis factor and melphalan for unresectable cancers confined to the liver. *J Clin Oncol* 1998;16:1479–1489. U.S. Government work, in public domain.)

are highly variable, however, and strategies that improve the duration of response are under evaluation. The mean duration of response in the liver after therapy is approximately 9 months and ranges from 6 to 48 months (Fig. 4).

The liver is subjected to significant physical manipulation, brief periods of eschemia, and the effects of perfusion using high-dose TNF and melphalan. Most patients have significant but transient elevations in hepatic function tests, which typically return towards baseline within 7 to 10 days of treatment (211). The systemic effects of IHP with high-dose TNF and melphalan may occur primarily as a result of the release of proinflammatory cytokines presumably from the liver after hepatic perfusion. IL-6 and IL-8 levels have been routinely detected in patients after hepatic perfusion. The release of vasoactive cytokines from the liver transiently after perfusion may be responsible for some of the hemodynamic alterations that are typically observed after treatment. Leak of perfusate TNF into the systemic circulation is extremely rare when a complete and systematic preparation of the liver is performed before IHP. Systemic TNF concentrations are not measurable in patients after hepatic perfusion and were only detectable in 2 of 34 patients who also had a small (<3%) leak of perfusate during treatment.

IHP with TNF and melphalan may be ideally suited for patients with ocular melanoma metastatic to liver because of the

Pre-op MRI

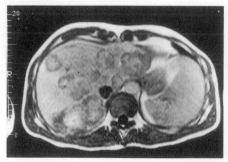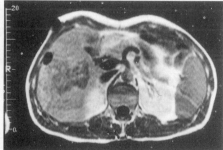

10 Months Post-IHP MRI

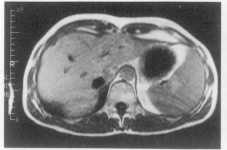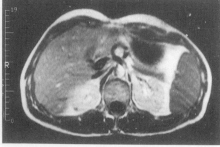

FIGURE 4. Pre– and post–isolated hepatic perfusion (IHP) magnetic resonance imaging (MRI) in a patient treated with 1-mg tumor necrosis factor and 1.5 mg per kg melphalan at the National Cancer Institute in Bethesda, Maryland. The patient did not respond to systemic and intraarterial chemotherapy. The patient had a stable response in the liver but developed new pulmonary metastases 13 months after treatment.

Pre-IHP

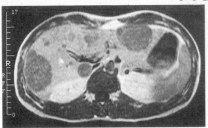
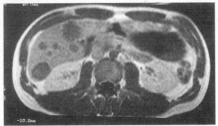

2 years post-IHP

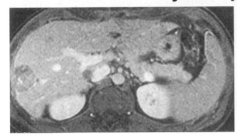
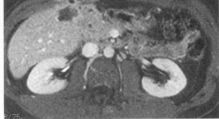

FIGURE 5. Pre– and post–isolated hepatic perfusion (IHP) magnetic resonance imaging (MRI) in a patient with metastatic ocular melanoma to the liver. The patient was treated with 1-mg tumor necrosis factor and 1.5 mg per kg melphalan at the National Cancer Institute in Bethesda, Maryland. The patient had a solitary site of extra hepatic intraabdominal recurrence resected 2 years after treatment and has an ongoing response in the liver 2.5 years after IHP.

selective uptake of melphalan by melanocytes (212). The response rate in this subgroup of patients treated with TNF and melphalan is more than 80%, and, in some cases, has been durable, extending beyond 2 to 3 years (Fig. 5).

The initial results with hepatic perfusion in various centers have been encouraging. With additional application, IHP may be a more routinely considered option for people with extensive metastatic or primary unresectable cancers confined to the liver. The exact contribution of TNF in IHP when combined with melphalan has not been established. In the initial phase 1 study of escalating-dose TNF alone, the overall response rates in that cohort of patients was only 20% and occurred in patients treated with the lowest doses of TNF, suggesting transient antitumor effects may have been caused by some other nonspecific effects of the perfusion, such as eschemia or acidosis.

Because TNF has presumed effects of the tumor neovasculature (82,205), the effect of TNF on capillary leak in tumor during IHP was evaluated and reported by Alexander et al. (213). In this study, patients were administered iodine-131–radiolabeled albumin as part of the leak monitoring system. Biopsies of liver and tumor before and after therapy and interstitial concentrations of iodine-131–radiolabeled albumin were determined. A significant increase in capillary leak was observed in tumor at the end of treatment compared with liver. This augmentation and capillary leak were comparable in patients who received TNF and in those who did not, suggesting that the augmentation in capillary leak must occur via other unknown TNF-independent mechanisms. The exact contribution of TNF administered via hepatic perfusion deserves continued and critical clinical evaluation.

Isolated Lung or Liver Perfusion with Tumor Necrosis Factor

A phase 1 trial was reported by Pass and colleagues from the National Cancer Institute of isolated lung perfusion with esca-

lating-dose TNF under conditions of moderate hyperthermia for patients with unresectable pulmonary metastases (214). Twenty patients were treated with doses of up to 6 mg of TNF. A short-term (6 to 9 months) decrease in nodules was noted in only three patients. No long-term sequelae of high-dose TNF perfusion occurred in the pulmonary parenchyma and all patients except one were extubated immediately or within 24 hours of the procedure. Consistent with the findings of TNF alone, perfusion of the limb or liver and minimal antitumor efficacy was observed in this trial. Further application of isolated lung perfusion combining TNF with chemotherapeutics is necessary to determine the use of isolated lung perfusion for pulmonary metastases.

A case report of isolated kidney perfusion using TNF has been reported by Walther and colleagues from the National Cancer Institute (215). The application of TNF via isolated kidney perfusion may be limited to unusual circumstances when renal-sparing surgery is indicated, such as in familial multifocal bilateral renal cell cancer syndrome.

SUMMARY

In conclusion, although enthusiasm for the use of TNF administered via isolated perfusion for regionally advanced cancer of the extremity or liver has been considerable, several major issues remain unanswered. With respect to ILP for intransit melanoma, the use of TNF has focused concern on the potential systemic toxicities of TNF and has heightened awareness of the importance of the technical aspects of isolation perfusion; most notably, the need for continuous leak monitoring systems to ensure complete vascular isolation with minimal leak of perfusate. These technical refinements may be responsible in part for the relatively high complete response rate observed in both arms of a single phase 3 random assignment trial comparing melphalan alone with melphalan, TNF, and IFN. These data suggest that the ability to define a role for TNF in ILP for intransit melanoma may be difficult. For patients with a small or limited number of lesions, melphalan alone may be efficacious as the combination therapy. For high-grade extremity sarcoma, the weight of data from the multiinstitutional European trial has been sufficient to result in the licensing of TNF for this indication in Europe. The experience with TNF-based ILP for high-grade extremity sarcoma in the United States is limited.

IHP for unresectable cancers confined to the liver using TNF-based regimens at a small number of centers around the world is under active evaluation. Many patients with unresectable cancers confined to the liver have conditions based on the size and number of lesions for which IHP may be ideally suited. Data suggest that IHP can be conducted safely. Continued clinical evaluation is warranted to define those patients best suited for TNF-based treatment.

REFERENCES

1. Frei E, Spriggs D. Tumor necrosis factor: still a promising agent. *J Clin Oncol* 1989;7:291–294.
2. Coley WB. The treatment of malignant tumors by repeated inoculums of erysipelas. *Am J Med Sci* 1893;105:487–511.
3. Coley WB. Late results of the treatment of inoperable sarcoma by the mixed toxins of erysipelas and bacillus prodigiosus. *Am J Med Sci* 1906;131:375–430.
4. Coley WB. The therapeutic value of the mixed toxins of the streptococcus of erysipelas and the bacillus prodigiosus. *Am J Med Sci* 1896;112:251–281.
5. Shear MJ, Turner FC, Perrault A, Shorelton J. Chemical treatment of tumors. V. Isolation of the hemorrhage-producing fraction from serratia marcescens (Bacillus prodigiosus) culture filtrate. *J Natl Cancer Inst* 1943;3:81–97.
6. Shear MJ. Chemical treatment of tumors, IX. Reactions of mice with primary subcutaneous tumors to injection of a hemorrhage-producing bacterial polysaccharide. *J Natl Cancer Inst* 1944;4:461–476.
7. O'Malley WE, Achinstein B, Shear MJ. Action of bacterial polysaccharide on tumors. II. Damage of sarcoma 37 by serum of mice treated with serratia marcescens polysaccharide, induced tolerance. *J Natl Cancer Inst* 1962;29:1169–1175.
8. Carswell EA, Old LJ, Kassel RL, Green S, Fiore N, Williamson B. An endotoxin-induced serum factor that causes necrosis of tumors. *Proc Natl Acad Sci U S A* 1975;72:3666–3670.
9. Helson L, Green S, Carswell E, Old LJ. Effect of tumour necrosis factor on cultured human melanoma cells. *Nature* 1975;258:731–732.
10. Pennica DG, Nedwin GE, Hayflick JS, et al. Human tumor necrosis factor: precursor structure, expression and homology to lymphotoxin. *Nature* 1984;312:724–729.
11. Aggarwal BB, Kohr WJ. Human tumor necrosis factor. Production, purification, characterization. *J Biol Chem* 1985;260:2345–2354.
12. Liénard D, Ewalenko P, Delmotti JJ, Renard N, Lejeune FJ. High-dose recombinant tumor necrosis factor alpha in combination with interferon gamma and melphalan in isolation perfusion of the limbs for melanoma and sarcoma. *J Clin Oncol* 1992;10:52–60.
13. Kawakami M, Cerami A. Studies of endotoxin-induced decrease in lipoprotein lipase activity. *J Exp Med* 1981;154:631–639.
14. Granger GA, Williams TW. Lymphocyte cytotoxicity *in vitro*: activation and release of a cytotoxic factor. *Nature* 1968;218:1253–1254.
15. Gray PW. Cloning and expression of cDNA for human lymphotoxin, a lymphokine with tumour necrosis activity. *Nature* 1985;312:721–724.
16. Spies T, Blanck G, Bresnahan M, Sands J, Strominger JL. A new cluster of genes within the human major histocompatibility complex. *Science* 1989;243:214–217.
17. Kriegler M, Perez C, DeFay K, Albert I, Lu SD. A novel form of TNF/cachectin is a cell surface cytotoxic transmembrane protein: ramifications for the complex. *Cell* 1988;53:45–53.
18. Jones EY, Stuart DI, Walker NP. Structure of tumour necrosis factor. *Nature* 1986;338:225–228.
19. Rubin BY, Anderson SL, Sullivan SA, Williamson BD, Carswell EA, Old LJ. Nonhematopoietic cells selected for resistance to tumor necrosis factor produce tumor necrosis factor. *J Exp Med* 1986;164:1350–1355.
20. Degliantoni G, Murphy M, Kobayashi M, Francis MK, Perussia B, Trinshieri G. Natural killer (NK) cell-derived hematopoietic colony-inhibiting activity and NK cytotoxic factor. Relationship with tumor necrosis factor and synergism with immune interferon. *J Exp Med* 1985;162:1512–1530.
21. Beutler B, Krochin N, Milsark IW, Luedke C, Cerami A. Control of cachectin (tumor necrosis factor) synthesis: mechanisms of endotoxin resistance. *Science* 1986;232:977–980.
22. Balkwill FR. Tumor necrosis factor. *Br Med Bull* 1989;45:389–400.
23. Strieter RM, Remick DG, Ward PA, et al. Cellular and molecular regulation of tumor necrosis factor-alpha production by pentoxifylline. *Biochem Biophys Res Commun* 1988;155:1230–1236.
24. Chantry D, Turner M, Abney E, Feldman M. Modulation of cytokine production by transforming growth factor-beta. *J Immunol* 1989;142:4295–4300.
25. Hart PH, Vitti GF, Burgess DR, et al. Potential antiinflammatory effects of interleukin-4: suppression of human monocyte tumor necrosis factor alpha, interleukin-1, prostaglandin E2. *Proc Natl Acad Sci U S A* 1989;86:3803–3807.
26. Hohmann HP, Remy R, Brockhaus M, van Loon AP. Two different cell types have different major receptors for human tumor necrosis factor (TNF alpha). *J Biol Chem* 1989;264:14927–14934.
27. Tartaglia LA, Goeddel DV. Two TNF receptors. *Immunol Today* 1992;13:151–153.
28. Shalaby MR, Palladino MA Jr, Hirabayashi SE, et al. Receptor binding and activation of polymorphonuclear neutrophils by tumor necrosis factor-alpha. *J Leukoc Biol* 1987;41:196–204.
29. Munker R, DiPersio J, Koeffler HP. Tumor necrosis factor: receptors on hematopoietic cells. *Blood* 1987;70:1730–1734.
30. Smith RA, Kirstein M, Fiers W, Baglioni C. Species specificity of human and murine tumor necrosis factor. A comparative study of tumor necrosis factor receptors. *J Biol Chem* 1986;261:14871–14874.
31. Kramer SM, Aggarwal BB, Eessalo TE, et al. Characterization of the *in vitro* and *in vivo* species preference of human and murine tumor necrosis factor-alpha. *Cancer Res* 1988;48:920–925.
32. Rothe J, Bluethmann H, Gentz R, Lesslauer W, Steinmetz M. Genomic organization and promoter function of the murine tumor necrosis factor receptor beta gene. *Mol Immunol* 1993;30:165–175.
33. Bebo BF Jr, Linthicum DS. Expression of mRNA for 55-kDa and 75-kDa tumor necrosis factor (TNF) receptors in mouse cerebrovascular endothelium: effects of interleukin-1 beta, interferon-gamma and TNF-alpha on cultured cells. *J Neuroimmunol* 1995;62:161–167.
34. Wu PC, Alexander HR, Huang J, et al. *In vivo* sensitivity of human melanoma to tumor necrosis factor (TNF)-α is determined by tumor production of the novel cytokine endothelial-monocyte activating polypeptide II (EMAPII). *Cancer Res* 1999;59:205–212.
35. Berger AC, Alexander HR, Wu PC, et al. Tumor necrosis factor receptor I (p55) is upregulated on endothelial cells by exposure to the tumor-derived cytokine endothelial monocyte activating polypeptide II (EMAP-II). *Cytokine* 2000 (*in press*).
36. Tsujimoto M, Yip YK, Vilcek J. Interferon-gamma enhances expression of cellular receptors for tumor necrosis factor. *J Immunol* 1986;136:2441–2444.
37. Owen-Schaub LB, Crump WL III, Morin GI, Grimm EA. Regulation of lymphocyte tumor necrosis factor receptors by IL-2. *J Immunol* 1989;143:2236–2241.
38. Scheurich P, Kobrich G, Pfizenmaier K. Antagonistic control of tumor necrosis factor receptors by protein kinases A and C. Enhancement of TNF receptor synthesis by protein kinase A and transmodulation of receptors by protein kinase C. *J Exp Med* 1989;170:947–958.

39. Loetscher H, Steinmetz M, Lesslauer W. Tumor necrosis factor: receptors and inhibitors. *Cancer Cells* 1991;3:221–226.

40. Tartaglia LA, Rothe M, Hu Y-F, Goeddel DV. Tumor necrosis factor's cytotoxic activity is signaled by the p55 TNF receptor. *Cell* 1993;73:213–216.

41. Tartaglia LA, Ayres TM, Wong GHW, Goeddel DV. A novel domain within the 55 Kd TNF receptor signals cell death. *Cell* 1993;74:845–853.

42. Yamada Y, Webber EM, Kirillova I, Peschon JJ, Fausto N. Analysis of liver regeneration in mice lacking type 1 or type 2 tumor necrosis factor receptor: requirement for type 1 but not type 2 receptor. *Hepatology* 1998;28:959–970.

43. Vandenabeele P, Declercq W, Vercammen D, et al. Functional characterization of the human tumor necrosis factor receptor p75 in a transfected rat/mouse T cell hybridoma. *J Exp Med* 1992;176:1015–1024.

44. Tartaglia LA, Pennica D, Goeddel DV. Ligand passing: the 75-kDa tumor necrosis factor (TNF) receptor recruits TNF for signaling by the 55 kDa TNF receptor. *J Biol Chem* 1993;268:18542–18548.

45. Pinckard JK, Sheehan KC, Arthur CD, Schreiber RD. Constitutive shedding of both p55 and p75 murine TNF receptors *in vivo*. *J Immunol* 1997;158:3869–3873.

46. Belldegrun A, Pierce W, Sayah D, et al. Soluble tumor necrosis factor receptor expression in patients with metastatic renal cell carcinoma treated with interleukin-2-based immunotherapy. *J Immunother* 1993;13:175–180.

47. Aderka D. The potential biological and clinical significance of the soluble tumor necrosis factor receptors. *Cytokine Growth Factor Rev* 1996;7:231–240.

48. Ythier A, Gascon MP, Juillard P, Vesin C, Wallach D, Grau GE. Protective effect of natural TNF-binding protein on human TNF-induced toxicity in mice. *Cytokine* 1993;5:459–462.

49. Aderka D, Engelmann H, Maor Y, Brakebusch C, Wallach D. Stabilization of the bioactivity of tumor necrosis factor by its soluble receptors. *J Exp Med* 1992;175:323–329.

50. Ruggiero V, Lathan K, Bagliani C. Cytostatic and cytotoxic activities of tumor necrosis factor in human renal cell carcinoma cells. *J Immunol* 1987;138:2711–2717.

51. Schutze S, Schluter C, Ucer U, Pfizenmaier K, Kronke M. Tumor necrosis factor-induced changes of gene expression in U937 cells. Differentiation-dependent plasticity of the responsive state. *J Immunol* 1988;140:3000–3005.

52. Sugarman BJ, Aggarwal BB, Hass PE, Figari IS, Palladino MA, Shepard HM. Recombinant human tumor necrosis factor-α: effects on proliferation of normal and transformed cells *in vitro*. *Science* 1985;230:943–945.

53. Vilcek J, Palombella VJ, Henriksen-DeStefano D, et al. Fibroblast growth-enhancing activity of tumor necrosis factor and its relationship to other polypeptide growth factors. *J Exp Med* 1986;163:632.

54. Fiers W. Tumour necrosis factor. In: Sim E, ed. *The natural immune system: humoral factors.* Oxford, UK: IRL Press, 1993:65–119.

55. Krönke M, Schütze S, Scheurich P. TNF signal transduction and TNF-responsive genes. In: Aggarwal BB, Vilcek J, eds. *Tumor necrosis factors: structure, function and mechanism of action.* New York: Marcel Dekker, 1992:189–216.

56. Lin JX, Vilcek J. Tumor necrosis factor and interleukin-1 cause a rapid and transient stimulation of c-fos and c-myc mRNA levels in human fibroblasts. *J Biol Chem* 1987;262:11908–11911.

57. Brenner DA, O'Hara M, Angel P, Chojkier M, Karin M. Prolonged activation of jun and collagenase genes by tumour necrosis factor-alpha. *Nature* 1989;337:661–663.

58. Wong GHW, Goeddel DV. Induction of manganous superoxide dismutase by tumor necrosis factor: possible protective mechanism. *Science* 1988;242:941–944.

59. Broudy VC, Kaushansky K, Segal GM, Harlan JM, Adamson JW. Tumor necrosis factor type alpha stimulates human endothelial cells to produce granulocyte/macrophase colony-stimulating factor. *Proc Natl Acad Sci U S A* 1986;83:7467–7471.

60. Laster SM, Wood JG, Gooding LR. Tumor necrosis factor can induce both apoptic and necrotic forms of cell lysis. *J Immunol* 1988;141:2629–2634.

61. Mosselmans R, Hepburn A, Dumont JE, Fiers W, Galand P. Endocytic pathway of recombinant murine tumor necrosis factor in L-929 cells. *J Immunol* 1988;141:3096–3100.

62. Neale ML, Fiera RA, Matthews N. Involvement of phospholipase A2 activation in tumour cell killing by tumour necrosis factor. *Immunology* 1988;64:81–85.

63. Hayakawa M, Ishida N, Takeuchi K, et al. Arachidonic acid-selective cytosolic phospholipase A2 is crucial in the cytotoxic action of tumor necrosis factor. *J Biol Chem* 1993;268:11290–11295.

64. Matthews N, Neale L, Jackson SK, Stark JM. Tumour cell killing by tumor necrosis factor: inhibition by anaerobic conditions, free-radical scavengers and inhibitors of arachidonate metabolism. *Immunology* 1987;62:153–155.

65. Watanabe N, Niitsu Y, Neda H, et al. Cytocidal mechanism of TNF: effects of lysosomal enzyme and hydroxyl radical inhibitors on cytotoxicity. *Immunopharmacol Immunotoxicol* 1988;10:109–116.

66. Schutze S, Potthoff K, Machleidt T, Berkovic D, Wiegmann K, Kronke M. TNF activates NF-kappa B by phosphatidylcholine-specific phospholipase C-induced "acidic" sphingomyelin breakdown. *Cell* 1992;71:765–776.

67. Grooten J, Goossens V, Vanhaesebroeck B, Fiers W. Cell membrane permeabilization and cellular collapse, followed by loss of dehydrogenase activity: early events in tumour necrosis factor-induced cytotoxicity. *Cytokine* 1993;5:546–555.

68. Watanabe N, Niitsu Y, Umeno H, et al. Synergistic cytotoxic and anti-tumor effects of recombinant human tumor necrosis factor and hyperthermia. Cancer Res 1988;48:650–653.

69. Tracey KJ, Beutler B, Lowry SF, et al. Shock and tissue injury induced by recombinant human cachectin. *Science* 1986;234:470–474.

70. Beutler B, Cerami A. Tumor necrosis factor in cachexia, shock, inflammation: a common mediator. *Ann Rev Biochem* 1988;57:505–518.

71. Vassalli P. The pathophysiology of tumor necrosis factors. *Annu Rev Immunol* 1992;10:411–452.

72. Oliff A, Defeo-Jones D, Boyer M, et al. Tumors secreting human TNF/cachectin induce cachexia. *Cell* 1987;50:555–563.

73. Sherry BA, Gelin J, Fong Y, et al. Anticachectin/tumor necrosis factor-α antibodies attenuate development of cachexia in tumor models. *FASEB J* 1989;3:1956–1962.

74. Tracey KJ, Cerami A. Tumor necrosis factor: other cytokines and disease. *Ann Rev Cell Biol* 1993;9:317–343.

75. Kettelhut IC, Fiers W, Goldberg AL. The toxic effects of tumor necrosis factor *in vivo* and their prevention by cyclooxygenase inhibitors. *Proc Natl Acad Sci U S A* 1987;84:4273–4277.

76. Dinarello CA, Cannon JG, Wolff SM, et al. Tumor necrosis factor (cachectin) is an endogenous pyrogen and induces production of interleukin-1. *J Exp Med* 1986;163:1433–1450.

77. Kilbourn RG, Gross SS, Jubran A, et al. NG-methyl-L-arginine inhibits tumor necrosis factor-induced hypotension: implications for the involvement of nitric oxide. *Proc Natl Acad Sci U S A* 1990;87:3629–3632.

78. Nawroth PP, Stern DM. Modulation of endothelial cell hemostatic properties by tumor necrosis factor. *J Exp Med* 1986;163:740–745.

79. Nawroth P, Handley D, Matsueda G, et al. Tumor necrosis factor/cachectin-induced intravascular fibrin formation in meth A fibrosarcomas. *J Exp Med* 1988;168:637–647.

80. Brett J, Gerlach H, Nawroth P, Steinberg S, Godman G, Stern D. Tumor necrosis factor/cachectin increases permeability of endothelial cell monolayers by a mechanism involving regulatory G proteins. *J Exp Med* 1989;169:1977–1991.

81. Renard N, Liénard D, Lespagnard L, Eggermont A, Heimann R, Lejeune F. Early endothelium activation and polymorphonuclear cell invasion precede specific necrosis of human melanoma and sarcoma treated by intravascular high-dose tumour necrosis factor alpha (rTNF alpha). *Int J Cancer* 1994;57:656–663.

82. Olieman AFT, van Ginkel RJ, Hoekstra HJ, Mooyaart EL, Molenaar WM, Koops HS. Angiographic response of locally advanced soft-tissue sarcoma following hyperthermic isolated limb perfusion with tumor necrosis factor. *Ann Surg Oncol* 1997;4:64–69.

83. Asami T, Imai M, Tanaka Y, et al. *In vivo* antitumor mechanism of natural human tumor necrosis factor involving a T cell-mediated immunological route. *Jpn J Cancer Res* 1989;80:1161–1164.

84. Balkwill FR, Lee A, Aldam G, et al. Human tumor xenografts treated with recombinant human tumor necrosis factor alone or in combination with interferons. *Cancer Res* 1986;46:3990–3993.

85. Nosoh Y, Toge T, Nishiyama M, et al. Antitumor effects of recombinant human tumor necrosis factor against human tumor xenografts transplanted into nude mice. *Jpn J Surg* 1987;17:51–54.

86. Alexander RB, Nelson WG, Coffey DS. Synergistic enhancement by tumor necrosis factor of *in vitro* cytotoxicity from chemotherapeutic drugs targeted at DNA Topoisomerase II. *Cancer Res* 1987; 47:2403–2406.

87. Krosnick JA, Mulé JJ, McIntosh JK, Rosenberg SA. Augmentation of antitumor efficacy by the combination of recombinant tumor necrosis factor and chemotherapeutic agents *in vivo*. *Cancer Res* 1989;49:3729–3733.

88. Asher A, Mulé JJ, Reichert CM, Shiloni A, Rosenberg SA. Studies on the anti-tumor efficacy of systemically administered recombinant tumor necrosis factor against several murine tumors *in vivo*. *J Immunol* 1987;138:963–974.

89. Palladino MA, Shalaby MR, Kramer SM, et al. Characterization of the antitumor activities of human tumor necrosis factor-α and the comparison with other cytokines: induction of tumor-specific immunity. *J Immunol* 1987;138:4023–4032.

90. Blick M, Sherwin SA, Rosenblum M, Gutterman J. Phase I study of recombinant tumor necrosis factor in cancer patients. *Cancer Res* 1987;47:2986–2989.

91. Kimura K, Taguchi T, Urushizaki I, et al. Phase I study of recombinant human tumor necrosis factor. *Cancer Chemother Pharmacol* 1987;20:223–229.

92. Selby P, Hobbs S, Viner C, et al. Tumor necrosis factor in man: clinical and biological observations. *Br J Cancer* 1987;56:803–808.

93. Taguchi T. Phase I study of recombinant human tumor necrosis factor (rHu-TNF:PT-050). *Cancer Detect Prev* 1988;12:561–572.

94. Moritz T, Kloke O, Nagel-Hiemke M, et al. Tumor necrosis factor-α modifies resistance to interferon alpha *in vivo*: first clinical data. *Cancer Immunol Immunother* 1992;35:342–346.

95. Gamm H, Lindemann A, Mertelsmann R, Herrmann F. Phase I trial of recombinant human tumour necrosis factor-α in patients with advanced malignancy. *Eur J Cancer* 1991;27:856–863.

96. Ferraiolo BL, Moore JA, Crase D, Gribling P, Wilking H, Baughman RA. Pharmacokinetics and tissue distribution of recombinant human tumor necrosis factor-α in mice. *Drug Metab Dispos* 1988;16:270–275.

97. Bemelmans MHA, Gouma DJ, Buurman WA. Influence of nephrectomy on tumor necrosis factor clearance in a murine model. *J Immunol* 1993;150:2007–2017.

98. Spriggs DR, Sherman ML, Michie H, et al. Recombinant human tumor necrosis factor administered as a 24-hour intravenous infusion. A Phase I and Pharmacologic Study. *J Natl Cancer Inst* 1988;80:1039–1044.

99. Mittelman A, Puccio C, Gafney E, et al. A phase I pharmacokinetic study of recombinant human tumor necrosis factor administered by a 5-day continuous infusion. *Invest New Drugs* 1992;10:183–190.

100. Lantz M, Malik S, Slevin ML, Olsson I. Infusion of tumor necrosis factor (TNF) causes an increase in circulating TNF-binding protein in humans. *Cytokine* 1990;2:402–406.

101. Jakubowski AA, Casper ES, Gabrilove JL, Templeton M-A, Sherwin SA, Oettgen HF. Phase I trial of intramuscularly administered tumor necrosis factor in patients with advanced cancer. *J Clin Oncol* 1989;7:298–303.

102. Chapman PB, Lester TJ, Casper ES, et al. Clinical pharmacology of recombinant human tumor necrosis factor in patients with advanced cancer. *J Clin Oncol* 1987;5:1942–1951.

103. Bartsch HH, Mull R, Pfizenmaier K. Phase I study of recombinant human tumor necrosis factor-alpha in patients with advanced malignancies. *Mol Biother* 1988;1:21–29.

104. Aulitzky WE, Tilg H, Gastl G, et al. Recombinant tumour necrosis factor-alpha administered subcutaneously or intramuscularly for treatment of advanced malignant disease: a Phase I trial. *Eur J Cancer* 1991;27:462–467.

105. Walsh C, Chachoua A, Hochster H, et al. Phase I study of recombinant human tumor necrosis factor (rhTNF). *Proc ASCO* 1989; 8:193(abst).

106. Schiller JH, Storer BE, Witt PL, et al. Biological and clinical effects of intravenous tumor necrosis factor-α administered three times weekly. *Cancer Res* 1991;51:1651–1658.

107. Furman WI, Strother D, McClain K, Bell B, Leventhol B, Pratt CB. Phase I clinical trial of recombinant human tumor necrosis factor in children with refractory solid tumors: a pediatric oncology group study. *J Clin Oncol* 1993;11:2205–2210.

108. Creagan ET, Kovach JS, Moertel CG, Frytak S, Kvols LK. A phase I clinical trial of recombinant human tumor necrosis factor. *Cancer* 1988;62:2467–2471.

109. Feinberg B, Kurzrock R, Talpaz M, Blick M, Saks S, Gutterman JU. A Phase I trial of intravenously administered recombinant tumor necrosis factor-alpha in cancer patients. *J Clin Oncol* 1988;6:1328–1334.

110. Creaven PJ, Brenner DE, Cowers JW, et al. A phase I clinical trial of recombinant human tumor necrosis factor given daily for five days. *Cancer Chemother Pharmacol* 1989;23:186–191.

111. Creaven PJ, Plager JE, Dupere S, Huben RP, Takita H, Mittelman A, Proefrock A. Phase I clinical trial of recombinant human tumor necrosis factor. *Cancer Chemother Pharmacol* 1987;20:137–144.

112. Lenk H, Tanneberger S, Müller U, Shiga T. Human pharmacological investigation of a human recombinant tumor necrosis factor preparation (PAC-4D) A phase-I trial. *Arch Geschwulstforsch* 1988;58:89–97.

113. Fraker DL, Stovroff MC, Merino MJ, Norton JA. Tolerance to tumor necrosis factor in rats and the relationship to endotoxin tolerance and toxicity. *J Exp Med* 1988;168:95–105.

114. Takahashi N, Brouckaert P, Fiers W. Induction of tolerance allows separation of lethal and antitumor activities of tumor necrosis factor in mice. *Cancer Res* 1991;51:2366–2372.

115. Sherman ML, Spriggs DR, Arthur KA, Imamura K, Frei EI, Kufe DW. Recombinant human tumor necrosis factor administered as a five-day continuous infusion in cancer patients: phase I toxicity and effects of lipid metabolism. *J Clin Oncol* 1988;6:344–350.

116. Wiedenmann B, Reichardt P, Räth U, et al. Phase-I trial of intravenous continuous infusion of tumor necrosis factor in advanced metastatic carcinomas. *J Cancer Res Clin Oncol* 1989;115:189–192.

117. Bauer KA, ten Cate H, Barzegar S, Spriggs DR, Sherman ML, Rosenberg RD. Tumor necrosis factor infusions have a procoagulant effect on the hemostasis mechanism of humans. *Blood* 1989;74:165–172.

118. Steinmetz T, Schaadt M, Gähl R, Schenk V, Diehl V, Pfreundschuh M. Phase I study of 24-hour continuous intravenous infusion of recombinant human tumor necrosis factor. *J Biol Response Mod* 1988;7:417–423.

119. Brown TD, Goodman P, Fleming T, Macdonald JS, Hersh EM, Braun TJ. A Phase II trial of recombinant tumor necrosis factor in patients with adenocarcinoma of the pancreas: a Southwest oncology group study. *J Immunother* 1991;10:376–378.

120. Lenk H, Tanneberger S, Müller U, Ebert J, Shiga T. Phase II clinical trial of high-dose recombinant human tumor necrosis factor. *Cancer Chemother Pharmacol* 1989;24:391–392.

121. Aboulafia D, Miles SA, Saks SR, Mitsuyasu RT. Intravenous recombinant tumor necrosis factor in the treatment of AIDS-related Kaposi's sarcoma. *J Acquir Immune Defic Syndr* 1989;2:54–58.

122. Kemeny N, Childs B, Larchian W, Rosado K, Kelsen D. A Phase II trial of recombinant tumor necrosis factor in patients with advanced colorectal carcinoma. *Cancer* 1990;66:659–663.

123. Whitehead RP, Fleming T, Macdonald JS, et al. A phase II trial of recombinant tumor necrosis factor in patients with metastatic colorectal adenocarcinoma: a Southwest oncology group study. *J Biol Response Mod* 1990;9:588–591.

124. Schaadt M, Pfreundschuh M, Lorscheidt G, Peters KM, Steinmedtz T, Diehl V. Phase II study of recombinant human tumor necrosis factor in colorectal carcinoma. *J Biol Response Mod* 1990;9:247–250.

125. Budd GT, Green S, Baker LH, Hersh EP, Weick JK, Osborne CK. A Southwest oncology group Phase II trial of recombinant tumor necrosis factor in metastatic breast cancer. *Cancer* 1991;68:1694–1695.

126. Skillings J, Wierzbicki R, Eisenhauer E, Venner P, Letendre F, Stewart D, Weinerman B. A Phase II study of recombinant tumor necrosis factor in renal cell carcinoma: a study of the National Cancer Institute of Canada clinical trials group. *J Immunother* 1992;11:67–70.

127. Feldman ER, Creagan ET, Schaid DJ, Ahmann DL. Phase II trial of recombinant tumor necrosis factor in disseminated malignant melanoma. *Am J Clin Oncol* 1992;15:256–259.

128. Hersh EM, Metch BS, Muggia FM, et al. Phase II studies of recombinant human tumor necrosis factor alpha in patients with malignant disease: a summary of the Southwest oncology group experience. *J Immunother* 1991;10:426–431.

129. McIntosh JK, Mulé JJ, Merino MJ, Rosenberg SA. Synergistic antitumor effects of immunotherapy with recombinant interleukin-2 and recombinant tumor necrosis factor. *Cancer Res* 1988;48:4011–4017.

130. Zimmerman RJ, Gauny S, Chan A, Landre P, Winkelhake JL. Sequence dependence of administration of human recombinant tumor necrosis factor and interleukin-2 in murine tumor therapy. *J Natl Cancer Inst* 1989;81:227–231.

131. Regenass U, Müller M, Curschellas E, Matter A. Anti-tumor effects of tumor necrosis factor in combination with chemotherapeutic agents. *Int J Cancer* 1987;39:266–273.

132. Watanabe N, Niitsu Y, Umeno H, et al. Synergistic cytotoxic and antitumor effects of recombinant human tumor necrosis factor and hyperthermia. *Cancer Res* 1988;48:650–653.

133. Rosenberg SA, Lotze MT, Yang JC, et al. Experience with the use of high-dose interleukin-2 in the treatment of 652 cancer patients. *Ann Surg* 1989;210:474–485.

134. Yang SC, Grimm EA, Parkinson DR, et al. Clinical and immunomodulatory effects of combination innumotherapy with low-dose interleukin-2 and tumor necrosis factor-α in patients with advanced non-small cell lung cancer: a phase I trial. *Cancer Res* 1991;51:3669–3676.

135. Negrier MS, Pourreau CN, Palmer PA, et al. Phase I trial of recombinant interleukin-2 followed by recombinant tumor necrosis factor in patients with metastatic cancer. *J Immunother* 1992;11:93–102.

136. Schiller JH, Witt PL, Storer B, et al. Clinical and biologic effects of combination therapy with gamma-interferon and tumor necrosis factor. *Cancer* 1992;69:562–571.

137. Smith JW II, Urba WJ, Clark JW, et al. Phase I evaluation of recombinant tumor necrosis factor given in combination with recombinant interferon-gamma. *J Immunother* 1991;10:355–362.

138. Fiedler W, Zeller W, Peimann C-J, Weh H-J, Hossfeld DK. A phase II combination trial with recombinant human tumor necrosis factor and gamma interferon in patients with colorectal cancer. *Klin Wochenschr* 1991;69:261–268.

139. Orita K, Fuchimoto S, Murimoto MS, Minowada J. Early Phase II study of interferon-α and tumor necrosis factor-alpha combination in patients with advanced cancer. *Acta Med Okayama* 1992;46:103–112.

140. Niijima T, Akaza H, Koyanagi T, et al. Combination therapy with natural type human tumor necrosis factor (MHR-24) and human lymphoblastoid interferon-α (MOR-22) against renal cell carcinoma. *Hinyokika Kiyo* 1992;38:1201 1207.

141. Jones AL, O'Brien MER, Lorentzos A, Viner C, Hanrahan A, Moore J, Millar JL, Gore ME. A randomized phase II study of carmustine alone or in combination with tumour necrosis factor in patients with advanced melanoma. *Cancer Chemother Pharmacol* 1992;30:73–76.

142. Maeda M, Watanabe N, Yamauchi N, Tsuji Y, Niitsu Y. Successful treatment of a case of hepatocellular carcinoma with tumor necrosis factor and local hyperthermia. *Gastroenterol Jpn* 1991;26:774–778.

143. Ijzermans JNM, van der Schelling GP, Scheringa M, Splinter RAW, Marquet RL, Jeekel J. Local treatment of liver metastases with recombinant tumour necrosis factor (rTNF): a phase one study. *Neth J Surg* 1991;43:121–125.

144. Kahn JO, Kaplan LD, Volberding PA, et al. Intralesional recombinant tumor necrosis factor-α for AIDS-associated Kaposi's sarcoma: a randomized, double-blind trial. *J Acquir Immune Defic Syndr* 1989;2:217–223.

145. Bartsch HH, Pfizenmaier K, Schroeder M, Nagel GA. Intralesional application of recombinant human tumor necrosis factor alpha induces local tumor regression in patients with advanced malignancies. *Eur J Cancer Clin Oncol* 1989;25:287–291.

146. Pfreundschuh MG, Steinmetz HT, Tüschen R, Schenk V, Diehl V, Schaadt M. Phase I study of intratumoral application of recombinant human tumor necrosis factor. *Eur J Cancer Clin Oncol* 1989;25:379–388.

147. Tada M, Sawamura Y, Sakuma S, et al. Cellular and cytokine responses of the human central nervous system to intracranial administration of tumor necrosis factor-α for the treatment of malignant gliomas. *Cancer Immunol Immunother* 1993;36:251–259.

148. Talmadge JE, Bowersox O, Tribble H, Shepard M, Liggitt D. Therapeutic and toxic activity of tumor necrosis factor is synergistic with gamma-interferon. *Pathol Immunopathol Res* 1989;8:21–34.

149. Markman M, Reichman B, Ianotti N, et al. Phase I trial of recombinant tumor necrosis factor administered by the intraperitoneal route. *Reg Cancer Treat* 1989;2:174–177.

150. Rath U, Kaufmann M, Schmid H, et al. Effect of intraperitoneal recombinant human tumour necrosis factor-α on malignant ascites. *Eur J Cancer* 1991;27:121–125.

151. Hardy J, Jones A, Gore ME, Viner C, Selby P, Wiltshaw E. Treatment of advanced ovarian cancer with intraperitoneal tumour necrosis factor. *Eur J Cancer* 1990;26:771.

152. Rath U, Schmid H, Karck U, Kempeni J, Schlick E, Kaufmann M. Phase-II- trial of recombinant human tumor necrosis factor-alpha (rHuTNF) in patients with malignant ascites from ovarian carcinomas and non-ovarian tumors with intraperitoneal spread. *Proc ASCO* 1991;10:187.

153. Serretta V, Corselli G, Piazza B, et al. Intravesical therapy of superficial bladder transitional cell carcinoma with tumor necrosis factor-alpha: preliminary report of a Phase I-II study. *Eur Urol* 1992;22:112–114.

154. Sternberg CN, Arena MG, Pansadoro V, Calabresi F, et al. Recombinant tumor necrosis factor for superficial bladder tumors. *Ann Oncol* 1992;3:741–745.

155. Mavligit GM, Zukiwski AA, Charnsargavej C. Regional biologic therapy: hepatic arterial infusion of recombinant human tumor necrosis factor in patients with liver metastases. *Cancer* 1992;69:557–561.

156. Yoshida J, Wakabayashi T, Mizuno M, et al. Clinical effect of intra-arterial tumor necrosis factor-α for malignant glioma. *J Neurosurg* 1992;77:78–83.

157. del Giglio A, Zukiwski AA, Ali MK, Mavligit GM. Severe, symptomatic, dose-limiting hypophosphatemia induced by hepatic arterial infusion of recombinant tumor necrosis factor in patients with liver metastases. *Cancer* 1991;67:2459–2461.

158. Rosenberg SA, Aebersold P, Cornetta K, et al. Gene transfer into human-immunotherapy of patients with advanced melanoma using tumor-infiltrating lymphocytes modified by retroviral gene transduction. *N Engl J Med* 1990;323:570–578.

159. Rosenberg SA. Gene therapy of cancer. *Important Adv Oncol* 1992:17–38(abst).

160. Rosenberg S. Gene therapy for cancer. *JAMA* 1992;268:2416–2419.

161. Hwu P, Yannelli J, Kriegler M, et al. Functional and molecular characterization of tumor-infiltrating lymphocytes transduced with tumor necrosis factor-α cDNA for the gene therapy of cancer in humans. *J Immunol* 1993;150:4104–4115.

162. Cao G, Kuriyama S, Du P, Sakamoto T, Kong X, Masui K, Qi Z. Complete regression of established murine hepatocellular carcinoma by *in vivo* tumor necrosis factor-α gene transfer. *Gastroenterology* 1997;112:501–510.

163. Wright P, Zheng C, Moyana T, Xiang J. Intratumoral vaccination of adenoviruses expressing fusion protein RM4/tumor necrosis factor (TNF)-α induces significant tumor regression. *Cancer Gene Ther* 1998;5:371–379.

164. Marr RA, Hitt M, Muller WJ, Gauldie J, Graham FL. Tumour therapy in mice using adenovirus vectors expression human TNF alpha. *Int J Oncol* 1998;12:509–515.

165. Marr RA, Addison CL, Snider D, Muller WJ, Gauldie J, Graham FL. Tumour immunotherapy using an adenoviral vector expressing a membrane-bound mutant of murine TNF alpha. *Gene Ther* 1997;4:1181–1188.

166. Sparmann G, Walther W, Günzburg WH, Uckert W, Balmons B.

Conditional expression of human TNF-α: a system for inducible cytotoxicity. *Int J Cancer* 1994;59:103–107.

167. Mauceri HJ, Hanna NN, Wayne JD, Hallahan DE, Hellman S, Wiechselbaum RR. Tumor necrosis factor-α (TNF-α) gene therapy targeted by ionizing radiation selectively damages tumor vasculature. *Cancer Res* 1996;56:4311–4314.

168. Stabe M-J, Mauceri HJ, Kufe DW, Hallahan DE, Weichselbaum RR. Adenoviral TNF-α gene therapy and radiation damage tumor vasculature in a human malignant glioma xenograft. *Gene Therapy* 1998;5:293–300.

169. Walther W, Stein U, Pfeil D. Gene transfer of human TNF alpha into glioblastoma cells permits modulation of mdr1 expression and potentiation of chemosensitivity. *Int J Cancer* 1995;61:832–839.

170. Moriuchi S, Oligino T, Krisky D, et al. Enhanced tumor cell killing in the presence of ganciclovir by herpes simplex virus type 1 vector-directed coexpression of human tumor necrosis factor-α and herpes simplex virus thymidine kinase. *Cancer Res* 1998;58:5731–5737 (abst).

171. Mizuguchi H, Nakagawa T, Toyosawa S, et al. Tumor necrosis factor-α-mediated tumor regression by the *in vivo* transfer of genes into the artery that leads to tumors. *Cancer Res* 1998;58:5725–5730.

172. Klostergaard J, Leroux E, Siddik ZH, Khodadadian M, Tomasovic SP. Enhanced sensitivity of human colon tumor cell lines *in vitro* in response to thermochemoimmunotherapy. *Cancer Res* 1992;52:5271–5277.

173. Hachiya T, Okada K, Sakurai A, Satomi N, Haranaka K. Antitumor activity of recombinant human tumor necrosis factor in combination with hyperthermia against heterotransplanted human prostatic carcinoma and its lymph node metastasis in nude mice. *Mol Biother* 1992;4:34–39.

174. Kitamura K, Kuwano H, Matsuda H, Toh Y, Masuda H, Sugimachi K. Synergistic effects of intratumor administration of cis-diamminedichloroplatinum(II) combined with local hyperthermia in melanoma bearing mice. *J Surg Oncol* 1992;51:188–194.

175. Miller RC, Richards M, Baird C, Martin S, Hall EJ. Interaction of hyperthermia and chemotherapy agents; cell lethality and oncogenic potential. *Int J Hyperthermia* 1994;10:89–99.

176. Hahn GM. Metabolic aspects of the role of hyperthermia in mammalian cell inactivation and their possible relevance to cancer treatment. *Cancer Res* 1974;34:3117–3123.

177. Klaase JM, Kroon BBR, van Geel AN, Eggermont AMM, Franklin HR. Systemic leakage during isolated limb perfusion for melanoma. *Br J Surg* 1993;80:1124–1126.

178. Barker WC, Rich MP, Alexander HR, Fraker DL. Continuous intraoperative external monitoring of perfusate leak using I-131 human serum albumin during isolated perfusion of the liver and limbs. *Eur J Nucl Med* 1995;22:1242–1248.

179. Hoekstra HJ, Naujocks T, Schraffordt-Koops H, et al. Continuous leaking monitoring during hyperthermic isolated regional perfusion of the lower limb: techniques and results. *Reg Cancer Treat* 1992;4:301–304.

180. Alexander C, Omlor G, Berberich R, Gross G, Feifel G. Rapid measurement of blood leakage during regional chemotherapy. *Eur J Nucl Med* 1993;4:606–612.

181. Sorkin P, Abu-Abid S, Lev D, et al. Systemic leakage and side effects of tumor necrosis factor-alpha administered via isolated limb perfusion can be manipulated by flow rate adjustment. *Arch Surg* 1995;130:1079–1084.

182. Thom AK, Alexander HR, Rich MP, Barker WC, Rosenberg SA, Fraker DL. Cytokine levels and systemic toxicity in patients undergoing isolated limb perfusion (ILP) with high-dose TNF, interferon-gamma and melphalan. *J Clin Oncol* 1995;13:264–273.

183. Alexander HR, Bartlett DL, Libutti SK, Fraker DL, Moser T, Rosenberg SA. Isolated hepatic perfusion with tumor necrosis factor and melphalan for unresectable cancers confined to the liver. *J Clin Oncol* 1998;16:1479–1489.

184. Liénard D, Lejeune F, Ewalenko I. In transit metastases of malignant melanoma treated by high dose rTNF alpha in combination with interferon-gamma and melphalan in isolation perfusion. *World J Surg* 1992;16:234–240.

185. Aggarwal BB, Eessalu TE, Hass PE. Characterization of receptors for tumor necrosis factor and their regulation by gamma-interferon. *Nature* 1985;318:665–667.

186. Balkwill FR, Ward BG, Moodie E, Fiers W. Therapeutic potential of tumor necrosis factor-α and gamma-interferon in experimental human ovarian cancer. *Cancer Res* 1987;47:4755–4758.

187. Wieberdink J, Benckhuysen C, Braat RP, van Slooten EA, Olthuis GAA. Dosimetry in isolation perfusion of the limbs by assessment of perfused tissue volume and grading of toxic tissue reactions. *Eur J Cancer Clin Oncol* 1982;18:905–910.

188. Liénard D, Aggermont A, Koops HS, Kroon B, Lejeune FJ. The use of TNF in isolated limb perfusion for treatment of locally advanced melanoma: an update. *Cambridge Symp* 1996;1:12(abst).

189. Fraker DL, Alexander HR, Bartlett DL, Rosenberg SA. A prospective randomized trial of therapeutic isolated limb perfusion (ILP) comparing melphalan (M) versus melphalan, tumor necrosis factor (TNF) and interferon-gamma (IFN): an initial report. *Soc Surg Oncol* 1996;49:6(abst).

190. Vaglini M, Belli F, Ammatuna M, et al. Treatment of primary or relapsing limb cancer by isolation perfusion with high-dose alpha-tumor necrosis factor, gamma-interferon, melphalan. *Cancer* 1994;73:483–492.

191. Hill S, Thomas JM. Low-dose tumour necrosis factor-alpha (TNF-α) and melphalan in hyperthermic isolated limb perfusion. Results from a pilot study performed in the United Kingdom. *Melanoma Res* 1994;4:31–34.

192. Fraker DL, Alexander HR, Andrich M, Rosenberg SA. Treatment of patients with melanoma of the extremity using hyperthermic isolated limb perfusion with melphalan, tumor necrosis factor, interferon-gamma: results of a TNF dose escalation study. *J Clin Oncol* 1996;14:479–489.

193. Posner MC, Lienard D, Lejeune FJ, Rosenfelder D, Kirkwood J. Hyperthermic isolated limb perfusion with tumor necrosis factor alone for melanoma. *Cancer J Sci Am* 1995;1:274–280.

194. Alexander HR, Fraker DL, Bartlett DL. Isolated limb perfusion for malignant melanoma. *Semin Surg Oncol* 1996;12:416–428.

195. Carswell EA, Old LJ, Kassel RL, Green S, Fiore N, Williamson B. An endotoxin-induced serum factor that causes necrosis of tumors. *Proc Natl Acad Sci U S A* 1975;72:3666–3670.

196. Fraker DL, Alexander HR. Use of high-dose tumor necrosis factor in isolation perfusion of the limbs and liver. *Reg Cancer Treat* 1995;8:37–41.

197. Eggermont AMM, Koops HS, Liénard D, Kroon BBR, van Geel AN, Hoekstra HJ. Isolated limb perfusion with high dose tumor necrosis factor-α in combination with interferon-gamma and melphalan for irresectable extremity soft tissue sarcomas: a multicenter trial. *J Clin Oncol* 1996;14:2653–2665.

198. Eggermont AMM, Koops HS, Klausner JM, et al. Isolated limb perfusion with tumor necrosis factor and melphalan for limb salvage in 186 patients with locally advanced soft tissue extremity sarcomas. *Ann Surg* 1996;224:756–765.

199. Olieman AFT, Pras E, van Ginkel RJ, Molenaar WM, Koops HS, Hoekstra HJ. Feasibility and efficacy of external beam radiotherapy after hyperthermic isolated limb perfusion with TNF-α and melphalan for limb-saving treatment in locally advanced extremity soft-tissue sarcoma. *Int J Radiat Oncol Biol Phys* 1998;40:807–814.

200. Heslin MJ, Woodruff J, Brennan MF. Prognostic significance of a positive microscopic margin in high-risk extremity soft tissue sarcoma: implications for management. *J Clin Oncol* 1996;14:473–478.

201. Brennan MF, Shiu MH. Soft tissue sarcoma of the extremities. In: Shiu MH, Brennan MF, eds. *Surgical management of soft tissue sarcoma.* Philadelphia: Lea & Febiger, 1989:79–124.

202. Shiu MH, Castro EB, Hajdu SI, Fortner JG. Surgical treatment of 297 soft tissue sarcomas of the lower extremity. *Ann Surg* 1975;182:597–602.

203. Fraker D, Alexander HR, Ross M, Tyler D, Bartlett D, Bauer T. A Phase II trial of isolated limb perfusion with high dose tumor necrosis factor and melphalan for unresectable extremity sarcomas. *Soc Surg Oncol* 1999;53:22(abst).

204. Gutman M, Inbar M, Lev-Shlush D, Abu-Abid S, Mozes M,

Chaitchik S, Meller I, Klausner JM. High-dose tumor necrosis factor-alpha and melphalan administered via isolated limb perfusion for advanced limb soft tissue sarcoma results in a >90% response rate and limb preservation. *Cancer* 1997;79:1129–1137.

205. Wu PC, Alexander HR, Huang J, et al. *In vivo* sensitivity of human melanoma to tumor necrosis factor (TNF)-α is determined by tumor production of the novel cytokine endothelial-monocyte activating polypeptide II (EMAPII). *Cancer Res* 1999; 59:205–212.

206. Alexander HR, Bartlett DL, Fraker DL, Libutti SK. Regional treatment strategies for unresectable primary or metastatic cancer confined to the liver. In: DeVita VT Jr, Hellman S, Rosenberg SA, eds. *Cancer: principles and practice of oncology.* Philadelphia: JB Lippincott Co, 1996:1–19.

207. Fraker DL, Alexander HR Jr. Isolated perfusion of the liver. In: Lotze MT, Rubin JT, eds. *Regional therapy of advanced cancer.* Philadelphia: Lippincott–Raven, 1997;141–150.

208. de Vries MR, Rinkes IH, van de Velde CJ, et al. Isolated hepatic perfusion with tumor necrosis factor-alpha and melphalan: experimental studies in pigs and phase I data from humans. *Recent Results Cancer Res* 1998;147:107–119.

209. Hafström L, Naredi P. Isolated hepatic perfusion with extracorporeal oxygenation using hyperthermia TNF alpha and melphalan: Swedish experience. *Recent Results Cancer Res* 1998;147:120–126.

210. Oldhafer KJ, Lang H, Frerker M, et al First experience and technical aspects of isolated liver perfusion for extensive liver metastasis. *Surgery* 1998;123:622–631.

211. Alexander HR Jr, Bartlett DL, Libutti SK, Fraker DL, Moser T, Rosenberg SA. Isolated hepatic perfusion with tumor necrosis factor and melphalan for unresectable cancers confined to the liver. *J Clin Oncol* 1998;16:1479–1489.

212. Luck JM. Action of p-dichloroethyl amino-L-phenylalanine on Harding-Passey mouse melanoma. *Science* 1956;123:984–985.

213. Alexander HR, Brown CK, Bartlett DL, et al. Augmented capillary leak during isolated hepatic perfusion (IHP) occurs via tumor necrosis factor independent mechanisms. *Clin Cancer Res* 1998;4:23–62.

214. Pass HI, Mew DJY, Kranda KC, Temeck BK, Donington JS, Rosenberg SA. Isolated lung perfusion with tumor necrosis factor for pulmonary metastases. *Ann Thorac Surg* 1996;61:1609–1617.

215. Walther MM, Jennings SB, Choyke PL, et al. Isolated perfusion of the kidney with tumor necrosis factor for localized renal-cell carcinoma. *World J Urol* 1996;14:S2–S7.

9

INTERFERON-α AND -β: BASIC PRINCIPLES AND PRECLINICAL STUDIES

BRYAN R. G. WILLIAMS

Interferons (IFNs) are antiviral cytokines originally described by Issacs and Lindenman (1) as factors induced by viral infection that can inhibit the replication of other viruses. In fact, IFNs are synthesized and secreted by vertebrate cells in response to other stimuli in addition to viruses, including chemical compounds, microbial and cellular products, and even other cytokines. Cells exposed to IFNs respond by acquiring resistance to subsequent viral infection. IFNs are also able to inhibit the proliferation of cancer cells. IFNs are used as therapeutic agents for the treatment of viral infections and cancer because of their properties that induce antiviral resistance and regulate cell growth. IFNs are also able to modulate the immune response. This has led to their clinical use in diseases with underlying immunologic etiologies, including forms of multiple sclerosis. Although IFNs were discovered and named for their ability to induce resistance to viral infection, IFNs were the first described members of what is known to be a large family of biologically important regulatory cytokines. IFNs are the only members of this family with potent antiviral activity.

Studies on the mechanism of action of IFN have provided significant insight into the mechanism of action of other cytokines, including the characteristics of receptors, signal transduction pathways, and transcriptional regulation of inducible genes. In a physiologic context, however, it is important to remember that IFNs act in concert with a complex network of other cytokines. They are essential to the development of a normal immune response. IFNs provide a bridge from innate to specific immunity and are potent immunomodulators.

The therapeutic potential of IFNs was apparent from their mode of discovery. The subsequent description of antiproliferative and immunomodulatory activities spurred further interest, but early clinical use was limited to IFN produced from virus-induced buffy-coat leucocytes. These trials, particularly in osteogenic sarcoma, however, encouraged the molecular cloning of IFN, which radically changed its availability and paved the way for subsequent regulatory approval for use in different malignancies and other diseases. More than 40 years of basic and clinical research has produced a vast literature on the mechanisms of action of IFNs. Comprehensive reviews (2,3) are available, and, when consulted along with this chapter, offer a current picture of IFN-α and -β biology.

DISCOVERY AND DESCRIPTION OF INTERFERONS

IFNs were discovered in 1957 as antiviral agents synthesized in influenza virus–infected chick embryo cells (1). IFNs are produced by cells in response to viral infection and confer an antiviral state on cells exposed to them. In addition to avians, IFNs are also present in fish, reptiles, and mammals. The cloning and characterization of IFNs revealed the existence of two types: type I and type II. The type I IFN family predominately comprises IFN-α and -β but also includes two other subfamily members: IFN-ω and IFN-τ. Type II is comprised of only IFN-γ.

THE TYPE I INTERFERON GENE AND PROTEINS

IFN-α is induced mainly in leucocytes or in lymphoblastoid cell lines, whereas IFN-β is a fibroblast cell product. The genes and corresponding proteins of the type I IFN superfamily are structurally related, and the human genes are clustered within 400 kilobase (kb) on the short arm of chromosome 9. Fourteen genes comprise the human IFN-α family. Twelve IFN-α proteins of 165– or 166–amino acid residues are produced from these 14 genes (two of the genes are pseudogenes) (Table 1). In primates and rodents, only a single IFN-β gene exists. In humans, the IFN-β gene is located at the telomeric end of the α cluster. Six IFN-ω genes exist in humans, but only one is functional. IFN-ω (which has not been described in mice) is characterized by a 6–amino acid extension at the carboxyl terminal compared with IFN-α (4). The functional IFN-ω gene maps to the end of the IFN-α cluster between IFN-α2 and -β. IFN-τ (trophoblast) is unique to cattle and sheep, where it is essential for the development and maintenance of pregnancy. IFN-ω and -τ have 172 residues. IFN-τ, like IFN-ω, has a 6–amino acid carboxyl terminal extension when aligned with IFN-α. Four conserved cysteines exist in IFN-α proteins, forming two intramolecular disulfide bonds (cysteine 1 to cysteine 98 and cysteine 29 to cysteine 138). Human IFN-α proteins do not contain *N*-glycosylation sites and are not *N*-glycosylated. The solution of the crystal structures of IFN-α2 and IFN-β has placed them in a class of helical cytokines that is defined by five

TABLE 1. HUMAN INTERFERON GENES AND PROTEINS

Genes	Proteins
IFNA1	IFN-α_1, IFN-αD
IFNA2	IFN-α_2 (IFN-A$_{2B}$), IFN-αA (IFN-α_{2a}), IFN-α_{2c}
IFNA4	IFN-α_{4a} (IFN-α76), IFN-α_{4b}
IFNA5	IFN-α_5, IFNα-G, IFN-α61
IFNA6	IFN-α_6, IFN-αK, IFN-α54
IFNA7	IFN-α_7, IFN-αJ, IFN-αJ1
IFNA8	IFN-α_8, IFN-αB2, IFN-αB
IFNA10	IFN-αC, ψIFN-α10, ψIFN-αL, IFN-α6L
IFNA13	IFN-α13 (sequence identical to that of IFN-α_1)
IFNA14	IFN-α14, IFN-αH, IFN-αH1
IFNA16	IFN-α16, IFN-αWA, IFN-αO
IFNA17	IFN-α17, IFN-αI, IFN-α88
IFNA21	IFN-α21, IFN-αF
IFNA22	ψIFN-αE
IFNB1	IFN-β
IFNW1	IFN-ω

IFN, interferon.

short helices, labeled A to E. Two surfaces on opposite sides of the molecule are sensitive to amino acid substitutes, supporting a model for single ligand interaction with two receptor chains analogous to growth hormone–receptor interactions.

IFN-β has 166–amino acid residues, an *N*-glycosylation site at position 80, and is glycosylated as a mature protein. Both unglycosylated, *Escherichia coli*–derived, recombinant IFN-β and glycosylated products produced from mammalian cell–expression vectors are used in clinical applications.

INDUCTION OF INTERFERON SYNTHESIS

Inducers

Type I IFNs can be induced by different infectious agents in most vertebrate cell types, although viral infection is most commonly linked to IFN production. Bacteria, mycoplasma, and protozoa also induce IFNs in different cells. Low-molecular-weight molecules can induce IFNs in animals and remain under clinical investigation as IFN inducers (5). Bacterial lipopolysaccharide is an efficient inducer of type I IFNs in mononuclear phagocytes. The mechanisms of induction have been studied in detail only with viruses. Viral induction of IFN synthesis is mediated by double-stranded RNA (dsRNA), although, in some cases, constituents of viruses, such as hemagglutinin (influenza virus), may act as IFN inducers in animals and humans. Viral dsRNA, which is produced during the replication of DNA and RNA viruses, is an effective inducer of type I IFNs in cell culture. The type I IFN genes are usually transcriptionally silent unless activated through a signal transduction pathway mediated by dsRNA. The synthesis of IFN-β, however, has been detected in normal epithelial cells (6). The nature of the inducer is not known, but different cytokines and growth factors can induce IFNs in cell culture and may provide physiologic stimuli. In tumors, a downregulation of IFN-β exists at the tumor–epithelial cell interface, suggesting that maintenance of IFN-β expression in epithelial cells is important in maintaining homeostasis (7).

Type I IFN synthesis is regulated at the transcriptional and posttranscriptional levels. Transcriptional activation of the type I IFN genes requires the formation of active transcription factor complexes on enhancer elements located 5' of the transcriptional start sites of these genes. This is achieved by a combination of posttranscriptional activation of preexisting transcriptional factors and displacement of repressors, which, in the absence of inducer-mediated signals, silences the type I IFN genes. Type I IFN messenger RNAs (mRNAs) are unstable because they are rapidly degraded as a result of the presence of instability sequences in the 3' untranslated regions of their transcripts. Thus, mRNA synthesis in response to virus or dsRNA induction is transient and returns to basal levels within a few hours. Type I IFN induction can be enhanced by priming cells with small amounts of type I IFN. This results in a maximum response after exposure to inducers, such as dsRNA or viruses. Inhibitors of protein synthesis, such as cycloheximide, can superinduce IFN mRNA by inhibiting the synthesis of negative regulatory factors that act at the levels of transcription and mRNA stability. Overall, the molecular mechanisms regulating the transcriptional induction of type I IFN synthesis involve a complex interplay between *cis*-acting negative and positive regulatory DNA elements and their cognate transcription factors. The steady level of RNA product is dictated by host mRNA stability factors, which are themselves subject to poorly understood regulators factors.

Induction of Interferon-β Synthesis

IFN-β gene regulation has been studied in detail as a model for understanding the role of inducible enhancer elements in regulating gene expression. Approximately 200 base pairs of 5' regulatory sequences upstream of the transcriptional start site constitute the virus-responsive promoter of IFN-β. Overlapping positive regulatory domains (PRDI-IV) and a negative regulatory element (Fig. 1) originally identified by deletional and point mutation analyses (8) are key features of this promoter.

The transcriptional activation of the human IFN-β gene by viruses is dependent on the assembly of a higher-order transcription-enhancer complex, termed the *enhancersome* (9). The assembly of the enhancersome requires different transcription factors and is coordinated through specific interactions with the high mobility group protein, HMG1(Y). These proteins promote the cooperative binding of the transcription factors and mediate their synergistic action *in vivo*. PRDI, which overlaps with PRDII, binds IFN-regulatory factor 1 (IRF-1) and other IRF family members. PRD-II is recognized by nuclear factor kappa B (NF-κB) and PRDI-V binds a heterodimer consisting of activating transcription factor 2 and c-jun. The transcriptional activator proteins, IRF-3 and IRF-7, as well as the transcriptional coactivators P300 and Creb-binding protein (CBP), are also required for induction of IFN-β synthesis. The enhancersome complex includes activating transcription factor–2, C-jun, NF-κB, HMG1(Y), and IRFs and can be assembled *in vitro* to stimulate IFN-β gene transcription (9). Several other DNA-binding proteins have been described that have no transcription activation potential, but can still bind to the enhancer region. These include IRF-2, PRDI–binding factor 1, and

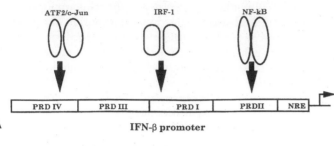

A
IFN-β promoter

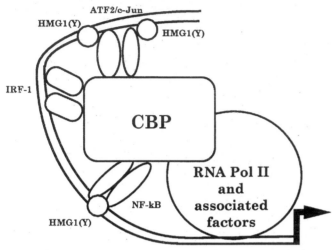

B
IFN-β promoter activated

FIGURE 1. Transcriptional activation of the interferon-β (IFN-β) promoter. **A:** Different transcription factors are activated as a result of viral infection and bind cognate DNA elements arranged in a unique pattern in the promoter region of the IFN-β gene. **B:** The high mobility group protein (HMG1)(Y) is required for assembly of the complex. The transcriptional coactivator Creb-binding protein (CBP) integrates the action of different transcription factors. (ATF, activating transcription factor; IRF, IFN regulatory factor; NF-κB, nuclear factor kappa B; PRD, positive regulatory domain.)

homodimers of the NF-κB component, p50. These proteins may repress the IFN promoter in the uninduced state. In virus induction, HMG1(Y) acts to cooperatively assemble the different transcriptional activators. Once assembled, the activation domains of these factors form a high-affinity binding site for the recruitment of the CBP/p300 coactivator. CBP/p300 interacts with the RNA polymerase II holoenzyme via its carboxyl terminal domain, whereas the activation domains of the other transcriptional activators contact components of the basal transcriptional apparatus. CBP/p300, which contains an intrinsic histone acetyltransferase, subsequently acetylates HMG1(Y), destabilizing the enhancersome, thereby terminating IFN-β gene transcription (10). Thus, the coordinate activation of a number of transcriptional-activated proteins and their cooperative assembly into a transcriptional-enhancer complex is required to drive transcription of the IFN-β gene after viral infection or dsRNA treatment of cells (see Fig. 1). In the mouse IFN-β promoter, the binding of histone H1 to an upstream adenosine thymidine–rich region of DNA appears to be responsible for the constitutive repression of the promoter. The dis-

placement of histone H1 by HMGI(Y) protein may convert the IFN-β promoter from a repressed state to an active state (11).

INTERFERON RECEPTORS

IFNs mediate their effects by binding and activating high–specific-affinity receptors on cell surfaces. This is a necessary first step in initiating a cellular response to IFNs and results in the generation of signals required for transcriptional induction of IFN-responsive genes, which encode the specific effectors for the different activities of IFNs. IFN-α and -β bind to the same type I receptor, whereas IFN-γ binds to a distinct type II receptor. IFNs exhibit host range restriction in their activities, mediated at the level of receptor binding. In general, human IFNs act on human cells and show only limited activity on cells from other species, although this varies among the several IFN-α subtypes.

The type I IFN receptor is present at only a few thousand binding sites per cell and exhibits an affinity for IFN in the subnanomolar range. Early investigations using radiolabeled recombinant type I IFNs revealed the cell surface expression of low-affinity and high-affinity receptors for type I IFNs (12–18). Studies on binding and cross-linking of radiolabeled IFNs to the cell surface suggested the existence of a multisubunit structure for the type I IFN receptors (19,20). This was subsequently demonstrated using specific monoclonal antibodies to receptor subunits (21). It is known that to elicit a cellular response, the type I IFN-α/β receptor requires two subunits, ifnar-1 and ifnar-2, which belong to the class II family of helical cytokine receptors (Fig. 2). Ifnar-1 was the first molecularly characterized subunit and was identified by an expression-cloning strategy using the species-specific recognition property of type I IFNs. This protein conferred resistance to vesicular somatitis virus replication in mouse cells in the presence of human IFN-α8 (22). The human ifnar-1 complementary DNA (cDNA) encodes a glycoprotein of 557 amino acids with a 436–amino acid extracellular region and a 21–amino acid transmembrane domain, followed by a cytoplasmic tail of 99 amino acids (22). When the human ifnar-1 cDNA was expressed in mouse cells, however, the protein could only bind to IFN-α8 at 37°C, but not to the other type I human IFNs (22). The human IFN-α8 was later found to possess some binding affinity for the mouse receptor. Therefore, ifnar-1 was not sufficient to confer responsiveness to all type I IFNs, indicating that another species-specific ligand-binding receptor subunit was required for signal transduction.

A human IFN-α binding protein was purified from urine and sequenced, leading to the identification of a novel subunit of 331 amino acids for the type I IFN receptor (23). This protein, termed *ifnar-2b* (or the β$_S$ subunit), was not a functional receptor subunit. A longer 515–amino acid form of human ifnar-2, termed the *ifnar-2c* (or β$_L$ subunit), was subsequently identified as the universal ligand-binding subunit of the type I IFN receptor (24). Neither ifnar-1 nor ifnar-2 alone binds to IFNs with high affinity, and the functional type I IFN receptor comprises ifnar-1 and ifnar-2c (25,26). Ifnar-1 and ifnar-2 are required to constitute a high-affinity α/β receptor, but only

Type I IFN receptor (ifnar) - a class II cytokine receptor

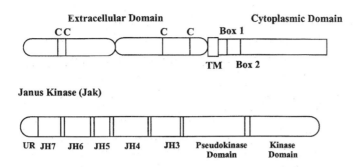

Janus Kinase (Jak)

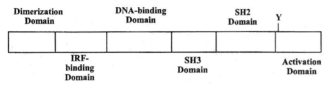

Signal Transducer and Activator of Transcription (Stat)

FIGURE 2. Essential components of interferon (IFN) signaling. In ifnar, C denotes conserved cysteine residues, and *TM* denotes the transmembrane domain. In the Janus kinase, *UR* refers to a unique region and *JH* refers to the Jak homology domain. In the signal transducers and activators of transcription proteins (STATs), *Y* denotes a regulatory tyrosine residue.

ifnar-2c is capable of transducing a signal after ligand binds to the receptor complex. The human ifnar-2 gene, located on chromosome 21, produces four transcripts, encoding the three different polypeptides through alternate splicing and differential usage of alternate polyadenylation sites (27). Ifnar-2a is probably secreted, whereas ifnar-2b and ifnar-2c are expressed as transmembrane proteins with identical extracellular and transmembrane domains but divergent cytoplasmic domains of 67 and 76 amino acids, respectively. When overexpressed, ifnar-2b can dominantly inhibit the IFN response (27).

The solution structure of other members of the helical cytokine receptors II family (IFNGR1 and tissue factor) has allowed the three-dimensional structure of the extracellular domains of ifnar-1 and ifnar-2 to be modeled (28). The domains are divided into two subdomains of approximately 100 amino acids (sd100A and 100B from the N-terminal), which each adopt an immunoglobulin-like fold with seven β strands (S1 to S7) in two β sheets. The ifnar-1 extracellular domain (317 amino acids) has a duplication of these subdomains. It is important to note that the structural integrity and formation of an active IFN-α/β binding site not only requires ifnar-1 and ifnar-2, but also requires the association of intracellular Janus kinases (Jaks) with the cytoplasmic domains. A binding site exists for the signal transducing Jak, Tyk2 (see Fig. 3), on the cytoplasmic tail of the ifnar-1 receptor subunit. The ifnar-2c subunit is 315 amino acids. The first 217 amino acids constitute the ligand-binding domain, followed by a transmembrane-spanning region of 22 amino acids and a cytoplasmic tail of 76 amino acids, which contains a binding site for another member of the Jak family,

Jak1. The high-affinity binding and signaling receptor for IFN-α/β requires ifnar-1 and ifnar-2c and their associated kinases.

IFN-β shares only 35% identity with the IFN-α subtypes and appears to engage the α/β receptor differently. This can result in the activation of selective subsets of genes (29,30) by IFN-β, even though it binds and activates the same receptor. Apparently, distinctive structural differences are transmitted through the membrane to the cytoplasmic domains of the receptors, which then mediate a differential response. Mutant cell lines lacking Tyk2, which are completely defective in their response to natural IFNs, IFN-α1, or IFN-α2, still respond to IFN-β or IFN-α8, albeit with reduced activity. In fact, by using these and other mutant cell lines reconstituted with different mutant proteins, three distinct modes of type I interaction with receptor subunits have been discerned: IFN-α with ifnar-1 and ifnar-2, IFN-β with ifnar-1 and ifnar-2, and IFN-β with ifnar-2 alone (28). Thus, IFN-α and -β signal differently through their receptors because they interact with the receptor in different ways.

A tight correlation exists between receptor occupancy and the transcriptional response to IFN. The degree of receptor occupancy is a rate-limiting step in determining the transcriptional response to IFN, which is transient and accompanied by the downregulation of receptors on the cell surface (31). Downregulation of type I IFN receptors is also seen *in vivo* on peripheral blood lymphocytes after IFN therapy (32). This is a temporary state. Receptors reappear on the cell surface 24 to 48 hours later.

SIGNALING PATHWAYS ACTIVATED BY INTERFERON-α AND -β

Type I IFNs can be induced ubiquitously, and most cells have a common response pathway initiated by the engagement of cellular receptors. The most well-characterized components required for this response are the receptor subunits themselves, Jaks and signal transducers and activators of transcription proteins (STATs) (see Fig. 2). IFN-receptor interactions result in the activation of the different components by phosphorylation of specific tyrosine residues. STATs form homodimers or heterodimers through mutual phosphotyrosine src homology region 2 (SH-2) interactions. STAT1 homodimers bind to DNA elements, termed *gamma activated sites* (GAS elements), which drive the expression of target genes. STAT1 and STAT2 heterodimers bind to p48, a member of the IRF family. The resulting complex, termed *IFN-stimulated gene factor 3* (ISGF3), binds to IFN-stimulated regulatory elements (ISREs) upstream of different IFN-responsive genes. The primary response to IFN-α/β can be divided into several distinct steps (see Fig. 3). These include (a) IFN-driven dimerization of the receptor subunits outside the cell, (b) initiation of a tyrosine phosphorylation cascade inside the cell, (c) dimerization of the phosphorylated STATs, (c) transport of the STATs into the nucleus, and (d) binding to specific DNA sequences and stimulation of transcription. It is important to note that other signaling cascades are also activated by type I IFNs. It is the combined actions of these different pathways, coupled with their downregulation in the continued presence of IFN, that lead to the over-

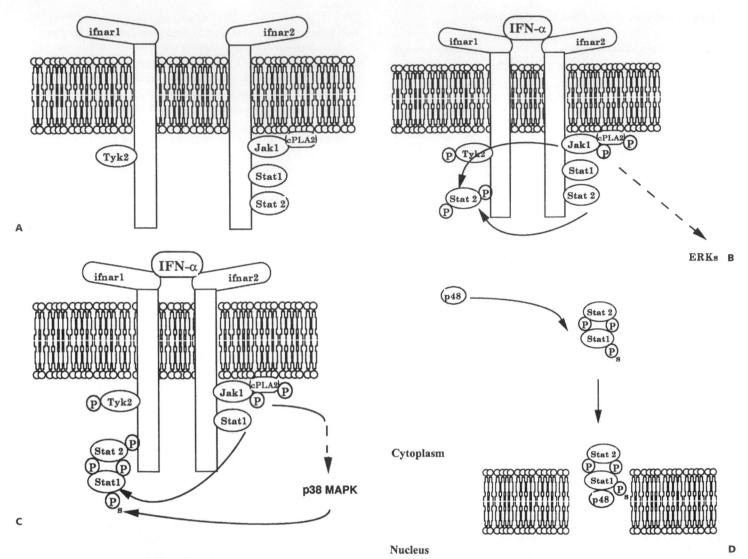

FIGURE 3. Interferon-α (IFN-α) signal transduction. **A:** Components of the signal transduction pathway are preassociated with the unliganded receptor. **B:** IFN-α binding activates Janus kinases (Jaks), resulting in phosphorylation of different components of the pathway. Signal transducers and activators of transcription proteins (STAT)2 moves to its docking site on ifnar1. **C:** Phosphorylated STAT1 interacts via SH-2 domains with STAT2, p38 mitogen-activated protein kinase (MAPK) phosphorylates serine 727 on STATs, and the heterodimers are released from the receptor and interact with p48 to form IFN-stimulated gene factor-3. **D:** IFN-stimulated gene factor-3 migrates to the nucleus.

all cellular response. For example, IFN-α/β treatment of cells causes the transient release of arachidonic acid, resulting from the phosphorylation and activation of cytosolic phospholipase A_2 (cPLA$_2$) (33,34). Inhibition of this enzyme blocks the formation of the transcription factor complex ISGF3. Mobilization of the phosphatidylinositol 3' kinase occurs in response to IFN-α/β in a Jak-dependent event. The mitogen-activated protein kinase (MAPK) cascade is also triggered by IFN-α/β (35,36). The latter may be differentially stimulated by the different IFN-α subtypes or by IFN-β, but this remains to be determined.

The IFN receptor subunits are primed to respond to the dimerization event driven by ligand binding. STAT1 and STAT2 are preassociated in latent form with the ifnar-2c

subunit of the IFN-α/β receptor. STAT1 binds well only when STAT2 is present, however, and functionally redundant phosphotyrosine-dependent and phosphotyrosine-independent binding sites for STAT2 also exist on ifnar-1 and ifnar-2 (37–39). The Jak kinases are also preassociated with receptor subunits, but in this case, a specificity of association exists. Tyk2 is associated with ifnar-1 and Jak1 with ifnar-2. The binding of IFN-α/β to ifnar-2c and receptor subunit dimerization brings the Jak kinases together, allowing cross-phosphorylation on tyrosine and kinase activation. Tyk2 is phosphorylated by Jak1, which, in turn, cross-phosphorylates Jak1 to increase its kinase activity. The tyrosine at residue 466 on ifnar-1 is phosphorylated. Latent STAT2 is then transferred to this docking site on ifnar-1 through an interaction requiring its specific SH-2 domain and the phosphotyrosine residue at 466 on ifnar-1. STAT2 then becomes tyrosine phosphorylated and provides a docking site for recruitment of STAT1 to ifnar-1, which is then tyrosine phosphorylated and activated. The arrangement of the IFN-α/β receptor preferentially results in the formation of heterodimers of STAT2 and STAT1, which are released from the receptor to interact with the IRF-1 family member p48 to form ISGF3, the major transcription factor activated in response to IFN-α/β. The heterodimers then translocate to the nucleus and form a high-affinity DNA-binding complex for the ISRE with p48. STAT1 and STAT2 heterodimers and STAT1 homodimers also form in response to IFN-α/β and can drive the transcription of a subset of genes through GAS elements. This action depends on the relative amounts of p48, which can vary among different cell types.

COMPONENTS OF THE INTERFERON SIGNAL TRANSDUCTION CASCADE

Janus Kinases

Jaks are a family of cytoplasmic protein tyrosine kinases that are essential for IFN action. As described in the section on Signaling Pathways Activated by Interferon-α and -β, two members of the Jak kinase family, Jak1, and Tyk2, are involved in IFN-α/β signaling (40). They each possess a tyrosine kinase activity mediated through a conserved catalytic domain and have seven highly conserved regions of shared homology, designated Jak homology (JH) domains 1 to 7 (see Fig. 2). The C-terminal JH-1 domain has conserved residues consistent with protein tyrosine kinase activity. The JH-2 kinase–like domain is the N-terminal to this site. This contains several amino acid substitutions, which render it inert for kinase activity. In the case of the JH-2 domain of Tyk2, however, it is essential for IFN-α signaling. The function of the other conserved domains remains to be established. After interaction of IFN with its receptor, the Jak kinases are phosphorylated on tyrosine and activated. The phosphotyrosine residue on Tyk2, activated as a result of IFN-α/β binding to ifnar-2c, maps to the JH-1 kinase domain. The specificity of Tyk2 and Jak1 is determined by their association with their particular IFN receptor subunits, not through a high degree of substrate specificity. Subtleties to the involvement of Jaks in the IFN response exist, however, that are still under investigation. For example, catalytic Tyk2 is required for the induction of the β-R1/I-TAC (IFN-inducible T-cell α-chemoattractant) gene, which is selectively induced by IFN-β compared with IFN-α, despite robust expression of other ISGFs induced by IFN-β through a Tyk2-independent pathway (41).

Signal Transducers and Activators of Transcription

IFN-induced receptor aggregation and activation of the Jak kinases results in the phosphorylation and assembly of STAT proteins (3). Phosphorylation of STATs on tyrosine permits the dimerization by reciprocal SH-2 phosphotyrosine interaction and entry into the nucleus to regulate the transcription of the different IFN-responsive genes. The STAT proteins most

closely associated with the IFN response include STAT1α/β and STAT2. STAT3 is also activated to a lesser extent. The STAT1α/β proteins are encoded by a single gene and are generated by alternative pre-mRNA splicing. They are identical through the first 712 amino acids, but STAT1α has additional 38 C-terminal residues. ISGF3 is composed of STAT1α, STAT2, or STAT1β/STAT2 heterodimers, along with p48. Single tyrosine residues (701 on STAT1 and 699 and STAT2) are phosphorylated after the activation of the Jak kinases. These tyrosine residues are situated in a phosphotyrosine-binding pocket of the SH-2 domains. They are essential for recruitment of the STAT proteins to the cytoplasmic tail of the activated receptor and for the formation of dimers either between STAT1 and STAT2, in the case of the formation of the complex ISGF3, or STAT1 homodimers that result from engagement of the IFN-γ receptor. In each case, dimerization occurs via association of the corresponding phosphotyrosine residues in the C-terminal of each partner with the SH-2 domain of the other member of the complex. Signal specificity in the IFN system is governed by localization of specific STATs to the cytoplasmic tails of the corresponding receptors. This is mediated by the SH-2 domains of the individual STAT molecules. The C-terminal domains of STATs are involved in transcriptional activation and in their ligand-dependent activation. As described previously in this section, the conserved tyrosine residue (701 on STAT1α) is responsible for the ability of STAT proteins to homodimerize. Phosphorylation of this residue is the hallmark of STAT activation. In STAT1α, the 38 C-terminal amino acids form an essential transcriptional activation domain. STAT1β lacks these residues and accordingly lacks transcriptional activation function. Serine residue 727 at the C-terminal of STAT 1α is required for full transcriptional activation and is phosphorylated by an unknown serine threonine kinase. STAT2 does not have a C-terminal serine phosphorylation site, but has a highly acidic transactivation domain downstream from the tyrosine phosphorylation site at residue 699. The terminal 181 amino acids of STAT2 are important for binding and association with the basal transcription machinery. The SH-2 of STAT proteins are the determinants of signaling specificity. STAT2 interacts specifically with the cytoplasmic domain of ifnar-2 through an SH-2 phosphotyrosine action. The SH-2 domain of STAT1 mediates an interaction with the phosphotyrosine 699 on STAT2, transmitting the signal through the IFN-α/β receptor.

Other functional domains on STATs include the amino-terminal domain, which is involved in binding protein tyrosine phosphatases and also in STAT dimer/dimer formation. The N-terminal domain of STAT2 is involved in binding to p48 via lysine residue 161. The N-terminal of STAT1 interacts with CBP-p300. Finally, the interaction of STAT2 and STAT1 is also mediated by the N-terminal domain of STAT2.

STAT1 is signaled through type I and type II IFN receptors. After type I receptor activation, STAT1 forms an essential component of ISGF3, along with STAT2 and p48. STAT1 and STAT2 heterodimers do not bind DNA strongly unless they are complexed with p48. STAT2 homodimers bind DNA weakly. Dimers of STAT1, however, are competent to bind DNA and drive the activation of transcription through GAS sites. In this case, phosphorylation of serine 727 is important for maximum transcriptional activation.

p48

p48 (earlier known as *ISGF3-γ*) is a member of a family of transcription factors, the IRFs (42). Different family members function as activators or repressors of transcription but share significant homology in their N-terminal DNA-binding domain. The signature feature of this domain is a cluster of five tryptophan residues, three of which are essential for contacting DNA. The C-terminal region of 398–amino acid p48 protein contains an IRF-association domain, which mediates the interaction between p48 and STAT1 and STAT2 heterodimers. As the essential DNA-binding domain subunit of ISGF3, p48 recognizes and binds to ISREs, usually located in the 5' upstream regions of IFN-stimulated genes. The association of p48 with STAT1 and STAT2 increases p48 DNA-binding activity 25-fold. Although the DNA-binding domain of p48 is sufficient for DNA binding, the first N-terminal 9 amino acids of p48 are essential for DNA target specificity.

Other Signaling Molecules in the Type I Interferon Response Pathway

Cytosolic Phospholipase A₂

The formation of ISGF3 after type I IFN signaling requires the enzymatic activity of $cPLA_2$ (33,34). Although type I and type II IFNs increase $cPLA_2$ activity, the formation of STAT1 homodimers by either type of IFN is unaffected by the inhibition of this enzyme. Activation of $cPLA_2$ is not seen in Jak1 mutant cells. Jak1 and $cPLA_2$ are physically associated in cells, even in the absence of IFN treatment. After IFN treatment, $cPLA_2$ is tyrosine phosphorylated, although it is not clear whether this affects its activity. In fact, $cPLA_2$ is known to be activated by serine phosphorylation by p38 MAPK. Specific inhibitors of p38 MAPK block IFN-induced ISGF3 formation and antiviral activity of IFN, suggesting that serine phosphorylation of $cPLA_2$ by p38 MAPK is an important event in type I IFN signaling (43). In accord with this, IFN-α induces the rapid activation of p38 MAPK, which can be blocked by dominant negative inhibitors of upstream kinase activators of p38 MAPK. Further analyses of this pathway also shows that IFN-activated p38 MAPK activity is necessary for serine phosphorylation of STAT1, which is required for maximum transcriptional activity of STAT1 homodimers.

Extracellular Signal-Regulated Kinase 2

The 42-kd MAPK or extracellular signal-regulated kinase 2 (ERK2) interacts with ifnar-1 *in vitro* and *in vivo* (36). Treatment of cells with IFN-β induces tyrosine phosphorylation and activation of ERK2 and causes it to associate with STAT1. The functional importance of ERK2 activation was shown by the inhibition of IFN-β–induced transcription of a transfected ISRE-dependent reporter by dominant negative MAPK (36). IFN-β also stimulates Raf-1 enzyme activity in a Ras-independent manner. Raf-1 activity can be coimmunoprecipitated with Jak1 or Tyk2 (44). In mutant cells lacking Jak1, IFN-β does not activate Raf-1. Transient expression of Jak1, however, reconstitutes the ability of IFN-β to activate Raf-1, indicating that Jak1 is required for Raf-1 activation by IFN-β (41).

IFN-γ also induces the activation of the MAPKs ERK1 and ERK2 in a Jak-dependent manner in several different cell types. It appears, however, that the proline-rich tyrosine kinase Pyk2 is required for IFN-γ, but not IFN-α–mediated activation of ERK2 (45).

INTERFERON-INDUCED PROTEINS

Treatment of cells with type I IFN induces the synthesis of many cellular RNAs and their corresponding proteins. The numbers of genes regulated by type I IFNs exceed 200 (27), but only a small number of the encoded proteins have been assigned specific IFN-regulated functions. IFN-α and -β induce the same set of proteins, but, in addition, IFN-β induces unique β-specific genes. The spectrum of proteins induced by IFNs depends on cell type, but most type I IFN-inducible mRNAs are transcribed as a primary response and do not require protein synthesis regulated through preexisting STAT1. The induction of protein synthesis by IFN is transient, peaking after several hours and then declining to uninduced levels. The element in the promoters of IFN-α/β–stimulated genes required for the response is the ISREs. GAS elements are also able to mediate a response to IFN-α, but to a lower level.

INTERFERON-INDUCED ANTIVIRAL PATHWAYS

The function of IFN-induced proteins has been most thoroughly studied in the antiviral response. Although IFN induces the synthesis and accumulation of many cellular RNAs and proteins that may differ in type and amount with different cells, only three IFN-regulated pathways have been definitively assigned an antiviral function. Two of these function at the level of protein synthesis inhibition, whereas the third selectively inhibits viral RNA transcription. IFNs are known to inhibit virus replication at different stages of infection, however, including entry into the cell and uncoating of the virus particle (e.g., SV40, retroviruses), DNA and RNA synthesis (e.g., influenza, vesicular stomatitis virus), protein synthesis (e.g., picornaviruses, adenovirus, vaccinia), and virus assembly and release from the cell (e.g., retroviruses, vesicular stomatitis virus). With the exception of protein synthesis and transcription, IFN-induced proteins that act specifically at different stages have not been described.

Three pathways that mediate the antiviral activity of IFNs have been characterized in detail; the Mx, PKR, and the 2-5A pathways (Fig. 4). The Mx pathway was discovered during the investigation of genetic resistance to influenza viral infection in mice. The latter two were discovered as a result of an investigation of the inhibitory effects of dsRNA on protein synthesis performed in extracts from IFN-treated cells. The key enzyme intermediates in both pathways require dsRNA for activation.

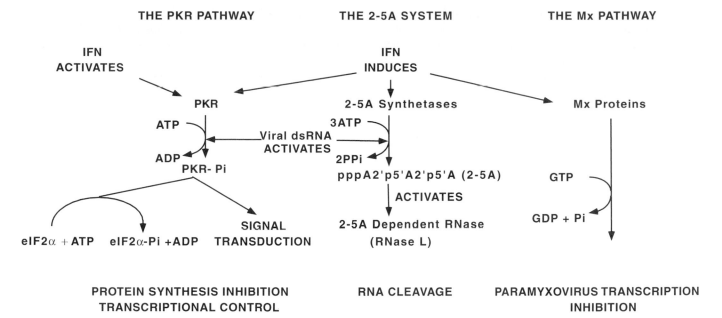

THE PKR PATHWAY   THE 2-5A SYSTEM   THE Mx PATHWAY

FIGURE 4. Three major pathways mediate the antiviral activities of interferons (IFNs). (ADP, adenosine diphosphate; ATP, adenosine triphosphate; GDP, guanosine diphosphate; GTP, guanosine triphosphate.)

During viral infection, dsRNA can be derived from the incoming viral RNA genome or from viral replication intermediates.

Mx Proteins

The Mx proteins are IFN-inducible 70- to 80-kd glutamyl transpeptidases, which belong to the Dynamin superfamily (46). Mx proteins, like other Dynamins, self assemble into horseshoe and ring-shaped helices and other helical structures. The Dynamins play important roles in transport processes, such as endocytosis and intracellular vesicle transport. In plants, Dynamins are important for cell formation. Transfected cells and transgenic mice expressing Mx proteins are resistant to Mx-sensitive viruses, demonstrating that Mx proteins are powerful antiviral agents. In humans, synthesis of MxA is observed during self-limiting viral infections and may thus promote recovery from disease. The human MxA protein is induced by type I IFNs and accumulates in the cytoplasm of cells, where it forms tight oligomeric complexes. MxA interferes with the multiplication and spread of orthomyxoviruses, rhabdoviruses, paramyxoviruses, and bunyaviruses. Synthesis of MxA is induced during acute viral infections and impairs the growth of influenza (a paramyxovirus) and other viruses at the level of transcription. MxA works in the cytoplasm to bind viral nucleocapsids and blocks their normal movement into the nucleus. This has been demonstrated for Thogoto virus, an influenza virus–like orthomyxovirus transmitted by ticks (47). This virus is susceptible to MxA, which blocks the transport of virus nucleocapsids into the nucleus, thereby preventing transcription of the viral genome. These reveal a novel antiviral mechanism, whereby an IFN-induced protein traps the incoming virus and interferes with proper transport of the viral genome to its ultimate target compartment within the infected cell.

Semliki Forest virus (SFV), a togavirus with a single-stranded RNA genome of positive polarity, has been found to be sensitive to MxA (48). Expression of MxA in different cell lines prevented the accumulation of 49S RNA and 26S RNA, indicating that SFV was inhibited early in its replication cycle. Thus, the antiviral spectrum of MxA is not restricted to negative-strand RNA viruses but also includes SFV, which contains an RNA genome of positive polarity. Importantly, the MxA protein can exert its inhibitory activity against SFV in the absence of viral structural proteins, suggesting that viral components other than the structural proteins are the target of MxA action. This could be a limitation in the use of SFV-based, self-replicating vectors in antitumor vaccine strategies. In contrast to the human MxA protein, the murine Mx-1 protein inhibits the primary transcription of viruses in the nucleus (49). Although the mechanisms of their action have not been established, the conservation of Mx proteins in vertebrates, including fish, suggest a broader spectrum of antiviral action (50).

The promoter of the MxA gene contains two functional ISREs near the transcription start site and one homologous ISRE-like element, which is apparently nonfunctional, further upstream (51). The two proximal ISRE sites are essential for IFN-α–induced transcription and bind ISGF3. The transcription factor Spl, which binds with high affinity to a region encompassing nucleotides 25 and 50, is most likely important for interacting with the basal transcriptional machinery (51). The highly responsive Mx promoter has proved useful for the induction of transgene expression by IFN in cell cultures and mice, including inducible gene targeting (52). The standard laboratory mouse strains carry deleted Mx-1 alleles and are susceptible to influenza virus, whereas mouse strains originating from wild mice carry the wild-type allele, which likely serves a protective function against orthomyxoviruses (49).

A novel function for MxA has been suggested in Fanconi anemia, a group of five autosomal recessive disorders that share common phenotypes of birth defects, hematopoietic failure, sensitivity to cross-linking agents, and predisposition to apoptosis. MxA is upregulated in the different complementation groups, but repressed when the Fanconi anemia complementation group C (FAC) gene cDNA (which encodes a 63-kd cytoplasmic protein thought to protect from DNA damage) is overexpressed in group C cells (53). This work suggests that MxA is a downstream target of FAC probably at the posttranscriptional level, although the presence or absence of FAC does not affect the expression of other IFN-regulated genes. Overexpression of MxA can lead to phenotypic abnormalities similar to those observed in Fanconi anemia group C cells, including sensitivity to mitomycin C and increased apoptosis.

Double-Stranded RNA-Dependent Protein Kinase

The IFN-inducible dsRNA-dependent kinase, PKR, is a serine-threonine kinase initially described as a mediator of protein synthesis inhibition by dsRNA. It has become apparent, however, that PKR plays roles in different cellular processes, including growth regulation, antiviral protection, and signal transduction and differentiation. Most cells express constitutive levels of PKR, but type I IFNs, through an ISRE, can induce the transcription of the PKR gene (54,55). PKR is normally inactive but, on binding dsRNA, undergoes a conformational change exposing the catalytic domain for activation. Autophosphorylation activates the kinase function, allowing phosphorylation downstream substrates independent of dsRNA. The binding of dsRNA requires the presence of two dsRNA-binding motifs present in the N-terminal regulatory domain of PKR. The first motif is the most critical for binding dsRNA and is highly conserved within a large family of dsRNA-binding proteins, most of which have no known functions. A single PKR dsRNA-binding motif can recognize as few as 11 base pairs of dsRNA. No sequence specificity exists to this recognition because this is based on interactions between conserved residues and hydroxyl groups of the minor groove of dsRNA (56). Most viruses present an opportunity to activate PKR during the infection cycle through the production of dsRNA. As dsRNA is also a structural feature of cellular RNAs, it is possible that these may activate PKR as part of a cellular regulatory control mechanism. In accord with this, exposure of cells to stress, such as heat shock, activates the transcription of cellular Alu RNAs, which can regulate PKR activity (57). PKR activity is also regulated during the cell cycle, although the nature of the endogenous activator has not been discerned (58).

The antiviral activity of PKR is largely mediated by its phosphorylation of the α-subunit of erythrocyte initiation factor (eIF2) (see Fig. 4). Phosphorylation of eIF2 prevents recycling of eIF2:guanosine diphosphate to eIF2:guanosine triphosphate, trapping the recycling factor eIF2α, inhibiting protein synthesis. PKR also mediates programmed cell death (apoptosis) induced by dsRNA (59). Consequently, a combination of protein synthesis inhibition and induction of apoptosis likely act to restrict viral replication and spread.

PKR can act as a signal transducing kinase for the transcription factor, NF-κB (60–63). Activation of PKR by dsRNA leads to the phosphorylation of IκB, the inhibitor of transcription factor NF-κB, causing its release from the inactive NFκB/IκB complex (60). This allows NF-κB to migrate to the nucleus and regulate the expression NF-κB–dependent genes, many of which are important in the development of an inflammatory response (62,63).

PKR is not constitutively active, but IFNs (and other cytokines) can directly activate latent PKR (63,64). Under these circumstances, the activation of PKR is a necessary step in a signal transduction pathway that eventually leads to the induction of expression of different genes involved in the cellular inflammatory response, including the synthesis of chemokines, class I major histocompatibility complex (MHC), and molecules involved in apoptosis. The loss of PKR function not only results in a decreased antiviral activity of IFNs, but also attenuates the cellular response to certain cytokines and growth factors.

To circumvent the antiviral effects of IFN and reduce an inflammatory reaction mediated by PKR, many viruses have elaborated mechanisms to inhibit this enzyme and other components of IFN-regulated pathways (65,66). These include the synthesis of inhibitory dsRNAs (e.g., adenoviruses, Epstein-Barr virus, human immunodeficiency virus) or the synthesis of proteins, which can bind and sequester dsRNA activators of PKR (e.g., reovirus, vaccinia). Other viruses synthesize protein inhibitors of PKR (e.g., hepatitis C virus, herpes simplex virus, vaccinia) or proteases that cleave PKR (e.g., poliovirus, encephalomyocarditis virus). In some cases, the inhibitors are normally sequestered but are activated in response to viral infection (e.g., influenza virus). Despite the fact that different viruses have targeted PKR, viral replication in PKR-null mice is accelerated, even in the absence of IFN, suggesting that PKR is important in restricting infection (62,67). In the context of an inflammatory response, PKR appears to be an important mediator of the synergy between cytokines. For example, synergy between tumor necrosis factor–α (TNF-α) and IFN-γ for induction of NF-κB is dependent on PKR (64). This may be an important role for PKR in a physiologic context.

PKR is a cell growth inhibitor. Transdominant mutants of the enzyme act as dominant oncogenes in NIH 3T3 cell assays (68,69). Some attempts have been made to link PKR dysregulation to cancer. It has been reported that PKR levels correlate inversely with proliferative activity in different human tumors and tumor cell lines (70–72). Human invasive ductal breast carcinomas, however, have high levels of PKR. In several breast carcinoma cell lines, PKR levels are high compared with those found in the normal breast cell lines (70,73). The activity of PKR from the carcinoma cells, however, is attenuated, although it remains capable of binding dsRNA. Mixing experiments suggest that carcinoma cells contain a transdominant inhibitor of PKR (73). Although this suggests a role for PKR in the pathogenesis of cancer, the underlying mechanism remains to be established. This could occur by disrupting the control of protein synthesis initiation by PKR. In support of this ribosomal protein, L18, a 22-kd protein that is overexpressed in colorectal cancer tissue, has been shown to bind to PKR through the first dsRNA-binding domain (74). L18 inhibits PKR autophosphorylation and PKR-mediated phosphorylation of eIF2-α *in vitro* and *in vivo*. It is speculated that overexpression of L18 in tumors may promote protein synthesis and cell growth through inhibition of PKR activity. A large number of dsRNA-binding proteins exist, however, that also bind PKR (75). Pinpointing any one of these as the crucial PKR regulator in tumorigenesis without more direct evidence is premature. Murine PKR has been shown to have undergone a rearrangement of one allele in a murine lymphocytic leukemia cell (76). Analyses of human acute lymphatic leukemia for PKR rearrangements could prove informative.

Although the regulation of eIF2 phosphorylation has remained a focus of several studies on the role of PKR in cell growth control, an interesting connection to regulation of the proto-oncogene c-Myc also exists that might prove to be of more fundamental importance in tumor development. IFN has been known for some time to suppress c-Myc expression. In M1, myeloid leukemia cells expressing inactive mutant forms of PKR can abrogate this (77). Transfection of M1 cells with wild-type human PKR inhibited proliferation in the absence of IFNs, but this could be rescued by the ectopic expression of deregulated c-Myc. Thus, a link appears to exist between PKR and c-Myc suppression. In accord with these results, transfection of breast carcinoma MCF-7 cells with a dominant negative mutant of PKR relieved c-Myc downregulation, occurring as a consequence of the synergistic inhibition of growth with all-trans-retinoic acid and IFN-α (78). Experiments show that PKR and STAT1 are required for IFN-mediated downregulation of c-Myc (79). In PKR or STAT1-null cells, c-Myc gene expression is stimulated, not repressed, by IFN. Moreover, in PKR-null cells, the phosphorylation of STAT1 on serine 727 is deficient (79). These results place PKR in pathways required for cell growth control and, potentially, tumor suppression.

2-5A Synthetase/Ribonuclease L System

Type I IFNs induce the 2-5A synthetase/ribonuclease (RNase) L system. This is a multienzyme cellular RNA degradation pathway that is activated by dsRNA (see Fig. 3). The 2-5A synthetases are transcribed from ISRE-containing genes in response to IFNs. The enzymes are activated by dsRNAs to polymerize short 2' and 5' oligoadenylates (2-5A). This unique oligomer activates the 2-5A–dependent ribonuclease RNase L. Thus, the enzymes in this pathway are present in all cells as inactive or latent forms and require first dsRNA as a cofactor in the case of the 2-5A synthetase enzymes and 2-5A as the activator for the latent ribonuclease, RNase L. IFNs can also stimulate the synthesis of RNase L by activating transcription. Latent RNase L is a monomer, but binding to 2-5A induces dimerization, activating the enzyme (80). Because 2-5A is rapidly degraded by phosphodiesterases and phosphatases, the activation of RNase L is reversible, resulting in deactivation of the 2-5A pathway. The three genes encoding the 2-5A synthetases map to a single locus (12q21) in humans (81). Although the individual enzymes reside in different subcellular locations, they are found in all cellular compartments. The different isoforms have differing activities. The largest 100-kd isoform is active as a monomer and

preferentially synthesizes dimers of 2-5A. The 69-kd enzyme and its alternatively spliced 71-kd isoform are myristylated and glycosylated and exist as membrane-bound homodimers. The small human 2-5A synthetase isoforms result from alternative splicing of the same gene, yielding 40- and 46-kd proteins. Although the amino terminal 346 residues of both proteins are identical, the 54 C-terminal unique residues of the 46-kd isoform are highly hydrophobic and allow the localization of this form to membranes. The 46-kd form, which lacks the hydrophobic C-terminal sequence, is cytoplasmic. The first 346 amino acids of 40- and 46-kd isoforms constitute a domain that is duplicated in the 69- and 71-kd isoforms and occurs three times in the 100-kd isoform. Unique antiviral functions for the different 2-5A synthetases have not been described. The only well-described function of these enzymes is to synthesize 2-5A, the activator of RNase L. Because the 100-kd form of the enzyme synthesizes predominantly dimers, which are not able to activate RNase L, it remains possible that other functions exist. The dsRNA-binding domains of the 2-5A synthetase isoforms bear no structural similarity to the dsRBD of PKR and require a higher concentration of dsRNA for activation than PKR. Thus, under situations when PKR can be inhibited by high concentrations of dsRNA, the 2-5A system becomes activated, providing a second line of defense against viral infection.

RNase L is single isozyme encoded by a unique gene mapping to human chromosome 1p31 (82,83). The human RNase L protein has 741 residues. The N-terminal is comprised of a repeated P-loop motif and 9 ankryin repeats, which are involved in 2-5A binding and function to repress RNase L activity in the absence of 2-5A (84). The C-terminal half of the protein contains a region of protein kinase homology, which consists of a cysteine-rich domain and a ribonuclease domain. The isolated C-terminal half of RNase L cleaves RNA in the absence of 2-5A. RNase L binds 2-5A with high affinity and the active ribonuclease activity is sequence nonspecific, but cleaves U-U and U-A bonds preferentially. Inhibition of RNase L activity by expression of dominant negative derivatives or deletion of the gene from mice result in a defective antiencephalomyocarditis virus effect of IFN-α (85).

RNase L is involved in cell growth control and apoptosis (85–88). Dominant negative inhibitors of RNase L block different apoptosis responses (e.g., staurosporine-induced apoptosis of NIH 3T3 cells and SV40-transformed BALB/c cells) (87,88). K562 cell lines expressing inactive RNase L are more resistant to apoptosis induced by decreased glutathione levels. When human RNase L cDNA is stably overexpressed in murine NIH 3T3 cells, the cell growth inhibitory activity of IFN and the proapoptotic activity of staurosporine are enhanced. The replication of different viruses are also inhibited. Inducible overexpression of human RNase L in NIH 3T3 fibroblasts decreases cell viability and triggers apoptosis (89). Activation of endogenous RNase L, specifically with 2-5A, also induces apoptosis, whereas inhibition of RNase L with a dominant negative mutant suppresses polyrI.rC-induced apoptosis in IFN-primed cells and suppresses apoptosis induced by poliovirus. Overproduced RNase L by recombinant vaccinia virus causes apoptotic death of mammalian cells, which can be prevented by the apoptosis antagonist Bcl-2 (90).

In accord with these results, RNase L–null mice exhibit enlarged thymuses resulting from a suppression of apoptosis (85). Apoptosis is also suppressed in RNase L-null thymocytes and fibroblasts treated with different apoptotic agents. Taken together, these results suggest that IFN action and apoptosis can be controlled at the level of RNA stability by RNase L.

In a study more directly connected to cancer, elevated levels of RNase L mRNA and activity were detected in colorectal tumors compared with corresponding normal mucosa (91). The occurrence of elevated levels of RNase L seems to be an early event in colorectal tumorigenesis, suggesting that control of RNA turnover is an important step in tumor progression (91). Clearly, these levels were insufficient to trigger apoptosis but, rather, suggest that activating RNase L activity, perhaps by delivery of 2-5A, may be a useful strategy in treating colorectal carcinomas.

The regulation of RNase L activity towards specific targets has been achieved by linking the 2-5A moiety to antisense oligonucleotides. Proof of principle for this was shown when the unaided uptake into HeLa cells of 2-5A linked to an antisense oligonucleotide, resulting in the selective ablation of mRNA for PKR (61). Cells depleted of PKR activity were unresponsive to activation of NF-κB by dsRNA (61). This strategy also works against cancer targets. For example, 2-5A antisense directed against the fusion site or against the translation start sequence in bcr/abl mRNA is selective in degrading this mRNA in chronic myelogenous leukemia cell lines and is accompanied by decreases of p210 (bcr/abl) kinase activity levels and suppression of cell growth (92). In primary chronic myelogenous leukemia cells isolated from bone marrow of patients, the 2-5A–antisense treatments suppressed proliferation of the leukemia cells and selectively depleted levels of bcr/abl mRNA. These findings suggest that these compounds may have potential as *ex vivo* purging agents of autologous hematopoietic stem-cell transplants from CML patients.

Telomerase is the RNA protein complex that elongates telomeric DNA and appears to play an important role in cellular immortalization. The almost exclusive expression of telomerase in tumor cells has offered an opportunity to exploit 2-5A antisense. This expression does not involve most normal cells. A 19-MER antisense oligonucleotide against human telomerase RNA linked to a 2-5A effectively suppressed glioma tumor cell growth and survival *in vitro* and inhibited survival of tumors grown in nude mice with the antisense possibly by the induction of apoptosis (93). Targeting telomerase RNA with 2-5A antisense could prove an effective treatment for a broad range of cancers.

The ability of IFNs to confer an antiviral state is a fundamental property that allows for classification and individual activity measurement. Different stages of virus replication may be inhibited by IFNs, including entry, uncoating, or both, and transcription initiation of translation, maturation, assembly, and release. Because the pathways described in this section are primarily directed towards translational control mechanisms, it is obvious that other IFN-regulated antiviral proteins exist to interfere with different stages of virus replication. Despite identification of a large number of IFN-regulated genes and pro-teins, however, the assignment of specific antiviral activities to these remains to be achieved.

INHIBITION OF CELL GROWTH AND IMMUNE REGULATION BY TYPE I INTERFERONS

The cell growth inhibitory properties of IFNs are assumed to contribute to their use as anticancer agents. IFNs also regulate cellular responses to inducers of apoptosis, however, and modulate the immune response. These effects underlie antitumor activity. The prolonged activation of STAT1 and the induction of synthesis of several proapoptotic genes by IFNs may sensitize cells to apoptosis inducers, including chemotherapeutic agents. Thus, the modulatory effects of IFNs influences the development of resistance to infection and antitumor activities. Direct inhibition of cell growth by IFN is displayed against a variety of cultured cells *in vitro*. This is partly caused by the promotion of differentiation, which is particularly apparent when used in combination with other agents, such as retinoids. Significant IFN-induced gene products have not been linked directly to antiproliferative activity. IFN-α does regulate properties of different components of the cell cycle, however, including c-Myc, pRB, cyclin D3, and cdc25A. The mechanisms by which the cell cycle is suppressed may differ in different cell types. Thus, the involvement of cyclin-dependent kinase inhibitors, such as p21, p27, and p57 kip, have been invoked in some cells, whereas in others these inhibitors are not involved.

A major problem in attributing the antiproliferative effects of IFNs on specific gene products is that they induce many hundreds of genes. This has been illustrated by determining mRNA profiles from IFN-α, -β, or -γ treatments of the human fibrosarcoma cell line, HT1080, using oligonucleotide arrays with probe sets corresponding to more than 6,800 human genes (30). Many novel IFN-stimulated genes were identified that were diverse in their known biologic functions. Moreover, several IFN-repressed genes also were identified. Until theses genes can be manipulated by overexpression or deletion, delineation of their role in the antiproliferative response of IFNs can only be speculative. It is noticeable that a number of genes induced by type I IFNs are involved in apoptosis, however, including RAP46/Bag-1, phospholipid scramblase, and hypoxia-inducible factor-1α (30). Consequently, it is likely the antitumor effects of IFNs in vivo can be augmented by combination with apoptosis-inducing agents. For example, the expression of TNF-related apoptosis-inducing ligand, a proapoptotic member of the TNF family of type II membrane proteins, is rapidly induced on the surface of CD4+ and CD8+ peripheral blood T cells on stimulation with anti-CD3 monoclonal antibody and type I IFNs, but not other cytokines (94). Most renal cell carcinoma cell lines are susceptible to TNF-related apoptosis-inducing ligand apoptosis. Type I IFNs can augment cytotoxic activity of anti–CD3-stimulated PBT cells against renal cell carcinoma cell lines in a TNF-related apoptosis-inducing ligand–dependent manner. This unique ability of type I IFNs to regulate TNF-related apoptosis-inducing ligand–mediated T-cell cytotoxicity may contribute to the antitumor effects of type I IFNs against various tumors. Type I IFNs also interfere with the rapid death of activated T cells without raising the levels of Bcl-2 or Bcl-XL, which distinguishes them from the interleukin-2 family or CD28 engagement (95). In some cases, for example, in hemopoietic progenitor cells, IFNs directly induce cell death. This requires the expression of PML to mediate Fas and caspase-dependent DNA damage–induced apoptosis. The PML-RAR α fusion protein of acute promyelocytic leukemia renders hemopoietic progenitor cells resistant to Fas-, TNF-, and IFN-induced apoptosis with a lack of caspase-3 activation by dominant negative inhibition of polymorphonuclear leukocytes (96). In most primary cell cultures, IFNs are not apoptotic by themselves but require the addition of dsRNA presumably to activate PKR and 2-5A–mediated apoptotic pathways. In the case of viruses, the dsRNA is generated during the course of infection, and the subsequent virus-induced apoptosis can be inhibited by anti type I IFN antibodies. This is not seen in cells lacking ifnar-1 or STAT1 (97). The selective promotion of apoptosis by IFN in virally infected cells could perhaps be exploited in cancer by combining IFN therapy with dsRNA analogues.

IFNs can have significant effects on all phases of innate and adaptive immune responses. Type I IFNs are largely responsible for increasing the effectiveness of the adaptive immune response to resist viral infection, including the stimulation of CD44 memory T cells (98). This bystander proliferation does not require T-cell receptor ligation but may result from IFN induction of macrophages to synthesize interleukin-15, which causes selective stimulation of CD44hi CD8⁺ (but not CD4⁺) cells.

Type I and type II IFNs enhance the expression of MHC class I proteins to promote the development of CD8⁺ T-cell responses (99). MHC class I expression is dependent on the transcription factor IRF-1. Mutations in genes linked to the IRF-1 signal transduction pathway result in failure to actively upregulate MHC class I proteins on cell surfaces in response to IFN. Both type I and type II IFNs are able to upregulate the expression of the different protein components, which constitute the proteosome-protein processing pathway responsible for generating antigenic peptides expressed by MHC class II (100). Accordingly, IFNs can enhance immunogenicity by increasing the quantity and repertoire of peptides displayed in association with MHC class I proteins, which are dependent on an active proteosome-mediated pathway .

Both type I and type II IFNs effect humoral immunity in complex ways by indirectly regulating the development of specific T-helper subsets or by directly regulating the specialized B-cell functions, including development and proliferation, immunoglobulin secretion, and immunoglobulin heavy chain switching. In immunoglobulin class switching, the type I IFNs can function redundantly to type II IFN (101).

CONCLUSION

Type I IFNs have proved to be remarkably pleiotropic cytokines with a broad range of clinical activities as antiviral and antitumor agents. The mechanisms underlying these activities are complex because of the large number of genes regulated by IFNs and also because of likely cell-type differences in responses. Although the introduction of recombinant IFN-α2

and IFN-β has enabled the evaluation and approval of these biologic response modifiers for different indications, natural IFN-α is a mixture of subtypes, some of which may have differing biologic activity. Further clinical evaluation of these different subtypes of IFNs alone or as adjuvant therapy is necessary. For example, early trials provided evidence for differing activity and lower side effects of IFN-α1 versus IFN-α2. This needs to be revisited using new methods for stabilizing IFN to increase its bioavailability and reduce side effects. The rapid protein clearance and systemic toxicities seen with unmodified IFNs can be modulated by conjugation with polyethylene glycol. Polyethylene glycol conjugation of proteins also makes them tolerogenic, inhibiting antibody responses, thus potentially overcoming the problem of developing neutralizing antibody. This has been reported in patients receiving IFN-α therapy. Although IFN therapy at therapeutic doses causes a number of dose-related side effects, these reactions are reversible on termination of therapy. The mechanisms underlying the most common adverse effects, such as flulike syndrome, fatigue, anorexia, and depression, are not well understood. IFNs can change the expression of more than 300 genes, including a number of proinflammatory cytokines. Thus, side effects may be unavoidable. Moreover, the use of antiinflammatory drugs to control side effects may be counterproductive because these drugs may also block IFN signaling. Alternatives, including the combination of systemic low-dose IFN administration with cytotoxic- or differentiation-inducing agents and gene therapeutic approaches, may deliver high concentrations of IFN into the tumor bed. Oral IFN therapies have shown efficacy in animal models and may be appropriate for treatment of diseases in which high-dose systemic administration and its associated toxicity are inappropriate.

REFERENCES

1. Issacs A, Lindenmann J. Virus Interference II. Some properties of interferon. *Proc R Soc Lond B Biol Sci* 1957;147:268–273.
2. Pfeffer LM, Dinarello CA, Herberman RB, et al. Biological properties of recombinant alpha-interferons: 40th anniversary of the discovery of interferons. *Cancer Res* 1998;58(12):2489–2499.
3. Stark GR, Kerr IM, Williams BRG, Silverman RH, Schreiber RD. How cells respond to interferons. *Ann Rev Biochem* 1998;67: 227–264.
4. Roberts RM, Liu L, Guo Q, Leaman D, Bixby J. The evolution of the type I interferons. *J Interferon Cytokine Res* 1998;18(10):805–816.
5. Goldstein D, Hertzog P, Tomkinson E, et al. Administration of imiquimod, an interferon inducer, in asymptomatic human immunodeficiency virus-infected persons to determine safety and biologic response modification. *J Infect Dis* 1998;178(3):858–861.
6. Bielenberg DR, McCarty MF, Bucana CD, et al. Expression of interferon-beta is associated with growth arrest of murine and human epidermal cells. *J Invest Dermatol* 1999;112(5):802–809.
7. Bielenberg DR, Bucana CD, Sanchez R, Mulliken JB, Folkman J, Fidler IJ. Progressive growth of infantile cutaneous hemangiomas is directly correlated with hyperplasia and angiogenesis of adjacent epidermis and inversely correlated with expression of the endogenous angiogenesis inhibitor, IFN-beta. *Int J Oncol* 1999;14(3): 401–408.
8. Goodbourn S, Zinn K, Maniatis T. Human beta-interferon gene expression is regulated by an inducible enhancer element. *Cell* 1985;41(2):509–520.

9. Thanos D, Maniatis T. Virus induction of human IFN beta gene expression requires the assembly of an enhanceosome. *Cell* 1995;83(7):1091–1100.

10. Parekh BS, Maniatis T. Virus infection leads to localized hyperacetylation of histones H3 and H4 at the IFN-beta promoter. *Mol Cell* 1999;3:125–129.

11. Bonnefoy E, Bandu MT, Doly J. Specific binding of high-mobility-group I (HMGI) protein and histone H1 to the upstream AT-rich region of the murine beta interferon promoter: HMGI protein acts as a potential antirepressor of the promoter. *Mol Cell Biol* 1999;4:2803–2816.

12. Joshi AR, Sarkar FH, Gupta SL. Interferon receptors. Cross-linking to human leukocytes interferon alpha-2 to its receptor on human cell. *J Biol Chem* 1982;257:13884–13887.

13. Hannigan GE, Gewert DR, Fish EN, Read SE, Williams BR. Differential binding of human interferon-alpha subtypes to receptors on lymphoblastoid cells. *Biochem Biophys Res Commun* 1983;110(2):537–544.

14. Aguet M, Grobke M, Dreiding P. Various human interferon alpha subclasses cross-react with common receptors: the binding affinities correlate with their specific biological activities. *Virology* 1984;132:211–216.

15. Merlin G, Falcoff E, Aguet M. 125-labeled human interferon alpha, beta and gamma: comparative receptor binding data. *J Gen Virol* 1985;66:1149–1152.

16. Faltynek CR, Branca AA, McCandless S, Baglioni C. Characterization of an interferon receptor on human lymphoblastoid cells. *Proc Natl Acad Sci U S A* 1993;80:3269–3273.

17. Hannigan GE, Lau AS, Williams BRG. Differential human interferon alpha receptor expression on proliferating and non-proliferating cells. *Eur J Biochem* 1996;157:187–193.

18. Hannigan GE, Fish EN, Williams BR. Modulation of human interferon-alpha receptor expression by human interferon-gamma. *J Biol Chem* 1984;259(13):8084–8086.

19. Hannigan GE, Gewert DR, Williams BR. Characterization and regulation of alpha interferon receptor expression in interferon-sensitive and -resistant human lymphoblastoid cells. *J Biol Chem* 1984;259(15):9456–9460.

20. Zhang ZQ, Fournier A, Tan YH. The isolation of human beta interferon receptor by wheat germ lectin affinity and immunosorbent column chromatographies. *J Biol Chem* 1986;261:8017–8021.

21. Colamonici OR, D'Alessandro F, Diaz MO, et al. Characterization of three monoclonal antibodies that recognize the IFN-α2 receptor. *Proc Natl Acad Sci U S A* 1990;87:7230–7234.

22. Uze G, Lutfalla G, Gresser I. Genetic transfer of a functional human interferon alpha receptor into mouse cells: cloning and expression of its cDNA. *Cell* 1990;60:225–234.

23. Novick D, Cohen B, Rubinstein M. The human interferon alpha/beta receptor: characterization and cloning. *Cell* 1994;77:391–400.

24. Domanski P, Witte M, Kellum M, et al. Cloning and expression of a long form of the beta subunit of the interferon alpha beta receptor that is required for signaling. *J Biol Chem* 1995;270:21606–21611.

25. Lutfalla G, Holland SJ, Cinato E, et al. Mutant U5A cells are complemented by an interferon-alpha beta receptor subunit generated by alternative processing of a new member of a cytokine receptor gene cluster. *EMBO J* 1995;14:5100–5108.

26. Uze G, Lutfalla G, Mogensen KE. Alpha and beta interferons and their receptor and their friends and relations. *J Interferon Cytokine Res* 1995;15:3–26.

27. Domanski P, Colamonici OR. The type I interferon receptor. The long and short of it. *Cytokine Growth Factor Rev* 1996;7:143–151.

28. Lewerenz M, Mogensen KE, Uze G. Shared receptor components but distinct complexes for alpha and beta interferons. *J Mol Biol* 1998;282(3):585–599.

29. Rani MR, Gauzzi C, Pellegrini S, Fish EN, Wei T, Ransohoff RM. Induction of beta-R1/I-TAC by interferon-beta requires catalytically active TYK2J. *J Biol Chem* 1999;274(4):1891–1897.

30. Der SD, Zhou A, Williams BR, Silverman RH. Identification of genes differentially regulated by interferon alpha, beta, or gamma using oligonucleotide arrays. *Proc Natl Acad Sci U S A* 1998;95(26):15623–15628.

31. Hannigan GE, Williams BRG. Transcriptional regulation of interferon responsive genes is closely linked to interferon receptor occupancy. *EMBO J* 1986;5:1607–1613.

32. Lau AS, Hannigan GE, Williams BRG. Regulation of interferon receptor expression in human body lymphocytes in vitro and during interferon therapy. *J Clin Invest* 1986;77:1632–1638.

33. Hannigan GE, Williams BRG. Signal transduction by interferon-alpha through phospholipase A$_2$-mediated arachidonic acid metabolism. *Science* 1991;251:204–207.

34. Flati V, Haque SJ, Williams BRG. Interferon-α-induced phosphorylation and activation of cytosolic phospholipase A$_2$ is required for the formation of interferon-stimulated gene factor three. *EMBO J* 1996;15:1566–1571.

35. Uddin S, Yenush L, Sun XJ, Sweet ME, White MF, Platanias LC. Interferon-alpha engages the insulin receptor substrate-1 to associate with the phosphatidylinositol 3'-kinase. *J Biol Chem* 1995;270(27):15938–15941.

36. David M, Petricoin E III, Benjamin C, Pine R, Weber MJ, Larner AC. Requirement for MAP kinase (ERK2) activity in interferon alpha- and interferon beta-stimulated gene expression through STAT proteins. *Science* 1995;269(5231):1721–1723.

37. Leung S, Qureshi SA, Kerr IM, Darnell JE Jr, Stark GR. Role of STAT2 in the alpha-interferon signaling pathway. *Mol Cell Biol* 1995;15(3):1312–1317.

38. Nadeau OW, Domanski P, Usacheva A, et al. The proximal tyrosines of the cytoplasmic domain of the beta chain of the type I interferon receptor are essential for signal transducer and activator of transcription (Stat) 2 activation. Evidence that two STAT2 sites are required to reach a threshold of interferon alpha-induced STAT2 tyrosine phosphorylation that allows normal formation of interferon-stimulated gene factor 3. *J Biol Chem* 1999;274(7):4045–4052.

39. Stark GR, Kerr IM, Williams BRG, Silverman RH, Schreiber RD. How cells respond to interferons. *Ann Rev Biochem* 1998;l67:227–264.

40. Darnell JE Jr, Kerr IM, Stark GR. Jak-STAT pathways and transcriptional activation in response to IFNs and other extracellular proteins. *Science* 1994;264:1415–1421.

41. Rani MRS, Foster GR, Leung S, Leaman D, Stark GR, Ransohoff RM. Characterization of beta-R1, a gene that is selectively induced by interferon beta (IFN-beta) compared with IFN-alpha. *J Biol Chem* 1996;271(37):22878–22884.

42. Pitha PM, Au WC, Lowther W, et al. Role of the interferon regulatory factors (IRFs) in virus-mediated signaling and regulation of cell growth. *Biochimie* 1998;80(8–9):651–658.

43. Goh KC, Haque SJ, Williams BRG. An essential role for p38MAPK in interferon signaling and antiviral activity. 1999 (*submitted*). *EMBO J* 1999;18:5601–5608

44. Stancato LF, Sakatsume M, David M, et al. Beta-interferon and oncostatin M activate Raf-1 and mitogen-activated protein kinase through a JAK1-dependent pathway. *Mol Cell Biol* 1997;17(7):3833–3840.

45. Takaoka A, Tanaka N, Mitani Y, et al. Protein tyrosine kinase Pyk2 mediates the Jak-dependent activation of MAPK and Stat1 in IFN-gamma, but not IFN-alpha, signaling. *EMBO J* 1999;18(9):2480–2488.

46. Haller O, Frese M, Kochs G. Mx proteins: mediators of innate resistance to RNA viruses. *Rev Sci Tech* 1998(1):220–230.

47. Kochs G, Haller O. Interferon-induced human MxA GTPase blocks nuclear import of Thogoto virus nucleocapsids. *Proc Natl Acad Sci U S A* 1999;96(5):2082–2086.

48. Landis H, Simon-Jodicke A, Kloti A, et al. Human MxA protein confers resistance to Semliki Forest virus and inhibits the amplification of a Semliki Forest virus-based replicon in the absence of viral structural proteins. *J Virol* 1998;72(2):1516–1522.

49. Jin HK, Yamashita T, Ochiai K, Haller O, Watanabe T. Characterization and expression of the Mx1 gene in wild mouse species. *Science* 1995;269(5229):1427–1429.

50. Leong JC, Trobridge GD, Kim CH, Johnson M, Simon B. Interferon-inducible Mx proteins in fish. *Immunol Rev* 1998;166:349–363.

51. Ronni T, Matikainen S, Lehtonen A, et al. The proximal interferon-stimulated response elements are essential for interferon responsiveness: a promoter analysis of the antiviral MxA gene. *J Interferon Cytokine Res* 1998;18(9):773–781.

52. Kuhn R, Schwenk F, Aguet M, Rajewsky K. Inducible gene targeting in mice. *Biochem Genet* 1998;36(9–10):311–322.

53. Li Y, Youssoufian H. MxA over expression reveals a common genetic link in four Fanconi anemia complementation groups. *J Clin Invest* 1997;100(11):2873–2880.

54. Williams BRG. The role of the dsRNA-activated kinase PKR in cell regulation. *Biochem Soc Trans* 1997;25:509–513.

55. Clemens MJ, Elia A. The double-stranded RNA-dependent protein kinase PKR: structure and function. *J Interferon Cytokine Res* 1997;17(9):503–524.

56. Nanduri S, Carpick BW, Yang Y, Williams BRG, Qin J. Structure of the double-stranded RNA-binding domain of the protein kinase PKR reveals the molecular basis of its dsRNA-mediate activation. *EMBO J* 1998;17:5458–5465.

57. Zamanian-Daryoush M, Der SD, Williams BRG. Cell cycle regulation of the double stranded RNA activated protein kinase, PKR. *Oncogene* 1999;18:315–326.

58. Chu W-M, Ballard R, Carpick BW, Williams BRG, Schmid CW. Potential alu function: regulation of the activity of double-stranded RNA-activated kinase PKR. *Mol Cell Biol* 1998;18:58–68.

59. Der S, Yang Y-L, Weissmann C, Williams BRG. A PKR-dependent pathway mediating stress-induced apoptosis. *Proc Natl Acad Sci U S A* 1997;94:3279–3283.

60. Kumar A, Haque J, Locaste J, Hiscott J, Williams BRG. The dsRNA-dependent protein kinase, PKR, activates transcription factor NF-κB by phosphorylating IκB. *Proc Natl Acad Sci U S A* 1994;91:6288–6292.

61. Maran A, Maitra R, Kumar A, et al. Selective ablation of an mRNA target by 2-5A -antisense chimeras blocks NF-kB signaling. *Science* 1994;265:789–792.

62. Yang Y-L, Reis LFL, Pavlovic J, et al. Deficient signaling in mice devoid of double-stranded RNA-dependent protein kinase, PKR. *EMBO J* 1995;14:6095–6106.

63. Kumar A, Yang Y-L, Flati V, et al. Deficient cytokine signaling in mouse embryo fibroblasts with a targeted deletion in the PKR gene: role of IRF-1 and NFκB. *EMBO J* 1997;16:406–416.

64. Cheshire JL, Williams BR, Baldwin AS Jr. Involvement of double-stranded RNA-activated protein kinase in the synergistic activation of nuclear factor-kappaB by tumor necrosis factor-alpha and gamma-interferon in perineuronal cells. *J Biol Chem* 1999;19;274(8):4801–4806.

65. Katze MG. The war against the interferon-induced dsRNA-activated protein kinase: can viruses win? *Interferon Res* 1992;12(4):241–248.

66. Kalvakolanu DV. Virus interception of cytokine-regulated pathways. *Trends Microbiol* 1999;7(4):166–171.

67. Zhou AZ, Paranjape JM, Der SD, Williams BRG, Silverman RH. Interferon action in triply deficient mice reveals the existence of alternative pathways. *Virology* 1999;258:435–440.

68. Koromilas AE, Roy S, Barber GN, Katze MG, Sonenberg N. Malignant transformation by a mutant of the IFN-inducible dsRNA-dependent protein kinase. *Science* 1992;257(5077):1685–1689.

69. Meurs EF, Galabru J, Barber GN, Katze MG, Hovanessian AG. Tumor suppressor function of the interferon-induced double-stranded RNA-activated protein kinase. *Proc Natl Acad Sci U S A* 1993;90(1):232–236.

70. Haines GK, Cajulis R, Hayden R, Duda R, Talamonti M, Radosevich JA. Expression of the double-stranded RNA-dependent protein kinase (p68) in human breast tissues. *Tumour Biol* 1996;17(1):5–12.

71. Zhou Y, Gobl A, Wang S, et al. Expression of p68 protein kinase and its prognostic significance during IFN-alpha therapy in patients with carcinoid tumours. *Eur J Cancer* 1998;34(13):2046–2052.

72. Shimada A, Shiota G, Miyata H, et al. Aberrant expression of double-stranded RNA-dependent protein kinase in hepatocytes of chronic hepatitis and differentiated hepatocellular carcinoma. *Cancer Res* 1998;58(19):4434–4438.

73. Savinova O, Joshi B, Jagus R. Abnormal levels and minimal activity of the dsRNA-activated protein kinase, PKR, in breast carcinoma cells. *Int J Biochem Cell Biol* 1999;31(1):175–189.

74. Kumar KU, Srivastava SP, Kaufman RJ. Double-stranded RNA-activated protein kinase (PKR) is negatively regulated by 60S ribosomal subunit protein L18. *Mol Cell Biol* 1999;19(2):1116–1125.

75. Patel RC, Vestal DJ, Xu Z, Bandyopadhyay S, et al. DRBP76, a double-stranded RNA-binding nuclear protein, is phosphorylated by the interferon-induced protein kinase, PKR. *J Biol Chem* 1999;274(29):20432–20437.

76. Abraham N, Jaramillo ML, Duncan PI, et al. The murine PKR tumor suppressor gene is rearranged in a lymphocytic leukemia. *Exp Cell Res* 1998;244(2):394–404.

77. Raveh T, Hovanessian AG, Meurs EF, Sonenberg N, Kimchi A. Double-stranded RNA-dependent protein kinase mediates c-Myc suppression induced by type I interferons. *J Biol Chem* 1996; 271(41):25479–25484.

78. Shang Y, Baumrucker CR, Green MH. c-Myc is a major mediator of the synergistic growth inhibitory effects of retinoic acid and interferon in breast cancer cells. *J Biol Chem* 1998;273(46):30608–30613.

79. Ramana CK, Grammatikakis N, Chernov M, et al. Regulation of c-myc expression by IFN-gamma through stat1-dpendent and independent pathways. *EMBO J* 2000;19(2):263–272.

80. Dong B, Silverman RH. 2-5A-dependent RNase molecules dimerize during activation by 2-5A. *J Biol Chem* 1995;270(8):4133–4137.

81. Rebouillat D, Hovanessian AG. The human 2',5'-oligoadenylate synthetase family: interferon-induced proteins with unique enzymatic properties. *J Interferon Cytokine Res* 1999;19(4):295–308.

82. Zhou A, Hassel BA, Silverman RH. Expression cloning of 2-5A-dependent RNAase: a uniquely regulated mediator of interferon action. *Cell* 1993;72(5):753–765.

83. Squire J, Zhou A, Hassel BA, Nie H, Silverman RH. Localization of the interferon-induced, 2-5A-dependent Rnase gene (RNS4) to human chromosome 1q25. *Genomics* 1994;19(1):174–175.

84. Dong B, Silverman RH. A bipartite model of 2-5A-dependent RNase L. *J Biol Chem* 1997;272(35):22236–22242.

85. Zhou A, Paranjape J, Brown TL, et al. Interferon action and apoptosis are defective in mice devoid of 2',5'-oligoadenylate-dependent RNase L. *EMBO J* 1997;16(21):6355–6363.

86. Hassel BA, Zhou A, Sotomayor C, Maran A, Silverman RH. A dominant negative mutant of 2-5A-dependent Rnase suppresses antiproliferative and antiviral effects of interferon. *EMBO J* 1993;12(8):3297–3304.

87. Zhou A, Paranjape JM, Hassel BA, et al. Impact of RNase L over expression on viral and cellular growth and death. *J Interferon Cytokine Res* 1998;18(11):953–961.

88. Castelli JC, Hassel BA, Maran A, et al. The role of 2'-5' oligoadenylate-activated ribonuclease L in apoptosis. *Cell Death Differ* 1998; 5(4):313–320.

89. Castelli JC, Hassel BA, Wood KA, et al. A study of the interferon antiviral mechanism: apoptosis activation by the 2-5A system. *J Exp Med* 1997;186(6):967–972.

90. Diaz-Guerra M, Rivas C, Esteban M. Activation of the IFN-inducible enzyme RNase L causes apoptosis of animal cells. *Virology* 1997; 236(2):354–363.

91. Wang L, Zhou A, Vasavada S, et al. Elevated levels of 2',5'-linked oligoadenylate-dependent ribonuclease L occur as an early event in colorectal tumorigenesis. *Clin Cancer Res* 1995;1(11):1421–1428.

92. Maran A, Waller CF, Paranjape JM, et al. 2',5'-oligoadenylate-antisense chimeras cause RNase L to selectively degrade bcr/abl mRNA in chronic myelogenous leukemia cells. *Blood* 1998;92(11):4336–4343.

93. Kondo S, Kondo Y, Li G, Silverman RH, Cowell JK. Targeted therapy of human malignant glioma in a mouse model by 2-5A antisense directed against telomerase RNA. *Oncogene* 1998;16(25):3323–3330.

94. Kayagaki N, Yamaguchi N, Nakayama M, Eto H, Okumura K, Yagita H. Type I interferons (IFNs) regulate tumor necrosis factor-

related apoptosis-inducing ligand (TRAIL) expression on human T cells: a novel mechanism for the antitumor effects of type I IFNs. *J Exp Med* 1999;189(9):1451–1460.

95. Marrack P, Kappler J, Mitchell T. Type I interferons keep activated T cells alive. *J Exp Med* 1999;189(3):521–530.

96. Wang ZG, Ruggero D, Ronchetti S, et al. PML is essential for multiple apoptotic pathways. *Nat Genet* 1998;20(3):266–272.

97. Tanaka N, Sato M, Lamphier MS, et al. Type I interferons are essential mediators of apoptotic death in virally infected cells. *Genes Cells* 1998;3(1):29–37.

98. Sprent J, Zhang X, Sun S, Tough D. T-cell turnover *in vivo* and the role of cytokines. *Immunol Lett* 1999;65(1-2):21–25.

99. Boehm U, Klamp T, Groot M, Howard JC. Cellular responses to interferon-gamma. *Annu Rev Immunol* 1997;15:749–795.

100. York IA, Rock KL. Antigen processing and presentation by the class I major histocompatibility complex. *Annu Rev Immunol* 1996;14: 369–396.

101. van den Broek MF, Muller U, Huang S, Aguet M, Zinkernagel RM. Antiviral defense in mice lacking both alpha/beta and gamma-interferon receptors. *J Virol* 1995;69(8):4792–4796.

10.1

INTERFERON-α AND -β: CLINICAL APPLICATIONS

Leukemias, Lymphoma, and Multiple Myeloma

MOSHE TALPAZ
FARHAD RAVANDI
RAZELLE KURZROCK
ZEEV ESTROV
HAGOP M. KANTARJIAN

The description of the viral inhibitory factor termed *interferon* (IFN) by Isaacs and Lindenman in 1957 (1) can be considered one of the first steps in the development of the field of biotherapy in medicine. Considerable progress in understanding the biology and clinical effects of these agents has led to their increased applications in various fields of medicine, including oncology. Hematologic malignancies in which applications of IFN have been extensively studied include chronic myelogenous leukemia (CML), hairy cell leukemia (HCL), follicular lymphomas, cutaneous T-cell lymphoma, and multiple myeloma (2).

Three types of IFNs have been identified in humans and are designated as IFN-α, IFN-β, and IFN-γ. These are produced by a variety of cells but most specifically by leukocytes, fibroblasts, and T-lymphocytes, respectively. IFN-α and IFN-β, collectively known as *type I IFNs*, are coded by genes located on chromosome 9. They share approximately 40% homology and act on cells through a common receptor (3). IFN-γ has little homology to type I IFNs, is classed as type II IFN, and is coded by a gene on chromosome 12 (4).

Interferons have potent effects on cell proliferation, although the mechanisms responsible for their antiproliferative effects remain unclear. The downregulation of the proto-oncogene c-myc and the induction of the enzyme 2',5'-oligoadenylate synthetase may be involved (5,6). Various immunomodulatory effects of IFNs have been described, including enhancement of cytotoxic activity of natural killer (NK) cells, stimulation of release of other cytokines, and increased expression of major histocompatibility antigens on the cell surface (7–9).

Research into cellular effects of IFNs—in particular, IFN-α—has shed light into possible mechanisms of their antitumor activity. Type I IFNs have been shown to induce G_1 arrest in hematopoietic target cells. This arrest is mediated by a number of biochemical events, including inhibition of c-myc expression (10), inhibition of phosphorylation of retinoblastoma protein (11–14), and downmodulation of E2F activity (15). Cell cycle progression is regulated by proteins known as *cyclins*, which activate cyclin-dependent kinases (CDKs), a process counterbalanced by CDK inhibitors (16). IFN-α has been shown to induce the expression of CDK inhibitors, including p21/WAF1, p15, and p16^{INK4} (17–19). The upregulation of these inhibitors is responsible for the downregulation of phosphorylation of retinoblastoma protein and G_1 arrest of cells (17–19).

IFN-α has also been demonstrated to be an inducer of apoptosis in certain cell lines by a mechanism independent of its antiproliferative effects (20,21). The exact mechanism of IFN-induced apoptosis remains unclear, but it likely involves effects on various families of proteins involved in controlling programmed cell death, including the Bcl-2/Bax family of proteins, the ICE^4/Ced-3 proteases, and the tumor necrosis factor/Fas receptor family.

This chapter reviews the clinical applications of IFNs in hematologic malignancies.

INTERFERON THERAPY OF CHRONIC MYELOGENOUS LEUKEMIA

CML is a chronic myeloproliferative disorder with an initial, chronic course lasting 3 to 5 years (22–24). It eventually transforms into accelerated and blastic phases, which are generally fatal. CML was one of the first diseases in which a specific chromosomal abnormality was identified: (9;22) (q34;q11), or Philadelphia chromosome.

TABLE 1. OUTCOME OF M. D. ANDERSON CANCER CENTER INTERFERON-α THERAPY FOR PHILADELPHIA POSITIVE CHRONIC MYELOGENOUS LEUKEMIA

Patients treated	274 (100%)
Complete hematologic response	219 (80%)
Cytogenetic responses	159 (58%)
Complete	72 (26%) } 38%
Partial [≤35%, Philadelphia	32 (12%) major
chromosome (Ph)]	
Minor	55 (20%)

From Talpaz M, Kantarjian HM, O'Brien S, Kurzrock R. The M. D. Anderson Cancer Center experience with interferon-α therapy in chronic myelogenous leukemia. In: Goldman JM, ed. *Clinical haematology.* London: Baillière Tindall, 1997:291–305, with permission.

Until the introduction of IFN-α in 1981, CML was traditionally treated with hydroxyurea (25,26). After a large body of clinical studies, IFN-α became the mainstay of CML nontransplant–based therapy. In this chapter, clinical studies with IFN-α in CML are summarized, and possible mechanisms of action of IFN leading to this rewarding clinical effect are discussed.

Interferon-α in Chronic Myelogenous Leukemia: Single Agent Studies

The initial demonstration of IFN activity in newly diagnosed CML patients was published by a team from M. D. Anderson Cancer Center (MDACC) (27–30). This work was subsequently expanded with results that confirmed initial observations. Their update is summarized in Table 1 (31). In this study, patients were administered an intended 5 MU per m² treatment dose of IFN-α; these patients were monitored frequently (every 3 to 4 months) for hematologic and cytogenetic changes. Additional studies from other institutions confirmed the MDACC studies, but failed in general to demonstrate a similar response rate (Table 2) (32–35).

Although most of these early studies demonstrated lower hematologic and cytogenetic response rates, several centers were able to reproduce in full the MDACC experience by adhering to similarly intensive dose regimes. It appears that doses of IFN-α influence hematologic and cytogenetic response rates; this notion was challenged, however, by Schofield et al., who demonstrated a high response rate with low doses of IFN-α (32). Nevertheless, these studies failed to address disease prognostic features; thus, they may have introduced a patient selection bias that could have had a major impact on IFN-α response outcomes.

In the MDACC study, a high response rate was demonstrated in low-risk patients, shown in Table 3 (31). It is apparent, therefore, that responses to IFN-α are influenced by characteristics of a study's patient population (and, most likely, by treatment intensity as well). Accordingly, a metaanalysis of a series of phase II studies or a comparison of studies from different centers may be problematic, unless they adhere to strict analysis by disease prognostic features.

This observation applies to newly diagnosed patients, and initial studies indicated poor responses in long-standing disease. Although hematologic responses were frequently seen in patients with long-standing CML—albeit to a lesser extent than in newly diagnosed patients—major cytogenetic responses were uncommon. Thus, resistance to IFN-α is slow to develop, although failure to induce cytogenetic response occurs early in the disease. These findings imply that cytogenetic responses may depend on a pool of "normal" stem cells that are depleted at a rapid pace, whereas true resistance of malignant clones are slow to develop and occur much later in the course of disease.

Survival Outcome: Summary of M. D. Anderson Cancer Center Experience and Randomized Studies

The survival outcome of patients treated at MDACC has been published on several occasions and was updated with patient follow-ups exceeding 10 years (29–31). A median survival of 89 months and a survival rate of 40% were noted in patients at 10 years' follow-up, compared to a rather negligible number of patients alive at 10 years with standard chemotherapy (Fig. 1)

TABLE 2. RESULTS OF SINGLE-ARM INTERFERON-α STUDIES

Study (Reference)	No. of Patients	IFN Dose Intended	Complete Hematologic Response (%)	Cytogenetic Responses (%)		
				Any	Major	Complete
Kantarjian et al. (31) (MDACC)	274	5×10^6 U/m²	80	58	38	26
Mahon et al. (175)	52	5×10^6 U/m²	81	—	49	—
Ozer et al. (176)	107	5×10^6 U/m²ᵃ	59	21	18	—
Niederle et al. (177)	40	—	56	40	—	—
Alimena et al. (33)	63	5×10^6 U/m² t.i.w., and 2×10^6 U/m², t.i.w.	46	70	2	—
Freund et al. (34)	10	5×10^6 U/m² t.i.w.	33	0	0	0
Anger et al. (35)	9	3×10^6 U/m² t.i.w.	22	20	0	0
Schofield et al. (32)	27	2×10^6 U/m²/d for 1 mo, followed by 2×10^6 U/m² t.i.w.	70	33	22	7

MDACC, M. D. Anderson Cancer Center.
ᵃReport states significant dose reduction.
From Talpaz M, Kantarjian HM, O'Brien S, Kurzrock. R The M. D. Anderson Cancer Center experience with interferon-α therapy in chronic myelogenous leukemia. In: Goldman JM, ed. *Clinical haematology.* London: Baillière Tindall, 1997:291–305, with permission.

TABLE 3. RESPONSE AND SURVIVAL BY PROGNOSTIC RISK GROUPS

Prognostic Model	Risk Group	No. of Patients (%)[a]	Proportion with Major Cytogenetic Response (%)	p Value	Median Survival (mo)	p Value
MDACC overall	Good	115 (48)	48	.09	102	.01
	Intermediate	86 (36)	38		82	
	Poor	38 (16)	26		56	
MDACC clinical	Good	115 (49)	52	<.01	102	<.01
	Intermediate	85 (36)	36		90	
	Poor	37 (16)	14		47	
Synthesis	1	149 (59)	48	<.01	102	<.01
	2	57 (23)	32		95	
	3	35 (14)	20		62	
	4	10 (4)	0		41	
Sokal et al. (36)	Good	124 (52)	52	<.01	104	.01
	Intermediate	59 (25)	32		90	
	Poor	54 (23)	24		62	

MDACC, M. D. Anderson Cancer Center.

[a]Percentage of evaluable patients.

From Talpaz M, Kantarjian HM, O'Brien S, Kurzrock R. The M. D. Anderson Cancer Center experience with interferon-α therapy in chronic myelogenous leukemia. In: Goldman JM, ed. *Clinical haematology*. London: Baillière Tindall, 1997:291–305, with permission.

(36). This impact on survival was a result of excellent survival among complete cytogenetic and partial cytogenetic responders. The impact of these responses on survival was demonstrated in a landmark analysis (Fig. 2), a study that can be criticized for not being randomized against a control group, thereby allowing possible factors unrelated to therapy, such as change in time of initial diagnosis (earlier diagnosis), to influence survival outcome. This study does provide information on very long patient follow-up, however, and appears to complement survival data from randomized studies by demonstrating long follow-up data not available in randomized trial summaries. The data are, therefore, much less subjected to impact on survival by disease-related prognostic features.

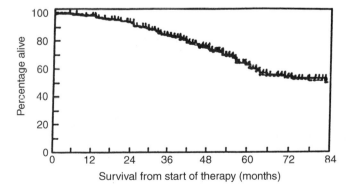

FIGURE 1. Survival of chronic myelogenous leukemia patients treated with interferon-α (total of patients, 274; number of patients who died, 92) (after censoring those who underwent allogeneic bone marrow transplantation—total number of patients, 274; number of patients who died, 104). (From Talpaz M, Kantarjian HM, O'Brien S, Kurzrock R. The M.D. Anderson Cancer Center experience with interferon-α therapy in chronic myelogenous leukemia. In: JM Goldman, ed. *Clinical haematology*. London: Baillière Tindall, 1997:291–305, with permission.)

Survival Outcome in Randomized Studies

Several randomized studies comparing IFN-α therapy with chemotherapy have been published; four are summarized in Table 4 (37–42). Three of these studies demonstrate survival advantage for patients treated with IFN-α. An average survival benefit of 20 months was demonstrated in Italian and United Kingdom studies. In a German study, IFN-α was found to be significantly superior to busulphan, although it only modestly prolonged survival over hydroxyurea (a difference that was not significant statistically). A difference in patient populations may explain some differences in these studies (such as inclusion of accelerated-disease patients in the German study), but differences in INF-α dosage may account for some of the differences. An update of the German study demonstrates that IFN-α is superior to hydroxyurea in low-risk patients.

Randomized studies were subjected to rigorous analysis by the CML Trialists' Collaborative Group (42). Using standard methods, these trials were analyzed individually and collectively. This analysis finds an overall improvement in survival among IFN- versus hydroxyurea-treated patients, with 26% reduction in odds of death (2p = .0001) [95%, confidence interval (CI) of 11% to 38%]. Furthermore, differences between different trial outcomes are consistent with chance effects. This analysis also indicates IFN-associated survival advantage for all disease prognostic groups.

Although many factors may contribute to survival prolongation with IFN-α, delay of blast crisis is probably the most significant one, demonstrated in the Italian study (37). Compared to the MDACC study, randomized studies resort to short follow-up, and early analysis focuses on a moderate gain in average survival (whereas a more significant impact on survival may be noted in a subset of patients at a much longer follow-up). Because survival benefits were noted even with low treatment doses, an erroneous conclusion may be reached that treatment intensity has only marginal significance. Its real benefit, however, may lie in complete and partial cytogenetic

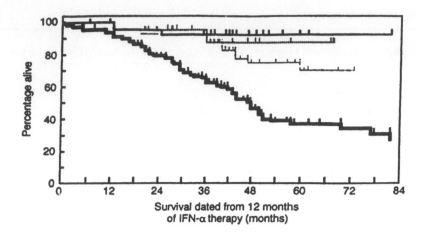

FIGURE 2. Estimated survival by response 12 months post–interferon-α (IFN-α) (landmark analysis). (From Talpaz M, Kantarjian HM, O'Brien S, Kurzrock R. The M. D. Anderson Cancer Center experience with interferon-α therapy in chronic myelogenous leukemia. In: Goldman JM, ed. *Clinical haematology.* London: Baillière Tindall, 1997:291–305, with permission.)

Total	Dead	Cytogenetic response at 12 months	
29	2	Complete	—————
22	2	Partial	··············
69	15	Minor	—————
138	67	None	—————

responses, whose survival benefits may be observed late in the course of disease and not detected when median survivals are compared in randomized studies [e.g., the duration-of-survival advantage with IFN in the Italian study is similar to that in the Medical Research Council (MRC) trials, which used much lower doses of IFN, although IFN-α dose intensity may actually have a dramatic impact on the incidence of long-term survivors]. Although the single-arm studies at MDACC are subjected to criticism, the analysis of survival outcome among the 274 patients treated with IFN-α as single-agent therapy demonstrates a median survival of 89 months (see Fig. 1). Perhaps more significant, however, are the unique survival patterns emerging for subsets of patients according to degrees of cytogenetic responses (see Fig. 2), and the notion that long-term survival of IFN-α–treated CML patients may be strongly influenced by degree of cytogenetic response. A substantial percentage of CML patients may live 10 years or more if the patterns of survival observed in Figs. 1 and 2 are maintained, representing a remarkable quantitative shift in the paradigm established by Sokal et al., who demonstrated only a negligible number of patients alive with CML at

10 years of follow-up when treated with standard chemotherapy (36).

Cytogenetic Responses

Cytogenetic responses have been observed in virtually all IFN-α studies in CML. Their incidences, however, varied greatly, from 22% of patients in the MRC trial to 58% of patients in the MDACC study (31,39). Incidences of complete and partial cytogenetic response also vary. Impacts of complete and partial cytogenetic responses on survival were demonstrated in most of the large studies. In the MRC study, the 5-year survival rates of complete, partial, minor, and no cytogenetic responders were 100%, 92%, 59%, and 47%, respectively ($p = .004$) (39). Similarly, the 3-year survival of the 7% of patients who achieved complete cytogenetic remission was 100%, compared with 72% survival for other patients ($p = .2$). In the Italian study, those patients who achieved cytogenetic response within 24 months had a 5-year survival of 88%, versus 65% survival for other patients ($p <.01$) (37). Impact of cytogenetic response is best demonstrated by the MDACC study (31). A

TABLE 4. COMPARISON OF SURVIVAL OUTCOME OF INTERFERON-α VERSUS CHEMOTHERAPY IN RANDOMIZED STUDIES

Study (Reference)	No. of Patients	Survival (Mo)		*p* Value
		Interferon	Chemotherapy	
Italian Cooperative Study Group on Chronic Myeloid Leukemia (37)	322	72	52	.002
Hehlmann et al. (38)	513	66	45 (busulphan)	.008
			56 (hydroxyurea)	.44
Allan et al. (39)	587	61	41	<.001
Ohnishi et al. (40)	159	54% at 5 yr	325 at 5 yr for busulphan	.029

From Talpaz M, Kantarjian HM, O'Brien S, Kurzrock R. The M. D. Anderson Cancer Center experience with interferon-α therapy in chronic myelogenous leukemia. In: Goldman JM, ed. *Clinical haematology.* London: Baillière Tindall, 1997:291–305, with permission.

TABLE 5. SUMMARY OF PROPORTIONAL HAZARDS REGRESSION MODEL RELATING FIXED AND TIME-VARYING COVARIATES TO SURVIVAL OUTCOMES

Factor	Multiplier (95% Confidence Interval)	p Value
Fixed		
Spleen size[a]	1.62 (1.05–2.49)	.029
Marrow basophils[b]	1.82 (1.18–2.80)	.007
Time-varying		
Complete or partial response[c]	0.21 (0.11–0.39)	.0001

[a]Baseline group: spleen size smaller than 5 cm.
[b]Baseline group: percentage of basophils less than 3%.
[c]Baseline group: other responses.
From Talpaz M, Kantarjian HM, O'Brien S, Kurzrock R. The M. D. Anderson Cancer Center experience with interferon-α therapy in chronic myelogenous leukemia. In: Goldman JM, ed. *Clinical haematology*. London: Baillière Tindall, 1997:291–305, with permission.

landmark analysis demonstrates the respective survival impacts of complete and partial cytogenetic remissions obtained at 12 months of IFN therapy (see Fig. 2). Furthermore, a multivariate regression analysis demonstrates the independent effect of cytogenetic responses on survival (Table 5). This impact is maintained in all pretherapy prognostic groups and overrides their impact on survival (Table 6). As is observed in Table 6, incidences of cytogenetic responses decrease with worsening of disease characteristics. Survival of all patients with cytogenetic responses is virtually constant regardless of prognostic groups, however.

Studies of Minimal Residual Disease and Interferon-α Therapy

Patients with complete cytogenetic remission were subjected to a series of studies that exploited the characterization of the molecular abnormality in Ph-positive CML.

Southern blot DNA hybridization with BCR probe confirmed that complete cytogenetic responses are also associated with disappearance of rearranged BCR bands (43). Neverthe-

less, standard cytogenetics and Southern blot have relatively low levels of sensitivity for detecting residual disease at a 3% to 5% level (44).

Western blot, which is conducted at MDACC with an antibody directed against an ABL epitope, provides information on the ratio between BCR-ABL and ABL protein, a ratio that correlates well with cytogenetic tests and perhaps has a higher level of sensitivity (45).

Fluorescent *in situ* hybridization (FISH) has become a useful technique after a modification developed at MDACC. Hypermetaphase FISH (HMF) is theoretically capable of detecting 0.2% of residual disease. Accordingly, we were able to detect residual disease among patients previously defined as complete cytogenetic responders by standard cytogenetics (Table 7) (45).

Finally, studies using reverse-transcriptase polymerase chain reaction (RT-PCR) amplification of the BCR-ABL RNA transcript were introduced to MDACC in the late 1980s. These tests possessed a theoretical level of resolution several thousandfold higher than the standard cytogenetic test. In the initial analysis, residual disease was detected in 17 of 18 studied patients (46). In an update, however, a reversal of this situation was observed, with 10 of 18 studied patients not demonstrating residual transcripts (47). The major difference between the current study and the previous one is the much longer follow-up of patients in complete cytogenetic remission [42 months for polymerase chain reaction (PCR)–negative patients; 21 months for PCR-positive patients] (Table 8). RT-PCR data in CML vary with different laboratories; at least one reason for this variance is a marked difference in sensitivity of assays (48). The achievement of BCR-ABL negativity by RT-PCR is not necessarily consistent with disease elimination. Based on cytogenetic results, treatment with IFN-α was discontinued in 30 patients at MDACC. Disease relapse occurred in ten of these patients; the remaining 20 patients remained in unmaintained and sustained complete cytogenetic response for an average period of 6 years (1+ to 11+ years) (49). Samples from seven of these patients were tested by high-sensitivity PCRs; residual disease was detected in four of them, despite long and uninter-

TABLE 6. CYTOGENETIC RESPONSE STATUS AT 12 MONTHS AND SURVIVAL WITHIN PROGNOSTIC GROUPS (SYNTHESIS MODEL)

Prognostic Risk Group	Cytogenetic Response	No. of Patients	No. Deceased	Estimated Percentage Surviving[a]		
				At 2 Yr	At 4 Yr	p Value
Good	Yes	73	13	93	79	<.01
	No	68	29	86	62	
Intermediate	Yes	25	4	95	82[b]	<.01
	No	31	18	76	35[b]	
High	Yes	9	1	100[b]	83[b]	<.01
	No	31	18	68	39	

Note: Survival rate from 1 yr after start of interferon-α therapy. p Values are from logarithmic rank tests comparing differences in survival curves of different cytogenetic response groups within prognostic groups.
[a]Estimated percentages of patients surviving 3 and 5 yr after starting interferon-α therapy.
[b]Estimate based on fewer than ten patients at risk.
From Talpaz M, Kantarjian HM, O'Brien S, Kurzrock R. The M. D. Anderson Cancer Center experience with interferon-α therapy in chronic myelogenous leukemia. In: Goldman JM, ed. *Clinical haematology*. London: Baillière Tindall, 1997:291–305, with permission.

TABLE 7. NUMBER OF PATIENTS IN CYTOGENETIC RESPONSE CATEGORIES AS DETERMINED BY STANDARD KARYOTYPE ANALYSIS AND THEIR CLASSIFICATION AS DETERMINED BY HYPERMETAPHASE FLUORESCENCE *IN SITU* HYBRIDIZATION

| | No. | Cytogenetic Response (Standard Cytogenetics) | | Cytogenetic Response (HMF) | |
		None	Minor	Partial	Complete
None	16	11	5	—	—
Minor	9	2	7	—	—
Partial	6	—	2	4	—
Complete	19	—	—	3	16
Unknown	8	—	2	2	4

HMF, hypermetaphase FISH.
From Talpaz M, Kantarjian HM, O'Brien S, Kurzrock R. The M. D. Anderson Cancer Center experience with interferon-α therapy in chronic myelogenous leukemia. In: Goldman JM, ed. *Clinical haematology*. London: Baillière Tindall, 1997:291–305, with permission.

rupted remissions (M Talpaz, *unpublished data*). These results support our observations on detectable residual disease in these patients, and provide findings consistent with establishment of tumor dormancy.

Analytic methods used greatly improved understanding of residual disease after IFN-α therapy, especially with active changes in quantity of residual disease occurring post–cytogenetic remission. They suggest an ongoing process of residual disease depletion occurs that requires several additional years of therapy. This information implies there is a need to continue IFN-α therapy for several years beyond complete remission. It is apparent, however, that a quantitative assessment of residual disease (in addition to qualitative assessment by PCR) is required to evaluate the impact of residual disease on disease relapse patterns.

Information that the association between residual disease and sustained remission is not purely quantitative exists, however. Residual disease was demonstrated in patients with ongoing sustained complete remission. Furthermore, residual disease was also demonstrated in PCR–negative remission when myeloid and erythroid colonies from the same patients were analyzed by PCR (50). We postulated, therefore, that mechanisms such as specific immune recognition may operate at that particular disease setting.

Interferon-α Combination Therapy of Chronic Myelogenous Leukemia

The effect of IFN combined with low-dose cytosine arabinoside (ARA-C) was examined at MDACC in two separate studies in which IFN was administered at 5 MU per m^2, whereas ARA-C

TABLE 8. CYTOGENETIC REMISSION DURATION AND POLYMERASE CHAIN REACTION STATUS OF 18 CHRONIC MYELOGENOUS LEUKEMIA PATIENTS WITH LONG-TERM RESPONSES

| Patient | Bone Marrow (BM) or Blood (Bl)[b] | RT-PCR Results[a] | | Continuous Complete Cytogenetic Remission Duration (Mo) |
		Positive vs. Negative	Junction Found to Be Positive (b2–a2 or b3–a2)	
1	BM	Positive	b3–2a	34
2	BM–Bl	Negative–negative	NA	85
3	BM–Bl	Negative–negative	NA	48
4	BM	Positive	b3–a2	63
5	Bl	Positive	b3–a2	23
6	BM–Bl	Negative–negative	NA	58
7	BM	Positive	b3–a2	17
8	BM–Bl	Negative–negative	NA	31
9	BM	Negative	NA	41
10	BM	Positive	b2–a2	12
11	BM	Negative	NA	69
12	BM–Bl	Negative–negative	NA	43
13	BM–Bl	Negative–negative	NA	24
14	Bl	Negative	NA	13
15	BM	Positive	b2–a2 and b3–a2	24
16	BM	Positive	b2–a2	19
17	Bl	Negative	NA	29
18	Bl	Positive	b3–a2	16

NA, not applicable; PCR, polymerase chain reaction; RT, reverse transcriptase.
[a]All samples listed showed positive results for PCR amplification of normal antigen-binding lymphocyte.
[b]Where BM–Bl is listed, both bone marrow and blood from the same date were available and tested.
From Talpaz M, Kantarjian HM, O'Brien S, Kurzrock R. The M. D. Anderson Cancer Center experience with interferon-α therapy in chronic myelogenous leukemia. In: Goldman JM, ed. *Clinical haematology*. London: Baillière Tindall, 1997:291–305, with permission.

TABLE 9. INTERFERON (IFN)-α PLUS LOW-DOSE CYTOSINE ARABINOSIDE IN PH-POSITIVE EARLY CHRONIC PHASE CHRONIC MYELOGENOUS LEUKEMIA

Parameter	IFN + LD ARA-C, 7 D/Mo	IFN + LD ARA-C, Daily
CHR (%)	84	95
CG response (%)		
Overall	64	78, *p* = .08
Major	38	53, *p* = .10
Complete	20	30
3-yr survival (%)	78	84

ARA-C, cytosine arabinoside; CG, cytogenic; CHR, complete hematologic response; IFN, interferon; LD, low-dose; Ph, Philadelphia chromosome.

was administered at two different doses and schedules: In study I (1989), ARA-C was administered at 15 mg per m^2 daily × 7 days, every 30 days. In study II (1993), ARA-C was administered at 10 mg daily. Results of the study indicate an improvement in hematologic and cytogenetic responses of IFN-α single therapy and are summarized in Table 9 (51). These results were also demonstrated in a large randomized French study that noted survival benefit for combination therapy (52,53).

The combination does not worsen IFN-α–induced toxicities because it frequently requires dose reduction due to myelosuppression. Although additional studies may be required, the combination is likely to become the standard of care in CML.

The effect of combining IFN-α and intensive chemotherapy was examined in a study at MDACC (Kantarjian et al., *unpublished data*). Seventy-four patients were included in the study; all were administered a standard dose of IFN-α (5 mIU per m^2). For 16 patients who failed to achieve hematologic or cytogenetic responses, however, at lease one course of intensive chemotherapy was added to treatment. This chemotherapy consisted of daunorubicin, vincristine, a standard dose of ARA-C, and prednisone. Although only a minority of patients received this additional therapy, an impact on survival occurred. Fifty-five percent of patients were alive at 10 years and beyond, implying (although it requires confirmation) that the intensive chemotherapy probably delayed transition to blastic crisis among the high-risk patients subjected to this treatment.

Interferon-α: Mechanism of Action

Although several groups of investigators have studied the role of IFN-α in CML, its mechanism of action in CML remains largely unknown. The reasons for these problems may lie with the unique growth features of CML, which behaves more like a premalignant disease. CML Ph-positive cell lines can be established only from the blast crisis phase of the disease, a stage mostly resistant to IFN-α. Other *in vitro* systems, such as short-term clonogenic growth assays or long-term bone marrow culture assays, failed to simulate the disease pattern of benign-phase CML; therefore, their usefulness may be limited. Animal models, either BCR-ABL transgenic mice or severe combined immunodeficiency mice xenotransplanted with human CML, develop hematopoietic abnormalities that follow only in part the typical phenotype of CML in humans.

A number of mechanisms of IFN-α action have been proposed to play a role in CML, including induction of FAS and its ligand on CML progenitors, thereby facilitating cell death of early stem-cell populations (54,55). Adhesion defects of CML progenitors that disrupt their ability to adhere to bone marrow stromal layers were proposed as major pathophysiologic defects in CML. These defects were attributed to an abnormal function of integrin α4α5/β1 receptors that affects their binding to fibronectin, a defect shown to be partially corrected with IFN-α (56). Suppression of CML cells by a cellular immune system has also been proposed to be a possible mode of action of IFN-α, and may explain long-term complete cytogenetic remission in spite of the presence of residual disease (50). IFN-α may possess all of these activities, which may operate at different times during the course of therapy. Understanding this mechanism of action is critical to the rational development of the next therapeutic modality for CML because it allows exploitation of the unique activities demonstrated by IFN-α.

INTERFERON THERAPY IN HAIRY CELL LEUKEMIA

HCL, a malignant proliferation of cells of lymphoid lineage associated with splenomegaly, pancytopenia, and recurrent infections, was the initial U.S. Food and Drug Administration–approved indication for IFN therapy. HCL was first described by Bouroncle et al., who referred to it as *leukemic reticuloendotheliosis* (57). The name *hairy cell leukemia* was coined by Schreck and Donelly to describe its characteristic morphology (58). Approximately 90% of patients with HCL require treatment during the course of their disease. Quesada et al. first reported on achievement of remission in seven patients with HCL using partially purified IFN-α, with three patients obtaining complete remissions and four obtaining partial remissions (59). Similar results were later obtained with recombinant IFN-α preparations (60,61). In these reports, nine and 22 patients, respectively, were treated with IFN-α-2b, 2 MIU per m^2, subcutaneously, three times per week, and frequent partial responses were observed. Other studies using IFN-α-2a reported major response rates together with significant complete responses (62–65). These studies demonstrated an overall response rate of 89%, including 9% complete response, 71% partial response, and 10% minor response (66) (Table 10).

IFN-α is effective as initial therapy and as therapy in patients with disease progression after splenectomy. Although the majority of these responses are partial responses, most patients with remissions have normal blood counts, with only a few residual hairy cells in the bone marrow and without predisposition to infections, the factors responsible for disease morbidity and mortality. Normalization of platelet count usually occurs after 2 months; normalization of hemoglobin and neutrophil counts usually takes longer, 4 to 5 months. Recovery of immune status accompanies the increases in blood counts with restoration of NK-cell and T-lymphocyte activity; these are associated with a decrease in incidence of infections.

In a small number of patients (5% to 10%) developments of neutralizing antibodies to recombinant preparations results in

TABLE 10. SELECTED TRIALS OF RECOMBINANT INTERFERON-α THERAPY IN HAIRY CELL LEUKEMIA

Study (Reference)	Patient (No.)	Response (%)			
		Complete	Partial	Minor	None
Quesada et al. (62)	30	30	60	10	0
Foon et al. (75)	14	7	86	0	7
Rai et al. (65)	25	28	24	48	0
Golomb (64)	195	4	78	5	13
Total	264	9	71	10	10

IFN-resistance (67,68). This resistance can be overcome using the partially pure IFN-α preparations (69).

Necessary duration of IFN-α therapy was examined by several studies (64,70); 12 months of IFN-α therapy was recommended as optimal. Most investigators have suggested that discontinuation of IFN-α results in relapse in most patients, however, with relapses responding to a reinstitution of IFN-α (2).

Because IFN-α therapy is associated with significant toxic side effects, low-dose IFN-α (0.2 MIU per m²) was administered and examined for 6 to 12 months to minimize toxicity (71). Although toxicity was minimal, only 54% of patients had responses. Also, low-dose IFN-α was shown to be an ineffective regimen in treatment of relapse after previous IFN therapy (72). Therefore, low-dose regimens cannot be recommended in therapy of patients with HCL. At least 23 different IFN-α alleles have been identified, coding for 15 different proteins. Two approved IFN-α preparations are IFN-α-2a (Roferon-A) (Hoffman-La Roche, Nutley, NJ) and IFN-α-2b (Intron A) (Schering, Kenilworth, NJ). These differ only in amino acid residue at position 23, with IFN-α-2a having a cysteine residue and IFN-α-2b having an arginine residue at this position. The current suggested regimen for treatment of HCL is IFN-α, 2 MIU per m², three times per week for 12 to 18 months. Few studies of IFN-β and IFN-γ in the therapy of HCL exist, and they do not appear to have any advantage over IFN-α in response or toxicity (73,74).

The exact mechanisms of action of IFNs in HCL are not clear. NK cells are known to be deficient in HCL, and efficacy of IFNs in inducing NK cell activity may be important (75–77). HCL cells have been shown to be resistant to NK cell lysis; therefore, recovery of NK cell function cannot be the only mechanism of IFN effects (75,76). The antiproliferative and differentiating effects of IFNs demonstrated in other cell lines are also likely to be important (78,79). Interferons stimulate HLA-deoxyribose (DR) antigen expression in HCL cells. Increased expression of class II major histocompatibility antigens facilitates T-cell–mediated cytotoxic activity, which may be important in the antitumor effects of IFNs. Several different mechanisms of action, therefore, may account for the therapeutic effect of IFN-α.

The use of nucleoside analogues pentostatin (2-deoxycoformycin [DCF]) and cladarabine (2-chlorodeoxyadenosine [2CDA]) has changed the management of HCL. Pentostatin, an adenine deaminase inhibitor, administered at a dose of 4 mg per m² every 2 weeks, produced complete responses and partial responses in 50% and 25% of patients, respectively (80,81). Toxicity associated with this therapy is generally mild and remissions are durable. Patients who have not experienced success with previous IFN therapy do respond to pentostatin (81).

Cladarabine, an adenine-deaminase–resistant purine analogue, has been administered at a dose of 0.1 mg per kg per day by continuous infusion for 7 days, achieving an 80% complete response rate, with most of the remaining 20% of patients experiencing good partial responses (66,82). Again, toxicity of the drug is mild and limited to transient fevers and neutropenia. The responses, including partial responses, are durable, and the few patients who relapse respond to a second course of cladarabine. These drugs have been approved by the U.S. Food and Drug Administration for the treatment of HCL. At present, therefore, IFNs, although effective agents in therapy of HCL, should be considered as second-line agents used for the few patients who do not respond to one or two courses of cladarabine and pentostatin.

With the use of these effective treatments, relevance of long-term outcome in patients with HCL has become more significant. Kurzrock et al. compared survival of patients referred to a single institution before and after the availability of IFN-α and 2CDA therapy and noted significantly different 5- and 10-year rates (67% versus 89% and 64% versus 84%, respectively, *p* = .0009) (Fig. 3) (83). Overall mortality, however, still exceeded that in the general population, due to neutropenia-related infections (83).

Previous epidemiologic studies suggested that HCL patients were twice as likely as other cancer patients to have second malignancies (84). It has been postulated that their impaired immune functions, including impaired NK cell activity, may predispose these patients to a second cancer. It has been suggested also that the immune impairments associated with treat-

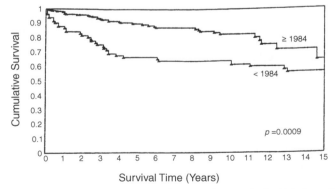

FIGURE 3. Kaplan-Meier analysis of actuarial survival of 265 hairy cell leukemia patients referred after January 1, 1984, compared with 85 patients referred before that date. (From Kurgrock R, Strom SS, Estey E, et al. Second cancer risk in hairy cell leukemia: analysis of 350 patients. *J Clin Oncol* 1997;15:1803–1810, with permission.)

TABLE 11. TRIALS OF COMBINED INTERFERON (IFN)–CHEMOTHERAPY INDUCTION IN MULTIPLE MYELOMA

Study (Reference)	No. of Patients		Chemotherapy	IFN Dose (MIU/m^2/wk)	Response (CR + PR)	
	IFN	Controls			IFN (%)	Controls (%)
Aitchison (107)	15	16	CP	3.8	53	25
Aviles (108)	52	51	VMCP/V-MTZ-CP/BepiVDex	9.4	81	47
Capnist (109)	15	14	MP	3.8	58	64
Casassus (110)	102	99	VMCP/VBAP	6.0	52	36
Cooper (111)	138	134	MP	3.0	38	44
Corrado (112)	33	29	MP	7.5	45	48
Galvez (113)	24	23	VABP	9.4	63	39
Garcia-Larana (114)	26	28	MP	11.7	62	54
Joshua (115)	59	54	PCAB	9.4	41	48
Ludwig (174)	125	131	VMCP	6.3	67	62
Montuoro (116)	51	44	MP	4.7	86	68
Nordic Myeloma Study Group (117)	297	286	MP	9.4	44	45
Osterborg (118)	164	171	MP	11.7	68	42
Scheithauer (119)	15	17	VMCP	6.3	67	35
Vela Ojeda (120)	18	18	VMCP	7.0	94	78
Vela Ojeda (120)	20	17	MP	7.0	80	71
Total	**1,154**	**1,132**	—	—	**54.4**	**45.9**

BepiVDex, BCNU, epirubicin, vincristine, dexamethasone; CR, complete response; CP, cyclophosphamide; IFN, interferon; PCAB, prednisone, cyclophosphamide, actinomycin D, bleomycin; PR, partial response; VABP, vincristine, actinomycin D, bleomycin, and prednisone; VMCP, vincristine, melphalan, cyclophosphamide, and prednisone; V-MTZ-CP, vincristine, mitoxantrone, cyclophosphamide, and prednisone.

ment with IFN-α, 2CDA, and DCF could contribute to this tendency (83,85). Kurzrock et al. studied 350 HCL patients treated in a 27-year period and found 26 patients (7.4%) with a second cancer developing at least 6 months after the HCL diagnosis (83). This increase, however, did not reach statistical significance and was not associated with therapy with IFN-α, 2CDA, or DCF (83). Other smaller studies have been conflicting in their results (86–88).

INTERFERON THERAPY IN MULTIPLE MYELOMA

Multiple myeloma is a malignant proliferation of plasma cells that has remained incurable despite considerable progress in understanding its biology. Several numeric and structural chromosomal abnormalities (particularly involving chromosomes 13 and 14) have been identified (89); it is believed that these abnormalities prevent the normal processes of differentiation and apoptosis of the myeloma cells, thus resulting in their accumulation in the bone marrow. In this process, deregulation of the c-myc oncogene is believed to be important (90). The role of interleukin-6 (IL-6) and bone marrow microenvironment have been extensively studied, and it has been shown that IL-6, produced by the stromal cells of marrow, promotes tumor growth and prevents dexamethasone-induced apoptosis (91–93).

After demonstrations in preclinical trials of the antitumor activity of IFNs in myeloma cell lines, considerable interest in examining this activity in patients was generated. Mellstedt et al. first reported the antitumor activity of IFN in myeloma (94). *In vitro* studies have demonstrated a direct and dose-dependent inhibitory effect on the proliferation of myeloma cells by IFNs (95,96). This growth inhibition is seen in IL-6–dependent and IL-6–independent cell lines (97). Interferons

have also been reported to downregulate expression of c-myc and N-ras oncogenes (98,99).

Initial pilot studies in patients with relapsing or refractory myeloma found evidence of activity; IFN-α as a single agent was not shown to be superior to conventional chemotherapy in previously untreated patients (94,100,101). It was concluded that the activity of IFN in multiple myeloma is comparable to that of several other agents, but is inferior to that of melphalan.

Because of the reported synergistic activities of IFNs and several cytostatic drugs (102,103), combinations of IFN-α with chemotherapy were examined, and initial phase 1/2 studies showed promising results. In a study combining IFN-α with melphalan and prednisone, a response rate of 75% was observed (104); in an alternating regimen—IFN-α combined with vincristine, bischloroethyl-nitrosourea, melphalan, cyclophosphamide, and prednisone—a response rate of 80% (including 30% complete responses) was reported (105). Subsequent prospective randomized trials, however, have not confirmed unequivocally that regimens combining chemotherapy with IFN are superior to chemotherapy alone (106–120) (Table 11). The IFN arms in these trials have produced outcomes ranging from substantially higher response rates or disease-free and overall survival to no difference from standard chemotherapy protocols (106).

The rationale for use of IFN-α as maintenance therapy in patients responding to conventional induction regimens was the finding that at the end of induction, myeloma cells in responding patients enter a plateau phase similar to the G phase of the cell cycle (121). Therefore, the antiproliferative activity of IFNs can be used to maintain responses obtained with chemotherapy. The first randomized trial using IFN-α for remission maintenance was reported by Mandelli et al. (122). During a period of 3 years, 101 patients with multiple myeloma who had responded to induction chemotherapy were

TABLE 12. TRIALS OF INTERFERON (IFN)-α THERAPY CONCURRENT WITH CHEMOTHERAPY FOR INDUCTION OF FOLLICULAR LYMPHOMAS

Study (Reference)	Chemotherapy	Patient (No.)	Remission (CR + PR)	5-Yr DFS (%)	5-Yr OS (%)
Chisesi (140)	Cb	29	62	55	58
	Cb + IFN-α	34	65	71	73
Price (141,146)	Cb	59	71	21	75
	Cb + IFN-α	49	55	78	75
Peterson (142)	CP	265	89	53	80
	CP + IFN-α	266	84	54	78
Solal-Celigny (143,147)	CHVP	134	58	27	69
	CHVP + IFN-α	137	76	47	86
Arranz (145)	CVP	71	53	24[a]	70[a]
	CVP + IFN-α	73	59	60[a]	82[a]
Smally (144,148)	COPA	127	86	21	61
	COPA + IFN-α	122	86	40	78

Cb, chlorambucil; CHVP, cyclophosphamide, doxorubicin, teniposide, prednisone; COPA, cyclophosphamide, Oncovin (vincristine), prednisone, Adriamycin (doxorubicin); CP, cyclophosphamide; CR, complete remission; CVP, cyclophosphamide, vincristine, prednisone; DFS, disease-free survival; IFN-α, interferon-α; OS, overall survival; PR, partial remission.
[a]Six-year data.

randomized to receive IFN-α-2a three times weekly (n = 50) or observation (n = 51) (122). Median duration of response from time of randomization was 26 months in the IFN-treated group versus 14 months in controls (p = .0002). Median survival was 52 months in the IFN arm and 39 months in controls (p = .035) (122). Other randomized trials have produced differing results; although relapse-free survival was usually prolonged in the IFN-treated patients, prolongation of disease-free and overall survival was substantial in some trials but minimal in others (106). In the Swedish study reported by Westin et al., induction therapy with melphalan and prednisone was followed by randomization to IFN-α therapy or observation in 120 patients achieving a plateau phase (123). Interferon-α-2b, 5 MIU, three times per week was administered subcutaneously to 59 patients until relapse. A prolongation of the plateau phase for the IFN-treated patients occurred (60 versus 25 weeks, p <.0001), but no improvement was observed in overall survival (123). In the study by the Southwest Oncology Group, however, no differences in response or overall survival duration were seen in patients treated with IFN-α-2b, 3 MIU, three times weekly, after achieving a response with conventional induction regimens (124).

Combination of IFN and dexamethasone has also been investigated because dexamethasone has been reported to reduce the toxicity of IFN without affecting its efficacy. A considerable response (57%) was noted in newly diagnosed patients (125), but a reported 68% response rate with this combination in refractory patients (126) could not be confirmed (127). This combination has resulted in the improvement of quality of partial responses (128,129).

IFN therapy has also been examined after high-dose chemotherapy and autologous bone marrow or stem-cell transplantation on the assumption that it may be more effective in patients with minimal residual disease (130–132). In one study, disease-free survival was found to be significantly prolonged in the IFN-treated patients (130).

IFN-α therapy cannot be considered as the standard in induction therapy or a way to maintain remission produced by conventional chemotherapy. Because no standard treatment for myeloma exists, however, the decision to incorporate IFN-α into a patient's regimen should be individualized, with the most consideration being given to younger patients with minimal residual disease who are able to tolerate the therapy.

INTERFERON THERAPY IN LYMPHOMAS

IFNs have little significant activity in aggressive-histology lymphomas, but their roles in therapy of follicular lymphomas and cutaneous T-cell lymphoma has been extensively investigated. Foon et al. reported four complete responses and nine partial responses among 24 patients with advanced non-Hodgkin's lymphoma treated with IFN-α-2a, 50 MIU per m^2, three times weekly (133). These responses were short-lived and were only maintained by continuing the toxic regimen. Using a lower dose of IFN-α-2a, 6 MIU per m^2, three times per week, Mantovani et al. reported a 52% response rate (134). VanderMolen et al. were unable to demonstrate a clear dose-response relationship in a trial of low-dose (3 MIU daily) versus high-dose (50 MIU per m^2, twice weekly) IFN-α-2a (135). Responses were generally of greater magnitude and longer duration using the higher dose (135). Several groups have clearly demonstrated the activity of IFNs in relapsed and refractory low-grade lymphomas, with responses of 30% to 40% (135–139).

IFN has been demonstrated to exhibit synergistic activity against follicular lymphomas when administered concomitantly with chemotherapy and has been investigated with conventional regimens in the hope of maintaining remission and prolonging disease-free survival. Several prospective randomized trials have been reported that assessed benefits of the addition of IFN to induction chemotherapy (Table 12) (140–148). In trials combining IFN with a single alkylating agent (chlorambucil or cyclophosphamide), no beneficial effect was

TABLE 13. TRIALS OF INTERFERON (IFN)-α MAINTENANCE THERAPY IN FOLLICULAR LYMPHOMAS

Study (Reference)	Patients without Progression of Disease			Follow-Up Time	p Value
	IFN-α	Observation	Total		
Peterson (150)	53	441	94	4 yr	.06
Hagenbeck (151)	44	38	82	3 yr	.12
Unterhalt (152)	49	27	76	4 yr	.003
Aviles (149)	62	25	87	8 yr	<.001
Dana (154)	?	?	279	4 yr	.18
Rohatiner (153)	68	28	96	4 yr	.05

demonstrated (140–142). Price et al. randomized patients with previously untreated stage III or IV follicular lymphoma to chlorambucil, with or without IFN-α-2b, for an 18-week induction period. Responding patients were next randomized to maintenance therapy with IFN-α-2b or observation (141). No improvements in response rate or overall survival were noted, but significantly lower recurrence rates were noted in a follow-up report (146). In the trial by Peterson et al., 581 previously untreated patients with stage III or IV follicular lymphoma were randomized to receive cyclophosphamide alone or with low-dose IFN-α-2b, followed by further randomization of responders to IFN maintenance or observation (142). No differences in response rate, estimated time to treatment failure, or overall survival for the two induction regimens occurred. Patients who received IFN maintenance showed a trend toward prolongation of time to treatment failure (p = .06) but no difference in survival.

In contrast, significant improvements in response rate and duration were observed by adding IFN to anthracycline-containing combination chemotherapy (143,144). In these studies, significant prolongation of overall survival was also noted for combination therapy. In the trial by the Groupe d'Etude des Lymphomes Folliculaires, reported by Solal-Celigny et al., patients received either cyclophosphamide, doxorubicin, teniposide, and prednisone alone or with IFN-α-2b, 5 MIU three times per week for 18 months. A higher response rate (85% versus 69%), event-free survival (34 months versus 19 months), and overall survival at 3 years (86% versus 69%) was observed in the IFN-treated group (143,147). An increase in incidence of some adverse events in the IFN-treated group occurred; a quality-adjusted time without symptoms of disease or toxicity of treatment analysis, however, suggested that the IFN-treated patients had more time without symptoms of disease or toxicity of therapy. The Eastern Cooperative Oncology Group investigated the effect of adding IFN-α-2a to cyclophosphamide, vincristine, prednisone, and doxorubicin (COPA) for patients with stage III or IV low-grade non-Hodgkin's lymphoma (144). Overall response rates were comparable in both groups (86%), as were complete remission rates (COPA, 29%; IFN-COPA, 32%). Time to treatment failure was significantly longer for the IFN-treated group, however, with 34% disease-free survival at a median of 5 years versus 19% (p = .0013). At 5-year follow-up, median survivals of the two groups were not significantly different (148).

The role of IFNs in maintaining remissions achieved by conventional cytoreductive chemotherapy has been investigated in

six prospective randomized trials using IFN maintenance without further chemotherapy (Table 13) (149–154). In four of these studies, the benefit of IFN therapy in prolonging disease-free survival was not statistically significant or could be seen only in patients in complete remission after initial chemotherapy. It has been argued that the low dose and short duration of IFN therapy in these trials may be the reason for suboptimal results (155). In a study by the German Low Grade Lymphoma Study Group using a relatively high dose of IFN-α (5 MIU, three times weekly) with no restriction on duration of therapy, a significant prolongation of median disease-free survival was observed (152). Using IFN maintenance, 49% of patients remained relapse-free at 4 years, versus 27% in the control arm (152). IFN therapy was well tolerated, an important consideration in a disease with a long natural history. A metaanalysis of these studies, including a total of 1,756 patients, showed a survival difference favoring IFN therapy (156). When dividing the trials into those with more intensive anthracycline-containing regimens versus those that used less intensive initial chemotherapy with alkylating agents, a large survival advantage for IFN-treated patients was observed in the more intensive trials (5-year survival, 74%, versus 60%, 2p = 0.00001). In the less intensive trials, no survival differences occurred between the two groups (2p = 0.89). The advantage for IFN was limited to patients achieving a response (2p = 0.00004) (156). Use of IFN in maintaining remission after minimal residual disease is achieved as a result of myeloablative therapy is currently under investigation. The European Organization for Research and Treatment of Cancer has initiated a randomized, controlled, multicenter, phase III trial to evaluate the role of IFN-α as maintenance treatment after autologous bone marrow or stem-cell transplant for previously untreated patients with stage III or IV follicular lymphoma.

It appears that IFN-α is a useful addition to the treatment of follicular lymphomas in combination with anthracycline-containing regimens for induction and for the maintenance of remissions after initial cytoreductive therapy.

IFN has been used effectively in the treatment of cutaneous T-cell lymphoma. IFN-α-2a at a dose of 50 MIU per m^2, three times weekly, achieved two complete responses and seven partial responses among 20 previously treated patients (157). Other investigators have reported even higher response rates in previously untreated patients (158). Combination of IFN-α with extracorporeal photopheresis (ECP) was investigated by Dipple and colleagues (159). Nine patients with advanced cutaneous T-cell lymphoma were treated with the combination, and ten patients received ECP alone. Of the patients treated with ECP alone, one achieved a complete remission, one showed a minor response, and eight patients had stable disease. When using the combination, four patients had complete remissions, two had partial responses, two patients had stable disease, and one patient had progressive disease (159). Combination of IFN-α with retinoids has also been investigated in several studies (160–163). These studies combined relatively low doses of IFN-α with etretinate or 13-*cis*-retinoic acid, reporting significant improvements in patient outcomes.

The role of IFN-α in Hodgkin's lymphoma has also been investigated. Although the use of current regimens of combination chemotherapy cures a high proportion of patients with untreated Hodgkin's disease (HD), 30% to 35% of these patients relapse. Despite the use of aggressive regimens, including bone marrow or stem-cell transplant, the prognosis of patients with relapsed or refractory disease is generally poor. IFN-α has been used with benefit in some cases of refractory HD (164–168). Mazza et al. randomized patients with high-risk HD who were treated with combination chemotherapy to receive maintenance therapy with IFN-α-2b or no further treatment (169). IFN was administered at a dose of 3 MIU per day for 3 months, followed by 3 MIU, three times per week for 9 months (169). They observed that IFN maintenance could improve duration of complete remission, but follow-up was too short to arrive at definitive conclusions. Aviles and colleagues reported 135 patients with stage IIIB-IVB HD who were initially treated with epirubicin, bleomycin, vinblastine, and dacarbazine (170). After the achievement of complete remission, the patients were randomized to either maintenance therapy with IFN-α, 5 MIU, three times per week for 1 year, or no further therapy. After a median follow-up of 74.3 months (range, 49 to 108 months), 91% of IFN-treated patients remained in remission (as compared to 58% of controls). Overall survival was also better in IFN-treated patients (92% at 7 years, compared to 67% in controls, *p* <.01) (170). Therefore, IFN-α appears to have activity in HD and may be beneficial in prolonging duration of remission—and possibly survival—in patients treated with combination chemotherapy.

INTERFERON THERAPY IN OTHER HEMATOLOGIC MALIGNANCIES

Interferon therapy has been investigated in other hematologic malignancies, albeit infrequently. Montserrat and colleagues reviewed the experience in chronic lymphocytic leukemia (CLL) (171), reporting that responses to IFN in CLL appeared to be transient, rarely complete, and more significant in early-stage disease. They concluded that IFN-α is not effective in previously treated patients or patients with more advanced disease. With the advent of more effective regimens in CLL, the role of IFNs in CLL may be limited to maintaining minimal residual disease.

The role of IFN therapy has also been examined in Waldenstrom's macroglobulinemia (WM), a differentiated B-cell malignancy that is usually less responsive to standard chemotherapeutic agents because of slow proliferating cells. Rotoli et al. examined the efficacy of IFN-α in 88 patients with an immunoglobulin M

monoclonal protein greater than 10 g per L (172). Thirty-eight patients were classified as WM. Response to therapy was based on a reduction in monoclonal protein in two consecutive measurements. They concluded that IFN-α produced a significant improvement in 50% of patients with immunoglobulin-M monoclonal protein greater than 30 g per L, including occasional complete remissions. In patients with a low protein (immunoglobulin M–monoclonal gammopathies of undetermined significance), therapy was, however, ineffective (172). Legouffe and colleagues used IFN-α in 14 patients with progressive WM manifested by a high level of monoclonal component (>10 g per L), severe anemia (hemoglobin <8.5 g per L), and a high tumor mass (lymphadenopathy or hepatosplenomegaly, or both) (173). Interferon-2α, 1 MIU, three times a week, was administered for a mean duration of 10.3 months (range, 2 to 44 months). An increase in hemoglobin level was observed in 42% of patients, and a significant reduction in monoclonal protein was observed in 28% of patients (173).

REFERENCES

1. Isaacs A, Lindermann J. Viral interference: I. The interferon. *Proc R Soc Lond B Biol Sci* 1957;147:258–267.
2. Mandelli F, Arcese W, Avvisati G. The interferons in hematological malignancies. *Bailliere's Clin Haematol* 1994;7:91–113.
3. Ruzicka FJ, Jach ME, Borden EC. Binding of recombinant-produced interferon βser to human lymphoblastoid cells. *J Biol Chem* 1987;262:16142–16149.
4. Stewart WE, Blalock JE, Burke DC, et al. Interferon nomenclature. *J Immunol* 1980;125:2353.
5. Kimci A. Autocrine interferon and the suppression of the c-myc nuclear oncogene. *Interferon* 1987;8:86–110.
6. Bishoff JR, Samuel CE. Mechanism of interferon action. *J Biol Chem* 1985;260:8237–8239.
7. Edwards BS, Hawkins MJ, Borden EC. Comparative *in vitro* and *in vivo* action of human NK cells by two recombinant α-interferons differing in antiviral activity. *Cancer Research* 1984;44:3135–3139.
8. DeMaeyer-Guinard J, DeMaeyer E. Immunomodulation by interferons: recent developments. *Interferon* 1985;6:69–86.
9. Fertsch D, Vogel SN. Recombinant interferons increase macrophage Fc receptor capacity. *J Immunology* 1984;132:2436–2439.
10. Einat M, Resnitzky D, Kimchi A. Close link between reduction of c-myc expression by interferon and G^0/G^1 arrest. *Nature* 1985;313: 597–600.
11. Resnitsky D, Tiefenbrun N, Berissi H, Kimchi A. Interferons and interleukin-6 suppress phosphorylation of the retinoblastoma protein in growth-sensitive hematopoietic cells. *Proc Natl Acad Sci U S A* 1992;89:402–406.
12. Kumar R, Atlas I. Interferon–α induces the expression of the retinoblastoma gene product in human Burkitt's lymphoma Daudi cells: role in growth regulation. *Proc Natl Acad Sci U S A* 1992;89:6599-6603.
13. Burke LC, Bybee A, Thomas NS. The retinoblastoma protein is partially phosphorylated during early G1 in cycling cells but not in G1 cells arrested with alpha-interferon. *Oncogene* 1992;7:783–788.
14. Thomas NS, Burke LC, Bybee A, Linch DC. The phosphorylation state of the retinoblastoma (RB) protein in G^0/G^1 is dependent on growth status. *Oncogene* 1991;6:317–322.
15. Melamed D, Tiefenbrun N, Yarden A, Kimchi A. Interferons and interleukin-6 suppress the DNA-binding activity of E2F in growth-sensitive hematopoietic cells. *Mol Cell Biol* 1993;13:5255–5265.
16. Sherr CJ. Mammalian G1 cyclins. *Cell* 1993;73:1059–1065.
17. Hobeika AC, Subramaniam PS, Johnson HM. IFN induces the expression of the cyclin-dependent kinase inhibitor p21 in human prostate cancer cells. *Oncogene* 1997;14:1165–1170.
18. Arora T, Jelinek F. Differential myeloma cell responsiveness to inter-

feron-α correlates with differential induction of p19^{INK4d} and cyclin D2 expression. *J Biol Chem* 1998;273:11799–11805.

19. Subramaniam PS, Johnson HM. A role for the cyclin-dependent kinase inhibitor p21 in the G1 cell cycle arrest mediated by the type I interferons. *J Interferon Cytokine Res* 1997;17:11–15.

20. Sangfelt O, Erickson S, Castro J, Heiden T, Einhorn S, Grander D. Induction of apoptosis and inhibition of cell growth are independent responses to interferon-α in hematopoietic cell lines. *Cell Growth Diff* 1997;8:343–352.

21. Jewell AP. Interferon-alpha, Bcl-2 expression and apoptosis in B-cell chronic lymphocytic leukemia. *Leuk Lymphoma* 1996;21:43–47.

22. Silver RT. Chronic myeloid leukemia. A perspective of the clinical and biologic issues of the chronic phase. *Hematol Oncol Clin North Am* 1990;4:319–335.

23. Champlin RE, Golde DW. Chronic myeloid leukemia: recent advances. *Blood* 1985;65:1039–1047.

24. Kantarjian HM, Deisseroth A, Kurzrock R, Estrov Z, Talpaz M. Chronic myelogenous leukemia: a concise update. *Blood* 1993;82: 691–703.

25. Cortes JE, Talpaz M, Kantarjian H. Chronic myelogenous leukemia: a review. *Am J Med* 1996;100:555–569.

26. Wetzler M, Kantarjian H, Kurzrock R, Talpaz M. Interferon-α therapy for chronic myelogenous leukemia. *Am J Med* 1995;99:402–411.

27. Talpaz M, McCredie KB, Mavligit GM, Gutterman JU. Leukocyte interferon–induced myeloid cyto reduction in chronic myelogenous leukemia. *Blood* 1983;62:689–692.

28. Talpaz M, Kantarjian H, McCredie KB, et al. Hematologic remission and cytogenetic improvement induced by recombinant human interferon alpha A in chronic myelogenous leukemia. *N Engl J Med* 1986;314:1065–1069.

29. Talpaz M, Kantarjian H, McCredie KB, et al. Clinical investigation of human alpha-interferon in chronic myelogenous leukemia. *Blood* 1987;69:1280–1288.

30. Talpaz M, Kantarjian H, Kurzrock R, et al. Interferon–alpha produces sustained cytogenetic responses in chronic myelogenous leukemia. *Ann Intern Med* 1991;114:532–538.

31. Kantarjian HM, Smith TL, O'Brien S, et al. Prolonged survival following achievement of cytogenetic response with alpha interferon therapy in chronic myelogenous leukemia. *Ann Intern Med* 1995;122:254–261.

32. Schofield JR, Robinson WA, Murphy JR, Rovira DK. Low doses of interferon-α are as effective as higher doses in inducing remissions and prolonging survival in chronic myeloid leukemia. *Ann Intern Med* 1994;121:736–744.

33. Alimena G, Morra E, Lazzarino M, et al. Recombinant interferon alpha 2-b as therapy for Philadelphia positive chronic myelogenous leukemia: a study of 82 patients treated with intermittent or daily administration. *Blood* 1988;72:542–647.

34. Freund M, von Wussow P, Dietrich H, et al. Recombinant human interferon alpha–2b in chronic myelogenous leukemia: dose dependency of response and frequency of neutralizing antibodies. *Br J Haematol* 1989;72:350–356.

35. Anger B, Porzolt F, Leichte R, et al. A phase 1-2 study of recombinant interferon alpha 2a and hydroxyurea for chronic myelocytic leukemia. *BLUT* 1989;58:275–278.

36. Sokal JE, Cox EB, Baccarani M, et al. Prognostic discrimination in "good risk" chronic granulocytic leukemia. *Blood* 1984;63:789–799.

37. Italian Cooperative Study Group on Chronic Myeloid Leukemia. Interferon alfa-2a compared with conventional chemotherapy for the treatment of chronic myeloid leukemia. *N Engl J Med* 1994;330: 820–825.

38. Hehlmann R, Heimpel H, Hasford J, et al. Randomized comparison of interferon-α with busulfan and hydroxyurca in chronic myelogenous leukemia (CML). *Blood* 1994;84:4064–4077.

39. Allan N, Richards S, Shepherd P, et al. UK Medical Research Council randomized, multicentre trial of interferon-α n1 for chronic myeloid leukaemia: improved survival irrespective of cytogenetic response. *Lancet* 1995;345:1392–1397.

40. Ohnishi K, Ohno R, Tomonaga M, et al. A randomized trial comparing interferon-α with busulfan for newly diagnosed chronic myelogenous leukemia in chronic phase. *Blood* 1995;86:906–916.

41. Benelux CML Study Group. Low dose interferon-alpha 2b combined

with hydroxyurea versus hydroxyurea alone for chronic myelogenous leukemia. *Bone Marrow Transplant* 1996;17[Suppl 3]:S19–S20.

42. Chronic Myeloid Leukemia Trialists' Collaborative Group. Interferon alfa versus chemotherapy for chronic myeloid leukemia: a meta-analysis of seven randomized trials. *J Natl Cancer Inst* 1997;89:1616.

43. Yoffe G, Blick M, Kantarjian H, et al. Molecular analysis of interferon-induced suppression of Philadelphia chromosome in patients with chronic myeloid leukemia. *Blood* 1987;69:961–963.

44. Verschraegen CF, Talpaz M, Hirsch-Ginsberg CF, et al. Quantification of the breakpoint cluster region rearrangement for clinical monitoring in Philadelphia chromosome-positive chronic myeloid leukemia. *Blood* 1995;85:2704–2710.

45. Guo JQ, Liang JY, Xian YM, et al. BCR-ABL protein expression in peripheral blood cells of chronic myelogenous leukemia patients undergoing therapy. *Blood* 1994;12:3629–3637.

46. Dhingra K, Kurzrock R, Baine R, et al. Minimal residual disease in interferon treated chronic myelogenous leukemia: results and pitfalls of analysis based on polymerase chain reaction. *Leukemia* 1992;6:754–760.

47. Kurzrock R, Estrov Z, Kantarjian H, Talpaz M. Conversion of interferon-induced long-term cytogenetic remissions in chronic myelogenous leukemia to polymerase chain reaction negativity. *J Clin Oncol* 1998;16:4:1526.

48. The Benelux CML Study Group. Randomized study on hydroxyurea alone versus hydroxyurea combined with low-dose interferon-α2b for chronic myeloid leukemia. *Blood* 1998;91:2713.

49. Talpaz M, Kurzrock R, O'Brien S, Kantarjian H. Unmaintained complete remissions (cures?) among interferon treated Philadelphia positive chronic myelogenous leukemia patients. *Amer Society of Hematol* 1998:317a(abst).

50. Talpaz M, Estrov Z, Kantarjian H, et al. Persistence of dormant leukemic progenitors during interferon-induced remission in chronic myelogenous leukemia: analysis by polymerase chain reaction of individual colonies. *J Clin Invest* 1994;94:1383–1389.

51. Kantarjian HM, O'Brien S, Smith TL, et al. Treatment of Philadelphia chromosome-positive early chronic phase chronic myelogenous leukemia with daily doses of interferon alpha and low-dose cytarabine. *J Clin Oncol* 1999;17:284–292.

52. Guilhot F, Dreyfus B, Brizard A, Huret JL, Tanzer J. Cytogenetic remissions in chronic myelogenous leukemia using interferon alpha-2a and hydroxyurea with or without low-dose cytosine arabinoside. *Leuk Lymphoma* 1991;4:49.

53. Guilhot F, Chastang C, Michallet M. Interferon alfa-2b combined with cytarabine versus interferon alone in chronic myelogenous leukemia. *N Engl J Med* 1997;337:223.

54. Miyamura K, Iijima N, Itou T, et al. Functional expression of FAS receptor on the progenitor cells of chronic myelogenous leukemia: induction by interferon alpha, gamma and Ubenimex. *Blood* 1996;88[Suppl 1]:232a(abst).

55. Selleri C, Sato T, Del Vecchio L, et al. Involvement of fas-mediated apoptosis in the inhibitory effects of interferon-α in chronic myelogenous leukemia. *Blood* 1996;88[Suppl 1]:231a(abst).

56. Bhatia R, McCarthy JB, Verfaillie CM. Interferon-α restores normal negative regulation of CML progenitor proliferation by the marrow microenvironment by restoring normal β1 integrin mediated proliferation inhibition. *Blood* 1996;87(9):3883–3891.

57. Bouroncle BA, Wiseman BK, Doan CA. Leukemic reticuloendotheliosis. *Blood* 1958;13:609–630.

58. Schreck R, Donelly WJ. Hairy cells in blood in lymphoreticular neoplastic and flagellated cells of normal lymph nodes. *Blood* 1966;27:199–211.

59. Quesada JR, Reuben J, Manning JT, Hersh EM, Gutterman JU. Alpha-interferon for induction of remission in hairy cell leukemia. *N Engl J Med* 1984;310:15.

60. Ratain MJ, Golomb HM, Vardiman JW, Vokes EE, Jacobs RH, Daly K. Treatment of hairy cell leukemia with recombinant alpha-2 interferon. *J Clin Oncol* 1985;65:644.

61. Jacobs AD, Champlin RE, Golde DW. Recombinant alpha-2 interferon for hairy cell leukemia. *J Clin Oncol* 1985;65:1017.

62. Quesada JR, Hersh EM, Manning JT, et al. Treatment of hairy cell leukemia with recombinant alpha-interferon. *Blood* 1986;68:493.

63. Golomb HM, Jacobs A, Fefer A, et al. Alpha-2 interferon therapy of

hairy cell leukemia: a multicenter study of 64 patients. *J Clin Oncol* 1986;4:900.

64. Golomb HM, Fefer A, Golde DW, et al. Update of a multi-institutional study of 195 patients with hairy cell leukemia (HCL) treated with interferon alfa-2b. *Proc Am Soc Clin Oncol* 1990;6:215.

65. Rai K, Mick R, Ozer H, et al. Alpha-interferon therapy in untreated active hairy cell leukemia: a cancer and leukemia group B (CALGB) study. *Proc Am Soc Clin Oncol* 1987;6:159.

66. Saven A, Piro LD. Treatment of hairy cell leukemia. *Blood* 1992;79:1111–1120.

67. Berman E, Heller G, Kempin S, Gee T, Tran LL, Clarkson B. Incidence of response and long-term follow-up in patients with hairy cell leukemia treated with recombinant interferon alfa-2a. *Blood* 1990;75:839–845.

68. Bekisz JB, Zur Nedden DL, Enterline JC, Zoon KC. Antibodies to interferon-α2 in patients treated with interferon-α2 for hairy cell leukemia. *J Interferon Res* 1989;9:51–57.

69. Kurzrock R, Talpaz M, Gutterman JU. Hairy cell leukemia: review of treatment. *Br J Haematol* 1991;79:17–20.

70. Golomb HM, Ratain MJ, Fefer A, et al. Randomized study of the duration of treatment with interferon alfa-2b in patients with hairy cell leukemia. *J Natl Cancer Inst* 1988;80:369.

71. Mooemeier JA, Ratain MJ, Westbrook CA, Vardiman JW, Daly KM, Golomb HM. Low-dose interferon alpha-2b in the treatment of hairy cell leukemia. *J Natl Cancer Inst* 1989;81:1172.

72. Thompson JA, Kidd P, Rubin E, Fefer A. Very low dose α-2b interferon for the treatment of hairy cell leukemia. *Blood* 1989;73:1440.

73. Michalevicz R, Aderka D, Frisch B, Revel M. Interferon beta induced remission in a hairy cell leukemia patient resistant to interferon-alpha. *Leuk Res* 1988;12:845–851.

74. Quesada JR, Alexanian R, Kurzrock R, et al. Recombinant interferon gamma in hairy cell leukemia, multiple myeloma and Waldenström's macroglobulinemia. *Am J Hematol* 1988;29:1–4.

75. Foon KA, Maluish AE, Abrams PG, et al. Recombinant leukocyte A interferon therapy for advanced hairy cell leukemia. Therapeutic and immunologic results. *Am J Med* 1986;80:351.

76. Ruco LP, Procapio A, Maccallini V, et al. Severe deficiency of natural killer activity in peripheral blood of patients with hairy cell leukemia. *Blood* 1983;61:1132.

77. Lee SH, Kelly S, Chin H, Stebbing N. Stimulation of natural killer cell activity and inhibition of proliferation of various leukemic cells by purified human leukocyte interferon subtypes. *Cancer Res* 1982;42:1312.

78. Taylor-Papadimitriou J. Effects of interferons on cell growth and function. In: Gresser I, ed. *Interferon 1980*, Vol 2. New York, NY: Academic 1980:13.

79. Lieberman D, Voloch Z, Aviv H, et al. Effects of interferon on hemoglobin synthesis and leukemia virus production of friend cells. *Mol Biol Rep* 1974;1:447.

80. Spiers SDC, Moore D, Cassileth PA, et al. Hairy cell leukemia: complete remission with pentostatin (2′ deoxycoformycin). *N Engl J Med* 1987;316:825.

81. Foon KA, Nakano GM, Koller CA, et al. Response to 2′-deoxycoformycin after failure of interferon-α in nonsplenectomized patients with hairy cell leukemia. *Blood* 1986;68:297.

82. Piro LD, Carrera CJ, Carson DA, Beutler E. Lasting remission in hairy cell leukemia induced by a single infusion of 2-chlorodeoxyadenosine. *N Engl J Med* 1990;322:117.

83. Kurzrock R, Strom SS, Estey E, et al. Second cancer risk in hairy cell leukemia: analysis of 350 patients. *J Clin Oncol* 1997;15:1803–1810.

84. Bernstein L, Newton P, Ross RK. Epidemiology of hairy cell leukemia in Los Angeles County. *Cancer Res* 1990;50:3605–3609.

85. Seymour JF, Talpaz M, Kurzrock R. Response duration and recovery of CD4+ lymphocytes following deoxycoformycin in interferon-α-resistant hairy cell leukemia: 7-year follow-up. *Leukemia* 1997;11:42–47.

86. Kampmeier P, Spielberger R, Dickstein J, et al. Increased incidence of second neoplasms in patients treated with interferon-α2b for hairy cell leukemia: a clinicopathologic assessment. *Blood* 1994;83:2931–2938.

87. Troussard X, Henry-Amar M, Flandrin G. Second cancer risk after interferon therapy? *Blood* 1994;84:3242–3244.

88. Jacobs RH, Vokes EE, Golomb HM. Second malignancies in hairy cell leukemia. *Cancer* 1985;56:1462–1467.

89. Dewald GW, Kyle RA, Hicks GA, Greipp PR. The clinical significance of cytogenetic studies in 100 patients with multiple myeloma, plasma cell leukemia, or amyloidosis. *Blood* 1985;66:380–390.

90. Greil R, Fasching B, Loidl P, Huber H. Expression of the c-myc proto-oncogene in multiple myeloma and chronic lymphocytic leukemia: an in situ analysis. *Blood* 1991;78:180–191.

91. Kawano M, Hirano T, Matsuda T, et al. Autocrine generation and requirement of BSF-2/IL-6 for human multiple myelomas. *Nature* 1988;332:83–85.

92. Klein B, Zhang XG, Jourdan M, et al. Paracrine but not autocrine regulation of myeloma cell growth and differentiation by interleukin-6. *Blood* 1989;73:517–526.

93. Hardin J, MacLeod S, Grigorieva I, et al. Interleukin-6 prevents dexamethasone-induced myeloma cell death. *Blood* 1994;84:3063–3070.

94. Mellstedt H, Aher A, Bjorkholm M, et al. Interferon therapy in myelomatosis. *Lancet* 1979;1:245–247.

95. Brenning G, Jernberg H, Gidlund M, et al. The effect of alpha and gamma-interferon on proliferation and production of IgE and beta-2-microglobulin in the human myeloma cell line U-266 and in the alpha-interferon resistant U-266 subline. *Scand J Haematol* 1986;37:280–288.

96. Ludwig H, Sweatly P. *In vitro* inhibitory effect of interferon on multiple myeloma stem cells. *Cancer Immunol Immunother* 1980;9:139–143.

97. Jernberg-Wiklund H, Pettersson M, Nilsson K. Recombinant interferon-gamma inhibits the growth of IL-6-dependent human multiple myeloma cell lines in vitro. *Eur J Haematol* 1991;46:231–239.

98. Kimchi A. Autocrine interferon and the suppression of the c-myc nuclear oncogene. *Interferon* 1987;8:85–110.

99. Samid D, Chang EH, Friedman RM. Development of transformed phenotype induced by a human ras oncogene is inhibited by interferon. *Biochem Biophy Res Commun* 1985;126:509–516.

100. Aher A, Bjorkholm M, Mellstedt H, et al. Human leukocyte interferon and intermittent high dose melphalan/prednisone administration in the treatment of multiple myeloma: a randomized clinical trial. *Cancer Treat Rep* 1984;68:1331–1338.

101. Ludwig H, Cortelezzi A, Scheithauer W, et al. Recombinant interferon alpha-2c versus polychemotherapy (VMCP) for treatment of multiple myeloma: a prospective randomized trial. *Eur J Cancer Clin Oncol* 1986;22:1111–1116.

102. Aapro MS, Alberts DS, Salmon SE. Interactions of human leukocyte interferon with vinca alkaloids and other chemotherapeutic agents against human tumors in clonogenic assay. *Cancer Chemother Pharmacol* 1983;10:161–166.

103. Balkwill FR, Moody EM. Positive interactions between human interferon and cyclophosphamide or adriamycin in a human tumor model system. *Cancer Res* 1985;44:906–908.

104. Cooper MR, Fefer A, Thompson J, et al. Alpha-2 interferon/melphalan/prednisone in previously untreated patients with multiple myeloma: a phase I-II trial. *Cancer Treat Rep* 1986;70:473–476.

105. Oken MM, Kyle RA. Strategies for combining interferon with chemotherapy for the treatment of multiple myeloma. *Semin Oncol* 1991;18[Suppl 7]:30–32.

106. Ludwig H, Fritz E. Should alpha-interferon be included as standard treatment in multiple myeloma? *Eur J Cancer* 1998;34:12–24.

107. Aitchison R, Williams A, Schey S, et al. A randomized trial of cyclophosphamide with or without low dose alpha-interferon in the treatment of newly diagnosed myeloma. *Leuk Lymphoma* 1993;9:243–246.

108. Aviles A, Alatriste S, Talavera A, et al. Alternative combination chemotherapy and interferon improves survival in poor prognosis multiple myeloma. *Clin Oncol* 1995;7:97–101.

109. Capnist G, Spirano M, Damasio EE, et al. Is IFN helpful in the treatment of multiple myeloma? Preliminary results of a multi-center study of Italian NHLCSG. *Proc Am Soc Clin Oncol* 1993;12:407(abst).

110. Casassus PH, Mahe B, Sadoun A, et al. Alpha interferon is not able to improve VMCP/VABP chemotherapy response rates in induction phase of untreated multiple myeloma: results in the first 201 patients included in a prospective randomized study (KIF protocol). International conference: multiple myeloma, from biology to therapy. *Mulhouse* (France) 1994:69(abst).

111. Cooper MR, Dear K, McIntyre OR, et al. A randomized clinical trial comparing melphalan/prednisone with or without interferon-alfa-2b in newly diagnosed patients with multiple myeloma: a cancer and

leukemia group B study. *J Clin Oncol* 1993;11:155–160.

112. Corrado C, Pavlovsky S, Saslasky J, et al. Randomized trial comparing melphalan-prednisone with or without recombinant alpha-2-interferon (r-alpha2IFN) in multiple myeloma. *Proc Am Soc Clin Oncol* 1989;8:258(abst).

113. Galvez CA, Pire R, Bonamassa, et al. Multiple myeloma: treatment with VABP with or without recombinant alpha-2b interferon in multiple myeloma. 18th International Congress of Chemotherapy, Stockholm, Sweden 1993:321 (abst).

114. Garcia-Larana J, Steegmann JL, Perez Oteyza J, et al. Treatment of multiple myeloma with melphalan/prednisone (MP) versus melphalan/prednisone and alpha-2b-interferon (MP-IFN). Results of a cooperative Spanish group. *Cong Int Soc Haematol ISH* 1992;24:301(abst).

115. Joshua DE, Penny R, Baldwin R, et al. The study of combination therapy plus or minus Roferon A in multiple myeloma. *Blood* 1994;84[Suppl 1]:179a(abst).

116. Montuoro A, De Rosa L, De Blasio A, et al. Alpha-2a-interferon/melphalan/prednisone versus melphalan/prednisone in previously untreated patients with multiple myeloma. *Br J Haematol* 1990;76:365–368.

117. The Nordic Myeloma Study Group. Interferon-α2b added to melphalan-prednisone for initial and maintenance therapy in multiple myeloma. *Ann Intern Med* 1996;124:212–222.

118. Osterborg A, Bjorkholm M, Bjoreman M, et al. Natural interferon-alpha in combination with melphalan/prednisone versus melphalan/prednisone in the treatment of multiple myeloma stages II and III: a randomized study from the myeloma group of central Sweden. *Blood* 1993;81:1428–1434.

119. Scheithauer W, Cortelezzi A, Fritz E, et al. Combined α-2c-interferon/VMCP polychemotherapy versus VMCP polychemotherapy as induction therapy in multiple myeloma: a prospective randomized trial. *J Biol Res Mod* 1989;8:109–115.

120. Vela Ojeda J, Vazquez V, Garcia Ruiz EM, et al. A randomized clinical trial comparing chemotherapy with or without interferon alpha-2b in newly diagnosed patients with multiple myeloma. IV International workshop on multiple myeloma. Rochester, MN 1993:150(abst).

121. Durie BGM, Russel DH, Salmon SE. Reappraisal of plateau phase in myeloma. *Lancet* 1980;2:65–67.

122. Mandelli F, Avvisati G, Amadori S, et al. Maintenance treatment with recombinant interferon alpha-2b in patients with multiple myeloma responding to conventional induction chemotherapy. *N Engl J Med* 1990;322:1430–1434.

123. Westin J, Rodjer S, Turesson I, et al. Interferon alfa-2b versus no maintenance therapy during the plateau phase in multiple myeloma: a randomized study. *Br J Haematol* 1995;89:561–568.

124. Salmon SE, Crowley JJ, Grogan TM, et al. Combination chemotherapy, glucocorticoids and interferon alfa in the treatment of multiple myeloma: a Southwest oncology group study. *J Clin Oncol* 1994;12: 2405–2414.

125. Alexanian R, Barlogie B, Gutterman J. Alpha-interferon combination therapy for multiple myeloma. Proceedings of the 5th Hannover interferon workshop. 1990:43(abst).

126. San Miguel JF, Moro M, Blade J, et al. Combination of interferon and dexamethasone in refractory multiple myeloma. *Haematol Oncol* 1990;8:185–189.

127. Alexanian R, Barlogie B, Gutterman J. Alpha-interferon combination therapy of resistant myeloma. *Am J Clin Oncol* 1991;14:188–192.

128. Salmon SE, Beckord J, Pugh RP, Barlogie B, et al. Alpha-interferon for remission maintenance: preliminary report on the Southwest oncology group study. *Semin Oncol* 1991;18[Suppl 7]:33–36.

129. Palumbo A, Boccadoro M, Garino LA, et al. Multiple myeloma: intensified maintenance therapy with recombinant interferon-alpha-2b plus glucocorticoids. *Eur J Haematol* 1992;49:93–97.

130. Cunningham D, Powels R, Malpas JS, et al. A randomized trial of maintenance therapy with intron-A following high dose melphalan and ABMT in myeloma. *J Clin Oncol* 1993;12:364(abst).

131. Attal M, Huguet F, Schlaifer D, et al. Maintenance treatment with recombinant alpha interferon after autologous bone marrow transplantation for aggressive myeloma in first remission after conventional chemotherapy. *Bone Marrow Transplant* 1991;8:125–128.

132. Anderson KC, Barut BA, Ritz J, et al. Monoclonal antibody-purged autologous bone marrow transplantation therapy for multiple myeloma. *Blood* 1991;77:712–720.

133. Foon KA, Sherwin SA, Abrams PG, et al. Treatment of advanced non-Hodgkin's lymphoma with recombinant leukocyte A interferon. *N Engl J Med* 1984;311:1148–1152.

134. Mantovani L, Guglielmi C, Martelli M, et al. Recombinant alpha interferon in the treatment of low grade non-Hodgkin's lymphoma: result of a cooperative phase II trial in 313 patients. *Haematologica* 1990;74:571–575.

135. VanderMolen LA, Steis RG, Duffey PL, et al. Low- versus high-dose interferon alfa-2a in relapsed indolent non-Hodgkin's lymphoma. *J Natl Cancer Inst* 1990;82:235–238.

136. Gutterman JU, Blumenschein GR, Alexanian R, et al. Leukocyte interferon-induced tumor regression in human metastatic breast cancer, multiple myeloma, and malignant lymphoma. *Ann Intern Med* 1980;93:399–406.

137. Foon KA, Roth MS, Bunn PA Jr. Alpha interferon treatment of low grade B-cell non-Hodgkin's lymphomas, cutaneous T-cell lymphomas, and chronic lymphocytic leukemia. *Semin Oncol* 1986;13[Suppl 2]:35–42.

138. Horning SJ, Merigan TC, Krown SE, et al. Human interferon alpha in malignant lymphoma and Hodgkin's disease: result of the American Cancer Society trial. *Cancer* 1985;56:1305–1310.

139. Wagstaff J, Loyds P, Crowther D. A phase II study of human rDNA alpha-2 interferon in patients with low-grade non-Hodgkin's lymphoma. *Cancer Chemother Pharmacol* 1986;18:54–58.

140. Chisesi T, Congiu M, Contu A, et al. Randomized study of chlorambucil (CB) compared to interferon alfa-2b combined with CB in low-grade non-Hodgkin's lymphoma: an interim report of a randomized study. *Eur J Cancer* 1991;27[Suppl 4]:31–33.

141. Price CG, Rohatiner AZ, Steward W, et al. Interferon-alpha 2b in the treatment of follicular lymphoma: preliminary results of a trial in progress. *Ann Oncol* 1991;2[Suppl 2]:141–145.

142. Peterson BA, Petroni G, Oken MM, et al. Cyclophosphamide plus interferon alfa-2b in follicular low-grade lymphomas: a preliminary report of an intergroup trial (CALGB 8691 and EST 7489). *Proc Am Soc Clin Oncol* 1993;12:366(abst).

143. Solal-Celigny P, Lepage E, Brousse N, et al. Recombinant interferon alfa-2b combined with a regimen containing doxorubicin in patients with advanced follicular lymphoma. *N Engl J Med* 1993; 329:1608–1614.

144. Smalley RV, Andersen JW, Hawkins MF, et al. Interferon alfa combined with cytotoxic chemotherapy for patients with non-Hodgkin's lymphoma. *N Engl J Med* 1992;327:1336–1341.

145. Arranz R, Garcia-Alfonso P, Sobrino P, et al. Role of interferon alfa-2b in the induction and maintenance treatment of low-grade non-Hodgkin's lymphoma: results from a prospective multicenter trial with double randomization. *J Clin Oncol* 1998;16:1538–1546.

146. Rohatiner A, Crowther D, Radford J, et al. The role of interferon in follicular lymphoma. *Proc Am Soc Clin Oncol* 1996;15:418(abst).

147. Solal-Celigny P, Lepage E, Brousse N, et al. A doxorubicin containing regimen with or without interferon alpha-2b for advanced follicular lymphomas: final analysis of survival and toxicity in the GELF 86 trial. *J Clin Oncol* 1998;16:2332–2338.

148. Andersen JW, Smalley RV. Interferon alfa plus chemotherapy for non-Hodgkin's lymphoma: five-year follow-up. *N Engl J Med* 1993; 329:1821–1822.

149. Aviles A, Duque G, Talavera A, et al. Interferon alpha 2b as maintenance therapy in low-grade malignant lymphoma improves duration of remission and survival. *Leuk Lymph* 1996;20:495–499.

150. Peterson BA, Petroni GR, Oken MM, et al. Cyclophosphamide versus cyclophosphamide plus interferon alfa-2b in follicular low-grade lymphomas: an intergroup phase III trial (CALGB 8691 and EST 7486). *Proc Am Soc Clin Oncol* 1997;16:14a(abst).

151. Hagenbeek A, Carde P, Meerwaldt JH, et al. Maintenance of remission with human recombinant alfa-2a in patients with stage III and IV low-grade malignant non-Hodgkin's lymphoma. *J Clin Oncol* 1998;16:41–47.

152. Unterhalt M, Herrmann R, Koch P, et al. Prognostic determinants for long-term outcome of low-grade follicular lymphomas after cytoreductive chemotherapy and interferon alpha maintenance. Results of the German Low Grade Lymphoma Study Group (GLSG). *Blood* 1997;10[Suppl. 1]:392a(abst).

153. Rohatiner AZ, Crowther D, Radford J, et al. The role of inter-

feron in follicular lymphoma. *Proc Annu Meet Am Soc Clin Oncol* 1996;15:418(abst 1285).

154. Dana BW, Unger J, Fisher RI. A randomized study of alpha-interferon consolidation in patients with low-grade lymphoma who have responded to Pro-MACE-MOPP (Day 1-8)(SWOG 8809). *Proc Am Soc Clin Oncol* 1998;17:3a(abst).

155. Hiddermann W, Griesinger F, Unterhalt M. Interferon alfa for the treatment of follicular lymphomas. *Cancer J Sci Am* 1998;4[Suppl 2]:13–18.

156. Rohatiner AZS, Gregory W, Petersen B, et al. A meta-analysis of randomized trials evaluating the role of interferon as treatment for follicular lymphoma. *Proc Am Soc Clin Oncol* 1998;17:4a(abst)

157. Bunn PA, Foon KA, Ihde DC, et al. Recombinant leukocyte A interferon: an effective agent in advanced cutaneous T-cell lymphomas. *Ann Intern Med* 1984;101:484–487.

158. Dreno B, Celerier P, Litoux P. Roferon-A in combination with Tigason in cutaneous T-cell lymphomas. *Acta Haematol* 1993;89[Suppl 1]:28–32.

159. Dippel E, Schrag H, Goerdt S, et al. Extracorporeal photopheresis and interferon-α in advanced cutaneous T-cell lymphoma. *Lancet* 1997;350:32–33.

160. Thestrup-Pedersen K, Hammer R, Kaltoft K, et al. Treatment of mycosis fungoides with recombinant interferon-alpha-2a alone and in combination with etretinate. *Br J Dermatol* 1988;118:811–818.

161. Dreno B, Claudy A, Meynadier J, et al. The treatment of 45 patients with cutaneous T-cell lymphoma with low doses of interferon-α2a and etretinate. *Br J Dermatol* 1991;125:456–459.

162. Braathen LS, McFadden N. Successful treatment of mycosis fungoides with the combination of etretinate and human recombinant interferon alfa-2a. *J Dermatol Treatment* 1989;1:29–32.

163. Knobler RM, Trautinger F, Radaszkiewicz T, et al. Treatment of cutaneous T-cell lymphoma with a combination of low-dose interferon alfa-2b and retinoids. *J Am Acad Dermatol* 1991;24:247–252.

164. Leavitt RD, Ratanatharatorn V, Ozer J, et al. Alfa-2b interferon in the treatment of Hodgkin's disease and non-Hodgkin's lymphoma. *Semin Oncol* 1987;14[Suppl 2]:8–23.

165. Ryback M, McCarroll K, Bernard S. Interferon therapy of relapsed and refractory Hodgkin's disease. *J Biol Respons Mod* 1990;9:1–4.

166. DelCarmen M, Koziner B, Nibroski R. Recombinant interferon alfa-2b in patients with progressive and/or recurrent Hodgkin's disease. *Leuk Lymph* 1991;3:439–441.

167. Atspodier J, Kircher H. The outpatient use of human interleukin-2 and interferon alfa-2b in advanced malignancies. *Eur J Cancer* 1991;27[Suppl 4]:88–92.

168. Maloisel F, Voillat L, Chenard MP, et al. Interferon-alpha-2b in the management of patients with relapsed and/or refractory Hodgkin's disease. *Ann Oncol* 1997;8:405–406.

169. Mazza P, Tura S, Bocchia M, et al. Alpha-2b recombinant interferon (Intron) in Hodgkin's lymphoma: therapeutic perspective. *Eur J Haematol* 1990;45[Suppl 52]:22–24.

170. Aviles A, Diaz-Maqueo JC, Talavera A, et al. Maintenance therapy with interferon alfa-2b in Hodgkin's disease. *Leuk Lymph* 1998;30:651–656.

171. Montserrat E, Villamor N, Urbano-Ipizua A, et al. Alpha interferon in chronic lymphocytic leukemia. *Eur J Cancer* 1991;27[Suppl 4]:74–77.

172. Rotoli B, De Renzo A, Frigeri F, et al. A phase II trial on alpha-interferon (α-IFN) effect in patients with monoclonal IgM gammopathy. *Leuk Lymph* 1994;13:463–469.

173. Legouffe E, Rossi JF, Laporte JP, et al. Treatment of Waldenström's macroglobulinemia with very low doses of alpha interferon. *Leuk Lymph* 1995;19:337–342.

174. Ludwig H, Cohen AM, Polliack A, et al. Interferon-alpha for induction and maintenance in multiple myeloma: results of two multicenter randomized trials and summary of other studies. *Ann Oncol* 1995;6:467–476.

175. Mahon FX, Montastruc M, Faberes C, Reiffers J. Predicting complete cytogenetic response in chronic myelogenous leukemia patients treated with recombinant interferon alpha. *Blood* 1994;84:3592–3594.

176. Ozer H, George ST, Schiffer CA, et al. Prolonged subcutaneous administration of recombinant alpha-2b interferon in patients with previously untreated Philadelphia-chromosome-positive chronic-phase myelogenous leukemia: effect on remission duration and survival. Cancer and Leukemia Group B Study 8583. *Blood* 1993;82:2975–2984.

177. Niederle N, Kioke O, Wandl UB, et al. Long-term treatment of chronic myelogenous leukemia with different interferons: Results from three studies. *Leuk Lymph* 1993;9:111–119.

10.2

INTERFERON-α AND -β: CLINICAL APPLICATIONS

Melanoma

JOHN M. KIRKWOOD

DIRECT EFFECTS: INTERFERONS BINDING RECEPTORS OF TYPE I: INTERFERON-α, -β, -τ, AND -Ω

Human interferon-α (IFN-α) is comprised of a complex array of subspecies of approximately 165 to 166 amino acids, each encoded by a superfamily of closely related genes located with the IFN-α and IFN-β genes on the short arm of human chromosome 9 that are variably modified by posttranslational glycosylation (1–3). In humans, 14 nonallelic IFN-α genes and four pseudogenes are clustered together with genes for IFN-α. A variable mixture of IFN-α species is induced in leukocytes and other host cells by stimuli classically including viruses or nucleic acids. A remarkable number of biologic effects of these separate subspecies are held in common, despite variable relative antiviral, antiproliferative, antigen-modulating, and immunomodulating effects (4,5).

IFNs α and β bind with high affinity (dissociation constant of 10^{-10} to 10^{-12} M per L) to single receptors of 110 kd that are specified on chromosome 21 and range in density from 100 to 10,000 receptors per cell (6,7). A range of cellular processes induced by IFNs follow the production of a new set of proteins after binding and internalization. Knowledge of events that occur after the binding of IFN to its receptors has advanced significantly in the 1990s (8–10). A multimeric transcription activator, interferon-stimulated growth factor 3 (ISGF3), is stimulated to translocate to the nucleus, where it binds *cis* to the IFN-response element of DNA, inducing genes that comprise the array of IFN-stimulated genes (10–14). When the cytoplasmic and nuclear components of ISGF3 associated with IFN-α are activated, ISGF3-γ, the component of the complex specifically recognizing the interferon-stimulated response element (ISRE), and ISGF3, which contains three polypeptides activated specifically on phosphorylation, interact and translocate to the nucleus without the requirement of protein synthesis to activate the IFN response element.

INTERFERON BINDING RECEPTOR OF TYPE II: INTERFERON-GAMMA

IFN-γ binds a receptor that is discrete from that which is reactive with type I IFNs. Evidence for two classes of receptors, one with low affinity (10^{-9} M) and one with high affinity (10^{-11} M), have been reported (15). Most melanomas have been found to express high-affinity receptors (16). The *in vitro* and preclinical *in vivo* immunomodulatory activity of IFN-γ has been one of the most potent of all interferons, leading to expectations that IFN-γ may also be the most therapeutically active interferon against cancer. Trials of IFN-γ in patients with advanced melanoma, as well as in patients with a high risk of relapse, have been conducted systematically as for interferon-α-2 (IFN-α-2), as detailed below.

Preclinical Effects of the Interferons Relevant to Melanoma

The pleiotropism of IFNs has posed a significant problem in their quantification. The specific activity of various IFN preparations may be expressed in terms of differing functions (e.g., antiviral, antiproliferative, differentiative, effector cell activating, antigen augmenting, and enzyme inducing). Antiviral activity has been accepted as the basis of IFN standardization, although it is not clear that this function is related to the effects of IFN-γ in cancer therapy. Units of antiviral activity determined against reference standards of the Center for Biologics in Washington, DC, are commonly used to quantify IFNs α and β; recombinant IFN-γ and newly developed polyethylene glycol (PEG)–bound forms of IFN-α-2 are generally reported in terms of mass. The various species, subspecies, and molecular variants (muteins) of IFNs argue for the adoption of functional standardization in terms of alternative mechanisms relevant to antitumor activity for clinical trials.

Pleiotropic actions of IFNs may be separated into several categories that are useful in analyzing preclinical and clinical data, as summarized in Table 1. Direct effects of IFNs include antiproliferative and differentiative effects that may be demonstrated against fresh melanoma tissues or cultured cell lines *in vitro*. Effects that result in alterations in tumor cell surface antigen expression without direct impact on tumor cell growth, invasion, or metastasis, or all three, have been designated as *composite*. These effects may permit host recognition and response *in vivo*. Three major categories of IFN effects that are potentially relevant to melanoma have been studied in some detail and may provide a basis for understanding the outcome of therapeutic trials. Indirect effects of IFNs are those mediated by the host immune system, including cellular elements such as large granular lymphocyte, natural killer (NK) or lymphokine-activated killer (LAK) cells, macrophage or dendritic cells, neutrophils, and T and B cells (17–20).

Direct Effects

Actual mechanisms of antitumor action of IFNs in human cancer remain uncertain. Nonrecombinant IFNs α and β and recombinant subspecies of IFN-α-2, -β, and -γ have been evaluated *in vitro* for antiproliferative activity against cultured

TABLE 1. PLEIOTROPY OF INTERFERONS: DIRECT, COMPOSITE, AND INDIRECT EFFECTS

Direct (Tumor Cell)	Composite (Tumor Cell Antigens)	Indirect (Immune)	Indirect (Vascular)
Antiproliferative	MHC class I and MHC class II cell surface antigens	Nonantigen-specific effector activation	Antiangiogenic
Differentiative	Tumor-restricted cell surface antigens	Macrophage-monocyte/dendritic cell	
Antiviral	Adhesion molecules	Large granular lymphocyte	
	ICAM-1	FcR expression	
		MHC class I/II expression	
		Antigen-specific effector modulation	
		T cell	
		B cell	

FcR, Fc receptor; ICAM-1, intercellular adhesion molecule-1; MHC, major histocompatibility complex.

and fresh melanoma. These IFNs demonstrate comparable growth-inhibitory activity, and one may draw from them three general observations: (a) a direct dose-response tumor-inhibiting relationship exists for each, (b) heterogeneity among different tumors regarding sensitivity to inhibition occurs, and (c) a sensitivity of a majority of melanomas to high levels (greater than 500 U per mL) of IFN *in vitro* exists. Molecular probes for the dissection of pathways of IFN signaling are available, allowing their analysis beyond measurement of IFN-induced enzymes such as oligoadenylate synthetase (see below), and more distal effects on target-cell major histocompatibility complex antigen expression. Some of these studies conducted with tumor cells suggest that acquired defects in the signal transducers and activators of transcription (STAT) pathway exist that may lend to combined IFN-α-2 therapy. Clinical trials to test these possibilities are underway. Analysis of signal transduction intermediates of IFNs in cells of the melanocytic series (such as atypical and dysplastic nevi) is feasible as a surrogate for effects on tumor cells remaining in patients after surgery for high-risk melanoma. These studies have revealed unexpected evidence of constitutive activation of some elements of the STAT pathway in precursor atypical nevi, arguing for the prospective evaluation and correlation of these intermediates and the markers of progression in prospective trials (21).

Enzyme Induction

A number of enzyme pathways are activated after induction of the IFN response element, including some that have been evaluated in clinical trials. These include 2'5' oligo adenylate synthetase (2'5' oligo-As), and protein kinase (p67) (22). Two molecular forms of 2'5' oligo-As of 33 kd and 110 kd have been identified, differing in subcellular localization and activation requirements (23,24). Roles of different forms of 2'5' oligo-As in relation to antitumor effects of IFN have not been established. Indoleamine 2,3,-dioxygenase is induced by IFNs in a dose- and time-dependent fashion; this enzyme alters tryptophan metabolism (25) and, with xanthine oxidase, generates superoxides that may relate to therapeutic and toxic effects of IFN, as well as to depression of cytochrome P-450 enzyme levels (26,27). IFN-γ–induced neopterin production may provide an additional biochemical tool for analyzing intermediate effects of IFN-γ *in vivo*.

Direct Effects: Antiproliferative Effects of Interferons in Combination with Chemotherapy and Other Biologic Agents *In Vitro*

The presence of additive or synergistic effects of chemotherapeutic agents have been examined with IFNs *in vitro*, using isobologram plots to assess comparing agents in combination with one another for synergistic, additive, or subadditive effects against melanoma lines (28). Synergistic effects between IFN-α-2a, doxorubicin, and bleomycin against SKMel-28 have been identified; additive effects between IFN-γ and doxorubicin have also been reported (29). Synergism between IFN-β and vinblastine, using melanoma line CRL

1424 (30), have been reported, as have negative interactions between vinblastine and IFN-α (29).

Synergistic antiproliferative interactions of IFNs α, β, and γ have been noted against murine B16 melanoma (31) and a human melanoma line (32), as well as fresh and cryopreserved human melanomas (33). At low levels of 1 to 10 U per mL, IFN-γ has been shown to increase the induction of enzyme 2'5' oligo by IFN-α and -β (34). IFN-γ has been shown to potentiate apoptotic cell death and DNA fragmentation induced by tumor necrosis factor (TNF) (35), whereas IFNs α and γ potentiate the tumor-cytotoxic activity of TNF in clonogenic stem cell assays (36).

Direct Effects: Differentiation *In Vitro* and *In Vivo*

Differentiative and growth regulatory, or apoptotic, effects of IFNs became focal points of interest in the 1990s. A number of adhesion molecules, growth factors, and receptors have been identified in malignant melanoma but not in normal nevi. Receptor-ligand pairs may serve as paracrine or autocrine growth-stimulating circuits in melanoma. A progression cascade has been proposed (37) in which precursor atypical (and histologically dysplastic) nevi evolve through discrete stages that culminate with invasive melanoma. Growth factor receptors, ligands, adhesion molecules, and other progression factors that distinguish the later phases in this melanocytic progression sequence may serve as ideal targets for interventions to prevent melanoma (38). Epidermal growth-factor receptor (EGFR) expression plays an uncertain role in melanoma. TNF, IFN-γ (or a combination of these cytokines) enhance expression of EGFR in melanoma line DX3 *in vitro*. In contrast, IFN-α and retinoic acid inhibit EGFR expression in other systems. Retinoids, as well as IFNs, are studied as potential inhibitors of melanoma induction in which the molecular impact of these agents on discrete mediators of progression provides the strongest preclinical rationale for their use in long-term melanoma prevention efforts.

All three species of IFN modulate melanocyte-stimulating hormone (MSH) receptor expression and have been reported to influence the response to MSH *in vitro*, with production of tyrosinase and melanization (39). In the absence of MSH, no prodifferentiative effect, augmented tyrosinase, or melanin production was demonstrable for any IFN. The differentiative effects of MSH *in vivo* provide one rationale for consideration of IFNs in treatment of melanoma precursors. Paradoxically, the induction of differentiation (melanization) by IFN-γ in experimental melanoma has been reported to be associated with increased metastatic potential of murine B16 melanoma (40).

Human IFN-α (N1) and IFN-γ have been tested against human DX3 melanoma, which metastasizes in the nude athymic mouse. Metastatic lung disease is reduced, and survival of mice is significantly prolonged without apparent effects on differentiation (pigmentation), NK activity, or macrophage activity in this model, in which therapeutic benefit has been attributed to direct antimetastatic effects of IFN-γ (41). Intercellular adhesion molecule-1 (ICAM-1) expressed in metastatic melanoma and associated with invasion in primary melanoma is induced by exposure of melanoma cells to IFN-γ (42,43). Effects on ICAM-1 and other molecules associated with progression may explain the untoward results obtained in some clinical trials.

Composite (Antigenic) Antitumor Mechanisms: Modulation of Melanoma-Associated Cell Surface Antigens

The effects of IFNs have been related to their impacts on cell surface antigens of melanoma in several systems. The histocompatibility complex is among the most consistent and sensitive targets of IFNs (see Composite Effects: Modulation of Major Histocompatibility Complex Antigens). The effects of IFNs on expression of melanoma-associated gangliosides or receptors for growth factors, or both, have been studied, in the hope that these effects may result in enhanced tumor cell susceptibility to host immune recognition and rejection by effector cells or antibodies.

IFNs modulate the expression of many cell surface molecules, not all of which have been assigned physiologic functions in the melanocyte, although some may play a role in the progression from premalignant process to metastasis-competent invasive disease, as noted in Table 1 (44–48). Markers found to be expressed in melanoma but not—or significantly less—in normal nevic melanocytes include antigens of class II major histocompatibility complex, ICAM-1, nerve cell adhesion molecule (N-CAM)–like molecule Muc-18, and growth factors like basic fibroblast growth factor (bFGF) and transforming growth factor-alpha (TGF-α), as well as gangliosides such as GD_2 (49–57). The molecular events of tumor progression may potentially be targeted immunologically or modulated by agents such as IFNs, retinoids, or antisense RNA, or all of these, to prevent evolution of melanoma. The ability of IFNs to modulate markers that distinguish melanoma from other tissues also lends to their use in combined-modality therapy.

Combined Use of Interferons and Antibodies

The expression of the melanoma-associated antigen p96 has been shown to be augmented by IFN-γ, but not by IFNs α or β. IFN-α and IFN-β have been reported to enhance the expression of the transferrin receptor–like glycoprotein p97, although neither affects the high-molecular-weight melanoma proteoglycan–associated glycoprotein antigen p240. Diagnostic and therapeutic results obtained with the corresponding antibody (96.5 anti-p97) were reported to be improved when combined with IFN and associated with a significantly prolonged plasma half-life and increased volume of distribution of radiolabeled 96.5 antibody administered 24 hours after IFN. Improved localization of antibody to tumor with threefold increased tumor: blood distribution was suggested, although direct evidence from tumor and normal tissue biopsies is lacking.

The monosialoganglioside G_{M2} and the disialoganglioside G_{D3} are recognized cell surface antigens of melanoma. G_{D3} is reported to be modulated in some cell lines by IFN-α and -β without apparent synergy or additive effects between IFN types. These effects of IFN have served as a rationale for trials of IFN in conjunction with antibodies to melanoma. In early series, the

anti-G_{D3} antibody R_{24} is reported to induce objective remissions in 10% to 20% of patients with metastatic melanoma (59–61), but these results have not been confirmed in larger subsequent studies studied to identify immunologic dose-response correlates and maximal tolerable dosage (62,63). IFN-α administered concomitantly with R_{24} has been reported to decrease circulating T-suppressor cell and NK cell numbers in patients (64).

Composite Effects: Modulation of Major Histocompatibility Complex Antigens

The modulation of major histocompatibility complex (MHC) class I HLA-A, -B, or -C antigens has been described for all classes of IFN. IFN-γ, and to a lesser extent, IFN-β, regulate MHC class II [HLA deoxyribose (DR), DP, and DQ], as well as class I antigens (45,65–69).

Human melanoma cells express class I and class II MHC antigens; class II MHC antigens are expressed hierarchically (with HLA-DR > DQ > DP) in melanoma (70). Expression of HLA-DR antigens is demonstrable in the majority of primary melanomas, whereas HLA-DQ antigens are detected in only 38% (71). Variable loss or alteration in expression or membrane transport of HLA-A, -B, or -C has been reported in dysplastic and congenital melanocytic lesions, as well as melanoma (72,73). The prognosis of primary melanoma has been correlated with the expression of MHC class I and II antigens. Melanomas expressing HLA-A, -B, or -C antigens in greater than 50% of tumor cells concomitantly, with HLA-DR expressed in less than 50% of cells, are noted to have a better prognosis.

Clinical implications of altered MHC antigen expression relate to their pivotal functions in intercellular immunologic recognition and communication at multiple levels. Antigen presentation to T cells by macrophages, Langerhans' or dendritic cells, and B cells are associated with the expression of MHC class I and II antigens, adhesion molecules, and costimulating molecules (e.g., B7) as recognition structures for helper and cytotoxic T cells. The expression of HLA-DR was recognized to be necessary but insufficient for recognition and response to melanoma by autologous T lymphocytes (71,74). Antitumor effects of IFNs α and β may thus occur through their augmentation of melanoma MHC class I antigen expression, whereas differing therapeutic effects of IFN-γ may relate to its broader impact on MHC class I and II antigens in melanoma and other tumors (75,76). Although induction of class II MHC antigens in primary melanoma cells may increase their immunologic reactivity, the treatment of metastatic melanoma cells *in vitro* with IFN-γ does not enhance autologous T-cell recognition, mitotic burst, or cytotoxic function. Decreased susceptibility to NK cells is associated with induction of increased class I major histocompatibility antigen expression (77,78). IFN-γ protects human melanoma cells from lysis by LAK or activated NK cells; exposure of melanoma cells to as little as 1 to 10 U per mL of IFN-γ decreases tumor cell sensitivity to LAK cell lysis within hours (79,80).

The induction of MHC class I and II antigens by IFN-γ may increase the immunogenicity of melanoma cells used for vaccination, outweighing effects on susceptibility to NK or LAK effector cells in a murine model (81). IFN-γ–treated B16 melanoma cells elicit improved host immune resistance to subsequent tumor

TABLE 2. RECOMBINANT INTERFERON (IFN)-α IN METASTATIC MELANOMA

Study (Reference)	Dose (MU)	Route/Schedule	Entered/ Evaluable	Response CR	PR	Percent	Median Duration (Mo)
IFN-α-2a							
Creagan (156)	$12/m^2$	i.m. t.i.w. × 12 wk	30/30	1	5	20	12.9+, 1.9, 3.0, 3.2, 19.6, 9.6+
Creagan (155)	$50/m^2$	i.m. t.i.w. × 12 wk	31/31	3	4	23	6.4, 10.0+, 11.2, 3.0; 3.0, 4.6, 7.0
Coates (157)	$20/m^2$	i.v. daily × 5–14 d	16/15	0	0	0	—
Hersey (93)	$50/m^2$	i.m. t.i.w.	20/18	1	1	11	12.0; 6.5
Legha (128)	3–36	i.m. daily	35/31	0	3	10	6.2, 6.7, 6.9, 10.0, 20.3
		i.m. 3 × wk	31/31	0	2	6	
Elsasser-Beile (159)	18	i.m. daily × 10 wk, then t.i.w.	21/21	3	0	14	6.0+, 7.8+, 12.0+
Steiner (160)	18	i.m. daily	12/12	1	0	8	4+
IFN-α-2a subtotal			**196/189**	**9**	**15**	**12.6**	**—**
IFN-α-2b							
Kirkwood (161)	10–100	i.m. or i.v. daily × 28 d	23/23	3	2	22	36+, 36+, 60+, 3, 4
Dorval (162)	$10/m^2$	s.c. t.i.w.	22/22	2	4	27	1.5, 4.6, 2.0, 4.0, 4.0, 4.0, 5.0
Robinson (163)	$30/m^2$	s.c. t.i.w. × 12+ wk	51/40	4	6	25	5, 13+, 15, 32+; 1, 1, 2, 5, 6, 6
Sertoli (158)	$10/m^2$	i.m. t.i.w.	21/21	0	3	14	7.0, 12.5, 13.0
IFN-α-2b subtotal			**117/106**	**9**	**15**	**22.6**	**—**
IFN-α-2 total			**313/295**	**18**	**30**	**16.3**	**—**

CR, complete response; PR, partial response.

challenge through effects attributed to an enhanced T-cell response (82). Thus, induction of increased MHC class I and II tumor-cell surface–antigen expression may account for the enhanced efficacy of host T-cell–mediated immunity or tumor cell elimination by means of a composite mechanism, irrespective of the modulation of effector cell functions.

INDIRECT IMMUNOMODULATORY EFFECTS

Macrophage, Natural Killer, T, and B Cells

The macrophage is a key target of IFN-γ, which is described as a macrophage-activating factor (83–85). The large granular lymphocyte known as the *NK cell* is a well-recognized target of IFNs *in vitro* (86,87). Clinical relevance of the effects of IFNs on NK activity has been sought *in vitro* and *in vivo* with IFNs α, β, and γ. NK activity measurements in multiple trials has depended on assay conditions, effector cell manipulation, and delay from blood-drawing to assay (rest period). No convincing evidence of a relationship between NK cell activity *in vivo* and therapeutic activity of IFNs in patients with melanoma or other solid tumors has been documented (88–91). Antibody-dependent cellular cytotoxicity (ADCC) function of peripheral blood lymphocytes is mediated in part by NK cells, and has been augmented *in vitro* and *in vivo* by IFN-α, as well as interleukin-2 (IL-2) (92). As trials of antitumor antibodies are further developed, the optimization of NK activity and ADCC with IFNs, IL-2, IL-12, and other biologics continues to be important.

T Cell

Specific T-cell–mediated immunity has been implicated as the basis of antitumor effects of IFNs in human melanoma. Durable complete responses have been reported in multiple clinical trials of IFN-α (Table 2). Population shifts in T-cell subsets has

been noted during therapy with IFNs α and γ, and clinical antitumor response to IFN-α and IFN-γ have been correlated with reproducible shifts in T-cell subset distribution, but not with other mechanisms examined to date (93–99). IFN-α modulates mixed leukocyte reactions *in vitro* (100), and the presence of T-cell infiltrates *in situ* has been correlated with favorable prognosis (101). The modulation of specific cytotoxic T-cell immune responses to melanoma by IFN-α-2 remains a leading hypothetical basis of durable antitumor effects observed with IFN-α-2 in multiple trials; prospectively, this observation is being evaluated in cooperative group trials that have sufficient numbers to permit correlation with treatment and outcome (18,19,102–107). The definition of MHC class I–restricted and MHC class II (DR)–restricted epitopes recognized by CD4+ T cells adds a new dimension to the expanse of CD8+ T-cell–defined MHC class I–restricted epitopes for analyzing IFN-modulated effector functions (108).

In preclinical systems, Belardelli, Gresser, and colleagues (109–111) have shown that IFN prevents the outgrowth of experimental murine tumors treated shortly after tumor challenge. Antitumor activity of murine type I IFN in this system critically depends on the presence of an intact immune system in the host and the participation of the CD4+ subset of T cells. Tumor response does not correlate with the tumor cell susceptibility to direct tumor growth inhibition by IFN in this model; rather, tumor regression induced by IFN in this system appears to be associated with immunologic effects of IFN on the tumor and host.

B Cell

In relation to the B cell response to tumor, IFN-γ increases production of immunoglobulin G (IgG)–2a and decreases that of IgG-3, IgG-1, IgG-2b, and IgE by human B cells (112). The last several years have seen the initiation of trials of several whole-cell tumor vaccines administered in conjunction

TABLE 3. SYSTEMICALLY ADMINISTERED INTERFERON (IFN)-γ ALONE AND IN COMBINATION WITH OTHER BIOLOGICS AND CHEMOTHERAPEUTIC AGENTS

Study (Reference)	Dose MU	Route/Schedule	Entered/ Evaluable	Response			Median Duration (Mo)
				CR	PR	Percent	
IFN-γ							
Creagan (180)	0.25 mg–0.5 mg/m^2	i.v. daily	27/27	0	3	11	3.7, 3.9, 8.3
Perez (181)[a]	0.01–2.00 mg/m^2	i.v. bolus daily, then i.m. or s.c. daily for 5 d/wk, 2 wk of every 4	12/12	0	0	0	—
Ernstoff (279)[b]	0.003–3.000 mg/m^2	i.v. 2 hr daily for 14 d out of every 28 d	15/15	1	1	13	4, 4
		i.v. 24 hr continuous infusion for 14 d out of every 28 d	15/15	0	0	0	—
Schiller (280–282)[a]	0.01–0.90 mg/m^2	i.v. t.i.w. for 3 mo	98/95/81	1	3	5	NA
IFN-γ + IFN-β$_{Ser}$							
Schiller (185)[b]							
rIFN-γ	2 mg	i.v. over 2 h, t.i.w.	15/15	0	0	0	—
+rIFN-β$_{ser}$	30 MU/m^2	i.v. t.i.w.					
IFN-β + IFN-α-2a							
Creagan (186)[a]							
rIFN-β	0.010–0.025–0.05 mg/m^2	i.m. daily	20/20	0	1	0	7+
+rIFN-α-2a	2–10 MU/m^2	i.m. daily for 7 d at each tier					
IFN-γ + IFN-α-2c							
Osanto (187)[b]							
rIFN-γ	0.05 mg/m^2	s.c. t.i.w.	15/15	0	0	0	—
	0.1 mg/m^2	Escalated every 2 wk					
	0.2 mg/m^2	s.c. 3 × wk					
+rIFN-α-2c	2 MU/m^2						

CR, complete response; PR, partial response; rIFN, recombinant interferon.
[a]Genentech, San Francisco, CA.
[b]Biogen, Inc., Cambridge, MA.

with IFN-α-2. The Eastern Cooperative Oncology Group (ECOG) trial E2696 analyzed immunomodulatory effects of IFN-α-2b administered together with or after the (GM2) vaccine [GM2–KLH plus QS 21 (GMK)] (Progenics, Tarrytown, NY), establishing the feasibility of this combination without loss of serologic response to GM2 (as detected by enzyme-linked immunoadsorbent assays for IgM and IgG) and paving the way for a GM2 plus IFN combination (see Adjuvant Combinations). A further phase 3 trial of Melacine (Ribi Immuno Chem, Inc.) is also in progress, testing vaccine plus IFN versus IFN at lower dosages.

Specific effects of IFNs α, β, and γ on specific immune function against autologous melanoma have not been examined, however. Difficulty measuring immune response to autologous tumor cell-surface antigens has impeded this analysis in clinical trials of IFNs, and it may be no less important than in the interpretation of therapeutic response to vaccine trials.

MULTIPARAMETER ANALYSIS OF IMMUNOMODULATION IN VIVO DURING PHASE 1B TRIALS FOR MELANOMA

Effects of IFN-α on elements of the immune system have been summarized. The activity of IFN-α and IFN-γ on several effector cell populations (potentially related to clinical antitumor

effects of IFN-α) has been reported by many authors (19,88,92,104,113,114).

Two single-institution dose-response studies of IFN-γ focusing on melanoma have been reported (Table 3). One phase 1–2 trial (105,115) of 30 patients with measurable metastatic melanoma conducted at the Pittsburgh Cancer Institute Melanoma Center evaluated the immunomodulatory effects of five different dosages of IFN-γ (Biogen, Inc., Cambridge, MA), ranging from 3 to 30 to 300 to 1,000 to 3,000 μg per m^2 per day intravenously, in groups of six patients each. Phenotypic markers of host effector–cell activation, NK cell activity, and IFN-induced enzyme activation reveal no major differences in the effects of 2-hour daily and 24-hour continuous intravenous infusions (115,116). The most potent and consistent augmentation of host mononuclear cell 2′5′ oligo-As enzyme and NK cell activity, as well as relative T helper: suppressor cell shifts at 2 weeks of treatment has been reported between dosages of 300 and 1,000 μg per m^2 per day.

The Biological Response Modifier Program of the National Cancer Institute has carried out a phase 1B trial (117) of IFN-γ in patients without measurable known metastatic disease. Twenty-five patients with resected stage I to III melanoma were treated for 15 days with one of five dosages ranging from 0.1 to 1 to 10 to 100 to 250 μg per m^2 per day intramuscular (i.m.) IFN-γ (Genentech, Inc., San Francisco, CA). NK activity, monocyte H$_2$O$_2$ release, Fc receptor expression, and HLA-DR expression were evaluated serially during the 15-day treatment cycles (118). A daily dosage of 100 μg per m^2 was found to induce maximally monocyte Fc receptor density, hydrogen peroxide production, and MHC class II DR antigen expression. These investigators recommended pursuing a three-times-weekly regimen of 0.2 mg IFN-γ, administered subcutaneously (see Adjuvant Application of Interferon). Kleinerman et al. have studied IFN-γ administered by 6-hour intravenous (i.v.) infusion in terms of monocyte tumoricidal activity; i.m. inoculations of 0.25 to 0.5 mg per m^2 per day were effective, but higher doses of 1.0 mg per m^2 per day did not activate monocytes (118).

Together, the data of the Melanoma Center of the Pittsburgh Cancer Institute and the Biologic Response Modifier Program of the National Cancer Institute suggest that intermediate dosages of IFN-γ, ranging from 100 to 1,000 mg, induce optimal activation of NK activity, CD4/CD8 ratio, DR expression, and 2'5' A synthetase on one hand, and NK activity, monocyte H$_2$O$_2$ release, and Fc receptor/DR antigen expression on the other (105,115,118,119). These studies have been limited in numbers, however; they included a total of only 25 to 30 patients each, with only three to seven patients per dose tier. Furthermore, IFN produced by two different pharmaceutical sources—Biogen and Genentech, respectively—were evaluated. In neither study were the immunologic effects of dose evaluated over intervals generally considered adequate for determining clinical antitumor effects (i.e., 1 to 3 months).

The ECOG reported a dose-seeking phase 2 study of seven dosages of IFN-γ (E4687) ranging from 0.01 to 0.90 mg (0.01, 0.03, 0.10, 0.30, 0.50, 0.70, and 0.90 mg per m^2, i.v., three times weekly). The dosages tested in this trial bracketed the suggested optimal immunomodulatory dosages of previous studies and extended to lower and higher dosages than previously evaluated. The clinical trial was complemented by a laboratory study of immunomodulatory effects measured in serial blood samples drawn over a 29-day interval from a majority of participants in the clinical study (118,120,121). Ninety-eight patients entered this therapeutic trial, with 11 to 16 per dose tier, several times the number studied in previous dose-response analyses. One-half of the patients treated during the clinical study E4687 entered the laboratory immunologic corollary study E4987, nested within the clinical trial.

The immunomodulatory impact of IFN-γ was found to be significant and durable at 29 days of treatment. Immune effects of IFN-γ were most pronounced in the T-cell compartment at the lowest dosages tested, whereas effects on the NK/monocyte compartment were maximal at the mid-to-higher dosages tested. This multiparameter analysis of immune response to IFN-γ produced results more complex than originally envisioned: rises in CD4/CD8 ratio and suppression of CD8 T-cell subset numbers occurred early in treatment and were durable through day 29 in only the lowest-dose (0.01 mg per m^2 per day) tier. NK and monocyte activation, determined either by functional assays or by phenotypic markers, were most notable earlier and correlated significantly with IFN-γ dosage for all dose groups over the lowest dosage (0.03→0.9 mg per m^2 per day). The results of this study differ according to time of assessment and dosage regarding phenotypic shifts (at low dosages) and NK cell/monocyte activation (at high dosages), suggesting that results of previously reported clinical trials must be interpreted with caution.

ROLE OF INTERFERON-γ AS A MEDIATOR OF CLINICAL EFFECTS OF OTHER CYTOKINES

IFN-γ induction by IL-2 has been documented in several trials (122) in which ambient levels of 1 to 7 U per mL were shown to be induced after continuous i.v. infusion of IL-2 at dosages of 1.5 to 20 MIU per m^2. IFN-γ induced during therapy with IL-2 may play a role in therapeutic, as well as toxic effects of IL-2. Other cytokines that are T-cell activators and modulators, including IL-4, IL-7, and IL-12, may also achieve their effects in part through IFN-γ or its modulation. The effects of IL-12 are closely related to the induction of IFN-α, in which the toxicity of induced IFN-α has proven to be problematic (123).

ANTIANGIOGENIC ACTIONS OF IFN-α

IFN-α was one of the earliest available antiangiogenic agents for clinical exploration. Based on seminal observations in B16 murine melanoma, angiogenesis is recognized as a factor in tumor progression (124). Despite the large clinical trial experience with IFNs α, β, and γ, no direct evidence of a role for antiangiogenic effects in clinical benefits exists for IFN-α or IFN-β in human melanoma and other solid tumors. The observation that IFN-α is able to cause regression of hemangiomas of childhood stands as a clinical basis for exploration of this mechanism in relation to the clinical antitumor activity of IFN in malignant neoplasms (125). Signaling through bFGF and its receptor, FGFR-1, is demonstrated to be relevant to human melanoma growth *in vitro* and in explant tumors of nude mice. The application of antisense ligand- and receptor-specific oligonucleotides is required for significant inhibition of tumor growth (126,127). Delivery of antisense nucleotides is an issue for extrapolation of this observation to clinical trials; the relevance of bFGF and VEGF to vascularization of human melanoma has not been documented directly, although studies now in progress may resolve this question. A balance between proangiogenic (bFGF) and antiangiogenic (IFN-2) effects have been proposed, based on preclinical studies that require evaluation.

TOXICITY AND PHARMACOKINETICS OF THE INTERFERONS: RESULTS OF PHASE 1 TRIALS

The clinical toxicity of different IFN species involves a similar range of target organs, although relative components of toxicity differ from species to species (128,129). Acutely, a flulike constitutional syndrome with fever, chills, headache, malaise, myalgias, arthralgias, and fatigue occurs in the majority of patients and is diminished over time with continued daily or alternate-daily administration (best at bedtime). Long-term toxicity of IFN consists of constitutional flulike symptoms compounded by anorexia, weight loss, and fatigue. These late toxicities are complex results of dysgeusia, low-grade fever, and nutritional compromise and may be difficult to differentiate from the appearance of thyroid dysfunction or other endocrine pathology on the basis of the autoimmune processes recognized for IFN-α as for IL-2. Neuropsychiatric toxicity ranges from mild cognitive deficits to frank depression and psychosis. Low back pain and headache with severe rigors have been associated with IFN-α in particular. Metabolic alterations in the blood–lipid profile and elevated low-density lipoproteins (LDLs), owing to inhibition of lipoprotein lipase, have been noted with hypertriglyceridemia (130). IFN-α may depress plasma cholesterol by 15% to 40%, with a parallel decrement in high- and low-density cholesterol (although very low-density lipoproteins are not altered) (131–133).

Leukopenia is a hematologic toxicity of the IFNs; less frequently, thrombocytopenia and anemia result. Infections are a recognized complication of leukopenia, but bleeding complications have been rare. Diminished colony-forming capacity and hypocellularity have been noted in the bone marrow, which are rapidly reversible on withdrawal of IFN (134,135).

Hepatotoxicity observed at high doses frequently includes elevated circulating transaminase enzyme levels that are dose-related and reversible on withdrawal of the agent without evidence of cholestasis. Rarely, subacute hepatic necrosis and cholestatic liver failure resulting in death have been observed when IFN is administered in the face of hepatotoxicity with hyperbilirubinemia or history of antecedent viral or alcoholic liver disease. Careful observation of hepatic function generally permits the avoidance of such problems, with treatment modified according to signs and symptoms of toxicity (18,136). After the initial report of two cases of fatal hepatotoxicity of high-dose IFN in the pivotal E1684 adjuvant trial for high-risk melanoma (137), the confirmatory intergroup trial E1690 was completed without any instance of life-threatening hepatotoxicity; the only two toxic fatalities noted were cardiovascular and cerebrovascular, occurring on low-dose IFN.

Cardiovascular, renal, and central nervous system (CNS) toxicity is less common. Supraventricular tachyarrhythmias noted with IFNs may be direct effects or related to fever, nutritional, and fluid imbalances. Complex conduction disturbances have been observed with IFN-γ, including bradycardia with high-grade heart block (105). Cardiotoxicity is increased among elderly patients and patients with underlying heart disease or previous exposure to cardiotoxic agents, but the mechanism has not been defined (138,139). Hypotension occurs through at least two separate mechanisms: acute hypotension 1 to 2 hours after IFN administration may be related to peripheral vasodilatation and responds to a fluid repletion (or, rarely, may require pressors); hypotension during chronic administration of IFNs is related to subclinical low-grade fever with insidious fluid losses, anorexia, dysgeusia, and diminished fluid intake. Proteinuria is the most common renal manifestation of IFN and is generally reversible on its withdrawal (140–143). Rarely, interstitial nephritis and nephrotic syndrome have been reported with IFNs α and γ (138,144).

CNS toxicity associated with global changes in mentation is often subtle. Although cognitive dysfunction induced by IFN may be documented in formal testing, it is often more apparent to families and friends of patients. Stupor and coma with diffuse slowing of electroencephalogram pattern has been reported infrequently and is reversible on discontinuation of IFN (139,145). Mild peripheral neuropathy has also been noted, with paraesthesia and slowing of nerve conduction velocity.

Reversible retinal microvascular toxicity has been noted during studies of IFN-α administered for macular degeneration that may indicate the need for ophthalmologic evaluation of IFN-α therapy in other settings (146).

Rhabdomyolysis has rarely been reported in association with IFN-α-2 at high dosages (147). The significance and attribution of such occurrences is difficult to resolve, however, because it has been reported to occur less than a week into IFN-α-2 therapy in patients who are postoperative. Although monitoring for elevations in creatine phosphokinase enzymes has been suggested, it is not an adopted practice because the event is rare and occurs early, precluding use of laboratory values to monitor treatment and supportive care. The maximum tolerated dose for IFN-α lies between 10 and 20 MU per m^2 daily and 50 MU per m^2 alternate-daily for periods of weeks to months, regardless of subspecies. The half-life of IFN is 6 hours in the blood and allows alternate-daily schedules of outpatient administration by i.m. and subcutaneous (s.c.) routes. The maximum tolerated dose for IFN-α varies according to industrial preparation used, schedule, and route; acceptable absorption and activity have been reported with IFN-γ administered intravenously or intramuscularly (148,149). Early pharmacokinetic studies of IFN-α-2 have demonstrated that peak levels at 5 MU per m^2 obtained by the intravenous (i.v.) route do not reach 100 U per mL, whereas by the i.m. and s.c. routes generally adopted for therapy, they remain less than 50 U per mL. By contrast, the administration of doses of 20 MU per m^2 (or 36 MU per dose in early pharmacodynamic studies) achieves serum levels approaching 10,000 U per mL. This difference in the pharmacodynamics and peak levels has been the focus of considerable interest as the positive results of trials using the i.v. administration of 20 MU per m^2 have shown the first survival benefits in melanoma, whereas lower dosages administered by alternative routes have yielded less clinically meaningful results. The maximum tolerated dose of IFN-γ ranges between 1,000 to 5,000 μg per m^2 for daily and alternate-daily (three times weekly) schedules and differs for the several preparations of IFN-γ (Biogen, Inc., Cambridge, MA; Genentech, San Francisco, CA; Schering Plough, Kenilworth, NJ) (105,143).

INTERFERON-γ AS A SINGLE AGENT FOR METASTATIC DISEASE: PHASE 1–2 TRIALS OF INTERFERON-α-2

The reference agent for treatment of melanoma, and the only chemotherapeutic agent approved by the U.S. Food and Drug Administration since 1976, is dacarbazine (dimethyl triazine imidazole carboxamide). Dacarbazine therapy is associated with response rates of 15% to 25% (20%, mean) in collected series and median duration of response is 5 to 6 months (151–153). Few patients with metastatic melanoma treated with dacarbazine achieve a complete response. Temozolomide is an orally well absorbed and widely distributed prodrug that has wider tissue distribution than dacarbazine and spontaneously converts rather than requiring hepatic anabolism to mitozolomide, the active agent in dacarbazine. Temozolomide has received accelerated approval from the U.S. Food and Drug Administration

Oncologic Drug Advisory Committee for use in anaplastic astrocytoma, and has shown equivalence to dacarbazine in large international phase 3 trials against melanoma with greater ease of administration of the potential for CNS antitumor activity (154). The nitrosoureas, vinca alkaloids, taxanes, and platinum coordination compound have exhibited activity against metastatic melanoma, although the response rate for each of these classes has generally been less than 15%.

Against this background, IFN-α was initially brought to clinical trial against melanoma in 1978, when the American Cancer Society began a series of trials of buffy-coat leukocyte IFN produced by K. Cantell from the Finnish Red Cross. These trials were limited by the extremely short supply of the agent, and trials that therefore endured for only 6 weeks; therefore, no firm conclusions can be drawn. The trials served as an important impetus for the pharmaceutical industry to begin commercial production of IFNs α, β, γ, and other biologics, using recombinant DNA (rDNA) technology. The large-scale production of IFNs by rDNA technology enabled the first systematic evaluation of appropriate dose, route, and schedule of IFN-α-2, as well as the other major subspecies of IFNs α, β, and γ.

Phase 2 trials that document the antitumor activity of recombinant IFN-α-2 in melanoma are summarized in Table 2 (93,128,155–163). The overall response rate with IFN-α-2 is 15.4% in these collected series, with one-third of those responses complete in the longest-followed series (5% overall), irrespective of IFN-α-2 subtype. No cross-resistance to IFN after unsuccessful previous chemotherapy, radiation therapy, hormonal therapy, IL-2, bacille Calmette-Guérin, or other non-IFN biologics has been reported. The comparable antitumor activity of IFN-α-2 in metastatic disease, whether administered early (as initial therapy) or late (after other modalities were unsuccessful), has led to its early exploration for advanced disease. It has been argued, however, that the best opportunity for additive or synergistic curative immunologic effects is available in initial treatment with the smallest tumor burden (see Combined Modality Therapy). The median duration of partial responses with recombinant IFN-α-2 is 4 months, whereas the duration of complete responses sustained off all therapy for as long as 7 years in results from several centers. A summary of long-term responders has shown in these patients no distinguishing features of disease that might allow prediction of response or any role of maintenance therapy with IFN after induction of complete response. The median interval to complete response in melanoma and other solid tumors may be as long as 3 months, with some responses noted as late as 6 months on therapy.

Predictors of Favorable Response

The best therapeutic results with IFN-α-2 have been reported with uninterrupted schedules of therapy, regardless of the route (s.c., i.m., or i.v.), and no clear advantage of lower or higher dosages exists in the range between 10 MU per m^2 daily and 50 MU per m^2, administered daily or alternate-daily (97,129,163). Intermittent cyclic treatment with IFN-α-2a administered 5 out of every 14 days, or IFN-α-2b, administered 5 of every 21 (163,165) days, are inactive (157,163,165). IFN-α-2 adminis-

tered alone at dosage ranges below 10 MU per m^2 three times weekly have not been studied adequately to date in metastatic measurable disease to allow firm conclusions.

Response to IFN-α-2 has been associated with cutaneous and soft tissue, pulmonary sites of disease, and low tumor bulk. Responses in visceral disease have been reported with IFNs in multiple series, however (128,129,163,164). In contrast to chemotherapy with dacarbazine, in which women appear to have a significant advantage, no influence of gender on response to IFN-α has been observed (129).

Predictors of Unfavorable Outcome

Creagan et al. (129,156,166) have prospectively stratified patient accrual for potential prognostic factors in several different trials. A logistic regression analysis of the effect of performance status (0 to 1), previous chemotherapy, site of dominant tumor involvement (visceral), age (older than 55 years), male gender, and treatment dosage, has demonstrated that response was not correlated with performance status, previous chemotherapy exposure, age, or gender. Only the site of dominant metastatic disease (and, in particular, the presence of visceral involvement) was associated with reduced response rate (129). The presence of visceral disease in this series may have served as a surrogate for increased tumor burden, which has also been correlated with diminished likelihood of objective response.

Visceral disease in the CNS has been a major problem with biologic modalities in general, and IFNs in particular. The occurrence of metastatic disease in the CNS (167) after remission of peripheral disease has been attributed to the presence of an immunologic sanctuary in the CNS (167), and anecdotal studies have demonstrated poor penetration of IFNs into the CNS. Observed activities of IFN-β in chronic relapsing multiple sclerosis suggest that IFN may mediate effects on disease sites in the brain, even if the IFN molecule has not been demonstrated to penetrate the CNS in significant levels during therapy.

The development of anti-IFN neutralizing serum antibodies has been correlated with loss of antitumor effects in other diseases (e.g., chronic myelogenous leukemia) and appears to vary with disease state and species of IFN used. In representative series, antibodies have been detected in up to 5% of subjects after 2 to 6 months of therapy (157,168) without demonstrable adverse consequences for therapeutic effects in patients with melanoma. Strategies to reduce immunogenicity and increase the likelihood of tolerance to recombinant IFN-α have included the initial use of i.v. (as opposed to s.c. or i.m.) routes and continuous (as opposed to interrupted) schedules.

REGIONAL THERAPY WITH INTERFERON-α OR INTERFERON-γ

Intralesional administration of IFN-α (169) at 6 to 10 MU twice or three times weekly is reported to improve tumor response in treated lesions. Three complete responses and six partial responses were noted in 51 patients, with some responses in lung lesions remote from the sites of intralesional IFN administration (170). However, the overall response rate for uninjected lesions among patients treated intralesionally in this series (18%) does not differ from that observed with systemic parenteral, i.m., or s.c. administration.

Regional therapy with IFN-γ has focused on two disease settings: malignant ascites and *in transit* involvement of extremities. In the former setting, Edington et al. (171) have demonstrated the feasibility of infusing large numbers of IFN-γ–activated autologous blood monocytes intraperitoneally and have shown the stable localization of radiolabeled monocytes in the peritoneum for 5 days. In the setting of regional *in transit* disease of extremities, Liénard and LeJeune (172,173) have reported striking efficacy of hyperthermic isolated limb perfusion with combinations of melphalan, TNF, and IFN-γ. IFN-γ was administered for the purpose of modulating TNF receptor expression during the subsequent isolated limb perfusion in this trial, but the role of IFN-γ has not been formally established in this setting. Response rates approaching 90% have been reported from Switzerland using this multimodal approach. These results have been confirmed by investigators in the United States (174,175) and the Netherlands (176,177). A more limited exploration of hyperthermic isolated limb perfusion with TNF alone at comparable doses has shown only brief and limited antitumor activity (178), arguing that melphalan, or melphalan and IFN-γ, may be critical to this therapeutic effect. Fraker and colleagues have undertaken a controlled study of isolated limb perfusion with and without IFN-γ that may allow more definitive conclusions (174,179).

PHASE 1 AND 2 TRIALS WITH SYSTEMIC INTERFERON-γ

Phase 1 and 2 studies of IFN-γ have been more limited in number than those of IFN-α but have systematically developed the agent based on preclinical evidence of immunomodulatory activity for IFN-γ (105,180–183). IFN-γ has exhibited the greatest immunomodulatory activity of any IFN studied; in view of this potent immunologic activity (90,115,120), it has been studied intensively in a number of single-institution and cooperative group trials, as therapy for melanoma. Published trials of IFN-γ administered alone or in combination with other biologics are summarized in Table 3. Phase 1 and 2 experience with IFN-γ has shown minimal antitumor activity against melanoma. Phase 1 and 2 studies by the i.v., i.m., and s.c. routes (105,148) have yielded one complete and three partial responses among 75 patients in phase 1–2 trials. A major dose-seeking phase 2 randomized trial of ECOG (E4697) has tested the antitumor activity of seven different dosages of therapy in a total of 98 patients with soft tissue or nodal-dominant disease. Even in this select group of patients with relatively favorable stage i.v. disease, only four responses were obtained (out of 81 evaluable subjects) (2 out of 16 at 0.01 mg per m^2, 1 out of 12 at 0.5 mg per m^2, and 1 out of 13 at 0.9 mg per m^2), for an overall response rate of 4.2%. Antitumor responses occurred at low and high dosages tested, not supporting the hypothetical bell-shaped dose-response relationship for anticancer effects of IFN-γ in humans. The immunomodulatory effects of IFN-γ in the dose-

response evaluation by ECOG (E4987) (120,121) establish a potent direct dose-response relationship for NK and monocyte activation; modulation of T-cell subset distribution followed a different dose-response pattern that was greatest at the lowest tested doses of IFN-γ 0.01 mg per m^2 per day) and durable for the 1-month interval studied in this trial. Neither the impact of IFN-γ on NK cells and monocytes nor its impact on T cells have followed patterns observed in earlier murine models (184), and no correlation has occurred between immunomodulatory and clinical antitumor effects of IFN in this large clinical-laboratory evaluation. Given the evidence for immunomodulation by IFN-γ in this trial, these effects may have little relationship to clinical antitumor outcomes or the pleiotropy of IFN-γ may include counterbalancing regulatory effects that outflank primary postulated effector systems. The impact of IFN-γ on specific host T-cell responses to tumors was not evaluated in this or any other trial of the IFNs; therefore, the correlation between the tumor-specific immunomodulatory effects of IFN and responses of metastatic disease have not been evaluated.

PHASE 2 TRIALS OF COMBINATIONS OF BIOLOGICS—TYPES I AND II: INTERFERON-α-2 PLUS INTERFERON-γ

Combinations of IFNs of types I and II (IFN-α-2, IFN-β, and IFN-γ, respectively) have been of theoretical interest, given the potential synergism of IFNs interacting through the two separate classes of IFN receptors. The modulation of receptors for IFN-α-2 by IFN-γ and elucidation of signal transduction modulated by IFN-α and IFN-γ (11) provide a further impetus for the exploration of combined-IFN therapy. Cytoplasmic and nuclear gene-regulatory mechanisms induced by these different IFNs may achieve molecular synergism through transcriptional activators of the IFN response elements summarized by Darnell (8,10–14).

Clinical studies of combinations of IFNs α and γ have followed two strategies, concurrent and sequenced administration. Concurrent programs of treatment have revealed increased toxicity without apparent therapeutic benefit in several trials (see Table 3) (185–188). Studies using sequenced delivery of IFNs α and γ suggest improved therapeutic and immunomodulatory activity in renal cell carcinoma (98,113) and deserve examination in melanoma (98,189).

MODULATION OF ANTITUMOR AND IMMUNOLOGIC EFFECTS OF INTERFERONS BY BIOLOGICS, CYTOTOXIC DRUGS, AND NONSTEROIDAL ANTIINFLAMMATORY DRUGS

The pleiotropic effects of IFN-α-2 include the induction of a variety of feedback mechanisms, including immunosuppressive mechanisms that may be associated with histamines and prostaglandins, for which cimetidine and nonsteroidal antiinflammatory drugs might be effective. In addition, it is hoped that these agents might alleviate the significant constitutional toxicity and flulike syndrome of IFN therapy. A large number of

TABLE 4. CLINICAL TRIALS OF INTERFERON (IFN)-α-2 IN COMBINATION WITH CIMETIDINE

Study (Reference)	Dose	Route/Schedule	Entered/ Evaluable	Response CR	PR	Percent	Duration (Mo)
Flodgren (272) IFN-α Le + cimetidine	4–12 MU/m^2; 250 mg	i.m./i.t. daily; 5 of 7 d, p.o. q.i.d.	20/20	5	1	30	5+, 6+ 12+, 18, 19, 23
Creagan (190) IFN-α-2a + cimetidine	50 MU/m^2; 50 mg	i.m. t.i.w.	35/35	0	8	22	2.0–4.1
Steiner (160) IFN-α-2a + cimetidine	9–36 MU/m^2; 250 mg	i.m. daily; p.o. q.i.d.	11/11	1	2	27	1, 23, 36+
Mughal (192) IFN-α-2b + cimetidine	10 MU/m^2; 300 mg	s.c. t.i.w.; p.o. q.i.d.	31/31[a]	0	2	6.4	6, 6
Ernstoff (288) IFN-α-2b + cimetidine	10–100 MU/m^2; 300 mg	i.v. daily; 5 of 7 d, p.o. q.i.d.	14/14[a]	0	0	0	—

CR, complete response; PR, partial response.
[a]All patients treated after failure of IFN-α-2 alone.

studies of IFN-α, administered with a variety of dosages and schedules of cimetidine, have not yielded convincing evidence of improved outcome (Table 4).

Clinical trials have explored difluoromethylornithine to modify polyamine-mediated pathways of immunosuppression, as well as low-dose cyclophosphamide, administered to inhibit suppression mediated by suppressor T cells. Neither of these approaches has altered clinical antitumor outcome significantly in small phase 2 trials (160,164–166,190–192). Analyses of intermediate end points relevant to postulated mechanisms being exploited have generally been omitted, so it is difficult to draw firm conclusions from these trials.

Miller (193) has conducted a more extensive study of the potential impact of indomethacin, demonstrating neither significant immunologic interactions, nor any durable amelioration of chronic toxicity of IFN-α-2 therapy, in this randomized controlled trial. Dexamethasone has been assiduously avoided in trials of IFN-α, IFN-β, and IFN-γ as a consequence of its potent immunosuppressive effects. Corticosteroids have been demonstrated to abrogate the benefit of other biologic interventions in experimental animals, and until clearer evidence of the mechanism of antitumor benefit has been obtained, are to be avoided on this basis (193,194).

MODULATION OF ANTITUMOR AND IMMUNOLOGIC EFFECTS OF INTERFERON-α BY RETINOIDS

Broad interest has developed regarding the potential applications of retinoids for therapy and prevention of a range of cancers. Unexpected and dramatic clinical responses of acute promyelocytic leukemia with retinoids (and the discovery that this disorder is associated with a lesion in the chromosomal region coding for the retinoic acid receptor) have led to studies in a number of epithelial neoplasms. Retinoic acid receptors exhibit sequence homology with the steroid hormone receptor superfamily, suggesting that both may function in the regulation of gene transcription through specific response elements

and promoters. The affinities of retinoic acid receptors α, β, and γ differ for the various retinoids currently under exploration in cancer therapy (e.g., all-*trans*-retinoic acid binds retinoic acid receptor-α, with fivefold higher affinity than 13-*cis*-retinoic acid) (195).

Clinical trials of 13-*cis*-retinoic acid (13cRA) as a single agent have not generally shown activity in solid tumors and have been unrewarding in melanoma in particular. The effects of fenretinoin or topical tretinoin (Retin-A), or both, on dysplastic nevi are of interest and currently under exploration in patients with multiple large atypical or dysplastic nevi and personal or a familial histories of melanoma (ECOG trial E2695). Based on the different antitumor mechanisms and nonoverlapping toxicities of these agents, retinoids and IFNs have been explored for therapy of a number of other solid tumors. Combined modality therapy of squamous cell carcinoma with 13cRA and IFN-α-2 has provided responses in 19 of 28 patients (68%; seven complete responses). On this basis, IFN-α-2 has been combined with either 13cRA or all-*trans*-retinoic acid in a larger series of trials against other solid tumors, including melanoma. The combinaion of IFN-α-2 and 13cRA, however, has shown no benefit in a limited series of patients with melanoma (196).

MODULATION OF INTERFERON-α-2 BY PROSTAGLANDIN SYNTHETASE INHIBITION WITH PIROXICAM

Piroxicam, an inhibitor of prostaglandin synthetase, has been evaluated as a means to inhibit suppression of peripheral blood mitogen responses after IFN therapy, thereby potentially improving the antitumor activity of IFN-α against melanoma. In patients with renal cell carcinoma, *in vitro* immunologic responses were improved with enhanced antitumor activity (197–199). In a clinical trial against melanoma, neither antitumor effects nor immunosuppressive effects of IFN-α were benefited by the use of piroxicam combined with IFN-α (Table 5) (199).

TABLE 8. RANDOMIZED CONTROLLED TRIALS OF POSTOPERATIVE ADJUVANT THERAPY IN INTERMEDIATE-RISK MELANOMA

Cooperative Group (PI)	Agent	Investigational Treatment
Austrian (Pehamberger)	IFN-α-2a	Low-dose (3 MU/d) s.c. qd × 3 wk, then t.i.w. × 12 mo
French (Grob)	IFN-α-2a	Low-dose (3 MU/d) s.c. t.i.w. × 18 mo vs. obs
UK–AIM High (Hanford)	IFN-α-2b	Low-dose (3 MU/d) s.c. t.i.w. × 18 mo vs. obs
ECOG 1697 (Agarwala/Kirkwood)	IFN-α-2b	High-dose (20 MU/m^2/d × 5 d/wk × 4 wk) vs. obs 20

AIM, adjuvant interferon in melanoma; ECOG, Eastern Cooperative Oncology Group; IFN, interferon; obs, observation; PI, principal investigator.

section. All new trials optimally specify manners of nodal staging using the most precise techniques available. Although the therapeutic value of the procedure has not been proven, its increased precision is widely accepted. Future trials should specify the pursuit of sentinel node mapping or stratify patients for this parameter to assure balance in treated and reference populations.

Melanoma risk may be categorized as very high, high, intermediate, and low, according to 5-year relapse and mortality. The prognosis of clinically localized primary melanoma may be estimated rather precisely by Breslow depth of primary tumor invasion at site of origin and presence or absence of ulceration. Very low relapse risk is associated with lesions thinner than 0.76 mm (T1) or less than 1.50 mm (T2). Risk of metastasis is incremental with increasing depth until the risk of lesions over 4.0 mm (T4) approaches that of overt lymph node metastatic disease. Patients without evident distant disease after primary surgical management for T3 primary melanoma have intermediate relapse risks, whereas those with deep (T4) primary lesions or already apparent regional lymph node metastases have high risks of distant relapse and death (greater than 50% at 5 years). The uniformly poor prognosis for cure after distant hematogenous metastasis has provided the rationale for postoperative adjuvant therapy of high-risk patients (235,236).

Adjuvant Therapy of High-Risk Resected Primary and Regionally Metastatic Melanoma

On the basis of antitumor activity of IFN-α-2 in metastatic melanoma and the response gradient of patients with the smallest sizes and numbers of metastases who exhibit the highest response rates, multiple trials of IFN-α-2 for prevention of melanoma relapse were begun in the United States and international cooperative groups during the 1980s (Table 8). Entry criteria for these trials has varied slightly in some groups, including deeper T3 primary melanomas (Breslow depth, 1.5 to 4.0 mm) among groups at high risk [North Central Cancer Treatment Group (NCCTG)/Southwest Oncology Group], and in other groups accepting only node-positive disease [e.g., the World Health Organization

(WHO)]. The three largest and most mature studies of IFN-α-2 conducted to date adopted similar entry criteria, including patients with T4 primaries or pathologically proven involvement of regional lymph nodes (NCCTG, ECOG, and WHO).

The therapeutic regimens tested in these major randomized trials may be divided according to the dosage, route, and duration of therapy, as well as the subspecies of IFN-α-2 used.

TRIAL OF HIGH DOSE IFN-α-2B VERSUS OBSERVATION IN HIGH-RISK RESECTED

Two-hundred eighty-seven patients were accrued in a trial conducted between 1984 and 1990 (E1684) that was unblinded and reported to the American Society of Clinical Oncology in 1993 at 5 years of median follow-up (237); the trial was published in 1996 at 6.9 years median follow-up (Table 9). This trial used a year-long aggressive therapy of IFN-α-2b, 20 MU per m^2 i.v., daily for 5 days per week for 1 month, then 10 MU per m^2 s.c., three times weekly for the balance of the year. Of the 287 patients enrolled, 252 were evaluable. Patients were observed as reference standards of care or received IFN-α-2b at maximally tolerable dosages intravenously and subcutaneously for 1 year. Risk groups were defined at lymph node pathology (reviewed in all cases) and stratified to allow analysis of therapeutic impact in homogeneous groups of patients whose susceptibility to this therapy was postulated potentially to be related to tumor burden and disease extent (101,238).

The dosage of IFN-α-2b selected for this study was based on phase 1 and 2 studies reported by Kirkwood et al. (95,161,239) that demonstrated that 20 MU per m^2 i.v., daily, and 10 MU per m^2 s.c., three times weekly, approach the maximum tolerated dosages for these two routes. Initial i.v. therapy was chosen to provide peak dosage intensity approaching 10,000 U per mL and to minimize potential anti-IFN antibody responses (based on a lack of antibody formation against IFN-α-2b observed in patients studied in several phase 1 and 2 trials) (95,161).

A group sequential design was used for the analysis of this trial with one-sided log rank tests. Distribution of patients entered onto the two arms of this trial was well balanced for all prognostic factors evaluated. Toxicity observed in this trial was considerable, with dosage reductions required in one-half of subjects during the first month of i.v. dosing; reductions in dosage were required during the s.c. maintenance treatment in more than one-half of patients, especially during the first month of s.c. treatment.

The analysis of treatment impact for high-dose IFN-α-2b (HDI) on relapse for the overall trial revealed a highly significant reduction of relapse rate at each of the interim analyses (p = <.005) and on final intention-to-treat analysis (p = .002). A significant benefit on survival was demonstrated in the intention-to-treat analysis, as well (p = .046). A Cox multivariate analysis demonstrated significant improvement in disease-free and OS (p = .001 to .010) and estimated the relative improvement in continuous relapse-free survival (RFS) to be 50%.

TABLE 9. RANDOMIZED CONTROLLED TRIALS OF POSTOPERATIVE ADJUVANT THERAPY IN HIGH-RISK INTERFERON (IFN) MELANOMA

Cooperative Group (PI)	Agent	Eligible Subjects	No. of Subjects	Investigational Treatment	Study Status
ECOG 1684 (Kirkwood)	IFN-α-2b	$T_4{}^a$,$N_1{}^b$	287	High-dose (20 MU/m²/d) i.v. × 1 mo, followed by high-dose s.c. t.i.w. regimen × 11 mo	Disease-free and survival benefit 6.9-yr follow-up
NCCTG 83-7052 (Creagan)	IFN-α-2a	T_4,N_1	273	High-dose 20 MU/m², limited-duration i.m. regimen × 3 mo	RFS trend stage III
SWOG (Meyskins)	IFN-β	T_3,T_4,N_1	134	Low-dose (0.2 mg/d), s.c. t.i.w. × 1 yr	Closed, negative
EORTC 18871 (Kleeberg)	IFN-β vs. IFN-α	$T_{3-4}{}^c$,N_1	900	Low-dose IFN-α (1 MU/d) vs. low-dose IFN-γ immunology action (0.2 mg/d) IFN-γ × 1 yr	Closed, negative
WHO 16 (Cascinelli)	IFN-α-2a	$N_1{}^d$	426	Low-dose (3 MU/d) s.c. t.i.w. regimen × 3 yr	Closed, negative
EORTC 18952 (Eggermont)	IFN-α-2b	T_4,N_1	1,000	Intermediate dose for 1 or 2 yr	Open
ECOG 1690 (Kirkwood)	IFN-α-2b	T_4,N_1	42	High-dose (20 MU/m²/d) i.v. × 1 mo plus s.c. × 11 mo (total, 1 yr) vs. low-dose prolonged s.c. t.i.w. (2+ yr) regimen	Closed, RFS benefit but non-OS benefit
ECOG 1694 (Kirkwood)	IFN-α-2b	T_4,N_1	880	High-dose IFN-α-2b vs. GM2 ganglioside	Closed, analysis pending
ECOG 3697 (Rosenstein)	IFN-α-2b + RT vs. IFN-α-2b	N + ECE	200	High-dose IFN-α-2b + RT vs. high-dose IFN	Open

ECE, extracapsular extension; ECOG, Eastern Cooperative Oncology Group; EORTC, European Organization for Research and Treatment of Cancer; IFN, interferon; NCCTG, North Central Cancer Treatment Group; OS, overall survival; RFS, relapse-free survival; RT, radiation therapy; SWOG, Southwestern Oncology Group; WHO, World Health Organization Melanoma Programme.
[a]Deep primary >4 mm, without satellites.
[b]Regional node involvement without extracapsular soft tissue extension.
[c]Regional nodal involvement, including extracapsular extension.
[d]Deep primary >3 m.

Subgroup Analyses

The impact of therapy was analyzed in four stratification subgroups according to estimated risk: (a) patients with clinical stage I with deep primary tumors (> 4 mm; Breslow depth, ~T4) and pathologically proven absence of nodal disease (11% of accrual, clinical stage 1[CS1], pathological stage 1 [PS1]); (b) patients with clinically inapparent but pathologically proven regional lymph nodal disease (10% of accrual, CS1 PS2); (c) patients with clinically apparent regional lymph node disease, post lymphadenectomy (14% of accrual, CS2 PS2); and (d) patients with clinical and pathologic evidence of regional lymph node recurrence at some time after adequate surgery for primary melanoma (64% of accrual, CS2 PS2R). Given a significant overall betterment of relapse and death rates, subset analyses were performed to identify whether treatment benefit was general or restricted to particular subsets of disease. The greatest impact of therapy was noted in patients who presented with overt nodal metastatic disease; in this small subset of only 41 patients, RFS was improved for the treated patients, who achieved nominal statistical significance (p <.01). Curiously, the small subset of patients with T4 primary lesions who were without nodal disease at elective dissection did not appear to benefit from HDI (n = 31). This group was unbalanced for the presence of ulceration in treated and observed populations and was too small to permit further analysis. Analysis of node-positive patients demonstrated highly significant relapse-free and OS benefits for IFN-α-2, driving the pursuit of nodal evaluation by sentinel node mapping to select patients that would benefit most from administration of HDI. The original trial did not gather information regarding the numbers of nodes involved in the 89% of node-positive patients; Smith et al. subsequently performed a retrospective analysis of this data in more than 90% of patients, however, demonstrating excellent balance between treated and observed populations for numbers of nodes involved at original pathology and demonstrating the most remarkable benefits of IFN in patients with single positive lymph nodes (107).

The median interval to relapse with IFN-α-2b adjuvant therapy was prolonged from 0.9 to 1.6 years, whereas the median survival of treated patients was prolonged from 2.62 to 3.78 years. Relapse-free survival in E1684 was 37% at 5 years for treated patients and 26% for observed patients. The continuous RFS advantage of 11% (a relative improvement of 40% over observation) has been durable, suggesting a curative potential for IFN-α-2 in patients with high-risk melanoma.

Quality of Life and Cost Efficacy

The impact of high-dose IFN-α-2b on quality of life (QOL) was evaluated in a retrospective quality-adjusted analysis of time spent without symptoms or toxicity (i.e., Q-TWiST study) (240). This study was developed by Goldhirsch et al. (241) in 1989 to allow a balanced evaluation of side effects and benefits of therapy. Time spent during and after treatment with treatment-related toxicity, relapse, and quality-adjusted analysis of time spent without symptoms or toxicity were analyzed for patients, weighted according to accepted indices that have been validated in a time–utility analysis (242). After 84 months of follow-up, the group of patients receiving IFN-α-2b gained a mean of 8.9 months without relapse (p = .03) and 7 months of OS time (p = .02) compared to the observation group. The treated group experienced at least one episode of severe treatment-related toxicity over a period averaging less than 5.8 months. As an overall result, the IFN-α-2b–treated group had more QOL–adjusted survival time than the observation group, regardless of relative valuations placed on time with toxicity and time with relapse.

The cost of IFN-α-2b in E1684 has raised serious societal questions about patient and insurer costs of the regimen. An economic analysis of the E1684 regimen was published by Hillner et al. (243), performed with coinvestigators of the E1684 trial; a separate analysis also has been published in Europe by Messori (244,245) with remarkably consistent results. The projected incremental cost gained in the IFN cohort of patients (in 1996 U.S. dollars per life-year) ranged from $13,700 (after 35 years) to $32,600 (at 7 years, the median follow-up of E1684). The benefits of IFN, projected over a lifetime, yield incremental costs per life-year or quality-adjusted life-years that are both less than $16,000. This figure is less than the rigorous Canadian benchmark of $20,000 per QOL-year gained and is comparable to other accepted adjuvant therapies of breast and colorectal cancer. Given the significant and durable benefit of this therapy, it has been approved for resected high-risk melanomas rapidly by regulatory authorities across North and South America, Europe, and Australia.

United States Intergroup Trial of High-Dose and Low-Dose Interferon versus Observation for Resected High-Risk Melanoma

To confirm and extend the preliminary results of the E1684 trial, the E1690 intergroup trial was initiated in 1990, just as the first striking relapse-free interval benefits of HDI in E1684 became available (but before any survival advantage had become apparent). This randomized three-arm study compared the same high-dose regimen of IFN-α-2b as was administered in E1684 to a low-dose, 3 MU s.c., three-times-weekly regimen of IFN-α-2b, chosen in conjunction with the WHO Trial 16 in Europe. Because this trial was initiated before maturity of E1684, the control arm remained observation. Targeted accrual of 642 patients was completed in June 1995. Entry criteria for this study were the same as for E1684, except the requirement for elective lymphadenectomy for patients with pT4cN0, clinically node-negative disease, was eliminated. Primary end points were relapse-free and OS, using a two-sided log-rank statistic comparing high-dose and low-dose arms versus observation. The statistic design used a mixed cure-rate model, seeking to establish a 10% cure rate and 50% improvement in time to relapse or death among those patients not cured with a power greater than 80% at maturity.

Six hundred forty-two patients entered the study between 1990 and 1995, with 608 evaluable patients at 52 months median follow-up when the study was unblinded in 1998. The study was unblinded at 91% of the projected number of events stipulated in the original protocol due to a reduction in event rate and a projected time of more than 2 years (which is the period that would have been required to reach the numbers of events originally specified in the protocol). The study population, comprised by stage groupings, included 25% deep primary, clinically node-negative patients (versus 11% in E1684); only 51% had recurrent nodal involvement (162 T4cN0, 68 T14pN1cN0, 83 T14cN1, and 326 recurrent node-positive). An improvement in RFS for the high-dose arm over observation (hazard ratio, 1.28; *p* = .05) was noted; the benefit for node-negative and node-positive populations was consistent overall.

Improvement in RFS was significant by Cox multivariate analysis for the high-dose arm (*p* = .03) but not for the low-dose arm (*p* = .16). Neither the high-dose arm nor the low-dose arm showed an improvement in OS compared with observation. OS was not prolonged in the face of results, corroborating a benefit on continuous RFS that has been attributed to post-relapse salvage with IFN, which became widely available during the trial interval. IFN was used extensively in patients whose observations were unsuccessful, more than after treatment with adjuvant IFN (*p* = .004) and among these patients the use of IFN was associated with significantly improved OS.

OTHER TRIALS OF HIGH-DOSE INTERFERON-α-2A AND LOW-DOSE INTERFERON-α-2A IN HIGH-RISK RESECTED MELANOMA: NORTH CENTRAL CANCER TREATMENT GROUP 83-7052 AND WORLD HEALTH ORGANIZATION TRIAL 16

The NCCTG adjuvant trial 83-7052 used IFN-α-2a, a short, 3-month treatment period, and a lowered dose of 10 MU per m^2 i.m., three times weekly, throughout. The NCCTG study randomized 273 patients to receive 3 months of treatment with IFN-α-2a at moderately high dosages by i.m. route or observation; the trial, conducted between 1984 and 1990, was reported at a follow-up interval of more than 5 years. The trial included 162 patients with nodal involvement and 111 patients with T3/T4 primary disease (>3.69 mm). No advantage in terms of RFS or OS was observed in the overall study, but a trend to improvement in the RFS was reported for the node-positive population (*p* = .03, by Cox analysis).

WHO's Melanoma Programmed Trial 16 evaluated 3 years of treatment with IFN-α-2a at the same dosage that the intergroup–ECOG E1690 trial tested for the U.S. intergroup trial (versus standard observation). WHO accrued patients with regional lymph node involvement (largely at recurrence), excluding deep primary (T4) node-negative or electively dissected, clinically node-negative populations. An early report of the findings of WHO Trial 16 suggested a lack of any durable impact of IFN-α-2a at low dosage on RFS intervals or OS (246). If these findings are borne out in a more formal complete analysis of the trial, they have important implications for the optimal integration of IFN-α-2b therapy in melanoma treatment.

HIGH-DOSE IFN-α-2B FOR ABBREVIATED INTERVAL INDUCTION THERAPY: E1697

On the basis of previous considerations, and the strong evidence of early impact for high-dose IFN-α regimens in E1684 and E1690, ECOG and the National Cancer Institute of Canada have designed a trial to test the benefit of 1 month of high-dose i.v. IFN-α-2b administered 5 out of 7 days per week for 4 weeks in T3N0M0 stage IIA patients with resected cutaneous melanoma. This study requires 1,444 patients to detect a cure rate benefit of 7.5% with a power of greater than 85% in a mixed–cure-rate model. This study was opened to accrual in December 1998 and is anticipated to accrue patients through 2001. This trial provides the first test of the hypothesis that peak-dose exposure is important to the therapeutic benefit of the E1684 regimen. Given the importance of preservation of QOL for such patients, a module evaluating QOL is incorporated into this study.

HIGH-DOSE INTERFERON-α-2B IN CONJUNCTION WITH RADIOTHERAPY FOR PATIENTS WITH GROSS EXTRACAPSULAR EXTENSION

Neither the completed E1684 and E1690/S9111/C9190 studies, nor the current E1694/S9512 intergroup trials have allowed entry of any patient with gross extracapsular extension of disease at the regional lymph node basin. The local-regional relapse rate is substantially elevated for this group, as was first noted in relation to melanoma of the head and neck by the group at the M. D. Anderson Cancer Center (247). It is uncertain whether a benefit of IFN-α-2 is manifest in this population; uncontrolled pilot data from the M. D. Anderson Cancer Center has suggested a potential role of hypofractionated radiotherapy for these patients (247). ECOG has therefore undertaken a test of the role of IFN-α-2b at high dosage administered with hypofractionated radiotherapy, versus IFN-α-2b at high dosage for 1 year alone in this group of patients (D. Wazer, principal investigator). This study began in October 1998, seeking accrual of 167 subjects to the evaluation of this combination, hoping for an improvement in local-regional relapse and the first evaluation of IFN-α-2b at high dosage with radiotherapy in this population.

LOW-DOSE INTERFERON IN INTERMEDIATE-RISK MELANOMA: AUSTRIAN AND FRENCH MULTICENTER TRIALS

Pehamberger (248) reported a study of IFN-α-2a administered 3 MU s.c., three times weekly, for 1 year after a period of 3 weeks of daily administration in 310 patients with intermediate-risk clinically node-negative patients. Excellent tolerance of this regimen has been noted, and an early outcome reported a significant reduction in frequency of relapse, although median follow-up was short (3 years). No survival data have been reported as initially published; therefore, the results of this experience must hear further follow-up. Grob et al. (249) have reported the significant prolongation of RFS interval but not OS for intermediate-risk (clinically node-negative AJCC stage II AB) melanoma patients treated with low-dose IFN-α-2a administered subcutaneously for 18 months at a median follow-up of 5 years (117). This trial entered 499 subjects and is relatively early in follow-up, given the intermediate-risk profiles of its subjects. The observed prolongation of RFS interval with these two low-dose regimens suggests a qualitatively different effect than that obtained with high-dose IFN, as tested by ECOG in E1684 and intergroup trials E1690 and NCCTG 83-77052. The low-dose effects reported in these two trials for immediate-risk patients (and in WHO Trial 16 for high-risk patients) appear to develop more gradually over time on therapy and wane over months after cessation of therapy. The curves plotting the treatment and

observation differential described by Grob suggest a transient relapse-free benefit rather than a durable curative advantage for the low-dose regimen.

The benefit of low-dose IFN-α in intermediate-risk patients is significant in terms of relapse-free interval at 3 to 5 years follow-up, although not in terms of survival. Pressing questions relate to the mechanism by which these results were induced and how they might be improved. One option is to protract the treatment interval, either to a fixed interval (e.g., 5 years) or indefinitely. The intermediate-risk population has a limit (risk of relapse is less than 50%); it poses difficulties with consideration of indefinite therapy, therefore, because therapy would be given needlessly to one-half of this population for an indefinite interval. Trials that would use IFN-α-2 at low dosages for more protracted intervals are being designed or discussed in several cooperative groups.

INTERGROUP EVALUATION OF VACCINE GM2–KLH PLUS QS 21 VERSUS HIGH-DOSE INTERFERON IN HIGH-RISK MELANOMA

ECOG and Southwest Oncology Group Melanoma committees have undertaken a trial to build on the results of E1684 and E1690, evaluating effects of the chemically defined vaccine composed of the immunogenic ganglioside GM2 coupled with the carrier molecule KLH (i.e., GMK), administered with the potent adjuvant agent QS 21 (in comparison to IFN-α-2b at high dosage). The rationale for the use of the GMK vaccine is drawn from a study conducted at the University of California, Los Angeles, by Jones et al. (250), who demonstrated that patients with native anti-GM2 antibody relapse less frequently than those without the antibody; the studies of Livingston et al. (251–253) corroborated this observation, demonstrating a trend to improved relapse-free OS in high-risk, node-positive stage III patients vaccinated with GM2 and bacille Calmette-Guérin (as opposed to bacille Calmette-Guérin alone) after resection of melanoma. The E1694/S9512 trial seeks to define the superiority of GMK over HDI in terms of RFS and OS of high-risk melanoma, and has completed accrual of 880 patients in 1999. The E1694 intergroup study tests the first of a potential series of vaccines that may induce either humoral or cellular immune response to defined antigens of melanoma, in which the opportunity to evaluate intermediate end points of antibody or cellular response to the immunogen exists.

With the recognition that combinations of GMK and IFN-α-2b are desirable for administration—provided the combination does not abrogate antibody response to GM2—ECOG trial E2696 (conducted with Memorial Sloan-Kettering) tested the induction of the anti-GM2 antibodies IgG and IgM by vaccine alone (as opposed to vaccine combined with or followed by IFN-α-2b at high dosage, as in E1684 and E1690). Completion and analysis of this trial demonstrated no significant inhibition of immunogenicity of the GMK vaccine in terms of IgG and IgM (254). Thus, it is reasonable to consider the combined use of this vaccine and HDI in adjuvant trials, once efficacy of the vaccine has been demonstrated.

RATIONALE FOR STUDY OF INTERFERON MECHANISM

The lack of a fundamental understanding of key mechanisms of therapeutic benefit with IFN in patients with melanoma has served as the impetus for developing laboratory corollary analyses of immune mechanisms modulated by IFN, tumor and MHC antigen expression, and direct antiproliferative effects that might explain antitumor activity of IFN against melanoma in humans (e.g., U.S. Intergroup Cooperative Trial E1690, WHO Trial 16, and Austrian/French Multicenter Studies).

In the context of the intergroup–ECOG E1690 trial, as well as WHO Trial 16, the opportunity has been taken to examine the potential mechanisms of specific T-cell–mediated antitumor actions of this therapy. The underlying goals of laboratory corollary studies are to identify the mechanisms of IFN-α-2 in melanoma therapy that correlate with therapeutic benefit. Successful trials allow future investigations to refine and heighten impacts on appropriate mechanisms, ideally permitting selection of candidates most likely to benefit from treatment. This has obvious relevance to high-risk populations (and compelling significance for the larger population of intermediate-risk patients); more long-term treatment is considered.

The therapeutic impact against melanoma is being evaluated in terms of direct tumor inhibition or antigen modulation, MHC-restricted cytotoxic T-cell function, and non-MHC restricted effector cell activation. The Melanoma Cancer Center of the Pittsburgh Cancer Institute (for the intergroup–ECOG E1690 trial) and Istituto Nazionale dei Tumori Experimental Oncology D Laboratories (for WHO Trial 16) have evaluated autologous tumors obtained at regional lymph node dissection and HLA-matched, cultured tumor cell lines of participating patients in treatment and control arms of these large ongoing studies. These laboratory corollaries are being analyzed; their respective clinical trials have now just been unblinded.

Although potent immunomodulatory activity of IFN-γ provided ample initial justification to prevent melanoma relapse in adjuvant settings, where immunologic activity may be optimally assessed, the observation of minimal antitumor activity in large phase 2 dose-seeking trials (ECOG E4687/E4987) makes it unlikely that further trials of IFN-γ will be undertaken in high-risk melanoma.

ADJUNCTIVE USE OF INTERFERONS WITH VACCINES

Peptide antigens recognized by the host T-cell response will be more relevant antigenic targets for specific vaccine immunization against melanoma in years to come. The assessment of host–response end points relevant for peptide and for ganglioside immunologic therapies differ: response to peptide and protein immunizations are defined by T-cell responses, either proliferative, cytokine-inductive, or cytotoxic; in contrast, serologic outcomes are critical covariates of ganglioside immunization strategies, and some data suggest that the production of antibodies against gangliosides is associated with favorable outcome of melanoma (251,255). The analysis of mechanisms of synergism with the interferons will likely also differ but will depend on the outcome of current and future trials of vaccine strategies as single interventions.

EPIDEMIOLOGY, ETIOLOGIC, AND BIOLOGIC HETEROGENEITY: FUTURE POTENTIAL FOR EARLIER BIOLOGIC INTERVENTION

The rising incidence of melanoma and the lack of effective treatment for distant metastatic and high-risk resectable disease has raised issues regarding the preventive role of available modalities. In the United States alone, incidence of cutaneous melanoma has tripled since 1950 and nearly doubled in the 1990s. More than 41,000 new melanoma cases were identified in 1998, with 7,500 deaths attributable to melanoma. One in every 75 whites will contract melanoma by the end of the 1990s, based on current incidence projections.

NONFAMILIAL (SPORADIC) AND FAMILIAL MELANOMA AND THEIR PRECURSORS

Approximately 10% of cutaneous melanomas are familied, linked with a syndrome of clinically atypical and histologically dysplastic nevi described by Clark et al. (257). A larger fraction of up to 40% of melanoma occurring outside the familial setting (258,259) is also associated with the presence of clinically atypical and histologically dysplastic nevi that closely resemble precursor lesions of the familial syndrome. Atypical (dysplastic) nevi may therefore serve as intermediate markers of nevi or patients at high risk for melanoma. The syndrome of atypical dysplastic nevi has been described in terms of increased numbers of larger-than-normal (i.e., >5 mm) nevi of irregular or indistinct margins, variegated pigmentation, and macular surfaces. Histopathologically, these lesions may be hyperplastic, with bridging or fusion of rete ridges manifesting cytologic or nuclear atypia, or both, and elicit a host lymphocytic response. IFNs have been shown to regulate a number of cellular genes in normal and neoplastic cells of the melanocytic lineage and have demonstrated activity in the advanced metastatic and adjuvant settings. Therefore, the evaluation of IFNs and retinoids as modulators of tumor progression is a reasonable goal and one that is in progress in clinical laboratory protocols of ECOG and University of Pittsburgh Cancer Institue.

IFNs are the best-studied biologic antineoplastic agents in melanoma. There are no compelling bases for choosing one over another species for investigation of melanoma-preventive activity. rDNA–produced IFNs of all three subspecies have shown activity against melanoma *in vitro*; antiproliferative activity has been related to their abilities to inhibit protein synthesis after binding to specific membrane receptors. IFN modulation of effector cell function, MHC class I and II antigens, and tumor-associated antigens, as well as receptors for growth factors, such as melanocyte-stimulating hormone, suggests a variety of potential mechanisms of action for clinical antitumor activity. Enhanced immunogenicity and altered susceptibility to T-cell–

mediated cytotoxicity or differentiate effects are of major interest. Immunomodulatory effects on NK-cell activation appear to be related to antitumor activity in experimental animals, but no clear evidence for a role of similar mechanisms in human cancer exists.

SUMMARY OF ADJUVANT EXPERIENCE IN HIGH- AND INTERMEDIATE-RISK MELANOMA

The only current evidence for a therapeutic benefit in patients with high-risk operable melanoma has been observed with maximally tolerable dosages of IFN-α-2b. Regarding high-risk melanoma, the E1684 regimen remains state-of-the-art, and its impact on continuous RFS has been corroborated by the E1690/S9111/C9190 intergroup trial, unblinded at 52 months' follow-up. Low-dosage IFN-α in high-risk disease (as pursued by WHO) has no durable relapse interval or survival impact of significance. In E1690, the only head-to-head comparison of high and low dosage regimens, the benefit of high-dose IFN differed quantitatively and quantitatively from that of low-dose IFN.

In patients with node-negative melanoma at higher risks as consequences of primary depth (Breslow depth, > 4 mm), the E1684 and NCCTG 83-7052 trials contained populations too small to derive meaningful conclusions regarding efficacy of high-dose IFN therapy. The Austrian and French Multicenter Trials have reported relapse interval prolongation with low-dose IFN-α-2a therapy administered for 1 to 1.5 years at median follow-ups of 3 and 5 years. Effects in these trials were only significant regarding RFS intervals. The larger and more mature French multicenter trial suggests a benefit that is not durable after withdrawal of treatment. This therapy did not significantly impact OS, and the basis of this difference has not been determined. In intermediate-risk disease, the French and Austrian trials have achieved transient relapse delays but not the stable durable impacts of high-dose regimens. Alternative trials of longer duration, either with previously administered low dosage or using newer formulations of polyethylene-glycol conjugated IFN-α-2, are of great interest. Is the impact of this therapy manifest only in certain limited (i.e., node-negative) spheres of disease? Neither Austrian nor French trials evaluated nodal involvement more precisely than by more precise sentinel or elective nodal staging techniques than clinical examination, however. RFS interval prolongation is achieved with low-dose IFN therapy administered for 12 to 18 months, occurring gradually on treatment, and lost gradually after discontinuation of therapy. Further studies of IFN at low doses for longer periods or with high doses for shorter intervals are reasonable and in progress. As surrogate markers of risk for the stage II population and the population susceptible to benefits for stage II and III patients, the therapeutic index for IFN-α-2 and its yield may improve. In conjunction with radiotherapy and vaccines, and as an earlier prevention strategy, much more remains to be explored using tools available for dissection of the molecular pathways of IFN-α-2 action, as well as specific host–immune response to potentially relevant tumor antigens.

REFERENCES

1. Zoon KC, Bekisz J, Miller D. Human interferon alpha family: protein structure and function. In: Baron S, Coppenhaver DH, Dianzani F, et al, eds. *Interferon: principles and medical applications*, 1st ed. Galveston: The University of Texas Medical Branch, 1992:95–105.
2. Dron M, Tovey MG. Interferon α/β, gene structure and regulation. In: Baron S, Coppenhaver DH, Dianzani F, et al, eds. *Interferon: principles and medical applications*, 1st ed. Galveston: The University of Texas Medical Branch, 1992:33–45.
3. Mariano TM, Donnelly RJ, Soh J, Pestka S. Structure and function of the type I interferon receptor. In: Baron S, Coppenhaver DH, Dianzani F, et al, eds. *Interferon: principles and medical applications*, 1st ed. Galveston: The University of Texas Medical Branch, 1992:129–138.
4. DeGrado WF, Wasserman ZR, Chowdry V. Sequence and structural homologies among type I and II interferons. *Nature* 1982;300:379.
5. Revel M. The interferon system in man: nature of the interferon molecules and mode of action. In: Becker Y, ed. *Antiviral drugs and interferon*. Nijhoff: Martinus, 1988:358–433.
6. Epstein LB, Epstein CJ. Localization of the gene AVG for the antiviral expression of immune and classical interferon to the distal part of the long arm of chromosome 21. *J Invest Dermatol* 1976;133[Suppl]:56.
7. Weil J, Tucker G, Epstein LB, Epstein CJ. Interferon induction of (2'-5') oligoisoadenylate synthetase in diploid and trisomy 21 human fibroblasts: relation to dosage of the interferon receptor gene (IRFC). *Human Genetics* 1983;65(2):108–111.
8. Levy DE. Cytoplasmic events in signal transduction leading to IFN α-induced gene expression. In: Baron S, Coppenhaver DH, Dianzani F, et al, eds. *Interferon: principles and medical applications*, 1st ed. Galveston: The University of Texas Medical Branch, 1992:161–173.
9. Fuchs E. Clues to β-cell memory. *Nature Medicine* 1996;2:743–744.
10. Darnell JE Jr. STATs and gene regulation. *Science* 1997;277:1630–1635.
11. Schindler C, Shuai K, Prezioso VR, Darnell JE Jr. Interferon-dependent tyrosine phosphorylation of a latent cytoplasmic transcription factor. *Science* 1992;257:809–813.
12. Pine R, Decker T, Kessler DS, Levy DE, Darnell JE. Purification and cloning of interferon-stimulated gene factor 2 (ISGF2): ISGF2 (IRF-1) can bind to the promoters of both beta interferon- and interferon-stimulated genes but is not a primary transcriptional activator of either. *Mol Cell Biol* 1990;10(6):2448–2457.
13. Fu X-Y, Kessler DS, Veals SA, Levy DE, Darnell JE Jr. ISGF3, the transcriptional activator induced by interferon α, consists of multiple interacting polypeptide chains. *Proc Natl Acad Sci U S A* 1990;87: 8555–8559.
14. Levy D, Darnell JE Jr. Interferon-dependent transcriptional activation: signal transduction without second messenger involvement? *New Biol* 1990;2(10):923–928.
15. Aiyer RA, Serrano LE, Jones PP. Interferon-gamma binds to high and low affinity receptor components on murine macrophages. *J Immunol* 1986;136:3329–3334.
16. Ucer U, Bartsch H, Scheurich P, Berkovic D, Ertel C, Pfizenmaier K. Quantitation and characterization of gamma interferon receptors on human tumor cells. *Cancer Res* 1986;46(10):5339–5343.
17. Herberman RB. *Natural cell-mediated immunity against tumors*. New York: Academic Press, 1980.
18. Müllbacher A. The long-term maintenance of cytotoxic T cell memory does not require persistence of antigen. *J Exp Med* 1994;179: 317–321.
19. Ernstoff MS, Fusi S, Kirkwood JM. Parameters of interferon action: II. immunological effects of recombinant leukocyte interferon (IFN alpha-2) in phase I/II trials. *J Biol Res Mod* 1983;2:540–547.
20. Ortaldo JR, Woodhouse C, Morgan AC, Herberman RB, Cheresh DA, Reisfeld R. Analysis of effector cells in human antibody-dependent cellular cytotoxicity with murine monoclonal antibodies. *J Immunol* 1987;138(10):3566–3572.
21. Kirkwood JM, Farkas DL, Chakraborty A, et al. Systemic interferon-alpha (IFN-alpha) treatment leads to Stat3 inactivation in melanoma precursor lesions. *Mol Med* 1999;5:11–20.

22. Merritt JA, Borden EC, Ball LA. Measurement of 2',5'-oligoadeny-late synthetase in patients receiving interferon-alpha. *J Interferon Res* 1985;5:191–198.
23. St. Laurent G, Yoshie U, Floyd-Smith G. Interferon action: two (2′5′) A (A)n synthetase specified by distinct mRNAs in Erhlich ascites tumor cells treated with interferon. *Cell* 1983;33:95.
24. Ilson DH, Torrence PF, Vilcek J. Two molecular weight forms of human 2'5'-oligoadenylate synthetase have different activation requirements. *J Interferon Res* 1986;6:5–12.
25. Yoshida R, Imanishi J, Oku T, Kishida T, Hayaishi O. Induction of pulmonary indoleamine 2,3, dioxygenase by interferon. *Proc Natl Acad Sci U S A* 1981;78:129.
26. Yasui H, Takai K, Yoshida R, Hayaishi O. Interferon enhances tryptophan metabolism by inducing pulmonary indoleamine 2,3-dioxygenase: its possible occurrence in cancer patients. *Proc Natl Acad Sci U S A* 1986;83:6622–6626.
27. Ghezzi P, Bianchi M, Montovani A, Spreafico F, Salmona M. Enhanced xanthine oxidase activity in mice treated with interferon and interferon inducers. *Biochem Biophys Res Commun* 1984;119:144.
28. Berens ME, Saito T, Welander CE, Modest EJ. Antitumor activity of new anthracycline analogues in combination with interferon alfa. *Cancer Chemother Pharmacol* 1987;19:301–306.
29. Saito T, Berens ME, Welander EC. Characterization of the indirect antitumor effect of gamma-interferon using ascites-associated macrophages in a human tumor clonogenic assay. *Cancer Res* 1987;47(3):673–679.
30. Nachbaur DM, Denz HA, Gastl G, Thaler J, Lechleitner M, Braunsteiner H. Combination effects of human recombinant interferon (alpha-2-arg, gamma) and cytotoxic agents on colony formation of human melanoma and hypernephroma cell lines. *Cancer Letters* 1989;44(1):49–53.
31. Fleischmann WR. Potentiation of the direct anti-cellular activity of mouse interferons: mutual synergism and interferon concentration dependence. *Cancer Res* 1982;42:869–875.
32. Czarniecki CW, Fennie CW, Powers DB, Estell DA. Synergistic antiviral and antiproliferative activities of Escherichia coli-derived human alpha, beta, and gamma interferons. *J Virol* 1984;49(2):490–496.
33. Schiller JH, Willson JKV, Bittner G, Wolberg WH, Hawkins MJ, Borden EC. Antiproliferative effects of interferons on human melanoma cells in the human tumor colony-forming assay. *J Interferon Res* 1986;6:615–625.
34. Justesen J, Berg K. Synergistic effects of HuIFN-gamma of 2'5'-oligoadenylate synthetase induction by HuIFN-alpha. *J Interferon Res* 1986;6:445–454.
35. Dealtry GB, Naylor MS, Fiers W, Balkwill FR. DNA fragmentation and cytotoxicity caused by tumor necrosis factor is enhanced by interferon-gamma. *Eur J Immunol* 1987;17:689–693.
36. Bregman MD, Meyskens FL, Jr. Human recombinant alpha- and gamma-interferons enhance the cytotoxic properties of tumor necrosis factor on human melanoma. *J Biol Res Mod* 1988;7(4):384–389.
37. Wang Y, Rao U, Mascari R, Richards TJ, et al. Molecular analysis of melanoma precursor lesions. *Cell Growth Differ* 1996;7:1733–1740.
38. Elder DE, Rodeck U, Thurin J, et al. Antigenic profile of tumor progression in human melanocytic nevi and melanomas. *Cancer Res* 1989;49:5091–5096.
39. Kameyama K, Tanaka S, Ishida Y, Hearing VJ. Interferons modulate the expression of hormone receptors on the surface of murine melanoma cells. *J Clin Invest* 1989;83:213–221.
40. Bennett DC, Dexter TJ, Ormerod EJ, Hart IR. Increased experimental metastatic capacity of a murine melanoma following induction of differentiation. *Cancer Res* 1986;46(7):3239–3244.
41. Ramani P, Balkwill FR. Human interferons inhibit experimental metastases of a human melanoma cell line in nude mice. *Br J Cancer* 1988;58(3):350–354.
42. Ruiter DJ. Clinical and pathologic diagnosis, staging and prognostic factors of melanoma, and management of primary disease. *Curr Opin Oncol* 1992;4:357–367.
43. Weyand EH, Bryla P, Wu Y, He Z-M. LaVoie EJ. Detection of B(j)F:DNA adducts arising from nonclassical dihydrodiol epoxides. *Proc Am Assoc Cancer Res* 1992;33:A832(abst).
44. Graf LH Jr, Rosenberg CD, Mancino VA, Ferrone S. Transfer and co-amplification of a gene encoding a 96-kDa immune IFN-inducible human melanoma-associated antigen. Preferential expression by mouse melanoma host cells. *J Immunol* 1988;141(3):1054–1060.
45. Matsui M, Temponi M, Ferrone S. Characterization of a monoclonal antibody-defined human melanoma-associated antigen susceptible to induction by immune interferon. *J Immunol* 1987;139(6):2088–2095.
46. Friess GG, Brown TD, Wrenn RC. Improvement in cardiac ectopy during gamma interferon infusion: a case report. *Cancer Treat Rep* 1986;70(12):1463–1464.
47. Murray JL, Stuckey SE, Pillow JK, Rosenblum MG, Gutterman JU. Differential *in vitro* effects of recombinant α-interferon and recombinant gamma-interferon alone or in combination on the expression of melanoma-associated surface antigens. *J Biol Res Mod* 1988;7:152–161.
48. Maio M, Gulwani B, Langer JA, et al. Modulation for interferons of HLA antigen, high-molecular-weight melanoma-associated antigen, and intercellular adhesion molecule 1 expression by cultured melanoma cells with different metastatic potential. *Cancer Res* 1989;49:2980–2987.
49. Elder DE, Clark WH, Jr, Elenitsas R, Guerry DIV, Halpern AC. The early and intermediate precursor lesions of tumor progression in the melanocytic system: common acquired nevi and atypical (dysplastic) nevi. *Semin Diagn Pathol* 1993;10:18–35.
50. Fountain JW, Karayiorgou M, Ernstoff MS, et al. Homozygous deletions within human chromosome band 9p21 in melanoma. *Proc Natl Acad Sci U S A* 1992;89.10557–10561.
51. Iliopoulos D, Ernst C, Steplewski Z, et al. Inhibition of metastases of a human melanoma xenograft by monoclonal antibody to the GD^2/GD^3 gangliosides. *J Natl Cancer Inst* 1989;81(6):440–444.
52. Lehmann JM, Riethmüller G, Johnson JP. MUC18, a marker of tumor progression in human melanoma, shows sequence similarity to the neural cell adhesion molecules of the immunoglobulin superfamily. *Proc Natl Acad Sci U S A* 1989;86:9891–9895.
53. Hersey P, Edwards A, Coates A, Shaw H, McCarthy W, Milton G. Evidence that treatment with vaccinia melanoma cell lysates (VMCL) may improve survival of patients with stage II melanoma: treatment of stage II melanoma with viral lysates. *Cancer Immunol Immunother* 1987;25:257–265.
54. Scott G, Stoler M, Sarkar S, Halaban R. Localization of basic fibroblast growth factor mRNA in melanocytic lesions by in situ hybridization. *J Invest Dermatol* 1991;96:318–322.
55. Tsuchida T, Saxton RE, Morton DL, Irie RF. Gangliosides of human melanoma. *Cancer* 1989;63:1166–1174.
56. Albelda SM, Mette DA, Elder DE, et al. Integrin distribution in malignant melanoma: association of the β_3 subunit with tumor progression. *Cancer Res* 1990;50:6757–6764.
57. Derynck R, Roberts AB, Winkler ME, Chen EY, Goeddel DV. Human transforming growth factor-alpha: precursor structure and expression in E. coli. *Cell* 1984;38:287–297.
58. Murray JL, Rosenblum MG. Modulation of melanoma antigens by interferons. In: Nathanson L, ed. *Melanoma research: genetics, growth factors, metastases, and antigens.* Boston: Kluwer Academic Publishers, 1991:153–167.
59. Houghton AN, Mintzer D, Cordon-Cardo C, et al. Mouse monoclonal IgG3 antibody detecting G_{D3} ganglioside: a phase I trial in patients with malignant melanoma. *Proc Natl Acad Sci U S A* 1985;82:1242–1246.
60. Vadhan-Raj S, Cordon-Cardo C, Carswell E, et al. Phase I trial of a mouse monoclonal antibody against G_{D3} ganglioside in patients with melanoma: induction of inflammatory responses at tumor sites. *J Clin Oncol* 1988;6:1636–1648.
61. Kirkwood JM, Vlock D, Day R, Waggoner A, Rabkin M, Whiteside T, et al. A phase Ib trial of murine monoclonal antibody R24 (anti-GD3) in metastatic melanoma. *Proc Am Assoc Cancer Res* 1992.
62. Kirkwood JM, Sosman J, Ernstoff M, et al. E2690: a study of the mechanism of IFN alfa-2b in high risk melanoma in the ECOG/intergroup trial E1690. *Proc Am Assoc Cancer Res* 1995;36:641(abst).
63. Bajorin DF, Chapman PB, Wong GY, et al. Treatment with high dose mouse monoclonal (anti-Gd3) antibody R24 in patients with metastatic melanoma. *Melanoma Res* 1992;2:355–362.

64. Caulfield MJ, Barna B, Murthy S, et al. Phase Ia-Ib trial of an anti-G_{D3} monoclonal antibody in combination with interferon-alpha in patients with malignant melanoma. *J Biol Res Mod* 1990;9:319–328.

65. Giacomini P, Aguzzi A, Pestka S, Fisher PB, Ferrone S. Modulation by recombinant DNA leukocyte (α) and fibroblast (β) interferons of the expression and shedding of HLA- and tumor-associated antigens by human melanoma cells. *J Immunol* 1984;133(3):1649–1655.

66. Giuffré L, Isler P, Mach J-P, Careel S. A novel IFN-gamma regulated human melanoma associated antigen gp33-38 defined by monoclonal antibody Mel4-D12. I. Identification and immunochemical characterization. *J Immunol* 1988;141(6):2072–2078.

67. Audette M, Carrel S, Hayoz D, Giuffre L, Mach J-P, Kuhn LC. A novel interferon-gamma regulated human melanoma-associated antigen, gp33-38, defined by monoclonal antibody Me14-D12. II. Molecular cloning of a genomic probe. *Mol Immunol* 1989;26(6):515–522.

68. Dolei A, Ameglio F, Capobianchi MR, et al. Human β-type interferon enhances the expression and shedding of Ia-like antigens, comparison to HLA-A, B, C and β_2-microglobulin. *Antiviral Res* 1981;1:367–381.

69. Basham TY, Bourgeade MF, Creasey AA, Merigan TC. Interferon increases HLA synthesis in melanoma cells: interferon-resistant and -sensitive cell lines. *Proc Natl Acad Sci U S A* 1982;79:3265–3269.

70. Anichini A, Mortarini R, Fossati G, Parmiani G. Phenotypic profile of clones from early cultures of human metastatic melanomas and its modulation by recombinant interferon-gamma. *Int J Cancer* 1986;38:505–511.

71. Taramelli D, Fossati G, Balsari A, Marolda R, Parmiani G. The inhibition of lymphocyte stimulation by autologous human metastatic melanoma cells correlates with the expression of HLA-DR antigens on the tumor cells. *Int J Cancer* 1984;34(6):797–806.

72. Ruiter DJ, Bröcker E-B, Ferrone S. Expression and susceptibility to modulation by interferons of HLA Class I and II antigens on melanoma cells. Immunohistochemical analysis and clinical relevance. *J Immunogenet* 1986;13:229–234.

73. Ernstoff MS, Duray PH, Steenn K, Kirkwood JM. Antigenic phenotype of pigmented lesions. *J Invest Dermatol* 1984;84:430–432.

74. Stötter H, Wiebke EA, Tomita S, et al. Cytokines alter target cell susceptibility to lysis. II. Evaluation of tumor infiltrating lymphocytes. *J Immunol* 1989;142(5):1767–1773.

75. Houghton AN, Thomson TM, Gross D, Oettgen HF, Old LJ. Surface antigens of melanoma and melanocytes. Specificity of induction of Ia antigens by human gamma-interferon. *J Exp Med* 1984;160:255.

76. Anichini A, Castelli C, Sozzi G, Fossati G, Parmiani G. Differential susceptibility to recombinant interferon-gamma-induced HLA-DQ antigen modulation among clones from a human metastatic melanoma. *J Immunol* 1988;140(1):183–191.

77. Taniguchi K, Petersson M, Höglund P, Kiessling R, Klein G, Kärre K. Interferon gamma induces lung colonization by intravenously inoculated B16 melanoma cells in parallel with enhanced expression of class I major histocompatibility complex antigens. *Proc Natl Acad Sci U S A* 1987;84:3405–3409.

78. Gorelik E, Gunji Y, Herberman RB. H-2 antigen expression and sensitivity of BL6 melanoma cells to natural killer cell cytotoxicity. *J Immunol* 1988;140(6):2096–2102.

79. Taramelli D, Fossati G, Mazzocchi A, Delia D, Ferrone S, Parmiani G. Classes I and II HLA and melanoma-associated antigen expression and modulation on melanoma cells isolated from primary and metastatic lesions. *Cancer Res* 1986;46:433–439.

80. De Fries RU, Golub SH. Characteristics and mechanism of IFN-gamma-induced protection of human tumor cells from lysis by lymphokine-activated killer cells. *J Immunol* 1988;140(10):3686–3693.

81. Zöller M, Strubel A, Hämmerling G, Andrighetto G, Raz A, Ben-Ze'ev A. Interferon gamma treatment of B16 melanoma cells: opposing effects for non-adaptive and adaptive immune defense and its reflection by metastatic spread. *Int J Cancer* 1988;41:256–266.

82. Zoller M. IFN-treatment of B16-F1 versus B16-F10: relative impact of non-adaptive and T-cell-mediated immune defense in metastatic spread. *Clin Exp Metastasis* 1988;6(5):411.

83. Kleinschmidt WJ, Schultz RM. Similarities of murine gamma interferon and the lymphokine that renders macrophages cytotoxic. *J Interferon Res* 1982;2:291–295.

84. Talmadge KW, Gallati H, Sinigaglia F, Walz A, Garotta G. Identity between human interferon-gamma and "macrophage-activating factor" produced by human T lymphocytes. *Eur J Immunol* 1986;16:1471–1477.

85. Spear GT, Paulnock DM, Jordan RL, Meltzer DM, Merritt JA, Borden EC. Enhancement of monocyte class I and II histocompatibility antigen expression in man by *in vivo* β-interferon. *Clin Exp Immunol* 1987;69:107–115.

86. Sayers TJ, Mason AT, Ortaldo JR. Regulation of human natural killer cell activity by interferon-gamma: lack of a role in interleukin 2-mediated augmentation. *J Immunol* 1986;136(6):2176–2180.

87. Platsoucas CD. Regulation of natural killer cytotoxicity by Escherichia coli-derived human interferon gamma. *Scand J Immunol* 1986;24:93–108.

88. Maluish AE, Ortaldo JR, Conlon JC, et al. Depression of natural killer cytotoxicity after *in vivo* administration of recombinant leukocyte interferon. *J Immunol* 1983;131(1):503–507.

89. Silver HK, Connors JM, Kong S, Karim KA, Spinelli JJ. Survival, response and immune effects in a prospectively randomized study of dose strategy for alpha-N1 interferon. *Br J Cancer* 1988;58(6):783–787.

90. Kirkwood JM, Bryant J, Schiller J, et al. Determination of phenotypic and functional correlates of interferon gamma (IFNγ) therapy of metastatic melanoma in a multi-institutional phase Ib trial (ECOG 4987/4687). *Proc Am Soc Clin Oncol* 1991;10:A733(abst).

91. Seitz DE. Trimetrexate: a critical appraisal of the phase II clinical trial experience: evidence of drug discovery—clinical development disjunction. *Cancer Invest* 1994;12(6):657–661.

92. Herberman RB, Ortaldo JR, Bonnard GD. Augmentation by interferon of human natural and antibody-dependent cell-mediated cytotoxicity. *Nature* 1979;227(5693):221–223.

93. Hersey P, Hasic E, MacDonald M, et al. Effects of recombinant leukocyte interferon (rIFN-αA) on tumour growth and immune responses in patients with metastatic melanoma. *Br J Cancer* 1985;51(6):815–826.

94. Mittleman A, Krown SE, Cirrincione C, Safai B, Oettgen HF, Koziner B. Analysis of T cell subsets in cancer patients treated with interferon. *Am J Med* 1983;75:966.

95. Kirkwood JM, Ernstoff MS. The role of interferons in the management of melanoma. In: Nathanson L, ed. *Management of advanced melanoma*. New York: Churchill Livingstone, 1986:209–223.

96. Creagan ET, Ahmann DL, Frytak S, Long HJ, Itri LM. Recombinant leukocyte A interferon (rIFN-αA) in the treatment of disseminated malignant melanoma: analysis of complete and long-term responding patients. *Cancer* 1986;58:2576–2578.

97. Neefe JR, Phillips EA, Treat J. Augmentation of natural immunity and correlation with tumor response in melanoma patients treated with human lymphoblastoid interferon. *Diagn Immunol* 1986;4:299.

98. Ernstoff MS, Nair S, Bahnson RR, et al. A phase IA trial of sequential administration recombinant DNA-produced interferons: combination recombinant interferon gamma and recombinant interferon alfa in patients with metastatic renal cell carcinoma. *J Clin Oncol* 1990;8:1637–1649.

99. Fuchs HJ, Debs R, Patton JS, Liggitt HD. The pattern of lung injury induced after pulmonary exposure to tumor necrosis factor-α depends on the route of administration. *Diag Microbiol Infect Dis* 1990;13:397–404.

100. Chen BP, Sondel PM. Recombinant DNA-derived interferons-α and -β modulate the alloactivated proliferative response of bulk and cloned human lymphocytes. *J Biol Res Mod* 1985;4:287–297.

101. Day CL Jr, Lew RA, Mihm MC Jr, et al. A multivariate analysis of prognostic factors for melanoma patients with lesions ≥ 3.65 mm in thickness: the importance of revealing alternate Cox models. *Ann Surg* 1982;195(1):44–49.

102. Laszlo J, Huang AT, Brenckman WD, et al. Phase I study of pharmacological and immunological effects of human lymphoblastoid interferon given to patients with carcinoma. *Cancer Res* 1983;43:4458.

103. Maluish AE, Ortaldo JR, Sherwin SA, Oldham RK, Herberman RB. Changes in immune function in patients receiving natural leukocyte interferon. *J Biol Res Mod* 1983;2:418.

104. Edwards BS, Merritt JA, Fuhlbrigge RC, Borden EC. Low doses of interferon-alpha result in more effective clinical natural killer cell activation. *J Clin Invest* 1985;75:1908–1913.

105. Ernstoff MS, Trautman T, Davis CA, et al. A randomized phase I/II study of continuous versus intermittent intravenous interferon-gamma in patients with metastatic melanoma. *J Clin Oncol* 1987;5(11):1804–1810.

106. Zarour H, Richards T, Whiteside T, et al. E2690: intergroup immunological evaluation of IFNα2b dose-response in patients (Pts) with high-risk melanoma. *Proc Am Soc Clin Oncol* 1999 (abst).

107. Kirkwood JM, Ibrahim J, Sondak V, et al. Preliminary analysis of the E1690/S9111/C9190 intergroup postoperative adjuvant trial of high- and low-dose IFNα2b (HDI and LDI) in high-risk primary or lymph node metastatic melanoma. *Proc Am Soc Clin Oncol* 1999;18:537A(abst).

108. Zarour H, Kirkwood JM, Salvucci-Kierstead L, et al. Melan-A/MART-1 represents an immunogenic HLA-DR4-restricted epitope recognized by melanoma-reactive CD4⁺Tcells. *Proc Natl Acad Sci U S A* 1999.

109. Belardelli F, Gresser I, Maury C, Maunoury MT. Anti-tumor effects of interferon in mice injected with interferon-sensitive and interferon-resistant Friend leukemia cells. II. Role of host mechanisms. *Int J Cancer* 1982;30:821–825.

110. Gresser I, Maury C, Belardelli F. Anti-tumor effects of interferon in mice injected with interferon-sensitive and interferon-resistant Friend leukemia cells. VI. Adjuvant therapy after surgery in the inhibition of liver and spleen metastases. *Int J Cancer* 1987;39:789–792.

111. Gresser I, Maury C, Carnaud C, DeMaeyer D, Maunoury MT, Belardelli F. Anti-tumor effects of interferon in mice injected with interferon-sensitive and interferon-resistant friend erythroleukemia cells. VIII. Role of the immune system in the inhibition of visceral metastases. *Int J Cancer* 1990;46(3):468–474.

112. Snapper CM, Paul WE. Interferon-gamma and B cell stimulatory factor-1 reciprocally regulate Ig isotype production. *Science* 1987;236(4804):944–947.

113. Ernstoff MS, Gooding W, Nair S, et al. Immunological effects of treatment with sequential administration of recombinant interferon-gamma and -alpha in patients with metastatic renal cell carcinoma during a phase I trial. *Cancer Res* 1992;52:851–856.

114. Ernstoff MS, Fusi S, Kirkwood JM, et al. Parameters of interferon action. I. Immunological effects of whole cell leukocyte interferon (IFN alpha) in phase I/II trials. *J Biol Res Mod* 1983;2:528–539.

115. Kirkwood JM, Ernstoff MS, Trautman T, et al. *In vivo* biological response to recombinant interferon gamma during a phase I dose-response trial in patients with metastatic melanoma. *J Clin Oncol* 1990;8(6):1070–1082.

116. Trautman T, Kirkwood, JM, Ernstoff MS, et al. Phase I-II trial of recombinant interferon-gamma (IFN-gamma) by 2 or 24 hour infusion in 30 melanoma patients. *Proc Am Soc Clin Oncol* 1985;4:C905(abst).

117. Herberman RB. Design of clinical trials with biological response modifiers. *Cancer Treat Reports* 1985;69:1161.

118. Maluish AE, Urba WJ, Longo DL, et al. The determination of an immunologically active dose of interferon-gamma in patients with melanoma. *J Clin Oncol* 1988;6:434–445.

119. Kleinerman ES, Kurzrock R, Wyatt D, Quesada JR, Gutterman JU, Fidler IJ. Activation or suppression of the tumoricidal properties of monocytes from cancer patients following treatment with human recombinant gamma-interferon. *Cancer Res* 1986;46:5401–5405.

120. Schiller JH, Pugh M, Kirkwood J. Phase II/III trial of interferon-gamma in metastatic melanoma: an innovative trial design. *Clin Cancer Res* 1996;2:29–36.

121. Kirkwood JM, Bryant J, Schiller JH, Strawderman MH, Borden EC, Whiteside TL. Immunomodulatory function of interferon gamma in patients with metastatic melanoma: results of a phase I trial in subjects with metastatic melanoma (EST 4987). *J Immunother* 1997;20:146–157.

122. Konrad MW, DeWitt SK, Bradley ED, et al. Interferon-gamma induced by administration of recombinant interleukin-2 to patients with cancer: kinetics, dose dependence, and correlation with physiological and therapeutic response. *J Immunother* 1992;12:55–63.

123. Atkins MB, Lotze M, Wiernick P, et al. High-dose IL-2 therapy alone results in long-term durable complete responses in patients with metastatic melanoma. *Proc Am Soc Clin Oncol* 1997;16:494A(abst).

124. Hanahan D, Folkman J. Patterns and emerging mechanisms of the angiogenic switch during tumorigenesis. *Cell* 1996;86:353–364.

125. Folkman J. Successful treatment of an angiogenic disease. *N Engl J Med* 1989;320:1211–1212.

126. Wang Y, Becker D. Antisense targeting of basic fibroblast growth factor and fibroblast growth factor receptor-1 in human melanomas blocks intratumoral angiogenesis and tumor growth. *Nature Med* 1997;3:887–893.

127. Becker JC, Brabletz T, Czerny C, Termeer C, Brocker EB. Tumor escape mechanisms from immunotherapy: induction of unresponsiveness in a specific MHC-restricted CD4⁺ human T cell clone by autologous MHC class II⁺ melanoma. *Int Immunol* 1996;5:1501–1508.

128. Legha SS, Papadopoulos NEJ, Plager C, et al. Clinical evaluation of recombinant interferon alfa-2a (Roferon-a) in metastatic melanoma using two different schedules. *J Clin Oncol* 1987;5(8):1240–1246.

129. Creagan ET, Ahmann DL, Frytak S, Long HJ, Chang MN, Itri LM. Phase II trials of recombinant leukocyte A interferon in disseminated malignant melanoma: results in 96 patients. *Cancer Treat Reports* 1986;70(5):619–624.

130. Creagan ET, Buckner JC, Hahn RG, Richardson RR, Schaid DJ, Kovach JS. An evaluation of recombinant leukocyte A interferon with aspirin in patients with metastatic renal cell cancer. *Cancer* 1988;61:1787–1791.

131. Massaro ER, Borden EC, Hawkins MJ, Wiebe DA, Shrago E. Effects of recombinant interferon-alpha$_2$ treatment upon lipid concentrations and lipoprotein composition. *J Interferon Res* 1986;6:655–662.

132. Ehnholm C, Aho K, Huttunen JK, et al. Effect of interferon on plasma lipoproteins and on the activity of postheparin plasma lipases. *Arterioscler: J Vasc Biol Thromb* 1982;2:68.

133. Dixon RM, Borden EC, Keim NL, et al. Decreases in serum high-density-lipoprotein cholesterol and total cholesterol resulting from naturally produced and recombinant DNA derived leukocyte interferons. *Metabolism* 1982;2:68.

134. Ernstoff MS, Kirkwood JM. Changes in the bone marrow of cancer patients treated with recombinant interferon alpha-2. *Am J Med* 1984;76:593.

135. Ernstoff MS, Gallicchio V, Kirkwood JM. Analysis of granulocyte macrophage progenitor cells in patients treated with recombinant interferon alpha-2. *Am J Med* 1985;79:167.

136. Krown SE, Burk MW, Kirkwood JM, Kerr D, Morton DL, Oettgen HF. Human leukocyte (alpha) interferon in metastatic malignant melanoma: the American Cancer Society phase II trial. *Cancer Treat Reports* 1984;68;5:723–726.

137. Kirkwood JM, Strawderman MH, Ernstoff MS, Smith TJ, Borden EC, Blum RH. Interferon alfa-2b adjuvant therapy of high-risk resected cutaneous melanoma: the Eastern Cooperative Oncology Group Trial EST 1684. *J Clin Oncol* 1996;14:7–17.

138. Kirkwood JM, Ernstoff MS. Interferons in the treatment of human cancer. *J Clin Oncol* 1984;2(4):336–352.

139. Mattson K, Niiranen A, Levanainen M, et al. Neurotoxicity of interferon. *Cancer Treat Reports* 1983;67:958.

140. Sumpio BE, Ernstoff MS, Kirkwood JM. Urinary excretion of interferon, albumin, and β$_2$-microglobulin during interferon treatment. *Cancer Res* 1984;44(8):3599–3603.

141. Ault BH, Stapleton FB, Gaber L, Martin A, Roy SI, Murphy SB. Acute renal failure during therapy with recombinant human gamma interferon. *N Engl J Med* 1988;319:1397–1400.

142. Taylor AE, Wiltshaw E, Gore ME, Fryatt I, Fisher C. Long-term follow-up of the first randomized study of cisplatin versus carboplatin for advanced epithelial ovarian cancer. *J Clin Oncol* 1994;12(10):2066–2070.

143. Kurzrock R, Quesada JR, Rosenblum MG, Sherwin SA, Gutterman JU. Phase I study of iv administered recombinant gamma interferon in cancer patients. *Cancer Treat Reports* 1986;70:1357–1364.

144. McDermott DF, Mier JW, Lawrence DP, Clancy M, King D, Atkins MBA. Phase II pilot trial of concurrent biochemotherapy with cisplatin, vinblastine, dacarbazine (CVD), interleukin-2 (IL-2) and interferon alpha-2b (IFN) in patients with metastatic melanoma. *Proc Am Soc Clin Oncol* 1997;16:490a(abst).

145. Rohatiner AZS, Balkwill FR, Griffin DB, et al. A phase I study of human lymphoblastoid interferon administered by continuous intravenous infusion. *Cancer Chemother Pharmacol* 1982;9:97.

146. Guyer DR, Tiedeman J, Yannuzzi LA, et al. Interferon-associated retinopathy. *Arch Ophthalmol* 1993;111(3):350–356.

147. Reinhold U, Hartl C, Hering R, Hoeft A, Kreysel HW. Fatal rhabdomyolysis and multiple organ failure associated with adjuvant high-dose interferon alfa in malignant melanoma. *Lancet* 1997;349: 540–541.

148. Thompson JA, Cox WW, Lindgren CG, et al. Subcutaneous recombinant gamma interferon in cancer patients: toxicity, pharmacokinetics, and immunomodulatory effects. *Cancer Immunol Immunother* 1987;25:47–53.

149. Wagstaff J, Smith D, Nelmes P, Loynds P, Crowther D. A phase I study of recombinant interferon gamma administered by s.c. injection three times per week in patients with solid tumours. *Cancer Immunol Immunother* 1987;25:54–58.

150. Wheeler A, Rubenstein EB. Current management of disseminated intravascular coagulation. *Oncology* 1994;8:69–79.

151. Balch CM, Houghton A, Peters L. Cutaneous melanoma. In: DeVita VT Jr, Hellman S, Rosenberg SA, eds. *Cancer principles & practice of oncology*, 3rd ed. Philadelphia: JB Lippincott Co, 1989:1499–1542.

152. Kirkwood JM, Ernstoff MS. Interferons—Clinical applications: cutaneous melanoma. In: DeVita VT Jr, Hellman S, Rosenberg SA, eds. *Biologic therapy of cancer*. Philadelphia: JB Lippincott Co, 1991:311–333.

153. Kirkwood JM, Agarwala S. Systemic cytotoxic and biologic therapy melanoma. *Cancer Principles and Practice of Oncology* 1993;7:1–16.

154. Newlands ES, Stevens MFG, Wedge SR, Wheelhouse RT, Brock C. Temozolomide: a review of its discovery, chemical properties, preclinical development and clinical trials. *Cancer Treat Reviews* 1997;23:35–61.

155. Creagan ET, Ahmann DL, Green SJ, et al. Phase II study of recombinant leukocyte A interferon (rIFN-αA) in disseminated malignant melanoma. *Cancer* 1984;54(12):2844–2849.

156. Creagan ET, Ahmann DL, Green SJ, et al. Phase II study of low-dose recombinant leukocyte A interferon in disseminated malignant melanoma. *J Clin Oncol* 1984;2(9):1002–1005.

157. Coates A, Rallings M, Hersey P, Swanson C. Phase II study of recombinant alpha 2-interferon in advanced malignant melanoma. *J Interferon Res* 1986;6:1–4.

158. Sertoli MR, Bernengo MG, Ardizzoni A, et al. Phase II trial of recombinant alpha-2b interferon in the treatment of metastatic skin melanoma. *Oncology* 1989;46(2):96–98.

159. Elsasser-Beile U, Drees N, Neumann HA, Schopf E. Phase II trial of recombinant leukocyte A interferon in advanced malignant melanoma. *J Cancer Res Clin Oncol* 1987;113(3):273–278.

160. Steiner A, Wolf C, Pehamberger H. Comparison of the effects of three different treatment regimens of recombinant interferons (r-IFN alpha, r-IFN gamma, and r-IFN alpha + cimetidine) in disseminated malignant melanoma. *J Cancer Res Clin Oncol* 1987;113: 459–465.

161. Kirkwood JM, Ernstoff MS, Davis CA, Reiss M, Ferraresi R, Rudnick SA. Comparison of intramuscular and intravenous recombinant alpha-2 interferon in melanoma and other cancers. *Ann Intern Med* 1985;103(1):32–36.

162. Dorval T, Palangie T, Jouve M, et al. Clinical phase II trial of recombinant DNA interferon (interferon alfa 2b) in patients with metastatic malignant melanoma. *Cancer* 1986;58(2):215–218.

163. Robinson WA, Mughal TI, Thomas MR, Johnson M, Spiegel RJ. Treatment of metastatic malignant melanoma with recombinant interferon alpha-2. *Immunobiology* 1986;172:275–282.

164. Kirkwood JM, Ernstoff MS. Melanoma: therapeutic options with recombinant interferons. *Semin Oncol* 1985;12(4-5):7–12.

165. Hawkins MJ, McCune CS, Speyer JL, Sorell M. Recombinant alpha 2 interferon (IFN alpha 2)(SCH 30500) in patients with metastatic malignant melanoma (MMM): an ECOG pilot study. *Proc Am Soc Clin Oncol* 1984;3:C195(abst).

166. Creagan ET, Ahmann DL, Green SJ, Long HJ, Frytak S, Itri LM. Phase II study of recombinant leukocyte A interferon (IFN-rA) plus cimetidine in disseminated malignant melanoma. *J Clin Oncol* 1985;3(7):977–981.

167. Mitchell MS. Relapse in the central nervous system in melanoma patients successfully treated with biomodulators. *J Clin Oncol* 1989;7(11):1701–1709.

168. Breslow A. Thickness, cross-sectional areas and depth of invasion in the prognosis of cutaneous melanoma. *Ann Surg* 1970;172:902–909.

169. Fogler WE, Sun LK, Klinger MR, Ghrayeb J, Daddona PE. Biological characterization of a chimeric mouse-human IgM antibody directed against the 17-1A antigen. *Cancer Immunol Immunother* 1989;30:43–50.

170. von Wussow P, Block B, Hartmann F, Deicher H. Intralesional interferon-alpha therapy in advanced malignant melanoma. *Cancer* 1988;61(6):1071–1074.

171. Edington HD, Stevenson HC, Sugarbaker PH. *In vitro* and *in vivo* models for monitoring the adoptive immunotherapeutic effects of recombinant gamma-interferon-activated human monocytes. *Curr Surg* 1987;44:210–213.

172. Lienard D, Ewalenko P, Delmotte JJ, et al. High dose recombinant tumor necrosis factor alpha in combination with interferon gamma and melphalan in isolation perfusion of the limbs for melanoma and sarcoma. *J Clin Oncol* 1992;10:52–60.

173. Lejeune FJ, Liénard D, Mirimanoff RO. Regional therapy of melanoma. *Eur J Cancer* 1993;29A:606–612.

174. Fraker DL, Alexander HR. The use of tumor necrosis factor in isolated limb perfusions for melanoma and sarcoma. *Cancer Principles and Practice of Oncology* 1993;7:1–10.

175. Lejeune FJ. Administration of high-dose tumor necrosis factor alpha by isolation perfusion of the limbs: rationale and results. *J Infusional Chemother* 1994.

176. Lienard D, Eggermont AM, Schraffordt Koops H, Lejeune FJ. High dose of rTNF-alpha, rINF-gamma and melphalan in isolation perfusion produce 90% CR in melanoma in-transit metastasis (Meeting abstract). *Ann Oncol* 1992;3[Suppl 5]:160.

177. Buzaid AC, Bedikian A, Houghton AN. Systemic chemotherapy and biochemotherapy. In: Balch CM, Houghton AN, Sober AJ, Soong SJ, eds. *Cutaneous melanoma*, 3rd ed. St. Louis: Quality Medical Publishing, Inc., 1998:405–418.

178. Posner M, Lienard D, Lejeune F, Rosenfelder D, Kirkwood J. Hyperthermic isolated limb perfusion (HILP) with tumor necrosis factor (TNF) alone for metastatic intransit melanoma. *Cancer J Sci Am* 1995;1(4):274.

179. Thom AK, Alexander HR, Andrich MP, Barker WC, Rosenberg SA, Fraker DL. Systemic toxicity and cytokine levels in patients undergoing isolated limb perfusion (ILP) with dose TNF, IFN-gamma and melphalan. *Proc Am Soc Clin Oncol* 1993;12:A1329(abst).

180. Creagan ET, Ahmann DL, Long HJ, Frytak S, Sherwin SA, Chang MN. Phase II study of recombinant interferon-gamma in patients with disseminated malignant melanoma. *Cancer Treat Reports* 1987;71(9):843–844.

181. Perez R, Lipton A, Harvey HA, et al. A phase I trial of recombinant human gamma interferon (IFN-γ_{4A}) in patients with advanced malignancy. *J Biol Res Mod* 1988;7:309–317.

182. Sarna GP, Figlin RA, Pertcheck M. Phase II study of Betaseron (βser^{17}-interferon) as treatment of advanced malignant melanoma. *J Biol Res Mod* 1987;6:375–378.

183. Kowalzick L, Weyer U, Lange P, Breitbart EW. Systemic therapy of advanced metastatic malignant melanoma with a combination of fibroblast interferon-beta and recombinant interferon-gamma. *Dermatologica* 1990;181:298–303.

184. Talmadge JE, Tribble HR, Pennington RW, Phillips H, Wiltrout RH. Immunomodulatory and immunotherapeutic properties of

recombinant gamma interferon and recombinant tumor necrosis factor in mice. *Cancer Res* 1987;47:2563–2570.

185. Schiller JH, Storer B, Bittner G, Willson JKV, Borden EC. Phase II trial of a combination of interferon-β$_{ser}$ and interferon-Γ in patients with advanced malignant melanoma. *J Interferon Res* 1988;8(5):581–589.

186. Creagan ET, Loprinzi CL, Ahmann DL, Schaid DJ. A phase I-II trial of the combination of recombinant leukocyte A interferon and recombinant human interferon-gamma in patients with metastatic malignant melanoma. *Cancer* 1988;62:2472–2474.

187. Osanto S, Jansen R, Naipal AMIH, Gratama J-W, van Leeuwen A, Cleton FJ. *In vivo* effects of combination treatment with recombinant interferon-gamma and -alpha in metastatic melanoma. *Int J Cancer* 1989;43:1001–1006.

188. Kurzrock R, Rosenblum MG, Quesada JR, Sherwin SA, Itri LM, Gutterman JU. Phase I study of a combination of recombinant interferon-alpha and recombinant interferon-gamma in cancer patients. *J Clin Oncol* 1986;4(11):1677–1683.

189. Furukawa K, Thampoe IJ, Yamaguchi H, Lloyd KO. The addition of exogenous gangliosides to cultured human cells results in the cell type-specific expression of novel surface antigens by a biosynthetic process. *J Immunol* 1989;142:848–854.

190. Creagan ET, Ahmann DL, Green SJ, Long HJ, Frytak S, Itri LM. Phase II study of leukocyte A interferon (IFN Alfa a) plus cimetidine in disseminated malignant melanoma (DMM). *J Clin Oncol* 1985;3:977–981.

191. Borgstrom S, von Eyben FE, Flodgren P, Axelsson B, Sjogren HO. Human leukocyte interferon and cimetidine for metastatic melanoma [letter]. *N Engl J Med* 1982;307(17):1080.

192. Mughal TI, Robinson WA, Thomas MR, Spiegel R. Role of recombinant interferon alpha$_2$ and cimetidine in patients with advanced melanoma. *J Cancer Res Clin Oncol* 1988;114(1):108–109.

193. Miller RL, Steis RG, Clark JW, et al. Randomized trial of recombinant α2b-interferon with or without indomethacin in patients with metastatic malignant melanoma. *Cancer Res* 1989;49(7):1871–1876.

194. Eddy B, Ernstoff MS, Logan T, et al. A randomized phase I trial of recombinant interferon gamma (IFNγ, Biogen, Inc., Cambridge, MA) with indomethacin (I), dexamethasone (D) or acetaminophen (A) in patients (PT) with melanoma (M) and renal cell carcinoma (RCC). *Proc Am Soc Clin Oncol* 1987;6:A955 (abst).

195. Cretaz M, Baron A, Siegenthaler G, Hunziker W. Ligand specificities of recombinant retinoic acid receptors RAR-α and RAR-β. *Biochem J* 1990;27:391–397.

196. Dhingra K, Papadopoulos N, Lippman S, Lotan R, Legha SS. Phase II study of alpha-interferon and 13-cis-retinoic acid in metastatic melanoma. *Invest New Drugs* 1993;11:39–43.

197. Braun DP, Harris ZL, Harris JE, et al. Effect of interferon therapy on indomethacin-sensitive immunoregulation in the peripheral blood mononuclear cells of renal cell carcinoma patients. *J Biol Res Mod* 1983;2:3:251–262.

198. Braun DP, Bonomi PD, Taylor ST, Harris JE. Modification of the effects of cytotoxic chemotherapy on the immune responses of cancer patients with a non-steroidal anti-inflammatory drug, piroxicam. *J Biol Res Mod* 1987;6:331–345.

199. Harris J, Bines S, Das Gupta T. Therapy of disseminated malignant melanoma with recombinant alfa-2b interferon and piroxicam: clinical results with a report of an unusual response-associated feature (vitiligo) and unusual toxicity (diffuse pulmonary interstitial fibrosis). *Med Pediatr Oncol* 1994;22:103–106.

200. Nordlund JJ, Kirkwood JM, Forget BM. Vitiligo in patients with metastatic melanoma: a good prognostic sign. *J Am Acad Dermatol* 1983;9(5):689–696.

201. Richards JM, Mehta N, Ramming K, et al. Sequential chemoimmunotherapy in the treatment of metastatic melanoma. *J Clin Oncol* 1992;8:1338–1343.

202. McLeod GRC, Thomson DB, Hersey P. Recombinant interferon alfa-2a in advanced malignant melanoma: a phase I-II study in combination with DTIC. *Int J Cancer* 1987;[Suppl 1]:31–35.

203. Kirkwood JM, Ernstoff MS, Guiliano A, et al. Clinical trials of interferon alfa-2B (Intron A, alpha-IFN) in melanoma: review of phase I, II, and III studies. *Proc XIV Int Cancer Congress (Budapest)* 1986.

204. Kirkwood JM, Ernstoff MS, Guiliano A, et al. Interferon α-2a and dacarbazine in melanoma [Letter]. *J Natl Cancer Inst* 1990;82:1062–1063.

205. Thompson D, Adena M, McLeod GRC, et al. Interferon alpha-2a does not improve response or survival when added to dacarbazine in metastatic melanoma: results of a multi-institutional Anstrahan randomized trial. *Proc Am Soc Clin Oncol* 1992;11:343(abst).

206. Bajetta E, Negretti E, Giannotti B, et al. Phase II study of interferon α-2a and dacarbazine in advanced melanoma. *Am J Clin Oncol* 1990;13(5):405–409.

207. Gundersen S, Flokkmann A. Interferon plus dacarbazine in advanced malignant melanoma: a phase I-II study. *Eur J Cancer* 1991;27(2):220–221.

208. Mulder NH, deVries EGE, Sleijfer DT, Schraffordt Koops H, Willemse PHB. Dacarbazine (DTIC), human recombinant interferon alpha 2a (roferon) and 5-fluorouracil for disseminated malignant melanoma. *Br J Cancer* 1992;65:303–304.

209. Sertoli MR, Queirolo P, Bajetta E, et al. Dacarbazine with or without recombinant interferon alpha-2a at different dosages in the treatment of stage IV melanoma patients. *Proc Am Soc Clin Oncol* 1992;11:345(abst).

210. Bajetta E, Zampino MG, Di Leo A, et al. A phase III study with dacarbazine (DTIC) ± r-interferon alpha-2a (r-IFN) at different doses in advanced melanoma. *Ann Oncol* 1992;3(5):612(abst).

211. Falkson CI, Falkson G, Falkson HC. Improved results with the addition of interferon alfa-2b to dacarbazine in the treatment of patients with metastatic malignant melanoma. *J Clin Oncol* 1991;9(8):1403–1408.

212. Cocconi G, Bella M, Calabresi F, et al. DTIC versus DTIC plus tamoxifen in metastatic malignant melanoma. *Proc Am Soc Clin Oncol* 1990;9:278(abst).

213. Cocconi G, Bella M, Calabresi F, et al. Treatment of metastatic malignant melanoma with dacarbazine plus tamoxifen. *N Engl J Med* 1992;327:516–523.

214. McClay EF, Mastrangelo MJ. Systemic chemotherapy for metastatic melanoma. *Semin Oncol* 1988;15(6):569–577.

215. Falkson CI, Ibrahim J, Kirkwood JM, Coates AS, Atkins MB, Blum RH. Phase III trial of dacarbazine versus dacarbazine with interferon α–2b versus dacarbazine with tamoxifen versus dacarbazine with interferon α-2b and tamoxifen in patients with metastatic malignant melanoma: an Eastern Cooperative Oncology Group Study (E3690). *J Clin Oncol* 1998;16:1743–1751.

216. Khayat D, Borel C, Tourani JM, et al. Sequential chemoimmunotherapy with cisplatin, interleukin-2, and interferon alfa-2a for metastatic melanoma. *J Clin Oncol* 1993;11(11):2173–2180.

217. Rixe O, Benhammouda A, Antoine E, et al. Final results of a prospective multicentric study on 91 metastatic malignant melanoma (MMM) patients treated by chemo-immunotherapy (CH-IM) with cisplatin interleukin 2 (IL2) interferon-α (IFN). *Proc Am Soc Clin Oncol* 1994(abst).

218. Keilholz U, Conradt C, Legha SS, et al. Results of interleukin-2-based treatment in advanced melanoma: a case record-based analysis of 631 patients. *J Clin Oncol* 1998;16:2921–2929.

219. Keilholz U, Stoter G, Punt CJA, Scheibenbogen C, Lejeune F, Eggermont AMM. Recombinant interleukin-2 based treatments for advanced melanoma: the experience of the European organization for research and treatment of cancer melanoma cooperative group. *Cancer J* 1998;3:S22–S28.

220. Keilholz U, Goey SH, Punt CJA, et al. Interferon alfa-2a and interleukin-2 with or without cisplatin in metastatic melanoma: a randomized trial of the European organization for research and treatment of cancer melanoma cooperative group. *J Clin Oncol* 1997;15:2579–2588.

221. Walsh C, Speyer JL, Wernz J, et al. A phase I study of the combination of alpha-2 interferon and cisplatinum. *J Biol Res Mod* 1989;8(1):11–15.

222. Schuchter LM, Wohlganger J, Fishman EK, MacDermott ML, McGuire WP. Sequential chemotherapy and immunotherapy for the treatment of metastatic melanoma. *J Immunother* 1992;12:272–276.

223. Richner J, Joss RA, Goldhirsch A, Brunner KW. Phase II study of continuous subcutaneous interferon-alfa combined with cisplatin in

advanced malignant melanoma. *Eur J Cancer* 1992;28A:1044–1047.

224. Hamblin TJ, Davies B, Sadullah S, Oskam R, Palmer P, Franks CR. A Phase II study of the treatment of metastatic malignant melanoma with a combination of dacarbazine, cisplatin, interleukin-2 (IL-2) and alfa-interferon (IFN). *Proc Am Soc Clin Oncol* 1991;10:294(abst).

225. Legha S, Plager C, Ring S, Eton O, Talpaz M, Gutterman J, Benjamin RS. A phase II study of biochemotherapy using interleukin-2 (IL-2) + interferon alfa-2A (IFN) in combination with cisplatin (C) Vinblastine (V) and DTIC (D) in patients with metastatic melanoma. *Proc Am Soc Clin Oncol* 1992;11:1179(abst).

226. Pyrhonen S, Hahka-Kemppinen M, Muhonen T. A promising interferon plus four-drug chemotherapy regimen for metastatic melanoma. *J Clin Oncol* 1992;10:1919–1926.

227. Thompson JA, Shulman KL, Benyunes MC, et al. Prolonged continuous intravenous infusion interleukin-2 and lymphokine-activated killer-cell therapy for metastatic renal cell carcinoma. *J Clin Oncol* 1992;10(6):960–968.

228. Balch CM, Soong S-J, Shaw HS, Urist MM, McCarthy WH. An analysis of prognostic factors in 8500 patients with cutaneous melanoma. In: Balch CM, Houghton AN, Sober AJ, Soong S-J, eds. *Cutaneous melanoma*, 2nd ed. Philadelphia: JB Lippincott Co 1992:165–187.

229. Buzaid AC, Ross MI, Balch CM, et al. Critical analysis of the current American joint committee on cancer staging system for cutaneous melanoma and proposal of a new staging system. *J Clin Oncol* 1997;15:1039–1051.

230. Slingluff CL Jr, Vollmer RT, Reintgen DS, Seigler HF. Lethal "thin" malignant melanoma: identifying patients at risk. *Ann Surg* 1988:150–161.

231. Parmiter AH, Nowell PC. The cytogenetics of human malignant melanoma and premalignant lesions melanoma. In: Nathanson L, ed. *Malignant melanoma: biology, diagnosis, and therapy.* Boston: Kluwer Academic Publishers, 1988:47–61.

232. Creagan ET, Dalton RJ, Ahmann DL, et al. Randomized, surgical adjuvant clinical trial of recombinant interferon alfa-2a in selected patients with malignant melanoma. *J Clin Oncol* 1995;13:2776–2783.

233. Cascinelli N. Evaluation of efficacy of adjuvant rIFNa 2A in melanoma patients with regional node metastases. *Proc Am Soc Clin Oncol* 1995;14: A1296–A1296 (abst).

234. Figlin RA. Biotherapy with interferon in solid tumors. *Oncol Nurs Forum* 1987;14:23–26.

235. Karjalainen S, Hakulinen T. Survival and prognostic factors of patients with skin melanomas. *Cancer* 1988;62:2274–2280.

236. Ryan L, Kramar A, Borden E. Prognostic factors in metastatic melanoma. *Cancer* 1993;71(10):2995–3005.

237. Kirkwood J, Hunt M, Smith T, Ernstoff M, Borden E, Blum R. A randomized controlled trial of high-dose IFN alfa-2b for high-risk melanoma: the ECOG trial EST-1684. *Proc Am Soc Clin Oncol* 1993;12:390(abst).

238. Day CL Jr, Sober AJ, Lew RA, et al. Malignant melanoma patients with positive nodes and relatively good prognoses: microstaging retains prognostic significance in clinical stage I melanoma patients with metastases to regional nodes. *Cancer* 1981;47:955–962.

239. Ernstoff MS, Rudnick S, and Kirkwood JM. Comparative toxicity of two alpha interferon preparations given by two different routes in three phase I-II trials. *Clin Res* 1983;31(2):406A–406A(abst).

240. Cole BF, Gelber RD, Kirkwood JM, Goldhirsch A, Barylak E, Borden E. A quality-of-life-adjusted survival analysis of interferon alfa-2b adjuvant treatment for high-risk resected cutaneous melanoma: an Eastern Cooperative Oncology Group Study (E1684). *J Clin Oncol* 1996;14:2666–2673.

241. Goldhirsch A, Gelber RD, Simes RJ, Glasziou P, Coates AS. Costs and benefits of adjuvant therapy in breast cancer: a quality-adjusted survival analysis. *J Clin Oncol* 1989;7:36–44.

242. Kilbridge KL, Sock D, Kirkwood J, et al. Patient utilities for adjuvant interferon (IFN) treatment for high-risk melanoma. *Proc Am Soc Clin Oncol* 1999;(abst).

243. Hillner BE, Kirkwood JM, Atkins MB, Johnson ER, Smith TJ. Economic analysis of adjuvant interferon alfa-2b in high-risk melanoma based on projections from ECOG 1684. *J Clin Oncol* 1997;15:2351–2358.

244. Messori A, Becagli P, Trippoli S, Tendi E. A retrospective cost-effectiveness analysis of interferon as adjuvant therapy in high-risk resected cutaneous melanoma. *Eur J Cancer* 1997;33:1373–1379.

245. Messori A, Becagli P, Trippoli S. Cost-effectiveness of interferon-alpha as maintenance therapy in chronic myelogenous leukemia. *Ann Intern Med* 1997;126:664–665.

246. Cascinelli N, Bufalino R, Morabito A, MacKie R. Results of adjuvant interferon study in WHO melanoma programme. *Lancet* 1994;343:913–914.

247. Ang KK, Byers RM, Peters LJ, et al. Regional radiotherapy as adjuvant treatment for head and neck malignant melanoma. *Arch Otolaryngol Head Neck Surg* 1990;116:169–172.

248. Pehamberger H, Soyer P, Steiner A, et al. Adjuvant interferon alfa-2a treatment in resected primary stage II cutaneous melanoma. *J Clin Oncol* 1998;16:1425–1429.

249. Grob JJ, Dreno B, de la Salmonière P, et al. Randomised trial of interferon α-2a as adjuvant therapy in resected primary melanoma thicker than 1–5 mm without clinically detectable node metastases. *Lancet* 1998;351:1905–1910.

250. Owen-Schaub LB, Gutterman JU, Grimm EA. Synergy of tumor necrosis factorα and interleukin-2 in the activation of human cytotoxic lymphocytes: effect of tumor necrosis factor α and interleukin-2 in the generation of human lymphokine-activated killer cell cytotoxicity. *Cancer Res* 1988;48:788–792.

251. Livingston PO, Wong GYC, Adluri S, et al. Improved survival in stage III melanoma patients with GM2 antibodies: a randomized trial of adjuvant vaccination with GM2 ganglioside. *J Clin Oncol* 1994;12(5):1036–1044.

252. Scheibenbogen C, Keilholz U, Mytilineos J, Suciu S, Manasterski M, Hunstein W. HLA class I alleles and responsiveness of melanoma to immunotherapy with interferon-alpha (IFN-α) and interleukin-2 (IL-2). *Melanoma Res* 1994;4:191–194.

253. Livingston PO, Adluri S, Helling F, et al. Phase 1 trial of immunological adjuvant QS-21 with a GM2 ganglioside-keyhole limpet hemocyanin conjugate vaccine in patients with malignant melanoma. *Vaccine* 1994;12:1275–1280.

254. Chapman PB, Morrissey D, Ibrahim J, et al. Eastern Cooperative Oncology Group phase II randomized adjuvant trial of GM2-KLH + QS21 (GMK) vaccine ± high dose interferon-α2b (HD IFN) in melanoma (MEL). *Proc Am Soc Clin Oncol* 1999:538a(abst).

255. Vlock DR, DerSimonian R, Kirkwood JM. Prognostic role of antibody reactivity to melanoma. *J Clin Invest* 1986;77(4):1116–1121.

256. Riegel DS, Kopf AN, Friedman RJ. The rate of malignant melanoma in the US: are we making an impact? *J Am Acad Dermatol* 1987;17:1050.

257. Itoh K, Shiba K, Shimizu Y, Suzuki R, Kumagai K. Generation of activated killer (AK) cells by recombinant interleukin-2 (rIL-2) in collaboration with interferon-gamma (IFN-gamma). *J Immunol* 1985;134(5):3124–3129.

258. McGovern VJ. *Malignant melanoma: clinical and histological diagnosis.* New York: John Wiley and Sons, 1976:47–48.

259. Elder DE, Goldman LI, Goldman SC, Greene MH, Clark WH Jr. Dysplastic nevus syndrome: a phenotypic association of sporadic cutaneous melanoma. *Cancer* 1980;46:1787–1794.

260. Nordlund JJ, Kirkwood JM, Forget BM, et al. Demographic study of clinically atypical (dysplastic) nevi in patients with melanoma and comparison subjects. *Cancer Res* 1985;45:1855–1861.

261. Roush GC, Schymura MJ, Holford TR. Patterns of invasive melanoma in the Connecticut tumor registry. *Cancer* 1988;61:2586–2595.

262. Roush GC, Nordlund JJ, Forget B, Gruber SB, Kirkwood JM. Independence of dysplastic nevi from total nevi in determining risk for nonfamilial melanoma. *Prev Med* 1988;17:273–279.

263. Titus-Ernstoff L, Duray PH, Ernstoff MS, Barnhill RL, Horn PL, Kirkwood JM. Dysplastic nevi in association with multiple primary melanoma. *Cancer Res* 1988;48:1016–1018.

264. Stewart T. *The interferon system.* New York: Academic Press, 1979.

265. Lengyel P. Biochemistry of interferons and their actions. *Annu Rev*

Biochem 1982;51:251.

266. Carrel S, Schmidt-Kessen A, Giuffrè L. Recombinant interferon-gamma can induce the expression of HLA-DR and -DC on DR-negative melanoma cells and enhance the expression of HLA-ABC and tumor-associated antigens. *Eur J Immunol* 1985;15:118–123.

267. Wadler S, Einzig AI, Dutcher JP, Ciobanu N, Landau L, Wiernik PH. Phase II trial of recombinant alpha-2b-interferon and low-dose cyclophosphamide in advanced melanoma and renal cell carcinoma. *Am J Clin Oncol* 1988;11(1):55–59.

268. Rosenberg SA, Mule JJ. Immunotherapy of cancer with lymphokine-activated killer cells and recombinant interleukin-2. *Surgery* 1985;98:437–444.

269. Ythier A, Abbud-Filho M, Williams JM, et al. Interleukin 2-dependent release of interleukin 3 activity by T4$^+$ human T-cell clones. *Proc Natl Acad Sci U S A* 1985;82:7020–7024.

270. Rapp UR, Cleveland JL, Brightman K, Scott A, Ihle JN. Abrogation of IL-3 and IL-2 dependence by recombinant murine retroviruses expressing v-myc oncogenes. Editorial. *Nature* 1985;317:434–438.

271. Kirkwood JM, Ernstoff MS, Guiliano A, et al. Clinical trials of interferon alfa-2B (Intron A, alpha-IFN) in melanoma: review of phase I, II, and III studies. *Proc XIV Intl Cancer Congress.* Budapest, 1986.

272. Flodgren P, Borgstrom S, Jonsson PE, Lindstrom C, Sjogren HO. Metastatic malignant melanoma: regression induced by combined treatment with interferon [HuIFN-alpha(Le)] and cimetidine. *Int J Cancer* 1983;32(6):657–665.

273. Robinson WA, Kirkwood J, Harvey H, et al. Effective use of recombinant human alpha-2 interferon (IFN-alpha$_2$) in metastatic malignant melanoma (MMM): a comparison of two regimens. *Proc Am Soc Clin Oncol* 1984;3:C234(abst).

274. Talpaz M, Kantarjian HM, McCreedie K, Trujillo JM, Keating MJ, Gutterman JU. Hematologic remission and cytogenetic improvement induced by recombinant human interferon alpha in chronic myelogenous leukemia. *N Engl J Med* 1986;314:1065–1069.

275. Croghan MK, Booth A, Meyskens FL Jr. A phase I trial of recombinant interferon-α and α-difluoromethylornithine in metastatic melanoma. *J Biol Res Mod* 1988;7(4):409–415.

276. Creagan ET, Long HJ, Ahmann DL, Schaid DJ. Phase II assessment of recombinant leukocyte A interferon with difluoromethylornithine in disseminated malignant melanoma. *Am J Clin Oncol* 1990;13: 218–220.

277. Morton RF, Creagan ET, Schaid DJ, et al. Phase II trial of recombinant leukocyte A interferon (IFN-α2A) plus 1,3-bis(2-chloroethyl)-1-nitrosurea (BCNU) and the combination cimetidine with BCNU in patients with disseminated malignant melanoma. *Am J Clin Oncol* 1991;14(2):152–155.

278. Rustin GJS, Dische S, De Garis ST, Nelstrop A. Treatment of advanced malignant melanoma with interferon alpha and etretinate. *Eur J Cancer Clin Oncol* 1988;24(4):783–784.

279. Ernstoff MS, Titus-Ernstoff L, Kirkwood JM. The utility of prophylactic dissection in the treatment and evaluation of patients with clinical stage I cutaneous melanoma: an argument against routine procedure. In: Duffy T, ed. *Debates in medicine,* 1st ed. Chicago: Year Book, 1988:192–202.

280. Schiller JH, Morgan-Ihrig C, Levitt ML. Concomitant administration of interleukin-2 plus tumor necrosis factor in advanced non-small cell lung cancer. 1994(unpublished).

281. Schiller JH, Storer B, Tutsch K, et al. Phase I trial of 3-hour infusion of paclitaxel with or without granulocyte colony-stimulating factor in patients with advanced cancer. *J Clin Oncol* 1994;12:241–248.

282. Clark WH Jr, Elder DE, Guerry D IV, Epstein MN, Greene MH, Van Horn M. A study of tumor progression: the precursor lesions of superficial spreading and nodular melanoma. *Hum Pathol* 1984;15:1147–1165.

283. Mulder NH, Willemse PHB, Schraffordt Koops H, de Vries EGE, Sleijfer DT. Dacarbazine (DTIC) and human recombinant interferon alpha 2a (Roferon) in the treatment of disseminated malignant melanoma. *Br J Cancer* 1990;62:1006–1007.

284. Bajetta E, Di Leo A, Zampino MG, et al. Multicenter randomized trial of dacarbazine alone or in combination with two different doses and schedules of interferon alfa-2a in the treatment of advanced melanoma. *J Clin Oncol* 1994;12:806–811.

285. Richards JM, Gilewski TA, Ramming K, Mitchel B, Doane LL, Vogelzang NJ. Effective chemotherapy for melanoma after treatment with interleukin-2. *Cancer* 1992;69:427–429.

286. Legha SS, Ring S, Eton O, Buzaid AC, Plager C, Papadopoulos N. Development of a biochemotherapy regimen with concurrent administration of cisplatin, vinblastine, dacarbazine, interferon alfa, and interleukin-2 for patients with metastatic melanoma. *J Clin Oncol* 1998;16:1752–1759.

287. Rosenberg SA, Yang JC, Schwartzentruber DJ, et al. Prospective randomized trial of the treatment of patients with metastatic melanoma using chemotherapy with cisplatin, dacarbazine, and tamoxifen alone or in a combination with interleukin-2 and interferon alfa-2b. *J Clin Oncol* 1999;17:968–975.

288. Ernstoff MS, Davis CA, Kirkwood JM. Cimetidine plus IFN-alpha-2 does not remit metastatic melanoma which has failed IFN alone. *Proc Am Soc Clin Oncol* 1984;3:62 (abst).

10.3

INTERFERON-α AND -β: CLINICAL APPLICATIONS

Renal Cell Cancer

CHRISTOPHER TRETTER
PAUL D. SAVAGE
HYMAN B. MUSS
MARC S. ERNSTOFF

Epithelial kidney tumors, comprised of seven morphologic types arising from the proximal tubule or collecting duct, are collectively known as *renal cell carcinoma* (1). An estimated 30,000 new cases of renal cell cancer (RCC) resulting in 11,900 deaths will occur in the United States in 1999 (2). Common risk factors for RCC do not distinguish patient populations that may benefit from screening, except in cases of rare inherited disorders, such as von Hippel–Lindau disease. Although many patients present with local symptoms, such as hematuria, flank pain, a palpable mass, or signs and symptoms of metastasis, an increasing number of patients have asymptomatic renal tumors identified serendipitously when undergoing radiologic evaluation of the abdomen (e.g., computed tomography scan, ultrasound) for unrelated reasons. Approximately 50% to 60% of patients have surgically resectable disease at the time of diagnosis. Five-year survival rates are approximately 61% for all stages and 62% to 89% for local regional disease (2). Metastatic disease carries a bleak prognosis with a 74% mortality rate at 1 year and a 96% mortality rate at 3 years (3). Even those patients with resectable disease have a risk of recurrence of at least 10% over a 10-year period (4,5). When metastases develop, they are most commonly seen in the lungs (approximately 65% of patients), followed by bone (40%), liver (14%), adrenals (8%), peritoneum (8%), and brain (5%) (3).

RCCs can secrete a variety of biologically active substances, which accounts for RCC-associated paraneoplastic syndromes. Common paraneoplastic syndromes include cachexia, anemia, fever, and hypercalcemia. Polycythemia and hepatitis are less frequently observed (6). These paraneoplastic syndromes have not been found to have a significant impact on prognosis except when overall performance status is compromised.

Spontaneous or unexplained regression of RCC metastases have been observed in a variety of patients. Initially thought to occur after nephrectomy, spontaneous regression was commonly used as a rationale for removal of the primary neoplasm in the setting of metastatic disease. Spontaneous regressions are infrequent, occurring in less than 1% of patients, and are not necessarily associated with resection of the primary (7–9) neoplasm. Thus, nephrectomy in patients with metastatic disease should be reserved for those with symptoms directly caused by their renal mass. These patients may benefit from palliative resection. A randomized study of interferon-γ (IFN-γ) versus placebo in metastatic RCC patients reported a response rate of 6.6% in the placebo group, suggesting that unexplained regressions may be more common than once thought (10). The documented cases of spontaneous regression most often occurred in pulmonary metastases and were usually short-lived (a few months), although a small percentage of patients have remained disease-free for years (7,9).

In general, the failure of established endocrine therapy and chemotherapy to significantly impact clinical response or overall survival has led to the abandonment of these approaches as first-line therapy. Although the benefit of single-agent immunotherapies, including IFN-α and interleukin-2 (IL-2), is modest, clinical response rates of 10% to 20% in RCC patients have been seen and long-term survivors have been reported. Thus, cytokine therapies have become the foundation of modern treatment strategies for RCC patients.

It is well established that prognostic groups of patients with metastatic RCC can be defined by clinical criteria. Performance status, time from nephrectomy at initial diagnosis, the number of metastatic sites, prior cytotoxic chemotherapy, and recent weight loss can be used as important indicators of survival, predicting as much as a sixfold difference in survival between good and poor prognostic groups (2.1 to 12.8 months) (11). Furthermore, these factors can be used to predict the likelihood of response to biologic therapies. Performance status, recurrence at the renal bed, weight loss, history of nephrectomy, sarcomatoid histology, and bone metastasis correlated with response to biologic treatment on univariate analysis with only bone metastasis, sarcomatoid histology, and performance status significant predictors in a multivariate analysis (12). This may explain the variation in responses reported in many series. It is therefore critical that carefully controlled randomized studies be conducted before adopting new strategies for treatment of this disease.

ENDOCRINE THERAPY AND CHEMOTHERAPY

Initial reports by Bloom described a response rate of 16% with little toxicity for medroxyprogesterone (13). When evaluated in randomized studies, medroxyprogesterone has had little to no activity (14). Although other endocrine therapies have been used, true complete and partial response rates using objective response criteria are less than 5% (15). Progestins have also been used as adjuvant therapy for patients with high-risk, resectable primary lesions but have not been effective (16). A trial of high-dose tamoxifen demonstrated a 10% response rate in hormone refractory patients, but patient numbers were small (17). Combination hormonal therapy has not increased the efficacy of this modality (17). The lack of significant clinical benefit from hormonal therapy in RCC and the lack of evidence that human RCC is under hormonal regulation does not support the use of this approach in the treatment of RCC today.

Chemotherapy for RCC has also been unsatisfactory. Reviews of chemotherapy and endocrine therapy for advanced disease confirm the poor response to systemic treatment (15,18–22). Almost all single-agent trials have been associated with response rates less than 10%. Part of this difficulty arises from the high prevalence of expression of multidrug resistance (MDR) mechanisms present in *de novo* RCC at diagnosis (23). Overexpression of p-glycoprotein (MDR1) with associated drug resistance has been described in more than 80% of primary RCCs (24). Traditionally, vinblastine has been used for therapy of metastatic disease, but phase 2 studies failed to confirm significant single-agent activity. One explanation of vinblastine's poor response rates is the expression of MDR1 in RCC. The addition of MDR1 inhibitors, such as tamoxifen, quinidine, and cyclosporin, have also failed to enhance vinblastine activity in RCC patients (25,26). Given as a chronobiologically defined continuous infusion, floxuridine (FUdR) has been associated with response rates of 28% (27), although it is not clear that this route offers any advantage over constant infusion FUdR (28). This issue continues to be evaluated in an ongoing randomized trial of circadian versus flat infusion of FUdR. Combining vinblastine with other chemotherapeutic or endocrine agents has not resulted in superior response rates and has been associated with greater toxicity. Although vinblastine is still used as a single-agent therapy, the response rates and overall survival are poor. This poor response rate to chemotherapy and endocrine therapy has led many physicians, including some urologists and surgical and medical oncologists, to offer only supportive care to patients with metastatic RCC. The lack of an effective treatment for metastatic RCC has led to clinical trials with numerous agents, including IFNs. A review of the basic principles and preclinical studies of IFN therapy is presented in Chapter 9.

INTERFERON THERAPY

Overview of Interferon-α and -β Clinical Trials

Of the three types of IFNs (α, β, and γ) commercially available, only IFN-α has shown significant single-agent clinical response rates in RCC to warrant consideration for use. Table 1 represents the list of clinical investigations involving single-agent IFN-α or IFN-β (29–67). Results are presented according to IFN type and include six trials using leucocyte preparations, nine trials using lymphoblastoid (partially purified) IFNs, 19 trials using recombinant IFN-α (rIFN-α), and three trials using IFN-β. When possible, response criteria following World Health Organization guidelines and calculated 95% confidence intervals (CIs) are reported for these trials to explore the effect of selected covariables on response, duration of response, and survival. We attempt to formulate meaningful recommendations from interpretation of this data, although small numbers of patients, dose and schedule variations, and nonrandomized study designs make it difficult to draw firm conclusions (68). Doses of IFN are presented as MU (1 MU = 1×10^6 IU).

Initial IFN trials used crude preparations of leukocyte IFN produced by methods described by Cantell et al. at the Finnish Red Cross Blood Center (69). These preparations likely contained other cytokines capable of augmenting response, and dose was limited by volume of subcutaneous (s.c.) injections. Response rates of 18% (95% CI of 13% to 25%) were observed. Nine trials reported the use of partially purified lymphoblastoid IFN; in at least seven of these trials, the IFN studied was obtained from the Namalwa strain of lymphoblasts originally derived from a young female with Burkitt's lymphoma. This partially purified IFN developed by Burroughs-Wellcome contains eight different IFN-αs. An overall response rate of 16% (95% CI of 13% to 20%) were noted in these nine trials.

The development of recombinant DNA techniques made it possible to produce highly purified preparations of IFN with high specific activity, as measured by antiviral U per mg of protein (70). This allowed for the expansion of clinical trials, which began in 1981. At least 19 trials have involved rIFN-αs. rIFNα-2a (Roferon, Hoffman LaRoche Laboratories) has been used in nine trials with an overall response rate of 15% (95% CI of 12% to 19%). rIFNα-2b (Intron, Schering Plough Laboratories), a second rIFNα-2, has displayed an overall response rate of 16% (95% CI of 12% to 22%). Porzsolt and colleagues noted only a 6% response rate in 47 patients using rIFNα-2c (52). rIFN-β has been studied by three groups, each with small numbers of patients; the overall response rate of 7% has a 95% CI of 1% to 24%.

These data do not suggest the superiority of one IFN-α preparation over another. Cantell-derived IFN preparations and lymphoblastoid IFN have been associated with higher response rates than their recombinant counterparts. Without randomized studies, however, these minor differences do not provide support of one preparation over another. The most commonly used preparations of IFN-α include rIFNα-2a and rIFNα-2b, which currently represent the "standard" of comparison for future clinical trials.

TABLE 1. SINGLE-AGENT INTERFERON COLLECTED SERIES

Author	Reference	Dose	Route	Schedule	Evaluable Patients	CR + PR	Percent	95% CI
Leucocyte IFN-Cantell type								
Quesada et al.	29,30	3[a]	i.m.	q.d.	50	3 + 10	26	15–40
De Kernion et al.	31	3[a]	i.m.	q.d. × 5, qwk	43	1 + 6	16	7–31
Kirkwood et al.[b]	32	1[a]	i.m.	q.d.	14	—	—	0–19
		10[a]	i.m.	q.d.[c]	16	1 + 2	19	4–46
Edsmyr et al.	33	3[a]	i.m.	q.d.	11	1 + 2	27	6–61
Medencia and Slack	34	6	i.m.	q.d. × 3, q4wk	4	1 + 1	50	7–93
Bengtsson et al.	58	2[a] → 7[a]	s.c.	q.d.	28	2 + 0	7	1–24
Subtotal					166	9 + 21	18	13–25
Lymphoblastoid IFN (partially purified)								
Neidhart et al.	35	5	i.m.	t.i.w.	33	0 + 5	15	5–32
Neidhart et al.[d]	36	3 → 20[a]	i.m.	q.d. × 10, q3wk	23	1 + 4[e]	22	7–44
		5 → 50[a]	i.m.	q.d. × 5, q3wk	9	0 + 2	22	3–60
Marumo et al.	37	3[a]	i.m.	q.d.	18	1 + 0	6	0–27
Trump et al.	38	3 → 20	i.m.	q.d. × 10, q3wk	39	0 + 5	13	4–27
Vugrin et al.	39	3	i.m.	t.i.w.	21	0 + 1	5	0–24
Eisenhauer et al.	40	3 → 100	i.v.	q wk	37	0 + 4	11	3–25
Fujita et al.	41	3[a]	i.m.	q.d.	24	2 + 4	25	10–47
Umeda and Niijima	42	5[a]	i.m.	b.i.w.→ t.i.w.→ q.d.	73	1 + 16	23	14–35
Oliver et al.[d]	8	2.5	n.s.	q.d. × 5, qwk	34	0 + 5	15	5–31
		5 → 30	n.s.	q.d.	31	2 + 4	19	7–37
		3[a]	n.s.	t.i.w.	17	0 + 1	6	0–29
Subtotal					359	7 + 51	16	13–20
rIFN-α–2a								
Enzig et al., Krown	43,44	3 → 36[a]	i.m.	q.d.	62	0 + 7	11	5–22
Quesada et al.[b]	45	2	i.m.	q.d.	15[f]	0 + 0	0	0–18
		20	i.m.	q.d.	41	1 + 11	29	16–46
Buzaid et al.	46	3 → 36[a]	i.m.	q.d.	22	0 + 5	23	8–45
Figlin et al.	47	3 → 36[a]	i.m.	q.d. × 5, qwk	19	1 + 4	26	9–51
Umeda and Niijima	42	3 → 36[a]	i.m.	q.d.	108	2 + 13	24	8–22
Schnall et al.	48	3 → 36[a]	i.m.	q.d.	22	0 + 1	5	0–23
Fossa	49	18–36	i.m.	t.i.w.	17	0 + 2	11	1–36
Marshall et al.	59	1[a]	s.c.	q.d.	16	0 + 4	25	7–52
Minasian et al.[d]	60	3 → 36[a]	s.c.	q.d.	59	2 + 5	12	5–23
			i.m.	t.i.w.	39	0 + 7	18	7–34
Subtotal					420	6 + 59	15	12–19
rIFN-α–2b								
Muss et al.[b]	50	2	s.c.	t.i.w.	51	1 + 4	10	3–21
Umeda and Niijima	42	6-10[a]	i.m.	q.d. × 3, q5wk	45	1 + 7	18	8 + 32
Foon et al.	51	2	s.c.	t.i.w.	21	0 + 1	5	0–24
Levens et al.	61	10[a]	s.c.	q.d.	15	1 + 3	27	
Bono et al.	62	3	s.c.	t.i.w.	61	2 + 16	30	—
Subtotal					239	6 + 33	16	12–22
Other α or subtype not specified								
Porzsolt et al. (α-2c)	52	2[a]	s.c.	q.d. × 5 , qwk	47	1 + 2	6	1–18
Otto et al.	53	18[a]	i.m.	t.i.w.	30	0 + 3	10	2–27
Abratt et al. (rIFN-α)	63	3[a]	s.c.	t.i.w.	12	2 + 0	17	—
Rosenthal et al. (rIFN-α2)	64	2 → 5	s.c.	t.i.w.	20	0 + 1	5	0–14
Subtotal					109	3 + 6	8	4–15
rIFN-β								
Rinehart et al.	55,65	0.01 → 150	i.v.	b.i.w.	13	0 + 2	15	2–45
Nelson et al.	66	90 → 720	i.v.	t.i.w.	15	0	0	—
Subtotal					28	0 + 2	7	1–24
IFN-β–serine								
Kinney et al.	67	45 → 990	i.v.	t.i.w.	25	1 + 4	20	7–41

CI, confidence interval; CR, complete remission; IFN, interferon; PR, partial response; rIFN, recombinant IFN.
Note: Dose in MU/m^2 unless specified.
[a]Total dose.
[b]Randomized study; results of each arm(s) given, when possible.
[c]Given 4 to 8 weeks only; responders given maintenance.
[d]Nonrandomized (usually sequential studies): results of each arm(s) given, when possible.
[e]No response in ten patients with prior IFN.
[f]Initial 15 patients randomized.

Response by Dose and Type of Interferon

The dose, route, and schedule of IFN administration are presented in Table 1. In an attempt to determine the relationship of response versus dose, available data for phase 2 studies were converted into an average daily dose when possible; no attempt was made to calculate cumulative doses of therapy (Table 2). These data must be interpreted cautiously because of major scheduling differences (many of the trials used an escalating induction sequence), variable dose modification procedures, and different IFN preparations.

Three randomized studies have evaluated dosage (32,45,50). Kirkwood and colleagues performed a randomized trial of 1 MU versus 10 MU of leukocyte IFN. The trial allowed for a cross-over from low-dose to high-dose arms. None of 14 patients responded to low-dose therapy, whereas 3 of 16 patients responded to high-dose therapy. As responses to IFN may take several months, many of these patients may not have had an adequate trial at a low dose. Of four patients initially treated with low-dose therapy who subsequently received 10 MU daily, one partial response occurred.

Quesada and colleagues performed a randomized trial of rIFNα-2a comparing 2 MU per m^2 with 20 MU per m^2 given daily for a minimum of 8 weeks; none of 15 patients randomized to the low-dose arm responded, whereas 22 of 41 patients receiving high-dose therapy responded (39). These results differed from a previous study by Quesada and colleagues (29,30) using Cantell-type IFN in which a response rate of 26% was noted at the daily 3-MU dose. It was speculated that the differences in response rates may have been the result of other IFNs and lymphokines with potential antitumor activity present in the Cantell-type preparation. Like Kirkwood (32), however, it is also possible that their initial induction phase using the low-dose treatment was too short.

Of the five trials using rIFNα-2b, Muss and colleagues randomized patients to receive rIFNα-2 at 2 MU per m^2 subcutaneously three times weekly or 30 to 50 MU per m^2 given intravenously for 5 consecutive days every 3 weeks (50). A 10% response rate occurred in the low-dose regimen (5 of 51 patients). A 7% response rate occurred in the high-dose regimen (3 of 46 patients). Differences in the two groups may be related to schedule, route of administration, or both. Intermittent dosing, as used in the high-dose group, may be inferior to continuous dosing schedules. The pharmacokinetic profile of IFNs differs significantly between the s.c. and intramuscular (i.m.) route and the i.v. (intravenous) route. The s.c. and i.m. route provides more prolonged systemic exposure.

In general, no clear dose-response relationship is supported by published data. Randomized data are incomplete but suggest that doses greater than 3 MU per m^2 given in a continuous dosing schedule are therapeutic. As IFN toxicity is directly related to dose, a dose of 5 to 10 MU given at least three times per week appears to have the best therapeutic index. Route does not seem to be a major factor in determining response, as i.m. and s.c. administration appear equivalent (an observation supported by pharmacologic data). i.v. regimens are more difficult to administer and are not superior to i.m. or s.c. treatment.

Time to Response and Response Durability

Time to response, duration of response, and the number of patients responding for longer than 12 months are presented in Table 3. The time to achieve a partial response was generally 1 to 3 months; however, on occasion, responses were seen after 6 months or longer (62). Once response was obtained, the median duration of response ranged from 2.5 to 35 months with an average duration of approximately 6 months. Of the 159 responders, 77 had long-term follow-up data concerning response duration. Twenty-eight of these 77 patients (36%) had response durations longer than 1 year, representing about 3% of all patients treated with IFN; Minasian et al., however, reported that 3% of their patients had survival durations that exceeded 5 years (60).

Characteristics of Interferon Responders

Pretreatment characteristics, including age, gender, disease-free interval, performance status, prior treatment, sites of metastasis, and nephrectomy, as well as toxicity secondary to treatment, were analyzed to determine their effect on response. No obvious relationship existed between age and gender to response. In most trials, males predominated and responded more frequently, reflecting the increased incidence of RCC in males. Disease-free interval was not associated with response. Responses were more frequent in patients with good performance status; however, most protocols restricted eligibility to patients who had favorable or normal performance-activity levels. Several investigators noted higher response rates in patients without prior chemotherapy or radiation (32,42), whereas others reported no major differences. Again, many trials restricted entry to patients without prior chemotherapy, and most studies were too small and had too few responders for major analyses. Leukopenia secondary to IFN treatment significantly correlated with response in two series (29,42), but not in four other studies (32,41,46,50). In a univariate and multivariate analysis of response to biologic therapy in metastatic RCC, Mani et al. (14) confirmed that performance status was the most important predictor of responses. The univariate analysis revealed that nephrectomy, histology, weight loss, and local recurrence were predictors of response as well. Indeed, the best responses were seen in patients with pulmonary or lymph node metastases only. Bone metastases, performance status, and sarcomatoid histology

TABLE 2. PHASE 2 STUDIES: AVERAGE DAILY DOSE INTERFERON-α

	<5 MU	>5 MU
No. in series	15	6
Reference	8,29,31–33,35,37,39,41, 45,50,52,59,62,63	32,41,43,48,53,61
Total no. of patients	471	187
CR	14	4
PR	60	28
CR/PR (%)	16	17
95% CI	13–19	12–22

CI, confidence interval; CR, complete remission; PR, partial response.

TABLE 3. TIME TO RESPONSE AND DURATION OF RESPONSE

Author	Reference	No. of Responders	Time to Response		Duration of Response		Responders >12 Mo.	
			Median	Range	Median	Range[a]	Number	Duration
Quesada et al.	29	13	3	1–6	6+	2–16	NA	—
DeKernion et al.	31	7	NA[b]	NA	7	2–19+	2	12+,19+
Kirkwood et al.	32	3	2	1–7	15	4–28	2	15,28
Edsmyr et al.	33	3	NA	NA	6	2–28+	1	28+
Medencia and Slack	34	2	NA	NA	NA	13+,18+	2	13+,18+
Neidhart et al.	35,36	5	NA	0.7–6.2	7.6	3–14+	2	12+,14+
Marumo et al.	37	1	3	—	24+	—	1	24+
Trump et al.	38	5	4.7	1.6–5.6	8.1+	2.8–14.6	1	14.6
Eisenhauer et al.	40	4	NA	>3	8.1	2.8–12+	2	12+,12+
Fujita et al.	41	6	2.8	1–8	6+	1–20+	1	20+
Umeda and Niijima	42	15	NA	0.7–7.0	2.5	1–12	NA	—
Quesada et al.	45	12	NA	1–3	3	1–12+	NA	—
Buzaid et al.	46	5	2	1–3	8	1–17+	2	12+,17+
Figlin et al.	47	5	1	1–5	9.5	1–18.3	NA	
Muss et al.	50	8	NA	2–13	17	3–26	5	13,16,17,26
Porzsolt et al.	52	3	NA	2–6	5+	3–21+	1	21+
Kinney et al.	67	5	2.3	1.8–8.9	3.7	1.9–7.7	NA	—
Levens et al.	61	4	NA	<3	8	5–20+	1	20+
Marshall et al.	59	4	NA	NA	9.5+	2+–20+	1	20+
Oliver et al.	8	12	NA	<4	4.5	1+–18	2	18,18
Abratt et al.	63	2	3.4	NA	NA	23+,45+	2	23+,45+
Bengtsson et al.	58	2	3.5	1–7	NA	11,14	1	14
Rosenthal et al.	64	1	3.5	—	1.25	—	NA	—
Fossa et al.	73	9	NA	NA	8	4–20	4	15+,21,24,30
Minasian et al.	60	14	NA	NA	12.2	2.6–98.6+	NA	—

NA, not available.
[a]Median, range, and duration in months.
[b]Median and/or range not stated in reference.

remained predictive in the multivariate model. In review of RCC patient characteristics, performance status, minimal disease in the soft tissue or lung only, and survival greater than 1 year postnephrectomy were associated with a better likelihood of response to treatment. Bone metastases and sarcomatoid histology predicted a poor outcome.

The relationship of response to sites of metastases may help the clinician identify patients more likely to respond to IFN-α therapy. Approximately 80% of patients in published trials have had nephrectomy. It is unlikely to observe response in primary RCC, even when distant metastases have responded to treatment. Although trials of patients with nephrectomy report response rates of 17% and an 11% response rate has been observed in patients without nephrectomy, it is erroneous to conclude that a potential advantage may exist in patients who had nephrectomy. The data should be interpreted cautiously, as other patient characteristics are likely to confound this type of analysis. Approximately 20% of patients with lung metastases displayed a complete or partial response, a rate almost double that of patients with other metastatic sites. Of 143 patients who had metastases confined only to the lung, 51 (36%) displayed response. Few authors presented detailed data on sites of metastases; nevertheless, only a small percentage of patients with liver or bone metastases displayed objective responses. Responses were described in at least ten patients with primary lesions in the kidney and in others with soft tissue lesions,

including the skin and retroperitoneal lymph node metastases. Caution is advised, however, when interpreting these results. Pulmonary lesions were usually easily measured, and, in most trials, chest x-rays were obtained more frequently than liver scans, bone scans, or computed tomography scans. For these reasons, brief responses were more likely to be seen in the lung. In addition, measurement of bone metastases is frequently indirect (i.e., bone scan), whereas skeletal x-rays may require long periods to show improvement. Also, patients with bone and liver metastases are more likely to have poor performance status, making them less likely to be eligible for study or tolerate the side effects of IFN therapy.

Toxicity

Patients receiving IFN therapy for RCC display similar toxicity profiles to those receiving IFN for other malignant diseases. Even at lower doses, almost all patients display fever, taste change, lassitude, myalgia, loss of appetite, and other flulike symptoms. For most patients, this represents the most distressing aspect of treatment. As the dosage is increased, depression, anorexia, leukopenia, transient elevation of liver function tests, and increasing lassitude become more common and more pronounced. Nausea, vomiting, diarrhea, and atrial tachyarrhythmias are uncommon side effects, even at higher doses. Moderate to severe symptoms are especially frequent at

TABLE 4. ANTIINTERFERON ANTIBODIES

Author	Reference	IFN Type	Patients Positive	Patients Tested	Patients Positive (%)	Assay	Comments
Tuttle et al.	77	Ly	—	267	—	NS	Analysis of six phase 2 trials
Umeda and Niijima	42	α-2a	13	108	14	Bioassay[a]	No effect on response
Krown et al.	126	α-2a	4	10	40	NS	One PR progressed when antibody detected
Quesada et al.	45	α-2a	20	53	38	Bioassay	Response and toxicity abated in antibody
Buzaid et al.	46	α-2a	8	21	83	EIA	No effect of antibody on response
Figlin et al.	47	α-2a	12	19	63	EIA	No effect of antibody on response survival
			6	19	32	Bioassay	—
Muss et al.	50	α-2a	7	131	5	EIA	No effect of antibody on response
Fossa et al.	73	α-2a	8	26[b]	31	EIA	—
			2	8[b]	25	Bioassay	—
Prummer	78	α-2a	40	86	47	EIA	Adjuvant study; no effect
			25	86	29	Bioassay	of antibody on relapses

EIA, enzyme-linked immunoassay; IFN, interferon; Ly, lymphoblastoid IFN; NS, method not stated; PR, partial response.
[a]Bioassay is viral challenge in cell culture to detect neutralizing antibody.
[b]Bioassay only performed on EIA-positive patient.

doses greater than 10 MU per day. For patients receiving IFN for long periods, fatigue frequently becomes the most distressing symptom, resulting in marked reduction of physical activity. Neuropsychiatric manifestations of IFN may result in moderate to severe changes in behavior, possibly a result of direct effects of IFN on the brain (71,72). Discontinuation of IFN generally results in the resolution of toxicity after several days to several weeks. Frequently, IFN-induced tachyphylaxis for fever and chills develop, making treatment better tolerated. In addition, the use of acetaminophen may help ameliorate mild symptoms. Although corticosteroids can control the flulike symptoms related to IFN and do not appear to adversely affect response, we generally do not use them (73–75). Aspirin, however, does not control the flulike symptoms (76). Newer approaches to ameliorate toxicity have focused on different preparations of IFN (see the section on Response and Antiinterferon Antibodies). Once recognized, depression can be treated with antidepressant agents with good response.

Response and Antiinterferon Antibodies

Several investigators have monitored patients for the development of anti-IFN antibodies during the course of therapy. An overview of these data are presented in Table 4. An analysis of six phase 2 trials using human lymphoblastoid IFN (Wellferon, Burroughs Wellcome Company) failed to show antibody development in 267 patients (77). This is likely due to the fact that the preparation of IFNs are genetically identical to natural forms. Antibodies have frequently been demonstrated in patients receiving rIFNα-2a, however, and less frequently in patients receiving rIFNα 2b. The most frequently detected antibodies are IFN-binding antibodies, which are detected by enzyme-linked immunoassay; neutralizing antibodies, demonstrable by decreased inhibition of virally induced cytopathic changes in cell cultures, are also frequently found. Thirty-eight percent of patients treated by Quesada et al. (45) and 32% of patients treated by Figlin et al. (47) developed neutralizing antibodies. In Quesada's series, the development of such antibodies was associated

with relapse in all seven patients who developed them. The median duration of response in antibody-positive patients was 2 months versus 10 months in those who were antibody negative (p = .009). Median survival was also shorter (12 months) in antibody-positive than in antibody-negative (19 months) patients. Of note, antibody development was associated with a decrease in fatigue, anorexia, and IFN levels; an increase in white blood cell counts; and normalization of liver function tests. The authors concluded that such antibody production neutralized the biologic effects of IFN, abrogating response and toxicity. In contrast, Figlin et al., using an identical rIFNα-2a preparation at a similar dosage, noted the appearance of antibody before response in two patients and found no relationship between antibody formation and response duration. Buzaid et al. noted neutralizing antibodies in one partial responder who continues in remission for 17+ months (46). Fossa and colleagues were unable to demonstrate any difference in clinical outcome between antibody-positive and antibody-negative patients, although patient numbers were small; a reduction in serum levels of IFN correlated with the presence of neutralizing antibodies (73). An adjuvant study reported by Prommer for the Delta P Study Group did not demonstrate any difference in disease-free interval nor relapse rate based on anti-IFN antibody status (78). The reasons for these discrepancies are not clear. Using rIFNα-2a, Muss et al. detected antibodies in three of seven responders (50). Anti-IFN antibody production in this series was low and had no effect on response. A summary of neutralizing antibodies in a combined series of trials using rIFNα-2b revealed a neutralizing antibody rate of 2.4% (10 out of 423 patients) (79). The development of such antibodies was not associated with amelioration of IFN toxicity when compared with antibody-negative patients and had no discernible effect on response (80). In summary, the role of neutralizing antibodies in the development of clinical IFN resistance occurs rarely. Patients receiving IFN with chemotherapy have not been studied for antibody information to determine whether chemotherapy can prevent antibody development; prednisone may be capable of blunting forma-

TABLE 5. COMBINATIONS OF INTERFERON OR INTERFERONS AND OTHER BIOLOGICS[a]

Author	Reference	Dose[b]	Route	Schedule	Evaluable Patients	CR + PR	Percent	95% CI
Foon et al.	51	α/2 γ/2	s.c.	t.i.w.	47	0 + 2	—	1–15
Quesada et al.	56	α-2a/2	i.m.	q.d.	10	—	—	0–26
		γ/2	i.m.	q.d.				
		α-2a/2	i.m.	q.d.	23	0 + 4	17	5–39
		γ/0.2	i.m.	q.d.				
		γ/5[c]	i.m.	q.d. × 7	13	0 + 1	8	0 + 36
		α-2a/10	i.m.	q.d. × 7				
Geboers et al.	57	α-2c/2	s.c.	b.i.w.[c]	38	0 + 5	13	4–28
		γ/2	s.c.	b.i.w.				
De Mulder et al.	84	α-2a/2–36	s.c.	b.i.w.	31	2 + 6	26	12–45
		γ/2	s.c.	b.i.w.				
Ernstoff et al.	81	α-2a/2–20	s.c.	q.d.	36	2 + 6	22	10–39
		γ/0.6–20	s.c.	q.d. × 5; q3wk				
Mulder et al.	127	γ/100 μg	s.c.	t.i.w.	14	0	0	0–23
				Total	212	28 (13)		(8.5–175)
		RNA/1–3,000 mg	i.v.	b.i.w.				
		TNF[d]-α/50 μg	i.m.	t.i.w.				
Strayer et al.	128	α[e]/1.5–3.0	i.m.	q.d.	12	0 + 4	33	10–65
Marumo et al.	129	Ly/3 OK–432[f]	i.m.	q.d.	12	1	8	1–38

CI, confidence interval; CR, complete response; Ly, lymphoblastoid interferon; PR, partial response; TNF, tumor necrosis factor.
[a]Excludes combinations with interleukin-2.
[b]Interferon type noted before dose.
[c]Five responses seen in 24 patients with escalation of interferon-α.
[d]Tumor necrosis factor.
[e]Leukocyte interferon; mismatched double-stranded RNA (Ampligen).
[f]A streptococcal preparation.

tion of anti-IFN antibodies (81), although a randomized trial has not been performed.

The data strongly suggest that successful treatment of metastatic RCC with single-agent IFN-α is related to clinical characteristics, IFN dose, and schedule. In this regard, convenience of administration and flulike symptoms are major barriers to therapy. To reduce toxicity and provide prolonged serum levels of IFN-α, IFNα-2b has been coupled to polyethylene glycol (polyethylene glycol–IFNα-2b, Schering) and has been tested in a phase 1 setting (82). A maximum tolerated dose of 6 μg per kg is well tolerated with significantly less toxicity than antiviral equivalents of IFNα-2b. Responses have been noted in a variety of tumors, including RCC. A phase 2 trial has been initiated and is currently under way.

Interferon Combined with Other (Non Interleukin-2) Biotherapies

rIFN-γ has been extensively studied in patients with metastatic RCC and has demonstrated a low response rate of 6% to 10% (95% CI of 6% to 14%) in 236 patients. The observation that IFN-α and IFN-γ can exhibit synergy *in vitro* has prompted several clinical trials of rIFN-α and rIFN-γ used together (83). IFN-α and IFN-γ bind to different cell surface receptors and enhance expression of different classes of histocompatibility antigens. Although initial studies of combined IFN-γ and IFN-α were limited by toxicity, a sequential trial design allowed for higher combined doses to be administered (81). A hint of greater activity was seen in a single institution study of sequential IFN-γ followed by IFN-α, which was not confirmed in a later multiinstitutional trial (46,56,57,81,84).

Two small trials of IFN-α in combination with tumor necrosis factor or mismatched double-stranded RNA are listed in Table 5. Although *in vitro* data have suggested a synergistic effect for combinations of IFNs (85) and tumor necrosis factor (86), the pilot clinical trials have not supported this approach. Another approach for enhancing response is to use recombinant hybrid IFNs, but this has not shown promise in clinical trials (87).

Interferon Combined with Chemotherapy

The combination of vinblastine and IFN have been the most extensively studied combination of IFN and chemotherapy. In addition to demonstrable synergism *in vitro* (88), vinblastine represents the most used single agent for metastatic RCC. The results of published trials of this combination are presented in Table 6. Response rates for this combination have ranged from 7% to 43%. In general, vinblastine was given in a dose of 0.1 mg per kg every 3 weeks combined with i.m. IFN given three times weekly. Also, time to response and response duration of the vinblastine/IFN combination are similar to that of IFN alone. In a randomized trial of 178 patients comparing rIFNα-2a (18 MU t.i.w.) plus vinblastine (0.1 mg per kg every 3 weeks) with IFN alone, an improvement in the overall response rate (11% vs. 24%) occurred, but no difference in survival between the treatment arms (89) was detected. Another phase 3 trial reported by Pyrhonen et al. also compared vinblastine with IFNα-2a plus vinblastine (90). The combination therapy improved overall response rates (16% vs. 25%), as well as overall survival (15.8 months vs. 8.8 months). Although direct comparison between vinblastine and IFN-α has not been performed,

TABLE 6. INTERFERON PLUS VINBLASTINE

Author	Reference	Interferon[a]	Vinblastine	Evaluable Patients	CP + PR	CR + PR (%)	95% CI
Figlin et al.	130	Le/3±/i.m. q.d. × 5 q wk	0.15 mg/kg q wk	23	0 + 3	13	3–34
Fossa et al.	49	α-2a/18–36 ±/i.m. t.i.w.	0.1–0.15 mg/kg q2–3wk	40	10	25	13–41
Fossa and DeGaris	131,132						
Cetto et al.	133	α-2b/3–10 s.c. t.i.w.	0.1 mg/kg q3wk	26	1 + 7	31	14–52
Killokumpu-Lehtinen et al.	134	α-2a/18 ± i.m. t.i.w.	0.075–0.15 mg/kg q3wk	20	3 + 3	20	12–54
Bergerat et al.	135	α-2a/10–20/i.m. t.i.w.	0.075–0.15 mg/kg q3wk	40	1 + 16	43	23–59
Sertoli et al.	136	α-2a/18±/i.m. t.i.w.	0.1 mg/kg q3wk	20	0 + 2	10	1–32
Otto et al.	53	α/18/i.m. t.i.w.	0.1 mg/kg q3wk	34	2 + 4	18	7–35
Schornagel et al.	137	α-2a/18 ± t.i.w.	0.1. mg/kg q3wk	56	0 + 9	16	8–28
Trump et al.	138	Ly/e-5 × 10 d q4wk	1.5/q.d. × 5 c.i.v. 2	18	0 +1	7	1–27
Neidhart et al.	139	Ly/2–20 × 5 d q2wk	10/mg q4wk	83	3 + 4	8	3–17

CI, confidence interval; CP, cardiac performance; CR, complete remission; Le, leucocyte interferon; Ly, lymphoblastoid interferon; PR, partial response.
[a]Type/dose in MU/m^2 unless otherwise specified.

the data suggest that single-agent IFN-α has significant clinical activity in patients with metastatic RCC. In the opinion of these investigators, the addition of vinblastine to IFN has not improved response and has resulted in substantially higher hematologic toxicity; its use outside the setting of a clinical trial is not justified.

Combinations of IFN-α and pyrimidine antimetabolites have been explored in metastatic RCC based on preliminary clinical data in other diseases and *in vitro* studies. *In vitro* data suggests that IFN-α enhances 5-FU thymidylate synthetase inhibition (91,92). In addition, 5-FU may enhance host cell–mediated immunity (93). Table 7 summarizes some key studies that evaluated the effects of the combination of 5-FU and IFN-α in metastatic RCC.

Of these 11 studies, only two did not include IL-2 in the treatment regimen. Elias et al. (92) combined IFN-α (3 × weekly) with 5-day continuous infusion of 5-FU every 3 weeks and reported 5 out of 34 partial responses. Gebroskey et al. (94), using lower doses of daily 5-FU and daily IFN-α, reported a response rate of 43% after 6 months of therapy. Again, large controlled studies have yet to be completed, and the optimal dose and schedule of this regimen has not been identified.

Other regimens have used IL-2 in combination with 5-FU and IFN-α. Hanninen et al. reported a trial comparing the three-drug regimen (IL-2, IFN-α, 5-FU) with low-dose IL-2 (95). Triple therapy resulted in an improved overall response rate (39% vs. 28% for combined cytokine therapy) and a better complete response rate (13 complete responses vs. 2 complete responses). Patients with good prognostic characteristics had a survival benefit to three-drug therapy. Subsequent phase 2 trials confirmed the response rates of the three-drug regimen (96). A limited randomized phase 3 trial comparing the three-drug combination with tamoxifen (97) confirmed a 39% response rate and an improved overall median survival of at least 28 months. The M. D. Anderson group further attempted to optimize this regimen by using continuous infusion 5-FU, continuous infusion IL-2, and IFNα-2a. This therapy demonstrated a 31% response rate, but more than 50% of patients needed blood pressure support and 25% of patients developed gram-positive bacteremia.

Two reports raise questions about response rates and toxicity. Using bolus 5-FU combined with s.c. IL-2 and IFN-α, Subcutaneous Administration Propeukin Program Cooperative Group investigators reported only a 19% response rate in 62 patients; 43% of patients required dose reduction, delay, or termination

TABLE 7. INTERFERON-α/5-FLUOROURACIL COMBINATION THERAPY SELECTED TRIALS

Author (Year)	Reference	N[a]	IL-2	5-FU Dose[b]	ORR (%)
Lopez Hanninen et al. (1996)	95	120	+	750 q wk × 4	39.0
Hofmackel et al. (1996)	96	33	+	750 q wk × 4	38.0
Elias et al. (1996)	140	34/40	–	750 c.i.v. × 5 d	15.0
Atzpodien et al. (1997)	97	41	+	1,000 q wk × 4	39.0
Ellerhorst et al. (1997)	141	52/56	+	600 c.i.v. × 5 d	31.0
Gebrosky et al. (1997)	94	21	–	200–300 c.i.v.	43.0
Olencki et al. (1997)	142	39/41	+	250–350 dL–5	8.0
Kirchner et al. (1998)	143	246	+	1,000 q wk × 4	33.0
Tourani et al. (1998)	98	62	+	750 q wk × 2	19.0
Ravaud et al. (1998)	99	105/111	+	600 c.i.v. × 5 d	1.8

IL-2, interleukin-2; ORR, objective response rate; 5-FU, 5-fluorouracil; +, present; –, not present.
[a]Number of patients evaluable/number of patients enrolled.
[b]In mg/m^2/d.

TABLE 8. INTERFERON PLUS OTHER THERAPIES

Author	Reference	Interferon[a]	Other Treatment[a]	Evaluable Patients	CR + PR	CR + PR (%)	95% CI
Wadler et al.	144	α-2b/10 s.c. t.i.w.	Cyclophosphamide 25 mg/p.o. b.i.d.	25	1	4	0–20
Muss et al.	145	α-2b/20/s.c. + i.v. qwk	Doxorubicin 20/m² qwk	15	—	—	0–18
Dexeus et al.	101	Le(10) α-2a (6)/3[c] –10 q.d. × 5 wk 1 and 3	"FAMP" wk 4 and 8[b]	16	0 + 2	13	2–38
Dimopoulos et al.	103	α-2b/2 q.d.	FUdR/0.125 d q.d. × 14 d, q4wk[c]	13	0 + 4	31	9–61
Falcone et al.	106	α-2b/10/i.m. t.i.w.	FUdR, 0.075–0.175 mg/mg/d c.i.v. × 14d, q28d	15	1 + 4	33	12–62
Stadler et al.	105	α-2b/30/s.c. q.d. × 6, q28d	FUdR, 0.1 mg/kg/d c.i.v. × 5 d LV, 100 mg p.o. q4h × 6 d, q28d	20	—	—	0–17
Murphy et al.	104	α-2a/9 s.c. t.i.w.	FU/750 q.d. × 5qwk	14	—	—	0–23
Sella et al.	100	α-2a/5/s.c./q.d.	FU/750/dL–5 Mito/5/dL–2 q4wk	49	0 + 17	35	22–50
Konig et al.	146	α-2b/5 s.c. d 7–19	Ifos/1.5 g dL–5 + Vind/3 mg dL q3wk	29	1 + 6	24	10–44
Pasccon et al.	147	α-2/10/s.c./t.i.w.	Vind/3/q3wk	11	0 + 2	18	2–52
Creagan et al.	148	α-2a/20/i.m. t.i.w.	Aspirin 600 mg/p.o. q.i.d.	29	2 + 3	17	6–36
	76	α-2a/20/i.m. t.i.w.	Aspirin 600 mg/p.o. q.i.d.	89	1 + 3	4	1–11
Kotake et al.	107	Ly/5 q.d.	Cimetidine 800 mg/d	20	3 + 3	30	12–54
Fossa	149	α-2a/18–36[d]/i.m. t.i.w.	Prednisone 5–20 mg/p.o. q.d.	5	0 + 1	20	1–72
Abdi	75	α-2b/10[d]/i.m. t.i.w.	Prednisone 10 mg/p.o. q.d.	4	0 + 1	25	1–81
Fossa et al.[f]	69	α-2a/18/i.m. t.i.w.	Prednisone, 20–10 mg/p.o. q.d.	23	1 + 4	22	8–44
Porzsolt et al.	52	α-2c/2/s.c. q.d. × 5 qwk	Medroxyprogesterone 750 mg/p.o. q.d.	46	1 + 1	4	1–15
Hartlapp	152	α-2b/18–21/s.c./t.i.w.	Flutamide 250 t.i.d.	52	2 + 12	27	16–41
Tapazoglou et al.	102	alpha/3[e]	Whole body hyperthermia	8	—	—	0–37

CI, confidence interval; CR, complete response; "FAMP," 5-fluorouracil, adriamycin, mitomycin and cisplatin; FUdR, floxuridine; FU, fluorouracil; Ifos, ifosfamide; Le, leukocyte interferon; Ly, lymphoblastoid interferon; Mito, mitomycin; PR, partial response; Vind, vindesine.
[a]Type of interferon/dose per m²/route/schedule.
[b]Ten patients treated with leukocyte IFN; 6 with α2a; fluorouracil, doxorubicin, mitomycin, cisplatin.
[c]Given as circadian-modified continuous infusion.
[d]Dose in MU, not MU/m².
[e]Given 1 to 2 hours before hyperthermia.
[f]Nonrandomized (sequential studies); results of each study given.

of therapy because of toxicity (98). Furthermore, Ravaud et al. (99) reported only a 1.8% response rate when continuous 5-FU was combined with s.c. IFN-α and IL-2. Forty-nine percent of patients experienced greater than a grade 3 toxicity and five deaths occurred. Thus, the role of three-drug therapy in metastatic RCC remains unclear. Dose, schedule, and route have not been optimized for clinical benefit and limited toxicity. Further evaluation of the "Atzpodien regimen" in larger multiinstitutional trials are needed.

Several small trials of IFN and other agents in RCC are presented in Table 8. Most of the trials of IFN and chemotherapeutic agents included small numbers of patients. The addition of IFN to 5-FU and mitomycin (100) and to ifosfamide and vindesine appears somewhat higher than for IFN alone, but not convincingly so; further trials are necessary to confirm these data. Dexeus et al. noted that of 12 patients who received prior IFN therapy, seven subsequently responded to combination chemotherapy with 5-FU, doxorubicin, mitomycin, and cisplatin (101). To determine if IFN exposure increased the likelihood of response to chemotherapy, they conducted a randomized trial comparing chemotherapy alone with chemotherapy alternating with IFN (101). Four responses occurred in 32 patients, two in each arm. This small trial failed to show that alternating IFN with chemotherapy improved response. To the limited extent one can compare trials, it would appear that the addition of the fluorinated pyrim-

idines may only be useful when infused for longer durations (102–105). Further, it is not clear whether circadian-modified infusions of FUdR are essential (103,106). Clearly, randomized trials are needed to resolve these issues.

Combinations of IFN and substances intended to ameliorate the flulike symptoms of IFN (i.e., steroids, aspirin) have not affected response rates, although only corticosteroids have been useful against the flulike side effects of IFN (73–76). Neither agent prevents hepatic or other toxicities associated with IFN. Nevertheless, we recommend nonsteroidal antiinflammatory drugs and acetaminophen as palliative approaches. In addition, we consider antidepressant agents to treat the depression associated with IFN therapy.

Kotake and colleagues studied the combination of IFN and cimetidine and noted responses in 6 of 20 patients (107). Previous data suggested that cimetidine might inactivate suppressor T cells by binding to the histamine receptor present on such cells. One study comparing IFN and medroxyprogesterone acetate with IFN alone showed no benefit for this combination (52). Another trial combining IFN with the antiandrogen flutamide demonstrated a response rate of 27% in 52 patients, warranting further investigations of this combination.

The continued development of trials using combinations of biologics, as well as biologics and chemotherapy based on encouraging laboratory data, is justified. Also, several *in vitro* systems have been extensively studied and provide a major resource for studying IFNs in combination with other agents (108–113).

Interest in combining IFNs with *cis*-retinoic acid is derived from data that demonstrated synergistic interaction against tumor cell lines *in vitro* (114). An initial trial performed in 1997 by Motzer and colleagues achieved a 29% response rate with combined therapy in a series of 24 patients with metastatic RCC (115). Duration of response in some of these patients lasted as long as 9 months. Another series was able to demonstrate increased time to progression and increased 1-year survival in patients who responded to a combination regimen of *cis*-retinoic acid and IFN-α (116). Other small studies have been conducted with response rates ranging from 18% to 29% (116,117), including one study that examined IL-2 (118). These results are promising and await larger trials to properly test these preliminary findings.

SUMMARY

Newer therapies are needed for the treatment of metastatic RCC. IFN represents a small but significant advance in this area, and numerous trials have confirmed an objective response rate of approximately 15%. The side effects of IFN may be considerable, but may be limited by supportive care, including hydration, antipyretics, and antidepressants. Newer preparation of IFN-α may allow higher doses with less toxicity.

The lack of major long-term toxicity of IFN led to a clinical trial comparing rIFN with observation in the adjuvant setting by the Eastern Cooperative Oncology Group (protocol, 2,886), which is closed to accrual. Outcomes are awaiting data analysis. Another study of adjuvant therapy compares 6 months of combination rIFNα–2b with 5-FU versus observation for patients with resected stage III or IV RCC. Lack of significant myelosuppression with lower doses of IFN also makes it ideal for trial in combination regimens with myelosuppressive agents. In addition, the discovery and cloning of new cytokines and the potential for combined cytokine therapy are promising.

The ideal candidate for IFN therapy is a patient with good performance status and pulmonary lesions, as one-third of such patients may respond to IFN; liver, bone, and other visceral metastases are more resistant, although responses in all metastatic sites have been reported. Age, gender, disease-free interval, and prior therapy do not clearly affect response. Patients with favorable or normal performance appear to respond more frequently.

The effect of IFN therapy on the survival of patients with RCC is unclear. Trump et al. reported a median survival of 7.1 months for their IFN-treated patients with metastases, a similar survival duration to their prior phase 2 studies of chemotherapeutic agents (38). Buzaid et al. (46) noted a median survival in excess of 18.6 months in his trial; his patients, however, may have been more highly selected for favorable prognostic factors. Porzsolt and colleagues noted a median survival of 7 months in their series (52). Our review of the literature indicates that approximately 3% of patients treated with IFN have a sustained clinical response lasting longer than a year; this number may be an underestimate given the data from Minasian and colleagues of a 5-year survival rate of 3% (60). Two reports have evaluated prognostic

factors. In a data-based study of 610 patients with metastatic RCC, multivariate analysis identified five variables related to survival: (a) performance status, (b) disease-free interval, (c) prior cytotoxic chemotherapy, (d) number of metastatic sites, and (e) recent weight loss (11). Five risk groups were defined by these variables. The most favorable group had a median survival of 12.8 months. The least favorable group had a median survival of 2.1 months. It is not possible to draw firm conclusions on possible improvement in survival related to IFN, but it is likely that the influence of IFN on survival for most patients with RCC is small. Nevertheless, a subset of patients (3%) may have prolonged survival secondary to such therapy, which is comparable with the long-term survival rates reported for the more toxic IL-2. Manni et al. reported histology, performance status, and base disease as prognostic factors for response to biologic therapy (12).

Finding new biologic parameters that may help select patients most likely to respond to IFN in the adjuvant or advanced setting would be of major clinical importance. In one trial, flow cytometry analysis of renal cell tumor specimens suggested that patients with aneuploid tumors had a higher risk of recurrence after potentially curative resection than patients with diploid tumors (119). In another study, the risk of distant metastases was similar for patients with aneuploid and diploid tumors, but multiple metastases and lung metastases were more common with aneuploid lesions (120). Cytogenetic and molecular abnormalities involving 3p, 17p, and other regions are recognized in hereditary renal carcinoma (121) and sporadic RCC (122), but no correlation to clinical outcome, response to IFN, or other treatment is known (123,124). Further investigations are needed.

The selection of patients for IFN therapy frequently poses a dilemma for the oncologist. The best candidates are usually those who may be candidates for more toxic or investigational therapies, yet it is these same patients who may remain asymptomatic for long periods. The benefit of a response in such patients must be carefully weighed against treatment toxicity. Quality of life issues obviously are of paramount importance in making such decisions, and the risks and benefits of therapy should be discussed carefully with the patient. Improved therapy, however, can only result from the continued development of clinical trials. The increased availability of such trials in the community makes it possible to accrue patients and complete important studies in shorter periods. Computerized databases of active protocols are available through the Protocol Data Query System (125) and other sources. This information is readily available to physicians who manage such patients. IFN therapy represents an appropriate standard of care for the treatment of patients with metastatic RCC. Fundamental research related to the biology of RCC, as well as exploration of new therapies, will undoubtedly improve the outlook for patients in the future.

REFERENCES

1. Storkel SF. Pathology of Renal Cell Carcinomas. In: Ernstoff MS, Heaney JH, Peschel R, eds. *Urologic cancer.* Cambridge, MA: Blackwell Science, 1997.
2. American Cancer Society Web page (www.cancer.org), Facts and Figures, 1999.

3. Patel NP, Livengood RW. Renal cell cancer: natural history and results of treatment. *J Urol* 1977;119:722–726.
4. Myers M, Gloeckler L. Cancer patient survival rates: SEER program results for 10 years of follow-up. *KCA Cancer J Clin* 1989;39(1):21–32.
5. McNichols DW, Seguar JW, DeWeerd JH. Renal cell carcinoma: long-term survival and late recurrence. *J Urol* 1981;126:17–23.
6. Stewart, AF, Soifer NE. Endocrine paraneoplastic syndromes associated with renal carcinoma. In: Ernstoff MS, Heaney JH, Peschel R, eds. *Urologic cancer.* Cambridge, MA: Blackwell Science, 1997.
7. Marcus SG, Choyke PL, Reiter R, et al. Regression of metastatic renal cell carcinoma after cytoreductive nephrectomy. *J Urol* 1993; 150:463–466.
8. Oliver RTD, Nethersell ABW, Bottomley JM. Unexplained spontaneous regression and alpha-interferon as treatment for metastatic renal carcinoma. *Br J Urol* 1989;63:128–131.
9. Vogelzang NJ, Priest ER, Borden L. Spontaneous regression of histologically proved pulmonary metastases from renal cell carcinoma: a case with 5-year followup. *J Urol* 1992;148:1247–1248.
10. Gleave ME, Elhilali M, Fradet Y, et al. Interferon gamma-1b compared with placebo in metastatic renal-cell carcinoma. Canadian Urol Oncol Group. *N Engl J Med* 1998;338(18):1265–1271.
11. Elson PJ, Witte RS, Trump DL. Prognostic factors for survival in patients with recurrent or metastatic renal cell carcinoma. *Cancer Res* 1988;48:7310–7313.
12. Mani S, Todd MB, Katz K, Poo WJ. Prognostic factors for survival in patients with metastatic renal cancer treated with biological response modifiers. *J Urol* 1995;154(1):35–40.
13. Bloom HJG. Medroxyprogesterone Acetate (Provera) in the treatment of metastatic renal cancer. *Br J Cancer* 1971;25:250–265.
14. Kriegmair M, Oberneder R, Hofstetter A. Interferon alfa and vinblastine versus medroxyprogesterone acetate in the treatment of metastatic renal cell carcinoma. *Urology* 1995;45(5):758–762.
15. Hrushesky WJ, Murphy GP. Current status of the therapy of advanced renal carcinoma. *J Surg Oncol* 1977;9:277–288.
16. Pizzocaro G, Piva L, DiFronzo G. Adjuvant medroxyprogesterone acetate to radical nephrectomy in renal cancer: 5-year results of a prospective randomized study. *J Urol* 1987;138:1379–1381.
17. Papac RJ, Keohane MF. Hormonal therapy for metastatic renal cell carcinoma combined androgen and provera followed by high dose tamoxifen. *Eur J Cancer* 1993;29A(7):997–999.
18. Torti FM. Treatment of metastatic renal cell carcinoma. *Recent Results Cancer Res* 1983;85:123–142.
19. Talley R. Chemotherapy of adenocarcinoma of the kidney. *Cancer* 1973;32:1062–1065.
20. Lokich J, Harrison J. Renal cell carcinoma. Natural history and chemotherapeutic experience. *J Urol* 1975;114:371–374.
21. Harris DT. Hormonal therapy and chemotherapy of renal cell carcinoma. *Semin Oncol* 1984;10:422–430.
22. Logan TF, Trump DL. The role of cytotoxic chemotherapy in the management of renal cancer. In: Ernstoff MS, Heaney JH, Peschel R, eds. *Urologic cancer.* Cambridge, MA: Blackwell Science, 1997.
23. Volm M, Mattern J, Efferth T, et al. Expression of several resistance mechanisms in untreated human kidney and lung carcinomas. *Anticancer Res* 1992;12:1063–1068.
24. Naito S, Sakamoto N, Kotoh S, Goto K, Matsumoto T, Kumazawa J. Expression of P-glycoprotein and multidrug resistance in renal cell carcinoma. *Eur Urol* 1993;24(1):156–160.
25. Samuels BL, Hollis DR, Rosner GL, et al. Modulation of vinblastine resistance in metastatic renal cell carcinoma with cyclosporin A or tamoxifen: a Cancer and Leukemia Group B study. *Clin Cancer Res* 1997;3:1977–1984.
26. Agarwala SS, Bahnson RR, Wilson JW, et al. Evaluation of the combination of vinblastine and quinidine in patients with metastatic renal cell carcinoma. *Am J Clin Oncol* 1995;18:211–215.
27. Von Roemeling R, Rabatin JT, Fraley EE, et al. Progressive metastatic renal cell carcinoma controlled by continuous 5-fluoro-2-deoxyuridine infusion. *J Urol* 1988;139:259–262.
28. Wilkinson MJ, Frye JW, Small EJ, et al. A phase II study of constant-infusion floxuridine for the treatment of metastatic renal cell carcinoma. *Cancer* 1993;71(11):3601–3604.
29. Quesada JR, Swanson DA, Gutterman JU. Phase II study of interferon alpha in metastatic renal-cell carcinoma: a progress report. *J Clin Oncol* 1985;3:1086–1092.
30. Quesada JR, Swanson DA, Trindade A, et al. Renal cell carcinoma: antitumor effects of leukocyte interferon. *Cancer Res* 1983;43:940–947.
31. DeKernion JB, Sarna G, Figlin R, et al. The treatment of renal cell carcinoma with human leukocyte-alpha-interferon. *J Urol* 1983;130:1063–1066.
32. Kirkwood JM, Harris JE, Vera R, et al. A randomized study of low and high doses of leukocyte-α-interferon in metastatic renal cell carcinoma. The American Cancer Society Collaborative Trial. *Cancer Res* 1985;45:863–871.
33. Edsmyr F, Esposti PL, Andersson L, et al. Interferon therapy in disseminated renal cell carcinoma. *Radiother Oncol* 1985;4:21–26.
34. Medencia R, Slack N. Clinical results of leukocyte interferon-induced tumor regression in resistant human metastatic cancer resistant to chemotherapy and/or radiotherapy-pulse therapy schedule. *Cancer Drug Deliv* 1985;2–53.
35. Neidhart J, Gagen M, Young D. Interferon-α therapy of renal cancer. *Cancer Res* 1984;44:4140–4143.
36. Neidhart J, Gagen M, Kisner R. Therapy of renal cancer with low (LD), intermediate (ID), and high (HD) dose regimens of human lymphoblastoid interferon (HBLI; Wellferon). *Proc Am Soc Clin Oncol* 1984;3:60.
37. Marumo K, Murai M, Hayakawa M, et al. Human lymphoblastoid interferon therapy for advanced renal cell carcinoma. *Urology* 1984;24:567–571.
38. Trump DL, Elson PJ, Borden EC, et al. High dose lymphoblastoid interferon in advanced renal cell carcinoma: an Eastern Cooperative Oncology Group Study. *Cancer Treat Rep* 1987;71:165–169.
39. Vugrin D, Hood L, Taylor W, et al. Phase II study of human lymphoblastoid interferon in patients with advanced renal carcinoma. *Cancer Treat Rep* 1985;69:817–820.
40. Eisenhauer EA, Silver HK, Venner PM, et al. Phase II study of high dose weekly intravenous human lymphoblastoid interferon in renal cell carcinoma. A study of the National Cancer Institute of Canada Clinical Trials Group. *Br J Cancer* 1987;55:5541–5542.
41. Fujita T, Asano H, Naide Y, et al. Antitumor effects of human lymphoblastoid interferon on advanced renal cell carcinoma. *J Urol* 1988;139:256–258.
42. Umeda T, Niijima N. Phase II study of alpha interferon on renal cell carcinoma: summary of three collaborative trials. *Cancer* 1986;58:1231–1235.
43. Einzig A, Krown S, Oettgen H. Recombinant leukocyte α interferon (γIFN-α) in renal cell cancer, abstracted. *Proc Am Soc Clin Oncol* 1984;4:54.
44. Krown SE. Therapeutic options in renal cell carcinoma. *Semin Oncol* 1985;12:13–17.
45. Quesada JR, Rios A, Swanson D, et al. Antitumor activity of recombinant-derived interferon alpha in metastatic renal cell carcinoma. *J Clin Oncol* 1985;3:1522–1528.
46. Buzaid AC, Robertyone A, Kisala C, et al. Phase II study of interferon alfa-2a, recombinant (Rogeron-A) in metastatic renal cell carcinoma. *J Clin Oncol* 1987;5:1083–1089.
47. Figlin RA, deKernion JB, Mukamel E, et al. Recombinant interferon alfa-2a in metastatic renal cell carcinoma: assessment of antitumor activity and anti-interferon antibody formation. *J Clin Oncol* 1988;6:1604–1610.
48. Schnall S, Davis C, Kirkwood J. Treatment of metastatic renal cell carcinoma (RCC) with intramuscular (IM) recombinant alpha A (IFN, Hoffman-La Roche). *Proc Am Soc Clin Oncol* 1986;5:227.
49. Fossa SD. Is interferon with or without vinblastine the "treatment of choice" in metastatic renal cell carcinoma? The Norwegian Radium Hospital's experience 1983–1986. *Semin Surg Oncol* 1988; 4:178–183.
50. Muss HB, Costanzi JJ, Leavitt R, et al. Recombinant alfa interferon in renal cell carcinoma; a randomized trial of two routes of administration. *J Clin Oncol* 1987;5:286–291.
51. Foon K, Doroshow J, Bonnem E, et al. A prospective randomized trial of alpha 2B-interferon/gamma-interferon or the combination in

advanced metastatic renal cell carcinoma. *J Biol Response Mod* 1988;7:540–545.

52. Porzsolt F, Messerer D, Hautmann R, et al. Treatment of advanced renal cell cancer with recombinant interferon alpha as a single agent and in combination with medoxyrogesterone acetate. A randomized multicenter trial. *J Cancer Res Clin Oncol* 1988;114:95–100.

53. Otto U, Bauer H, Jager N. Alpha-2 recombinant interferon treatment of metastatic renal cell cancer. International symposium on the status and treatment of metastatic renal cell carcinoma. Presented to the International Union Against Cancer, Vienna, Austria, 1987.

54. Machida T, Koiso K, Takaku F, et al. Phase II study of recombinant human interferon gamma (S-6810) in renal cell carcinoma. Urological Cooperative Study Group of Recombinant Human Interferon Gamma (S-6810). *Gan To Kagaku Ryoho* 1987;14:440–445.

55. Rinehart J, Malspeis L, Young D, et al. Phase I/II trial of human recombinant beta-interferon serine in patients with renal cell carcinoma. *Cancer Res* 1986;46:5364–5367.

56. Quesada JR, Evans L, Saks SR, et al. Recombinant interferon alpha and gamma in combination as treatment for metastatic renal cell carcinoma. *J Biol Response Mod* 1988;7:234–239.

57. Geboers AD, de Mulder PH, Debruyne FM, et al. Alpha and gamma interferon in the treatment of advanced renal cell carcinoma. *Semin Surg Oncol* 1988;4:191–194.

58. Bengtsson N-O, Lenner P, Sjodin M, et al. Metastatic renal cell carcinoma treated with purified leukocyte interferon. Clinical response in relation to tumor DNA content. *Acta Oncologica* 1991;30(6): 713–717.

59. Marshall ME, Simpson W, Butler K, et al. Treatment of renal cell carcinoma with daily low-dose alpha-interferon. *J Biol Response Mod* 1989;8:453–461.

60. Minasian LM, Motzer RJ, Gluck L, et al. Interferon alfa-2a in advanced renal cell carcinoma: treatment results and survival in 159 patients with long-term follow-up. *J Clin Oncol* 1993;11(7):1368–1375.

61. Levens W, Rubben H, Ingenhag W. Long-term interferon treatment in metastatic renal cell carcinoma. *Eur Urol* 1989;15:378–381.

62. Bono AV, Reali L, Benvenuti C, et al. Recombinant alpha interferon in metastatic renal cell carcinoma. A cooperative phase II study. *Urology* 1991;38(1):60–63.

63. Abratt RP, Pontin AR, Ball HS. Activity of a short course of interferon alpha for metastatic renal cell carcinoma—a phase-2 study. *Cancer Immunol Immunother* 1993;37:140–141.

64. Rosenthal MA, Cox K, Raghavan D, et al. Phase II clinical trial of recombinant alpha-2 interferon for biopsy-proven metastatic or recurrent renal carcinoma. *Br J Urol* 1992;69:491–494.

65. Rinehart JJ, Young D, Laforge J, et al. Phase I/II trial of interferon-beta-serine in patients with renal cell carcinoma: immunological and biological effects. *Cancer Res* 1987;47:2481–2485.

66. Nelson KA, Wallenberg JC, Todd MB. High-dose intravenous therapy with beta-interferon in patients with renal cell cancer. *Proc Am Assoc Cancer Res* 1989;30:260.

67. Kinney P, Triozzi P, Young D, et al. Phase II trial of interferon-beta-serine in metastatic renal cell carcinoma. *J Clin Oncol* 1990;8(5): 881–885.

68. Simon R. Confidence intervals for reporting results in clinical trials. *Ann Intern Med* 1986;105:429–435.

69. Cantrell K, Hervonen S, Mogensen KE. Human leukocyte interferon production, purification, and animal experimental results *in vitro. In Vitro* 1975;25–38.

70. Pestka S. The purification and manufacturing of human interferons. *Sci Am* 1983;249:36–43.

71. Adams F, Quesada J, Gutterman J. Neuropsychiatric manifestations of leukocyte interferon therapy in patients with cancer. *JAMA* 1984;252:938–941.

72. Renault P, Hoofnagle J, Park Y. Psychiatric complications of long-term interferon alfa therapy. *Arch Int Med* 1987;14k7:1577–1580.

73. Fossa SD, Lehne G, Gunderson R, et al. Recombinant interferon alpha-2A combined with prednisone in metastatic renal-cell carcinoma: treatment results, serum interferon levels and the development of antibodies. *Int J Cancer* 1992;50:868–870.

74. Fossa SD, Gunderson R, Moe B. Recombinant interferon-alpha combined with prednisone in metastatic renal cell carcinoma. Reduced toxicity without reduction of the response rate—a phase II study. *Cancer* 1990;65:2451–2454.

75. Abdi EA. Combination of interferon and prednisone in human cancer. *Eur J Cancer Clin Oncol* 1988.

76. Creagan ET, Twito DI, Johansson SL, et al. A randomized prospective assessment of recombinant leukocyte A human interferon with or without aspirin in advanced renal adenocarcinoma. *J Clin Oncol* 1991;9(12):2104–2109.

77. Tuttle R, Wold D, Neidhart J. Analysis of human lymphoblastoid interferon, Wellcome (Wellferon) in the treatment of advanced renal cell carcinoma (ARCC), abstracted. *Antiviral Res* 1984;3:95.

78. Prummer O. Interferon-alpha antibodies in patients with renal cell carcinoma treated with recombinant interferon-alpha-2A in an adjuvant multicenter trial. The Delta-P Study Group. *Cancer* 1993;71(5):1828–1834.

79. Spiegel RJ, Spicehandler JR, Jacobs SL, et al. Low incidence of serum factors in patients receiving recombinant alfa-2b interferon (Intron-A). *Am J Med* 1986;80:223.

80. Figlin RA, Itri LM. Anti-interferon antibodies: a perspective. *Semin Hematol* 1988;25:9–15.

81. Ernstoff MS, Nair S, Hahnson RR, et al. A phase IA trial of sequential administration recombinant DNA-produced interferons: combination recombinant interferon gamma and recombinant interferon alpha in patients with metastatic renal cell carcinoma. *J Clin Oncol* 1990;8:1637–1649.

82. Bukowski R, Ernstoff MS, Gore M, et al. Phase I study of polyethylene glycol (PEG) interferon alpha-2B (PEG INTRON) in patients with solid tumors. *Proc Am Soc Clin Oncol* 1999 *(in press).*

83. Bonnem EM. Alpha interferon: combinations with other antineoplastic modalities. *Semin Oncol* 1987;14:48–60.

84. DeMulder PH, Debruyne FM, Franssen MP, et al. Phase I/II study of recombinant interferon alpha and gamma in advanced progressive renal-cell carcinoma. *Cancer Immunol Immunother* 1990;31:321–324.

85. Schiller J, Groveman D, Schmid S. Synergistic antiproliferative effects of human recombinant α54- or βser interferon with γ-interferon on human cell lines of various histogenesis. *Cancer Res* 1986;46:483–488.

86. Beniers AJ, Peelen WP, Hendriks BT, et al. Effects of alpha- and gamma- and tumor necrosis factor on colony formation of two human renal tumor xenografts in vitro. *Semin Surg Oncol* 1988;4:195–198.

87. Fidler I, Heicappel R, Saiki I. Direct antiproliferative effects of recombinant human interferon-α B/D hybrids on human tumor cell lines. *Cancer Res* 1987;47:2020–2027.

88. Aapro MS, Alberts DS, Salmon SE. Interactions of human leukocyte interferon with vinca alkaloids and other chemotherapeutic agents against human tumors in clonogenic assay. *Cancer Chemother Pharmacol* 1983;10:161–168.

89. Fossa SD, Martinelli G, Otto U, et al. Recombinant interferon alfa-2a with or without vinblastine in metastatic renal cell carcinoma: results of a European multi-center phase III study. *Ann Oncol* 1992;3(4):301–305.

90. Pyrhonen S, Hahka-Kemppinen M, Muhonen T. A promising interferon plus four-drug therapy regimen for metastatic melanoma. *J Clin Oncol* 1992;10(12):1919–1926.

91. Elias L, Crissman HA. Interferon effects upon the adenocarcinoma 38 and HL-60 cell lines: antiproliferative responses and synergistic interactions with halogenated pyrimidine antimetabolites. *Cancer Res* 1988;48(17):4868–4873.

92. Warrell RP. Differentiation agents. In: DeVita VT Jr, Hellman S, Rosenberg SA, eds. *Cancer principles and practice of oncology.* Philadelphia: Lippincott-Raven, 1997:483–490.

93. Reister Z, Ozes ON, Blott LM, et al. A dual anti-tumor effect of interferon-alpha or interleukin-2 and 5-fluorouracil on natural killer cell-mediated cytotoxicity. *Clin Immunol Immunopathol* 1992;62:103.

94. Gebrosky NP, Koukol S, Nseyo UO, et al. Treatment of renal cell carcinoma with 5-fluorouracil and alfa-interferon. *Urology* 1997;50(6):863–867.

95. Lopez Hanninen E, Kirchner H, Atzpodien J. Interleukin-2 based home therapy metastatic renal cell carcinoma: risks and benefits in

215 consecutive single institution patients. *J Urol* 1996;155(1): 19–25.

96. Hofmackel G, Langer W, Theiss M, Gruss A, Frohmuller HG. Immunochemotherapy for metastatic renal cell carcinoma using a regimen of interleukin-2 and 5-fluorouracil. *J Urol* 1996;156(1):18–21.

97. Atzpodien J, Kirchner H, Duensing S, et al. Biochemotherapy of advanced metastatic renal-cell carcinoma: results of the combination of interleukin-2, alpha-interferon, 5-fluorouracil, vinblastine, and 13-cis-retinoic acid. *World J Urol* 1995;13(3):174–177.

98. Tourani JM, Pfister C, Berdah JF, et al. Outpatient treatment with subcutaneous interleukin-2 and interferon alfa administration in combination with fluorouracil in patients with metastatic renal cell carcinoma: results of a sequential nonrandomized phase II study. Subcutaneous Admin Propeukin Program Cooperative Group. *J Clin Oncol* 1998;16(7):2505–2513.

99. Ravaud A, Audhuy B, Gomez F, et al. Subcutaneous interleukin-2, interferon alfa-2a, and continuous infusion of fluorouracil in metastatic renal cell carcinoma: a multicenter phase II trial. Groupe Francais d'Immunotherapie. *J Clin Oncol* 1998;16(8):2728–2732.

100. Sella A, Logothetis CJ, Fitz K, et al. Phase II study of interferon-alpha and chemotherapy (5-fluorouracil and mitomycin C) in metastatic renal cell cancer. *J Urol* 1992;147:573–577.

101. Dexeus FH, Logothetis CJ, Sella A, et al. Interferon alternating with chemotherapy for patients with metastatic renal cell carcinoma. *Am J Clin Oncol* 1989;12:350–354.

102. Tapazoglou E, et al. Whole-body hyperthermia (wbh) and human lymphoblastoid interferon (IFN-alpha) in the treatment of renal cell cancer (rcc). Presented at the thirty-eighth annual meeting of the Radiation Research Society, 1993.

103. Dimopoulos MA, Dexeus FH, Jones E, et al. Evidence for additive antitumor activity and toxicity for the combination of FudR and interferon alpha2b[(IRNα), (Intron)] in patients (pts) with metastatic renal cell carcinoma (RCC). *Proc Am Assoc Cancer Res* 1991;32:186.

104. Murphy BR, Rynard SM, Einhorn LH, et al. A phase II trial of interferon alpha-2A plus fluorouracil in advanced renal cell carcinoma. A Hoosier Oncology Group study. *Invest New Drugs* 1992; 10:225–230.

105. Stadler WM, Vogelzang NJ, Vokes EE, et al. Continuous-infusion fluorodeoxyuridine with leucovorin and high-dose interferon: a phase II study in metastatic renal-cell cancer. *Cancer Chemother Pharmacol* 1992;31:213–216.

106. Falcone A, Cianci C, Ricci S, et al. Alpha-2B interferon plus floxuridine in metastatic renal cell carcinoma. A phase I-II study. *Cancer* 1993;72(2):564–568.

107. Kotake T, Kinouchi T, Saiki S, et al. Treatment of metastatic renal cell carcinoma with a combination of human lymphoblastoid interferon-alpha and cimetidine. *Jpn J Clin Oncol* 1991;21:46–51.

108. Bradley E, Ruscetti F. Effect of fibroblast, lymphoid, and myeloid interferons on human tumor colony formation *in vitro*. *Cancer Res* 1981;41:244–249.

109. Borden E, Hogan T, Voelkel J. Comparative antiproliferative activity *in vitro* of natural interferon α and β for diploid and transformed human cells. *Cancer Res* 1982;42:4948–4953.

110. Kataoka T, Oh-hashi F, Sakurai Y. Characteristics of *in vitro* anti-proliferation activity of human interferon-β. *Cancer Chemother Pharmacol* 1982;9:75–80.

111. Yamaoka T, Takada H, Yanagi Y. Effects of cloned human leucocyte interferons in the human tumor stem cell assay. *J Clin Oncol* 1983;1:217–225.

112. Yamaoka T, Takada H, Yanagi Y, et al. The antitumor effects of human lymphoblastoid interferon on human renal cell carcinoma in athymic nude mice. *Cancer Chemother Pharmacol* 1985;14:184–187.

113. Saito T, Berens M, Welander C. Direct and indirect effects of human recombinant γ-interferon on tumor cells in a clonogenic assay. *Cancer Res* 1986;46:1142–1147.

114. Motzer RJ, Bajorin DF, Schwartz LH, et al. Antitumor activity of interferon alfa-2a and 13-cis-retinoic acid in patients with advanced renal cell carcinoma. *Proc Am Soc Clin Oncol* 1994;13:713.

115. Campus D, et al. Interferon alfa-2a and 13-cis-retinoic acid in

116. Jacobs AD, et al. Alpha-interferon and cis-retinoic acid in patients with metastatic renal cell cancer. *Proc Am Soc Clin Oncol* 1997:16:1197.

117. Casali A, Sega FM, Casali M, et al. 13-cis-retinoic acid and interfereon alpha-2a in the treatment of metastatic renal cell carcinoma. *J Exp Clin Cancer Res* 1998;17(2):227–229.

118. Stodler WM, et al. Interleukin-2, interferon-α and cis-retinoic acid: an effective outpatient regimen for metastatic renal cell carcinoma. *Proc Am Soc Clin Oncol* 1996;15:602.

119. Otto U, Baisch H, Huland H. Tumor cell deoxyribonucleic acid content and prognosis in human renal cell carcinoma. *J Urol* 1984;1332:237–239.

120. Ljungberg B, Stenling R, Roos G. Tumor spread and DNA content in human renal cell carcinona. *Cancer Res* 1988;48:3165–3167.

121. Cohen A, Li F, Berg S. Hereditary renal-cell carcinoma associated with a chromosomal translocation. *N Engl J Med* 1979;301:592–595.

122. Meloni AM, Bridge J, Sandberg AA. Reviews on chromosome studies in urological tumors. I. Renal tumors. *J Urol* 1992;148:253–265.

123. Savage PD. Renal cell carcinoma. *Curr Opin Oncol* 1993;5:538–545.

124. Savage PD. Renal cell carcinoma. *Curr Opin Oncol* 1994;6:301–307.

125. Perry D, Sloane E, Hubbard S. Keeping up with the cancer literature. *J Clin Oncol* 1988;10:1649–1652.

126. Krown S, Einzig A, Abramson J. Treatment of advanced renal cell cancer (RCC) with recombinant leukocyte A interferon (rIRN-αA), abstracted. *Proc Am Soc Clin Oncol* 1983;2:58.

127. Mulder P, DeBruyne F, Rikken G. Recombinant® tumor necrosis factor alpha (TNF-α) and interferon (IFN)-gamma (γ) in the treatment of advanced renal cell carcinoma (RCC). *Soc Clin Oncol* 1989;8:144.

128. Strayer DR, Carter WA, Crilley P, et al. Phase I-II study of mismatched double-stranded RNA (Ampligen) in combination with interferon-α-(Le) in renal cell carcinoma (RCC). *Proc Am Assoc Cancer Res* 1989;30:258.

129. Marumo K, Mura M, Deguchi N, et al. Sequential combination therapy with alpha interferon and OK-432 (streptococcal preparation) against advanced renal cell carcinoma. *Gan to Kagaku Ryoho* 1986;13:2434–2439.

130. Figlin RA, deKernion JB, Maldazys J, et al. Treatment of renal cell carcinoma with alpha (human leukocyte) interferon and vinblastine in combination: a phase I-II trial. *Cancer Treat Rep* 1985;69:263–267.

131. Fossa SD, De Garis ST, Heier MS, et al. Recombinant interferon alfa-2a with or without vinblastine in metastatic renal cell carcinoma. *Cancer* 1986;57:1700–1704.

132. Fossa SD, DeGaris ST. Further experience with recombinant interferon alfa-2a with vinblastine in metastatic renal cell carcinoma; a progress report. *Int J Cancer Suppl* 1987;1:36–40.

133. Cetto GL, Franceschi T, Turrina G, et al. Recombinant alpha-interferon and vinblastine in metastatic renal cell carcinoma: efficacy of low doses. *Semin Surg Oncol* 1988;4:184–190.

134. Kellokumpu-Lehtinen P, Nordman E. Recombinant interferon-alpha 2a and vinblastine in advanced renal cell cancer: a clinical phase I-II study. *J Biol Res Mod* 1990;9:439–444.

135. Bergerat JP, Herbrecht R, Dufour P, et al. Combination of recombinant interferon alpha-2a and vinblastine in advanced renal cell cancer. *Cancer* 1988;62:2320–2324.

136. Sertoli MR, Brunetti I, Ardizzoni A, et al. Recombinant alpha-2a interferon plus vinblastine in the treatment of metastatic renal call carcinoma. *Am J Clin Oncol* 1989;12:43–45.

137. Schornagel JH, Verweij J, ten Bokkel Huinink WW, et al. Phase II study of recombinant interferon alpha-2a and vinblastine in advanced renal cell carcinoma. *J Urol* 1989;142:253–256.

138. Trump DL, Ravdin PM, Borden EC, et al. Interferon-alpha-nl and continuous infusion vinblastine for treatment of advanced renal cell carcinoma. *J Biol Response Mod* 1990;9:108–111.

139. Neidhart JA, Anderson SA, Harris JE, et al. Vinblastine fails to improve response of renal cancer to interferon alfa-nl: high response rate in patients with pulmonary metastases. *J Clin Oncol* 1991;9(5): 832–837.

140. Elias L, Blumenstein BS, Kish J, Flanigan RC, et al. A phase II trial of interferon-alpha and 5-fluorouracil in patients with advanced renal cell carcinoma. *Cancer* 1996;78(5):1085–1088.

141. Ellerhorst JA, Sella A, Amato RJ, et al. Phase II trial of 5-fluorouracil, interferon-alpha and continuous infusion interleukin-2 in patients with metastatic renal cell carcinoma. *Cancer* 1997;80(11): 2128–2132.

142. Olencki T, Budd GT, Peereboom D, et al. Phase I/II trial of subcutaneous (sc) interleukin-2 and interferon-alpha with or without 5-flourouracil in metastatic renal cell carcinoma: clinical results and effects on acquired immune dysfunction. *Proc Am Soc Clin Oncol* 1997;15:1209.

143. Kirchner GI, Franzke A, Buer J, et al. Pharmacokinetics of recombinant human interleukin-2 in advanced renal cell carcinoma patients following subcutaneous application. *Br J Clin Pharmacol* 1998; 46(1):5–10.

144. Wadler S, Einzig AI, Dutcher JP, et al. Phase II trial of recombinant alpha-2b-interferon and low-dose cyclophosphamide in advanced melanoma and renal cell carcinoma. *Am J Clin Oncol* 1988:11: 55–59.

145. Muss HB, Welander C, Caponera M, et al. Interferon and doxorubicin in renal cell carcinoma. *Cancer Treat Rep* 1985;69:721–722.

146. Konig HJ, Gutmann W, Weissmuller J. Ifosfamide, vindesine and recombinant alpha-interferon combination chemotherapy for metastatic renal cell carcinoma. *J Cancer Res Clin Oncol* 1991;117[Suppl 4]:S221–S223.

147. Pasccon G, Koliren L, Levin R, et al. Recombinant alfa2 interferon (IFN), with or without chemotherapy (CT) for melanoma and renal cancer (CA) patients (pt). A preliminary report. *Proc Am Soc Clin Oncol* 1990;9:198.

148. Creagan ET, Buckner JC, Hahn RG, et al. An evaluation of recombinant leukocyte A interferon with aspirin in patients with metastatic renal cell cancer. *Cancer* 1988;61:1787–1791.

149. Fossa SD. Improved subjective tolerability of interferon by combination with prednisone [Letter]. *Eur J Cancer Clin Oncol* 1987;23: 875–876.

150. Harlapp JHS. Interferon-alpha/flutamide combination in renal cell carcinoma. *Proc Am Soc Clin Oncol* 1992;11:A678(abst).

10.4

INTERFERON-α AND -β: CLINICAL APPLICATIONS

Kaposi's Sarcoma

SUSAN E. KROWN

Kaposi's sarcoma (KS), the most common malignancy associated with human immunodeficiency virus type-1 (HIV-1) infection, was one of the first recognized clinical manifestations of the acquired immune deficiency syndrome (AIDS) (1–3). Although interferon-α (IFN-α) has been used to treat KS since 1981, only recently have advances in understanding KS pathogenesis and relevant IFN actions provided a strong rationale for IFN use and supported its use in conjunction with modern antiretroviral drug regimens. In addition, IFN dosages have been modified in recent years as treatment of coexisting HIV-1 infection has evolved. This chapter reviews pertinent information on KS pathogenesis and IFN actions, use of type I IFNs to treat AIDS-associated KS, and potential applications of IFN therapy.

KAPOSI'S SARCOMA: PATHOGENESIS AND THE RATIONALE FOR USING INTERFERON

When IFN was first used to treat KS, its antiproliferative activity was thought to play a major role in mediating tumor regres-

sion, although poorly characterized immunomodulatory and antiviral activities were also considered to have potential roles. In the earliest studies of IFN-α in KS, it appeared that very high IFN-α doses were required to induce tumor regression, whereas low doses rarely induced responses (4,5). This was usually interpreted to mean that direct inhibitory effects on cell proliferation were essential for tumor regression to occur, although an alternative explanation may be that other antitumor effector mechanisms were optimally activated at high IFN doses. Because KS had been shown to occur with increased frequency in immunosuppressed individuals, including recipients of solid organ transplants, and to occasionally regress when immunosuppressive drugs were withdrawn (6–10), a link between tumor and immune function had been established. Although changes in immune function were observed in some IFN-α–treated patients with KS, consistent effects were not documented, even in patients whose lesions regressed. In addition, although neither HIV nor human herpesvirus 8 (HHV-8) had yet been discovered when IFN-α's activity against KS was first described, earlier studies implicated a link between cytomegalovirus

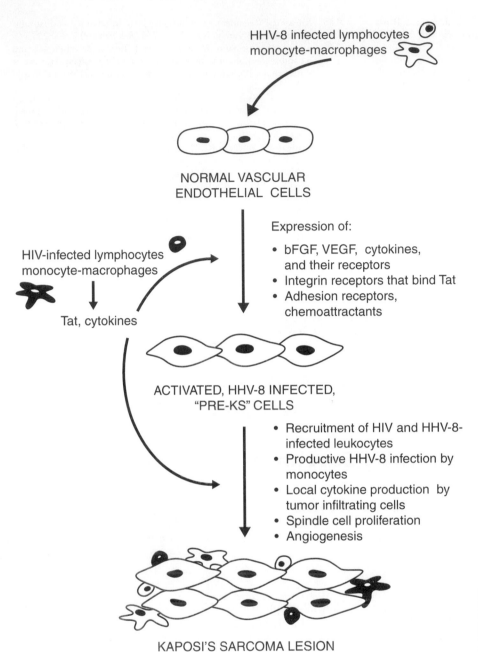

HHV-8 infected lymphocytes
monocyte-macrophages

NORMAL VASCULAR
ENDOTHELIAL CELLS

HIV-infected lymphocytes
monocyte-macrophages

Tat, cytokines

Expression of:

• bFGF, VEGF, cytokines,
  and their receptors
• Integrin receptors that bind Tat
• Adhesion receptors,
  chemoattractants

ACTIVATED, HHV-8 INFECTED,
"PRE-KS" CELLS

• Recruitment of HIV and HHV-8-
  infected leukocytes
• Productive HHV-8 infection by
  monocytes
• Local cytokine production by
  tumor infiltrating cells
• Spindle cell proliferation
• Angiogenesis

KAPOSI'S SARCOMA LESION

FIGURE 1. Factors in the development of acquired immunodeficiency syndrome–associated Kaposi's sarcoma. (bFGF, basic fibroblast growth factor; HHV-8, human herpesvirus 8; HIV, human immunodeficiency virus; VEGF, vascular endothelial growth factor.)

(CMV) infection and KS (11). It was suggested, therefore, that antiviral effects of IFN-α might be important in mediating tumor regression.

In recent years, a multistep model for KS pathogenesis in HIV-infected individuals emerged that is depicted in simplified form in Fig. 1. An essential element of the model is exposure to an infectious agent, HHV-8, that infects B cells and vascular endothelial cells (the latter being the likely cell of origin of KS). The model also includes altered expression and response to cytokines and stimulation of KS growth by an HIV-1 gene product, often in the setting of at least moderate immunosuppression. These factors contribute to the development of a lesion comprised of elongated spindle cells organized into slitlike vascular spaces containing extravasated

erythrocytes and surrounded by a variable cellular infiltrate. This model does not completely explain the interplay of factors that leads to the development of KS in some, but not all, HHV-8–infected individuals. It does, however, not only help to explain the frequent occurrence and unusually aggressive behavior of KS in HIV-infected individuals but also provides a stronger rationale for the therapeutic use of IFNs than the one proposed in the early 1980s.

Major advances in understanding factors involved in the development and growth of KS lesions were made possible in the late 1980s when techniques to establish KS-derived spindle cell cultures were first developed (12,13). Cultured KS-derived spindle cells were subsequently shown to secrete a variety of cytokines and growth factors that included, among others, interleukin-6 (IL-6), interleukin-1 (IL-1), basic fibroblast growth factor (bFGF), and vascular endothelial growth factor/vascular permeability factor (VEGF/VPF) (14–16), and to express receptors for these factors. In addition to secreting factors with potential autocrine and paracrine activities, KS-derived spindle cells were also shown to proliferate in response to exogenous cytokines and growth factors. These KS growth factors include tumor necrosis factor (TNF), IL-1, IL-6, IFN-α, platelet-derived growth factor, bFGF, VEGF/VPF, oncostatin M, and granulocyte-macrophage colony-stimulating factor (GM-CSF) (15,17–22). Many of these factors were present in the retrovirus-infected T-cell–conditioned media that were found to support KS spindle cell growth *in vitro* (17–19). Many of these cytokines, in particular TNF, IFN-α, IL-1, and IL-6, are also produced in excess in patients with advanced HIV infection (23–25), can stimulate HIV expression *in vitro* in infected cells (17,26), and can induce normal vascular endothelial cells to acquire a spindle morphology, secrete bFGF, and express $\alpha_v\beta_3$, a cell surface adhesion protein of the integrin family required for angiogenesis (17,21,22).

Although HIV has not been found within KS spindle cells and is not required for the development of KS, several observations suggest that the virus may contribute indirectly to the development of KS and its unusually aggressive course in HIV-infected individuals. A role for HIV was originally suggested by the observation that transgenic mice bearing the HIV transactivation gene, *tat*, transiently developed KS-like angiogenic lesions (28). In addition to being associated with the excess production of KS-stimulatory cytokines, active HIV infection results in the secretion by infected CD4 cells and monocytes of a biologically active form of the *tat* gene product, Tat (29). Extracellular Tat binds to $\alpha_v\beta_3$ and $\alpha_5\beta_1$, which are strongly expressed on KS-derived spindle cells (30). IFN-γ, which is increased in KS lesions (20), has been shown to upregulate the expression and activation of Tat-binding integrins and to induce endothelial cells to proliferate and invade the extracellular matrix in response to Tat (21). Tat has also been shown to stimulate proliferation of KS-associated spindle cells *in vitro* (31) and to synergistically stimulate KS cell proliferation when combined with bFGF or inflammatory cytokines (32). In addition, in the presence of bFGF and cytokines, normal vascular endothelial cells become responsive to the stimulatory effects of Tat on proliferation, cell migration, and angiogenic differentiation (15,27). Tat also induces the expression *in vitro* of the adhesion molecules VCAM-1 and ICAM-1, the monocyte chemoattractant protein MCP-1, and IL-6 in KS-derived cells (33), which could help recruit leukocytes to a developing KS lesion.

Epidemiologic studies have long suggested that exposure to a transmissible or environmental cofactor distinct from HIV might be required for the development of AIDS-associated KS (34,35). A sexually related factor was implicated by the high incidence of KS in HIV-infected homosexual men (compared to men from other risk groups), a higher incidence in women who acquired their HIV infection through sex with bisexual men (compared to women from other transmission groups) (34), and anecdotal reports of a higher than expected frequency of KS in homosexual HIV-seronegative men (35). Although many of the factors previously investigated for their possible etiologic role in KS (e.g., CMV, human papillomavirus, HHV-6, inhaled nitrites) have been eliminated from serious consideration, studies performed over the past 5 years have conclusively demonstrated a central role for a newly described HHV in the development of KS. Sequences of the virus, called HHV-8 or Kaposi's sarcoma–associated herpesvirus (KSHV), have been shown to be present in virtually all KS tissue, whether from HIV-infected individuals or those with the classic, endemic African or organ transplant–associated forms of the disease (36–39). HHV-8 sequences have also been identified in a limited number of other pathologic conditions, in some normal cells of patients with KS, and in the cells of some HIV-infected patients without KS who subsequently developed KS (40–43).

The precise mechanisms by which HHV-8 leads to KS development are incompletely understood. It has been shown, however, that HHV-8 can infect and transform human primary endothelial cells *in vitro* (44) and that in KS tissue, the virus can be found in the flat endothelial cells lining vascular spaces of KS lesions as well as in KS spindle cells (45). HHV-8 has also been found to encode an array of functional homologues of cellular proteins, including bcl-2, IL-6, the IL-8 receptor, interferon regulatory factor, chemokine-like macrophage inflammatory proteins (MIP-I and MIP-II), and a D-type viral cyclin that can direct phosphorylation of the retinoblastoma tumor suppressor protein (pRB) (46–50). In addition, viral MIP-I and MIP-II were highly angiogenic in the chorioallantoic membrane assay, suggesting a possible role in KS pathogenesis (49).

With this model for KS pathogenesis in mind, a more robust and multifaceted rationale for the use of IFN and possible explanations for its activity can be proposed (Table 1). Current knowledge of the multiplicity of IFN actions suggest that several steps in KS pathogenesis can be considered potential targets for IFN, although many of these activities have not been specifically studied in patients with KS or KS cell cultures. In addition to their direct inhibitory effects on cell proliferation, IFNs have been shown *in vitro* to increase natural killer cell and monocyte-mediated cytotoxicity against KS targets (51–53). IFNs α and β have also been shown to downregulate steady-state bFGF messenger ribonucleic acid (mRNA) expression and protein production in certain tumor cell lines by proliferation-independent mechanisms (54,55). Additionally, IFN treatment has been shown to increase circulating levels of the soluble TNF receptor and the IL-1 receptor antagonist (56,57), which are endogenous downregulators of the KS-stimulatory cytokines TNF and IL-1. IFNs have also been shown to have direct inhibitory effects against HIV (58) and to synergistically inhibit HIV when used in combination with other antiretroviral agents (59–61). HIV inhibition could directly affect KS growth by decreasing release of the HIV Tat protein and could act indirectly by decreasing the production of inflammatory and angiogenic cytokines associated with poorly controlled HIV infection. The relatively recent observation that KS sometimes regresses when effective, multiagent antiretroviral therapy is intro-

TABLE 1. TARGETS FOR INTERFERON TREATMENT OF ACQUIRED IMMUNODEFICIENCY SYNDROME–ASSOCIATED KAPOSI'S SARCOMA

Target	Relevant Interferon Action
Angiogenic growth factors	Inhibits basic fibroblast growth factor production
Inflammatory cytokines	Increases levels of endogenous down-regulators of tumor necrosis factor (sTNF-R) and interleukin-1 (IL-1RA)
Endothelial cell proliferation	Inhibits proliferation
Human immunodeficiency virus	Inhibits replication
Human herpesvirus-8	Inhibits replication
Immune effector cells	Stimulates natural killer and mono-cyte cytotoxicity versus Kaposi's sarcoma targets

IL-1RA, ; sTNF-R, soluble tumor necrosis factor receptor.

duced (62,63) suggests that these actions may be important, although enhanced immune function may also result in more effective control of HHV-8 infection. A direct inhibitory effect of IFN on HHV-8 is also possible and has been demonstrated in a preliminary *in vitro* study (64). In one patient with classic KS, however, IFN-α treatment reportedly led to complete tumor regression, but HHV-8 sequences remained detectable in the lesional skin (65).

INTERFERON-α THERAPY

Monotherapy

Monotherapy refers to IFN treatment in the absence of other antitumor or antiretroviral drugs. IFN-α's single-agent activity against AIDS-associated KS was initially demonstrated in the early 1980s, long before the availability of specific antiretroviral therapy directed against HIV. Tumor regression was documented in various studies in which either recombinant IFN-α-2a or -α-2b or lymphoblastoid IFN (IFN-α-n1) was administered daily or three times a week (4,5,66–75). A common feature of these studies was the superiority of very high IFN-α doses ($\geq$20 MU per m^2 body surface area) over lower doses. Objective tumor response rates averaging 30% were observed in patients treated with high IFN-α doses (4,5,66,67,69,71–75), whereas an average response rate of less than 10% was observed among patients treated at doses ranging from 1.0 MU to 7.5 MU per m^2 (4,5,67).

These studies also documented superior response rates among patients with CD4-positive T-lymphocyte counts of 200 per μL or more and no previous AIDS-defining opportunistic infections (OIs) or lymphoma-like "B" symptoms than among patients with lower CD4 counts or histories of OIs or B symptoms, or both. For example, a cross-study analysis of patients without previous OIs or B symptoms who were treated with high-dose IFN-α-2a revealed response rates of 7.2%, 27.5%, and 45.4% among patients with <200, 200–400, and >400 CD4-positive T lymphocytes per μL, respectively (66). Only one of 28 patients (3.6%) with previous

OIs or B symptoms responded (66). Other factors reported to be associated with a higher likelihood of response to IFN-α include the absence of cutaneous anergy, relatively high proliferative responses of PBMC to mitogens and microbial antigens, the absence of endogenous, acid-labile IFN-α in the serum, and relatively low serum levels of β_2-microglobulin and neopterin (76–79). Although various markers of immune function or activation, or both, have been shown to correlate with the response of KS to IFN-α, neither tumor stage nor gastrointestinal KS were associated with response (4,66–68,76,77).

Although evidence for tumor regression often occurs within the first 4 to 8 weeks of treatment, maximum responses often require continued treatment for 6 months or more. The relatively slow response of KS to IFN-α makes this treatment inappropriate for highly symptomatic patients in whom rapid cytoreduction is required—for example, patients with lung lesions, symptomatic gastrointestinal KS, or severe tumor-associated edema. The optimal duration of treatment in responding patients is not known. Before the availability of effective antiretroviral treatment, discontinuation of IFN-α therapy was usually followed within 6 to 8 months by tumor progression. Although it has not been systematically studied, some indications suggest that successful systemic therapy for KS may be discontinued in some patients in whom HIV replication is well controlled. Response duration with IFN-α monotherapy has not been well studied. The few published data indicate that partial responses last, on average, from 6 to 12 months, and complete responses persist for an average duration of 2 years (4). In some cases, responses persist for over a decade.

Interferon with Chemotherapy

In the 1980s, several trials were conducted in which IFN-α was combined with chemotherapeutic agents in an attempt to increase KS response rates (66,73,80–83). IFN-α was combined with vinblastine, etoposide, or a combination of actinomycin-D, vinblastine, and bleomycin. Little or no evidence for increased efficacy was found, and the combination regimens led almost uniformly to greater toxicity. In a randomized trial that compared IFN-α alone to IFN-α with vinblastine, objective response rates in the two groups were almost identical, but dose-limiting hematologic and constitutional toxicity was twice as frequent in the combination therapy arm than with IFN-α alone (66,83). In a nonrandomized trial of the IFN-α and vinblastine combination in patients with advanced KS, 12 of 27 patients (44%) required dose attenuation or discontinuation of therapy because of severe toxicity (73). Sequential administration of IFN-α followed by etoposide induced a response rate of only 8% (80), whereas concurrent administration of these drugs was toxic and ineffective; only one of 14 patients (7%) showed an objective response (80). Maintenance of chemotherapy-induced response with IFN-α was also unsuccessful in a small group of patients (84).

All of the studies cited were conducted well before the widespread availability of effective antiretroviral therapy, and all used IFN-α doses associated with significant constitutional, hematologic, and hepatic toxicities. It is not known whether IFN-α would be an effective and less toxic adjunct to chemotherapy if it were used at lower, better tolerated doses in patients whose HIV infection was well-controlled and for whom supportive therapies (e.g., hematopoietic colony-stimulating factors or appetite stimulants) were available.

Interferon with Antiretroviral Therapy

High-dose monotherapy with IFN-α-2a and IFN-α-2b received U.S. Food and Drug Administration approval in 1989 for treatment of patients with AIDS-associated KS. At that time, zidovudine (ZDV) was the only antiretroviral agent approved for treatment of a subset of HIV-infected individuals. Several studies were already underway in 1989 to evaluate the IFN-α and ZDV combination in KS, and subsequent trials to evaluate IFN-α with ZDV and other antiretroviral agents have been completed or are in progress. Current standards for antiviral treatment do not support the use of IFN monotherapy for HIV-infected individuals with KS. Nonetheless, despite safety and efficacy data indicating that lower doses of IFN-α than those originally recommended for monotherapy should be used in conjunction with other antiretroviral agents, the approved doses of IFN-α were not modified in the 1990s.

The rationale for combined IFN-α and antiretroviral therapy was originally based on *in vitro* studies showing synergistic suppression of HIV replication when IFN-α was combined with ZDV (59). These observations were later extended to the combinations of IFN-α with didanosine and zalcitabine (60,61). In addition, the combination of IFN-α and ZDV induced synergistic suppression of retrovirus-induced splenomegaly and viremia in mice (85,86). Single-agent nucleoside reverse transcriptase inhibitor therapy is no longer the standard of care for HIV-infected individuals and has shown no significant activity against KS (87,88). These drugs sometimes induced improvements in the levels of markers associated with responsiveness of KS to IFN-α, however, including enhanced CD4 T-lymphocyte counts and skin test reactivity, and decreased serum levels of β_2-micro-

globulin and neopterin (89,90). Furthermore, it was suggested that IFN-α, which inhibits HIV at a step in virus replication distinct from that of other antiretroviral agents (91), might overcome or inhibit the development of nucleoside resistance. Indeed, combinations of IFN-α with ZDV or didanosine induced synergistic inhibition *in vitro* of ZDV-resistant clinical isolates of HIV-1 (61).

The results of ten published clinical trials of the IFN-α and ZDV combination are summarized in Table 2 (92–101). Although it is difficult to compare the results of one study with another because of nonuniform trial design, drug dosages, and patient prognostic features (including the duration of previous ZDV treatment), the majority documented response rates of 40% or more. In some, but not all, of these studies, objective tumor regression was attained at IFN-α doses significantly lower than those shown to be effective without concurrent antiretroviral therapy. Also, some of these studies documented response rates of up to 30% in patients with pretreatment CD4 T-lymphocyte counts below 200 per μL (92,95,100,101), a group with a low probability of response to high-dose IFN-α monotherapy. Patients with higher CD4 counts also showed higher response rates with combination therapy than previously reported for high-dose IFN monotherapy (92–97,99–101).

The combination of IFN-α with ZDV often induces neutropenia and anemia, along with other side effects typically associated with single agents. These hematologic side effects were anticipated by the known toxicities of the two drugs and by *in vitro* studies showing synergistic suppression of granulocyte-monocyte (colony-forming unit, granulocyte-monocyte) and erythroid (burst-forming unit, erythroid) precursors when the two drugs were combined (102). Two strategies have been used to reduce the hematologic toxicity associated with combination therapy. In two clinical studies in patients with KS, low doses of GM-CSF were shown to prevent or ameliorate neutropenia induced by the IFN-α and ZDV combination (103,104). The improved hematologic tolerance was offset in some cases by the toxicities of GM-CSF (104), and there was

TABLE 2. RESULTS OF COMBINED INTERFERON-α (IFN-α) AND ZIDOVUDINE (ZDV) THERAPY FOR KAPOSI'S SARCOMA

IFN-α Dose (MU) and Schedule	Total Daily ZDV Dose (mg)[a]	Evaluable Patients (n)	Response Rate (CR + PR) (%)	Reference
4.5–18 q.d.	600–1,200	37	46	92
9–27 q.d.	600–1,200	43	47	93
<5 to >25 q.d.	300–1,200	26	42	94
18 q.d.	600	62	40	95
10 q.d.	500	15	27	96
1 q.d.	500	53	8	97
8 q.d.	500	54	31	97
9–18 q.d.	600	20	5	98
3 t.i.w.	500	17	65	99
10–20 q.d.	500–800	40	45	100
18 q.o.d.	800–1,200	15	46	101

CR, complete response; PR, partial response.
[a]Administered as divided doses, two to six times daily.

no indication that nonhematologic toxicities were affected or that maximally tolerated IFN-α doses or response rates were substantially increased. The use of less myelosuppressive nucleoside analog reverse transcriptase inhibitors has also been investigated. In one randomized trial, the AIDS Clinical Trials Group has evaluated didanosine in combination with either 1 MU or 10 MU of IFN-α daily. These doses are approximately three- to 30-fold less than the IFN-α doses considered effective as monotherapy. Although the final trial results are still under analysis, KS regression has been observed at both IFN-α doses and in patients with low CD4 T-lymphocyte counts (S. Krown, *unpublished results*). In a phase 1 trial, the AIDS Malignancy Consortium is investigating the clinical and pharmacologic interactions between IFN-α and protease inhibitor–based combination antiretroviral regimens.

Interferon Effects on Human Immunodeficiency Virus

No question exists that type I IFNs inhibit HIV replication *in vitro* (58–61,105). The data in patients are conflicting, however, and their relevance to KS regression is unclear. Many studies of high-dose IFN-α monotherapy were conducted before the discovery of HIV and before standardized, sensitive methods were available to evaluate viral burden. By the late 1980s, two studies had documented a decrease in serum levels of the HIV p24 antigen in KS patients whose tumors regressed during high-dose IFN-α monotherapy (74,75), whereas patients whose KS did not regress showed no virus suppression. Those patients whose KS regressed and whose p24 antigen levels decreased were more likely than nonresponders to have high CD4 T-lymphocyte counts. These concordant effects suggested that common mechanisms were involved in IFN's antitumor and antiviral activities, and that intact immunologic effector mechanisms might be required for both. Of the 21 patients in one of these studies, three with CD4 T-lymphocyte counts above 500 cells per μL showed clearance of HIV from cultured peripheral blood mononuclear cells (74). These observations led to a randomized clinical trial of high-dose IFN-α versus placebo in asymptomatic HIV-seropositive patients with CD4 counts of 400 per μL or more and positive PBMC cultures for HIV (106). Sixty-four percent of the patients who received IFN-α for 12 or more weeks had consistently negative HIV cultures during treatment, whereas negative cultures were documented in only 13% of placebo recipients (106). The combination of IFN-α and ZDV was also reported to synergistically suppress p24 antigen levels in HIV-infected patients who had CD4 counts above 200 per μL and measurable p24 antigen levels before treatment (107), but clinical end points were not monitored in this study. Suppression of serum p24 antigen levels and inhibition of HIV recovery from peripheral blood cells was also reported in several trials of the IFN-α and ZDV combination in patients with KS (92,94–97,100), but the effect was not limited to patients whose KS regressed. In one study, however, an undetectable p24 antigen level at baseline was associated with a greater likelihood of KS regression (101). Finally, a randomized study compared the efficacy of combination therapy with IFN-α (5

MU, three times a week) with ZDV (500 mg daily) to ZDV alone in 250 evaluable HIV-seropositive patients who were asymptomatic or minimally symptomatic and who had a baseline CD4 count of 200 to 500 cells per μL (108). The concomitant administration of IFN-α with ZDV had no effect on the development of AIDS-defining clinical events, viral burden (measured by serum p24 antigen and quantitative PBMC microcultures), or the development of phenotypic resistance to ZDV (108).

In the late 1990s, sensitive polymerase chain reaction–based assays have been developed to quantitate HIV viral load and have proved more useful than p24 antigen or quantitative microculture for monitoring patients receiving antiviral therapy. These methods are currently being applied to patients with KS in a variety of clinical studies, including those involving IFN-α treatment. It should eventually be possible to determine whether baseline viral load or changes associated with the administration of IFN-α–containing regimens predict the response of KS to therapy.

Intralesional Interferon

IFN-α has been reported to induce local regression of directly injected KS lesions in patients with HIV-associated and classic KS (109–112). Neither the dose nor the administration schedule of IFN have been optimized; individual doses ranging from 50,000 U to 1 MU were injected into or around each lesion two to three times a week for up to 8 weeks. In one study, intralesional IFN and a sterile water placebo were found equally effective (109).

Interferon Toxicity

The side effects induced by IFN-α in patients with AIDS-associated KS are not unique. They may, however, be exacerbated by the many other drugs used to treat HIV-infected patients and by the presence of coexisting conditions (e.g., chronic hepatitis, neutropenia, distal sensory peripheral neuropathy, and cognitive defects) commonly observed in such patients. When IFN treatment is initiated at relatively high doses, high fever, chills, and labile blood pressure are common. These side effects can be ameliorated, although not always eliminated, by gradual dosage escalation and pretreatment with either acetaminophen or nonsteroidal antiinflammatory agents. The severity of these side effects diminishes over time and is less in patients who receive low IFN-α doses (≤5 MU). The more chronic side effects of IFN-α include a flulike syndrome characterized by low-grade fever, myalgias, arthralgias, general malaise, and anorexia. Neutropenia is common and may be dose limiting but responds to administration of low intermittent doses of granulocyte- or GM-CSF. Hepatic enzyme elevations are common, particularly early in the course of treatment. Although in many cases hepatic enzyme abnormalities have resolved without interruption of treatment or a decrease in IFN dose, they were found to be dose-limiting in one phase 1 study in which IFN-α and ZDV were combined (93). A reversible congestive cardiomyopathy was reported in three patients with KS after prolonged high-dose IFN-α treatment (113). Additional side effects may include rash, thrombocytopenia, headache, depression, minor cognitive impairment, thyroid abnormalities, autoimmune diseases, decreased libido, and distal paraesthesias. Because many IFN side effects mimic the signs and symptoms of other HIV-associated complications, particular care must be taken in evaluating new symptoms and laboratory abnormalities so that inter-current illnesses are not overlooked. In addition, because IFNs have the potential to influence hepatic microsomal enzymes involved in the metabolism of a variety of drugs (114), including HIV protease inhibitors, the possibility of drug interactions is a concern.

INTERFERON-β

A role for IFN-β in the treatment of KS has not been defined. Despite *in vitro* studies that demonstrate inhibition of HIV replication (105) and inhibition of HIV Tat-induced angiogenesis by IFN-β (115), scant clinical data are published. Furthermore, all published studies were conducted well before the availability of highly effective combination antiretroviral regimens. In one study, recombinant IFN-β_{ser} induced a major response rate of 16% without inducing significant hematologic toxicity (116). Dose-limiting toxicity included injection-site necrosis. In another trial, the combination of IFN-β_{ser} with ZDV was studied at IFN doses of 22.5, 45.0, and 90.0 MU administered by daily subcutaneous injection (117). Although the combination was described as "generally well-tolerated," constitutional symptoms and local skin necrosis were dose-limiting; the maximum tolerated dose was 45 MU daily. Despite the presence of limited KS, only two of 15 patients (13%) showed objective tumor responses (117). Rapid progression of KS was observed in three of four patients treated with a combination of recombinant IFN-β and IL-2 (118).

POTENTIAL FUTURE APPLICATIONS OF INTERFERON IN KAPOSI'S SARCOMA THERAPY

IFN-α was the first drug to receive U.S. Food and Drug Administration approval for treatment of KS and is currently the only biologic approved for this indication. Although IFN-α activity against KS has been demonstrated in many clinical trials, several factors have limited its use. The requirement for frequent, long-term self-injection of IFN-α has been a disincentive for many patients. Occasional patients have developed painful reactions or infections at injection sites, and most patients are also receiving complex drug regimens for which adherence is often a problem. Chronic side effects, especially malaise and flulike syndrome, have also been troublesome, especially for patients treated at moderate to high doses. These side effects have generally not presented major obstacles for patients treated at lower IFN-α doses, particularly those patients who show objective tumor regression. Many patients and their physicians are aware of the significant toxicities associated with high-dose monotherapy, however, and are reluctant to use even low-dose IFN-α when alternative treatments are available.

Despite these obstacles, reasons to believe that IFN-α can still be a valuable therapeutic agent for KS exist, especially when it is used at better tolerated doses and schedules, probably in conjunction with other agents that inhibit angiogenesis by different mechanisms. Fidler and colleagues found that optimal tumor growth inhibition and down-regulation of bFGF mRNA and protein were achieved when low IFN-α doses were administered twice daily to mice bearing orthotopic implants of human bladder cancer (119,120). When the same total weekly dose of IFN-α was administered less often (i.e., once, twice, or three times per week, or once a day), or if the daily doses of IFN-α were increased, tumor growth inhibition was decreased (119,120). These findings suggest that IFN-α's effectiveness as an angiogenesis inhibitor may depend not only on its administration at an optimal dose (which may be well below the maximum tolerated dose) but also on its administration at an optimal schedule (120). Admittedly, the idea of twice-daily injection of IFN is unlikely to be met with great enthusiasm by patients, even if a very low and nontoxic dose is proved optimal. The use of pegylated IFN preparations may, however, eventually allow less frequent parenteral dosing while maintaining optimal angiogenesis inhibitory effects.

Angiogenesis is a multistep process stimulated by a variety of regulatory factors released by tumor and host cells (many of which may be involved in the development and progression of KS). Although IFNs have the potential to influence many of these factors, other agents may prove more powerful than IFN against some of these factors, or may act synergistically with IFN to suppress angiogenesis. A number of such agents are now under study in KS. These include thalidomide (which may affect KS growth through inhibition of TNF and through TNF-independent mechanisms) (121–123), inhibitors of endothelial cell proliferation (124–127), and inhibitors of matrix metalloproteinases, enzymes that facilitate capillary budding and invasion by disrupting the extracellular matrix. Other potential approaches include agents that abrogate tyrosine kinase–mediated transmembrane receptor signals for VEGF/VPF (128), antisense oligonucleotides directed against angiogenic growth factors (129), and agents directed against endothelial cell surface molecules expressed on proliferating vasculature, such as $\alpha_v\beta_3$ (130). Once clinically active agents of this type are identified, a reasonable approach would be to design studies to investigate them in combination with IFN-α and effective antiretroviral therapy.

Finally, a better understanding of the expression of HHV-8–encoded genes in KS lesions may make it possible to further optimize the antitumor effects of IFN. Although many HHV-8 gene products have been implicated in the promotion of KS by a variety of mechanisms, it is not clear that the respective genes are expressed in the tumor cells of all KS lesions (131). Perhaps pertinently, however, HHV-8 encodes an IFN regulatory factor homologue capable of repressing transcriptional activation induced by all classes of IFNs (132–134). If expression of the viral interferon regulatory factor gene in KS cells was found to be associated with a poor response to IFN, this might provide a method for selecting appropriate patients for treatment and a target for therapy.

REFERENCES

1. Centers for Disease Control and Prevention. Kaposi's sarcoma and Pneumocystis pneumonia among homosexual men—New York City and California. *MMWR Morb Mortal Wkly Rep* 1981;30: 305–308.
2. Jacobson LP, Munoz AP, Fox R, et al. Incidence of Kaposi's sarcoma in a cohort of homosexual men infected with the human immunodeficiency virus type 1. The Multicenter AIDS Cohort Study Group. *J Acquir Immune Defic Syndr* 1990;3[Suppl 1]:S24–S31.
3. Lyter DW, Bryant J, Thackeray R, et al. Incidence of human immunodeficiency virus-related and nonrelated malignancies in a large cohort of homosexual men. *J Clin Oncol* 1995;13:2540–2546.
4. Real FX, Krown SE, Oettgen HF. Kaposi's sarcoma and the acquired immunodeficiency syndrome: treatment with high and low doses of recombinant leukocyte A interferon. *J Clin Oncol* 1986;4:544–551.
5. Groopman JE, Gottlieb MS, Goodman J, et al. Recombinant alpha-2-interferon therapy for Kaposi's sarcoma associated with the acquired immunodeficiency syndrome. *Ann Intern Med* 1984;100: 671–676.
6. Safai B, Good RA. Kaposi's sarcoma: a review and recent developments. *Cancer* 1981;31:2–12.
7. Myers BD, Kessler E, Levi J, et al. Kaposi's sarcoma in kidney transplant recipients. *Arch Intern Med* 1974;133:307–311.
8. Penn I. Kaposi's sarcoma in organ transplant recipients: report of 20 cases. *Transplantation* 1979;27:8–11.
9. Kapadia SB, Krause JR. Kaposi's sarcoma after long-term alkylating agent therapy for multiple myeloma. *South Med J* 1977;70: 1011–1013.
10. Klein MB, Pereira FA, Kantor I. Kaposi's sarcoma complicating systemic lupus erythematosus treated with immunosuppression. *Arch Dermatol* 1974;110:602–604.
11. Giraldo G, Beth E, Henle W, et al. Antibody patterns to herpes viruses in Kaposi's sarcoma. II. Serological association of American Kaposi's sarcoma with cytomegalovirus. *Int J Cancer* 1978;22:126–131.
12. Nakamura S, Salahuddin SZ, Biberfeld P, et al. Kaposi's sarcoma cells: long-term culture with growth factor from retrovirus infected CD4+ T cells. *Science* 1988;242:426–430.
13. Salahuddin SZ, Nakamura S, Biberfeld P, et al. Angiogenic properties of Kaposi's sarcoma-derived cells after long-term culture *in vitro*. *Science* 1988;242:430–433.
14. Ensoli B, Nakamura S, Salahuddin SZ, et al. AIDS Kaposi's sarcoma derived cells express cytokines with autocrine and paracrine growth effects. *Science* 1989;243:223–226.
15. Miles SA, Rezai AR, Salazar-Gonzales JF, et al. AIDS Kaposi sarcoma-derived cells produce and respond to interleukin-6. *Proc Natl Acad Sci U S A* 1990;87:4068–4072.
16. Weindel K, Marme D, Weich HA. AIDS-associated Kaposi's sarcoma cells in culture express vascular endothelial growth factor. *Biochem Biophys Res Commun* 1992;183:1167–1174.
17. Barillari G, Bunoaguro L, Fiorelli V, et al. Effects of cytokines from activated immune cells on vascular cell growth and HIV-1 gene expression. *J Immunol* 1992;149:3727–3734.
18. Miles SA, Martinez-Maza O, Rezai A, et al. Oncostatin M as a potent mitogen for AIDS-Kaposi's sarcoma derived cells. *Science* 1992;255:1432–1434.
19. Nair BC, DeVico AL, Nakamura S, et al. Identification of a major growth factor for AIDS-Kaposi's sarcoma cells as Oncostatin M. *Science* 1992;255:1430–1432.
20. Sirianni MC, Vincenzi L, Fiorelli V, et al. γ-Interferon production in peripheral blood mononuclear cells and tumor infiltrating lymphocytes from Kaposi's sarcoma patients: correlation with the presence of human herpesvirus-8 in peripheral blood mononuclear cells and lesional macrophages. *Blood* 1998;91:968–976.
21. Fiorelli V, Barillari G, Toschi E, et al. IFN-γ induces endothelial cells to proliferate and to invade the extracellular matrix in response to HIV-1 Tat protein: implications for AIDS-Kaposi's sarcoma pathogenesis. *J Immunol* 1999;162:1165–1170.
22. Samaniego F, Markham PD, Gendleman R, et al. Vascular endothelial growth factor and basic fibroblast growth factor present in Kaposi's sarcoma (KS) are induced by inflammatory cytokines and synergize to promote vascular permeability and KS lesion development. *Am J Pathol* 1998;152:1433–1443.
23. Roux-Lombard P, Modoux C, Cruchaud A, Dayer JM. Purified blood monocytes from HIV 1-infected patients produce high levels of TNF alpha and IL-1. *Clin Immunol Immunopathol* 1989;50:374–384.
24. Jassoy C, Harrer T, Rosenthal T, et al. Human immunodeficiency virus type 1-specific cytotoxic T lymphocytes release gamma interferon, tumor necrosis factor alpha (TNF-alpha), and TNF-beta when they encounter their target antigens. *J Virol* 1993;67:2844–2852.
25. Graziosi C, Gantt KR, Vaccarezza M, et al. Kinetics of cytokine expression during primary human immunodeficiency virus type 1 infection. *Proc Natl Acad Sci U S A* 1996;93:4386–4391.
26. Poli G, Fauci AS. The effect of cytokines and pharmacologic agents on chronic HIV infection. *AIDS Res Hum Retroviruses* 1992;8: 191–197.
27. Fiorelli V, Gendelman R, Samaniego F, et al. Cytokines from activated T cells induce normal endothelial cells to acquire the phenotypic and functional features of AIDS-Kaposi's sarcoma spindle cells. *J Clin Invest* 1995;95:1723–1734.
28. Vogel J, Hinrichs SH, Reynolds RK, et al. The HIV *tat* gene induces dermal lesions resembling Kaposi's sarcoma in transgenic mice. *Nature* 1988;335:606–611.
29. Ensoli B, Buonaguro L, Barillari G, et al. Release, uptake, and effects of extracellular human immunodeficiency virus type 1 Tat protein on cell growth and viral transactivation. *J Virol* 1993;67:277–287.
30. Barillari G, Gendelman R, Gallo RC, et al. The Tat protein of human immunodeficiency virus type I, a growth factor for AIDS Kaposi sarcoma and cytokine-activated vascular cells, induces adhesion of the same cell types by using integrin receptors recognizing the RGD amino acid sequence. *Proc Natl Acad Sci U S A* 1993;90:7941–7945.
31. Ensoli B, Barillari G, Salahuddin SZ, et al. Tat protein of HIV-1 stimulates growth of cells derived from Kaposi's sarcoma lesions of AIDS patients. *Nature* 1990;345:84–86.
32. Ensoli B, Gendelman R, Markham P, et al. Synergy between basic fibroblast growth factor and HIV-1 Tat protein in induction of Kaposi's sarcoma. *Nature* 1994;371:674–680.
33. Kelly GD, Ensoli B, Gunthel CJ, Offermann MK. Purified Tat induces inflammatory response genes in Kaposi's sarcoma cells. *AIDS* 1998;12:1753–1761.
34. Beral V, Peterman TA, Berkelman RL, et al. Kaposi's sarcoma among persons with AIDS: a sexually transmitted infection. *Lancet* 1990; 335:123–128.
35. Friedman-Kien AE, Saltzman BR, Cao Y, et al. Kaposi's sarcoma in HIV-negative homosexual men. *Lancet* 1990;335:168–169.
36. Chang Y, Cesarman E, Pessin MS, et al. Identification of herpes virus-like DNA sequences in AIDS-associated Kaposi's sarcoma. *Science* 1994;266:1865–1869.
37. Chang Y, Ziegler J, Wabinga H, et al. Kaposi's sarcoma-associated herpesvirus and Kaposi's sarcoma in Africa: Uganda Kaposi's sarcoma study group. *Arch Intern Med* 1996;156:202–204.
38. Moore PS, Chang Y. Detection of herpes virus-like DNA sequences in Kaposi's sarcoma in patients with and without HIV infection. *N Engl J Med* 1995;332:1181–1185.
39. Schalling M, Ekman M, Kaaya E, et al. A role for a new herpes virus (KSHV) in different forms of Kaposi's sarcoma. *Nat Med* 1995;1:707–708.
40. Ambrosziak JA, Blackburn D, Herndier BG, et al. Herpes-like sequences in HIV-infected and uninfected Kaposi's sarcoma patients. *Science* 1995;268:582–583.
41. Cesarman E, Chang Y, Moore PS, et al. Kaposi's sarcoma-associated herpes virus-like DNA sequences are present in AIDS-related body cavity B-cell lymphomas. *N Engl J Med* 1995;332:1186–1191.
42. Soulier J, Grollet L, Oksenhendler E, et al. Kaposi's sarcoma-associated herpes virus-like DNA sequences in multicentric Castleman's disease. *Blood* 1995;86:1276–1280.
43. Whitby D, Howard MR, Tenant-Flowers M, et al. Detection of Kaposi sarcoma associated herpesvirus in peripheral blood of HIV-

infected individuals and progression to Kaposi's sarcoma. *Lancet* 1995;346:799–802.

44. Flore O, Rafii S, Ely S, et al. Transformation of primary human endothelial cells by Kaposi's sarcoma-associated herpesvirus. *Nature* 1998;394:588–592.

45. Boshoff C, Schulz TF, Kennedy MM, et al. Kaposi's sarcoma-associated herpesvirus infects endothelial and spindle cells. *Nat Med* 1995;1:1274–1278.

46. Sarid R, Wiezorek JS, Moore PS, Chang Y. Characterization and cell cycle regulation of the major Kaposi's sarcoma-associated herpesvirus (human herpesvirus 8) latent genes and their promoter. *J Virol* 1999;73:1428–1436.

47. Russo JJ, Bohenzky RA, Chien MC, et al. Nucleotide sequence of the Kaposi sarcoma-associated herpesvirus (HHV8). *Proc Natl Acad Sci U S A* 1996;93:14862–14867.

48. Whitby D, Boshoff C. Kaposi's sarcoma herpesvirus as a new paradigm for virus-induced oncogenesis. *Curr Opin Oncol* 1998;10: 405–412.

49. Boshoff C, Endo Y, Collins PD, et al. Angiogenic and HIV-inhibitory functions of KSHV-encoded chemokines. *Science* 1997;278: 290–294.

50. Moore PS, Chang Y. Kaposi's sarcoma-associated herpesvirus-encoded oncogenes and oncogenesis. *J Natl Cancer Inst Monogr* 1998;23:65–71.

51. Reiter Z, Ozes ON, Blatt LM, et al. A possible role for interferon-alpha and activated natural killer cells in remission of AIDS-related Kaposi's sarcoma: in vitro studies. *J Acquir Immune Defic Syndr* 1992;5:469–476.

52. Lebbé C, de Crémoux P, Millot G, et al. Characterization of in vitro culture of HIV-negative Kaposi's sarcoma-derived cells. *In vitro* responses to alfa interferon. *Arch Dermatol Res* 1007;289:421–428.

53. Philip R, Debs R. Cytokine-activated human monocytes show differential cytotoxicity toward fresh and cultured Kaposi's sarcoma cells. *J Acquir Immune Defic Syndr* 1991;4:1254–1257.

54. Dinney CP, Bielenberg DR, Perrotte P, et al. Inhibition of basic fibroblast growth factor expression, angiogenesis, and growth of human bladder carcinoma in mice by systemic interferon-alpha administration. *Cancer Res* 1998;58:808–814.

55. Fidler IJ, Singh RK, Gutman M, et al. Interferons alpha and beta down regulate the expression of basic fibroblast growth factor (bFGF) in human carcinomas (abstr) *Proc Am Assoc Cancer Res* 1994;35:47.

56. Tilg H, Mier JM, Vogel W, et al. Induction of circulating IL-1 receptor antagonist by IFN treatment. *J Immunol* 1993;150:4687–4692.

57. Tilg H, Vogel W, Dinarello CA. Interferon-α induces circulating tumor necrosis factor receptor in humans. *Blood* 1995;85.433–435.

58. Ho DD, Hartshorn KL, Rota TR, et al. Recombinant human interferon alpha-A suppresses HTLV-III replication in vitro. *Lancet* 1985;1:602–604.

59. Hartshorn KL, Vogt MW, Chou TC, et al. Synergistic inhibition of human immunodeficiency virus in vitro by azidothymidine and recombinant interferon alpha A. *Antimicrob Agents Chemother* 1987;31:168 172.

60. Vogt MW, Durno AG, Chou TC, et al. Synergistic interaction of 2'3'-dideoxycytidine (ddCyd) and recombinant interferon alpha A (rIFN-αA) on HIV-1 replication. *J Infect Dis* 1988;158:378–385.

61. Johnson VA, Merrill DP, Videler JA, et al. Two-drug combinations of zidovudine, didanosine, and recombinant interferon-α A inhibit replication of zidovudine-resistant human immunodeficiency virus type 1 synergistically *in vitro. J Infect Dis* 1991;164:646–655.

62. Krischer J, Rutschmann O, Hirschel B, et al. Regression of Kaposi's sarcoma during therapy with HIV-1 protease inhibitors: a prospective pilot study. *J Am Acad Dermatol* 1998;38:594–598.

63. Lebbé C, Blum L, Pellet C, et al. Clinical and biological impact of antiretroviral therapy with protease inhibitors on HIV-related Kaposi's sarcoma. *AIDS* 1998;12:F45–49.

64. Monini P, Franco M, Carlini F, et al. αIFN and HIV-1 protease inhibitors (PI) inhibit HHV-8 infection: possible therapeutic approaches for Kaposi's sarcoma (KS). *J Acquir Immune Defic Syndr Hum Retrovirol* 1998;17:A17(abst).

65. Pfrommer C, Tebbe B, Tidona CA, et al. Progressive HHV-8-positive classic Kaposi's sarcoma: rapid response to interferon alpha-2a but persistence of HHV-8 DNA sequences in lesional skin. *Br J Dermatol* 1998;139:516–519.

66. Evans LM, Itri LM, Campion M, et al. Interferon alfa-2a in the treatment of acquired immunodeficiency syndrome-related Kaposi's sarcoma. *J Immunother* 1991;10:39–50.

67. Gelmann EP, Preble OT, Steis R, et al. Human lymphoblastoid interferon treatment of Kaposi's sarcoma in the acquired immunodeficiency syndrome. *Am J Med* 1985;78:737–741.

68. Kern P, Meigel W, Racz P, et al. Interferon-alpha in the treatment of AIDS-associated Kaposi's sarcoma. *Onkologie* 1987;10:50–52.

69. Krown SE, Real FX, Cunningham-Rudles S, et al. Preliminary observations on the effect of recombinant leukocyte A interferon in homosexual men with Kaposi's sarcoma. *N Engl J Med* 1983;308: 1071–1076.

70. Rozenbaum W, Gharakhanian S, Navarette M-S, et al. Long-term follow-up of 120 patients with AIDS-related Kaposi's sarcoma treated with interferon alpha-2A. *J Invest Dermatol* 1990;95: S161–S165.

71. Volberding PA, Mitsuyasu RT, Golando JP, et al. Treatment of Kaposi's sarcoma with interferon alfa-2b (Intron A). *Cancer* 1987;59:620–625.

72. Rios A, Mansell PWA, Newell GR, et al. Treatment of acquired immunodeficiency syndrome-related Kaposi's sarcoma with lymphoblastoid interferon. *J Clin Oncol* 1985;3:506–512.

73. Fischl MA, Gorowski E, Koch G, et al. Interferon alfa-n1 Wellferon® in Kaposi's sarcoma: single agent or combination with vinblastine. In: Cantell K, Schellekens H, eds. *The biology of the interferon system 1986.* Boston: Martinus Nijhoff 1987: 355–362.

74. Lane HC, Kovacs JA, Feinberg J, et al. Anti-retroviral effects of interferon-α in AIDS-associated Kaposi's sarcoma. *Lancet* 1988;2: 1218–1222.

75. deWit R, Schatenkerk JKME, Boucher CAB, et al. Clinical and virological effects of high-dose recombinant interferon-α in disseminated AIDS-related Kaposi's sarcoma. *Lancet* 1988;2:1214–1217.

76. Vadhan-Raj S, Wong G, Gnecco C, et al. Immunological variables as predictors of prognosis in patients with Kaposi's sarcoma and the acquired immunodeficiency syndrome. *Cancer Res* 1986;46: 417–425.

77. Mitsuyasu RT, Taylor JMG, Glaspy J, et al. Heterogeneity of epidemic Kaposi's sarcoma. Implications for therapy. *Cancer* 1986;57: 1657–1661.

78. Krown SE, Niedzwiecki D, Bhalla RB, et al. Relationship and prognostic value of endogenous interferon-alpha, beta₂-microglobulin, and neopterin serum levels in patients with Kaposi sarcoma and AIDS. *J Acquir Immune Defic Syndr* 1991;4:871–880.

79. Rasokat H, Haussermann L, Minnemann M. Response of AIDS-related Kaposi's sarcoma to treatment with recombinant interferon alpha depends on the stage of underlying immunodeficiency. *J Invest Dermatol* 1987;67:531–534.

80. Krigel RL, Slywotzky CM, Lonberg M, et al. Treatment of epidemic Kaposi's sarcoma with a combination of interferon-alpha 2b and etoposide. *J Biol Response Mod* 1988;7:359–364.

81. Rios A, Mansell P, Newell G, et al. The use of lymphoblastoid interferon HuIFN-α (Ly) and vinblastine in the treatment of acquired immune deficiency syndrome (AIDS) related Kaposi's sarcoma (KS). *Proc Am Soc Clin Oncol* 1985;5:6(abst).

82. Shepherd FA, Evans WK, Garvey B, et al. Combination chemotherapy and α-interferon in the treatment of Kaposi's sarcoma associated with acquired immune deficiency syndrome. *Can Med Assoc J* 1988;139:635–639.

83. Krown SE, Real FX, Lester T, et al. Interferon alfa-2a (IFN-α2a) ± vinblastine (VLB) in AIDS-related Kaposi's sarcoma (KS/AIDS): a prospective randomized trial. *Proc Am Soc Clin Oncol* 1986; 5:6(abst).

84. Gill PS, Rarick MU, Bernstein-Singer M, et al. Interferon-alpha maintenance therapy after cytotoxic chemotherapy for treatment of acquired immunodeficiency syndrome-related Kaposi's sarcoma. *J Biol Response Mod* 1990;9:512–516.

85. Ruprecht RM, Bernard LD, Gama Sosa MA, et al. Murine models for evaluating antiretroviral therapy. *Cancer Res* 1990;50:S5618–S5627.

86. Ruprecht RM, Chou TC, Chipty F, et al. Interferon-alpha and 3′-azido-3′-deoxythymidine are highly synergistic in mice and prevent viremia after acute retrovirus exposure. *J Acquir Immune Defic Syndr* 1990;3:591–600.

87. Lane HC, Falloon J, Walker RE, et al. Zidovudine in patients with human immunodeficiency virus (HIV) infection and Kaposi sarcoma. A phase II randomized, placebo-controlled trial. *Ann Intern Med* 1989;111:41–50.

88. de Wit R, Reiss P, Bakker PJ, et al. Lack of activity of zidovudine in AIDS-associated Kaposi's sarcoma. *AIDS* 1989;3:847–850.

89. Mildvan D, Machado SG, Wilets I, Grossberg SE. Endogenous interferon and triglyceride concentrations to assess response to zidovudine in AIDS and advance AIDS-related complex. *Lancet* 1992;339:453–456.

90. Jacobson MA, Bacchetti P, Kolokathis A, et al. Surrogate markers for survival in patients with AIDS and AIDS-related complex. *BMJ* 1991;302:73–78.

91. Pitha PM. Multiple effects of interferon on the replication of human immunodeficiency virus type 1. *Antiviral Res* 1994;24:205–219.

92. Krown SE, Gold JWM, Niedzwiecki D, et al. Interferon-α with zidovudine: safety, tolerance, and clinical and virologic effects in patients with Kaposi's sarcoma associated with the acquired immunodeficiency syndrome (AIDS). *Ann Intern Med* 1990;112:812–821.

93. Fischl MA, Uttamchandani RB, Resnick L, et al. A phase I study of recombinant human interferons-alfa-2a or human lymphoblastoid interferon alfa-n1 and concomitant zidovudine in patients with AIDS-related Kaposi's sarcoma. *J Acquir Immune Defic Syndr* 1991;4:1–10.

94. Kovacs JA, Deyton L, Davey R, et al. Combined zidovudine and interferon-α therapy in patients with Kaposi's sarcoma and the acquired immunodeficiency syndrome (AIDS). *Ann Intern Med* 1989;111:280–287.

95. Fischl MA, Finkelstein DM, He W, et al. A phase II study of recombinant human interferon-α 2a and zidovudine in patients with AIDS-related Kaposi's sarcoma. *J Acquir Immune Defic Syndr Hum Retrovirol* 1996;11:379–384.

96. Baumann R, Tauber MG, Opravil M, et al. Combined treatment with zidovudine and lymphoblast interferon-alpha in patients with HIV-related Kaposi's sarcoma. *Klin Wochenschr* 1991;69:360–367.

97. Shepherd FA, Beaulieu R, Gelmon K, et al. Prospective randomized trial of two dose levels of interferon alfa with zidovudine for the treatment of Kaposi's sarcoma associated with human immunodeficiency virus infection: a Canadian HIV clinical network study. *J Clin Oncol* 1998;16:1736–1742.

98. de Wit R, Danner SA, Bakker PJ, et al. Combined zidovudine and interferon-alpha treatment in patients with AIDS-associated Kaposi's sarcoma. *J Intern Med* 1991;229:35–40.

99. Mauss S, Jablonowski H. Efficacy, safety, and tolerance of low-dose, long-term interferon-alpha 2b and zidovudine in early-stage AIDS-associated Kaposi's sarcoma. *J Acquir Immune Defic Syndr Hum Retrovirol* 1995;10:157–162.

100. Podzamczer D, Bolao F, Clotet B, et al. Low-dose interferon alpha combined with zidovudine in patients with AIDS-associated Kaposi's sarcoma. *J Intern Med* 1993;233:247–253.

101. Stadler R, Bratzke B, Schaart F, Orfanos CE. Long-term combined rIFN-alpha-2a and zidovudine therapy for HIV-associated Kaposi's sarcoma: clinical consequences and side effects. *J Invest Dermatol* 1990;95:S170–S175.

102. Berman E, Duigou-Osterndorf R, Krown SE, et al. Synergistic cytotoxic effect of azidothymidine and recombinant interferon alpha on normal human bone marrow progenitor cells. *Blood* 1989;74: 1281–1286.

103. Scadden DT, Bering HA, Levine JD, et al. Granulocyte-macrophage colony-stimulating factor mitigates the neutropenia of combined interferon alfa and zidovudine treatment of acquired immune deficiency syndrome-associated Kaposi's sarcoma. *J Clin Oncol* 1991;9:802–808.

104. Krown SE, Paredes J, Bundow D, et al. Interferon-α, zidovudine and granulocyte macrophage colony-stimulating factor: a phase I trial in patients with Kaposi's sarcoma associated with the acquired immunodeficiency syndrome (AIDS). *J Clin Oncol* 1992;10: 1344–1351.

105. Williams GJ, Colby CB. Recombinant human interferon-beta suppresses the replication of HIV and acts synergistically with AZT. *J Interferon Res* 1989;9:709–718.

106. Lane HC, Davey V, Kovacs JA, et al. Interferon-alpha in patients with asymptomatic human immunodeficiency virus (HIV) infection. A randomized, placebo-controlled trial. *Ann Intern Med* 1990;112:805–811.

107. Mildvan D, Bassiakos Y, Zucker ML, et al. Synergy, activity and tolerability of zidovudine and interferon-alpha in patients with symptomatic HIV-1 infection: ACTG 068. *Antivir Ther* 1996;1: 77–88.

108. Krown SE, Aeppli D, Balfour HH Jr. Phase II, randomized, open-label, community-based trial to compare the safety and activity of combination therapy with recombinant interferon-α2b and zidovudine versus zidovudine alone in patients with asymptomatic to mildly symptomatic HIV infection. *J Acquir Immune Defic Syndr Hum Retrovirol* 1999;20:245–254.

109. Depuy J, Price M, Lynch G, et al. Intralesional interferon-alpha and zidovudine in epidemic Kaposi's sarcoma. *J Am Acad Dermatol* 1993;28:966–972.

110. Sulis E, Floris C, Sulis ML, et al. Interferon administered intralesionally in skin and oral cavity lesions in heterosexual drug addicted patients with AIDS-related Kaposi's sarcoma [Letter]. *Eur J Cancer Clin Oncol* 1989;25:759–761.

111. Trattner A, Reizis Z, David M, et al. The therapeutic effect of intralesional interferon in classical Kaposi's sarcoma. *Br J Dermatol* 1993;129:590–593.

112. Ghyka G, Alecu M, Halalau F, Coman G. Intralesional human leukocyte interferon treatment alone or associated with IL-2 in non-AIDS related Kaposi's sarcoma. *J Dermatol* 1992;19:35–39.

113. Deyton LR, Walker RE, Kovacs JA, et al. Reversible cardiac dysfunction associated with interferon-alfa therapy in AIDS patients with Kaposi's sarcoma. *N Engl J Med* 1989;321:1246.

114. Mannering GJ, Renton KW, El Azhary R, et al. Effect of interferon-inducing agents on hepatic cytochrome p-450 drug metabolizing systems. *Ann N Y Acad Sci* 1980;350:314–331.

115. Iurlaro M, Benelli R, Masiello L, et al. β Interferon inhibits HIV-1 Tat-induced angiogenesis: synergism with 13-cis retinoic acid. *Eur J Cancer* 1998;34:570–576.

116. Miles SA, Wang HJ, Cortes E, et al. Beta-interferon therapy in patients with poor-prognosis Kaposi sarcoma related to the acquired immunodeficiency syndrome (AIDS). A phase II trial with preliminary evidence of antiviral activity and low incidence of opportunistic infections. *Ann Intern Med* 1990;112:582–589.

117. Miles S, Levine A, Feldstein M, et al. Open-label phase I study of combination therapy with zidovudine and interferon-beta in patients with AIDS-related Kaposi's sarcoma: AIDS clinical trials group protocol 057. *Cytokines Cell Mol Ther* 1998;4:17–23.

118. Krigel RL, Padavic SK, Rudolph AR, et al. Exacerbation of epidemic Kaposi's sarcoma with a combination of interleukin-2 and beta-interferon: results of a phase 2 study. *J Biol Response Mod* 1989; 8:359–365.

119. Slaton JW, Perotte P, Bielenberg D, et al. Dosing interval of alpha-interferon (IFN-α) is critical to the down-regulation of angiogenesis and invasive factors in orthotopically implanted human transitional cell carcinoma. *Proc Am Assoc Cancer Res* 1998;39:148(abst).

120. Fidler IJ, Slaton J, Perrotte P, et al. Host factors in neoplastic angiogenesis. *Proc Am Assoc Cancer Res* 1999;40:770.

121. Karp JE, Pluda JM, Yarchoan R. AIDS-related Kaposi's sarcoma: a template for the translation of molecular pathogenesis into targeted therapeutic approaches. *Hematol Oncol Clin North Am* 1996;10: 1031–1049.

122. Welles L, Little R, Wyvill K, et al. Preliminary results of a phase II study of oral thalidomide in patients with HIV infection and Kaposi's sarcoma (KS). *J Acquir Immune Defic Syndr Hum Retrovirol* 1997;14:A21(abst).

123. Bower M, Howard M, Gracie F, et al. A phase II study of thalidomide for Kaposi's sarcoma: activity and correlation with KSHV DNA load. *J Acquir Immune Defic Syndr Hum Retrovirol* 1997;14:A35.
124. Dezube BJ, vonRoenn JH, Holden-Wiltse J, et al. Fumagillin analog in the treatment of Kaposi's sarcoma: a phase I AIDS clinical trial group study. *J Clin Oncol* 1998;16:1444–1449.
125. Pluda JM, Wyvill KK, Lietzau J, et al. A phase I trial administering the angiogenesis inhibitor TNP-470 (AGM-1470) to patients (pts) with HIV-associated Kaposi's sarcoma (KS). *J Acquir Immune Defic Syndr Hum Retrovirol* 1997;14:A19(abst).
126. O'Reilly MS, Holmgren L, Shing Y, et al. Angiostatin: a novel angiogenesis inhibitor that mediates the suppression of metastases by a Lewis lung carcinoma. *Cell* 1994;79:315–328.
127. O'Reilly MS, Boehm T, Shing Y, et al. Endostatin: an endogenous inhibitor of angiogenesis and tumor growth. *Cell* 1997;88:277–285.
128. Fong TAT. Development of small molecule inhibitors of the VEGF receptor (flk-1/KDR) for treatment of human cancers. *J Acquir Immune Defic Syndr Hum Retrovirol* 1998;17:A41(abst).
129. Ensoli B, Markham P, Kao V, et al. Block of AIDS-Kaposi's sarcoma (KS) cell growth, angiogenesis and lesion formation in nude mice by antisense oligonucleotide targeting basic fibroblast growth factor. *J Clin Invest* 1994;94:1736–1746.
130. Brooks PC, Montgomery AMP, Rosenfeld M, et al. Integrin $\alpha_v\beta_3$ antagonists promote tumor regression by inducing apoptosis of angiogenic blood vessels. *Cell* 1994;79:1157–1164.
131. Sturzl M, Ensoli B. Big but weak: how many pathogenic genes does human herpesvirus-8 need to cause Kaposi's sarcoma? *Int J Oncol* 1999;14:287–289.
132. Gao SJ, Boshoff C, Jayachandra S, et al. KSHV ORF K9 (vIRF) is an oncogene which inhibits the interferon signaling pathway. *Oncogene* 1997;15:1979–1985.
133. Zimring JC, Goodbourn S, Offermann MK. Human herpesvirus 8 encodes an interferon regulatory factor (IRF) homolog that represses IRF-1-mediated transcription. *J Virol* 1998;72:701–707.
134. Li M, Lee H, Guo J, et al. Kaposi's sarcoma-associated herpesvirus viral interferon regulatory factor. *J Virol* 1998;72:5433–5440.

10.5

INTERFERON-α AND -β: CLINICAL APPLICATIONS

Epithelial Cancers

SANJIV S. AGARWALA

Interferon-α (IFN-α) has not been effective as single-agent therapy for most epithelial tumors, with no responses observed in phase 2 trials for cancers of the gastrointestinal tract and non–small-cell lung cancer (1–4). Efforts at exploiting the unique antineoplastic effects of IFN-α are based on the concept of biomodulation and preclinical data of synergy between it and other chemotherapeutic agents.

Biomodulation is the enhancement of the antitumor activity of a cytostatic agent by a drug (the biomodulator) that per se has no direct antiproliferative effect against the tumor of interest. Biomodulators act by manipulating the intracellular metabolic pathways of antineoplastic agents, with subsequent enhancement of antitumor activity or protection of the normal tissues of the host, or both. The interaction between 5-fluorouracil (5-FU) and IFN-α is an example of biomodulation. This chapter discusses the role of IFN as a biomodulator in various epithelial cancers, with emphasis on gastrointestinal cancers and squamous cell carcinoma of the lungs, head, and neck.

COLORECTAL CANCER

Rationale for Use of Interferon in Colorectal Cancer

Interferons as single agents have not shown activity in colorectal cancer. Investigations with IFN in this disease have concentrated on exploiting the biologic synergy between IFN and 5-FU. In concert with 5-FU, IFN-α acts as a biomodulator by inhibiting thymidylate synthetase, a key enzyme in the metabolic pathway of 5-FU. IFN-α also decreases the clearance of 5-FU, thereby increasing plasma levels and the area under the curve (5).

Biomodulation of 5-Fluorouracil by Interferon (Phase 2 Studies)

Wadler et al. were the first to report the encouraging results of a phase 2 trial of IFN-α and 5-FU in 30 patients with metastatic colorectal cancer (6). Of the 17 previously untreated patients,

TABLE 1. FLUOROURACIL AND INTERFERON-α IN ADVANCED COLORECTAL CANCER

Author (Reference)	No. of Patients	Response (%)	Survival (Mo)
Wadler et al. (6)	17	64	16
Kemeny and Younes (7)	38	26	13
Pazdur et al. (32)	45	35	16
Weh et al. (33)	59	31	10
Diaz et al. (34)	35	24	NR
Wadler et al. (35)	38	42	18
John et al. (36)	18	33	11
Barzacchi et al. (8)	31	10	7.5

NR, not reported.

TABLE 2. DOUBLE MODULATION OF 5-FLUOROURACIL BY LEUCOVORIN AND INTERFERON IN METASTATIC COLORECTAL CANCER

Author (Reference)	No. of Patients	Response (%)	Survival (Mo)
Grem et al. (37)	46	54	7.8
Schmoll et al. (38)	43	10	NR
Punt (39)	45	25	11
Sobrero et al. (40)	15	20	NR
Cascinu (41)	45	51	NR
Labianca et al. (42)	63	24	13
Marshall et al. (43)	46	13	17
Buter (44)	53	58	16.6
Moore (45)	43	24	10
Kohne et al. (46)	71	15	9.9
		17	11.4
Tournigand et al. (47)	50	44	25

NR, not reported.

13 responded; no patient who had received previous chemotherapy had a response. Toxicity was manageable with one toxic death. Median survival was in excess of 16 months.

Subsequent phase 2 trials showed less encouraging results and are summarized in Table 1. Response rates (RRs) varied from 10% to 64% and median survival ranged from 8 to 18 months. Most patients in these trials had not received previous chemotherapy for metastatic disease. Clinical toxicities typical of IFN (fever, myalgia, and fatigue) were universally seen. Neurotoxicity in the form of memory disturbance, sensory neuropathy, confusion, and tardive dyskinesia was noted in one study, affecting 13 of 38 patients (34%), 9 of whom were 60 years of age or older (7). All studies used recombinant IFN; lymphoblastoid interferon was used in one trial with a low (10%) RR (8).

Biomodulation of 5-FU has also been investigated as second-line therapy in patients with advanced or metastatic colorectal cancer, or both. To assess the ability of IFN to modulate 5-FU in patients refractory to protracted venous infusion 5-FU, Findlay and coworkers added IFN-α, 5 MU subcutaneous (s.c.), three times weekly, to a regimen of protracted venous infusion 5-FU, 200 to 300 mg per m^2 per day, in patients determined to become refractory to the latter. An 8% RR was observed in 60 patients (9). Perez et al. reported the results of FU and IFN in 34 patients refractory to previous therapy with FU with methotrexate or leucovorin, or both (10). Only two responses were observed, with a median survival of 5 months. Hepatic arterial infusion of 5-FU and IFN was tested in 48 patients with unresectable liver metastases from colorectal carcinoma refractory to systemic FU and leucovorin. Fifteen responses [three complete responses, 12 partial responses (PRs)] were seen in 45 evaluable patients; median survival was 15 months. Notable was the lack of hepatobiliary toxicity (11).

Double and Triple Modulation of 5-Fluorouracil (Phase 2 Studies)

Leucovorin and IFN modulate the activity of 5-FU, using different mechanisms of action. Several trials designed to test this potential synergy have been completed. *In vitro* data suggest a minimum dose of 5 MU per m^2 of IFN is necessary for adequate modulation (12,13), but various doses and schedules have been used. Phase 2 clinical trials of so-called double modulation of FU are summarized in Table 2. Response rates vary between

months. Toxicity was mainly in the form of mucositis and diarrhea and tended to be more severe than with single modulation.

Randomized Phase 3 Trials

Several large, randomized phase 3 trials have matured and helped better define the role of biomodulation of 5-FU in advanced and metastatic colorectal cancer. Results of five randomized trials comparing a combination of 5-FU and IFN to 5-FU alone are available and summarized in Table 3. Patients entered into these trials had not received previous chemotherapy for metastatic disease. The regimen used in three of these studies used the initial regimen described by Wadler et al. (Table 4). One used lower doses of both drugs (14); one used a slightly higher dose of IFN (10 MU) (15); and another used protracted venous infusion of 5-FU (16).

Greco and colleagues reported the results of a protocol (N-3411) designed to evaluate the RR, time to progression, survival, and toxicity of a combination of 5-FU and IFN-α-2a versus 5-FU alone in patients with chemotherapy-naïve, advanced colorectal cancer (17). Two hundred forty-five patients were randomized to either 5-FU, 750 mg per m^2 per day continuous intravenous infusion, days 1 through 5, followed by a weekly bolus of the same dose 9 days later or the same regimen concurrent with IFN-α-2a, 9 MU s.c., three times weekly throughout treatment. The overall RR was 24% for the IFN/FU arm and 17% for the FU arm (*p* = not significant). Neither time to progression nor survival were different in the two arms of the trial. Toxicity was greater on the combination arm. Dufour et al. tested an identical regimen in a randomized trial of 105 patients. Although a higher RR was observed for the IFN-treated group (19.6% versus 6.1%), no significant difference in overall survival (OS) occurred (18). The trial reported by Palmieri and colleagues randomized 235 patients in a similar fashion. No significant difference in the RR (25% versus 21%) or survival (48.5 weeks versus 43.7 weeks) was observed for the IFN-treated patients. A prospective, randomized phase 2 trial was conducted by Piga et al. of a lower dose of FU (500 mg per m^2) and IFN (6 MU per day, later lowered further to 3 MU per

TABLE 3. RANDOMIZED TRIALS OF 5-FLUOROURACIL (5-FU) ALONE VERSUS 5-FU AND INTERFERON (IFN)

Author (Reference)	No. of Patients	Response (%) (5-FU/5-FU and IFN)	Survival (Mo) (5-FU/5-FU and IFN)	Comment
Dufour (18)	105	6.1/19.6	9/12	*p* = NS
Hill (15)	106	25/25	8/8	*p* = NS
Hill (16)	160	33/22	12/11	PVI FU; *p* = NS
Palmeri et al. (19)	235	21/25	43.7/48.5	*p* = NS
Piga et al. (14)	142	12.5/8.7	12/12	*p* = NS
Greco (17)	245	17/24	13.2/13.9	*p* = NS
O'Dwyer et al. (20)	1,118 (5 arms)	Awaited	14.8/15.3	Trial yet to mature

NS, not significant; PVI FU, protracted venous infusion 5-FU.

day due to toxicity) in 142 patients. No difference in response or survival occurred and the trial was stopped early (14).

The Royal Marsden Group in the United Kingdom tested a similar combination of 5-FU and IFN-α (10 MU s.c. three times weekly) to 5-FU alone in 106 eligible patients who had not previously received chemotherapy. No improvement in RR, duration of response, or survival was observed for the combination (15). A significantly greater number of patients on the IFN arm had to discontinue therapy due to toxicity (leukopenia, lymphopenia, depression, and alopecia). In another trial conducted by the same group, protracted venous infusion 5-FU, 300 mg per m^2 per day for 10 weeks, was substituted for the 5-day regimen and the IFN-α dose was reduced to 5 MU s.c. three times weekly. Once again, RR did not differ significantly between the two arms of the study. Although the treatment was in general well-tolerated, mucositis, alopecia, and leukopenia were significantly worse for the IFN-treated group. At a median follow-up at 1 year, no difference in time to progression or survival occurred (16).

The Eastern Cooperative Oncology Group and the Cancer and Leukemia Group B conducted a large phase 3 randomized, five-arm trial involving 1,118 patients with previously untreated metastatic colorectal carcinoma. The design of this trial is depicted in Table 5. Preliminary results from this large study were available in 1996 for 1,021 patients (20). The addition of IFN-α to 5-FU was not superior to the reference arm of single-agent 5-FU (2,600 mg/m^2/week) and was more toxic.

Randomized trials of double modulation of 5-FU with IFN and leucovorin have also been conducted (Table 6). The results of a large, multicenter, randomized trial designed to identify the most effective biomodulating agent of 5-FU have been reported (21). 5-FU was administered as a weekly 24-hour infusion of 2,600 mg per m^2 per week in combination with either leucovorin or IFN, or both. After a preliminary toxicity assessment, the double modulation arm was halted. Response rates for

TABLE 4. WADLER REGIMEN FOR METASTATIC COLORECTAL CANCER

5-Fluorouracil, 750 mg/m^2
    Continuous i.v. infusion, d 1–5
    i.v. bolus starting d 15, q weekly
Interferon-α, 9 MU
    s.c., t.i.w., continuously

patients who received 5-FU and leucovorin were significantly higher than for those who received 5-FU and IFN (44% versus 18%; *p* <.05), as was median survival (16.2 months versus 12.7 months; *p* = .02). Toxicity was worse for the IFN-treated patients.

The Hellenic Cooperative Oncology Group trial randomized 106 previously untreated patients with metastatic colorectal cancer to either bolus 5-FU, 450 mg per m^2, and leucovorin, 200 mg per m^2 or the same regimen with IFN-α-2b, 5 MU s.c. three times weekly (22). Objective responses were 7.8% and 9.8%, respectively. Not only was median survival significantly better for the single modulation arm (10.1 months versus 7.2 months), but toxicity was also worse for the patients treated with IFN. The authors concluded that double modulation of 5-FU with IFN and leucovorin is worse than single modulation with leucovorin. The Colorectal Working Party of the United Kingdom Medical Council conducted a randomized, multi-center trial of 5-FU and leucovorin on a 2-week cycle with or without IFN-α-2a administered every other day throughout the treatment period. In 205 assessable patients, the overall RRs and survival were virtually identical (23). A quality-of-life analysis showed a worse quality-of-life for IFN-treated patients. Another trial using IFN-α-2c also showed no significant difference in RRs or survival in an interim analysis.

5-FU and IFN was compared to 5-FU and leucovorin in a randomized trial of 142 patients. A trend to improved survival was noted for the leucovorin-treated patients (25). A larger trial of 496 patients with a similar design showed similar RRs for the two regimens and similar OS (26). Of note, more patients treated with IFN withdrew from treatment due to side effects.

TABLE 5. INTERGROUP TRIAL OF BIOMODULATION OF 5-FLUOROURACIL (5-FU)

A. 5-FU, 2,600 mg/m^2/wk (24-hr infusion)
B. PALA, 250 mg/m^2/d
    5-FU, 2,600 mg/m^2/wk (24-hr infusion), b.i.d.
C. 5-FU, 600 mg/m^2/wk
    Leucovorin (oral), 125 mg/m^2/hr × 4 before FU
D. 5-FU, 600 mg/m^2/wk
    Leucovorin, 600 mg/m^2/wk
E. 5-FU, 750 mg/m^2/d × 5 d, c.i.v., followed by 750 mg/m^2/wk, i.v.
    IFN-α-2a, 9 MU t.i.w., s.c.

c.i.v., continuous intravenous infusion; IFN, interferon; PALA, *N*-phosphonacetyl-L-aspartic acid.

TABLE 6. OTHER RANDOMIZED TRIALS OF MODULATION OF 5-FLUOROURACIL IN ADVANCED COLORECTAL CANCER

Author (Reference)	Regimen	Patients	Response (%)	Survival	Comment
Kreuser (52)	FU/FA	129	—	55 d	p = .06, preliminary results
	FU/IFN			185 d	
Di Costanzo (53)	FU/HU/FA	232	29	NR	Preliminary results
	FU/HU/IFN		9		
Man et al. (26)	FU/IFN	496	21	11 mo	p = NS
	FU/FA		18	11.3 mo	
Moser (24)	FU/FA	218	25	13	p = .07
	FU/FA/IFN		38	10	
Colucci (54)	FU/FA	203	23	NR	Preliminary results
	FU/FA/IFN		30		
Barone (55)	FU/FA	67	18	18 mo	Preliminary results
	FU/FA/IFN	58	26	Overall	
Kosmidis et al. (22)	FU/FA	106	7.8	10.1 mo	p = .0189
	FU/FA/IFN		9.8	7.2 mo	
Seymour et al. (23)	FU/FA	260	27	10 mo	p = NS
	FU/FA/IFN		28	Overall	
Kohne et al. (21)	FU/FA	236	44	16.2 mo	p = NS
	FU/IFN		18	12.7 mo	Arm C dropped early for
	FU/FA/IFN		27	19.6 mo	toxicity

FA, folinic acid; FU, fluorouracil; HU, hydroxyurea; IFN, interferon; NR, not reported; NS, not significant.

As expected, second-line therapy for metastatic colorectal cancer with 5-FU and IFN combinations with or without leucovorin have been uniformly unsuccessful (Table 7) (10,29). Hepatic arterial infusion of IFN-α-2b and 5-FU was tested in 48 patients with liver metastases from colorectal cancer refractory to systemic 5-FU and leucovorin. A response was obtained in 33% of patients (median response duration, 7 months) (28).

Based on the results of these mature, randomized trials, it is evident that the initial promise of combination therapy 5-FU and IFN has not been confirmed, and this regimen can no longer be recommended for metastatic colorectal cancer. It also appears that regimens of 5-FU modulation using leucovorin are either superior to (or no better than) regimens of double modulation with IFN and leucovorin. Most trials have shown worse toxicity or quality-of-life for IFN-treated patients.

Few data regarding other IFN-containing biologic regimens for colorectal cancer exist. IFN-based therapy has been combined with IL-2 in two small phase 2 trials with disappointing results (Table 8). Other chemotherapy regimens with IFN also have been unsuccessful (29).

TABLE 7. SALVAGE THERAPY FOR ADVANCED COLORECTAL CANCER

Author (Reference)	No. of Patients	Response (%)	Duration (Mo)
John (36)	9	11	4
Ridolfi et al. (27)	21	1	8
Findlay (9)	64	8	2.5
Bracarda (50)	31	23	4.8
Loffler (51)	55	34	5.2
Patt et al. (28)	48	33	7
Perez et al. (10)	34	6	3

Adjuvant Therapy of Colorectal Cancer

Based on the initial promising phase 2 results of 5-FU biomodulation with IFN and the benefit from leucovorin-modulated 5-FU adjuvant therapy shown in National Surgical Adjuvant Breast and Bowel Project protocol C-03, the NSABP initiated a randomized trial of 5-FU and leucovorin with or without IFN in 1991 (NSABP Trial C0-5). Data are available for 2,176 patients with Dukes' B or C colon carcinoma who were entered through February 1994. The study design is shown in Table 4. At 4 years of follow-up, disease-free survival is virtually identical for the two arms (70% for the experimental arm versus 69% for the controls), as is OS (81% versus 80%). Apart from toxicity, which was worse for patients treated with IFN, no other significant differences between the two treatment groups occurred (30). The only other randomized trial of biomodulation in the adjuvant setting was conducted by the Italian Cooperative Oncology Group in 1995. The aim of this study was to evaluate the impact of the addition of levamisole or IFN-α-2b to the combination of 5-FU and leucovorin on the OS and disease-free survival of Dukes' B and C colon cancer. The 5-FU/leucovorin arm was dropped halfway through the trial secondary to poor patient accrual. Only toxicologic data have to date been reported and are worse for the patients who received IFN (31).

TABLE 8. INTERFERON AND INTERLEUKIN-2 IN ADVANCED COLORECTAL CARCINOMA

Author (Reference)	No. of Patients	Response (%)	Survival (Mo)
Hjelm (48)	15	0	13
Goey (49)	43	14	11

TABLE 9. CISPLATIN- AND INTERFERON-BASED CHEMOTHERAPY FOR ESOPHAGUS CANCER

Author (Reference)	Regimen	No. of Patients	Response (%)	Survival (Mo)
Ilson et al. (60)	C/FU/IFN	27	50	NR
Temeck et al. (58)	C/FU/FA/IFN	11	27	11.8
Wadler et al. (59)	C/FU/IFN	23	65	8.6
Pai et al. (61)	C/FU/IFN	26	73	6

C, cisplatin; FA, folinic acid; FU, fluorouracil; IFN, interferon; NR, not reported.

ESOPHAGUS CANCER

Two groups of patients have been the focus of IFN-based modulation of chemotherapy for carcinoma of the esophagus. In addition to the more traditional group with metastatic or unresectable disease, there are those patients in whom a neoadjuvant chemotherapy approach before to planned surgery has been attempted. The goal in this latter group is ostensibly to improve pathologic cure rates and OS by eradicating micrometastatic disease.

IFN combined with 5-FU in a regimen identical to that originally described for colorectal cancer has been tested in two phase 2 studies (56,57). Responses were noted 26% of the time on the average and lasted approximately 6 months. The demonstrated single-agent activity of cisplatin has led to its incorporation in combination regimens with IFN-α. Results from at least four phase 2 trials are available (Table 9) (58–61). Although RRs as high as 73% have been reported, small numbers of patients have been treated, and follow-up is short. Toxicity has been considerable. No difference appears to exist between adenocarcinomas and squamous cell carcinomas with regard to response or survival. The activity of *cis*-retinoic acid in squamous cell carcinoma of the skin and cervix was the impetus behind its combination with IFN-α. No responses were observed in 23 patients, many of whom had previously received chemotherapy (60,62).

An aggressive phase 1–2 trial of neoadjuvant cisplatin, 5-FU, IFN-α-2b, and radiation therapy was tested in 45 patients with potentially resectable adeno- or squamous-cell carcinoma (63). Forty-one patients completed chemoradiotherapy; all but four went on to attempted curative resection. Thirty-six of these 37 patients underwent curative esophagectomy, 80% of whom

were pathologically free of tumors. Median survival for the group as a whole was 27 months with a 2-year survival of 52%. The authors concluded that although this was an effective regimen, the contribution of IFN was unclear.

In summary, it is not known if IFN has an impact on the treatment of resectable or metastatic esophageal cancer.

GASTRIC CANCER

As with other malignancies of the gastrointestinal tract, IFN has no single-agent activity in gastric cancer. A phase 1 trial of FU and IFN-α in this disease established a lower dose of IFN (3 MU s.c., three times weekly) in combination with FU as compared with the original regimen for colorectal cancer (64). Experience with IFN-chemotherapy combinations in gastric cancer is limited to small phase 2 trials reported mainly in abstract form (Table 10). An Eastern Cooperative Oncology Group trial of FU, folinic acid, and IFN in 27 patients with metastatic gastric carcinoma produced three PRs of 16, 23, and 33 weeks' duration (25). Grade III and IV toxicities occurred in up to 36% of patients. Median progression-free survival and OS were 2.5 and 7.8 months, respectively. The addition of etoposide to FU, IFN, and folinic acid produced a 73% RR in one trial (65) and 22% in another (66). Other regimens have included cisplatin, epidoxorubicin, and *N*-phosphonacetyl-L-aspartic acid (67–69). Once again, no conclusions regarding the efficacy of IFN-α in gastric cancer can be drawn.

CANCER OF THE PANCREAS AND NEUROENDOCRINE TUMORS

The outlook for advanced or metastatic pancreatic cancer remains dismal. Several investigators have attempted FU-based regimens in this disease without major success. FU has been combined with IFN in two studies (73,74). In 52 previously untreated patients, three PRs (5%) were observed. Toxicity was substantial, with 19 of 49 patients in one study experiencing grade III or IV mucositis, diarrhea, granulocytopenia, and fatigue. Both studies concluded that this regimen had no efficacy in advanced pancreatic cancer.

TABLE 10. INTERFERON AND CHEMOTHERAPY IN GASTRIC CANCER

Author (Reference)	Regimen	No. of Patients	Response (%)	Survival (Mo)
Lee et al. (64)	FU/IFN	14	31	—
Pazdur et al. (70)	FU/IFN	44	25	—
Jager-Arand et al. (71)	FU/FA/IFN	41	41	—
Loffler et al. (65)	FU/FA/IFN/E	30	73	15.1
Maiello et al. (68)	FU/IFN/F	39	33	6 (duration of response)
Hudes et al. (72)	FU/FA/IFN	27	13	7.8
Wadler et al. (69)	FU/IFN/PALA	23	18	14
Ajani et al. (67)	FU/C/IFN	30	40	NR
Alabiso et al. (66)	FU/FA/IFN/E	24	26	NR

C, cisplatin; E, etoposide; FA, folinic acid; FU, fluorouracil; IFN, interferon; PALA, *N*-phosphonacetyl-L-aspartic acid.

TABLE 11. FLUOROURACIL, INTERFERON, AND LEUCOVORIN IN PANCREATIC CANCER

Author (Reference)	No. of Patients	Response (%)
Pazdur et al. (73)	13	23
Knuth et al. (81)	32	12
Scheithauer et al. (82)	24	8
Schneider et al. (83)	21	0
Bernhard et al. (75)	57	14

Experience with FU, IFN, and leucovorin in pancreatic cancer is summarized in Table 11. One hundred and forty-seven patients were treated on these trials, with RRs of 0% to 23%. In the largest of these trials (57 patients), eight partial responses lasting 2 to 10 months were reported; median survival for all patients was 10 months (75). Lung metastases appeared to be the most responsive to therapy. Although side effects of IFN (fever and fatigue) occurred in up to 56% of patients, 22 out of 36 patients (60%) with preexisting tumor-related pain experienced significant symptom palliation, regardless of response. Oral *cis*-retinoic acid was combined with IFN-α in a phase 2 trial of 26 patients with unresectable adenocarcinoma of the pancreas; one PR was observed (76).

Interferon has been used singly or in combination with FU or octreotide for the treatment of advanced neuroendocrine carcinoma (77–80). It is difficult to judge efficacy in these trials because several have used biochemical parameters (50% reduction in hormone secretion) as surrogate markers for response. Data are preliminary and no conclusions regarding survival can be drawn.

HEPATOCELLULAR CARCINOMA AND CANCER OF THE BILIARY TRACT

Initial enthusiasm for the use of IFN-α in hepatocellular carcinoma was kindled by a randomized controlled trial of IFN-α versus best supportive care in 71 patients with inoperable hepatocellular carcinoma (84). A doubling of survival (14 weeks versus 7 weeks) was reported for the treated group, with 31% objective responses. Phase 2 data for IFN-based therapy for hepatocellular carcinoma has, however, been less than favorable. Two trials reported results of FU with IFN. One used a continuous infusion of FU (750 mg per m^2 per day for 5 days) with IFN-α, 5 MU (days 1, 3, and 5) once every 14 days (85). The other tested a 500 mg per m^2 weekly bolus and the same dose of IFN-α (87). PRs were observed in four of 35 patients. Combining doxorubicin with IFN has also not been rewarding, with three PRs in 46 patients (87,88).

Experience with cancers of the biliary tract (gallbladder and bile duct) is even more limited. Thirty-five patients were treated with a 5-day continuous infusion of 5-FU and IFN-α-2b, 5 MU per m^2 every other day (89). One PR was observed in 11 patients and median survival time was 12 months.

HEAD AND NECK CANCER

The combination of cisplatin and 5-FU is still the most widely used chemotherapeutic regimen for recurrent and metastatic head and neck cancer (HNC). In addition to its ability to modulate FU, IFN-α has also potentiated the effects of cisplatin in a xenograft mouse model, leading to several phase 2 trials evaluating the combination of IFN-α, cisplatin, and 5-FU for HNC, with initially encouraging results. A 47% RR was reported in a phase 1–2 pilot study with acceptable toxicity. Cisplatin, 20 mg per m^2 per day; 5-FU 200 mg per m^2 per day; and IFN, 3 MU per day for 5 days, were administered to 14 patients with recurrent or metastatic HNC. Two complete responses and two PRs were observed (90). A slight variation of the same regimen was tested in 29 patients with an overall RR of 30% (91). A more prolonged infusion of FU (1,000 mg per m^2 per day for 96 hours) with cisplatin, 100 mg per m^2 on day 1, and IFN-α-2a, 5 MU s.c. days 1 through 4, repeated every 21 days, was reported for 52 patients with advanced HNC. Nine responses were reported, with an estimated median survival of 5 months. The authors concluded that this regimen did not appear to be superior to chemotherapy alone (92). Other phase 2 regimens have included PALA, FU, IFN (93), and the cisplatin, fluorouracil, and leucovorin–induction regimen followed by hydroxyurea, fluorouracil, and concurrent radiation therapy (94). The latter trial included 65 patients with previously untreated disease and reported an overall RR of 86% (complete response, 51%; PR, 35%). As expected, toxicity was considerable and led to treatment-related death in five patients.

A randomized trial of cisplatin, 100 mg per m^2 on day 1, 5-FU, 1,000 mg per m^2 per day for 96 hours, without (arm A) or with (arm B) IFN-α, 3 MU per day s.c. days 1 through 5, was conducted in 244 patients with recurrent or metastatic HNC (95). No significant difference in RRs (47% versus 38%) or survival (6.3 months versus 6.0 months, arm A versus arm B, respectively) was reported. Based on the results of this large phase 3 trial and the added toxicity of IFN in this patient population, the enthusiasm for IFN-containing regimens for this disease has waned.

LUNG CANCER

Phase 2 data in non–small-cell lung cancer is summarized in Table 12. Combinations have in general included variations of cisplatin, ifosfamide, and mitomycin with IFN. Most are small phase 2 studies with immature data. The largest experience is from a European multicenter trial of cisplatin with IFN in which a 27% RR and a median survival of 6.4 months was observed in 55 patients with non–small-cell lung cancer (96). IFN also has been combined with retinoids (*cis*-retinoic acid and all *trans*-retinoic acid). Data are available for 111 patients and

TABLE 12. INTERFERON (IFN) IN HEPATOCELLULAR CARCINOMA

Author (Reference)	Regimen	No. of Patients	Response
Patt et al. (85)	FU/IFN	18	3/18
Mughal et al. (86)	FU/IFN	17	1/17
Kardinal et al. (87)	FU/A	31	1/31
Sangro et al. (88)	FU/D	15	2/15

A, adriamycin; D, doxorubicin; FU, fluorouracil.

TABLE 13. INTERFERON-α IN NON–SMALL-CELL LUNG CANCER

Author (Reference)	Regimen	No. of Patients	Response (%)
Bowman (99)	C/IFN-α	60	30
Adizzoni (100)	MIP	23	8.8
	MIP/IFN-α-2b	27	7.4
	C/carboplatin	43	14
Garaci et al. (101)	C/E/thymosin-α/ IFN-α-2a	60	40
Hasturk et al. (102)	C/E/IFN-α	38	34
Kataja (96)	C/IFN-α-2a	55	27

C, cisplatin; E, etoposide; IFN, interferon; MIP, mitomycin, ifosfamide, cisplatin.

only a few responses were noted (Table 13). Results of two randomized trials have not indicated a benefit for IFN-containing regimens over chemotherapy alone. A phase 3 trial of 60 patients treated with cyclophosphamide, epirubicin, and cisplatin, with or without IFN-α, showed an inferior survival for the IFN-treated patients (5.5 versus 6.0 months, p = .045) (97), despite an increased RR (19% versus 8%, p = .042). A three-arm randomized phase 2 trial of chemotherapy with cisplatin (60 mg per m^2 on day 1) and etoposide (100 mg per m^2 on days 1, 3, and 5) once every 28 days or the same chemotherapy with IFN-γ (0.2 mg per m^2 three times weekly) or IFN-α-2c (6 MU s.c. three times weekly) did not show a difference in responses (6/22, 5/21, and 6/18, respectively) or survival (7, 6, and 7 months, respectively) between the different treatments (98).

Efforts in small-cell lung cancer have looked mainly at maintenance IFN in patients who respond to induction chemotherapy. Results of four large, randomized trials are available; only one showed a benefit for IFN treatment (Table 14).

BLADDER CANCER

Research with the use of IFN in bladder cancer has addressed two areas: prevention of recurrence of superficial bladder cancer after resection and the combination of IFN with chemotherapy for advanced disease. The presence of IFN-α receptors has been demonstrated in normal bladder urothelium and with increased frequency in malignant tissue (107), providing a rationale for its use in intravesical therapy for bladder cancer. Bacillus Calmette-Guérin (BCG) has been widely adopted as the standard prophylactic treatment for superficial bladder cancer to prevent recurrence. IFN-α has been shown to synergize with BCG in bladder cancer cell lines, which has led to efforts to combine the two agents in phase 2 trials. Several randomized trials comparing IFN to BCG and other agents have been completed and analyzed (Table 15). In general, results have not been encouraging and seem to indicate that intravesical BCG and other chemotherapeutic agents are superior to IFN in the prevention of superficial bladder cancer. Doses and schedules of intravesical IFN have ranged from 50 MU to 100 MU, usually administered once a week and retained in the bladder for 2 hours. Intravesical IFN-α-2b, 50 MU per week, was compared to mitomycin, 40 mg per week, in 287 patients with superficial bladder cancer after transurethral resection (109). Mitomycin was superior with regard to recurrence rate and median time to recurrence (36 months versus 21 months). Local toxicity was higher for patients treated with mitomycin. BCG (150 mg in 50 mL saline) was compared to IFN-α-2a (54 MU) in a prospective, randomized multicenter trial of 122 patients with recurrent superficial transitional cell cancer of the bladder (110). A statistically significant advantage in terms of recurrence and time to progression was found for the BCG group (p = .001).

CONCLUSIONS

Despite provocative initial results in phase 2 trials, the promise of IFN-α–mediated biomodulation has not been substantiated by randomized phase 3 studies. It appears that in epithelial tumors in general, the added toxicity of this agent does not justify its use outside the context of clinical trials. Further research into the mechanism of action of the IFNs and elucidation of the molecular and immunologic basis behind biomodulation may help provide a rationale for a more tailored approach to therapy with this drug in epithelial cancers.

TABLE 14. RANDOMIZED TRIALS OF INTERFERON (IFN) IN SMALL-CELL LUNG CANCER

Author (Reference)	Regimen	No. of Patients	Survival (Mo)	Comment
Kelly et al. (103)	C/E/RT, followed by IFN or obs	140	16 (obs) 13 (IFN)	Patients randomized after response to induction p = NS
Mattson et al. (104)	C/E C/E/nIFN-α (Finniferon) C/E/IFN-α-2a	130	NR	Up-front randomization
Mattson et al. (105)	Cy/V/E/RT Followed by IFN or Cy/A/C or obs	237	11 (IFN) 11(Cy/A/C) 10 (obs)	Patients randomized after response to induction. No difference in survival.
Prior et al. (106)	Cy/A/C alternating with E/C is followed by IFN or obs	77	11 (IFN) 9 (obs)	p = .02 for survival

A, adriamycin; C, cisplatin; Cy, cyclophosphamide; E, epidoxorubicin; obs, observation; RT, radiation therapy; V, vincristine.

TABLE 15. RANDOMIZED INTRAVESICAL INTERFERON (IFN) TRIALS FOR SUPERFICIAL BLADDER CANCER

Author (Reference)	Regimen	No. of Patients	Result
Boccardo (111)	IFN	287	TTP: 21 mo
	Mitomycin		TTP: 36 mo
Jimenez-Cruz (110)	BCG	122	RFS: 61%
	IFN		RFS: 44% (*p* = .001)
Kalble (112)	BCG	78	Recurrence: 15.6%
	IFN		Recurrence: 60% (*p* = .03)
Raitanen (113)	Observation	81	
	Epirubicin		RFS: 44%
	Epirubicin + IFN		RFS: 63%
Portillo (72)	IFN	90	Recurrence: 53.8%
	Placebo		Recurrence: 51.3% (*p* = NS)
Tizzani (114)	Mitomycin	210	More recurrences in sequential group (*p* <.05)
	Mitomycin + IFN (sequential)		
Rajala (115)	Observation	283	Recurrence: 54%
	IFN (single-dose)		Recurrence: 54.5%
	Epirubicin (single-dose)		Recurrence: 29% (*p* <.01)

BCG, bacillus Calmette-Guerin; NS, not significant; RFS, relapse-free survival; TTP, time to peak.

REFERENCES

1. Agarwala SS, Kirkwood JM. Interferons in the therapy of solid tumors. *Oncology* 1994;51:129–136.
2. Neefe JR, Silgals R, Schein PS. Minimal activity of recombinant clone α-interferon in metastatic colon cancer. *J Biol Res Mod* 1984;3(4):366–370.
3. Gilewski TA, Golomb HM. Interferon in the treatment of malignant disease. In: Zenser TV, Coe RM, eds. *Cancer and aging: progress in research and treatment.* New York: Springer, 1989:46–85.
4. Foon KA. Biological response modifiers: the new immunotherapy. *Cancer Res* 1989;49:1621–1639.
5. Schulman J, Czejka MJ, Schernthaner G, Fogl U, Jager W, Micksche M. Influence of interferon alfa-2b with or without folinic acid on pharmacokinetics of fluorouracil. *Semin Oncol* 1992;19:93–97.
6. Wadler S, Schwartz EL, Goldman M, et al. Fluorouracil and recombinant alfa-2a-interferon: an active regimen against advanced colorectal carcinoma. *J Clin Oncol* 1989;7(12):1769–1775.
7. Kemeny N, Younes A. Alfa-2a interferon and 5-fluorouracil for advanced colorectal carcinoma: the Memorial Sloan-Kettering experience. *Semin Oncol* 1992;19:171–175.
8. Barzacchi MC, Nobile MT, Sanguineti O, Rosso R. Treatment of metastatic colorectal carcinoma with lymphoblastoid interferon and 5-fluorouracil: data of a phase II study. *Anticancer Res* 1994;14:2147–2150.
9. Findlay M, Hill A, Cunningham D, Carter R. Protracted venous infusion 5-fluorouracil and interferon-alpha in advanced and refractory colorectal cancer. *Ann Oncol* 1994;5(3):239–243.
10. Perez JE, Lacava JA, Dominguez ME, Romero AO, et al. Biomodulation with sequential intravenous IFN-alfa-2b and 5-fluorouracil as second-line treatment in patients with advanced colorectal cancer. *J Interferon Cytokine Res* 1998;18:565–569.
11. Patt YZ, Hoque A, Lozano R, et al. Phase II trial of hepatic arterial infusion of flourouracil and recombinant human interferon alfa-2b for liver metastases of colorectal cancer refractory to systemic flourouracil and leucovorin. *J Clin Oncol* 1997;15:1432–1438.
12. Grem JL, McAtee N, Murphy RF, et al. A pilot study of interferon alfa-2a in combination with fluorouracil plus high-dose leucovorin in metastatic gastrointestinal carcinoma. *J Clin Oncol* 1991;9(10): 1811–1820.
13. Yee LK, Allegra CJ, Steinberg SM. Decreased catabolism of 5-fluorouracil in peripheral blood monocytes during therapy with 5-fluorouracil, leucovorin and interferon alpha-2a. *J Natl Cancer Inst* 1992;84:1820–1825.
14. Piga A, Cascinu S, Latini L, et al. A Phase II randomized trial of 5-fluorouracil with or without interferon-alpha-2a in advanced colorectal cancer. *Br J Cancer* 1996;74:971–974.
15. Hill M, Norman A, Cunningham D, Hickish T. Royal Marsden phase III trial of fluorouracil with or without interferon alfa-2b in advanced colorectal cancer. *J Clin Oncol* 1995;13:1297–1302.
16. Hill M, Norman A, Cunningham D, Evans C. Impact of protracted venous infusion fluorouracil with or without interferon alfa-2b on tumor response, survival, and quality of life in advanced colorectal cancer. *J Clin Oncol* 1995;13:2317–2323.
17. Greco F, Figlin R, York M, Yap AKL. Phase III randomized study to compare interferon alfa-2a in combination with fluorouracil versus fluorouracil alone in patients with advanced colorectal cancer. *J Clin Oncol* 1996;14:2674–2681.
18. Dufour P, Husseini F, Dreyfus B, Oberling F. 5-fluorouracil versus 5-fluorouracil plus alpha-interferon as treatment of metastatic colorectal carcinoma. A randomized study. *Ann Oncol* 1996;7(6):575–579.
19. Palmeri S, Meli M, Danova M, et al. 5-Fluorouracil plus interferon alfa-2a compared to 5-fluorouracil alone in the treatment of advanced colon carcinoma: a multicentric study. *J Cancer Res Clin Oncol* 1998;124:191–198.
20. O'Dwyer PJ, Ryan LM, Valone FH, et al. Phase III trial of biochemical modulation of 5-fluorouracil by iv or oral leucovorin or by interferon in advanced colorectal: an ECOG/CALGB phase III trial. *Proc Am Soc Clin Oncol* 1996;15:207.
21. Kohne C-H, Schoffski P, Wilke H, et al. Effective biomodulation by leucovorin of high-dose infusion fluorouracil given as weekly 24-hour infusion: results of a randomized trial in patients with advanced colorectal cancer. *J Clin Oncol* 1998;16:418–426.
22. Kosmidis PA, Tsavaris N, Skarlos D, et al. Fluorouracil and leucovorin with or without interferon alfa-2b in advanced colorectal cancer: analysis of a prospective randomized phase III trial. *J Clin Oncol* 1996;14:2682–2687.
23. Seymour MT, Slevin ML, Kerr DJ, et al. Randomized trial assessing the addition of interferon alfa-2a to fluorouracil and leucovorin in advanced colorectal cancer. *J Clin Oncol* 1996;14:2280–2288.
24. Moser R, Hausmaninger H, Ludwig H, Samonigg H. 5-Fluorouracil and folinic acid with or without alpha-2c interferon in the treatment of metastatic colorectal cancer: preliminary results of multicenter prospective randomized phase III trial. *Onkologie* 1995;18:131–135.
25. Kreuser E-D, Streit M, Kuchler T, et al. A multicenter randomized trial with the assessment of the quality of life in patients with meta-

static colorectal carcinoma given with folinic acid or interferon-alfa-2b as a modulator of 5-fluorouracil. *Proc Am Soc Clin Oncol* 1995;14:202.

26. Man A, Levi J, Bell D, Cockey L, et al. Phase III randomized study of two fluorouracil combinations with either interferon alfa-2a or leucovorin for advanced colorectal cancer. *J Clin Oncol* 1995;13:921–928.

27. Ridolfi R, Maltoni R, Ricobon A, et al. A Phase II study of advanced colorectal cancer patients treated with combination 5-fluorouracil plus leucovorin and subcutaneous interleukin-2 plus alpha interferon. *J Chemother* 1994;6:265–271.

28. Patt YZ, Hoque A, Lozano R, et al. Phase II trial of hepatic arterial infusion of fluorouracil and recombinant human interferon alfa-2b for liver metastases of colorectal cancer refractory to systemic fluorouracil and leucovorin. *J Clin Oncol* 1997;15:1432–1438.

29. Ajani JA, Abbruzzese JL, Markowitz AB, Patt YZ, Daugherty K. Phase II study of etoposide and alpha-interferon in patients with advanced measurable colorectal carcinoma. *Invest New Drugs* 1993;11:67–69.

30. Wolmark N, Bryant J, Smith R, et al. Adjuvant 5-fluorouracil and leucovorin with or without interferon alfa-2a in colon carcinoma: National Surgical Adjuvant Breast and Bowel Project Protocol C-05. *J Natl Cancer Inst* 1998;90:1810–1816.

31. Tonelli F, Periti P, Mazzei T, et al. Adjuvant therapy of colorectal carcinoma with 5-fluorouracil (5-FU) and L-folinic acid (L-LV) alone or combined with levamisole (LEV) or interferon-alfa 2a (IFN-alfa 2a). Preliminary toxicological results of a multicenter study of the gruppo oncologico-chirurgio cooperativo Italian (GOCCI). *Proc Am Soc Clin Oncol* 1995;14:219.

32. Pazdur R, Moore FD Jr, Bready B. Modulation of fluorouracil with recombinant alfa interferon: MD Anderson clinical trial. *Semin Oncol* 1992;19:176–179.

33. Weh HJ, Platz D, Braumann D, et al. Phase II trial of 5-fluorouracil and recombinant interferon alfa-2b in metastatic colorectal carcinoma. *Eur J Cancer* 1992;28A:1820–1823.

34. Diaz Rubio E, Jimeno J, Comps C, et al. Treatment of advanced colorectal cancer with recombinant interferon alpha and fluorouracil: activity in liver metastasis. *Cancer Invest* 1992;10:259–264.

35. Wadler S, Lembersky B, Atkins M, Kirkwood J, Petrelli N. Phase II trial of fluorouracil and recombinant interferon alfa-2a in patients with colorectal carcinoma: an Eastern Cooperative Oncology Group study. *J Clin Oncol* 1991;19:1806–1810.

36. John WJ, Neefe JR, Macdonald JS, Cantrell J Jr, Smith M. 5-fluorouracil and interferon-alpha-2a in advanced colorectal cancer. *Cancer* 1993;72:3191–3195.

37. Grem JL, Jordan E, Robson ME, et al. Phase II study of fluorouracil, leucovorin, and interferon alfa-2a in metastatic colorectal carcinoma. *J Clin Oncol* 1993;11(9):1737–1745.

38. Schmoll HJ, Kohne-Wompner CH, Hiddemann W, et al. Interferon alpha-2b, 5-fluorouracil, and folinic acid combination therapy in advanced colorectal cancer: preliminary results of a phase I/II trial. *Semin Oncol* 1992;19(2)[Suppl 3]:191–196.

39. Punt CJ, Burbouts JT, Croles JJ, van Liessum PA, de Mulder PH, Kamm Y. Continuous infusion of high-dose 5-fluorouracil in combination with leucovorin and recombinant interferon-alpha-2b in patients with advanced colorectal cancer: a multicenter phase II study. *Cancer* 1993;72:2111.

40. Sobrero A, Nobile MT, Guglielmi A, et al. Phase II study of 5-fluorouracil plus leucovorin and interferon alpha-2b in advance colorectal cancer. *Eur J Cancer* 1992;28A:850–852.

41. Cascinu S, Fedeli A, Fedeli SL, Catalano G. Double modulation of 5-fluorouracil leucovorin and cyclic low dose interferon alpha-2b in advanced colorectal cancer patients. *Ann Oncol* 1992;3:491.

42. Labianca R, Giaccone G, Barni S, et al. Double modulation of 5-fluorouracil in advanced colorectal cancer with low-dose interferon-alfa-2b and folinic acid. The Giscad Experience. *Eur J Cancer* 1994;30A:1611–1616.

43. Marshall ME, Tangen CM, Berenberg JL, et al. Treatment of advanced colorectal carcinoma with 5 fluorouracil, leucovorin and Roferon-A: a Southwest Oncology Study Group study. *Cancer Bio-ther* 1994;9:301–304.

44. Buter J, Sinnige HAM, Sleijfer DT, Mulder NH. 5-fluorouracil/leucovorin/interferon alpha-2a in patients with advanced colorectal cancer. *Cancer* 1995;75(5):1072–1076.

45. Moore MJ, Kaizer L, Erlichman C, Fine S. A clinical and pharmacological study of 5-fluorouracil, leucovorin and interferon alfa in advanced colorectal cancer. *Cancer Chemother* 1995;37:86–90.

46. Kohne C-H, Wilke H, Hiddemann W, et al. Phase II evaluation of 5-fluorouracil plus folinic acid and alpha 2b-interferon in metastatic colorectal cancer. *Oncology* 1997;54:96–101.

47. Tournigand C, Louvet C, de Gramont A, et al. Bimonthly high dose leucovorin and 5-fluorouracil 48-hour infusion with interferon-alpha-2a in patients with advanced colorectal carcinoma. *Cancer* 1997;79:1094–1099.

48. Hjelm AL, Ragnhammar P, Fagerberg J, Wersäll JP. Subcutaneous interleukin-2 and alpha interferon in advanced colorectal carcinoma. A phase II study. *Cancer Biother* 1995;10:5–12.

49. Goey SH, Gratama JW, Primorse JN, Stoter G. Interleukin-2 and interferon alpha-2a do not improve anti-tumour activity of 5-fluorouracil in advanced colorectal cancer. *Br J Cancer* 1996;74: 2018–2023.

50. Contu A, Bracarda S, Crino L, Tonato M II. Chemotherapy with cisplatin, 5-fluorouracil, L-folinic acid and r-interferon-alpha-2a in advanced, 5-FU pretreated, colorectal carcinoma, phase I/II trial. *Ann Oncol* 1994;5[Suppl 8]:50.

51. Loffler TM, Huck L, Hausamen TU. Weekly high-dose continuous infusion 5-fluorouracil, leucovorin and interferon-alpha (LIF) as second-line chemotherapy in metastatic colorectal cancer. *Ann Oncol* 1994;5:55.

52. Kreuser ED, Kuchler T, Zwingers T, Thiel E. A multicenter prospective randomized trial with assessment of quality of life in patients with metastatic colorectal carcinoma comparing interferon alfa-2b and folinic acid as modulators of 5-fluorouracil. *Onkologie* 1994;17:78–84.

53. Di Costanzo F, El-Taani H, Marzola M, Angiona S. Hydroxyurea (HU), high dose folinic acid (L-FA) ABD 5-FU vs. HU, 5-FU and interferon-alfa-2b (IFN) in advanced colorectal cancer (ACRC): a randomized trial of the Italian oncology group for clinical research (GOIRC). *Proc Am Soc Clin Oncol* 1995;14:208.

54. Colucci G, Maiello E, Gebbia V, Gebbia N. Fluorouracil (FU) and folinic acid (FA) alone or with alpha-2b interferon (IFN) in advanced colorectal cancer (ACC), a multicentric randomized study of the southern Italy oncology group (GOIM). *Eur J Cancer* 1995;31A[Suppl 5]:154–155.

55. Barone C, Cassano A, Pozzo C, Gasbarrini GB. The role of interferon-alpha-2b in the treatment of advanced colorectal cancer with folinic acid and 5-fluorouracil: a randomized study. *Gastroenterology* 1999;110(4):A488.

56. Kelsen D, Lovett D, Wong J, et al. Interferon alfa-2a and fluorouracil in the treatment of patients with advanced esophageal cancer. *J Clin Oncol* 1992;10:269–274.

57. Walder S, Fell S, Haynes H, Kaleya R, Rosenblit A, Wiernik PH. Treatment of carcinoma of the esophagus with 5-fluorouracil and recombinant alfa-2a-interferon. *Cancer* 1993;71:1730.

58. Temeck BK, Liebmann JE, Theodossiou C, et al. Phase II trial of 5-fluorouracil, leucovorin, interferon-alpha-2a and cisplatin as neoadjuvant chemotherapy for locally advanced esophageal carcinoma. *Cancer* 1996;77:2432–2439.

59. Wadler S, Haynes H, Beitler JJ, Wiernik PH, et al. Phase II clinical trial with 5-fluorouracil, recombinant interferon-alfa-2b, and cisplatin for patients with metastatic or regionally advanced carcinoma of the esophagus. *Cancer* 1996;78:30–34.

60. Ilson DH, Sirott M, Saltz L, Kelsen DP. A phase II trial of interferon alpha-2a, 5-fluorouracil, and cisplatin in patients with advanced esophageal carcinoma. *Cancer* 1995;75:2197–2202.

61. Pai C, Bazarbashi S, Rahal M, Ezzat A. Phase II study of cisplatinum, 5-fluorouracil and interferon-alfa-2b in advanced/metastatic epidermoid esophageal carcinoma. *Proc Am Soc Clin Oncol* 1998;17:301A.

62. Falkson G, Falkson G, Burger W, et al. A phase II study of 13-cis ret-

inoic acid and interferon alpha-2a in patients with inoperable squamous carcinoma of the esophagus. *Ann Oncol* 1994;5:84.

63. Posner MC, Gooding WE, Landreneau RJ, et al. Preoperative chemoradiotherapy for carcinoma of the esophagus and gastroesophageal junction. *Cancer J Sci Am* 1998;4:237–246.

64. Lee KH, Lee JS, Suh C, et al. Combination of fluorouracil and recombinant interferon alpha-2b in advanced gastric cancer. A phase I trial. *Am J Clin Oncol* 1992;15:141–145.

65. Loffler TM, Lohlein D, Hausamen TU. Chemotherapy of metastatic gastric carcinoma with weekly continuous infusion 5-fluorouracil, leucovorin, etoposide and interferon-alpha (LIFE). *Ann Oncol* 1994;5:79.

66. Alabiso O, Castiglione F, Destefanis M, Zanon C. Double modulation of 5-FU (F) made with leucovorin (L) and alpha-interferon (I) in combination with etoposide (E) (ELFI regimen) in the treatment of advanced gastric cancer (AGC). A phase II trial. *Preliminary Report Ann Oncol* 1999;7:51.

67. Ajani JA, Mansfield PF, Dumas P, et al. All chemotherapy (CT) preoperatively with cisplatin 5-FU and intron, (CFI) in patients (PTS) with potentially resectable gastric carcinoma (PRGC). *Proc Am Soc Clin Oncol* 1999;15:208.

68. Maiello E, Cifarelli RA, Gebbia V, et al. Folinic acid (FA), 5-fluorouracil (FU), epidoxorubicin (EPI) and interferon (IFN) in advanced gastric carcinoma. *Ann Oncol* 1994;5:87.

69. Walder S, Gleissner B, Hilgenfeld RU, et al. Phase II trial of N-(Phosphonoacetyl)-L-aspartate (PALA), 5-fluorouracil and recombinant interferon-alfa-2b in patients with advanced gastric carcinoma. *Eur J Cancer* 1996;32A:1254–1256.

70. Pazdur R, Ajani JA, Winn R, et al. A phase II trial of 5-fluorouracil and recombinant alpha-2a-interferon in previously untreated metastatic gastric carcinoma. *Cancer* 1992;69:882.

71. Jager-Arand E, Bernhard H, Klein O, et al. Combination 5-fluorouracil (FU), folinic acid (FA), and alpha-interferon-2b (IFN) in advanced gastric cancer. *Proc Am Soc Clin Oncol* 1993;12:192 (abst).

71a. Hudes G, Lipeitz S, Grem J, et al. Phase II study of interferon-alfa 2a (IFN) in combination with 5-fluorouracil (5-FU) plus calcium leucovorin (LV) in metastatic of recurrent gastric carcinoma: an Eastern Cooperative Oncology Group study. *Proc Am Clin Oncol* 1995;14:197.

72. Portillo J, Martin B, Hernandez R, et al. Results at 43 months' follow-up of a double-blind, randomized, prospective clinical trial using intravesical interferon alpha-2b in the prophylaxis of stage pT1 transitional cell carcinoma of the bladder. *Urology* 1997;49:187–190.

73. Pazdur R, Ajani JA, Abbruzzese JL, et al. Phase II evaluation of fluorouracil and recombinant alpha-2a-interferon in previously untreated patients with pancreatic adenocarcinoma. *Cancer* 1992;70:2073–2076.

74. John WJ, Flett MQ. Continuous venous infusion 5-fluorouracil and interferon-alpha in pancreatic carcinoma. *Am J Clin Oncol* 1998;21:146–150.

75. Bernhard H, Jager-Arand E, Knuth A, et al. Treatment of advanced pancreatic cancer with 5-fluorouracil, folinic acid and interferon alpha-2a: results of a phase II trial. *Br J Cancer* 1995;71:102–105.

76. Brembeck FH, Schoppmeyer K, Leupold U, et al. A phase II pilot trial of 13-cis retinoic acid and interferon-alpha in patients with advanced pancreatic carcinoma. *Cancer* 1998;83:2317–2323.

77. Fiasse S, Deprez P, Pauwels S. Is alpha-interferon (IF) useful in the treatment of metastatic neuro-endocrine tumors? *Gastroenterology* 1996;110(4):A511.

78. Nold R, Frank M, Kajdan U, et al. Combined treatment of metastatic endocrine gastroenteropancreatic tumors with octreotide and interferon-alpha. *Z Gastroenterol* 1994;32:193–197.

79. Saltz L, Kemeny N, Schwartz G, Kelsen D. A phase II trial of alpha-interferon and 5-fluorouracil in patients with advanced carcinoid and islet cell tumors. *Cancer* 1994;74:958–961.

80. Hughes MJ, Kerr DJ, Cassidy J, et al. A pilot study of combination therapy with interferon-alpha-2a and 5-fluorouracil in metastatic carcinoid and malignant endocrine pancreatic tumours. *Ann Oncol* 1996;7:208–210.

81. Knuth A, Bernhard H, Klein O, Meyer zum Buschenfelde KH. Combination fluorouracil, folinic acid, and interferon-alfa-2a: an active regimen in advanced pancreatic carcinoma. *Semin Oncol* 1992;19:211–214.

82. Scheithauer W, Pfeffel F, Kornek G, Marczell A, Wiltshke C, Funovics J. A phase II trial of 5-fluorouracil, leucovorin, and recombinant alpha-2b-interferon in advanced adenocarcinoma of the pancreas. *Cancer* 1992;70:1864–1866.

83. Schneider CJ, Vaughn DJ, Holroyde C, et al. Phase II trial of 5-FU, leucovorin, and interferon alpha 2a in metastatic pancreatic carcinoma: a Penn cancer clinical trials group (PCCTG) trial. *Proc Am Soc Clin Oncol* 1995;14:189.

84. Lai CL, Lau JY, Wu PC, et al. Recombinant interferon-alpha in inoperable hepatocellular carcinoma: a randomized controlled trial. *Hepatology* 1993;17:394.

85. Patt YZ, Noonan C, Pazdur R, Smith R, Levin B, Yoffe B. Phase II trial of 5-FU and R interferon-alpha (RIFN) in hepatocellular carcinoma (HCC). *Proc Am Soc Clin Oncol* 1991;10:(abst).

86. Mughal TI, Koreich OM. Interferon and 5-fluorouracil in the management of advanced hepatomas. *Can J Infect Dis* 1995;6:458.

87. Kardinal CG, Moertel CG, Wieand HS, et al. Combined doxorubicin and alpha-interferon therapy of advanced hepatocellular carcinoma. *Cancer* 1993;71:2190.

88. Sangro B, Herrero JI, Betes M, et al. Phase II trial of doxorubicin and interferon for hepatocellular carcinoma—(HCC). *J Hepatol* 1995;23:231.

89. Patt YZ, Jones DV, Hoque A, Charnsangavej C. Phase II trial of intravenous fluorouracil and subcutaneous interferon alfa-2b for biliary tract cancer. *J Clin Oncol* 1996;14:2311–2315.

90. Benasso M, Merlano M, Blengio F, et al. Concomitant alpha-interferon and chemotherapy in advanced squamous cell carcinoma of the head and neck. *Cancer Treat Update* 1994:234–236.

91. Huber MH, Shirinian M, Lippman SM, et al. Phase I/II study of cisplatin, 5-fluorouracil and alpha-interferon for recurrent carcinoma of the head and neck. *Invest New Drugs* 1994;12:223–229.

92. Hussain M, Benedetti J, Smith RE, et al. Evaluation of 96-hour infusion fluorouracil plus cisplatin in combination with alpha interferon for patients with advanced squamous cell carcinoma of the head and neck. *Cancer* 1995;76:1233–1237.

93. Langer CJ, Schaebler D, Sauter E, et al. Phase II study of N-phosphonoacetyl-L-aspartate, recombinant interferon-alpha, and fluorouracil infusion in advanced squamous cell carcinoma of the head and neck. *Head Neck Surg* 1998;20:385–391.

94. Vokes EE, Kies M, Haraf DJ, et al. Induction chemotherapy followed by concomitant chemoradiotherapy for advanced head and neck cancer: impact on the natural history of the disease. *J Clin Oncol* 1995;13:876–883.

95. Schrijvers D, Johnson J, Jiminez U, et al. Phase III trial of modulation of cisplatin/fluorouracil chemotherapy by interferon alfa-2b in patients with recurrent or metastatic head and neck cancer. *J Clin Oncol* 1998;16:1054–1059.

96. Kataja V, Yap A. Combination of cisplatin and interferon-alpha-2a (ROFERON-A) in patients with non-small cell lung cancer (NSCLC). An open phase II multicentre study. *Eur J Cancer* 1995;31A:35–40.

97. Ardizzoni A, Salvati F, Rosso R. Combination of chemotherapy and recombinant alpha-interferon in advanced non-small cell lung cancer: multicenter randomized FONICAP trial report. *Cancer* 1993;72:2929–2935.

98. Halme M, Maasilta PK, Pyhonen SO, Mattson KV. Interferons combined with chemotherapy in the treatment of stage III-IV non-small cell lung cancer—a randomized study. *Eur J Cancer* 1994;30A:11–15.

99. Bowman A, Fegusson RJ, Allan SG. Potentiation of cisplatin by alpha-interferon in advanced non-small cell lung cancer (NSCLC): a phase II study. *Ann Oncol* 1990;1:351–353.

100. Ardizzoni A, Addamo GF, Baldini E, Salvati F. Mitomycin-ifosfamide-cisplatinum (MIP) vs. MIP-interferon vs. cisplatinum-carboplatin in metastatic non-small-cell lung cancer: a FONICAP randomized phase II study. *Br J Cancer* 1995;71:115–119.

101. Garaci E, Lopez M, Bonsignore G, et al. Sequential chemo-immunotherapy for advanced non-small cell lung cancer using cisplatin,

etoposide, thymosin-alpha1 and interferon-alpha-2a. *Eur J Cancer* 1995;31A:2403–2405.

102. Hasturk S, Kurt B, Ozyildirim A, et al. Combination of chemotherapy and recombinant interferon-alpha in advanced non-small cell lung cancer. *Eur Respir J Suppl* 1995;8:S528.

103. Kelly K, Crowley JJ, Bunn PA, et al. Role of recombinant interferon alfa-2a maintenance in patients with limited-state small-cell lung cancer responding to concurrent chemoradiation. *J Clin Oncol* 1995;13:2924–2930.

104. Mattson K, Nijranen A, Pyrhonen S, et al. Concomitant chemotherapy (CT) and interferon alpha (IFN-Alpha) for SCLC. *Am J Respir Crit Care Med* 1995;151:848.

105. Mattson K, Ruotsalainen T, Tamminen K, et al. Interferon-alpha and retinoic acid maintenance therapy for small cell lung cancer. *Chest* 1996;110:S104.

106. Prior C, Oroszy S, Oberaigner W, et al. Adjunctive interferon-alpha-2c in stage IIIB/IV small-cell lung cancer: a phase III trial. *Eur Respir J* 1997;10:392–396.

107. Giannopoulos A, Constantinides C, Kortsaris A, et al. Determination of interferon-alpha receptors in urothelial cancer and in normal urothelium. *J Urol* 1997;157:82.

108. Bazarbashi S, Kattan S, Lindestedt E, et al. Phase II trial of intravesical instillation of bacillus Calmette Guerin (BCG) and interferon alpha-2b (IFN) on alternate weeks in the prevention of treatment of superficial transitional cell carcinoma (TCC) of the urinary bladder. *Proc Am Soc Clin Oncol* 1998;17:A326.

109. Bystryn J-C, Oratz R, Roses DF, Harris MN, Henn M, Lew R. Improved survival of melanoma patients with delayed type hypersensitivity response to melanoma vaccine immunization. *Clin Res* 1991;39:A503(abst).

110. Jimenez-Cruz JF, Vera-Donoso CD, Leiva O. Intravesical immunoprophylaxis in recurrent superficial bladder cancer (stage T1): multicenter trial comparing bacille Calmette-Guerin and interferon-alpha. *Urology* 1997;50:529–535.

111. Boccardo F, Cannata D, Rubagotti A, et al. Prophylaxis of superficial bladder cancer with mitomycin or interferon alfa-2b: results of a multicentric Italian study. *J Clin Oncol* 1994;12:7–13.

112. Kalble T, Beer M, Staehler G. Intravesical prophylaxis with BCG versus interferon-α for superficial bladder cancer. *J Urol* 1994;151:233A.

113. Raitanen MP, Lukkarinen O. A controlled study of intravesical epirubicin with or without alpha-2b-interferon as prophylaxis for recurrent superficial transitional cell carcinoma of the bladder. *Br J Urol* 1995;76:697–701.

114. Tizzani A, Bertetto O, Gontero P. Effectiveness of intravesical chemophylaxis with mitomycin alone vs. sequential mitomycin and interferon alpha-2b. A randomized, multicentric study on 210 patients with superficial bladder carcinoma. *J Urol* 1998;159:144.

115. Rajala P, Raitanen M, Rintala E, et al. Single dose interferon alpha or epirubicin plus transurethral resection compared with transurethral resection alone in the prophylaxis of recurrence of primary superficial bladder cancer: a prospective randomized multicentre study, Finnbladder II. *Eur Urol* 1998;33[Suppl 1]:124.

11

INTERFERON-γ: BASIC PRINCIPLES AND CLINICAL APPLICATIONS

VIJAY SHANKARAN
ROBERT D. SCHREIBER

Our understanding of interferon-γ (IFN-γ) has increased greatly since its initial description in 1965 as an antiviral activity produced by phytohemagglutinin-activated human leukocytes. Progress has been especially rapid in the 1980s and 1990s, during which time the genes encoding IFN-γ and its receptor chains have been cloned and expressed. The production of large amounts of recombinant IFN-γ and soluble IFN-γ receptors and the generation of specific monoclonal antibodies to these proteins have facilitated their molecular definition and yielded insights into their *in vivo* function. Structure-function studies of these proteins have identified the key regions required for their biologic activity; these insights have been supported by the solving of the crystal structures of IFN-γ and the IFN-γ–IFN-γ receptor complex. Mice lacking expression of IFN-γ, the IFN-γ receptor chains, or IFN-γ signaling components have been generated and have confirmed and extended the results from previous studies using anti-IFN-γ–neutralizing antibodies concerning the physiologic roles of these proteins. In addition, our understanding of the role of IFN-γ in preventing human disease has been advanced by the identification of human patients with IFN-γ production or signaling deficiencies and the demonstration that IFN-γ plays a critical role in promoting tumor surveillance in immunocompetent hosts. Therefore, we now have a relatively clear view of the biochemistry and biology of the IFN-γ system in mice and humans. This chapter reviews key aspects of the IFN-γ system and discusses data supporting its central role in modulating immune system activity and its ability to coordinate host defense to microbial pathogens and tumors.

STRUCTURE OF INTERFERON-γ GENES AND PROTEINS

IFN-γ is a member of a family of proteins that were originally described as antiviral activities produced by virally infected cells or mitogen-stimulated leukocytes (1,2). These proteins have been divided into two classes on the basis of structural and functional criteria, as well as the stimuli that induce their expression. The first class, termed type I IFNs, is primarily induced in response to viral infection of cells and has been further subdivided into two groups, IFN-α and IFN-β, based on cellular origin (3). The IFN-α family consists of more than 22 structurally related polypeptides that are encoded by distinct genes and produced largely by leukocytes (4,5). IFN-β is the product of a single distinct gene and is produced by fibroblasts (3). The second class of IFNs, termed *type II IFN*, *immune IFN*, or *IFN-γ*, is the product of a single gene and is produced by T lymphocytes and natural killer (NK) cells after activation with immune and inflammatory stimuli rather than viral infection (6,7).

IFN-γ is unrelated to IFN-α or IFN-β at genetic and protein levels and is encoded by a single 6-kb gene that resides on human chromosome 12 and murine chromosome 10 (8,9). The gene is organized in an identical manner in humans and mice and contains four exons and three introns. The human IFN-γ gene encodes a 1.2-kb messenger ribonucleic acid (mRNA) that is translated into a 166–amino acid polypeptide. After removal of its 23–amino acid signal sequence, the mature human IFN-γ polypeptide consists of 143 amino acids. Differential glycosylation at two *N*-linked glycosylation sites gives rise to mature human IFN-γ polypeptides of molecular mass (Mr) of 17, 20, and 25 kd (10). The murine IFN-γ gene encodes a 1.2-kb mRNA that gives rise to a 134–amino acid mature polypeptide, which, depending on its glycosylation state, displays Mr of 15.4, 20, or 25 kd. In both species, the fully glycosylated IFN-γ polypeptide predominates. Human and murine IFN-γ coding sequences display 60% identity, whereas the polypeptides share only 40% identity. This primary amino acid sequence diversity is the basis for the strict species specificity that human and murine IFN-γ display in binding to and inducing responses in human and murine cells, respectively (6). Under physiologic conditions, two IFN-γ polypeptides self-associate to form a noncovalent homodimer with a molecular mass of 50 kd (11,12). The IFN-γ homodimer is a labile molecule that can be denatured by extremes of temperature (>65°C) or pH (pH <4 or >9). Only the homodimeric form of IFN-γ is fully capable of binding to the IFN-γ receptor on cells and inducing biologic responses. The crystal structure of the IFN-γ dimer has been solved and indicates that two IFN-γ monomers associate in an antiparallel fashion to form a symmetric dimer (13). Subsequent crystallographic studies of the complex of IFN-γ bound to the ligand-binding chain of the IFN-γ receptor indicate that the IFN-γ homodimer contains two identical receptor binding sites and interacts with two receptor molecules (14).

INTERFERON-γ BIOSYNTHESIS

In hosts with normal function, IFN-γ production is restricted to appropriately stimulated T lymphocytes and NK cells (6,7). CD8+ T cells and the CD4+ T-helper (Th)-0 and -1 subsets secrete IFN-γ and other T-cell–derived cytokines in response to antigens presented in the context of the proper major histocompatibility (MHC) protein and costimulation. Agents that mimic T-cell activation, such as antibodies that cross-link the T-cell receptor (TCR), mitogens, or pharmacologic agents (such as the combination of phorbol myristate acetate and calcium ionophore), can also stimulate IFN-γ production in these cells. Neither IFN-γ message nor protein can be detected in resting T cells. IFN-γ transcripts can be detected within 6 to 8 hours of T-cell activation, however, reaching maximum levels by 12 to 24 hours and then subsequently declining to baseline values. The IFN-γ protein is secreted immediately after synthesis and reaches maximal extracellular levels 18 to 24 hours after T-cell stimulation (6). A second, TCR-independent pathway has been shown to induce robust IFN-γ production by T cells. This pathway involves the cytokines interleukin-12 (IL-12) and interleukin-18 (IL-18), which synergize to induce IFN-γ production through mechanisms involving transcription factors STAT4 and nuclear factor kappa B (15–21). Activation of these transcription factors is not sufficient to induce IFN-γ transcription in T cells, however, and additional protein synthesis is required (21). Further work is needed to define these other proteins that regulate IFN-γ production.

Activated NK cells comprise the other cellular source of IFN-γ. Unlike T cells, NK cells produce IFN-γ solely in an MHC-unrestricted manner. Analysis of lymphocyte-deficient severe combined immunodeficiency disease (SCID) mice infected with the gram-positive bacteria *Listeria monocytogenes* identified a cytokine amplification loop that leads to the production of large amounts of IFN-γ by NK cells (22,23). On interaction with bacterial products, tissue macrophages produce small amounts of tumor necrosis factor–α (TNF-α) and IL-12, which together stimulate NK cells to secrete low levels of IFN-γ. This NK-cell–derived IFN-γ in turn stimulates the macrophages to increase their production of TNF-α and IL-12, which subsequently leads to enhanced production of IFN-γ by NK cells. This reciprocal stimulation forms a positive amplification loop that results in the rapid production of substantial quantities of IFN-γ early in the course of infection and facilitates the generation of large numbers of activated macrophages with antimicrobial activity. Therefore, the interdependent synergistic effects of IFN-γ, IL-12, and TNF-α on macrophages and NK cells provides the host with an innate mechanism for IFN-γ production and macrophage activation that facilitates early control of infection (24).

Interleukin-10 (IL-10) is a cytokine produced late in the course of infection that, through indirect mechanisms, downreg-ulates the production of IFN-γ by NK and T cells (20,23,25). IL-10 functions by preventing macrophage secretion of TNF-α and IL-12, although its mechanism of action is undefined.

INTERFERON-γ RECEPTOR

IFN-γ interacts with a distinct high affinity (Ka = 10^{10}–10^{11}M^{-1}) receptor that is expressed on nearly all cell surfaces (14,26). IFN-γ receptors consist of two species-matched polypeptides. The first is a 90-kd protein known as the *IFN-γ receptor–α chain, IFNGR1, IFN-γ-R1,* or *CDw119* and is encoded by a gene on human chromosome 6 and murine chromosome 10. The IFNGR1 subunit is responsible for ligand binding and ligand trafficking through the cell and is required (but not sufficient) for signal transduction. The second is a 62-kd protein termed the *IFN-γ receptor–β chain, IFNGR2, IFN-γ-R2,* or *accessory factor-1* and is encoded by a gene on human chromosome 21 and murine chromosome 16. The IFNGR2 subunit plays only a minor role in ligand binding but is required for IFN-γ signaling.

The two IFN-γ receptor subunits differ significantly in terms of their cell-surface expression. IFNGR1 is expressed constitutively at moderate levels on the surface of nearly all cells (200 to 25,000 sites per cell), and its expression does not appear to be modulated by external stimuli. In contrast, IFNGR2 is expressed on cells at very low levels, and its expression is regulated in certain cell types (such as T lymphocytes) by external stimuli (27,28). In some cells, expression of the IFNGR2 gene is a critical factor in determining IFN-γ responsiveness.

The human IFNGR1 gene encodes a 489–amino acid precursor that contains a 17–amino acid signal sequence (29), whereas the murine IFNGR1 gene encodes a 477–amino acid polypeptide containing a 26–amino acid signal peptide (30–34). The human and murine proteins are organized in a similar manner; both contain a 228–amino acid extracellular and a 23–amino acid transmembrane domain and relatively large, serine- and threonine-rich intracellular domains that also contain several tyrosine residues. Despite this organizational similarity, however, the two polypeptides exhibit only 52.5% overall sequence identity, which applies to extracellular and intracellular domains. The Mr of mature human IFNGR1 proteins from different cells range from 80 to 95 kd due to cell-specific differences in glycosylation (35–37).

Human and murine IFNGR2 subunits are also structurally similar to one another. Human IFNGR2 is a 337–amino acid type I transmembrane polypeptide that contains a 21–amino acid signal sequence, an extracellular domain of 226 amino acids, a single 24–amino acid transmembrane domain, and a relatively short intracellular domain of only 66 amino acids (38). Murine IFNGR2 consists of an 18–amino acid signal sequence, a 224–amino acid extracellular domain, a 24 amino acid transmembrane domain, and a 64–amino acid intracellular domain (39). Although human and murine IFNGR2 exhibit only 58% overall identity, their cytoplasmic domains display 73% identity. The human and murine complementary DNAs (cDNAs) encode polypeptides of 38 kd. Mature forms of human and murine IFNGR2 display an Mr of 62 kd, however (28). This difference is most likely explained

TABLE 1. PHENOTYPES OF MICE LACKING JAK-STAT PATHWAY PROTEINS

Gene Deleted	Knockout Mouse Phenotype	Cytokine Receptors Affected	Reference
Jak1	Perinatal lethality, T- and B-cell deficits, innate immunity defect, neuronal survival deficit	IFN-α and -β, IFN-γ, IL-10, γ_c family, gp130 family	46
Jak2	Early embryonic lethality, no blood formation, lack of IFN-γ signaling	IFN-γ, Epo	47, 48
Jak3	T- and B-cell deficits	γ_c family	142–144
Tyk2	ND	ND	—
STAT1	Innate immunity defect, poor Th1 response	IFN-α and -β, and IFN-γ	50, 51
STAT2	Enhanced viral susceptibility	IFN-α and -β	C Schindler, *personal communication*, 1999
STAT3	Early embryonic lethality, dysregulated macrophage production of inflammatory cytokines	IL-10, gp130 family	145–147
STAT4	Th1 defect	IL-12	148, 149
STAT5A	Lactation defect	Prolactin	150, 151
STAT5B	Dwarfism	GH	151, 152
STAT5A × STAT5B	T-cell defect	IL-2	151
STAT6	Th2 defect	IL-4	153, 154

Epo, erythropoietin; GH, growth hormone; IFN, interferon; IL, interleukin; Jak, Janus protein tyrosine kinase; ND, no data; STAT, signal transducers and activators of transcription proteins; Th, T-helper cell.

by the postsynthetic glycosylation of polypeptides, although the composition and location of IFNGR2–associated carbohydrates has not been established.

SIGNAL TRANSDUCTION THROUGH THE INTERFERON-γ RECEPTOR

Janus Protein Tyrosine Kinases and Signal Transducers and Activators of Transcription Proteins

Work performed in many laboratories during the 1990s has demonstrated that the IFN-γ receptor, as well as many other cytokine and growth factor receptors, functions as a result of the ligand-induced coupling of the cognate cell surface receptor to a signal transduction pathway termed the *Jak-STAT pathway* (14,40–44). The Jak-STAT pathway rapidly transfers signals directly from the cell surface to the nucleus. To do so, the pathway uses two families of molecules. The first is a family of related protein tyrosine kinases known as *Janus kinases*, or *Jaks* (Table 1). The second is a family of latent cytosolic transcription factors termed *signal transducers and activators of transcription*, or *STATs* (see Table 1).

The Janus kinase family currently consists of four molecules: Jak1, -2, and -3 and Tyk2 (40,43,45). The Jak family members are structurally distinguished from other protein tyrosine kinases in that they contain dual kinase domains at their carboxy-terminus, although only the most extreme C-terminal kinase domain has documented kinase activity. The Jaks associate with cytokine receptor subunits in a specific and constitutive manner, and, on ligand addition, are able to phosphorylate activated cytokine receptors and STAT proteins (46–49).

The STAT protein family currently consists of seven distinct polypeptides: STAT1, -2, -3, -4, -5A, -5B, and -6 (41,43). This family of transcription factors is unusual in that its members possess src homology-2 (SH2) domains capable of binding to phosphotyrosine-containing sequences. Studies using cells and mice engineered to lack particular STAT proteins have demonstrated that the STATs play a major role in determining cytokine receptor signaling specificity (40,50,51). This property derives

from sequence differences within the SH2 domains of the STAT proteins, enabling the selective recruitment of distinct STATs to different activated, tyrosine-phosphorylated cytokine receptor subunits, and allows for the subsequent specific pairing that occurs between two tyrosine-phosphorylated STAT proteins that form the functionally active transcription factor complex.

Interferon-γ Receptor Signaling

Detailed structure/function analyses performed on the IFN-γ receptor and its signaling proteins has defined proximal IFN-γ signal transduction events and facilitated the construction of a model of IFN-γ signal transduction that currently serves as a paradigm for cytokine receptor signaling (Fig. 1). In unstimulated cells, the IFN-γ receptor subunits are not preassociated with one another (52) but rather associate constitutively via their intracellular domains with inactive forms of specific Janus kinases (52–55). Jak1 binds to a $_{266}$LPKS$_{269}$ sequence in the membrane proximal portion of the intracellular domain of the human IFNGR1 chain, and Jak2 associates with a 12–amino acid sequence ($_{263}$PPSIPLQIEEYL$_{274}$) in the intracellular domain of the human IFNGR2 chain. Signal transduction is initiated when a homodimeric IFN-γ molecule binds to two IFNGR1 subunits, leading to the formation of a complex to which two IFNGR2 proteins subsequently bind. Within the ligand-assembled receptor complex, the inactive subunit-associated kinases are brought into close juxtaposition with one another and are activated by mechanisms involving auto- and transphosphorylation. The activated kinases then phosphorylate a key tyrosine residue within a $_{440}$YDKPH$_{444}$ sequence near the carboxy-terminus of the human IFNGR1 chain, thereby forming the phosphorylated sequence that is specifically recognized by the SH2 domain of STAT1 (56,57). Two STAT1 molecules then bind to the paired docking sites on the activated receptor complex, are brought into close proximity with the receptor-associated, activated tyrosine kinases, and are themselves phosphorylated at a specific tyrosine residue (Y701) near their C-terminus (58,59). The two phosphorylated STAT1 proteins then dissociate from the

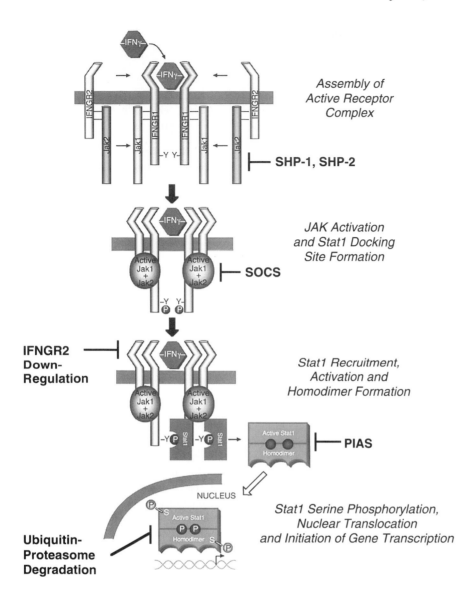

FIGURE 1. Model of IFN-γ signaling. (IFN, interferon; IFNGR2, interferon gamma-receptor 2; Jak, Janus tyrosine kinase; PIAS, proteins that inhibit activated signal transducers and activators of transcription proteins; SHP, SH2 domain containing protein tyrosine phosphatase; SOCS, suppressor of cytokine signaling; STAT, signal transducers and activators of transcription proteins.)

IFNGR1 subunits, form reciprocal homodimers which have also been serine-phosphorylated during the activation process, and then translocate to the nucleus. In the nucleus, the STAT1 homodimers bind to specific promoter elements (known as *gamma-interferon–activated sites*, or *GAS elements*) and thereby effect transcription of IFN-γ–induced genes (14,40). Studies using cells and mice with induced genetic deficiencies of different Jaks and STATs have demonstrated that most IFN-γ–induced biologic responses require Jak1, Jak2, and STAT1 (see Table 1) (46–48,50,51). These studies therefore establish the physiologic relevance of this IFN-γ signaling model.

Regulation of Interferon-γ–Dependent Janus Protein Tyrosine Kinase Signal Transducers and Activators of Transcription Proteins Signaling

Role of Phosphatases

Several different mechanisms have been proposed to regulate IFN-γ signaling. Experiments demonstrating the transient nature of IFN-γ receptor and STAT protein tyrosine phosphorylation inspired the straightforward hypothesis that IFN-γ signaling is regulated directly by specific protein tyrosine phosphatases. Several groups have studied this issue, and some initial data have emerged. The SH2-domain–containing protein tyrosine phosphatase, SHP-2, was reported to interact constitutively with the IFN-γ receptor (60). Embryonic fibroblasts from SHP-2–deficient mice displayed hyperactive STAT activation after IFN-γ stimulation, indicating that SHP-2 plays a negative role in regulating IFN-γ signaling (60). Another group proposed an opposite, positive role for SHP-1 (a different protein tyrosine phosphatase) in regulating IFN-γ signaling, based on the observation that overexpression of a catalytically inactive SHP-1 protein in HeLa cells led to a 30% to 50% increase in STAT1 activation in response to IFN-γ (61). Detailed analyses of the magnitude of IFN-γ–dependent biologic responses in the phosphatase-deficient cells should be performed to establish the importance of tyrosine phosphatases in regulating IFN-γ signaling.

Role of Janus Protein Tyrosine Kinase Inhibitors

Three groups independently cloned a family of proteins, termed *suppressors of cytokine signaling* (SOCS), *Jak-binding proteins* (JABs), or *STAT-induced STAT inhibitors* (SSIs), whose production is induced by many different cytokines; these proteins appear to function by binding via their SH2 domains to activated Jaks and inhibiting their catalytic activity (62–64). One member of this family, cytokine-inducible SH2 protein (CIS), appears to function in a different manner because it binds directly to activated receptors that contain phosphorylated STAT5 recruitment sequences [such as erythropoietin and interleukin-3 (IL-3) receptors] and thereby blocks STAT5 recruitment and activation at the receptor (65). The SOCS proteins contain an N-terminal region that is variable in length and sequence, a central SH2 domain, and a 40–amino acid region at the C-terminus termed the SOCS box. The formal SOCS family includes eight proteins, SOCS-1 through SOCS-7, and CIS. However, 12 other proteins have also been identified that contain the SOCS box (66). The function of these related proteins remains unknown. The induction of SOCS gene transcription by cytokines appears to be mediated by STAT transcription factors. The time course of induction of many of the SOCS family genes is rapid and transient (transcript appears within 20 minutes of cytokine stimulation and disappears 2 to 4 hours later); for some (such as SOCS-5 and CIS), however, the time course of induction is delayed or prolonged (67). Because many of the functional analyses of the SOCS proteins have relied on overexpression approaches in intact cells and cell-free systems, and because many of the SOCS family members are promiscuously induced by many different cytokines, the *in vivo* role of the SOCS proteins remains unclear. However, an initial view of the physiologic role of these proteins has come from the work of two different groups that generated mice devoid of SOCS-1/SSI-1 (68,69). SOCS-1/SSI-1 gene-targeted mice display retarded growth and die within 3 weeks of age. These mice exhibit fatty liver degeneration and accelerated apoptosis of lymphocytes with aging, which correlates with an upregulation of Bax in the thymus and spleen. Further work, including the generation of mice lacking expression of other SOCS family members, should be done to place the role of these proteins in proper perspective. Key questions that should be addressed are whether the different SOCS proteins specifically regulate distinct cytokine-signaling responses and if they function as a generalized mechanism to affect the return of activated cytokine signaling pathways to their homeostatic baselines.

Role of Signal Transducers and Activators of Transcription Protein Inhibitors

Another family of novel inhibitory proteins termed *proteins that inhibit activated STATs* (PIAS) have been identified and appear to function downstream of the activated receptor complex. The first of these proteins to be described (PIAS-1) was cloned using a yeast two-hybrid screen for STAT1 interacting proteins; another four PIAS family members were subsequently cloned on the basis of homology to PIAS-1 (70,71). The PIAS proteins, which contain a putative zinc-binding motif, are expressed con-stitutively and are thought to specifically associate with activated STAT molecules upon cytokine stimulation of cells. The PIAS proteins show a high degree of specificity for a particular activated STAT complex. Of the two family members that have been characterized, PIAS-1 binds selectively to activated STAT1 molecules, whereas PIAS-3 binds selectively to activated STAT3 molecules. Whether other PIAS proteins display specificity for other activated STAT molecules should be determined.

Role of the Ubiquitin-Proteasome Pathway

A fourth mechanism proposed to control the amount of activated STAT after IFN-γ stimulation is degradation via the ubiquitin-proteasome pathway. One group showed that an inhibitor of the proteasome MG132 stabilized STAT1 phosphorylation after IFN-γ treatment of HeLa cells. Phosphorylated STAT1 was ubiquitinated *in vivo*, implying that at some time after activation, STAT1 is targeted for degradation by the proteasome (72). However, these data do not exclude the possibility that signaling intermediates upstream of the STATs are also targeted for proteasome degradation. In fact, another group, using ^{35}S-labeling to study the distribution of total STAT1 and activated STAT1 after IFN-γ treatment of cells showed that STAT1 molecules translocate into the nucleus as tyrosine-phosphorylated molecules, later returning quantitatively to the cytoplasm as nonphosphorylated molecules (73). This result indicates that phosphorylated STAT1 molecules are not the main targets of proteasome degradation. Interestingly, a third group reported that the SOCS box of SOCS family proteins mediates interactions with elongins B and C, which may target SOCS-bound proteins (i.e., Jaks or cytokine receptor chains) to the proteosomal degradation pathway (74).

Role of Receptor Downregulation

Finally, IFN-γ signaling can be regulated by a mechanism involving inhibition of expression of particular receptor subunits. IFNGR2 has been shown to be downregulated (probably at the transcriptional level) in T cells as they differentiate to the Th1 CD4$^+$ subset (27,28). In newly developing T-cell clones, exposure of the cells to IFN-γ leads to a loss of IFNGR2 message and protein. In long-term Th1 clones, IFNGR2 expression is permanently suppressed. The generality and molecular basis of the mechanism underlying this unusual type of homologous desensitization remains poorly understood.

INTERFERON-γ–INDUCIBLE GENES

The rapid signaling of the Jak-STAT pathway makes it an ideal system to regulate the activation of immediate early genes that provide the host with a rapid mechanism to respond to an infectious agent. In fact, it has been possible to identify a large number of IFN-γ–stimulated genes that are induced rapidly (i.e., within 15 to 30 minutes) after IFN-γ treatment of cells and whose transcription does not depend on new protein synthesis (75,76). The promoter regions of these IFN-γ–stimulated genes contain the GAS element that functions to promote transcription. The GAS site is a nine-nucleotide sequence with a consensus motif of TTNCNNNAA and is specifically bound by STAT1 homodimers.

Examples of IFN-γ–induced immediate early genes include interferon regulatory factor-1 (IRF-1), guanylate binding protein-1 (GBP-1), and the type I Fcγ receptor (FcγR-I), which encode proteins that participate in inflammatory and immune responses. Several IFN-γ–regulated intermediate genes have also been identified. These genes are induced within 6 to 8 hours of stimulation and require additional protein synthesis for transcriptional activation to occur. Examples of these genes include those that encode class I and class II MHC proteins, which play a central role in determining adaptive immune responses. Studies using STAT1-, Jak1-, or Jak2-deficient mice have shown that these proteins play an obligate role in activating most IFN-γ–inducible genes (47,48,50,51). More than 100 IFN-γ–regulated genes have been identified. This subject has been reviewed elsewhere and the reader is referred to several excellent reviews on the subject (7,75,77).

INTERFERON-γ BIOLOGIC ACTIVITIES

Antiviral and Antiproliferative Activities

The molecular basis of the antiviral effects of IFNs has been extensively studied since the mid 1980s. IFN-γ promotes antiviral responses that are either intrinsic to the infected cell itself or extrinsic (in that they effect recognition and destruction of infected cells by components of either the innate or specific limbs of the host immune response).

IFN-γ induces several proteins in cells that promote intrinsic mechanisms of resistance to viral infection, thus functioning in a manner similar to IFN-α and -β (78). Two distinct mechanisms have been identified. The first relies on the actions of a family of enzymes known as 2′5′ oligoadenylate synthetases, which are induced by IFN-γ and activated by double-stranded RNA (intermediates or byproducts of viral RNA replication) (79). The activated enzymes polymerize adenosine triphosphate into 2′5′-linked oligomers that in turn activate ribonuclease-L, a latent constitutively expressed endoribonuclease. Activated ribonuclease-L degrades single-stranded RNA, thereby inhibiting protein synthesis in cells. The second antiviral mechanism depends on the protein PKR (also known as *double-stranded RNA-dependent kinase, P1 kinase, p68 kinase*, or *eukaryotic protein synthesis initiation factor–2 kinase*), a serine/threonine kinase also induced by IFN-γ and activated by double-stranded RNA (80,81). PKR phosphorylates and inactivates the eukaryotic protein synthesis initiation factor-2, thereby blocking protein synthesis in cells. Thus, these two mechanisms produce their antiviral effects by inhibiting cellular protein synthesis (82).

Extrinsic antiviral mechanisms induced by IFN-γ are largely those that direct the development of innate and specific immune responses. IFN-γ promotes antigen processing and presentation and plays a key role in the induction of antiviral cellular and humoral immune responses. These actions are discussed in more detail in the section Antigen Processing and Presentation.

IFN-γ has been shown also to manifest antiproliferative effects on cells. Although these biologic effects are well docu-

mented, their molecular bases are not yet well defined. Several studies have revealed that at least some of the antiproliferative actions of IFN-γ are due to the induction of proteins that inhibit enzymes involved in cell cycle progression. IFN-γ, for example, has been shown to induce expression of the protein p21$^{WAF1/CIP1/CAP1}$, an inhibitor of CDK2, via the Jak-STAT pathway (83,84). This process occurs in a relatively cell-specific manner, however, and it is unclear whether other cell cycle inhibitors may also be involved in this process. Nevertheless, this negative biologic response can still be attributed to a positive induction of a particular gene product.

Macrophage Activation and Innate Immunity

IFN-γ is the major physiologic macrophage activating factor (MAF); thus, it plays a critical role in promoting nonspecific host-defense mechanisms against a number of pathogens (85–87). Data supporting this concept comes from *in vitro* and *in vivo* studies that have demonstrated that IFN-γ can induce in macrophages the capacity to nonspecifically kill a variety of intracellular and extracellular parasites, as well as neoplastic cells (6,88). In addition, IFN-γ reduces the susceptibility of macrophages to microbial infection and enhances recognition of targets during the early innate phase of immunity through regulation of undefined macrophage cell-surface proteins (89). The physiologic significance of IFN-γ's role in macrophage activation and host defense against microbial pathogens has been established by several *in vivo* murine infection models. Mice pretreated with neutralizing antibodies to IFN-γ lose the ability to resist a sublethal challenge of a variety of microbial pathogens such as *L. monocytogenes* (22,86), *Toxoplasma gondii* (90), or *Leishmania major* (91). In addition, mice with disrupted genes for IFN-γ, the IFNGR1 chain, or the IFN-γ signaling protein STAT1, die when challenged with sublethal doses of microbial pathogens such as *Mycobacterium bovis*, *L. monocytogenes*, or *L. major* (50,92,93).

Activated macrophages kill microbial targets using a variety of toxic substances, such as reactive oxygen and nitrogen intermediates induced by IFN-γ. Much of the antimicrobial function of IFN-γ–activated macrophages can be attributed to the actions of nitric oxide (NO) or reactive oxygen intermediates, or both (94,95). NO is produced in activated macrophages by the inducible form of NO synthase (iNOS or NOS2). The gene encoding iNOS is transcriptionally activated after treatment of cells with IFN-γ plus a variety of second signals that activate transcription factor nuclear factor kappa B [such as TNF-α, interleukin-1 (IL-1), or bacterial endotoxin]. The enzyme catalyzes the conversion of L-arginine to L-citrulline, giving rise to large amounts of NO. NO is thought to kill target cells by one of two mechanisms. First, it can form an iron-nitrosyl complex with Fe-S groups of aconitase and complex I and complex II, thereby causing the inactivation of the mitochondrial electron transport chain. Alternatively, NO may react with superoxide anion [a reactive oxygen intermediate formed by the IFN-γ–induced enzyme nicotinamide adenine dinucleotide phosphate (NADPH) oxidase] to form peroxynitrite, which decays rapidly once protonated, to form the highly toxic compound hydroxyl radical. Evidence that NO is responsible for macrophage killing of intracellular parasites comes from a number of studies with *Listeria* and *Leishmania*. Mice pretreated with the L-arginine analogue *N*-monomethyl- L-arginine, an iNOS inhibitor, were unable to resolve footpad infection with *Leishmania* parasites. Similarly, mice treated with another iNOS inhibitor (aminoguanidine) died due to sublethal *Listeria* infection (96). Furthermore, mice lacking the iNOS gene are highly susceptible to infection with microbial pathogens (94,95,97).

Antigen Processing and Presentation

One of the major immunoregulatory roles of IFN-γ is its ability to promote the inductive phase of immune responses. This cytokine significantly influences the generation and presentation of antigenic peptides on cell surfaces (6,7). IFN-γ can regulate the expression of MHC class II proteins on cells, thereby regulating CD4$^+$ T-cell responses (7,98). IFN-γ induces MHC class II protein expression on many cells, such as mononuclear phagocytes, endothelial cells, and epithelial cells. IFN-γ can also inhibit IL-4–dependent class II expression on B cells (99), although the molecular basis for this apparently discordant effect is unknown. It is known that type I IFN, TNF, bacterial endotoxin, and immune complexes can either inhibit or enhance IFN-γ's ability to induce MHC class II. In the case of mononuclear phagocytes, for example, preexposure of cells to type I IFNs induces a state of unresponsiveness to IFN-γ. In contrast, treatment of cells with IFN-α and -β either together with or after IFN-γ treatment leads to enhanced class II expression. Thus, a cell's ability to express MHC class II in response to IFN-γ is influenced by the composition of the microenvironment (6).

IFN-γ also regulates the expression of molecules involved in the MHC class I antigen processing and presentation pathway (7). Some of these effects are at the level of regulating cell surface molecules. IFN-γ enhances the expression of MHC class I proteins and beta$_2$-microglobulin in a wide variety of cell types. This cytokine also enhances the expression of several cell surface proteins, such as ICAM-1 and B7, which are responsible for increasing target-cell–T-cell contact and T-cell costimulation, respectively (100,101).

IFN-γ also promotes antigen processing by regulating expression of many intracellular proteins required for antigenic peptide generation (7,101). IFN-γ has been shown to play a key role in modifying the activity of the proteasome, a multisubunit enzyme complex responsible for generating the peptides that bind to MHC class I proteins. It does so in part by modulating the expression of the enzymatic proteasome subunits. IFN-γ increases expression of the inducible subunits LMP2, LMP7, and MECL1 while decreasing expression of constitutive subunits x, y, and z, thereby altering proteasome composition and specificity (101–103). In addition, IFN-γ enhances the production of nonenzymatic proteasome components, such as the α and β subunits of PA28 (i.e., the 11S regulator of the proteasome), which function to regulate proteasome enzymatic activity (104). Purified 20S and 26S proteosomes from IFN-γ–treated cells show an increased capacity to cleave peptides after hydrophobic and basic residues, revealing that IFN-γ alters the proteasome in a way that changes the types of antigenic peptides that it produces (102).

IFN-γ additionally increases expression of the peptide transporters associated with antigen processing-1 and -2 (TAP-1 and TAP-2), which transfer peptides that have been generated in the cytoplasm by the proteasome into the endoplasmic reticulum where they can bind to nascently produced MHC class I proteins (100,101). Moreover, IFN-γ increases expression of the heat shock protein gp96, which may play a role in transferring peptide within the cell from the TAPs to MHC class I and between cells from nonprofessional antigen-presenting cells to a subset of macrophages (105). Taken together, these data strongly suggest that IFN-γ plays an important role in enhancing immunogenicity by increasing the quantity and the repertoire of peptides displayed on MHC class I.

Helper T-Cell Phenotype Development

Human and murine CD4$^+$ T cells can be divided into two subsets based on their pattern of cytokine secretion after stimulation (20,106). Th1 cells promote cell-mediated immunity and delayed-type hypersensitivity responses through their production of IFN-γ, lymphotoxin, and IL-2. In contrast, Th2 cells predominantly produce interleukin-4 (IL-4), interleukin-5 (IL-5), and IL-10, thereby providing help for humoral immune responses. IFN-γ plays an important role in Th1 development. *In vitro*, antibody neutralization of IFN-γ greatly reduces the development of Th1 cells and augments the development of Th2 cells. Importantly, administration of exogenous IFN-γ either *in vitro* or *in vivo* does not drive a Th1 response. Thus, IFN-γ is necessary but is not sufficient for Th1 development.

In vitro and *in vivo* studies have demonstrated that IL-12 is the single most important cytokine that drives T cells to the Th1 pole (107,108). Bacterial products promote Th1 cell development by inducing IL-12 production from antigen-presenting cells such as macrophages. In addition, mice deficient in either the gene for IL-12 or the IL-12–signaling protein STAT4 are unable to generate Th1 cells and display reduced delayed-type hypersensitivity responses.

The role of IFN-γ in Th development has been shown to be due to its effects at the level of the macrophage and the CD4$^+$ T cell. The effects of IFN-γ on macrophages were elucidated in studies that used transgenic mice lacking IFN-γ sensitivity specifically in the macrophage compartment. IFN-γ–insensitive macrophages were unable to support efficient Th1 development due to a severely reduced capacity to produce IL-12 (109). IFN-γ has been shown to have direct effects on the developing Th cells themselves. IFN-γ maintains expression of the β2 subunit of the IL-12 receptor on developing T cells thereby preserving sensitivity of these cells to IL-12 and promoting their development into a Th1 phenotype (110). IFN-γ also blocks development of Th2 phenotype through two mechanisms. First, it inhibits synthesis of IL-4 from undifferentiated, antigen-stimulated T cells, thereby inhibiting production of the cytokine required for Th2 development (111). Second, it inhibits Th2 cell expansion by directly inhibiting proliferation of Th2 cells (112). The antiproliferative effects of IFN-γ are not observed on

Th1 cells because these cells do not express the IFNGR2 subunit (27,28). Thus, IFN-γ simultaneously promotes cell-mediated immunity (through facilitating Th1 cell formation) and inhibits development of humoral immunity (through blockade of Th2 cell expansion).

Humoral Immunity

IFN-γ plays a complex role in regulating humoral immunity, exerting its effects either indirectly by regulating the development of specific T-helper cell subsets (as described above) or directly at the level of the B cell. In the latter case IFN-γ is predominantly responsible for regulating three specialized B-cell functions: B-cell development and proliferation, immunoglobulin (Ig) secretion, and Ig-heavy chain switching.

IFN-γ has been shown to negatively regulate B-cell differentiation by inhibiting IL-4–dependent induction of MHC class II protein expression and proliferation of murine B cells stimulated with anti-Ig and IL-4. In contrast, IFN-γ enhances proliferative responses in human B cells activated with anti-Ig. IFN-γ can also enhance or inhibit Ig secretion by either murine or human B cells. In this process, however, IFN-γ's effects depend on the differentiation state of the B cell, the timing of IFN-γ stimulation, and the nature of the activating stimulus.

The best characterized B-cell–directed effect of IFN-γ is its ability to influence Ig heavy chain switching. Ig class switching is significant because the different Ig isotypes promote distinct effector functions in the host. Immunoglobulin E (IgE) is the only isotype that can bind to Fc-ε receptors on mast cells and basophils and thereby promotes immediate type hypersensitivity and allergic reactions. IgG2a fixes complement and can bind (in monomeric form) to FcγR-I on murine macrophages, a high-affinity Fc receptor upregulated during IFN-γ–induced macrophage activation. Activated macrophages can efficiently use antibodies of the IgG2a isotype to mediate antibody-dependent cellular cytotoxicity. IgG3 is an isotype that can self-aggregate, a process that may enhance its opsonic activity. Along with IgG2a, IgG3 can also bind to the NK-cell–IgG receptor CD16 and effect NK-mediated antibody-dependent cellular cytotoxicity. IFNs, by favoring the production of IgG2a and IgG3 and inhibiting the production of IgE isotypes, can facilitate the interaction between the humoral and cellular effector limbs of the immune response and enhance host defense against certain bacteria and viruses.

In vitro IFN-γ is able to direct immunoglobulin class switching from IgM to the IgG2a subtype in lipopolysaccharide (LPS)-stimulated murine B cells and to IgG2a and IgG3 in murine B cells which have been stimulated with activated T cells (113,114). Moreover, IFN-γ blocks IL-4 induced Ig class switching in murine B cells to IgG1 or IgE (115). The validity of these observations has been stringently tested in experiments in which Ig subclass production was monitored in mice that were injected with immunoglobulin-D (IgD)–specific antiserum to achieve polyclonal activation of B cells. Mice treated in this manner produced large quantities of IgG1 and IgE. When IFN-γ was administered to the mice before anti-IgD treatment, however, they produced high levels of IgG2a and decreased levels of IgG1. Thus IFN-γ is clearly an important regulator of Ig class switching *in vivo* (116).

Tumor Immunity

An accumulating body of evidence suggests that IFN-γ plays an important role in promoting host defense to tumors. IFN-γ has been proposed to inhibit tumor generation by directly increasing expression of several tumor suppressor genes such as IRF-1 and PKR. IFN-γ also possesses properties that may inhibit the growth of already-transformed cells. *In vitro*, IFN-γ can exert direct antiproliferative and antimetabolic effects on a wide variety of tumor cells. IFN-γ is also able to activate macrophages to nonspecifically lyse certain tumor cells through mechanisms involving the generation of reactive oxygen and nitrogen intermediates and the production of cytotoxic ligands of the tumor necrosis family, such as TNF, Fas ligand (FasL), and TNF-related apoptosis-inducing ligand (88,117,118). In addition, IFN-γ is required for robust IL-12 secretion by macrophages. IL-12 has been shown in several studies to possess potent antitumor activities, even in mice with preestablished tumors (108). Injection of recombinant IL-12 into tumor-bearing mice reduces the rate of metastasis, slows tumor growth, and, in some cases, effects complete tumor regression. IFN-γ is required for IL-12–mediated antitumor effects. This conclusion is based on the observation that neutralizing IFN-γ–specific monoclonal antibodies ablate the effects of IL-12 on tumors *in vivo* (119,120).

Many experiments indicate that the major mechanism of IFN-γ's antitumor effects involve its ability to promote the generation of specific immune responses to tumors. IFN-γ upregulates MHC class I and class II molecules on a wide variety of cells and increases the magnitude and changes the nature of MHC class I antigen processing. IFN-γ treatment of a wide variety of nonantigenic tumors made them highly antigenic and correlated with an increase in expression levels of IFN-γ–inducible genes that regulate MHC class I processing and presentation including LMP2, LMP7, Tap1, and Tap2 (121,122). Another study showed that the ability of lymphocytes harvested from draining lymph nodes of mice harboring the fibrosarcoma MCA-105 adoptively transfer immunity to MCA-105 was abrogated by *in vivo* administration of neutralizing IFN-γ antibodies to the recipient mice (123). Together, these studies suggest that a major effect of IFN-γ is to increase the antigenicity of tumors and augment tumor immunity.

A clear demonstration of a role for IFN-γ in immune-mediated tumor rejection comes from a series of studies using chemically induced fibrosarcomas, such as the Meth-A tumor cell line (124). Meth-A is an MCA-induced fibrosarcoma of BALB/c mice that grows progressively when transplanted intradermally in syngeneic mice. Although the tumor is highly aggressive and eventually kills the host, a tumor-bearing mouse can be induced to reject the tumor by administration of LPS. Using neutralizing mAb specific for murine IFN-γ, it was determined that IFN-γ is obligatorily required for LPS-induced tumor rejection. In addition, Meth-A tumors grew significantly more rapidly in anti–IFN-γ treated syngeneic mice.

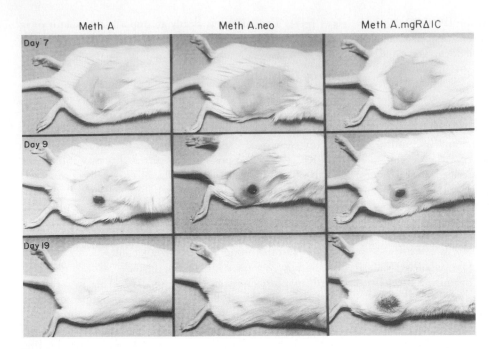

FIGURE 2. Effects of lipopolysaccharide (LPS) injection on BALB/c mice bearing IFN-γ–sensitive or –insensitive Meth-A tumor cells. Mice were injected on day 0 with 5×10^5 Meth-A, mock-transfected Meth-A (Meth A.neo), or dominant-negative IFNGR1–transfected Meth-A (Meth-A.mgRΔIC) cells. In top panels, day 7 tumors are shown. Intraperitoneal treatment with LPS (3 mg/kg) was administered on day 7 and the middle panels show mice 48 hours post-LPS treatment (day 9). The bottom panels show the mice on day 19, 12 days after LPS treatment. (IFN-γ, interferon-γ.)

Although these results established the importance of IFN-γ in Meth-A growth regulation, they did not identify the cellular target of IFN-γ's actions. By introducing a mutant nonfunctional IFNGR1 protein into Meth-A tumor cells, it was possible to specifically ablate tumor cell responsiveness to the cytokine and demonstrate that the tumor itself was a major target of IFN-γ's actions. IFN-γ–insensitive Meth-A grew more rapidly in naive syngeneic mice than did control tumors and were not rejected when the tumor-bearing mice were treated with LPS (Fig. 2). In addition, the IFN-γ–insensitive tumors neither primed naive mice for induction of Meth-A immunity nor were rejected in mice with preestablished immunity to the wild-type tumor cell (Figs. 3 and 4). This effect was not due to the antiproliferative actions of IFN-γ. Similar studies using different murine fibrosarcomas have yielded similar results. Thus, the ability of the immune system to recognize and reject certain tumors is critically dependent on the tumor's ability to respond to IFN-γ (124).

A subsequent study suggests that IFN-γ may also exert its antitumor effects in tumor transplant models through a mechanism involving the inhibition of blood vessel recruitment by tumors (125). Overexpression of a mutant nonfunctional IFNGR1 chain in tumor cells rendered them relatively insensitive to IFN-γ, highly tumorigenic, and relatively unresponsive to IL-12 therapy *in vivo*. IL-12 was found to induce ischemic damage only in IFN-γ–responsive tumors. *In vivo* Matrigel assays showed that whereas IFN-γ–sensitive and –insensitive tumors recruited blood vessels equally well, IL-12 therapy only inhibited angiogenesis in the IFN-γ–responsive tumors. IFN-γ induces the expression of a number of angiostatic molecules in target cells, including the chemokines IP-10 and Mig, which may mediate its antiangiogenic activity.

Although the tumor transplantation studies described above identified a critical role for IFN-γ in promoting rejection of transplantable tumors, they did not address the question of whether IFN-γ participates in the elimination of primary developing tumor cells (126). To examine this question, IFN-γ-R$^{-/-}$ mice, STAT1$^{-/-}$ mice and wild-type mice, all of which were derived on a pure inbred 129/Sv/Ev background, were treated with different doses of the chemical carcinogen methylcholanthrene (MCA) and tumor development followed through 165 days. At every MCA dose examined, IFN-γ–insensitive mice developed tumors significantly more rapidly and with greater frequency compared to wild-type mice (Fig. 5). IFN-γ–insensitive mice also displayed enhanced tumor development in a model of spontaneous tumor formation. Mice lacking the p53 tumor suppressor gene were bred onto either a wild-type 129/Sv/Ev background or onto either IFN-γ-R$^{-/-}$ or STAT1$^{-/-}$ backgrounds, and tumor development in the single or double knockout offspring was assessed (Fig. 6). IFN-γ–insensitive p53$^{-/-}$ mice developed spontaneous tumors significantly earlier than did their IFN-γ–sensitive counterparts. Furthermore, the two groups of mice displayed differences in the types of tumors that formed. Whereas all of the IFN-γ–sensitive p53$^{-/-}$ mice developed lymphoid tumors, 35% of the IFN-γ-R$^{-/-}$ × p53$^{-/-}$ mice and 38% of the STAT1$^{-/-}$ × p53$^{-/-}$ formed nonlymphoid tumors without concomitant lymphoid tumors.

Two series of studies indicate that the increased tumor incidence in IFN-γ unresponsive hosts is due to IFN-γ unresponsiveness at the level of the transformed cell itself. First, tumor cells derived from MCA-treated IFN-γ–insensitive mice grew progressively with identical kinetics when transplanted into either wild-type mice or the corresponding IFN-γ–insensitive mouse strain. Second, introduction of the missing IFN-γ signaling protein into these cells by gene transfer reconstituted their capacity to respond to IFN-γ and converted them into immunogenic tumors that were rejected in wild-type 129/Sv/Ev mice but not Rag2$^{-/-}$ mice devoid of lymphocytes. Together, these results thus demonstrate that the interplay between IFN-γ and the specific immune system forms the basis of an effective tumor surveillance system in the host. In addition, these observations indicate that a major target of IFN-γ's antitumor functions is the tumor cell

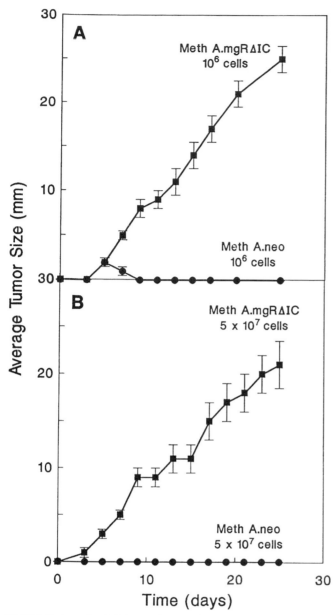

FIGURE 3. Growth of IFN-γ–sensitive and –insensitive Meth-A tumors in Meth-A–immune mice. **A:** BALB/c mice were inoculated twice with 1 × 10^7 irradiated (8,000 rads) Meth-A cells. Immunized mice were rested for 2 weeks and then injected subcutaneously on day 0 with either Meth-A, Meth A.neo or Meth A.mgRΔIC cells at the inocula shown. **B:** BALB/c mice were injected with 2 × 10^5 live wild-type Meth-A tumor cells and cured of Meth-A tumors by lipopolysaccharide administration 7 days later. Immunized mice were rested for 2 weeks and then injected subcutaneously on day 0 with either Meth-A neoadjuvant or Meth A.mgRΔIC at the inocula shown. Data are represented as mean tumor size ± SE of six mice per group.

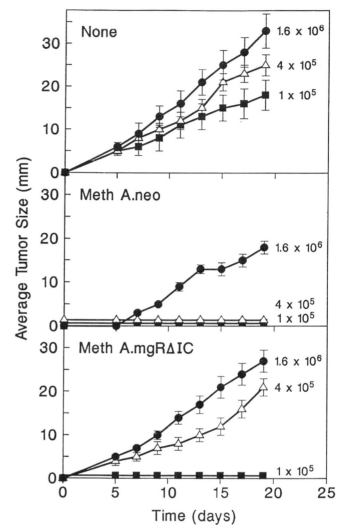

FIGURE 4. Immunogenicity of IFN-γ–sensitive and –insensitive Meth-A tumors. BALB/c mice were left untreated (top panel) or were intradermally inoculated with either Meth A.neo (middle panel) or Meth A.mgRΔIC (lower panel) at a dose of 5 × 10^5 cells. After 7 days of *in vivo* growth, the tumors were surgically resected. Immunized mice were rested for 10 days, then challenged on day 0 by subcutaneous inoculation of wild-type Meth-A at the inocula shown. Data are represented as mean tumor size ± SE of six mice per group.

itself. A critical role for lymphocytes in this process has been confirmed by studies showing that lymphocyte-deficient Rag2$^{-/-}$ mice are highly susceptible to tumor induction by MCA and that tumors that develop in the absence of lymphocytes are strongly immunogenic.

The existence of an IFN-γ–dependent antitumor system is further supported by the identification of tumor cells that have

developed spontaneous and specific insensitivity to IFN-γ (126). A screen of human tumor cell banks revealed that lung adenocarcinomas show a tendency to spontaneously develop permanent IFN-γ unresponsiveness. Four out of seventeen lines tested failed to initiate IFN-γ–dependent signaling (as measured using an electrophoretic mobility shift assay) and failed to develop biologic responses to human IFN-γ as determined by monitoring-enhanced MHC class I expression. Using immunochemical and molecular genetic approaches, the IFN-γ unresponsiveness in each cell line was determined to be the result of a discrete lesion in a proximal IFN-γ signaling component. One tumor cell line lacked the IFNGR1 chain, two others produced abnormal forms of Jak2, and the fourth lacked Jak1. A subset of primary MCA-induced murine tumors have also been identified that develop quantitative insensitivity to IFN-γ. These IFN-γ–

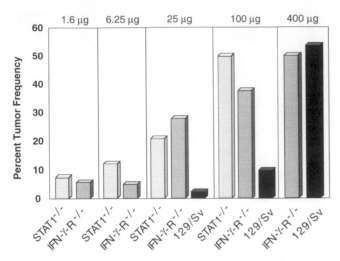

FIGURE 5. IFN-γ–insensitive mice demonstrate an increased susceptibility to development of chemically induced tumors. Groups of wild-type, IFN-γ-R⁻/⁻, and STAT1⁻/⁻ mice were injected with one of a range of doses of methylcholanthrene; tumor development was monitored for 165 days. Values represent the composite of four independent experiments. (IFN-γ-R, interferon-γ receptor; STAT, signal transducers and activators of transcription proteins.)

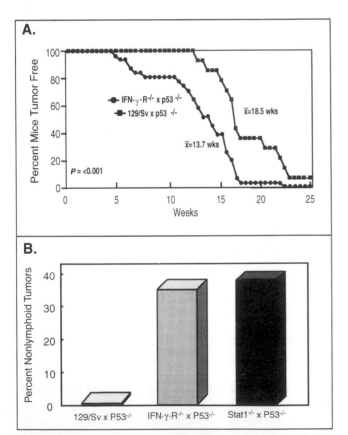

FIGURE 6. IFN-γ–insensitive mice demonstrate an increased susceptibility to development of spontaneous tumors. **A:** Spontaneous tumor development in IFN-γ-R⁻/⁻ × p53⁻/⁻ and 129/Sv/Ev × p53⁻/⁻ mice. The difference in average tumor development times between 129/Sv/Ev × p53⁻/⁻ (18.5 weeks) and IFN-γ-R⁻/⁻ × p53⁻/⁻ (13.7 weeks) is statistically significant by the Wilcoxon rank sum test (*p* = .001). **B:** Percent 129/Sv/Ev × p53⁻/⁻, IFN-γ-R⁻/⁻ × p53⁻/⁻ and STAT1⁻/⁻ × p53⁻/⁻ mice developing nonlymphoid tumors without concomitant lymphoid tumors. (IFN-γ-R, interferon-γ receptor; STAT, signal transducers and activators of transcription proteins.)

insensitive tumors grow in a highly aggressive manner when transplanted into syngeneic immunocompetent mice.

IN VIVO DYSFUNCTION OF IFN-γ SIGNALING

Mice with Targeted Disruption of Genes Involved in Interferon-γ Signaling

The physiologic consequences of global *in vivo* inactivation of the IFN-γ signaling pathway in mice were originally uncovered using neutralizing monoclonal antibodies specific for IFN-γ. However, the physiologic role of IFN-γ has been more fully elucidated using mice with engineered disruptions in either the IFN-γ structural gene (92), the genes encoding the two IFN-γ receptor subunits (IFNGR1 and IFNGR2) (93,127,128), or the genes encoding either of the three signaling proteins required by IFN-γ for biologic response induction—that is, STAT1 (50,51), Jak1 (46), and Jak2 (47,48). As a group, these mice display a greatly impaired ability to resist infection by a variety of microbial pathogens including *Leishmania monocytogenes*, *L. major*, and several mycobacterial species, including *M. bovis* and *Mycobacterium avium*. Importantly, mice lacking either IFNGR1 or IFNGR2 are able to mount a curative response to many viruses, whereas mice lacking the IFN-α and -β receptor or STAT1 and cells of mice deficient in Jak1 are not. These results thus demonstrate that under physiologic conditions, the majority of the antiviral effects of the IFN system are largely mediated via type I IFNs (129).

Identification of Human Patients with Defects in Interferon-γ Signaling or Production

Results obtained from IFNGR1–deficient mice suggest that individuals with inactivating mutations in the human IFN-γ receptor genes might suffer from recurrent microbial but not viral infections. Three years ago, two research groups identified children from three unrelated families with such mutations who manifest a severe susceptibility to weakly pathogenic mycobacterial species (130,131). Genetic analysis of these patients' families revealed that susceptibility to atypical mycobacterial infection was inherited in an autosomal recessive manner. Sequence analysis of the patients' IFNGR1 alleles identified missense mutations in genetic regions coding for the extracellular domain of the IFNGR1 polypeptide, leading to the production of truncated receptor proteins that are not able to be retained at the cell surface. The clinical syndromes of these patients were similar. In one study, a group of related Maltese children were identified that showed extreme susceptibility to infection with *Mycobacterium fortuitum*, *M. avium*, and *Mycobacterium chelonei* (130). In another study, a Tunisian child was identified with disseminated *M. bovis* infection after bacille Calmette-Guérin (BCG) vaccination (131). A third study identified a child of distinct ancestry who had a similar immunocompromised phenotype (132). Biopsies from these patients revealed the presence of multibacillary, poorly defined granulomas, which contained scattered macrophages but lacked epithelioid and giant cells and surrounding lymphocytes. Importantly, these patients showed enhanced susceptibility to mycobacteria and occasionally to *Salmonella* but not to other typical bacteria or other common microbial pathogens or fungi. Moreover, in all three kindred, the patients were able to mount antibody or curative responses, or both, to several different viruses.

Subsequently, a number of patients were identified who develop less severe mycobacterial disease than the children described above. These patients were successfully treated with IFN-γ and antibiotics. On analysis of their IFN-γ-R genes, some of the patients were found to display distinct mutations in the IFNGR1 gene, leading to reduced but not ablated receptor function (133). A Portuguese family was identified in which one child developed disseminated BCG infection and a sibling who had not been vaccinated with BCG developed clinical tuberculosis. Both patients were homozygous for a point mutation in the extracellular domain-encoding region of the IFNGR1 subunit gene that produced an isoleucine-to-threonine amino acid substitution. The mutant receptors were found to require 100- to 1,000-fold higher concentrations of IFN-γ than normal receptors to activate STAT1 (133).

Another set of 19 patients from 12 unrelated families were found to inherit partial IFN-γ insensitivity in an autosomal dominant manner (134). All of these patients were found to be heterozygous for a wild-type IFNGR1 allele and an IFNGR1 allele with a frameshift mutation that produced an IFNGR1 protein that lacked most of the intracellular domain, including the Jak1 and STAT1 binding sites. Interestingly, in this group of patients, 12 independent mutation events occurred at a single site, defining a small deletion hotspot in the IFNGR1 gene. The truncated receptor chain accumulated on cell surfaces and was shown to act in a dominant negative manner to inhibit IFN-γ responses in cells. The definition of the molecular basis for this defect was facilitated by the observation that these patients phenotypically resembled IFN-γ–insensitive cells and transgenic mice generated earlier that overexpressed a genetically engineered truncated IFNGR1 subunit (124,135). In all of these patients, defects in IFN-γ responsiveness were partial, and cells from the patients retained some degree of sensitivity to IFN-γ. This correlates with the milder infections in these patients, and their positive responses to exogenous IFN-γ therapy.

A case of a child with severe, disseminated infections due to *M. fortuitum* and *M. avium* who lacked mutations in the IFNGR1 gene was described (136). This child was found to be homozygous for mutations in the IFNGR2 gene. The mutation resulted in a premature stop codon in the extracellular domain-encoding region and led to the production of IFNGR2 proteins that could not be expressed at the cell surface. The clinical and histopathologic phenotype of this patient closely resembled that of patients lacking expression of the IFNGR1 chain.

An additional group of patients were identified whose clinical syndromes resembled partial IFN-γ-R deficiency but on analysis were found to express normal IFN-γ-R polypeptides. Seven of these patients lacked functional IL-12 receptor complexes due to null mutations in the IL-12R-β1 gene (137,138). Lymphocytes from these patients were deficient in producing IFN-γ. This defect could not be corrected by addition of recombinant IL-12. One case of an individual with a homozygous frameshift deletion encompassing two exons of the IL-12 p40 gene was also reported (139). This patient's lymphocytes had a reduced capacity to secrete IFN-γ, which could be complemented by exogenous IL-12. All of these patients with functional defects in IFN-γ production developed atypical mycobacterial infections that could be cured by exogenous IFN-γ therapy. As a group, the patients with defects in either IFN-γ signaling or IL-12–induced IFN-γ production have taught us that IFN-γ plays a critical role in host defense to mycobacterial infections in humans. We must determine why IFN-γ receptor defects in humans lead almost exclusively to enhanced susceptibility to mycobacterial infection.

CLINICAL USES OF INTERFERON-γ

Despite expectations that IFN-γ would be used in the therapy of a wide variety of infectious diseases and malignancies, this cytokine has been shown to be effective in treating only a limited number of human diseases. Clinical trials of IFN-γ for treatment of many different solid and hematologic tumors have been disappointing. One of the few cancers that have been shown to regress in response to IFN-γ therapy is chronic myelogenous leukemia, a hematologic malignancy (140).

IFN-γ has been shown to be somewhat more effective as an adjuvant to antibiotic therapy in decreasing the severity and frequency of infections in patients with chronic granulomatous disease (141). Chronic granulomatous disease patients suffer from chronic bacterial infections as a result of defects in the phagocyte-specific NADPH oxidase system that generates superoxide radicals during the respiratory burst. IFN-γ was selected as a candidate therapeutic for chronic granulomatous disease because it is known to increase superoxide production and the microbicidal activity of phagocytes. IFN-γ's mechanism of therapeutic action appears to be independent of these direct effects on the NADPH oxidase system, however, because cells from patients who responded to IFN-γ therapy did not display enhanced superoxide production or *in vitro* bacterial killing (141).

Type I IFNs have been found to have more clinical efficacy in general than IFN-γ. This is somewhat surprising because of the more potent immunomodulatory activity of IFN-γ versus IFN-α and -β. These results thus suggest that more research should be conducted before these cytokines can be used most effectively in a clinical setting.

ACKNOWLEDGMENTS

Vijay Shankaran is supported by a predoctoral training award from the Cancer Research Institute. Work from Robert D. Schreiber's laboratory, quoted in this review, was supported by grants from the National Institutes of Health (CA43039 and CA76464) and Genentech, Inc. (San Francisco, CA).

REFERENCES

1. Isaacs A, Lindenmann J. Virus interference. I. The interferon. *Proc R Soc Lond Biol Sci* 1957;147:258.
2. Wheelock EF. Interferon-like virus-inhibitor induced in human leu-

kocytes by phytohemagglutinin. *Science* 1965;149:310–311.

3. Pestka S, Langer JA, Zoon KC, Samuel CE. Interferons and their actions. *Annu Rev Biochem* 1987;56:727–777.

4. Henco K, Brosius J, Fujisawa A, et al. Structural relationships of human interferon alpha genes and pseudogenes. *J Mol Biol* 1985;185:227–260.

5. Zoon KC, Miller D, Bekisz J, et al. Purification and characterization of multiple components of human lymphoblastoid interferon alpha. *J Biol Chem* 1992;267:15210–15216.

6. Farrar MA, Schreiber RD. The molecular cell biology of interferon-γ and its receptor. *Annu Rev Immunol* 1993;11:571–611.

7. Boehm U, Klamp T, Groot M, Howard JC. Cellular responses to interferon-γ. *Annu Rev Immunol* 199715:749–795.

8. Naylor SL, Sakaguchi AY, Shows TB, Law ML, Goeddel DV, Gray PW. Human immune interferon gene is located on chromosome 12. *J Exp Med* 1983;157:1020–1027.

9. Naylor SL, Gray PW, Lalley PA. Mouse immune interferon (IFNγ) gene is on human chromosome 10. *Somat Cell Mol Genet* 1984;10: 531–534.

10. Kelker HC, Le J, Rubin BY, Yip YK, Nagler C, Vilcek J. Three molecular weight forms of natural human interferon-gamma revealed by immunoprecipitation with monoclonal antibody. *J Biol Chem* 1984;259:4301–4304.

11. Scahill SJ, Devos R, Van der Heyden J, Fiers W. Expression and characterization of the product of a human immune interferon cDNA gene in Chinese hamster ovary cells. *Proc Natl Acad Sci U S A* 1983;80:4654–4658.

12. Chang TW, McKinney S, Liu V, Kung PC, Vilcek J, Le J. Use of monoclonal antibodies as sensitive and specific probes for biologically active human gamma-interferon. *Proc Natl Acad Sci U S A* 1984;81:5219–5222.

13. Ealick SE, Cook WJ, Vijay-Kumar S, et al. Three-dimensional structure of recombinant human interferon-γ. *Science* 1991;252: 698–702.

14. Bach EA, Aguet M, Schreiber RD. The IFNγ receptor: a paradigm for cytokine receptor signaling. *Annu Rev Immunol* 1997; 15:563–591.

15. Wolf SF, Temple PA, Kobayashi M, et al. Cloning of cDNA for natural killer cell stimulatory factor, a heterodimeric cytokine with multiple biologic effects on T and natural killer cells. *J Immunol* 1991;146:3074–3080.

16. Stern AS, Podlaski FJ, Hulmes JD, et al. Purification to homogeneity and partial characterization of cytotoxic lymphocyte maturation factor from human B-lymphoblastoid cells. *Proc Natl Acad Sci U S A* 1990;87:6808–6812.

17. Jacobson NG, Szabo SJ, Weber-Nordt RM, et al. Interleukin 12 signaling in T helper type 1 (Th1) cells involves tyrosine phosphorylation of signal transducer and activator of transcription (Stat)3 and Stat4. *J Exp Med* 1995;181:1755–1762.

18. Okamura H, Tsutsul H, Komatsu T, et al. Cloning of a new cytokine that induces IFN-γ production by T cells. *Nature* 1995;378:88–91.

19. Robinson D, Shibuya K, Mui A, et al. IGIG does not drive Th1 development, but synergizes with IL-12 for IFN-γ production, and activates IRAK and NF-kB. *Immunity* 1997;7:571–581.

20. O'Garra A. Cytokines induce the development of functionally heterogeneous T helper cell subsets. *Immunity* 1998;8:275–283.

21. Yang J, Murphy TL, Ouyang W, Murphy KM. Induction of interferon-gamma production in Th1 CD4+ T cells: evidence for two distinct pathways for promoter activation. *Eur J Immunol* 1999;29: 548–555.

22. Bancroft GJ, Schreiber RD, Unanue ER. Natural immunity, a T-cell-independent pathway of macrophage activation, defined in the SCID mouse. *Immunol Rev* 1991;124:5–24.

23. Tripp CS, Wolf SF, Unanue ER. Interleukin-12 and tumor necrosis factor alpha are co-stimulators of interferon-gamma production by natural killer cells in severe combined immunodeficiency mice with listeriosis, and interleukin-10 is a physiologic antagonist. *Proc Natl Acad Sci U S A* 1993;90:3725–3729.

24. Unanue ER. Interrelationship among macrophages, NK cells and neutrophils in early stages of Listeria resistance. *Curr Opin Immunol*

1997;9:35–43.

25. Fiorentino DF, Zlotnik A, Mosmann TR, Howard M, O'Garra A. IL-10 inhibits cytokine production by activated macrophages. *J Immunol* 1991;147:3815–3822.

26. Pestka S, Kotenko SV, Muthukumaran G, Izotova LS, Cook JR, Garotta G. The interferon gamma (IFN-γ) receptor: A paradigm for the multichain cytokine receptor. *Cytokine Growth Factor Rev* 1997;8:189–206.

27. Pernis A, Gupta S, Gollob KJ, et al. Lack of interferon-γ receptor β chain and the prevention of interferon-γ signaling in T_H1 cells. *Science* 1995;269:245–247.

28. Bach EA, Szabo SJ, Dighe AS, et al. Ligand-induced autoregulation of IFN-γ receptor β chain expression in T helper cell subsets. *Science* 1995;270:1215–1218.

29. Aguet M, Dembic Z, Merlin G. Molecular cloning and expression of the human interferon-γ receptor. *Cell* 1988;55:273–280.

30. Gray PW, Leong S, Fennie EH, et al. Cloning and expression of the cDNA for the murine interferon gamma receptor. *Proc Natl Acad Sci U S A* 1989;86:8497–8501.

31. Kumar CS, Muthukumaran G, Frost LJ, et al. Molecular characterization of the murine interferon-γ receptor cDNA. *J Biol Chem* 1989;264:17939–17946.

32. Munro S, Maniatis T. Expression and cloning of the murine interferon-γ receptor cDNA. *Proc Natl Acad Sci U S A* 1989;86: 9248–9252.

33. Hemm S, Peghini P, Metzler M, Merlin G, Dembic Z, Aguet M. Cloning of murine interferon gamma receptor cDNA: expression in human cells mediates high-affinity binding but is not sufficient to confer sensitivity to murine interferon gamma. *Proc Natl Acad Sci U S A* 1989;86:9901–9905.

34. Cofano F, Moore SK, Tanaka S, Yuhki N, Landolfo S, Appella E. Affinity purification, peptide analysis, and cDNA sequence of the mouse interferon-γ receptor. *J Biol Chem* 1990;265:4064–4071.

35. Hershey GK, Schreiber RD. Biosynthetic analysis of the human interferon-gamma receptor. Identification of N-linked glycosylation intermediates. *J Biol Chem* 1989;264:11981–11988.

36. Mao C, Aguet M, Merlin G. Molecular characterization of the human interferon-gamma receptor: analysis of polymorphism and glycosylation. *J Interferon Res* 1989;9:659–669.

37. Fischer T, Thoma B, Scheurich P, Pfizenmaier K. Glycosylation of the human interferon-gamma receptor. N-linked carbohydrates contribute to structural heterogeneity and are required for ligand binding. *J Biol Chem* 1990;265:1710–1717.

38. Soh J, Donnelly RO, Kotenko S, et al. Identification and sequence of an accessory factor required for activation of the human interferon-γ receptor. *Cell* 1994;76:793–802.

39. Hemmi S, Bohni R, Stark G, DiMarco F, Aguet M. A novel member of the interferon receptor family complements functionality of the murine interferon γ receptor in human cells. *Cell* 1994;76:803–810.

40. Darnell JE Jr, Kerr IM, Stark GR. Jak-STAT pathways and transcriptional activation in response to IFNs and other extracellular signaling proteins. *Science* 1994;264:1415–1421.

41. Schindler C, Darnell JE Jr. Transcriptional responses to polypeptide ligands: the JAK-STAT pathway. *Annu Rev Biochem* 1995;64:621–651.

42. Darnell JE Jr. STATs and gene regulation. *Science* 1997;277: 1630–1635.

43. O'Shea JJ. Jaks, STATs, cytokine signal transduction, and immunoregulation: are we there yet? *Immunity* 1997;7(1):1–11.

44. Stark GR, Kerr IM, Williams BRG, Silverman RH, Schreiber RD. How cells respond to interferons. *Annu Rev Biochem* 1998;67:227–264.

45. Ihle JN, Witthuhn BA, Quelle FW, Yamamoto K, Silvennoinen O. Signaling through the hematopoietic cytokine receptors. *Annu Rev Immunol* 1995;13:369–398.

46. Rodig SJ, Meraz MA, White JM, et al. Disruption of the Jak1 gene demonstrates obligatory and nonredundant roles of the Jaks in cytokine-induced biologic responses. *Cell* 1998;93:373–383.

47. Paraganas E, Wang D, Stravopodis D, et al. Jak2 is essential for signaling through a variety of cytokine receptors. *Cell* 1998;93:385–395.

48. Neubauer H, Cumano A, Muller M, Wu H, Huffstadt U, Pfeffer K. Jak2 deficiency defines an essential developmental checkpoint in

definitive hematopoiesis. *Cell* 1998;93:397–409.

49. Kotenko SV, Izotova LS, Pollack BP, et al. Other kinases can substitute for Jak2 in signal transduction by interferon-γ. *J Biol Chem* 1996;271:17174–17182.

50. Meraz MA, White JM, Sheehan KCF, et al. Targeted disruption of the STAT1 gene in mice reveals unexpected physiologic specificity in the Jak-STAT signaling pathway. *Cell* 1996;84:431–442.

51. Durbin JE, Hackenmiller R, Simon MC, Levy DE. Targeted disruption of the mouse Stat1 gene results in compromised innate immunity to viral infection. *Cell* 1996;84:443–450.

52. Bach EA, Tanner JW, Marsters SA, et al. Ligand-induced assembly and activation of the gamma interferon receptor in intact cells. *Mol Cell Biol* 1996;16:3214–3221.

53. Kaplan DH, Greenlund AC, Tanner JW, Shaw AS, Schreiber RD. Identification of an interferon-γ receptor α chain sequence required for JAK-1 binding. *J Biol Chem* 1996;271:9–12.

54. Kotenko S, Izotova L, Pollack B, et al. Interaction between the components of the interferon gamma receptor complex. *J Biol Chem* 1995;270:20915–20921.

55. Sakatsume M, Igarashi K, Winestock KD, Garotta G, Larner AC, Finbloom DS. The Jak kinases differentially associate with the α and β (accessory factor) chains of the interferon-gamma receptor to form a functional receptor unit capable of activating STAT transcription factors. *J Biol Chem* 1995;270:17528–17534.

56. Greenlund AC, Farrar MA, Viviano BL, Schreiber RD. Ligand induced IFNγ receptor phosphorylation couples the receptor to its signal transduction system (p91). *EMBO J* 1994;13:1591–1600.

57. Greenlund AC, Morales MO, Viviano BL, Yan H, Krolewski J, Schreiber RD. STAT recruitment by tyrosine-phosphorylated cytokine receptors: an ordered reversible affinity-driven process. *Immunity* 1995;2:677–687.

58. Schindler C, Shuai K, Prezioso VR, Darnell JE Jr. Interferon-dependent tyrosine phosphorylation of a latent cytoplasmic transcription factor. *Science* 1992;257:809–813.

59. Shuai K, Stark GR, Kerr IM, Darnell JE Jr. A single phosphotyrosine residue of stat 91 required for gene activation by interferon-γ. *Science* 1993;261:1744–1746.

60. You M, Yu D, Feng G. SHP-2 tyrosine phosphatase functions as a negative regulator of the interferon-stimulated JAK/STAT pathway. *Mol Cell Biol* 1999;19:2416–2424.

61. You M, Zhao Z. Positive effects of SH2 domain-containing tyrosine phosphatase SHP-1 on epidermal growth factor- and interferon-gamma-stimulated activation of STAT transcription factors in HeLa cells. *J Biol Chem* 1997;272:23376–23381.

62. Starr R, Wilson TA, Viney EM, et al. A family of cytokine-inducible inhibitors of signaling. *Nature* 1997;387:917–920.

63. Endo TA, Masuhara M, Yokouchi M, et al. A new protein containing an SH2 domain that inhibits JAK kinases. *Nature* 1997;387:921–924.

64. Naka T, Narazaki M, Hirata M, et al. Structure and function of a new STAT-induced STAT inhibitor. *Nature* 1997;387:924–928.

65. Matsumoto A, Masuhara M, Mitsui K, et al. CIS, a cytokine inducible SH2 protein, is a target of the JAK-STAT5 pathway and modulates STAT5 activation. *Blood* 1997;89:3148–3154.

66. Hilton DJ, Richardson RT, Alexander WS, et al. Twenty proteins containing a C-terminal SOCS box form five structural classes. *Proc Natl Acad Sci U S A* 1998;95:114–119.

67. Starr R, Hilton DJ. Negative regulation of the JAK/STAT pathway. *Bioessays* 1999;21:47–52.

68. Starr R, Metcalf D, Elefanty AG, et al. Liver degeneration and lymphoid deficiencies in mice lacking suppressor of cytokine signaling-1. *Proc Natl Acad Sci U S A* 1998;95:14395–14399.

69. Naka T, Matsumoto T, Narazaki M, et al. Accelerated apoptosis of lymphocytes by augmented induction of Bax in SSI-1 (STAT-induced STAT inhibitor-1) deficient mice. *Proc Natl Acad Sci U S A* 1998;95:15577–15582.

70. Chung CD, Liao JY, Liu B, et al. Specific inhibition of Stat3 signal transduction by PIAS3. *Science* 1997;278:1803–1805.

71. Liu B, Liao J, Rao X, et al. Inhibition of Stat1-mediated gene activation by PIAS1. *Proc Natl Acad Sci U S A* 1998;95:10626–10631.

72. Kim TK, Maniatis T. Regulation of interferon-gamma-activated Stat1

73. Haspel RL, Salditt-Georgieff M, Darnell JE. The rapid inactivation of nuclear tyrosine phosphorylated Stat1 depends upon a protein tyrosine phosphatase. *EMBO J* 1996;15:6262–6268.

74. Zhang J, Farley A, Nicholson SE, et al. The conserved SOCS box motif in suppressors of cytokine signaling binds to elongins B and C and may couple bound proteins to proteasomal degradation. *Proc Natl Acad Sci U S A* 1999;96:2071–2076.

75. Kerr IM, Stark GR. The control of interferon-inducible gene expression. *FEBS Lett* 1991;285:194–198.

76. Lewin AR, Reid LE, McMahon M, Stark GR, Kerr IM. Molecular analysis of a human interferon-inducible gene family. *Eur J Biochem* 1991;199:417–423.

77. Der SD, Zhou A, Williams BR, Silverman RH. Identification of genes differentially regulated by interferon alpha, beta, or gamma using oligonucleotide arrays. *Proc Natl Acad Sci U S A* 1998;95:15623–15628.

78. Vilcek J, Sen GC. Interferons and other cytokines. In: Fields BN, Knipe DM, Howley PM, eds. *Fields virology*, 3rd ed. Philadelphia: Lippincott–Raven Publishers, 1996:375.

79. Silverman RH, Cirino NM. In: Morris DR, Harford JB, eds. *mRNA metabolism and post-transcriptional gene regulation*. New York: John Wiley and Sons, 1997:295.

80. Meurs E, Chong K, Galabru J, Thomas NS, Kerr IM, Williams BR, Hovanessian AG. Molecular cloning and characterization of the human double-stranded RNA-activated protein kinase induced by interferon. *Cell* 1990;62:379–390.

81. McMillan NAJ, Williams BRG. Structure and function of the interferon-induced protein kinase, PKR, and related enzymes. In: Clemens MJ, ed. *Protein phosphorylation in cell growth regulation*. London: Harwood Academic Publishers, 1996;225.

82. Arnheiter H, Frese M, Kambadur R, Meier E, Haller O. Mx transgenic mice—animal models of health. *Curr Top Microbiol Immunol* 1996;206:119–147.

83. Chin YE, Kitagawa M, Su WS, You Z, Iwamoto Y, Fu X. Cell growth arrest and induction of cyclin-dependent kinase inhibitor p21 mediated by Stat1. *Science* 1996;272:719–722.

84. Bromberg JF, Horvath CM, Wen Z, Schreiber RD, Darnell JE. Transcriptionally active Stat1 is required for the antiproliferative effects of both interferon alpha and interferon gamma. *Proc Natl Acad Sci U S A* 1996;93:7673–7678.

85. Schreiber RD, Pace JL, Russell SW, Altman A, Katz DH. Macrophage-activating factor produced by a T cell hybridoma: physiochemical and biosynthetic resemblance to gamma-interferon. *J Immunol* 1983;131:826–832.

86. Buchmeier NA, Schreiber RD. Requirement of endogenous interferon-gamma production for resolution of Listeria monocytogenes infection. *Proc Natl Acad Sci U S A* 1985;82:7404–7408.

87. Nathan CF, Murray HW, Wiebe ME, Rubin BY. Identification of interferon-gamma as the lymphokine that activates human macrophage oxidative metabolism and antimicrobial activity. *J Exp Med* 1983;158:670–689.

88. Schreiber RD, Celada A. Molecular characterization of interferon gamma as a macrophage activating factor. *Lymphokines* 1985;11:87–118.

89. Belosevic M, Davis CE, Meltzer MS, Nacy CA. Regulation of activated macrophage antimicrobial activities. Identification of lymphokines that cooperate with IFN-gamma for induction of resistance to infection. *J Immunol* 1988;141:890–896.

90. Suzuki Y, Orellana MA, Schreiber RD, Remington JS. Interferon-gamma: the major mediator of resistance against Toxoplasma gondii. *Science* 1988;240:516–518.

91. Nacy CA, Fortier AH, Meltzer MS, Buchmeier NA, Schreiber RD. Macrophage activation to kill Leishmania major: activation of macrophages for intracellular destruction of amastigotes can be induced by both recombinant interferon-gamma and non-interferon lymphokines. *J Immunol* 1985;135:3505–3511.

92. Dalton DK, Pitts-meek S, Keshav S, Figari IS, Bradley A, Stewart TA. Multiple defects of immune function in mice with disrupted interferon-γ genes. *Science* 1993;259:1739–1742.

93. Huang S, Hendriks W, Althage A, et al. Immune response in mice

by the ubiquitin-proteasome pathway. *Science* 1996;273:1717–1719.

that lack the interferon-γ receptor. *Science* 1993;259:1742–1745.

94. Nathan C. Natural resistance and nitric oxide. *Cell* 1995;82:873–876.

95. MacMicking J, Xie Q-W, Nathan C. Nitric oxide and macrophage function. *Annu Rev Immunol* 1997;15:323–350.

96. Beckerman KP, Rogers HW, Corbett JA, Schreiber RD, McDaniel ML, Unanue ER. Release of nitric oxide during the T cell-independent pathway of macrophage activation. Its role in resistance to Listeria monocytogenes. *J Immunol* 1993;150:888–895.

97. Shiloh MU, MacMicking JD, Nicholson S, et al. Phenotype of mice and macrophages deficient in both phagocyte oxidase and inducible nitric oxide synthase. *Immunity* 1999;10:29–38.

98. Mach B, Steimle V, Martinez-Soria E, Reith W. Regulation of MHC class II genes: lessons from a disease. *Annu Rev Immunol* 1996;14: 301–331.

99. Mond JJ, Carman J, Sarma C, Ohara J, Finkelman FD. Interferon-gamma suppresses B cell stimulation factor (BSF-1) induction of class II MHC determinants on B cells. *J Immunol* 1986;137:3534–3537.

100. Germain RN. Antigen processing and presentation. In: Paul WE, ed. *Fundamental immunology*, 3rd ed. New York: Raven Press, 1993:629.

101. Pamer E, Cresswell P. Mechanisms of MHC class I restricted antigen processing. *Annu Rev Immunol* 1998;16:323–358.

102. Gaczynska M, Rock KL, Spies T, Goldberg AL. Peptidase activities of proteasomes are differentially regulated by the major histocompatibility complex-encoded genes for LMP2 and LMP7. *Proc Natl Acad Sci U S A* 1994;91:9213–9217.

103. York IA, Rock KL. Antigen processing and presentation by the class I major histocompatibility complex. *Annu Rev Immunol* 1996;14: 369–396.

104. Groettrup M, Soza A, Eggers M, et al. A role for the proteasome regulator PA28α in antigen presentation. *Nature* 1996;381:166–168.

105. Suto R, Srivastava PK. A mechanism for the specific immunogenicity of heat shock proteins-chaperoned peptides. *Science* 1995;269:1585–1588.

106. Abbas AK, Murphy KM, Sher A. Functional diversity of helper T lymphocytes. *Nature* 1997;383:787–793.

107. Hsieh C-S, Macatonia S, Tripp CS, Wolf SF, O'Garra A, Murphy KM. Development of Th1 CD4$^+$ T cells through IL-12 produced by Listeria-induced macrophages. *Science* 1993;260:547–549.

108. Gately MK, Renzetti LM, Magram J, et al. Interleukin-12/Interleukin-12-receptor system: role in normal and pathologic immune responses. *Annu Rev Immunol* 1998;16:495–521.

109. Dighe AS, Campbell D, Hsieh C-S, et al. Tissue specific targeting of cytokine unresponsiveness in transgenic mice. *Immunity* 1995;3: 657–666.

110. Szabo SJ, Dighe AS, Gubler U, Murphy KM. Regulation of the interleukin (IL)-12R β2 subunit expression in developing T helper 1 (Th1) and Th2 cells. *J Exp Med* 1997;185:817–824.

111. Szabo SJ, Jacobson NG, Dighe AS, Gubler U, Murphy KM. Developmental commitment to the Th2 lineage by extinction of IL-12 signaling. *Immunity* 1995;2:665–675.

112. Gajewski TF, Fitch FW. Anti-proliferative effect of IFN-gamma in immune regulation. IV. Murine CTL clones produce IL-3 and GM-CSF, the activity of which is masked by the inhibitory action of secreted IFN-gamma. *J Immunol* 1990;144:548–556.

113. Snapper CM, Peschel C, Paul WE. IFN-gamma stimulates IgG2α secretion by murine B cells stimulated with bacterial lipopolysaccharide. *J Immunol* 1988;140:2121–2127.

114. Snapper CM, McIntyre TM, Mandler R, et al. Induction of IgG3 secretion by interferon gamma: a model for T cell-independent class switching in response to T cell-independent type 2 antigens. *J Exp Med* 1992;175:1367–1371.

115. Snapper CM, Paul WE. Interferon-gamma and B cell stimulatory factor-1 reciprocally regulate Ig isotype production. *Science* 1987;236:944–947.

116. Snapper CM. Interferon-gamma. In: Snapper CM, ed. *Cytokine regulation of humoral immunity*. West Sussex, UK: John Wiley and Sons, 1996:325.

117. Adams DO, Hamilton TA. The cell biology of macrophage activation. *Annu Rev Immunol* 1984;2:283–318.

118. Griffith TS, Wiley SR, Kubin MZ, Sedger LM, Maliszewski CR, Fanger NA. Monocyte-mediated tumoricidal activity via the tumor necrosis fac-tor-related cytokine, TRAIL. *J Exp Med* 1999;189:1343–1354.

119. Nastala CL, Edington HD, McKinney TG, et al. Recombinant IL-12 administration induces tumor regression in association with IFN-gamma production. *J Immunol* 1994;153:1697–1706.

120. Brunda MJ. Interleukin-12. *J Leukoc Biol* 1994;55:280–288.

121. Restifo NP, Esquivel F, Asher AL, et al. Defective presentation of endogenous antigens by a murine sarcoma. *J Immunol* 1991;147:1453–1459.

122. Restifo NP, Esquivel F, Kawakami Y, et al. Identification of human cancers deficient in antigen processing. *J Exp Med* 1993;177:265–272.

123. Tuttle TM, McCrady CW, Inge TH, Salour M, Bear HD. Gamma interferon plays a key role in T-cell-induced tumor regression. *Cancer Res* 1993;53:833–839.

124. Dighe AS, Richards E, Old LJ, Schreiber RD. Enhanced *in vivo* growth and resistance to rejection of tumor cells expressing dominant negative IFNγ receptors. *Immunity* 1994;1:447–456.

125. Coughlin CM, Salhany KE, Gee MS, et al. Tumor cell responses to IFNγ affect tumorigenicity and response to IL-12 therapy and antiangiogenesis. *Immunity* 1998;9:25–34.

126. Kaplan DH, Shankaran V, Dighe AS, et al. Demonstration of an IFNγ dependent tumor surveillance system in immunocompetent mice. *Proc Natl Acad Sci U S A* 1998;95:7556–7561.

127. Kamijo R, Le J, Shapiro D, et al. Mice that lack the interferon-γ receptor have profoundly altered responses to infection with bacillus Calmette-Guérin and subsequent challenge with lipopolysaccharide. *J Exp Med* 1993;178:1435–1440.

128. Lu B, Ebensperger C, Dembic Z, et al. Targeted disruption of the interferon-gamma receptor 2 gene results in severe immune defects in mice. *Proc Natl Acad Sci U S A* 1998;95:8233–8238.

129. Müller U, Steinhoff U, Reis LFL, et al. Functional role of type I and type II interferons in antiviral defense. *Science* 1994;264:1918–1921.

130. Newport MJ, Huxley CM, Huston S, et al. A mutation in the interferon-γ-receptor gene and susceptibility to mycobacterial infection. *N Engl J Med* 1996;335:1941–1949.

131. Jouanguy E, Altare F, Lamhamedi S, et al. Interferon-γ-receptor deficiency in an infant with fatal bacille Calmette-Guérin infection. *N Engl J Med* 1996;335:1956–1961.

132. Pierre-Audigier C, Jouanguy E, Lamhamedi S, et al. Fatal disseminated mycobacterium smegmatis infection in a child with inherited interferon γ receptor deficiency. *Clin Infect Dis* 1997;24:982–984.

133. Jouanguy E, Lamhamedi-Cherradi S, Altare F, et al. Partial interferon-gamma receptor 1 deficiency in a child with tuberculoid bacillus Calmette-Guérin infection and a sibling with clinical tuberculosis. *J Clin Invest* 1997;100:2658–2664.

134. Jouanguy E, Lamhamedi-Cherradi S, Lammas D, et al. A human IFNGR1 small deletion hotspot associated with dominant susceptibility to mycobacterial infection. *Nat Genet* 1999;21:370–378.

135. Dighe AS, Farrar MA, Schreiber RD. Inhibition of cellular responsiveness to interferon-γ (IFNγ) induced by overexpression of inactive forms of the IFNγ receptor. *J Biol Chem* 1993;268:10645–10653.

136. Dorman SE, Holland SM. Mutation in the signal-transducing chain of the interferon-gamma receptor and susceptibility to mycobacterial infection. *J Clin Invest* 1998;101:2364–2369.

137. Altare F, Durandy A, Lammas D, et al. Impairment of mycobacterial immunity in human interleukin-12 receptor deficiency. *Science* 1998;280:1432–1435.

138. de Jong R, Altare F, Haagen I, et al. Severe mycobacterial and salmonella infections in interleukin-12 receptor-deficient patients. *Science* 1998;280:1435–1438.

139. Altare F, Lammas D, Revy P, et al. Inherited interleukin-12 deficiency in a child with bacille Calmette-Guérin and salmonella enteritidis disseminated infection. *J Clin Invest* 1998;102:2035–2040.

140. Kurzrock R, Talpaz M, Kantarjian H, et al. Therapy of chronic myelogenous leukemia with recombinant interferon-gamma. *Blood* 1987;70:943–947.

141. Dinauer MC, Orkin SH. Chronic granulomatous disease. *Ann Rev Med* 1992;43:117–124.

142. Nosaka T, van Deursen JMA, Tripp RA, et al. Defective lymphoid development in mice lacking Jak3. *Science* 1995;270:800–802.

143. Thomis DC, Gurniak CB, Tivol E, Sharpe AH, Berg LJ. Defects in B lymphocyte maturation and T lymphocyte activation in mice lack-

ing Jak3. *Science* 1995;270:794–797.

144. Park SY, Saijo K, Takahashi T, et al. Developmental defects of lymphoid cells in Jak3 kinase-deficient mice. *Immunity* 1995;3: 771–782.

145. Takeda K, Noguchi K, Shi W, et al. Targeted disruption of the mouse Stat3 gene leads to early embryonic lethality. *Proc Natl Acad Sci U S A* 1997;94:3801–3804.

146. Takeda K, Kaisho T, Yoshida N, Takeda J, Kishimoto T, Akira S. Stat3 activation is responsible for IL-6-dependent T cell proliferation through preventing apoptosis: generation and characterization of T cell-specific Stat3-deficient mice. *J Immunol* 1998;161:4652–4660.

147. Takeda K, Clausen BE, Kaisho T, et al. Enhanced Th1 activity and development of chronic enterocolitis in mice devoid of Stat3 in macrophages and neutrophils. *Immunity* 1999;10:39–49.

148. Thierfelder WE, van Deursen JM, Yamamoto K, et al. Requirement for Stat4 in interleukin-12-mediated responses of natural killer and T cells. *Nature* 1996;382:171–174.

149. Kaplan MH, Sun Y-L, Hoey T, Grusby MJ. Impaired IL-12 responses and enhanced development of Th2 cells in Stat4-deficient mice. *Nature* 1996;382:174–177.

150. Feldman GM, Rosenthal LA, Liu X, et al. STAT5A-deficient mice demonstrate a defect in granulocyte-macrophage colony-stimulating factor-induced proliferation and gene expression. *Blood* 1997;90:1768–1776.

151. Teglund S, McKay C, Schuetz E, et al. Stat5a and Stat5b proteins have essential and nonessential, or redundant, roles in cytokine responses. *Cell* 1998;93:841–850.

152. Udy GB, Towers RP, Snell RG, et al. Requirement of STAT5b for sexual dimorphism of body growth rates and liver gene expression. *Proc Natl Acad Sci U S A* 1997;94:7239–7244.

153. Shimoda K, van Deursen J, Sangster MY, et al. Lack of IL-4-induced Th2 response and IgE class switching in mice with disrupted Stat6 gene. *Nature* 1996;380:630–633.

154. Kaplan MH, Schindler U, Smiley ST, Grusby MJ. Stat6 is required for mediating responses to IL-4 and for the development of Th2 cells. *Immunity* 1996;4:313–319.

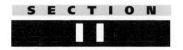

PRINCIPLES AND PRACTICE
OF CELL TRANSFER THERAPY

12

CELL TRANSFER THERAPY: BASIC PRINCIPLES AND PRECLINICAL STUDIES

MARK E. DUDLEY

The cellular arm of the immune system plays a central role in the destruction of tumor cells, regression of established tumor deposits, and maintenance of antitumor immunity. Adoptive transfer therapy aims to promote these cellular immune functions in cancer patients by the administration of cells that have been cultured *ex vivo*. In adoptive transfer approaches, immune effector cells are collected and cultured, circumventing normal immune regulatory constraints and potential tumor suppression. Desirable cellular characteristics can be enhanced in cell culture, even by agents that are toxic or would otherwise compromise the patient's health *in vivo*. Finally, the activated and expanded effector-cell population is used to treat the autologous patient. Adoptive transfer therapy can be simply a passive treatment aimed at direct lysis of tumor targets *in vivo*. Many approaches, however, aim to use adoptive transfer as an active immunization strategy in which the administered immune cells undergo amplification *in vivo*, elaborate cytokines that regulate host immune responses, and recruit endogenous immune effector cells to eliminate tumor cells.

Preclinical models have helped define the critical parameters of adoptive transfer therapy and have laid the groundwork for designing clinical trials. Early studies relied on immunization of tumor-free donor mice for the generation of potent effector cells that were subsequently transferred into syngeneic, tumor-bearing recipients. These studies proved effective for determining the attributes of transferred lymphocytes that contributed to therapeutic efficacy, as well as for evaluating adjuvant treatments to the recipient animals that could impact disease outcome. The approach of using cells from immunized donor animals to treat tumor-bearing recipients, however, is not easily translated to human tumor therapy. In most clinical settings, each patient must be the donor, as well as the recipient of transferred cells. With technical advances in cell culture methodology and *ex vivo* activation of human cells, studies were undertaken to directly model the clinical application of the new technique. Mouse models helped to evaluate multiple parameters of transfer that could not easily be resolved in clinical trials and defined the *in vitro* characteristics of the transferred cell relevant to therapeutic benefit *in vivo*. The influence of tumor immunogenicity, methods of cell expansion, and other parameters of treatment have been investigated in these preclinical models and have impacted clinical trial design and interpretation.

ADOPTIVE TRANSFER IN MICE USING SYNGENEIC IMMUNE SPLENOCYTES

Established Tumors Suppress Adoptive Immunotherapy

Many virally or chemically induced tumors of mice have been used to immunize syngeneic mice against challenge by the same tumor. Methods of antitumor immunization have included injection of irradiated tumors (often mixed with *Corynebacterium parvum*) or surgical removal of a transplanted tumor mass. Mice who have undergone a primary immunization *in vivo* ("primed" mice) could subsequently reject a lethal challenge of the immunizing tumor. Furthermore, splenocytes derived from immunized animals could be secondarily stimulated *in vitro* to specifically lyse tumor cells. The same methods of immunization that readily generated protective immunity, however, were generally ineffective for treatment of established tumors. Similarly, although adoptively transferred immune splenocytes conferred protective immunity when transferred before tumor challenge, they did not eradicate established tumors (1–3).

The result that adoptive transfer of immune splenocytes was less effective in treatment of established tumors than in protection against tumor challenge suggested that established tumors could suppress an antitumor immune response. This hypothesis fueled a search for mechanisms of tumor-generated immune suppression. Multiple factors have been proposed to account for tumor suppression of adoptively transferred cells. One proposed mechanism involves systemically active, soluble factors that nonspecifically interfere with immune function in tumor-bearing mice. North et al. (4) reported that a low-molecular-weight factor in the circulation of tumor-bearing mice severely impaired the capacity of the host to resist experimental bacterial infection. Ting et al. (5) similarly reported a humoral factor in the ascitic fluid of tumor-bearing mice that could suppress primary *in vivo* immunization against tumors, as well as the induction of cell-mediated cytotoxic responses *in vitro*. Subsequently, several tumor-produced suppressors of immune function have

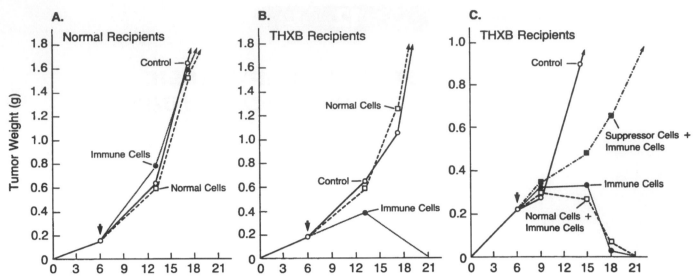

FIGURE 1. Evidence that transplantable suppressor T cells prevent tumor elimination by immune spleen cells. **A:** Normal mice treated by infusion of *in vitro* sensitized or normal splenocytes 6 days after challenge with an intradermal Meth A tumor demonstrate progressive tumor growth. **B:** Infusion of immune cells into T-cell–depleted (THXB) mice 6 days after challenge with an intradermal Meth A tumor caused complete tumor rejection. THXB mice treated with normal splenocytes showed progressive growth. **C:** Prior infusion of suppressor splenocytes from a mouse with progressively growing Meth A tumor abrogated the effect of immune cell transfer. Normal splenocytes had no effect on immune cell–mediated tumor regression. [Adapted from Berendt MJ and North RJ. T-cell–mediated suppression of antitumor immunity. An explanation for progressive growth of an immunogenic tumor. *J Exp Med* 1980;151(1):69.]

been identified at the molecular level, including soluble tumor necrosis factor receptor (6), transforming growth factor–β (7), and prostaglandins (8), as well as additional unidentified factors (9,10). Soluble suppressive molecules produced by the tumor could directly inhibit T-cell function or interfere with macrophage or other immune cell functions.

In addition to systemic, nonspecific suppression of immunity, a T-cell–mediated mechanism of immune suppression was described by Berendt and North (11). These authors investigated treatment of the highly immunogenic Meth A fibrosarcoma by adoptive transfer of T cells from immunized donors. They showed that it was possible to invoke the regression of large, established Meth A tumors by intravenous infusion of immune T cells, but only if the tumors were growing in T-cell–deficient mice. Furthermore, tumor treatment in T-cell–deficient mice was prevented by prior infusion of splenic T cells from T-cell–intact, tumor-bearing donors (Fig. 1). These studies support a role for suppressor T cells in the resistance of established tumors to adoptive transfer therapy. North and his collaborators extended these results to other immunogenic murine tumors, including the SA-1 sarcoma and the L5178Y lymphoma, and defined a CD4+ subset of T cells as the effector-cell population (12–14). Similarly, Greenberg et al. demonstrated that a suppressive population of T cells was generated when FBL-3–immune splenocytes were cultured *in vitro* for 5 days without antigen stimulation (15). The mechanism of T-cell–mediated suppression in these murine models and the relevance of these findings to poorly immunogenic tumors (including most human tumors) remains to be determined. Whatever the mechanisms involved, an established growing tumor interacts

differently with the host immune system than a newly transplanted tumor.

Systemic Immunosuppression and Interleukin-2 Administration Augment Adoptive Therapy

Although tumor suppression of adoptive immunotherapy has been proposed to occur by many mechanisms, some immunogenic tumors proved to be susceptible to treatment with transferred cells. In 1975, Berenson et al. (16) showed that the immunogenic Friend virus–induced lymphoma, FBL-3, could be successfully treated by adoptive transfer therapy. An intraperitoneal challenge of 1×10^4 FBL-3 cells was treated with immune splenocytes administered intravenously within 1 day of tumor challenge. Although treatment using 1×10^7 immune cells alone was successful only with a relatively unimpressive tumor burden, manipulation of the tumor-bearing host greatly improved the efficacy of adoptive transfer. Mice inoculated intraperitoneally with as many as 1×10^7 FBL-3 cells and treated as late as 5 days after inoculation with cyclophosphamide plus 1×10^6 immune spleen cells survived tumor free (Fig. 2). The effectiveness of adoptive transfer treatments for many different murine tumors has been greatly improved by immunosuppressive regimens, such as cyclophosphamide administration or radiation treatment. The mechanisms by which cyclophosphamide enhanced adoptive transfer therapy were unclear. For the FBL-3 tumor, cyclophosphamide had a significant tumoricidal effect, but cyclophosphamide alone in this model was not curative. North and his coworkers (12,17) indirectly demonstrated that elimination of CD4+ cells from an L5178 lym-

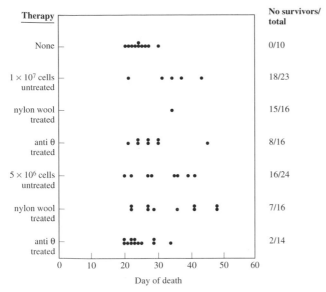

Therapy		No survivors/ total
None		0/10
1 × 10⁷ cells untreated		18/23
nylon wool treated		15/16
anti θ treated		8/16
5 × 10⁶ cells untreated		16/24
nylon wool treated		7/16
anti θ treated		2/14

FIGURE 2. Adoptive immunotherapy cures mice of large tumor burden after pretreatment with cyclophosphamide. Mice received intraperitoneal inoculation with 1×10^7 FBL-3 leukemia cells. Five days later, cyclophosphamide mice received cyclophosphamide followed 6 hours later by the indicated number of immune splenocytes. Each dot represents survival of one mouse. (From Berenson JR, Einstein AB, Fefer A. Syngeneic adoptive immunotherapy and chemotherapy of a Friend leukemia: requirement for T cells. *J Immunol* 1975;115:234, with permission.)

phoma-bearing host augmented adoptive therapy by CD8⁺ immune cells. The researchers championed a hypothesis of suppressor cell abrogation of immune cell function.

In contrast, Cameron et al. (18) concluded that suppressor T cells could not account for the results of experiments with MCA-38 tumors. They investigated the synergistic effects of local irradiation with adoptive therapy of hepatic metastasis of the weakly immunogenic murine adenocarcinoma, MC-38. Mice underwent radiation treatment that included only the right side of the liver, followed by adoptive immunotherapy. When the number of right- and left-sided metastases were individually counted, tumor reduction compared with controls was seen only on the right (irradiated) side. The presence of left-sided tumor did not affect the reduction in the number of right-sided metastases. The authors concluded that these data failed to support a role for suppressor T cells in the abrogation of adoptive immunotherapy. Other possible mechanisms by which cyclophosphamide and radiation augment adoptive transfer therapy include activation of macrophages in the tumor bed or reduction of the tumor burden before immune cell transfer. Additional studies are required to resolve the mechanisms involved. In any case, the use of an immunosuppressive agent before adoptive therapy is a highly effective strategy. This strategy has been used to augment adoptive cell treatment in many of the mouse tumor models described below.

In addition to immune suppression, other manipulations of the tumor-bearing recipient can augment adoptive therapy with immune cells. Interleukin-2 (IL-2) support of transferred T cells *in vivo* can be critical to T-cell efficacy. Cheever et al. (19) investigated the role of IL-2 in the adoptive immunother-

apy of the FBL-3 leukemia. When immune splenocytes were specifically activated by *in vitro* culture with FBL-3 and then expanded in culture with IL-2, the resulting T lymphocytes specifically lysed FBL-3. They also mediated specific adoptive therapy of disseminated FBL-3 *in vivo* when used with cyclophosphamide. In this model, IL-2 was highly effective in augmenting the *in vivo* efficacy of these IL-2–dependent, cultured T lymphocytes in adoptive therapy. IL-2 did not augment the *in vivo* efficacy of noncultured immune splenocytes in the FBL-3 model. Shu and Rosenberg (20) reported similar results with a weakly immunogenic transplantable sarcoma, MCA-105. In this study, fresh immune spleen cells were not cytotoxic to MCA-105 tumor targets in a 4-hour chromium-release assay. Adoptive transfer of fresh immune splenocytes, however, mediated the regression of established MCA-105 tumors. The therapeutic efficacy of these cells was not augmented by IL-2 administration *in vivo*. In contrast to fresh cells, secondary *in vitro* sensitization (IVS) by culture of immune cells with irradiated MCA-105 tumors generated cytotoxic cultures that lysed MCA-105 tumors. Effective adoptive immunotherapy with these secondarily sensitized immune cells required the *in vivo* administration of IL-2 (Fig. 3).

One mechanism by which IL-2 treatment may augment adoptive transfer therapy *in vivo* is by promoting the survival and proliferation of transferred cells. Evidence for this proposal was collected using immune effector cells and Thy-1 congenic mice (21). Fluorescence activated cell sorting with an antibody specific for the Thy-1 marker of donor origin was used to identify and enumerate the transferred T cells in the host after adoptive transfer. When cultured T-cell lines immune to the FBL-3 leukemia were transferred into FBL-3–bearing hosts in a manner that was effective in tumor therapy, the T cells proliferated *in vivo* even in the absence of IL-2. The growth rate of donor T cells, however, was augmented by administration of exogenous IL-2. Further work showed that IL-2 and the availability of antigen *in vivo* affected the persistence of T cells after transfer (22). Again, T cells and mice congenic for the Thy-1 marker were used to examine immune cells after transfer. Cultured T cells specific for FBL-3 tumors were adoptively transferred into normal mice and then induced to proliferate *in vivo* by specific stimulation with irradiated FBL-3 and IL-2. The growth of antigen-activated donor T cells, rather than host lymphocytes, was preferentially stimulated (Fig. 4). Additionally, IL-2 administration increased the long-term (day 35) survival of transferred lymphocytes.

A poorly understood variable in studies of adoptive transfer therapy is the inflammatory context of antigen *in vivo*. In a nontumor model, Jenkins et al. demonstrated that the fate of adoptively transferred naïve T cells is critically dependent on encountering their cognate antigen (23). When naïve CD4⁺ T cells from T-cell receptor transgenic mice were transferred to syngeneic recipients, the donor cells could be followed by a clonotype-specific, anti–T-cell receptor monoclonal antibody. Without administration of cognate antigen, the transferred T cells disappeared within weeks. If cognate antigen was administered by an "inflammatory route" (i.e., by subcutaneous injection in adjuvant), transferred T cells in the draining lymph node underwent activation, rapid proliferation, and large

FRESH IMMUNE SPLEEN CELLS

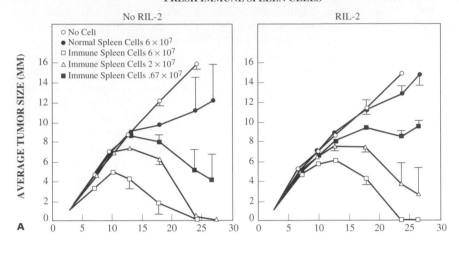

A

5 DAY IVS IMMUNE CELLS

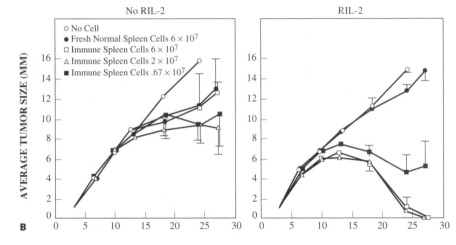

B

FIGURE 3. Adoptive immunotherapy of MCA-105 tumors with *in vitro* sensitized (IVS) immune cells **(B)**, but not with fresh immune splenocytes **(A)**, is augmented by recombinant interleukin-2 (rIL-2). Preirradiated mice received intradermal inoculation of MCA-105 tumor. Three days later, immune effectors were transferred intravenously and rIL-2 was given intraperitoneally twice a day for 6 days. (From Shu S and Rosenberg SA. Adoptive immunotherapy of a newly induced sarcoma: immunologic characteristics of effector cells. *J Immunol* 1985; 135:2895, with permission.)

numerical expansion within 3 days. If the antigen was administered by a "tolerogenic route" (i.e., by intravenous injection), then the transferred T cells underwent a brief period of activation, followed by apoptosis and anergy. Other studies using T-cell receptor transgenic mice and transplantable tumors have shown that tumor-specific cells in a tumor-bearing animal were also sensitive to the inflammatory environment of the antigen (24–26). In each of these reports, tumor cells survived and tumors grew, despite the presence in the host of many tumor-specific T cells. The persistence and function of lymphocytes *in vivo*, and ultimately their ability to eradicate tumors, were affected by the availability and the inflammatory context of their specific antigen.

These studies demonstrated that the tumor-bearing host can affect the outcome of adoptive transfer therapy. Several systemic treatments of tumor-bearing mice were effective in augmenting adoptive therapy. Host immune suppression by using cyclophosphamide or radiation before immune cell transfer was critical to the treatment of some tumors. Large, well-established, weakly immunogenic tumor deposits (analogous to human tumors) were most dependent on immunosuppressive treatment. Similarly, IL-2 administration after lymphocyte transfer was shown to augment antitumor therapy and increase trans-

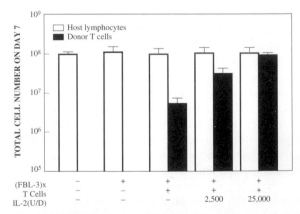

FIGURE 4. Adoptively transferred donor T cells rather than host lymphocytes preferentially expand after administration of interleukin-2 (IL-2) and antigen *in vivo*. Mice were left untreated or injected with irradiated FBL-3 leukemia cells. Concurrently, mice received no additional treatment or administration of cultured FBL-3–specific, Thy-1–congenic T cells. IL-2 was administered by intraperitoneal injection for 7 days. On day 7, the total number of host lymphocytes and donor-derived T cells within the ascites and spleen of each group of mice were identified and enumerated. Mean of donor T cells (*closed bars*) and host lymphocytes (*open bars*) with standard deviations are shown. (From Chen W and Cheever MA. Donor T cells can be induced to grow and survive long term in vivo without previous host immunosuppression. *J Immunol* 1994;152:4767, with permission.)

ferred cell persistence. IL-2–dependent effector cells derived the most benefit from *in vivo* IL-2 support. Although the use of systemic treatments could increase the morbidity and expense of adoptive transfer protocols, these preclinical studies strongly support a role for systemic treatment with chemotherapy, IL-2, or both, for patients receiving adoptive cell transfer therapy.

In Vitro Sensitization Generates Potent Effector Cells

From the first successful reports of adoptive therapy, attempts to characterize the origin and function of immune cells mediating tumor rejection were undertaken. Early work in the FBL-3 lymphoma model demonstrated that T cells constituted the immune population in transferred splenocytes (16). Cheever et al. (27) demonstrated that transferred splenocytes mediated tumor treatment by an antigen-specific mechanism. Cytolytic assays *in vitro* demonstrated that FBL-3 and EL-4, a chemically induced virus-negative tumor, were antigenically distinct. *In vitro* immune spleen cells lysed the tumor to which they were immunized, but did not lyse the unrelated tumor. Immune cells demonstrated similar specificity when used in adoptive therapy studies. Mice with established FBL-3 or EL-4 tumors were cured by treatment on day 5, consisting of cyclophosphamide plus 2×10^7 immune spleen cells. Mice given 2×10^7 normal cells or cells sensitized to the other tumor did not demonstrate cures. The *in vivo* specificity of adoptively transferred cells strongly suggested that specific antigens expressed by each tumor were being targeted.

To generate effector cells with better tumor specificity, enhancement of primary immune cells by secondary IVS was investigated. Early studies relied on mixed lymphocyte and tumor cultures for secondary IVS. Typical of these studies was a report by Cheever et al., who examined the generation of therapeutically effective cells during secondary IVS of FBL-3–immune splenocytes. IVS of FBL-3–immune cells with FBL-3 tumors generated lytic cultures with improved therapeutic activity. The generation of maximum lytic activity and maximum therapeutic activity were chronologically disparate, suggesting different effector-cell populations mediating each function. Greenberg et al. (29) eventually showed that therapeutic efficacy was largely mediated by transfer of Lyt-1+2− (CD8−) T cells, whereas *in vitro* cytotoxicity was derived from the Lyt-2+ (CD8+) subset. Thus, when effector cells were derived using this *in vitro* culture system, the predominant cell required to eradicate FBL-3 *in vivo* was not cytolytic to the tumor *in vitro*. In retrospect, secondary IVS alone rarely added much to primary immunization for highly immunogenic tumors, such as FBL-3. For weakly or nonimmunogenic tumors, however, IVS dramatically improved the efficacy of adoptively transferred cells.

The identification of T-cell growth factor (30) and the subsequent production of recombinant IL-2 (31), its active component, facilitated IVS and improved the effectiveness of lymphocyte cultures in treating established tumors. Using the FBL-3 tumor model, Eberlein et al. (32) demonstrated that adoptive immunotherapy could result in curing mice of the established local tumor, as well as the established disseminated

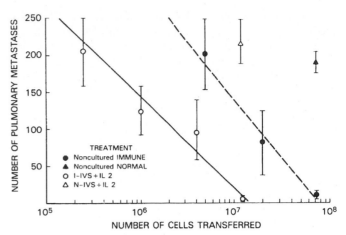

FIGURE 5. *In vitro* sensitized (IVS)-immune splenocytes are more effective in adoptive immunotherapy of pulmonary metastasis than fresh splenocytes. Mice with established 3-day-old MCA-105 pulmonary metastases were treated with the indicated number of fresh or IVS splenocytes from immune or normal mice. Three to 9 days later, mice received twice-daily interleukin-2 (IL-2) administration. Pulmonary metastases were counted on day 14. Lines of linear regression are shown for different types of cells. (From Shu S et al. In vitro sensitization and expansion with viable tumor cells and interleukin-2 in the generation of specific therapeutic effector cells. *J Immunol* 1986;136:3891, with permission.)

tumor. These authors showed for the first time that when immune splenocytes were secondarily sensitized to the FBL-3 tumor *in vitro*, they could be expanded in IL-2 and grown for multiple generations while retaining their ability to cure mice. Shu et al. (33) used IVS with IL-2 to examine adoptive immunotherapy of experimentally induced pulmonary metastases from the weakly immunogenic MCA-105 sarcoma. Using IL-2 during IVS, nonimmune or MCA-105–immune spleen cells increased in numbers up to 94-fold in 15 days. Only the IVS cultures of animals primed *in vivo*, however, were therapeutically effective. Immunotherapy with expanded MCA-105–immune cultures led to the reduction of established 3-day-old pulmonary metastases, prolongation of survival, and tumor cure in the majority of animals. Administration to tumor-bearing hosts of exogenous IL-2 improved the efficacy of the adoptive cellular therapy with cultured, but not fresh, immune cells. On a per-cell basis, the IVS-immune cells were eight to tenfold more effective when compared with fresh, noncultured MCA-105–immune cells in eliminating established pulmonary metastases (Fig. 5).

Many other studies reported improved adoptive immunotherapy using IVS cells. Peng et al. (34) reported on the eradication of subcutaneous MCA-205 sarcoma by immune T cells. Successful therapy in this difficult treatment model was dependent on transfer of a large number of secondary IVS-immune T cells, as well as pretreatment of the tumor-bearing mice with radiation. Additionally, the therapeutic effect of the adoptively transferred T cells was eliminated if CD4 cells or CD8 cells were depleted. In another difficult treatment model, the T-cell subsets mediating therapy of the nonimmunogenic MCA-102 sarcoma were identified (35). IVS of immune cells with IL-2 was required to generate therapeutically effective cultures. Selective depletion of T-cell subsets *in vivo* was used to show a requirement for CD4+ (L3T4+) and CD8+ (Lyt-2+) T cells in mediating tumor regression. The depletion of CD4+ cells was circumvented by administration of exogenous IL-2 in this model. Taken as a group, these studies indicated that IVS of immune cells and culture expansion with IL-2 significantly increased therapeutic efficacy of immune cell cultures. The number of cells available for adoptive transfer and the "per cell" therapeutic efficacy of the transferred cells were improved by IVS methods.

Selection of Effector-Cell Attributes Impacts Therapeutic Efficacy

Lymphocytes are a highly heterogeneous group of cells. Questions remain regarding which T-cell traits should be selected and which T-cell traits should be abandoned for optimum efficacy in adoptive transfer. Specific tumor lysis by IVS cultures has been widely used as a surrogate marker of the therapeutic value of T-cell cultures. Direct evidence for a correlation between lytic ability and therapeutic effectiveness was collected by Matsumura et al (36). In this study, cloned T-cell lines were generated by IVS with tumor and IL-2. Experiments using these clones demonstrated that the *in vitro* cytotoxic specificity of the clones correlated with their *in vivo* infiltration into metastatic tumor deposits, as well as their *in vivo* antitumor specificity.

Specific cytokine secretion by transferred cell cultures may be a more valuable surrogate marker for therapeutic efficacy than lysis. Several reports document the capability of T-cell cultures from cancer patients to specifically secrete cytokines when stimulated with autologous tumor cells. For instance, Schwartzentruber et al. (37) described T-cell lines derived from tumor-infiltrating lymphocytes (TILs) from two melanoma patients and one breast carcinoma patient that specifically secreted interferon-γ (IFN-γ), tumor necrosis factor–α, and granulocyte-macrophage colony-stimulating factor when stimulated with the autologous tumor. Similarly, Maccalli et al. (38) reported that tumor-specific T-cell clones derived from melanoma patients exhibited heterogeneous lytic activity and expressed multiple cytokines. Importantly, cytokine secretion has been implicated in the antitumor mechanisms used by T-cell cultures in the elimination of metastatic tumor deposits in mice. Barth et al. (39) investigated the mechanisms whereby adoptively transferred murine CD8+ lymphocytes mediate tumor regressions. They found that noncytolytic CD8+ cultures from TILs eradicated pulmonary metastasis in irradiated mice. Many of these cultures specifically secreted IFN-γ and tumor necrosis factor when stimulated with tumor cells *in vitro*. The *in vivo* effectiveness of cultures for treatment of mice bearing pulmonary micrometastases correlated better with specific cytokine secretion than with cytotoxicity *in vitro*. Only 8 of 15 therapeutically effective TILs were cytolytic, whereas 14 of 15 therapeutically effective TILs specifically secreted IFN-γ *in vitro*. Additionally, antibodies to IFN-γ abrogated the ability of four different CD8+ cultures to mediate tumor regression, indicating that secretion of IFN-γ was an essential part of their mechanism of action. Nagoshi et al. (40) investigated the role of cytokine secretion *in vivo* during adoptive immunotherapy of pulmonary metastases of the MCA-105 murine sarcoma. T-cell cultures

were transferred into Thy-1 congenic mice and immunohistochemistry was performed to identify donor cells that produced cytokines. The authors propose a model in which cytokine secretion by the transferred tumor-specific effector cells caused tumor inflammation and recruitment of host cells. Host cells, especially dendritic cells and macrophages, were essential for therapeutic efficacy. Additional work needs to be done to understand the roles played in tumor eradication by host immune cells and inflammatory cytokines produced by transferred cells.

Other T-cell phenotypes may also predict therapeutic efficacy, including tumor-specific proliferation of transferred cells. Klarnet et al. (41) described helper cell–independent cytotoxic T lymphocytes (CTLs). These cloned, antigen-driven, helper cell–independent CTL cells were specifically cytolytic to FBL-3. Furthermore, activation with FBL-3 induced secretion of IL-2, expression of IL-2 receptors, and *in vitro* proliferation. Cloned helper cell–independent CTL cells administered to cyclophosphamide-treated tumor-bearing mice were effective in the elimination of disseminated FBL-3. Even 125 days after therapeutic transfer, the cloned cells in these mice could be recovered. Similarly, Rosenstein and Rosenberg (42) examined T-cell clones that exhibited lytic activity and proliferation when stimulated by the syngeneic FBL-3 lymphoma. T-cell clones exhibiting proliferation and cytotoxic activity were more effective in adoptive therapy of FBL-3 tumors than clones exhibiting lytic activity but no proliferation.

Summary of Adoptive Transfer Using Immune Splenocytes

In summary, several qualities of T-cell cultures measured *in vitro* were correlated with the outcome of adoptive transfer therapy *in vivo*. First, virtually all models of adoptive transfer, including those described here, demonstrated a direct correlation between the number of transferred cells and their therapeutic efficacy. Second, the *in vitro* specificity of effector cells for tumors was generally correlated with their therapeutic efficacy. *In vitro* specificity of T cells has been measured by several criteria, including tumor-specific proliferation, cytokine secretion, and lysis. The most relevant of these *in vitro* characteristics for prediction of therapeutic efficacy in a clinical setting remains to be determined. Third, for most murine tumor models, including large, established, and poorly immunogenic tumors, IVS and culture with IL-2 increased immune cell numbers, as well as therapeutic efficacy of the cultured cells. Other important features of the effector cells may include the CD4/CD8 phenotype, the ability to traffic to tumors, and the capability of recruiting host cells into an antitumor inflammatory response.

NONSPECIFIC LYMPHOCYTE ACTIVATION AND LYMPHOKINE-ACTIVATED KILLER CELLS

The models of adoptive transfer in mice discussed so far have in common the prior immunization of donor mice to obtain immune splenocytes for transfer. Immunization of patients to obtain antitumor immune cells, however, was not technically

TABLE 1. LYMPHOKINE-ACTIVATED KILLER CELLS ACTIVATED BY INTERLEUKIN-2 LYSE A VARIETY OF FRESH NATURAL KILLER–RESISTANT TUMOR TARGETS

	Effector: Target					
	LAK-Cell Effector				Fresh PBML Effector	
	40:1	10:1	2.5:1.0	0.6:1.0	60:1	15:1
Target Cells	% Specific Lysis ± SEM					
Fresh tumor						
Sarcoma (autologous)	76 ± 6	73 ± 1	52 ± 3	73 ± 13	−4 ± 10	−9 ± 1
Sarcoma	88 ± 3	78 ± 2	67 ± 2	44 ± 2	7 ± 2	1 ± 1
Sarcoma	57 ± 3	48 ± 3	37 ± 1	20 ± 3	−8 ± 1	−12 ± 2
Sarcoma	85 ± 1	70 ± 5	57 ± 2	42 ± 5	9 ± 8	2 ± 5
Sarcoma	98 ± 1	87 ± 1	77 ± 4	62 ± 5	1 ± 2	1 ± 2
Sarcoma	64 ± 2	54 ± 7	38 ± 4	23 ± 5	−4 ± 3	−11 ± 8
Sarcoma	67 ± 3	57 + 2	48 ± 4	34 ± 3	−6 ± 4	−3 ± 1
Colon carcinoma	62 ± 1	41 ± 3	18 ± 3	15 ± 4	−16 ± 1	−14 ± 1
Adrenal carcinoma	68 ± 2	41 ± 3	18 ± 3	15 ± 4	−16 ± 1	−20 ± 2
Esophageal carcinoma	78 ± 5	62 ± 2	38 ± 1	23 ± 2	0 ± 4	−1 ± 1
Pancreas carcinoma	28 ± 5	17 ± 2	16 ± 2	8 ± 1	−5 ± 1	−2 ± 1
PBML						
Sarcoma patient 1	4 ± 1	9 ± 6	1 ± 2	1 ± 5	−9 ± 3	−8 ± 2
Sarcoma patient 2	9 ± 2	5 ± 3	0 ± 1	−1 ± 3	−5 ± 1	−3 ± 3
Cultured tumor						
K562	105 ± 6	89 ± 2	86 ± 1	75 ± 2	46 ± 3	15 ± 1
Daudi	85 ± 5	101 ± 18	89 ± 3	77 ± 1	2 ± 2	3 ± 3

LAK, lymphokine-activated killer; PBML, peripheral blood mononuclear leukocyte; SEM, standard error of the mean.
From Rayner AA et al. Lymphocyte-activated killer (LAK) cells. Analysis of factors relevant to the immunotherapy of human cancer. *Cancer* 1985;55:1327, with permission.

feasible. The application of adoptive transfer therapy to a clinical setting relied on the development of other sources of autochthonous cells. The availability of recombinant IL-2 (31) allowed for the activation and *ex vivo* expansion of large numbers of lymphocytes. Grimm et al. (43) examined human peripheral blood lymphocytes from cancer patients and normal donors that were cultured in a high concentration (1,000 U per mL) of IL-2. Within 2 to 3 days, these cultures exhibited cytotoxicity toward 20 of 21 natural killer (NK)-resistant, fresh tumor cells tested. The cells mediating this nonspecific cytotoxicity were termed *lymphokine-activated killer* (LAK) *cells*. LAK-cell lysis was not major histocompatibility complex restricted, and LAK cells mediated lysis of autologous tumors and allogeneic tumors derived from multiple histologies (43–45). Low-level lysis of cultured fibroblasts and cultured normal cell lines were also observed, but fresh, unstimulated peripheral blood mononuclear cells (PBMC) from humans were not lysed (Table 1).

IL-2 was determined to be the only lymphokine absolutely required for elaboration of LAK cells (46). LAK-cell precursors were virtually ubiquitous in lymphoid tissues; lymphocytes from mouse and human sources, including PBMC, lymph nodes, spleen, thymus, and even solid tissue digests, could evolve LAK-cell activity (46,47). Human LAK cells could be readily generated in culture with recombinant IL-2 grown for several months without loss of activity and expanded *in vitro*, potentially to more than 10^{20} cells (44). LAK cells fulfilled one prerequisite for clinical trials of adoptive transfer therapy by providing a potent effector cell population from the autochtho-

nous source. LAK cells abrogated the need for a second, immune host as a source of transferred cells.

Demonstration of the therapeutic potential of LAK cells *in vivo* was accomplished using mouse metastatic tumor models. Mazumder and Rosenberg (48) showed that established pulmonary metastases of the B16 melanoma were successfully treated and survival time was increased in mice that received 1×10^8 LAK cells. LAK cells generated from tumor-bearing mice were equally effective as cells from naïve mice. With this experimental model, the therapeutic effect of LAK cells was independent of prior cyclophosphamide treatment of the host. IL-2 administered *in vivo* had a small therapeutic effect in reducing B16 pulmonary metastases, but IL-2 and LAK cells administered together were highly effective.

The therapeutic effect of LAK-cell administration with IL-2 support was characterized using mouse sarcomas, melanoma, and adenocarcinoma metastatic to the lungs or liver (48–51). In murine tumor models metastatic to the liver, IL-2 alone also had a significant effect at high dose, but only a small effect at lower doses. LAK cells alone were ineffective. The combination of LAK cells with IL-2 treatment, however, mediated significant reductions in the number and size of liver nodules (Fig. 6). In a lung tumor model, IL-2 administration alone also had a dose-dependent effect on lung metastasis. When LAK cells and IL-2 were administered together, LAK cells added significantly to tumor reduction at all doses of IL-2. High-dose IL-2 may act by supporting the growth of transferred cells and by inducing the formation of host LAK-like cells *in vivo*, even in the absence of

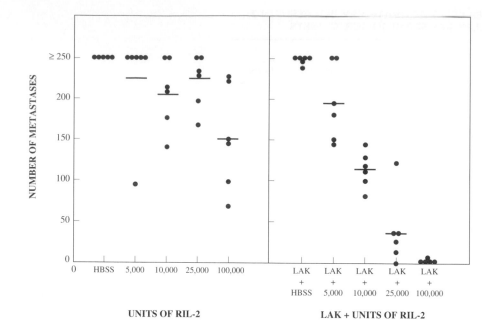

FIGURE 6. Lymphokine-activated killer (LAK) cells augment the effect of recombinant interleukin-2 (rIL-2) for therapy of MCA-38 adenocarcinoma liver metastases. Experimentally induced 3-day-old liver metastases of the MCA-38 adenocarcinoma were treated with rIL-2 three times a day at the indicated dose for 4 or 7 consecutive days, starting on day 3. LAK cells were administered at 1×10^8 cells per treatment on days 3 and 6. Each dot represents a measure of liver metastases in a single mouse. (HBSS, Hanks' balanced salt solution.) (From Lafreniere R and Rosenberg SA. Adoptive immunotherapy of murine hepatic metastases with lymphokine-activated killer (LAK) cells and recombinant interleukin-2 (rIL-2) can mediate the regression of both immunogenic and nonimmunogenic sarcomas and an adenocarcinoma. *J Immunol* 1985;135:4273, with permission.)

transferred cells (52). IL-2 administration at low doses was shown to support the growth of transferred LAK cells. Using a DNA labeling technique for monitoring cell proliferation *in vivo*, Ettinghausen et al. (53) showed that transferred LAK cells failed to proliferate *in vivo* in the absence of IL-2. When IL-2 was administered after LAK-cell transfer, however, increased proliferation of the transferred cells was seen in the lungs and liver and, to a lesser extent, at other sites.

To improve LAK-cell efficacy, many studies attempted to identify a LAK precursor cell and determine the mechanism of LAK-cell antitumor activity *in vivo*. Using complement and antibody-mediated lysis, Yang et al. (54) demonstrated that the majority of LAK-cell precursor activity in mice resided in the "null" cell population (i.e., Thy-1⁻, CD3⁻, FcR⁺). Yang et al. suggested an NK precursor. This hypothesis was supported by additional studies, which showed that LAK-cell activity could be greatly reduced by depletion of splenocytes with anti-asialo-GM antibody before culture with IL-2. Similar studies using antibody depletion of human peripheral blood lymphocytes before culture in IL-2 concluded that LAK-cell precursors were found predominantly in the NK compartment. LAK-cell precursors manifested potent NK activity before IL-2 stimulation and expressed NK markers, including CD56 (55). In addition to NK-cell precursors, some contribution to LAK-cell activity was derived from CD3⁺ cells. Raynor et al. (56) examined limiting dilution clones of LAK-cell cultures and identified CD3⁻ clones with high LAK-cell activity and CD3⁺ clones with intermediate LAK-cell activity. Similarly, Roussel et al. (57) defined culture condition for the production of long-term LAK-cell cultures comprised predominantly of CD3⁺ large granular lymphocytes.

Studies of LAK-cell precursors *in vitro* were mirrored by studies of therapeutic efficacy in mouse metastatic tumor models. Mulé et al. (58) showed that LAK-cell cultures derived from Thy-1–depleted cells were as effective for treating sarcoma lung metastases as standard cultures, indicating that T cells were not a predominant LAK-cell precursor population. Furthermore, host

T cells were not necessary for *in vivo* LAK-cell activity because irradiated mice and T-depleted bone marrow chimeric mice showed no diminution of LAK-cell effectiveness. Further experiments investigating LAK-cell activity *in vivo* were performed by depleting mice of LAK-cell subsets after transfer (59). These studies demonstrated that only the asialo-GM–sensitive cells were required for elimination of metastatic deposits from a nonimmunogenic tumor. In contrast, LAK-cell activity *in vivo* against a weakly immunogenic tumor was mediated by anti-asialo-GM–sensitive and Lyt-2–sensitive (CD8) components.

Principles of LAK-cell activity and LAK-cell behavior have translated well from murine models to the clinical setting (see Chapter 13). Investigators continue to probe the clinical potential of nonspecific LAK cells derived by the *ex vivo* activated of PBMC for tumor therapy. Augmentation of LAK-cell activity by coadministration of tumor-specific monoclonal antibodies *in vivo* is being studied. LAK cells demonstrated potent antibody-dependent cellular cytotoxicity *in vitro* (60). *In vivo*, antibody administration was shown to act synergistically with LAK cells and IL-2 treatment in some experimental tumor models (61–63). Other studies are focusing on a role for LAK cells in regional local therapy by isolated perfusion techniques (64,65). Preclinical models continue to guide the clinical application of these approaches.

In summary, the discovery and recombinant production of IL-2 provided the means to generate highly activated cells with nonspecific killer activity for adoptive transfer. Preclinical mouse models elucidated principles of LAK cells that were exploited for clinical adoptive transfer trials. LAK cells were generated from PBMC and other lymphocyte sources by culture in 1,000 U per mL of IL-2. LAK cells developed within 2 to 3 days and LAK-cell activity was manifested as nonspecific lysis of fresh and cultured tumor targets. Transfer of LAK cells could treat established murine liver and lung tumors in a dose-dependent manner, and treatment efficacy was dependent on or greatly enhanced by coadministration of IL-2. In most tumor models, prior immune

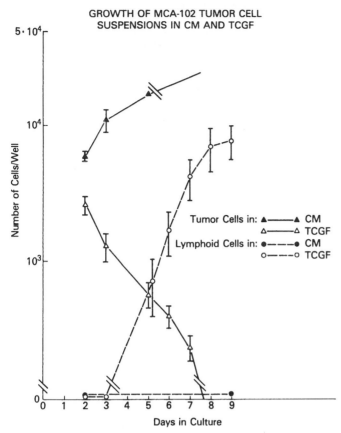

FIGURE 7. Growth of nonimmunogenic MCA-102 sarcoma tumor-cell suspensions with or without T-cell growth factor (TCGF). 1×10^4 cells were plated in microtiter plate wells with or without TCGF. At the indicated times, cells were counted. Each point represents mean ± standard error of eight replicates. Lymphocytes predominated in cultures with TCGF, whereas tumor cells grew in wells without TCGF. (CM, complete media.) (From Yron I et al. In vitro growth of murine T cells. V. The isolation and growth of lymphoid cells infiltrating syngeneic solid tumors. *J Immunol* 1980;125:238, with permission.)

suppression of the transfer recipient by cyclophosphamide or radiation could greatly augment LAK-cell efficacy.

TUMOR ANTIGEN SPECIFICITY AND TUMOR-INFILTRATING LYMPHOCYTES

Studies of Murine Tumor-Infiltrating Lymphocytes

A major improvement to adoptive transfer therapy was obtained by using TILs as the precursor population for LAK-cell generation. Single-cell suspensions of mouse sarcoma digests cultured without IL-2 generated cultures in which the tumor cells grew, whereas the lymphocyte population rapidly disappeared. When cultured in the presence of 1,000 U per mL of IL-2, the tumor cells in the single-cell digest specifically disappeared, however, whereas the lymphocytes proliferated (Fig. 7) (66). Speiss et al. (67) used adoptive transfer into animals bearing 3-day-old established pulmonary micrometastases to investigate the *in vivo* specificity and therapeutic activity of mouse TILs. In this metastatic model, TILs were 50- to 100-fold more effective than

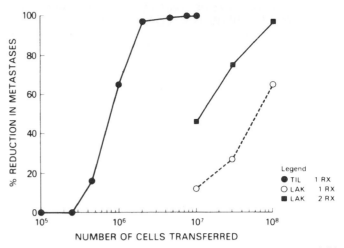

FIGURE 8. Tumor-infiltrating lymphocytes (TILs) are 50- to 100-fold better than lymphokine-activated killer (LAK) cells at treating MCA-105 pulmonary metastases. Three-day-old pulmonary metastases of MCA-105 sarcoma were treated with infusion of TILs or LAK cells. LAK cells were given in one or two doses separated by 3 days. All mice received interleukin-2 three times a day for 5 days. (From Spiess PJ, Yang JC, and SA Rosenberg. In vivo antitumor activity of tumor-infiltrating lymphocytes expanded in recombinant interleukin-2. *J Natl Cancer Inst* 1987;79:1067, with permission.)

LAK cells at mediating clearance of autologous tumors (Fig. 8). IL-2 was not required absolutely, but did enhance the therapeutic effect of transferred TILs approximately fivefold. Using the simple method of culturing tumor digests in high-dose IL-2, therapeutically effective TIL cultures were successfully established from mouse tumors of diverse histology, including sarcomas, a melanoma, a colon carcinoma, and a bladder tumor (Table 2). The *in vivo* specificity of TILs was determined by comparing the therapeutic capacity of TILs from two chemically induced sarcomas, MCA-105 and MCA-106, which did not cross-protect in immunization and challenge experiments. TILs from the MCA-105 sarcoma eliminated autologous MCA-105 lung metastases, but not MCA-106 metastases. TILs from

TABLE 2. TUMOR-INFILTRATING LYMPHOCYTES FROM FIVE DIFFERENT TUMORS EFFICIENTLY TREAT PULMONARY METASTASES

| | Mean No. of Metastases[a] for Treatment Groups[b] with: | | |
Tumor	HBSS	IL-2	TILs + IL-2 (*p* Value)
MCA-38 colon adenocarcinoma	≥250	>250	0 (<.01)
B16 melanoma	≥250	>250	3.2 (<.01)
1660 bladder carcinoma	63	64	0.2 (<.01)
MCA-105 sarcoma	≥250	248	0 (<.01)
MCA-106 sarcoma	≥250	≥250	1 (<.01)

HBSS, Hanks' balanced salt solution; IL-2, interleukin 2; TILs, tumor infiltrating lymphocytes.
[a]Enumerated on day 15.
[b]Mice bearing 3-day-old pulmonary metastases were treated with either HBSS or 7,500 U IL–2 in 0.5 mL HBSS three times a day on days 3 through 8 or with a single i.v. injection of 4×10^6 TILs in addition to IL-2.
From Spiess PJ, et al. In vivo antitumor activity of tumor-infiltrating lymphocytes expanded in recombinant interleukin-2. *J Natl Cancer Inst* 1987;79:1067, with permission.

TABLE 3. TREATMENT OF LIVER METASTASES FROM THE MC-38 COLON ADENOCARCINOMA WITH TUMOR-INFILTRATING LYMPHOCYTES

Treatment			Experiment 1				Experiment 2			
			No. of Mice				No. of Mice			
Cy	IL-2	TILs	Total	Cured	Survival (Days)	Median Survival Time (Days)	Total	Cured	Survival (Days)	Median Survival Time (Days)
—	—	—	6	—	17, 17, 18, 18, 19, 22	18	6	—	16, 16, 16, 17, 18, 18	17
—	—	+	6	—	18, 19, 20, 22, 23, 24	21	5	—	16, 17, 18, 19, 19	18
—	+	—	5	—	19, 20, 21, 22, 28	21	6	—	18, 18, 18, 18, 20, 21	18
—	+	+	5	—	21, 21, 22, 22, 24	22	5	—	17, 17, 17, 18, 19	17
+	—	—	12	—	24, 25, 25, 26, 27, 28, 29, 29, 29, 30, 32, 86	29	5	—	24, 25, 28, 28, 29	28
+	+	—	6	2	27, 27, 40, 44, >100, >100	42	6	—	24, 25, 28, 28, 29, 30	28
+	—	+	6	2	45, 51, 67, 91, >100, >100	79[a]	6	—	30, 30, 35, 41, 43, 62	38[a]
+	+	+	6	6	>100, >100, >100, >100, >100, >100	>100[a]	6	6	>100, >100, >100, >100, >100, >100	>100[a]
+	+	LAK[b]	5	—	28, 29, 29, 29, 30	29	—		—	—

Cy, cyclophosphamide; IL-2, interleukin-2; LAK, lymphokine-activated killer; TILs, tumor-infiltrating leukocytes.
Note: Tumor induction was by intrasplenic injection. Treatment with TILs began on day 8 with 1.2×10^7 or 1.4×10^7 TILs (experiment 1 and 2, respectively). IL-2 was given three times a day from days 8 to 12. Only the combination of cyclophosphamide with TILs and IL-2 was highly effective at curing mice.
[a]$p < .01$ compared with Cy alone; $p = .02$ and $p < .01$ with Cy + TIL compared with Cy + TIL + IL-2.
[b]The LAK-cell dose was 10^8 cells intravenously.
From Rosenberg SA et al. A new approach to the adoptive immunotherapy of cancer with tumor-infiltrating lymphocytes. *Science* 1986;233:1318, with permission.

MCA-106 eliminated MCA-105 metastases and autologous MCA-106 metastases. In these studies, TILs generated in 1,000 U per mL of IL-2 could show tumor-specific or nonspecific effects *in vivo*.

The ease of generation of TIL cultures and their striking therapeutic potential in murine models suggested that TILs from human tumors could be a useful effector-cell population for adoptive therapy. To investigate clinically relevant questions, investigators turned to more difficult tumor models. Rosenberg et al. (68) examined the effectiveness of systemic treatments of tumor-bearing animals for enhancement of TIL activity. These studies showed that murine TILs could mediate the treatment of large established lung and liver metastases of transplantable sarcomas in mice. In this setting, TILs were not effective alone, but TILs could enhance the effects of cyclophosphamide and IL-2 to promote complete tumor regression (Table 3). Another model was developed by Yang et al. (69) to address the problem that TILs were not routinely generated from nonimmunogenic murine tumors. They optimized the culture conditions for generating tumor-reactive lymphocyte cell lines, including IVS, with irradiated autologous tumor and growth in low-dose IL-2 (10 U per mL). These culture changes increased the *in vivo* efficacy of TILs from the weakly immunogenic carcinoma, MC-38, and the sarcoma, MCA-105 (Fig. 9). When used with the nonimmunogenic sarcoma, MCA-102, the improved culture conditions enabled the generation of therapeutically effective TILs, whereas standard bulk-culture conditions did not.

TILs constitute a unique source of T cells in terms of cell trafficking and persistence because, by definition, TILs are derived from lymphocytes that found their way into and persisted within the tumor. It is possible that TILs express cell sur-

face receptors or other features that render them well suited to the tumor microenvironment compared with other lymphocytes. Ames et al. (70) provided support for this hypothesis with evidence that TILs preferentially home to tumor deposits in mammary tumor-bearing mice. TILs, normal splenocytes, or LAK and NK cells from splenocytes were labeled with indium-111 and injected via a tail vein into female mice bearing one or more mammary tumors. Only TILs were found to be more concentrated in tumors than in corresponding normal mammary tissue. Wong et al. (71) studied the uptake of a radiolabeled thymidine analogue into the DNA of dividing cells to study the *in vivo* proliferation and migration patterns of transferred TILs. Twenty hours after injection of label, tissues were removed and radioactivity was determined. Animals receiving TILs and high-dose IL-2 showed high-level of label uptake in the lungs, liver, kidneys, and spleen compared with controls. Experiments with TIL transfer in Thy-1 congenic mice confirmed that TILs were localized in these organs. These studies in mice indicate that TILs can traffic into and persist in solid tissues of mice and may preferentially home to tumor.

Human Tumor-Infiltrating Lymphocytes

Based on the results in mouse models, a host of experiments to characterize the *in vitro* reactivity of human TIL cultures were performed. Unique among human tumors investigated, TILs from human melanoma consistently and reproducibly exhibited specific lysis of autologous tumors. In contrast, when single-cell digests from nonmelanoma human tumors were cultured with IL-2 to generate TILs, specific recognition of autologous tumor by lysis or cytokine-release assays could only rarely be demon-

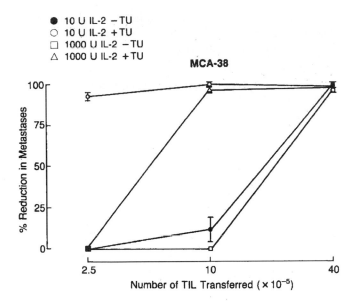

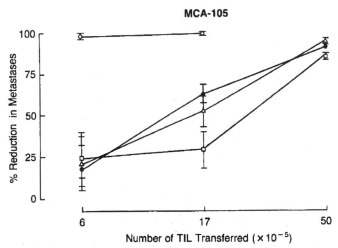

FIGURE 9. The effect of tumor and interleukin-2 (IL-2) doses during culture of tumor-infiltrating lymphocytes (TILs) on therapeutic efficacy. Three-day-old pulmonary metastases of MCA-105 or MCA-38 tumors were treated with TILs grown under different conditions. Pulmonary nodules were enumerated on day 14. Results are reported as the reduction in metastasis by mice given the indicated number of TILs and IL-2 compared with mice given IL-2 alone. The greatest antitumor effect was obtained with TILs grown in low-dose IL-2 with tumor stimulation. (Filled circles, 10 U per mL IL-2, no tumor; open circles, 10 U per mL IL-2 with tumor; open squares, 1,000 U per mL IL-2, no tumor; open triangles, 1,000 U per mL IL-2 with tumor.) (TU, tumor.) (From Yang JC et al. An improved method for growing murine tumor-infiltrating lymphocytes with in vivo antitumor activity. *J Biol Response Mod* 1990;9:149, with permission.)

strated. Sporadic reports of specific TILs have been published for tumors of many different histologies, including ovarian carcinoma (72), colon carcinoma (73,74), breast carcinoma (75), cervical carcinoma (76), renal cell carcinoma (77,78), and gastric carcinoma (79). Even when specificity to the autologous tumor was documented, in many cases the responsible TIL was not typical of mouse TIL lines. And, despite these sporadic reports of specific TIL recognition, most reports indicate that TILs from nonmelanoma tumors are nonlytic or express LAK-like nonspecific lysis. In fact, even LAK-cell activity has been

difficult to generate from some tumors. Low TIL-derived LAK-cell activity has been directly attributed to a low LAK-cell precursor, low "null" cell components, or both, in several reports. Lymphocytes infiltrating carcinomas of the lung and colon were low in CD16+ (NK) cells and deficient in their ability to generate LAK-cell activity compared with PBMC (80,81). Similarly, TILs from breast carcinoma exhibited poor proliferation when stimulated with IL-2 compared with PBMC and were low in LAK-cell precursors (82,83). The examples cited reflect a broad spectrum of different experimental approaches and conclusions. In general, most human tumors do not harbor a highly selected and highly reactive population of lymphocytes.

In marked contrast to TILs from most tumor histologies, TILs derived from melanoma exhibited nonspecific LAK-cell activity and specific autologous tumor recognition. Almost unique among human tumors, TILs from melanomas matched the general immunologic features of lymphocytes cultured from mouse transplantable tumors. Itoh et al. (84) reported that four of nine TIL cultures from melanoma lesions generated typical nonspecific LAK-cell activity, but five of nine TILs were preferentially lytic for autologous tumors. In this report, autologous tumor-specific TIL cultures expressed typical T-lymphocyte markers, including CD8, but not the NK marker, CD16. Autologous tumor lysis was blocked by antibodies specific for the major histocompatibility complex or the T-cell receptor. Similarly, Muul et al. (85) reported that six of six TILs from melanoma patients preferentially lysed autologous melanoma. Three TIL cultures were specific for autologous tumors and failed to lyse allogeneic tumors or fresh cells, whereas three TIL cultures demonstrated specific autologous tumor lysis and some lysis of nonautologous tumor cells. These trials and subsequent studies indicated that melanoma TILs cultured in IL-2 could consistently evolve CD8+ CTLs that were readily expanded in culture and demonstrated specific lysis of autologous tumors. These features indicated that TILs from melanoma constituted an ideal effector-cell population for clinical adoptive transfer studies. In fact, melanoma TIL cultures have been clinically evaluated for efficacy in treatment of metastatic melanoma and were shown to be therapeutically effective in some patients (see Chapter 13).

The reasons for the unique immunologic properties of melanoma compared with other human tumors are not clear. One possibility is that some melanomas are more immunogenic than tumors from other tumor histologies and can mediate immune priming against melanoma antigens *in situ*. In fact, TIL-like activity could be derived from PBMC of melanoma patients after repeated *in vitro* stimulations with tumors (86), suggesting that systemic immunization against tumor antigens had occurred. Similarly, Marincola et al. (87) concluded that melanoma patients exhibited evidence of *in vivo* priming against melanoma antigens based on secondary *in vitro* stimulation of patient and normal donor peripheral blood lymphocytes with defined melanoma antigens. Whatever the mechanism of *in vivo* priming in melanoma patients, the high frequency of tumor-reactive cells in melanoma TILs served as an excellent source of cells for adoptive transfer.

The specific recognition of autologous melanomas by TIL cultures invited the exploration of the tumor antigens recognized by TIL-derived T cells. A fair number of melanoma-associated antigens were discovered and their genes identified by the ability to stimulate melanoma TILs. These and other tumor antigens are described in Chapter 16. TILs from melanoma patients continue to provide a rich source of reagents for tumor antigen discovery. One possibility for future research involves identification using melanoma TILs of antigens expressed not only by melanomas, but also by tumors of other histologies. The first example of such an antigen was reported by Wang et al. (88), who demonstrated that a TIL-derived, T-cell clone specific for an epitope of the NY-ESO-1 protein also recognized HLA-31$^+$, ESO-1$^+$, melanoma, and breast carcinoma cells.

The diversity of TIL-recognized tumor antigens presents an embarrassment of riches and a conundrum for adoptive transfer therapy: Which tumor antigen should be targeted? Therapeutically effective TILs from human and mouse tumors were shown to recognize shared, as well as unique, tumor antigens. Shared antigens (i.e., antigens expressed in common by multiple HLA-matched tumors) are generally derived from nonmutated genes. These are tempting targets for immunotherapy because of the logistical ease of administering a single therapeutic agent to multiple patients. Questions about the absolute strength and persistence of an immune response against an antigen from a normal "self" protein, however, remain a vexing problem for approaches that target shared antigens. In contrast, uniquely expressed tumor antigens would require herculean efforts for clinical application because each new patient requires an essentially new therapeutic agent. Uniquely expressed antigens, however, might prove beneficial by provoking a strong inflammatory response that is not muted by self tolerance.

Another critical question involves the role of CD4$^+$ cells in antitumor therapeutic efficacy. Many TILs administered to patients in the Surgery Branch of the National Cancer Institute exhibited a CD4$^+$, HLA class II–restricted recognition of autologous tumors (89). Antigens stimulating several CD4$^+$ TILs have been identified and their genes have been cloned. These genes include shared antigens from the tyrosinase protein (90,91), as well as unique antigens, such as a mutation in the triosephosphate isomerase gene (92), a mutated form of human CDC27 (93), and a novel fusion protein derived from the translocation of the LDLR and FUT genes (94). The identification of unique and shared antigens recognized by CD4$^+$ TILs, as well as other evidence (95), indicates that the CD4$^+$ T-cell response to melanoma may be as diverse as the CD8$^+$ response. The individual contributions of CD4$^+$ and CD8$^+$ T cells and their potential for synergy in the treatment of solid tumor deposits are actively being investigated.

A final question concerns whether TILs in humans preferentially traffic back to tumor deposits. In a large series of patients treated with indium-111–labeled TILs in the Surgery Branch of the National Cancer Institute, TIL localization and *in vivo* kinetics were analyzed (96). In these studies, TILs from responsive and nonresponsive patients showed preferential homing to tumor deposits. TIL trafficking to tumors was significantly correlated with patient objective responses. No objective responses were seen in patients who received nontrafficking TILs. Trafficking to tumor deposits was also significantly correlated with the dose of TILs administered and the prior administration of cyclophosphamide. These and additional studies in melanoma

patients receiving TILs provided evidence that therapeutically effective TILs preferentially trafficked to the tumor, participated in tumor destruction, and persisted in the patient.

Summary of Preclinical Experience with Tumor-Infiltrating Lymphocytes

For immunogenic tumors, such as transplanted mouse sarcomas and human melanoma, TILs have proven to be a rich source of tumor-specific lymphocytes. Isolation of efficacious TILs from nonimmunogenic tumors was only variably successful. Culture of tumor digests in IL-2 resulted in tumor destruction and lymphocyte outgrowth with concomitant elaboration of tumor-specific T-cell functions, including lysis and cytokine secretion. Mouse TILs exhibited greatly improved specific lysis of autologous tumors when cultured under conditions of IVS to tumors. Adoptive transfer of specific TIL cells could mediate destruction of metastatic tumor deposits in the lung and liver from a variety of tumor types in mouse models. Adoptive transfer of TILs in melanoma patients was associated with objective responses (see Chapter 13). Therapeutic benefit in mouse models was directly dependent on the transferred cell number. T cells from therapeutic TILs homed to tumor deposits and persisted *in vivo*. TIL treatment was augmented by pretreatment of tumor-bearing mice with cyclophosphamide or radiation and by systemic IL-2 support.

IN VITRO–SENSITIZED T-CELL CLONES

T cells that mediate tumor destruction are crucial to the success of adoptive therapy approaches in mouse models and in the clinic. Rapid advances in tumor immunology and molecular genetics have identified a host of tumor-specific genes that potentially encode T-cell recognizable tumor antigens. The discovery of these genes and their production as synthetic peptides and recombinant proteins provides possibilities for adoptive transfer therapy. Patients could be primarily sensitized *in vivo* by antigen immunization. Then, peripheral blood lymphocytes or vaccine-draining lymph nodes could be secondarily sensitized *in vitro* with the same antigen. To improve the tumor reactivity of bulk IVS cultures, T-cell clones with the appropriate characteristics, such as antigen specificity and tumor reactivity, could be identified. Once isolated from bulk cultures, these clones could be expanded *in vitro* to therapeutic levels and finally transferred to the autologous patient. Several reasons exist to believe that cloned T cells can be highly effective for adoptive transfer. First, cloned T cells were effective in elimination of tumors in several mouse models (97,98). Second, the technical feasibility of growing clones for patient treatment has been proven in a clinical trial for prophylaxis of cytomegalovirus-associated disease in bone marrow transplant recipients (99). Third, the phenotype of the transferred cells can be manipulated by selecting a clone for transfer with the appropriate phenotype. Thus, the potential for transfer of cloned T cells for cancer therapy incorporates many features of previously successful adoptive transfer approaches.

The ability to select a specific T-cell phenotype for adoptive transfer led to the initiation of a clinical trial with gp100:209–217 (referred to as *g209*) peptide-specific T-cell clones for treat-

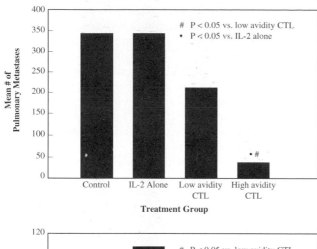

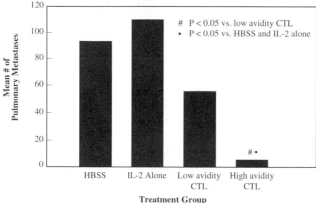

A

B

FIGURE 10. Treatment of day 4 pulmonary metastases of B16 melanoma by high- and low-avidity cytotoxic T lymphocyte (CTL) lines. Mice were injected intravenously with B16 melanoma on day 0 to induce pulmonary micrometastases. On day 4, 3×10^6 TRP-2–specific CTL (**A**) or 7×10^4 p15E-specific CTL (**B**) were given intravenously and interleukin-2 (IL-2) was given three times a day for 3 days. On day 14, pulmonary metastases were counted. Only the high-avidity CTLs significantly treated the tumor. (HBSS, Hank's balanced salt solution.) (From Zeh HJ III et al. High avidity CTLs for two self-antigens demonstrate superior in vitro and in vivo antitumor efficacy. *J Immunol* 1999;162:989, with permission.)

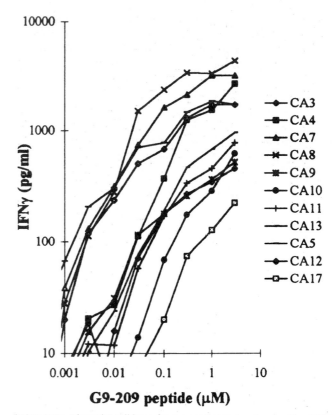

FIGURE 11. Cloned T-cell lines from a patient immunized with g209-2M were tested for peptide avidity. Interferon-γ (IFN-γ) secretion (pg per mL per 10,000 cells) by individual clones in an overnight assay is plotted as a function of the concentration of g209 peptide pulsed onto the T2 stimulators. Clones differ by two orders of magnitude in the minimum peptide concentration recognized. (From Dudley ME et al. High-avidity CTLs for two self-antigens demonstrate superior in vitro and in vivo antitumor efficacy. *J Immunotherapy* 1999;22:288, with permission.)

ment of patients with metastatic melanoma. Using defined antigens in mouse models, several reports have shown a correlation between T-cell avidity *in vitro* and efficacy on adoptive transfer *in vivo* (100–102). For instance, Zeh et al. (100) used different concentrations of defined peptide antigens expressed by B16 melanoma to generate CTL cultures. CTLs expanded in low concentrations of purified antigens demonstrated higher avidity for peptide-pulsed targets and better tumor recognition when compared with CTLs generated in the presence of high concentrations of antigens. More important, high-avidity CTLs demonstrated superior *in vivo* efficacy in adoptive transfer experiments (Fig. 10). These results suggest that selection and expansion of a clone with high avidity could generate a highly therapeutic CTL culture.

Patients who received a primary immunization with a modified 9–amino acid peptide, gp100:209–217(210M) (referred to as *209-2M*), exhibited increased frequency of g209-specific, tumor-reactive T cells (103). Tumor-reactive, g209-specific CTLs were cloned by limiting dilution. Their function was then analyzed. Individual CD8+ clones displayed wide diversity in

peptide-antigen avidity and tumor recognition (Fig. 11). Clones differed by more than two logs in the minimum concentration of antigens that they recognized. Clones displayed a similar variation in their ability to recognize tumor cells (104). This functional variation was mirrored at the structural level, whereas sequence analysis of T-cell receptor β chains revealed 11 different receptors from 13 clones analyzed in one patient. The analysis of functional activity of individual clones confirmed that the ability to recognize tumors is highly correlated with the recognition of the native gp100:209–217 epitope. In all patients examined, the cells that demonstrated the highest avidity for peptide antigens also exhibited the best tumor recognition. In addition, although the apparent frequency of high-avidity clones varied from patient to patient, all patients examined had at least one clone that was high avidity. Clinical evaluation of the therapeutic potential of high-avidity clones is under way.

The approach outlined above could be used with virtually any synthetic peptide or recombinant protein identified as a tumor antigen. Antigen-specific CTLs could potentially be derived from each patient after immunization. Clones with the most suitable characteristics, such as high avidity for tumor antigens, could be expanded and administered by adoptive transfer. The generation of CTLs for adoptive immunotherapy from nonimmunized patients presents additional challenges. Its feasibility remains to be evaluated. CTL epitopes have been identified for a large number of tumor-encoded proteins, including her2/neu, CEA, and p53 (105–109). Although the therapeutic potential of each of these antigens is unproved, any of these antigens could be used for IVS of patient lymphocytes for clone isolation and adoptive transfer therapy.

Recipients of allogeneic bone marrow transplants for treatment of leukemia constitute another patient population that could benefit from clonal adoptive transfer. The evaluation of patients who have undergone allogeneic bone marrow transplants provides some of the strongest evidence that adoptive transfer can cure patients with advanced cancer. Graft-versus-host disease in these patients is a serious problem; however, patients with this condition may actually benefit from the development of concomitant graft-versus-leukemia (110). This observation led to strategies for augmenting the graft-versus-leukemia effect of allogeneic donor cells without aggravating graft-versus-host disease. One such strategy involves immunizing the marrow donor before marrow harvest. Several reports indicate that CTL immunity is transferred with marrow transplantation in mouse models (111,112). Another strategy involves the cloning of IVS donor lymphocytes to identify T cells that are specific for leukemia cells or purified leukemia antigens but do not react with recipient normal tissues. Tumor-specific antigens in this setting would include clonotype-specific immunoglobulins produced by some B-cell malignancies (111), the unique junction sequences of translocation fusion proteins (113), or the viral proteins produced by Epstein-Barr virus in some leukemias. Some of these potential applications for adoptive transfer therapy are presented in detail in Chapter 13.

SUMMARY

Transplantable tumors of mice represent an imperfect but highly useful model to elucidate the basic principles of adoptive cellular therapy. Small, recently transplanted, and highly immunogenic mouse tumors were artificially "easy" targets for immunotherapy, but were useful for testing novel technologies and poorly understood principles. Large, established, and poorly immunogenic tumors in mice were more representative of human disease and comprised a gold standard of adoptive therapy. Whether tumors were actively interfering with immune effector-cell function or passively subverting the existing host mechanisms for maintenance of self tolerance, immunosuppressive treatment of the tumor-bearing transfer recipient generally augmented adoptive cellular transfer. Similarly, administration of systemic IL-2 to tumor-bearing mice supported the transferred cells and improved therapeutic outcome.

Several effector-cell populations demonstrated therapeutic benefit in mouse adoptive transfer studies. The potent lytic activity of LAK cells *in vitro* emphasized the inherent antitumor destructive power of immune effector cells when removed from *in vivo* regulatory constraints. LAK-cell therapeutic efficacy in some preclinical models demonstrated the importance of effector-cell activation for adoptive transfer. The use of TILs extended the power of *ex vivo* lymphocyte activation to include

tumor-specific cells that were primed *in vivo*. Specificity of transferred cells by *in vitro* measures correlated with their efficacy *in vivo*. Different *in vitro* effector-cell functions, including lysis, cytokine secretion, and proliferation, have been accented in different studies. *In vivo*, TILs may act through direct tumor-cell destruction or through the elaboration of inflammatory cytokines and the recruitment of host immune effectors to the tumor site. Therapeutically effective TILs from mouse tumors and human melanomas are a highly enriched source of reagents for tumor-antigen identification.

Cloned T cells represent the ultimate in antigen specificity for adoptive transfer. Cloning of tumor antigen-specific lymphocytes from mice produced monospecific cultures that were effective in adoptive transfer experiments. High-avidity cloned T cells with defined *in vitro* characteristics can be obtained from immunized cancer patients. These reactive clones can be expanded *in vitro* and evaluated in clinical trials. In addition, T-cell clones with different *in vitro* qualities need to be further evaluated in preclinical models to resolve basic questions of tumor immunology. The therapeutic value of different antigens, the role of CD4 cells in tumor immunity, and the importance of inflammation at the tumor site are a few examples of the unsettled issues that adoptive transfer experiments could address. The ability to immunize patients with synthetic tumor antigens provides the capability of extending clinical studies of adoptive transfer from melanoma to other tumor types. Preclinical and basic studies in mouse models of adoptive transfer should continue to guide clinical practice and resolve the underlying biology of tumor immunotherapy.

REFERENCES

1. Klein G. Tumor antigens. *Annu Rev Microbiol* 1966;20:223–252.
2. Borberg H, Oettgen HF, Choudry K, Beattie EJ Jr. Inhibition of established transplants of chemically induced sarcomas in syngeneic mice by lymphocytes from immunized donors. *Int J Cancer* 1972;10:539.
3. Fass L, Fefer A. Studies of adoptive chemoimmunotherapy of a Friend virus-induced lymphoma. *Cancer Res* 1972;32:997.
4. North RJ, Kirstein DP, Tuttle RL. Subversion of host defense mechanisms by murine tumors. I. A circulating factor that suppresses macrophage-mediated resistance to infection. *J Exp Med* 1976;143:559.
5. Ting CC. Humoral regulation of cell-mediated immunity to syngeneic tumor. *Cancer Res* 1976;36:3695.
6. Selinsky CL, Boroughs KL, Halsey WA Jr, Howell MD. Multifaceted inhibition of anti-tumour immune mechanisms by soluble tumour necrosis factor receptor type I. *Immunology* 1998;94:88.
7. Wahl SM, Hunt DA, Wong HL, et al. Transforming growth factor-beta is a potent immunosuppressive agent that inhibits IL-1-dependent lymphocyte proliferation. *J Immunol* 1988;140:3026.
8. Roth MD, Golub SH. Human pulmonary macrophages utilize prostaglandins and transforming growth factor beta 1 to suppress lymphocyte activation. *J Leukoc Biol* 1993;53:366.
9. Somers SS, Dye JF, Guillou PJ. Comparison of transforming growth factor beta and a human tumour-derived suppressor factor. *Cancer Immunol Immunother* 1991;33:217.
10. Tsunawaki S, Sporn M, Nathan C. Comparison of transforming growth factor-beta and a macrophage-deactivating polypeptide from tumor cells. Differences in antigenicity and mechanism of action. *J Immunol* 1989;142:3462.
11. Berendt MJ, North RJ. T-cell-mediated suppression of anti-tumor immunity. An explanation for progressive growth of an immunogenic tumor. *J Exp Med* 1980;151:69.

12. North RJ, Awwad M. Elimination of cycling CD4+ suppressor T cells with an anti-mitotic drug releases non-cycling CD8+ T cells to cause regression of an advanced lymphoma. *Immunology* 1990;71:90.

13. Awwad M, North RJ. Immunologically mediated regression of a murine lymphoma after treatment with anti-L3T4 antibody. A consequence of removing L3T4+ suppressor T cells from a host generating predominantly Lyt-2+ T cell-mediated immunity. *J Exp Med* 1988;168:2193.

14. Dye ES, North RJ. T cell-mediated immunosuppression as an obstacle to adoptive immunotherapy of the P815 mastocytoma and its metastases. *J Exp Med* 1981;154:1033.

15. Greenberg PD, Cheever M, Fefer A. Suppression of the in vitro secondary response to syngeneic tumor and of in vivo tumor therapy with immune cells by culture-induced suppressor cells. *J Immunol* 1979;123:515.

16. Berenson JR, Einstein AB Jr, Fefer A. Syngeneic adoptive immunotherapy and chemoimmunotherapy of a Friend leukemia: requirement for T cells. *J Immunol* 1975;115:234.

17. Awwad M, North RJ. Cyclophosphamide-induced immunologically mediated regression of a cyclophosphamide-resistant murine tumor: a consequence of eliminating precursor L3T4+ suppressor T-cells. *Cancer Res* 1989;49:1649.

18. Cameron RB, Spiess PJ, Rosenberg SA. Synergistic antitumor activity of tumor-infiltrating lymphocytes, interleukin 2, and local tumor irradiation. Studies on the mechanism of action. *J Exp Med* 1990;171:249.

19. Cheever MA, Greenberg PD, Fefer A, Gillis S. Augmentation of the anti-tumor therapeutic efficacy of long-term cultured T lymphocytes by in vivo administration of purified interleukin-2. *J Exp Med* 1982;155:968.

20. Shu S, Rosenberg SA. Adoptive immunotherapy of a newly induced sarcoma: immunologic characteristics of effector cells. *J Immunol* 1985;135:2895.

21. Cheever MA, Thompson DB, Klarnet JP, Greenberg PD. Antigen-driven long term-cultured T cells proliferate in vivo, distribute widely, mediate specific tumor therapy, and persist long-term as functional memory T cells. *J Exp Med* 1986;163:1100.

22. Chen W, Cheever MA. Donor T cells can be induced to grow and survive long term in vivo without previous host immunosuppression. *J Immunol* 1994;152:4767.

23. Kearney ER, Pape KA, Loh DY, Jenkins MK. Visualization of peptide-specific T cell immunity and peripheral tolerance induction in vivo. *Immunity* 1994;1:327.

24. Wick M, Dubey P, Koeppen H, et al. Antigenic cancer cells grow progressively in immune hosts without evidence for T cell exhaustion or systemic anergy. *J Exp Med* 1997;186:229.

25. Hermans IF, Daish A, Yang J, Ritchie DS, Ronchese F. Antigen expressed on tumor cells fails to elicit an immune response, even in the presence of increased numbers of tumor-specific cytotoxic T lymphocyte precursors. *Cancer Res* 1998;58:3909.

26. Prevost-Blondel A, Zimmermann C, et al. Tumor-infiltrating lymphocytes exhibiting high ex vivo cytolytic activity fail to prevent murine melanoma tumor growth in vivo. *J Immunol* 1998;161:2187.

27. Cheever MA, Greenberg PD, Fefer A. Specificity of adoptive chemoimmunotherapy of established syngeneic tumors. *J Immunol* 1980;125:711.

28. Cheever MA, Greenberg PD, Fefer A. Chemoimmunotherapy of a Friend leukemia with cells secondarily sensitized in vitro: effect of culture duration on therapeutic efficacy. *J Natl Cancer Inst* 1981;67:169.

29. Greenberg PD, Cheever MA, Fefer A. Eradication of disseminated murine leukemia by chemoimmunotherapy with cyclophosphamide and adoptively transferred immune syngeneic Lyt-1+2-lymphocytes. *J Exp Med* 1981;154:952.

30. Morgan DA, Ruscetti FW, Gallo R. Selective in vitro growth of T lymphocytes from normal human bone marrows. *Science* 1976;193:1007.

31. Rosenberg SA, Grimm EA, McGrogan M, et al. Biological activity of recombinant human interleukin-2 produced in Escherichia coli. *Science* 1984;223:1412.

32. Eberlein TJ, Rosenstein M, Rosenberg SA. Regression of a disseminated syngeneic solid tumor by systemic transfer of lymphoid cells expanded in interleukin 2. *J Exp Med* 1982;156:385.

33. Shu S, Chou T, Rosenberg SA. In vitro sensitization and expansion with viable tumor cells and interleukin-2 in the generation of specific therapeutic effector cells. *J Immunol* 1986;136:3891.

34. Peng L, Shu S, Krauss JC. Treatment of subcutaneous tumor with adoptively transferred T cells. *Cell Immunol* 1997;178:24.

35. Sakai K, Chang AE, Shu S. Effector phenotype and immunologic specificity of T-cell-mediated adoptive therapy for a murine tumor that lacks intrinsic immunogenicity. *Cell Immunol* 1990;129:241.

36. Matsumura T, Sussman JJ, Krinock RA, Chang AE, Shu S. Characteristics and in vivo homing of long-term T-cell lines and clones derived from tumor-draining lymph nodes. *Cancer Res* 1994;54:2744.

37. Schwartzentruber DJ, Topalian SL, Mancini M, Rosenberg SA. Specific release of granulocyte-macrophage colony-stimulating factor, tumor necrosis factor alpha, and IFN-gamma by human tumor-infiltrating lymphocytes after autologous tumor stimulation. *J Immunol* 1991;146:3674.

38. Maccalli C, Mortarini R, Parmiani G, Anichini A. Multiple sub-sets of CD4+ and CD8+ cytotoxic T-cell clones directed to autologous human melanoma identified by cytokine profiles. *Int J Cancer* 1994;57:56.

39. Barth RJ Jr, Mulé JJ, Spiess PJ, Rosenberg SA. Interferon gamma and tumor necrosis factor have a role in tumor regressions mediated by murine CD8+ tumor-infiltrating lymphocytes. *J Exp Med* 1991;173:647.

40. Nagoshi M, Goedegebuure PS, Burger UL, Sadanaga N, Chang MP, Eberlein TJ. Successful adoptive cellular immunotherapy is dependent on induction of a host immune response triggered by cytokine (IFN-gamma and granulocyte/macrophage colony-stimulating factor) producing donor tumor-infiltrating lymphocytes. *J Immunol* 1998;160:334.

41. Klarnet JP, Matis LA, Kern DE, et al. Antigen-driven T cell clones can proliferate in vivo, eradicate disseminated leukemia, and provide specific immunologic memory. *J Immunol* 1987;138:4012.

42. Rosenstein M, Rosenberg SA. Generation of lytic and proliferative lymphoid clones to syngeneic tumor: in vitro and in vivo studies. *J Natl Cancer Inst* 1984;72:1161.

43. Grimm EA, Mazumder A, Zhang HZ, Rosenberg SA. Lymphokine-activated killer cell phenomenon. Lysis of natural killer-resistant fresh solid tumor cells by interleukin 2-activated autologous human peripheral blood lymphocytes. *J Exp Med* 1982;155:1823.

44. Rayner AA, Grimm EA, Lotze MT, Chu EW, Rosenberg SA. Lymphokine-activated killer (LAK) cells. Analysis of factors relevant to the immunotherapy of human cancer. *Cancer* 1985;55:1327.

45. Rosenstein M, Yron I, Kaufmann Y, Rosenberg SA. Lymphokine-activated killer cells: lysis of fresh syngeneic natural killer-resistant murine tumor cells by lymphocytes cultured in interleukin-2. *Cancer Res* 1984;44:1946.

46. Grimm EA, Robb RJ, Roth JA, et al. Lymphokine-activated killer cell phenomenon. III. Evidence that IL-2 is sufficient for direct activation of peripheral blood lymphocytes into lymphokine-activated killer cells. *J Exp Med* 1983;158:1356.

47. Hogan PG, Hapel AJ, Doe WF. Lymphokine-activated and natural killer cell activity in human intestinal mucosa. *J Immunol* 1985;135:1731.

48. Mazumder A, Rosenberg SA. Successful immunotherapy of natural killer-resistant established pulmonary melanoma metastases by the intravenous adoptive transfer of syngeneic lymphocytes activated in vitro by interleukin-2. *J Exp Med* 1984;159:495.

49. Mulé JJ, Shu S, Schwarz SL, Rosenberg SA. Adoptive immunotherapy of established pulmonary metastases with LAK cells and recombinant interleukin-2. *Science* 1984;225:1487.

50. Lafreniere R, Rosenberg SA. Adoptive immunotherapy of murine hepatic metastases with lymphokine activated killer (LAK) cells and recombinant interleukin-2 (RIL 2) can mediate the regression of both immunogenic and nonimmunogenic sarcomas and an adenocarcinoma. *J Immunol* 1985;135:4273.

51. Lafreniere R, Rosenberg SA. Successful immunotherapy of murine experimental hepatic metastases with lymphokine-activated killer cells and recombinant interleukin-2. *Cancer Res* 1985;45:3735.

52. Rosenberg SA, Mulé JJ, Spiess PJ, Reichert CM, Schwarz SL. Regression of established pulmonary metastases and subcutaneous tumor mediated by the systemic administration of high-dose recombinant interleukin-2. *J Exp Med* 1985;161:1169.

53. Ettinghausen SE, Lipford EH III, Mulé JJ, Rosenberg SA. Recombinant interleukin-2 stimulates in vivo proliferation of adoptively transferred lymphokine-activated killer (LAK) cells. *J Immunol* 1985;135:3623.

54. Yang JC, Mulé JJ, Rosenberg SA. Murine lymphokine-activated killer (LAK) cells: phenotypic characterization of the precursor and effector cells. *J Immunol* 1986;137:715–722.

55. Roberts K, Lotze MT, Rosenberg SA. Separation and functional studies of the human lymphokine-activated killer cell. *Cancer Res* 1987;47:4366.

56. Rayner AA, Grimm EA, Lotze MT, Wilson DJ, Rosenberg SA. Lymphokine-activated killer (LAK) cell phenomenon. IV. Lysis by LAK cell clones of fresh human tumor cells from autologous and multiple allogeneic tumors. *J Natl Cancer Inst* 1985;75:67.

57. Roussel E, Gerrard JM, Greenberg AH. Long-term cultures of human peripheral blood lymphocytes with recombinant human interleukin-2 generate a population of virtually pure CD3+ CD16– CD56– large granular lymphocyte LAK cells. *Clin Exp Immunol* 1990;82:416.

58. Mulé JJ, Yang J, Shu S, Rosenberg SA. The anti-tumor efficacy of lymphokine-activated killer cells and recombinant interleukin 2 in vivo: direct correlation between reduction of established metastases and cytolytic activity of lymphokine-activated killer cells. *J Immunol* 1986;136:3899.

59. Mulé JJ, Yang JC, Afreniere RL, Shu SY, Rosenberg SA. Identification of cellular mechanisms operational in vivo during the regression of established pulmonary metastases by the systemic administration of high-dose recombinant interleukin-2. *J Immunol* 1987;139:285.

60. Shiloni E, Eisenthal A, Sachs D, Rosenberg SA. Antibody-dependent cellular cytotoxicity mediated by murine lymphocytes activated in recombinant interleukin-2. *J Immunol* 1987;138:1992.

61. Schultz KR, Klarnet JP, Peace DJ, et al. Monoclonal antibody therapy of murine lymphoma: enhanced efficacy by concurrent administration of interleukin-2 or lymphokine-activated killer cells. *Cancer Res* 1990;50:5421.

62. Pendurthi TK, Schlom J, Primus FJ. Human lymphokine-activated killer cells augment immunotherapy of human colon carcinoma xenografts with monoclonal antibody D612. *J Immunother* 1991;10:2.

63. Eisenthal A, Cameron RB, Uppenkamp I, Rosenberg SA. Effect of combined therapy with lymphokine-activated killer cells, interleukin-2 and specific monoclonal antibody on established B16 melanoma lung metastases. *Cancer Res* 1988;48:7140.

64. Keilholz U, Scheibenbogen C, Brado M, et al. Regional adoptive immunotherapy with interleukin-2 and lymphokine-activated killer (LAK) cells for liver metastases. *Eur J Cancer* 1994;30A:103.

65. Sacchi M, Vitolo D, Sedlmayr P, et al. Induction of tumor regression in experimental model of human head and neck cancer by human A-LAK cells and IL-2. *Int J Cancer* 1991;47:784.

66. Yron I, Wood TA Jr, Spiess PJ, Rosenberg SA. In vitro growth of murine T cells. V. The isolation and growth of lymphoid cells infiltrating syngeneic solid tumors. *J Immunol* 1980;125:238.

67. Spiess PJ, Yang JC, Rosenberg SA. In vivo antitumor activity of tumor-infiltrating lymphocytes expanded in recombinant interleukin-2. *J Natl Cancer Inst* 1987;79:1067.

68. Rosenberg SA, Spiess P, Lafreniere R. A new approach to the adoptive immunotherapy of cancer with tumor-infiltrating lymphocytes. *Science* 1986;233:1318.

69. Yang JC, Perry-Lalley D, Rosenberg SA. An improved method for growing murine tumor-infiltrating lymphocytes with in vivo antitumor activity. *J Biol Response Mod* 1990;9:149.

70. Ames IH, Gagne GM, Garcia AM, et al. Preferential homing of tumor-infiltrating lymphocytes in tumor-bearing mice. *Cancer Immunol Immunother* 1989;29:93.

71. Wong RA, Alexander RB, Puri RK, Rosenberg SA. In vivo proliferation of adoptively transferred tumor-infiltrating lymphocytes in mice. *J Immunother* 1991;10:120.

72. Peoples GE, Goedegebuure PS, Andrews JV, Schoof DD, Eberlein TJ. HLA-A2 presents shared tumor-associated antigens derived from endogenous proteins in ovarian cancer. *J Immunol* 1993;151:5481.

73. Hom SS, Rosenberg SA, Topalian SL. Specific immune recognition of autologous tumor by lymphocytes infiltrating colon carcinomas: analysis by cytokine secretion. *Cancer Immunol Immunother* 1993;36:1.

74. Gohara R, Nakao M, Ogata Y, Isomoto H, Oizumi K, Itoh K. Histocompatibility leukocyte antigen-A2402-restricted cytotoxic T lymphocytes recognizing adenocarcinoma in tumor-infiltrating lymphocytes of patients with colon cancer. *Jpn J Cancer Res* 1997;88:198.

75. Schwartzentruber DJ, Solomon D, Rosenberg SA, Topalian SL. Characterization of lymphocytes infiltrating human breast cancer: specific immune reactivity detected by measuring cytokine secretion. *J Immunother* 1992;12:1.

76. Hilders CG, Ras L, van Eendenburg JD, Nooyen Y, Fleuren GJ. Isolation and characterization of tumor-infiltrating lymphocytes from cervical carcinoma. *Int J Cancer* 1994;57:805.

77. Finke JH, Rayman P, Hart L, et al. Characterization of tumor-infiltrating lymphocyte subsets from human renal cell carcinoma: specific reactivity defined by cytotoxicity, interferon-gamma secretion, and proliferation. *J Immunother Emphasis Tumor Immunol* 1994;15:91.

78. Schendel DJ, Gansbacher B, Oberneder R, et al. Tumor-specific lysis of human renal cell carcinomas by tumor-infiltrating lymphocytes. I. HLA-A2-restricted recognition of autologous and allogeneic tumor lines. *J Immunol* 1993;151:4209.

79. Hoshino T, Seki N, Kikuchi M, et al. HLA class-I-restricted and tumor-specific CTL in tumor-infiltrating lymphocytes of patients with gastric cancer. *Int J Cancer* 1997;70:631.

80. Staren ED, Economou SG, Harris JE, Braun DP. Lymphokine-activated killer cell induction in tumor-infiltrating leukocytes from colon cancer patients. *Cancer* 1989;64:2238.

81. Yano T, Yasumoto K, Togami M, et al. Properties of recombinant interleukin-2-cultured tumor-infiltrating lymphocytes in human lung cancer. *Int J Cancer* 1989;43:619.

82. Whiteside TL, Miescher S, MacDonald HR, Von Fliedner V. Separation of tumor-infiltrating lymphocytes from tumor cells in human solid tumors. A comparison between velocity sedimentation and discontinuous density gradients. *J Immunol Methods* 1986;90:221.

83. Whiteside TL, Miescher S, Hurlimann J, Moretta L, Von Fliedner V. Clonal analysis and in situ characterization of lymphocytes infiltrating human breast carcinomas. *Cancer Immunol Immunother* 1986;23:169.

84. Itoh K, Tilden AB, Balch CM. Interleukin-2 activation of cytotoxic T-lymphocytes infiltrating into human metastatic melanomas. *Cancer Res* 1986;46:3011.

85. Muul LM, Spiess PJ, Director EP, Rosenberg SA. Identification of specific cytolytic immune responses against autologous tumor in humans bearing malignant melanoma. *J Immunol* 1987;138:989.

86. Stevens EJ, Jacknin L, Robbins PF, et al. Generation of tumor-specific CTLs from melanoma patients by using peripheral blood stimulated with allogeneic melanoma tumor cell lines. Fine specificity and MART-1 melanoma antigen recognition. *J Immunol* 1995;154:762.

87. Marincola FM, Rivoltini L, Salgaller ML, Player M, Rosenberg SA. Differential anti-MART-1/MelanA CTL activity in peripheral blood of HLA-A2 melanoma patients in comparison to healthy donors: evidence of in vivo priming by tumor cells. *J Immunother Emphasis Tumor Immunol* 1996;19:266.

88. Wang RF, Johnston SL, Zeng G, Topalian SL, Schwartzentruber DJ, Rosenberg SA. A breast and melanoma-shared tumor antigen: T cell responses to antigenic peptides translated from different open reading frames. *J Immunol* 1998;161:3598.

89. Markus NR, Rosenberg SA, Topalian SL. Analysis of cytokine secretion by melanoma-specific CD4+ T lymphocytes. *J Interferon Cytokine Res* 1995;15:739.

90. Topalian SL, MI Gonzales, Parkhurst M, et al. Melanoma-specific CD4+ T cells recognize nonmutated HLA-DR-restricted tyrosinase epitopes. *J Exp Med* 1996;183:1965.

91. Topalian SL, Rivoltini L, Mancini M, et al. Human CD4+ T cells specifically recognize a shared melanoma-associated antigen encoded by the tyrosinase gene. *Proc Natl Acad Sci U S A* 1994;91:9461.

92. Pieper R, Christian RE, Gonzales MI, et al. Biochemical identification of a mutated human melanoma antigen recognized by CD4(+) T cells. *J Exp Med* 1999;189:757.

93. Wang RF, Wang X, Atwood AC, Topalian SL, Rosenberg SA. Cloning genes encoding MHC class II-restricted antigens: mutated CDC27 as a tumor antigen. *Science* 1999;284:1351.

94. Wang RF, Wang X, Rosenberg SA. Identification of a novel major histocompatibility complex class II-restricted tumor antigen resulting from a chromosomal rearrangement recognized by CD4(+) T cells. *J Exp Med* 1999;189:1659.

95. Nishimura MI, Custer MC, Schwarz SL, et al. T cell-receptor V gene use by CD4+ melanoma-reactive clonal and oligoclonal T-cell lines. *J Immunother* 1998;21:352.

96. Pockaj BA, Sherry RM, Wei JP, et al. Localization of 111 indium-labeled tumor infiltrating lymphocytes to tumor in patients receiving adoptive immunotherapy. Augmentation with cyclophosphamide and correlation with response. *Cancer* 1994;73:1731.

97. Shilyansky J, Yang JC, Custer MC, et al. Identification of a T-cell receptor from a therapeutic murine T-cell clone. *J Immunother* 1997;20:247.

98. Overwijk WW, Tsung A, Irvine KR, et al. gp100/pmel 17 is a murine tumor rejection antigen: induction of "self"-reactive, tumoricidal T cells using high-affinity, altered peptide ligand. *J Exp Med* 1998;188:277.

99. Walter EA, Greenberg PD, Gilbert MJ, et al. Reconstitution of cellular immunity against cytomegalovirus in recipients of allogeneic bone marrow by transfer of T-cell clones from the donor [see comments]. *N Engl J Med* 1995;333:1038.

100. Zeh HJ III, Perry-Lalley D, Dudley ME, Rosenberg SA, Yang JC. High avidity CTLs for two self-antigens demonstrate superior in vitro and in vivo antitumor efficacy. *J Immunol* 1999;162:989.

101. Alexander-Miller MA, Leggatt GR, Berzofsky JA. Selective expansion of high- or low-avidity cytotoxic T lymphocytes and efficacy for adoptive immunotherapy. *Proc Natl Acad Sci U S A* 1996;93:4102.

102. Romieu R, Baratin M, Kayibanda M, et al. Passive but not active CD8+ T cell-based immunotherapy interferes with liver tumor progression in a transgenic mouse model. *J Immunol* 1998;161:5133.

103. Rosenberg SA, Yang JC, Schwartzentruber DJ, et al. Immunologic and therapeutic evaluation of a synthetic peptide vaccine for the treatment of patients with metastatic melanoma [see comments]. *Nat Med* 1998;4:321.

104. Dudley ME, Nishimura MI, Holt AKC, Rosenberg SA. Antitumor immunization with a minimal peptide epitope (G9-209-2M) leads to a functionally heterogeneous CTL response. *J Immunother* 1999;22:288.

105. McCarty TM, Liu X, Sun JY, Peralta EA, Diamond DJ, Ellenhorn JD. Targeting p53 for adoptive T-cell immunotherapy. *Cancer Res* 1998;58:2601.

106. Nukaya I, Yasumoto M, Iwasaki T, et al. Identification of HLA-A24 epitope peptides of carcinoembryonic antigen which induce tumor-reactive cytotoxic T lymphocyte. *Int J Cancer* 1999;80:92.

107. Kawashima I, Tsai V, Southwood S, Takesako K, Sette A, Celis E. Identification of HLA-A3-restricted cytotoxic T lymphocyte epitopes from carcinoembryonic antigen and HER-2/neu by primary in vitro immunization with peptide-pulsed dendritic cells. *Cancer Res* 1999;59:431.

108. Kawashima I, Hudson SJ, Tsai V, et al. The multi-epitope approach for immunotherapy for cancer: identification of several CTL epitopes from various tumor-associated antigens expressed on solid epithelial tumors. *Hum Immunol* 1998;59:1.

109. Goedegebuure PS, Douville CC, Doherty JM, et al. Simultaneous production of T helper-1-like cytokines and cytolytic activity by tumor-specific T cells in ovarian and breast cancer. *Cell Immunol* 1997;175:150.

110. Dazzi F, Goldman JM. Adoptive immunotherapy following allogeneic bone marrow transplantation. *Annu Rev Med* 1998;49:329–340.

111. Kwak LW, Pennington R, Longo DL. Active immunization of murine allogeneic bone marrow transplant donors with B-cell tumor-derived idiotype: a strategy for enhancing the specific antitumor effect of marrow grafts. *Blood* 1996;87:3053.

112. Slifka MK, Whitmire JK, Ahmed R. Bone marrow contains virus-specific cytotoxic T lymphocytes. *Blood* 1997;90:2103.

113. Osman Y, Takahashi M, Zheng Z, et al. Generation of bcr-abl specific cytotoxic T-lymphocytes by using dendritic cells pulsed with bcr-abl (b3a2) peptide: its applicability for donor leukocyte transfusions in marrow grafted CML patients. *Leukemia* 1999;13:166.

CELL TRANSFER THERAPY: CLINICAL APPLICATIONS

Melanoma

STEVEN A. ROSENBERG

Cell transfer therapy (or *adoptive immunotherapy*) refers to the transfer of immune cells with antitumor activity that can mediate, directly or indirectly, antitumor effects in the tumor-bearing host. The successful application of cell transfer therapy for the treatment of patients with cancer depends on a variety of factors, including the lymphocyte subtype used for cell transfer, the presence on the tumor cell of the target antigen to which the lymphocytes are reactive, the avidity of the lymphocytes for recognition of the target antigen, the ability of lymphocytes to traffic to tumor deposits, the specific effector function of immune lymphocytes necessary for tumor destruction, and the ability of lymphocytes to overcome any suppressive or tolerizing factors that might exist in the host or at the tumor site to prevent the transferred cells from reacting with the tumor.

Most studies of cell transfer therapies in cancer have involved patients with melanoma because of the relative ease of generating immune cells directed against melanoma antigens, as well as the substantial progress made in the identification and characterization of melanoma antigens that can serve as targets for this therapy. A variety of cell types have been used for cell transfer, including tumor-infiltrating lymphocytes (TILs), peripheral lymphocytes sensitized *in vitro* to tumor antigens, and lymphocytes obtained from sites of tumor vaccinations. Cells with major histocompatibility complex (MHC)–restricted or non–MHC-restricted recognition of tumor cells have been used. Although these treatments remain experimental, antitumor effects have been seen in patients receiving the adoptive transfer of cells. These studies provide important biologic information about the functional characteristics of lymphocytes, as well as the target antigens required for tumor destruction.

BRIEF HISTORICAL PERSPECTIVE

In the early 1960s, increasing information from immunologic studies indicated that the cellular arm of the immune response was a predominant factor in the *in vivo* rejection of tissue, such as organ allografts and experimental tumors, in mice. These find-ings led to attempts to transfer cells to tumor-bearing patients with the hope of mediating antitumor effects (1). Moore and Gerner developed techniques for the large-scale cultivation of human B lymphocytes and treated 28 patients with 1 to 236 g of allogeneic-cultured B cells without therapeutic benefit (2).

Many workers attempted to treat cancer patients with fresh cells immunized against cancer tissue. Nadler and Moore cross-immunized cancer patients by reciprocal subcutaneous implantation of tumor into the thigh (3,4). Leukocytes were then cross-transfused between the patients daily for 3 weeks. Similar cross-immunization studies were also performed by Marsh et al. (5). Feneley et al. treated patients with lymph node cells from pigs immunized with tumor (6). Cheema and Hersh treated 15 patients with injections of phytohemagglutinin-activated autologous lymphocytes directly into cutaneous cancer nodules (7), and Frenster and Rogoway described techniques for activating large numbers of human lymphocytes with phytohemagglutinin before infusion into patients (8). Although minor antitumor responses were claimed, no reproducible antitumor effects were seen. These approaches to immunotherapy were therefore largely abandoned.

The ability to grow lymphocytes *in vitro* using interleukin-2 (IL-2) and other cytokines and the ability to identify lymphocytes with unique antitumor activity opened new possibilities for the development of highly specific cell transfer therapies for the treatment of patients with cancer. These developments have renewed interest in the application of this approach.

TUMOR-INFILTRATING LYMPHOCYTES

TILs are lymphoid cells that infiltrate solid tumors and can be grown from single-cell suspensions of tumors by incubation in IL-2–containing media. Interest in the use of TILs for the adoptive immunotherapy of patients with metastatic melanoma was stimulated by the study of TILs obtained from transplantable mouse tumors (9,10). TILs able to recognize specific tumor-associated antigens from a variety of experimental tumors could

TABLE 1. MELANOMA ANTIGENS RECOGNIZED BY TUMOR-INFILTRATING LYMPHOCYTES

Name of Antigen	TILs Used for Identification	HLA Restriction	Immunodominant Epitopes	Characteristics
MART-1	1235 and others	A2	AAGIGILTV	Normal differentiation antigen
gp100	1200 and others	A2	KTWGQYWQV	Normal differentiation antigen
			ITDQVPFSV	
			YLEPGPVTA	
	1351	A3	LIYRRLMK	
	888	A24	VYFFLPDHL	Intronic sequence
Tyrosinase	1138 and 1374	A2	YMDGTMSQV	Normal differentiation antigen
	1138	A1	SSDYVIPIGTY	
	888 and 1413	A24	AFLPWHRLF	
	1088	DR4	QNILLSNAPLGPQFP	
p15	1290	A24	AYGLDFYIL	Posttranscriptional control
TRP-1	586	A31	MSLQRQFLR	Translated from alternate open reading frame
TRP-2	586	A31	LLGPGRPYR	Normal differentiation antigen
ESO-1	586	A31	ASGPGGGAPR	Translated from normal and alternate open reading frames
			LAAQERRVPR	
β-catenin	1290	A24	SYLDSGIHF	Single base mutation
TP1	1558	DR4	ELIGILNAAKVPAD	Single base mutation
CDC-27	1359	DR4	FSWAMDLDPKGA	Aberrant processing
LDL-FUT	1363	DR1	WRRAPAPGA	Chromosomal rearrangement
			PVTWRRAPA	

TILs, tumor-infiltrating lymphocytes.

be expanded in culture and exhibited specific killing, as well as specific cytokine secretion, when cocultivated with the syngeneic tumor (11,12). *In vivo* studies using the adoptive transfer of syngeneic murine TILs, often in association with cyclophosphamide administration or whole-body irradiation, demonstrated that established lung and liver metastases from a variety of murine tumor models could be successfully treated (9,10). In these studies, there was a correlation between the therapeutic effectiveness of TILs and the ability of TILs to specifically lyse or secrete cytokines, such as interferon (IFN)-γ, when cocultivated with syngeneic tumor (13).

These studies of murine TILs lead to attempts to derive TILs from a variety of histologic types of human cancer, including metastatic melanoma, lung cancer, breast cancer, colon cancer, renal cell cancer, and ovarian cancer (14–24). TILs grown from approximately 50% of patients with melanoma exhibit specific tumor lysis or specific cytokine secretion when stimulated *in vitro* with tumor from the autologous patient (25). A variety of techniques were developed for the expansion of TILs *in vitro* to the large numbers required for the adoptive therapy of cancer patients (25–27). In one study, 206 melanoma biopsies were processed from a variety of metastatic sites, and attempts were made to grow TILs to therapeutic levels (25). TIL cultures were initiated from single-cell suspensions of tumors obtained by enzymatic digestion. These cultures were first grown in culture plates. Later, when sufficient numbers were reached, the cultures were grown in gas-permeable bags. Of these 206 biopsies, 124 (60%) grew to levels of more than 10^{10} cells, usually within 45 days of initiating the culture. Eighty-nine TIL cultures were grown to levels of 10^{11} cells or more. TILs could be successfully grown from tumors obtained from a variety of metastatic sites, including involved lymph nodes, lungs, muscles, intestines, and subcutaneous tissues. The cytotoxicity of 115 TIL cultures were tested. Preferential

lysis of autologous tumor cells was seen in 43 cultures (25). This preferential lysis of fresh autologous tumor cells was obtained more frequently from subcutaneous tumors (50%) than tumor-involved lymph nodes (18%) ($p < .05$). In another study, melanoma metastases were harvested from 82 patients for the purpose of growing TILs (28). Cells were incubated in IL-2 followed by repeated exposure to tumor and, in some cases, by the use of anti-CD3 monoclonal antibody bound to plastic culture vessels. In this study, more than 10^{10} cells could be grown in 23 of 26 attempted cultures (88%).

TILs from melanoma patients recognize a wide variety of melanoma-associated antigens, including melanoma and melanocyte differentiation antigens (i.e., MART-1, gp100, tyrosinase, TRP-1, TRP-2), antigens that represent unique mutations of intracellular proteins (i.e., beta-catenin), and proteins that are expressed in a variety of cancers, as well as the testes (i.e., NY-ESO-1 antigen) (29–31). Antigens have been identified that are encoded not only by the primary open reading frame of the gene, but by alternative open reading frames, as well as intronic regions. A list of the class I– and class II–restricted antigens recognized by TILs is shown in Table 1. Each of these antigens is recognized by TILs in an MHC-restricted fashion. TILs can recognize a broad array of epitopes, even within a single protein. All MART-1 reactive TILs thus far obtained from patients with melanoma recognize the MART-1:27–35 peptide, AAGIGILTV, although ten different peptides are recognized by TILs reactive with the gp100 antigen (32,33).

TILs have been identified that recognize melanoma antigens restricted by HLA-A1, HLA-A2, HLA-A3, HLA-A24, HLA-A31, B44, DR1, and DR4 (34–46). A study of TIL cultures grown from 123 patients with melanoma is shown in Table 2 (34). Six of 38 TILs that express HLA-A1 recognized shared antigens, including one TIL that recognized gp100, one TIL that recognized tyrosinase, and four TILs that recognized

TABLE 2. SUMMARY OF TUMOR-INFILTRATING LYMPHOCYTE RECOGNITION OF SHARED MELANOMA ANTIGENS

HLA Class I Restriction Element	Number of Shared Antigen-Specific CTLs/Total TILs Expressing HLA (%)	Number of CTLs that Recognized Melanocyte Antigens					
		MART-1	gp100	Tyrosinase	TRP-1	TRP-2	Unidentified
HLA-A1	6/38 (16)	0	1	1	0	0	4
HLA-A2	32/57 (57)	22	13	2	0	0	2
HLA-A3	2/28 (7)	0	1	0	0	0	2
HLA-A24	3/23 (13)	0	1[a]	2	0	0	1
HLA-A31	3/11 (27)	0	0	0	1[b]	1	2

CTLs, cytotoxic T lymphocytes; TILs, tumor-infiltrating lymphocytes.
[a]Peptide encoded by an intron sequence of the gp100 gene was recognized by TILs.
[b]Peptide encoded by an alternative open reading frame of the TRP-1 gene was recognized by TILs.

unidentified antigens. The HLA-A2 molecule is found in approximately 50% of whites. Thirty-two of 57 TILs that expressed HLA-A2 recognized shared melanoma antigens. Twenty-two of these cultures recognized MART-1, 13 recognized gp100, two recognized tyrosinase, and two recognized unidentified antigens. Similar observations were made for TILs restricted by HLA-A3, HLA-A24, and HLA-A31 (as shown in Table 2).

Clinical Effect of Transfer of Tumor-Infiltrating Lymphocytes to Patients with Metastatic Melanoma

The largest reported series of patients with melanoma treated with TILs included 86 patients with metastatic melanoma treated in the Surgery Branch at the National Cancer Institute (NCI) with TILs plus high-dose intravenous bolus IL-2 at 720,000 IU per kg every 8 hours (47). Two treatment cycles were administered approximately 2 weeks apart. Fifty-seven of the 86 patients received a single intravenous dose of 25 mg per kg cyclophosphamide before the infusion of TILs plus IL-2 based on data from animal models indicating that immunosuppression before adoptive transfer could improve the immunotherapeutic effect (48–50). The characteristics of the patients in this trial, as well as the characteristics of the adoptively transferred TILs, are shown in Table 3. In this study, the overall objective clinical response rate was 34% and was similar in patients receiving TILs and IL-2 alone (31%) or in conjunction with cyclophosphamide (35%) (Tables 4 and 5). The objective response rate was similar in patients who received prior treatment with high-dose IL-2 (32%) compared with patients not previously treated with IL-2 (34%). This overall response rate of 34% was approximately twice the response rate seen in 134 consecutive melanoma patients treated using the same regimen of high-dose IL-2 alone, although the duration of responses was often short (51).

A collaborative study from multiple institutions of 21 patients with metastatic melanoma who received adoptive transfer of TILs plus IL-2 was published by the National Biotherapy Study Group (28). TILs were grown in IL-2 followed by repeated exposure to tumor antigen and, sometimes, with stimulation by immobilized anti-OKT3 monoclonal antibody. Patients received 1 g per m² of cyclophosphamide and 36 hours later began a constant infusion of 18×10^6 IU per

kg of IL-2 daily for 4 days. Four hours after initiation of IL-2, TIL cells were infused. Some patients with stable or responding disease were retreated at 3- to 4-week intervals. Objective responses were seen in 24% of patients. Two of ten patients who had previously failed treatment with IL-2 exhibited a response compared with 3 of 11 patients who had not previously received IL-2.

Kradin et al. reported the treatment of 13 patients with melanoma treated by TILs in conjunction with relatively low doses of IL-2 administered by constant infusion (1 to 3×10^6 IU per kg for 24 hours) (52). Objective responses were seen in three patients. The doses of IL-2 used in this trial would not be expected to mediate antitumor responses when administered alone. In a study by Arienti et al., 12 evaluable patients with metastatic melanoma were treated by the adoptive transfer of TILs followed by the administration of IL-2 by continuous infusion at 12×10^6 IU per kg for 5 days (53). In this study, patients also received 3×10^6 IU of IFN-α as an intramuscular injection for 3 consecutive days and a single intravenous injection of 350 mg per m² of cyclophosphamide 1 day before TIL administration. Four of these 12 evaluable patients exhibited an objective response to treatment. Similarly, Queirolo et al. saw two complete responses in 19 melanoma patients treated with TILs plus IL-2 and IFN-α (54). The small number of patients in these trials makes it difficult to determine whether the antitumor effects were attributable to the TILs or to the administration of IL-2 and IFN-α.

Although one large study suggested that the response rates of patients with metastatic melanoma receiving the adoptive transfer of TIL cells plus IL-2 is twice that of patients treated with IL-2 alone (47), a prospective randomized trial in which patients with metastatic melanoma receive TIL cells plus IL-2 or the identical regimen of IL-2 alone is required to determine the clinical effectiveness of TILs. Several other factors, however, suggest that TIL cells played a therapeutic role in these patients. In the NCI Surgery Branch study (47) and the National Biotherapy Study Group trial (28), similar response rates were seen after treatment with TIL cells plus IL-2, regardless of whether patients had previously failed treatment with IL-2. This result is in contrast to reports that repeat treatments with IL-2 alone could not mediate therapeutic responses, even in patients who previously responded to IL-2 and then recurred (55,56). Thus, the responses to TILs plus IL-2 in patients who previously did not respond to IL-2

TABLE 3. TREATMENT WITH TILS PLUS INTERLEUKIN-2

Patient Characteristics	No. (%)	TIL Characteristics		Total (%)
Total	86	Days of growth	11–20	1 (1)
Sex:			21–30	17 (20)
Male	48 (56)		31–40	33 (38)
Female	38 (44)		41–50	19 (22)
Age:			51–60	11 (13)
11–20	1 (1)		61–70	4 (5)
21–30	13 (15)		71–80	1 (1)
31–40	26 (30)		**Total**	86
41–50	18 (21)	Doubling time (days)	1.0–1.9	7 (10)
51–60	24 (28)		2.0–2.9	29 (43)
61–70	4 (5)		3.0–3.9	21 (31)
Performance Status (ECOG):			4.0–4.9	2 (3)
0	68 (79)		5.0–5.9	5 (7)
1	15 (17)		6.0–6.9	3 (4)
2	2 (2)		**Total**	67
3	1 (1)	Lysis of autologous melanoma	<10%	31 (50)
			≥10%	31 (50)
Previous Treatment:			**Total**	62 (**100**)
None	3 (3)	Lysis of Daudi lymphoma	<10%	54 (82)
Surgery	80 (93)		≥10%	12 (18)
Chemotherapy	20 (23)		**Total**	66
Radiotherapy	10 (12)	CD3$^+$	70%–79%	2 (3)
Hormonal	1 (1)		80%–89%	4 (6)
Immunotherapy	43 (50)		≥90%	60 (91)
Any two or more	48 (56)		**Total**	66
Any three or more	19 (22)	CD4$^+$	0%–19%	37 (56)
			20%–39%	7 (11)
			40%–59%	7 (11)
			60%–79%	5 (8)
			≥80%	10 (15)
		CD8$^+$	0%–19%	13 (20)
			20%–39%	6 (9)
			40%–59%	6 (9)
			60%–79%	7 (11)
			≥80%	34 (52)
		CD56$^+$	0%–9%	29 (44)
			10%–19%	13 (20)
			20%–29%	8 (12)
			≥30%	5 (8)

ECOG, Eastern Cooperative Oncology Group; TILs, tumor-infiltrating lymphocytes.
Note: Effector to target ratio of 40:1 in a 4-hour CR-51 release assay. Measurement of CD3$^+$, CD4$^+$, CD8$^+$, and CD56$^+$ cells based on 26 patients receiving no cyclophosphamide and 40 patients receiving cyclophosphamide. From Rosenberg SA, Yannelli JR, Yang JC, et al. Treatment of patients with metastatic melanoma using autologous tumor-infiltrating lymphocytes and interleukin 2. *J Natl Cancer Inst* 1994;86:1159, with permission.

TABLE 4. TREATMENT WITH TUMOR-INFILTRATING LYMPHOCYTES PLUS INTERLEUKIN-2: RESPONSE TO TREATMENT

	No CY				Plus CY				Total			
	Total number of patients	CR	PR	CR + PR (%)	Total number of patients	CR	PR	CR + PR (%)	Total number of patients	CR	PR	CR + PR (%)
Prior IL-2	11	1	2	27	17	—	6	35	28	1	8	32
No prior IL-2	18	3	3	33	40	1	13	35	58	4	16	34
Total	**29**	**4**	**5**	**31**	**57**	**1**	**19**	**35**	**86**	**5**	**24**	**34**

CR, complete response; CY, cyclophosphamide; IL-2, interleukin-2; PR, partial response.
From Rosenberg SA, Yannelli JR, Yang JC, et al. Treatment of patients with metastatic melanoma using autologous tumor-infiltrating lymphocytes and interleukin-2. *J Natl Cancer Inst* 1994;86:1159, with permission.

TABLE 5. TREATMENT WITH TUMOR-INFILTRATING LYMPHOCYTES PLUS INTERLEUKIN-2: DURATION OF RESPONSE

	No CY		Plus CY	
	CY (Mo)	PR (Mo)	CR (Mo)	PR (Mo)
Prior IL-2	23	4,1	—	8,7,6,5,5,1
No prior IL-2	46+,38,21+	7,4,2	20	53 + 9,7,7,4,4,4,4,4, 3,3,3,3

CR, complete response; CY, cyclophosphamide; PR, partial response.
From Rosenberg SA, Yannelli JR, Yang JC, et al. Treatment of patients with metastatic melanoma using autologous tumor-infiltrating lymphocytes and interleukin-2. *J Natl Cancer Inst* 1994;86:1159, with permission.

TABLE 6. TREATMENT WITH TUMOR-INFILTRATING LYMPHOCYTES PLUS INTERLEUKIN-2: CHARACTERISTICS OF TUMOR-INFILTRATING LYMPHOCYTES ASSOCIATED WITH RESPONSE

	Responders (Mean ± SEM)	Nonresponders (Mean ± SEM)	p_2
Time in culture (d)	33 ± 1	43 ± 2	0.0001
Doubling time (d)	2.4 ± 0.2	3.5 ± 0.4	0.03
Percent lysis (E:T of 40:1) autologous tumor target	25 ± 4	10 ± 2	0.0008
Daudi lymphoma target	11 ± 6	6 ± 2	0.6
Phenotype (% of cells)			
CD3$^+$	96 ± 1	95 ± 1	0.9
CD4$^+$	24 ± 8	32 ± 5	0.3
CD8$^+$	71 ± 8	62 ± 5	0.3
CD56$^+$	9 ± 3	13 ± 2	0.3

SEM, standard error of the mean.
From Rosenberg SA, Yannelli JR, Yang JC, et al. Treatment of patients with metastatic melanoma using autologous tumor-infiltrating lymphocytes and interleukin-2. *J Natl Cancer Inst* 1994;86:1159, with permission.

strongly suggest that TILs were a factor in the beneficial response. Furthermore, several characteristics of TILs strongly correlate with their ability to manifest therapeutic responses. The specific reactivity of TILs, the reactivity of TILs against particular antigens, and the ability of TILs to traffic to tumor sites are correlated with clinical response. Although it is possible that patients who give rise to TILs with these characteristics are patients more likely to respond to IL-2 alone, it appears more likely that TILs play a direct role in the antitumor responses. Definite resolution of this question must await prospective randomized trials.

Characteristics of Tumor-Infiltrating Lymphocytes Associated with Antitumor Responses in Patients

In a detailed study of melanoma patients who underwent treatment with TILs and IL-2, multiple patient and treatment characteristics were evaluated for correlation with clinical response (Tables 6 and 7) (47,56). TIL characteristics, such as doubling time, cell surface phenotype, autologous tumor lysis, and cytokine secretion after autologous tumor stimulation, were assayed within 7 days of infusion. A statistically significant increase in clinical response was seen when TILs were obtained from subcutaneous sites compared with TILs obtained from lymph nodes (p_2 = .006). TILs that were cultured for a shorter duration and TILs with shorter doubling times also were associated with higher responses (p_2 = .0001 and .03, respectively). A significant increase in clinical response was seen for TILs able to lyse autologous tumor cells (p_2 =.0008). In another study, clinical response was associated with the ability of TILs to secrete cytokines (especially granulocyte-macrophage colony-stimulating factor) when cocultivated with autologous tumor cells (p = .04) (57). The correlation of clinical response with the ability of TILs to specifically recognize tumors was a major factor that stimulated attempts to clone individual TIL populations with high levels of antitumor reactivity for use in cell transfer therapies.

The molecular identification of antigens recognized by transferred TILs has enabled an analysis of the specific reactivity of TILs against known antigens and their correlation with clinical response (34). Twenty-one HLA-A2 patients were treated with TIL cells that recognized shared melanoma antigens. Twelve of these TILs recognized the gp100 antigen, 16

recognized the MART-1 antigen, and two recognized the tyrosinase antigen. Nine TIL populations recognized gp100 and MART-1. A significant correlation existed between gp100 recognition by TILs and objective tumor regression after the adoptive transfer of TILs plus IL-2 (p = .024). No correlation of clinical responsiveness existed with recognition by TILs of the MART-1 antigen (p = .61).

Traffic of Adoptively Transferred Tumor-Infiltrating Lymphocytes to Tumor Sites

Although the mechanism of action of TILs in mediating antitumor effects is not known, it is hypothesized that adoptively transferred TILs traffic to tumor sites and, on encountering

TABLE 7. TREATMENT WITH TUMOR-INFILTRATING LYMPHOCYTES PLUS INTERLEUKIN-2: SITE OF TUMOR HARVEST

Site of Tumor Harvest	Total	Responders	Nonresponders	%
Lymph node	35	6	29	17[a]
Subcutaneous	37	18	19	49[a]
Muscle	3	0	3	0
Lung	3	1	2	33
Intraperitoneal mass	2	0	2	0
Pleural effusion	1	0	1	0
Colon	1	1	0	100
Liver	1	1	0	100
Spleen	1	0	1	0
Ovary	1	1	0	100
Bone	1	1	0	100
Total	**86**	**29**	**57**	**34**

[a]Difference in response rates comparing lymph nodes with subcutaneous harvest sites, p = .006.
From Rosenberg SA, Yannelli JR, Yang JC, et al. Treatment of patients with metastatic melanoma using autologous tumor-infiltrating lymphocytes and interleukin-2. *J Natl Cancer Inst* 1994;86:1159, with permission.

TABLE 8. FACTORS INFLUENCING INDIUM-111–LABELED TUMOR-INFILTRATING LYMPHOCYTE LOCALIZATION TO TUMOR

	Number of Patients		
	Negative Nuclear Scan	Positive Nuclear Scan	p^a
Cyclophosphamide administration			
Yes	5	21	
No	7	5	.026
IL-2 doses given			
2–7	9	18	
≥8	3	8	NS
IL-2 concentration in culture medium			
10–20 U/mL	1	2	
1,000 U/mL	10	20	NS
TIL culture media			
AIM V	6	12	
RPMI + human serum	2	4	
Half AIM V + RPMI + serum	3	8	NS
Lysis of autologous tumor			
≤9%	3	8	
≥10%	3	11	NS
Phenotype: CD8+			
≤50%	2	4	
>50%	7	14	NS

IL-2, interleukin-2; NS, not significant; TIL, tumor-infiltrating lymphocyte.
[a]Fisher's Exact Test.
From Pockaj BA et al. Localization of 111 indium-labeled tumor infiltrating lymphocytes to tumor in patients receiving adoptive immunotherapy. Augmentation with cyclophosphamide and correlation with response. *Cancer* 1994;73:1731–1737, with permission.

tumor antigens, directly lyse tumor cells or secrete cytokines, or both, which can amplify local antitumor immune responses. Studies to determine whether transferred TILs can traffic to sites of tumors have used TILs radiolabeled with indium-111-oxine (58–60). In a study of 38 patients with metastatic melanoma receiving high-dose IL-2 and TILs labeled with indium-111, significant localization of TILs to metastatic tumor deposits was seen in 26 of 38 patients (68%), as measured by gamma camera imaging or biopsies of tumors and normal tissue (60) (Table 8 and Fig. 1). In a univariate analysis of factors influencing TIL traffic, administration of cyclophosphamide (25 mg per kg) 24 to 36 hours before TIL infusion was significantly associated with the ability to localize to tumors. Twenty-one of 26 (80.8%) treatment courses given with cyclophosphamide demonstrated tumor localization compared with 5 of 12 (41.7%) treatment courses given without cyclophosphamide ($p_2 = .026$). Biopsy of cutane

IMAGING OF MELANOMA PATIENT WITH INDIUM-111 LABELED TIL

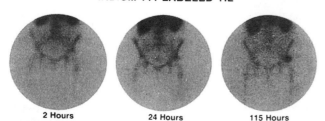

2 Hours   24 Hours   115 Hours

FIGURE 1. Nuclear scan of a patient infused with indium-111–labeled tumor-infiltrating lymphocytes. Areas of tumor show enhanced uptake of labeled cells

ous tumors, as well as nearby normal skin, showed a significantly greater accumulation of indium-111–labeled TILs at tumor sites ($p_2 > .001$) (Fig. 2). Clinical response was also correlated with localization of TILs to sites of tumors (60) (Table 9). Ten of twenty-six (38.5%) patients who exhibited tumor localization by radionuclide scans had an objective clinical response, whereas no responses were noted in 12 patients whose tumors did not image ($p_2 = .022$). It thus appears that the traffic of TILs to tumor deposits is an important part of the mechanism involved in the antitumor response of TILs in melanoma patients.

The short half-life of indium-111 (2.8 days) and the spontaneous loss of indium-111 from lymphocytes made it difficult to determine the long-term survival of TIL cells. Adoptive transfer studies of T cells in patients with acquired immunodeficiency syndrome suggested that the limited survival of transferred lymphocytes was a result of rapid apoptosis of the infused cells (61). Other studies in recipients of allogeneic bone marrow transfer who received T-cell clones directed against cytomegalovirus suggested that CD4+ cells were important for maintaining the prolonged survival of transferred CD8+ cells that recognized the same antigen (62). Similar data have been obtained in animal models, indicating the importance of CD4+ cells for the survival of CD8+ cells (63). Other factors, such as the expression of L-selectin on the T-cell surface, may impact on the traffic and survival of these cells (64).

To study the long-term survival of T cells after adoptive transfer, ten patients with metastatic melanoma received autologous TIL cells retrovirally transduced with the gene for neomycin phosphotransferase (65). Polymerase chain reaction assays demonstrated that the transferred TILs persisted in the circula-

¹¹¹INDIUM RECOVERY IN BIOPSIES

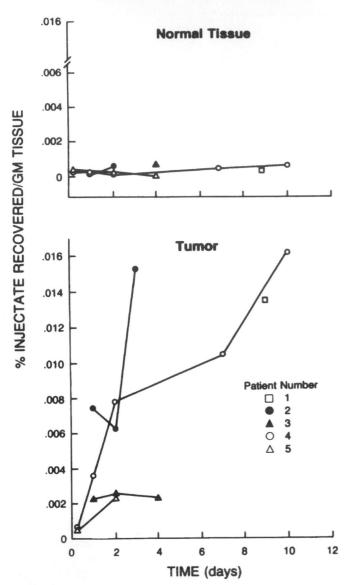

FIGURE 2. Results of sequential biopsies of patients receiving indium-111–labeled tumor-infiltrating lymphocytes. An increased accumulation of tumor-infiltrating lymphocytes with time was found in tumor deposits, but not in normal tissue.

TABLE 9. RELATIONSHIP BETWEEN CLINICAL RESPONSE AND LOCALIZATION OF TUMOR-INFILTRATING LYMPHOCYTES TO TUMOR

Clinical Response (CR or PR)	Localization of Indium-111–Labeled Tumor-Infiltrating Lymphocytes to Tumor by Scan	
	No	Yes
Yes	—	10
No	12	16

CR, complete response; PR, partial response.
Note: Localization of tumor-infiltrating lymphocytes to melanoma metastases is associated with responses to tumor-infiltrating lymphocytes and interleukin-2 adoptive immunotherapy (p_2 = .022, Fisher's Exact Test). No patients responded without tumor-infiltrating lymphocyte localization. From Pockaj BA et al. Localization of 111 indium-labeled tumor infiltrating lymphocytes to tumor in patients receiving adoptive immunotherapy. Augmentation with cyclophosphamide and correlation with response. *Cancer* 1994;73:1731–1737, with permission.

cells (66). In animal models, the adoptive transfer of LAK cells plus IL-2 was capable of mediating the regression of established micrometastases (67,68). Mechanistic studies indicated that the LAK cells could expand *in vivo* under the influence of IL-2 administration and maintain their antitumor activity (69).

Because IL-2 was available only in tiny amounts in the 1980s, studies began with the adoptive transfer of phytohemagglutinin-activated killer cells, a cell type quite similar to LAK cells (70). The adoptive transfer of these phytohemagglutinin-activated cells alone or in combination with cyclophosphamide or activated macrophages was performed in 21 patients between 1981 and 1983 (71). When recombinant IL-2 became available, a clinical trial was performed at the NCI Surgery Branch for patients with advanced cancer using the combined administration of LAK cells and IL-2. Published in 1985, this study provided evidence that adoptive immunotherapy with LAK cells and IL-2 could mediate antitumor effects (72,73). These clinical trials used a preinfusion of IL-2 for 3 to 5 days, which resulted in profound lymphocytosis when IL-2 administration ceased. Repeated leukophereses were performed during this period of lymphocytosis to increase the yield of lymphocytes. These harvested lymphocytes were then cultured in the presence of IL-2 for 3 to 4 days to produce LAK cells, which were then reinfused along with the administration of IL-2. In these studies, patients received IL-2 by intravenous bolus infusion every 8 hours, usually at a dose of 720,000 U per kg. In early trials, patients with renal cell cancer and melanoma showed the most significant anticancer responses, and, thus, patients with these diagnoses accounted for the majority of patients treated. The patients entering these trials had advanced cancer that did not respond to standard effective therapy, no treatment other than this protocol for 30 days before or throughout the follow-up period, evaluable disease, and life expectancies longer than 3 months.

After the initial reports of tumor regressions using LAK cells and IL-2 by the NCI Surgery Branch, other groups began clinical studies using LAK cells (Table 10). In these studies, responses were reported in patients with lymphoma, ovarian cancer, and lung cancer, although few patients with these histologies were treated.

tion of patients for 3 weeks and, in some cases, for as long as 2 months, although only a small fraction of the infused cells could be detected. Cells bearing the neomycin phosphotransferase gene could also be recovered from tumor deposits. The unique rearranged sequences of the T-cell receptor can also be used to follow the survival of transferred cloned lymphocytes (62).

CELLULAR IMMUNOTHERAPY WITH LYMPHOKINE-ACTIVATED KILLER CELLS

Lymphokine-activated killer (LAK) cells are lymphocytes that develop the ability to lyse fresh tumors but not fresh normal

TABLE 10. TREATMENT OF PATIENTS WITH ADVANCED CANCER USING LYMPHOKINE-ACTIVATED KILLER (LAK) CELLS PLUS INTERLEUKIN-2 (IL-2)

Author	Year	IL-2, Dose and Schedule	LAK Cells, No. Cells (Mean)	Diagnosis	Total No. Patients	CR (No. Patients)	PR (No. Patients)	CR + PR (%)	Comments
Schoof et al. (26)	1988	30,000 U/kg q8h	4.3×10^{10}	Renal	10	1	4	50	Duration, 1+ to 9+ mo
				Melanoma	9	1	4	56	Minimal toxicity (no vasopressors)
				Lymphoma	3	1	1	67	
				Colorectal	4	0	0	0	
				Ovarian	1	1	0	100	
				Sarcoma	1	0	0	0	
Dutcher et al. (27)	1989	100,000 U/kg q8h	8.9×10^{10}	Melanoma	32	1	5	19	Duration, 31+ mo; 36 patients, 1 death
Thompson et al. (28)	1989	1×10^6 U/m^2 q8h	3.4×10^{10}	Melanoma	4	0	0	0	
				Renal	3	0	0	0	
				Colorectal	4	0	0	0	
		3×10^6 U/m^2/d c.i.	4.3×10^{10}	Melanoma	4	0	0	0	
				Renal	8	1	0	13	CR at 7+ mo
				Lymphoma	1	0	0	0	
West et al. (25)	1987	1 to 7×10^6 U/m^2/d c.i.		Melanoma	10	0	5	50	Duration, 1 to 7+ mo
				Renal	6	0	3	50	1 death
				Lung	5	0	1	20	
				Parotid	2	0	1	50	
				Ovary	1	0	1	100	
				Breast	1	0	0	0	
				Lymphoma	2	0	2	100	
				Colon	13	0	0	0	
Paciucci et al. (29)	1989	1 to 5×10^6 U/m^2/d c.i.	5.6×10^9	Melanoma	5	0	1	20	LAK cells incubated for only 1 d in IL-2
				Renal	9	0	1	20	
				Lymphoma	4	0	1	25	
				Chronic myelocytic leukemia	3	0	0	0	Duration, 1–12 mo
				Sarcoma	2	0	1	100	
				Colorectal	1	0	1	100	
Neqrier et al. (30)	1989	3×10^6 U/m^2/d 1.2 $\times 10^{10}$ c.i.	1.2×10^{10}	Renal	51	5	9	27	
Stahel et al. (31)	1989	3×10^4 U/kg q8h	5.1×10^{10}	Renal	14	0	3	21	Duration, 1–6 mo
				Melanoma	7	0	1	14	
					3	0	0	0	
				Colon	2	0	0	0	
Hawkins (24)	1989	10^5 U/kg q8h		Melanoma	32	1	5	19	
				Colorectal	19	1	2	16	
Dutcher et al. (32)	1991	3×10^4/m^2 c.i.		Melanoma	33	0	1	3	

c.i., continuous i.v. infusion; CR, complete response; PR, partial response.

As experience with the use of high-dose IL-2 evolved, significant responses were seen in cancer patients treated with high-dose IL-2 alone. To evaluate the role of LAK cells in antitumor responses, the Surgery Branch at the NCI conducted a prospective trial in 181 patients with advanced cancer randomized to receive LAK cells and IL-2 or IL-2 alone (74). The results of this trial were reported in 1993 with a median follow-up of 63.2 months. A trend toward improved survival was seen for patients with melanoma who received IL-2 plus LAK cells, compared with those who received IL-2 alone (24-month survival: 32% vs. 15%; 48-month survival: 18% vs. 4%; p_2 = .064). No difference in survival was seen in patients with renal cell cancer in the two treatment groups (p_2 = .52). Because of the suggestion that treatment with LAK cells and IL-2 improved survival in patients with metastatic melanoma, a second randomized clinical trial was initiated in the Surgery Branch at the NCI among 128 patients with melanoma comparing treatment with LAK cells and IL-2 or IL-2 alone. This trial did not reveal a difference in survival between the two treatment groups. Thus, systemic treatment with LAK cells is no longer recommended.

Clinical studies did not demonstrate that LAK cells traffic to tumor deposits. Therefore, attempts were made to administer LAK-cell therapy locally to increase the concentration of tumor-reactive cells at the tumor site (75–80). LAK cells were instilled at the site of brain tumors by directly injecting the LAK cells into a tumor cavity after resection of recurrent disease. Jacobs et al. (75) treated 15 patients with recurrent glioblastoma by injecting LAK cells and IL-2 directly into the brain tissue surrounding the resection site intraoperatively. Others have instilled LAK cells and IL-2 through an Ommaya reservoir inserted intraoperatively or by using a plasma clot containing LAK cells placed into a resected tumor bed (76–79). Nitta et al. (80) reported tumor regression after the direct injection of LAK cells plus bispecific (anti–CD3-antiglioma) antibody into the tumor site after "debulking" surgery. In most of these studies, no measurable tumor was present at the time of treatment. Indications of successful therapy could be obtained only by following the survival of treated patients. It is difficult to interpret these studies because no randomized studies of patients receiving and not receiving LAK cells after resection of brain tumors have been performed.

Others have instilled LAK cells or IL-2 directly into a body cavity, such as the peritoneal or pleural space (81–84). Steis et al. (83) reported objective responses in patients with peritoneal carcinomatosis from ovarian and colorectal cancer who were treated with LAK cells and IL-2 administered intraperitoneally. Yasumoto et al. (85) reported the administration of LAK cells and IL-2 into the pleural cavity of patients with malignant pleural effusion. The intrathecal administration of IL-2 and LAK cells for the treatment of patients with leptomeningeal carcinomatosis has also been reported (86).

In an attempt to improve the traffic of LAK cells to tumor deposits, LAK cells have been infused directly into the hepatic artery of patients with liver metastases or introduced into the isolation-perfusion extracorporeal circulation of patients with intransit metastases from melanoma (87–90). Although these studies suggest that higher response rates are obtained, direct comparative studies using conventional modes of administration are required before conclusions can be drawn.

OTHER CELLS USED IN CELL TRANSFER THERAPY

The TIL populations used for cell transfer therapy were heterogeneous populations grown from the lymphocytes infiltrating into tumor deposits, many of which may have been bystander cells with no reactivity against tumors. Attempts to transfer improved populations of cells with increased antitumor activity have used a variety of *in vitro* and *in vivo* techniques. Sporn et al. treated 14 patients with metastatic melanoma using autologous peripheral blood lymphocytes that had been cocultured with irradiated autologous tumor cells for 1 week followed by expansion in IL-2–containing medium (91). These lymphocytes were then infused into patients followed by the administration of IL-2 at relatively low doses (2×10^6 IU per kg per day). Patients received a single dose of 300 mg per m^2 of cyclophosphamide 4 days before each treatment. In this protocol, approximately 10^9 cells were given per treatment and from one to five cell infusions were given to patients. The infused lymphocytes exhibited some degree of specificity for the autologous target cell in only 2 of the 14 patients. No significant therapeutic responses were seen in this trial.

Chang et al. attempted to increase the effectiveness of adoptively transferred cells by obtaining lymphocytes from lymph node draining sites of vaccination (92,93). These studies were based on preclinical studies in mice showing that immune T cells from lymph nodes primed by *in vivo* vaccination could be successfully used for the immunotherapy of transplantable tumors (94). In this study, irradiated autologous tumor cells mixed with bacillus Calmette-Guérin were used to vaccinate patients. Seven days later, draining lymph nodes were removed, activated with anti-CD3 monoclonal antibody, and expanded in IL-2. Eleven patients were treated with a mean of 3.4×10^{10} expanded lymphocytes and the bolus administration of IL-2 at 360,000 IU per kg every 8 hours for up to 5 days. Three of these melanoma patients developed delayed-type hypersensitivity skin tests to autologous tumor. One of the 11 melanoma patients had an objective tumor response.

Techniques for the effective immunization of patients using immunodominant peptides from tumor antigens have improved the prospects for isolating cells with specific antitumor reactivity. After immunization of melanoma patients with the modified gp100 peptide [gp100:209–217(210M)], more than 80% of patients developed circulating peripheral blood lymphocytes capable of reacting with unique melanoma antigens (95). Techniques for cloning these cells have been developed (96,97), and more than 1,000-fold differences in the affinity of these cells for tumor antigens were seen when individual clones were examined (98). In addition, techniques for the isolation of specifically reactive cells using peptide-MHC tetramers have enabled the rapid identification and isolation of lymphocytes with high levels of antitumor activity (99–101) that can potentially be used for cell transfer. This represents an exciting area for the future development of cell transfer therapies. The T-cell receptors from antitumor immune cells have been characterized and successfully transferred into OKT-3–stimulated human lymphocytes (102). These lymphocytes then exhibit the antitumor activity conveyed by the retrovirally transduced T-cell receptors and represent cells suitable for therapy.

REFERENCES

1. Rosenberg SA, Terry W. Passive immunotherapy of cancer in animals and man. *Adv Cancer Res* 1977;25:323.
2. Moore GE, Gerner RE. Cancer immunity-hypothesis and clinical trial of lymphocytotherapy for malignant diseases. *Ann Surg* 1970;172:733.
3. Nadler SH, Moore GE. Clinical immunologic study of malignant disease: response to tumor transplants and transfer of leukocytes. *Ann Surg* 1966;164:482.
4. Nadler SH, Moore GE. Immunotherapy of malignant disease. *Arch Surg* 1969;99:376.
5. Marsh B, Flynn L, Enneking W. Immunologic aspects of osteosarcoma and their application to therapy. *J Bone Joint Surg Br* 1972;7:1367.
6. Feneley RCL, Eckert H, Riddell AG. The treatment of advanced bladder cancer with sensitized pig lymphocytes. *Br J Surg* 1974;61:825.
7. Cheema AR, Hersh EM. Local tumor immunotherapy with *in vitro* activated autochthonous lymphocytes. *Cancer* 1972;29:982.
8. Frenster JH, Rogoway WM. Immunotherapy of human neoplasms with autologous lymphocytes activated in-vitro. Fifth Leukocyte

Culture Conference. 1999;359.

9. Rosenberg SA, Spiess P, Lafreniere R. A new approach to the adoptive immunotherapy of cancer with tumor-infiltrating lymphocytes. *Science* 1986;233:1318–1321.

10. Spiess PJ, Yang JC, Rosenberg SA. In vivo antitumor activity of tumor infiltrating lymphocytes expanded in recombinant interleukin-2. *J Natl Cancer Inst* 1987;79:1067.

11. Barth RJ, Bock SN, Mule JJ, Rosenberg SA. Unique murine tumor associated antigens identified by tumor infiltrating lymphocytes. *J Immunol* 1990;144:1531.

12. Barth RJ, Mule JJ, Asher AL, Sanda MG, Rosenberg SA. Identification of unique murine tumor associated antigens by tumor infiltrating lymphocytes using tumor specific secretion of interferon-gamma and tumor necrosis factor. *J Immunol Methods* 1991;140:269.

13. Barth RJ, Mule JJ, Spiess PJ, Rosenberg SA. Interferon gamma and tumor necrosis factor have a role in tumor regressions mediated by murine CD8+ tumor-infiltrating lymphocytes. *J Exp Med* 1991;173:647.

14. Muul LM, Spiess PJ, Director EP, Rosenberg SA. Identification of specific cytolytic immune responses against autologous tumor in humans bearing malignant melanoma. *J Immunol* 1987;138:989.

15. Topalian SL, Solomon D, Rosenberg SA. Tumor-specific cytolysis by lymphocytes infiltrating human melanomas. *J Immunol* 1989;142:3714.

16. Belldegrun A, Muul LM, Rosenberg SA. Interleukin-2 expanded tumor infiltrating lymphocytes in human renal cell cancer: isolation, characterization and antitumor activity. *Cancer Res* 1988;48:206.

17. Itoh K, Tilden AB, Balch CM. Interleukin-2 activation of cytotoxic T-lymphocytes infiltrating into human metastatic melanomas. *Cancer Res* 1986;46:3011.

18. Kurnick JT, Kradin RL, Blumberg R. Functional characterization of T lymphocytes propagated from human lung carcinoma. *Clin Immunol Immunopathol* 1986;38:367.

19. Whiteside TL, Miescher S, Hurlimann J. Clonal analysis and in situ characterization of lymphocytes infiltrating human breast carcinomas. *Cancer Immunol Immunother* 1986;23:169.

20. Whiteside TL, Miescher S, Hurlimann J. Separation, phenotyping, limiting dilution analysis of T-lymphocytes infiltrating human solid tumors. *Int J Cancer* 1986;23:169.

21. Melioli G, Ratto G, Guastella M, et al. Isolation and *in vitro* expansion of lymphocytes infiltrating non-small cell lung carcinoma: functional and molecular characterization for their use in adoptive immunotherapy. *Eur J Cancer* 1994;30A:97.

22. Schendel DJ, Gansbacher B, Obemeder R, et al. Tumor-specific lysis of human renal cell carcinomas by tumor infiltrating lymphocytes: I. HLA-A2-restricted recognition of autologous and allogeneic tumor lines. *J Immunol* 1993;151:4209.

23. Dadmarz RD, Ordoubadi A, Mixon A, et al. Tumor infiltrating lymphocytes from human ovarian cancer patients recognize autologous tumor in an MHC-class II restricted fashion. *Cancer Immunol Immunother* 1995;40:1.

24. Schwartzentruber DJ, Solomon D, Rosenberg SA, Topalian SL. Characterization of lymphocytes infiltrating human breast cancer: specific immune reactivity detected by measuring cytokine secretion. *J Immunother* 1992;12:1.

25. Yannelli JR, Hyatt C, McConnell S, et al. Growth of tumor-infiltrating lymphocytes from human solid cancers: summary of a 5-year experience. *Int J Cancer* 1996;65:413.

26. Topalian SL, Muul LM, Solomon D, Rosenberg SA. Expansion of human tumor infiltrating lymphocytes for use in immunotherapy trials. *J Immunol Methods* 1987;102:127.

27. Knazek RA, Wu YW, Aebersold PM, Rosenberg SA. Culture of human tumor infiltrating lymphocytes in hollow fiber bioreactors. *J Immunol Methods* 1990;127:29.

28. Dilman RO, Oldham RK, Barth NM, et al. Continuous interleukin-2 and tumor-infiltrating lymphocytes as treated of advanced melanoma. *Cancer* 1991;68:1.

29. Rosenberg SA. Development of cancer immunotherapies based on identification of the genes encoding cancer regression antigens. *J Natl Cancer Inst* 1996;88:1635.

30. Rosenberg SA. Cancer vaccines based on the identification of genes encoding cancer regression antigens. *Immunol Today* 1997;18:175.

31. Rosenberg SA. Mini review: a new era for cancer immunotherapy based on the genes that encode cancer antigens. *Immunity* 1999;10:281.

32. Kawakami Y, Eliyahu S, Sakaguchi K, et al. Identification of the immunodominant peptides of the MART-1 human melanoma antigen recognized by the majority of HLA-A2 restricted tumor infiltrating lymphocytes. *J Exp Med* 1994;180:347.

33. Kawakami Y, Eliyahu S, Jennings C, et al. Recognition of multiple epitopes in the human melanoma antigen gp100 by tumor infiltrating T-lymphocytes associated with *in vivo* tumor regression. *J Immunol* 1995;154:3461.

34. Kawakami Y, Dang N, Wang X, et al. Recognition of shared melanoma antigens in association with major HLA-A alleles by tumor infiltrating lymphocytes from 123 patients with melanoma. *J Immunother* 1999 (*in press*).

35. Kawakami Y, Eliyahu S, Delgado CH, et al. Identification of a human melanoma antigen recognized by tumor infiltrating lymphocytes associated with *in vivo* tumor rejection. *Proc Natl Acad Sci U S A* 1994;91:6458.

36. Kawakami Y, Eliyahu S, Delgado CH, et al. Cloning of the gene coding for a shared human melanoma antigen recognized by autologous T cells infiltrating into tumor. *Proc Natl Acad Sci U S A* 1994;91:3515.

37. Brichard V, Van Pel A, Wolfel T, et al. The tyrosinase gene codes for an antigen recognized by autologous cytolytic T lymphocytes on HLA-A2 melanomas. *J Exp Med* 1993;178:489.

38. Brichard VG, Herman J, Van Pel A. A tyrosinase nonapeptide presented by HLA-AB44 is recognized on a human melanoma by autologous cytolytic T lymphocytes. *Eur J Immunol* 199626:224.

39. Wolfel T, Van Pel A, Brichard V, et al. Two tyrosinase nonapeptides recognized on HLA-A2 melanomas by autologous cytolytic T lymphocytes. *Eur J Immunol* 1994;24:759.

40. Skipper JCA, Hendrickson RC, Gulden PH, et al. An HLA-A2-restricted tyrosinase antigen on melanoma cells results from post-translational modification and suggests a novel pathway for processing of membrane proteins. *J Exp Med* 1996;183:527.

41. Skipper JCA, Kittleson DJ, Hendrickson RC, et al. Shared epitopes for HLA-A3-restricted melanoma-reactive human CTL include a naturally processed epitope from Pmel-17/gp100. *J Immunol* 1996;157:5027.

42. Robbins PF, El-Gamil M, Li Y, et al. Cloning of a new gene encoding an antigen recognized by melanoma-specific HLA-A24-restricted tumor-infiltrating lymphocytes. *J Immunol* 1995;154:5944.

43. Robbins PF, El-Gamil M, Li YF, et al. A mutated B-catenin gene encodes a melanoma-specific antigen recognized by tumor infiltrating lymphocytes. *J Exp Med* 1996;183:1185.

44. Wang RF, Robbins PF, Kawakami Y, Kang XQ, Rosenberg SA. Identification of a gene encoding a melanoma tumor antigen recognized by HLA-A31-restricted tumor-infiltrating lymphocytes. *J Exp Med* 1995;181:799.

45. Pieper R, Christian RE, Gonzales MI, et al. Biochemical identification of a mutated human melanoma antigen recognized by CD4+ T cells. *J Exp Med* 1999;189:757.

46. Wang R-F, Wang X, Rosenberg SA. Identification of a novel major histocompatibility complex class II-restricted tumor antigen resulting from a chromosomal rearrangement recognized by CD4+ T cells. *J Exp Med* 1999;189:1659.

47. Rosenberg SA, Yannelli JR, Yang JC, et al. Treatment of patients with metastatic melanoma using autologous tumor-infiltrating lymphocytes and interleukin-2. *J Natl Cancer Inst* 1994;86:1159.

48. Berendt MJ, North RJ. T-cell-mediated suppression of anti-tumor immunity: an explanation for progressive growth of an immunogenic tumor. *J Exp Med* 1980;151:69.

49. Greenberg PD, Cheever MA. Treatment of disseminated leukemia with cyclophosphamide and immune cells: tumor immunity reflects long-term persistence of tumor-specific donor T cells. *J Immunol* 1984;133:3401.

50. Eberlein TJ, Rosenstein M, Rosenberg SA. Regression of a disseminated syngeneic solid tumor by systemic transfer of lymphoid cells

expanded in IL-2. *J Exp Med* 1982;156:385.

51. Rosenberg SA, Yang JC, Topalian SL, et al. Treatment of 283 consecutive patients with metastatic melanoma or renal cell cancer using high-dose bolus interleukin-2. *JAMA* 1994;271:907.

52. Kradin RL, Lazarus DS, Dubinett SM. Tumor-infiltrating lymphocytes and interleukin-2 in treatment of advanced cancer. *Lancet* 1989;1:577.

53. Arienti F, Belli F, Rivoltini L, et al. Adoptive immunotherapy of advanced melanoma patients with interleukin-2 (IL-2) and tumor-infiltrating lymphocytes selected *in vitro* with low doses of IL-2. *Cancer Immunol Immunother* 1993;36:315.

54. Queirolo P, Ponte M, Gipponi M, et al. Adoptive immunotherapy with tumor-infiltrating lymphocytes and subcutaneous recombinant interleukin-2 plus interferon alfa-2a for melanoma patients with nonresectable distant disease: a phase I/II pilot trial. *Ann Surg Oncol* 1999;6:272.

55. Sherry RM, Rosenberg SA, Yang JC. Relapse after response to IL-2 based immunotherapy: patterns of progression and response to retreatment. *J Immunother* 1991;10:371.

56. Lee DS, White DE, Hurst R, Rosenberg SA, Yang JC. Patterns of relapse and response to retreatment in patients with metastatic melanoma or renal cell carcinoma who responded to interleukin-2-based immunotherapy. *Cancer J Sci Am* 1998;4:86.

57. Schwartzentruber DJ, Hom SS, Dadmarz R, et al. In vitro predictors of therapeutic response in melanoma patients receiving tumor infiltrating lymphocytes and interleukin-2. *J Clin Oncol* 1994;12:1475.

58. Fisher B, Packard BS, Read EJ, et al. Tumor localization of adoptively transferred Indium-111 labeled tumor infiltrating lymphocytes in patients with metastatic melanoma. *J Clin Oncol* 1989;7:250.

59. Griffith KD, Read EJ, Carrasquillo JA, et al. *In vivo* distribution of adoptively transferred indium-111 labeled tumor infiltrating lymphocytes and peripheral blood lymphocytes in patients with metastatic melanoma. *J Natl Cancer Inst* 1989;81:1709.

60. Pockaj BA, Sherry R, Wei J, et al. Localization of Indium-111-labeled tumor infiltrating lymphocytes to tumor in patients receiving adoptive immunotherapy: augmentation with cyclophosphamide in association with response. *Cancer* 1994;73:1731.

61. Tan R, Xu X, Ogg GSHP, et al. Rapid death of adoptively transferred T cells in acquired immunodeficiency syndrome. *Blood* 1999;93:1506.

62. Walter EA, Greenberg PD, Gilbert MJ, et al. Reconstitution of cellular immunity against cytomegalovirus in recipients of allogeneic bone marrow by transfer of T-cell clones from the donor. *N Engl J Med* 1995;333:1038.

63. Matloubian M, Concepcion RJ, Ahmed R. CD4+ T cells are required to sustain CD8+ cytotoxic T-cell responses during chronic viral infection. *J Virol* 1994;68:8056.

64. Kjaergaard J, Shu S. Tumor infiltration by adoptively transferred T cells is independent of immunologic specificity but requires downregulation of L-selectin expression. *J Immunol* 1999;163:751.

65. Rosenberg SA, Aebersold PM, Cornetta K, et al. Gene transfer into humans: immunotherapy of patients with advanced melanoma, using tumor-infiltrating lymphocytes modified by retroviral gene transduction. *N Engl J Med* 1990;323:570.

66. Rosenberg SA. The development of new immunotherapies for the treatment of cancer using interleukin-2: a review. *Ann Surg* 1988;208:121.

67. Mule JJ, Shu S, Schwarz SL, Rosenberg SA. Adoptive immunotherapy of established pulmonary metastases with LAK cells and recombinant interleukin-2. *Science* 1984;225:1487.

68. Lafreniere R, Rosenberg SA. Successful immunotherapy of murine experimental hepatic metastases with lymphokine-activated killer cells and recombinant interleukin-2. *Cancer Res* 1985;45:3735.

69. Ettinghausen SE, Lipford EH, Mule JJ, Rosenberg SA. Recombinant interleukin-2 stimulates in vivo proliferation of adoptively transferred lymphokine activated killer (LAK) cells. *J Immunol* 1985;135:3623.

70. Mazumder A, Grimm EA, Rosenberg SA. Characterization of the lysis of fresh human solid tumors by autologous lymphocytes activated in vitro with phytohemagglutinin. *J Immunol* 1983;130:958.

71. Mazumder A, Eberlein TJ, Grimm EA, et al. Phase I study of the adoptive immunotherapy of human cancer with lectin activated

autologous mononuclear cells. *Cancer* 1984;53:896.

72. Rosenberg SA, Lotze MT, Muul LM, et al. Observations on the systemic administration of autologous lymphokine-activated killer cells and recombinant interleukin-2 to patients with metastatic cancer. *N Engl J Med* 1985;313:1485.

73. Rosenberg SA, Lotze MT, Muul LM, et al. A progress report on the treatment of 157 patients with advanced cancer using lymphokine activated killer cells and interleukin-2 or high dose interleukin-2 alone. *N Engl J Med* 1987;316:889.

74. Rosenberg SA, Lotze MT, Yang JC, et al. Prospective randomized trial of high-dose interleukin-2 alone or in conjunction with lymphokine-activated killer cells for the treatment of patients with advanced cancer. *J Natl Cancer Inst* 1993;85:622.

75. Jacobs SK, Wilson DJ, Kornblith PL. Interleukin-2 or autologous lymphokine-activated killer cell treatment of malignant glioma: phase I trial. *Cancer Res* 1986;46:2101.

76. Yoshida S, Tanaka R, Takai N. Local administration of autologous lymphokine-activated killer cells and recombinant interleukin-2 to patients with malignant brain tumors. *Cancer Res* 1988;48:5011.

77. Ingram M, Jacques S, Freshwater DB. Salvage immunotherapy of malignant glioma. *Arch Surg* 1987;122:1483.

78. Merchant RE, Merchant LH, Cook SHS. Intralesional infusion of lymphokine-activated killer (LAK) cells and recombinant interleukin-2 (rIL-2) for the treatment of patients with malignant brain tumor. *Neurosurgery* 1988;23:725.

79. Barba D, Sarvis SC, Holder C. Immunotherapy of human gial tumors: report of multiple dose intratumoral infusions of lymphokine-activated killer cells and interleukin-2. *J Neurosurg* 1988;70:175.

80. Nitta T, Sato K, Yagita H. Preliminary trial of specific targeting therapy against malignant glioma. *Lancet* 1990;335:368.

81. Lotze MT, Custer MC, Rosenberg SA. Intraperitoneal administration of interleukin-2 in patients with cancer. *Arch Surg* 1986;121:1373.

82. Chapman PB, Kolitz JE, Hakes TB. A phase I trial of intraperitoneal recombinant interleukin-2 (IL-2) in patients with ovarian cancer. *Invest New Drugs* 1988;6:179.

83. Steis R, Bookman M, Clark J. Intraperitoneal lymphokine activated killer (LAK) cell and interleukin-2 (IL-2) therapy for peritoneal carcinomatosis: toxicity, efficacy, and laboratory results (abstract). *Proc Annu Meet Am Soc Clin Oncol* 1987;6:250.

84. Urba WJ, Clark JW, Steis RG. Intraperitoneal lymphokine-activated killer cell/interleukin-2 therapy in patients with intraabdominal cancer: immunologic considerations. *J Natl Cancer Inst* 1989;81:602.

85. Yasumoto K, Miyazaki K, Nagashima A. Induction of lymphokine-activated killer cells by intrapleural instillations of recombinant interleukin-2 in patients with malignant pleurisy due to lung cancer. *Cancer Res* 1987;47:2184.

86. Shimizu K, Okamoto Y, Miyao Y. Adoptive immunotherapy of human meningeal gliomatosis and carcinomatosis with LAK cells and recombinant interleukin-2. *J Neurosurg* 1987;66:519.

87. Belli F, Arienti F, Rivoltini L, et al. Treatment of recurrent in transit metastases from cutaneous melanoma by isolation perfusion in extracorporeal circulation with interleukin-2 and lymphokine activated killer cells. A pilot study. *Melanoma Res* 1992;2:263.

88. Keilholz U, Scheibenbogen C, Brado M, et al. Regional adoptive immunotherapy with interleukin-2 and lymphokine-activated killer (LAK) cells for liver metastases. *Eur J Cancer* 1994;30A:103.

89. Keilholz U, Schlag P, Tilgen W, et al. Regional administration of lymphokine-activated killer cells can be superior to intravenous application. *Cancer* 1992;69:2172.

90. Okuno K, Takagi H, Nakamura T, Nakamura Y, Iwasa Z, Yasutomi M. Treatment for unresectable hepatoma via selective hepatic arterial infusion of lymphokine-activated killer cells generated from autologous spleen cells. *Cancer* 1986;58:1001.

91. Sporn JR, Ergin MT, Robbins GR, Cable RG, Silver H, Mukherji B. Adoptive immunotherapy with peripheral blood lymphocytes cocultured in vitro with autologous tumor cells and interleukin-2. *Cancer Immunol Immunother* 1993;37:175.

92. Chang AE, Yoshizawa H, Sakai K, Cameron MJ, Sondak VK, Shu S. Clinical observations on adoptive immunotherapy with vaccine-primed T-lymphocytes secondarily sensitized to tumor in vitro. *Can-*

cer Res 1993;53:1043.

93. Chang AE, Aruga A, Cameron MJ, et al. Adoptive immunotherapy with vaccine-primed lymph node cells secondarily activated with anti-CD3 and interleukin-2. *J Clin Oncol* 1997;15:796.

94. Shu S, Chou T, Rosenberg SA. Generation from tumor-bearing mice of lymphocytes with in vivo therapeutic efficacy. *J Immunol* 1987;139:295.

95. Rosenberg SA, Yang JC, Schwartzentruber DJ, et al. Immunologic and therapeutic evaluation of a synthetic vaccine for the treatment of patients with metastatic melanoma. *Nat Med* 1998;4:321.

96. Riddell SR, Watanabe KS, Goodrich JM, Li CR, Agha ME, Greenberg PD. Restoration of viral immunity in immunodeficient humans by the adoptive transfer of T cell clones. *Science* 1992;257:238.

97. Yee C, Gilbert MJ, Riddell SR. Isolation of tyrosinase-specific CD8+ and CD4+ T cell clones from the peripheral blood of melanoma patients following in vitro stimulation with recombinant vaccinia virus. *J Immunol* 1996;157:4079.

98. Dudley ME, Nishimura MI, Czopik AK, Rosenberg SA. Anti-tumor immunization with a minimal epitope (G9-209-2M) leads to a functionally heterogeneous CTL response. *J Immunother* 1999 (*in press*).

99. Yee C, Savage PA, Lee PP, Davis MM, Greenberg PD. Isolation of high avidity melanoma-reactive CTL from heterogeneous populations using peptide-MHC tetramers. *J Immunol* 1999;162:2227.

100. Lee PP, Yee C, Savage PA, et al. Characterization of circulating T cells specific for tumor-associated antigens in melanoma patients. *Nat Med* 1999;5:677.

101. Dunbar PR, Chen J-L, Chao D, et al. Cutting edge: rapid cloning of tumor-specific CTL suitable for adoptive immunotherapy of melanoma. *J Immunol* 1999;162:6959.

102. Clay TM, Custer MC, Sachs J, Hwu P, Rosenberg SA, Nishimura MI. Efficient transfer of a tumor antigen-reactive TCR to human peripheral blood lymphocytes confers anti-tumor reactivity. *Nat Med* 1999 (*in press*).

13.2

CELL TRANSFER THERAPY: CLINICAL APPLICATIONS

Renal Cell Carcinoma

ARIE S. BELLDEGRUN
ROBERT A. FIGLIN
BELUR PATEL

Adoptive immunotherapy has evolved with improved understanding of tumor biology, as well as the rapid growth in genetic engineering. This mode of treatment involves the transfer of soluble messengers and cytolytic cells that stimulate the host immune system toward tumor cells. The activation of the immune system leads to tumor regression by direct antitumor effects or by an indirect cytokine-mediated pathway that ends in tumor destruction (1). Most methods use four distinct forms of cellular immunotherapy: lymphokine-activated killer (LAK) cells, autolymphocyte therapy (ALT), tumor-infiltrating lymphocytes (TILs), and dendritic cell (DC)–based therapy.

The basis of cellular immunotherapy began with mice models immunized with chemically induced tumors, which prevented the growth of transplanted tumors (2). The mechanism for this process involves T lymphocytes, which have been shown to cause the rejection of not only virally or chemically induced tumors in murine mice (3), but also allogeneic tumors in normal mice (4). T lymphocytes have also been implicated in the

antitumor activity seen with cytokine therapy (5,6). These findings have also led to the notion that suppressive factors are present around the tumor, preventing an effective immune response (7). Adoptive immunotherapy has overcome this problem by infusing the host with cells capable of mediating tumor regression. These cells have the capability to cause tumor regression by cytokine-mediated mechanisms (i.e., using host cells to destroy tumor cells) or by direct antitumor effects.

Another major advancement in adoptive cellular immunotherapy has been the discovery of interleukin-2 (IL-2) (discussed in Chapter 2), which has shown enhanced therapeutic effect when administered in conjunction with cellular therapy (8,9). IL-2 has not only allowed the expansion of *in vitro* lymphocytes, but has also been shown to cause *in vivo* proliferation and prolonged survival of cells used in adoptive immunotherapy (10). Thus, IL-2 is routinely administered with some form of cellular therapy.

Difficulties with adoptive cellular therapy in humans include the identification of specific cells that have antitumor effects and the generation of these cells in numbers large enough for clinical use. Over the years, however, more information on specific cellular immunology and biotechnology has evolved, opening the avenue for application of cellular therapy for renal cell carcinoma (RCC) in the clinical setting.

LYMPHOKINE-ACTIVATED KILLER CELLS

One of the first cell types to be implemented for adoptive immunotherapy were LAK cells. LAK cells were described in the 1970s by Rosenberg et al., who were investigating lymphoid cells capable of lysing neoplastic cells at the National Cancer Institute (NCI) (11). LAK cells appear to be part of the primitive immunosurveillance system and are capable of recognizing and destroying altered cells (12). LAK cells cause a nonspecific natural killer–like cytotoxicity in contrast to cytotoxic T lymphocytes because LAK-cell activity is major histocompatibility complex (MHC)–nonrestricted and causes lysing of tumor target cells derived from syngeneic, allogeneic, or xenogeneic sources regardless of target expression of MHC antigens (13).

The distinct characteristic of LAK-cell activity is the ability to differentiate tumor cells and normal cells. The characteristics and mechanisms of LAK-cell effects have been described in another chapter, as have preclinical studies. Preclinical studies using LAK cells and IL-2 demonstrated that this form of adoptive cellular therapy was capable of mediating tumor regression of micrometastases. Preclinical studies also demonstrated that both treatments provided better antitumor effects than either therapy alone (14–17). In addition, these studies exhibited the effect of IL-2 on LAK cells by causing *in vivo* expansion and proliferation of LAK cells and the death of LAK cells when IL-2 was discontinued (18). Further studies also showed that LAK cells were effective in the treatment of immunogenic and nonimmunogenic murine tumors (19). These animal studies led to the first clinical use of LAK cells and recombinant IL-2 in six patients and proved cell transfer to be feasible with only a few side effects (20).

The feasibility of LAK cells and IL-2 led to a clinical trial at the NCI in patients with advanced cancer (21). Of the 25 patients, 11 had an objective tumor response (1 complete response and 10 partial responses). These responses were seen in metastatic disease to the lung, liver, and subcutaneous tissues in patients with RCC, melanoma, lung adenocarcinoma, or colorectal carcinoma who did not respond to standard therapy. On follow-up, it was noted that patients with RCC and melanoma had the most significant tumor response and accounted for the majority of patients receiving this treatment (22,23). Of the 178 patients, 72 had metastatic kidney cancer. Complete regression of metastases was seen in eight patients, as well as a partial regression in 17 patients, with a combined response of 35%.

LAK cells are generated by initially treating patients with IL-2 to induce lymphopenia, followed by rebound lymphocytosis 2 to 3 days after infusion of high-dose (23) and low-dose IL-2 (24). Leukopheresis is then performed at the peak of the rebound lymphocytosis. Peripheral blood mononuclear cells (PBMCs) are then isolated. The cells are cultured *in vitro* using high concentrations of IL-2 (400 to 1,000 IU per mL) to generate approximately 10^{10} to 10^{11} LAK cells and are then infused

into the patient together with high- or low-dose IL-2. The high-dose IL-2 is administered by intravenous bolus infusion every 8 hours for 4 to 5 days, whereas the low-dose IL-2 is administered by continuous intravenous infusion over 4 or more days. Most of the side effects of concomitant therapy with LAK cells plus IL-2 were from toxicities related to the dose of IL-2. The optimal dose and schedule of IL-2 administration with LAK cells are not clearly defined. Studies have found less clinical toxicity with lower-dose continuous intravenous IL-2 infusion regimens when compared with bolus IL-2 infusions (25). In addition, schedules using continuous infusion of IL-2 also showed an improved response rate (26). A randomized phase 2 trial by the NCI Extramural IL-2/LAK Working Group, however, found equivalent anticancer activity and toxicity when using high-dose IL-2 as a bolus or continuous infusion in the treatment of patients with metatastic RCC (mRCC) (27). Gold et al. (28) have also shown that continuous infusion of IL-2 is associated with less toxicity than high-dose bolus IL-2.

The favorable results reported by early NCI studies led to a number of subsequent clinical studies at various institutions using LAK cells plus IL-2 for the treatment of mRCC. These trials used a variety of preparative and treatment regimens with response rates ranging from 9% to 35% and a combined objective response rate of approximately 22%. A list of studies is shown in Table 1 (22,26–41,44). Randomized trials have also been conducted to determine whether adoptive cellular therapy with LAK cells plus IL-2 could improve the clinical response rather than the use of IL-2 alone. In one study by investigators from the Modified Group C Program, a total of 167 patients from 13 institutions, including 69 patients with mRCC, were enrolled (42). The response rates for the treatment of mRCC with LAK cells and IL-2 and IL-2 alone were 13% and 8%, respectively. These results suggested that LAK cells did not contribute to higher response rates than IL-2 alone. The Surgery Branch at the NCI conducted another prospective randomized study. In this study, 181 patients with advanced cancer were randomized, including 97 patients with mRCC, to receive LAK cells plus IL-2 or IL-2 alone. The results for the 46 assessable patients with mRCC showed complete response in eight patients and a partial response in seven patients who received LAK cells plus IL-2. For the patients who received IL-2 alone, only four complete responses and six partial responses occurred. The overall response rate was 33% for LAK cells plus IL-2 versus 24% for IL-2 alone, showing no statistical difference between the two therapies. Moreover, no statistically significant difference was seen in survival at 48 months; 29% for LAK cells plus IL-2 versus 25% for IL-2 alone ($p = .52$) (23). Similarly, in Bajorin and colleagues' trial of 49 patients randomized to receive IL-2 with or without LAK cells reinfused on days 13 through 15, no significant difference was found (43). Two responses occurred (one complete response and one partial response) in 21 patients randomized to receive IL-2 plus LAK cells. Three responses occurred (one complete response and two partial responses) in 28 patients who received IL-2 alone. Results from a study by Law et al. (44) involved 71 randomized patients with advanced RCC; 36 patients received IL-2 alone and 35 patients received LAK cells plus IL-2. Of the 66 eligible patients, objective responses (complete responses and partial responses) were seen in 9% and 3% of patients receiving IL-2 alone and

TABLE 1. STUDIES AND RESPONSE RESULTS USING LYMPHOKINE-ACTIVATED KILLER CELLS AND CYTOKINE IMMUNOTHERAPY FOR THE TREATMENT OF METASTATIC RENAL CELL CARCINOMA

Source	No. of Patients	No. of CRs	No. of PRs	No. of Overall Responses (CR + PR) (%)
Schoof et al. (26)	10	1	4	5 (50)
Rosenberg et al. (22)	54	7	10	17 (54)
Weiss et al. (27)[a]	48	2	5	7 (15)
Thompson et al. (29)	42	4	10	14 (33)
Margolian et al. (30)	35	2	3	5 (16)
West et al. (31)	6	—	3	3 (50)
	12	2	2	4 (33)
Paciucci et al. (32)	9	—	1	1 (11)
Negrier et al. (33)	51	5	9	14 (27)
Stahl et al. (34)	14	—	3	3 (21)
Davis et al. (35)	31	3	11	14 (39)
Fujioka et al. (36)	10	1	3	4 (40)
Palmer et al. (37)	102	5	12	17 (18)
Parkinson et al. (38)	47	2	2	4 (9)
Gold et al. (28)	76	6	11	17 (22)
Foon et al. (39)	23	2	4	6 (17)
Kruit et al. (40)[b]	51	6	13	19 (37)
	17	3	2	4 (24)
Law et al. (44)	32	1	3[c]	4 (13)
Tomita et al. (41)	9	3	4[d]	7 (78)
Total	**679**	**55**	**114**	**169 (25)**

CR, complete response; PR, partial response.
[a]From the IL-2/LAK Working Group: IL-2/LAK Working Group included six institutions: City of Hope, CA; Albert Einstein College of Medicine of Yeshiva University, NY; Loyola University of Chicago Stritch School of Medicine, Chicago; New England Medical Center, Boston; University of California, San Francisco School of Medicine; and University of Texas Medical School at San Antonio.
[b]Results of two protocols. Protocol 1 involved 17 patients treated with interleukin-2 and lymphokine-activated killer cells. Protocol 2 involved 51 patients treated with interleukin-2, interferon-α, and lymphokine-activated killer cells.
[c]These are the patients with minor responses. No partial responses were seen.
[d]Includes one patient with minor response.

LAK cells plus IL-2, respectively. No significant differences were found in the overall median survival for the two groups (IL-2–alone arm, 11 months; LAK-cell–arm, 13 months; $p = .47$). Gold et al. reported results that confirmed these findings. Although not randomized, this report included 123 patients with mRCC who received recombinant IL-2 and 76 patients who received LAK cells. In the patients who were treated with LAK cells plus IL-2, the overall response rate was 22% with six complete responses (8%) and 11 partial responses (14%). The overall survival at 5 and 9 years was 19% and 17%, respectively, with a median survival of 22 months (range, 1.5 to 109+ months). Comparing these results with those of the patients treated with IL-2 alone, the overall response rate was 13% (three complete responses and partial responses). The overall survival rate was 28% at 4 years with a median survival of 14 months (range, 1 to 49+ months). Although the influence of each study on its own is not convincing, the overall data available strongly suggest that the combination of LAK cells plus IL-2 does not offer any significant advantage over IL-2 therapy alone in the treatment of mRCC.

AUTOLYMPHOCYTE CELLULAR THERAPY

ALT is a form of adoptive immunotherapy based on the activation and expansion of autologous memory T cells in patients with metastatic cancer. The memory T cells are presumed to have been exposed to tumor antigens and thus may have the potential for mediating tumor regression after nonspecific activation (45). Memory T cells are activated *ex vivo* by mitogenic monoclonal antibody directed against the invariant region of the CD3 component of the T-cell antigen receptor in a combination of autologous cytokines, resulting in polyclonal activation of heterogeneous memory T cells (46,47).

The preparation of autolymphocytes for immunotherapy involves two steps (48). The first step involves the preparation of an autologous cytokine mixture by harvesting approximately 2×10^9 PBMCs by pheresis from patients. These cells are then exposed to anti-CD3 monoclonal antibody and incubated for 3 days. Supernatant fluid is then collected and frozen. The supernatant is important because it contains a variety of cytokines, including a number of ILs, tumor necrosis factors (TNFs), interferon (IFN)-γ, and granulocyte-macrophage colony-stimulating factor (GM-CSF). The second step consists of *ex vivo* activation of the memory T cells 2 weeks after initial pheresis. Patients undergo another pheresis to collect PBMCs that contain the memory T cells for activation. The cells are incubated for 5 days in media containing 25% supernatant, indomethacin, and cimetidine, then irradiated. Indomethacin, cimetidine, and radiation are used to decrease the suppressor T-cell activity (49–51). The activated T cells are then infused back into the patients with oral cimetidine on a monthly outpatient basis over 6 months.

The initial clinical use of ALT in the treatment of mRCC has proved this form of adoptive cellular therapy to be safe and feasible (52,53). In a phase 2 trial for treatment of mRCC using ALT and cimetidine, Krane et al. (54) showed a delayed progression of disease in 33% of the patients. The median survival was 32 months, with a survival estimate of 56% and 36% at 1 and 2 years, respectively. These early results have prompted a multicenter phase 3 trial comparing ALT plus cimetidine with cimetidine alone in patients with mRCC (55). Initial results from this trial reported a 2.5-fold survival advantage for the ALT group (21 months vs. 8.5 months). Updated results showed a median survival of 29% at 46 months for the patients who received ALT. This phase 3 trial also revealed some interesting findings in the patients treated with ALT. First, a fourfold survival advantage was seen only in men, whereas women showed no advantage. This survival advantage was seen only in patients with anti-CD3–activated supernatant containing high levels of IL-1. Secondly, a lack of correlation existed between response (21%) and survival, and these were only partial responses. The results from these clinical trials initiated the use of ALT in the clinical practice setting at three sites: Boston; Orange, California; and Atlanta (56,57). The results from 335 patients with mRCC treated with ALT and cimetidine continued to show a survival advantage.

A randomized trial conducted with only 45 patients compared ALT with observation for the adjuvant treatment of RCC (58). A significant difference was found in favor of ALT versus observation for the overall median time to progression of disease. In addition, further subgroup analysis revealed an advantage in median time to recurrence of disease in patients with stage T3 and node-positive disease (59). Updated results from this trial continued to show a delay in progression of disease in the ALT group (18.5 months) compared with the observation group (11.9 months) (60). Even with these results, no randomized trial comparing ALT with high-dose IL-2 therapy has been implemented to validate the feasibility of ALT to improve survival in patients with mRCC.

TUMOR-INFILTRATING LYMPHOCYTES

The continued interest in adoptive cellular immunotherapy led to the evaluation of more potent lymphoid cells, designated *tumor-infiltrating lymphocytes*, for the treatment of mRCC. The biologic principles and preclinical aspects of TILs have been discussed earlier. Human RCC possesses a high number of TILs that can be cultured *ex vivo* from surgically resected tumors (61). The preparation of TILs involves the digestion of the tumor specimen mechanically and enzymatically to grow a single-cell suspension. After several weeks in culture, the tumor cells died, leaving a culture of pure lymphocytes, predominantly T lymphocytes (10,62,63). TILs can be selectively grown in single-cell tumor suspensions when cultured with IL-2. These activated TIL cells proliferate and induce the destruction of RCC tumor cells, resulting in a pure culture of TILs (63).

In preclinical studies, murine tumor models with pulmonary and liver micrometastasis tumors exhibited from 50- to 100-fold greater effectiveness of TILs when compared with LAK cells (64). TILs and LAK cells also differ in their *in vitro* tumor-lytic specificity. LAK cells react nonspecifically to a broad spectrum of tumors. In contrast, TILs display tumor-specific reactivity to distinct murine tumors (62,64,65). Numerous TIL cultures have been successfully established from different human tumors, including RCC, melanoma, colon and breast cancer, lymphoma, and other tumor types. These TIL cultures have shown *in vitro* antitumor reactivity (11,63,66). Most of the bulk TILs contain a heterogeneous population of cells, consisting of CD3$^+$CD8$^+$ cytotoxic/suppressor T cells, CD3$^+$CD4$^+$ helper/inducer T cells, and natural killer cells (67). The subset of TILs responsible for tumor lysis is debatable, but all subsets have been active against RCC in *in vitro* studies (68). Several studies have determined that CD8$^+$ TILs possess most of the antitumor effect, and studies have shown the same for RCC (69–71), demonstrating that antigen-specific cytotoxicity against autologous tumors does exist within RCC tumors.

The preparation of TILs for adoptive cellular immunotherapy is conducted in a sterile fashion (72). The primary tumor from patients' radical nephrectomy specimens are mechanically and enzymatically disrupted to obtain single-cell suspensions containing viable mononuclear and tumor cells. The cells are expanded *ex vivo* in the presence of IL-2. After approximately 2 weeks in culture, the tumor cells die, and the TIL cells continue to proliferate and overgrow. After 3 to 5 weeks in culture, the initial 10^8 to 10^9 mononuclear cells proliferate and expand to approximately 10^{10} to 10^{11} TIL cells. During this time, the patients have recovered from their surgery, and the TILs can be infused into patients together with IL-2.

Treatment of mRCC with TILs is still in its early stages. Only a limited number of patients are receiving this therapy. Table 2 summarizes some of the clinical studies using TILs in mRCC (73–79). The two largest studies were conducted at the Cleveland Clinic and the University of California at Los Angeles (UCLA). At the Cleveland Clinic, patients were treated according to two types of clinical protocols. The first protocol involved 18 patients and the second protocol involved 16 patients. In the first protocol, TILs were obtained from the primary tumor or metastatic sites and infused into the patients using three different IL-2 doses (0.0, 3.0, and 4.5×10^6 U per m^2). The second protocol involved 16 patients with mRCC treated with TILs isolated from the primary tumor, activated, and expanded in IL-2 and IL-4. The response rate was 0% (0 out of 18 patients) and 25% (4 out of 16 patients) in the first and second trials, respectively. The overall response rate at the Cleveland Clinic for both groups was 12% of the 34 patients who had mRCC. In the large study conducted at UCLA, a different regimen and technique for cell expansion were used, and the results were encouraging. The UCLA study was a single trial that involved 55 patients with mRCC, and their primary tumor in place, and TILs were obtained from primary tumors. A total of 23 patients received TILs that had been generated and expanded after enrichment in the CD8$^+$ population of cells using CD8 capture flasks (i.e., flasks coated with anti-CD8 monoclonal antibody). The other 32 patients received TILs that were primed *in vivo*, expanded *in vitro*, and harvested for infusion. The *in vivo* priming of the TILs was conducted by administering cytokines to the patients

TABLE 2. SUMMARY OF RESPONSES IN STUDIES USING TUMOR-INFILTRATING LYMPHOCYTES AND INTERLEUKIN-2 FOR THE TREATMENT OF METASTATIC RENAL CELL CARCINOMA

Source	No. of Patients	No. of CRs	No. of PRs	No. of Overall Responses (CR + PR) (%)
Dillman et al. (75)	6	0	0	0
Topalian et al. (73)	4	0	1	1 (25)
Kradin et al. (74)	7	0	2	2 (29)
Goedegebuure et al. (79)	8	0	0	0
Bukowski et al. (76), Olencki et al. (77)	34	2	2	4 (12)
Figlin et al. (78)	55	5	14	19 (35)
Ridolfi et al. (89)	1	0	0	0
Total	**115**	**7**	**19**	**26 (23)**

CR, complete response; PR, partial response.

before their nephrectomies. Of these 32 patients, 15 received IFN-α, four received TNF-α, four received IL-2, four received IL-6, and five received IFN-γ. All the patients received intravenous IL-2 during the treatment period, and an additional 48 patients also received IFN-α. Complete response was achieved in five (9.1%) patients and a partial response in 14 (25.5%) patients, for an overall response in 19 (34.6%) patients. The results are shown in Table 3 and Figure 1. Figure 1 shows computed tomographic scans of complete response in a patient who presented with mRCC involving the lung parenchyma, pleural base, hilar, and vena caval extension. The patient underwent radical nephrectomy and thrombectomy, followed by immunotherapy with TILs, IL-2, and IFN-α. The patient remains disease free at 5-year follow-up. These responses were noted to be durable with a median duration of response of 14 months (range, 0.8+ to 64+ months). The overall median survival was 22 months (range, 2 to 70+ months) with actuarial survival rates at 1 and 2 years as 65% and 43%, respectively (Fig. 2A and B). This study also demonstrated promising results with the use of low-dose IL-2 with or without IFN combined with TILs for adoptive immunotherapy for mRCC. The overall response rate of 34.6% in 55 patients compares favorably with those seen with high-dose IL-2. At UCLA, we have also studied the effect

of adoptive immunotherapy in a subgroup of patients with sarcomatoid RCC tumors (80). Sarcomatoid RCCs have been found to be associated with local aggressiveness, high metastatic potential, and poor prognosis (81,82). In this evaluation of nine patients with sarcomatoid RCC, an 11% complete response rate and 22% partial response rate were seen when patients were treated with TILs, IL-2, and IFN-α. In a separate study at UCLA, 23 patients received CD8$^+$ lymphocytes selected by using CD8 capture flasks coated with anti-CD8 antibodies. The flasks positively selected adherent CD8$^+$ cells by immunogenicity. The expanded cells were harvested and suspended in 10% human serum albumin. One hour after IL-2 therapy, patients received a single intravenous infusion of purified CD8$^+$ lymphocytes. Of the 23 patients who received therapy, the overall response rate was 43.5% (83). A multicenter phase 3 trial has been conducted by Rhône-Poulenc Rorer (Agoura, CA) to compare CD8$^+$ TILs plus low-dose IL-2 with low-dose IL-2 (84). Patients with mRCC were randomized to receive low-dose IL-2 plus CD8$^+$-selected TILs or low-dose IL-2 alone. In this study, a total of 178 patients with mRCC were initially enrolled and underwent radical nephrectomy. One hundred-sixty patients were randomized to the two groups—81 patients in the TIL and IL-2 group, and 79 patients in the

TABLE 3. CLINICAL RESPONSE, DURATION OF RESPONSE, AND DURATION OF SURVIVAL IN RESPONDING PATIENTS WITH METASTATIC RENAL CELL CARCINOMA TREATED WITH NEPHRECTOMY, TUMOR-INFILTRATING LYMPHOCYTES, AND INTERLEUKIN-2

Variable	Total	Primed TILs	CD8$^+$ TILs	p Value[a]
No. of CR (%)	5 (9.1)	3 (9.4)	2 (8.7)	—
No. of PR (%)[b]	14 (25.5)	6 (18.8)	8 (34.8)	—
No. of overall response (CR + PR)	19 (34.6)	9 (28.1)	10 (43.5)	0.26 (Fisher's two tailed test)
Median duration of response (range)	14 (0.8–64+)	24 (0.8–64+)	12 (3–48+)	0.73 (Log rank test)
Median overall survival (range)	22+ (2–70+)	24+ (3–53+)	21 (2–70+)	0.94 (Log rank test)

CR, complete response; PR, partial response; TILs, tumor-infiltrating lymphocytes.
[a]p values are for comparison between primed TILs and CD8$^+$ TIL results.
[b]Two cases of partial response were converted to complete surgical remission and pathologic remission, respectively, on surgical resection.

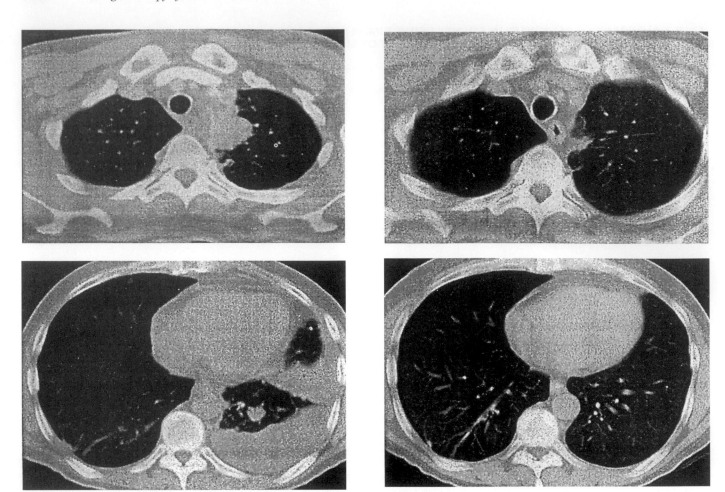

FIGURE 1. Computed tomographic scans of complete response in a patient who presented with metastatic renal cell carcinoma involving the lung parenchyma, pleural base, hilar, and venal caval extension. The patient underwent radical nephrectomy and thrombectomy, followed by immunotherapy with tumor-infiltrating lymphocytes, interleukin-2, and interferon-α. The patient remains disease free at 5-year follow-up.

IL-2–alone group. Each group had comparable characteristics. From these two groups, 20 patients could not receive IL-2 because of surgical complications or failure to meet eligibility criteria. Results were thus analyzed in the remaining patients, 72 of whom received TIL and IL-2 and 68 of whom received IL-2 alone. On initial intent to treat analysis, the overall response rate, according to the Eastern Cooperative Oncology Group (ECOG) performance status (ps), showed eight responders in the TIL and IL-2 group. Three (7.9%) of the patients had ECOG ps = 0 and five (11.6%) had ECOG ps = 1 with an overall response rate of 9.9%. In the IL-2–alone group, nine patients responded. Five (14.3%) patients had ECOG ps = 0 and four (9.1%) patients had ECOG ps = 1, for an overall response rate of 11.4%. Statistical analysis of the two groups revealed no significant difference between the two treatment groups (p = .894), as well as an odds ratio of 0.851, indicating a similar likelihood of response regardless of TIL treatment or ECOG ps. Overall survival rates were also similar for both groups with 1-year survival rates of 55% for the TIL and IL-2 group and 47% for the IL-2–alone group, showing median survival of 12.8 months and 11.5 months, respectively (Fig. 3). In addition, only 39 of the 81 patients randomized to the TIL and

IL-2 group actually received TILs because of technical problems encountered with TIL generation. The study was therefore terminated early because of lack of efficacy, as determined by the Data Safety Monitoring Board; thus, long-term results are not available. Although the 1-year survival rates in both groups in this study compared favorably with other studies, no demonstrable difference was found in response rate or survival between the TIL and IL-2 group and the low-dose IL-2–alone group.

Interest in the role of radical nephrectomy in the presence of metastatic disease has increased in the 1990s, especially with the advance of modern of immunotherapy. In an analysis at UCLA, 203 patients were consecutively treated with IL-2 (85). The study compared patients without nephrectomies who received IL-2 therapy with patients who had nephrectomies performed less than 6 months before or more than 6 months after administration of IL-2 or TIL. The results are summarized in Table 4. Overall, the median survival was 18 months, which is comparable with that reported with the 255-patient database of bolus IL-2 treatment alone. Survival at 1, 2, and 3 years was 61%, 40%, and 31%, respectively. Patients who had nephrectomies more than 6 months before IL-2 therapy had a 46% 3-year survival rate compared with 9% for patients who underwent nephrectomies less than 6 months before

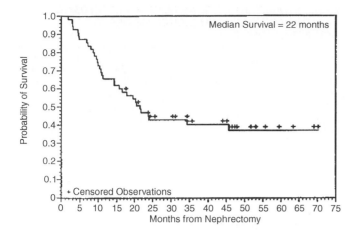

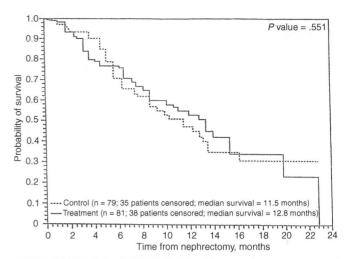

FIGURE 3. Overall survival for all patients by treatment group, based on the intent to treat analysis.

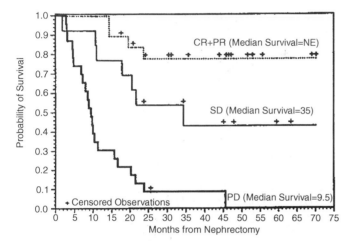

FIGURE 2. A: Overall survival of patients with metastatic renal cell carcinoma treated with tumor-infiltrating lymphocytes and interleukin-2. **B:** Effect of response to combined therapy with tumor-infiltrating lymphocytes, interleukin-2, and nephrectomy on survival. (CR, complete response; PD, progressive disease; PR, partial response; SD, stable disease.)

TILs could not be grown in one patient, and the other patient had transitional cell carcinoma. In addition, many of these patients underwent extensive and complicated operations, including resection of caval thrombus, partial hepatectomy, and splenectomy. The results revealed an overall response of 33.9% (12.5% complete response and 21.4% partial response), as well as a 43% and 38% survival rate at 2 and 3 years, respectively (see Table 4). Although these results do not explain these observations (i.e., whether nephrectomy alone or the combination of nephrectomy and cellular therapy was responsible for the responses), radical nephrectomy before systemic immunotherapy is still an attractive alternative in select patients. The overall contribution of adjuvant nephrectomy for the therapy of patients with metastatic disease must be determined by prospective randomized trials. One such study is being addressed in a randomized phase 3 Southwest Oncology Group trial comparing IFN-α alone versus nephrectomy followed by

IL-2 therapy, and 4% for patients who received IL-2 therapy and had no nephrectomies. The 3-year survival for patients treated with TIL was 38%, which was significantly better than the 3-year survival for patients treated with IL-2 who had no nephrectomy or a nephrectomy less than 6 months before treatment. To receive TIL therapy, patients must undergo radical nephrectomy to obtain tumor specimens for TIL generation. The question remains, however, whether surgery and its associated morbidities allow any further therapeutic benefits. Studies from other institutions have shown that as many as 40% of patients with mRCC undergoing nephrectomy are unable to receive adjuvant systemic immunotherapy because of morbidity, mortality, and deterioration caused by progressive disease (86,87). At UCLA, we have reported more favorable results for patients with mRCC undergoing cytoreductive surgery and subsequent TIL and IL-2 therapy (88). Of the 63 patients, 56 (88%) were able to receive TILs. Seven patients were unable to receive treatment with TILs because of postoperative complications—including myocardial infarction, transient ischemic attack, mild chronic renal failure, and deterioration of ps—in five patients. The other two patients were excluded because

TABLE 4. RESPONSE AND SURVIVAL TO INTERLEUKIN-2 PLUS TILS FOR TREATMENT OF METASTATIC RENAL CELL CARCINOMA WITH OR WITHOUT NEPHRECTOMY AT THE UNIVERSITY OF CALIFORNIA AT LOS ANGELES

Treatment Received	No. of Patients	No. of Overall Response (%)	% Survival at 2 Years	% Survival at 3 Years
TILs and nephrectomy	56	19 (35)	43	38
No nephrectomy	24	4 (17)	13	4
Nephrectomy >6 months[a]	76	15 (19)	60	46
Nephrectomy <6 months[a]	47	10 (21)	21	9
All patients	203	48 (24)	40	31

TILs, tumor-infiltrating lymphocytes.
[a]Nephrectomy performed either less than or more than 6 months before administration of interleukin-2 therapy.

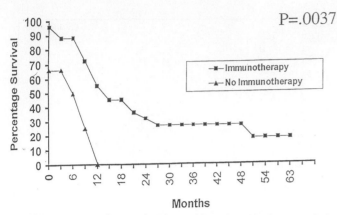

P=.0037

FIGURE 4. Percent of survival with or without immunotherapy administration in patients with inferior vena cava tumors who underwent surgery.

TABLE 5. MULTIVARIATE ANALYSIS: PROGNOSTIC FACTORS FOR THE OCCURRENCE OF DEATH AFTER TREATMENT

	p Value	Relative Risk of Death
With or without immunotherapy	.042	3.18
Pulmonary vs. extrapulmonary metastasis	.058	3.38
Low-grade vs. high-grade tumor	.077	2.68

IFN-α therapy. Another aspect of surgery and adjuvant TIL and IL-2 treatment is being studied by Ridolfi et al. (89), who are evaluating the feasibility of TIL and IL-2 therapy in patients who undergo resection of metastatic disease. The initial report on 22 patients with metastatic disease, including one patient with mRCC, shows the latter patient to be disease free at 22 months. The question of extensive surgery for metastatic disease coupled with postoperative adjuvant immunotherapy, including TIL therapy, has also been studied at UCLA (90). We identified 31 patients with the primary tumor in place and extension of the tumor into the inferior vena cava, as well as other metastatic sites. These patients all underwent radical nephrectomy and inferior vena cava thrombectomy followed by adjuvant immunotherapy. Of the 31 patients, a total of 80% received received IFN plus isotretinoin (Accutane). The overall survival was 17% with a mean follow-up of 18 months (range, 1+ to 88+ months). The correlation between survival and the ability to administer postoperative immunotherapy was statistically significant on univariate and multivariate analysis ($p = .0037$), as shown in Figure 4. Similar analysis also demonstrated a positive correlation between survival and site of metastases or histologic grade of tumor (Table 5). In addition, multivariate analysis based on the Cox Proportional Hazards model also suggested that the use of immunotherapy ($p = .042$) acts independently in reducing the risk of death in these patients. This result indicates that patients with inferior vena cava tumor and metastatic disease can benefit from thrombectomy and immunotherapy with survival, which is comparable to previous survival data in patients who underwent caval thrombectomy without other metastases (91). We therefore continue to favor the use of aggressive treatment with tumor debulking and immunotherapy, including adoptive cellular therapy (TILs), for advanced RCC. We believe that selected patients immunotherapy, 42% received IL-2, 26% received TILs, and 10%exhibit an overall improved survival with this treatment.

TUMOR-DRAINING LYMPH NODE LYMPHOCYTES

Another intriguing approach to adoptive cellular therapy is the use of lymphocytes obtained from tumor-draining lymph nodes (TDLNs). Preclinical studies have established methods to activate and expand tumor-reactive T cells from lymph nodes, and these cells demonstrated the ability to cure visceral tumors in animals (92–95). In view of these results, a clinical study was initiated by Chang et al. (96) in patients with advanced RCC (all had prior nephrectomies) and melanoma. Patients were initially vaccinated with irradiated autologous tumor cells admixed with bacille Calmette-Guérin. After 7 days, TDLNs were removed and activated with anti-CD3 antibody and cells expanded with IL-2. The activated lymph node cells were then infused into the patients with concomitant IL-2. Of the 12 patients with advanced RCC, complete and partial responses were seen in two patients with an overall response of 33%, with duration of 12+ to 36+ months and 12 to 20 months, respectively. This study shows the feasibility of using vaccines with adoptive immunotherapy—using cells from other sites when no primary tumor is available.

FUTURE PROSPECTS OF CELLULAR THERAPY

Dendritic Cells

DCs are the primary antigen-presenting cells responsible for *in situ* stimulation of T-cell mediated immune response, including antitumor immunity (97,98). DCs are leukocytes derived from bone marrow and lack cell surface markers typical for B cells, T cells, natural killer cells, or monocyte and macrophage lineage. DCs are derived in large numbers from PBMCs with the aid of the cytokines GM-CSF and IL-4 (97,99,100). GM-CSF and IL-4 allow the proliferation and maturation of DCs from monocyte precursors (Fig. 5). As many as 8% of circulating mononuclear cells can be recovered as functional DCs using these cell-culturing techniques. These cultured cells possess all the necessary functional, morphologic, and phenotypical antigen-presenting cell features and are crucial for the stimulation of T-cell subsets CD4 and CD8. More specifically, they express high levels of MHC classes I and II, adhesion molecules ICAM-1 and LFA-3, as well as other important costimulatory molecules, such as CD40, CD80, and CD86, that are essential to the process of proper antigen presentation. A phase 1 trial at UCLA showed that DCs can also be generated *in vivo* by administering GM-CSF plus IL-4 subcutaneously to patients with advanced cancer (101). This trial showed that patients had minimally detectable DCs at baseline and a marked increase in circulating DCs after 7 days of cytokine administration. An interesting point of these results may be the application of forming an antigen-based vaccination trial without the need for *ex vivo* processing of PBMCs to generate DCs.

Kidney Cancer Treatment Using Dendritic Cell (DC) Loaded With Tumor Antigen

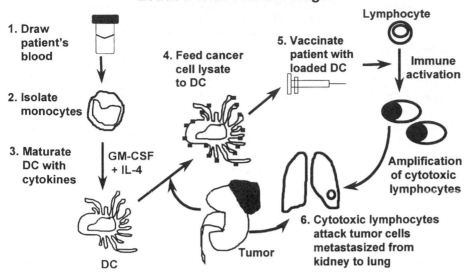

FIGURE 5. Schematic diagram of dendritic cell (DC) generation and activation for application in the treatment of metastatic renal cell carcinoma. (GM-CSF, granulocyte-macrophage colony-stimulating factor; IL-4, interleukin-4.)

The discovery of DCs has stimulated interest in using DCs for the treatment of cancer. This interest stems from the ability to induce a specific antitumor response using DCs isolated from patients loaded with tumor antigens. Phase 1 clinical trials using DCs have already shown promising results in patients with B-cell lymphoma, melanoma, and prostate cancer (102–104). Interest in DCs also lies in the ability to pulse DCs with various forms of antigens, including peptide-specific antigens, whole proteins in the form of tumor lysates (103,105), and even RNA encoding for antigens (106). At UCLA, large numbers of functional DCs have been generated from the PBMCs of patients with mRCC using IL-4 and GM-CSF (107). These DCs induce a rapid proliferation of CD8$^+$ and CD4$^+$ T lymphocytes, cytokine release, and enhancement of autologous tumor lysis in a TIL-based culture system on loading with unfractionated RCC tumor proteins in the form of crude tumor lysate (TuLy). This *in vitro* data led to a phase 1 clinical trial for patients with mRCC using TuLy obtained from the patients' primary RCC. The protocol is shown in Table 6. The TuLy is used to produce an autologous lysate-loaded DC vaccination (108). Thus far, DC cultures have been consistently obtained from patients' PBMCs for 3 consecutive TuLy-loaded DC vaccinations without any dose-limiting toxicities.

The capability to arm DCs with target-specific tumor-associated antigens (TAAs) has been the basis of many ongoing studies. The association of DCs and TAAs has led to efforts in discovering TAAs in RCC because of common antigenic determinants demonstrated in RCC that can be expressed and are recognized by MHC-restricted cytotoxic T lymphocytes. Isolation of TAAs is a laborious process that involves classification of antigens that can be used *in vitro* to generate an MHC-restricted cytotoxic T-lymphocyte response (109), followed by peptide mapping and cloning. A number of TAAs have been identified and are being assessed for their frequency of expression in human RCC. The possible TAAs include RAGE-1, PRAME, gp75 messenger RNA, and, most recently, G250. These are expressed in adequate, although heterogeneous, frequency in surgically removed tumor specimens, but not in the adjacent normal epithelium (110,111). The RCC-TAA G250 has gained increased interest for use as possible target immunotherapy for RCC. Studies have shown that monoclonal antibody G250 reacts with more than 75% of primary and metastatic RCCs with no cross-reactivity to normal kidneys. In addition, further imaging studies using biodistribution of iodine-131–labeled chimeric monoclonal antibody G250 in patients with RCC revealed several areas of previously unrecognized metastases and also excellent tumor localization (112). These findings suggest that monoclonal antibody G250 can recognize RCC-TAA and

TABLE 6. PROTOCOL OUTLINE FOR PHASE 1 STUDY AT THE UNIVERSITY OF CALIFORNIA AT LOS ANGELES IMPLEMENTING DENDRITIC CELL THERAPY FOR METASTATIC RENAL CELL CARCINOMA

Cohort	No. of Patients	Immunization	Route	Day
A	6	Irradiated autologous TuLy[a]	i.d.	0
		Irradiated autologous TuLy-loaded DCs[b]	i.d.	7
		Irradiated autologous TuLy-loaded DCs	i.d.	14
		Irradiated autologous TuLy-loaded DCs	i.d.	21
B	6	Irradiated autologous TuLy[a]	i.v.	0
		Irradiated autologous TuLy-loaded DCs[b]	i.v.	7
		Irradiated autologous TuLy-loaded DCs	i.v.	14
		Irradiated autologous TuLy-loaded DCs	i.v.	21

DCs, dendritic cells; TuLy, tumor lysate.
[a]Amount of TuLy irradiated depends on the number of DCs, usually 30% of the amount of DCs generated.
[b]Ideal number of DCs is 9 x 10^6.

may be applied in strategies for adoptive immunotherapy or vaccine therapy in the treatment of RCC.

Future Trends in Gene Modification

One of the major problems encountered with cellular therapy involves the generation and expansion of adequate numbers of potent effector cells. To overcome this problem, genetic approaches have been implemented to alter tumor cells to enable enhanced cellular immune response to TAAs expressed on the primary tumor. The majority of the work has focused on the use of cytokine genes introduced into tumor cells. Animal studies using genetically modified tumor cells that secrete IL-4 or IFN-γ have shown tumor regression in established tumors when administered as a vaccine for active specific immunotherapy (113–115). These early animal studies led to the development of gene-modified tumors that can be used to generate various cells for adoptive cellular therapy. Two of these cell types are TILs and vaccine-primed lymph node cells or TDLNs that have been generated using gene-modified tumors.

Tumors that are genetically engineered to produce certain cytokines, such as IFN-γ and TNF-α, have been discovered to contain TILs with enhanced antitumor activity *in vitro* and *in vivo*, even in poorly immunogenic tumors (116,117). These TILs showed increased antitumor activity when compared with TILs generated from wild-type tumors. Another cytokine, IL-7, has also been shown to enhance recovery of TILs from tumors and showed a fivefold increase in T cells, as well as enhanced *in vitro* cytotoxicity (118). In the case of vaccine-primed lymph node cells, antitumor activity is accomplished by secondary activation *in vitro* by coculturing with irradiated tumors and IL-2 or by sequential activation with anti-CD3 monoclonal antibody and expansion with IL-2 (93,94,119,120). These cells have antitumor effects with immunogenic tumors, but not with nonimmunogenic tumors. To overcome this problem, draining lymph nodes are primed by potent immunologic adjuvants, like *Corynebacterium parvum*, and then secondarily activated *in vitro*, leading to an increased antitumor effect (121). This increased activity has encouraged the exploration of genes to modify sensitization of T cells in TDLNs. Transfection of tumor B16-Bl6 melanoma with allogeneic MHC class I genes and then activation of TDLNs in anti-CD3 monoclonal antibody and IL-2 have significant antitumor effects compared with parental TDLNs when adoptively transferred into animals with pulmonary metastases (122). Genetic modification of tumor cells with other cytokines, such as IL-4, GM-CSF, and IFN-γ, have generated TDLNs that have mediated significant regression of established, poorly immunogenic tumors (123–125). These results show a promising avenue in enhancing antitumor activity of TILs and TDLNs that can be applied in clinical studies using cell transfer therapy for RCC.

Another path involving genetic modification in adoptive immunotherapy is to enhance the therapeutic efficacy of the cells being transferred. Initial application was addressed by Rosenberg et al. (126) using retroviral transduced TILs in patients with advanced melanoma. The ability of TILs to induce *in vitro* cytolysis or cause tumor regression was not affected. Moreover, TILs were detected in tumor deposits for as many as 64 days and in the circulation for as many as 189 days. The other strategies involve the use of various promoters and modification of cytokines such as TNF-α and IL-2 to enhance secretion of these cytokines. Possible methods that may be implemented in the future include modification of effector cells with signal transduction to enhance propagation or the introduction of chimeric receptor genes to specifically redirect TIL cells to specific tumors. Finally, the future in enhancing the efficacy of cellular transfer therapy may lie in the genetic engineering of naïve cells to become immunocompetent effector cells. These methods are still in their early stages but may provide future directions in the application of cellular transfer therapy in RCC.

REFERENCES

1. North RJ, Havell EA. The antitumor function of tumor necrosis factor (TNF). II. Analysis of the role of endogenous TNF in endotoxin-induced hemorrhagic necrosis and regression of an established sarcoma. *J Exp Med* 1988;167:1086–1099.
2. Algire OH, Weaver JM, Prehn RT. Growth of cells *in vivo* in diffusion chambers. I. Survival of homografts in immunized mice. *J Natl Cancer Inst* 1954;15:493–507.
3. Tevethia SS, Blasecki JW, Vaneck G, Goldstein AL. Requirement of thymus-derived theta-positive lymphocytes for rejection of DNA virus (SV4O) tumors in mice. *J Immunol* 1974;113:1417–1423.
4. Mulé JJ, Yang JC, Afreniere RL, Shu SY, Rosenberg SA. Identification of cellular mechanisms operational *in vivo* during the regression of established pulmonary metastases by the systemic administration of high-dose recombinant interleukin-2. *J Immunol* 1987;139:285–294.
5. Rosenberg SA, Schwarz SL, Spiess PJ. Combination immunotherapy for cancer: synergistic antitumor interactions of interleukin-2, alpha-interferon, and tumor-infiltrating lymphocytes. *J Natl Cancer Inst* 1988;80:1393–1397.
6. Fujimoto S, Greene ML, Sehon AH. Regulation of the immune response to tumor antigens. I. Immunosuppressor cells in tumor-bearing hosts. *J Immunol* 1976;116:791–799.
7. Cheever MA, Greenberg PD, Fefer A, et al. Augmentation of the anti-tumor therapeutic efficacy of long-term cultured lymphocytes by *in vivo* administration of purified interleukin 2. *J Exp Med* 1982;155:968–980.
8. Donohue JH, Rosenstein M, Chang AE, et al. The systemic administration of purified interleukin-2 enhances the ability of sensitized murine lymphocytes to cure a disseminated syngeneic lymphoma. *J Immunol* 1984;132:2123–2128.
9. Cheever MA, Greenberg PD, Irle C, et al. Interleukin-2 administered *in vivo* induces the growth of cultured T cells in vivo. *J Immunol* 1984;132:2259–2265.
10. Yron I, Wood TA, Spiess P, Rosenberg SA. *In vitro* growth of murine T cells. V. The isolation and growth of lymphoid cells infiltrating syngeneic solid tumors. *J Immunol* 1980;125:238–245.
11. Rosenberg SA. Karnofsky Memorial Lecture: the immunotherapy and gene therapy of cancer. *J Clin Oncol* 1992;75:1578–1583.
12. Rosenberg SA, Lotze MT. Cancer immunotherapy using interleukin 2-activated lymphocytes. *Annu Rev Immunol* 1986;4:681–709.
13. Mulé JJ, Shu S, Schwarz SL, et al. Adoptive immunotherapy of established pulmonary metastases with LAK cells and recombinant interleukin-2. *Science* 1984;225:1487–1489.
14. Lafreniere R, Rosenberg SA. Successful immunotherapy of murine experimental hepatic metastases with lymphokine-activated killer cells and recombinant interleukin-2. *Cancer Res* 1985;45:3735–3741.
15. Lafreniere R, Rosenberg SA. Adoptive immunotherapy of murine hepatic metastases with lymphokine-activated killer cells and recombinant interleukin-2 can mediate the regression of both immuno-

genic and nonimmunogenic sarcomas and an adenocarcinoma. *J Immunol* 1985;135:4273–4280.

16. Mulé JJ, Shu S, Rosenberg SA. The anti-tumor efficacy of lymphokine-activated killer cells and recombinant interleukin-2 *in vivo*. *J Immunol* 1985;135:646–652.

17. Ettinghausen SE, Lipford EH, Mulé JJ, et al. Recombinant interleukin-2 stimulates *in vivo* proliferation of adoptively transferred lymphokine-activated killer cells. *J Immunol* 1985;135:3623–3635.

18. Papa MZ, Mulé JJ, Rosenberg SA. Antitumor efficacy of lymphokine-activated killer cells and recombinant interleukin-2 *in vivo*: successful immunotherapy of established pulmonary metastases from weakly immunogenic and nonimmunogenic tumors of three distinct histological types. *Cancer Res* 1986;46:4973–4978.

19. Rosenberg SA. Immunotherapy of cancer by systemic administration of lymphoid cells plus interleukin-2. *Biol Resp Mod* 1984;3:501–511.

20. Rosenberg SA, Lotze MT, Muul LM, et al. Observations on the systemic administration of autologous lymphokine-activated killer cells and recombinant interleukin 2 to patients with metastatic cancer. *N Engl J Med* 1985;313:1485–1492.

21. Rosenberg SA, Lotze MT, Yang JC, et al. Experience with the use of high-dose interleukin-2 in the treatment of 652 cancer patients. *Ann Surg* 1989;210:474–485.

22. Rosenberg SA, Lotze MT, Muul LM, et al. A progress report on the treatment of 157 patients with advanced cancer using lymphokine activated killer cells and interleukin-2 or high-dose interleukin-2 alone. *N Engl J Med* 1987;316:889–905.

23. Rosenberg SA, Lotze MT, Aebersold PM, et al. Prospective randomized trial of high dose interleukin-2 alone or in conjunction with lymphokine-activated killer cells for the treatment of patients with advanced cancers. *J Natl Cancer Inst* 1993;85:622–632.

24. Sznol M, Clark JW, Smith JW, et al. Pilot study of interleukin-2 and lymphokine-activated killer cells combined with immunomodulatory doses of chemotherapy and sequenced with interferon alpha-2A in patients with metastatic melanoma and renal cell carcinoma. *J Natl Cancer Inst* 1992;84:929–937.

25. Clark JW, Smith JW, Steis RG, et al. Interleukin-2 and lymphokine-activated killer cell therapy: analysis of a bolus interleukin-2 and a continuous infusion interleukin 2 regimen. *Cancer Res* 1990;50:7343–7350.

26. Schoof DD, Gramolini BA, Davidson DL, et al. Adoptive immunotherapy of human cancer using low dose recombinant interleukin-2 and lymphokine-activated killer cells. *Cancer Res* 1988;48:5007–5010.

27. Weiss GR, Margolin KA, Aronson FR, et al. A randomized phase II trial of continuous infusion interleukin-2 or bolus injection interleukin-2 plus lymphokine-activated killer cells for advanced renal cell carcinoma. *J Clin Oncol* 1992;10:275–281.

28. Gold PJ, Thompson JA, Markowitz DR, et al. Metastatic renal cell carcinoma: long-term survival after therapy with high-dose continuous-infusion interleukin-2. *Cancer J Sci Am* 1997;3[Suppl l]:S85–S91.

29. Thompson JA, Shulman KL, Benyunes MC, et al. Prolonged continuous intravenous infusion interleukin-2 and lymphokine-activated killer cell therapy for metastatic renal cell carcinoma. *J Clin Oncol* 1992;10:960–980.

30. Margolian KA, Rayner AA, Hawkins MJ, et al. Interleukin-2 and lymphokine-activated killer cell therapy of solid tumors: analysis of toxicity and management guidelines. *J Clin Oncol* 1989;7:489–498.

31. West WH, Tauer KW, Yanneli JR, et al. Multiple cycles of constant infusion recombinant interleukin-2 adoptive cellular therapy of metastatic renal cell carcinoma. *Mol Biother* 1989;1:268–274.

32. Paciucci PA, Holland JF, Gildewell O, et al. Recombinant interleukin-2 by continuous infusion and adoptive transfer of interleukin-2 activated cells in patient with advanced cancer. *J Clin Oncol* 1989;7:869–878.

33. Negrier S, Philip I, Stoter G, et al. Interleukin-2 with or without LAK cells in metastatic renal cell carcinoma: a report of a European multi-center study. *Eur J Cancer Clin Oncol* 1989;23:21–28.

34. Stahl RA, Sculier J, Jost LM, et al. Tolerance and effectiveness of recombinant interleukin-2 (r-met Hu IL-2 (ala 125)) and lymphokine-activated killer cells in patients with metastatic solid tumors. *Eur J Clin Oncol* 1989;25:965–972.

35. Davis SD, Berkmen YM, Wang JCL. Interleukin-2 therapy for advanced renal cell carcinoma: radiographic evaluation of response and complications. *Radiology* 1990;177:127–131.

36. Fujioka I, Nomura K, Hasegawa M, et al. Combination of lymphokine-activated killer cells and interleukin-2 in treating metastatic renal cell carcinoma. *Br J Urol* 1994;73:23–31.

37. Palmer PA, Vinke J, Evers P, et al. Continuous infusion of recombinant interleukin-2 with or without autologous lymphokine-activated killer cells for the treatment of advanced renal cell carcinoma. *Eur J Cancer* 1992;28A:1038–1044.

38. Parkinson DR, Fisher RI, Rayner AA, et al. Therapy of renal cell carcinoma with interleukin-2 and lymphokine-activated killer cells: phase II experience with a hybrid bolus and continuous infusion interleukin-2 regimen. *J Clin Oncol* 1990;8:1630–1636.

39. Foon KA, Waither PJ, Bernstein ZP, et al. Renal cell carcinoma treated with continuous-infusion interleukin-2 with *ex vivo*-activated killer cells. *J Immunother* 1992;11:184–190.

40. Kruit WII, Goey SH, Lamers CH, et al. High-dose regimen of interleukin-2 and interferon-alpha in combination with lymphokine-activated killer cells in patients with metastatic renal cell cancer. *J Immunother* 1997;20:312–320.

41. Tomita Y, Katagiri A, Saito K, et al. Adoptive immunotherapy of patients with metastatic renal cell cancer using lymphokine-activated killer cells, interleukin-2 and cyclophosphamide: long-term results. *Int J Urol* 1998;5:16–21.

42. McCabe M, Stablein D, Hawkins MJ. The Modified Group C experience—phase III randomized trials of IL-2 versus IL-2/LAK in advanced renal cell cancer and advanced melanoma. *Proc Am Soc Oncol* 1991;10:213(abst).

43. Bajorin D, Sell KW, Richards JM, et al. A randomized trial of interleukin-2 plus lymphokine-activated killer cells versus interleukin-2 alone in renal cell carcinoma. *Proc Am Assoc Cancer Res* 1990;31:186(abst).

44. Law TM, Motzer RJ, Mazumdar M, et al. Phase III randomized trial of interleukin-2 with or without lymphokine-activated killer cells in the treatment of patients with advanced renal cell carcinoma. *Cancer* 1995;76:824–832.

45. Gray D, Sprent J. Immunological memory. *Curr Top Microbiol Immunol* 1990;159:1.

46. Cavagnaro J, Osband ME. Successful *in vitro* primary immunization of human peripheral blood mononuclear cells and its role in the development of human-derived monoclonal antibodies. *Biotechniques* 1983;1:30–36.

47. Osband ME, Plummer J. Antigen-specific secondary ex vivo immunization does not require antigen. *Pediatr Res* 1989;45:155a(abst).

48. Sawczuk IS. Auto lymphocyte therapy in the treatment of metastatic renal cell carcinoma. *Urol Clin North Am* 1993;20:297–301.

49. Waymack JP, Guzman RF, Burleson DG, et al. Effect of prostaglandin E in multiple experimental models. *Prostaglandins* 1989;38:345–353.

50. Khan MM, Sansone P, Englemen EG, et al. Pharmacologic effects of autocoids on subsets of T cells: regulation of expression function of histamine-2 receptors by a subset of suppressor cells. *J Clin Invest* 1985;75:1578–1583.

51. Wasserman J, Petrini B, Blomgren H. Radiosensitivity of T lymphocyte subpopulations. *J Clin Lab Immunol* 1982;7:139–140.

52. Carpentino GA, Levine S, Hamiltom D, et al. Successful adoptive immunotherapy of cancer using *ex vivo* immunized autologous lymphocytes and cimetidine. *Surg Forum* 1986;27:418–422.

53. Osband ME, Carpentino GA, Levine SI, et al. Successful adoptive immunotherapy of metastatic renal cell carcinoma with *ex vivo* immunized autologous lymphocytes and cimetidine. *Word J Urol* 1987;4:2173–2177.

54. Krane RJ, Carpinito GA, Ross SD, et al. Treatment of metastatic renal cell carcinoma with autolymphocyte therapy. *Urology* 1990;35:417–422.

55. Osband ME, Lavin PT, Babayan RK, et al. Effect of autolymphocyte therapy on survival and quality of life in patients with metastatic renal cell carcinoma. *Lancet* 1990;335:994–998.

56. Lavin PT, Maar R, Franklin M, et al. Autolymphocyte therapy for metastatic renal cell carcinoma: initial clinical results from 335

patients treated in a multisite clinical practice. *Transplant Proc* 1992;24:3057–3062.

57. Graham S, Babayan RK, Lamm DL, et al. The use of ex vivo activated memory T cells (autolymphocyte therapy) in the treatment of metastatic renal cell carcinoma: final results from a randomized controlled multisite study. *Semin Urol* 1993;11:27–34.

58. Sawczuk IS, Graham SD Jr, Miesowicz F and the ALT Adjuvant Study Group, Cellcor Inc., Newton MA, Emory Clinic, Atlanta GA, and Columbia University, NY, NY. Randomized, controlled trial of adjuvant therapy with ex vivo activated T cells (ALT) in $T_{1.3a,b,c}$ or T_4N+M_0 renal cell carcinoma. *Proc Am Soc Clin Oncol* 1997;16:326a.

59. Sawczuk IS, Arnientrout S, Babayan RK, et al. Adjuvant autolymphocyte therapy in the treatment of $T_{1-3a,b,c}$ or T_4N+M_0 renal cell carcinoma. *J Urol* 1998;159[Suppl]:653(abst).

60. Saidi JA, Newhouse JH, Sawzuk IS. Radiologic follow-up of patients with $T_{1-3a,b,c}$ or T_4N+M_0 renal cell carcinoma after radical nephrectomy. *Urology* 1998;52:1000–1003.

61. Balch CM, Riley LB, Bae YJ, Salermon MA, et al. Patterns of human tumor-infiltrating lymphocytes in 120 cancers. *Arch Surg* 1990;125:200–205.

62. Speiss PJ, Yang JC, Rosenberg SA. *In vivo* antitumor activity of tumor infiltrating lymphocytes expanded in recombinant interleukin-2. *J Natl Cancer Inst* 1987;79:1067–1075.

63. Belldegrun A, Muul LM, Rosenberg SA. Interleukin 2 expanded lymphocytes in human renal cell cancer: isolation, characterization, and antitumor activity. *Cancer Res* 1988;48:206–214.

64. Rosenberg SA, Speiss PJ, Lafreniere R. A new approach to the adoptive immunotherapy of cancer with tumor-infiltrating lymphocytes. *Science* 1986;233:1318–1321.

65. Barth RI, Bock SN, Mulé JJ, et al. Unique murine tumor-associated antigens identified by tumor infiltrating lymphocytes. *J Immunol* 1990;144:1531–1537.

66. Yannelli JR, Hyatt C, McConnell S, et al. Growth of tumor-infiltrating lymphocytes from human solid cancers: summary of a 5-year experience. *Int J Cancer* 1996;65:413–421.

67. Itoh K, Hayakawa K, von Eschenbach AC, Morita T. Natural killer cells in human cell carcinoma. In: Klein EA, Bukowski RM, Finke JH, eds. *Renal cell carcinoma: immunotherapy and cellular biology.* New York: Dekker, 1993:96–97.

68. Finke JH, Rayman P, Alexander J, et al. Characterization of the cytolytic activity of CD4+ and CD8+ tumor-infiltrating lymphocytes in human renal cell carcinoma. *Cancer Res* 1990;50:2263–2370.

69. Morecki S, Topalian SL, Myers WW, et al. Separation and growth of human CD4+ and CD8+ tumor-infiltrating lymphocytes and peripheral blood mononuclear cells by direct positive panning on covalently attached monoclonal antibody-coated flasks. *J Biol Res Mod* 1990;9:463–472.

70. Okada Y, Yahata G, Shoshchi I, et al. A correlation between the expression of CD8 antigen and specific cytotoxicity of tumor-infiltrating lymphocytes. *Jpn J Cancer Res* 1989;80:249–255.

71. Linna TI, Moody DI, Tso CL, et al. Tumor microenvironment and immune effector cells: isolation, large-scale propagation and characterization of CD8+ tumor infiltrating lymphocytes from renal cell carcinomas. In: RH Goldfarb, TL Whiteside, eds. *Tumor immunology and cancer therapy.* New York: Dekker, 1994.

72. Belldegrun A, Pierce WC, Kaboo R, et al. Interferon alpha-primed tumor-infiltrating lymphocytes combined with interleukin-2 and interferon alpha as a therapy for metastatic renal cell carcinoma. *J Urol* 1993;150:1384–1390.

73. Topalian SL, Solomon D, Frederick P, et al. Immunotherapy of patients with advanced cancer using tumor-infiltrating lymphocytes and recombinant interleukin-2: a pilot study. *J Clin Oncol* 1988;6:839–853.

74. Kradin RL, Lazarus DS, Dubinett SM, et al. Tumour-infiltrating lymphocytes and interleukin-2 in treatment of advanced cancer. *Lancet* 1989;1:577–580.

75. Dillman RO, Church C, Oldham RK, et al. A randomized phase II trial of continuous infusion interleukin-2 in 788 patients with cancer. The National Biotherapy Study Group Experience. *Cancer* 1993;71:2358–2370.

76. Bukowski RM, Sharfman W, Murthy S, et al. Clinical results and characterization of tumor-infiltrating lymphocytes with or without recombinant interleukin 2 in human metastatic renal cell carcinoma. *Cancer Res* 1991;51:4199–4206.

77. Olencki I, Finke I, Lorenzi V, et al. Adoptive immunotherapy (AIT) for renal cell carcinoma (RCC) tumor infiltrating lymphocytes (TILs) cultured *in vitro* with rIL-2, rhIL-4, and autologous tumor: a phase II trial. *Proc Am Soc Clin Oncol* 1994;13:244(abst).

78. Figlin RA, Pierce WC, Kaboo R, et al. Treatment of metastatic renal cell carcinoma with nephrectomy, interleukin-2 and cytokine-primed or CD8(+) selected tumor infiltrating lymphocytes from primary tumor. *J Urol* 1997;158:740–745.

79. Goedegebuure PS, Douville LM, Li H, et al. Adoptive immunotherapy with tumor-infiltrating lymphocytes and interleukin-2 in patients with metastatic malignant melanoma and renal cell carcinoma: a pilot study. *J Clin Oncol* 1995;13:1939–1949.

80. Cangiano I, Liao I, Naitoh I, et al. Sarcomatoid renal cell carcinoma: biological behavior, prognosis, and response to combined surgical resection and immunotherapy. *J Clin Oncol* 1999;17:523–528.

81. Oda H, Machinami R. Sarcomatoid renal cell carcinoma: a study of its proliferative activity. *Cancer* 1993;71:2292–2298.

82. Juhasz J, Sebok J, Galambos J, et al. Renal carcinosarcoma (mixed tumors) of the kidney. *Int Urol Nephrol* 1980;122:103–108.

83. Belldegrun A, Pierce W, deKernion J, et al. Clinical activity of purified CD8+ tumor-infiltrating lymphocytes (CD8+TIL) and low dose IL-2 in the treatment of metastatic renal cell carcinoma. *J Urol* 1994;151:315A.

84. Figlin R, Thompson C, Bukowski RM, et al. A multicenter, randomized, phase III trial of CD8+ tumor infiltrating lymphocyte in combination with recombinant interleukin-2 in metastatic renal cell carcinoma. *J Clin Oncol* 1999;17:2521.

85. Figlin R, Gitlitz B, Franklin J, et al. Interleukin-2 based immunotherapy for the treatment of metastatic renal cell carcinoma: an analysis of 203 consecutively treated patients. *Cancer J Sci Am* 1997;3:S92–S97.

86. Walther MM, Alexander RB, Weiss GH, et al. Cytoreductive surgery prior to interleukin-2 based therapy in patients with metastatic renal cell carcinoma. *Urology* 1993;42:250–258.

87. Flanigan RC. Role of surgery in patients with metastatic renal cell carcinoma. *Semin Urol Oncol* 1996;14(4):227–229.

88. Franklin JR, Figlin RA, Rauch J, et al. Cytoreductive surgery in the management of metastatic renal cell carcinoma: the UCLA experience. *Semin Urol Oncol* 1996;14(4):230–236.

89. Ridolfi R, Flamini E, Riccobon A, et al. Adjuvant adoptive immunotherapy with tumour-infiltrating lymphocytes and modulated doses of interleukin-2 in 22 patients with melanoma, colorectal and renal cancer, after radical metastasectomy, and in 12 advanced patients. *Cancer Immunol Immunother* 1998;46:185–193.

90. Naitoh J, Kaplan A, Dorey F, et al. Metastatic renal cell carcinoma with concurrent inferior vena cava invasion: long-term survival following combination therapy using radical nephrectomy, vena cava thrombectomy, and postoperative immunotherapy. *J Urol* 1999;162:46.

91. Neves RJ, Ziacke H. Surgical treatment of renal cell cancer with vena cava extension. *Br J Urol* 1987;59:390–394.

92. Shu S, Chou C, Sakai K. Lymphocytes generated by *in vivo* priming and *in vitro* sensitization demonstrate therapeutic efficacy against a murine tumor that lacks apparent immunogenicity. *J Immunol* 1989;143:740–748.

93. Yoshizawa H, Chang AE, Shu S. Specific adoptive immunotherapy mediated by tumor-draining lymph node cells sequentially activated with anti-CD3 and IL-2. *J Immunol* 1991;147:729–737.

94. Chou T, Bertera S, Chang AE, et al. Adoptive immunotherapy of microscopic and advanced visceral metastases with *in vitro* sensitized lymphoid cells from mice bearing progressive tumors. *J Immunol* 1988;141:1775–1781.

95. Aruga A, Shu S, Chang AE. Tumor-specific granulocyte/macrophage colony-stimulating factor and interferon gamma secretion is associated with *in vivo* therapeutic efficacy of activated tumor-draining lymph node cells. *Cancer Immunol Immunother* 1995;41(5):317–324.

96. Chang AE, Aruga A, Cameron MJ, et al. Adoptive immunotherapy with vaccine-primed lymph node cells secondarily activated with anti-CD3 and IL-2. *J Clin Oncol* 1997;15(2):796–807.

97. Kiertcher S, and Roth M. Human CD 14+ leukocytes acquire the phenotype and function of antigen-presenting dendritic cells when cultured in GM-CSF and IL-4. *J Leukoc Biol* 1996;59:208–218.

98. Enaba K, Metlay JP, Crowley MT, et al. Dendritic cells as antigen presenting cells in vivo. *Int Rev Immunol* 1990;6:197–206.

99. Sallusto F, Cella M, Danieli C, et al. Efficient presentation of soluble antigen by cultured human dendritic cells is maintained by GM-CSF plus IL-4 and down regulated by tumor necrosis factor-alpha. *J Exp Med* 1994;179:1109–1118.

100. Romani N, Gruner S, Brang D. Proliferating dendritic cell progenitors in human blood. *J Exp Med* 1994;180:83–93.

101. Gitlitz B, Roth M, Kiertscher S, et al. *In vivo* generation of dendritic cells by the combination of interleukin-4 and granulocyte macrophage colony stimulating factor in patients with metastatic cancer—a phase 1 trial. *Proc Am Soc Clin Oncol* 1998;17:429a.

102. Hsu FJ, Benike C, Fagnoni F, et al. Vaccination of patients with B-cell lymphoma using autologous antigen-pulsed dendritic cells. *Nat Med* 1996;2(1):52–58.

103. Nestle FO, Alijagic S, Gilliet M, et al. Vaccination of melanoma patients with peptide or tumor lysate-pulsed dendritic cells. *Nat Med* 1998;4(3):328–332.

104. Tjoa BA, Simmons SJ, Bowes VA, et al. Evaluation of phase I/II clinical trials in prostate cancer with dendritic cells and PSMA peptides. *Prostate* 1998;36:39–44.

105. Fields RC, Shimizu K, Mulé JJ. Murine dendritic cells pulsed with whole tumor lysates mediate potent antitumor immune responses *in vitro* and *in vivo. Proc Natl Acad Sci U S A* 1998;95:9482–9487.

106. Gilboa E, Nair SK, Lyerly HK. Immunotherapy of cancer with dendritic-cell-based vaccines. *Cancer Immunol Immunother* 1998;46:82–87.

107. Mulders P, Tso CL, Gitlitz BJ, et al. Presentation of renal tumor antigens by human dendritic cells activates tumor-infiltrating lymphocytes against autologous tumor: implications for live kidney cancer vaccines. *Clin Cancer Res* 1999;5:445–454.

108. Hinkel A, Gitlitz B, Mulders P, et al. Dendritic cells therapy for metastatic renal cell carcinoma—a translational phase 1 clinical trial. *Proc Am Soc Clin Oncol* 1998;17:432a.

109. Rosenberg, SA. The immunotherapy of solid cancers based on cloning the genes encoding tumor-rejection antigens. *Ann Rev Med* 1996;46:481–491.

110. Neumann E, Engelsberg A, Decker J, et al. Heterogeneous expression of the tumor-associated antigens RAGE-I, PRAME, and glycoprotein 75 in human renal cell carcinoma: candidates for T-cell-based immunotherapies? *Cancer Res* 1998;58:4090–4095.

111. Oosterwijk E, de Weijert M, van Bokhoven, et al. Molecular characterization of the renal cell carcinoma-associated antigen G250. *J Cancer Res* 1996;37:A3147.

112. Steffens MG, Boerman OC, Oosterwijk-Wakka JC, et al. Targeting of renal cell carcinoma with iodine-131-labeled chimeric monoclonal antibody G250. *J Clin Oncol* 1997;15:1529–1537.

113. Gansbacher B, Bannerji R, Daniels B, et al. Retroviral vector mediated γ-interferon gene transfer into tumor cells generates potent and long lasting antitumor immunity. *Cancer Res* 1990;50:7820–7825.

114. Golumbek PT, Lazenby AJ, Levitsky HI, et al. Treatment of established renal cell cancer by tumor cells engineered to secrete interleukin-2. *Science* 1991;254:713–716.

115. Tepper RJ, Coffiuian RL, Leder P. An eosinophil dependent mechanism for the antitumor effect of interleukin-2. *Science* 1992;257: 548–551.

116. Restifo NP, Speiss PJ, Karp SE, et al. A nonimmunogenic sarcoma transduced with the cDNA for interferon gamma elicit CD8+ T cells against wild-type tumor: correlation with antigen presentation capability. *J Exp Med* 1992;175:1423–1431.

117. Marincola FM, Ettinghausen S, Cohen PA, et al. Treatment of established lung metastases with tumor infiltrating lymphocytes derived from a poorly immunogenic tumor engineered to secrete human TNF-alpha. *J Immunol* 1994;152:3500–3513.

118. McBride WH, Thacker JD, Comora S, et al. Genetic modification of a murine fibrosarcoma to produce interleukin-7 stimulates host cells infiltration and tumor immunity. *Cancer Res* 1992;52:3931–3937.

119. Chou T, Chang AE, Shu S, et al. Generation of therapeutic T lymphocytes from tumor-bearing mice by *in vitro* sensitization: culture requirements and characterization of immunologic specificity. *J Immunol* 1988;141:1775–1781.

120. Yoshizawa H, Sakai K, Chang AE, et al. Activation by anti-CD3 of tumor draining lymph node cells for specific adoptive immunotherapy. *Cell Immunol* 1991;134:473–479.

121. Geiger JD, Wagner PD, Cameron MJ, et al. Generation of T cells reactive to the poorly immunogenic B16-BL6 melanoma with efficacy in the treatment of spontaneous metastases. *J Immunother* 1993;13:153–165.

122. Wahl WL, Strome SE, Nabel GJ, et al. Generation of therapeutic T lymphocytes after *in vivo* tumor transfection with an allogenic class I major histocompatibility complex gene. *J Immunother* 1995;17:1–11.

123. Krauss JC, Strome SE, Chang AE, et al. Enhancement of immune reactivity in the lymph nodes draining a murine melanoma engineered to elaborate interleukin-4. *J Immunother* 1994;16:77–84.

124. Arca MJ, Krauss JC, Aruga A, et al. Therapeutic efficacy of T cells derived from lymph nodes draining a poorly immunogenic tumor transduced to secrete GM-CSF. *Cancer Gene Ther* 1996;3(1):39–47.

125. Shiloni E, Karp SE, Custer MC, et al. Retroviral transduction of interferon-gamma cDNA into a nonimmunogenic murine fibrosarcoma: generation of T cells in draining lymph nodes capable of treating established parental metastatic tumor. *Cancer Immunol Immunother* 1993;37:286–292.

126. Rosenberg SA, Aebersold P, Cornetta K, et al. Gene transfer into humans—immunotherapy of patients with advanced melanoma, using tumor–infiltrating lymphocytes modified by retroviral gene transudation. *N Engl J Med* 1990;323:570–578.

13.3

CELL TRANSFER THERAPY: CLINICAL APPLICATIONS

Allogeneic Graft-Versus-Leukemia and Antitumor Effects

JOHN BARRETT

Perhaps the only positive outcome after the use of atomic bombs in 1945 was the stimulus given to research aimed at protecting individuals from the lethal effects of ionizing radiation. This research paved the way for bone marrow transplantation (BMT) (1). In 1951, two investigators, Jacobson and Lorenz, independently showed that infusions of hematopoietic tissues could rescue rodents from bone marrow failure induced by radiation. It was subsequently found that transplanted cells from different mouse strains or different species could cause a lethal "secondary" disease, called *graft-versus-host disease* (GVHD). Although details of the immune mechanisms involved were unknown, Barnes and colleagues in Harwell, England, suspected that the GVHD reaction induced by the use of "foreign" (i.e., alloreacting) transplants might also affect malignant cells. In 1956, these investigators were the first to prove the existence of a graft-versus-leukemia (GVL) effect (2). They showed that transplants of hematopoietic cells and splenic lymphocytes into mice delayed death from a transplanted lymphosarcoma. In Paris, Georges Mathé carried out similar experiments and went on to apply the adoptive transfer of alloimmune reactivity as a form of immunotherapy for cancer and leukemia. He used bone marrow transplants and lymphocyte transfusions in attempts to obtain a GVL effect in patients with advanced malignancies with some early but inconclusive successes (3). At that time, it became apparent that the GVHD induced after allogeneic BMT was a highly dangerous complication, requiring prophylactic immunosuppression and intensive treatment of established disease. Because GVL appeared to be inseparably linked to GVHD, its deliberate induction was considered to be impracticable in a clinical setting. This perception changed at the beginning of the 1990s, after the publication by the International Bone Marrow Transplant Registry (IBMTR) of a large analysis that showed that a GVL effect mediated by T lymphocytes was demonstrable in the absence of GVHD (4). Any doubts about the clinical potential of the GVL effect were dispelled by reports from Slavin, working in Israel, and Kolb,

working in Germany, who showed that adoptively transferred donor lymphocytes given to patients relapsing with leukemia after transplant could induce stable remissions, sometimes without any accompanying GVHD (5). The cellular mechanisms mediating GVL responses have become better defined in the 1990s, as a result of animal experimental research and clinical studies. We are beginning to identify the antigens presented by major histocompatibility complex (MHC) molecules on malignant cells that serve as the target of T-cell attack. A natural killer (NK) cell alloresponse to leukemia is also beginning to be defined. With these developments, it is reasonable to anticipate the successful treatment of otherwise refractory malignant diseases, using alloreacting lymphocytes from closely matched healthy donors specifically targeted against the malignant cell. In this chapter, we describe the experimental and clinical basis of the GVL effect, the cellular mechanisms and antigens involved in the GVL response, and clinical results and developments in the application of GVL and graft-versus-tumor (GVT) effects.

IMMUNOLOGY OF THE GRAFT-VERSUS-LEUKEMIA EFFECT

Experimental Evidence for Graft-Versus-Leukemia in Animal Models

Research into the GVL effect progressed rapidly after the introduction of transplantable leukemias, such as the AKR leukemic mouse, and the establishment of cell lines, such as EL4 and L1210 leukemia. Rodent GVL models using these well-defined malignancies have been used to elucidate the major features of the GVL response (6). These experiments have repeatedly shown that allogeneic lymphocytes have a powerful antileukemic effect. This GVL effect is greatest in the presence of strong allogeneic differences and is least, or absent, in syngeneic transplant models. Depending on the experimental conditions, T

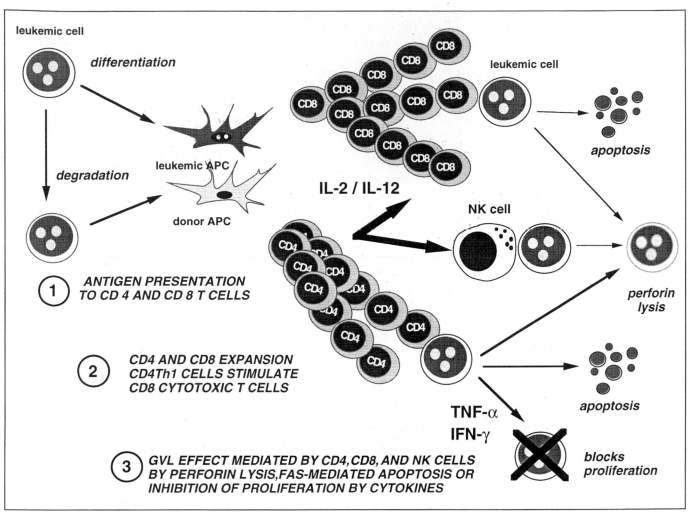

FIGURE 1. Cellular and cytokine mechanisms of the immune response.

lymphocytes and NK cells can be shown to exert GVL reactivity. Experimental leukemias and lymphomas differ widely in their susceptibility to alloimmune attack. Using a mouse AKR leukemia transplant model, Bortin and colleagues (who coined the term *graft-versus-leukemia*) were the first to show that it was possible to generate leukemia-specific T cells capable of inducing GVL without GVHD (7). The ability to separate antihost alloresponses from antileukemic responses varies: Leukemias induced by viruses are good models for leukemia-specific GVL reactions, whereas a rat model of acute myelogenous leukemia showed only GVHD-induced GVL activity (8,9). The role of cytokines, such as interleukin-2 (IL-2) in GVL and GVHD reactions, has been extensively studied in murine transplant models (10). The effect is schedule-dependent, inducing tolerance and GVL. Studies have focused on the role of T-cell subsets in GVL and GVHD reactions and on methods to separate the two by delayed T-cell add-back, induction of specific tolerance, use of specific lymphocyte subsets and leukemia-specific T-cell clones. Two techniques have further increased the potential of animal models for the study of GVL. First, gene knockout mice have given insight into the cytokines and surface molecules critical for the alloresponse (11). Second, the severe combined

immunodeficiency disease nonobese diabetic mouse strain accepts transplanted human malignancies and malignant cell lines and allows the *in vivo* expansion of human lymphocytes. Immunodeficient mice can therefore be used to develop *in vivo* immunotherapy models of human malignancies (12).

Cellular and Cytokine Basis of the Graft-Versus-Leukemia Response

The mechanisms involved in the generation of the alloresponse after bone marrow stem-cell transplantation form the basis for understanding GVL. The process, traced from the initiation of the alloresponse through a phase of clonal expansion to the effector phase, involves interactions between many cell types and the cytokines they produce (13) (Fig. 1).

Initiation of the Alloresponse

The allogeneic T-cell response involves the interaction between class I and class II MHC on antigen-presenting cells with CD8+ and CD4+ lymphocytes, respectively. MHC molecules interact with the CD3 and CD4/8 molecules on the T cell and present their antigens to the T-cell receptor. The antigens seen by T cells are peptides brought to the cell surface bound to MHC molecules. Just as antigens interact with their specific antibody, these peptide antigens interact with specific T cells bearing a specific matching configuration of the hypervariable CDR3 region of their T-cell receptor. Antigens can be presented by many cell types, including leukemia cells and donor and host antigen-presenting cells. Some myelogenous leukemias can differentiate into functional dendritic cells and monocyte macrophages to become competent antigen-presenting cells. Furthermore, donor macrophages and dendritic cells can present leukemia antigens derived from engulfed or disintegrating leukemia cells.

Clonal Expansion Phase

After antigen recognition, T-cell activation is required for the continuation of the immune response. The activation of the costimulatory molecules CD28 and CTLA4 on the T cell by B7.1 and B7.2 (CD80 and CD86) molecules on the stimulator cell governs whether the T cell undergoes clonal expansion or, in the absence of a signal, becomes anergic. Interaction of $CD4^+$ cells with dendritic cells activates CD40 and provides the signal for $CD8^+$ activation, whereas IL-2 and IL-12 production by $CD4^+$ cells provides the proliferative stimulus to $CD8^+$ cells and NK cells. The process of clonal expansion to alloantigens can be rapid; acute GVHD occurs within 7 to 10 days of the transplant. In contrast, the GVL process is slower: After donor lymphocyte transfusion (DLT), months may pass before an antileukemic response is seen. This may represent the time taken to expand an effector population from a low frequency of T-cell precursors.

Effector Phase

Three mechanisms appear to be responsible for the GVL effect:

1. Direct killing of leukemia cells by perforin and granzyme attack from cytotoxic lymphocytes ($CD4^+$, $CD8^+$, and NK cells)
2. Apoptotic death through the fas/fas ligand pathway ($CD4^+$ and $CD8^+$ T cells)
3. Cytokine-mediated leukemia cell death or control of proliferation ($CD4^+$ and $CD8^+$ cells)

Leukemia-reactive T-cell clones derived from healthy donors responding to HLA-identical or closely identical leukemia cells have been used to study GVL mechanisms. Leukemia-specific T cells inhibit the clonal growth of leukemic progenitors in colony-inhibition assays and induce apoptosis in leukemia cells expressing fas through fas/fas-ligand interaction. T cells can inhibit leukemic proliferation by producing interferon-γ (IFN-γ) and tumor necrosis factor-α.

Lymphocyte Subsets and Graft-Versus-Leukemia

The GVL response involves many effector cell types. After allogeneic BMT or DLT, an early rise in activated T cells and NK cells occurs and the frequency of leukemia-reactive cytotoxic T

lymphocyte precursors increases (14,15). A general association exists between prolonged remission and full recovery of $CD4^+$ and NK cells (16). It is now clear that NK cells are capable of powerful but poorly characterized alloresponses to leukemia through recognition of foreign MHC molecules on the leukemia target (17). The relative contribution of $CD4^+$ and $CD8^+$ T cells to GVL has been studied in animal models and in humans. Mice receiving CD8-depleted marrow or marrow with addition of purified $CD4^+$ T cells had a low incidence of GVHD with high leukemia-free survival, supporting a role for $CD4^+$ cells in GVL. In other murine models, however, the addition of purified $CD8^+$ T cells to the graft had an antitumor effect and facilitated engraftment without inducing GVHD (13). We can conclude that $CD4^+$ and $CD8^+$ T-cell subsets contribute to GVL reactions. The dominant mechanism, however, is strain specific and varies with the degree of donor-recipient histocompatibility and the type of leukemia. In humans, $CD4^+$ and $CD8^+$ alloreactive cells with antileukemia activity have been generated *in vitro*.

Susceptibility of Leukemia to Graft-Versus-Leukemia

To be immunogenic, leukemia cells must express critical surface molecules that render them susceptible to attack from donor lymphocytes. To be killed, they must be susceptible to apoptosis, induction, or lysis by perforin-granzyme systems of NK cells or T lymphocytes. To elicit T-lymphocyte responses, leukemia cells must express MHC class I or class II adhesion molecules, such as ICAM-1, and costimulatory molecules, such as CD80 and CD81 (13). Donor T cells recognize small peptide antigens presented by the leukemia cell through MHC class I and class II molecules. We can define three functional categories of antigens: ubiquitous, tissue-specific, and leukemia-specific (Table 1). The first two categories comprise the minor histocompatibility antigen (mHA) system (18). Although only a handful have so far been characterized, hundreds of mHA are believed to exist. They are allelic peptide sequences of numerous polymorphic proteins scattered throughout the genome. From analysis of natural pep-

TABLE 1. ANTIGENS INDUCING T-CELL–MEDIATED GRAFT-VERSUS-LEUKEMIA RESPONSES

Minor histocompatibility antigens (mHA)
  Ubiquitously distributed
    HA-3, HA-4, HA-5, HA-6, HA-7
    Y chromosome–derived proteins
  Restricted to hematopoietic tissue
    HA-1, HA-2, HB-1
    Some Y chromosome–derived proteins
Normal but aberrantly expresses proteins restricted to hematopoietic tissue
    PR-1 (proteinase-3), alleles of proteinase-2
    PRAME
Leukemia-specific proteins
    Fusion proteins from chromosomal translocation
    (e.g., BCR-ABL, PML-RARA)
    Single point or frame-shift mutations of oncogenes
    (e.g., p53, RAS)

BCR-ABL, B-cell reactivity–antigen-binding lymphocyte.

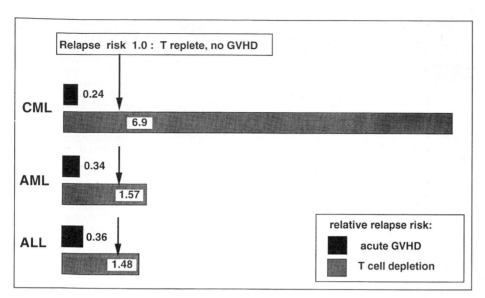

FIGURE 2. The graft-versus-leukemia effect in chronic myelogenous leukemia (CML), acute myelogenous leukemia (AML), and acute lymphoblastic leukemia (ALL). The bars indicate the relative relapse risk for each disease compared with the relapse rate of a T-cell–replete transplant not developing acute or chronic graft-versus-host disease. The figure illustrates the different impact of T-cell depletion in each disease (greatest in CML) and the powerful antileukemic effect of acute graft-versus-host disease. (Data adapted from Horowitz MM, Gale RP, Sondel PM, et al. Graft-versus-leukemia reactions after bone marrow transplantation. *Blood* 1990;75:555–562.)

tides present in MHC molecules, it appears that self peptides can be derived from all parts of the cell. Ubiquitous antigens are those that are widely distributed in recipient tissues, such as the gut, skin, liver, and marrow cells. Alloresponses against these antigens are thought to induce a nonspecific response, causing GVHD in addition to any GVL effect. In contrast, tissue-restricted antigens are derived from proteins with a limited tissue distribution (19). Three hematopoietic tissue-restricted mHA are known: HA-1, HA-2 (on lymphoid and myeloid cells), and HB-1 (on B lymphocytes) (20). These mHA are of particular interest because T-cell clones specific for these antigens should induce GVL responses without causing GVHD. The identification of tissue-restricted antigens is an active area of research because of their potential to initiate specific GVL responses.

The third category of leukemia antigens are those that are truly leukemia specific (21). These are antigens unique to the leukemia because they are derived from leukemia-specific chromosomal translocations and point and frame-shift mutations and deletions. Peptide sequences from the area of mutation or fusion region of translocations could function as neoantigens. Several translocations and mutations have been extensively studied, notably the BCR-ABL transcript from chronic myelogenous leukemia (CML) and mutations of the p53 gene in many myeloid malignancies. Despite almost a decade of research using fusion peptide sequences representing the recombined region of the gene, no definitive evidence exists proving fusion proteins or mutated genes induce GVL in stem-cell transplant recipients. From what is already known about tumor-specific antigens, overexpressed or aberrantly expressed normal tissue-restricted proteins (e.g., MAGE, MART, and tyrosinase in melanomas) represent a more likely category of potent leukemia-specific antigens. Peptides from these proteins induce autologous and allogeneic cytotoxic T-cell responses against the tumor. It is clear that similar overexpressed proteins occur in marrow-derived cells. PRAME, an antigen expressed by several solid tumors, is also expressed in some hematologic malignancies (22). Primary granule proteins, such as proteinase-3, overexpressed in many myeloid leukemias and in myelodysplastic syndrome, are the source of powerful leukemia-

specific antigens. Cytotoxic T cells recognizing proteinase 3 peptides that show cytotoxicity specifically to leukemia cells and their progenitors but not to normal marrow cells can readily be produced *in vitro* from healthy individuals (23).

Nevertheless, despite great progress in the identification of target antigens on leukemia cells, it should be emphasized that no direct evidence exists that any of the antigens thus far described are instrumental in causing GVL responses after allogeneic stem-cell transplantation.

GRAFT-VERSUS-LEUKEMIA IN CLINICAL PRACTICE

Therapeutic Potential of the Graft-Versus-Leukemia Response

An analysis by the IBMTR of 2,030 HLA-identical sibling transplant recipients demonstrated two clinical characteristics of the GVL effect (4): (a) GVL was greatest in CML, less in acute myeloid leukemia, and least in ALL; and (b) the relapse rate after T-cell depletion was significantly greater than that observed in a comparable patient group who received non–T-cell–depleted transplants and did not develop acute GVHD (Fig. 2). A further study from the IBMTR showed that relapse rates are higher in transplants between identical twin transplants compared with HLA-identical sibling transplants (24). These observations provide indisputable evidence for a GVL effect mediated by allogeneic, but not syngeneic, BMTs and implicate T lymphocytes in the mechanism. These studies were the first to quantitate the strength of the GVL response. Further evidence of the power of the GVL effect of allogeneic lymphocytes comes from widely confirmed observations by Slavin et al. (25) and Kolb et al. (26) that DLTs given after allogeneic BMT induce permanent remissions in patients whose leukemia relapses after allogeneic BMT. This finding is all the more striking because it implies that donor lymphocytes alone in these circumstances can be more effective at eradicating leukemia than the original transplant involving myeloablative chemoradiotherapy and a T-

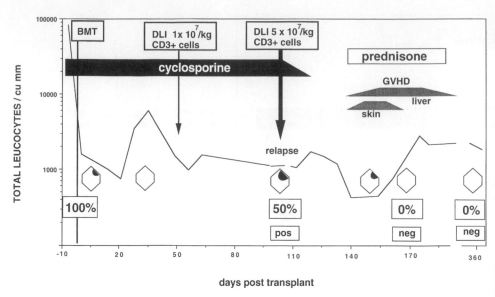

FIGURE 3. Hematologic course after allogenic bone marrow transplantation for chronic phase chronic myelogenous leukemia in a 24-year-old woman. After a T-cell–depleted stem-cell transplant from an HLA-identical sibling and a planned delayed add-back of 1×10^7 per kg of CD3 donor lymphocytes, she entered hematologic remission. On day 100, however, the spleen was enlarged. The bone marrow appearance suggested chronic myelogenous leukemia, and karyotyping showed 50% Ph+ metaphases. She was treated by withdrawal of cyclosporine and a further donor lymphocyte transfusion (DLT) of 5×10^7 CD3+ cells per kg. Within 4 weeks, hematologic recovery occurred, the spleen returned to normal size, and she became Ph+ chromosome negative and negative for the B-cell receptor–antigen-binding lymphocyte marker by RT-PCR. At the same time, she developed skin and liver graft-versus-host disease (GVHD), which was successfully treated with prednisone. She remains in complete molecular remission 1 year posttransplant.

cell–replete marrow transplant. It therefore appears that a major component of the curative potential of the allogeneic transplant is the establishment of a donor immune system that permits the survival of transfused alloreacting lymphocytes from the same donor, exerting a GVL effect. Figure 3 illustrates a complete remission of CML persisting after allogeneic BMT after transfusion of donor lymphocytes.

The realization that the GVL effect can be powerful is beginning to bring about a fundamental change in transplant strategy. First, the old perception that immunotherapy with lymphocytes can be successful only in eradicating malignancy at the level of minimal residual disease has been overturned by the observation that, after BMT, full hematologic relapse of leukemia can respond completely to DLT. Secondly, new transplant approaches are emerging based on the idea that in malignancies in remission or with slow progression, it may be possible to rely exclusively on the GVL effect to achieve disease control and subsequent cure. This is the basis for nonmyeloablative stem-cell transplants (27). Patients receive an immunosuppressive, but not myeloablative, preparative regimen (usually a combination of an alkylating agent and fludarabine or low-dose radiation), followed by a lymphocyte-rich peripheral blood stem-cell transplant and short posttransplant immunosuppression. After such low-intensity preparative regimens, the malignancy initially persists. Approximately 2 to 3 months posttransplant, regression of disease coincides with donor immune recovery. Experience with this type of stem-cell allograft is still limited, but it is already clear that the approach holds promise for cure of otherwise untreatable lymphoid and myeloid malignancies and, possibly, solid tumors.

Factors Determining the Strength of the Graft-Versus-Leukemia Effect

Type of Malignancy

GVL effects are being demonstrated in a variety of hematologic malignancies. Table 2 lists the conditions where clinical evidence exists for a GVL effect. Two methods exist for measuring the

strength of GVL effects from clinical data: comparisons of relapse rates between allogeneic transplants and syngeneic transplants (where no GVL effect is seen) and analysis of remission rate and duration after DLT to treat leukemia relapsing after BMT. Several factors govern susceptibility of leukemia to GVL effects:

1. Disease progression—Early relapse is more favorable than later relapse or relapse of progressing leukemia. Thus, CML in molecular or cytogenetic relapse is more likely to respond than relapse into hematologic chronic phase. Relapse in accelerated or blast phase is the least likely to respond.

2. Leukemia type—Myeloid leukemias are more susceptible to GVL effects than acute lymphoblastic leukemia after BMT and DLT.

3. Pace of disease—Reports of responses of relapsed myeloma to DLT suggest that, together with CML, myeloma is susceptible to GVL effects because of a slower pace of proliferation and progression than the acute leukemias.

TABLE 2. MALIGNANCIES WITH CLINICAL EVIDENCE OF A GRAFT-VERSUS-LEUKEMIA EFFECT

Hematologic malignancies
  Myeloid malignancies
    Chronic myelogenous leukemia
     Chronic phase >accelerated phase >blast phase
    Acute myelogenous leukemia
    Myelodysplastic syndrome
    Myeloproliferative disorders
  Lymphoid malignancies
    Acute lymphoblastic leukemia
    Chronic lymphocytic leukemia
    Prolymphocytic leukemia
    Non-Hodgkin's lymphomas, including mantle cell lymphoma
    Multiple myeloma
Nonhematologic malignancies
  Breast cancer
  Renal cell cancer

Graft-Versus-Host Disease

Numerous clinical observations have linked regression of leukemia with the onset of acute or chronic GVHD. The Seattle marrow transplant group were the first to study a large enough leukemia transplant series to show that leukemic relapse was significantly reduced in patients who developed acute or chronic GVHD (28). An IBMTR study came to similar conclusions: The relative risk of relapse in recipients developing acute or chronic GVHD was significantly reduced, and the combination of grade II or greater acute GVHD with any degree of chronic GVHD conferred the greatest protection against relapse in all leukemia types studied (4). A similar correlation of GVHD with leukemic relapse has been shown in patients given DLT to treat leukemia relapsing after BMT. In CML patients, the chance of achieving a further remission developing acute GVHD was 80% compared with 40% for those who did not (26).

Minor Histocompatibility Antigen Differences

The importance of mHA differences in exerting GVL effects can be studied by comparing outcome of HLA-identical sibling BMT in genetically homogeneous and genetically diverse populations. In this situation, patient and donor are genotypically matched at the MHC loci, but the genetically homogeneous group should have a lower diversity of the mHA gene repertoire. The effect of mHA disparity on GVL was studied in comparable CML patients transplanted with HLA-identical siblings in Japan (genetically homogeneous) and the United Kingdom (genetically diverse) (29). The U.K. BMT recipients had twice as much acute GVHD (50% vs. 25%) and became polymerase chain reaction negative for the BCR-ABL transcript more rapidly than comparable Japanese patients. The overall relapse rate, however, was low (10% vs. 12%) and comparable in the two groups.

Major Histocompatibility Antigen Differences

Comparison of relapse rates between HLA-identical siblings and haploidentical family transplants should define the contribution of MHC-antigen differences to the GVL effect. The preparative regimens and GVHD prophylaxis used, however, differ widely between HLA-matched and HLA-mismatched transplants. No comparative data exist to determine whether the degree of MHC disparity modulates the GVL effect.

HLA-Identical Unrelated Transplants

The GVL potential of HLA-identical unrelated donor transplants should be greater than that of HLA-identical sibling transplants because of a greater mHA disparity in the unrelated transplants, as well as differences in nonclassical MHC antigens and cryptic variations in DNA sequences of HLA molecules apparently identical by serotyping. The assumption that relapse rates after unrelated donor BMT are lower than comparable transplants from HLA-identical sibling donors remains unconfirmed. Comparisons are complicated by the greater degree of immunosuppression given to unrelated transplant recipients. Nevertheless, one report of T-cell depleted unrelated BMT for leukemia suggests that the effect on GVL of histocompatibility differences outweighs the deleterious effect of T-cell depletion on relapse (30). A comparison of unrelated versus related donor DLT to treat relapse of CML showed a more rapid disappearance of residual disease but a similar overall response rate with the unrelated donor transplants, indicating that the GVL effect in unrelated donor BMT may be more rapid but has comparable strength to identical sibling BMT (31).

Immunosuppression

As indicated previously, GVHD is a two-edged sword that, while protecting against leukemic relapse, confers a high mortality. Inevitably, therefore, patients developing GVHD are given immunosuppression with steroids alone or in combination with other immunosuppressive agents. Furthermore, to prevent GVHD, patients receive cyclosporine, FK506, or mycophenolate mofetil, often in association with methotrexate, steroids, or ATG. Such powerful immunosuppressive regimens clearly impact on the ability of the transplanted donor immune system to recognize and respond to residual malignant disease in the BMT recipient. Good evidence exists that cyclosporine is permissive for leukemic relapse. Numerous observations link the disappearance of residual disease or the reversal of incipient relapse with the withdrawal of cyclosporine immunosuppression (32,33). The leukemic regression may occur without development of GVHD. Steroid treatment has not been clearly linked with relapse and the routine use of steroids to treat clinically significant GVHD does not seem to abrogate the powerful GVL effect associated with this complication.

Source of Transplanted Stem Cells

Allogeneic peripheral blood progenitor cells (PBPCs) and cord blood (CB) stem-cell transplants are increasingly used in leukemia treatment. PBPC transplants contain approximately tenfold more lymphocytes and at least as many stem cells as a BMT. PBPC transplants have similar rates of acute GVHD, but probably confer a greater risk of chronic GVHD. It has therefore been of interest to look for differences in leukemic relapse rates in bone marrow and PBPC transplants. Several uncontrolled comparative studies suggest that PBPC transplants confer a better GVL effect than BMT, but these results have not yet been confirmed in a large prospective trial (34). Even less experience exists in the use of CB transplants in leukemia; however, *in vitro* evidence exists suggesting that lymphocytes from CB have greater GVL reactivity than lymphocytes from older donors. Because few CB transplants have so far been carried out, it is not clear to what degree this stem-cell source differs in its GVL potential from BMT and PBPC transplant. Sustained remissions of CB transplants in high-risk leukemias do, however, suggest the presence of a strong GVL effect (35).

Stem-Cell Dose

Differences in the GVL potential of stem cells from different sources could be explained by differences in the quality or quantity of lymphocytes contained in the transplant. Evidence also exists that the stem-cell dose itself affects relapse. Animal and clinical studies have shown a powerful effect of high CD34⁺ cell doses, conferring resistance to leukemic relapse (36). Even patients at high risk have significantly lower relapse rates if given more than 3×10^6 CD34 cells per kg. The mechanism is independent of a GVL effect from transplanted lymphocytes. The protective effect against relapse is unknown.

Preparative Regimens, Chimerism, and Tolerance

The degree to which the donor T lymphocytes engraft depends in part on the efficiency of the preparative regimen to immunosuppress the recipient's immunity and in part on the number and alloreactivity of the lymphocytes given in the transplant. Consequently, poorly immunosuppressive preparative regimens and T-cell–depleted transplants predispose to a state of mixed chimerism in which donor and recipient lymphocytes coexist after transplant. Prolonged mixed chimerism is strongly associated with an increased rate of leukemic relapse (37,38). One reason that T-cell–depleted transplants incur a higher rate of relapse is that they predispose to mixed chimerism and a state of tolerance between donor and recipient, which abrogates the GVL effect.

T-Cell Depletion and Lymphocyte Add-Back

Although T-cell–depleted transplants increase the risk of relapse, the effect can be overcome by transfusing donor lymphocytes at the first sign of leukemic relapse or in a prophylactic approach to prevent relapse. Both strategies are effective. In CML, where residual disease can be easily monitored using a polymerase chain reaction technique to measure the BCR-ABL transcript, DLT reverses incipient relapse in more than 80% of cases (39). In another study, a scheduled DLT on days 45 and 100 after transplant successfully prevented leukemic relapse in 85% of transplanted CML patients (40). The method used to deplete the transplant of T cells also has an impact on relapse. Nonspecific techniques that remove NK cells and T cells indiscriminately have a greater risk of provoking relapse than more selective T-cell depletion (41). Depletion of CD8 cells alone, at least in CML transplants, results in strong protection against relapse with little GVHD (42).

Cytokines

Several investigators have used IL-2 to boost the antileukemic response in patients relapsing after transplant. Anecdotal evidence exists that IL-2 enhances GVL responses and, when given in conjunction with DLT, can induce remission in leukemias relapsing after transplant. IFN-α has been used with and without DLT to treat CML relapsing after BMT with some success, but it is not clear whether the regression of the leukemia is a result of an antiproliferative effect of IFN or an enhancement of the GVL response. A better understanding of the mechanisms whereby cytokines can alter the immunogenicity of the leukemia and the donor's immune response may permit the intelligent use of cytokine combinations to treat and prevent relapse (43).

Graft-Versus-Leukemia and Leukemic Relapse after Bone Marrow Transplantation

Mechanisms of Relapse

Case reports in which leukemic relapse after BMT was reversed by stopping immunosuppression support the idea that residual leukemia is often under the control of a competent donor immune system. In other instances in which relapse follows rapidly after transplant, it is more likely that leukemic cytoreduction from the preparative regimen was inadequate and that residual leukemia outstripped the developing GVL response. A third possibility is that leukemic relapse after BMT represents a form of immune escape. Data supporting this possibility comes from a paired study of leukemia samples obtained before marrow transplant and at relapse posttransplant (44). Many of the relapsed leukemias showed alterations in surface phenotype, including downregulation of MHC class I and II antigens associated with a decreased ability to stimulate allogeneic proliferative T-cell responses and decreased susceptibility to lysis by cytotoxic T lymphocytes or NK cells. These findings, coupled with evidence of clonal progression in relapsed leukemias, suggested that the allograft selected leukemia subclones that were resistant to the GVL effect.

Treatment of Relapse with Donor Lymphocyte Transfusions

It is well established that DLT can induce remission in leukemia relapsing after BMT. Two large DLT series from Europe and North America have been reported (26,45). Both groups found that patients with CML in cytogenetic relapse or CML relapsing into chronic phase had the best response to DLT with complete cytogenetic remission rates of 84% and 76% for the European and American cohorts, respectively. These responses were not only complete at the cytogenetic level, but were also complete by molecular criteria because nearly all patients studied were negative for BCR-ABL messenger RNA by sensitive two-step polymerase chain reaction techniques. The majority of remissions were stable with second relapse rates of only 6% to 12%. The results for transformed-phase CML, however, were considerably worse in both series, with complete response rates of only 13% (European group) and 28% (American group). The time to cytogenetic remission after DLT is usually 3 to 4 months, but it may be longer. The delay between infusion of donor lymphocytes and hematologic response presumably reflects the period required for the activation and expansion of the GVL effector cells. More rapid responses occur when DLT is given for Epstein-Barr virus (EBV) lymphoproliferative disorders (46). This is presumed to be related to the high precursor frequency of EBV-specific cytotoxic T lymphocytes present in the donor.

In acute leukemias, the contribution of DLT to remission induction is unclear because many patients receive DLT and chemotherapy. Whatever approach is used, acute myeloid leukemia and myelodysplastic syndromes respond poorly to DLT. In the European and North American series, only 15% and 29% of patients given DLT achieved remissions, which were often short lived. Only a few patients have received DLT for myelodysplastic syndrome, but only approximately 20% of patients respond. Individual case reports of successful therapy with DLT in acute lymphoblastic leukemia (ALL) exist, including the high-risk subtype Ph$^+$ ALL. Overall, results of DLT in relapsed ALL are poor, with response rates of 3% to 18%. Donor lymphocytes also mediate an antitumor effect in chronic lymphoid disorders. Hematologic responses coinciding with the onset of GVHD have been observed in patients with persistent chronic lymphoid leukemia, prolymphocytic leukemia, and non-Hodgkin's lymphoma (47,48). A graft-versus-myeloma effect was demonstrated in three patients with progressive myeloma treated with DLT after T-cell–depleted transplants (49,50). Complete remission coincided with the development of GVHD. Responses are also reported in mantle cell lymphoma, as well as dramatic regressions of EBV lymphoproliferative disease. DLT, however, has little efficacy in non-Hodgkin's lymphoma and Hodgkin's disease. The antileukemic effect of DLT may be enhanced by cytokines and growth factors. IFN-α may increase the rate of hematologic remission in CML; IL-2 and granulocyte-macrophage colony-stimulating factor may improve responses in ALL and acute myeloid leukemia relapse, respectively. The T-lymphocyte dose also determines the response rate. For CML relapse, approximately 10^7 CD3$^+$ cells per kg are needed to achieve remissions (39).

Separating Graft-Versus-Leukemia and Graft-Versus-Host Disease

Allogeneic stem-cell transplants require some method of preventing GVHD. Both T-cell depletion and posttransplant immunosuppression, however, are nonselective, diminishing GVL as much as GVHD reactions. To optimize the GVL effect, techniques that selectively reduce GVHD while conserving or enhancing GVHD are needed. Several approaches are being explored.

Delayed T-Cell Add-Back

In animal experiments, T-cell depletion followed by delayed add-back of immune-competent donor cells confers GVL with only a low incidence of acute GVHD. Clinical studies confirm experimental predictions: Although DLTs used to treat leukemia relapsing after BMT can cause GVHD, approximately 25% of patients with CML achieve a remission without clinical GVHD. In HLA-matched sibling BMT for CML, T-cell depletion followed by cyclosporine treatment and graded add-back of donor T cells from as early as day 30 confers protection from relapse with a low incidence of severe acute GVHD (40). Smaller T-cell doses given after 100 days from BMT without cyclosporine cover also achieve a GVL effect with a low risk from GVHD (51).

T-Cell Subset Depletion

Some promising results of selective CD8 depletion of donor marrow have been reported in transplants for CML. In clinical trials in CML using CD8-depleted marrow transplants, the presence of CD4 cells alone prevented relapse after BMT. In one report, CD8-depleted DLT were also effective in treating CML relapsing after BMT with 60% complete remission and only a 20% incidence of clinically significant GVHD (42). Although this technique has produced some favorable results in CML patients, it is possible that other hematologic malignancies require CD4 and CD8 T cells for the GVL effect. Because CD4$^+$ and CD8$^+$ subsets are involved in GVHD and GVL reactions, selective T-cell subset depletion does not appear likely to completely separate GVL from GVHD.

Thymidine Kinase "Suicide Genes"

In this approach, T cells marked with a "suicide gene" (viral thymidine kinase) that renders the cells susceptible to elimination by ganciclovir are given to the recipient to induce a GVL effect (52). At the onset of a serious GVHD reaction, the alloreacting T cells can be eliminated by administering ganciclovir to the recipient. Although this strategy appears attractive, it remains to be seen whether GVL responses can be effective in the brief window between the infusion of gene-marked T cells and their removal at the onset of the GVHD reaction.

Selective Depletion of Alloreacting Donor T Cells

Selective depletion of alloreacting donor T cells involves the *in vitro* stimulation of donor T cells with nonleukemic cells from the recipient (usually lymphocytes). Responding donor cells are eliminated by the addition of antibodies to CD25 activation markers coupled to toxins or immunomagnetic beads. Remaining cells conserve reactivity to recipient leukemia, EBV-transformed B cells, and third-party stimulators. Clinical trials with this selective immunodepletion are under way (53).

Generating Leukemia-Specific T Cells

It is technically possible to generate leukemia-specific donor T-cell clones in many, but not all, HLA-matched donor-recipient pairs. One group of investigators in Leiden, Netherlands, have successfully generated sufficiently large numbers of leukemia-specific donor-derived T-cell lines by expanding them *in vitro* using the patient's leukemia cells as stimulators. They have successfully used these T-cell lines to induce permanent remission in patients relapsing with CML after BMT. Although this is clear proof of principle, better and more reliable techniques for selecting and expanding leukemia-specific T cells are needed before this approach can have general application (54).

Graft-Versus-Tumor Effects

By extension, it can be hypothesized that an allogeneic GVT response analogous to the GVL effect could be used to treat solid tumors. Evidence supporting the possibility of an allogeneic GVT effect is summarized in Table 3. Malignancies arising in skin, the gastrointestinal tract, and biliary tree, which are targets of the GVHD response, might be similarly susceptible to immune damage from donor immune cells. Conversely, tissues uninvolved in GVHD reactions (e.g., muscles and the nervous system) may, by the same argument, be immune to GVT effects. A useful

TABLE 3. ARGUMENTS FOR AND AGAINST A GRAFT-VERSUS-TUMOR EFFECT

Arguments in favor of a graft-versus-tumor effect:

Tumors arising in tissues that are targets of cytotoxic damage in graft-versus-host disease could also be susceptible to immune-mediated apoptosis.

Tumors possessing major histocompatibility class I and class II, ICAM-1, B7.1, and fas should be targets of T-cell attack.

Evidence exists of autologous antitumor immune responses in some malignancies. Alloresponses are likely to be at least as powerful.

Alloreacting T cells can recognize a wide range of antigens on the recipient's malignant cells (e.g., minor histocompatibility antigens, alleles of tissue-specific antigens).

Clinical graft-versus-malignancy effects are being demonstrated in a widening range of diseases (e.g., leukemias, lymphomas, myeloma, and some solid tumors).

Arguments against a graft-versus-tumor effect:

Tumors arising in tissues not involved in graft-versus-host disease are less likely to be suitable targets of alloreacting T cells.

Tumors are notoriously adapted to escape from immune control.

Posttransplant immune deficiency may favor tumor progression.

Graft-versus-tumor effects may be abrogated after the establishment of tolerance posttransplant.

Large tumor masses may limit complete infiltration by tumor-infiltrating lymphocytes.

Delayed second malignancies develop after bone marrow transplants.

ICAM-1, intracellular adhesion molecule-1.

approach to identifying susceptible tumors would be the demonstration that allogeneic cytotoxic T lymphocytes or NK cells and lymphokine-activated killer cells are cytotoxic to the tumor cells. The tumor characteristics required for a GVT response would include slow proliferation (matching the relatively slow pace of the T-cell response) and surface expression of MHC class I and II, costimulatory molecules (CD80, CD86) and adhesion molecules, such as the ICAM molecules and fas. Many malignancies possess some or all of these characteristics. It should also be noted, however, that many solid tumors have developed mechanisms to escape immune-mediated killing. Locus or allele-specific downregulation of MHC molecules is a common mechanism used by tumor cells to escape T-cell attack. In addition, aberrations in the number of MHC molecules on the surface of melanomas affect their susceptibility to lysis by cytotoxic T lymphocytes. Solid tumors may escape host immune surveillance by upregulating fas-ligand expression, leading to direct cytotoxicity of those lymphocytes that may have targeted the tumor.

Malignant melanoma and renal cell carcinoma deserve special consideration. The occurrence of autologous T cells that recognize and kill the tumor in these malignancies strongly supports the possibility of a therapeutic effect from a T-cell allograft.

Stem-Cell Transplants for Solid Tumors in Humans

The clinical experience of stem-cell allografts in solid tumors is limited and, at best, anecdotal. At this stage, proof that clini-

cally measurable GVT effects occur is scanty. Inevitably, in these experimental techniques, patients with advanced disease with no other conventional treatment options have been selected for treatment. The following accounts provide the first proof of principle that allogeneic GVT effects may have a place in the treatment of cancer.

Breast Cancer

To evaluate the feasibility of allogeneic PBPC transplantation and to assess GVT effects in patients with metastatic breast cancer, investigators at the M. D. Anderson Cancer Center evaluated allogeneic PBPC transplantation in ten women (median age, 42 years) with metastatic breast cancer involving the liver or bone marrow. The patients were prepared with a myeloablative regimen of cyclophosphamide, carmustine, and thiotepa. GVHD prophylaxis was achieved with cyclosporine or tacrolimus. All patients engrafted with full hematologic recovery. Three patients developed grade II acute GVHD, and four patients had chronic GVHD. After transplantation, one patient was in complete remission, five patients achieved a partial remission, and four patients had stable disease. In two patients, metastatic liver lesions regressed in association with skin GVHD after withdrawal of immunosuppression. The regression of tumor associated with GVHD suggests a GVT effect. Because of the slow progression of some patients with metastatic breast cancer, however, longer follow-up and larger studies are required to fully evaluate a beneficial effect of PBPC allografts in this disease (55). A further case report of a regression of breast cancer metastases coincident with acute GVHD has been reported in Germany (56).

Renal Cell Cancer

In renal cell cancer, some evidence exists that autologous T lymphocytes exert an immune antitumor response: Tumor-infiltrating lymphocytes can be readily isolated from some renal cell carcinomas and have been shown *in vitro* to have HLA-restricted specific cytotoxicity against tumor cells (57). Because renal cell cancer has been shown *in vitro* to be a target for T-cell cytotoxicity and potential renal tissue–restricted mHAs have been described, we carried out an experimental study of allogeneic PBPC transplants in patients with advanced metastatic renal cell carcinoma (58). To minimize the complications of transplantation, we used a nonmyeloablative preparative regimen of cyclophosphamide (120 mg per kg), followed by fludarabine (125 mg per m^2), to immunosuppress, but not myeloablate, the recipient. Three patients with metastatic renal cell cancer have received PBPC transplants from HLA-identical or near-identical siblings. All three patients showed a response with diminution of pulmonary and hepatic metastases beginning approximately 2 to 4 months posttransplant. Figure 4 illustrates the resolution of pulmonary metastases in the first patient treated. Two patients are currently well and disease free; the third patient continues to show tumor regression on successive computed tomography scans. The preparative regimen was well tolerated, and GVHD was readily controlled with combinations of steroids and cyclosporine. These promising results

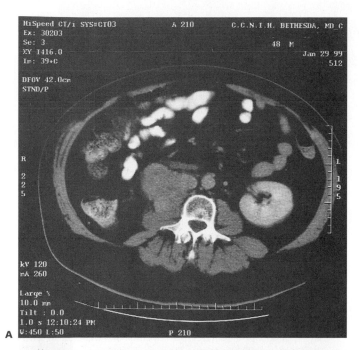

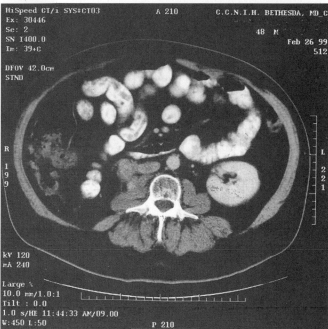

FIGURE 4. Regression of metastatic renal cell carcinoma after non-myeloablative stem-cell transplant in a 48-year-old man. **A:** Computed tomography scan on day 100 posttransplant with stable retroperitoneal disease. (The original tumor in the right kidney was surgically removed 1 year previously.) At this point, cyclosporine treatment for graft-versus-host disease was withdrawn. **B:** Repeat computed tomography scan at the same level on day 129 shows marked tumor regression.

suggest that some patients with renal cell carcinoma may benefit from allogeneic stem-cell transplantation. The results encourage further exploration of a GVT effect from allogeneic stem-cell transplantation in the treatment of other advanced malignant diseases.

FUTURE PROSPECTS

The GVL effect is emerging as the most powerful form of T-cell–mediated immunotherapy in use in clinical practice. Furthermore, the full potential of alloreacting lymphocytes to control an increasing variety of malignant diseases is becoming apparent. The challenge for the future is to characterize the nature of the alloimmune response against the malignant disease, to refine the approach to alloimmunotherapy, and to avoid the unwanted aspect of GVHD. Ultimately, it should be possible to use healthy donors to provide *in vitro*–expanded lymphocytes, specific for a given malignancy to augment the immune response to the disease after transplant. It is also possible that, in the future, improved transplant preparative regimens will allow the use of adoptive T-cell immunotherapy without the toxicity associated with intensive myeloablative transplants.

REFERENCES

1. Van Bekkum DW, de Vries MJ. *Radiation chimeras*. London: Academic Press, 1967:4–123.
2. Barnes DWH, Loutit JF. Treatment of murine leukemia with X-rays and homologous bone marrow. BMJ 1956;2:626–627.
3. Mathé G. Lessons from past experience in cancer immunotherapy and their application to cancer and AIDS treatment and prophylaxis. *Biomed Pharmacother* 1989;43:551–561.
4. Horowitz MM, Gale RP, Sondel PM, et al. Graft-versus-leukemia reactions after bone marrow transplantation. *Blood* 1990;75:555–562.
5. Van Rhee F, Kolb H-J. Donor leukocyte transfusions for leukemic relapse. *Curr Opin Hematol* 1995;2:423–429.
6. Van Bekkum DW, de Vries MJ. *Radiation chimeras*. London: Academic Press, 1967:214–227.
7. Bortin MM, Truitt RL, Rimm AA, Bach FH. Graft-versus-leukaemia reactivity induced by alloimmunization without augmentation of graft-versus-host reactivity. *Nature* 1979;281:490–491.
8. Glass B, Uharek L, Gassmann W, et al. Graft-versus-leukemia activity after bone marrow transplantation does not require graft-versus-host disease. *Ann Hematol* 1992;64:255–259.
9. Kloosterman TC, Martens AC, van Bekkum DW, Hagenbeek A. Graft-versus-leukemia in rat MHC-mismatched bone marrow transplantation is merely an allogeneic effect. *Bone Marrow Transplant* 1995;15:583–590.
10. Sykes M, Pearson DA, Szot GL. IL-2-induced GVHD protection is not inhibited by cyclosporine and is maximal when IL-2 is given over a 25-hour period beginning on the day following bone marrow transplantation. *Bone Marrow Transplant* 1995;15:395–399.
11. Murphy WJ, Welniak LA, Taub DD, et al. Differential effects of the absence of interferon-gamma and IL-4 in acute graft-versus-host disease after allogeneic bone marrow transplantation in mice. *J Clin Invest* 1998;102:1742–1748.
12. Malkovska V, Cigel F, Storer BE. Human T cells in hu-PBL-SCID mice proliferate in response to Daudi lymphoma and confer antitumor immunity. *Clin Exp Immunol* 1994;96:158–165.
13. Barrett AJ. Mechanisms of graft-versus-leukemia in man. *Stem Cells* 1997;15:248–258.
14. Rettie JE, Gottleib D, Heslop H, et al. Endogenously generated activated killer cells circulate after autologous and allogeneic bone marrow transplantation but not after chemotherapy. *Blood* 1989;73:1351–1358.
15. Jiang YZ, Cullis JO, Kanfer EJ, Goldman JM, Barrett AJ. T cell and NK cell mediated graft versus leukemia reactivity following donor buffy coat transfusion to treat relapse after marrow transplantation for chronic myeloid leukemia. *Bone Marrow Transplant*

1993;11:133–138.

16. Jiang YZ, Barrett AJ, Goldman JM, Mavroudis DA. Association of natural killer cell immune recovery with a graft-versus-leukemia effect independent of graft-versus-host disease following allogeneic bone marrow transplantation. *Anna Hematol* 1997;74:1–6.

17. Kurago ZB, Smith KD, Lutz CT. NK cell recognition of MHC class I. *J Immunol* 1995;153:2631–2641.

18. Perreault C, Decary F, Brochu S, Gyger M, Belanger R, Roy DC. Minor histocompatibility antigens. *Blood* 1990;76:1269–1277.

19. de Bueger M, Bakker A, van Rood JJ, van der Woude F, Goulmy E. Tissue distribution of minor histocompatibility antigens. *J Immunol* 1992;149:1788–1794.

20. Dolstra H, Fredrix H, Preijers F, et al. Recognition of a B cell leukemia-associated minor histocompatibility antigen by CTL. *J Immunol* 1997;158:560–565.

21. Gambacorti-Passerini C, Bertazzoli C, Dermime S, Scardino A, Schendel D, Parmiani G. Mapping of HLA class I binding motifs in forty-four fusion proteins involved in human cancers. *Clin Cancer Res* 1997,5:675–683.

22. van Barn N, Chambost H, Ferrant A, et al. PRAME, a gene encoding an antigen recognized on a human melanoma by cytolytic T cells is expressed in acute leukemias. *Br J Haematol* 1998;102:1376–1379.

23. Molldrem JJ, Clave E, Jiang YZ, et al. Cytotoxic T lymphocytes specific for a non-polymorphic proteinase 3 peptide preferentially inhibit chronic myeloid leukemia colony forming units. *Blood* 1997;90:2529–2534.

24. Gale RP, Horowitz MM, Ash RC, et al. Identical twin bone marrow transplants for leukemia. *Ann Intern Med* 1994,120:646–652.

25. Slavin S, Naparstek E, Nagler A, et al. Allogeneic cell therapy with donor peripheral blood cells and recombinant human interleukin-2 to treat leukemia relapse post allogeneic bone marrow transplantation. *Blood* 1996;87:2195–2204.

26. Kolb HJ, Schattenberg A, Goldman JM, et al. Graft-versus-leukemia effect of donor lymphocyte transfusions in marrow grafted patients. *Blood* 1995;86:2041–2050.

27 Slavin S, Nagler A, Naparstek E, et al. Nonmyeloablative stem cell transplantation and cell therapy as an alternative to conventional bone marrow transplantation with lethal cytoreduction for the treatment of malignant and nonmalignant hematologic diseases. *Blood* 1998;91:756–763.

28 Weiden P, Flournoy N, Thomas E, et al. Antileukemic effects of graft-versus-host disease in human recipients of allogeneic marrow grafts. *N Engl J Med* 1979;300:1068–1073.

29 Miyamura K, Barrett AJ, Kodera Y, Saito H. Minimal residual disease after bone marrow transplantation for chronic myelogenous leukemia and implications for graft-versus-leukemia effect: a review of recent results. *Bone Marrow Transplant* 1994;14:201–210.

30. Hessner M, Endean D, Casper J, et al. Use of unrelated marrow grafts compensates for reduced graft-versus-leukemia reactivity after T-cell-depleted allogeneic marrow transplantation for chronic myelogenous leukemia. *Blood* 1995;86:3987–3996.

31. Van Rhee F, Feng L, Cullis JO, et al. Relapse of chronic myeloid leukemia after allogeneic bone marrow transplantation: the case for giving donor leucocyte transfusions before the onset of hematological relapse. *Blood* 1994;83:3377–3383.

32. Collins RH Jr, Rogers ZR, Bennett M, Kumar V, Niekein A, Fay JW. Hematologic relapse of chronic myelogenous leukemia following allogeneic bone marrow transplantation: apparent graft-versus-leukemia effect following abrupt discontinuation of immunosuppression. *Bone Marrow Transplant* 1992;10:391–395.

33. Higano CS, Brixey M, Bryant EM, et al. Durable complete remission of acute non-lymphoblastic leukaemia associated with discontinuation of immunosuppression following relapse after allogeneic bone marrow transplantation. A case report of a probable graft-versus-leukaemia effect. *Transplantation* 1990;50:175–177.

34. Russell JA. Allogeneic blood stem cell transplantation for hematological malignancies: preliminary comparison of outcome with bone marrow transplantation. *Bone Marrow Transplant* 1996;17:703–709.

35. Kurtzberg J, Laughlin M, Graham ML, et al. Placental blood as a source of hematopoietic stem cells for transplantation into unrelated recipients. *N Engl J Med* 1996;335:157–161.

36. Bahçeci E , Barrett AJ , Childs R, Leitman S, Read EJ. CD34+ dose predicts survival and relapse following T cell depleted HLA-identical bone marrow or blood stem cell transplantation for hematologic malignancies. *Br J Haematol* 2000 (in press).

37. Mackinnon S, Barnett L, Bourhis JH, et al. Myeloid and lymphoid chimerism after T-cell depleted bone marrow transplantation: evaluation of conditioning regimens using the polymerase chain reaction to amplify human minisatellite regions of genomic DNA. *Blood* 1992;l80:3235–3241.

38. Roux E, Helg C, Dumont-Girard F, Chapuis B, Jeannet M, Roosnek E. Analysis of T-cell repopulation after allogeneic bone marrow transplantation: significant differences between recipients of T-cell depleted and unmanipulated grafts. *Blood* 1996;87:3984–3992.

39. Mackinnon S, Papadopoulos EB, Carabasi MH, Reich L, Collins NH, O'Reilly RJ. Adoptive immunotherapy using donor leukocytes following bone marrow transplantation for chronic myeloid leukemia: is T cell dose important in determining biological response? *Bone Marrow Transplant* 1995;15:591–594.

40. Barrett AJ, Mavroudis D, Tisdale J, et al. T-cell depleted bone marrow transplantation and delayed T-cell add-back to control severe acute GVHD and conserve a GVL effect. *Bone Marrow Transplant* 1998;21:543–551.

41 Champlin RE, Passweg JR, Zhang M-J, et al. T-cell depletion of bone marrow transplants for leukemia from donors other than HLA-identical siblings: advantages of T-cell antibodies with narrow specificities. *Blood* 1999 (in press).

42. Nimer SD, Giorgi J, Gajewski JL, et al. Selective depletion of CD8+ cells for prevention of graft-versus-host disease after bone marrow transplantation. *Transplantation* 1994;57:82–87.

43. Mehta J, Powles RL, Singhal S, Tait D, Sawnsbury J, Treleaven J. Cytokine-mediated immunotherapy with or without donor leukocytes for poor-risk acute myeloid leukemia relapsing after allogeneic bone marrow transplantation. *Bone Marrow Transplant* 1995;16:133–138.

44. Dermime S, Mavroudis D, Jiang YZ, Hensel N, Molldrem J, Barrett AJ. Immune escape from a graft-versus-leukemia effect may play a role in the relapse of myeloid leukemias following allogeneic bone marrow transplantation? *Bone Marrow Transplant* 1997;19:989–999.

45. Collins RH, Shpilberg O, Drobyski WR, et al. Donor leukocyte infusions in 140 patients with relapsed malignancy after allogeneic bone marrow transplantation. *J Clin Oncol* 1997;15:433–444.

46. Papadopoulos EB, Carabasi MH, Castro-Malaspina H, et al. T-cell-depleted allogeneic bone marrow transplantation as postremission therapy for acute myelogenous leukemia: freedom from relapse in the absence of graft-versus-host disease. *Blood* 1998;91:1083–1090.

47. van Biesen KW, de Lima M, Giralt SA, et al. Management of lymphoma recurrence after allogeneic transplantation: the relevance of graft-versus-lymphoma effect. *Bone Marrow Transplant* 1997;19:977–982.

48. Giralt S, Estey E, Albitar M, van Biesen K, et al. Engraftment of allogeneic hematopoietic progenitor cells with purine analog containing chemotherapy: harnessing graft-versus-leukemia without myeloablative therapy. *Blood* 1997;89:12–20.

49. Tricot G, Vesole D, Jagannath S, Hilton J, Munshi N, Barlogie B. Graft-versus-myeloma effect: proof of principle. *Blood* 1996;87:1196–1198.

50. Verdonck L, Lokhorst H, Dekker A, et al. Graft-versus myeloma effect in two cases. *Lancet* 1996;347:800–801.

51. Naparstek E, Or R, Nagler A, et al. T-cell depleted allogeneic bone marrow transplantation for acute leukaemia using Campath-1 antibodies and post-transplant administration of donor's peripheral blood lymphocytes for prevention of relapse. *Br J Haematol* 1995;89:506–515.

52. Bonini C, Ferrari G, Verzeletti S, et al. HSV-TK gene transfer into donor lymphocytes for control of allogeneic graft versus leukemia. *Science* 1997;276:1719–1724.

53. Mavroudis DA, Dermime S, Molldrem JJ, et al. Specific depletion of alloreactive T cells in HLA-identical siblings—a method for separating graft-vs-host and graft-vs-leukaemia reactions. *Br J Haematol* 1998;101:565–570.

54. Falkenberg JHF, Faber LM, van der Elshout M, et al. Generation of donor-derived antileukemic cytotoxic T-lymphocyte responses for

treatment of relapsed leukemia after allogeneic HLA-identical bone marrow transplantation. *J Immunother* 1993;14:305–309.

55. Ueno NT, Rondon G, Mirza NQ, et al. Allogeneic peripheral-blood progenitor-cell transplantation for poor-risk patients with metastatic breast cancer. *J Clin Oncol* 1998;16:986–993.

56. Eibl B, Schwaighofer H, Nachbaur D, et al. Evidence for a graft-versus-tumor effect in a patient treated with marrow ablative chemotherapy and allogeneic bone marrow transplantation for breast cancer. *Blood* 1996;88:1501–1508.

57. Poindexter N, Shenoy S, Howard T, et al. Allograft infiltrating cytotoxic T lymphocytes recognize kidney-specific human minor histocompatibility antigens. *Clin Transplant* 1997;11:174–177

58. Childs R, Clave E, Plante M, Tisdale J, Barrett AJ. Successful treatment of metastatic renal-cell carcinoma with a non-myeloablative allogeneic peripheral blood progenitor cell transplant: evidence for a graft-versus-tumor effect. *J Clin Oncol* 1999;17:2044.

13.4

CELL TRANSFER THERAPY: CLINICAL APPLICATIONS

Adoptive Cellular Immunotherapy for Epstein-Barr Virus–Associated Malignancies

MALCOLM K. BRENNER
HELEN E. HESLOP
CLIONA M. ROONEY

Epstein-Barr virus (EBV) is a latent herpesvirus that infects more than 90% of the world's population. The primary infection usually begins in the oropharynx, where mucosal epithelial cells become productively infected. The virus produced in these cells may then infect neighboring epithelial cells and B cells circulating through the mucosa-associated lymphoid tissues (MALTs). Primary infection most often results in a mild, self-limiting illness that is followed by lifelong virus latency in oral epithelial cells and in B cells (1,2). B cells infected with EBV *in vitro* undergo transformation as a result of the expression of latency-associated transforming protein (2). In normal seropositive individuals, B cells that express these proteins are tightly controlled by the abundant EBV-specific T cells present in the circulation (3). Although cell-mediated responses to the immunogenic proteins prevents outgrowth in the immunocompetent host, reactivation of EBV in severely immunocompromised individuals can lead to uncontrolled lymphoproliferation and the development of frank B-immunoblastic lymphoma (2,4). The proliferating EBV-infected B cells seen in lymphoproliferative disease (LPD) have a phenotype and pattern of EBV gene expression identical to that of lymphoblastoid cell lines generated by infecting normal peripheral blood mononuclear cells (PBMCs) with EBV. This type III latency (Tables 1 and 2) involves the expression of nine latency-associated viral proteins: Epstein-Barr nuclear antigens (EBNAs) 1, 2, 3a, 3b, 3c, and EBNA leader protein (EBNA-LP); the latent membrane proteins (LMP)1, 2a, and 2b; and the cytosolic protein RK-BARFO. Because the cells express viral antigens and are rich in cell adhesion and costimulatory molecules, they are highly immunogenic (Fig. 1) and are normally susceptible to immune-mediated killing.

In immunocompetent individuals, latent EBV is associated with other types of malignancy (see Table 2). In approximately 50% of patients with Hodgkin's disease, EBV antigens can be detected in the pathognomonic Reed-Sternberg cells (5), whereas patients with endemic nasopharyngeal carcinoma express EBV antigens in the epithelial tumor cells. In both of these malignancies, a more restricted array of EBV antigens (EBNA1, RK-BARFO, LMP1, 2) are expressed in a pattern termed *type II latency* (see Table 1). A number of other virus-associated malignancies—in particular, carcinomas of mucosal epithelium and mucosa-associated lymphoid tissue (MALT) lymphomas—also express type II EBV-latency antigens. In endemic Burkitt lym-

TABLE 1. TYPES OF EPSTEIN-BARR VIRUS (EBV) LATENCY

EBV Genes	Latency Type
LMP2a	0
EBNA1, BARTs, EBERs, ± LMP2a	I
EBNA1, BARTs, EBERs, LMP1, LMP2a	II
EBNA1, 2, 3a, 3b, 3c, LP; LMP1 and 2; BARTs and EBERs	III

BARTs, a rightward transcript encoding at least one protein (RK-BARFO); EBERs, EBV small RNAs; EBNA, EBV nuclear antigen; LMP, latent membrane protein.

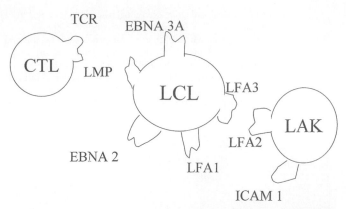

FIGURE 1. Phenotype and pattern of Epstein-Barr virus (EBV) gene expression of a lymphoblastoid cell line (LCL) that is identical to the cells that outgrow in EBV lymphoproliferative disease after bone marrow transplant. These cells express all latent cycle EBV antigens [Epstein-Barr nuclear antigens (EBNA)1, EBNA2, EBNA3A, EBNA3B, EBNA3C, latent membrane protein (LMP)1, LMP2a, and LMP2b], as well as a number of adhesion and costimulatory molecules that enhance cytotoxic T lymphocyte (CTL) generation and target recognition. (ICAM-1, intracellular adhesion molecule-1; LAK, lymphokine-activated killer cell; LFA, lymphocyte functional antigen ; TCR, T-cell receptor.)

phoma (West and North Africa, Papua New Guinea), the B cells are also infected with latent EBV but express only two latency-associated antigens, EBNA1 and RK-BARFO, and are termed *type I latent cells* (see Table 1). Other malignancies, such as smooth muscle leiomyosarcomas common in children with acquired immunodeficiency syndrome and in organ transplant recipients, also carry the EBV genome, although their latency type is unclear (4). In principle, all of these tumors should be suitable targets for immunotherapy directed against the appropriate EBV-associated latency antigens. In this chapter, we describe the successes and limitations of this strategy.

EPSTEIN-BARR VIRUS–RELATED LYMPHOPROLIFERATIVE DISEASE

Pathogenesis

The onset of EBV-LPD seems to be preceded by a large increase in EBV load, as well as the proliferation of EBV-infected B cells. Rises in EBV levels have been observed before the onset of LPD in solid organ transplant patients (6–8) and in stem-cell transplant patients; a 2- to 3-log increase in EBV DNA was found to be highly predictive of the subsequent development of EBV-related lymphoproliferation (9). These observations were confirmed by Lucas et al. (10), who reported high EBV-DNA levels (>40,000 copies per μg DNA) in the peripheral blood leukocytes

of patients with T-cell–depleted transplants, as compared with low levels (40 to 4,000 copies per μg) in recipients of unmanipulated stem-cell transplants and healthy seropositive individuals. The increase in EBV load was associated with an increased risk of LPD. The disease begins as a polyclonal lymphoproliferation but may evolve into an oligoclonal or even a monoclonal true immunoblastic lymphoma.

Several viral factors that may be important in the pathogenesis of LPD have been elucidated. The transforming protein EBNA2 functions through interaction with the cellular DNA-binding protein human C protein–binding factor (CBF1) to control the expression not only of viral genes, but also of cellular genes, such as CD21, CD23 (11), and c-fgr (12). EBNA3a, 3b, 3c, and LP appear to be important in regulating the activity of EBNA2. The growth-promoting effect of LMP1 in LPD was

TABLE 2. EPSTEIN-BARR VIRUS (EBV)—ASSOCIATED DISEASES

EBV-Related Disease	Cell Type	Latency Type	Reference
Burkitt lymphoma	B lymphocyte	I	83
Gastric carcinoma	Mucosal epithelium	I	84
Nasal natural killer lymphoma	Natural killer	II	85,86
Pleural cavity lymphoma	B lymphocyte	I/II	87
Parotid carcinoma	Mucosal epithelium	II	88
Hodgkin's lymphoma	B lymphocyte	II	89
Nasopharyngeal carcinoma	Mucosal epithelium	II	90
T-cell lymphoma	T lymphocyte	II	91
Midline granuloma	T lymphocyte	II	86
Thymic carcinoma	Epithelium	III	92
Pyothorax-associated lymphoma	B lymphocyte	III	93
Infectious mononucleosis	B lymphocyte	III	94
Lymphoproliferative disorders	B lymphocyte	III	95
Leiomyosarcoma	Smooth muscle	N/A	5
Sjögren's syndrome	—	N/A	97
Adrenal lymphoma	B lymphocyte	N/A	96

N/A, not applicable.

TABLE 3. INCIDENCE OF EPSTEIN-BARR VIRUS–RELATED LYMPHOPROLIFERATIVE DISEASE AFTER DIFFERENT T-CELL DEPLETION METHODS

Center	T-Cell Depletion Method	Incidence (%)	Reference
Memorial Sloan-Kettering Cancer Center	E-rosetting	11.0	21
St. Jude Children's Research Hospital	CD6/CD8 or T10/B9 monoclonal antibodies	11.5	26
Indiana University School of Medicine	E-rosetting or CD34 selection	26.0	10
University of Wisconsin, Madison, Medical School	CT-2 antibody	11.0	22
Medical College of Wisconsin	CD3 monoclonal antibodies and complement	8.0	98
Leiden University	E-rosetting	14.0	21
Multicenter (Europe)	CAMPATH (CD52) antibody	<2.0	28

shown to be mediated by binding to cytoplasmic tumor necrosis factor receptor–associated factors, leading to activation of the NF-κB transcription factor (13,14). The constitutive activity of LMP1 can replace activation of CD40 ligand, upregulating the epidermal growth factor receptor and preventing apoptosis (15). EBV relies on a number of mechanisms for modulating host immune responses, some of which may play a role in the pathogenesis of LPD. Viral interleukin-10 (IL-10) expressed as a late protein and cellular IL-10 induced in B cells by LMP1 not only act as autocrine growth factors for B cells but also inhibit the activation of macrophages and inflammatory responses (16–18). The CD8⁺ T-cell response to EBV includes γ-interferon–secreting cytotoxic T lymphocytes (CTLs) and cells secreting the type II cytokines IL-4 and IL-13, which can activate EBV-infected B cells (19). Thus, although the CTL response to EBV is an important factor in host control of EBV infection and the proliferation of EBV-infected B cells (2), the virus may also manipulate the immune response, allowing viral persistence. In the setting of transplantation and immunosuppression, this complex regulatory balance is disturbed, allowing uncontrolled growth of EBV-infected B cells and reactivation of latent EBV infection (20,21).

Incidence and Risk Factors

In general, the incidence of EBV-LPD rises as the level of host immunosuppression increases (Table 3). For example, after stem-cell transplantation, EBV-LPD is highest in recipients of grafts from mismatched family members or closely matched unrelated donors, when the stem-cell preparations have also been depleted of donor T cells to prevent graft-versus-host disease (GVHD), a severe and frequent complication of such transplants. The incidence of EBV-LPD is lowest in recipients of autologous stem cells. Several reports, however, suggest an increasing incidence of EBV-LPD in these patients because of more ablative preparatory regimens used in conjunction with stem-cell transplants depleted of T cells by procedures such as CD34 selection (22) or *in vitro* purging (23). There has even been a documented case developing after intensive chemotherapy for a B-cell malignancy, not followed by transplantation (24). After solid organ transplantation, the incidence of LPD is highest in recipients of heart–lung or gut grafts and lowest in those with renal transplants. Overall, the incidence after T-cell depletion ranges from less than 2% to as high as 26% (see Table 3), representing a devastatingly frequent and lethal problem in some groups of patients (10,21,25–27). After allogeneic stem-cell transplantation, the proliferating B cells are almost always of donor origin (>95%),

and methods that deplete not only donor T cells but also donor B cells appear to reduce the disease incidence. In a large review of patients whose transplants were treated with the Campath series of antibodies, the incidence of EBV-LPD was less than 2% (28). A similar low incidence was seen after elutriation, which removes more than 90% of B cells from the donor graft (29). In a French series, addition of a monoclonal antibody–depleting B cells to the T-cell–depletion regimen resulted in no cases of EBV lymphoma in 19 patients compared with 7 in 19 historical controls (30). After solid organ grafting, EBV-related lymphomas more often derive from host B cells and are correspondingly harder to prevent by manipulation of the graft (31).

Conventional Treatment

Because EBV-induced LPD is driven by latent virus, drugs such as acyclovir that interfere with viral replication have been of little benefit in prevention and of no benefit in treatment. Indeed, several reports suggest that in fact the EBV thymidine kinase gene does not phosphorylate acyclovir to the active agent, although this drug clearly inhibits virus replication *in vivo* and *in vitro* (32–35). In organ transplant recipients, the disease usually involves transmission of donor virus to recipient B cells, so that this transmission phase should be susceptible to inhibitors of virus replication. The timing of drug administration may be critical.

Because of the limitations of drug therapy, the treatment of EBV-LPD has largely been focused on strategies that boost the immune response to EBV. In solid organ transplant patients, simply withdrawing immunosuppressive therapy has proven effective but carries a high risk of graft rejection (31,36). Because of the more pronounced immunodeficiency after bone marrow transplantation, withdrawal of immune suppression does not usually result in a rapid enough immune recovery to eradicate EBV-infected B cells, although anecdotal reports of responses occurred in some patients who had developed lymphoma as their immune response was recovering (37,38). Therapy with interferon-α plus intravenous immune globulin after solid organ grafting and in a small number of hemopoietic stem cell recipients have elicited responses in some cases (31,38).

Anti–B-cell antibodies, a third approach for treating LPD, have been used clinically with some success in hemopoietic stem cell and organ transplant patients (39), although responses were often incomplete or transient. The anti-CD21 and anti-CD24 antibodies used in these studies are not clinically available, but anti-CD20 conjugated to ritoxylin has been approved for clinical use and may be warranted in some patients (40). Hydroxyurea and EBV-specific ribozymes are two other agents used in preclinical studies (41,42). Low concentrations of hydroxyurea eradicated latent EBV infection and inhibited proliferation of EBV-infected cell lines *in vitro* (41). Because hydroxyurea has been used clinically for other applications and has an acceptable toxicity profile at the doses suggested, it may be useful in patients for whom adoptive immunotherapy is not available. Adenoviral vectors encoding a ribozyme directed to EBNA1, an EBV protein required for viral replication, inhibited the growth of EBV-infected cells *in vitro* and in severe combined immunodeficiency disease mice (42). This strategy would likely be limited *in vivo*, however, because of low gene transfer efficiency.

UNMANIPULATED DONOR T CELLS

Overall, the failure of available treatments for EBV-LPD, coupled with an improved understanding of the biology of the disease, has stimulated interest in cellular immunotherapies. Most people infected with EBV have persistent infections, so that a significant proportion of peripheral blood T lymphocytes (from 1 in 300 to 1 in 4,000) are specific for the virus. It was therefore postulated that adaptively transferred PBMCs would include small numbers of EBV-specific T lymphocytes, which may proliferate *in vivo* and restore the patients' ability to respond to the virus and extirpate the lymphoma. Papadopoulos et al. (43) from Memorial Sloan-Kettering Cancer Center originally reported on five patients with EBV-LPD, all of whom responded to donor leukocyte infusion. These patients received less than 10^7 total T cells per kg, so that their response can be credited to EBV-specific T cells that originally numbered only in the tens of thousands and presumably underwent massive expansion *in vivo*. Although the percentage of EBV-specific T cells in peripheral blood is relatively small, a much higher proportion of T lymphocytes may be alloreactive, and these, too, can expand if the host expresses the relevant alloantigens. As might be predicted, therefore, three of these patients developed GVHD. Unexpectedly, two died from respiratory insufficiency (43), presumably because of the inflammatory reactions that occurred when EBV-specific T cells entered pulmonary tissue infiltrated by large numbers of EBV-positive immunoblasts. In an update of the Sloan-Kettering experience, 17 out of 19 patients responded to donor T cells (21). Other centers have also reported success with this strategy (10,44,45) while emphasizing the risk of GVHD (10,44). Still, others have had only poor rates of response to donor T cells (Table 4). Lucas et al. (10) described the Indiana University experience in treating LPD (10). In a comparison of outcomes among recipients of T-cell–depleted allogeneic stem-cell transplants who were treated with donor leukocytes and ten patients treated by observation, interferon-α plus intravenous immune globulin, chemotherapy, or surgery (10), only one of the control patients (surgery only) survived. By contrast, complete responses were induced in 4 out of 13 (31%) patients in the group receiving donor leukocytes, although 31% also experienced severe GVHD. One of the two patients who survived was actually treated with EBV-specific

TABLE 4. THERAPY FOR EPSTEIN-BARR VIRUS (EBV) LYMPHOPROLIFERATIVE DISEASE WITH DONOR T CELLS OR EBV–SPECIFIC CYTOTOXIC T LYMPHOCYTES (CTLs)

Cell Product	Responses	GVHD	Reference
Therapy			
Donor T cells	17/19	3 acute, 8 chronic	21
Donor T cells	1/1	1/1	44
Donor T cells	0/3	Not reported	38
Donor T cells	4/13[a]	4/13	10
Donor T cells	0/1	0/1	46
EBV-specific CTLs and donor T cells	0/1	0/1	45
EBV-specific CTLs	2/3	0/3	58
Prophylaxis			
EBV-specific CTLs	0/39 developed LPD	1/39	58

GVHD, graft-versus-host disease; LPD, lymphoproliferative disease.
[a]One responder received EBV-specific CTLs.

CTLs (see the section Virus-Specific Cytotoxic T Lymphocytes later in this chapter) (10). The Indiana investigators noted that five of the nine patients with disease progression died within 10 days of receiving donor leukocytes, most likely because of advanced LPD at the time of treatment, and therefore advocated earlier diagnosis and therapy. Two case reports from Japan describe patients who failed to respond to donor T cells (46,47), and none of three patients treated at the University of Minnesota responded (38). The reasons for these differences in response rate are unclear, but they may reflect different types of disease or a better outcome with early diagnosis.

Two strategies have been used to reduce the risk of GVHD after immunotherapy with donor T cells. The first, evaluated by Bonini and colleagues (48), is to transduce T cells with a "suicide gene," so that cell death may be induced if adverse effects occur after treatment of EBV-LPD or leukemic relapse (48). After a brief 24- to 48-hour primary stimulation with antigen, lymphocytes were transduced with a construct containing the thymidine kinase gene, which phosphorylates ganciclovir and renders host cells sensitive to the cytotoxic effects of the active drug. The construct also encoded a truncated version of the low-molecular-weight nerve growth factor gene, whose expression on the lymphocyte surface allows its use as a selectable marker. Eight patients have been reported, and, in three, ganciclovir treatment abolished the signs and symptoms of GVHD (48). A multicenter trial is in progress. The second strategy, adopted by our own center, is to administer EBV-antigen–specific CTLs (26) rather than unmanipulated polyspecific donor T cells with the intent of avoiding alloreactivity.

VIRUS-SPECIFIC CYTOTOXIC T LYMPHOCYTES

Virus-specific CTLs were first used by investigators in Seattle, who administered cytomegalovirus-specific CD8 T-cell clones to three recipients of matched sibling grafts (49,50). No adverse effects from the adoptive transfer of these clones occurred. Moreover, cytomegalovirus-specific immune responses were reconstituted, and none of the patients developed cytomegalovirus disease (49). Because the tumor cells of posttransplant EBV-LPD express all latent-cycle virus-encoded antigens (EBNA1, 2, 3a, 3b, 3c, and LMP1, 2a, 2b), it should be an excellent model in which to evaluate the efficacy of adoptively transferred antigen-specific CTL therapy. Moreover, EBV-transformed B-lymphoblastoid cell lines (LCLs) can readily be prepared from any donor and could provide a source not only of antigen-presenting cell expressing the appropriate viral antigens, but also of autologous target cells bearing the tumor antigens for CTL testing. Finally, most donors are immune to EBV, and because the virus persists in latent form, the EBV-specific CTL precursors persist long term in higher frequency than precursors specific for acutely infectious viruses. All of these features simplify the technical aspects of preparing EBV-CTL.

Functional CTL epitopes have been identified in seven of the nine EBV latency-associated proteins (51,52) and could be used to generate T-cell clones specific for each epitope. We elected to prepare polyclonal T-cell lines, however, because we did not know which epitopes are protective *in vivo* and because of fear that mutations in single viral epitopes would permit escape from monospecific T-cell clones. Hence, donor-derived EBV-specific CTL lines were generated by culturing donor T cells with donor-derived EBV-infected LCLs using techniques that have been described in detail (53). To determine how long these cells would persist in the recipient and to evaluate adverse or therapeutic effects, we marked the CTLs with a retroviral vector encoding the neomycin resistance gene.

Since our study opened, we have been able to establish cell lines from the CTLs of more than 120 normal donors, failing in only two cases (one seronegative and the other a recent seroconversion). CTL lines were predominantly CD3$^+$ (median, 99%) and contained CD4$^+$ and CD8$^+$ T cells. Both subsets were retained in the infused lines because CD4$^+$ cells may play an important role in maintaining long-term CD8$^+$ cytotoxic effector cells (54). The median percentages of CD4$^+$ and CD8$^+$ cells were 19% and 75%, respectively, but with wide variation among individual lines (55). All lines readily killed autologous LCL but showed variable activity against HSB-2 cells, targets of activated natural killer cells (55).

Clinical Trial of Cytotoxic T Lymphocytes as Prophylactic Therapy

We determined if adoptively transferred EBV-specific CTLs might be effective in preventing or treating EBV-LPD in recipients of mismatched or unrelated donor transplants who were at high risk for this complication (56). Patients were eligible for the study beginning at day 45 posttransplantation if they had engrafted, did not have severe GVHD (>grade II), had normal liver function, and had no severe intercurrent infection. The initial design was a dose-escalation study, but after six patients had been treated at the first two dose levels (4×10^7 and 1.2×10^8 cells per m^2 over 4 weeks), evidence existed of both persistence and efficacy (58). The study was then modified so that the remaining patients received just two injections of 2×10^7 cells per m^2 4 weeks apart. Subsequently, a single injection proved

effective, emphasizing how few EBV-specific T cells are needed to reconstitute the host defense against EBV.

Safety and Toxicity

As of January 1999, 54 patients were enrolled on the prophylaxis arm of this study. No immediate adverse effects of CTL administration occurred. Of particular importance, no evidence existed of acute GVHD within the first 3 months after CTL administration. This is significant because CTLs that recognize certain EBV-derived peptides in the context of a particular HLA molecule can cross-react with alloantigen (58). In two patients, preexisting GVHD continued; however, a biopsy specimen from one patient who had received gene-marked CTLs showed no evidence of selective accumulation of marked cells. Four other patients developed limited chronic GVHD, although the incidence was somewhat lower than in a comparable transplant group who did not receive CTLs (57).

Persistence of Immune Response

Reconstitution of immunity to EBV after adoptive transfer of CTL lines was demonstrated by a rise in virus-specific CTL activity in peripheral blood and by an increase in CTL precursor frequencies to the high end of the normal range (59). The level of marker gene detection in CD4$^+$ and CD8$^+$ components ranged from 0.1% to 1%, corresponding to levels in the infused lines. T cells in peripheral blood that were positive for the neo marker gene were not detectable by polymerase chain reaction (PCR) at 18 weeks' postinfusion. Antigen-reactive precursors persisted at a subthreshold level, however, and readily could be expanded to a detectable level by stimulation with EBV-LCL *in vitro*. Indeed, in these studies, it was possible to detect CTLs by this method more than 4 years after their administration (26). Additional evidence for long-term persistence of *in vivo* immunity is available from a boy with late reactivation of EBV (more than a year after CTL infusion) (59). He presented with fever and had an elevated EBV-DNA level in his peripheral blood. The marker gene, which had been undetectable in peripheral blood for 9 months, reappeared at this time, suggesting that the transferred CTLs had expanded in response to an increased viral load. The patient received no specific therapy, EBV-DNA levels returned to baseline, and the neo signal again disappeared from peripheral blood. The long-term persistence of antigen-specific CTLs may relate to the continued presence of EBV antigen and to the presence of CD4$^+$ cells and CD8$^+$ cells in the infused line.

Clinical Effects

None of the 54 patients in the prophylaxis study developed EBV-LPD, compared with 6 (11%) of 52 controls (*p* <.03) (58). The latter group consisted of patients who received T-cell–depleted marrow from mismatched-related or matched-unrelated donors but not prophylactic CTLs, owing to transplantation before the current study opened, ineligibility, or refusal to participate. Additional data also suggest the efficacy of CTL prophylaxis. We and others have shown that high EBV-DNA levels in peripheral blood are strongly predictive of the development of EBV-LPD (6,7,9). Thus, the initial presence of such levels in seven patients scheduled to receive CTLs might be expected to produce a high incidence of EBV-LPD. But, in fact, the EBV-DNA level in each of these patients returned to normal within 1 to 2 weeks after CTL infusion, and none of this subgroup developed EBV-LPD (58). These findings suggest that EBV-specific CTLs are effective therapy for "incipient" lymphoma, in addition to preventing the disease in patients without unfavorable presenting features.

Cytotoxic T Lymphocytes for Established Epstein-Barr Virus–Related Lymphoma

We also treated four patients who did not receive CTLs prophylactically and who subsequently developed frank EBV-related immunoblastic lymphoma. In three cases, CTL infusion produced disease resolution. Two of the patients presented with nodal disease and attained remission uneventfully after receiving 1.2×10^8 or 2×10^7 CTLs per m^2 (74 and *unpublished data*). A third patient presented with high fever and bulky cervical and nasopharyngeal disease causing respiratory compromise at 7 months after transplantation of cells from an unrelated donor (58). After the diagnosis of EBV-LPD was confirmed, he received 2×10^7 CTLs per m^2. Over the next week, cervical and oropharyngeal swelling increased, necessitating tracheostomy. A biopsy of sample nasopharyngeal tumor taken at that time showed an infiltrate of small lymphocytes, the majority of which stained with antibodies to T-cell markers; a few residual B cells were also found. Both *in situ* PCR and semiquantitative PCR analysis of DNA extracted from nasopharyngeal tissue showed that 1% of the infiltrating lymphocytes were positive for the neo marker gene, a marking efficiency similar to that in the adoptively transferred line. These data suggest that the gene-marked EBV-specific T cells had selectively accumulated at the tumor site. Because of evidence that the tissue swelling represented an inflammatory response during therapy rather than disease progression, this boy received no further specific therapy and remains in remission 3 years later. The complexity of this case provides a clear illustration of why prophylactic or early treatment (i.e., when elevated EBV-DNA levels are detected) is more desirable than treatment of established disease.

The fourth patient in this series illustrates another reason why CTL prophylaxis is preferable to treatment of overt disease. This 17-year-old girl received a T-cell–depleted unrelated donor transplant. She was admitted to the hospital on day 45 with fever, and repeated computed tomography scans showed progressive pulmonary infiltrates and nodules (61). Her EBV-DNA levels were high, and she received CTLs on day 56. Her lung disease progressed, and a lymph node biopsy revealed persisting lymphoblasts. She died on day 80 with an autopsy showing widespread EBV-positive lymphoma. Why did treatment fail? Analysis of her CTL line showed that almost all activity was directed towards a single EBV antigen, EBNA3b, and to two epitopes within that antigen (61). Sequencing of the viral DNA within the tumor revealed a deletion affecting precisely those two epitopes recognized by the CTL line. The loss of the two immunodominant epitopes thereby caused resistance to killing by the CTLs (61). The occurrence of escape mutants argues for treating patients when they have a low viral/tumor burden and, hence, a lower probability of mutation. The result also argues against attempting to substitute T-cell clone(s) for polyclonal lines because the escape phenomenon is more likely to occur when there is a limited range of target epitopes to be recognized.

Cytotoxic T Lymphocytes for Recipients of Solid Organ Transplants

The successful use of anti-EBV CTL in solid organ recipients requires identification of recipients at high risk of disease. Several groups fall into this category:

1. Seronegative recipients are at particularly high risk of post-transplant lymphoma because they frequently fail to mount an effective primary immune response to virus associated with the graft or other blood products. Although it is not possible to generate anti-EBV CTL from the T cells of seronegative recipients using EBV-transformed B-cell lines as antigen presenters, dendritic cells have the capacity to induce primary immune responses *in vitro*, and thus may be able to recruit naive CTL precursors *in vitro* to become EBV-specific effector cells. For example, dendritic cells can be induced to express EBV peptides by transducing them with recombinant vectors or pulsing them with apoptotic LCL, after which they are capable of inducing EBV-specific CTL, even from naive donors (CM Rooney, *unpublished data*).

2. Patients whose grafts (e.g., pancreas or intestine) contain high B-cell numbers are also at high risk of EBV-LPD.

3. Individuals who have received prolonged or intensive immunosuppression to overcome repeat rejection episodes may be at exceptionally high risk if they are also in the first two categories. Of note, CTLs can still be generated from such patients by *ex vivo* culture, even when the patients are receiving intensive immunosuppressive therapy.

4. Few reports of treatment of organ recipients with anti-EBV CTLs exist, but Comoli et al. (personal communication, 1999) have shown that liver transplant recipients with EBV-LPD respond to autologous CTL infusions with dramatic decreases in virus load and tumor regression. As with bone marrow recipients, the successful use of CTLs in organ recipients requires careful monitoring of virus load and may work best with early or prophylactic administration. Although most investigators who have studied CTL therapy after solid organ transplantation propose using autologous T cells, two alternative treatments, EBV-reactive CTLs from HLA-matched or haploidentical related donors, are being evaluated at the Johns Hopkins Medical School (61).

Improving the Feasibility of Cytotoxic T Lymphocyte Therapy

The feasibility of making CTL treatment available for patients with active EBV-LPD would be increased if it were possible to shorten the time required to prepare the activated lymphocytes. Four to 6 weeks are needed to generate LCL lines and an additional 4 to 6 weeks to generate specific CTLs. It may be possible to simplify and accelerate the production of CTLs by substitut-

32. Datta AK, Colby BM, Shaw JE, Pagano JS. Acyclovir inhibition of Epstein-Barr virus replication. *Proc Natl Acad Sci U S A* 1980; 77:5163–5166.
33. Pagano JS, Sixbey JW, Lin JC. Acyclovir and Epstein-Barr virus infection. *J Antimicrob Chemother* 1983;12:113–121.
34. Datta AK, Pagano JS. Phosphorylation of acyclovir *in vitro* in activated Burkitt somatic cell hybrids. *Antimicrob Agents Chemother* 1999;24(1):10–14.
35. Gustafson EA, Chillemi AC, Sage DR, Fingeroth JD. The Epstein-Barr virus thymidine kinase does not phosphorylate ganciclovir or acyclovir and demonstrates a narrow substrate specificity compared to the herpes simplex virus type 1 thymidine kinase. *Antimicrob Agents Chemother* 1998;42:2923–2931.
36. Starzl TE, Naleskin MA, Porter KA, et al. Reversibility of lymphomas and lymphoproliferative lesions developing under cyclosporin-steroid therapy. *Lancet* 1984;1:583.
37. Heslop HE, Li C, Krance RA, Loftin SK, Rooney CM. Epstein-Barr infection after bone marrow transplantation. *Blood* 1994;83: 1706–1708.
38. Gross TG, Steinbuch M, DeFor T, et al. B cell lymphoproliferative disorders following hematopoietic stem cell transplantation: risk factors, treatment and outcome. *Bone Marrow Transplant* 1999;23:251–258.
39. Leblond V, Sutton L, Dorent R, et al. Lymphoproliferative disorders after organ transplantation: a report of 24 cases observed in a single center. *J Clin Oncol* 1996;13:961–968.
40. Faye A, Van Den Abeele T, Peuchmaur M, Matheu-Boue A, Vilmer E. Anti-CD20 monoclonal antibody for post-transplant lymphoproliferative disorders. *Lancet* 1998;352:1285.
41. Chodosh J, Holder VP, Gan Y-J, Belgaumi A, Sample J, Sixbey JW. Eradication of latent Epstein-Barr virus by hydroxyurea alters the growth-transformed cell phenotype. *J Infect Dis* 1998;177:1194–1201.
42. Huang S, Stupack D, Mathias P, Wang Y, Nemerow GR. Growth arrest of Epstein-Barr virus immortalized B lymphocytes by adenovirus-delivered ribozymes. *Proc Natl Acad Sci U S A* 1997;94:8156–8161.
43. Papadopoulos EB, Ladanyi M, Emanuel D, MacKinnon S, Boulad F, Carabasi MH, et al. Infusions of donor leukocytes to treat Epstein-Barr virus-associated lymphoproliferative disorders after allogeneic bone marrow transplantation. *N Engl J Med* 1994;330:1185–1191.
44. Heslop HE, Brenner MK, Rooney CM. Donor T cells to treat EBV-associated lymphoma. *N Engl J Med* 1994;331:679–680.
45. Sasahara Y, Kawai S, Itano M, et al. Epstein-Barr virus-associated lymphoproliferative disorder after unrelated bone marrow transplantation in a young child with Wiskott-Aldrich syndrome. *Pediatr Hematol Oncol* 1998;15:347–352.
46. Nagafuji K, Eto T, Hayashi S, et al. Donor lymphocyte transfusion for the treatment of Epstein-Barr virus-associated lymphoproliferative disorder of the brain. *Bone Marrow Transplant* 1998;21:1155–1158.
47. Imashuku S, Goto T, Matsumura T, et al. Unsuccessful CTL transfusion in a case of post-BMT Epstein-Barr virus-associated lymphoproliferative disorder (EBV-LPD). *Bone Marrow Transplant* 1998;20:337–340.
48. Bonini C, Ferrari G, Verzeletti S, et al. HSV-TK gene transfer into donor lymphocytes for control of allogeneic graft versus leukemia. *Science* 1997;276:1719–1724.
49. Walter EA, Greenberg PD, Gilbert MJ, et al. Reconstitution of cellular immunity against cytomegalovirus in recipients of allogeneic bone marrow by transfer of T-cell clones from the donor. *N Engl J Med* 1995;333:1038–1044.
50. Riddell SR, Watanabe KS, Goodrich JM, Li CR, Agha ME, Greenberg PD. Restoration of viral immunity in immunodeficient humans by the adoptive transfer of T cell clones. *Science* 1992;257:238–241.
51. Murray RJ, Kurilla MG, Brooks JM, et al. Identification of target antigens for the human cytotoxic T cell response to Epstein-Barr virus (EBV): implications for the immune control of EBV-positive malignancies. *J Exp Med* 1992;176:157–168.
52. Khanna R, Burrows SR, Kurilla MG, et al. Localization of Epstein-Barr virus cytotoxic T cell epitopes using recombinant vaccinia: implications for vaccine development. *J Exp Med* 1992;176:169–176.
53. Smith CA, Ng CYC, Heslop HE, et al. Production of genetically modified EBV-specific cytotoxic T cells for adoptive transfer to patients at high risk of EBV-associated lymphoproliferative disease. *J Hematother* 1995;4:73–79.
54. Matloubian M, Concepcion RJ, Ahmed R. CD4+ T cells are required to sustain CD8+ cytotoxic T cell responses during chronic viral infection. *J Virol* 1994;68:8056–8063.
55. Smith CA, Ng CYC, Loftin SK, et al. Adoptive immunotherapy for Epstein-Barr virus-related lymphoma. *Leuk Lymphoma* 1996;23: 213–220.
56. Heslop HE, Brenner MK, Rooney CM, et al. Administration of neomycin-resistance-gene-marked EBV-specific cytotoxic T lymphocytes to recipients of mismatched-related or phenotypically similar unrelated donor marrow grafts. *Hum Gene Ther* 1994;5: 381–397.
57. Rooney CM, Smith CA, Ng CYC, et al. Infusion of cytotoxic T cells for the prevention and treatment of Epstein-Barr virus-induced lymphoma in allogeneic transplant recipients. *Blood* 1998;92: 1549–1555.
58. Burrows SR, Khanna R, Burrows JM, Moss DJ. An allo response in humans is dominated by cytotoxic T lymphocytes (CTL) cross-reactive with a single Epstein-Barr virus CTL epitope: implications for graft-versus-host disease. *J Exp Med* 1994;179:1155–1161.
59. Heslop HE, Ng CYC, Li C, et al. Long-term restoration of immunity against Epstein-Barr virus infection by adoptive transfer of gene-modified virus-specific T lymphocytes. *Nat Med* 1996;2:551–555.
60. Rooney CM, Smith CA, Ng C, et al. Use of gene-modified virus-specific T lymphocytes to control Epstein-Barr virus-related lymphoproliferation. *Lancet* 1995;345:9–13.
61. Gottschalk S, Ng CYC, Perez M, Brenner MK, Heslop HE, Rooney CM. Mutation in EBV produces immunoblastic lymphoma unresponsive to CTL immunotherapy. *Blood* 1998;[Suppl 1]:(abst).
62. Orentas RJ, Lemas MV, Mullin MJ, Colombani PM, Schwartz K, Ambinder R. Feasibility of cellular adoptive immunotherapy for Epstein-Barr virus-associated lymphomas using haploidentical donors. *J Hematother* 1998;7:257–261.
63. Romani N, Gruner S, Brang D, et al. Proliferating dendritic cell progenitors in human blood. *J Exp Med* 1994;180:83–93.
64. Rooney CM, Roskrow MA, Smith CA, Brenner MK, Heslop HE. Immunotherapy of EBV lymphoma. *J Natl Cancer Inst Monogr* 1998;23:89–93.
65. Beaty O, Hudson MM, Greenwald C, et al. Subsequent malignancies in children and adolescents after treatment for Hodgkin's disease. *J Clin Oncol* 1995;13:603–609.
66. Herbst H, Dallenback F, Hummel M, et al. Epstein-Barr virus latent membrane protein expression in Hodgkin and Reed-Sternberg cells. *Proc Natl Acad Sci U S A* 1991;88:4766–4770.
67. Levitskaya J, Coram M, Levitsky V, et al. Inhibition of antigen processing by the internal repeat region of the Epstein-Barr virus nuclear antigen-1. *Nature* 1995;375:685–688.
68. Kienzle N, Sculley TB, Poulson L, et al. Identification of a cytotoxic T-lymphocyte response to the novel BARFO protein of Epstein-Barr virus: a critical role for antigen expression. *J Virol* 1998;72:6614–6620.
69. Lee SP, Thomas WA, Murray RJ, et al. HLA A2.1-restricted cytotoxic T cells recognizing a range of Epstein-Barr virus isolates through a defined epitope in latent membrane protein LMP2. *J Virol* 1993;67:7428–7435.
70. Hsu SM, Lin J, Xie SS, Hsu PL, Rich S. Abundant expression of transforming growth factor-beta 1 and -beta 2 by Hodgkin's Reed-Sternberg cells and by reactive T lymphocytes in Hodgkin's disease. *Hum Pathol* 1993;24:249–255.
71. Slivnick DJ, Ellis TM, Nawrocki JF, Fisher RI. The impact of Hodgkin's disease on the immune system. *Semin Oncol* 1990;17: 673–682.
72. Renner C, Ohnesorge S, Held G, et al. T cells from patients with Hodgkin's disease have a defective T-cell receptor zeta chain expression that is reversible by T-cell stimulation with CD3 and CD28. *Blood* 1996;88:236–241.
73. Roskrow MA, Suzuki N, Gan Y-J, et al. EBV-specific cytotoxic T lymphocytes for the treatment of patients with EBV positive relapsed Hodgkin's disease. *Blood* 1998;91:2925–2934.
74. Sing AP, Ambinder RF, Hong DJ, et al. Isolation of Epstein-Barr

ing dendritic cells expressing EBV antigens for the LCLs. Because dendritic cells can be prepared in only 3 to 7 days (63), their use would markedly reduce the total preparation time. Moreover, dendritic cells can be used to stimulate CTL responses to the more restricted set of EBV antigens expressed by Hodgkin's disease and nasopharyngeal carcinoma cells (64). Their value would therefore be especially high in extending adoptive immunotherapy to the EBV-related malignancies described below (see the section Immunotherapy for Epstein-Barr Virus-Related Hodgkin's Disease).

IMMUNOTHERAPY FOR EPSTEIN-BARR VIRUS–RELATED HODGKIN'S DISEASE

Although the origin of Hodgkin's disease remains unclear, approximately 50% of cases in North America and Europe are associated with EBV (4). In South America, Kenya, and parts of Asia, a 90% to 100% association exists. Thus, CTLs could prove a valuable addition to conventional therapy for EBV and Hodgkin's disease, if they could be marshaled against this disease as effectively as against EBV-LPD. Although 80% or more of patients with Hodgkin's disease are cured with available treatments, 50% of the minority who relapse do not respond to salvage chemotherapy or relapse a second time. Furthermore, the unacceptably high level of therapy-related secondary malignancies (18% at 5 years) and other serious medical complications in those who are "cured" also underscores the need to improve current therapeutic options (65).

A number of obstacles could diminish the effectiveness of EBV-specific CTLs in Hodgkin's disease. First, the malignant cells express a restricted set of viral genes, namely, EBNA1, RK-BARFO, and LMP1 and 2 (66). In the majority of cases, memory CTL responses are preferentially directed against the highly immunogenic EBNA3a, 3b, and 3c antigens, irrespective of the patient's HLA type. By comparison, EBNA-1, RK-BARFO, and LMP1 and 2 are poorly immunogenic. EBNA1 contains a repeating glycine-alanine amino acid sequence that inhibits its ubiquitination and subsequent processing and presentation of EBNA1 peptides by HLA class I antigens (67). RK-BARFO-specific CTLs can be generated *in vitro* from seropositive individuals, but they do not kill target cells naturally expressing the protein (68). The mechanism for this immune evasion is unclear. The reason for the limited immunogenicity of LMP1 and 2 is similarly unclear, because LMP1 or 2 epitopes are presented in the context of the HLA A2.1, B24, B40, B51, and B55 alleles (51,69). This lack of immunogenicity is particularly disappointing because EBV and Hodgkin's tumors express costimulatory molecules, such as HLA DR, CD40, CD80, and CD86, and should therefore be excellent antigen-presenting cells. They also secrete the Th2 cytokines IL-10 and tumor growth factor-β, however, as well as thymus and activation-regulated chemokine (TARC), a chemoattractant for $CD4^+$ T cells of the Th2 biotype (70). This overwhelmingly Th2 phenotype likely helps the antibody response and inhibits the CTL response. IL-10 may also act as an autocrine growth factor for Reed-Sternberg cells. Patients with Hodgkin's disease also have T-cell abnormalities, such as low expression of the zeta chain of the T-cell receptor (71), which further reduce the effectiveness of the host immune response to the tumor (72).

To assess the feasibility of using EBV-specific CTLs as therapy for Hodgkin's disease, we generated EBV-specific CTLs from the peripheral blood of patients with this lymphoma, with the notion of expanding the cells *in vitro* in the absence of *in vivo* immunosuppressive effects. We then compared them phenotypically and functionally with CTLs generated from normal donors (53). To discover whether autologous EBV-specific CTLs could persist and produce antiviral activity *in vivo*, we genetically marked the cells and then adoptively transferred them to three patients with relapsed disease.

Cytotoxic T Lymphocytes from Patients with Hodgkin's Disease Compared with Those from Healthy Epstein-Barr Virus–Positive Donors

In the presence of IL-2 and B-LCL, cell counts of cultures from healthy donors (n = 15) typically increased by tenfold every 2 weeks, so that after 16 weeks in culture, CTLs from normal donors had expanded approximately 1,500-fold. During the same 16-week period, CTL cultures from patients in remission expanded by only approximately 150-fold, whereas those from patients with relapsed disease increased by just 80-fold. In more than 75% of patients, however, it was still possible to generate at least 10^8 CTLs, a number suggested by previous studies of EBV-LPD to be well in excess of that required to establish EBV immunity (59,60). Phenotypically, the patient lines were essentially identical to the lines from normal donors, except that the level of the T-cell receptor–zeta chain was abnormally low (73). The cytoplasmic portion of the T-cell receptor–zeta chain is involved in signal transduction and subsequent activation and proliferation of T cells, so that downregulation of this chain may contribute to the decreased proliferative response of patient T cells. Nonetheless, the lines produced had strong activity against HLA-matched EBV-positive targets. Of particular note, lines from Hodgkin's disease patients had activity against cells expressing Hodgkin's-associated viral antigens, including LMP1 and LMP2. This effect was demonstrated by the cells' ability to kill HLA-matched fibroblasts infected with vaccinia recombinants, each expressing one of the EBV-latent cycle proteins. Both HLA class I– and class II–restricted CTLs could be detected. The presence of the class II–restricted cells may be of benefit because approximately 50% of Hodgkin's tumor cells downregulate HLA class I molecules, and may therefore be protected from conventional CTL killing. They generally maintain class II major histocompatibility complex (MHC) expression, however.

Biologic and Clinical Study of Cytotoxic T Lymphocytes

Encouraged by our ability to generate CTLs with activity against at least one of the Hodgkin's-associated antigens, we asked whether these cells would have antiviral and antimalignant properties *in vivo*. To track the persistence of infused CTLs, we marked the cells with a neo-containing retroviral vector. The neo gene was detectable in PBMCs for 4 to 12 weeks after the initial dose of 3.2×10^7 EBV-specific CTLs (73). The

levels of marking indicated that approximately 1 of every 1,000 circulating PBMCs was derived from the infused cell line.

The infused CTLs had cytotoxic antiviral activity. Thus, the proportion of circulating EBV-specific cytotoxic precursor cells was increased 10- to 100-fold, indicating an enhanced cell-mediated immune response to EBV. The number of MHC-unrestricted cytotoxic effector precursors remained constant, as demonstrated by the minimal change in the proportion of cytotoxic precursor cells that killed HLA-mismatched LCLs. In addition to the rise in cytotoxic precursor cell frequency, the CTL activity tested after 2 weeks of culture with the autologous LCLs also increased *in vivo*, from less than 3% killing of autologous LCLs at an effector:target ratio of 40:1 to more than 25% killing at the same effector:target ratio. Again, little effect on the activity of MHC-unrestricted cytotoxic effector cells occurred, suggesting that an increase in classical MHC-restricted CTL activity was responsible for the observed increase in autologous LCL target killing.

The observed increase in cytotoxic function was associated with measurable antiviral activity. We used semiquantitative PCR analysis to calculate the viral burden in peripheral blood before and after CTL infusion. The number of EBV-DNA genomes in normal donors ranges from less than 20 to 2,000 copies per 10^6 PBMCs (9). Before CTL infusion, the level of EBV DNA in patient 1 was 30,000 EBV genomes per 10^6 PBMCs, which is 15-fold higher than in normal individuals and within the range seen for stem-cell transplant recipients with immunoblastic lymphoma (9,58). After CTL infusion, the level of EBV DNA decreased dramatically and was undetectable at 4 weeks' postinfusion. Associated with this drop in EBV DNA, the patient showed improvement of stage B symptoms with increased appetite and resolution of fever and sweats; stabilization of his pulmonary disease also occurred. These effects were apparent even though the patient had received no chemotherapy for 4 weeks before or 6 weeks after infusion. In fact, the viral load in the peripheral blood of this patient increased only during readministration of chemotherapy at 6 weeks' postinfusion (the end of the evaluation period). Patient 2 had insufficient blood counts to allow measurement of EBV-DNA levels but also showed improvement in stage B symptoms before the institution of further chemotherapy and disease progression. Although the EBV burden was not supranormal in the third patient, an initial level of 400 EBV genomes per 10^6 PBMCs fell to undetectable levels by 19 days after the first infusion. These effects were again produced in the absence of chemotherapy (>6 weeks before and after). This patient had an initial worsening of his pleural effusion, and gene-marked CTLs were detected in pleural biopsies of diseased areas (73). His disease then stabilized and no further pleural effusions occurred for more than a year. The tumor ultimately progressed in all three patients, who died of their disease 10 to 13 months later.

Improving the Clinical Outcome

These preliminary studies show:

1. It is feasible to obtain substantial *ex vivo* expansion of EBV-specific T cells from patients with advanced Hodgkin's disease.
2. These cells have *in vivo* cytotoxic activity against EBV-infected cells and are detectable *in vivo* for up to 12 weeks.
3. These cells can be targeted to Hodgkin's disease–associated antigens.

Our efforts are directed at enhancing the component of the anti-EBV response that is directed to the Hodgkin's-associated antigens LMP1 and 2 by using dendritic cells expressing the appropriate proteins (see the section Cytotoxic T Lymphocytes for Recipients of Solid Organ Transplants). The CTLs generated will be given to patients with minimal residual disease to reduce the immunosuppressive effects associated with bulky tumors. An alternative approach is to develop CTL clones directed against Hodgkin's-associated antigens. Such an approach is possible (74) but is time consuming because the frequency of cells with such specificity is low. Moreover, many Hodgkin's tumors have mutations within the 3' region of the LMP1 oncogene, including a 30–base pair deletion and a high frequency of nonrandom point mutations (75,76). As we have already found in our EBV-LPD patients, these mutations may destroy the epitopes recognized by CTLs specific for wild-type LMP1, a problem that can only be accentuated if monospecific CTL clones, rather than polyspecific CTL lines, are used. It may also be possible to vaccinate patients directly using polypeptides, DNA, or dendritic cells as immunogens. The capacity to induce an immune response *in vivo*, however, may be limited by tumor-mediated immune escape mechanisms that subvert the induction or expansion of a cytotoxic response.

OTHER EPSTEIN-BARR VIRUS–ASSOCIATED MALIGNANCIES

EBV is associated with an increasing number of frequently rare and geographically associated malignancies (see Table 2). Lethal midline granulomas involving natural killer–like T-cell lymphomas, gastric carcinomas, and pyothorax-associated lymphoma seem to have an increased frequency in Japan, whereas parotid carcinomas are found predominantly in American Eskimos. EBV-positive smooth muscle tumors (leiomyosarcomas) are the second most prevalent malignancy of children with acquired immunodeficiency syndrome, and have an increased frequency after organ transplantation. In nonimmunosuppressed individuals, leiomyosarcomas rarely carry the EBV genome. EBV has also been found in carcinomas of the thymus and salivary gland. With the exception of gastric carcinoma and pyothorax-associated lymphoma, these tumors all express the intermediate type II latency and therefore are potential targets for immunotherapies targeting viral proteins, although the success of such therapies may depend on the immune-evasion strategies used by the tumor.

The type I tumors, Burkitt lymphoma and gastric carcinoma, pose a greater challenge for immunotherapy. The only viral proteins expressed in type I tumors are EBNA1 and RK-BARFO, which, as described in the preceding paragraph, do not provide target epitopes for HLA class I–restricted CTLs. Burkitt lymphoma cells have been shown to use additional antiimmune response mechanisms. They have defects in their expression of TAP I transporter proteins and HLA class I molecules (77,78). Moreover, they have the immunophenotype of a resting B cell and do not express costimulatory molecules necessary for the induction of an effective immune response. It may be possible to use $CD4^+$ HLA class II–restricted EBNA-1 or RK-BARFO–specific CTL to target tumor cells expressing type-I latency (81,82).

CONCLUSIONS

EBV-associated malignancies provide an investigational bridge between viral diseases and classic malignancies. As increasing numbers of tumor-associated antigens are identified, the effectiveness and limitations of CTL therapies in EBV-related diseases should provide an invaluable guide for improving immunotherapies for an ever broader range of cancers.

ACKNOWLEDGMENTS

We would like to thank John Gilbert for scientific editing and Gloria Levin for word processing. This work was supported in part by grants HL 55703, CA 74126, and CA 61384 from the National Institutes of Health.

REFERENCES

1. Rickinson AB, Kieff E. Epstein-Barr virus. In: Fields BN, Knipe DM, Howley PM, eds. *Fields virology.* Philadelphia: Lippincott–Raven Publishers, 1996:2397–2446.
2. Rickinson AB, Moss DJ. Human cytotoxic T lymphocyte responses to Epstein-Barr virus infection. *Annu Rev Immunol* 1997;15:405–431.
3. Bourgault I, Gomez A, Gomard E, Levy JP. Limiting-dilution analysis of the HLA restriction of anti-Epstein-Barr virus-specific cytolytic T lymphocytes. *Clin Exp Immunol* 1991;84:501–507.
4. Jenson H, Montalvo EA, McClain K, et al. Characterization of natural Epstein-Barr virus infection and replication in smooth muscle cells from a leiomyosarcoma. *J Med Virol* 1999;57:(1)36–46.
5. Weiss LM, Movahed LA, Warnke RA, Sklar J. Detection of Epstein-Barr viral genomes in Reed-Sternberg cells of Hodgkin's disease. *N Engl J Med* 1989;320:502–506.
6. Savoie A, Perpete C, Carpentier L, Joncas J, Alfieri C. Direct correlation between the load of Epstein-Barr virus-infected lymphocytes in the peripheral blood of pediatric transplant patients and risk of lymphoproliferative disease. *Blood* 1994;83:2715–2722.
7. Riddler SA, Breinig MC, McKnight JLC. Increased levels of circulating Epstein-Barr virus (EBV)-infected lymphocytes and decreased EBV nuclear antigen antibody responses are associated with the development of posttransplant lymphoproliferative disease in solid-organ transplant recipients. *Blood* 1994;84:972–984.
8. Fontan J, Bassignot A, Mougin C, Cahn JY, Lab M. Detection of Epstein-Barr virus DNA in serum of transplanted patients: a new diagnostic guide for lymphoproliferative diseases. *Leukemia* 1998;12:772.
9. Rooney CM, Loftin SK, Holladay MS, Brenner MK, Krance RA, Heslop HE. Early identification of Epstein-Barr virus-associated post-transplant lymphoproliferative disease. *Br J Haematol* 1995;89:98–103.
10. Lucas KG, Burton RL, Zimmerman SE, et al. Semiquantitative Epstein-Barr virus (EBV) polymerase chain reaction for the determination of patients at risk for EBV-induced lymphoproliferative disease after stem cell transplantation. *Blood* 1998;91:3654–3661.
11. Cordier-Bussat M, Billaud M, Calender A, Lenoir GM. Epstein-Barr virus (EBV) nuclear-antigen-2-induced up-regulation of CD21 and CD23 molecules is dependent on a permissive cellular context. *Int J Cancer* 1993;53:153–160.
12. Kempkes B, Pawlita M, Zimber-Strobl U, Eissner G, Laux Bornkamm GW. Epstein-Barr virus nuclear antigen 2-estrog receptor fusion proteins transactivate viral and cellular genes a interact with RBP-J kappa in a conditional fashion. *Virolo* 1995;214:675–679.
13. Miller WE, Mosialos G, Kieff E, Raab-Traub N. Epstein-Barr viru LMP1 induction of the epidermal growth factor receptor is mediate through a TRAF signaling pathway distinct from NF-kappaB activation. *J Virol* 1997;71:586–594.
14. Izumi KM, Kieff ED. The Epstein-Barr virus oncogene product latent membrane protein 1 engages the tumor necrosis factor receptor-associated death domain protein to mediate B lymphocyte growth transformation and activate NF-kappaB. *Proc Natl Acad Sci U S A* 1997;94:12592–12597.
15. Eliopoulos AG, Dawson CW, Mosialos G, et al. CD40-induced growth inhibition in epithelial cells is mimicked by Epstein-Barr virus-encoded LMP1: involvement of TRAF3 as a common mediator. *Oncogene* 1996;13:2243–2254.
16. Stuart AD, Stewart JP, Arrand JR, Mackett M. The Epstein-Barr virus encoded cytokine viral interleukin-10 enhances transformation of human B lymphocytes. *Oncogene* 1995;11:1711–1719.
17. Moore KW, O'Garra A, de Waal M, Vieira P, Mosmann TR. Interleukin-10. *Annu Rev Immunol* 1993;11:165–190.
18. Caux C, Massacrier C, Vanbervliet B, Barthelemy C, Liu YJ, Banchereau J. Interleukin 10 inhibits T cell alloreaction induced by human dendritic cells. *Int Immunol* 1994;6:1177–1185.
19. Nazaruk RA, Rochford R, Hobbs MV, Cannon MJ. Functional diversity of the CD8+ T-cell response to Epstein-Barr virus (EBV): implications for the pathogenesis of EBV-associated lymphoproliferative disorders. *Blood* 1998;91:3875–3883.
20. Mathur A, Kamat D, Filipovitch A, Steinbuch M, Shapiro R. Immunoregulatory abnormalities in patients with Epstein-Barr virus-associated B cell lymphoproliferative disorders. *Transplantation* 1994;57:1042–1045.
21. O'Reilly RJ, Small TN, Papadopoulos E, Lucas K, Lacerda J, Koulova L. Biology and adoptive cell therapy of Epstein-Barr virus-associated lymphoproliferative disorders in recipients of marrow allografts. *Immunol Rev* 1997;157:195–216.
22. Peniket AJ, Perry AR, Williams CD, et al. A case of EBV-associated lymphoproliferative disease following high-dose therapy and CD34-purified autologous peripheral blood progenitor transplantation. *Bone Marrow Transplant* 1998;22:307–309.
23. Briz M, Fores R, Regidor C, et al. Epstein-Barr virus associated B-cell lymphoma after autologous bone marrow transplantation for T-cell acute lymphoblastic leukemia. *Br J Haematol* 1997;98:485–487.
24. Buckingham SC, Benaim E, Sandlund JT, et al. Primary central nervous system lymphoma in a child with acute B-cell lymphoblastic leukaemia: consecutive Epstein-Barr virus-related malignancies. *Br J Haematol* 1998;101:345–348.
25. Deeg HJ, Socie G. Malignancies after hemopoietic stem cell transplantation: many questions, some answers. *Blood* 1998;91:1833–1844.
26. Heslop HE, Rooney CM. Adoptive immunotherapy of EBV lymphoproliferative diseases. *Immunol Rev* 1997;157:217–222.
27. Gerritsen EJ, Stam ED, Hermans J, et al. Risk factors for developing EBV-related B cell lymphoproliferative disorders (BLPD) after non-HLA-identical BMT in children. *Bone Marrow Transplant* 1996;18:377–382.
28. Hale G, Waldmann H, for CAMPATH users. Risks of developing Epstein-Barr virus-related lymphoproliferative disorders after T-cell-depleted marrow transplants. *Blood* 1998;91:3079–3083.
29. Gross TG, Hinrichs SH, Davis JR, Mitchell D, Bishop MR, Wagner JE. Depletion of EBV-infected cells in donor marrow by counterflow elutriation. *Exp Hematol* 1998;26:395–399.
30. Cavazzana-Calvo M, Bensoussan D, Jabado N, et al. Prevention of EBV-induced B-lymphoproliferative disorder by ex vivo marrow B-cell depletion in HLA-phenoidentical or non-identical T-depleted bone marrow transplantation. *Br J Haematol* 1998;103:543–551.
31. Swinnen LJ. Treatment of organ transplant-related lymphoma. *Hematol Oncol Clin North Am* 1998;11:963–973.

virus (EBV)-specific cytotoxic T lymphocytes that lyse Reed-Sternberg cells: implications for immune-mediated therapy of EBV Hodgkin's disease. *Blood* 1997;89:1978–1986.

75. Knecht H, Bachmann E, Joske JL. Molecular analysis of the LMP (latent membrane protein) in Hodgkin's disease. *Leukemia* 1993;7:580–584.

76. Knecht H, Bachmann E, Brousset P, et al. Deletions within the LMP1 oncogene of EBV are clustered in Hodgkin's disease and identical to those observed in nasopharyngeal carcinoma. *Blood* 1993;82: 2937–2942.

77. Swaminathan S, Tomkinson B, Kieff E. Recombinant Epstein-Barr virus with small RNA (EBER) genes deleted transforms lymphocytes and replicates *in vitro*. *Proc Natl Acad Sci U S A* 1991;88:1546–1548.

78. Zeidler R, Eissner G, Meissner P, et al. Down-regulation of TAP1 in B lymphocytes by cellular and Epstein-Barr virus-encoded interleukin-10. *Blood* 1997;90:2390–2397.

79. Khanna R, Burrows SR, Steigerwald-Mullen PM, Moss DJ, Kurilla MG, Cooper L. Targeting Epstein-Barr virus nuclear antigen 1 (EBNA1) through the class II pathway restores immune recognition by EBNA1-specific cytotoxic T lymphocytes: evidence for HLA-DM-independent processing. *Int Immunol* 1997;9:1537–1543.

80. Khanna R, Burrows SR, Thomson SA, et al. Class I processing-defective Burkitt's lymphoma cells are recognized efficiently by CD4+ EBV-specific CTLs. *J Immunol* 1997;158:3619–3625.

81. Tao Q, Robertson KD, Manns A, Hildesheim A, Ambinder RF. Epstein-Barr virus (EBV) in endemic Burkitt's lymphoma: molecular analysis of primary tumor tissue [published erratum appears in *Blood* 1998;91(8):3091]. *Blood* 1998;91:1373–1381.

82. Sugiura M, Imai S, Tokunaga M, et al. Transcriptional analysis of Epstein-Barr virus gene expression in EBV-positive gastric carcinoma: unique viral latency in the tumour cells. *Br J Cancer* 1996;74:625–631.

83. Aozasa K, Ohsawa M, Tomita Y, Tagawa S, Yamamura T. Polymorphic reticulosis is a neoplasm of large granular lymphocytes with CD3+ phenotype [see comments]. *Cancer* 1995;75:894–901.

84. Chiang AK, Tao Q, Srivastava G, Ho FC. Nasal NK- and T-cell lymphomas share the same type of Epstein-Barr virus latency as nasopharyngeal carcinoma and Hodgkin's disease. *Int J Cancer* 1996;68:285–290.

85. Horenstein MG, Nador RG, Chadburn A, et al. Epstein-Barr virus latent gene expression in primary effusion lymphomas containing Kaposi's sarcoma-associated herpesvirus/human herpesvirus-8. *Blood* 1997;90:1186–1191.

86. Raab-Traub N, Rajadurai P, Flynn K, Lanier AP. Epstein-Barr virus infection in carcinoma of the salivary gland. *J Virol* 1991;65: 7032–7036.

87. Pallesen G, Hamilton-Dutoit SJ, Rowe M, Young LS. Expression of Epstein-Barr virus latent gene products in tumour cells of Hodgkin's disease. *Lancet* 1991;337:320–322.

88. Gilligan KJ, Rajadurai P, Lin JC, et al. Expression of the Epstein-Barr virus BamHI A fragment in nasopharyngeal carcinoma: evidence for a viral protein expressed *in vivo*. *J Virol* 1991;65: 6252–6259.

89. Chen CL, Sadler RH, Walling DM, Su IJ, Hsieh HC, Raab-Traub N. Epstein-Barr virus (EBV) gene expression in EBV-positive peripheral T-cell lymphomas. *J Virol* 1993;67:6303–6308.

90. Patton DF, Ribeiro RC, Jenkins JJ, Sixbey JW. Thymic carcinoma with a defective Epstein-Barr virus encoding the BZLF1 trans-activator. *J Infect Dis* 1994;170:7–12.

91. Aozasa K. Pyothorax-associated lymphoma. *Int J Hematol* 1996;65: 9–16.

92. Niedobitek G, Agathanggelou A, Herbst H, Whitehead L, Wright DH, Young LS. Epstein-Barr virus (EBV) infection in infectious mononucleosis: virus latency, replication and phenotype of EBV-infected cells. *J Pathol* 1997;182:151–159.

93. Oudejans JJ, Jiwa M, van den Brule AJ, et al. Detection of heterogeneous Epstein-Barr virus gene expression patterns within individual post-transplantation lymphoproliferative disorders. *Am J Pathol* 1995;147:923–933.

94. Jones DT, Monroy D, Ji Z, Atherton SS, Pflugfelder SC. Sjogren's syndrome: cytokine and Epstein-Barr viral gene expression within the conjunctival epithelium. *Invest Ophthalmol Vis Sci* 1994;35:3493–3504.

95. Ohsawa M, Tomita Y, Hashimoto M, Yasunaga Y, Kanno H, Aozasa K. Malignant lymphoma of the adrenal gland: its possible correlation with the Epstein-Barr virus. *Mod Pathol* 1996;9:534–543.

96. Casper J, Camitta B, Truitt R, et al. Unrelated bone marrow donor transplants for children with leukemia or myelodysplasia. *Blood* 1995;85:2354–2363.

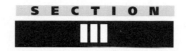

PRINCIPLES AND PRACTICE
OF MONOCLONAL
ANTIBODY THERAPY

MONOCLONAL ANTIBODIES: BASIC PRINCIPLES

Basic Concepts and Antigens Recognized

KENNETH A. FOON

This chapter is designed to overview basic concepts of monoclonal antibody diagnosis and therapy. The focus of this chapter is on those targeted antigens that have been used in the clinic for diagnostic and therapeutic applications. Monoclonal antibodies have emerged as the dominant reagent for *in vitro* diagnostics and immunohistopathology. Serologic assays, such as carcinoembryonic antigen (CEA) levels, CA125, and the prostate-specific antigen, are such examples. Monoclonal antibody reagents are used for flow cytometry in immunodiagnostic laboratories and for immunohistochemistry and have a critical role in the classification of leukemias and lymphomas.

MONOCLONAL ANTIBODIES FOR DIAGNOSIS AND THERAPY

The concept of monoclonal antibody–guided therapy and diagnosis has been studied for more than 20 years. One of the major limitations for *in vivo* diagnostics and therapeutics has been that murine antibodies generate immune response in immunocompetent patients. Therefore, the vast majority of patients injected with murine antibodies generate immunity that neutralizes the antibodies for future injections. A variety of strategies to overcome this obstacle are discussed in the section Genetic Engineering of Monoclonal Antibodies.

Another feature of the immunoglobulin molecule is size. Comparisons of the intact immunoglobulin G (IgG) and the F(ab')$_2$, Fab, and sFv molecules have been studied in animal models (Fig. 1). The concept is that the smaller molecules leave the circulation more rapidly and penetrate tumors more evenly than the whole immunoglobulin (1). The longer residence in the blood of whole IgG, however, has advantages in that the longer the antibody is in the blood, the greater opportunity for delivery of a higher percent of the injected dose to the tumor. This might be an advantage for unlabeled antibodies, but for the purposes of delivering radiolabeled antibodies to tumor, smaller molecules appear to be advantageous. Radiolabeled

F(ab')$_2$, Fab, and sFv are cleared from the bloodstream much more rapidly than the whole immunoglobulin, and this should lead to less bone marrow toxicity. The more rapid serum clearance, however, could lead to less uptake in the tumor. Another approach for more rapid clearance of the immunoglobulin is to remove the CH2 domain (Fig. 2), which allows the immunoglobulin to clear from the bloodstream more quickly than the intact IgG (2,3). Other characteristics of the various immunoglobulin molecules are that the Fab$_2$, Fab, and sFv molecules accumulate in kidney tubules; IgG does not accumulate in the kidneys (4). These patterns must be considered when conjugating antibodies to toxins, drugs, and isotopes.

Antibody administration has typically been by the intravenous route. Other approaches have been considered—in particular, the peritoneal route when tumors are primarily confined to the peritoneal cavity, such as ovarian cancer. The peritoneal route targets smaller peritoneal tumors more efficiently than does the intravenous route, and also the injected dose per gram in the blood pool is reduced, leading to potentially less systemic toxicity (5).

A variety of toxins, radionuclide drugs, and cytokines have been coupled to monoclonal antibodies. Diagnostic isotopes, such as indium-111 (^{111}In) and technetium-99m (^{99m}Tc) conjugated to monoclonal antibodies, have been used in clinical trials (6–9). For the intraoperative hand-held probe, iodine-125–labeled monoclonal antibodies are typically used (10). Most therapeutic trials have included iodine-131 (^{131}I)–labeled monoclonal antibodies because of its low cost, wide availability, and relatively simple chemistry. Disadvantages of ^{131}I include its long-range gamma emissions requiring lead-lined rooms and longer inpatient treatment. In addition, iodine is volatile and special hood precautions are required. Other isotopes, such as yttrium 90, lutetium-177, and rhenium-186, offer advantages because of the abundance of beta-emitting versus gamma-emitting energy. Patients can be treated as outpatients and special precautions are less stringent. Alpha emitters, such as bismuth-212 and copper-67, which have short half-lives and short path lengths, also have distinctive advantages. A variety of linker

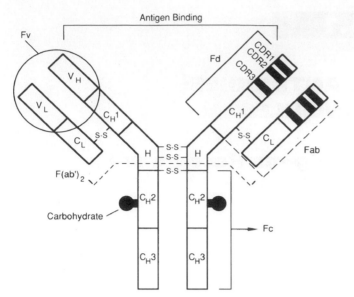

FIGURE 1. Binding regions and domains of an immunoglobulin molecule.

chemistries have been developed to couple these isotopes to monoclonal antibodies. No ideal isotope or linker system exists, and a variety of approaches continue to be studied.

Ricin is probably the most widely studied toxin conjugated to monoclonal antibodies. Ricin has both an A and B chain. The B chain is responsible for binding cell receptors but can be removed so that the A chain is coupled directly to the monoclonal antibody. Other toxins that have been studied in animal models and in the clinic include gelonin, saporin, and *Pseudomonas* exotoxin. Patients recognize these toxins as foreign, however, and antitoxin immune responses are common. Antibodies coupled to chemotherapy agents are also under investigation but

have been less successful in animal models. Passive immunotherapy with unconjugated or naked monoclonal antibodies has been focused primarily on chimerized or humanized antibodies. Two monoclonal antibodies approved for therapy by the U.S. Food and Drug Administration are rituximab, which is a human-chimerized anti-CD20 antibody (11,12) used for the treatment of follicular low-grade lymphomas, and herceptin, a humanized anti-Her-2/neu antibody, which is used in combination with chemotherapy for the treatment of advanced breast cancer (13). Unlabeled murine monoclonal antibodies are being studied in the clinic in the form of antiidiotype antibodies to generate active immunity in patients. This is discussed in the section Antiidiotype Monoclonal Antibodies.

TUMOR-ASSOCIATED ANTIGENS

This section focuses on three separate areas of tumor-associated antigens: (a) epithelial tumor–associated antigens, (b) melanoma-associated antigens, and (c) hematopoietic tumor–associated antigens. The antigens that are focused on are those that are most commonly used in clinical and laboratory studies.

Epithelial Tumor–Associated Antigens

The Her-2/neu oncogene protein is a member of the tyrosine kinase family of growth factor receptors (14,15). It is frequently overexpressed in adenocarcinomas of the breast, ovary, and colorectum and other histologies for which overexpression appears to correlate with a poor prognosis (16). A number of studies have demonstrated the importance of Her-2/neu in the tumorigenic and metastatic phenotype (17–19). It has therefore become an attractive target for cancer immunotherapy. A small subset of patients develop IgG antibody responses to Her-2/neu and, in some cases, CD4⁺ T-cell responses have been demonstrated

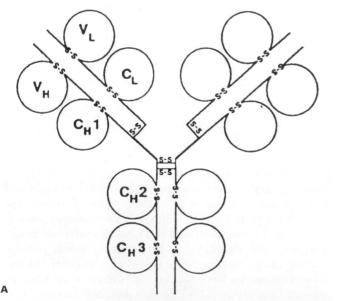

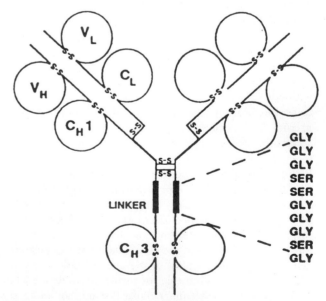

FIGURE 2. Diagram of an intact immunoglobulin molecule **(A)** and CH2 domain–deleted molecule **(B)**.

(20,21). Herceptin is a humanized monoclonal antibody that has been approved by the U.S. Food and Drug Administration for treatment of metastatic breast cancer (13). Her-2/neu is a growth factor receptor and herceptin mediates cell killing by apoptosis.

Another antigen that has been commonly targeted for immunotherapy is the nonsecreted MR40,000 glycoprotein CD17-1A antigen, which is overexpressed on most epithelial tumors. The murine monoclonal antibody that binds to this antigen, designated *171A*, is an IgG2A antibody that has been studied in patients with a variety of cancers, particularly colorectal cancers. Rare clinical responses have been described after the intravenous infusion of unlabeled murine 171A antibody in patients with metastatic disease (22–24). The mechanism remains unknown, but it has been hypothesized that responses were secondary to activation of the idiotypic network or antibody-dependent cellular cytotoxicity (ADCC), or both.

The most impressive and important 171A clinical trial was reported in 189 patients with Dukes' C colorectal cancer who were assigned to postoperative observation or treatment with 500 mg of 171A antibody, followed by four 100-mg monthly infusions. After a median follow-up of 7 years, the antibody-treated patients had an improved survival by 30% over patients in the control arm (25,26). Studies are underway in the United States and Europe to confirm these results.

The murine monoclonal antibody L6 is an IgG2A antibody that binds to a poorly characterized antigen on adenocarcinoma cells and is expressed on more than 90% of breast, colorectal, and non–small-cell lung cancer (27,28). This antibody has also been shown to mediate ADCC and complement-dependent cytotoxicity. Unlabeled chimeric antibody did not have clinical responses, whereas responses were seen in three of four patients treated with ^{131}I-labeled chimeric L6 (29).

Monoclonal antibody D612 is a murine IgG2A antibody directed at a membrane glycoprotein expressed on gastrointestinal tumors (30,31). This antibody has also been shown to mediate ADCC and its effects could be enhanced when combined with macrophage colony-stimulating factor (32).

TAG72 is expressed on most epithelial tumors, including colorectal cancer, ovarian cancer, and prostate cancer. The B72.3 monoclonal antibody binds to TAG72 and has been studied in a number of clinical trials. ^{111}In-B72.3, termed *Oncoscint*, has been approved for commercial use for the detection of colorectal cancer (6–8). This immunoconjugate was demonstrated to improve the detection of intraabdominal sites of tumor over computed axial tomography of the abdomen and pelvis.

The CEA gene has been sequenced and is part of the human immunoglobulin supergene family located on chromosome 19 (33,34). CEA is highly expressed on colorectal cancers and a variety of other epithelial cancers and is thought to be involved in cell–cell interactions. CEA is considered an adhesion molecule and may play an important role in the metastatic process by mediating attachment of tumor cells to normal cells (35,36). CEA has been a target for passive immunotherapy by monoclonal antibodies, monoclonal antibody imaging, as well as vaccine therapy. A Fab' antibody fragment of an anti-CEA antibody, designated *IMMU-4*, labeled with ^{99m}Tc has been approved commercially for radioimaging colorectal cancer (9).

Similar to ^{111}In-B72.3, ^{99m}Tc-IMMU-4 Fab' was superior to conventional diagnostic modalities in the extrahepatic abdomen and pelvis and complemented conventional modalities in the liver.

MUC1 is a highly glycosylated high-molecular protein abundantly expressed in human cancer of epithelial origin (37–39). The MUC1 gene is overexpressed and aberrantly glycosylated in a variety of cancers, including colorectal cancer, breast cancer, and ovarian cancer. Much of the glycosylation is found within regions of tandemly repeated sequences of 20 amino acids per repeat (40–42). Tumors derived from cells of epithelial origin often lose the carbohydrate side chains exposing the tandemly repeated protein core, resulting in antigenically active epitopes exposed to the cell surface membrane (40). A closely related antigen is the human milk fat globule antigen, which has the same tandemly repeated sequences of 20 amino acids as MUC1 (43). Both of these antigens have been the target of passive serotherapy, radioimmunoimaging, and vaccine therapies.

The monoclonal antibody OVB3 reacts with an ovarian cancer–associated antigen and has been linked to the pseudomonas exotoxin (44). Dose-limiting toxicity occurred as a result of reactivity with neural tissues, and no responses were reported.

A variety of clinical trials using antiferritin monoclonal antibodies and polyclonal sera have been reported for patients with hepatocellular carcinoma (45,46). Shrinkage of unresectable tumors has been reported.

A number of trials have been reported for monoclonal antibodies that target to the epithelial growth factor receptor (47,48). The epithelial growth factor receptor, similar to Her-2/neu, is a growth factor receptor and, therefore, binding to this receptor leads to apoptosis.

Melanoma Tumor–Associated Antigens

Gangliosides are sialic acid–containing glycosphingolipids and have increased surface membrane expression on cancers of neuroectodermal origin, including malignant melanoma. A number of immunotherapy studies have been targeted to gangliosides (49,50). The R24 antibody that targets the disialoganglioside GD3 has been the most widely studied with seven partial responses and one complete response among 58 patients (51–54). No response was reported among eight patients treated with the MG21 antibody that also recognizes the disialoganglioside GD3 (55). A number of studies with the disialoganglioside GD2 either alone or combined with R24 also reported two partial responses among nine patients with the 3F8 anti-GD2 antibody, but none of the other studies reported responses (56–58). Four partial and seven complete responses were reported, however, using the L72 antibody that also recognizes the disialoganglioside GD2 when injected intralesionally (59,60). Similar results were reported with intralesional injections of antibodies that bind to the GM2 and GM3 gangliosides (61,62). The high-molecular-weight melanoma-associated antigen, designated *mCSP*, is identified by a number of monoclonal antibodies, including 9.2.27. No responses were reported among 21 patients treated with intravenous therapy (63–65). Melanoma vaccines generated to a variety of melanoma-associated antigens recognized by T lymphocytes are presented in another chapter.

Hematopoietic Tumor–Associated Antigens

A variety of antigens that identify antigens on non-Hodgkin's lymphoma have been used as unlabeled monoclonal antibodies. The antigens targeted are the CD19, CD20, and CD22 antigens; the CD5 antigen has been targeted for chronic lymphocytic leukemia (CLL) and cutaneous T-cell lymphoma and the CD25 antigen [interleukin-2 (IL-2) receptor] has been targeted for certain non-Hodgkin's lymphoma and adult T-cell leukemia (66–72). Rare responses have been reported using these unlabeled murine antibodies. Antiidiotype antibodies that are custom made for individual patients that target the immunoglobulin on the surface of B-cell lymphomas have also been used as therapeutics. Antiidiotypes have been the most successful form of unlabeled murine monoclonal antibody therapy in that 40% of patients respond to antiidiotype antibodies with approximately 10% complete responses (73,74). Because of the difficulty of tailor-making individual antibodies for patients, this approach has largely been abandoned.

The most successful trials with unlabeled antibodies have been with chimerized and humanized antibodies. The anti-CD20 chimerized antibody rituximab has been the most extensively studied unconjugated antibody, and is the only antibody approved for therapy by the U.S. Food and Drug Administration for lymphomas (11,12). This antibody consists of a murine variable region from the parent antibody grafted onto a human IgG1 constant region backbone. The CD20 antigen is a more ideal target for unconjugated antibody therapy because it is not expressed on precursor B cells or stem cells but has high-density expression on mature B cells, including malignant B cells. CD20 does not shed and does not undergo modulation after antibody binding. *In vitro* data suggest that rituximab binding to CD20 may trigger apoptosis, as well as mediate complement-dependent cytoxicity and ADCC. Patients with follicular center cell low-grade lymphomas respond to rituximab in the 50% range with approximately 10% complete responses. Another monoclonal antibody that has been studied in the clinic is CAMPATH-1, which targets the CD52 antigen that is expressed on lymphocytes, monocytes, and granulocytes, but is not found on stem cells. The humanized version of this antibody, designated *CAMPATH-1H*, has shown responses in CLL and lymphoma (75–77).

Antibodies conjugated to radioisotopes have had considerable success. The most impressive responses have been with the ^{131}I-labeled anti-B1, which is an anti-CD20 antibody (78–81). Complete responses were reported in the majority of previously treated lymphoma patients. Another promising antibody is Lym-1, which binds to a DR-related antigen. ^{131}I-labeled Lym-1 therapy had excellent responses in the majority of treated lymphoma patients (82). Similar responses have been reported for ^{131}I-labeled OKB7 and LL2 (83,84).

Immunotoxins involve the linkage of monoclonal antibodies to a protein toxin. Growth factors and other ligands, such as IL-2, can also carry toxins (85,86). Toxins, such as ricin and diphtheria toxin, are natural products that disrupt protein synthesis. Immunotoxins must be internalized after antigen binding to allow the toxin entry into the cytosol for cell death. One methodology to fuse the toxin protein to the monoclonal antibody is to eliminate the binding domain of the toxin and to link the toxic domain directly to the antibody. Thus, without the nonspecific binding domain of the native protein, the antibody directs the toxin to the tumor cell. Another approach is to retain but modify the binding domain (87). An alternative approach is to fuse the DNA sequences that encode a toxin to the DNA elements that encode the antigen-binding site (Fv). This creates a small molecule that retains binding and cytotoxic properties (88–90). Clinical trials with immunotoxins have shown tumor cell cytoreduction in a variety of hematologic malignancies but with limited responses (91–95). Toxicity is characterized by a vascular leak syndrome with peripheral and pulmonary edema, hypotension, and hypoalbuminemia (91,92). There is also a high incidence of host immune responses to the antibody and the toxin.

More limited literature exists on monoclonal antibody studies with unconjugated and radiolabeled antibodies for the treatment of acute myelogenous leukemia (AML). In one trial, using the unlabeled humanized HuM195 antibody that targets the CD33 antigen, one of 13 patients had a transient clinical response with decreased circulating blasts (96). ^{131}I-labeled monoclonal antibody M195 demonstrated three complete responses among 24 AML and blastic chronic myelogenous leukemia patients treated with antibody alone (97). When combined as a conditioning regimen with chemotherapy before allogeneic bone marrow transplantation, 18 of 19 patients had complete remissions (98).

IMMUNE FLOW CYTOMETRY

Immune flow cytometry using monoclonal antibodies has become a critical tool in the diagnosis of leukemias and lymphomas. Correlating immunophenotype with molecular and cytogenetic data has delineated biologically important subgroups. This data was reviewed by Jennings and Foon in 1997 and is briefly discussed (99). Critical requirements for flow cytometry are viable cells that can be prepared in a single-cell suspension. This, of course, is not a problem for liquid tumors that invade the peripheral blood and bone marrow, but it may be a problem for certain solid tumors where it is more difficult to prepare single-cell suspensions. Lymphomas have generally not been a problem, even when they do not invade the peripheral blood and bone marrow, as a lymph node is more easily separated into a single-cell suspension. For AML, the critical antigenic markers that differentiate the Fab subtypes M0, M1, M2, M3, M4, M5, M6, and M7 include DR, CD13, CD14, CD15, CD33, and CD34. These markers help differentiate myeloid from monocytic leukemias. The M7 megakaryoblastic leukemia is differentiated by the CD41 and CD61 platelet-associated antigens. Detection of the cytoplasmic enzyme myeloperoxidase is more sensitive than CD13 and CD33 combined to detect AML, and may be particularly useful in differentiating M0 from acute lymphoblastic leukemia (ALL) (100). For the B-cell ALL, the critical markers are DR, CD10, CD19, CD20, CD22, CD24, and CD34. Markers for surface and cytoplasmic immunoglobulin differentiate more mature from more primitive B cells. T-

ALL is differentiated by T-cell antigens, which include CD1, CD2, cytoplasmic and surface membrane CD3, CD5, CD7, CD4, CD8, CD10, and CD34. Using combinations of the above markers, it is extremely rare for ALL to be confused with AML. To differentiate the B-lymphoproliferative disorders, the same monoclonal antibodies that differentiate the B-cell ALL are used. Subtle differences exist between some of these disorders. For instance, CLL shares many of the same markers with mantle cell lymphoma, including the B-cell antigens, CD19, CD20, and the putative T-cell antigen CD5. In mantle cell lymphoma, however, the CD5 antigen, as well as CD20, are much more intensely expressed than is typically seen with CLL. Follicular lymphomas typically express B-cell markers in addition to CD10, which is not typically expressed by the other B-lymphoproliferative disorders. Hairy cell leukemia expresses B-cell markers but also expresses CD103, which is unique to hairy cell leukemia among the B-cell disorders. T-cell lymphoproliferative disorders also incorporate the same surface markers as T-ALL, but again, subtle differences may differentiate subclassifications. For instance, adult T-cell leukemia lymphoma expresses the T-cell markers CD3, CD4, and CD5, but also have a bright CD25 expression, which is uncommon for the other T-cell malignancies. Natural killer cell lymphocytic leukemias are subclassified by their expression of the natural killer–associated antigens CD16, CD56, and CD57.

IMMUNOHISTOCHEMISTRY

Traditional morphology is not always adequate for poorly differentiated tumors. For decades, pathologists have relied on histochemical techniques to differentiate a variety of tumors using enzymes, mucin, reticulum, and so forth. Monoclonal antibodies have greatly expanded this specificity. This section only presents examples of some of the more useful differentiation markers studied by immunohistochemistry, and the reader is referred to reference 101.

One common problem is diagnosing poorly differentiated lymphomas and carcinomas. The leukocyte common antigens distinguish hematopoietic malignancies from nonhematopoietic malignancies (102). A variety of antibodies that can be used in paraffin-embedded tissue to differentiate lymphomas have been described, including L26, which identifies the CD20 antigen common to B-cell malignancies (103). Immunoglobulins are the most reliable B-cell markers and can be used in paraffin-embedded tissue. CD3 identifies the T-cell receptor (104) and differentiates T-cell malignancies. Leu-M1 identifies the CD15 antigen common to Reed-Sternberg cells (105), CD30 identifies the Ki-1 antigen found in Reed-Sternberg cells and anaplastic large-cell lymphoma cells. Anti-T6 (CD1a) reacts with cortical thymocytes and Langerhans' cells and identifies Langerhans' tumors (106).

Common epithelial tumor antigens include the epithelial membrane antigen (107), keratin (108,109), and CEA (110). Monoclonal antibodies against lung tumor cells may be useful in differentiating lung cancers and may also be useful for the detection of metastasis. For example, the monoclonal antibody SM-1 reacts with small-cell carcinoma of the lung and can be

TABLE 1. GENETIC MODIFICATION OF THE IMMUNOGLOBULIN MOLECULE

Recombinant Immunoglobulin	Purpose
Chimeric	Reduce immunogenicity
CDR grafting	
Veneering	
Phage display technology	
Deletions in At 2 domain	Alter size
F(ab')2 or Fab'	
sFv	
Hinge alterations	Increase affinity
CDR modification	
Changes in glycosylation	

CDR, complementarity-determining regions.

used to detect bone marrow metastasis (111). The HMB-45 is widely used in the diagnosis of malignant melanoma (112). This antibody reacts with immature melanosomes and stains cutaneous melanocytes, retinal pigment epithelium, and melanocytic tumors (113). Antibodies to the S100 protein identify malignant melanoma, neurogenic tumors, chondrosarcomas, meningiomas, tumors of the breast and salivary glands, and neuroendocrine tumors. The demonstration of S100 protein, vimentin, and HMB-45 in the absence of staining for keratin distinguishes malignant melanoma from poorly differentiated carcinomas (114). Some antigens, such as prostate-specific antigen and thyroglobulin, are specific markers for prostate cancer and thyroid cancer, respectively.

GENETIC ENGINEERING OF MONOCLONAL ANTIBODIES

Genetically modifying murine immunoglobulin molecules to enhance desired characteristics and eliminate undesirable characteristics is common practice (115–117). One approach is chimerization of the immunoglobulin molecules in which the murine variable region is linked to a human Fc molecule. This involves the inclusion of possible immunogenic mouse sequences (Table 1). Another approach is CDR grafting in which the six murine hypervariable regions or CDRs are grafted onto a human antibody (118–120). This procedure may lead to loss of affinity. A second approach involves veneering the murine immunoglobulin (121). The murine sequences of the immunoglobulin molecule are analyzed via computer programs, and potential sequences distinguishing mouse from human immunoglobulins are eliminated and substituted with human-like sequences. Another approach is the derivation of completely human antibodies with an expected minimal immunogenicity in humans using phage-display technology (122). Repertoires of human sFv or Fab fragments are cloned for display on the surface of filamentous phage, and antigen-specific "phage antibodies" are enriched on immobilized antigen (123). From libraries of millions to a few billion antibody fragments derived from an IgM pool of naïve human B cells, it is possible to isolate high-affinity human antibodies. One approach to enhance this methodology is using cells from patients that are immunized with specific tumor-associated gene products. Another approach to generate human antibodies is to use transgenic mice that generate human immunoglobulin. These animals can be immunized with any desired antigen.

Another advantage of genetic manipulation of monoclonal antibodies is to alter pharmacokinetic properties, metabolic properties, and affinity. Advantages may exist for immunoglobulins to have shorter half-lives, which would lead to more rapid clearance from the body, more rapid tumor penetrance and, possibly, lower immunogenicity. Deleting the CH2 domain (see Fig. 2) results in enhanced clearance of immunoglobulin from the plasma with a limited loss of tumor uptake (2,3). sFv molecules (Fig. 3) have the advantage of reduced size, more rapid clearance, and better tumor penetration (4,124). Other genetic modifications include hinge modifications, modifications of single domains, and alterations in V regions.

Another genetic modification is ligating of genes coding for various biologic response modifiers to the immunoglobulin molecules. Molecules such as interferon-α, interferon-γ, and IL-6 upregulate certain tumor antigens. Such molecules have been constructed using IL-2. Engineering recombinant Fv immunotoxins was reviewed by Reiter and Pastan in 1996 (125). The antigen-binding and targeting domains in recombinant immunotoxins are typically single-chain sFv or Fab connected by a flexible peptide binder and fused directly to a bacterial toxin. Because of problems with stability and binding of some sFv immunotoxins, new recombinant Fv immunotoxins have been developed, in which the targeting variables of the Fv are stabilized by an interchain disulfide bond located in framework positions of the V_H and V_L domains.

ANTIIDIOTYPE MONOCLONAL ANTIBODIES

The idiotype network hypothesis of Lindenmann (126) and Jerne (127) offers an elegant approach to transforming epitope structures into idiotypic determinants expressed on the surface of antibodies. According to the network concept, immunization with a given tumor-associated antigen will generate production of antibodies against this tumor-associated antigen, which are termed *Ab1*; Ab1 is then used to generate a series of antiidiotype antibodies against the Ab1, termed *Ab2*. Some of these Ab2 molecules can effectively mimic the three-dimensional structure of the tumor-associated antigen identified by the Ab1. These particular antibodies, called *Ab2β*, fit into the paratopes of Ab1 and express the internal image of the tumor-associated antigen. The Ab2β can induce specific immune responses similar to those induced by the original tumor-associated antigen and, therefore, can be used as surrogate tumor-associated antigens. Immunization with Ab2 can lead to the generation of anti-

antiidiotypic antibodies (Ab3) that recognize the corresponding original tumor-associated antigen identified by Ab1. Because of this Ab1-like reactivity, the Ab3 is also called *Ab1'* to indicate that it might differ in its other idiotopes from Ab1. The putative immune pathways for antiidiotype vaccines are presented in Figure 4. The antiidiotype antibody represents an exogenous protein that should be endocytosed by antigen-presenting cells and degraded to 14- to 25-MER peptides to be presented by class II antigens to activate CD4 helper T cells. Activated Th2 CD4 helper T cells secrete cytokines, such as IL-4, which stimulate B cells that have been directly activated by the Ab3 to produce antibody that binds to the original antigen identified by the Ab1. In addition, activation of Th1 CD4 helper T cells secrete cytokines that activate T cells, macrophages, and natural killer cells, which directly lyse tumor cells and, in addition, contribute to ADCC. Th1 cytokines, such as IL-2, also contribute to the activation of a CD8 cytotoxic T-cell response. This represents a second putative pathway of endocytosed antiidiotype antibody. The antiidiotype antibody may be degraded to 9/10-MER peptides to present in the context of class I antigens to activate CD8 cytotoxic T cells (128,129), which are also stimulated by the IL-2 from Th1 CD4 helper T cells.

Several antiidiotype antibodies that mimic tumor-associated antigens on colorectal cancer cells have been reported. One such antibody was generated against the murine 17-1A antibody, described in the section Epithelial Tumor–Associated Antigens. After surgery for colorectal cancer, six patients were immunized with this human antiidiotype antibody, which mimics the GA733-2 antigen (130). All of the patients developed a long-lasting T-cell immunity against GA733-2 and five mounted a specific IgG antibody response against GA733. Another group, using a rat antiidiotype antibody generated to the 17-1A antibody, immunized nine colorectal cancer patients with aluminum hydroxide–precipitated 17-1A; none of the nine patients developed specific antibodies, although four patients developed delayed-type hypersensitivity (131). Another group of investigators has developed both murine and human monoclonal antiidiotype antibodies that mimic the gp72 antigen (132–135). They demonstrated delayed-type hypersensitivity reactions when murine antiidiotype antibody was injected without adjuvant (135). When the antiidiotype was linked to keyhole limpet hemocyanin in the presence of Freund's adjuvant, anti-gp72 antibodies were detected. Using the human equivalent antiidiotype antibody precipitated in aluminum hydroxide, 9 of 13 patients with advanced colorectal cancer produced blastogenic responses to gp72-expressing tumor cells or produced detectable levels of IL-2 in their plasma (133). They suggested that survival correlated with immune responses. In another study with the same human antiidiotype antibody, six patients with rectal cancer were immunized preoperatively (134). This study demonstrated significant killing of autologous tumor cells using cryopreserved lymphocytes or lymph node cells from patients 1 to 2 weeks postimmunization.

CeaVac is an antiidiotype murine monoclonal antibody to an antibody designated *8019*, which identifies a specific epitope on CEA that is highly restricted to tumor cells and is not found on normal tissues (136). CeaVac generated antiidiotypic (Ab3)

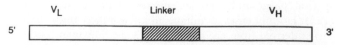

FIGURE 3. Single-chain antigen-binding protein (sFv) shows a linker connecting the V_L and V_H.

Potential Immune Pathways for Anti-Idiotype Vaccines

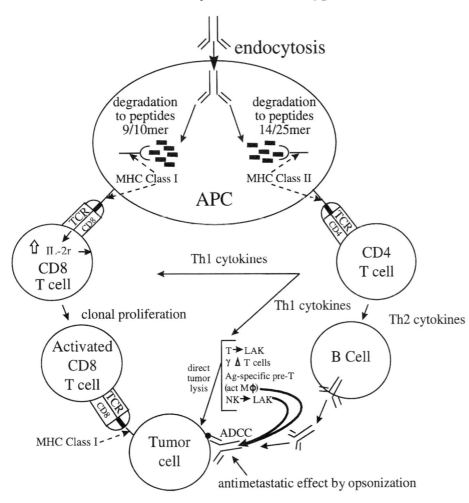

FIGURE 4. Antiidiotype antibodies are endocytosed by antigen-presenting cells (APCs). They may be degraded to 14/25-MER peptides and presented on major histocompatibility complex (MHC) class II molecules to CD4 helper T cells. Activated Th2 CD4 helper T cells secrete Th2 cytokines that stimulate B cells that have been directly activated by the antiidiotype antibody to produce the anti-antiidiotypic antibody or Ab3 (Ab1') that binds directly to tumor cells. This antibody can mediate complement- and antibody-dependent cellular cytotoxicity (ADCC), as well as a direct antimetastatic effect by opsonization. In addition, Th1 CD4 helper T cells secrete Th1 cytokines that activate T cells, natural killer cells, and macrophages. The activated macrophages and lymphokine-activated killer (LAK) cells may also serve as effector cells for ADCC. All of these cells may mediate direct tumor lysis. Data also suggest that exogenously processed proteins can be degraded to 9/10-MER peptides that can be presented by MHC class I molecules to activate CD8 cytotoxic T cells. This is enhanced by Th1 cytokines, such as interleukin-2 (IL-2). Activated CD8 cytotoxic T cells make contact with tumor cells, leading to direct tumor cell lysis. (TCR, T-cell receptor.)

responses that recognize CEA in mice, rabbits, and monkeys, and had a major antitumor effect in a murine tumor model (137). Among 23 patients with advanced colorectal cancer, 17 generated anti-antiidiotypic Ab3 responses (138,139).

Thirty-two patients with resected colorectal cancer were treated with 2 mg of CeaVac every other week × 4, then monthly until recurrent disease (140). Four patients were Dukes' B2, 11 were Dukes' C, eight were completely resected Dukes' D, and nine were incompletely resected Dukes' D. The incompletely resected Dukes' D were those with positive margins after surgery. Fourteen of the patients received 5-fluorouracil–based chemotherapy regimens (11 leucovorin, 3 levamisole) concurrently with CeaVac. Two of nine patients with Dukes' B and C disease progressed at 19 and 24 months, and one patient developed a second primary at 18 months. Seven of eight patients with completely resected Dukes' D remain on study from 10 to 31 months; one resected Dukes' D patient relapsed at 9 months. Two patients with incompletely resected Dukes' D remain on study at 12 and 29 months without evidence of progression; seven progressed at 6 to 30 months. All 32 patients had high-titer polyclonal anti-CEA responses (50 to 300 μg per mL) that mediated ADCC. The predominant Ab3 immunoglobulin was IgG, and the major subclasses were

IgG1 and IgG4. All 32 patients generated idiotypic-specific T-cell responses, and 75% were CEA-specific. A linear peptide derived from the CDR2 light-chain region stimulated a Th1 CD4 proliferative response *in vitro* (141). These data demonstrate that 5-fluorouracil–based chemotherapy regimens do not adversely affect the immune response to CeaVac. In addition, high-titer anti-CEA immunoglobulin and Th1 helper-cell response can be maintained indefinitely with monthly boosts with CeaVac. Injections were well tolerated with only minor local reactions and minimal systemic side effects. Although longer follow-up is required, a biologic effect on tumor progression is apparent, suggested by the ten patients with resected and incompletely resected Dukes' D disease who continue on study from 10 to 31 months.

A number of antiidiotype antibody vaccines exist for malignant melanoma. Two of these have been the gangliosides GD2 and GD3 (142,143). Immune responses with high-titer anti-GD2 polyclonal responses were reported in one study using an antiidiotype antibody designated *TriGem* that mimics the disialoganglioside GD2 (142). Forty-seven patients with advanced melanoma received four weekly injections with TriGem and then monthly injections until disease progression. Hyperimmune sera from 40 of 47 patients revealed an anti–anti-Id (Ab3) response (144). The isotypic specificity of the Ab3 antibody consisted of predominantly IgG with only minimal IgM. All of the IgG subclasses were represented with IgG1 as the most abundant. A T-cell clone-specific for the idiotypic portion of TriGem was identified that was a Th2 CD4⁺ cell as it secreted IL-4 and IL-10. One patient had a complete response to the Tri-Gem vaccine. Seventeen patients are stable on study from 8+ to 34+ months (median, 13+ months). Twenty-seven patients have progressed on study from 1 to 9 months (median, 13+ months), and 20 have died from 1 to 16 months (median, 6 months). The Kaplan-Meier–derived overall median survival has not been reached but, at 16 months, was 52%. For the 26 patients with soft tissue–only disease, the median survival has not been reached. For 18 patients with visceral metastasis, the median survival was 15 months. Toxicity consisted of local reaction at the site of the injection, mild fever, and chills. No additional toxicity, such as abdominal pain, that was seen previously with infusion of murine monoclonal anti-GD2 antibody occurred.

Another trial with antiidiotype antibodies that mimic the melanoma-associated chondroitin sulfate proteoglycan (MPG) have been used. In one study, 26 patients with metastatic melanoma were treated with an antiidiotype antibody that mimics the MPG antigen (145). These authors did not report whether an anti-MPG immune response was identified in these patients, but they did correlate antiidiotypic responses with clinical responses. Similar results were reported for another antiidiotype antibody that mimics MPG (146,147).

Antiidiotype vaccines are capable of inducing prophylactic and therapeutic immunity in animal models (148,149). It has been suggested that they may not be ready for the clinic because murine antibodies induce neutralizing antibody responses in humans, idiotype vaccines do not induce long-lasting immunity, and the predominant immune response to antiidiotypes is IgM (150). These data clearly demonstrate that monthly injections of murine antiidiotype antibodies can generate and maintain high-titer IgG antibody and proliferative T-cell responses (151).

REFERENCES

1. Yokota TM, Milenic DE, Whitlow M, et al. Rapid tumor penetrance of a single chain Fv and comparison with other immunoglobulin forms. *Cancer Res* 1992;52:3402–3408.
2. Mueller BM, Reisfeld RA, Gillies SD. Serum half-life and tumor localization of a chimeric antibody deleted for the CH2 domain and directed against the disialoganglioside GD2. *Proc Natl Acad Sci U S A* 1990;87:5702–5705.
3. Slavin-Chiorini DC, Horan Hand P, Kashmiri SVS, et al. Biologic properties of a C$_H$2 domain-deleted recombinant immunoglobulin. *Int J Cancer* 1993;53:97–103.
4. Milenic DE, Yokota T, Filpula DR, et al. Construction, binding properties metabolism, and tumor targeting of a single-chain Fv derived from the pancarcinoma monoclonal antibody CC49. *Cancer Res* 1991;51:6363–6371.
5. Colcher D, Esteban J, Carrasquillo JA, et al. Complementation of intracavitary and intravenous administration of a monoclonal antibody (B72.3) in patients with carcinoma. *Cancer Res* 1987;47:4218–4224.
6. Doerr RJ, Abdel-Nabi H, Krag D, Mitchell E. Radiolabeled antibody imaging in the management of colorectal cancer. Results of a multicenter clinical study. *Ann Surg* 1991;2:118–124.
7. Winzelberg GG, Grossman SJ, Rizk S, et al. Indium-111 monoclonal antibody B72.3 scintigraphy in colorectal cancer. Correlation with computed tomography, surgery, histopathology, immunohistology, and human immune response. *Cancer* 1992;7:1656–1663.
8. Neal CE, Swan, TL, Baker MR, Ellis MR, Katterhagen JG. Immunoscintigraphy of colorectal carcinoma utilizing. In-labeled monoclonal antibody conjugate CYT-103. *Gastrointest Radiol* 1991;16: 251–255.
9. Moffat FL Jr, Pinsky CM, Hammershaimb NJ, et al. for the Immunomedics Study Group. Clinical utility of external immunoscintigraphy with the IMMU-4 technetium-99m Fab′ antibody fragment in patients undergoing surgery for carcinoma of the colon and rectum: results of a pivotal, phase II trial. *J Clin Oncol* 1996;8:2295–2305.
10. Martin EW, Mojzisik CM, Hinkle GM, et al. Radioimmunoguided surgery: a new approach to the intraoperative detection of tumor using monoclonal antibody B72.3. *Am J Surg* 1988;156:386–392.
11. Maloney DG, Grillo-Lopez AJ, White CA, et al. IDEC-C2B8 (rituximab) anti-CD20 monoclonal antibody therapy in patients with relapsed low-grade non-Hodgkin's lymphoma. *Blood* 1997;90:2188–2195.
12. McLaughlin P, Grillo-Lopez AJ, Link BK, et al. Rituximab chimeric anti-CD20 monoclonal antibody therapy for relapsed indolent lymphoma: half of patients respond to a four-dose treatment program. *J Clin Oncol* 1998;16:2825–2833.
13. Slamon D, Leyland-Jones B, Shak S, et al. Addition of Herception™ (Humanized Anti-Her2 Antibody) to first line chemotherapy for Her2 overexpressing metastatic breast cancer (Her2+/MBC) markedly increases anticancer activity: a randomized, multinational controlled phase III trial. *Proc Am Soc Clin Oncol* 1998;17:98a.
14. Coussens L, Yang-Feng TL, Liao YC, et al. Tyrosine kinase receptor with extensive homology to EGF receptor shares chromosomal location with neu oncogene. *Science* 1985;230:1132–1139.
15. Bargmann CI, Hung MC, Weinberg RA. The neu oncogene encodes an epidermal growth factor receptor-related protein. *Nature* 1986;319:226–230.
16. Slamon DJ, Clark GD, Wong SG, et al. The HER-2/neu oncogene. *Science* 1987;235:177–182.
17. Guy CT, Webster MA, Schaller M, Parsons TJ, Cardiff RD, Muller WJ. Expression of the neu proto-oncogene in the mammary epithelium of transgenic mice induces metastatic disease. *Proc Natl Acad Sci U S A* 1992;89:10578–10582.
18. Katsumata M, Okudaira T, Samanta A, et al. Prevention of breast tumour development *in vivo* by downregulation of the p185neu receptor. *Nat Med* 1995;1:644–648.
19. Schlegel J, Trenkle T, Stumm G, Kiessling M. Growth inhibition by dominant-negative mutations of the neu-encoded oncoprotein. *Int J Cancer* 1997;70:78–83.
20. Disis ML, Calenoff E, McLaughlin G, et al. Existent T-cell and antibody immunity to HER-2/neu protein in patients with breast cancer. *Cancer Res* 1994;54:16–20.
21. Fisk B, Hudson JM, Kavanagh J, et al. Extensive proliferative responses of peripheral blood mononuclear cells from healthy donors and ovarian cancer patients to HER-2 peptides. *Anticancer Res* 1997;17:45–53.
22. Sears HF, Steplewski A, Herlyn D, Koprowski H. Effects of monoclonal antibody immunotherapy on patients with gastrointestinal adenocarcinoma. *J Biol Res Mod* 1983;3:138–150.
23. Sears HF, Atkinson B, Herlyn D, et al. The use of monoclonal antibody in a phase I clinical trial of human gastrointestinal tumors. *Lancet* 1982;1:762–765.
24. Sears HF, Herlyn D, Steplewski A, Koprowski H. Phase II clinical trial of a murine monoclonal antibody cytotoxic for gastrointestinal adenocarcinoma. *Cancer Res* 1985;45:5910–5913.
25. Riethmuller G, Schneider-Gadicke E, Schlmok G, et al. and the German Cancer Aid 17-1A Study Group. Randomized trial of monoclonal antibody for adjuvant therapy of resected Dukes' C colorectal carcinoma. *Lancet* 1994;343:1177–1183.
26. Riethmuller G, Holz E, Schlimok G, et al. Monoclonal antibody therapy for resected Dukes' C colorectal cancer: seven-year outcome of a multicenter randomized trial. *J Clin Oncol* 1998;16:1788–1794.

27. Hellstrom I, Horn D, Linsley P, et al. Monoclonal mouse antibodies raised against human lung carcinoma. *Cancer Res* 1986;46:3917–3923.

28. Hellstrom I, Beaumier PL, Hellstrom KE. Antitumor effects of L6, an IgG2a antibody that reacts with most human carcinomas. *Proc Natl Acad Sci U S A* 1986;83:7059–7063.

29. DeNardo SJ, Warhoe KA, O'Grady LF, et al. Radioimmunotherapy with I-131 chimeric L-6 in advanced breast cancer. In: Ceriani RL (ed). *Breast epithelial antigens.* New York: Plenum Press, 1991.

30. Murara R, Wunderhih D, Thor A, Cunningham R, Mogenchi P, Schlom J. A monoclonal antibody (D612) with selective reactivity for malignant and normal gastrointestinal epithelium. *Int J Cancer* 1989;43:598–607.

31. Pendurthi TK, Schlom J, Primus FJ. Human lymphokine-activated killer cells augment immunotherapy of human colon carcinoma xenografts in monoclonal antibody D612. *J Immunother* 1991;10:2–12.

32. Qi C, Nieroda C, De Filippi R, et al. Macrophage colony-stimulating factor enhancement of antibody-dependent cellular cytotoxicity against human colon carcinoma cells. *Immunol Lett* 1995;47:15–24.

33. Thompson J, Zimmerman W. The carcinoembryonic antigen gene family: structure, expressions and evolution. *Tumour Biol* 1988;9:63–83.

34. Paxton RJ, Mooser G, Pande H, Lee TD, Shivley JF. Sequence analysis of carcinoembryonic antigen: identification of glycosylation sites and homology with the immunoglobulin super-gene family. *Proc Natl Acad Sci U S A* 1987;84:920–924.

35. Bechimol S, Fuks A, Jothy S, Beauchemia N, Shirota K, Standers C. Carcinoembryonic antigen, a human tumor marker, functions as an intercellular adhesion molecule. *Cell* 1989;57:327–334.

36. Oikawa S, Inuzuka C, Kuroki M, Matsuoka Y, Kosaki G, Nakazato H. Cell adhesion activity of non-specific cross-reacting antigen (NCA) and carcinoembryonic antigen (CEA) expressed on CHO cell surface: homophilic and heterophilic adhesion. *Biochem Biophys Res Commun* 1989;164:39–45.

37. Kotera Y, Fontenot JD, Pecher G, Metzgar RS, Finn OJ. Human immunity against a tandem repeat epitope of human mucin MUC-1 in sera from breast, pancreatic and colon cancer patients. *Cancer Res* 1994;54:2856–2860.

38. Devine PL, Layton GT, Clark BA, Birrell GW, Ward BG, Xing PX, McKenzie FC. Production of MUC-1 and MUC-2 mucins by human tumor cell lines. *Biochem Biophys Res Commun* 1991;178:593–599.

39. Hollingsworth MA, Strawhecker JM, Caffrey TC, Mack DR. Expression of MUC-1, MUC-2, MUC-3 and MUC-4 mucin nRNAs in human pancreatic and intestinal tumor cell lines. *Int J Cancer* 1994;57:198–203.

40. Gendler SJ, Spicer AP, Lalani E-N, et al. Structure and biology of a carcinoma-associated mucin, MUC-1. *Am Rev Respir Dis* 1991;144:S42–S47.

41. Burchell J, Taylor-Papadimitriou J, Boshell M, Gendler S, Duhig T. A short sequence, within the amino acid tandem repeat of a cancer-associated mucin, contains immunodominant epitopes. *Int J Cancer* 1989;44:691–696.

42. Fontenot JD, Tjandra N, Bu D, Ho C, Montelaro RC, Finn OJ. Biophysical characterization of one-, two-, and three-tandem repeats of human mucin (MUC-1) protein core. *Cancer Res* 1993;53:5386–5394.

43. Peterson JA, Zava DT, Duwe AK, Blank EW, Battifora H, Ceriani RL. Biochemical and histological characterization of antigens preferentially expressed on the surface and cytoplasm of breast carcinoma cells identified by monoclonal antibodies against the human milk fat globule. *Hybridoma* 1990;9:221–235

44. Pai LH, Bookman MA, Ozols RF, et al. Clinical evaluation of intraperitoneal pseudomonas exotoxin immunoconjugate OVB3-PE in patients with ovarian cancer. *J Clin Oncol* 1991;9:2095–2103.

45. Order SE, Stillwagon GB, Klein JL, et al. Iodine antiferritin, a new treatment modality in hepatoma: a Radiation Therapy Oncology Group study. *J Clin Oncol* 1985;3:1573–1582.

46. Mendelsohn J. Epidermal growth factor receptor as a target for therapy with antireceptor monoclonal antibodies. *Monogr Natl Cancer Inst* 1992;13:125–131.

47. Mendelsohn J. Epidermal growth factor receptor inhibition by a monoclonal antibody as anticancer therapy. *Clin Cancer Res* 1997;12:2703–2707.

48. Mendelsohn J, Fan Z. Epidermal growth factor receptor family and chemosensitization. *J Natl Cancer Inst* 1997;89:341–343.

49. Hamilton WB, Helling F, Lloyd KO, Livingston PO. Ganglioside expression on human malignant melanoma assessed by quantitative immune thin-layer chromatography. *Int J Cancer* 1993;53:566–573.

50. Tsuchida T, Saxton RE, Morton DL, Irie RF. Gangliosides of human melanoma. *Cancer* 1989;63:1166–1174.

51. Kirkwood JM, Day R, Mascari RA, et al. Phase Ib trial of murine R24 anti-GD3 antibody in 37 patients with metastatic melanoma. *Proc Am Assoc Cancer Res* 1994;35:218(abst).

52. Houghton AN, Elsinger M, Albino AP, et al. Surface antigens of melanocytes and melanoma. Markers of melanocyte differentiation and melanoma subsets. *J Exp Med* 1982;156:1755.

53. Dippold W, Bernhard H, Meyer zum Buschenfelde KH. Immunological response to intrathecal and systemic treatment with ganglioside antibody R-24 in patients with malignant melanoma. *Eur J Cancer* 1994;30A:137.

54. Vadhan-Raj S, Cordon-Cardo C, Carswell E, et al. Phase I trial of a mouse monoclonal antibody against GD3 ganglioside in patients with melanoma: induction of inflammatory responses at tumor sites. *J Clin Oncol* 1988;6:1636.

55. Goodman GE, Hellstrom I, Hummel D, et al. Phase I trial of monoclonal antibody MG-21 directed against a melanoma-associated GD3 ganglioside antigen. *Proc Am Soc Clin Oncol* 1987;6:823.

56. Cheung NK, Lazarus H, Miraldi FD, et al. Ganglioside GD2-specific monoclonal antibody 3F8: a phase I study in patients with neuroblastoma and malignant melanoma. *J Clin Oncol* 1987;5:1430.

57. Lonberg M, Bajorin D, Cheung N-K, et al. Phase I trial of a combination of two mouse monoclonal antibodies, anti-GD3 and anti-GD2, in patients with melanoma and soft tissue sarcoma. *Proc Am Soc Clin Oncol* 1988;7:668(abst).

58. Lichtin A, Iliopoulos D, Guerry D, et al. Therapy of melanoma with an antimelanoma ganglioside monoclonal antibody: a possible mechanism of a complete response. *Proc Am Soc Oncol* 1988;7:247(abst).

59. Irie RF, Morton DL. Regression of cutaneous metastatic melanoma by intralesional injection with human monoclonal antibody to ganglioside GD2. *Proc Natl Acad Sci U S A* 1986;83:86–94.

60. Irie RF, DeNunzio FD. Immunotherapy of melanoma: current status and prospects for the future. *J Dermatol* 1993;20:65.

61. Irie RF, Matsuki T, Morton DL. Human monoclonal antibody to ganglioside GM2 for melanoma treatment. *Lancet* 1989;1:786.

62. Hoon DS, Wang Y, Sze L, et al. Molecular cloning of a human monoclonal antibody reactive to ganglioside GM3 antigen on human cancers. *Cancer Res* 1993;53:5244.

63. Oldham RK, Foon KA, Morgan AC, et al. Monoclonal antibody therapy of malignant melanoma: *in vivo* localization in cutaneous metastasis after intravenous administration. *J Clin Oncol* 1984;2:1235.

64. Schroff RW, Morgan AC, Woodhouse CS, et al. Monoclonal antibody therapy in malignant melanoma: factors effecting *in vivo* localization. *J Biol Response Mod* 1987;6:457.

65. Schroff RW, Woodhouse CS, Foon KA, et al. Intratumoral localization of monoclonal antibody in patients with melanoma treated with antibody to a 250,000-dalton melanoma-associated antigen. *J Natl Cancer Inst* 1985;74:299.

66. Multani PS, Grossbard ML. Monoclonal antibody-based therapies for hematologic malignancies. *J Clin Oncol* 1998;16:3691–3710.

67. Hekman A, Honselqaar A, Vuist WM, et al. Initial experience with treatment of human B-cell lymphoma with anti-CD19 monoclonal antibody. *Cancer Immunol Immunother* 1991;32:364–372.

68. Waldmann TA, Goldman CK, Bongiovanni KF, et al. Therapy of patients with human T-cell lymphotrophic virus I-induced adult T-cell leukemia with anti-Tac, a monoclonal antibody to the receptor for interleukin-2. *Blood* 1988;72:1805–1816.

69. Miller RA, Oseroff AR, Stratte PT, et al. Monoclonal antibody therapeutic trials in seven patients with T-cell lymphoma. *Blood* 1983;62:988–995.

70. Foon KA, Schroff RW, Bunn PA, et al. Effects of monoclonal anti-

body therapy in patients with chronic lymphocytic leukemia. *Blood* 1984;64:1085–1093.

71. Dillman RO, Beauregard J, Shawler DL, et al. Continuous infusion of T101 monoclonal antibody in chronic lymphocytic leukemia and cutaneous T-cell lymphoma. *J Biol Res Mod* 1986;5:394–410.

72. Press OW, Appelbaum F, Ledbetter JA, et al. Monoclonal antibody 1F5 (anti-CD20) serotherapy of human B-cell lymphomas. *Blood* 1987;69:584–591.

73. Miller RA, Maloney DG, Warnke R, et al. Treatment of B-cell lymphoma with monoclonal anti-idiotype antibody. *N Engl J Med* 1982;306:517–522.

74. Meeker TC, Lowder J, Maloney DG, et al. A clinical trial of anti-idiotype therapy for B-cell malignancy. *Blood* 1985;65:1349–1363.

75. Osterborg LA, Brittinger G, Crowther D, et al. for the European Study Group of CAMPTH-1H treatment in low-grade non-Hodgkin's lymphoma. *J Clin Oncol* 1998;16:3257–3263.

76. Osterborg A, Dyer MJ, Bunjes D, et al. Phase II multicenter study of human CD52 antibody in previously treated chronic lymphocytic leukemia. European Study Group of CAMPATH-1H treatment in chronic lymphocytic leukemia. *J Clin Oncol* 1997;15:1567–1574.

77. Bowen AL, Zomas A, Emmett E, et al. Subcutaneous CAMPATH-1H in fludarabine-resistant/relapsed chronic lymphocytic and B-pro-lymphocytic leukaemia. *Br J Haematol* 1997;96:617–619.

78. Kaminski MS, Zasadny KR, Francis IR, et al. Radioimmunotherapy of B-cell lymphoma with I anti-B1 (anti-CD20) antibody. *N Engl J Med* 1993;329:459–465.

79. Kaminski MS, Fig LM, Zasadny KR, et al. Imaging, dosimetry, and radioimmunotherapy with iodine 131-labeled anti-CD37 antibody in B-cell lymphoma. *J Clin Oncol* 1992;10:1696–1711.

80. Press OW, Eary JF, Appelbaum FR, et al. Radiolabeled-antibody therapy of B-cell lymphoma with autologous bone marrow support. *N Engl J Med* 1993;329:1219–1224.

81. Press OW, Eary JF, Appelbaum FR, et al. Phase II trial of I-B1 (anti-CD20) antibody therapy with autologous stem cell transplantation for relapsed B-cell lymphomas. *Lancet* 1995;346:336–340.

82. DeNardo GL, DeNardo SJ, Goldstein DS, et al. Maximum-tolerated dose, toxicity and efficacy of I-Lym-1 antibody for fractionated radioimmunotherapy of non-Hodgkin's lymphoma. *J Clin Oncol* 1998;16:3246–3256.

83. Czuczman MS, Straus DJ, Divgi CR, et al. Phase I dose-escalation trial of iodine 131-labeled monoclonal antibody OKB7 in patients with non-Hodgkin's lymphoma. *J Clin Oncol* 1993;11:2021–2029.

84. Juweid M, Sharkey RM, Markowitz A, et al. Treatment of non-Hodgkin's lymphoma with radiolabeled murine, chimeric, or humanized LL2, an anti-CD22 monoclonal antibody. *Cancer Res* 1995;55:S5899–S5907.

85. Tepler I, Schwartz G, Parker K, et al. Phase I trial of an interleukin-2 fusion toxin (DAB$_{486}$IL-2) in hematologic malignancies: complete response in a patient with Hodgkin's disease refractory to chemotherapy. *Cancer* 1994;73:1276–1285.

86. LeMaistre CF, Rosenblum MG, Reuben JM, et al. Therapeutic effects of genetically engineered toxin (DAB$_{486}$IL-2) in patients with chronic lymphocytic leukaemia. *Lancet* 1991;337:1124–1125.

87. Lambert JM, McIntyre G, Gauthier MN, et al. The galactose-binding sites of the cytotoxic lectin ricin can be chemically blocked in high yield with reactive ligands prepared by chemical modification of glycopeptides containing triantennary N-linked oligosaccharides. *Biochemistry* 1991;30:3234–3247.

88. Kreitman RJ, Chaudhary VK, Waldmann T, et al. The recombinant immunotoxin anti-Tac(Fv)-Pseudomonas exotoxin 40 is cytotoxic toward peripheral-blood malignant cells from patients with adult T-cell leukemia. *Proc Natl Acad Sci U S A* 1990;87:8291–8295.

89. Kreitman RJ, Chaudhary VK, Kozak RW, et al. Recombinant toxins containing the variable domains of the anti-Tac monoclonal antibody to the interleukin-2 receptor kill malignant cells from patients with chronic lymphocytic leukemia. *Blood* 1992;80:2344–2352.

90. Chaudhary VK, Gallo MG, Fitzgerald DJ, et al. A recombinant single-chain immunotoxin composed of anti-Tac variable regions and a truncated diphtheria toxin. *Proc Natl Acad Sci U S A* 1990;87:9491–9494.

91. Vitetta ES, Stone M, Amlot P, et al. Phase I immunotoxin trial in patients with B-cell lymphomas. *Cancer Res* 1991;51:4052–4058.

92. Stone MJ, Sausville EA, Fay JW, et al. A phase I study of bolus versus continuous infusion of the anti-CD19 immunotoxin, IgG-HD37-dgA, in patients with B-cell lymphoma. *Blood* 1996;88:1188–1197.

93. Engert A, Diehl V, Schnell R, et al. A phase I study of an anti-CD25 ricin A-chain immunotoxin (RFT5-SMPT-dgA) in patients with refractory Hodgkin's lymphoma. *Blood* 1997;89:403–410.

94. Falini B, Bolognesi A, Flenghi L, et al. Response of refractory Hodgkin's disease to monoclonal anti-CD30 immunotoxin. *Lancet* 1992;339:1195–1196.

95. Kuzel T, Olsen E, Martin A, et al. Pivotal phase III trial of two dose levels of DAB$_{486}$IL-2 (Ontak) for the treatment of mycosis fungoides. *Blood* 1997;90:A2607(abst).

96. Caron PC, Jurcic JG, Scott AM, et al. A phase IB trial of humanized monoclonal antibody ^{131}M195 (anti-CD33) in myeloid leukemia: specific targeting without immunogenicity. *Blood* 1994;83:1760.

97. Schwartz MA, Lovett DR, Redner A, et al. Dose-escalation trial of M195 labeled with I for cytoreduction and marrow ablation in relapsed or refractory myeloid leukemias. *J Clin Oncol* 1993;11:294.

98. Papadopoulos EB, Caron P, Castro-Malaspina H, et al. Results of allogeneic bone marrow transplant following ^{131}I-M195/busulfan/cyclophosphamide in patients with advanced myeloid malignancies. *Blood* 1993;82[Suppl]:309.

99. Jennings CD, Foon KA. Recent advances in flow cytometry: application to the diagnosis of hematologic malignancies. *Blood* 1997;90: 2863–2892.

100. Venditti A, Del Poeta G, Buccisano F, et al. Minimally differentiated acute myeloid leukemia (AML-M0). Comparison of 25 cases with other French-American-British subtypes. *Blood* 1997;89:621.

101. Bhan AK. Diagnostic strategies based on differentiation antigens. In: Colvin RB, Bhan AK, McCluskey RT, eds. *Diagnostic immunopathology*, 2nd ed. New York: Raven Press, 1995:455–478.

102. Battifora H, Trowbridge IS. A monoclonal antibody useful for the differential diagnosis between malignant lymphomas and non-hematopoietic neoplasms. *Cancer* 1983;51:816–821.

103. Cartun RW, Coles FB, Pastuszak WT. Utilization of monoclonal antibody L26 in the identification and confirmation of B-cell lymphomas: a sensitive and specific marker applicable to formalin and B5 fixed paraffin embedded tissue. *Am J Pathol* 1987;129:415–421.

104. West KP, Warford A, Fray L, Allen M, Campbell AC, Lauder I. The demonstration of B-cell, T-cell and myeloid antigens in paraffin sections. *J Pathol* 1986;150:89–101.

105. Hsu SM, Yang K, Jaffe ES. Phenotypic expressions of Hodgkin's and Reed-Sternberg cells in Hodgkin's disease. *Am J Pathol* 1985;118: 209–217.

106. Murphy GF, Bhan AK, Soto S, Harrist TJ, Mihm MC Jr. Characterization of Langerhans cells by the use of monoclonal antibodies. *Lab Invest* 1981;95:465–468.

107. Arklie J, Taylor-Papadimitriou J, Bodmar W, Egan M, Millis R. Differentiation antigens expressed by epithelial cells in the lactating breast are also detectable in breast cancer. *Int J Cancer* 1981;28: 23–29.

108. Denk H, Krepler R, Artlieb U, et al. Proteins of intermediate filaments, an immunohistochemical and biochemical approach to the classification of soft tissue tumors. *Am J Pathol* 1983;110:193–208.

109. Gabbiani G, Kapanci Y, Barazzone P, Franke WW. Immunochemical identification of intermediate-sized filaments in human neoplastic cells: a diagnostic aid for the surgical pathologist. *Am J Pathol* 1981;104:206–216.

110. Ahen DJ, Nakane PK, Brown WR. Ultrastructural localization of carcinoembryonic antigen in normal intestine and colon cancer: abnormal distribution of CEA on the surfaces of colon cancer cells. *Cancer* 1982;49:2077–2090.

111. Statiel RA, Mabry M, Skanu AT, Speak J, Bernal SD. Detection of bone marrow metastasis in small cell lung cancer by monoclonal antibody. *J Clin Oncol* 1985;3:455–461.

112. Kapur RP, Bigler SA, Skelly M, Gown AM. Anti-melanoma monoclonal antibody HMB45 identifies an oncofetal glycoconjugate associated with immature melanosomes. *J Histochem Cytochem* 1992;40: 207–212.

113. Kahn HJ, Marks A, Thom H, Baumal R. Role of antibody to S100

protein in diagnostic pathology. *Am J Clin Pathol* 1983;79:341.

114. Ramackers FCS, Puts JJG, Moesker O, Kant A, Vooijs GP, Jap PHK. Intermediate filaments in malignant melanomas. Identification and use as marker in surgical pathology. *J Clin Invest* 1983;71:635–643.

115. Morrison SL, Oi T. Genetically engineered antibody molecules. *Adv Immunol* 1989;44:65–92.

116. Morrison SL, Schlom J. Recombinant chimeric monoclonal antibodies. In: DeVita VT, Hellman S, Rosenberg SA (eds). *Important advances in oncology*. Philadelphia: JB Lippincott Co., 1990:3–18.

117. Winter G, Milstein C. Man-made antibodies. *Nature* 1991;349: 293–299.

118. Baker TS, Bose CC, Caskey-Finney HM, et al. Humanization of an anti-mucin antibody for breast and ovarian cancer therapy. *Adv Exp Med Biol* 1994;353:61–82.

119. Couto JR, Padlan EA, Blank EW, Peterson JA, Ceriani RL. Humanization of KC4G3, an anti-human carcinoma antibody. *Hybridoma* 1994;13:215–219.

120. Fiorentini S, Matczak E, Gallo RC, Reitz MS, Keydar I, Watkins BA. Humanization of an antibody recognizing a breast cancer specific epitope by CDR-grafting. *Immunotechnology* 1997;3:45–59.

121. Padlan EA. Anatomy of the antibody molecule. *Mol Immunol* 1994;31:169–217.

122. Winter G, Griffiths AD, Hawkins RE, Hoogenboom HR. Making antibody by phage display technology. *Annu Rev Immunol* 1994;12:433–455.

123. Marks JD, Hoogenboom HR, Bonnert TP, McCafferty J, Griffiths AD, Winter G. By-passing immunization. Human antibodies from V-gene libraries displayed on phage. *J Mol Biol* 1991;222:581–597.

124. Bird RE, Hardman KD, Jacobson JW. Single-chain antigen-binding proteins. *Science* 1988;242:423–426.

125. Reiter Y, Pastan I. Antibody engineering of recombinant Fv immunotoxins for improved targeting of cancer: disulfide-stabilized Fv immunotoxins. *Clin Can Res* 1996;2:245–252.

126. Lindenmann J. Speculations on idiotypes and homobodies. *Ann Immunol (Paris)* 1973;124:171–184.

127. Jerne NK. Towards a network theory of the immune system. *Ann Immunol (Paris)* 1974;125C:373–389.

128. Rock KL, Gamble S, Rothstein L. Presentation of exogenous antigen with class major histocompatibility complex molecules. *Science* 1990;249:918–921.

129. Grant EP, Rock KL. MHC class I-restricted presentation of exogenous antigen by thymic antigen-presenting cells *in vitro* and *in vivo*. *J Immunol* 1992;148:13–18.

130. Fagerberg J, Steinitz M, Wigzell H, Askelöf P, Mellstedt H. Human anti-idiotypic antibodies induced a humoral and cellular immune response against a colorectal carcinoma-associated antigen in patients. *Proc Natl Acad Sci U S A* 1995;92:4773–4777.

131. Herlyn D, Harris D, Zaloudik J, et al. Immunomodulatory activity of monoclonal anti-idiotypic antibody to anti-colorectal carcinoma antibody CO17-1A in animals and patients. *J Immunother* 1994;15:303–311.

132. Robins RA, Denton GWL, Hardcastle JD, Austin EB, Baldwin RW, Durrant LG. Antitumor immune response and interleukin-2 production induced in colorectal cancer patients by immunization with human monoclonal anti-idiotypic antibody. *Cancer Res* 1991;51: 5425–5429.

133. Denton GWL, Durrant LG, Hardcastle JD, Austin EB, Sewell HF, Robins RA. Clinical outcome of colorectal cancer patients treated with human monoclonal anti-idiotypic antibody. *Int J Cancer* 1994;57:10–17.

134. Durrant LG, Buckley TJD, Denton GWL, Hardcastle JD, Sewell HF, Robins RA. Enhanced cell-mediated tumor killing in patients immunized with human monoclonal anti-idiotypic antibody 105AD7. *Cancer Res* 1994;54:4837–4840.

135. Durrant LG, Doran M, Austin EB, Robins RA. Induction of cellular immune responses by a murine monoclonal anti-idiotypic antibody recognizing the 791Tgp72 antigen expressed on colorectal, gastric and ovarian human tumours. *Int J Cancer* 1995;61:62–66.

136. Bhattacharya-Chatterjee M, Mukerjee S, Biddle W, Foon KA, Köhler H. Murine monoclonal anti-idiotype antibody as a potential network antigen for human carcinoembryonic antigen. *J Immunol* 1990;145:2758–2765.

137. Pervin S, Chakraborty M, Bhattacharya-Chatterjee M, Zeytin H, Foon KA, Chatterjee S. Induction of antitumor immunity by an anti-idiotype antibody mimicking carcinoembryonic antigen. *Cancer Res* 1997;57:728–734.

138. Foon KA, Chakraborty M, John WJ, Sherratt A, Köhler H, Bhattacharya-Chatterjee M. Immune response to the carcinoembryonic antigen in patients treated with an anti-idiotype antibody vaccine. *J Clin Invest* 1995;96:334–342.

139. Foon KA, John WJ, Chakraborty M, et al. Clinical and immune responses in advanced colorectal cancer patients treated with anti-idiotype monoclonal antibody vaccine that mimics the carcinoembryonic antigen. *Clin Cancer Res* 1997;3:1267–1276.

140. Foon KA, John WJ, Chakraborty M, Garrison J, Bard V, Bhattacharya-Chatterjee. Clinical and immune responses in surgically resected colorectal cancer (CRC) patients treated with an anti-idiotype (Id) monoclonal antibody that mimics carcinoembryonic antigen (CEA) with or without 5-fluorouracil. *Proc Am Soc Clin Oncol* 1998;17:435a.

141. Chatterjee SK, Tripathi PK, Chakraborty M, et al. Molecular mimicry of carcinoembryonic antigen by peptides derived from the structure of an anti-idiotype antibody. *Cancer Res* 1998;58:1217–1224.

142. Foon K, Sen G, Hutchins L, et al. Antibody responses in melanoma patients immunized with an anti-idiotype antibody mimicking disialoganglioside GD2. *Clin Cancer Res* 1998;4:1117–1124.

143. Chapman PB, Livingston PO, Morrison ME, Williams L, Houghton AN. Immunization of melanoma patients with anti-idiotypic monoclonal antibody BEC2 which mimics GD3 ganglioside: pilot trials using no immunological adjuvant. *Vaccine Res* 1994;3:59–69.

144. Foon KA, Lutzky J, Baral RN, et al. Clinical and immune responses in advanced melanoma patients immunized with an anti-idiotype mimicking disialoganglioside GD2. *J Clin Oncol* 2000;18:376.

145. Quan WDY, Dean GE, Spears CP, Groshen S, Merritt JA, Mitchell MS. Active specific immunotherapy of metastatic melanoma with an anti-idiotype vaccine: a phase I/II trial of I-Mel-2 plus SAF-m. *J Clin Oncol* 1997;15:2103–2110.

146. Mittelman A, Chen ZJ, Kageshita T. Active specific immunotherapy in patients with melanoma. A clinical trial with mouse anti-idiotypic monoclonal antibodies elicited with syngeneic anti-high-molecular-weight melanoma-associated antigen monoclonal antibodies. *J Clin Invest* 1990;86:2136–2144.

147. Mittelman A, Chen ZJ, Yang H, Wong GY, Ferrone S. Human high molecular weight melanoma-associated antigen (HMW-MAA) mimicry by mouse anti-idiotypic monoclonal antibody MK2-23: induction of humoral anti-HMW-MAA immunity and prolongation of survival in patients with stage IV melanoma. *Proc Natl Acad Sci U S A* 1992;89:466–470.

148. Magliani W, Polonelli L, Conti S, et al. Neonatal mouse immunity against group B streptococcal infection by maternal vaccination with recombinant anti-idiotypes. *Nat Med* 1998;4:705–709.

149. Ruiz PJ, Wolkowicz R, Waisman A, et al. Idiotypic immunization induces immunity to mutated p53 and tumor rejection. *Nat Med* 1998;4(6):7102.

150. Bona CA. Idiotype vaccines. Forgotten but not gone. *Nat Med* 1998;4:668–669.

151. Foon KA, Bhattacharya-Chatterjee M. Idiotype vaccines in the clinic [Letter]. *Nat Med* 1998;4:870.

14.2

MONOCLONAL ANTIBODIES: BASIC PRINCIPLES

Immunotoxins and Recombinant Immunotoxins

LEE H. PAI-SCHERF
ROBERT J. KREITMAN
IRA PASTAN

Approximately 100 years ago, Paul Ehrlich first suggested the concept of targeted drug delivery (1). By linking a tumor-specific antibody to a toxin, these magic bullets would seek out and kill cancer cells without being toxic to normal tissues. It was not until 1975, with the invention of the hybridoma technique by Kohler and Milstein (2), that monoclonal antibodies (MAb) with well-defined specificity and purity could be obtained in large amounts and used for the production of these magic bullets.

MAb coupled to bacterial or plant toxins are termed *immunotoxins*. Much progress has been made in the field since the first *in vitro* study was reported in the 1970s (3). First-generation immunotoxins were made by chemically coupling MAb to a native plant or bacterial toxin. The experience gained from laboratory and clinical studies using these first-generation molecules led scientists to produce more specific and potent molecules that are now being tested in humans. Two major advances in the immunotoxin field have been the use of the recombinant DNA technique to produce recombinant toxins with better clinical properties and the production of single-chain immunotoxins by fusing the DNA elements encoding combining regions of antibodies, growth factors, or cytokines to a toxin gene.

In this chapter, we give a brief overview of the current status of immunotoxins and recombinant toxins in cancer therapy. The structure and function of plant and bacterial toxins and advances in design and manufacture of immunotoxins are reviewed. A summary of major clinical trials and their problems are presented. The rationale and approaches used to design the new generation of recombinant toxins (single-chain immunotoxins and disulfide-linked immunotoxins) and prospects for the future are discussed.

TOXINS—STRUCTURE AND FUNCTION

Several plant and bacterial toxins have been used in the construction of immunotoxins (Table 1). These toxins belong to a group of polypeptide enzymes that catalytically inactivate protein synthesis leading to cell death. Some of these toxins have been shown to induce apoptosis (4,5).

Plant Toxins

Ricin, or the ricin A chain fragment, has been a commonly used toxin for conjugation to antibodies. Ricin is synthesized as single polypeptide chains and processed posttranslationally into two subunits, A and B, linked though a disulfide bond. Ricin is a 65-kd glycoprotein purified from the seeds of the castor bean (*Ricinus communis*). It is composed of an A subunit, which kills cells by catalytically inactivating ribosomes. The A subunit is linked by a disulfide bond to a B subunit, which is responsible for cell binding. The B chain is a galactose-specific lectin that binds to galactose residues present on cell-surface glycoproteins and glycolipids (6). Once the B subunit of ricin binds to the cell membrane, the protein enters the cell through coated pits and endocytic vesicles. The A and B subunits of ricin are separated by a process involving disulfide bond reduction. The A subunit of ricin translocates across an intracellular membrane to the cell cytosol, probably with the assistance of the B subunit. In the cytosol, it arrests protein synthesis by enzymatically inactivating the 28S subunit of eukaryotic ribosomes (7,8). Because native ricin is highly toxic and lacks specificity, several modified forms of ricin have been developed to prepare immunotoxins that are better tolerated by patients.

TABLE 1. COMMON TOXINS USED IN THE CONSTRUCTION OF IMMUNOTOXINS

Toxins	Source	Molecular Weight	Intracellular Target	Structure
Plant Toxins				
Ricin	Seeds of castor bean *Ricinus communis*	62 kd	Inactivates 28s rRNA	
Saporin	*Saponaria officinalis*	30 kd	Same	
PAP	*Phytolacca americana* pokeweed	30 kd	Same	
Bacterial Toxins				
Pseudomonas exotoxin	*Pseudomonas aeruginosa*	66 kd	Adenosine diphosphate–ribosylation of EF2	
Diphtheria toxin	*Corynebacterium diphtheriae*	58 kd	Adenosine diphosphate–ribosylation of EF2	

Ricin A Chain

To decrease the nonspecific binding of whole ricin, the A chain alone has been coupled to antibodies. The A chain is obtained by reducing the disulfide bond that links it to the B chain. Immunotoxins composed of the ricin A chain coupled to well-internalized antibodies can be highly cytotoxic (9). In the absence of B chain (the binding subunit), however, immunotoxins made with poorly internalized antibodies are not cytotoxic.

Deglycosylated Ricin A Chain

Immunotoxins containing ricin A chain are rapidly cleared from the circulation by the liver by the binding of mannose and fucose residues of the A chain to receptors present on the reticuloendothelial system and hepatocytes. To circumvent this problem, these carbohydrate residues were chemically modified (10), resulting in a deglycosylated A chain (dgA) molecule. In preclinical studies, dgA-containing immunotoxins were found to have longer half-lives in the circulation and better antitumor efficacy *in vivo* (11). Also, recombinant A chain produced in *Escherichia coli* can be used in place of dgA because it is devoid of carbohydrate and is not rapidly cleared by the liver.

Blocked Ricin

Another strategy to decrease the nonspecific toxicity of native ricin is to block the galactose-binding sites of the B chain by cross-linking with glycopeptide (12) or to use short cross-linkers to connect the antibody to the toxin so that the galactose-binding site is sterically blocked by the antibody (13). Blocked ricin retains a low affinity for galactose-binding sites, which enhances internalization and cytotoxicity of an antibody that binds to a poorly internalized antigen.

Other plant toxins commonly used for clinical immunotoxin construction are also shown in Table 1. Saporin and pokeweed antiviral protein are single polypeptide chains that inactivate ribosomes in similar fashion to ricin. Because these toxins lack the binding chain (B chain), they are relatively nontoxic to cells and are used for immunotoxin production (14–17).

Bacterial Toxins

Both *Pseudomonas* exotoxin (PE) and diphtheria toxin (DT) have been used in constructing immunotoxins (18,19). PE is a 613–amino acid (66 kd) single-chain protein secreted by *Pseudomonas aeruginosa*. X-ray crystallography (20) and mutational studies (21) have shown that PE is composed of three major structural and functional domains (see Table 1): an amino terminal cell-binding domain (domain Ia, composed of amino acids 1 through 252), a central translocation domain (domain II, amino acids 253 through 364), and a carboxyl terminal domain (domain III, amino acids 395 through 613). The latter catalyzes the adenosine diphosphate ribosylation and inactivation of elongation factor 2 and thereby inhibits protein synthesis and leads to cell death. Domain III contains a carboxyl terminal sequence (REDLK). After lysine is removed, the REDL binds within the cell to the KDEL receptor, which directs endocytosed toxin to the endoplasmic reticulum. Substitution of REDLK with a KDEL sequence, which is known to retain newly synthesized proteins in the endoplasmic reticulum (22), results in a PE molecule that is more toxic to cells (23). Domain Ib is composed of amino acids 365 to 395 and has no known function; deleting part or all of this domain results in no loss of activity.

Cell killing is initiated when PE binds to a multifunctional high molecular-weight cell-surface glycoprotein. This protein is

TABLE 2. STRUCTURE AND ACTIVITY OF RECOMBINANT TOXINS DERIVED FROM *PSEUDOMONAS AERUGINOSA*

Name	Structure	Target Cells	Size (Molecular Weight)	Reference
PE		Most mammalian cells	66 kd	20,21
PE40/PE38		—	40/38 kd	21
B3-LysPE38 (LMB-1)		Lewis Y carbohydrate carcinomas: gastrointestinal, breast, lung, ovary, bladder	200 kd	74,75
B3(Fv)PE38 (LMB-7)		Same	65 kd	76
B3(dsFv)PE38 (LMB-9)		Same	65 kd	79
e23(dsFv)PE38		Her2/neu carcinomas: breast, gastric, lung, ovary	64 kd	83,84
AntiTac (Fv)PE38 (LMB-2)		Human IL-2 receptor Leukemia/lymphomas	65 kd	41,76
RFB4(dsFv)-PE38 (BL22)		CD22 Leukemia/lymphomas	65 kd	48
TGF-PE40/38		Epidermal growth factor receptor Epidermoid carcinoma Adenocarcinoma Glioblastoma	46 kd	88,92,93
IL-4(38-37)-PE38KDEL		IL-4 receptor Glioblastoma	56 kd	102,103

IL, interleukin; PE, *Pseudomonas* exotoxin.

the receptor for α_2-macroglobulin and a low-density lipoprotein (24). PE is then internalized by the pathway of receptor-mediated endocytosis (25). Either before entry into the cell or on reaching the endocytic compartment, the PE proenzyme is activated by a cleavage between amino acids 279 and 280, followed by reduction of a disulfide bond connecting amino acids 265 through 287. This generates a 37-kd fragment composed of a portion of domain II and all of domain III. The 37-kd fragment is ultimately translocated to the cytosol, where it inactivates elongation factor 2 and produces cell death (26). Translocation to the cytosol probably occurs from the endoplasmic reticulum. The structure and activity of various recombinant toxins and immunotoxins derived from PE are depicted in Table 2.

DT is produced by *Corynebacterium diphtheriae*. It is a single-chain polypeptide of 535 residues. Like PE, it is also made up of three domains (27). Fragment A, the 21-kd amino terminal catalytic domain, catalyses the transfer of the adenosine diphosphate-ribosyl group of NAD^+ to elongation factor 2, arresting protein synthesis and, thus, killing the target cell. Fragment B (37 kd) consists of two domains, a receptor-binding domain (amino acids 386 to 535) and a transmembrane domain (amino acids 205 to 378), which is responsible for membrane insertion and translocation of the A fragment to the cytosol. After binding to a receptor on the cell surface, DT is internalized through coated pits into endocytic vesicles, where it is proteolytically cleaved into A and B fragments. The low pH in the vesicular compartment (approximately pH 5) initiates the translocation process, but reduction of the disulfide bond is required for translocation into the cytosol (28,29).

CONSTRUCTION OF IMMUNOTOXINS

How Immunotoxins Are Attached to Antibodies

First-generation immunotoxins were constructed by coupling toxins to MAb or antibody fragments using a heterobifunctional cross-linking agent. All the immunotoxins containing plant toxins that are described in this review have been produced in this manner. Subsequently, it was discovered that genetic engineering could be used to replace the cell-binding domains of bacterial toxins with the Fv portions of antibodies or with growth factors (30,31). Because bacterial toxins have no carbohydrates and are naturally produced by bacteria, production of recombinant immunotoxins and growth factor toxin–fusion proteins in *E. coli* has been successful. Initially, single-chain Fvs were used to fuse to toxins in which the heavy and light chains are connected together by a peptide linker. Because the majority of single-chain Fvs cloned from MAb are unstable and cannot be used to make recombinant immunotoxins, it was necessary to find a method of stabilizing the Fvs. This was accomplished by replacing the peptide linker with a disulfide bond connecting framework residues in the V_H and V_L. Residues that can be used to introduce disulfide bonds for almost all antibodies were identified by protein modeling (32). Recombinant immunotoxins containing truncated PE are most commonly 38 kd in molecular weight and include B3(Fv)-PE38, anti-Tac(Fv)-PE38, etc., or if a growth factor is used, transforming growth factor–α (TGF-α)–PE38, etc. The mechanism of cell killing by a single-chain immunotoxin containing an Fv fragment and a portion of PE is depicted in Figure 1. With DT, the ligand is inserted at the carboxyl end of the toxin and the number of amino acids in the toxin (including the initiator methionine) is noted [e.g., DAB_{486},-interleukin-2 (IL-2) or DAB_{389}-IL-2].

Recombinant immunotoxins have several advantages over chemical conjugates with antibodies or antibody fragments. One is that they are homogeneous with respect to the toxin-ligand junction, whereas chemical conjugates are heterogeneous. Second, they are less immunogenic. Third, they are less costly to produce. Their most important attribute, however, is that they are often more active than chemical conjugates, probably because they closely resemble the parental toxin from which they are derived and are activated by the target cell more efficiently.

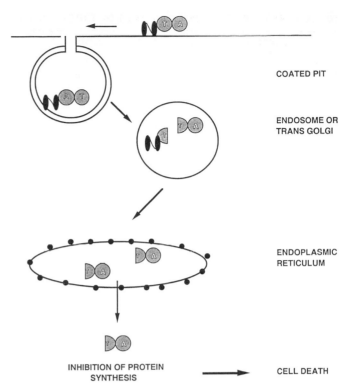

FIGURE 1. Mechanism of cell killing by a single-chain immunotoxin containing an antibody Fv fragment and a portion of *Pseudomonas* exotoxin. Domain I (the binding domain of *Pseudomonas* exotoxin) is replaced with the variable regions of an antibody. *T* indicates translocation domain (II) and *A* indicates the adenosine diphosphate ribosylation domain (III) of *Pseudomonas* exotoxin. After binding to a cell-surface antigen, the toxin-receptor complex is internalized via coated pits into the endocytic vesicle and trans Golgi compartments, where the low pH environment causes toxin unfolding and facilitates proteolysis; the cleaved toxin is then reduced into two fragments. The 37-kd carboxyl terminal fragment is transported to the endoplasmic reticulum and from there to the cytosol. The toxin fragment inactivates elongation factor 2, arrests protein synthesis, and causes cell death.

CLINICAL TRIALS

Immunotoxins Targeting Hematologic Malignancies

Many of the initial immunotoxins were directed toward hematologic tumors, which are easier to target than solid tumors for several reasons, including direct access of the immunotoxin to intravascular tumor cells and better penetration into lymphomatous tumor–cell masses. Moreover, fresh cells can be obtained and tested for immunotoxin binding and cytotoxic activity. Immunotoxins also have been developed for the indirect treatment of malignancies by targeting T cells that mediate graft-versus-host disease (GVHD) in the setting of allogeneic transplantation. Table 3 summarizes some of the immunotoxin clinical trials in hematologic malignancies from the mid-1990s.

Immunotoxins Targeting CD5

CD5 is a T-cell antigen that is present in T-cell and some B-cell malignancies, particularly B-cell chronic lymphocytic leukemia (CLL) (33). In one of the earliest clinical trials of immunotox-

ins, the anti-CD5 MAb T101 was conjugated to ricin A chain (RTA) and T101-RTA was tested in patients with GVHD and CLL with some responses reported (34). A related immunotoxin H65-RTA (also called *XomaZyme-CD5*), showed some activity in patients with GVHD and other autoimmune disorders. A randomized double-blind trial comparing steroids with or without H65-RTA in 243 patients with acute GVHD, however, showed control of clinical manifestations of GVHD for the first 5 weeks but no lasting significant difference in the complete response rate, incidence of chronic extensive GVHD, or survival (35). Toxicities included fever and vascular leak syndrome (VLS), and patients treated for GVHD had a high mortality rate from infections because of the late return of CD4- and CD8-positive T cells (36).

Immunotoxins Targeting Interleukin-2 Receptor

The IL-2 receptor (IL-2R) binds IL-2 with high affinity (kd = 10^{-11} M) if all three subunits of the receptor are present (α, β, γc). IL-2 binds with intermediate affinity (kd = 10^{-9} M) to the complex of β and γc and with low affinity (kd = 10^{-8} M) to α

TABLE 3. RESULTS OF CLINICAL TRIALS OF TARGETED TOXINS IN HEMATOLOGIC MALIGNANCIES

Target Toxin	Phase	Target	Patients	Response	Frequent Toxicities	References
H65-RTA	2	CD5	41	GVHD prevention	N/A	35
Anti-CD6-bRicin	1	CD6	5	CTCL	Ongoing	54
DAB$_{389}$IL-2	1–3	IL-2R	144	13 CR, 24 PR	Asthenia, mild VLS	38,39
Anti-Tac(Fv)-PE38(LMB-2)	1	CD25	32	1 CR, 7 PR	Transaminases, fever	37,41
RFT5-dgA	1	CD25	20	2 PR	VLS	43
RFB4-IgG-dgA	1	CD22	42	1 CR, 9 PR	VLS	44,46
Bispecific αCD22/αSAP	1	CD22	5	0 PR	Preliminary data	118
RFB4(dsFv)-PE38 (BL22)	1	CD22	—	—	Ongoing	48
B43-PAP	1	CD19	17	4 CR, 1 PR	Preliminary data	51
HD37-dgA	1	CD19	40	1 CR, 2 PR	VLS	52
Anti-B4-bRicin	1–2	CD19	95 Measurable	4 CR, 5 PR	Transaminases, platelets	53,54
Anti-B4-bRicin	1–3	CD19	143 Adjuvant	DFS unchanged	N/A	55,56
Ber-H2-Sap6	1	CD30	12 HD	4 PR	—	57
Anti-My9-bRicin	1	CD33	18 AML	0 PR VLS	Platelets	54

AML, acute myelogenous leukemia; CTCL, cutaneous T-cell lymphoma; CR, complete remission; DFS, disease-free survival; dgA, deglycosylated A chain; GVHD, graft-versus-host disease; HD, Hodgkin's disease; IL-2, interleukin-2; IL-2R, interleukin-2 receptor; N/A, not applicable; PE, *Pseudomonas* exotoxin; PR, partial remission; VLS, vascular leak syndrome.

(CD25) alone. CD25 is overexpressed on the malignant cells in adult T-cell leukemia, peripheral T-cell leukemia/lymphomas, cutaneous T-cell lymphoma (CTCL), B-cell non-Hodgkin's lymphomas, Hodgkin's disease (HD), hairy cell leukemia, and CLL, as well as on activated T cells (37).

The high-affinity IL-2R has been targeted using single-chain fusions of truncated DT with IL-2. DAB$_{486}$IL-2 contains the first 485 amino acids of DT; it was tested in 112 patients with hematologic malignancies in several phase 1 trials (38). Responses (mostly partial) were observed in 4 of 46 patients with B-cell non-Hodgkin's lymphoma, one of nine patients with HD, 5 of 36 patients with CTCL, 1 of 13 patients with CLL, and no patients with Kaposi's sarcoma, adult T-cell leukemia, acute myelogenous leukemia, prolymphocytic leukemia, and acute lymphocytic leukemia. Dose-limiting toxicity when given as bolus injections was usually from transaminase elevations, and when given as a 90-minute infusion, toxicity was caused by renal insufficiency, hemolysis, and thrombocytopenia.

An improved derivative, DAB$_{389}$IL-2, containing the first 388 amino acids of DT, was subsequently produced. In a phase 1 trial, it produced five complete remissions (CRs) and eight partial remissions (PRs) in 35 patients with CTCL, one CR and two PRs in 17 patients with non-Hodgkin's lymphoma, and no responses in 21 patients with HD (39,40). The maximum tolerated dose (MTD) was 27 μg per kg per day × 5 days, and the dose-limiting toxicity was asthenia. Common toxicities included transaminase elevations (62%), hypoalbuminemia (86%), hypotension (32%), rashes (32%), other allergic reactions (21%), and mild VLS comprised of hypotension, hypoalbuminemia, and edema (8%). The average overall half-life was 72 minutes. A phase 3 trial of DAB$_{389}$IL-2 was performed in 71 patients with CTCL who were randomized between receiving 9 and 18 μg per kg per day × 5. Overall, seven CRs and 14 PRs were observed (39). Slightly more responses occurred in the high-dose arm (36% vs. 23%), which became more significant (10% vs. 38%, p = .03) when patients with at least stage IIb disease were considered.

An alternative strategy for IL-2R targeting is to target CD25 directly, and this is particularly useful for targeting malignant cells that express CD25 alone or with low expression of the other IL-2R chains. Anti-Tac(Fv)-PE38 (LMB-2) is a recombinant immunotoxin that targets CD25. It is composed of the V$_H$ domain of anti-Tac fused via a 15–amino acid linker to V$_L$, which, in turn, is fused to a PE38 (30,37,41). In a phase 1 trial, 35 patients with chemotherapy refractory hematologic malignancies have been treated with doses of LMB-2 ranging from 2 to 63 μg per kg q.o.d. × 3. One CR and seven PRs were observed in 19 evaluable patients treated with 30 to 63 μg per kg q.o.d. × 3, including four of four patients with hairy cell leukemia, one of three patients with CLL, one of one patient with CTCL, one of two patients with adult T-cell leukemia, and one of six patients with HD. One hairy cell leukemia patient had a clinical CR lasting longer than 9 months. The MTD of LMB-2 is 40 μg per kg q.o.d. × 3 with the most common toxicities being transient transaminase elevations and fever. A phase 2 trial is planned for 1999. LMB-2 is also being developed for the prevention of GVHD. One strategy is to react donor T cells with radiated patient cells to selectively upregulate CD25 only on those donor T cells that are potentially reactive with patient cells. Using LMB-2 *ex vivo*, these patient-reactive donor T cells are killed, leaving a graft more suitable for haplotype-mismatched transplantation (42). This should represent an improvement over nonspecific T-cell depletion from the donor graft, which has been associated with impaired engraftment when antigens, such as CD3, are targeted. A chemical conjugate of the anti-CD25 MAb RFT5 with dgA has also been tested in a phase 1 trial in which 2 of a total of 20 patients with HD responded (43). This immunotoxin, RFT5-dgA, is also being administered to patients immediately after allogeneic transplantation in an effort to prevent GVHD.

Immunotoxins Targeting CD22

Because approximately 70% of B-cell lymphomas and leukemias are CD22$^+$, these disorders have been targeted by a variety of immunotoxins, the most successful of which have contained the anti-CD22 MAb RFB4 or its Fab' fragment conjugated chemically to dgA (44–46). RFB4-Fab'-dgA produced PRs in 5 of 13 patients and RFB4-IgG-dgA produced one CR and nine PRs in 30 evaluable patients. Another durable CR was reported with RFB4-IgG-dgA (47). The dose of RFB4-dgA is limited by VLS, which in several cases has been fatal (44–46). RFB4(dsFv)-PE38 is a PE-based recombinant immunotoxin targeted at CD22 (48) that has just entered clinical trials. It contains the Fv portion of the RFB4 antibody, so it targets the same epitope as RFB4-dgA. It could potentially have fewer side effects than RFB4-dgA, however, because PE38 is much less toxic than dgA toward human endothelial cells (49) and RFB4(dsFv)-PE38 is well tolerated in preclinical studies done in mice and monkeys.

Immunotoxins Targeting CD19

CD19 is the most ubiquitously expressed protein in the B-lymphocyte lineage and is present on B cells from the time stem cells begin B-cell commitment until the time of plasma-cell differentiation (50). Pokeweed antiviral protein has been targeted using the anti-CD19 MAb B43. In a phase 1 trial in relapsed patients with childhood acute lymphocytic leukemia, the MTD was found to be more than 1.25 mg per kg, and toxicities included VLS and myalgias. To date, responses in 17 evaluable patients have been reported, including four CRs and one PR (51). Another anti-CD19 antibody, HD37, was conjugated to dgA and administered to lymphoma patients in various schedules. HD37-dgA produced one CR and two PRs in 40 evaluable patients. Dose-limiting toxicity was caused by VLS (52). The anti-CD19 MAb anti-B4 was conjugated to blocked ricin (bR). When anti-B4-bR was administered by five daily bolus injections or by continuous infusion, a total of three CRs and five PRs were observed in 59 patients, but, in a follow-up phase 2 trial, no responses were observed (53). Anti-B4-bR was also tested by continuous infusion in patients with B-cell lymphoma in CR after autologous bone marrow transplantation, where residual disease was minimal. Although phase 1 and 2 trials appeared promising, in a phase 3 trial, 82 patients randomized to anti-B4-bR showed no benefit in disease-free survival (54–56).

Immunotoxins Targeting Other Hematologic Antigens

The T-cell antigen CD6 is present on CTCL cells, and a clinical trial of anti-CD6-bR is under way in this disease (54). Because CD30 is expressed in HD, an anti-CD30 immunotoxin was made by coupling MAb Ber-H2 to saporin. Ber-H2-Sap6 produced four PRs in 12 patients (57). CD33 is expressed on acute myelogenous leukemia cells and has been targeted using the chemical conjugate anti-My9-bR, but it produced no major responses in 18 patients in a trial in which the dose was limited by VLS and thrombocytopenia (54). Recombinant toxins targeted at the granulocyte-macrophage colony-stimulating factor receptor on acute myelogenous leukemia (58) and CD40 on B-cell malignancies (59) are under development with the former agent, DT$_{388}$-granulocyte-macrophage colony-stimulating factor, already in clinical testing.

Immunotoxins Targeting Solid Tumors

Although encouraging results have been observed in the treatment of patients with leukemia and lymphomas, the efficacy of immunotoxins in the treatment of epithelial carcinomas has been limited. A major obstacle has been the difficulty in finding MAb without cross-reactivity to essential normal tissues. The first immunotoxin studies designed to target breast and ovarian carcinomas were hampered by unexpected neurotoxicities as a result of cross-reactivity with cells of the central nervous system (60,61). Another barrier has been the inability of these macromolecules to reach the target cell in adequate quantities because of physiologic factors well described by Jain et al (62). The heterogeneous blood supply, elevated interstitial pressure within the tumor, and large transport distances in the interstitium (63) play a role in decreasing the therapeutic window of these agents. These physiologic barriers do not represent a problem for treating leukemias, lymphomas, and micrometastasis in which the interstitial pressure is low and diffusion distances are small (64).

Valuable clinical experience was gained from first-generation immunotoxins. They are listed in Table 4 (60,61,65–71). Progress in the understanding of tumor physiology and biology has also led to the development of newer-generation recombinant immunotoxins with better properties. The advent of computer protein design and modeling has been instrumental in many of these improvements. Some of the new-generation immunotoxins developed during the past few years are described.

Anti-Lewis Y Recombinant Immunotoxins

MAb B3 is a murine antibody that reacts with several human epithelial carcinomas with limited expression in normal tissue (72). The hybridoma that produces MAb B3 (IgG1k) was isolated from the spleen of a mouse immunized with MCF-7 (human breast carcinoma) cells. Immunohistochemical studies of a panel of human carcinomas show that MAb B3 react strongly and homogeneously in more than 90% of the colorectal carcinomas. Other gastrointestinal malignancies, such as esophageal (80%) and gastric carcinomas (75%), showed similar strong reactivity, as do 70% of non–small-cell carcinomas of the lung. MAb B3 also reacts strongly with as many as 70% of breast carcinomas tested and mucinous adenocarcinomas of the ovary.

Peroxidase immunohistochemistry with frozen sections of normal tissues demonstrated that MAb B3 reacts with the glands of the stomach, the differentiated cell layer of the esophagus, and the epithelia of the trachea and bladder. One of the important characteristics of this antibody is that similar reactivity was found in normal monkey and normal human tissues, so that monkeys could be used for toxicology studies. Biochemical analysis indicated that MAb B3 reacts with a carbohydrate antigen of the Lewis^y (Le^y) family that is present on many cell-surface glycoproteins. These range in molecular weight from more than 200,000 kd to less than 40,000 kd. Because many of these glycoproteins are internalized, they represent good targets for immunotoxin therapy.

TABLE 4. CLINICAL TRIALS OF IMMUNOTOXINS AND RECOMBINANT IMMUNOTOXINS FOR SOLID TUMORS

Immunotoxin	Target/Toxin Moiety	Disease (Mode of Delivery)	Major Side Effect	Reference
Systemic Delivery				
Xomazyme-Mel	Proteoglycan/A chain	Melanoma (i.v.)	VLS	65,66,67
Xomazyme-791	gp72/ A chain	Colon cancer (i.v.)	VLS, renal, neurologic	68,69
260F9-rRTA	Anti-gp55/rA chain	Breast cancer (i.v.)	Neuropathy, VLS	60,70
N901-bB	Anti-NCAM/blocked R	Small-cell lung cancer (i.v.)	VLS, hepatic, hematologic	85
LMB-1 (B3LysPE38)	Anti-Le^y/PE38	Epithelial carcinoma (i.v.)	VLS	75
LMB-7 (B3FvPE38)	Anti-Le^y/PE38	Epithelial carcinoma(i.v.)	Gastrointestinal	78
LMB-9 (B3dsFvPE38)	Anti-Le^y/PE38	Epithelial carcinoma (i.v.)	Ongoing	Ongoing
erb-38	Her2-neu/PE38	Her2neu-positive tumors (i.v.)	Hepatic	84
DAB$_{389}$EGF	EGF/DT	EGF-positive tumors (i.v.)	Hepatic	86,87
Regional Immunotoxin Delivery				
454A12-rRTA	Anti-transf./r A chain	Epithelial cancer (i.p.)	VLS, encephalopathy	71
OVB3-PE	OVB-3/PE	Ovarian cancer (i.p.)	Encephalopathy	61
TP40	EGF/ PE40	Bladder cancer (intravesical)	None	93
45A12-rRA	Anti-transf./r A chain	Leptomeningeal carcinomatosis (intrathecal)	Neurologic	95
TF-CRN1-7	Transferrin/DT (CRM107)	Brain tumors (intratumoral)	Hepatic, neurologic	99
IL-4(38-37)-PE38KDEL	IL-4 receptor/PE38	Glioblastoma (intratumoral)	Ongoing	102–104

Anti-transf./r A, anti-transferrin ricin A; DT, diphtheria toxin; EGF, epidermal growth factor; PE, *Pseudomonas* exotoxin; VLS, vascular leak syndrome.

LMB-1 (B3-LysPE38) is an immunotoxin in which MAb B3 is chemically coupled to LysPE38 (73,74). Thirty-eight patients with advanced solid tumors were entered in a phase 1 clinical trial (16 male, 22 female) with a mean age of 47 years (age range, 30 to 70 years). All patients had B3 antigen on the surface of their tumor cells and no preexisting neutralizing antibodies to LMB-1 (75). Twenty-six patients had colorectal cancer, eight had breast cancer, one had cancer of the esophagus, one had cancer of the stomach, one had ovarian cancer, and one had cancer of the ampulla of Vater. LMB-1 was administered intravenously over 30 minutes on days 1, 3, and 5. Patients received doses ranging from 10 mg per kg per day to 100 mg per kg every day. The MTD is 75 mg per kg given on days 1, 3, and 5. The dose-limiting toxicity is VLS, manifested by hypoalbuminemia, fluid retention, and peripheral edema. In severe cases, hypotension and pulmonary edema were observed. Other side effects include "flulike" symptoms, fever, malaise, skin rash, headache, and nonspecific electrocardiogram changes. Antitumor activity was observed in four patients (one CR, one PR, two minor responses), 20 patients had stable disease, and 15 patients progressed. Thirty-three of 38 (90%) patients developed antibodies against LMB-1 3 weeks after treatment.

The evidence of antitumor activity observed with LMB-1 proves that it is possible to target epithelial malignancies in humans. Although immunotoxin therapy has been shown to be active in hematologic malignancies, this is the first time that objective antitumor activity against metastatic colon and breast cancers has been documented. At the MTD, side effects of LMB-1 were well tolerated and transient. The major side effect, VLS, is secondary to targeting of LMB-1 to antigen-positive endothelial cells (49).

Single-Chain Immunotoxins [B3(Fv)-PE38 and B3(dsFV)-PE38]

LMB-7

Inadequate distribution of drug within tumors is probably one of the major obstacles for the efficacy of LMB-1 and other high-molecular-weight immunotoxins. Although this is a problem that affects drugs in general, it is particularly troublesome for macromolecules, such as LMB-1 (molecular weight, approximately 200 kd). The differences in the blood flow within the tumor and the elevation of interstitial pressure greatly slows the penetration of molecules like LMB-1 into the interior of tumors. Successful therapy may not be possible, unless this barrier can be circumvented. The production of small, genetically engineered single-chain (Fv) immunotoxins (65 kd) helps overcome the tumor distribution problem (76). B3(Fv)-PE38 or LMB-7 is a single-chain immunotoxin composed of the variable regions (Fvs) of the light (V$_L$) and heavy (V$_H$) chains of B3, connected by a flexible linker to form a single-chain antigen-binding protein B3(scFv), which, in turn, is fused to PE38 (77). It has a molecular weight of 63 kd. Because LMB-7 lacks the Fc portion of the murine MAb and is smaller in size, it was expected to be less immunogenic than LMB-1.

Fifty-one patients were entered into a phase 1 clinical trial at doses ranging from 2 μg per kg per day to 48 μg per kg per day given as a 30-minute bolus on days 1, 3, and 5 (78). At 7 μg per kg, the first signs of nausea, vomiting, and diarrhea were noted. The dose-limiting toxicity was 30 μg per kg, and the MTD was defined as 24 μg per kg. Upper gastrointestinal endoscopy revealed severe gastritis and ulcers. This side effect was expected because the B3 antigen is also expressed on the surface of the human gastric mucosa. The etiology of the diarrhea is unclear. Our hypothesis is that the targeting of the gastric mucosa by LMB-7 leads to increased gastric secretion, which, in turn, stimulates intestinal movement. Based on this hypothesis, the clinical protocol was amended to circumvent the gastrointestinal toxicity. Patients are now pretreated with antiemetics and omeprazole to suppress gastric acid secretion. Loperamide is administered to patients as needed. Using this regimen, the LMB-7 dose has been escalated up to 48 μg per kg with marked improvement of the gastrointestinal symptoms. Other non–dose-limiting side effects thus far include VLS, transient elevation of transaminases, and transient elevation of creatinine. A minor response (<50% tumor shrinkage) was observed in one patient with colon cancer (78).

Preliminary pharmacokinetic data indicates that LMB-7 is cleared monoexponentially from the circulation with a half-life of 60 minutes (± 38); the area under the curve, 2.2 µg per hour per mL (± 14); the Vd = volume of distribution, 3.2 liters (± 1.6); and the Cl = clearance, 2.2 liters per hour (± 0.6). LMB-7 is cleared from the circulation more rapidly than the chemical conjugate LMB-1 (half-life, 1 hour vs. 8 hours). Sixty-five percent (33 of 51) of the patients developed neutralizing antibodies against LMB-7 after one cycle of treatment. This result indicates that, as predicted, LMB-7 is less immunogenic than the chemical conjugate LMB-1.

LMB-9

Single-chain (Fv) immunotoxins, such as LMB-7, were created to overcome the poor tumor penetration of large immunotoxins made with whole IgG. Although LMB-7 is smaller in size than LMB-1 and should penetrate more readily into tumor, LMB-7 is unstable in serum. When incubated at 37°C in human serum, it loses 50% of its activity after 2 to 4 hours. Dissociation of V_L and V_H leads to aggregation and inactivation. To overcome the instability of LMB-7, a method was developed to stabilize the Fv fragment of the B3 antibody by producing genetically altered forms of V_L and V_H in which a disulfide bond connects the two chains (79). LMB-9 was synthesized using this new approach. B3(dsFv)PE38 or LMB-9 is extremely stable (80). When incubated at 37°C in phosphate-buffered saline or human serum, it remains fully active for more than 14 days. This property renders LMB-9 superior to LMB-7. Because LMB-9 is much more stable in physiologic conditions than LMB-7, LMB-9 should remain active within the tumor interstitium as it slowly distributes and binds to the cancer cells. Preclinical experiments indicate that, when given by slow intraperitoneal infusion, LMB-9 has superior antitumor activity than LMB-7 (81).

Preclinical pharmacokinetic studies of LMB-7 and LMB-9 indicate that these molecules are cleared rapidly from the circulation in mice (half-life, 20 to 23 minutes) and Cynomolgus monkeys (half-life, 30 to 180 minutes). The plasma clearances of LMB-7 and LMB-9 in humans are expected to be similar. Because of the improved stability of LMB-9, however, its behavior within the tumor interstitium is expected to be superior. A phase 1 clinical trial using the improved disulfide-stabilized immunotoxin LMB-9 is ongoing.

Recombinant Immunotoxins Targeting Her2/neu (Erb-38)

To exploit the overexpression of erbB-2 in many human cancers (breast, stomach, lung, and ovary), a recombinant immunotoxin was made using MAb e23 (82) that reacts with erbB-2. Erb-38 is a recombinant immunotoxin in which the Fv portion of an MAb recognizing erbB2 is fused to a 38-kd fragment of PE A. This immunotoxin is specifically cytotoxic to cells expressing erbB-2 and causes regression of the human gastric cancer cells (N87) growing as tumors in immunodeficient mice (83). We conducted a phase 1 study of erb-38 in adult cancer patients with carcinomas that express Her2/neu

(84). Erb-38 was administered as a 30-minute intravenous bolus on days 1, 3, and 5. Six patients (five breast, one esophageal cancer) were entered at doses of 1 or 2 µg per kg. Transient transaminase elevation was observed in all patients. Erb-38 was cleared monoexponentially from the circulation with a half-life of 2.4 to 10.3 hours at 2 µg per kg; the maximum plasma concentration achieved was 47 to 105 ng per mL. One of five patients developed antibodies against erb-38 (84). The toxicity observed with erb-38 is most likely caused by the presence of erbB2 on hepatocytes. This finding led us to conclude that the toxicity observed with erb-38 is most likely caused by the presence of erbB2 on hepatocytes because recombinant immunotoxins targeting other antigens (Le^y or CD25) did not produce the same liver toxicity when given much higher doses. The targeting of tumors with antibodies to erbB2 that are armed with radioisotopes, chemotherapy drugs, and other toxic agents may also result in unexpected organ toxicities caused by erB2 expression on normal tissues.

Immunotoxin for Small-Cell Lung Cancer (N901-bR, anti-NCAM-Blocked Ricin)

bR was coupled to N901, a murine IgG anti-NCAM (CD56), which is expressed in more than 95% of small-cell lung cancer cell lines. This antigen is also present in cardiac muscle, peripheral nerve, and human natural killer cells. In preclinical toxicity studies, monkeys were able to tolerate up to 1 mg per kg of intravenous N901-bR, but myocardial inflammation and mild nerve conduction alterations were observed in animals treated with N901-bR. In a phase 1/2 study, N901-bR was given by continuous intravenous infusion × 7 days to 21 patients with small-cell lung cancer who had failed standard therapy (85). Patients were treated with doses ranging from 5 to 40 µg per kg per day. The MTD was 30 mg per kg lean body weight per day with VLS as the dose-limiting toxicity. Other side effects included transaminase elevation, fever, myalgia, weight gain, and thrombocytopenia. Fifteen of the 21 patients were evaluated pre- and posttreatment with detailed neurologic examinations, electromyelogram, and nerve conduction studies. No clinical symptoms or changes in the neurologic examination were noted, although there was a trend for amplitude decline in nerve conduction for both sensory motor and motor neurons. No evidence of clinically significant myocardial dysfunction was observed, but cardiac events occurred in three patients: one patient had a "silent" myocardial infarction with a change of ejection fraction from 66% to 36%, one patient with a previous history of fibrillation had an episode of atrial fibrillation, and one patient had an asymptomatic elevation of creatine phosphokinase. Sinus tachycardia was noted in 15 of 21 patients. These events were probably related to the specific binding of the antibody to neural and cardiac cells. Specific binding of the immunotoxin to tumor cells in bone marrow, liver, and lung was documented. One patient achieved a PR. Fifty percent of the patients developed human antimouse antibody (HAMA) and 85% developed human antiricin antibody. A phase 2 study after induction radiochemotherapy in patients with small-cell lung cancer will address the role of N901-bR in patients with a small tumor burden.

Epidermal Growth Factor Immunotoxin (DAB$_{389}$ Epidermal Growth Factor)

Two phase 1 studies using DAB$_{389}$ epidermal growth factor (EGF) (86) in patients with EGF receptor (EGF-R) expressing solid tumors has been conducted in patients with EGF-R–expressing malignancies. Two different dosing schedules repeated every 28 days (daily, 1 to 5 and days 1, 8, 9, 15, and 16) were examined. A total of 52 patients with metastatic disease were entered, receiving doses ranging from 0.3 to 15 μg per kg per day. The dose-limiting toxicity was renal tubular acidosis and back and chest pain. The toxicities include reversible hepatic transaminase elevation, renal toxicity, hypoalbuminemia, fever, chills, nausea, blood pressure alterations, and anorexia.

A PR was observed in one patient with lung cancer (6 μg per kg per day on the episodic schedule) (38,87). A phase 1/2 study is ongoing for patients with non–small-cell lung cancer with a starting dose of 6 μg per kg per day every other day for three doses.

REGIONAL IMMUNOTOXIN DELIVERY

Regional drug delivery is an approach designed to exploit dose-response effects by delivering more drug to locally confined tumors. When compared with intravenous administration, regional delivery of drugs can presumably increase drug concentration at tumor sites, decrease systemic exposure and, therefore, decrease toxicities. Modes of regional delivery include administration into an existing cavity (e.g., cerebrospinal, peritoneal, bladder, pleural) and direct instillation of drug into a tumor or intraarterial infusion. The general pharmacokinetic principles guiding regional therapy is that the rate of drug clearance from the local compartment is smaller than total body clearance, resulting in a higher drug concentration at the tumor site for a longer period. Regional delivery of immunotoxins might therefore help overcome the physiologic resistance to therapy of solid tumors and minimize systemic toxicities.

Intravesical Therapy of Transitional Cell Carcinoma with TP40

To exploit the EGF-R overexpression on neoplastic cells, the DNA encoding TGF-α has been fused to PE40 to form the chimeric toxin TGFα-PE40 (88). TGFα-PE40 specifically kills cells that overexpress EGF-Rs (89,90). Because several normal organs and, particularly, the liver express the EGF-R, the therapeutic window for TGFα-PE40 is narrow when delivered systemically. To circumvent liver toxicity, this agent has been used for the regional therapy of superficial bladder cancer in patients. Transitional cell cancer of the bladder is known to overexpress EGF-Rs, and tumors with a high density of EGF-R have been shown to correlate with poor clinical outcome (91). A phase 1 trial using a genetically modified form of TGFα-PE40, termed *TP40* (92), was carried out in patients with superficial bladder cancer. Forty-three patients were entered in

this study (93). Therapy was given weekly × 6 by intravesical administration at doses ranging from 0.15 mg per 60 mL to 9.6 mg. No toxicities were observed in this study. Eleven patients had evaluable Ta or T1 lesions, 19 patients had resected Ta or T1 lesions, seven patients had carcinoma *in situ* only, and six patients had mixed carcinoma *in situ* and Ta/T1 disease. One CR occurred in a patient with carcinoma *in situ*; five of seven (70%) patients with carcinoma *in situ* were found to have visual resolution of the lesions during follow-up cystoscopy. None of the patients in this trial developed antibodies against TP40. The absence of systemic toxicity and antibody formation against the toxin indicate that TP40 is not absorbed through the bladder mucosa. Further trials using prolonged bladder irrigation, daily intravesical administrations, or other schemes of delivery might help improve the efficacy of this agent for patients with superficial bladder cancer.

Treatment of Central Nervous System Malignancies with Immunotoxins

Several immunotoxins and recombinant immunotoxins are being tested in clinical studies for the treatment of malignancies of the central nervous system. Although normal blood–brain barrier represents an impediment for the delivery of large molecules, such as immunotoxins, it is known that this barrier is frequently disrupted at the tumor site. Although systemic administrations might have potential benefit for treatment of central nervous system malignancies, regional delivery of immunotoxins in this "self-contained" compartment is appealing, particularly in the setting of meningeal carcinomatosis. Furthermore, the immunoprotective environment of the central nervous system may also allow for repeated administration of immunotoxin without the development of neutralizing antibodies frequently observed in systemic delivery.

Anti-Transferrin-Ricin A Chain Immunotoxin

454A12-rRA is an immunotoxin made of an MAb against the human transferrin receptor and ricin A chain (94). Eight patients with leptomeningeal carcinomatosis were treated in a pilot study of intraventricular therapy (95). Patients received doses ranging from 1.2 to 1,200 μg. Doses of more than 120 μg were associated with headache, vomiting, and altered mental status. More than 50% reduction of tumor cell counts in the lumbar cerebrospinal fluid was observed in four of eight patients; however, no patients had their cerebrospinal fluid cleared of tumors, and clinical or magnetic resonance imaging evidence of tumor progression was demonstrated in seven of eight patients. Tumoricidal concentrations of 454A12-rRA were obtained. Pharmacokinetic studies showed that the early phase half-life in the cerebrospinal fluid was 44 ± 21 minutes and the late phase half-life was 237 ± 86 minutes.

LMB-1 and LMB-7

A mouse model of human meningeal carcinomatosis was developed by Bigner et al. using athymic rats bearing the human epidermoid carcinoma A431. The efficacy of anti–Lewis Y immunotoxins LMB-1 and LMB-7 were evaluated using this model (96,97).

Immunotoxins were injected intrathecally 3 days after tumor implantation. Without treatment, median survival was 10 days. When LMB-1 was administered at 40 or 200 μg given on days 3, 6, and 8, significant increase in median survival was observed (40.5 and 33 days, respectively). With two long-term survivors in each group (191-day survival), non–tumor-bearing athymic rats showed no toxicity with a single dose of either 40 μg or 200 μg, or three doses of 40 μg. Weight loss, neurologic deficit, and death (two of eight patients) occurred. LMB-1 had no therapeutic effect on the treatment of two B3 antigen–negative neoplastic meningitis models. Similarly, CR and long-term survivors were observed in animals given 10 μg of LMB-7 on days 3, 5, and 7. A phase 1 clinical study to determine the MTD and side effects of LMB-7 in patients with meningeal carcinomatosis is being carried out.

Treatment of High-Grade Astrocytomas with Immunotoxins

Glioblastoma multiforme is the most malignant tumor of the glial series. Despite technical advances in neurosurgery and radiation therapy, the median survival for glioblastoma multiforme remains dismal. Presently available chemotherapy agents provide little to no survival advantage. The average survival of patients with this tumor ranges from 6 to 12 months. Because death is most often caused by local failure after conventional therapy, regional delivery with highly potent agents, such as immunotoxins, is an attractive treatment modality that warrants consideration.

Clinical Trial with Transferrin-CRM107

Human transferrin (Tf) chemically coupled to a mutant of diphtheria toxin (CRM107) (98) has been evaluated and tested in a clinical trial in patients with recurrent malignant tumors. Tf-CRM107 was delivered by interstitial infusion in a dose-escalation schedule (99). After a computed tomography–guided tumor biopsy, one to three silastic infusion catheters were placed at selected sites in the tumor using stereotactic guidance. To distribute the immunotoxin in the tumor and the infiltrated brain surrounding the tumor, Laske and colleagues adapted a microinfusion technique in which a pressure gradient was maintained during interstitial brain infusion to establish convective flow in the extracellular space (100,101). Eighteen patients (ten male, eight female) ages 24 to 61 years (median, 48 years) with confirmed radiographic evidence of tumor progression were entered in the trial. Ten patients had glioblastoma multiforme, five patients had anaplastic astrocytoma, two patients had adenocarcinoma of the lung, and one patient had oligodendroglioma. The primary variables of this clinical trial were the drug concentration and the volume infused. Patients received doses ranging from 0.1 to 3.2 μg per mL (total dose, 0.5 to 199 μg). The total volume infused varied from 5 to 180 mL (duration of infusion, 2 to 15 days). Drug concentration and volume were escalated as tolerated. Doses of 1 mg per mL or more resulted in local toxicity, specifically peritumoral local brain injury, attributed to binding of the immunotoxin to transferrin receptors on endothelial cells. Objective tumor response was observed in 9 of 15 evaluable patients. Seven PRs (≥50% decrease in the enhancing volume of the tumor) and two CRs occurred. Tumor shrinkage occurred no earlier than 1 month. Time to maximum response was observed from 6 to 14 months in four patients after the first treatment. The median time to progression was 38 weeks. Transient worsening of neurologic deficit occurred three times in a total of 44 infusion treatments. This was attributed to increased cerebral edema in patients with preexisting significant edema and mass effect caused by the tumor. Four patients with history of seizure had seizure during infusion. Systemic toxicity included mild decrease in serum albumin (n = 12) and transient grade 1 to 3 elevation of transaminases (n = 14). Anti-DT antibody was detected in all patients before therapy. Six of 14 patients tested had more than a twofold increase in serum titers after treatment. Overall, at doses below 1 μg per mL, Tf-CRM107 was well tolerated with transient local and systemic toxicities.

Interleukin-4 Toxin

IL-4(38-37)-PE38KDEL (102,103) is a fusion protein consisting of a circularly permuted form of IL-4 fused to PE38KDEL. This chimeric toxin, composed of IL-4 residues 38-129, the linker GGNGG, and IL-4 residues 1-37, is highly cytotoxic to glioblastoma cell lines, as determined by clonogenic and protein synthesis inhibition assay. The IL-4 ligand in this toxin was circularly permuted to allow the toxin-ligand junction to be switched from the carboxyl terminus of IL-4, where the toxin interferes with IL-4R binding to residue 37 of IL-4. Human glioblastoma cells express high-affinity IL-4 receptors. IL-4 toxin, when administered directly into U251 tumors implanted in the flank of athymic mice, was capable of causing complete regressions (104). Significant antitumor activity was also observed in mice when IL-4 toxin was administered via intraperitoneal or intravenous routes. The potential advantage of IL-4 toxin over less tumor-specific immunotoxins is that IL-4R is not expressed on normal brain tissue (102), which allowed high concentrations to be well tolerated after intrathecal injections in monkeys or after intracerebral injection in rats. IL-4(38-37)-PE38KDEL is being tested in a phase 1/2 study in patients with glioblastoma, where the drug is administrated intratumorally.

Transforming Growth Factor–α–PE40 and Transforming Growth Factor–α–PE38

To exploit the overexpression of EGF-R in glioblastoma (105,106), we tested the activity of TGFα-PE40 (87) on tumor cells derived from patients diagnosed with glioblastoma multiforme. These cells were found to be highly sensitive to the recombinant toxin with an IC_{50} of 0.4 ng per mL for U-251 and 1.5 ng per mL for the T-98G cell line (90). Most significant, when given by continuous infusion over 7 days, TGFα-PE40 caused significant tumor regressions in nude mice bearing U-215 human glioblastoma xenografts (90). Preclinical toxicity experiments using a close derivative TGFα-PE38 indicate that this agent is well tolerated by rats (MTD, 666 ng) and monkeys (MTD, 2,000 ng) when administered intracerebrally. Higher doses lead to necrosis with microhemorrhage in the region of infusion. A phase 1 clinical study is being planned for patients with high-grade astrocytomas using TGFα-PE38.

PROBLEMS

Several problems that limit the clinical efficacy of immunotoxins have been identified. One is toxicity caused by antigen present on essential normal tissues. This can be circumvented by the selection of antibodies or growth factors that are more specific for tumor cells. A second is nonspecific toxicity caused by an uptake of the immunotoxin by antigen-negative cells, such as in the liver or kidney. This can occur because of low-affinity binding of the immunotoxin to normal cells. For example, bR retains some affinity for normal liver cells and causes liver damage. In addition, nonspecific dose-limiting toxicities have been observed with several agents. The most severe is VLS (see next section). Immunogenicity is another problem. The toxins are products of plants of bacteria, which are immunogenic in humans. Finally, it is important to have molecules that are small and stable because proteins that are the size of antibodies or larger penetrate into tumors poorly.

Vascular Leak Syndrome

Damage to endothelial cells that manifest as VLS is a major dose-limiting toxicity for several immunotoxins presently in clinical trials. This syndrome has been observed with immunotoxins made of various toxins, including ricin, saporin, pokeweed antiviral protein, and PE. This toxicity was observed in the preclinical testing of some, but not all, of these agents in rodents and monkeys. VLS in humans is characterized by a decreased serum albumin and accumulation of fluid in the interstitial space, leading to weight gain and edema. In the most severe cases, excess fluid accumulates in the lungs, resulting in pulmonary edema. Acute and severe fluid leakage into the interstitium leads to intravascular depletion with hemodynamic consequences, such as sinus tachycardia, hypotension, oliguria, and prerenal azotemia. Similar toxicity has been reported in patients after administration of IL-2 therapy (107), although the mechanisms of action of IL-2 and immunotoxins are probably different.

The mechanisms involved in immunotoxin-mediated VLS are complex and poorly understood. *In vitro* and animal studies indicate that several different mechanisms might be involved in endothelial cell damage; furthermore, the pathogenesis of the endothelial cell damage may also differ from immunotoxin to immunotoxin. Soler-Rodriguez et al. have shown that human umbilical vein endothelial cells undergo rapid and dramatic changes in morphology after treatment with ricin A chain and ricin A chain containing immunotoxins (108). Rounding of the endothelial cells results in the formation of gaps between them; subsequently, protein synthesis is arrested and the cells die. VLS caused by LMB-1 appears to be due in large part to the presence of a small amount of Le^Y on endothelial cells and is a specific effect of the immunotoxin (49). Because LMB-1 leaves the circulation slowly (half-life in humans is 8 ± 2 hours), endothelial cells are exposed to a high concentration of LMB-1 for extended periods. Smaller recombinant immunotoxins (e.g., LMB-7 and LMB-9) that leave the circulation more rapidly may not produce this side effect.

In vitro and animal studies have shown that leukocytes (109,110) and cytokine and inflammatory mediators (111) are involved in endothelial cell damage. In 1998, Rafi et al.

showed that perforin and Fas ligand may actively participate in IL-2–induced endothelial cell injury and induction of VLS in a variety of organs (112). It is possible that these mechanisms might also play a role in immunotoxin-mediated toxicity in humans. Prophylactic administration of corticosteroids and nonsteroidal antiinflammatory drugs has been shown to prevent PE-immunotoxin–mediated VLS in rats (113).

Clinical management of the capillary leak syndrome is mainly supportive. Pulmonary edema and hypotension are the most troublesome toxicity and have produced major morbidity and mortality in some trials. These patients require close monitoring, oxygen supplementation, fluid reconstitution, and, if necessary, ventilatory support and vasopressors. Judicious use of diuretics if hypotension is not present may be warranted. Serum albumin and steroids have been given to occasional patients in the event of acute VLS with no clear beneficial effects (44,45).

In an attempt to study the usefulness of corticosteroids in preventing immunotoxin-induced VLS, eight cancer patients received immunotoxin LMB-1 at 60 μg per kg on days 1, 3, and 5 and oral prednisone at 60 mg per m^2 for 2 weeks starting 4 days before the first dose of LMB-1. Eight patients received immunotoxin alone. No statistical differences were observed in the incidence of VLS, maximum decrement of serum albumin, weight gain, or development of HAMA/human antitoxin antibody (HATA) among the two groups.

Immunogenicity

Murine antibodies and toxins are highly immunogenic foreign proteins. HAMA and HATA can generally be detected 7 to 14 days after the initial exposure. Approximately 90% of patients with epithelial carcinomas and 30% of lymphoma patients have detectable HAMA and HATA after one cycle of immunotoxin. These antibodies neutralize the activity of the immunotoxin, precluding a multiple course therapy. Although the formation of HAMA is overcome by the use of single-chain recombinant immunotoxins, formation of antitoxin antibodies continues to represent a major problem.

Traditional immunosuppressive agents have been evaluated as a means of decreasing the antibody formation to the immunotoxins. Cyclophosphamide and cyclosporin (66,67) have been tested and were unsuccessful in reducing antibody formation at the doses administered. Newer agents, such as 15-deoxyspergualin, a metabolite of *Bacillus laterosporus*, were tested in a phase 1 study as immunosuppressive agent on HAMA formation (114,115) with encouraging effectiveness. The effectiveness of these agents was in part limited by the dose that could be administered without significant systemic toxicity.

A phase 2 study to explore the ability of the anti-CD20 antibody rituximab to suppress HAMA and HATA formation after treatment with immunotoxin LMB-1 is being conducted at the National Cancer Institute. Rituximab is used to treat B-cell lymphomas (116). It mediates complement and antibody-dependent cell-mediated cytotoxicity (ADCC) and has direct antiproliferative effects against malignant B-cell lines (117). In addition, a single dose of rituximab is able to completely clear normal B cells from the peripheral circulation. By giving an immunotoxin at the time of maximum B-cell depletion post-rituximab, it might be possible to reduce or eliminate the host antibody response to the immunotoxin LMB-1, which permits repeated cycles to be administered. It is clear that to improve the efficacy of the immunotoxins and their clinical usefulness, this and other strategies to inhibit the immune response to foreign proteins need to be explored.

CONCLUSION

The concept of targeting cancer cells with toxins attached to antibodies is more than two decades old. Several clinical trials have clearly documented antitumor activity in humans. The most promising and exciting results have been with hematopoietic tumors and in brain tumors using direct intratumoral infusion. Progress in the treatment of epithelial tumors has been slower because tumor-specific antibodies have been more difficult to identify, and first-generation immunotoxins have had difficulty penetrating into solid tumor masses because of their large size. Ongoing clinical trials using recombinant immunotoxins that are smaller, more active, and more stable in human circulation (e.g., LMB-9) may prove to be superior to the first-generation immunotoxins. Future clinical trials should select patients with minimal residual disease in whom target therapy with immunotoxin should be most effective. Strategies to reduce the immunogenicity and nonspecific toxicity are presently explored. These obstacles need to be overcome before immunotoxins can become an effective treatment modality for cancer.

REFERENCES

1. Ehrlich P. *Collected studies on immunity*. New York: John Wiley and Sons, 1906.
2. Kohler G, Milstein C. Continuous cultures of fused cell secreting antibody of predefined specificity. *Nature* 1975;256:495–497.
3. Moolten FL, Cooperband SR. Selective destruction of target cells by diphtheria toxin conjugated to antibody directed against antigens on the cells. *Science* 1970;169:68–70.
4. Komatsu N, Oda T, Muramatsu T. Involvement of both caspase-like proteases and serine proteases in apoptotic cell death induced by ricin, modeccin, diphtheria toxin, and pseudomonas toxin. *J Biochem (Tokyo)* 1998;124:1038–1044.
5. Bolognesi A, Tazzari PL, Olivieri F, et al. Induction of apoptosis by ribosome-inactivating proteins and related immunotoxins. *Int J Cancer* 1996;68:349–355.
6. Olsnes S, Pihl A. Toxic lectins and related proteins. In: Cohen P, van Heyningen S, eds. *Molecular action of toxins and viruses*. New York: Elsevier Science, 1982:51.
7. Eiklid K, Olsnes S, Pihl A. Entry of lethal doses of abrin, ricin and modeccin into the cytosol of HeLa cells. *Exp Cell Res* 126;321:1980.
8. Endo Y, Tsurigi K. RNA N-glycosidase activity of ricin A-chain. Mechanism of action of the toxic lectin ricin on eukaryotic ribosomes. *J Biol Chem* 1987;262:8128–8130.
9. Shen G-L, Li J-L, Ghetie MA, Ghetie V, et al. Evaluation of four CD22 antibodies as ricin A-chain containing immunotoxins for the *in vivo* therapy of human B-cell leukemias and lymphomas. *Int J Cancer* 1988;42:792–797.
10. Blakey DS, Watson GJ, Knowles PP, et al. Effect of chemical deglycosylation of ricin A-chain on the *in vivo* fate and cytotoxic activity of an immunotoxin composed of ricin A-chain and anti-Thy 1.1 antibody. *Cancer Res* 1987;47:947–952.
11. Thorpe PE, Wallace PM, Knowles PP, et al. Improved anti-tumor effects of immunotoxins prepared with deglycosylated ricin-A chain and hindered disulfide linkages. *Cancer Res* 1988;48:6396–6403.
12. Moroney SE, D'Alarcao LJ, Goldmacher VS, et al. Modification of the binding site(s) of lectins by an affinity column carrying an activated galactose-terminated ligand. *Biochemistry* 1987;26:8390–8398.
13. Thorpe PE, Ross WCJ, Brown ANF, et al. Blockade of the galactose-binding sites of ricin by its linkage to antibody. Specific cytotoxic effects of the conjugates. *Eur J Biochem* 1984;140:63–71.
14. Pasqualucci L, Wasik M, Teicher BA, et al. Antitumor activity of anti-CD30 immunotoxin (Ber-H2/saporin) *in vitro* and in severe combined immunodeficiency disease mice xenografted with human CD30+ anaplastic large-cell lymphoma. *Blood* 1995;85:2139–2146.
15. Flavell DJ. Saporin immunotoxins. *Curr Top Microbiol Immunol* 1998;234:57–61.
16. Uckun FM, Reaman GH. Immunotoxins for treatment of leukemia and lymphoma. *Leukoc Lymphoma* 1995;18:195–201.
17. Irvin JD, Uckun FM. Pokeweed antiviral protein: ribosome inactivation and therapeutic applications. *Pharmacol Ther* 1992;55:279–302.
18. Gary GL, Smith DH, Baldridge JS, et al. Cloning, nucleotide sequence and expression in *Escherichia coli* of the exotoxin A structural gene of *Pseudomonas aeruginosa*. *Proc Natl Acad Sci U S A* 1984;8:2645–2649.
19. Greenfield L, Bjorn MJ, Horn G, et al. Nucleotide sequence of the structural gene for diphtheria toxin carried by corynebacteriophage beta. *Proc Natl Acad Sci U S A* 1983;80:6853–6857.
20. Allured VS, Collier RJ, Carroll SF, et al. Structure of exotoxin A of *Pseudomonas aeruginosa* at 3.0 Angstrom resolution. *Proc Natl Acad Sci U S A* 1986;83:1320–1324.
21. Hwang J, FitzGerald DJ, Adhya S, et al. Functional domains of *Pseudomonas* exotoxin identified by deletion analysis of the gene expressed in *E. coli*. *Cell* 1987;48:129–136.
22. Munro S, Pellham HRB. A C-terminal signal prevents secretion of luminal ER proteins. *Cell* 1987;48:899–907.
23. Seetharam S, Chaudhary VT, FitzGerald D, et al. Increased cytotoxic activity of *Pseudomonas* exotoxin and the chimeric toxins ending in KDEL. *J Biol Chem* 1991;266:17376–17381.
24. Kounnas MZ, Morris RE, Thompson MR, et al. The α_2-macroglobulin receptor/low density lipoprotein receptor-related protein binds and internalizes *Pseudomonas* exotoxin A. *J Biol Chem* 1992;267:12420–12423.
25. FitzGerald DJ, Morris RE, Saelinger CB. Receptor-mediated internalization of *Pseudomonas* toxin by mouse fibroblasts. *Cell* 1980;21:867–873.
26. Iglewski BH, Kabat D. NAD-dependent inhibition of protein synthesis by *Pseudomonas aeruginosa* toxin. *Proc Natl Acad Sci U S A* 1975;72:2284–2288.
27. Choe S, Bennet MJ, Fujii G, et al. The crystal structure of diphtheria toxin. *Nature* 1992;357:216–222.
28. Papini E, Schiavo G, Tomasi M, et al. Lipid interaction of diphtheria toxin and mutants with altered fragment B2. Hydrophobic photolabeling and cell intoxication. *Eur J Biochem* 1987;169:637–644.
29. Moskaug JO, Stenmark H, Olsnes S. Insertion of diphtheria toxin B-fragment into the plasma membrane at low pH. *J Biol Chem* 1991;266:2652–2659.
30. Chaudhary VK, Queen C, Junghans RP, et al. A recombinant immunotoxin consisting of two antibody variable domains fused to *Pseudomonas* exotoxin. *Nature* 1989;339;394–397.
31. Murphy JR, Bishai W, Borowski M, et al. Genetic construction, expression, and melanoma-selective cytotoxicity of a diphtheria toxin-related alpha-melanocyte-stimulating hormone fusion protein. *Proc Natl Acad Sci U S A* 1986;83:8258–8262.
32. Chowdhury PS, Vasmatzis G, Beers R, et al. Improved stability and yield of a Fv-toxin fusion protein by computer design and protein engineering of the Fv. *J Mol Biol* 1998;281:917–928.
33. Foon, KA, Rai KR, Gale RP. Chronic lymphocytic leukemia: new insights into biology and therapy. *Ann Intern Med* 1990;113:525–539.
34. Hertler AA, Frankel AE. Immunotoxins: a clinical review of their use

in the treatment of malignancies. *J Clin Oncol* 1989;7:1932–1942.

35. Martin PJ, Nelson BJ, Appelbaum FR, et al. Evaluation of a CD5-specific immunotoxin for treatment of acute graft-versus-host disease after allogeneic marrow transplantation. *Blood* 1996;88:824–830.

36. Koehler M, Hurwitz CA, Krance RA, et al. XomaZyme-CD5 immunotoxin in conjunction with partial T cell depletion for prevention of graft rejection and graft-versus-host disease after bone marrow transplantation from matched unrelated donors. *Bone Marrow Transplant* 1994;13:571–575.

37. Kreitman RJ, Pastan I. Targeting *Pseudomonas* exotoxin to hematologic malignancies. *Semin Cancer Biol* 1995;6:297–306.

38. Foss FM, Saleh MN, Krueger JG, Nichols JC, Murphy JR. Diphtheria toxin fusion proteins. In: Frankel AE, ed. *Clinical applications of immunotoxins.* Berlin: Springer 1998:63–81.

39. LeMaistre CF, Saleh MN, Kuzel TM, et al. Phase I trial of a ligand fusion-protein (DAB$_{389}$IL-2) in lymphomas expressing the receptor for interleukin-2. *Blood* 1998;91:399–405.

40. Duvic M, Kuzel T, Olsen E, et al. Quality of life is significantly improved in CTCL patients who responded to DAB$_{389}$IL-2 (ONTAK) fusion protein. *Blood* 1998;92[Suppl 1]:2572a.

41. Kreitman RJ, Bailon P, Chaudhary VK, et al. Recombinant immunotoxins containing anti-Tac(Fv) and derivatives of *Pseudomonas* exotoxin produce complete regression in mice of an interleukin-2 receptor-expressing human carcinoma. *Blood* 1994;83:426–434.

42. Mavroudis DA, Juang YZ, Hensel N, et al. Specific depletion of alloreactivity against haplotype mismatched related individuals: a new approach to graft-versus-host disease prophylaxis in haploidentical bone marrow transplantation. *Bone Marrow Transplant* 1996;17:793–799.

43. Schnell R, Vitetta E, Schindler J, et al. Clinical trials with an anti-CD25 ricin A-chain experimental and immunotoxin (RFT5-SMPT-dgA) in Hodgkin's lymphoma. *Leukoc Lymphoma* 1998;30:525–537.

44. Amlot PL, Stone MJ, Cunningham D, et al. A phase I study of an anti-CD22-deglycosylated ricin A chain immunotoxin in the treatment of B-cell lymphomas resistant to conventional therapy. *Blood* 1993;82:2624–2633.

45. Vitetta ES, Stone M, Amlot P, et al. Phase I immunotoxin trial in patients with B-cell lymphoma. *Cancer Res* 1991;51:4052–4058.

46. Sausville EA, Headlee D, Stetler-Stevenson M, et al. Continuous infusion of the anti-CD22 immunotoxin IgG-RFB4-SMPT-dgA in patients with B-cell lymphoma: a phase I study. *Blood* 1995;85:3457–3465.

47. Senderowicz AM, Vitetta E, Headlee D, et al. Complete sustained response of a refractory, post-transplantation, large B-cell lymphoma to an anti-CD22 immunotoxin. *Ann Intern Med* 1997;126:882–885.

48. Kreitman RJ, Wang Q-C, FitzGerald DJP, Pastan I. Complete regression of human B-cell lymphoma xenografts in mice treated with recombinant anti-CD22 immunotoxin RFB4(dsFv)-PE38 at doses tolerated by cynomolgus monkeys. *Int J Cancer* 1999;81:148–155.

49. Kuan C-T, Pai LH, Pastan I. Immunotoxins containing *Pseudomonas* exotoxin targeting Le^Y damage human endothelial cells in an antibody specific mode: relevance to vascular leak syndrome. *Clin Cancer Res* 1995;1:1589–1594.

50. Scheuermann RH, Racila E. CD19 antigen in leukemia and lymphoma diagnosis and immunotherapy. *Leukoc Lymphoma* 1995;18:385–397.

51. Uckun F. Immunotoxins for the treatment of leukaemia. *Br J Haematol* 1993;85:435–438.

52. Stone MJ, Sausville EA, Fay JW, et al. A phase I study of bolus versus continuous infusion of the anti-CD19 immunotoxin, IgG-HD37-dgA, in patients with B-cell lymphoma. *Blood* 1996;88:1188–1197.

53. Multani PS, O'Day S, Nadler LM, Grossbard ML. Phase II clinical trial of bolus infusion anti-B4 blocked ricin immunoconjugate in patients with relapsed B-cell non-Hodgkin's lymphoma. *Clin Cancer Res* 1998;4:2599–2604.

54. O'Toole JE, Esseltine D, Lynch TJ, Lambert JM, Brossbard ML. Clinical trials with blocked ricin immunotoxins. *Curr Top Microbiol Immunol* 1998;234:35–56.

55. Grossbard ML, Niedzwiecki D, Nadler LM, et al. Anti-B4-blocked ricin (Anti-B4bR) adjuvant therapy post-autologous bone marrow transplant (ABMT) (CALGB 9254): a phase III intergroup study. *Proc Am Soc Clin Oncol* 1998;17:3a.

56. Grossbard ML, Gribben JG, Freedman AS, et al. Adjuvant immunotoxin therapy with anti-B4-blocked ricin after autologous bone marrow transplantation for patients with B-cell non-Hodgkin's lymphoma. *Blood* 1993;81:2263–2271.

57. Winkler U, Barth S, Schnell R, et al. The emerging role of immunotoxins in leukemia and lymphoma. *Ann Oncol* 1997;1[Suppl]:139–146.

58. Hogge DE, Willman CL, Kreitman RJ, et al. Malignant progenitors from patients with acute myelogenous leukemia are sensitive to a diphtheria toxin-granulocyte-macrophage colony-stimulating factor fusion protein. *Blood* 1998;92:589–595.

59. Francisco JA, Siegall CB. Single-chain immunotoxins targeted to CD40 for the treatment of human B-lineage hematologic malignancies. *Leuk Lymphoma* 1998;30:237–245.

60. Gould BJ, Borowtz MJ, Groves ES, et al. Phase I study of an anti-breast cancer immunotoxin by continuous infusion: report of a targeted toxic effect not predicted by animal studies. *J Natl Cancer Inst* 1989;81:775–781.

61. Pai LH, Bookman MA, Ozols RF, et al. Clinical evaluation of intraperitoneal *Pseudomonas* exotoxin immunoconjugate OVB3-PE in patients with ovarian cancer. *J Clin Oncol* 1991;9:2095–2103.

62. Jain RK. The next frontier of molecular medicine: delivery of therapeutics. *Nat Med* 1998;6:655–657.

63. Jain RK, Baxter LT. Mechanisms of heterogeneous distribution of monoclonal antibodies and other macromolecules in tumors: significance of elevated interstitial pressure. *Cancer Res* 1988;48:7022–7032.

64. Jain RK, Ward-Hartley KA. Tumor blood flow—characterization, modifications, and tolerance in hyperthermia. *IEEE Trans Son Ultrason* 1984;31:504–526.

65. Spitler L, del Rio M, Khentigan A, et al. Therapy of patients with malignant melanoma using a monoclonal anti-melanoma antibody ricin-A chain immunotoxin. *Cancer Res* 1987;47:1717–1723.

66. Oratz R, Speyer JL, Wernz JC, et al. Antimelanoma monoclonal antibody-ricin-A-chain immunoconjugate (XMMME-001-RTA) plus cyclophosphamide in the treatment of metastatic malignant melanoma: results of a phase II trial. *J Biol Resp Mod* 1990;9:345–354.

67. Selvaggi K, Saria EA, Schwarta R, et al. Phase I/II study of murine monoclonal antibody ricin A chain (XOMAZYME-Mel) immunoconjugate plus cyclosporine A in patients with metastatic melanoma. *J Immunother* 1993;3;201–207.

68. Byers VS, Rodvien R, Grant K, et al. Phase I study of monoclonal antibody-ricin A chain immunotoxin XomaZyme-791 in patients with metastatic colon cancer. *Cancer Res* 1989;49:6153–6160.

69. LoRusso PM, Lomen PL, Redman BG, et al. Phase I study of monoclonal antibody-ricin A chain immunoconjugate Xomazyme 791 in patients with metastatic colon cancer. *Am J Clin Oncol* 1995;18:307–314.

70. Weiner LM, O'Dwyer J, Kitson J, et al. Phase I evaluation of an anti-breast carcinoma monoclonal antibody 260F9-recombinant ricin A chain immunoconjugate. *Cancer Res* 1989;49;4062–4067.

71. Bookman MA, Godfrey S, Padavic K, et al. Anti-transferrin receptor immunotoxin (IT) therapy: phase I intraperitoneal (i.p.) trial. *Proc Am Soc Clin Oncol* 1990;9:187.

72. Pastan I, Lovelace ET, Gallo MG, et al. Characterization of monoclonal antibodies B1 and B3 that react with mucinous adenocarcinomas. *Cancer Res* 1991;51:3781–3787.

73. Pai LH, FitzGerald DJ, Willingham MC, et al. Antitumor activities of immunotoxins made of monoclonal antibody B3 and various forms of *Pseudomonas* exotoxin. *Proc Natl Acad Sci U S A* 1991;88:3358–3362.

74. Pai LH, Batra JK, FitzGerald DJ, et al. Anti-tumor effects of B3-PE and B3-LysPE40 in a nude mouse model of human breast cancer and the evaluation of B3-PE toxicity in monkeys. *Cancer Res* 1992;52:3189–3193.

75. Pai LH, Wittes RE, Setser A, et al. Phase I study of the immunotoxin LMB-1 (B3-LysPE38). *Nat Med* 1996;2:350–353.

76. Chaudhary VK, Batra JK, Gallo M, et al. A rapid method of cloning functional variable region antibody genes in *E. coli* as single-chain immunotoxins. *Proc Natl Acad Sci U S A* 1990;87:1066–1070.

77. Brinkmann U, Pai LH, FitzGerald DJ, et al. B3(Fv)-PE38KDEL, a single-chain immunotoxin that causes complete regression of a human carcinoma in mice. *Proc Natl Acad Sci U S A* 1991;88: 8616–8620.

78. Pai LH, Wittes RE, Setser A, et al. Phase I trial of recombinant immunotoxin LMB-7 (B3(Fv)PE38) for adult solid tumors. *Proc Am Assoc Cancer Res* 1997;38:85.

79. Brinkmann U, Reiter Y, Jung S-H, et al. A recombinant immunotoxin containing a disulfide-stabilized Fv fragment (dsFv). *Proc Natl Acad Sci U S A* 1993;90:7538–7545.

80. Reiter Y, Brinkmann U, Kreitman R, et al. Stabilization of the Fv fragments in recombinant immunotoxins by disulfide bonds engineered into conserved framework regions. *Biochemistry* 1994;33: 5451–5459.

81. Reiter R, Pai LH, Brinkmann U, Wang Q-C, Pastan I. Anti-tumor activity and pharmacokinetics in mice of a recombinant immunotoxin containing a disulfide-stabilized Fv fragment. *Cancer Res* 1994;54:2714–2718.

82. Kasprzyk PG, Song SV, DiFiore PP, King CR. Therapy of an animal model of human gastric cancer using a combination of anti-erbB2 monoclonal antibodies. *Cancer Res* 1992;52:2771–2776.

83. Batra JK, Kasprzyk PG, Bird RE, et al. Recombinant anti-erbB2 immunotoxins containing *Pseudomonas* exotoxin. *Proc Natl Acad Sci U S A* 1992;89:5867–5871.

84. Pai-Scherf LH, Villa J, Pearson P, et al. Hepatotoxicity in cancer patients receiving erb-38, a recombinant immunotoxin that targets the erbB2 receptor. *Clin Cancer Res* 1999;5:2311–2315.

85. Ariniello PD, Braman G, Cook S, et al. Immunotoxin therapy of small-cell lung cancer: a phase I study of N901-blocked ricin. *J Clin Oncol* 1997;15:723–734.

86. Shaw JP, Akiyoshi DE, Arrigo DA, et al. Cytotoxic properties of DAB$_{486}$EGF and DAB$_{389}$EGF, epidermal growth factor (EGF) receptor-targeted fusion toxins. *J Biol Chem* 1991;266:21118–21124.

87. Theodoulou M, Baselga J, Scher H, et al. Phase I dose escalation study of safety, tolerability and pharmacokinetics of DAB389EGF in patients with solid malignancies expressing EGF receptor. *Proc Am Soc Clin Oncol* 1995;14:480.

88. Chaudhary VK, FitzGerald DJ, Adhya S, et al. Activity of a recombinant fusion protein between transforming growth factor type alpha and *Pseudomonas* toxin. *Proc Natl Acad Sci U S A* 1987;84:4538–4542.

89. Pai LH, Gallo MG, FitzGerald DJ, et al. Anti-tumor activity of a transforming growth factor alpha-*Pseudomonas* exotoxin fusion protein (TGFalpha-PE40). *Cancer Res* 1991;51:2808–2812.

90. Kunwar S, Pai LH, Pastan I. Cytotoxicity and antitumor effects of growth factor-toxin fusion proteins on human glioblastoma multiforme cells. *J Neurosurg* 1993;79:569–576.

91. Neal DE, Sharples L, Smith K, et al. The epidermal growth factor receptor and the prognosis of bladder cancer. *Cancer* 1990;65:1619–1625.

92. Heimbrook DC, Stirdivant SM, Ahern JD, et al. Transforming growth factor-alpha-*Pseudomonas* exotoxin fusion protein prolongs survival of nude mice bearing tumor xenografts. *Proc Natl Acad Sci U S A* 1990;87:4697–4701.

93. Goldberg MR, Heimbrook DC, Russo P, et al. Phase I clinical study of the recombinant oncotoxin TP40 in superficial bladder cancer. *Clin Cancer Res* 1995;1:57–61.

94. Muraszko K, Sung C, Walbridge S, et al. Pharmacokinetics and toxicology of immunotoxins administered into the subarachnoid space in nonhuman primates and rodents. *Cancer Res* 1993;53:3752–3757.

95. Laske DW, Muraszko KM, Oldfield EH, et al. Intraventricular immunotoxin therapy for leptomeningeal neoplasia. *Neurosurgery* 1997;41:1039–1049.

96. Pastan IH, Archer GE, McLendon RE, et al. Intrathecal administration of single-chain immunotoxin LMB-7 [B3(Fv)-PE38], produces cures of carcinomatous meningitis in a rat model. *Proc Natl Acad Sci U S A* 1995;92:2765–2769.

97. Bigner DD, Archer GE, McLendon RE, et al. Efficacy of compartmental administration of immunotoxin LMB-1 (B3-LysPE38) in a rat model of carcinomatous meningitis. *Clin Cancer Res* 1995;12:1545–1555.

98. Greenfield L, Johnson VG, Youle RJ. Mutations in diphtheria toxin separated binding from entry and amplify immunotoxin selectivity. *Science* 1987;238:536–539.

99. Laske DW, Youle RJ, Oldfield EH. Tumor regression with regional distribution of the targeted toxin TFCRM107 in patients with malignant brain tumors. *Nat Med* 1994;3:1362–1368.

100. Bobo RH, Laske DW, Akbasak A, et al. Convection-enhanced delivery of macromolecules in the brain. *Proc Natl Acad Sci U S A* 1994;91:2076–2080.

101. Lieberman DM, Laske DW, Morrison PF, Bankiewicz KS, Oldfield EH. Convection-enhanced distribution of large molecules in gray matter during interstitial drug infusion. *J Neurosurg* 1995;82:1021–1029.

102. Puri RK, Hoon DS, Leland P, et al. Preclinical development of a recombinant toxin containing circularly permuted interleukin 4 and truncated *Pseudomonas* exotoxin for therapy of malignant astrocytoma. *Cancer Res* 1996;56:5631–5637.

103. Kreitman RJ, Puri RK, Pastan I. Increased antitumor activity of a circularly permuted interleukin 4 toxin in mice with interleukin 4 receptor-bearing human carcinoma. *Cancer Res* 1995;55:3357–3363.

104. Husain SR, Behari N, Kreitman RJ, et al. Complete regression of established human glioblastoma tumor xenograft by interleukin-4 toxin therapy. *Cancer Res* 1998;58:3649–3653.

105. Ekstrand AJ, James CD, Cavenee WK, et al. Genes for epidermal growth factor receptor, transforming growth factor alpha and epidermal growth factor and their expression in human gliomas *in vivo*. *Cancer Res* 1991;51:2164–2172.

106. Torp SH, Helseth E, Dalen A, et al. Epidermal growth factor receptor expression in human gliomas. *Cancer Immunol Immunother* 1991;33:61–64.

107. Siegel JP, Puri RK. Interleukin-2 toxicity. *J Clin Oncol* 1991;9: 694–704.

108. Soler-Rodriguez AM, Ghetie MA, Oppenheimer-Marks N, et al. Ricin A-chain and ricin A-chain immunotoxins rapidly damage human endothelial cells: implications for vascular leak syndrome. *Exp Cell Res* 1993;206:227–234.

109. Cotran RS, Pober JS, Gimbrone MA Jr, et al. Endothelial activation during interleukin-2 immunotherapy. A possible mechanism for the vascular leak syndrome. *J Immunol* 1988;140:1883–1888.

110. Lentsch AB, Miller FN, Edwards MJ. Mechanisms of leukocyte-mediated interleukin-2. *Cancer Immunol Immunother* 1999;47:243–248.

111. Cotran RS, Pober JS. Cytokine-endothelial interactions in inflammation, immunity, and vascular injury. *J Am Soc Nephrol* 1990;1: 225–235.

112. Rafi AQ, Zeytun A, Bradley MJ, et al. Evidence for the involvement of Fas ligand and perforin in the induction of vascular leak syndrome. *J Immunol* 1998;161:3077–3086.

113. Siegall CB, Liggitt D, Chac D, et al. Prevention of immunotoxin-mediated vascular leak syndrome in rats with retention of antitumor activity. *Proc Natl Acad Sci U S A* 1994;91:9514–9518.

114. Pai LH, FitzGerald DJ, Tepper M, et al. Inhibition of antibody response to *Pseudomonas* exotoxin and an immunotoxin containing *Pseudomonas* exotoxin by 15-deoxyspergualin in mice. *Cancer Res* 1990;50:7750–7753.

115. Dhingra K, Fritsche H, Murray JL, et al. Phase I clinical and pharmacological study of suppression of human antimouse antibody response to monoclonal antibody L6 by deoxyspergualin. *Cancer Res* 1995;55:3060–3067.

116. Reff ME, Carner K, Chambers KS, et al. Depletion of B cells *in vivo* by a chimeric mouse human monoclonal antibody to CD20. *Blood* 1994;83:435–445.

117. Maloney DG, Grillo-Lopez AJ, White CA, et al. IDEC-C2B8 (Rituximab) anti-CD20 monoclonal antibody therapy in patients with relapsed low-grade non-Hodgkin's lymphoma. *Blood* 1997;90: 2188–2195.

118. French RR, Bell AJ, Hamblin TU, Tutt AL, Glennie MJ. Response of B-cell lymphoma to a combination of bispecific antibodies and saporin. *Leukoc Res* 1996;20:607–617.

14.3

MONOCLONAL ANTIBODIES: BASIC PRINCIPLES

Radioisotope Conjugates

STEVEN M. LARSON
CHAITANYA DIVGI
GEORGE SGOUROS
NAI-KONG V. CHEUNG
DAVID A. SCHEINBERG

In this review, we focus primarily on the emerging promise of radiolabeled antibodies as therapeutic agents. Long-lasting major responses have been observed using radiolabeled antibody as the sole treatment in hematopoietic tumors refractory to chemotherapy. Responses to solid tumors have been fewer. Progress in this area depends on the success of new approaches under investigation, such as the use of alpha emitters for intracavitary therapy and micrometastases. Advances in the radiochemistry of antibody labeling, genetic engineering–based production methods, and better understanding of tumor and normal tissue dosimetry provide a strong, fundamental, scientific basis for the development of new reagents and approaches to improve treatment applications in human tumors.

HISTORICAL PERSPECTIVE

Radioisotopes can be conjugated to antibodies to tumor-specific antigens, and when administered parenterally, the radioimmunoconjugates serve as a carrier for radioactivity, targeting tumor sites deep within the human body. The specific antibody binds to its antigen at the tumor site, much like a key fits into a lock and, over time, there is progressive concentration at the antigen-binding site with catabolism and clearance of conjugate through non–antigen-bearing tissues. In this way, a radioactivity concentration gradient can be developed between tumor and surrounding tissue, serving as a basis for focused radiation therapy to the tumor site.

An attractive feature of radioimmunotherapy is that most normal tissues are spared intensive radiation. In addition, the same radiolabeled antibody may be initially used to determine appropriate dosimetry and subsequently used for radioimmunotherapy labeled with larger quantities of radioisotope. Further-more, because most tumor types have been shown to have characteristic tumor-associated antigens, such targeted radiotherapy can, in principle, be applied broadly to human cancers.

Pressman and collaborators discovered the elegant principle of immune-specific targeting of tumors in the late 1940s and 1950s (1–3). Over the next 50 years, many challenges were overcome to permit clinical applications. Throughout the 1960s and 1970s, incremental advances in immunologic methods gradually led to more reproducible methods of preparation of radiolabeled (polyclonal) antitumor antibodies, and targeting of human tumors significantly improved (4,5).

Interest in this field is largely due to the development of the hybridoma technology of Kohler and Milstein (6), whereby monospecific antibodies (monoclonal) can be produced. The hybridoma method of producing antibody lends itself readily to the manufacture of pharmaceutical grade reagents. Also based on these methods, it is likely that, in the future, still greater improvements in tumor targeting will be achieved through the use of specially tailored hybrid antibodies that have been created through genetic engineering. Examples of such molecules include humanized antibodies, genetically engineered sFv fragments, Fab', F(ab)'$_2$, diabodies, and minibodies (7).

Radioisotope conjugates of antitumor antibodies are being slowly introduced for diagnosis and therapy of human neoplasms. In regard to diagnostic use, four new drug applications have been issued by the U.S. Food and Drug Administration in the last 5 years for radiolabeled antibodies: an indium-111– (^{111}In) labeled form of B72.3 for colorectal and ovarian cancer imaging (satumomab pendetide, Cytogen Corp.); an ^{111}In-labeled antibody against the prostate-specific membrane antigen for imaging of prostate cancer (capromab pendetide, Cytogen Corp.), a technetium-99m (^{99m}Tc)–labeled anti-CEA Fab' fragment (arcitumomab, Immunomedics Inc.), and Tc-99m–

labeled NR-LU-10 ("Verluma," an anti–small-cell lung cancer Fab' antibody, NeoRx Corp.).

The toxicity associated with radioimmunotherapy has been predominantly hematopoietic and relatively mild under the conditions of use. As doses are increased in clinical trials, however, "second organ" toxicities are likely to emerge in radiosensitive organs, such as the lungs, or along the route of excretion of the radionuclide, in the gut and kidney. Principal problems encountered have been the rapid development of immunity against the murine antibodies used and the fact that only a relatively small fraction of the total radioactivity injected is actually concentrated in tumor. Technical problems associated with radioimmunotherapy include inaccurate dosimetry for estimating radiation-absorbed dose to tumor and radiation-sensitive tissues, such as red marrow. Symposia address dosimetry (8) and other technical issues (9,10). Dosimetric considerations are presented in detail in the section Modeling and Dosimetry for Radioimmunotherapy. Reviews have appeared (11–14).

No radiolabeled antibodies have yet been approved by the Food and Drug Administration for therapeutic use. Pivotal clinical trials leading to Food and Drug Administration approval have nearly been completed for therapy of non-Hodgkin's lymphoma using radiolabeled anti-CD20 antibodies [iodine-131 (^{131}I)–labeled anti-B1, Bexxar, Coulter Pharmaceuticals, and Y-90 IDEC-Y2B8, IDEC Laboratories]. Although both of these antibodies are of murine origin, they do not evoke an antimurine antibody response in most patients with established disease, presumably because the B lymphocyte is the principal modulator of the immune response.

RADIOISOTOPE-ANTIBODY CONJUGATES

Future prospects for improving radioimmunotherapy are based on firmly conjugating relatively nonimmunogenic antibodies with nuclides with especially favorable radioactive decay properties. Radionuclides that offer specific advantages due to their nuclear decay properties, including auger emitters, negatron (beta) emitters, and alpha emitters, are being explored.

The special chemistry for preparation of radioisotope-antibody conjugates is a branch of applied chemistry (15). Some radioisotopes, such as iodine and other halogens, can be directly attached to the antibodies; the most commonly used for this purpose are the radioiodine isotopes, particularly ^{131}I and ^{125}I. Other radioisotope-antibody conjugates are formed by indirect labeling, in which a linker is first attached to the antibody and the radioisotope is conjugated to the antibody by binding via the linker. This approach is widely used for radiometals [e.g., ^{111}In and yttrium-90 (^{90}Y)] (15,16). Alpha-emitting radionuclides have been linked to monoclonal antibodies and should be excellent for some applications (17–19). The recent implementation of the alpha-emitting radionuclides, bismuth-213 (^{213}Bi) and astatine-211 (^{211}At) (a halogen), into clinical trials is important because of the enormous potency of radiation delivery by alpha emission over the range of a few cell diameters. This offers the prospect of killing single tumor cells and greatly increases the chances that radioimmunotherapy will be useful in treating leukemia and solid tumor micrometastases. These

agents are discussed more completely in the section Alpha Particle Emitters.

Radiolabeling by whatever method should be optimized so the immunobiologic properties of the antibody are retained because the ability of the radioisotope conjugate to bind to antigen (radioimmunoreactivity) is of major importance to optimal *in vivo* tumor uptake (20).

RADIONUCLIDES FOR RADIOIMMUNOTHERAPY

Table 1 lists some of the radioisotopes that are being used for radioimmunotherapy. Therapeutic nuclides may be broadly divided into beta-minus emitters, which deposit low-level radiation over relatively long (millimeter) distances, and alpha emitters, which deposit high-level radiation over short (micron) distances. Auger emitters, such as ^{125}I, fall into the latter category; these have been rarely explored, presumably because they are cytocidal only when they decay in the nucleus. Beta-plus or positron emitters are useful for quantitative imaging of targeted therapy, particularly when the radionuclide is an isotope of a therapeutic radionuclide, such as ^{124}I, copper-64 (^{64}Cu), or ^{86}Y.

A limited number of beta particle emitters are suitable for the successful application of radioimmunotherapy. Beta particle emitters [e.g., ^{131}I, ^{90}Y, rhenium-188 (^{188}Re)] with long-range (1–10 mm) emissions are generally restricted to settings of large tumor burden or when bone marrow transplant is possible because of their considerable bystander cell killing. In contrast, the physical characteristics of alpha particle–emitting radionuclides make them attractive for radioimmunotherapy:

1. High linear energy transfer make alpha particles up to 100 times as potent as beta particles.
2. The nonspecific irradiation of normal tissue around the target cell is greatly reduced. The path lengths of typical alpha particles are on the order of 60 μm.
3. The damage to DNA and induction of apoptosis from alpha particle irradiation is difficult to repair, which makes alpha particles extremely cytotoxic.

The uses of alpha-emitting radionuclides for the treatment of disease have appeared in several reviews (21–23).

ALPHA EMITTERS

Alpha particles are high-energy helium nuclei (He-4) with high linear energy transfer in the range of 100 keV per μm. The mean linear energy transfer value for the beta particle–emitting ^{90}Y is 0.2 keV per μm, whereas that of ^{211}At (an alpha emitter) is 97 keV per μm. Tissue penetration ranges differ greatly, from 70 μm for the ^{211}At alpha particle to 3,960 μm for the ^{90}Y beta particle. Therefore, the cytotoxicity induced by alpha particles is far more selective. Daughter nuclides that may be metabolized differently from the parent isotope must also be taken into account, especially if the daughter is long lived.

TABLE 1. SELECTED RADIOISOTOPES FOR RADIOIMMUNOTHERAPY

Radionuclide	Decay Mode (Energy, MeV)	Half-Life
Iodine-131 (^{131}I)	Beta minus (0.182)	8.0 d
Yttrium-90 (^{90}Y)	Beta minus (0.934)	64.0 hr
Iodine-124 (^{124}I)	E.C., beta plus (0.188)	4.2 d
Copper-64 (^{64}Cu)	E.C., beta plus (0.656)	12.8 hr
Copper -67 (^{67}Cu)	Beta minus (0.142)	62.0 hr
Gallium-67 (^{67}Ga)	E.C.	3.3 d
Iodine-125 (^{125}I)	E.C.	60.2 d
Rhenium-188 (^{188}Re)	Beta minus	17.0 hr
Rhenium-186 (^{186}Re)	E.C., beta minus (0.323)	3.8 d
Bismuth-212 (^{212}Bi)	Alpha (2.17), beta minus (0.492)	1.0 hr
Bismuth-213 (^{213}Bi)	Alpha and beta (multiple)	45.0 mo
Actinium-225 (^{225}Ac)	Alpha (multiple)	10.0 d
Astatine-211 (^{211}At)	Alpha decay (2.447)	7.2 hr

E.C., electron capture.
Note: For beta decay, average energy is given.
From Browne E, Firestone RB. *Table of radioactive isotopes.* Wiley-Interscience, New York, 1976. Reprinted by permission of John Wiley & Sons, Inc.

Using a two-step labeling method, Zalutsky et al. (24) have successfully attached ^{211}At to monoclonal antibodies and fragments. Only a few research centers have the capability for production of ^{211}At. This remains a potential drawback to the widespread use of this radionuclide. The 7.2-hour half-life, however, makes ^{211}At attractive for radioimmunotherapy. This half-life is appropriate for moderate diffusion of the targeting molecule to gain access to the tumor cells. The thorium-228 decay chain yields ^{212}Bi, an alpha particle–emitting radiometal with a short half-life (60 minutes). Bifunctional metal chelating moieties have been extensively investigated (25) that can be readily attached covalently to protein molecules, such as immunoglobulin G (IgG). These stably bind bismuth radionuclides.

This decay scheme also yields lead-212 (^{212}Pb) (10.6-hour half-life). Both ^{212}Bi and ^{212}Pb nuclides can be produced using a radium-224 (^{224}Ra) generator system. When administered clinically, a monoclonal antibody labeled with ^{212}Pb would serve as an *in situ* ^{212}Bi generator (25). One difficulty in chelating ^{212}Pb results from the electron capture branch in the decay scheme, which through the concomitant charge build-up after Auger electron emission would destroy the chelating moiety.

The natural decay of uranium-233 or the neutron irradiation of ^{226}Ra by successive n,β capture decay reactions will yield actinium-225 (^{225}Ac) (26). Six daughters of ^{225}Ac are produced in its cascade, and five alpha and three beta disintegrations are produced before stable ^{209}Bi is reached. The high-energy alpha particle emission, the favorable rapid decay chain to stable ^{209}Bi, and the 10-day half-life make ^{225}Ac an excellent candidate for use in cancer therapy. No suitable chelating agent exists, however, that is able to withstand the immense alpha particle recoil energies for the actinium ion. Thus, the major application of ^{225}Ac is a source for the generation of ^{213}Bi.

^{213}Bi (45.6-minute half-life) is a decay product of ^{225}Ac. A clinically proven ^{213}Bi generator has been developed that pro-

vides up to 925 MBq (25 mCi) of pure chemically reactive ^{213}Bi (27). ^{213}Bi is bound to antibody with the C-functionalized *trans*-cyclohexyldiethylenetriamine pentaacetic acid moiety, CHX-A-DTPA (28). Clinical trials using a ^{213}Bi-labeled anti-CD33 construct are in progress. The ^{213}Bi 440-keV photon emission allows *in vivo* patient imaging, and detailed pharmaco-kinetic and dosimetry information in patients with leukemia have been obtained (29).

MODELING AND DOSIMETRY FOR RADIOIMMUNOTHERAPY

Radiation damage is the result of ionization along the emitted particle track, which disrupts critical biomolecules. Tumor cell kill is most closely associated with damage to the nuclear material of the cell, so it is the nucleus and, more precisely, the DNA within the nucleus, which is the target for tumor killing. A single "hit" from an alpha particle emitter is usually sufficient to kill a cell (30). A variety of methods have been developed to estimate the amount of energy deposited in tissues; this is usually expressed in terms of rad or gray. Internally administered radio-isotopes and the radiation-absorbed dose from their use is computed by the medical internal radiation dose (MIRD) schema, a method for obtaining whole body and organ radiation doses (31). This method is suitable for estimating doses when the distributions of radioisotopes are relatively homogeneous throughout volumes in the order of a few grams or greater.

A single alpha particle track, originating from the cell's surface and traversing the nucleus, is capable of resulting in cell death (32). Thus, the conventional methodologies for estimating mean absorbed dose may not always yield physically or biologically meaningful information when estimating alpha doses. Instead, stochastic or microdosimetric methodologies may be required. Pharmacokinetics of alpha particle emitters may not be extrapolated from experience obtained using ^{131}I or other longer-lived beta emitters. With longer-lived radionuclides, the pharmacokinetics are dominated by biologic clearance of the antibody. This is in contrast to ^{213}Bi (half-life = 45.6 minutes) (e.g., in which 94% of the total alpha particle emissions occur within the first 3 hours after injection).

Systemically administered radiolabeled antibodies against tumor cell–specific or tumor cell–associated antigen must equilibrate within a distribution volume that contains the tumor, bind to tumor cell antigen, and remain attached to tumor while excess unbound antibody clears from the body. If the antibody remains attached to the antigen for a sufficiently long period of time, a radionuclide with an appropriate half-life delivers most of the radiation dose to antigen-positive cells without delivering a toxic dose to normal organs. Selective irradiation of target cells is contingent on using a radiolabel with appropriately ranged emissions, so that the majority of the energy per radionuclide decay is delivered to antigen-positive cells rather than to adjacent normal tissue. If the absorbed dose delivered to all sites of a tumor meets the radiobiologic requirements for tumor kill without inducing intolerable normal tissue damage, then the radiolabeled antibody selectively targets and eradicates the tumor.

ing dendritic cells expressing EBV antigens for the LCLs. Because dendritic cells can be prepared in only 3 to 7 days (63), their use would markedly reduce the total preparation time. Moreover, dendritic cells can be used to stimulate CTL responses to the more restricted set of EBV antigens expressed by Hodgkin's disease and nasopharyngeal carcinoma cells (64). Their value would therefore be especially high in extending adoptive immunotherapy to the EBV-related malignancies described below (see the section Immunotherapy for Epstein-Barr Virus-Related Hodgkin's Disease).

IMMUNOTHERAPY FOR EPSTEIN-BARR VIRUS–RELATED HODGKIN'S DISEASE

Although the origin of Hodgkin's disease remains unclear, approximately 50% of cases in North America and Europe are associated with EBV (4). In South America, Kenya, and parts of Asia, a 90% to 100% association exists. Thus, CTLs could prove a valuable addition to conventional therapy for EBV and Hodgkin's disease, if they could be marshaled against this disease as effectively as against EBV-LPD. Although 80% or more of patients with Hodgkin's disease are cured with available treatments, 50% of the minority who relapse do not respond to salvage chemotherapy or relapse a second time. Furthermore, the unacceptably high level of therapy-related secondary malignancies (18% at 5 years) and other serious medical complications in those who are "cured" also underscores the need to improve current therapeutic options (65).

A number of obstacles could diminish the effectiveness of EBV-specific CTLs in Hodgkin's disease. First, the malignant cells express a restricted set of viral genes, namely, EBNA1, RK-BARFO, and LMP1 and 2 (66). In the majority of cases, memory CTL responses are preferentially directed against the highly immunogenic EBNA3a, 3b, and 3c antigens, irrespective of the patient's HLA type. By comparison, EBNA-1, RK-BARFO, and LMP1 and 2 are poorly immunogenic. EBNA1 contains a repeating glycine-alanine amino acid sequence that inhibits its ubiquitination and subsequent processing and presentation of EBNA1 peptides by HLA class I antigens (67). RK-BARFO-specific CTLs can be generated *in vitro* from seropositive individuals, but they do not kill target cells naturally expressing the protein (68). The mechanism for this immune evasion is unclear. The reason for the limited immunogenicity of LMP1 and 2 is similarly unclear, because LMP1 or 2 epitopes are presented in the context of the HLA A2.1, B24, B40, B51, and B55 alleles (51,69). This lack of immunogenicity is particularly disappointing because EBV and Hodgkin's tumors express costimulatory molecules, such as HLA DR, CD40, CD80, and CD86, and should therefore be excellent antigen-presenting cells. They also secrete the Th2 cytokines IL-10 and tumor growth factor–β, however, as well as thymus and activation-regulated chemokine (TARC), a chemoattractant for CD4$^+$ T cells of the Th2 biotype (70). This overwhelmingly Th2 phenotype likely helps the antibody response and inhibits the CTL response. IL-10 may also act as an autocrine growth factor for Reed-Sternberg cells. Patients with Hodgkin's disease also have T-cell abnormalities, such as low expression of the zeta

chain of the T-cell receptor (71), which further reduce the effectiveness of the host immune response to the tumor (72).

To assess the feasibility of using EBV-specific CTLs as therapy for Hodgkin's disease, we generated EBV-specific CTLs from the peripheral blood of patients with this lymphoma, with the notion of expanding the cells *in vitro* in the absence of *in vivo* immunosuppressive effects. We then compared them phenotypically and functionally with CTLs generated from normal donors (53). To discover whether autologous EBV-specific CTLs could persist and produce antiviral activity *in vivo*, we genetically marked the cells and then adoptively transferred them to three patients with relapsed disease.

Cytotoxic T Lymphocytes from Patients with Hodgkin's Disease Compared with Those from Healthy Epstein-Barr Virus–Positive Donors

In the presence of IL-2 and B-LCL, cell counts of cultures from healthy donors (n = 15) typically increased by tenfold every 2 weeks, so that after 16 weeks in culture, CTLs from normal donors had expanded approximately 1,500-fold. During the same 16-week period, CTL cultures from patients in remission expanded by only approximately 150-fold, whereas those from patients with relapsed disease increased by just 80-fold. In more than 75% of patients, however, it was still possible to generate at least 10^8 CTLs, a number suggested by previous studies of EBV-LPD to be well in excess of that required to establish EBV immunity (59,60). Phenotypically, the patient lines were essentially identical to the lines from normal donors, except that the level of the T-cell receptor–zeta chain was abnormally low (73). The cytoplasmic portion of the T-cell receptor–zeta chain is involved in signal transduction and subsequent activation and proliferation of T cells, so that downregulation of this chain may contribute to the decreased proliferative response of patient T cells. Nonetheless, the lines produced had strong activity against HLA-matched EBV-positive targets. Of particular note, lines from Hodgkin's disease patients had activity against cells expressing Hodgkin's-associated viral antigens, including LMP1 and LMP2. This effect was demonstrated by the cells' ability to kill HLA-matched fibroblasts infected with vaccinia recombinants, each expressing one of the EBV-latent cycle proteins. Both HLA class I and class II–restricted CTLs could be detected. The presence of the class II–restricted cells may be of benefit because approximately 50% of Hodgkin's tumor cells downregulate HLA class I molecules, and may therefore be protected from conventional CTL killing. They generally maintain class II major histocompatibility complex (MHC) expression, however.

Biologic and Clinical Study of Cytotoxic T Lymphocytes

Encouraged by our ability to generate CTLs with activity against at least one of the Hodgkin's-associated antigens, we asked whether these cells would have antiviral and antimalignant properties *in vivo*. To track the persistence of infused CTLs, we marked the cells with a neo-containing retroviral vector. The neo gene was detectable in PBMCs for 4 to 12 weeks after the initial dose of 3.2×10^7 EBV-specific CTLs (73). The

levels of marking indicated that approximately 1 of every 1,000 circulating PBMCs was derived from the infused cell line.

The infused CTLs had cytotoxic antiviral activity. Thus, the proportion of circulating EBV-specific cytotoxic precursor cells was increased 10- to 100-fold, indicating an enhanced cell-mediated immune response to EBV. The number of MHC-unrestricted cytotoxic effector precursors remained constant, as demonstrated by the minimal change in the proportion of cyto-toxic precursor cells that killed HLA-mismatched LCLs. In addition to the rise in cytotoxic precursor cell frequency, the CTL activity tested after 2 weeks of culture with the autologous LCLs also increased *in vivo*, from less than 3% killing of autolo-gous LCLs at an effector:target ratio of 40:1 to more than 25% killing at the same effector:target ratio. Again, little effect on the activity of MHC-unrestricted cytotoxic effector cells occurred, suggesting that an increase in classical MHC-restricted CTL activity was responsible for the observed increase in autologous LCL target killing.

The observed increase in cytotoxic function was associated with measurable antiviral activity. We used semiquantitative PCR analysis to calculate the viral burden in peripheral blood before and after CTL infusion. The number of EBV-DNA genomes in normal donors ranges from less than 20 to 2,000 copies per 10^6 PBMCs (9). Before CTL infusion, the level of EBV DNA in patient 1 was 30,000 EBV genomes per 10^6 PBMCs, which is 15-fold higher than in normal individuals and within the range seen for stem-cell transplant recipients with immunoblastic lymphoma (9,58). After CTL infusion, the level of EBV DNA decreased dramatically and was undetectable at 4 weeks' postinfusion. Associated with this drop in EBV DNA, the patient showed improvement of stage B symptoms with increased appetite and resolution of fever and sweats; stabiliza-tion of his pulmonary disease also occurred. These effects were apparent even though the patient had received no chemother-apy for 4 weeks before or 6 weeks after infusion. In fact, the viral load in the peripheral blood of this patient increased only during readministration of chemotherapy at 6 weeks' postinfu-sion (the end of the evaluation period). Patient 2 had insuffi-cient blood counts to allow measurement of EBV-DNA levels but also showed improvement in stage B symptoms before the institution of further chemotherapy and disease progression. Although the EBV burden was not supranormal in the third patient, an initial level of 400 EBV genomes per 10^6 PBMCs fell to undetectable levels by 19 days after the first infusion. These effects were again produced in the absence of chemother-apy (>6 weeks before and after). This patient had an initial worsening of his pleural effusion, and gene-marked CTLs were detected in pleural biopsies of diseased areas (73). His disease then stabilized and no further pleural effusions occurred for more than a year. The tumor ultimately progressed in all three patients, who died of their disease 10 to 13 months later.

Improving the Clinical Outcome

These preliminary studies show:

1. It is feasible to obtain substantial *ex vivo* expansion of EBV-specific T cells from patients with advanced Hodgkin's disease.

2. These cells have *in vivo* cytotoxic activity against EBV-infected cells and are detectable *in vivo* for up to 12 weeks.
3. These cells can be targeted to Hodgkin's disease–associated antigens.

Our efforts are directed at enhancing the component of the anti-EBV response that is directed to the Hodgkin's-associated antigens LMP1 and 2 by using dendritic cells expressing the appropriate proteins (see the section Cytotoxic T Lymphocytes for Recipients of Solid Organ Transplants). The CTLs generated will be given to patients with minimal residual disease to reduce the immunosuppressive effects associated with bulky tumors. An alternative approach is to develop CTL clones directed against Hodgkin's-associated antigens. Such an approach is pos-sible (74) but is time consuming because the frequency of cells with such specificity is low. Moreover, many Hodgkin's tumors have mutations within the 3' region of the LMP1 oncogene, including a 30–base pair deletion and a high frequency of non-random point mutations (75,76). As we have already found in our EBV-LPD patients, these mutations may destroy the epitopes recognized by CTLs specific for wild-type LMP1, a problem that can only be accentuated if monospecific CTL clones, rather than polyspecific CTL lines, are used. It may also be possible to vaccinate patients directly using polypeptides, DNA, or dendritic cells as immunogens. The capacity to induce an immune response *in vivo*, however, may be limited by tumor-mediated immune escape mechanisms that subvert the induction or expansion of a cytotoxic response.

OTHER EPSTEIN-BARR VIRUS–ASSOCIATED MALIGNANCIES

EBV is associated with an increasing number of frequently rare and geographically associated malignancies (see Table 2). Lethal midline granulomas involving natural killer–like T-cell lympho-mas, gastric carcinomas, and pyothorax-associated lymphoma seem to have an increased frequency in Japan, whereas parotid carcinomas are found predominantly in American Eskimos. EBV-positive smooth muscle tumors (leiomyosarcomas) are the second most prevalent malignancy of children with acquired immunodeficiency syndrome, and have an increased frequency after organ transplantation. In nonimmunosuppressed individu-als, leiomyosarcomas rarely carry the EBV genome. EBV has also been found in carcinomas of the thymus and salivary gland. With the exception of gastric carcinoma and pyothorax-associated lym-phoma, these tumors all express the intermediate type II latency and therefore are potential targets for immunotherapies targeting viral proteins, although the success of such therapies may depend on the immune-evasion strategies used by the tumor.

The type I tumors, Burkitt lymphoma and gastric carci-noma, pose a greater challenge for immunotherapy. The only viral proteins expressed in type I tumors are EBNA1 and RK-BARFO, which, as described in the preceding paragraph, do not provide target epitopes for HLA class I–restricted CTLs. Burkitt lymphoma cells have been shown to use additional antiimmune response mechanisms. They have defects in their expression of TAP I transporter proteins and HLA class I molecules (77,78). Moreover, they have the immunophenotype of a resting B cell and do not express costimulatory molecules necessary for the induction of an effective immune response. It may be possible to use CD4$^+$ HLA class II–restricted EBNA-1 or RK-BARFO–specific CTL to target tumor cells expressing type-I latency (81,82).

CONCLUSIONS

EBV-associated malignancies provide an investigational bridge between viral diseases and classic malignancies. As increasing numbers of tumor-associated antigens are identified, the effectiveness and limitations of CTL therapies in EBV-related diseases should provide an invaluable guide for improving immunotherapies for an ever broader range of cancers.

ACKNOWLEDGMENTS

We would like to thank John Gilbert for scientific editing and Gloria Levin for word processing. This work was supported in part by grants HL 55703, CA 74126, and CA 61384 from the National Institutes of Health.

REFERENCES

1. Rickinson AB, Kieff E. Epstein-Barr virus. In: Fields BN, Knipe DM, Howley PM, eds. *Fields virology.* Philadelphia: Lippincott–Raven Publishers, 1996:2397–2446.
2. Rickinson AB, Moss DJ. Human cytotoxic T lymphocyte responses to Epstein-Barr virus infection. *Annu Rev Immunol* 1997;15:405–431.
3. Bourgault I, Gomez A, Gomard E, Levy JP. Limiting-dilution analysis of the HLA restriction of anti-Epstein-Barr virus-specific cytolytic T lymphocytes. *Clin Exp Immunol* 1991;84:501–507.
4. Jenson H, Montalvo EA, McClain K, et al. Characterization of natural Epstein-Barr virus infection and replication in smooth muscle cells from a leiomyosarcoma. *J Med Virol* 1999;57:(1)36–46.
5. Weiss LM, Movahed LA, Warnke RA, Sklar J. Detection of Epstein-Barr viral genomes in Reed-Sternberg cells of Hodgkin's disease. *N Engl J Med* 1989;320:502–506.
6. Savoie A, Perpete C, Carpentier L, Joncas J, Alfieri C. Direct correlation between the load of Epstein-Barr virus-infected lymphocytes in the peripheral blood of pediatric transplant patients and risk of lymphoproliferative disease. *Blood* 1994;83:2715–2722.
7. Riddler SA, Breinig MC, McKnight JLC. Increased levels of circulating Epstein-Barr virus (EBV)-infected lymphocytes and decreased EBV nuclear antigen antibody responses are associated with the development of posttransplant lymphoproliferative disease in solid-organ transplant recipients. *Blood* 1994;84:972–984.
8. Fontan J, Bassignot A, Mougin C, Cahn JY, Lab M. Detection of Epstein-Barr virus DNA in serum of transplanted patients: a new diagnostic guide for lymphoproliferative diseases. *Leukemia* 1998;12:772.
9. Rooney CM, Loftin SK, Holladay MS, Brenner MK, Krance RA, Heslop HE. Early identification of Epstein-Barr virus-associated posttransplant lymphoproliferative disease. *Br J Haematol* 1995;89:98–103.
10. Lucas KG, Burton RL, Zimmerman SE, et al. Semiquantitative Epstein-Barr virus (EBV) polymerase chain reaction for the determination of patients at risk for EBV-induced lymphoproliferative disease after stem cell transplantation. *Blood* 1998;91:3654–3661.
11. Cordier-Bussat M, Billaud M, Calender A, Lenoir GM. Epstein-Barr virus (EBV) nuclear-antigen-2-induced up-regulation of CD21 and CD23 molecules is dependent on a permissive cellular context. *Int J Cancer* 1993;53:153–160.
12. Kempkes B, Pawlita M, Zimber-Strobl U, Eissner G, Laux G, Bornkamm GW. Epstein-Barr virus nuclear antigen 2-estrogen receptor fusion proteins transactivate viral and cellular genes and interact with RBP-J kappa in a conditional fashion. *Virology* 1995;214:675–679.
13. Miller WE, Mosialos G, Kieff E, Raab-Traub N. Epstein-Barr virus LMP1 induction of the epidermal growth factor receptor is mediated through a TRAF signaling pathway distinct from NF-kappaB activation. *J Virol* 1997;71:586–594.
14. Izumi KM, Kieff ED. The Epstein-Barr virus oncogene product latent membrane protein 1 engages the tumor necrosis factor receptor-associated death domain protein to mediate B lymphocyte growth transformation and activate NF-kappaB. *Proc Natl Acad Sci U S A* 1997;94:12592–12597.
15. Eliopoulos AG, Dawson CW, Mosialos G, et al. CD40-induced growth inhibition in epithelial cells is mimicked by Epstein-Barr virus-encoded LMP1: involvement of TRAF3 as a common mediator. *Oncogene* 1996;13:2243–2254.
16. Stuart AD, Stewart JP, Arrand JR, Mackett M. The Epstein-Barr virus encoded cytokine viral interleukin-10 enhances transformation of human B lymphocytes. *Oncogene* 1995;11:1711–1719.
17. Moore KW, O'Garra A, de Waal M, Vieira P, Mosmann TR. Interleukin-10. *Annu Rev Immunol* 1993;11:165–190.
18. Caux C, Massacrier C, Vanbervliet B, Barthelemy C, Liu YJ, Banchereau J. Interleukin 10 inhibits T cell alloreaction induced by human dendritic cells. *Int Immunol* 1994;6:1177–1185.
19. Nazaruk RA, Rochford R, Hobbs MV, Cannon MJ. Functional diversity of the CD8+ T-cell response to Epstein-Barr virus (EBV): implications for the pathogenesis of EBV-associated lymphoproliferative disorders. *Blood* 1998;91:3875–3883.
20. Mathur A, Kamat D, Filipovitch A, Steinbuch M, Shapiro R. Immunoregulatory abnormalities in patients with Epstein-Barr virus-associated B cell lymphoproliferative disorders. *Transplantation* 1994;57:1042–1045.
21. O'Reilly RJ, Small TN, Papadopoulos E, Lucas K, Lacerda J, Koulova L. Biology and adoptive cell therapy of Epstein-Barr virus-associated lymphoproliferative disorders in recipients of marrow allografts. *Immunol Rev* 1997;157:195–216.
22. Peniket AJ, Perry AR, Williams CD, et al. A case of EBV-associated lymphoproliferative disease following high-dose therapy and CD34-purified autologous peripheral blood progenitor transplantation. *Bone Marrow Transplant* 1998;22:307–309.
23. Briz M, Fores R, Regidor C, et al. Epstein-Barr virus associated B-cell lymphoma after autologous bone marrow transplantation for T-cell acute lymphoblastic leukemia. *Br J Haematol* 1997;98:485–487.
24. Buckingham SC, Benaim E, Sandlund JT, et al. Primary central nervous system lymphoma in a child with acute B-cell lymphoblastic leukaemia: consecutive Epstein-Barr virus-related malignancies. *Br J Haematol* 1998;101:345–348.
25. Deeg HJ, Socie G. Malignancies after hemopoietic stem cell transplantation: many questions, some answers. *Blood* 1998;91:1833–1844.
26. Heslop HE, Rooney CM. Adoptive immunotherapy of EBV lymphoproliferative diseases. *Immunol Rev* 1997;157:217–222.
27. Gerritsen EJ, Stam ED, Hermans J, et al. Risk factors for developing EBV-related B cell lymphoproliferative disorders (BLPD) after non-HLA-identical BMT in children. *Bone Marrow Transplant* 1996;18:377–382.
28. Hale G, Waldmann H, for CAMPATH users. Risks of developing Epstein-Barr virus-related lymphoproliferative disorders after T-cell-depleted marrow transplants. *Blood* 1998;91:3079–3083.
29. Gross TG, Hinrichs SH, Davis JR, Mitchell D, Bishop MR, Wagner JE. Depletion of EBV-infected cells in donor marrow by counterflow elutriation. *Exp Hematol* 1998;26:395–399.
30. Cavazzana-Calvo M, Bensoussan D, Jabado N, et al. Prevention of EBV-induced B-lymphoproliferative disorder by ex vivo marrow B-cell depletion in HLA-phenoidentical or non-identical T-depleted bone marrow transplantation. *Br J Haematol* 1998;103:543–551.
31. Swinnen LJ. Treatment of organ transplant-related lymphoma. *Hematol Oncol Clin North Am* 1998;11:963–973.

32. Datta AK, Colby BM, Shaw JE, Pagano JS. Acyclovir inhibition of Epstein-Barr virus replication. *Proc Natl Acad Sci U S A* 1980; 77:5163–5166.

33. Pagano JS, Sixbey JW, Lin JC. Acyclovir and Epstein-Barr virus infection. *J Antimicrob Chemother* 1983;12:113–121.

34. Datta AK, Pagano JS. Phosphorylation of acyclovir *in vitro* in activated Burkitt somatic cell hybrids. *Antimicrob Agents Chemother* 1999;24(1):10–14.

35. Gustafson EA, Chillemi AC, Sage DR, Fingeroth JD. The Epstein-Barr virus thymidine kinase does not phosphorylate ganciclovir or acyclovir and demonstrates a narrow substrate specificity compared to the herpes simplex virus type 1 thymidine kinase. *Antimicrob Agents Chemother* 1998;42:2923–2931.

36. Starzl TE, Naleskin MA, Porter KA, et al. Reversibility of lymphomas and lymphoproliferative lesions developing under cyclosporin-steroid therapy. *Lancet* 1984;1:583.

37. Heslop HE, Li C, Krance RA, Loftin SK, Rooney CM. Epstein-Barr infection after bone marrow transplantation. *Blood* 1994;83: 1706–1708.

38. Gross TG, Steinbuch M, DeFor T, et al. B cell lymphoproliferative disorders following hematopoietic stem cell transplantation: risk factors, treatment and outcome. *Bone Marrow Transplant* 1999;23:251–258.

39. Leblond V, Sutton L, Dorent R, et al. Lymphoproliferative disorders after organ transplantation: a report of 24 cases observed in a single center. *J Clin Oncol* 1996;13:961–968.

40. Faye A, Van Den Abeele T, Peuchmaur M, Matheu-Boue A, Vilmer E. Anti-CD20 monoclonal antibody for post-transplant lymphoproliferative disorders. *Lancet* 1998;352:1285.

41. Chodosh J, Holder VP, Gan Y-J, Belgaumi A, Sample J, Sixbey JW. Eradication of latent Epstein-Barr virus by hydroxyurea alters the growth-transformed cell phenotype. *J Infect Dis* 1998;177:1194–1201.

42. Huang S, Stupack D, Mathias P, Wang Y, Nemerow GR. Growth arrest of Epstein-Barr virus immortalized B lymphocytes by adenovirus-delivered ribozymes. *Proc Natl Acad Sci U S A* 1997;94:8156–8161.

43. Papadopoulos EB, Ladanyi M, Emanuel D, MacKinnon S, Boulad F, Carabasi MH, et al. Infusions of donor leukocytes to treat Epstein-Barr virus-associated lymphoproliferative disorders after allogeneic bone marrow transplantation. *N Engl J Med* 1994;330:1185–1191.

44. Heslop HE, Brenner MK, Rooney CM. Donor T cells to treat EBV-associated lymphoma. *N Engl J Med* 1994;331:679–680.

45. Sasahara Y, Kawai S, Itano M, et al. Epstein-Barr virus-associated lymphoproliferative disorder after unrelated bone marrow transplantation in a young child with Wiskott-Aldrich syndrome. *Pediatr Hematol Oncol* 1998;15:347–352.

46. Nagafuji K, Eto T, Hayashi S, et al. Donor lymphocyte transfusion for the treatment of Epstein-Barr virus-associated lymphoproliferative disorder of the brain. *Bone Marrow Transplant* 1998;21:1155–1158.

47. Imashuku S, Goto T, Matsumura T, et al. Unsuccessful CTL transfusion in a case of post-BMT Epstein-Barr virus-associated lymphoproliferative disorder (EBV-LPD). *Bone Marrow Transplant* 1998;20:337–340.

48. Bonini C, Ferrari G, Verzeletti S, et al. HSV-TK gene transfer into donor lymphocytes for control of allogeneic graft versus leukemia. *Science* 1997;276:1719–1724.

49. Walter EA, Greenberg PD, Gilbert MJ, et al. Reconstitution of cellular immunity against cytomegalovirus in recipients of allogeneic bone marrow by transfer of T-cell clones from the donor. *N Engl J Med* 1995;333:1038–1044.

50. Riddell SR, Watanabe KS, Goodrich JM, Li CR, Agha ME, Greenberg PD. Restoration of viral immunity in immunodeficient humans by the adoptive transfer of T cell clones. *Science* 1992;257:238–241.

51. Murray RJ, Kurilla MG, Brooks JM, et al. Identification of target antigens for the human cytotoxic T cell response to Epstein-Barr virus (EBV): implications for the immune control of EBV-positive malignancies. *J Exp Med* 1992;176:157–168.

52. Khanna R, Burrows SR, Kurilla MG, et al. Localization of Epstein-Barr virus cytotoxic T cell epitopes using recombinant vaccinia: implications for vaccine development. *J Exp Med* 1992;176:169–176.

53. Smith CA, Ng CYC, Heslop HE, et al. Production of genetically modified EBV-specific cytotoxic T cells for adoptive transfer to patients at high risk of EBV-associated lymphoproliferative disease. *J Hematother* 1995;4:73–79.

54. Matloubian M, Concepcion RJ, Ahmed R. CD4+ T cells are required to sustain CD8+ cytotoxic T cell responses during chronic viral infection. *J Virol* 1994;68:8056–8063.

55. Smith CA, Ng CYC, Loftin SK, et al. Adoptive immunotherapy for Epstein-Barr virus-related lymphoma. *Leuk Lymphoma* 1996;23: 213–220.

56. Heslop HE, Brenner MK, Rooney CM, et al. Administration of neomycin-resistance-gene-marked EBV-specific cytotoxic T lymphocytes to recipients of mismatched-related or phenotypically similar unrelated donor marrow grafts. *Hum Gene Ther* 1994;5: 381–397.

57. Rooney CM, Smith CA, Ng CYC, et al. Infusion of cytotoxic T cells for the prevention and treatment of Epstein-Barr virus-induced lymphoma in allogeneic transplant recipients. *Blood* 1998;92: 1549–1555.

58. Burrows SR, Khanna R, Burrows JM, Moss DJ. An allo response in humans is dominated by cytotoxic T lymphocytes (CTL) cross-reactive with a single Epstein-Barr virus CTL epitope: implications for graft-versus-host disease. *J Exp Med* 1994;179:1155–1161.

59. Heslop HE, Ng CYC, Li C, et al. Long-term restoration of immunity against Epstein-Barr virus infection by adoptive transfer of gene-modified virus-specific T lymphocytes. *Nat Med* 1996;2:551–555.

60. Rooney CM, Smith CA, Ng C, et al. Use of gene-modified virus-specific T lymphocytes to control Epstein-Barr virus-related lymphoproliferation. *Lancet* 1995;345:9–13.

61. Gottschalk S, Ng CYC, Perez M, Brenner MK, Heslop HE, Rooney CM. Mutation in EBV produces immunoblastic lymphoma unresponsive to CTL immunotherapy. *Blood* 1998;[Suppl 1]:(abst).

62. Orentas RJ, Lemas MV, Mullin MJ, Colombani PM, Schwartz K, Ambinder R. Feasibility of cellular adoptive immunotherapy for Epstein-Barr virus-associated lymphomas using haploidentical donors. *J Hematother* 1998;7:257–261.

63. Romani N, Gruner S, Brang D, et al. Proliferating dendritic cell progenitors in human blood. *J Exp Med* 1994;180:83–93.

64. Rooney CM, Roskrow MA, Smith CA, Brenner MK, Heslop HE. Immunotherapy of EBV lymphoma. *J Natl Cancer Inst Monogr* 1998;23:89–93.

65. Beaty O, Hudson MM, Greenwald C, et al. Subsequent malignancies in children and adolescents after treatment for Hodgkin's disease. *J Clin Oncol* 1995;13:603–609.

66. Herbst H, Dallenback F, Hummel M, et al. Epstein-Barr virus latent membrane protein expression in Hodgkin and Reed-Sternberg cells. *Proc Natl Acad Sci U S A* 1991;88:4766–4770.

67. Levitskaya J, Coram M, Levitsky V, et al. Inhibition of antigen processing by the internal repeat region of the Epstein-Barr virus nuclear antigen-1. *Nature* 1995;375:685–688.

68. Kienzle N, Sculley TB, Poulson L, et al. Identification of a cytotoxic T-lymphocyte response to the novel BARFO protein of Epstein-Barr virus: a critical role for antigen expression. *J Virol* 1998;72:6614–6620.

69. Lee SP, Thomas WA, Murray RJ, et al. HLA A2.1-restricted cytotoxic T cells recognizing a range of Epstein-Barr virus isolates through a defined epitope in latent membrane protein LMP2. *J Virol* 1993;67:7428–7435.

70. Hsu SM, Lin J, Xie SS, Hsu PL, Rich S. Abundant expression of transforming growth factor-beta 1 and -beta 2 by Hodgkin's Reed-Sternberg cells and by reactive T lymphocytes in Hodgkin's disease. *Hum Pathol* 1993;24:249–255.

71. Slivnick DJ, Ellis TM, Nawrocki JF, Fisher RI. The impact of Hodgkin's disease on the immune system. *Semin Oncol* 1990;17: 673–682.

72. Renner C, Ohnesorge S, Held G, et al. T cells from patients with Hodgkin's disease have a defective T-cell receptor zeta chain expression that is reversible by T-cell stimulation with CD3 and CD28. *Blood* 1996;88:236–241.

73. Roskrow MA, Suzuki N, Gan Y-J, et al. EBV-specific cytotoxic T lymphocytes for the treatment of patients with EBV positive relapsed Hodgkin's disease. *Blood* 1998;91:2925–2934.

74. Sing AP, Ambinder RF, Hong DJ, et al. Isolation of Epstein-Barr

ing dendritic cells expressing EBV antigens for the LCLs. Because dendritic cells can be prepared in only 3 to 7 days (63), their use would markedly reduce the total preparation time. Moreover, dendritic cells can be used to stimulate CTL responses to the more restricted set of EBV antigens expressed by Hodgkin's disease and nasopharyngeal carcinoma cells (64). Their value would therefore be especially high in extending adoptive immunotherapy to the EBV-related malignancies described below (see the section Immunotherapy for Epstein-Barr Virus-Related Hodgkin's Disease).

IMMUNOTHERAPY FOR EPSTEIN-BARR VIRUS–RELATED HODGKIN'S DISEASE

Although the origin of Hodgkin's disease remains unclear, approximately 50% of cases in North America and Europe are associated with EBV (4). In South America, Kenya, and parts of Asia, a 90% to 100% association exists. Thus, CTLs could prove a valuable addition to conventional therapy for EBV and Hodgkin's disease, if they could be marshaled against this disease as effectively as against EBV-LPD. Although 80% or more of patients with Hodgkin's disease are cured with available treatments, 50% of the minority who relapse do not respond to salvage chemotherapy or relapse a second time. Furthermore, the unacceptably high level of therapy-related secondary malignancies (18% at 5 years) and other serious medical complications in those who are "cured" also underscores the need to improve current therapeutic options (65).

A number of obstacles could diminish the effectiveness of EBV-specific CTLs in Hodgkin's disease. First, the malignant cells express a restricted set of viral genes, namely, EBNA1, RK-BARFO, and LMP1 and 2 (66). In the majority of cases, memory CTL responses are preferentially directed against the highly immunogenic EBNA3a, 3b, and 3c antigens, irrespective of the patient's HLA type. By comparison, EBNA-1, RK-BARFO, and LMP1 and 2 are poorly immunogenic. EBNA1 contains a repeating glycine-alanine amino acid sequence that inhibits its ubiquitination and subsequent processing and presentation of EBNA1 peptides by HLA class I antigens (67). RK-BARFO-specific CTLs can be generated *in vitro* from seropositive individuals, but they do not kill target cells naturally expressing the protein (68). The mechanism for this immune evasion is unclear. The reason for the limited immunogenicity of LMP1 and 2 is similarly unclear, because LMP1 or 2 epitopes are presented in the context of the HLA A2.1, B24, B40, B51, and B55 alleles (51,69). This lack of immunogenicity is particularly disappointing because EBV and Hodgkin's tumors express costimulatory molecules, such as HLA DR, CD40, CD80, and CD86, and should therefore be excellent antigen-presenting cells. They also secrete the Th2 cytokines IL-10 and tumor growth factor–β, however, as well as thymus and activation-regulated chemokine (TARC), a chemoattractant for CD4$^+$ T cells of the Th2 biotype (70). This overwhelmingly Th2 phenotype likely helps the antibody response and inhibits the CTL response. IL-10 may also act as an autocrine growth factor for Reed-Sternberg cells. Patients with Hodgkin's disease also have T-cell abnormalities, such as low expression of the zeta

chain of the T-cell receptor (71), which further reduce the effectiveness of the host immune response to the tumor (72).

To assess the feasibility of using EBV-specific CTLs as therapy for Hodgkin's disease, we generated EBV-specific CTLs from the peripheral blood of patients with this lymphoma, with the notion of expanding the cells *in vitro* in the absence of *in vivo* immunosuppressive effects. We then compared them phenotypically and functionally with CTLs generated from normal donors (53). To discover whether autologous EBV-specific CTLs could persist and produce antiviral activity *in vivo*, we genetically marked the cells and then adoptively transferred them to three patients with relapsed disease.

Cytotoxic T Lymphocytes from Patients with Hodgkin's Disease Compared with Those from Healthy Epstein-Barr Virus–Positive Donors

In the presence of IL-2 and B-LCL, cell counts of cultures from healthy donors (n = 15) typically increased by tenfold every 2 weeks, so that after 16 weeks in culture, CTLs from normal donors had expanded approximately 1,500-fold. During the same 16-week period, CTL cultures from patients in remission expanded by only approximately 150-fold, whereas those from patients with relapsed disease increased by just 80-fold. In more than 75% of patients, however, it was still possible to generate at least 10^8 CTLs, a number suggested by previous studies of EBV-LPD to be well in excess of that required to establish EBV immunity (59,60). Phenotypically, the patient lines were essentially identical to the lines from normal donors, except that the level of the T-cell receptor–zeta chain was abnormally low (73). The cytoplasmic portion of the T-cell receptor–zeta chain is involved in signal transduction and subsequent activation and proliferation of T cells, so that downregulation of this chain may contribute to the decreased proliferative response of patient T cells. Nonetheless, the lines produced had strong activity against HLA-matched EBV-positive targets. Of particular note, lines from Hodgkin's disease patients had activity against cells expressing Hodgkin's-associated viral antigens, including LMP1 and LMP2. This effect was demonstrated by the cells' ability to kill HLA-matched fibroblasts infected with vaccinia recombinants, each expressing one of the EBV-latent cycle proteins. Both HLA class I and class II restricted CTLs could be detected. The presence of the class II–restricted cells may be of benefit because approximately 50% of Hodgkin's tumor cells downregulate HLA class I molecules, and may therefore be protected from conventional CTL killing. They generally maintain class II major histocompatibility complex (MHC) expression, however.

Biologic and Clinical Study of Cytotoxic T Lymphocytes

Encouraged by our ability to generate CTLs with activity against at least one of the Hodgkin's-associated antigens, we asked whether these cells would have antiviral and antimalignant properties *in vivo*. To track the persistence of infused CTLs, we marked the cells with a neo-containing retroviral vector. The neo gene was detectable in PBMCs for 4 to 12 weeks after the initial dose of 3.2×10^7 EBV-specific CTLs (73). The

levels of marking indicated that approximately 1 of every 1,000 circulating PBMCs was derived from the infused cell line.

The infused CTLs had cytotoxic antiviral activity. Thus, the proportion of circulating EBV-specific cytotoxic precursor cells was increased 10- to 100-fold, indicating an enhanced cell-mediated immune response to EBV. The number of MHC-unrestricted cytotoxic effector precursors remained constant, as demonstrated by the minimal change in the proportion of cytotoxic precursor cells that killed HLA-mismatched LCLs. In addition to the rise in cytotoxic precursor cell frequency, the CTL activity tested after 2 weeks of culture with the autologous LCLs also increased *in vivo*, from less than 3% killing of autologous LCLs at an effector:target ratio of 40:1 to more than 25% killing at the same effector:target ratio. Again, little effect on the activity of MHC-unrestricted cytotoxic effector cells occurred, suggesting that an increase in classical MHC-restricted CTL activity was responsible for the observed increase in autologous LCL target killing.

The observed increase in cytotoxic function was associated with measurable antiviral activity. We used semiquantitative PCR analysis to calculate the viral burden in peripheral blood before and after CTL infusion. The number of EBV-DNA genomes in normal donors ranges from less than 20 to 2,000 copies per 10^6 PBMCs (9). Before CTL infusion, the level of EBV DNA in patient 1 was 30,000 EBV genomes per 10^6 PBMCs, which is 15-fold higher than in normal individuals and within the range seen for stem-cell transplant recipients with immunoblastic lymphoma (9,58). After CTL infusion, the level of EBV DNA decreased dramatically and was undetectable at 4 weeks' postinfusion. Associated with this drop in EBV DNA, the patient showed improvement of stage B symptoms with increased appetite and resolution of fever and sweats; stabilization of his pulmonary disease also occurred. These effects were apparent even though the patient had received no chemotherapy for 4 weeks before or 6 weeks after infusion. In fact, the viral load in the peripheral blood of this patient increased only during readministration of chemotherapy at 6 weeks' postinfusion (the end of the evaluation period). Patient 2 had insufficient blood counts to allow measurement of EBV-DNA levels but also showed improvement in stage B symptoms before the institution of further chemotherapy and disease progression. Although the EBV burden was not supranormal in the third patient, an initial level of 400 EBV genomes per 10^6 PBMCs fell to undetectable levels by 19 days after the first infusion. These effects were again produced in the absence of chemotherapy (>6 weeks before and after). This patient had an initial worsening of his pleural effusion, and gene-marked CTLs were detected in pleural biopsies of diseased areas (73). His disease then stabilized and no further pleural effusions occurred for more than a year. The tumor ultimately progressed in all three patients, who died of their disease 10 to 13 months later.

Improving the Clinical Outcome

These preliminary studies show:

1. It is feasible to obtain substantial *ex vivo* expansion of EBV-specific T cells from patients with advanced Hodgkin's disease.

2. These cells have *in vivo* cytotoxic activity against EBV-infected cells and are detectable *in vivo* for up to 12 weeks.

3. These cells can be targeted to Hodgkin's disease–associated antigens.

Our efforts are directed at enhancing the component of the anti-EBV response that is directed to the Hodgkin's-associated antigens LMP1 and 2 by using dendritic cells expressing the appropriate proteins (see the section Cytotoxic T Lymphocytes for Recipients of Solid Organ Transplants). The CTLs generated will be given to patients with minimal residual disease to reduce the immunosuppressive effects associated with bulky tumors. An alternative approach is to develop CTL clones directed against Hodgkin's-associated antigens. Such an approach is possible (74) but is time consuming because the frequency of cells with such specificity is low. Moreover, many Hodgkin's tumors have mutations within the 3' region of the LMP1 oncogene, including a 30–base pair deletion and a high frequency of nonrandom point mutations (75,76). As we have already found in our EBV-LPD patients, these mutations may destroy the epitopes recognized by CTLs specific for wild-type LMP1, a problem that can only be accentuated if monospecific CTL clones, rather than polyspecific CTL lines, are used. It may also be possible to vaccinate patients directly using polypeptides, DNA, or dendritic cells as immunogens. The capacity to induce an immune response *in vivo*, however, may be limited by tumor-mediated immune escape mechanisms that subvert the induction or expansion of a cytotoxic response.

OTHER EPSTEIN-BARR VIRUS–ASSOCIATED MALIGNANCIES

EBV is associated with an increasing number of frequently rare and geographically associated malignancies (see Table 2). Lethal midline granulomas involving natural killer–like T-cell lymphomas, gastric carcinomas, and pyothorax-associated lymphoma seem to have an increased frequency in Japan, whereas parotid carcinomas are found predominantly in American Eskimos. EBV-positive smooth muscle tumors (leiomyosarcomas) are the second most prevalent malignancy of children with acquired immunodeficiency syndrome, and have an increased frequency after organ transplantation. In nonimmunosuppressed individuals, leiomyosarcomas rarely carry the EBV genome. EBV has also been found in carcinomas of the thymus and salivary gland. With the exception of gastric carcinoma and pyothorax-associated lymphoma, these tumors all express the intermediate type II latency and therefore are potential targets for immunotherapies targeting viral proteins, although the success of such therapies may depend on the immune-evasion strategies used by the tumor.

The type I tumors, Burkitt lymphoma and gastric carcinoma, pose a greater challenge for immunotherapy. The only viral proteins expressed in type I tumors are EBNA1 and RK-BARF0, which, as described in the preceding paragraph, do not provide target epitopes for HLA class I–restricted CTLs. Burkitt lymphoma cells have been shown to use additional antiimmune response mechanisms. They have defects in their expression of TAP I transporter proteins and HLA class I mole-

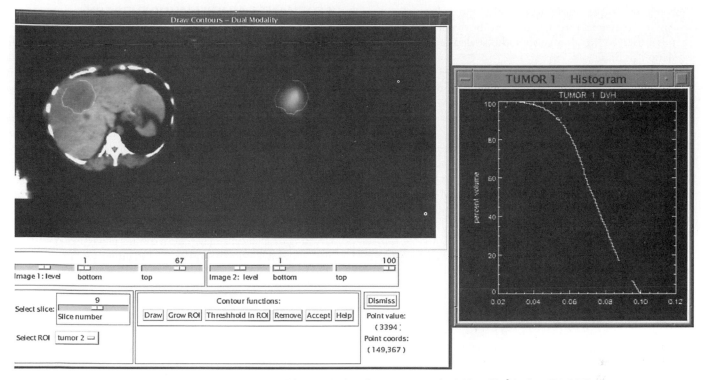

FIGURE 1. Dose contours. Patient with metastatic colon cancer received 90 mCi/m² iodine-131-CC49 intravenously. Coregistered computed tomography (left) and single-photon emission computed tomography (right) slices through the liver are shown; the box on the right demonstrates the dose received by tumor; most of the tumor received a relatively low dose.

Three-Dimensional Dosimetry

To evaluate the effectiveness and potential hazard of a particular radionuclide-antibody combination, the absorbed dose to target and normal organs must be calculated. This requires estimation of the total energy emitted per decay of the radionuclide and the fraction of the emitted energy that is absorbed in a source or in another (target) tissue. Using an idealized representation of human anatomy to mathematically define the coordinates, volumes, and compositions of organs, the MIRD Committee has performed such calculations for a large number of radionuclide and source-target organ combinations (31). The results are compiled in a series of "S-factor" tables. Given the time course of radioactivity in a particular organ, the S-factor tables may be used to determine the absorbed dose to other organs from radioactivity in the source organ.

The S-factor formalism was developed in the early to mid-1970s. This approach has proved adequate because most internally administered radiolabeled agents have been used for imaging and diagnosis; the absorbed dose to critical organs has usually been far below the level associated with tissue damage. Those cases in which radionuclides are used for nonantibody therapy (e.g., radioiodine therapy of thyroid disease), exhibit a high target-to-normal tissue activity concentration ratio. In radioimmunotherapy, however, the high levels of administered activity and the biodistribution of labeled antibody may lead to normal tissue morbidity. In such cases, the average absorbed dose over the volume of an idealized organ are misleading because information regarding the maximum dose to the organ is not provided.

The spatial distribution of absorbed dose for each patient's actual organ geometry is necessary to assess the potential for normal tissue morbidity.

To overcome these limitations, techniques that combine computed tomography and magnetic resonance images with single-photon emission computed tomography or positron emission tomography have been developed to account for each patient's anatomy and radioactivity distribution (32). The anatomic modalities, computed tomography, and magnetic resonance imaging are used to define tumor and normal organ geometry; single-photon emission computed tomography and positron emission tomography provide the spatial distribution of radioactivity. A series of images may be obtained by three-dimensional registration of these two image sets, such that the radioactivity distribution is superimposed on, and may be directly related to, patient anatomy (33). By way of illustration (Fig. 1), this approach has been combined into a dosimetry software package, called *3D-ID*, and is implemented for radiolabeled-antibody trials at Memorial Sloan-Kettering Cancer Center (34).

Red Marrow Dose

The red marrow is the dose-limiting organ in most implementations of radioimmunotherapy. Marrow vasculature is fenestrated and does not present a significant barrier to antibody penetration. The red marrow is composed of cells that are continuously undergoing cell division, and are therefore more radiosensitive. Early accessibility and enhanced radio-sensitivity are two factors that account for the marrow toxicity that is observed in almost all radiolabeled antibody dose-escalation studies.

Red marrow dosimetry introduces a number of difficulties that are not shared by other organs. Because of the distributed nature of this organ, it is difficult to obtain a time-activity curve from external imaging that is representative of all sites of active marrow.

Marrow dosimetry falls into two situations depending on the targeting properties and expected distribution of the antibody and the nature of the disease. If the antibody is not bound to antigen in the marrow, the radioactivity is distributed passively to the marrow based in the blood (passive distribution). If the antibody actively binds to antigen, a buildup of a higher concentration occurs on cellular components in the marrow (active distribution). Both situations fall within the MIRD S-factor formalism (31); their difference lies in the approach used to determine the cumulated activity in marrow.

Passive Distribution

The time-activity curve for intravenously administered antibody that does not target cellular components of the marrow, blood, or bone is obtained by assuming that the red marrow radioactivity concentration is equal to the radioactivity concentration in blood multiplied by a correction factor. After a review of the literature, the American Association of Physicists in Medicine Task Group on the Dosimetry of Radiolabeled Antibodies has recommended that a factor between 0.2 and 0.4 be used, and these general values have been rationalized by Sgouros (35).

These correction factors apply to blood activity concentration, and cumulated activity estimate for blood must be converted to cumulated activity concentration before the correction factor may be applied. The result must then be multiplied by the red marrow volume to give red marrow cumulated activity.

Active Distribution

In targeting hematologic disease or when the radiolabeled antibody cross-reacts with antigen that is associated with a cellular component of blood, marrow, or bone, antibody kinetics in marrow may not be approximated by blood kinetics. In this case, the time-activity curve of bone marrow concentration must be measured directly. The most widely adopted approach for obtaining the time-activity curve in marrow combines planar imaging with a single bone marrow biopsy. By drawing a region of interest around a marrow-rich, low-background area (e.g., ball of the femur or humerus), imaging may be used to determine the kinetics. The absolute radioactivity concentration in a bone marrow biopsy may then be used to "fix" the time-activity curve obtained from imaging to an absolute scale.

An increasing number of radioimmunotherapy protocols include a bone marrow transplant component. In such protocols, the red marrow is no longer the dose-limiting organ, and preliminary results suggest that lung or liver morbidity may limit the total dose that can be administered.

ADJUVANT RADIOIMMUNOTHERAPY

Although regional spread of cancer is associated with lymphatic invasion, distant metastases are generally thought to occur via hematologic spread. Such hematologic spread may arise from direct invasion of tumor vasculature or via the lymphatics to the thoracic duct and then into the circulation. That hematologic spread of micrometastatic cells is potentially important in the long-term course of the disease is suggested by studies that show a correlation between the number of tumor cells in marrow of breast cancer patients and their likelihood of developing distant metastases. The detection of hematologic micrometastases early in the course of disease has also been observed in prostate cancer. Although these studies have not demonstrated a cause-and-effect relationship, the possibility that radiolabeled antibody targeting of such cells may reduce distant metastases is enticing. The size distribution, number, and anatomic location of such micrometastases are critical in assessing the potential efficacy of radioimmunotherapy as an adjuvant treatment modality.

Using Monte Carlo–derived data regarding the size distribution and number of micrometastases that are present in a given prostate cancer patient population at the time of diagnosis and a mathematical model of antibody distribution and tumor cell cluster penetration, the potential efficacy of adjuvant radioimmunotherapy has been examined (27). The analysis suggests that a single administration of radiolabeled antibody could yield a potentially lethal dose ($\geq$20–38 Gy for ^{131}I) to 23% of micrometastases present at the time of initial diagnosis without inducing prohibitive red marrow morbidity (absorbed dose $\leq$2.5 Gy). Multiple courses of radioimmunotherapy designed to target micrometastases that are initially too small but that eventually reach a targetable size (i.e., 20 μm $\leq$ μm radius $\leq$200 μm) yields a potentially lethal dose to 87% of micrometastases. These results indicate that approximately 25% of "high-risk" prostate cancer patients (i.e., patients with occult metastases at the time of diagnosis) making up the population used for the Monte Carlo simulation would benefit from a single course of radioimmunotherapy; multiple courses could benefit 75% of these patients.

Alpha Particle Emitters

Although the extensive experience and easy availability of ^{131}I have made it the most commonly used radionuclide for antibody therapy, it is not ideal for targeting disseminated disease. Given the number of antigen sites per cell for most antibodies, the achievable specific activity, and the limitations on the amount of ^{131}I that may be administered because of red marrow toxicity, ^{131}I-labeled antibodies are not capable of single-cell kill (27).

Alpha particles are effective cytotoxic agents, capable of single-cell kill without limiting morbidity (28). The effectiveness of alpha particles arises because the amount of energy deposited per unit distance traveled (linear energy transfer) is approximately 400 times greater than that of beta particles (80 keV per μm vs. 0.2 keV per μm). Each traversal of an alpha particle through the nucleus results in a highly ionizing track. Cell survival studies have shown that alpha particle–induced killing is independent of oxygenation state or cell cycle during irradiation and that a single track across the nucleus may result in cell death (36–38). Most studies with alpha particle–emitting radionuclides for therapy have examined either ^{212}Bi or ^{211}At. Both radionuclides are short lived with 61-minute and 7.2-hour half-life, respectively. Both emit alpha particles whose range is 40–80 µm. In rapidly accessible, disseminated disease, these radionuclides have demonstrated a significant curative potential with minimal toxicity. In an ascites tumor mouse model, Macklis et al. (36) demonstrated specific targeting and 80% cure after injection of 5.6 to 8.5 MBq ^{212}Bi-labeled antibody. These results were observed after intraperitoneal administration.

The first human trial of an alpha particle emitter used systemically has been conducted with ^{213}Bi. ^{213}Bi is available in a generator system and has a half-life of 45.6 minutes. The highly stable CHXA-DTPA chelate has been used for labeling the anti-leukemia antibody, HuM195, with ^{213}Bi (19,21). Seventeen patients have participated in a phase 1 study of this agent without evidence of extra medullary toxicity. Dosimetry and pharmacokinetics associated with this trial have been described (27).

DOSIMETRY-BASED DESIGN OF RADIOIMMUNOTHERAPY TRIALS

Seminal studies carried out in human melanoma demonstrated the concept of using an initial tracer dose of radioactivity to predict organ-specific dose-limiting toxicity for subsequent calculation of maximum tolerated doses that could be safely administered. These studies also showed that there was an optimal mass amount of antibody for achieving the highest tumor radiation dose relative to the critical organ, which in most instances is the bone marrow (39). Using this same concept, Press et al. (40) and Kaminski et al. (41) showed that calculation of radiation-absorbed dose to the whole body (as a surrogate for red marrow) or to the next critical normal organ (42) permitted delivery of patient-specific amounts of radioactivity conjugated to antibody. All of these studies were possible in large part due to the relatively low immunogenicity of Fab murine fragments in the melanoma patients or to whole antibodies in patients with B-cell lymphoma using ^{131}I-labeled antibodies that permitted external measurement of whole-body radioactivity. In solid tumors, dosimetry-based measurements of optimum, patient-specific, therapeutic amounts of radioactivity were not possible because of the invariable development of an antimurine antibody response when whole antibody was used. Phase 1 solid tumor radioimmunotherapy trials with murine antibodies have used a radioactivity dose-escalation design based on weight or body surface area. Most ^{131}I-labeled antibody studies showed a maximum tolerated dose of 75 mCi per m^2, and comparable agreement was found in trials with other radionuclides, suggesting that estimation of radioactivity based on weight or body surface area was an adequate measure of maximum tolerated dose. Evaluation of these data, however, have conclusively shown that the amount of radioactivity administered is indeed a poor predictor of toxicity. Toxicity has been shown to be dependent, not surprisingly, on radiation-absorbed dose to the whole body and, correspondingly, to the

red marrow (43). Adequate prediction of toxicity, therefore, demands the estimation of clearance of radioactivity from each patient so that radiation-absorbed dose to critical normal organ(s) may be determined.

The development of relatively nonimmunogenic forms of antibody have allowed the possibility of treatment based on radiation-absorbed dose to critical normal organs. Clinical trials are increasingly based on estimation of whole body, red marrow, and other normal critical organ radiation-absorbed dose estimates to determine appropriate patient-specific amount of radioactive antibody that would deliver predictable toxicity to a known normal organ. These treatment schema are similar to those used to determine the maximum safe dose of ^{131}I for thyroid carcinoma (44), and to those used for ^{131}I-labeled antibody therapy for lymphoma (41). An initial dose of radiolabeled antibody is used to determine the biodistribution and pharmacokinetics of the radiolabeled antibody in the particular patient. These data are then used to determine the radiation-absorbed dose to normal organ(s) and a patient-specific radioactivity amount calculated. Initial prospective studies at the Memorial Sloan-Kettering Cancer Center have already demonstrated the wide range of radioactivity that would deliver comparable whole-body radiation-absorbed doses.

For such a schema to be feasible, however, the radionuclide needs to be measurable *in vivo* using external measuring devices; this is feasible for most nuclides with therapeutic potential, including ^{131}I, ^{186}Re, ^{188}Re, and lutetium-177 (^{177}Lu). For nuclides like ^{90}Y and ^{67}Cu, which cannot be measured in this manner, suitable surrogates need to be identified. Developments in radiochemistry have permitted the use of ^{111}In as a surrogate in most cases. Moreover, developments in cyclotron chemistry have allowed the use of the positron emitters ^{124}I, ^{86}Y, and ^{64}Cu as "true" surrogates; positron emission tomography of positron-labeled antibodies permits *in vivo* quantitation (45). It seems likely, therefore, that future radioimmunotherapy trials will increasingly use radiation-absorbed dose estimates for determination of toxicity, allowing optimal therapeutic delivery with minimal and predictable toxicity.

Single Large-Dose and Fractionated Radioimmunotherapy

The conventional wisdom that low-dose rate radiation, such as that delivered by radioimmunotherapy, is best administered as a single large dose may have important caveats. The twin limitations of antigen density and specific activity, for example, necessitate multiple treatments in radioimmunotherapy with ^{213}Bi-huM195 therapy. Studies by DeNardo et al. (46) have suggested that specific activity with ^{90}Y-labeled antibodies is also an important factor in therapy delivery that may necessitate fractionation.

Xenograft studies carried out, notably by Schlom et al. (47), Buchsbaum et al. (48), and Buchegger et al. (49), have suggested that fractionated radioimmunotherapy may have greater efficacy than single-dose therapy. This may be due to variability in tumor interstitial pressure and vascular flow, among other poorly understood factors. As in external beam radiotherapy, fractionated radioimmunotherapy may also permit recovery of radiation-injured normal cells. Theoretical models developed by O'Donoghue at the Memorial Sloan-Kettering Cancer Center (50) have suggested that although the tumor cell survival fraction is less after single large-dose radioimmunotherapy, repopulation of cells occurs at a slower rate after fractionated radioimmunotherapy. To test this hypothesis clinically, our group, in conjunction with colleagues at the Ludwig Institute for Cancer Research, are undertaking simultaneous radioimmunotherapy trials using the single large-dose and the fractionated models based on whole-body (or red marrow) radiation-absorbed dose. These studies should provide important information regarding the relative merits of each schedule of radioimmunotherapy. Needless to say, both methods have been made possible by the development of relatively nonimmunogenic antibody constructs, especially in nonlymphoid malignancies, as both require multiple administration of antibody.

CLINICAL TRIALS

To a certain extent, the development of radioimmunotherapy depends on the stepwise application of newly established biologic principles in the fields of radiation biology, immunology, and hematopoiesis to ongoing clinical protocols. The basic principles have been developed for *in vitro* systems and animal models in the laboratory and have progressed to clinical trials. The reader is referred to prior editions of this book for historical aspects. Review of progress since the last edition of this textbook is emphasized in this section, followed by examples from the experience of our group at the Memorial Sloan-Kettering Cancer Center. In particular, applications of ^{131}I-, ^{90}Y-, and ^{213}Bi-labeled huM195 (against CD33) in leukemia; ^{131}I-3F8 (against GD$_2$) in neuroblastoma; ^{131}I CC49 (against TAG-72) in prostate cancer; and ^{131}I-chimeric G250 in renal cancer illustrate the problems and promise of radioimmunotherapy.

Lymphomas/Leukemia

Reviews of the treatment of lymphomas/leukemia have appeared, which summarize the early history of treatment of lymphomas and leukemias (51,52). From the earliest studies, there were major responses in a variety of lymphoma types and clinical situations. Studies have been performed with ^{131}I, ^{90}Y, and ^{67}Cu (53). Antibodies have been used which target the differentiation antigens for white cells, CD5 (54), CD19, CD20, CD21, CD22 (55), CD33, and CD45 (56), as well as the HLA-DR (53) antigens. Each of these cellular targets provides tissue specificity to various subpopulations of myeloid and T-cell lineage and, as such, each cluster differentiation antigen has its proponents and detractors for the purpose of immune-specific targeting. In this review, we focus on radioimmunotherapy using anti-CD20 and anti-CD33 antibodies, which have been studied more extensively with less emphasis on CD37- and HLA-DR–targeting antibodies (57).

Treatment of Non-Hodgkin's Lymphoma: Myeloablative Dose Regimens and Autologous Bone Marrow Rescue

CD20 and CD37 Targeting

CD20 is a pan B-cell antigen that is broadly expressed on most B cells, whereas CD37 is an antigen found in late pre–B-cell precursors. Initial studies (40) used high doses of ^{131}I-labeled B1 and 1F5 anti-CD20 antibodies, as well as a few patients with anti-CD37 MB1 antibody. The study plan involved:

1. An antibody mass dose escalation in individual patients to determine "favorable dosimetry," defined as *tumor radiation-absorbed dose*, greater than the highest normal tissue (usually the lung)
2. Single massive doses of ^{131}I requiring hospitalization
3. Autologous bone marrow rescue

A tracer dose of ^{131}I B1 or MB1 was administered in patients with relapsed non-Hodgkin's lymphoma and radiation-absorbed dose to liver, lung, and kidney estimated by MIRD techniques (29). Favorable distribution was interpreted as preferential radiation dose to tumor compared with normal organs. Twenty-four (56%) patients showed preferential targeting of radioantibody to tumor ("favorable dosimetry"). Major responses were seen in 86% of patients, including 79% complete responses (CRs). Nonhematopoietic dose-limiting toxicity was cardiopulmonary with the estimated maximum tolerated radiation dose being 23.75 Gy (42).

Unmaintained CR has been seen in almost one-half of the patients for more than 7 years after therapy. The most common late toxicity was biochemical thyroid insufficiency in 60% of patients.

Nonmyeloablative Dose Regimens

Using smaller but multiple doses of ^{131}I B1 antibody in non-Hodgkin's lymphoma, ten patients (five low-grade lymphoma, five intermediate-grade lymphoma) were treated with a tracer dose to determine the optimal milligram amount of coadministered cold B1 to result in a whole-body dose of 25–45 cGy per injection. Thereafter, nine patients received 1–2 doses of 24–66 mCi ^{131}I B1, administered at 6- to 8-week intervals. Six of nine patients responded to the treatment; there were four CRs of 8, 11+, 9+, and 8+ months' duration. In this study, all known tumor greater than 2 cm was scan positive, and there was mild or no myelosuppression (41).

A summary of the experience with this nonmyeloablative regimen has been published using ^{131}I B1 antibody in doses that give whole-body radiation doses of 45–75 cGy. Fifty percent of the patients in the phase 1 trial of patients refractory to chemotherapy achieved a CR, and thrombocytopenia was dose limiting. The whole-body dose of 75 cGy is the maximum tolerated dose in patients who have not had a bone marrow transplant, and durable CRs were more likely to be seen in patients treated with the higher dose of radiation (65–75 cGy to whole body). Patients with low-grade and transformed

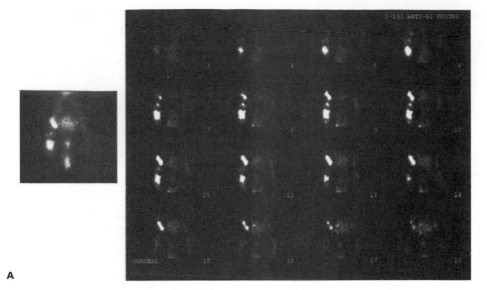

A

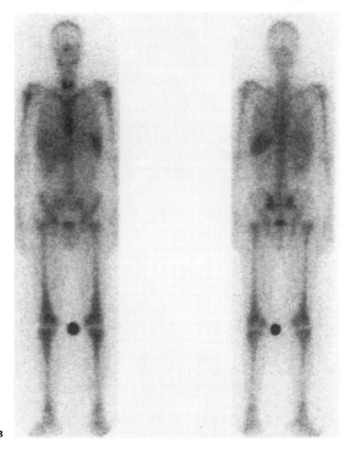

B

FIGURE 2. A: Therapy with iodine-131 (^{131}I)-anti-B-1. Anterior spot view of the pelvis (inset) and coronal single-photon emission computed tomography slices of the pelvis a week after therapy calculated to deliver no more than 0.75 Gy to whole body. There is excellent targeting to the right femoral lesion, as well as to the right inguinal adenopathy. **B:** Anterior and posterior whole body images 2 hours after ^{131}I-huM195 in a patient with acute promyelocytic leukemia. Targeting to marrow is clearly demonstrated.

low-grade non-Hodgkin's lymphoma appear most likely to respond (58).

This approach has developed into a phase 2/3 clinical trial, and initial results appear favorable. Of special interest was the fact that the ^{131}I-labeled B1 could be prepared centrally with the immunoreactivity maintained and shipped to clinical investigators around the country. Figure 2A demonstrates targeting of ^{131}I B1 to known nodal disease.

Yttrium-90 Anti-CD20 Antibodies in Lymphoma

^{90}Y is a high-energy beta emitter that may be more effective than ^{131}I for irradiating large tumor masses because of a longer mean range of beta particle penetration into tumor tissue *in vivo*. On a per-millicurie basis, ^{90}Y delivers 2.3 times as much radiation to tissue as ^{131}I. A phase 1/2 trial has been performed with an ^{90}Y-labeled anti-CD20 antibody in recurrent B-cell lymphoma. Again, myelosuppression was dose limiting, and the maximum tolerated dose was 50 mCi in this group of patients. Eighteen patients were studied with a major response rate of 72%, approximately one-half being CRs (59). In a phase 2 study using ^{111}In as a surrogate for ^{90}Y, the median bone marrow dose at the maximum tolerated dose of ^{90}Y was estimated to be 0.53 Gy. An overall response rate of 82% in low-grade non-Hodgkin's lymphoma was reported with 27% CRs (60). A phase 3 study is ongoing.

Monoclonal Antibody M195 (Anti-CD33)

Monoclonal antibody M195 (anti-CD33) is a murine IgG$_{2a}$ monoclonal antibody that reacts with most myeloid leukemic cells, monocytes, and hematopoietic progenitors. This antibody does not react with the pluripotent stem cell. [131]I M195 was studied as a therapeutic agent in acute and chronic leukemia. The chapter in the prior edition details phase 1 studies, which showed prompt targeting to tumor elements in the bone marrow; relatively low doses of antibody (4–6 mg) appeared to be optimal for targeting, presumably because of the low number of CD33 receptors per cell (61). [131]I M195 showed antileukemic activity in a subsequent phase 1/2 study; the invariable development of human antimouse antibody (HAMA), however, precluded multiple therapies, limiting efficacy (62).

Another group of patients studied were in clinical remission from acute promyelocytic leukemia after treatment with all-*trans*-retinoic acid in whom the status of the marrow was followed with a polymerase chain reaction technique designed to detect the particular gene translocation [t(15;17)] associated with acute promyelocytic leukemia. Disease-free survival appears to be increased by the use of the [131]I M195 at nonmyeloablative doses (50 mCi per m^2) to eliminate minimal disease. In relapsed patients with acute myelocytic leukemia for first transplants, patients were prepared for bone marrow transplant with ^{131}I-M195 cytoreduction instead of whole-body radiation therapy. Seven patients studied have achieved CR (initial doses were 120 mCi per m^2). Four patients were alive at 24 months after follow-up, and this approach compared favorably with prior treatment regimens (63). Figure 2B demonstrates targeting of ^{131}I-M195 to bone marrow in a patient with acute promyelocytic leukemia.

Humanized M195 consists of the murine complementarity–determining regions grafted to a human IgG1 backbone by genetic engineering methodology. Affinity of the humanized variant is approximately one order of magnitude higher than the murine monoclonal M195. In initial studies, biodistribution of the ^{131}I huG$_1$-M195 was similar to ^{131}I murine M195, and an anti-antibody response was absent (64).

Because the CD33 antigen is internalized subsequent to interaction with antibody, a phase 1/2 trial to evaluate the use of ^{90}Y-huM195 is being carried out at the Memorial Sloan-Kettering Cancer Center. The maximum tolerated dose of ^{90}Y-huM195 appears to be 0.25 mCi per kg body weight. Considerable cytoreduction has been seen in the majority of patients with no nonhematopoietic toxicity. Dose modifications are being continued for evaluation of toxicity and efficacy. No antihumanized antibody responses have been seen thus far.

Human trials with the short-lived [213]Bi required construction and operation of a [225]Ac/[213]Bi generator capable of producing 25–100 mCi of [213]Bi suitable for clinical antibody labeling (65). A generator has been designed to have an effective lifetime of several weeks and produces up to four therapeutic doses of radionuclide per day.

A phase 1 trial to determine the safety, pharmacology, dosimetry, and biologic activity of [213]Bi-HuM195 was completed (27). Eighteen patients with relapsed (n = 14) or refractory (n = 3) acute myelogenous leukemia or chronic myelomonocytic leukemia (n = 1) were treated with 0.28, 0.42, 0.56, 0.7, or 1 mCi per kg of [213]Bi-HuM195 in 3–6 fractions over 2–4 days. Total [213]Bi doses ranged from 17 mCi to 96 mCi; no acute toxicity was seen. Delayed toxicity was limited to myelosuppression, lasting 8 to 34 days. Biodistribution and dosimetry data were obtained by serial gamma camera images and blood samples after injection of [213]Bi-HuM195. Uptake of [213]Bi in the bone marrow, liver, and spleen occurred within 10 minutes of administration and was maintained throughout the half-life of the isotope. No significant uptake was seen in any other organ. Radiation doses to the bone marrow or spleen were up to 40,000 times higher than the estimated radiation doses to the kidneys or whole body. The absorbed-dose ratios between marrow, liver, and spleen and the whole body for [213]Bi-HuM195 were 1,000–10,000 times greater than those seen with beta-emitting nuclides, such as ^{131}I or [90]Y. Ten of 12 evaluable patients had reductions in peripheral blood leukemia cells, and 13 of the 18 patients had decreases in the percentage of bone marrow blasts. No CRs have been observed. This was the first study to show that systemic, targeted alpha particle therapy is safe and feasible in humans and has antileukemic activity.

Solid Tumors

One advance in this field has been the development of methods for assessing dosimetry of radioimmunotherapy based on quantitative imaging approaches. At Memorial Sloan-Kettering Cancer Center, for example, we have developed a three-dimensional dosimetry technique, 3D-ID (32). Using this method, we estimated that doses of up to 80 Gy could be delivered to selected tumor deposits using nonmyeloablative doses of ^{131}I-labeled CC49. HAMA occurs in virtually all patients by 3 weeks after a single injection of this murine IgG, however, and repeat injections were ineffective because the radioantibody is neutralized by the HAMA, and clearance into the reticuloendothelial system is accelerated. Moreover, even after a single injection, the uptake seen in the tumor is decidedly heterogeneous with a majority of the tumor volume receiving significantly less than the mean dose (32). Thus, it appears from these data that, to be successful in the treatment of solid tumors, repeated doses in this same range would be required. This depends on the development of less immunogenic reagents, probably humanized antibodies or some form of antibody fragment (66).

CC49 is one of the most widely studied of antibodies, and this antibody targets a mucinlike antigen, TAG-72, which is widely expressed on colon cancer (67) and a variety of other tumor types, including prostate. The chapter in the prior edition of this textbook details the experience with ^{131}I-CC49, an antibody directed against the sialyl-Tn antigen in colon and breast cancer. The antibody, conjugated with[177]Lu using a stable chelate, was subsequently studied in colon cancers by Carrasquillo et al.; as with the iodinated antibody, myelotoxicity was dose limiting, and responses were few and transient (68). A myeloablative regimen with ^{131}I CC49 was studied by Tempero et al.; they too found that responses were not lasting, and that at high doses of radioantibody, autologous rescue was not successful, precluding the use of this antibody even in a myeloablative setting (69). The development of an antimurine response precluded repeat therapies in these trials (66), although the response could be mitigated with immunosuppressive drugs (70).

Meredith et al. studied ^{177}Lu-CC49 in ovarian cancers (71). Administered via the intraperitoneal route, complete responses were seen in a few patients treated at the maximum tolerated dose. Rosenblum et al. similarly used ^{90}Y-labeled B72.3 (the "first-generation" anti-sialyl Tn antibody) intraperitoneally in patients with ovarian cancer (72). Again, an antimurine antibody response precluded multiple therapies; the study, however, confirmed the advantages of loco-regional delivery of radioimmunotherapy. Humanized CC49 is being developed and is expected to enter clinical trials shortly.

We (73) and others (74) have studied radiolabeled CC49 in prostate cancer (Fig. 3A). We used interferon to upregulate the antigen and to assess targeting and toxicity in phase 2 trials. Although targeting was good and minor responses, including pain relief, were seen in some patients, the results were not sufficiently promising to serve as a basis for more extensive clinical trials with these agents. A number of biologic insights have been offered from this work, however, including the extensive nature of bone marrow involvement of prostate cancer and the replacement of normal intramedullary marrow by tumor (see Fig. 2).

Pastan et al. have completed a phase 1 trial with ^{90}Y-labeled anti-Lewis[y] (Le[y]) antibody B1 (Carrasquillo J, *personal communication*, 1999). As with other radiolabeled antibodies, dose-limiting toxicity has been myelosuppression; as with other murine antibodies, the invariable occurrence of an antimurine antibody response has led to the development of humanized anti-Le[y] antibody, and we and other groups are initiating therapeutic trials with ^{90}Y-labeled humanized anti-Le[y] antibodies. Because the Le[y] complex is internalized, radiometals may be more suitable than radioiodine for therapy (75). Welt et al. developed A33 (Fig. 3B), an antibody against an antigen found in virtually all colon cancers with normal tissue reactivity limited to normal colon (76). Mixed responses were seen in patients treated with ^{131}I murine A33, which had a maximum tolerated dose comparable with other iodinated antibodies, with myelosuppression being dose limiting; development of HAMA again precluded multiple therapies (77). Unlike CC49, A33 is internalized subsequent to interaction with antigen. A33 internalization occurs by macropinocytosis (78); this allows the use of radioiodine as a therapeutic conjugate. We also carried out a study using ^{125}I-labeled murine A33; no toxicity was seen at ^{125}I doses of up to 400 mCi per m[2] (79). Even at these dose levels, however, the overall response rate was not different from that observed earlier. Serial external imaging was possible because of the large amounts of administered radioactivity; these showed that retention of radiolabeled

antibody in tumor was significant for up to 6 weeks with concomitant clearance from normal tissue, particularly large bowel. No bowel toxicity has been seen. The antibody has been humanized, and clinical trials with ^{131}I-A33 are under way.

G$_{D2}$ as Tumor Target

Gangliosides are acidic glycosphingolipids found on the outer surface of most cell membranes; they are particularly concentrated in gray matter and synaptic junctions in the nervous system, especially during brain development. During oncogenesis, major changes in the composition and distribution of cell-surface gangliosides can occur in tumors, including those of the central nervous system. G$_{D2}$ and G$_{D3}$ have been found in a wide spectrum of human tumors, including neuroblastoma, small-cell lung cancer, and brain tumors (80,81). In contrast, the only normal tissues with high ganglioside expression are restricted to tissues of the central nervous system and some peripheral nerves. A number of anti-G$_{D2}$ antibodies have been produced by hybridoma technique. 3F8 is a murine IgG$_3$ monoclonal antibody (80). In preclinical studies, [131]I-3F8 targeted to human neuroblastoma xenografts with exceptionally high %ID per gm (20%–40%). Intravenous ^{131}I-labeled murine IgG$_3$ 3F8 produced a substantial dose-dependent shrinkage of established neuroblastoma in preclinical studies. Dose calculations suggested that tumors that received more than 42 Gy rads were completely ablated.

Neuroblastoma

The biodistribution of [131]I-3F8 has shown excellent tumor targeting in patients with neuroblastoma (82), detecting more tumor sites than ^{131}I-MIBG (metaiodobenzylguanidine), ^{99m}Tc-MDP (technetium-labeled methylene diphosphonate) bone scan. The uptake that was observed was surgically confirmed to be in active neuroblastoma, and tumor uptake was high: 0.08%–0.1% injected dose per gm (83,84). This high tumor uptake was probably the result of the high antigen density (10[7] per cell) (85).

Radioimmunotherapy of Neuroblastoma

Next to lymphoid and brain tumors, neuroblastoma is the most common solid tumor of childhood. Large primaries and widespread metastatic disease at diagnosis, coupled with the early emergence of resistance to chemotherapy, magnified its management difficulties. Because neuroblastoma is a radiosensitive tumor, clinical applications of local radiotherapy and total-body irradiation have been incorporated into most "curative" strategies. Hyperfractionation at 150 cGy b.i.d. (total of 2,100 cGy) appears to be quite effective, especially for local control of microscopic disease. Long-term effects on growth and organ function plus the 1,200-cGy limit on total-body irradiation are two compelling reasons to develop alternative methods to deliver selective radiotherapy, both for bulky and microscopic disease. Neuroblastoma is suitable for testing radioimmunotherapy because:

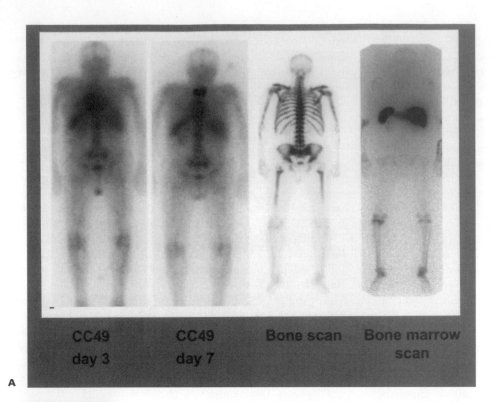

CC49
day 3

CC49
day 7

Bone scan

Bone marrow
scan

A

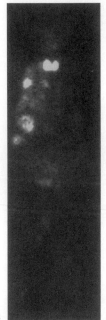

B

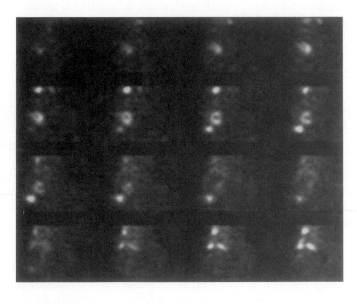

FIGURE 3. A: Anterior whole-body (left) and coronal slices through the thorax and liver in a patient with metastatic colon carcinoma treated with 140 mCi iodine-131 (^{131}I)-murine A33. Targeting to liver metastasis and pleural-based lung metastases is excellent; the patient had resolution of several pleural lesions with significant drop in serum carcinoembryonic antigen. Human antimouse antibody precluded further therapy. **B:** Posterior whole-body images in a patient with hormone-refractory prostate cancer treated with 140 mCi ^{131}I-CC49 administered after interferon therapy to upregulate antigen. From left: images 3 and 7 days after treatment with ^{131}I-CC49; bone marrow scan with technetium-99m–sulfur colloid. (*Continued*)

1. The shed antigen G_{D2} has not interfered with antibody delivery, especially in patients with small tumor load.
2. The tumor cells have a limited ability to repair radiation damage.
3. These tumors are generally vascular and their sites of metastases (liver, bone marrow, lymph nodes) are usually not perfusion limited.
4. Tumoricidal levels of radiation can be delivered by ^{131}I-labeled monoclonal antibody despite dehalogenation *in vivo*.

A radiation dose of more than 40 Gy is curative for neuroblastoma xenografts (86).

5. Radiolabeled antibodies with minimal extramedullary toxicities can be given over a short time to exploit the steep dose response of radiosensitive tumors, as long as the marrow can be rescued.

Toxicities

Acute side effects of pain, hypertension, hypotension, urticaria, and fever occur but can be controlled by appropriate premedica-

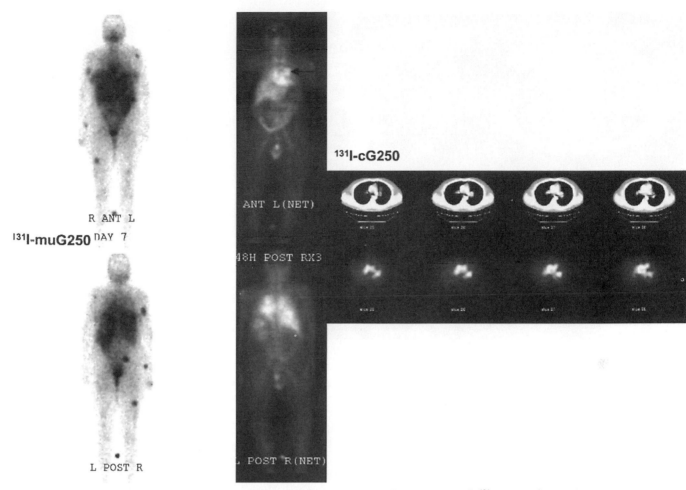

FIGURE 3. *Continued.* **C:** Treatment of metastatic renal cell carcinoma with ^{131}I-G250. Left: anterior (top) and posterior (bottom) images a week after 90 mCi ^{131}I-murine G250. Targeting to lesions in liver, lung, lymph nodes, bone, and subcutaneous lesions is excellent. Right: anterior and posterior whole body images and coregistered thoracic computed tomography and single-photon emission computed tomography images in a patient treated with ^{131}I-chimeric G250.

tion. No lethality has been reported in patients undergoing treatment with nonradioactive antibodies directed at G_{D2}. Severe, though reversible, neuropathy, however, was observed with the anti-G_{D2} antibodies 14.2a and ch14.18, thought to be associated with HAMA (87). This toxicity probably derived from antibody cross-reactivity with myelinated nerve fibers. More than 150 children have been treated with 3F8, and many have been followed for more than 4 years (maximum, 12 years) after treatment. None of the pediatric patients had obvious signs or symptoms of neuropathy, despite the finding of G_{D2} on peripheral nerves and previous reports of cross-reactivity of 3F8 with neurocellular adhesion molecule. This difference in toxicity spectrum may be caused by differences in antibody biodistribution in the child versus the adult. Because anti-G_{D2} antibodies may differ in their spectrum of reactivity with various gangliosides and their O-acetylated derivative, their fine specificities may determine their relative efficacy and toxicity.

The radiation toxicities of [131]I-3F8 were defined in a phase 1 dose-escalation study. Twenty-three patients (12 male and 12 female, 0.3 to 24.2 years of age at diagnosis) with refractory neuroblastoma (23, stage IV; 1, stage 3u) were treated with [131]I-3F8 at seven dose levels, namely 6, 8, 12, 16, 20, 24, and 28 mCi per kg. Radiation dose to the blood was calculated based on blood clearance, total-body dose based on MIRD, and the tumor/organ dose on regions of interest calculations from serial imaging. Twenty-two of 24 patients were rescued with cryopreserved autologous bone marrow; one patient received granulocyte-macrophage colony-stimulating factor and one patient died of progressive disease before marrow reinfusion. Marrow was infused when blood radioactivity decreased to less than 0.01 µCi per mL in the first 17 and less than 1 µCi per mL in the last five patients. Acute toxicities of [131]I-3F8 treatment included pain (20 of 24) during the infusion, fever (20 of 24), and mild diarrhea. All developed grade 4 myelosuppression. Thyroid uptake despite oral saturated solution of potassium iodine (SSKI), levothyroxine sodium (Synthroid), or liothyronine sodium (Cytomel) (or both) led to biochemical hypothyroidism in the majority. Among the six who survived more than 20 months after antibody treatment, no delayed extramedullary toxicities were encountered. Ten patients were evaluable for response to [131]I-3F8. There were two partial responses of soft tissue masses and two CRs of bone marrow disease. Average

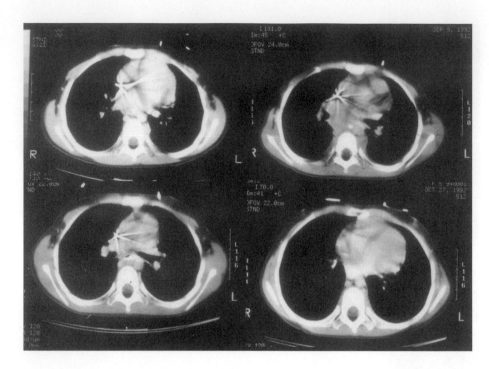

FIGURE 4. Computed tomography before and after therapy with iodine-131-3F8 (24 mCi per kg) in a patient with neuroblastoma.

tumor dose was calculated to be 150 rad per mCi per kg. Thus, when ^{131}I-3F8 was administered intravenously (6–28 mCi per kg), significant toxicities were encountered, including myelosuppression, and their infectious complications—pain, fever, and hypothyroidism. Autologous marrow rescue could reverse marrow aplasia. Although extramedullary toxicities in the acute phase were not severe, the late effects of this treatment modality have not yet been definitively defined (88,89).

In a subsequent study, the acute and delayed toxicities of this modality were confirmed in 25 patients with high-risk neuroblastoma treated with the N7 protocol (90). The N7 protocol uses dose-intensive chemotherapy for induction; surgical resection and 2,100 cGy hyperfractionated radiotherapy for local control; and, for consolidation, targeted radioimmunotherapy with ^{131}I-labeled anti-GD2 3F8 and immunotherapy with unlabeled/unmodified 3F8 (400 mg per m²). Intravenous ^{131}I-3F8 was given at 4 mCi per kg daily for 5 days (maximum, 1,000 mCi). Approximately 18 days after antibody treatment, autologous marrow or peripheral blood stem cells were infused. Among the first 25 consecutive previously untreated patients older than 1 year at diagnosis, 22 were stage 4 and two were unresectable stage 3 with n-myc amplification. Chemotherapy achieved complete or very good partial responses in 22 of 25 patients. All 25 patients engrafted, the major complications being myelosuppression plus infections with no lethal complications. Hypothyroidism was again noted despite aggressive thyroid protection using oral SSKI, liothyronine sodium, and Perchloracap. For dosimetry of both imaging (tracer) and therapeutic doses of ^{131}I-3F8, plasma time-activity curve was integrated over time to yield cumulated activity. Antibody clearance in normal organs generally closely followed that of blood. The plasma cumulative activity concentration was used to calculate activity in the liver, spleen, lungs, and red marrow according to each organ's extracellular fluid volume, which were estimates

adjusted for body weight. Conjugate planar images obtained on the day of injection (day 0) and on days 1, 2, and 4 were used to calculate tumor time-activity curves. Total-body cumulated activity obtained from imaging was within 5% of estimates based on external survey meter data. Computed tomography–based volume estimation technique was used to determine tumor volume. Using the DOSCAL program developed at Memorial Sloan-Kettering Cancer Center that implements the S-factor formalism, absorbed dose could be estimated (90). Figure 4 depicts the chest computed tomography scans of a patient before and after treatment with 24 mCi per kg of ^{131}I-3F8. Based on tracer dosimetry, the absorbed doses to liver, spleen, red marrow, lung, total body, and tumor were 537, 574, 445, 454, 499, and 4,926 cGy, respectively. The average cGy per mCi were 2.3, 2.5, 2, 2, 1.9, and 13.7, respectively.

Monoclonal Antibodies Against Renal Cancer

Monoclonal antibody G250 reacts against a cell surface antigen expressed in virtually all clear-cell renal carcinomas, and normal tissue expression is limited to large bile ducts and gastric epithelium. A presurgical study showed excellent tumor localization with uptake being among the highest reported in solid tumor. A phase 1/2 therapy study with murine ^{131}I-mG250 showed excellent targeting with mixed responses; development of an antimurine response precluded repeat therapy, underscoring the need for development of less immunogenic forms (91).

Chimeric G250 (cG250) was developed to circumvent the immunogenicity observed with mG250 and showed comparable targeting characteristics without immunogenicity (92). Radioimmunotherapy trials are being carried out to assess safety and efficacy; these have shown that the relative lack of immunogenicity of this chimeric antibody allows calculation of therapeutic dose based on radiation-absorbed dose to marrow estimated by measurement of clearance kinetics of an initial "scout" infusion of ^{131}I-cG250. Experimental data suggests that multiple administrations of radiolabeled antibody may have greater therapeutic effect than a single infusion; this has led to the study of single large-dose and fractionated radioimmunotherapy studies. Initial results indicate that calculation of absorbed dose based on scout data is reliable and that the low immunogenicity of cG250 permits multiple therapies (see Fig. 3C).

Intracavitary and Direct Intratumoral Injection Therapy

An additional situation of some promise for radioimmunotherapy is the use of intracavitary therapy for tumors, such as ovary and colon, which stay confined to the peritoneal surface. Greater concentrations of antibody can be achieved in tumor after intracavitary injection than intravenously (93,94). In addition, the use of antibodies directly injected into primary brain tumors appears to show some promise as well (95), especially with the alpha emitter ^{211}At (see Alpha Therapy).

Intraperitoneal Therapy

A clinical trial performed by Stewart and colleagues (96) gives cause for some optimism regarding the possible use of radiolabeled monoclonal antibodies in microscopic disease when given by the intraperitoneal route as adjunctive therapy for ovarian cancer post surgery. Nine of 15 patients with stage I ovarian cancer and small tumors (<2 cm) had complete responses, and three others had positive peritoneal washings only. On the other hand, in patients with tumor masses larger than 2 cm (eight patients in this group), no objective responses to therapy occurred (97). Such studies lend credence to the concept that intraperitoneal therapy as a surgical adjunct may reduce the rate of recurrence in patients with intraperitoneal metastases. These studies have formed the basis for prospective clinical trials in Europe and the United States. In 52 patients who received adjuvant antibody therapy after cytoreductive surgery and chemotherapy, 21 showed no evidence of recurrence during the median follow-up of 35 months (98).

In a follow-up study, the same group studied radioimmunotherapy in an adjuvant setting after successful debulking surgery for ovarian cancer. Twenty-five patients received 25 mg of antihuman milk fat globulin antibody (HFMG1) labeled with ^{90}Y to a dose of 18 mCi per m^2. In comparison with case-matched controls, there are survival advantages and a Cox proportional hazards model predicts that 10-year survival will be 70% in comparison with only 32% for controls treated with chemotherapy alone (99).

Intralesional Administration

Intralesional Therapy in Brain Tumors

Surgically created resection cavities provide an opportunity for direct intracavitary therapy. ^{131}I-labeled 81C6 has been injected into a surgically created cavity in the tumor site of patients with glioblastoma multiforme. At the maximum tolerated dose of 100 mCi injected, large doses of radiation can be delivered to the cyst wall (1,180 Gy) at 1-cm (71 Gy) and 2-cm (39 Gy) depths, with only approximately 6 Gy to normal brain tissue (99).

Alpha Therapy

Zalutsky et al. are performing a phase 1 trial to determine the maximum tolerated dose, pharmacokinetics, and objective responses for ^{211}At-labeled human/mouse chimeric antitenascin monoclonal antibody 81C6 administered into surgically created resection cavities of recurrent malignant glioma. Twelve patients have received a single injection of 10 mg of monoclonal antibody labeled with escalating doses of ^{211}At, ranging from 2 to 10 mCi. For 2 mCi ^{211}At monoclonal antibody, calculated radiation doses for the tumor cavity interface were 472 Gy compared with less than 0.02 Gy for normal brain, liver, spleen, and bone marrow. This study demonstrates that it is feasible to produce clinical levels of ^{211}At, administer ^{211}At-labeled chimeric 81C6 monoclonal antibody with minimal toxicity, and achieve high tumor:normal organ dose ratios (100,101).

SUMMARY

Radioimmunotherapy with radiolabeled monoclonal antibodies is increasingly effective for hematopoietic tumors with a number of investigators reporting persistent major responses. Radioimmunotherapy for solid tumors has been more difficult, and only an occasional major response has been reported; so far, these have not been persistent. Toxicity is predominantly hematopoietic with platelets being most sensitive to the effects of radiation. Even at ultra-high doses (up to 28 mCi per kg of ^{131}I), second organ toxicity has not been reached. Rational approaches to dose planning are becoming possible with improvements in dosimetry, based on quantitative single-photon emission computed tomography and positron electron tomography imaging. Therapeutic indices for tumor/marrow, the most radiosensitive organ, are in the range of 5–10 to 1. This is probably still too low for curative treatment of solid tumors, and further refinements, perhaps based on novel antibody formulations, are needed.

Several approaches are being investigated that may potentially result in an improvement in tumor response and a reduction in toxicity. These include enhancement of vascular permeability, regional administration, bifunctional antibodies, improved labeling chemistry, new radiolabels, and the use of mouse-human chimeric antibodies. In the future, further investigations of alternate radiolabels, the use of radiation dose–modifying agents, the identification of more reactive antigens, the use of antibody combinations, the alteration of routes of excretion of chelated antibodies, the investigation of human monoclonal antibodies, and biochemical modifications of antibodies to improve tumor deposition and reduce nonspecific targeting of normal tissues will be conducted. The number of clinical trials using radiolabeled antibodies to deliver radiation therapy is rapidly expanding. These studies should define the role of this modality in the cancer therapeutic armamentarium.

REFERENCES

1. Pressman D, Keighley G. The zone of activity of antibodies as determined by the use of radioactive tracers: the zone of activity of nephrotoxic antikidney serum. *J Immunol* 1948;59:141–146.

2. Pressman D, Day ED, Blau M. The use of paired labeling in the determination of tumor-localizing antibodies. *Cancer Res* 1948;17:845–850.

3. Bale WF, Spar IL. Studies directed toward the use of antibodies as carriers of radioactivity for therapy. *Adv Biol Med Phys* 1948;5:285–356.

4. Belitsky P, Ghose T, Aquino J, Norvell ST, Blair AH. Radionuclide imaging of primary renal-cell carcinoma by I-131-labeled antitumor antibody. *J Nucl Med* 1978;19:427–430.

5. Goldenberg DM, DeLand FH, Kim E, et al. Use of radiolabeled antibodies to carcinoembryonic antigen for the detection and localization of diverse cancers by external photoscanning. *N Engl J Med* 1978;298:1384–1388.

6. Kohler G, Milstein C. Continuous cultures of fused cells secreting antibody of predefined specificity. *Nature* 1975;256:495–497.

7. Winter G. Making antibody and peptide ligands by repertoire selection technologies. *J Mol Recognit* 1998;11:126–127.

8. Weber DA, Kassis AI. Radiolabeled Antibody Tumor Dosimetry. *Med Phys* 1993;20(2)[Suppl]:497–611.

9. Goldenberg DM (ed). Fifth conference on radioimmunodetection and radioimmunotherapy of cancer: October 6–7, 1994. *Cancer Res* 1995;55[Suppl]:S5708–S5990.

10. Goldenberg DM (ed). Sixth conference on radioimmunodetection and radioimmunotherapy of cancer: October 10–12, 1997. *Cancer* 1997;80[Suppl]:2343–2749.

11. Jurcic JG, Scheinberg DA, Houghton AN. Monoclonal antibody therapy of cancer. *Cancer Chemother Biol Response Modif* 1997;17:195–216.

12. Meredith RF, LoBuglio AF, Spencer EB. Recent progress in radioimmunotherapy for cancer. *Oncology* 1997;11(7):979–984(discussion 987–988).

13. Corcoran MC, Eary J, Bernstein I, Press OA. Radioimmunotherapy strategies for non-Hodgkin's lymphomas. *Oncology* 1997;8(1)[Suppl]:133–138.

14. Zalutsky MR (ed). *Antibodies in radiodiagnosis and therapy.* Boca Raton, FL: CRC Press, l989:240.

15. Gansow OA, Brechbiel MW, Mirzadeh S, Colcher DC, Roselli M. Chelates and antibodies: current methods and new directions. *Cancer Treat Res* 1990;51:153–171.

16. Meares CF, Moi MK, Diril H, et al. Macrocyclic chelates of radiometals for diagnosis and therapy. *Br J Cancer* 1990;10:21–26.

17. Zalutsky MR, Garg PK, Friedman HS, Bigner DD. Labeling monoclonal antibodies and F(ab′)2 fragments with the α-particle-emitting nuclide astatine-211: preservation of immunoreactivity and *in vivo* localizing capacity. *Proc Natl Acad Sci U S A* 1989;86:7149–7153.

18. Kozak RW, Atcher RW, Gansow OA, Friedman AM, Hines JJ, Waldmann TA. Bismuth-212 labeled anti-Tac monoclonal antibody: alpha-particle emitting radionuclides as modalities for radiotherapy. *Proc Natl Acad Sci U S A* 1986;83:474–478.

19. Nikula TK, McDevitt MR, Finn RD, et al. Alpha-emitting bismuth cyclohexylbenzyl DTPA constructs of recombinant humanized anti-CD33 antibodies: pharmacokinetics, bioactivity, toxicity and chemistry. *J Nucl Med* 1999;40:166–176.

20. Colcher D. Centralized radiolabeling of antibodies for radioimmunotherapy. *J Nucl Med* 1998;39[Suppl 8]:S11–S13.

21. McDevitt MR, Sgouros G, Finn RD, et al. Radioimmunotherapy with alpha-emitting nuclides. *Eur J Nucl Med* 1998;25:1341–1351.

22. Vaidyanathan GA, Zalutsky MR. Targeted therapy using alpha emitters. *Phys Med Biol* 1996;41:1915–1931.

23. Zalutsky MR, Bigner DD. Radioimmunotherapy with α-particle emitting radio-immunoconjugates. *Acta Oncol* 1996;35:373–379.

24. Zalutsky MR, Garg PK, Friedman HS, Bigner DD. Labeling monoclonal antibodies and F (ab)$_2$ fragments with the alpha particle emitting nuclide astatine-211: preservation of immunoreactivity with *in vivo* localizing capacity. *Proc Natl Acad Sci U S A* 1989;86:7149–7153.

25. Brechbiel MW, Pippin CG, McMurry TJ, et al. An effective chelating agent for labeling of monoclonal antibody with Bi-212 for alpha particle mediated radioimmunotherapy. *J Chem Soc Chem Commun* 1991:1169–1170.

26. Boll RA, Mirzadeh S, Kennel SJ, DePaoli DW, Webb OF. ^{213}BI for alpha-particle-mediated radioimmunotherapy. *J Lab Camp Radiopharm* 1997:341.

27. Sgouros G. Radioimmunotherapy of micrometastases: sidestepping the solid-tumor hurdle. *J Nucl Med* 1995;36(10):1910–1912.

28. Humm JL. A microdosimetric model of astatine-211 labeled antibodies for radioimmunotherapy. *Int J Radiat Oncol Biol Phys* 1987;13:1767–1773.

29. Jurcic JG, McDevitt MR, Sgouros G, et al. Phase I trial of targeted alpha-particle therapy for myeloid leukemias with bismuth-213-HuM195 (ANTI-CD33). *Proc Am Soc Clin Oncol* 1999.

30. Rao DV, Mara VR, Howell RW, Govelitz GF, Sastry KSR. *In vivo* radiotoxicity of DNA-incorporated ^{125}I compared with that of densely ionizing alpha particles. *Lancet* 1989:2:650–653.

31. Loevinger R, Budinger TF, Watson EE. *MIRD primer for absorbed dose calculations.* New York: The Society of Nuclear Medicine, 1989.

32. Raju MR, Eisen Y, Carpenter S, Inkret WC. Radiobiology of alpha particles. III. Cell inactivation by alpha-particle traversals of the cell nucleus. *Radiat Res* 1991;128:204–209.

33. Scott AM, Macapinlac HA, Divgi CR, et al. Clinical validation of SPECT and CT/MRI registration in radiolabeled monoclonal antibody studies of colorectal carcinoma. *J Nucl Med* 1993;34:94.

34. Kolbert KS, Sgouros G, Scott AM, et al. Implementation and evaluation of patient-specific three-dimensional internal dosimetry. *J Nucl Med* 1997;38(2):301–308.

35. Sgouros G. Bone marrow dosimetry for radioimmunotherapy: theoretical considerations. *J Nucl Med* 1993;34(4):689–694.

36. Macklis RM, Kinsey BM, Kassis AL, et al. Radioimmunotherapy with alpha-particle emitting immunoconjugates. *Science* 1988;240:1024–1026.

37. Macklis RM, Yin JY, Beresford B, Atcher RW, Hines JJ, Humm JL. Cellular kinetics, dosimetry and radiobiology of alpha-particle radioimmunotherapy: induction of apoptosis. *Radiat Res* 1992;130:220–226.

38. McDevitt MR, Nikula TN, Finn RD, et al. Bismuth labeled antibodies for therapy of leukemias, lymphomas and carcinomas: preclinical studies. *Tumor Targeting* 1996;2:182.

39. Larson SM, Carrasquillo JA, Krohn KA, et al. Localization of 131I-labeled p97 specific fab fragments in human melanoma as a basis for radiotherapy. *J Clin Invest* 1983;72:2101–2114.

40. Press OW, Eary JF, Appelbaum FR, et al. Radiolabeled-antibody therapy of B-cell lymphoma with autologous bone marrow support. *N Engl J Med* 1993;329:1219–1224.

41. Kaminski MS, Zasadny KR, Francis IR, et al. Radioimmunotherapy of B-cell lymphoma with [131I]anti-B1 (anti-CD20) antibody. *N Engl J Med* 1993;329:459–465.

42. Liu SY, Eary JF, Petersdorf SH, et al. Follow-up of relapsed B-cell lymphoma patients treated with iodine-131-labeled anti-CD20 antibody and autologous stem-cell rescue. *J Clin Oncol* 1998;16(10):3270–3278.

43. Larson SM, Raubitschek A, Reynolds JC, et al. Comparison of bone marrow dosimetry and toxic effect of high dose I-131 labeled monoclonal antibodies administered to man. *Nuc Med Biol Int J Appl Radiat Instrum* 1989;16(2):153–158.

44. Leeper RD. Thyroid cancer. *Med Clin North Am* 1985;69(5):1079–1096.

45. Larson SM, Pentlow KS, Volkow ND, et al. PET scanning of iodine-124-3F8 as an approach to tumor dosimetry during treatment planning for radioimmunotherapy in a child with neuroblastoma. *J Nucl Med* 1992;33:2020–2023.

46. Salako QA, O'Donnell RT, DeNardo SJ. Effects of radiolysis on yttrium-90-labeled Lym-1 antibody preparations. *J Nucl Med* 1998;39(4):667–670.

47. Schlom J, Molinolo A, Simpson JF, et al. Advantage of dose fractionation in monoclonal antibody-targeted radioimmunotherapy. *J Natl Cancer Inst* 1990;82:763–771.

48. Buchsbaum D, Khazaeli MB, Liu T, et al. Fractionated radioimmuno-

therapy of human colon carcinoma xenografts with 131I-labeled monoclonal antibody CC49. *Cancer Res* 1995;55[Suppl]:S5881–S5887.

49. Sun LQ, Vogel CA, Mirimanoff RO, et al. Timing effects of combined radioimmunotherapy and radiotherapy on a human solid tumor in nude mice. *Cancer Res* 1997;57:1312–1319.

50. O'Donoghue JA. The response of tumours with Gompertzian growth characteristics to fractionated radiotherapy. *Int J Radiat Biol* 1997;72:325–339.

51. Larson SM, Sgouros G, Cheung N-KV. Radioisotope conjugates. In: DeVita VT Jr, Hellman S, Rosenberg SA, eds. *Biologic therapy of cancer: principles and practice*. 2nd ed. Philadelphia: JP Lippincott Co 1995:534–552.

52. Jurcic JG, Scheinberg DA. Radioimmunotherapy of hematological cancer: problems and progress. *Clin Cancer Res* 1995;1(12):1439–1446.

53. DeNardo GL, Kukis DL, Shen S, DeNardo DA, Meares CF, DeNardo SJ. 67Cu-versus 131I-labeled Lym-1 antibody: comparative pharmacokinetics and dosimetry in patients with non-Hodgkin's lymphoma. *Clin Cancer Res* 1999;5(3):533–541.

54. Foss FM, Raubitscheck A, Mulshine JL, et al. Phase I study of the pharmacokinetics of a radioimmunoconjugate, 90Y-T101, in patients with CD5-expressing leukemia and lymphoma. *Clin Cancer Res* 1998;4(11):2691–2700.

55. Juweid M, Sharkey RM, Markowitz A, et al. Treatment of non-Hodgkin's lymphoma with radiolabeled murine, chimeric, or humanized LL2, an anti-CD22 monoclonal antibody. *Cancer Res* 1995;55[Suppl]:S5899–S5907.

56. Matthews DC, Appelbaum FR, Press OW, Eary JF, Bernstein ID. The use of radiolabeled antibodies in bone marrow transplantation for hematologic malignancies. *Cancer Treat Res* 1997;77:121–139.

57. Lamborn KR, DeNardo GL, DeNardo SJ, et al. Treatment-related parameters predicting efficacy of Lym-1 radioimmunotherapy in patients with B-lymphocytic malignancies. *Clin Cancer Res* 1997; 3(8):1253–1260.

58. Wahl RL, Zasadny KR, MacFarlane D, et al. Iodine-131 anti-B1 antibody for B-cell lymphoma: an update on the Michigan Phase I experience. *J Nucl Med* 1998;39[Suppl 8]:S21–S27.

59. Knox SJ, Goris ML, Trisler K, et al. Yttrium-90-labeled anti-CD20 monoclonal antibody therapy of recurrent B-cell lymphoma. *Clin Cancer Res* 1996;2(3):457–470.

60. Wiseman GA, White CA, Witzig TA, et al. Final dosimetry results of IDEC-Y2B8 Phase I/II Yttrium-90 radioimmunotherapy trial in non-Hodgkins Lymphoma (NHL). *J Nucl Med* 1999;40:64.

61. Scheinberg DA, Lovett D, Divgi CR, et al. A phase I trial of monoclonal antibody M195 in acute myelogenous leukemia: specific bone marrow targeting and internalization of radionuclide. *J Clin Oncol* 1991;9(3):478–490.

62. Caron PC, Schwartz MA, Co MS, et al. Murine and humanized constructs of monoclonal antibody M195 (anti-CD33) for the therapy of acute myelogenous leukemia. *Cancer* 1994;73[Suppl 3]:1049–1056.

63. Jurcic JG, Caron PC, Miller WH Jr, et al. Sequential targeted therapy for relapsed acute promyelocytic leukemia with all-trans retinoic acid and anti-CD33 monoclonal antibody M195. *Leukemia* 1995;9(2):244–248.

64. Caron PC, Jurcic JG, Scott AM, et al. A phase 1B trial of humanized monoclonal antibody M195 (anti-CD33) in myeloid leukemia: specific targeting without immunogenicity. *Blood* 1994;83(7):1760–1768.

65. McDevitt MR, Finn RD, Sgouros G, Ma D, Scheinberg DA. A 225 Ac/213 Bi generator system for therapeutic clinical applications: construction and operation. *Appl Radiat Isot* 1999;50:895–904.

66. Larson SM, El-Shirbiny AM, Divgi CR, et al. Single chain antigen binding protein (sFv CC49): first human studies in colorectal carcinoma metastatic to liver. *Cancer* 1997;80[Suppl 12]:2458–2468.

67. Divgi CR, Scott AM, Dantis L, et al. Phase 1 radioimmunotherapy trial with I-131 CC49 in metastatic colon carcinoma. *J Nucl Med* 1995;36:586–592.

68. Mulligan T, Carrasquillo JA, Chung Y, et al. Phase I study of intravenous Lu-labeled CC49 murine monoclonal antibody in patients with advanced adenocarcinoma. *Clin Cancer Res* 1995;1(12):1447–1454.

69. Tempero M, Leichner P, Dalrymple G, et al. High-dose therapy

with iodine-131-labeled monoclonal antibody CC49 in patients with gastrointestinal cancers: a phase I trial. *J Clin Oncol* 1997; 15(4):1518–1528.

70. Divgi CR, Scott AM, Gulec S, et al. Pilot radioimmunotherapy trial with 131I-labeled murine monoclonal antibody CC49 and deoxyspergualin in metastatic colon carcinoma. *Clin Cancer Res* 1995; 1(12):1503–1510.

71. Alvarez RD, Partridge EE, Khazaeli MB, et al. Intraperitoneal radioimmunotherapy of ovarian cancer with 177Lu-CC49: a phase I/II study. *Gynecol Oncol* 1997;65(1):94–101.

72. Rosenblum MG, Verschraegen CF, Murray JL, et al. Phase I study of 90Y-B72.3 intraperitoneal administration in patients with ovarian cancer: effect of dose and EDTA coadministration on pharmacokinetics and toxicity. *Clin Cancer Res* 1999;5:953–961.

73. Meredith RF, Bueschen AJ, Khazaeli MB, et al. Treatment of metastatic prostate carcinoma with radiolabeled antibody CC49. *J Nucl Med* 1994;35(6):1017–1022.

74. Slovin SF, Scher HI, Divgi CR, et al. Interferon-gamma and monoclonal antibody 131I-labeled CC49: outcomes in patients with androgen-independent prostate cancer. *Clin Cancer Res* 1998;4:643–651.

75. Carrasquillo JA, Mulshine JL, Bunn PA, et al. Tumor uptake of 111In T101 monoclonal antibody is superior to 131I T101 in cutaneous T cell lymphoma. *J Nucl Med* 1987;28(3):281–287.

76. Welt S, Divgi CR, Real FX, et al. Quantitative analysis of antibody localization in human metastatic colon cancer: a phase I study of monoclonal antibody A33. *J Clin Oncol* 1990;8:1894–1906.

77. Welt S, Divgi CR, Kemeny N, et al. Phase I/II study of iodine 131-labeled monoclonal antibody A33 in patients with advanced colon cancer. *J Clin Oncol* 1994;12:1561–1571.

78. Daghighian F, Barendswaard E, Welt S, et al. Enhancement of radiation dose to the nucleus by vesicular internalization of iodine-125-labeled A33 monoclonal antibody. *J Nucl Med* 1996;37(6):1052–1057.

79. Welt S, Scott AM, Divgi CR, et al. Phase I/II study of iodine-125 labeled monoclonal antibody A33 in patients with advanced colon cancer. *J Clin Oncol* 1996;14:1787–1797.

80. Cheung NK, Saarinen UM, Neely JE, Landmeier B, Donovan D, Coccia PF. Monoclonal antibodies to a glycolipid antigen on human neuroblastoma cells. *Cancer Res* 1985;45:2642–2649.

81. Schulz G, Cheresh DA, Varki NM, Yu A, Staffileno LK, Reisfeld RA. Detection of ganglioside GD2 in tumor tissues and sera of neuroblastoma patients. *Cancer Res* 1984;44:5914–5920.

82. Yeh SDJ, Larson SM, Burch L, et al. Radioimmunodetection of neuroblastoma with iodine-131-3F8: correlation with biopsy, iodine-131-metaiodobenzylguanidine (MIBG) and standard diagnostic modalities. *J Nucl Med* 1991;32:769–776.

83. Nelson AD, Miraldi F, Cheung NKV. Biodistribution and dosimetry of 3F8 neuroblastoma monoclonal antibody. *Am J Physiol* 1989;4:143–150.

84. Larson SM, Pentlow KS, Volkow ND, et al. PET scanning of iodine-124-3F8 as an approach to tumor dosimetry during treatment planning for radioimmunotherapy in a child with neuroblastoma. *J Nucl Med* 1992;33:2020–2023.

85. Wu Z, Schwartz E, Seeger RC, Ladisch S. Expression of GD2 ganglioside by untreated primary human neuroblastomas. *Cancer Res* 1986;46:440–443.

86. Cheung NKV, Landmeier B, Neely J, et al. Complete tumor ablation with iodine 131-radiolabeled disialoganglioside GD2 specific monoclonal antibody against human neuroblastoma xenografted in nude mice. *J Natl Cancer Inst* 1986;77:739–745.

87. Saleh MN, Khazaeli MB, Wheeler RH, et al. A phase I trial of the murine monoclonal anti-GD2 antibody 14.G2a in metastatic melanoma. *Cancer Res* 1992;52:4342–4347.

88. Cheung NKV, Kushner BH, Yeh SJ, Larson SM. 3F8 Monoclonal antibody treatment of patients with stage IV neuroblastoma: a phase II study. *Int J Oncol* 1998;12:1299–1306.

89. Cheung NKV, Kushner BH, Cheung IY, et al. Anti-GD2 antibody treatment of minimal residual stage 4 neuroblastoma diagnosed at more than 1 year of age. *J Clin Oncol* 1998;16:3053–3060.

90. Cheung NKV, Kushner BH, LaQuaglia M, et al. N7: a novel multimodality therapy of high risk neuroblastoma (NB) in children diag-

nosed over 1 year of age. *Eur J Cancer* 1999 (*in press*).

91. Divgi CR, Bander NH, Scott AM, et al. Phase I/II radioimmuno-therapy trial with iodine-131 labeled monoclonal antibody (MAb) G250 in metastatic renal cell carcinoma. *Clin Cancer Res* 1998;4: 2729–2739.

92. Steffens MG, Boerman OC, Oosterwijk-Wakka JC, et al. Targeting of renal cell carcinoma with iodine-131 labeled chimeric monoclonal antibody G250. *J Clin Oncol* 1997;15(4):1529–1537.

93. Lashford LS, Davies AG, Richardson RB, et al. A pilot study of ^{131}I monoclonal antibodies in the therapy of leptomeningeal tumors. *Cancer* 1988;61:857–868.

94. Courtenay-Luck NS, Epenetos AA, Halnan KE, et al. Antibody-guided irradiation of malignant lesions: three cases illustrating a new method of treatment: a report from the Hammersmith Oncology Group and the Imperial Cancer Research Fund. *Lancet* 1984; 1441–1443.

95. Riva P, Franceschi G, Frattarelli M, et al. 131I radioconjugated anti-bodies for the locoregional radioimmunotherapy of high-grade malig-nant glioma—phase I and II study. *Acta Oncol* 1999;38(3): 351–359.

96. Stewart JS, Hird V, Sullivan M, Snook D, Epenetos AA. Intraperito-neal radioimmunotherapy for ovarian cancer. *Br J Obstet Gynaecol* 1989;96(5):529–536.

97. Maraveyas A, Snook D, Hird V, Kosmas C, Meares CF, Lambert HE, Epenetos AA. Pharmacokinetics and toxicity of an yttrium-90-CITC-DTPA-HMFG1 radioimmunoconjugate for intraperitoneal radioim-munotherapy of ovarian cancer. *Cancer* 1994;73:1067–1075.

98. Hird V, Maraveyas A, Snook D, et al. Adjuvant therapy of ovarian cancer with radioactive monoclonal antibody. *Br J Cancer* 1993;68(2):403–406.

99. Nicholson S, Gooden CS, Hird V, et al. Radioimmunotherapy after chemotherapy compared to chemotherapy alone in the treatment of advanced ovarian cancer: a matched analysis. *Oncol Rep* 1998;5(1): 223–226.

100. Akabani G, Reist CJ, Cokgor I, et al. Dosimetry of 131I-labeled 81C6 monoclonal antibody administered into surgically created resection cavities in patients with malignant brain tumors. *J Nucl Med* 1999;40(4):631–638.

101. Zalutsky MR, Akabani G, Cokgor I, et al. Dose escalation study of compartmental deliver of astatine-211 labeled human/mouse chi-meric anti-tenascin monoclonal (MAb) antibody in patients with recurrent malignant gliomas. Proceedings of the 13th International Conference on Brain Tumors 1999(abst).

MONOCLONAL ANTIBODIES: CLINICAL APPLICATIONS

B-Cell Lymphomas

SCOTT M. SCHUETZE
DAVID G. MALONEY

Using monoclonal antibodies (MAb) to treat cancer has evolved through a long process of promise, hype, and now, finally, positive clinical trial results. Lymphoma has been an appealing target for immunotherapy in part due to the relative ease of acquiring tumor cells by biopsy and because of the extensive identification and characterization of B-lymphocyte antigen expression.

The goal of antibody therapy for the treatment of cancer is the selective destruction of tumor, while minimizing toxicity to normal host tissues. Two general approaches have been pursued. The first uses "naked" or unconjugated MAb against antigens on tumor cells to cause direct effects and to recruit the host's immune system to eliminate the MAb-coated tumor cells. The second approach uses MAb conjugated to toxins, drugs, or radioisotopes to concentrate these agents at sites of tumor, thereby improving their therapeutic index.

Elements critical to the success of MAb therapy include the target antigen, the MAb, and the type and characteristics of the tumor. In 1981, the first MAb-based treatments demonstrated antitumor activity and with the approval of rituximab (anti-CD20 MAb, Rituxan), the antibody-based treatment of B-cell non-Hodgkin's lymphoma (NHL) has entered clinical practice. Hopefully, the agents discussed here represent the tip of the iceberg as more specific cancer therapies continue to be refined and developed.

IMPORTANT ANTIGEN CHARACTERISTICS FOR ANTIBODY THERAPY

From a large number of preclinical and clinical trials since the early 1980s, many of the characteristics of antigens critical for successful antibody-based immunotherapy have been elucidated (Table 1). Of primary importance is the tissue distribution and expression of the antigen. The ideal tumor antigen would only be expressed on malignant cells and especially not on vital normal host cells. The B-cell surface immunoglobulin (Ig) is formed by genetic recombination and somatic mutation during development of B cells and the protein sequence and structure is unique to each mature lymphocyte and malignant clone. This surface Ig is tumor specific (Ig-idiotype), and treatment with antiidiotype antibodies causes minimal toxicity (1,2). In contrast, CD52 is expressed on most B and T cells, and treatment with anti-CD52 antibodies can cause profound immunosuppression (3,4). Many of the antigens targeted for B-cell lymphoma immunotherapy are restricted to expression in the B-cell or lymphoid lineage (Table 2). Thus, an effective therapy against a pan B-cell antigen would also deplete normal B cells. If the antigen were not expressed on stem cells or progenitor cells, however, normal lymphocytes would be expected to repopulate after the elimination of the MAb from the patient. This has been observed with anti-CD20 therapy (5). In some cases, the antibody (e.g., Lym-1) is more avid for HLA-DR10 on malignant cells than on normal lymphocytes, which may limit toxicity (6). Nonspecific binding of antibody can also result in toxicity to normal host tissues, especially with radioimmunoconjugate or immunotoxin.

A second critical issue is the degree of heterogeneity of antigen expression on the malignant cell. Unconjugated MAb need to bind to all of the tumor cells as they act by directing components of the immune system to the tumor or by inducing intracellular signals, or both. Toxin or drug-conjugated MAb also need to bind to every cell as they act by delivering the substance to the cell cytosol. Tumor cells not expressing the antigen at the cell surface would not be killed. In contrast, radioisotopes emit radiation or particles, or both, that can exert lethal damage over a distance. Thus, a theoretical advantage of radiolabeled antibodies is the ability to kill nearby antigen-negative cells by this "cross-fire" effect. A high antigen mutation rate or the loss of antigen expression may lead to the escape of epitope-negative clones under the selective pressure of targeted therapy. The more critical the biologic function of the antigen, the less likely antigen loss mutation should occur.

TABLE 1. IDEAL ANTIGEN CHARACTERISTICS FOR MONOCLONAL ANTIBODY THERAPY

Antigen Characteristic	Type of Antibody Therapy		
	Unconjugated	Immunotoxin	Radioimmunoconjugate
Expression on normal host cells	Disadvantage	Disadvantage	Disadvantage
Present on all tumor cells	Necessary	Necessary	Important
Mutation or loss of antigen variants	Disadvantage	Disadvantage	Disadvantage
High-density cell surface expression	Important	Important	Important
Shed from cell surface or secreted	Disadvantage	Disadvantage	Disadvantage
Internalization upon binding antibody	Disadvantage	Necessary	Disadvantage for [131]I
Biologic function	Important	Less important	Less important

Additional factors include antigen density and disposition of the antigen in the cell membrane. In most studies, higher density of the target antigen led to a greater clinical effect. Modulation or internalization of the MAb/antigen complex from the cell surface is required for immunotoxin constructs but is detrimental to unconjugated MAb therapy. Endocytosis of radioimmunoconjugate often leads to cleavage and secretion of the radioisotope-labeled fragments. Antigen shed or secreted from the cell into the serum can bind MAb and block interactions with the tumor. In some cases, this problem may be circumvented by infusing large doses of antibody (2).

Increasing importance is being given to the biologic function of the target antigen and to the intracellular molecular events arising from the interaction of antibody with antigen. These events may be crucial to the success of unconjugated MAb-based therapy. Interaction of the MAb with antigen may exert direct antitumor effects by blocking a natural ligand-ligand receptor interaction [anti–interleukin-6 (IL-6), anti-CD25], mimicking a natural ligand (antiidiotype antibody simulating antigen) or interfering with the function of a molecule. These interactions may have direct antiproliferative or apoptotic effects and are dependent on the antibody, the antigen, and the biology of the tumor cell. As an example, clinical trials of antiidiotype MAb found that the isotype of murine MAb used (thus, the ability of antibody to recruit effector cells) did not correlate with clinical outcome (2,7,8). However, the ability of antiidiotype MAb to induce tyrosine phosphorylation in the patient's lymphoma cells *in vitro* correlated with the clinical antitumor effectiveness of the antibody (9). The interaction of some anti-CD20 antibodies with CD20 directly induces growth arrest and apoptosis in some lymphoma cell lines (10–12). The degree to which these direct antitumor effects from antibody-antigen interactions influence the clinical outcome is still largely unknown. It is likely that the more successful antibody-based therapies (especially that of unconjugated MAb) will capitalize on these effects.

Selected characteristics of the antigens on B-cell lymphomas that have been targeted with MAb therapies are listed in Table 2. Some are widely expressed on most B-cell malignancies,

TABLE 2. CHARACTERISTICS OF SELECTED ANTIGENS ON B-CELL NEOPLASMS

Antigen	Normal Tissue Distribution	MAb-Targeted NHL Histology	Mutation	Internalization/ Modulation	Biologic Function
Immunoglobulin (idiotype)	Mature B cells	Low, intermediate, and high grades	Yes	Yes	Antigen receptor
CD5	T cells, B cells	CLL, mantle cell	No	Yes	CD72 ligand
CD19	Immature and mature B cells	Low, intermediate, and high grades	No	Yes	Signal transduction complex
CD20	Mature B cells	Low, intermediate, and high grades	No	No	Calcium channel
CD21	B cells, dendritic cells, neutrophils	PTLD	No	?	EBV/C3d receptor
CD22	B cells, T cells	Low, intermediate, and high grades	No	Yes	Adhesion receptor
CD24	B cells, T cells, neutrophils, neural tissue, red cells	PTLD	?	?	Cell adhesion and signaling
CD37	Mature B cells	Low, intermediate, and high grades	?	Yes	Tetraspanin
CD38	T cells, B cells, NK cells, monocytes	Multiple myeloma, PTLD	?	Yes	Ectoenzyme
CD40	B cells, T cells, dendritic cells	Low, intermediate, and high grades	No	Yes	Costimulatory molecule receptor
CD52	B cells, T cells, monocytes, platelets	Low, intermediate, and high grades, CLL	Yes	No	?
HLA-DR	B cells, T cells	Low, intermediate, and high grades	Yes	No	Antigen presentation
HM1.24	Plasma cells	Multiple myeloma	?	?	?

CLL, chronic lymphocytic leukemia; MAb, monoclonal antibody; NK, natural killer; PTLD, posttransplant lymphoproliferative disorder.

whereas others are more restricted to a specific developmental stage or B-cell lymphoma histology. Specific clinical trials are discussed in the following sections.

CLINICAL TRIALS OF UNCONJUGATED MONOCLONAL ANTIBODIES FOR THERAPY OF B-CELL LYMPHOMA

The development of MAb technology led to a large number of exploratory preclinical and clinical trials. Leukemia and lymphoma were often targeted for antibody therapy because of ease of access of antibody to tumor *in vivo*. Numerous preclinical models helped define the important interactions between antibodies, antigens, and the host environment. However, successful eradication of tumor in preclinical models was not always predictive of a response in human trials. More recently, clinical studies using genetically engineered MAb, combinations of antibodies, or combinations of antibody and chemotherapy have demonstrated significant activity in patients with NHL. This has renewed enthusiasm for the development and use of unconjugated antibodies for cancer therapy.

The greatest success in unconjugated antibody therapy for lymphoma has been with CD20-targeted treatment of follicular lymphoma. Substantial antibody activity has also been seen in posttransplant lymphoproliferative disorders (PTLDs), antiidiotype therapy of follicular lymphoma, and CD52-targeted therapy for chronic lymphocytic leukemia (CLL). Unconjugated MAb against other antigens, such as CD19 and HLA-DR, have been less successful. Table 3 lists selected informative clinical trials of unconjugated antibody therapy for the treatment of NHL. Therapy directed against CD20, surface Ig, CD21, CD24, and CD52 are discussed in detail.

Anti-CD20 Antibody Therapy

CD20 is a nearly ideal antigen for unconjugated antibody therapy. The antigen is expressed in high density on most malignant B cells, does not mutate or internalize, and is not shed from the cell surface (13). The binding of some anti-CD20 antibodies directly induces antiproliferative or apoptotic events in some lymphomas (10–12). An early clinical trial of immunotherapy for B cell lymphoma using the murine anti-CD20 MAb 1F5 was conducted by Press and colleagues in 1986 (14). Four patients with refractory, low-, and intermediate-grade NHL were treated with a continuous infusion of 1F5 over 5–10 days in a dose-escalation study. Total dosages ranged from 52 to 2,380 mg anti-CD20 MAb 1F5. Higher doses of antibody were required to penetrate extravascular tumor and to saturate binding sites. Most adverse events were asymptomatic low-grade fevers, transient reduction in neutrophil and platelet counts, and clearance of normal circulating B cells. The MAb was rapidly cleared from the blood after discontinuation of the infusion and partial remissions were observed in the two patients receiving the highest dosages.

A human/mouse chimeric anti-CD20 antibody rituximab (IDEC-C2B8) was developed to enhance tumor-cell lysis via complement fixation and antibody-dependent, cell-mediated cytotoxicity; reduce immunogenicity; and improve pharmacokinetics (15). Human IgG1k-constant regions were molecularly grafted onto the murine variable regions from anti-CD20 MAb IDEC-2B8 using recombinant DNA techniques. A dose-escalation clinical trial of rituximab in 15 patients with relapsed low-grade B-cell lymphoma established the safety in administering 10 to 500 mg per m^2 of this MAb in a 5- to 6-hour intravenous infusion (16). The mean serum half-life was 4.4 days, which was longer than that seen with the murine MAb 1F5. Moreover, 2 weeks after treatment, antibody bound to tumor could still be detected in excised lymph nodes and in the serum of most patients treated with more than 100 mg per m^2.

A trial of rituximab given as four weekly infusions in 20 patients with relapsed low- or intermediate/high-grade lymphoma confirmed the safety of the chimeric MAb (17). Side effects were similar to those seen in the initial study and were mostly related to the initial infusion. Grade I and II fevers, chills, asthenia, and nausea were the most frequent side effects. Skin rash, pruritus, urticaria, arthralgia, rhinitis, and night sweats were reported in 10% of patients. Peripheral B cells were rapidly depleted but repopulated the peripheral blood in 6 to 9 months. Mean Ig levels and T-cell subset numbers remained unchanged, and significant bacterial, viral, or opportunistic infections were not observed. Hematologic events included transient thrombocytopenia and neutropenia in a minority of patients and did not appear to be due to lymphoma involvement of the marrow, but may have been from clearance of cells with antibody bound to Fc-receptors or to release of cytokines. Only one patient treated in the phase 1 trials developed a human anti-chimeric antibody response. The mild toxicities and ease of administration in an outpatient setting helped move rituximab into larger multiinstitutional trials.

Two hundred and three patients with relapsed low-grade and follicular NHL were treated with four weekly infusions of 375 mg per m^2 rituximab [37 patients in a phase 2 single institution trial (5) and 166 patients in a phase 2 multicenter trial (18)]. On an intent-to-treat analysis, 46% to 48% of patients had an antitumor response [complete response (CR) or partial response (PR)] to therapy. The response of follicular lymphomas was better (53% to 60% CR + PR) than the response of small lymphocytic lymphoma (SLL) (0% to 13% CR + PR). The reason for the lower response in SLL is not known but may be due to the lower density of CD20. Additionally, response correlated with increasing MAb levels in the serum and patients with SLL had increased clearance of MAb (19). Collectively, there were 13 complete remissions using strict criteria (all lesions less than 1 cm × 1 cm). In the smaller study, the median time to onset of tumor response was 50 days and maximal tumor response occurred 3 to 4 months after therapy (5). Median time to progression in responders in both trials was 10 to 13 months. Forty percent of patients whose low-grade lymphoma progressed after a response to rituximab had another response to retreatment with rituximab (20). Forty-three percent of patients with bulky (more than 10 cm) low-grade NHL responded to treatment with rituximab, although most of the remissions were partial (21).

The single agent activity of rituximab for follicular NHL has encouraged trials of rituximab in other lymphomas that express

TABLE 3. SELECTED CLINICAL TRIALS USING UNCONJUGATED MONOCLONAL ANTIBODIES FOR TREATMENT OF B-CELL LYMPHOMA

Target	Antibody	Disease	Dose	Patients (n)	Response	Problems	Studies
CD20	C2B8 (Rituximab) (Chimeric)	Relapsed low-grade NHL	375 mg/m^2 qwk × 4	204	50% CR + PR	Mild infusional toxicity, fever, rare CD20 escape, rare HACA	Maloney et al. (5), McLaughlin et al. (18)
CD20	C2B8 (Chimeric)	Relapsed and refractory intermediate-grade NHL	375–500 mg/m^2 qwk × 8	54	5 CR, 12 PR	Mild infusional toxicity	Coiffier et al. (22)
CD20	C2B8 (Chimeric)	Untreated low-grade NHL	375 mg/m^2 6 doses + CHOP 6 cycles	38	22 CR, 16 PR	Mild infusional toxicity, no additive toxicity to CHOP	Czuczman et al. (23)
CD20	1F5 (Murine)	Refractory low- and intermediate-grade NHL	5–800 mg/m^2/d × 5–10 d	4	1 PR	Minimal toxicity	Press et al. (14)
Ig idiotype	Custom anti-idiotype (Murine)	Relapsed low-grade NHL	400–11,500 mg qod × 2–3 wk alone, with Chl, or with INF	34	18% CR, 50% PR	Mild infusional toxicity; Id negative escape	Meeker et al. (2), Brown et al. (8), Maloney et al. (7), Davis et al. (20)
CD21 + CD24	BL13 + ALB9 (Murine)	PTLD	0.2 mg/kg/d × 10 d	58	36 CR	Mild infusional toxicity, neutropenia in 46%, HAMA	Benkerrou et al. (38)
CD52	CAMPATH-1G (Rat)	NHL	25–50 mg/d × 10 d	13	1 CR, 3 PR	Moderate infusional toxicity, fever	Dyer et al. (39)
CD52	CAMPATH-1H (Humanized)	Relapsed and refractory NHL	30 mg t.i.w. × 12 wk	42	6 PR	Moderate infusional toxicity, immunosuppression	Lundin et al. (4)
CD52	CAMPATH-1H (Humanized)	CLL: No prior therapy	30 mg t.i.w. × 18 wk	9	3 CR, 5 PR	Moderate infusional toxicity, immunosuppression	Osterborg et al. (42)
CD52	CAMPATH-1H (Humanized)	CLL: Prior therapy	30 mg t.i.w. × 12 wk	29	1 CR, 11 PR	Moderate infusional toxicity, immunosuppression	Osterborg et al. (3)
CD5	T-101 (Murine)	CLL	1–140 mg b.i.w. × 4 wk	13	Transient	Mild infusional toxicity, fever, antigen modulation	Foon et al. (45)
CD5	T-101 (Murine)	CLL	Various	4	Transient	Mild infusional toxicity, fever, antigen modulation	Dillman et al. (44)
CD19	CLB-CD19 (Murine)	Progressive NHL	225–1,000 mg	6	1 PR	Minimal toxicity, antigen modulation	Hekman et al. (46)
CD19	CLB-CD19 (Murine)	Low-grade NHL	50 mg/m^2 b.i.d. × 12 wk + IL-2	7	1 PR	Mild toxicity due to IL-2, antigen modulation	Vlasveld et al. (47)
HLA-DR	LYM-1 (Murine)	Refractory low- and intermediate-grade NHL	58–465 mg qwk x 4	10	3 Minor	Mild infusional toxicity	Hu et al. (48)

Chl, chlorambucil; CHOP, cyclophosphamide, doxorubicin, vincristine, and prednisone; CLL, chronic lymphocytic leukemia; CR, complete response; HACA, human antichimeric antibody; HAMA, human antimouse antibody; Id, idiotype; IL-2, interleukin-2; INF, interferon; NHL, non-Hodgkin's lymphoma; PR, partial response; PTLD, posttransplant lymphoproliferative disorder.

CD20. Coiffier reported on a multicenter phase 2 trial of 54 patients with diffuse large-cell and mantle cell NHL (22). Patients received either eight weekly infusions of 375 mg per m^2 or one infusion of 375 mg per m^2 followed by seven weekly infusions of 500 mg per m^2. Eighty-three percent of patients had received earlier chemotherapy, including autologous bone marrow transplantation (ABMT) in nine patients. Previously untreated patients were older than 60 years of age. Five patients (9%) had a complete remission and 12 patients (22%) had a PR to therapy for an overall response in patients with either diffuse large-cell NHL or mantle-cell lymphoma of 35%. The majority of responses were observed in patients without bulky tumor (largest lesion smaller than 5 cm) and with disease that was responsive to earlier chemotherapy. The median time to progression in responding patients had not been reached at the time of publication but exceeded 8 months. In seven patients with progressive intermediate-grade NHL after high-dose chemotherapy with ABMT support, salvage therapy with rituximab resulted in one complete remission, five PRs, and one mixed response. This study demonstrates that there is single-agent activity of rituximab in aggressive NHL and provides rationale for sequential or combined trials with standard therapy.

In vitro data suggest that rituximab may act synergistically with some cytotoxic chemotherapeutics (11). Czuczman et al.

reported on the results of a clinical trial of rituximab given concurrently with cyclophosphamide, doxorubicin, vincristine, and prednisone (CHOP) chemotherapy (23). Thirty-eight patients with newly diagnosed or relapsed low-grade NHL were treated with six cycles of standard-dose CHOP and six cycles of rituximab. Two doses (375 mg per m^2) of rituximab were given before the first cycle of CHOP, one dose was given before the third and fifth cycles of CHOP, and two doses were given after the sixth cycle of CHOP. Thirty-five of 38 patients who began treatment completed the regimen. A CR occurred in 22 (58%) and a PR in 16 (42%) of the treated patients for an overall response rate of 100%. The mean time to response was similar to that seen in trials of rituximab alone, and median time to progression was more than 17 months. Toxicity was additive, and the more serious adverse events were attributable to CHOP. It is not known if responses to rituximab plus CHOP will be more durable than responses to chemotherapy alone, but the shape of the disease-free survival curve is encouraging, with 75% of patients remaining in remission with more than 30 months' median follow-up.

Multiple ongoing cooperative trials (SWOG 9800, ECOG 1496, and ECOG/CALGB 4494) are addressing the benefit of consolidation with rituximab after treatment with chemotherapy. Additionally, trials are taking advantage of the peripheral blood B-cell depletion observed with rituximab to "*in vitro* purge" peripheral blood stem cell collections before high-dose therapy and peripheral blood stem cell transplantation and evaluating rituximab posttransplant to eliminate minimal residual disease.

In general, therapy with rituximab has been well tolerated. Dose-limiting or cumulative toxicities have not been observed. However, infusion-related symptoms consisting of fevers, chills, and rigor are most commonly observed (17). Nausea, hypotension, and bronchospasm are occasionally seen and can be abated by temporary cessation of the antibody infusion along with administration of acetaminophen and diphenhydramine (16,17). Reinfusion of antibody at a reduced rate is usually tolerated. Side effects are often most pronounced during the initial infusion and are less problematic with subsequent doses. In some patients, more serious adverse events, including death, have been reported. In some cases, these may be associated with high numbers of circulating tumor cells, leading to severe bronchospasm, hypoxemia, biochemical evidence of rapid destruction of tumor, and thrombocytopenia (24). It is possible that initial infusions of lower doses of antibody may prevent this constellation of symptoms in patients with large, readily accessible tumor burdens (24).

Antiimmunoglobulin Idiotype Antibody Therapy

During B-cell development, Ig variable-region gene segments undergo recombination and somatic mutation, which results in an Ig sequence unique to each B cell. Thus, clonally derived mature B-cell lymphomas usually express unique Ig sequences. MAb against these unique sequences (antiidiotype) can be generated using hybridoma technology; however, this necessitates the development of a custom antibody for each patient. Treat-

ment with antiidiotype MAb can achieve potent antitumor activity. In a series of trials at Stanford University, 34 patients were treated with infusions of murine antiidiotype antibodies either alone, with chlorambucil, or with interferon (1,2,7,8). Tumor responses were observed in 68% of patients (CR in six patients). Responses occurred in patients who had failed earlier chemotherapy; who had large tumor burdens; and who had disease in blood, bone marrow, lymph nodes, spleen, liver and/or extranodal sites. *In vivo* antitumor activity correlated with the ability of antiidiotype antibodies to induce cell signaling through tyrosine phosphorylation *in vitro* in pretreatment tumor cells (9). This suggested that direct effects of the interaction of antiidiotype antibody with cell-surface Ig were important for antitumor activity. The addition of chlorambucil (7) or interferon (8) did not significantly improve disease response.

Most PRs lasted less than 1 year; however, in an update of long-term remissions induced by antiidiotype antibodies, six of eight CRs persisted longer than 4 years (25). Of interest, analysis of five patients in clinical complete remission 3 to 8 years after MAb therapy detected molecular markers of the tumor in all cases, suggesting the induction of a tumor dormancy state (25). Relapse, in these clinical trials, was usually owing to the outgrowth of idiotype-negative variant cells that expressed mutated Ig that did not bind the treatment antibody (26). Low levels of variant cells, a product of somatic mutation of the Ig hypervariable regions, could be detected in the pretreatment tumor-cell population, and treatment with monoclonal antiidiotype antibody allowed the outgrowth of these variants (26). In some cases of poor antitumor response, tumors secreted high levels of idiotype into the serum that bound to infused antiidiotype antibody and presumably blocked antibody from binding to lymphoma cells (2). Infusions of antiidiotype antibodies were generally well tolerated, with mild fever, chills, and rigor observed during the initial infusion (2,7). These studies first demonstrated that MAb could lead to tumor regression in patients with relapsed B-cell NHL.

Due to the expense and difficulty in developing custom antiidiotype MAb for each patient with follicular lymphoma and the frequent selection of idiotype-variant tumor cells, however, subsequent trials have explored vaccination with the idiotype protein to induce a polyclonal, *in vivo* immune response directed at multiple epitopes on tumor Ig idiotype, thus limiting the risk of variant idiotype tumor-cell outgrowth. For these trials, Ig is isolated from follicular lymphoma and used to formulate a custom antitumor vaccine. Long-term results from the Stanford idiotype-vaccine trial investigating the use of tumor-specific idiotype vaccination after standard chemotherapy in patients with follicular NHL has been reported (27). Forty-one patients were immunized with tumor idiotype chemically coupled to keyhole limpet hemocyanin and mixed with an immunologic adjuvant. Evidence of humoral or cellular antiidiotype immune responses could be detected in 20 patients postimmunization. Of 32 patients in first complete remission after standard chemotherapy, significant prolongation of time to tumor progression (7.9 years versus 1.3 years) and median survival from time of last chemotherapy was observed in patients with detectable antiidiotype immune responses compared to those not making an idiotype-specific immune response. Twenty patients had residual tumor at the time of immunization. Tumor regression occurred in two of five patients who mounted a detectable antiidiotype immune response, whereas no cases of tumor regression were observed in the 15 patients without a detectable response. Despite these promising results, a randomized trial is required to prove that the induction of a polyclonal antiidiotype response or an idiotype-specific T-cell response, or both, is responsible for the improved outcome.

Anti-CD21 and Anti-CD24 Antibody Therapy of Posttransplant Lymphoproliferative Disorders

The combined use of two MAb reactive to different cell-surface antigens for the treatment of B-cell lymphoma was first explored in PTLD. PTLD most often arises from Epstein-Barr virus–infected B lymphocytes and is associated with T-cell immunosuppression. PTLD may be an oligoclonal or a monoclonal process at the time of diagnosis, often arising in recipients of T-depleted allogeneic bone marrow or solid organ transplants on immunosuppressive therapy. PTLD occasionally remits after reduction of immunosuppressive therapy, but outcomes of treatment with chemotherapy are generally poor (28,29). CD21, the human complement receptor type 2, is also the receptor for Epstein-Barr virus and is expressed on mature B cells and follicular dendritic cells (30). CD24 is a glycosylphosphatidylinositol-linked, mucin-type molecule expressed on B cells, neutrophils, neural tissue, and numerous types of tumors (31).

Infusion of murine anti-CD21 and anti-CD24 MAb was used to treat two children with PTLD after T-cell depleted mismatched bone marrow transplants (32). Complete remissions were obtained in both cases, and an open, multicenter, prospective trial was initiated. An update of 58 patients with PTLD who did not respond to reduction in immunosuppressive therapy showed complete remissions in 36 of 59 treated cases (61%) (33). CR rates were similar between patients who had developed PTLD after bone marrow transplantation or solid organ transplant. The relapse rate for complete responders was 8% with a median follow-up of 61 months. Significant factors predicting a poor response to antibody therapy were greater than four involved sites of disease, central nervous system disease, onset greater than 1 year from transplant, and transplant performed for treatment of hematologic malignancy. Monoclonal PTLD was statistically less likely to respond (48% CR rate) than oligoclonal disease (80% CR rate); however, overall survival was not statistically different. Time to complete response from the initiation of therapy ranged from 5 days to 150 days, with a median of 15 days. The treatment consisted of infusions of 0.2 mg of antibody per kg of body weight over 4 to 6 hours per day for 10 days and was well tolerated. Mild fevers and chills occurred in 20% of patients, and transient neutropenia occurred in one-half of the patients, presumably due to the expression of CD24 on neutrophils (34). Circulating B cells were also depleted but began to repopulate peripheral blood within 15 days of the completion of antibody infusion. Episodes of infection were infrequent and occurred during periods of neutropenia. Human antimouse antibodies (HAMA) developed in 50% of the patients tested.

For unclear reasons, PTLD may be particularly sensitive to unconjugated MAb therapy. An anecdotal response of PTLD to the sequential administration of anti-CD37 and anti-CD38 has been described (35). Relatively little experience is available on the use of anti-CD20, although preliminary reports suggest significant activity (36). Multiple trials in PTLD are under way with rituximab.

Anti-CD52 (CAMPATH-1) Antibody Therapy

CD52 is a 21- to 28-kd glycosylphosphatidylinositol-linked glycoprotein that is expressed at high density on T cells, B cells, and most lymphoid malignancies and is the target for the CAMPATH-1 MAb (37). It is not shed from the cell surface and does not modulate on binding anti-CD52 antibodies (38,39). Antigen-negative normal T cells have been observed posttherapy (40), but antigen-negative escape by lymphoma has not been reported.

Initial studies used a rat IgM anti-CD52 (CAMPATH-1M) antibody that actively fixed complement but was rapidly cleared from serum. Depletion of circulating lymphoma cells was transient and may have been due to sequestration rather than lysis (39). An IgG2b-subclass anti-CD52 (CAMPATH-1G) was tested in 18 patients with lymphoid malignancies because of the *in vitro* ability of the antibody to fix complement and mediate antibody-dependent cellular cytotoxicity (39). During treatment with 25 to 50 mg of CAMPATH-1G per day for 10 days, normal and malignant lymphocytes were cleared from the circulation, and unlike trials using CAMPATH-1M, lymphocytopenias persisted after discontinuation of therapy. Responses in blood, marrow, and spleen were observed, but minimal effects on lymph nodes and extranodal masses occurred. Subsequent trials have used humanized anti-CD52 antibody (CAMPATH-1H) developed by molecularly splicing the rat hypervariable regions into the human-IgG1 Ig genes (41).

In a phase 2 multicenter study, 50 patients with relapsed or resistant low-grade NHL received 30 mg of CAMPATH-1H thrice weekly for up to 12 weeks (4). Forty-two of the 50 patients had B-cell lymphomas and in this group there were six PRs. The median time to progression in responders was 4 months. As seen with CAMPATH-1G, the overall response of disease in blood and bone marrow was higher than in spleen and lymph nodes.

CAMPATH-1H has increased activity for CLL and T-cell disorders (mycosis fungoides and T-cell prolymphocytic leukemia). In a report of nine previously untreated patients with CLL, three patients had a complete remission, five had a PR, one had progressive disease, and three patients had a CR of lymph–node-based disease (42). Response duration was greater than 20 months in four patients at the time of publication. A phase 2 trial of subcutaneous CAMPATH-1H for first-line therapy of CLL has been initiated. Therapy in patients with previously treated CLL has been less successful, possibly due to immune system dysfunction secondary to advanced disease or earlier chemotherapy, or both. In 29 previously treated CLL patients, intravenous administration of CAMPATH-1H induced a CR in one patient and PRs in 11 patients (3). Bone marrow, spleen, and lymph nodes were cleared of disease in 36%, 32%, and 7% of patients, respectively, with a median duration of response of 12 months.

These results have been accompanied by infusion-related toxicity and immunosuppression. Infusion-related adverse events include fevers, rigors, nausea, and rash and were observed in the majority of patients (3). Tachyphylaxis rapidly occurred, and dosages could be escalated from 3 to 30 mg without causing additional infusion-related side effects. Hypotension requiring temporary cessation of infusion was reported in 16% of patients. The side effects have been less common with subcutaneous administration and have consisted principally of fever and moderate local skin reactions (43). Hematologic toxicities were less severe and less frequent in patients with CLL than in patients with NHL (3,4). Profound T-cell depletion accompanied by complications, including viral reactivation and opportunistic infections, were observed (3,4). These were more frequent in heavily pretreated patients. Current trials of subcutaneous CAMPATH-1H include prophylactic treatment with acyclovir, trimethoprim/sulfamethoxazole, and fluconazole to prevent infections.

Other Unconjugated Antibody Therapy

Additional cell-surface antigens on B-cell lymphomas have been targeted but have proved to be poor candidates for unconjugated antibody therapy. CD5 is a 65-kd transmembrane protein found on T cells, CLL, and mantle-cell lymphoma. Infusion of an IgG2a-murine anti-CD5 antibody (T101) in patients with CLL resulted in only transient (24 to 48 hours) reductions in levels of circulating malignant cells (44,45). CD19 is a 90-kd transmembrane protein expressed during B-cell development and on most malignant B cells. Infusions of IgG2a murine anti-CD19 antibody (CLB-CD19) in patients with low- or intermediate-grade NHL has produced responses in only a small minority of patients (46,47). Both CD5 and CD19 internalize on binding antibody, and more recent trials have focused on immunotoxin conjugates. MAb have also been raised against a polymorphic variant of HLA-DR that is present on normal and malignant B cells. Infusions of IgG2a murine anti-HLA-DR antibody (Lym-1) in ten patients with refractory low- and intermediate-grade NHL failed to produce significant responses (48), but some trials using radiolabeled Lym-1 are more promising.

Multiple myeloma is a late B-cell stage malignancy that usually does not express CD19 or CD20. Clinical trials of rituximab are under way to target "putative" B cells that may be part of the malignant clone. Additional MAb under development include anti-HM1.24 (49) and anti-CD38 (50). Myeloma may in part be driven by IL-6 or an IL-6 like substance (51–53). Trials of chimeric anti-IL-6 antibody therapy in patients with multiple myeloma have substantially lowered serum levels of free, biologically active IL-6 and C-reactive protein and have inhibited myeloma-cell proliferation during therapy but have not demonstrated disease responses (54–56).

CLINICAL TRIALS OF TOXIN-CONJUGATED MONOCLONAL ANTIBODIES FOR THERAPY OF B-CELL LYMPHOMAS

Immunotoxin therapy takes advantage of selective binding of MAb to the target antigen to deliver potent toxins to the tumor cells. Toxins or drugs must typically reach the cytosol to have antitumor activity (inhibition of protein synthesis); therefore, useful cell surface antigens must internalize on binding antibody. Additionally, because toxins are lethal to any cell that internalizes them, the antigens should be expressed on few nonmalignant cells. Early clinical trials using immunotoxins for treatment of malignancy encountered multiple difficulties. The chemical links between toxins and antibodies were unstable *in vivo*, resulting in short immunotoxin half-life and poor delivery of toxin to tumor. Unmodified toxins bound to liver and endothelium, which rapidly decreased serum concentrations of the immunotoxins and contributed to toxicity in normal host tissues. Second-generation immunotoxins were developed with more stable toxin-antibody links that would still allow release of free toxin intracellularly. Additionally, toxins were modified to limit binding to liver and endothelium. Most trials of immunotoxin therapy of NHL have used either the deglycosylated ricin-A chain or a "blocked" heterodimeric ricin to reduce the nonspecific binding of the B chain to galactose residues on normal cells. A theoretical advantage exists to using a heterodimeric ricin conjugate because the B chain facilitates translocation of the protein into the cytosol after endocytosis.

CD19 and CD22 have been most extensively used as targets for immunotoxin-directed therapy of B-cell lymphoma (Table 4). Expression of these antigens is limited to lymphocytes, and both CD19 and CD22 internalize on MAb binding (57,58). CD19 is a B-cell differentiation transmembrane protein and part of the antigen receptor complex, and CD22 is a transmembrane adhesion receptor expressed on normal B cells and many B-cell malignancies.

Anti-CD22 Immunotoxin Therapy

CD22 has been targeted with F(ab')$_2$ fragments or intact murine IgG1 anti-CD22 antibody (RFB4) coupled to deglycosylated ricin-A chain (RFB4-dgA) in three separate trials (see Table 4). Forty-one patients with refractory or relapsed B-cell NHL received two to 12 doses of immunotoxin every 48 hours in dose-escalation studies (59,60). Immunotoxin was rapidly cleared from the serum [half-life 1.5 hours for F(ab')$_2$-RFB4 (60) and 7.8 hours for IgG-RFB4 (59)]. Thirty-eight percent of patients treated with the F(ab')$_2$ immunotoxin had a PR (60), and 25% of evaluable patients treated with the IgG immunotoxin responded (CR+PR) (59). In general, responses were rapid, and delayed tumor regression was not observed. The higher doses of immunotoxin were associated with fever, myalgia, and a vascular leak syndrome. Dose-limiting toxicity consisting of pulmonary edema, aphasia, and rhabdomyolysis was observed.

IgG-RFB4-dgA was given as an 8-day continuous infusion in an effort to increase the therapeutic index, because earlier results suggested that peak dosage rather than cumulative dosages contributed to toxicity. However, the maximum tolerated dose was similar to that obtained by bolus administration, and three of the four PRs occurred in patients receiving the highest dose level of immunotoxin (61). Toxicities were similar to those seen with bolus infusions. One-third of treated patients developed HAMA or human antiricin antibodies, or both.

TABLE 4. SELECTED CLINICAL TRIALS USING IMMUNOTOXINS FOR TREATMENT OF B-CELL LYMPHOMA

Target	Antibody	Toxin	Disease	Dose (MTD)	Patients (n)	Response	Problems	Studies
CD19	Anti-B4 (Murine)	Blocked ricin	Refractory B-ALL, B-CLL, NHL	1–60 µg/kg/d × 5 d (50 µg/kg/d)	25	1 CR, 2 PR	Elevated aminotransferase, fever, HAMA, HARA	Grossbard et al. (63)
CD19	Anti-B4 (Murine)	Blocked ricin	Refractory B-ALL, B-CLL, NHL	CI 10–70 µg/kg/d × 7 d (50 µg/kg/d)	34	2 CR, 3 PR	Elevated aminotransferase, fever, thrombocytopenia, HAMA, HARA	Grossbard et al. (64)
CD19	Anti-B4 (Murine)	Blocked ricin	NHL post ABMT	CI 20–50 µg/kg/d × 7d q28d × 2 (40 µg/kg/d)	12	11 CR (13–26 months post ABMT)	Elevated aminotransferase, thrombocytopenia, mild capillary leak syndrome, HAMA, HARA	Grossbard et al. (67)
CD19	HD37 (Murine)	dgA	Refractory low- and intermediate-grade NHL	Bolus 2–24 mg/m² / 8d (16 mg/m² / 8d)	23	1 CR, 1 PR	Vascular leak syndrome, aphasia, acrocyanosis HAMA, HARA	Stone et al. (66)
—	—	—	—	CI 9.6–19.2 mg/m² / 8d (19.2 mg/m² / 8d)	9	1 PR	Vascular leak syndrome, aphasia, acrocyanosis, HAMA, HARA	Stone et al. (66)
CD19	Anti-B4 (Murine)	Blocked ricin	AIDS-related NHL	CI 20 µg/kg/d × 7d 2 cycles + m-BACOD 8 cycles	44	13 CR, 12 PR	Elevated aminotransferase, fever, HAMA, HARA	Scadden et al. (72)
CD19	Anti-B4 (Murine)	Blocked ricin	Multiple myeloma	30–40 µg/kg LBW/ d × 5–7 d	5	none	Elevated aminotransferase, fatigue, thrombocytopenia	Grossbard et al. (70)
CD22	Fab'-RFB4 (Murine)	dgA	Refractory NHL	25–120 mg/m² (75 mg/m²)	15	38% PR	Vascular leak syndrome, fever, myalgia	Vitetta et al. (60)
CD22	IgG-RFB4 (Murine)	dgA	Relapsed NHL	5–142 mg/m² (32 mg/m²)	26	1 CR, 5 PR	Vascular leak syndrome, myalgia, fever, aphasia	Amlot et al. (59)
CD22	IgG-RFB4 (Murine)	dgA	Relapsed NHL	9.6–28.8 mg/m² (19 mg/m²)	18	4 PR	Vascular leak syndrome, fever, myalgia	Sausville et al. (61)
CD22	Bispecific F(ab')₂ (Murine)	Saporin	Relapsed or refractory low-grade NHL	1–3 mg saponin qwk × 3–6 wk	5	5 transient PR	Myalgia, malaise	French et al. (62)
IL-2R	IL-2 (Ligand)	DAB₃₈₉ (Diphtheria toxin)	NHL	3–27 mg/kg/d × 5 d q3–4 wk	17	1 CR, 2 PR	Fevers, asthenia, anorexia, anti-DT, anti-DAB₃₈₉IL-2	LeMaistre et al. (73)

ABMT, autologous bone marrow transplant; AIDS, acquired immunodeficiency syndrome; ALL, acute lymphocytic leukemia; CI, continuous infusion; CLL, chronic lymphocytic leukemia; CR, complete response; dgA, deglycosylated ricin-A chain; DT, diphtheria toxin; HAMA, human antimouse antibody; HARA, human anti-ricin antibody; IgG, immunoglobulin G; IL-2, interleukin-2; IL-2R, interleukin-2 receptor; LBW, lean body weight; m-BACOD, methotrexate, bleomycin, doxorubicin, cyclophosphamide, vincristine; MTD, maximal tolerated dose; NHL, non-Hodgkin's lymphoma; PR, partial response.

A novel approach to targeting toxin to CD22 has been described. Two distinct bispecific antibodies against CD22 and the ribosome-inactivating toxin, saponin, were used in combination in five patients with relapsed low-grade B-cell NHL (62). Each antibody recognized different epitopes on CD22 and saponin, resulting in a high-avidity double-attachment of saponin to CD22. Patients received weekly infusions of immunotoxin, and substantial but incomplete tumor response was seen in all five patients. Responses, however, were transient. Disease progressed in each patient between 2 and 4 weeks after completion of therapy. The immunotoxin was well tolerated, with mild weakness, myalgias, and malaise reported. HAMA occurred in only one patient.

A critical disadvantage to the use of CD22 alone as a target is the marked heterogeneity of antigen expression on lymphoma cells (59). Tumor cells lacking CD22 either constitutively or during a portion of the cell cycle escape the tumoricidal effects of the immunotoxin. In one report, patients with tumors that expressed CD22 in less than 50% of the lymphoma cells had a lower likelihood of responding to anti-CD22 immunotoxin therapy (60). Anti-CD19 immunotoxins have been developed, in part, due to the more ubiquitous and homogeneous expression of CD19 on B-cell lymphoma.

Anti-CD19 Immunotoxin Therapy

Early clinical trials of anti-CD19 immunotoxin therapy determined the dose-limiting toxicities and maximum tolerated dose of blocked ricin conjugated to a murine IgG1 anti-CD19 MAb (anti-B4-bR) given in either bolus or continuous intravenous infusions in patients with relapsed or refractory B-cell lymphoma. Dose-limiting toxicity was reversible elevation of serum aminotransferase without impairment of hepatic synthetic function, and the maximum tolerated doses were 50 µg per kg per day for both routes of administration (63,64). Other common adverse reactions included fevers, headache, malaise, and hypoalbuminemia, with occasional capillary leak syndrome. Marked thrombocytopenia occurred more frequently with continuous infusion of anti-B4-bR. HAMA and human antiricin antibodies occurred in the majority of patients between 12 and 92 days after initiation of therapy and increased clearance of MAb on rechallenge.

Collectively, results from 59 treated patients were reported with three CRs and five PRs (overall response rate, 14%) (63,64). Responding patients did not have bulky disease. Additional trials have been done with another immunotoxin consisting of deglycosylated ricin-A chain conjugated to murine IgG1 anti-CD19 antibody (HD37-dgA). In 40 patients with refractory NHL, two patients had CRs and two patients had PRs, although one CR was accompanied by fatal toxicities from HD37-dgA given at the highest dose (65,66). Similar serum concentrations of HD37-dgA and maximum tolerated doses were seen in patients receiving the drug via bolus or continuous infusion. The dose-limiting toxicities were vascular leak syndrome, aphasia, and rhabdomyolysis.

Because tumor response to immunotoxin therapy was observed more often in patients with lower burdens of lymphoma, clinical trials using immunotoxins as adjuvant treatment after chemotherapy have been performed. Anti-B4-bR was administered after ABMT in 12 patients with NHL in complete remission (67). The majority of patients had low-grade NHL. The maximum tolerated dose of a continuous infusion of the immunotoxin for 7 days was 20% lower than that seen in patients who had not undergone transplant, but the dose-limiting toxicities were similar. Based on this phase 2 trial, adjuvant posttransplant immunotoxin therapy was evaluated in a phase 3 multicenter trial. Patients in complete remission 2 to 4 months post-ABMT received two 7-day infusions of anti-B4-bR at 30 µg per kg per day. Seventy-five patients were randomized to observation and 82 were placed on immunotoxin therapy. Treatment with anti-B4-bR was well tolerated, but at interim analysis there was no statistically significant difference in disease-free survival between the treatment arms, although the trends in disease-free survival favored patients or the observation arm (68). This phase 3 trial has been closed due to the low likelihood of demonstrating benefit from the adjuvant immunotoxin therapy in this setting.

The response of NHL to a combination of anti-CD19 and anti-CD22 immunotoxins to overcome the problem of heterogeneous expression of B-cell antigens in lymphoma has been explored. A phase 1 trial of deglycosylated ricin-A chain linked to anti-CD19 mixed with deglycosylated ricin-A chain linked to anti-CD22 (Combotox) has been conducted and further trials using Combotox in states of minimal residual disease have been proposed (69). Published results of these trials, however, are not yet available.

The use of immunotoxin therapy has been investigated in a number of other areas. Anti-B4-bR has been infused into patients with multiple myeloma but too few patients have been treated to draw conclusions about rates of response (70). The use of anti-B4-bR to purge stem cells of lymphoma *in vitro* has also been explored (71).

Acquired immunodeficiency syndrome–related lymphomas have been treated with combinations of anti-B4-bR and che-

motherapy. In one report, 26 of 44 patients received up to two 7-day infusions of anti-B4-bR along with up to eight cycles of methotrexate, bleomycin, doxorubicin (Adriamycin), cyclophosphamide, vincristine (Oncovin), and dexamethasone (m-BACOD) (72). Elevated serum levels of liver transaminases, thrombocytopenia, and infusion-related flu-like symptoms were seen. The overall tumor response for the 44 patients treated with chemotherapy was 57%. It is not known if the 26 patients who received immunotoxin benefited from this combined approach because they also received chemotherapy. Among the 26 patients, 15 had measurable disease at the time of immunotoxin therapy. Two patients with a PR after two cycles of chemotherapy had a CR to anti-B4-bR and additional cycles of m-BACOD.

Numerous combinations of antibodies and toxins are in development and show disease activity in preclinical models. An alternative approach to the use of antibody for the selective targeting of toxin to tumor is the use of cell surface receptor ligands. A trial of IL-2 conjugated to diphtheria toxin as treatment of IL-2 receptor–expressing malignancies was performed in 73 patients (73). NHL was only minimally responsive, whereas 37% of patients with cutaneous T-cell lymphoma responded.

Although powerful antitumor activity has been observed *in vitro*, a number of obstacles have become apparent for the clinical application of immunotoxins. The first is that even with modification, most immunotoxins have nonspecific interactions, resulting in excessive toxicity at the doses required for antitumor effect. Second, the toxins are highly immunogenic, which limits retreatment options. Third, some antigens are heterogeneously expressed on B-cell lymphomas, which limits the extent of tumor-cell kill on exposure to the immunotoxin. As better drug/toxin conjugates become available, including the use of novel BsAb, these agents alone or in combination with or after chemotherapy may yet succeed.

CLINICAL TRIALS OF RADIOLABELED MONOCLONAL ANTIBODIES FOR THERAPY OF B-CELL LYMPHOMA

Radiolabeled MAb possess several properties that impart a theoretical advantage over other forms of immunotherapy for the treatment of NHL. These include the observation that lymphoma is usually sensitive to the ionizing effects of radiation. Beta particles emitted by commonly used radioisotopes [iodine-131 (^{131}I) and yttrium-90 (^{90}Y)] are tumoricidal over a distance greater than a cell diameter. Thus, internalization of the targeted antigen is not necessary, and antigen-negative cells may be killed by nearby bound radioimmunoconjugates. Unlike unconjugated antibodies, radioimmunoconjugates do not depend on immune effector systems or critical biologic events arising from the interaction of antibody with antigen. However, this increased antitumor activity occurs at the cost of dose-limiting toxicity. Because hematopoietic cells are sensitive to radiation, hematologic toxicity has been a significant problem and is dose limiting. Moreover, proper dosimetry determinations may require sophisticated imaging systems and nuclear medicine expertise. Last, treatment with radioimmunoconjugates may

TABLE 5. SELECTED CLINICAL TRIALS USING RADIOIMMUNOCONJUGATES FOR TREATMENT OF B-CELL LYMPHOMA

Target	Antibody	Disease	Isotope	Dose (mCi)	Patients (n)	Response	Problems	Studies
CD20	B1 (Murine)	Relapsed low- and intermediate-grade NHL	[131]I	34–161	28	14 CR, 8 PR	Minimal infusion toxicity, myelosuppression	Kaminski et al. (75), (76)
CD20	Y2B8 or B1 (Murine)	Relapsed low- and intermediate-grade NHL	[90]Y	14–53	18	6 CR, 7 PR	Myelosuppression requiring PBSC support in 2 patients, infection	Knox et al. (81)
CD20	B1 (Murine)	Relapsed NHL	[131]I	280–785	29	23 CR, 2 PR	With ABMT support, reversible cardiopulmonary toxicity	Press (95), Liu (96)
CD21	OKB7 (Murine)	Relapsed low- and intermediate-grade NHL	[131]I	90–200	18	1 PR, 13 mixed	Myelosuppression, HAMA	Czuczman (87)
CD22	IgG-LL2 or F(ab')$_2$-LL2 (Murine)	Refractory NHL	[131]I	15–343	21	2 CR, 2 PR	Myelosuppression, HAMA	Juweid et al. (97)
CD22	IgG-LL2 (Murine)	Refractory NHL	[131]I	90/m^2	3	2 PR	With ABMT support	Juweid et al. (97)
CD37	MB-1 (Murine)	Relapsed low- and intermediate-grade NHL	[131]I	234–628	6	6 CR	With ABMT support	Press et al. (92), (93)
CD37	MB-1 (Murine)	Relapsed low- and intermediate-grade NHL	[131]I	25–161	10	1 CR, 1 PR	Myelosuppression	Kaminski et al. (74)
HLA-DR	Lym-1 (Murine)	Relapsed diffuse large cell NHL	[131]I	37–384	25	3 CR, 10 PR	Mild infusion toxicity, HAMA	Lewis et al. (84)
HLA-DR	Lym-1 (Murine)	Refractory NHL	[131]I	52–290	21	7 CR, 4 PR	Myelosuppression, HAMA	Denardo et al. (85)
HLA-DR	Lym-1 (Murine)	Refractory CLL	[131]I	160–500	5	1 CR, 4 PR	Thrombocytopenia	Denardo et al. (86)
Ig idiotype	Anti-idiotype (Murine)	Relapsed low- and intermediate-grade NHL	[90]Y	10–54	9	2 CR, 1 PR	Myelosuppression, idiotype-negative escape	White et al. (91)

ABMT, autologous bone marrow transplant; CLL, chronic lymphocytic leukemia; CR, complete response; HAMA, human antimouse antibody; ^{131}I, iodine-131; Ig, immunoglobulin; NHL, non-Hodgkin's lymphoma; PBSC, peripheral blood stem cell; PR, partial response; ^{90}Y, yttrium-90.

require hospitalization for administration depending on state and local regulations.

Two general approaches to the treatment of NHL with radioimmunoconjugates have been pursued (Table 5). One approach has been to use a low dose of radioactive isotope administered at the maximum bone marrow tolerated dose. The other approach has been to use stem-cell transplantation to rescue patients from the hematologic toxicity of radiation and to treat with the maximum tolerated amount with respect to non-hematologic toxicity.

Clinical Trials Using Nonmyeloablative Doses of Radioimmunoconjugates

Anti-CD37 Radioimmunotherapy

Kaminski and colleagues initially studied the effects of nonmyeloablative doses of ^{131}I-labeled murine-IgG1, anti-CD37 (MB-1) in patients with relapsed or refractory NHL (74). To limit hematologic toxicity, patients were required to have less than 25% marrow involvement with lymphoma. Eleven of 12 patients who received antibody labeled with trace amounts of isotope had radioimmunoconjugate uptake in areas of lymphoma. Uptake in tumor masses, however, was heterogeneous

within patients, and doses of radiation to tumor were not much higher than doses delivered to normal organs. Ten patients subsequently received MB-1 labeled with a quantity of ^{131}I projected to deliver a whole-body radiation dose of 10 to 50 cGy. Most patients received a whole-body dose of 40 to 50 cGy. Thrombocytopenia and leukopenia were dose-limiting toxicities, and peripheral counts did not recover until 2 months posttherapy. Responses correlated with favorable imaging of tumor. One patient had a CR lasting 2 months, and one patient had a PR.

Anti-CD20 Radioimmunotherapy

The delivery of radiation to sites of tumor compared to normal organs was significantly improved by targeting CD20 with the murine IgG2a anti-B1 antibody and by pretreating patients with unlabeled (cold) antibody (75). The pretreatment with cold MAb blocked readily accessible CD20 in the blood, spleen, and marrow, allowing the radiolabeled MAb to penetrate lymph nodes and extranodal tumor masses. Infusion of 685 mg of cold anti-B1 before infusion of radioactive anti-B1 appeared optimal for targeting radioactivity to tumor (75,76). On average, tumors received 17 times the dose of radiation delivered to the whole body.

In a dose escalation study of ^{131}I-anti-B1, 34 patients with low- or intermediate-grade NHL received an initial trace radioisotope-labeled dose (76). Three patients developed HAMA and did not receive further antibody treatment, and three patients had rapid progression of lymphoma before receiving treatment doses of ^{131}I. Twenty-eight patients were given an infusion of radiolabeled antibody calculated to deliver 25 to 85 cGy to the whole body. The maximum tolerated dose was 75 cGy due to myelosuppression. Hematologic toxicity in patients receiving whole-body doses of 75 cGy or less was mild to moderate unless the patient had undergone earlier bone marrow transplantation. Infusions of radiotherapeutic dosages of antibody were accompanied by fever and chills in 31% and 14% of the treatments, respectively. Fourteen patients (41%) achieved a CR and eight patients (24%) a PR. Complete remissions were seen at all of the whole-body dose levels studied. All of the low-grade, 60% of transformed, and 33% of *de novo* intermediate-grade NHL responded. The median duration of response was 1 year, and the median survival from study entry was longer than 4 years (77).

Preliminary results of a multicenter, phase 2 trial of radiolabeled anti-B1 (tositumomab) for therapy of refractory low-grade or transformed NHL have been reported (78). Sixty patients received 450 mg of unlabeled antibody followed by 5 mCi of ^{131}I conjugated to 35 mg of anti-B1 to calculate biodistribution. One to 2 weeks later, patients received cold antibody followed by tositumomab labeled with a quantity of ^{131}I calculated to deliver a whole-body radiation dose of 65 cGy or 75 cGy, depending on the pretreatment platelet count. A CR to therapy was seen in ten patients (17%), and PRs occurred in 30 patients (50%). The duration of remission after radioimmunotherapy was significantly longer than the preceding cycle of chemotherapy. In one report, 13 patients with NHL relapsing after an initial response to ^{131}I-tositumomab were retreated with ^{131}I tositumomab (79). Eight patients (62%) responded with a median duration of response of 210 days, and three of six patients who had a CR to initial radioimmunotherapy had a CR to retreatment. One patient developed significant neutropenia and thrombocytopenia.

A phase 2 trial of ^{131}I-tositumomab in previously untreated patients with follicular lymphoma is ongoing. Preliminary results have been reported (80). The response rate in 21 evaluable patients was 100% with a 71% CR rate. Some patients in CR had no molecular evidence of lymphoma. Symptomatic HAMA developed in more than one-third of the patients.

Anti-CD20 antibodies labeled with ^{90}Y have also been evaluated in patients with NHL. Potential advantages include a greater path length of radiation from ^{90}Y compared to ^{131}I (5.3 mm versus 0.8 mm), decreased hazard of thyroid toxicity, and less exposure to staff due to the absence of gamma emissions. These advantages of ^{90}Y may result in more homogeneous doses of radiation delivered to tumor and allow for safer outpatient administration. In a phase 1/2 study, 18 patients with relapsed low- or intermediate-grade NHL were treated with 14 to 53 mCi of ^{90}Y-labeled anti-B1 or murine-IgG1 2B8 (81). Because ^{90}Y does not emit gamma radiation, biodistribution studies were performed with indium-111–labeled antibody before treatment. Patients received infusions of cold antibody before infusions of radioimmunoconjugates. Lymph node–based disease was poorly imaged in patients with splenomegaly. Fevers and rash were the most frequent nonhematologic toxicities. Thrombocytopenia and leukopenia occurred in most of the patients 3 to 6 weeks after treatment. Two of the four patients receiving 50 mCi of ^{90}Y met criteria for reinfusion of previously harvested, purged, and stored stem cells. CRs occurred in six patients (33%), and PRs were seen in seven patients. The median duration of response was 6 months. Patients without splenomegaly, bulky adenopathy, or large tumor burdens tended to have better responses. Current clinical trials are evaluating ^{90}Y-2B8 with rituximab, as the cold MAb and have demonstrated substantial activity in low-grade NHL (82). Another trial is exploring pretargeted radioimmunotherapy in NHL as a means to increase the therapeutic index of administered radioisotope. Rituximab conjugated to streptavidin was infused and allowed to penetrate tumor masses and lymph nodes. Circulating antibody was subsequently removed by a clearing agent and ^{90}Y conjugated to biotin was injected. In preliminary studies, the estimated tumor to marrow radiation dose was 75:1, suggesting that pretargeting antibody may allow delivery of significantly higher levels of radiation to tumor without myelosuppression (83).

Anti-HLA-DR Radioimmunotherapy

The murine IgG2a antibody Lym-1 recognizes an HLA-DR antigen on B-cell lymphomas and normal B-lymphocytes but has increased avidity for B-cell malignancies (6). Minimal activity was observed with weekly infusions of unconjugated Lym-1 (see Table 3). However, significant activity in aggressive B-cell NHL has been noted after treatment with ^{131}I or copper-67 radioconjugates of Lym-1 (84). One trial evaluated the effect of low doses of radiolabeled Lym-1 given in multiple infusions to simulate fractionated radiotherapy (84). Twenty-five patients with relapsed NHL received 20 to 60 mCi of ^{131}I-conjugated Lym-1 given every 2 to 6 weeks. Before infusions of radiolabeled antibody, patients were given 5 mg of cold Lym-1 to block nonspecific binding sites in the bloodstream. Three patients had a CR of disease and ten patients had PRs. Responses were observed only in patients who received cumulative doses of 180 mCi or more of ^{131}I. Median survival of responders was 18 months in contrast to a survival of 3 months in patients without a response. Infusion-related toxicities were mild.

A dose-escalation study was performed in 20 patients with relapsed NHL to determine the maximum tolerated amount of iodinated Lym-1 per infusion (85). One patient entered the study twice, thus 21 treatments were counted. Most of the patients had extranodal or bulky (>7 cm) disease, or both, but patients with more than 20% of marrow involved by lymphoma were excluded. Eleven patients received radiation therapy to sites of lymphoma. The dose of ^{131}I was escalated from 40 to 100 mCi per m^2 per infusion. Multiple infusions were given to 14 patients at 4-week intervals. Significant thrombocytopenia and neutropenia occurred in some patients at the higher doses, and 100 mCi was determined to be the maximum tolerated dose. Seven patients (33%) had a CR with a mean duration of 14 months. Four patients (19%) had PRs.

More low-grade and high-grade lymphomas responded than did intermediate-grade lymphomas (67%, 67%, and 42%, respectively). The median duration of survival in patients with responsive disease was 19.5 months compared to 1.9 months in patients without a response.

Approximately 40% of CLL cases demonstrate Lym-1 reactivity, but the percent of Lym-1–positive CLL cells in a patient can vary considerably (6,86). The effect of repeated infusions of low doses of iodinated Lym-1 on refractory CLL was studied in five patients (86). Patients received 30 to 60 mCi of ^{131}I-Lym-1 administered at 2- to 6-week intervals for a total dose of 160 to 500 mCi. One patient, who had a lower burden of disease, had a complete remission and survived more than 24 months after therapy. The four other patients had partially responding disease that relapsed quickly. Lymph-node based disease tended to respond better than circulating CLL cells. This may be related to the ability of radiation to kill nearby antigen-negative cells in lymph nodes, whereas circulating antigen-negative cells may be more likely to escape a radiation cross-fire effect.

Other Radioimmunoconjugates

A dose escalation trial of ^{131}I conjugated to murine-IgG2b anti-CD21 (OKB7) was conducted in 18 patients with relapsed or refractory low- or intermediate-grade NHL (87,88). Patients received doses of 30 or 50 mCi of ^{131}I conjugated to 25 mg of OKB7 given 2 to 3 days apart to a cumulative dose of 90 to 200 mCi. Myelosuppression was seen in four patients. HAMA developed in 12 of 16 assessable cases. One patient who received two courses of treatment of 90 mCi each achieved a PR after the second course. Most responses, however, were mixed and of short duration.

Exploratory trials of the anti-CD22 MAb LL2 labeled with low doses of ^{131}I have been performed in patients with refractory NHL (89). Six patients received infusions of murine IgG-LL2, 14 patients received murine F(ab')$_2$-LL2, and one patient received human-mouse chimeric LL2. Multiple infusions of antibody were given. The cumulative dose of ^{131}I administered ranged from 15 to 343 mCi. Lymphoma completely responded in two patients and partially responded in two patients. Duration of response was generally less than 6 months. Because CD22 internalizes after MAb binding, treatment with a radiometal-labeled (e.g., ^{90}Y) MAb may be preferable. Radiometals are trapped within the cell rather than being quickly excreted in the urine, as with ^{131}I (90).

Antiidiotype antibodies have been conjugated to ^{90}Y and infused into patients with relapsed follicular or diffuse, mixed small- and large-cell NHL (91). Patients also received large doses of unlabeled antibody before infusion of the ^{90}Y conjugate to block readily accessible Fc and nonspecific binding sites and to eliminate circulating idiotype protein. Two complete remissions and one PR were seen; however, the responses were not unequivocally due to effects of radiation because unconjugated antiidiotype antibodies also have antitumor activity (2). HAMA was seen in only one patient, but two of five assessable patients had progression of idiotype-negative tumors after therapy. The outgrowth of antigen-negative escape variants was pre-

viously shown to be a serious hindrance to successful antiidiotype therapy with unconjugated MAb (26).

Clinical Trials Using Myeloablative Doses of Radioimmunoconjugates

Anti-CD37 Radioimmunotherapy

Press and colleagues have explored the effects of high doses of radiolabeled MAb for the therapy of NHL (92). To overcome dose-limiting hematotoxicity, patients have been supported using ABMT. Initial trials used iodinated anti-CD37 antibodies (93). Biodistribution studies of MB-1 showed those patients with splenomegaly or large tumor burdens had poor localization of antibody to tumor compared to normal organs. Six patients with relapsed low- or intermediate-grade B-cell NHL were treated with therapeutic doses of radiolabeled MB-1. All six patients had low tumor burden; normal-sized spleens, or had undergone splenectomy; low amount of tumor in the marrow; and favorable biodistribution of antibody. Three patients, two patients, and one patient received an amount of ^{131}I calculated to deliver 10 Gy, 15 Gy, or 17 Gy or less, respectively, to the normal organ receiving the highest dose of radiation. Whole-body radiation dosages ranged from 100 cGy to approximately 300 cGy. Toxicities due to infusion of the antibody were mild nausea, urticaria, pruritus, and malaise. Myelosuppression occurred in all patients and was maximal 20 to 40 days after treatment. Hematopoiesis recovered spontaneously in three patients. Three patients were infused with previously harvested, purged, and cryopreserved autologous bone marrow because of neutropenia. All six patients had a complete remission of disease that lasted from 4 months to longer than 53 months.

Anti-CD20 Radioimmunotherapy

Press and colleagues found that the anti-CD20 antibody, anti-B1, was superior to MB-1 at targeting tumor more than normal tissue (93). Twelve patients with relapsed low- or intermediate-grade NHL were treated in a dose-escalation study with therapeutic doses of ^{131}I-labeled anti-B1 calculated to deliver 17 to 31 Gy of radiation to the organ receiving the highest dose of radiation in biodistribution studies. Eleven patients were supported with ABMT from 13 to 27 days after treatment. Mild nausea, fever, hyperbilirubinemia, and elevated levels of serum aminotransferase occurred frequently. Biochemical hypothyroidism and partial alopecia were also observed. Six cases of minor infection and three cases of serious infection occurred, but all resolved with antibiotic therapy. Life-threatening cardiopulmonary complications occurred in two patients who received a dose of 2,725 cGy or 3,075 cGy to the lungs. A CR of disease occurred in ten patients (83%), a PR was seen in one patient, and one patient had a minor response. Eight patients remain in continuous complete remission 46 to 95 months after therapy (94).

A phase 2 trial of myeloablative doses of ^{131}I-anti-B1 was performed to more closely define the maximum tolerated dose and efficacy in patients with relapsed low- and intermediate-grade B-cell NHL (95). Twenty-five patients were entered on study. Nineteen patients had favorable biodistribution of antibody to the tumor. Three patients presented with large tumor burdens but achieved favorable biodistribution of antibody after receiving cytoreductive chemotherapy. One patient developed a HAMA response and did not receive a therapeutic dose of iodinated anti-B1. Four patients who were treated in the preceding phase 1 trial were included in the analysis of the phase 2 study results. Twenty-one patients were administered therapeutic infusions of anti-B1 labeled with a quantity of ^{131}I calculated to deliver 25 to 27 Gy to the normal organ receiving the highest dose of radiation (lung in 20 cases and kidney in one case). Frequent nonhematologic toxicities included nausea, mucositis, partial alopecia, elevated serum aminotransferase levels, and asymptomatic hypothyroidism. All of the patients developed severe myelosuppression and were reinfused with previously harvested, purged, and stored marrow (19 patients) or with previously mobilized and stored peripheral blood progenitor cells (two patients). Seven minor infections and three serious infections, one that was fatal, were reported. A dose of radiolabeled anti-B1 calculated to deliver 27 Gy to the lungs was confirmed to be the maximum tolerated dosage.

Nearly all of the treated patients had a major response, CRs were seen in 16 cases (76%), and two additional patients achieved a PR. Extended follow-up of 29 patients treated with myeloablative doses of anti-B1 has been published (96). Twenty-three CRs (79%) and two PRs to therapy were reported. Disease remained in unmaintained remission in 14 patients 27 to 87 months posttherapy. The estimated progression-free survival and overall survival at 4 years were 42% and 68%, respectively, with a median time to treatment failure of 37 months. The majority of these patients had follicular or transformed histology. To improve on these results, a phase 1/2 trial combining high doses of etoposide and cyclophosphamide with ^{131}I-anti-B1 was initiated. Approximately 80% of treated patients are in complete remission 1 to 34 months after therapy (94).

Anti-CD22 Radioimmunotherapy

High-dose radioimmunotherapy using anti-CD22 has also been studied. In a preliminary report of a phase 1 trial of high doses of ^{131}I conjugated to LL2, three patients received 90 mCi per m^2 (97). Two patients were assessable for response. One patient had a PR of 2 months and one patient had a PR of 8-months' duration. A full report of this trial has not been published. However, the modulation of the cell surface CD22 that occurs after MAb binding likely results in rapid cleavage of the ^{131}I and elimination in the urine. Further trials using the radio metals (such as ^{90}Y), which tend to be retained within the cell on modulation, are ongoing (90).

CONCLUSION

Immunotherapy, and specifically MAb therapy, has emerged as a viable option for the treatment of patients with B-cell lymphoma. Unconjugated MAb-based treatments, such as rituximab (anti-CD20), have demonstrated significant single-agent activity with manageable toxicity that allows use alone, com-

bined with, or after current standard treatments with chemotherapy or radiotherapy. Although this antitumor activity is a benefit to patients, clinical trials are still required to determine if these combinations result in longer disease-free or overall survival. Additional unconjugated MAb, such as CAMPATH-1H, may also find a place in the treatment of small-lymphocytic or CLL histology.

Radiolabeled MAb have also demonstrated augmented antitumor activity, but with dose-limiting toxicity. It is likely that ^{131}I- or ^{90}Y-radiolabeled anti-CD20 MAb will soon be available for clinical use. The use of nonmyeloablative and myeloablative doses of these MAb with stem-cell support provide additional treatment options for patients with B-cell NHL. Toxin labeled MAb continues to show promise, but with significant obstacles yet to overcome. Again, clinical trial results are required to determine the optimal use of these new agents, their proper sequence, and proper combination with or after current treatments.

Overall, the future is bright, with these treatments entering expanded clinical trials and a myriad of new agents poised on the horizon. The concept attributed to Ehrlich (98) and made possible by the pioneering works of Kohler and Milstein (99) has finally begun to be realized through the antibody-based treatment of B-cell malignancies.

REFERENCES

1. Miller RA, Maloney DG, Warnke R, Levy R. Treatment of B-cell lymphoma with monoclonal anti-idiotype antibody. *N Engl J Med* 1982;306:517–522.
2. Meeker TC, Lowder J, Maloney DG, et al. A clinical trial of anti-idiotype therapy for B cell malignancy. *Blood* 1985;65:1349–1363.
3. Osterborg A, Dyer MJ, Bunjes D, et al. Phase 2 multicenter study of human CD52 antibody in previously treated chronic lymphocytic leukemia. European Study Group of CAMPATH-1H Treatment in Chronic Lymphocytic Leukemia. *J Clin Oncol* 1997;15:1567–1574.
4. Lundin J, Osterborg A, Brittinger G, et al. CAMPATH-1H monoclonal antibody in therapy for previously treated low-grade non-Hodgkin's lymphomas: a phase II multicenter study. European Study Group of CAMPATH-1H treatment in low-grade non-Hodgkin's lymphoma. *J Clin Oncol* 1998;16:3257–3263.
5. Maloney DG, Grillo-Lopez AJ, White CA, et al. IDEC-C2B8 (Rituximab) anti-CD20 monoclonal antibody therapy in patients with relapsed low-grade non-Hodgkin's lymphoma. *Blood* 1997;90:2188–2195.
6. Epstein AL, Marder RJ, Winter JN, et al. Two new monoclonal antibodies, Lym-1 and Lym-2, reactive with human B-lymphocytes and derived tumors, with immunodiagnostic and immunotherapeutic potential. *Cancer Res* 1987;47:830–840.
7. Maloney DG, Brown S, Czerwinski DK, et al. Monoclonal anti-idiotype antibody therapy of B-cell lymphoma: the addition of a short course of chemotherapy does not interfere with the antitumor effect nor prevent the emergence of idiotype-negative variant cells. *Blood* 1992;80:1502–1510.
8. Brown SL, Miller RA, Horning SJ, et al. Treatment of B-cell lymphomas with anti-idiotype antibodies alone and in combination with alpha interferon. *Blood* 1989;73:651–661.
9. Vuist WM, Levy R, Maloney DG. Lymphoma regression induced by monoclonal anti-idiotypic antibodies correlates with their ability to induce Ig signal transduction and is not prevented by tumor expression of high levels of bcl-2 protein. *Blood* 1994;83:899–906.
10. Maloney D, Smith B, Appelbaum F. The anti-tumor effect of monoclonal anti-CD20 antibody (mAb) therapy includes direct antiprolif-

erative activity and induction of apoptosis in CD20 positive non-Hodgkin's lymphoma (NHL) cell lines. *Blood* 1996;88:637a.

11. Demidem A, Lam T, Alas S, Hariharan K, Hanna N, Bonavida B. Chimeric anti-CD20 (Idec-C2b8) monoclonal antibody sensitizes a B cell lymphoma cell line to cell killing by cytotoxic drugs. *Cancer Biother Radiopharmaceuticals* 1997;12:177–186.

12. Shan D, Ledbetter JA, Press OW. Apoptosis of malignant human B cells by ligation of CD20 with monoclonal antibodies. *Blood* 1998;91:1644–1652.

13. Nadler LM, Ritz J, Hardy R, Pesando JM, Schlossman SF, Stashenko P. A unique cell surface antigen identifying lymphoid malignancies of B cell origin. *J Clin Invest* 1981;67:134–140.

14. Press OW, Appelbaum F, Ledbetter JA, et al. Monoclonal antibody 1F5 (anti-CD20) serotherapy of human B cell lymphomas. *Blood* 1987;69:584–591.

15. Reff ME, Carner K, Chambers KS, et al. Depletion of B cells in vivo by a chimeric mouse human monoclonal antibody to CD20. *Blood* 1994;83:435–445.

16. Maloney DG, Liles TM, Czerwinski DK, et al. Phase I clinical trial using escalating single-dose infusion of chimeric anti-CD20 monoclonal antibody (IDEC-C2B8) in patients with recurrent B-cell lymphoma. *Blood* 1994;84:2457–2466.

17. Maloney DG, Grillo-Lopez AJ, Bodkin DJ, et al. IDEC-C2B8: results of a phase I multiple-dose trial in patients with relapsed non-Hodgkin's lymphoma. *J Clin Oncol* 1997;15:3266–3274.

18. McLaughlin P, Grillo-Lopez AJ, Link BK, et al. Rituximab chimeric anti-CD20 monoclonal antibody therapy for relapsed indolent lymphoma: half of patients respond to a four-dose treatment program. *J Clin Oncol* 1998;16:2825–2833.

19. Berinstein NL, Grillo-Lopez AJ, White CA, et al. Association of serum Rituximab (IDEC-C2B8) concentration and anti-tumor response in the treatment of recurrent low-grade or follicular non-Hodgkin's lymphoma. *Ann Oncol* 1998;9:995–1001.

20. Davis T, Levy R, White C, et al. Rituximab: phase II (PII) retreatment (ReRx) study in patients (Pts) with low-grade or follicular (LG/F) NHL. *Blood* 1998;92:414a.

21. Davis T, White C, Grillo-Lopez A, et al. Rituximab: first report of a phase II (PII) trial in NHL patients (Pts) with bulky disease. *Blood* 1998;92:414a.

22. Coiffier B, Haioun C, Ketterer N, et al. Rituximab (anti-CD20 monoclonal antibody) for the treatment of patients with relapsing or refractory aggressive lymphoma: a multicenter phase II study. *Blood* 1998;92:1927–1932.

23. Czuczman M, Grillo-Lopez A, White C, et al. Treatment of patients with low-grade B-cell lymphoma with the combination of chimeric anti-CD20 monoclonal antibody and CHOP chemotherapy. *J Clin Oncol* 1999;17:268–276.

24. Byrd J, Waselenko J, Maneatis T, et al. Rituximab therapy in hematologic malignancy patients with circulating blood tumor cells: association with increased infusion-related side effects and rapid blood tumor clearance. *J Clin Oncol* 1999;17:791–795.

25. Davis TA, Maloney DG, Czerwinski DK, Liles TM, Levy R. Anti-idiotype antibodies can induce long-term complete remissions in non-Hodgkin's lymphoma without eradicating the malignant clone. *Blood* 1998;92:1184–1190.

26. Meeker T, Lowder J, Cleary ML, et al. Emergence of idiotype variants during treatment of B-cell lymphoma with anti-idiotype antibodies. *N Engl J Med* 1985;312:1658–1665.

27. Hsu FJ, Caspar CB, Czerwinski D, et al. Tumor-specific idiotype vaccines in the treatment of patients with B-cell lymphoma—long-term results of a clinical trial. *Blood* 1997;89:3129–3135.

28. Hanto DW, Frizzera G, Gajl-Peczalska KJ, Simmons RL. Epstein-Barr virus, immunodeficiency, and B cell lymphoproliferation. *Transplantation* 1985;39:461–472.

29. Leblond V, Sutton L, Dorent R, et al. Lymphoproliferative disorders after organ transplantation: a report of 24 cases observed in a single center. *J Clin Oncol* 1995;13:961–698.

30. Tolnay M, Tsokos GC. Complement receptor 2 in the regulation of the immune response. *Clin Immunol Immunopathol* 1998;88: 123–132.

31. Kay R, Rosten PM, Humphries RK. CD24, a signal transducer modulating B cell activation responses, is a very short peptide with a glycosyl phosphatidylinositol membrane anchor. *J Immunol* 1991;147:1412–1416.

32. Blanche S, Le Deist F, Veber F, et al. Treatment of severe Epstein-Barr virus-induced polyclonal B-lymphocyte proliferation by anti-B-cell monoclonal antibodies. Two cases after HLA-mismatched bone marrow transplantation. *Ann Intern Med* 1988;108:199–203.

33. Benkerrou M, Jais JP, Leblond V, et al. Anti-B-cell monoclonal antibody treatment of severe posttransplant B-lymphoproliferative disorder: prognostic factors and long-term outcome. *Blood* 1998;92: 3137–3147.

34. Fischer A, Blanche S, Le Bidois J, et al. Anti-B-cell monoclonal antibodies in the treatment of severe B-cell lymphoproliferative syndrome following bone marrow and organ transplantation. *N Engl J Med* 1991;324:1451–1456.

35. Antoine C, Garnier JL, Duboust A, Bariety J, Stevenson G, Glotz D. Successful treatment of posttransplant lymphoproliferative disorder with renal graft preservation by monoclonal antibody therapy. *Transplant Proc* 1996;28:2825–2826.

36. Faye A, Van Den Abeele T, Peuchmaur M, Mathieu-Boue A, Vilmer E. Anti-CD20 monoclonal antibody for post-transplant lymphoproliferative disorders. *Lancet* 1998;352:1285.

37. Hale G, Bright S, Chumbley G, et al. Removal of T cells from bone marrow for transplantation: a monoclonal antilymphocyte antibody that fixes human complement. *Blood* 1983;62:873–882.

38. Hale G, Swirsky DM, Hayhoe FG, Waldmann H. Effects of monoclonal anti-lymphocyte antibodies in vivo in monkeys and humans. *Mol Biol Med* 1983;1:321–334.

39. Dyer MJ, Hale G, Hayhoe FG, Waldmann H. Effects of CAMPATH-1 antibodies *in vivo* in patients with lymphoid malignancies: influence of antibody isotype. *Blood* 1989;73:1431–1439.

40. Riechmann L, Clark M, Waldmann H, Winter G. Reshaping human antibodies for therapy. *Nature* 1988;332:323–327.

41. Brett SJ, Baxter G, Cooper H, et al. Emergence of CD52-, glycosylphosphatidylinositol-anchor-deficient lymphocytes in rheumatoid arthritis patients following Campath-1H treatment. *Int Immunol* 1996;8:325–334.

42. Osterborg A, Fassas AS, Anagnostopoulos A, Dyer MJ, Catovsky D, Mellstedt H. Humanized CD52 monoclonal antibody Campath-1H as first-line treatment in chronic lymphocytic leukaemia. *Br J Haematol* 1996;93:151–153.

43. Mellstedt H, Osterborg A, Lundin J, et al. Campath-1H therapy of patients with previously untreated chronic lymphocytic leukemia (CLL). *Blood* 1998;92:490a.

44. Dillman RO, Shawler DL, Dillman JB, Royston I. Therapy of chronic lymphocytic leukemia and cutaneous T-cell lymphoma with T101 monoclonal antibody. *J Clin Oncol* 1984;2:881–891.

45. Foon KA, Schroff RW, Bunn PA, et al. Effects of monoclonal antibody therapy in patients with chronic lymphocytic leukemia. *Blood* 1984;64:1085–1093.

46. Hekman A, Honselaar A, Vuist WM, et al. Initial experience with treatment of human B cell lymphoma with anti-CD19 monoclonal antibody. *Cancer Immunol Immunother* 1991;32:364–372.

47. Vlasveld LT, Hekman A, Vyth-Dreese FA, et al. Treatment of low-grade non-Hodgkin's lymphoma with continuous infusion of low-dose recombinant interleukin-2 in combination with the B-cell-specific monoclonal antibody CLB-CD19. *Cancer Immunol Immunother* 1995;40:37–47.

48. Hu E, Epstein AL, Naeve GS, et al. A phase 1a clinical trial of LYM-1 monoclonal antibody serotherapy in patients with refractory B cell malignancies. *Hematol Oncol* 1989;7:155–166.

49. Ozaki S, Kosaka M, Wakatsuki S, Abe M, Koishihara Y, Matsumoto T. Immunotherapy of multiple myeloma with a monoclonal antibody directed against a plasma cell-specific antigen, HM1.24. *Blood* 1997;90:3179–3186.

50. Maloney DG, Donovan K, Hamblin TJ. Antibody therapy for treatment of multiple myeloma. *Semin Hematol* 1999;36:30–33.

51. Klein B, Zhang XG, Jourdan M, et al. Paracrine rather than autocrine regulation of myeloma-cell growth and differentiation by interleukin-6. *Blood* 1989;73:517–526.

52. Kawano M, Hirano T, Matsuda T, et al. Autocrine generation and requirement of BSF-2/IL-6 for human multiple myelomas. *Nature* 1988;332:83–85.

53. Tanabe O, Kawano M, Tanaka H, et al. BSF-2/IL-6 does not augment Ig secretion but stimulates proliferation in myeloma cells. *Am J Hematol* 1989;31:258–262.

54. Bataille R, Barlogie B, Lu ZY, et al. Biologic effects of anti-interleukin-6 murine monoclonal antibody in advanced multiple myeloma. *Blood* 1995;86:685–691.

55. van Zaanen HC, Koopmans RP, Aarden LA, et al. Endogenous interleukin 6 production in multiple myeloma patients treated with chimeric monoclonal anti-IL6 antibodies indicates the existence of a positive feed-back loop. *J Clin Invest* 1996;98:1441–1418.

56. van Zaanen HC, Lokhorst HM, Aarden LA, et al. Chimaeric anti-interleukin 6 monoclonal antibodies in the treatment of advanced multiple myeloma: a phase I dose-escalating study. *Br J Haematol* 1998;102:783–790.

57. Stein R, Belisle E, Hansen HJ, Goldenberg DM. Epitope specificity of the anti-(B cell lymphoma) monoclonal antibody, LL2. *Cancer Immunol Immunother* 1993;37:293–298.

58. Nadler LM, Anderson KC, Marti G, et al. B4, a human B lymphocyte-associated antigen expressed on normal, mitogen-activated, and malignant B lymphocytes. *J Immunol* 1983;131:244–250.

59. Amlot PL, Stone MJ, Cunningham D, et al. A phase I study of an anti-CD22-deglycosylated ricin A chain immunotoxin in the treatment of B-cell lymphomas resistant to conventional therapy. *Blood* 1993;82:2624–2633.

60. Vitetta ES, Stone M, Amlot P, et al. Phase I immunotoxin trial in patients with B-cell lymphoma. *Cancer Res* 1991;51:4052–4058.

61. Sausville EA, Headlee D, Stetler-Stevenson M, et al. Continuous infusion of the anti-CD22 immunotoxin IgG-RFB4-SMPT-dgA in patients with B-cell lymphoma: a phase I study. *Blood* 1995;85:3457–3465.

62. French RR, Bell AJ, Hamblin TJ, Tutt AL, Glennie MJ. Response of B-cell lymphoma to a combination of bispecific antibodies and saporin. *Leuk Res* 1996;20:607–617.

63. Grossbard ML, Freedman AS, Ritz J, et al. Serotherapy of B-cell neoplasms with anti-B4-blocked ricin: a phase I trial of daily bolus infusion. *Blood* 1992;79:576–585.

64. Grossbard ML, Lambert JM, Goldmacher VS, et al. Anti-B4-blocked ricin: a phase I trial of 7-day continuous infusion in patients with B-cell neoplasms. *J Clin Oncol* 1993;11:726–737.

65. Conry RM, Khazaeli MB, Saleh MN, et al. Phase I trial of an anti-CD19 deglycosylated ricin A chain immunotoxin in non-Hodgkin's lymphoma: effect of an intensive schedule of administration. *J Immunother Emphasis Tumor Immunol* 1995;18:231–241.

66. Stone MJ, Sausville EA, Fay JW, et al. A phase I study of bolus versus continuous infusion of the anti-CD19 immunotoxin, IgG-HD37-dgA, in patients with B-cell lymphoma. *Blood* 1996;88:1188–1197.

67. Grossbard ML, Gribben JG, Freedman AS, et al. Adjuvant immunotoxin therapy with anti-B4-blocked ricin after autologous bone marrow transplantation for patients with B-cell non-Hodgkin's lymphoma. *Blood* 1993;81:2263–2271.

68. Grossbard M, Niedzwiecki D, Nadler L, et al. Anti-B4-blocked ricin (Anti-B4-bR) adjuvant therapy post-autologous bone marrow transplant (ABMT) (CALGB 9254): a phase III intergroup study. *Proc Amer Soc Clin Oncol* 1998;17:3a.

69. Engert A, Sausville EA, Vitetta E. The emerging role of ricin A-chain immunotoxins in leukemia and lymphoma. *Curr Top Microbiol Immunol* 1998;234:13–33.

70. Grossbard ML, Fidias P, Kinsella J, et al. Anti-B4-blocked ricin: a phase II trial of 7 day continuous infusion in patients with multiple myeloma. *Br J Haematol* 1998;102:509–515.

71. Roy DC, Perreault C, Belanger R, et al. Elimination of B-lineage leukemia and lymphoma cells from bone marrow grafts using anti-B4-blocked-ricin immunotoxin. *J Clin Immunol* 1995;15:51–57.

72. Scadden DT, Schenkein DP, Bernstein Z, et al. Immunotoxin combined with chemotherapy for patients with AIDS-related non-Hodgkin's lymphoma. *Cancer* 1998;83:2580–2587.

73. LeMaistre CF, Saleh MN, Kuzel TM, et al. Phase I trial of a ligand fusion-protein (DAB389IL-2) in lymphomas expressing the receptor for interleukin-2. *Blood* 1998;91:399–405.

74. Kaminski MS, Fig LM, Zasadny KR, et al. Imaging, dosimetry, and radioimmunotherapy with iodine 131-labeled anti-CD37 antibody in B-cell lymphoma. *J Clin Oncol* 1992;10:1696–1711.

75. Kaminski MS, Zasadny KR, Francis IR, et al. Radioimmunotherapy of B-cell lymphoma with [131I]anti-B1 (anti-CD20) antibody. *N Engl J Med* 1993;329:459–465.

76. Kaminski MS, Zasadny KR, Francis IR, et al. Iodine-131-anti-B1 radioimmunotherapy for B-cell lymphoma. *J Clin Oncol* 1996;14: 1974–1981.

77. Wahl RL, Zasadny KR, MacFarlane D, et al. Iodine-131 anti-B1 antibody for B-cell lymphoma: an update on the Michigan Phase I experience. *J Nucl Med* 1998;39[Suppl]:S21–S27.

78. Kaminski M, Zelenetz A, Press O, et al. Multicenter, phase III study of iodine-131 tositumomab (anti-B1 antibody) for chemotherapy-refractory low-grade or transformed low-grade non-Hodgkin's lymphoma (NHL). *Blood* 1998;92:316a.

79. Wahl R, Tidmarsh G, Kroll S, Kaminski M. Successful re-treatment of non-Hodgkin's lymphoma (NHL) with iodine-131 anti-B1 antibody. *Proc Amer Soc Clin Oncol* 1998;17:40a.

80. Kaminski M, Gribbin T, Estes J, et al. I-131 anti-B1 antibody for previously untreated follicular lymphoma (FL): clinical and molecular remissions. *Proc Amer Soc Clin Oncol* 1998;17:2a.

81. Knox SJ, Goris ML, Trisler K, et al. Yttrium-90-labeled anti-CD20 monoclonal antibody therapy of recurrent B-cell lymphoma. *Clin Cancer Res* 1996;2:457–470.

82. Witzig T, White C, Wiseman G, et al. Idec-Y2B8 radioimmunotherapy: responses in patients with splenomegaly. *Blood* 1998;92:417a.

83. Weiden P, Breitz H, Press O, et al. Radioimmunotherapy (RIT) in the treatment of non-Hodgkin's lymphoma (NHL): advantage of pretargeted RIT (PRIT^R). *Blood* 1998;92:414a.

84. Lewis JP, Denardo GL, Denardo SJ. Radioimmunotherapy of lymphoma: a UC Davis experience. *Hybridoma* 1995;14:115–120.

85. DeNardo GL, DeNardo SJ, Goldstein DS, et al. Maximum-tolerated dose, toxicity, and efficacy of (131)I-Lym-1 antibody for fractionated radioimmunotherapy of non-Hodgkin's lymphoma. *J Clin Oncol* 1998;16:3246–3256.

86. DeNardo GL, Lewis JP, DeNardo SJ, O'Grady LF. Effect of Lym-1 radioimmunoconjugate on refractory chronic lymphocytic leukemia. *Cancer* 1994;73:1425–1432.

87. Czuczman MS, Straus DJ, Divgi CR, et al. Phase I dose-escalation trial of iodine 131-labeled monoclonal antibody OKB7 in patients with non-Hodgkin's lymphoma. *J Clin Oncol* 1993;11:2021–2029.

88. Scheinberg DA, Straus DJ, Yeh SD, et al. A phase I toxicity, pharmacology, and dosimetry trial of monoclonal antibody OKB7 in patients with non-Hodgkin's lymphoma: effects of tumor burden and antigen expression. *J Clin Oncol* 1990;8:792–803.

89. Goldenberg DM, Horowitz JA, Sharkey RM, et al. Targeting, dosimetry, and radioimmunotherapy of B-cell lymphomas with iodine-131-labeled LL2 monoclonal antibody. *J Clin Oncol* 1991;9:548–564.

90. Sharkey RM, Behr TM, Mattes MJ, et al. Advantage of residualizing radiolabels for an internalizing antibody against the B-cell lymphoma antigen, CD22. *Cancer Immunol Immunother* 1997;44:179–188.

91. White CA, Halpern SE, Parker BA, et al. Radioimmunotherapy of relapsed B-cell lymphoma with yttrium 90 anti-idiotype monoclonal antibodies. *Blood* 1996;87:3640–3649.

92. Press OW, Eary JF, Badger CC, et al. Treatment of refractory non-Hodgkin's lymphoma with radiolabeled MB-1 (anti-CD37) antibody. *J Clin Oncol* 1989;7:1027–1038.

93. Press OW, Eary JF, Appelbaum FR, et al. Radiolabeled-antibody therapy of B-cell lymphoma with autologous bone marrow support. *N Engl J Med* 1993;329:1219–1224.

94. Press OW. Prospects for the management of non-Hodgkin's lymphomas with monoclonal antibodies and immunoconjugates. *Cancer J Sci Am* 1998;4[Suppl 2]:S19–S26.

95. Press OW, Eary JF, Appelbaum FR, et al. Phase II trial of 131I-B1 (anti-CD20) antibody therapy with autologous stem cell transplantation for relapsed B cell lymphomas. *Lancet* 1995;346:336–340.

96. Liu SY, Eary JF, Petersdorf SH, et al. Follow-up of relapsed B-cell lymphoma patients treated with iodine-131-labeled anti-CD20 antibody and autologous stem-cell rescue. *J Clin Oncol* 1998;16:3270–3278.

97. Juweid M, Sharkey RM, Markowitz A, et al. Treatment of non-Hodgkin's lymphoma with radiolabeled murine, chimeric, or humanized LL2, an anti-CD22 monoclonal antibody. *Cancer Res* 1995;55[Suppl]:S5899–S5907.

98. Ehrlich P. On immunity with specific reference to cell life. *Proc Royal Soc London* 1900;66:424.

99. Kohler G, Milstein C. Continuous cultures of fused cells secreting antibody of predefined specificity. *Nature* 1975;256:495–497.

15.2

MONOCLONAL ANTIBODIES: CLINICAL APPLICATIONS

T-Cell Leukemia and Lymphoma

THOMAS A. WALDMANN

The hybridoma technique of Köhler and Milstein rekindled interest in the use of antibodies in cancer patients (1). Monoclonal antibodies (MAb) have been put to a broad array of uses in the clinical care of patients with T-cell leukemia and lymphoma (2). They have been used in conjunction with flow microfluorometry to define the immunologic phenotype of abnormal cells, thus providing an approach for the classification of T-cell malignancies. Radioimmunoassays and enzyme-linked immunosorbent assay procedures have been used to monitor the serum levels of the released form of T-cell surface peptides such as those identified by anti-CD4, CD8, and CD25 [anti–interleukin-2 receptor (anti-IL-2R)]. In particular, the assessment of the serum level of the Tac peptide (CD25) has proven to be of value in the diagnosis of certain lymphoreticular malignancies, in determining prognosis, and tracking the efficacy of therapy of these lymphomas (3,4). An additional diagnostic use of MAb involves the *in vivo* administration of a MAb radionuclide conjugate in conjunction with radioimmunoimaging or immunoscintigraphy to define tumor-bearing sites (5–8). This approach has been used with a number of tumors, including cutaneous T-cell lymphoma (CTCL), to obtain valuable staging information without resorting to a surgical procedure.

MAb have also been used with therapeutic intent to modulate the host's immune response, to purge autologous bone marrow of neoplastic cells, and, after intravenous administration, for the immune elimination of the neoplastic cells *in vivo*. The purging of malignant or normal T cells from bone marrow represents an *in vitro* use of MAb (9–14). Antibodies, including anti-CD2, CD5, and CD7 in conjunction with complement, and antibodies conjugated to toxins or to magnetizable compounds have been used to purge malignant cells, including malignant T cells, from bone marrow before autologous transplantation. Furthermore, they have been used to purge normal T cells from marrow to prevent graft-versus-host disease (GVHD) in allogeneic transplantation. Finally, MAb directed against tumor-associated antigens have been used as antitumor agents *in vivo*. This use of MAb as direct antitumor agents is the focus of the remainder of the chapter. Initially, such MAb had only modest effects against tumor cells in clinical trials (15). However, as noted by Dickman, 11 antibodies have received U.S. Food and Drug Administration (FDA) approval (16). At the present time, FDA approval has been achieved for rituximab (Rituxan, anti-CD20), trastuzumab (Herceptin, anti-HER-2/*neu*), and daclizumab (Zenapax, anti-IL-2Rα, CD25), among others (17–20). A number of factors underlie the improved efficacy of MAb therapy for cancer. First, human or humanized antibodies have been developed that manifest reduced immunogenicity, have augmented effector functions, and have markedly improved pharmacokinetics with prolonged *in vivo* survival when compared to unmodified murine antibodies. A second critical advance is that more effective antigenic targets have been identified, including growth factor (GF) and death pathway receptors. In the case of GF-receptor cytokine deprivation, mediated apoptotic cell death of the leukemic cells can be induced by interdicting the interaction of the GF with its receptor. In particular, receptors for IL-2 and IL-7 have been targeted in monoclonal antibody therapy of T-cell leukemia and lymphoma (19–23). A third advance involves the arming of antibodies with toxins or radionuclides, thereby enhancing their effector functions.

have been introduced, including (a) unmodified murine antibodies (Mu-anti-Tac) directed toward IL-2Rα, (b) humanized versions of the anti-Tac MAb prepared by genetic engineering, as well as (c) the anti-Tac MAb armed with toxins or radionuclides. Finally, receptors (e.g., IL-2/IL-15Rβ) shared by multiple cytokines (e.g., IL-2 and IL-15) as well as molecules in the signaling pathway (e.g., Jak3) used by diverse T-cell stimulatory interleukins (IL-2, IL-4, IL-7, IL-9, and IL-15) are being targeted for therapy of leukemia and lymphoma (20,61).

INTERLEUKIN-2 AND INTERLEUKIN-2 RECEPTOR SYSTEM AND ITS SIGNAL PATHWAY

An analysis of the structure and function of the multisubunit IL-2R and the disorders in IL-2R expression in HTLV-I–associated ATL provide the scientific basis for rational IL-2R–directed therapy (61,66,67). Successful T cell-mediated immune responses require that these cells change from a resting to an activated state. The sequence of events involved in the activation of T cells begins when a foreign pathogen encounters the antigenic-specific receptor on the surface of resting T cells. This antigen-stimulated activation induces the synthesis of the 15-kd lymphokine IL-2 (68,69). To exert its biologic effect, IL-2 must interact with specific high-affinity receptors. However, resting cells do not express high-affinity IL-2R, but they are rapidly expressed on T cells after activation with antigen or mitogen (59,66,67,70).

IL-2 is a glycoprotein with an apparent molecular mass of 15.5 kd that is made up of 133 amino acids (aa) in a short-chain four-helical bundle topology (66–70). Three forms of IL-2R can be distinguished based on their affinity for ligand, with IL-2–binding affinities of 10^{-11} mol/L, 10^{-9} mol/L, and 10^{-8} mol/L (67,70). Furthermore, there are three critical IL-2R subunits, IL-2Rα, IL-2Rβ, and IL-2Rγ (59,71,72). IL-2Rα, identified by the anti-Tac MAb, is a densely glycosylated structure with an apparent molecular mass of 55 kd composed of 251 aa (59,60,66,70,73). Using cross-linking methodology with radiolabeled IL-2, Sharon and coworkers (71,74) defined a second 70- to 75-kd IL-2 binding protein, now termed *IL-2Rβ*. Hatakeyama and coworkers (75) molecularly cloned the gene encoding IL-2Rβ and demonstrated that the mature protein is composed of 525 aa. Takeshita and colleagues (76) identified a third IL-2R subunit, the 64-kda γ chain, that binds IL-2 and plays a pivotal role in binding IL-2, in facilitating IL-2 binding by IL-2Rβ, and in receptor signaling. IL-2Rβ and IL-2Rγ are members of the cytokine receptor superfamily. Shared features of these receptors include four conserved cysteine residues located in an extracellular domain and a Trp-Ser-X-Trp-Ser motif (WSXWS) located just outside of the membrane-spanning domain (77). Cytokines, such as IL-2, manifest considerable redundancy that is explained by sharing of common receptor subunits among members of the cytokine receptor family. Each of these cytokines has its own private receptor, but IL-2 also shares two of its receptor subunits. In particular, the β chain (IL-2/15Rβ) is shared by IL-2 and IL-15 and the γc chain is shared by the five cytokines: IL-2, IL-4, IL-7, IL-9, and IL-15 that activate T cells (78–81). The IL-2Rα subunit associates

with IL-2/15Rβ and γc subunits to form a high-affinity IL-2R complex (20,70,82).

The IL-2R in T cells and natural killer (NK) cells, like most cytokine receptors, does not possess intrinsic protein tyrosine kinase domains. However, receptor stimulation evokes rapid tyrosine phosphorylation of intracellular proteins, including the receptors themselves. The IL-2R binds Jak1 and Jak3, members of the Janus kinase (Jak) family of protein tyrosine kinases (83,84). Jak activation by IL-2 in turn leads to phosphorylation and nuclear translocation of STAT3 and STAT5, two members of the transcription factor family known as *signal transducers and activators of transcription* (STATS) (84,85).

INTERLEUKIN-2 RECEPTOR EXPRESSION IN NORMAL INDIVIDUALS AND IN T-CELL LEUKEMIA AND LYMPHOMA

Resting T cells, B cells, large granular lymphocytes (LGLs), and monocytes do not express IL-2Rα; however, they can be induced to express this receptor (66,67). Most LGLs constitutively express only IL-2Rβ and IL-2Rγ of the IL-2 system as well as IL-15Rα, the private receptor for IL-15 (86). Addition of IL-2 to LGL enhances NK activity and leads to the generation of lymphokine-activated killer (LAK) activity and IL-2Rα expression (87). In contrast to the lack of IL-2Rα expression in normal resting cells, IL-2Rα is expressed by abnormal cells in patients with certain leukemias and autoimmune diseases and is associated with allograft rejection (62,66). That is, some of the abnormal cells in these diseases express the Tac antigen on their surface. Furthermore, Nelson, Rubin, and coworkers (4) demonstrated that the serum concentration of the soluble form of IL-2Rα (sIL-2Rα) is elevated in patients with these disorders. In terms of neoplasia, certain T cell, B cell, monocytic, and even granulocytic leukemias express the Tac antigen (62–65). In particular, the malignant T cells of patients with HTLV-I–induced ATL constitutively express IL-2Rα (62). Furthermore, the malignant T cells of the skin and lymph nodes of patients with CTCL (mycosis fungoides and the Sézary syndrome) express the Tac antigen (63). Additionally, virtually all of the malignant cells of patients with hairy cell B-cell leukemia and a proportion of other B-cell lymphomas are also Tac positive (65). Finally, true histiocytic leukemia cells and the Reed-Sternberg cells of Hodgkin's disease also manifest IL-2Rα (64). In addition to these Tac-expressing leukemias and lymphomas, our laboratory group has shown that there are certain leukemias (e.g., ALL and LGL leukemia) that do not express IL-2Rα yet express the IL-2Rβ subunit of the IL-2R (87). Autoimmune diseases may also be associated with disorders of IL-2Rα expression (88–91). A proportion of the mononuclear cells in the involved tissues express the Tac antigen, and the serum concentration of the soluble form of this receptor subunit is elevated. Such evidence of T-cell activation and disorders of IL-2Rα expression are present in more than 15 autoimmune diseases, including tropical spastic paraparesis/HTLV-I–associated myelopathy (TSP/HAM) (91). Finally, the Tac antigen is expressed by the T cells recognizing foreign transplantation antigens in individuals undergoing allograft rejection (20,66).

Our group focused its initial IL-2R immunotherapeutic studies on ATL, a distinct form of aggressive T-cell leukemia defined by Uchiyama and coworkers (92). ATL is an aggressive malignancy of lymphocytes displaying a multilobulated nucleus expressing a CD3$^+$, CD4$^-$, CD8$^-$, CD7$^-$, and CD25$^+$ phenotype that typically infiltrates the skin, lungs, and liver. The disease exhibits a striking clustering of cases in certain geographic regions, notably southwestern Japan, the Caribbean basin, northeastern South America, Central America, sub-Saharan Africa, and, to a lesser extent, the southeastern United States. The retrovirus HTLV-I is clearly associated with this disease and appears to play a major role in its pathogenesis (93–96). The majority of HTLV-I–infected individuals are asymptomatic carriers of the virus; however, an infected individual has approximately 0.1% per year risk of developing frank ATL. Although ATL has a wide range of clinical courses, in the majority of patients the principal clinical features include lymphadenopathy; hepatosplenomegaly; and skin, central nervous system, and pulmonary involvement. The occurrence of hypercalcemia is characteristic of ATL (97). Patients with acute ATL manifest a striking degree of immunosuppression and develop opportunistic infections such as *Pneumocystis pneumonia* and cryptococcal meningitis.

INTERLEUKIN-2 RECEPTOR α AS A TARGET FOR THERAPY IN PATIENTS WITH HUMAN T-CELL LYMPHOMA OR LEUKEMIA VIRUS TYPE I–ASSOCIATED ADULT T-CELL LEUKEMIA

All populations of leukemic cells my colleagues and I have examined from patients with HTLV-I–associated ATL constitutively express high- and low-affinity IL-2R, including large numbers of the IL-2Rα (CD25) defined by the anti-Tac MAb (62). An analysis of HTLV-I and its protein products suggests a potential mechanism for the association between HTLV-I and constitutive IL-2Rα expression (94). The retrovirus HTLV-I encodes a 42-kd protein (termed tax) that plays an important role in the early phases of HTLV-I–induced malignancy by deregulating the expression of the cellular genes that encode IL-2 and IL-2Rα, thereby establishing an autocrine stimulation of proliferation that can be inhibited by anti-Tac *ex vivo*.

No conventional treatment program is successful in inducing long-term disease-free survival in ATL patients. A total of 854 patients with HTLV-I antibody-positive ATL newly diagnosed from 1983 to 1987 were analyzed for prognostic factors and survival after combination chemotherapy by Shimoyama and the Japanese Lymphoma Study Group (98). The median survival time and projected 2- and 4-year survival rates of all patients were 10 months, 28%, and 12%, respectively. However, the HTLV-I–induced ATL cells constitutively express the IL-2Rα chain identified by the anti-Tac MAb, whereas normal resting cells do not. This observation provided the scientific basis for IL-2R–directed immunotherapy with this MAb. IL-2R–directed immunotherapeutic agents could theoretically eliminate IL-2Rα–expressing leukemic cells or abnormally activated T cells involved in other disease states while retaining the Tac-nonexpressing normal T cells and their precursors that express the antigen receptors for T-cell–mediated immune responses. In initial studies, my colleagues and I administered unmodified murine anti-Tac to patients with ATL (21). Our goal was to inhibit the interaction of IL-2 with its GF receptors expressed on the malignant cells. Six of the 19 treated patients had a partial (four patients), or complete (two patients) remission, lasting from 1 month to more than 9 years after anti-Tac therapy (21). This was assessed by the demonstration of the elimination of measurable skin and lymph nodal disease, normalization of serum calcium levels, and routine hematologic and phenotypic analysis of circulating cells. Furthermore, elimination of clonal malignant cells was shown by molecular genetic analysis of HTLV-I proviral integration and T-cell antigen receptor gene rearrangement.

HUMANIZED ANTIBODIES TO INTERLEUKIN-2 RECEPTOR α

Although murine antibodies, such as murine anti-Tac, are of value in the therapy of human disease, their effectiveness is limited because rodent MAb have a short *in vivo* survival in humans, induce an immune response that neutralizes their therapeutic effect, and, as is the case with anti-Tac, are ineffective at recruiting host-effector functions. We addressed these issues by joining with Cary Queen in the development and evaluation of humanized anti-Tac [Hu-anti-Tac (daclizumab)] (99,100). The Hu-anti-Tac molecules retain the complementarity-determining regions from the murine antibody but have virtually all of the remainder of the molecule derived from human IgG$_1$κ. Hu-anti-Tac had improved pharmacokinetics when compared with the murine version. Hu-anti-Tac *in vivo* survival was longer (terminal half-life 103 hours vs. 38 hours in Cynomolgus monkeys and 20 days vs. 40 hours in humans). In addition, Hu-anti-Tac was markedly less immunogenic than murine anti-Tac when administered to monkeys undergoing heterotopic cardiac allografting or to patients with leukemia or lymphoma or those receiving renal allografts (101,102). Furthermore, in contrast to the parent murine anti-Tac, Hu-anti-Tac participated in ADCC with human mononuclear cells (100).

TRIALS INVOLVING HU-ANTI-TAC (DACLIZUMAB) IN BENIGN CONDITIONS AND LEUKEMIA

On the basis of encouraging observations in preclinical trials and in phase 1 and 2 trials of Hu-anti-Tac, two double-blind (placebo-controlled) randomized trials involving 535 evaluated patients were conducted to determine the value of Hu-anti-Tac (daclizumab) in preventing renal allograft transplant rejection (19). In each trial, the patients received a standard immunosuppressive agent regimen (cyclosporin A and hydrocortisone in one study; cyclosporin A, hydrocortisone, and azathioprine in the other). The parallel treatment groups received either an intravenous placebo or a dose of 1.0 mg per kg of daclizumab before transplant and on four subsequent occasions separated by 2 weeks. No drug-specific adverse events or increased morbidity were observed. In particular, there was no increase in the inci-

dence of infections or of B-cell lymphoma in the group receiving daclizumab. Acute rejection episodes were reduced by 40% in patients treated with daclizumab ($p < .001$). Ninety-eight percent of the patients receiving triple immunotherapy and daclizumab retained their renal allograft for 6 months, whereas only 92% of the patients in the placebo control group retained their grafts ($p < .02$). On the basis of these phase 3 clinical trials, the FDA on December 10, 1997, approved daclizumab for use in humans (marketing clearance) to prevent acute kidney-transplant rejection (20). In addition to its use in the prevention of organ allograft rejection, daclizumab (Hu-anti-Tac) appears to be of value in the therapy of T-cell mediated autoimmune disorders such as T-cell mediated uveitis and TSP/HAM, a neurological disorder that results from HTLV-I infection leading to immune activation (103,104). In this disorder, as in ATL HTLV-I, encoded Tax transactivates the expression of IL-2 and the IL-2 receptor. Anti-Tac blocks the interaction of IL-2 with IL-2Rα. Finally, humanized anti-Tac therapy has been associated with remissions in patients with ATL, especially in patients with smoldering and chronic forms of the disease (T. Waldmann, unpublished observation).

BIFUNCTIONAL ANTIBODIES

Bispecific antibodies (BsAb) with two distinct binding activities have been generated to retarget cytotoxic NK cells or cytotoxic T-lymphocytes to tumor cells—that is, to induce cytotoxic cells to target and lyse cells they normally would not lyse (105,106). Such bifunctional antibodies have been prepared by chemical cross-linking, by disulfide exchange, or by the production of hybrid hybridomas. To be effective, the BsAb not only must be targeted to cytotoxic cells but also must activate these cells into functional effectors bypassing normal, major histocompatibility complex and antigen-specific restrictions. The most effective bispecific MAb used as their nontarget antigen specificity the CD3 peptide on cytotoxic T cells or the CD16 FcRIII receptor on NK cells. BsAb with specificity against tumor targets and against CD3- or CD16-effector cells were modestly effective in mediating tumor-cell killing *in vitro* and *in vivo*. For example, the murine anti-Tac MAb does not participate in ADCC with human mononuclear cells. In contrast, murine anti-Tac-CD3 and anti-Tac-CD16 bifunctional agents used in conjunction with peripheral blood mononuclear cells killed IL-2Rα–expressing targets (106). Thus, although problems associated with their manufacture remain to be resolved, BsAb show modest promise as therapeutic agents for ATL.

MONOCLONAL ANTIBODY AND CYTOTOXIC AGENT CONJUGATES

During the progression of ATL, the malignant cells continue to express IL-2Rα but no longer produce or require IL-2 for their proliferation and survival. Nevertheless, the signaling pathway involving Jak1 and Jak3 and STAT5 remains activated (107). A number of factors underlie this IL-2–independent activation. HTLV-I Tax transactivates IL-15, which acts on the private IL-

15Rα and on IL-2/15Rβ and $γ_c$ shared with IL-2 (108). Additionally, in IL-2–independent ATL cell lines there is a loss of the SH2-containing phosphatase (SHP-1), the phosphatase that normally inactivates Jak3 (109). Nevertheless, IL-2Rα is still expressed on the leukemic cells but not on the normal cells of the patients, thus providing a target for immunotherapy.

INTERLEUKIN-2 RECEPTOR–DIRECTED IMMUNOTOXINS

An additional IL-2R–directed approach to the therapy of ATL is based on the observation that ATL cells continue to express IL-2R during the late stages of the disease when they no longer require IL-2 and thus are no longer responsive to therapy with unmodified murine anti-Tac. In this approach, anti-Tac or IL-2 is used to deliver a toxin to IL-2R–expressing cells. In this strategy, one selects from nature a toxic protein and then modifies the toxin so that it no longer indiscriminately binds to and kills normal cells but instead targets and kills only cells expressing the receptor identified by the MAb or lymphokine. The majority of toxins targeted to cell surfaces by immunoconjugates act in the cytoplasm, where they inhibit protein synthesis. We have collaborated with Ira Pastan and Robert Kreitman and coworkers in the study of immunotoxins involving *Pseudomonas* exotoxin (PE) conjugated to agents that target the toxin to the IL-2R (110–112). PE is an enzyme that catalyzes adenosine diphosphate (ADP) ribosylation and inactivation of elongation factor II, a factor that is required for protein synthesis. A functional analysis by Hwang and coworkers (111) of deletion mutants of the PE structural gene demonstrated that domain I of the 66-kd PE molecule is responsible for cell recognition, domain II for translocation across membranes, and domain III for ADP ribosylation of elongation factor II, the step actually responsible for cell death. A PE molecule from which domain I had been deleted (PE40 or PE38) has full ADP-ribosylating activity but extremely low cell-killing activity when used without an associated targeting agent because of the deletion of the cell recognition domain. The PE40 was produced in *Escherichia coli*, purified, and conjugated to anti-Tac. The anti-Tac-PE conjugates inhibited the protein synthesis of Tac-expressing T-cell lines, but not that of lines not expressing IL-2Rα. However, immunotoxins made by chemically attaching a toxin to an intact antibody generate a protein that is heterogeneous with yields that are often poor. To circumvent this problem, IL-2-PE40, a chimeric protein composed of human IL-2 genetically fused to the amino terminus of the modified form of PE40, was constructed to provide an alternative (lymphokine-mediated) method of delivering PE40 to the surface of IL-2–expressing cells (112). IL-2-PE40 was produced by fusion of a complementary DNA encoding human IL-2 to the 5' end of a modified PE40 gene that lacks sequences encoding the cell recognition domain. The addition of IL-2-PE40 led to the inhibition of protein synthesis when added to a human T-cell line, HUT-102, expressing high-affinity IL-2R. IL-2-PE40 was effective in a series of rodent models; specifically, IL-2-PE40 inhibited the growth of murine T-cell lymphoma (113). Furthermore, by killing activated T cells, it prolonged the survival of cardiac allografts in mice and prevented the development of adjuvant arthritis in rats (114). However, IL-2-PE40 was much less active against primate- and human-activated T cells than against mouse T cells, even though its binding to the IL-2R of the two species was similar.

Bracha and associates (115) performed parallel studies in which the portion of the diphtheria toxin gene that encodes the receptor-binding domain was genetically replaced with the complementary DNA encoding IL-2. Using this agent, they achieved prolongation of allograft survival and suppression of delayed hypersensitivity. Furthermore, the diphtheria toxin/IL-2 fusion protein inhibited protein synthesis by 60% to 80% in lymph node ATL cells, whereas protein synthesis in peripheral blood was inhibited by 20% to 57% in acute type and 3% to 13% in chronic ATL (116). Recombinant fusion toxins containing truncated diphtheria toxin, including DAB_{486}-IL-2 and, more recently, DAB_{389}-IL-2, have been tested in clinical trials (117–120). DAB_{389}-IL-2, which appears to require high-affinity IL-2 receptors for cytotoxicity, produced five complete responses (CRs) and eight PRs in 35 patients with CTCL, one CR and two PRs in 17 patients with NHL, and no responses in 21 patients with Hodgkin's disease (119,120). In a phase 3 trial in CTCL patients, seven CRs and 14 PRs were observed in 71 patients. The more frequent toxicities included transaminase elevations (62%), hypoalbuminemia (86%), hypotension (32%), and rashes (32%). DAB_{389}-IL-2 has been approved by the FDA for salvage treatment of CTCL (119–120).

CD25 has been targeted using a chemical conjugate for anti-CD25 MAb RFT5 with dgA (121–122). RFT5-dgA has been tested in a phase 1 trial in which 2 of 20 patients with Hodgkin's disease responded. More than 50% of the patients treated for at least two cycles made high levels of antibodies to the infused agent after the second cycle. Similarly, patients with hematologic malignancies treated with DAB_{389}-IL-2 had high rates of seroconversion detected by enzyme-linked immunosorbent assay (119–122).

To address the limited activity of IL-2-PE40 against human T cells, alternative molecules have been constructed in a search for a more active agent. This required the observation that active single-chain Fv fragments of antibodies can be produced in *E. coli* by attaching the light- and heavy-chain variable domains together with a peptide linker (123). Single-chain antibody toxin fusion proteins [anti-Tac(Fv)-PE40 and anti-Tac(Fv)-PE38] in which the variable regions of anti-Tac are joined in peptide linkage to PE40 or PE38 was constructed and expressed in *E. coli* (110). Anti-Tac(Fv)-PE38 was very cytotoxic to IL-2R–bearing human malignant T-cell lines but was not cytotoxic to receptor-negative cell lines. Furthermore, this toxin fusion protein inhibited proliferative responses induced by the mixed leukocyte reaction and by CD3 antibodies. Finally, anti-Tac(Fv)-PE38 was cytotoxic to freshly obtained ATL cells (124). This agent is more than 100-fold more active against freshly obtained ATL cells than IL-2-PE38. Thus, this drug has characteristics that suggest that it may be a useful IL-2R–directed therapeutic agent in patients with ATL (124). The anti-Tac(Fv)-PE derivative produced complete regression in mice of an IL-2R expressing human carcinoma (125). Therefore, in collaboration with Pastan and Kreitman, a phase 1 trial of the immunotoxin

anti-Tac(Fv)-PE38 has been completed that evaluated the immunogenicity, toxicity, and efficacy of this oncotoxin in the treatment of patients with a wide variety of IL-2Rα–expressing leukemias and lymphomas, including hairy-cell leukemia (HCL) and ATL (126). Of the 35 patients treated, one HCL patient had a CR. Furthermore, there were seven PRs consisting of HCL (three), CLL (one), Hodgkin's disease (one), CTCL (one), and ATL (one). All five patients with HCL or CTCL and one of two patients with ATL responded.

ANTI-TAC ARMED WITH α- AND β-EMITTING RADIONUCLIDES

The action of toxins conjugated to MAb depends on their ability to be internalized by the cell and translocated to the cytoplasm. In fact, the toxin conjugates do not pass easily from the endosome to the cytosol. Furthermore, large protein toxins are immunogenic and thus provide only a narrow therapeutic window before the development of host antibodies directed toward the toxin. In the future, these problems should probably be resolved. To circumvent these limitations, however, radiolabeled MAb were developed as alternative immunoconjugates to deliver a cytotoxic agent to target cells. A number of advantages exist over other approaches in the use of radiolabeled MAb conjugates for therapy. One is that with the appropriate choice of radionuclide, radiolabeled MAb kill cells at distances of several cell diameters; therefore, a radiolabeled MAb binding to an antigen-expressing cell may kill adjacent antigen-nonexpressing cells, thereby overcoming the tumor-cell antigenic heterogeneity that presents a problem for most other MAb-mediated approaches. Furthermore, the radiolabeled antibody need not be internalized to kill the tumor cell. Nuclear chemistry has provided a selection of radioisotopes that could be linked to immunoproteins.

In studies performed in collaboration with Otto Gansow and Martin Brechbiel, we turned to α- and β-emitting radionuclides as cytotoxic agents that could be conjugated to anti-Tac (127–129). In initial studies, a series of linker agents was developed that did not compromise antibody specificity and did not permit premature release of the radionuclide *in vivo*. The choice of isotopes was based on the desire to have agents with a short distance of action that would act on the cell in question and on a small number of bystander cells without unwanted toxicity.

Radionuclides emitting α particles release high-energy emission (6 to 9 MeV) over a short distance (40 to 80 μm) and are efficient at killing individual target cells such as those found in patients with leukemia without significantly penetrating normal tissues. Suitable α-emitting radionuclides that are under investigation include ^{213}Bi, ^{212}Bi, ^{212}Pb, and ^{211}At. We have shown with *in vitro* studies that ^{212}Bi is well suited for immunotherapy (129). Activity levels of 0.5 μCi targeted by ^{212}Bi-labeled anti-Tac eliminated more than 98% of the proliferative capacity of HuT-102 cells, with only a modest effect on IL-2R–negative cells. In addition, an *in vivo* tumor model in nude mice was used to show that ^{212}Bi-labeled anti-Tac used at a dose that produced only modest toxicity was effective in preventing the

development of tumors expressing the Tac antigen (130). ^{211}At, with its longer physical half-life 7.2 hours versus 1 hour for ^{212}Bi and its almost pure α emission, appears to be even more suitable for therapy (128). Therefore, our group plans to initiate the clinical trials of ^{211}At-labeled anti-IL-2Rα MAb for the treatment of IL-2R–expressing leukemia and lymphoma.

The focus of the program involving IL-2R–directed MAb armed with radionuclides has been on the use of yttrium-90 (^{90}Y) linked to anti-Tac (22). We administered anti-Tac armed with ^{90}Y to 18 patients with ATL; initially, (the first nine patients) in a phase 1 dose-escalation trial and, subsequently, (the second group of nine patients) in a phase 2 trial involving a uniform 10-mCi dose of ^{90}Y-labeled anti-Tac. Patients undergoing a remission were permitted to receive up to eight additional doses (22). At the 5 to 15 µCi doses used, 9 of the 16 evaluable patients manifested PR (seven) or CR (two) induced by courses of ^{90}Y anti-Tac therapy. The duration of the seven PRs ranged from 1.6 to 22.4 months (mean, 9.2 months). Two additional patients developed a CR. The observations that support these conclusions concerning the favorable therapeutic responses include the demonstration of a reduction in size of all measurable lesions as assessed by physical examination, computed tomography scan, and γ-camera imaging studies after intravenous coadministration of indium-111 anti-Tac. Furthermore, the clinical responses in all patients with leukemia were associated with a reduction in the number of peripheral blood leukemic cells enumerated by fluorescence-activated cell-sorting analysis, by a decline in the serum IL-2Rα concentration, by a normalization of the Southern blot patterns of T-cell receptor β gene arrangement, and by HTLV-I integration. The responses observed represent an improved efficacy in terms of length of remission compared with previous results with unmodified anti-Tac. Clinically meaningful ($\geq$ grade 3) toxicity was limited largely to the hematopoietic system.

FUTURE DIRECTIONS

Although IL-2Rα–directed therapy has met with considerable success, there are limitations in approaches directed solely to this receptor subunit. Antibodies to IL-2Rα do not inhibit IL-2–mediated activation of NK cells, which, in their resting state, do not express IL-2Rα but do express IL-2/IL-15Rβ and γ_c (87). Furthermore, antibodies to IL-2Rα do not inhibit the action of IL-15 that utilizes its own private receptor (IL-15Rα) rather than IL-2Rα (131). Finally, anti-IL-2Rα antibodies alone do not provide the virtually complete immunosuppression of T-cell function that could be achieved if the actions of all the cytokines that stimulate T cells were inhibited. These limitations are relevant to leukemia therapy because certain leukemias, such as T-cell–type LGL leukemia, express IL-2/IL-15Rβ and γ_c, but not IL-2Rα.

As noted earlier, there is a sharing of receptor subunits and signaling pathway elements between IL-2 and its receptor plus those of the other cytokines that stimulate T cells (79–85). A major corollary of this sharing of cytokine receptor subunits and signaling pathways among the cytokines is that therapy directed toward a shared cytokine receptor (e.g., IL-2/IL-15Rβ or γ_c), or to a shared signal transduction element (e.g., Jak3) may yield more profound immunosuppression than can be achieved by an antibody directed toward a private receptor subunit such as IL-2Rα. Tinubu et al. (132) demonstrated that a humanized version of the Mikβ1 antibody directed toward the IL-2/IL-15Rβ that is shared by IL-2 and IL-15 prolongs renal allograft survival in Cynomolgus monkeys. Furthermore, we are evaluating the value of Mikβ1 in the therapy of patients with T-cell–type LGL associated with granulocytopenia.

Many groups have initiated programs directed toward developing and evaluating inhibitors of Jak3 as agents for controlled immunosuppression. Jak3 is involved in the signaling of some cytokines, including IL-2 and IL-15 that use γ_c but is not essential for signaling by other GFs (83–85). Jak3 expression is largely limited to lymphocytes and hematopoietic cells. Jak3 deficiency in the autosomal form of severe combined immunodeficiency disease (Jak3-deficient SCID) in humans yields immunodeficiency but no disorders in nonimmunologic systems (133,134). In parallel, mice made Jak3 deficient by gene targeting manifested an absence of NK cells and abnormalities of T and B cells but, like the Jak3-deficient humans, do not have disorders in nonimmunologic systems (135). Taken together, these observations suggest that agents that inhibit Jak3 action may be of value as therapeutic agents in patients with T-cell leukemia or lymphoma. In conclusion, the emerging understanding of the IL-2/IL-15R system opens the possibility for more specific immune intervention and for the therapy of T-cell leukemia and lymphoma.

SUMMARY

MAb are assuming an increasing role in diagnostic and therapeutic approaches to T-cell leukemias and lymphomas. An array of MAb, including CD3, CD4, CD5, CD7, CAMPATH-1, IL-7R, anti-T-cell antigen receptor, and CD25 (anti-Tac, anti-IL-2R) directed antibodies, have been evaluated as anti-T-cell leukemia agents. The anti-CD5 antibodies were generally well tolerated but were relatively ineffective. Factors in the low efficacy observed with the early use of MAb include the fact that murine MAb are immunogenic and that, in many cases, they were not cytocidal or cytostatic agents against human neoplastic cells. To circumvent the first of these problems, chimeric humanized forms of CAMPATH-1 that react with virtually all lymphoid cells and monocytes have been generated. Additionally, antiidiotypic antibodies directed toward the human T-cell receptor were evaluated as a therapeutic modality for human T-lymphoid malignancies. Furthermore, the IL-2R is proving to be an extraordinarily valuable target, because it is expressed by the T cells in individuals rejecting allografts and by the abnormal T cells in select patients with autoimmune disorders and with certain lymphoid malignancies, whereas it is not expressed by normal resting cells. To exploit this difference in IL-2R (Tac) expression, we have initiated therapeutic trials using unmodified murine anti-Tac, humanized anti-Tac, anti-Tac variable-region truncated toxin fusion proteins [anti-Tac(Fv)-PE38], and α- and β-emitting radionuclide-armed anti-Tac. Humanized hyperchimeric anti-Tac molecules have been prepared by genetic engineering in which the molecule is entirely human IgG$_1$, except for the small complementary determining regions that are retained from the mouse antibody. The humanized antibody manifests ADCC with human mononuclear cells that were absent in the parental mouse anti-Tac. Thirty percent to more than 50% of patients with HTLV-I–associated ATL developed a remission when treated with unmodified anti-Tac or with the antibody armed with the β-emitting radionuclide ^{90}Y. Thus, the developing understanding of receptors for antigen and for lymphokines on the surface of malignant T-lymphocytes, together with the capacity to produce humanized forms of receptor-directed monoclonal antibodies and to arm these antibodies with toxins or radionuclides, provide a new strategy for the treatment of human T-cell leukemias and lymphomas.

ACKNOWLEDGMENT

The author thanks Barbara Holmlund for her editorial assistance.

REFERENCES

1. Köhler G, Milstein C. Continuous cultures of fused cells secreting antibody of predefined specificity. *Nature* 1975;256:495–497.
2. Levy R, Miller RA. Tumor therapy with monoclonal antibodies. *Fed Proc* 1983;42:2650–2656.
3. Rubin LA, Kurman CC, Biddison WE, et al. A monoclonal antibody 7G7/B6, binds to an epitope on the human interleukin-2 (IL-2) receptor that is distinct from that recognized by IL-2 or anti-Tac. *Hybridoma* 1985;4:91–102.
4. Nelson DL, Rubin LA, Kurman CC, et al. An analysis of the cellular requirements for the production of soluble interleukin-2 receptors *in vitro. J Clin Immunol* 1986;6:114–120.
5. Bunn PA Jr, Carrasquillo JA, Keenan AM, et al. Imaging of T-cell lymphoma by radiolabeled monoclonal antibody. *Lancet* 1984;2:1219–1221.
6. Halpern SE, Dillman RO, Witztum KF, et al. Radioimmunodetection studies of prostate, colon and T-cell lymphoma using IN-111 labeled monoclonal anti-tumor antibodies (In-111-MoAb); preliminary studies. *Clin Nucl Med* 1984;9[Suppl]:38.
7. Carrasquillo JA, Bunn PA Jr, Keenan AM, et al. Radioimmunodetection of cutaneous T-cell lymphoma with ^{111}In-labeled T101 monoclonal antibody. *N Engl J Med* 1986;315:673–680.
8. Rosen ST, Zimmer AM, Goldman-Leikin R, et al. Radioimmunodetection and radioimmunotherapy of cutaneous T cell lymphomas using ^{131}I-labeled monoclonal antibody: an Illinois Cancer Council study. *J Clin Oncol* 1987;5:562–573.
9. Nadler LM, Takvorian T, Botnick L, et al. Anti-B1 monoclonal antibody and complement treatment in autologous for bone-marrow transplantation for relapsed B-cell non-Hodgkin's lymphoma. *Lancet* 1984;2:427–431.
10. Slavin S, Waldmann H, Or R, et al. Prevention of graft-versus-host disease in allogeneic bone marrow transplantation for leukemia by T-cell depletion *in vitro* prior to transplantation. *Transplant Proc* 1985;17:465–467.
11. Uckun FM, Gail-Peczalska K, Meyers DE, et al. Marrow purging in autologous bone marrow transplantation for T-lineage acute lymphoblastic leukemia: efficacy of *ex vivo* treatment with immunotoxins and 4-hydroperoxyl-cyclophosphamide against fresh leukemic marrow progenitor cells. *Blood* 1987;69:361–366.
12. Bast RC, Jr, DeFabritis P, Lipton J, et al. Elimination of malignant clonogenic cells from human bone marrow using multiple monoclonal antibodies and complement. *Cancer Res* 1985;45:499–503.
13. Preijers FWMB, DeWitte T, Wessels GC, et al. Autologous transplantation of bone marrow purged *in vitro* with anti-CD7-(WT-1)

14. Wang MY, Kvalheim G, Kvaloy S, et al. An effective immunomagnetic method for bone marrow purging in T cell malignancies. *Bone Marrow Transplant* 1992;9:319–323.
15. Catane R, Longo DL. Monoclonal antibodies for cancer therapy. *Isr J Med Sci* 1988;24:471–476.
16. Dickman S. Antibodies stage a comeback in cancer treatment. *Science* 1998;280:1196–1197.
17. Pegram MD, Baly D, Wirth C, et al. Antibody dependent cell mediated cytotoxicity in breast cancer patients in phase III clinical trials of humanized anti-HER2 antibody. *Proc Am Assoc Cancer Res* 1997;38:602(abst).
18. Maloney DG, Grillo-Lopez AJ, Bodkin DJ, et al. IDEC-C2B8: results of a phase I multiple-dose trial in patients with relapsed non-Hodgkin's lymphoma. *J Clin Oncol* 1997;15:3266–3274.
19. Vincenti F, Kirkman R, Light S, et al. Interleukin-2-receptor blockade with dacliximab to prevent acute rejection in renal transplantation. Dacliximab Triple Therapy Study Group. *N Engl J Med* 1998;338:161–165.
20. Waldmann TA, O'Shea J. The use of antibodies against the IL-2 receptor in transplantation. *Curr Opin Immunol* 1998;10:507–512.
21. Waldmann TA, Goldman CK, Bongiovanni KF, et al. Therapy of patients with human T-cell lymphotrophic virus I-induced adult T-cell leukemia with anti-Tac, a monoclonal antibody to the receptor for interleukin-2. *Blood* 1988;72:1805–1816.
22. Waldmann TA, White JD, Carrasquillo JA, et al. Radioimmunotherapy of interleukin-2R alpha-expressing adult T-cell leukemia with Yttrium-90-labeled anti-Tac. *Blood* 1995;86:4063–4075.
23. Sweeney EB, Foss FM, Murphy JR, et al. Interleukin 7 (IL-7) receptor-specific cell killing by DAB389 IL-7: a novel agent for the elimination of IL-7 receptor positive cells. *Bioconjug Chem* 1998;9:201–207.
24. Royston I, Majda JA, Baird SM, et al. Human T-cell antigen of T cells (T65) is also found on chronic lymphocytic leukemia cells bearing surface immunoglobulin. *J Immunol* 1980;125:725–731.
25. Miller RA, Maloney DG, McKillop J, et al. *In vivo* effects of murine hybridoma monoclonal antibody in a patient with T cell leukemia. *Blood* 1981;58:78–86.
26. Miller RA, Levy R. Response of cutaneous T cell lymphoma to therapy with hybridoma monoclonal antibody. *Lancet* 1981;2:226–340.
27. Miller RA, Osheroff AR, Stratte PT, et al. Monoclonal antibody therapeutic trials in seven patients with T-cell lymphoma. *Blood* 1983;62:988–995.
28. Dillman RO, Shawler DL, Dillman JB, et al. Therapy of chronic lymphocytic leukemia and cutaneous T-cell lymphoma with T101 monoclonal antibody. *J Clin Oncol* 1984;2:881–891.
29. Foon KA, Schroff RW, Mayer D, et al. Monoclonal antibody therapy of chronic lymphocytic leukemia and cutaneous T-cell lymphoma: preliminary observations. In: Boss BD, Langman RE, Trobridge IS, Dulbecco R, eds. *Monoclonal antibodies and cancer.* Orlando, FL: Academic Press, 1983:39–52.
30. Shawler DL, Batholomew RM, Smith LM, et al. Human immune response to multiple injections of murine monoclonal IgG. *J Immunol* 1985;135:1530–1535.
31. Schroff RW, Foon KA, Beatty SM, et al. Human anti-murine immunoglobulin responses in patients receiving monoclonal antibody therapy. *Cancer Res* 1985;45:879–885.
32. LeMaistre CF, Rosen S, Frankel A, et al. Phase I trial of H65-RTA immunoconjugate in patients with cutaneous T-cell lymphoma. *Blood* 1991;78:1173–1182.
33. Dyer MJS, Hale G, Hayhoe FGJ, et al. Effects of CAMPATH-1 antibodies *in vivo* in patients with lymphoid malignancies: influence of antibody isotype. *Blood* 1989;73:1431–1439.
34. Hale G, Hoang T, Prospero T, et al. Removal of T cells from bone marrow for transplantation: comparison of rat monoclonal antilymphocyte antibodies of different isotypes. *Mol Biol Med* 1983;1:305–319.
35. Waldmann H, Polliale A, Hale G, et al. Elimination of graft versus host disease by *in vitro* depletion of alloreactive lymphocytes with a monoclonal rat anti-human lymphocyte antibody (CAMPATH-1). *Lancet* 1984;2:483–486.

Ricin A immunotoxin in T-cell lymphoblastic leukemia and lymphoma. *Blood* 1989;74:1152–1158.

36. Hale G, Dyer MJS, Clark MR, et al. Remission induction in non-Hodgkin lymphoma with reshaped human monoclonal antibody CAMPATH-1H. *Lancet* 1988;2:1394–1399.

37. Pawson R, Dyer MJS, Barge R, et al. Treatment of T-cell prolymphocytic leukemia with human CD52 antibody. *J Clin Oncol* 1997;15:2667–2672.

38. Baum W, Steininger H, Blair HJ, et al. Therapy with CD7 monoclonal antibody TH-69 is highly effective for xenografted human T-cell ALL. *Br J Haematol* 1996;95:327–328.

39. Clynes R, Takechi Y, Morio Y, et al. Fc receptors are required in passive and active immunity to melanoma. *Proc Natl Acad Sci U S A* 1998;95:652–656.

40. Fishwild DM, Aberle S, Bernhard SL, et al. Efficacy of an anti-CD7-Ricin A chain immunoconjugate in a novel murine model of human T-cell leukemia. *Cancer Res* 1992;52:3056–3062.

41. Jansen B, Vallera DA, Jaszcz WB, et al. Successful treatment of human acute T-cell leukemia in SCID mice using the anti-CD7-deglycosylated ricin A-chain immunotoxin DA7. *Cancer Res* 1992;52:1314–1321.

42. Waurzyniak B, Schneider EA, Tumer N, et al. *In vivo* toxicity, pharmacokinetics, and antileukemic activity of TXU (anti-CD7)-pokeweed antiviral protein immunotoxin. *Clin Cancer Res* 1997;3:881–890.

43. Pausa ME, Doumbia SO, Pennell CA. Construction and characterization of human CD7-specific single-chain Fv immunotoxins. *J Immunol* 1997;158:3259–3269.

44. Byers VS, Carroll S, Fishwild D, et al. Use of an anti-CD7-Ricin A chain immunotoxin in the treatment of T-cell acute lymphocytic leukemia. *Exp Hematol* 1990;18:640.

45. Frankel AE, Laver JH, Willingham MC, et al. Therapy of patients with T-cell lymphomas and leukemias using an anti-CD7 monoclonal antibody-ricin A chain immunotoxin. *Leuk Lymphoma* 1997;26:287–298.

46. Knox SJ, Levy R, Hodgkinson S, et al. Observations on the effect of chimeric anti-CD4 monoclonal antibody in patients with mycosis fungoides. *Blood* 1991;77:20–30.

47. Lenardo MJ. Fas and the art of lymphocyte maintenance. *J Exp Med* 1996;183:721–724.

48. Wang R, Murphy KM, Loh DY, et al. Differential activation of antigen-stimulated suicide and cytokine production pathways in CD4+ T cells is regulated by the antigen-presenting cell. *J Immunol* 1993;150:3832–3842.

49. Parijs LV, Biukian A, Iloragimov A, et al. Functional responses and apoptosis of CD25 (IL-2Rα)-deficient T cell expressing a transgenic antigen receptor. *J Immunol* 1997;158:3738–3745.

50. Ashwell JD, Longo DL, Bridges SH. T-cell tumor elimination as a result of T-cell receptor-mediated activation. *Science* 1987;237:61–64.

51. Maecker HT, Takahashi S, Levy R. *Anti-idiotype antibody therapy of human T-cell malignancies: progress and questions.* Seventh International Congress of Immunology 1989. Stuttgart, New York: Gustav Fisher, 1989:890.

52. Miller RA, Maloney DG, Warnke R, et al. Treatment of B-cell lymphoma with monoclonal anti-idiotype antibody. *N Engl J Med* 1982;306:517–522.

53. Maecker HT, Lowder J, Maloney DG, et al. A clinical trial of anti-idiotype therapy for B-cell malignancy. *Blood* 1985;65:1349–1363.

54. Levy R. Monoclonal antibodies: clinical trials and new insights into tumor biology. In: Johnson IS, Rue Y, eds. *A perspective on biology and medicine in the 21st century.* London: Royal Society of Medicine Services Press, 1988:107–116.

55. Janson CH, Jeddi-Tehram MJ, Mellsredt H, et al. Anti-idiotype monoclonal antibody to a T-cell chronic lymphatic leukemia. *Cancer Immunol Immunother* 1989;28:225–232.

56. Gramatzki M, Strobel G, Burger R, et al. CD3 antibody therapy of a refractory T-cell leukemia led to *in vitro* responsiveness for interleukin (IL) 2. *Proc Ann Meet Am Soc Clin Oncol* 1992;11:267.

57. Gramatzki M, Burger R, Strobel G, et al. Therapy with OKT3 monoclonal antibody in refractory T cell acute lymphoblastic leukemia induces interleukin-2 responsiveness. *Leukemia* 1995;9:382–390.

58. Martin PJ, Hansen JA, Torok-Storb B, et al. Effects of treating marrow with a CD3-specific immunotoxin for prevention of acute graft-versus-host disease. *Bone Marrow Transplant* 1998;3:437–444.

59. Uchiyama T, Broder S, Waldmann TA. A monoclonal antibody (anti-Tac) reactive with activated and functionally mature human T cells. I. Production of anti-Tac monoclonal antibody and distribution of Tac (+) cells. *J Immunol* 1981;126:1393–1397.

60. Leonard WJ, Depper JM, Uchiyama T, et al. A monoclonal antibody that appears to recognize the receptor for human T-cell growth factor; partial characterization of the receptor. *Nature* 1982;300:267–269.

61. Waldmann TA. Multichain interleukin-2 receptor: a target for immunotherapy in lymphoma. *J Natl Cancer Inst* 1989;81:914–923.

62. Waldmann TA, Greene WC, Sarin PS, et al. Functional and phenotypic comparison of human T cell leukemia/lymphoma virus positive adult T cell leukemia with human T cell leukemia/lymphoma virus negative Sézary leukemia, and their distinction using anti-Tac: monoclonal antibody identifying the human receptor for T cell growth factor. *J Clin Invest* 1984;73:1711–1718.

63. Nasu K, Said J, Vonderheid E, et al. Immunopathology of cutaneous T-cell lymphomas. *Am J Pathol* 1985;119:436–447.

64. Sheibani K, Winberg CD, van de Velde S, et al. Distribution of lymphocytes with interleukin-2 receptors (TAC antigens) in reactive lymphoproliferative processes, Hodgkin's disease, and non-Hodgkin's lymphomas. An immunohistologic study of 300 cases. *Am J Pathol* 1987;127:27–37.

65. Korsmeyer SJ, Greene WC, Cossman J, et al. Rearrangement and expression of immunoglobulin genes and expression of Tac antigen in hairy cell leukemia. *Proc Natl Acad Sci U S A* 1983;80:4522–4526.

66. Waldmann TA. The interleukin-2 receptor. *J Biol Chem* 1991;266:2681–2684.

67. Waldmann TA. The multi-subunit interleukin-2 receptor. *Ann Rev Biochem* 1989;58:875–911.

68. Morgan DA, Ruscetti FW, Gallo RC. Selective *in vitro* growth of T-lymphocytes from normal human bone marrows. *Science* 1976;193:1007–1008.

69. Smith KA. T-cell growth factor. *Immunol Rev* 1980;51:337–357.

70. Kuziel WA, Greene WC. Interleukin-2 and the IL-2 receptor: new insights into structure and function. *J Invest Dermatol* 1990;94[Suppl]:S27–S32.

71. Tsudo M, Kozak RW, Goldman CK, et al. Demonstration of a non-Tac peptide that binds interleukin-2: a potential participant in a multichain interleukin-2 receptor complex. *Proc Natl Acad Sci U S A* 1986;83:9694–9698.

72. Takeshita T, Asao H, Ohtani K, et al. Cloning of the γ chain of the human IL-2 receptor. *Science* 1992;257:379–382.

73. Leonard WJ, Depper JM, Crabtree GR, et al. Molecular cloning and expression of cDNAs for the human interleukin-2 receptor. *Nature* 1984;311:626–631.

74. Sharon M, Klausner RD, Cullen BR, et al. Novel interleukin-2 receptor subunit directed by cross-linking under high-affinity conditions. *Science* 1986;243:859–863.

75. Hatakeyama M, Tsudo M, Minamoto S, et al. Interleukin-2 receptor β chain gene: generation of three receptor forms by cloned human α and β chain cDNAs. *Science* 1989;244:551–556.

76. Takeshita T, Asao H, Ohtani K, et al. Cloning of the γ chain of the IL-2 receptor. *Science* 1992;257:379–382.

77. Bazan JF. Structural design and molecular evolution of a cytokine receptor superfamily. *Proc Natl Acad Sci U S A* 1990;87:6934–6938.

78. Bamford RN, Grant AJ, Burton JD, et al. The interleukin (IL) 2 receptor β-chain is shared by IL-2 and a cytokine, provisionally designated IL-T, that stimulates T-cell proliferation and the induction of lymphokine-activated killer cells. *Proc Natl Acad Sci U S A* 1994;91:4940–4944.

79. Grabstein KH, Eisenman J, Shanebeck K, et al. Cloning of a T cell growth factor that interacts with the beta chain of the interleukin-2 receptor. *Science* 1994;264:965–968.

80. Noguchi M, Nakamura Y, Russell SM, et al. Interleukin-2 receptor α-chain: a functional component of the interleukin-7 receptor. *Science* 1993;262:1877–1880.

81. Kondo M, Takeshita T, Ishii N, et al. Sharing of the interleukin-2 (IL-2) receptor gamma chain between receptors for IL-2 and IL-4. *Science* 1993;62:1874–1877.

82. Damjanovich S, Bene L, Matko J, et al. Preassembly of interleukin-2 (IL-2) receptor subunits on resting Kit-255 K6 T cells and their modulation by IL-2, IL-7 and IL-15: a fluorescence resonance energy transfer study. *Proc Natl Acad Sci U S A* 1997;94:13134–13139.

83. Witthuhn BA, Silvennoinen O, Miura O, et al. Involvement of the Jak-3 Janus kinase in signalling by interleukins 2 and 4 in lymphoid and myeloid cells. *Nature* 1994;370:153–157.

84. Johnston JA, Bacon CM, Finbloom DS, et al. Tyrosine phosphorylation and activation of STAT5, STAT3, and Janus kinases by interleukins 2 and 15. *Proc Natl Acad Sci U S A* 1995;92:8705–8709.

85. Lin JX, Migone TS, Tsang M, et al. The role of shared receptor motifs and common Stat proteins in the generation of cytokine pleiotropy and redundancy by IL-2, IL-4, IL-7, IL-13, and IL-15. *Immunity* 1995;2:331–339.

86. Anderson DM, Kumaki S, Abdieh M, et al. Functional characterization of human interleukin-15 receptor α chain and close linkage of IL-15RA and IL-2RA genes. *J Biol Chem* 1995;270:29862–29869.

87. Tsudo M, Goldman CK, Bongiovanni KF, et al. The p75 peptide is the receptor for interleukin-2 expressed on large granular lymphocytes and is responsible for the interleukin-2 activation of these cells. *Proc Natl Acad Sci U S A* 1987;84:5394–5398.

88. Williams JM, Kelly VE, Kirkman RL, et al. T cell activation antigens: therapeutic implications. *Immunol Inv* 1988;16:687–723.

89. Diamantstein T, Osawa H. The interleukin-2 receptor, its physiology and a new approach to a selective immunosuppressive therapy by anti-interleukin-2 receptor monoclonal antibodies. *Immunol Rev* 1986;92:5–27.

90. Strom TB, Kelley VR, Woodworth TG, et al. Interleukin-2 receptor-directed immunosuppressive therapies: antibody- or cytokine-based targeting molecules. *Immunol Rev* 1992;129:131–163.

91. Tendler CL, Greenberg SJ, Blattner WA, et al. Transactivation of interleukin-2 and its receptor induces immune activation in HTLV-I associated myelopathy: pathogenic implications and a rationale for immunotherapy. *Proc Natl Acad Sci U S A* 1990;87:5218–5222.

92. Uchiyama T, Yodoi J, Sagawa K, et al. Adult T-cell leukemia: clinical and hematologic features of 16 cases. *Blood* 1977;50:481–492.

93. Poiesz BJ, Ruscetti FW, Gazdar AF, et al. Detection and isolation of type C retrovirus particles from fresh and cultured lymphocytes of a patient with cutaneous T cell lymphoma. *Proc Natl Acad Sci U S A* 1980;77:7415–7419.

94. Sodroski JG, Rosen CA, Haseltine WA. Trans-acting transcriptional activation of the long terminal repeat of human T lymphotropic viruses in infected cells. *Science* 1984;225:381–385.

95. Broder S, Bunn PA Jr, Jaffe ES, et al. NIH conference: T-cell lymphoproliferative syndrome associated with human T-cell leukemia/lymphoma virus. *Ann Intern Med* 1984;100:543–557.

96. Hinuma Y, Nagata K, Hanaoka M, et al. Adult T cell leukemia: antigen in an ATL cell line and detection of antibodies to the antigen in human sera. *Proc Natl Acad Sci U S A* 1981;78:6476–6480.

97. Watanabe T, Yamaguchi K, Takatsuki K, et al. Constitutive expression of parathyroid hormone-related protein gene in human T cell leukemia virus type 1 (HTLV-1) carriers and adult T cell leukemia patients that can be transactivated by HTLV-1 tax gene. *J Exp Med* 1990;72:759–765.

98. Shimoyama M, Lymphoma Study Group. Diagnostic criteria and classification of clinical subtypes of adult T-cell leukaemia-lymphoma. A report from the Lymphoma Study Group (1984–1987). *Br J Haematol* 1991;79:428–437.

99. Queen C, Schneider WP, Selick HE, et al. A humanized antibody that binds to the interleukin-2 receptor. *Proc Natl Acad Sci U S A* 1989;86:10029–10033.

100. Junghans RP, Waldmann TA, Landolfi NF, et al. Anti-Tac-H, a humanized antibody to the interleukin-2 receptor with new features for immunotherapy in malignant and immune disorders. *Cancer Res* 1990;50:1495–1502.

101. Hakimi J, Chizzonite R, Luke DR, et al. Reduced immunogenicity and improved pharmacokinetics of humanized anti-Tac in cynomolgus monkeys. *J Immunol* 1991;147:1352–1359.

102. Brown PS Jr, Parenteau GL, Dirbas FM, et al. Anti-Tac-H, a human-ized antibody to the interleukin-2 receptor, prolongs primate cardiac allograft survival. *Proc Natl Acad Sci U S A* 1991;88:2663–2667.

103. Nussenblatt RB, Schiffman R, Fortin E, et al. Treatment of noninfectious intermediate and posterior uveitis with the humanized anti-Tac monoclonal antibody: a phase I/II study. *Proc Natl Acad Sci U S A* 1999(in press).

104. Lehky TJ, Levin M, Kubota R, et al. Reduction in HTLV-I proviral load and spontaneous lymphoproliferation in HTLV-I-associated myelopathy/tropical spastic paraparesis patients treated with humanized anti-Tac. *Ann Neurol* 1998;44:942–947.

105. MacLean JA, Su Z, Guo Y, et al. Anti-CD3: anti-IL-2 receptor bispecific monoclonal antibody. *J Immunol* 1993;150:1619–1628.

106. Waldmann TA, Pastan IH, Gansow OA, et al. The multichain interleukin-2 receptor: a target for immunotherapy. Conference of the Combined Staff, NIH. *Ann Intern Med* 1992;116:148–160.

107. Migone TS, Lin JX, Cereseto A, et al. Constitutively activated Jak-STAT pathway in T cells transformed with HTLV-I. *Science* 1995;269:79–81.

108. Azimi N, Brown K, Bamford RN, et al. Human T-cell lymphotropic virus type I Tax protein trans-activates interleukin 15 gene transaction through an NF-κB site. *Proc Natl Acad Sci U S A* 1998;95:2452–2457.

109. Migone TS, Cacalano NA, Taylor N, et al. Recruitment of SH2-containing protein tyrosine phosphatase SHP-1 to the interleukin 2 receptor; loss of SHP-1 expression in human T-lymphotropic virus type I-transformed T cells. *Proc Natl Acad Sci U S A* 1998;95:3845–3850.

110. Chaudhary VK, Queen C, Junghans RP, et al. A recombinant immunotoxin consisting of two antibody variable domains fused to Pseudomonas exotoxin. *Nature* 1989;339:394–397.

111. Hwang J, FitzGerald DJ, Adya S, et al. Functional domains of Pseudomonas exotoxin identified by deletion analysis of the gene expressed in E. coli. *Cell* 1987:48:129–136.

112. Lorberboum-Galski H, Kozak R, Waldmann T, et al. IL-2-PE40 is cytotoxic to cells displaying either the p55 or p75 subunit of the IL-2 receptor. *J Biol Chem* 1988;263:18650–18656.

113. Kozak RW, Lorberboum-Galski H, Jones L, et al. IL-2PE40 prevents the development of tumors in mice injected with IL-2 receptor expressing EL4 transfected tumor cells. *J Immunol* 1990;145:2766–2771.

114. Lorberboum-Galski HL, Barrett V, Kirkman RL, et al. Cardiac allograft survival in mice treated with IL-2-PE40. *Proc Natl Acad Sci U S A* 1989;86:1008–1012.

115. Bracha P, Williams DP, Waters C, et al. Interleukin-2 receptor-targeted cytotoxicity: interleukin-2-receptor-mediated action of a diphtheria toxin-related interleukin-2 fusion protein. *J Exp Med* 1988;167:612–622.

116. Kiyokawa T, Shirono K, Hattori T, et al. Cytotoxicity of interleukin-2 toxin toward lymphocytes from patients with adult T-cell leukemia. *Cancer Res* 1989;49:4042–4046.

117. Platanias LC, Ratain MJ, O'Brien S, et al. Phase I trial of a genetically engineered interleukin-2 fusion toxin (DAB$_{486}$IL-2) as a 6 hour intravenous infusion in patients with hematologic malignancies. *Leuk Lymphoma* 1994;14:257–262.

118. Tepler I, Schwartz G, Parker K, et al. Phase I trial of an interleukin-2 fusion toxin (DAB486IL-2) in hematologic malignancies: complete response in a patient with Hodgkin's disease refractory to chemotherapy. *Cancer* 1994;73:1276–1285.

119. LeMaistre CF, Saleh MN, Kuzel TM, et al. Phase I trial of a ligand fusion-protein (DAB389IL-2) in lymphomas expressing the receptor for interleukin-2. *Blood* 1998;91:339–405.

120. Duvic M, Kuzel T, Olsen E, et al. Quality of life is significantly improved in CTCL patients who responded to DAB389IL-2 (ONTAK) fusion protein. *Blood* 1998;92[Suppl 1]:2572a.

121. Engert A, Diehl V, Schnell R, et al. A phase-I study of an anti-CD25 ricin A-chain immunotoxin (RFT5-SMPT-dgA) in patients with refractory Hodgkin's lymphoma. *Blood* 1997;89:403–410.

122. Schnell R, Vitetta E, Schindler J, et al. Clinical trials with an anti-CD25 ricin A-chain experimental and immunotoxin (RFT5-SMPT-dgA) in Hodgkin's lymphoma. *Leuk Lymphoma* 1998;30:525–537.

123. Bird RE, Hardman KD, Jacobson JW, et al. Single-chain antigen-binding proteins. *Science* 1988;242:423–426.

124. Kreitman RJ, Chaudhary VK, Waldmann TA, et al. Cytotoxic activities of recombinant toxins composed of *Pseudomonas* toxin or diphtheria toxin toward lymphocytes from patients with adult T-cell leukemia. *Leukemia* 1993;7:553–562.

125. Kreitman RJ, Bailon P, Chaudhary VK, et al. Recombinant immunotoxins containing anti-Tac (Fv) and derivatives of Pseudomonas exotoxins produce complete regression in mice of an interleukin-2 receptor-expressing human carcinoma. *Blood* 1994;83:426–434.

126. Kreitman RJ, Wilson WH, White JD, et al. Phase I trial of recombinant immunotoxin anti-Tac (Fv)-PE38 (LMB-2) in patients with hematologic malignancies. *J Clin Oncol* 1999(Submitted).

127. Kozak RW, Raubitschek A, Mirzadeh S, et al. Nature of the bifunctional chelating agent used for radioimmunotherapy with yttrium-90 monoclonal antibodies: critical factors in determining *in vivo* survival and organ toxicity. *Cancer Res* 1989;49:2639–2644.

128. Schwarz UP, Plascjak P, Beitzel MP, et al. Preparation of 211At-labeled humanized anti-Tac using 211At produced in disposable internal and external bismuth targets. *Nucl Med Biol* 1998;25:89–93.

129. Kozak RW, Atcher RW, Gansow OA, et al. Bismuth-212-labeled anti-Tac monoclonal antibody: α-particle-emitting radionuclides as modalities for radioimmunotherapy. *Proc Natl Acad Sci U S A* 1986;83:474–478.

130. Hartmann F, Horak EM, Garmestani K, et al. Radioimmunotherapy of nude mice bearing a human IL-2Rα-expressing lymphoma utilizing the α-emitting radionuclide-conjugated monoclonal antibody ^{212}Bi-anti-Tac. *Cancer Res* 1994;54:4362–4370.

131. Waldmann T, Tagaya Y. The multifaceted regulation of interleukin-15 expression and the role of this cytokine in NK cell differentiation and host response to intracellular pathogens. *Ann Rev Immunol* 1999;17:19–49.

132. Tinubu SA, Hakimi J, Kondas JA, et al. Humanized antibody directed to the IL-2 receptor β-chain prolongs primate cardiac allograft survival. *J Immunol* 1994;153:4330–4338.

133. Russell SM, Tayebi N, Nakajima H, et al. Mutation of Jak3 in a patient with SCID: essential role of Jak3 in lymphoid development. *Science* 1995;270:797–800.

134. Macchi P, Villa A, Gillani S, et al. Mutations of Jak-3 gene in patients with autosomal severe combined immune deficiency (SCID). *Nature* 1995;377:65–68.

135. Thomis DC, Gurniak CB, Tivol E, et al. Defects in B lymphocyte maturation and T lymphocyte activation in mice lacking Jak3. *Science* 1995;270:794–797.

15.3

MONOCLONAL ANTIBODIES: CLINICAL APPLICATIONS

Melanoma

PAUL B. CHAPMAN
ALAN N. HOUGHTON

THERAPY OF SYSTEMATIC METASTATIC MELANOMA

A need exists to establish new and improved treatments for metastatic melanoma. Only a few agents have demonstrated antitumor activity against metastatic melanoma. In a review of phase 2 trials supported by the National Cancer Institute, only 2 of 30 tested drugs demonstrated a response rate greater than 10% (with 80% confidence limits) (1). The best single agents for treatment of melanoma are dacarbazine, nitrosoureas, cisplatin, interleukin-2 (IL-2), and interferon-α (2–6). Higher responses have been reported in preliminary evaluations using combinations of chemotherapeutic drugs with IL-2 and interferon-α (7), but these studies need to be confirmed.

Monoclonal antibodies (MAb) have been used alone (unconjugated) or conjugated to cytotoxic agents for the investigational treatment of melanoma. Two general applications of unconjugated MAb are being explored:

1. Activation of components of the immune system (e.g., complement, effector cells), including mediation of cytotoxicity against target tumor cells
2. Induction of active immunity (vaccination) through an idiotype-antiidiotype network

MAb conjugated to radionuclides, toxins, chemotherapeutic drugs, and other cytotoxic agents are also being pursued. Phase 1 studies in patients with melanoma have demonstrated that

TABLE 1. CELL SURFACE ANTIGENS OF HUMAN MELANOMA: TARGETS FOR MONOCLONAL ANTIBODY THERAPY

Antigen	Type of Molecule	Description
GD3	Glycolipid	Disialoganglioside
GD2	Glycolipid	Disialoganglioside
p97	Glycoprotein	95–97 kd; melanotransferrin (homology to transferrin)
gp75	Glycoprotein	TRP-1; 75-kd melanosomal glycoprotein (member of the tyrosinase gene family, homology to mouse *brown* locus gene product)
mCSP	Glycoprotein	240-kd core protein; fully processed protein >400 kd; mCSP

mCSP, melanoma chondroitin sulfated proteoglycan; TRP-1, tyrosinase-related peptide–1.

mouse MAb can be safely administered to patients with cancer, and severe toxicity is uncommon. Objective responses have been observed. The major challenge is to develop more effective strategies for therapy.

ANTIGEN TARGETS FOR TREATMENT OF MELANOMA

Several extensive reviews of melanoma antigens have been conducted, including a National Cancer Institute workshop that analyzed and compared MAb generated in different laboratories (8–15). Five antigen systems expressed by melanoma cells have been most thoroughly investigated as targets for therapy (Table 1):

1. Melanotransferrin, also known as the *p97/gp95 antigen*
2. The melanoma chondroitin sulfated proteoglycan (mCSP), also known as the *high-molecular-weight melanoma-associated antigen*
3. The glycolipid antigens, GD2 and GD3
4. gp75, the most abundant glycoprotein in melanocytic cells

In all cases, the antigens are expressed on certain normal tissues, as well as melanoma. In general, however, the quantity of antigen expression by melanomas is considerably higher than normal cells, and this quantitative difference appears to be crucial for tumor targeting and selective antitumor effects.

Melanotransferrin (p97/gp95)

Melanotransferrin is a 95,000- to 97,000-d phosphorylated sialoglycoprotein that is identified by more than ten different MAb (16–21). At least five distinct epitopes on the antigen have been mapped (18). Using MAb against distinct epitopes on melanotransferrin, it has been possible to measure melanotransferrin expression on tumors and normal tissues (22–25). Small quantities of melanotransferrin are expressed on most normal adult tissues, particularly the uterus, bladder, muscle, colon, and liver. It appears that smooth muscle cells express the highest levels of melanotransferrin among adult tissues—as many as 8,000 molecules per cell. Certain fetal tissues have been found to have rela-

tively high expression, particularly fetal colon. Most melanomas express much higher levels than normal tissues—50,000 to 500,000 molecules per cell. Thus, there is a 10- to 1,000-fold higher expression on tumor compared with normal cells.

Melanoma Chondroitin Sulfate Proteoglycan

A series of MAb recognize a high-molecular-weight complex (>500 kd), which has the properties of a proteoglycan (20,26–35). The melanoma proteoglycan is comprised of a 240- to 280-kd sialylated core protein with *N*-linked carbohydrate chains, to which are added high-molecular-weight chondroitin sulfate glycosaminoglycan side chains. The mCSP antigen (also known as *high-molecular-weight melanoma-associated antigen*) is expressed on most melanomas and nevi. Reactivity by MAb has not been detected with normal epidermal melanocytes, but cultured melanocytes express the mCSP antigen (8,20). Although the expression of mCSP appears to be relatively restricted in normal tissues, small blood vessels also express the antigen.

The gene coding for the core protein of mCSP has been cloned (36) and appears to be encoded or regulated by a locus on chromosome 15 (37). In serum-free medium, melanoma cells readily shed mCSP into the culture medium, and the molecule has the properties of a peripheral membrane component rather than an integral membrane protein. In serum-containing medium, however, the antigen is not shed. The mCSP antigen is expressed on microspikes at the cell surface of melanoma cells, a domain at the cell periphery that is involved in cell–cell interactions and contact of cell footpads to substrate (38). These findings suggest that mCSP helps mediate melanoma cell attachment to other cells and to substrates in tissues and could play a role in metastasis. Contact with substrate can induce mCSP expression in mCSP-negative somatic cell hybrids (37), suggesting that contact with tissue substrates are involved in regulation of mCSP. Binding of anti-mCSP MAb to melanoma cells *in vitro* leads to marked decrease in colony formation in soft agar, presumably through interference with cell–cell interactions (39).

Gangliosides GD2 and GD3

Gangliosides are glycolipid molecules composed of a sialylated oligosaccharide chain linked to a ceramide core consisting of fatty acids linked to sphingosine derivatives. The ceramide portion is inserted into the cell membrane. The diversity of gangliosides is determined largely by the composition of the oligosaccharide chains and the number and position of sialic acids. Melanoma cells are rich in gangliosides; the most prominent melanoma gangliosides are GM3 and GD3, followed by GD2 and GM2 (40–42). One notable feature of melanoma gangliosides is that the ceramide portion has a predominance of long-chain fatty acids (C22:0 and C24:0) compared with normal brain gangliosides (C18:0) (43). Several MAb that bind to melanoma have been found to react with the disialogangliosides GD2 (44–46) and GD3 (19,20,43,46,47). The fine specificity of these MAb is remarkable; MAb can distinguish GD3 from GD2, even though the two molecules only differ by a single sugar moiety (GalNAc). MAb against GD3 can also distinguish between the form of sialic acid residues linked to the oligosaccharide (*N*-acetyl versus *N*-glycolyl sialic acids) (48).

GD3 is expressed on some normal tissues, including subpopulations of neurons, adrenal medulla, melanocytes, and connective tissue in a variety of organs (20,47,49,50). It appears that the expression of GD3 in most normal tissues is considerably lower than on melanoma cells. Cultured normal melanocytes express only low levels of GD3, whereas melanoma cells express much higher levels (51). Transformation of cultured normal melanocytes by expression of the oncogene v-ras leads to a marked upregulation of GD3 with levels increasing by 10- to 1,000-fold (52). The tissue distribution of GD2 appears to be more restricted, but GD2 is also present in normal brain and other neuroectoderm-derived tissues. Like GD3, GD2 expression appears to be upregulated by transformation of melanocytes (13,53). Both GD2 and GD3 appear to be present in the serum of healthy individuals; a study in a small number of patients with metastatic melanoma has suggested that levels of GD2 and GD3 are elevated (54). Gangliosides and other glycosphingolipids have been presumed to play a role in cell–cell and cell–substrate recognition and in regulation of cell surface molecules, such as growth factor receptors. A potential role for GD2 and GD3 has been suggested by studies that demonstrate an association of GD2 and GD3 with cell surface receptors for vitronectin and fibronectin (55,56). These disialogangliosides appear to modulate the binding of these receptors to [Arg-Gly-Asp]-containing substrates, including vitronectin and fibronectin. This suggests that these gangliosides may play a critical role in the attachment of melanoma cells to tissue substrate.

Other gangliosides are potential targets for therapy of melanoma. MAb are available against GM2 (57), which appears to be more restricted on normal tissues but only is expressed on a subset of melanomas (58). Gangliosides can be modified by acetylation, and an O-acetylated variant of GD3 has been detected in human melanoma cells by MAb (59,60). 9-O-acetylated-GD3 is generally expressed at lower levels than GD3 but also may be present in fewer normal tissues.

gp75

Also known as *tyrosinase-related peptide-1*, gp75 is a member of the tyrosinase gene family and was initially defined by antibodies from a patient with melanoma (61). gp75 is the most abundant glycoprotein in melanocytic cells and is expressed by both pigmented melanomas and normal melanocytes. Preclinical animal experiments using a B16 lung metastasis model have shown that anti-gp75 immunotherapy, either passive immunotherapy infusing MAb against gp75 or active immunotherapy immunizing against gp75, results in an inhibition of lung metastases (62,63). Clinical trials are planned in which melanoma patients will be immunized against gp75 using the gene encoding gp75.

THERAPEUTIC USES OF UNCONJUGATED MONOCLONAL ANTIBODY AGAINST MELANOMA ANTIGENS

Mechanisms of Antimelanoma Effects

A subset of MAb is able to induce killing of target tumor cells. Two basic mechanisms have been identified: (a) antibody-dependent cellular cytotoxicity (ADCC) and (b) complement-mediated cytotoxicity. ADCC is mediated by the Fab portion of the antibody molecule binding to the target tumor cell and the Fc portion binding to a receptor (Fc receptor) on an immune effector cell. Two features appear to be important for effective mediation of ADCC: (a) the immunoglobulin isotype, with mouse immunoglobulin G3 (IgG3) and IgG2a and human IgG1 and IgG3 being most effective, and (b) characteristics of the antigen target, particularly density on the cell surface. Mouse IgG3 antibodies directed against ganglioside antigens GD3 and GD2 have been particularly effective for mediating tumor lysis *in vitro* in ADCC assays (64–70). The ganglioside GD3 is generally expressed at high density on melanoma, and although level of expression is related to susceptibility to lysis (46,70), other undetermined properties of GD3 may exist that are crucial for effective killing. Several cell types, each characterized by the expression of Fc receptor, have been found to mediate ADCC. Natural killer cells and monocytes can mediate ADCC both *in vitro* and *in vivo* (68,71–73). IL-2, an activator of natural killer cells, can increase ADCC mediated by a natural killer cell population both *in vitro* and *in vivo* (74,75). Granulocyte-macrophage colony-stimulating factor can also increase ADCC mediated by peripheral blood mononuclear cells (76).

Complement activation can potentially induce a variety of events, including increased capillary permeability, edema, chemotaxis, activation of leukocytes, and local tissue destruction. Target tumor cells can be lysed by complement activation and deposition at the cell surface, leading to formation of pores in the cell membrane. Again, mouse IgG3 MAb against GD3 and GD2 have been particularly effective in activating human complement leading to killing of target melanoma cells (77,78). Combinations of MAb directed against different determinants on the same molecule or against distinct molecules on the same cell have been found to induce substantially more cytotoxicity *in vitro* than either MAb alone (79,80). An important property of tumor cells may be their ability to resist or inactivate complement-mediated cytotoxicity. Factors produced by cells, including decay-accelerating factor and homologous restriction factor, can inactivate the complement cascade before formation of cytotoxic complement complexes, and melanoma cells have been found to produce some of these inhibitors (81,82).

Several antigens, mCSP and the gangliosides GD2 and GD3, are probably involved in cell adhesion, and MAb against these antigens may interfere with melanoma cell adhesion. For example, MAb against the ganglioside GD3 on melanoma cells can effectively block adherence to surfaces (49) and inhibit cell proliferation. Thus, MAb against GD3 might act directly on melanoma cells to inhibit cell attachment and proliferation.

Clinical Trials Using Unconjugated Monoclonal Antibodies

Phase 1 studies of unconjugated MAb (Table 2) have shown that the MAb can reach tumor sites after systemic administration. Most of the experience using unconjugated MAb in melanoma has focused on two antigens—GD2 and GD3 ganglioside. Toxicity has generally been mild to moderate, although maximum tolerated doses have been established for MAb against GD2 and GD3. For these MAb, dose-limiting toxicity is related to cross-reactivity with normal tissues expressing the antigen. Phase 1

TABLE 2. PASSIVE IMMUNOTHERAPY CLINICAL TRIALS USING UNCONJUGATED MONOCLONAL ANTIBODY (MAb) ADMINISTERED INTRAVENOUSLY TO PATIENTS WITH MELANOMA

MAb	Antigen	MAb Doses Used	No. of Patients	Toxicity	HAMA (%)	Response	Reference
R24	GD3 ganglioside	8–1,200 mg/m^2	103	Urticaria, nausea, diarrhea, malignant HTN, vascular leak syndrome, hypotension	96	2 CR, 8 PR	89,167–171
MG21	GD3 ganglioside	5–100 mg/m^2	8	Urticaria, nausea	Most patients	1 PR	91 (and I. Hellstrom, *personal communication*)
14G2a	GD2 ganglioside	10–200 mg/m^2	30 (23 melanoma)	Pain syndrome, neurotoxicity, SIADH, fever	93	2 PR in neuroblastoma	172,173
Chimeric 14.18	GD2 ganglioside	5–100 mg/m^2	13	Pain syndrome, nausea	61	None	97
3F8	GD2 ganglioside	5–100 mg/m^2	17 (9 melanoma)	Pain syndrome	60	2 PR	90,174
R24 + 3F8	GD3/GD2 gangliosides	1–10 mg/m^2	14 (6 melanoma)	Pain syndrome	NR	None	95
ME 36.1	GD2/GD3 gangliosides	25–500 mg/m^2	13	None	NR	1 CR >3 yr	175
9.227	mCSP	361–1,000 mg	21	Fever, nausea, serum sickness	25–37	None	86,87
96.5 + 48.7	mCSP/ melanoTr	212 each mg	4	None	100	None	88

CR, complete response; HAMA, human antimouse antibody; HTN, hypertension; melanoTr, melanotransferrin; mCSP, melanoma chondroitin sulfate proteoglycan; NR, not reported; PR, partial response; SIADH, syndrome of inappropriate antidiuretic hormone secretion.

clinical studies carried out at a variety of research centers suggest that treatment with MAb against gangliosides can induce major tumor regressions. Treatment with R24 (antiGD3), 3F8 (antiGD2), 14G2a (anti-GD2), and ME36.1 (antiGD2/GD3) MAb have induced partial and complete responses in patients with melanoma and neuroblastoma. Generally, in these studies, MAb have been administered systemically by an intravenous route, but regional therapy has been explored with limb perfusion (83) and intrathecal administration for meningeal disease (84) with evidence of antitumor effects. There appeared to be less human IgG antimouse antibody (HAMA) response in patients treated by regional perfusion compared with systemic treatment (83). In addition, studies by Irie and Morton have shown regression of cutaneous melanoma metastases after intralesional injection of a human IgM MAb against GD2 (85). Human MAb potentially offer distinct advantages—they may be less immunogenic than mouse MAb but have been difficult to produce in large quantities.

A common feature of these trials is that the MAb used for treatment were immunologically active. The antiganglioside MAb efficiently mediated ADCC, complement-mediated cytotoxicity, or both. Several phase 1 trials in patients with melanoma using MAb that were less active in ADCC and complement killing have demonstrated no antitumor activity (86–88). These observations suggest an association between the *in vitro* immunologic effects of MAb and tumor responses observed in phase 1 trials. More studies, however, are needed to establish response rates, duration, and responsive sites for these MAb. Although direct cytotoxicity is an attractive mechanism for tumor killing, several clinical observations suggest that the antitumor effects of antiganglioside MAb are mediated by alternate or additional mechanisms: (a) tumor

regressions often begin 4–10 weeks (and as late as 16 weeks) after starting treatment (89), and (b) tumor sites are characteristically infiltrated by T lymphocytes after R24 and 3F8 MAb treatment (89,90). An important finding in all of the studies discussed is that mouse MAb reaches tumor sites without evident localization to surrounding normal tissues (83,87–89,91). It is possible that the foreign mouse protein at the tumor site elicits a strong immune response, leading to tumor cell lysis (92) or triggering an active immune response against weak tumor antigens (93). This simple explanation is unlikely because other mouse MAb that also localize to tumor sites have not induced tumor responses. Alternatively, treatment with mouse MAb could immunize the patient against the target tumor antigen by eliciting an antiidiotype response (94).

It is possible that combinations of MAb may offer advantages over single MAb. Combinations, however, must be chosen rationally. A combination of MAb against GD3 (R24) and MAb against GD2 (either 3F8 or chimeric 14.18, a human mouse chimeric version of the anti-GD2 MAb 14G2a) have been assessed clinically in a small number of patients based on the following observations:

1. The two MAb react with a higher proportion of tumor cells in melanoma biopsies than either MAb alone.
2. R24 plus 3F8 mediate additive or synergistic complement-dependent cytotoxicity of melanoma targets *in vitro*.
3. Both R24 and 3F8 have demonstrated major antitumor effects in phase 1 trials.

No tumor responses were observed in 14 patients (only six with melanoma) treated with a combination of R24 and 3F8 MAb

TABLE 3. PASSIVE IMMUNOTHERAPY CLINICAL TRIALS USING UNCONJUGATED MONOCLONAL ANTIBODY (MAb) IN COMBINATION WITH CYTOKINES IN PATIENTS WITH MELANOMA

MAb	Antigen	MAb Dose	Cytokine	No. of Patients	Response	Comments	Reference
R24	GD3	1–12 mg/m^2 qd, d 8–12	IL-2	20	1 PR, 2 MR	Increase LAK, ADCC, peripheral blood T cells	101
R24	GD3	5–100 mg/m^2	IL-2	32	10 PR	2 IL-2–related deaths	102
MG22	GD3	75 and 150 mg/m^2/d, d 8–15	IL-2	7	None	Increased NK, LAK activity	176
XMMME-001	GD3	0.5 and 1 mg/kg/d, d 8–12	IL-2	9	1 MR	Increased LAK, possibly ADCC	177
Ch14.18	GD2	2–10 mg/m^2/d	IL-2	24	1 CR, 1 PR	IL-2 decreased anti-id response to chimeric 14.18	98
Ch14.18 + R24	GD2, GD3	2–7.5 mg/m^2/d; 1–10 mg/m^2/d	IL-2	20	1 PR	Increased MAb-related toxicity	96
R24	GD3	8 mg/m^2/d, d 1–5 and 8–12	IFN-α	8	2 MR	Decreased NK activity	178
Ch14.18	GD2	15–60 mg/m^2	GM-CSF	16	None	4/15 patients developed anti-ch14.18 antibodies	179
R24	GD3	10 and 50 mg/m^2/d, d 8–15	GM-CSF	12	None	Enhanced ADCC	180
R24	GD3	1–50 mg/m^2/d d 1–5	M-CSF	19	None	—	181
R24	GD3	10 mg/m^2, d 1,3	TNF-α	8	None	Tumor lysis syndrome in one patient, almost no viable tumor remaining	103
^{111}In-96.5	melanoTr	10 mg/m^2 qd × 5 d	IFN-α	5	Not stated	IFN-α altered MAb biodistribution	182

ADCC, antibody-dependent cellular cytotoxicity; GM-CSF, granulocyte-macrophage colony stimulating factor; IL-2, interleukin-2; IFN-α, interferon-α; LAK, lymphokine-activated killer cells; MR, minor response; NK, natural killer cells; PR, partial response; TNF-α, tumor necrosis factor–α; id, idiotype; melanoTr, melano–transferrin.

(95). In 20 evaluable patients treated with R24 and chimeric 14.18 in combination with IL-2, only one partial response was observed (96). These observations suggest that, despite *in vitro* analysis, antitumor effects of a combination of these MAb were not synergistic.

Among trials in which it was assessed, 60% to 100% of patients developed a human antimouse antibody (HAMA) response. In the setting of circulating HAMA, the pharmacokinetics of mouse MAb are significantly altered, resulting in rapid clearance of MAb and reduced tumor targeting. In an attempt to reduce the immunogenicity of MAb, mouse MAb have been "humanized" by either grafting the mouse variable domains onto a human IgG backbone (termed *human-mouse chimeric MAb*) or by grafting only the mouse complementarity-determining regions (termed *CDR-grafted MAb*). Because CDR-grafted MAb do not contain murine framework regions, these MAb may be less immunogenic than the chimeric MAb.

Thirteen patients were treated with chimeric 14.18 alone (97). Chimeric 14.18 had a half-life β of 181 hours, which is significantly longer than its murine counterpart 14G2a (42 hours). Chimeric 14.18, however, was immunogenic in patients because 61% of patients developed detectable antibodies against the MAb, although chimeric 14.18 was less immunogenic than the corresponding murine 14G2a. Because only a single dose of chimeric 14.18 was administered, it was not possible to determine whether this antichimeric 14.18 response affected the pharmacokinetics. When patients were treated with chimeric 14.18 and IL-2, only 10 of 24 (42%) patients developed an antichimeric antibody response (98). It is not clear whether this decrease in immunogenicity in the setting of concomitant IL-2 treatment is reproducible and whether it can improve the therapeutic effect of MAb treatment.

THERAPEUTIC USES OF UNCONJUGATED MONOCLONAL ANTIBODY IN CONJUGATION WITH CYTOKINES

Another strategy to enhance immune effects of MAb is the administration of cytokines in combination with MAb. Cytokines can augment ADCC mediated by MAb (74,76) and increase antitumor effects of MAb in animal models (75). It is also possible that cytokines can modulate the expression of cell surface antigens on melanoma cells (99), making the cell more susceptible to MAb-mediated killing. Treatment in animal models has demonstrated an increase in tumor targeting of an antimelanotransferrin MAb (measured as the percent of injected dose of MAb per g of tumor) in animals treated with interferon-α (100).

Clinical trials have been conducted in melanoma patients in which MAb were combined with a variety of cytokines (IL-2, granulocyte-macrophage colony-stimulating factor, macrophage colony-stimulating factor, tumor necrosis factor–α) to evaluate toxicity, *in vitro* cytotoxicity by mononuclear cells, and antitumor effects (Table 3). Combining MAb with cytokines introduces an additional level of complexity in which dose, schedule, and relative timing of the MAb and cytokine are undoubtedly critical factors. This is illustrated by the two trials combining R24 and IL-2 (101,102). When R24 was administered before IL-2, only one partial response was observed in 20 patients (101). When R24 was infused 2 weeks after beginning IL-2 administration, however, 10 of 32 patients experienced a partial response (102).

In an attempt to recruit neutrophils to mediate ADCC against tumors, a pilot trial was conducted in which melanoma patients were treated with R24, followed 6 hours later with tumor necrosis factor–α on days 1 and 3 (103). One of the eight patients treated experienced a massive tumor lysis syndrome hours after treatment with almost complete lysis of bulky tumor in multiple visceral sites. The combination R24 and tumor necrosis factor–α certainly merits further investigation and suggests that this approach may provide a means to focus to power of the immune system against tumor sites.

MONOCLONAL ANTIBODIES CONJUGATED TO TOXINS

A popular strategy has been delivery of cytotoxic agents to tumor sites by linkage to MAb. Although a wide variety of cytotoxic agents have been considered for conjugation, three classes have been studied most intensively in preclinical models: (a) cytotoxic drugs, (b) toxins, and (c) radionuclides. Vindesine, daunomycin, neocarzinostatin, and purothionin conjugated to MAb have shown antitumor effects in animal melanoma models (104–107). Critical issues remain for the use of immunoconjugates for therapy of solid tumors. Although tumor:normal tissue ratios of radionuclide are typically favorable in patients with solid tumors, the absolute amount of injected dose that localizes to tumor is usually low. Specificity and affinity of the MAb are probably crucial for tumor localization, but a number of other factors could greatly impact on targeting, including:

1. Tumor blood flow
2. Vascular permeability
3. Circulating antigen
4. Tumor size
5. Antigen expression and antigenic heterogeneity in the tumor
6. Tumor necrosis

Thus, in some animal models and under some conditions, control MAb can show the same tumor localization (or even better) compared with a specific MAb.

Toxins are among the most potent cytotoxic molecules in nature (108). They come from two sources: plants (e.g., ricin, abrin) and bacteria (e.g., *Pseudomonas* exotoxin A, diphtheria toxin). The most widely studied plant toxin is ricin, a natural product of beans from the plant *Ricinus communis*, which is an extremely potent inhibitor of protein synthesis. The molecule is composed of two chains, A and B, that are disulfide linked. The A chain is able to inhibit protein synthesis while the B chain mediates binding to the cell surface. Ricin and other immunotoxins have demonstrated antitumor activity against cultured melanoma cells and melanoma tumors growing in mice (109–113), but resistance to the toxic effect of immunotoxins can be striking (114,115). For cytotoxicity to be effective, the toxin must be delivered by the MAb into the cell, and the efficiency of delivery depends on the properties of the antigen target. Once inside the cell, the toxin must be able to translocate across a membrane into the cytosol, where it can inhibit protein synthesis. Resistance to the effect of immunotoxins could occur at any of these steps. An additional obstacle is that ricin is relatively immunogenic, and patients readily develop antiricin antibodies that interfere

with tumor targeting of the immunotoxin. Despite these problems, immunotoxins remain an appealing strategy, particularly as understanding of the biologic properties of the MAb, antigen, and toxin increases.

Therapeutic Uses of Monoclonal Antibody Conjugated to Ricin

Immunotoxins constructed using ricin A chain conjugated to MAb against mCSP have been evaluated in clinical trials (116–120). Generally, mild toxicity (flulike symptoms and hepatic enzyme elevations) has been observed, allowing treatment to be administered in an outpatient setting in some cases (118). Antiricin antibodies were commonly observed (116,118–121). Treatment with cyclophosphamide alone or in combination with prednisone did not affect immunogenicity (119,120,122), but azathioprine plus prednisone seemed to decrease the immune response (121). Among the 64 reported patients, one complete response and three partial responses have been observed.

MONOCLONAL ANTIBODIES CONJUGATED TO RADIONUCLIDES

Radiolabeled MAb against melanotransferrin, GD3, mCSP, and other antigens have been shown to localize to human melanoma tumors growing as xenografts in rodents after systemic administration (49,123–131). The central nervous system appears to be a sanctuary because antibodies, which are large protein molecules, do not readily cross the blood-brain barrier. Treatment with high osmotic solution, however, can augment central nervous system uptake (132).

The diagnosis and therapy of melanoma with radiolabeled MAb has been reviewed (133). Important issues for clinical trials with radiolabeled MAb include:

1. Route of administration
2. MAb dose
3. Type and dose of radionuclide
4 Ability of MAb to react with antigen after labeling with radionuclide (immunoreactivity)
5. Biodistribution and pharmacokinetics of radiolabeled MAb
6. Ability of MAb to reach tumor (reported usually as percent of injected dose of MAb/gram of tumor)
7. The use of control MAb (because control MAb can often localize preferentially to tumor sites) (49)
8. Nonspecific uptake of MAb or isotope by organs, such as the liver
9. Stability of MAb-radionuclide complex *in vivo*

Each of these issues is important for diagnosis and therapy with radiolabeled MAb and, in many cases, diagnostic studies are used to gather information about therapeutic potential of MAb. Optimally, evaluation of radiolabeled MAb should also include dosimetry data derived from biopsies of tumor, bone marrow, and other tissues.

TABLE 4. THERAPY TRIALS USING RADIOLABELED MONOCLONAL ANTIBODY (MAb) IN MELANOMA PATIENTS ADMINISTERED INTRAVENOUSLY

MAb	Route of Administration	Antigen	MAb Dose	Isotope	Total Isotope Dose	No. of Patients	Toxicity	Response	Reference
96.5 Fab	i.v.	melanoTr	5–10 mg	^{131}I	132–529 mCi	7	Hematologic, chills, fever, hypotension	None	183
96.5 Fab	i.v.	melanoTr	10 mg	^{131}I	100–200 mCi	7	None	None	144
48.7 Fab	i.v.	mCSP	2–10 mg	^{131}I	142–374 mCi	2	Hematologic	1 PR	145

^{131}I, iodine-131; melanoTR, melanotransferrin; mCSP, melanoma chondroitin sulfated proteoglycan.

Clinical Studies Using Radiolabeled Monoclonal Antibody to Target Melanoma

Clinical trials using nontherapeutic doses of radionuclide for detection of melanoma lesions have investigated MAb labeled with indium-111, iodine-131, iodine-125, or technetium-99m. Blood or plasma half-lives after intravenous injection were relatively short for Fab fragments (ranging from 80 to 100 minutes) and longer for whole IgG molecules (20–100 hours). Up to 0.04% of the injected MAb could be detected per gram of tumor, but usually a much smaller proportion of the injected dose reached the tumor. Autoradiography of biopsied lesions has revealed that distribution of radiolabel within lesions can be uneven, in part because of antigenic heterogeneity, but primarily because of factors unrelated to antigen expression (134). Toxicity has been seen only rarely. Control MAb could often localize to melanoma lesions, although, in most cases, two to more than ten times lower concentrations than the test MAb. Antimelanoma MAb have not been found to target nonmelanoma tumors (135).

In imaging studies, sensitivity (number of tumor lesions detected/number of known lesions) range from 16% to 96%, although most studies demonstrated a sensitivity in the range of 43% to 96%. In anecdotal case, previously unsuspected sites of disease were detected (136,137) with the potential for altering therapy (138). Interest exists in the effect of unlabeled ("cold") MAb on the biodistribution and tumor targeting of radiolabeled MAb (129). In several studies, imaging of tumor sites was improved when high doses of cold MAb were injected (139–143). In addition to evaluation for systemic disease, radiolabeled MAb have been evaluated as agents to detect regional metastases by lymphoscintigraphy after injection subcutaneously (144). It is not possible to determine the diagnostic role of radiolabeled MAb in the evaluation of patients for metastatic melanoma, although it is clear that, in individual patients, radiolabeled MAb can detect unsuspected metastatic sites. Imaging with radiolabeled MAb has not proved superior to conventional imaging techniques in patients with melanoma. Further clinical trials to compare radiolabeled MAb imaging with physical examination and standard diagnostic procedures is necessary to assess the role of diagnostic imaging with radiolabeled MAb.

Therapeutic Uses of Radiolabeled Monoclonal Antibody in Melanoma

Clinical experience with radiolabeled MAb for therapy of melanoma is limited (Table 4). For radiolabeled MAb, bone marrow toxicity (thrombocytopenia, neutropenia) appears to be dose-limiting, although this may have to be reassessed with the availability of bone marrow transplant techniques and hematopoietic growth factors. One partial response has been observed in intraabdominal lymph nodes lasting 3 months after two doses of 181 and 193 mCi of MAb 48.7 (145).

REGIONAL ADMINISTRATION OF MONOCLONAL ANTIBODY

Several investigators have explored the possibility of administering MAb into isolated regions rather than injecting the MAb intravenously (Table 5). This was done to achieve high local concentrations of MAb (e.g., regional perfusion, intralesional injection) or to deliver MAb into regions where MAb would generally not have access (e.g., central nervous system). The largest experience is from Coit and colleagues, who used isolated limb perfusion in 12 patients to achieve high local concentrations of the anti-GD3 MAb R24 (83). Only one partial response was observed. Irie et al. reported that among eight patients injected intralesionally with a human anti-GD2 antibody, four partial responses occurred (85).

A small number of patients have received MAb administered directly into the central nervous system, either via the intrathecal route or injected directly into the ventricle or a surgically prepared cavity. Although this type of treatment can clear malignant cells from the cerebrospinal fluid as assessed by cytologic examination, no objective antitumor responses have occurred.

ANTIIDIOTYPE MONOCLONAL ANTIBODIES AS VACCINES

The antigen-binding or complementarity-determining region of antibodies can be antigenic. Thus, an immune response can be directed against determinants within or near the antigen-binding site, and the term *idiotype* refers to the collection of these determinants. Idiotype determinants are uniquely expressed on antibodies directed against a single antigen or are shared by small families of related antibodies. Antibodies directed against idiotypic determinants are called *antiidiotypic antibodies*. Some antiidiotype MAb bind directly within the antigen-binding site, forming an image of the antigen. This subgroup of antiidiotype MAb can mimic the antigen and provide an alterna-

TABLE 5. REGIONAL ADMINISTRATION OF MONOCLONAL ANTIBODY (MAb) IN PATIENTS WITH MELANOMA

MAb	Route of Administration	Antigen	MAb Dose	No. of Patients	Response	Reference
R24	Regional limb perfusion	GD3	10–25–50 mg/m^2	12	1 PR	83
R24	i.t.	GD3	92/8 mg	2	1 CR (>6 yr)	170
Human L72	Intralesional	GD2	0.6–6.0 mg	8	4 PR	85
^{131}I-Mel 14 F(ab')$_2$	i.t.	mCSP	7.7–10.2 mg (42–80 mCi)	7	Clearance of malignant cells from CSF; no objective tumor responses	184
454A12-ricin A chain	Intraventricular	Transferrin receptor	380 µg	1	None	185
^{131}I-81C6	Intracavitary, brain	Tenascin	9.8 mg (40 mCi)	1	None	184

CR, complete response; CSF, cerebrospinal fluid; ^{131}I, iodine-131; mCSP, melanoma chondroitin sulfated proteoglycan; PR, partial response.

tive source of "antigen" for immunization. Antiidiotype antibodies have been used to immunize against a wide spectrum of viral (146–151), bacterial (152–155), and parasitic (156,157) antigen agents, as well as against tumor antigens (158–161). Antiidiotype vaccines offer potential advantages over purified antigen:

1. They are a reproducibly pure source of "antigen," particularly where antigen is either hard to purify or is potentially dangerous (e.g. viruses).
2. Antiidiotype antibodies may be able to induce an immune response or break immunologic tolerance in circumstances in which immunization with antigen is poorly immunogenic.

Antiidiotype MAb have been produced that mimic melanotransferrin (161), mCSP (160,162), GD3 ganglioside (158), GD2 ganglioside (163–165), and GM3 ganglioside (166). Immunization of animals with these antiidiotype MAb induce immune responses against purified antigen or antigen-positive melanoma cells. These mouse anti-id MAb are the basis for a novel strategy for antimelanoma vaccines.

Clinical trials have been carried out in melanoma patients using antiidiotypic MAb that mimic mCSP, GD3 ganglioside, or GD2 ganglioside (Table 6). These patients have had either metastatic melanoma or were at high risk for recurrence after being rendered free of disease after complete surgical resection. Experimental end points have generally been safety, induction of antibody responses against antigen (mCSP, GD3, or GD2), and tumor shrinkage in patients with active disease.

Several general conclusions are suggested by these data. First, these vaccines have been safe and have resulted in only minor toxicity. Second, it is possible to induce antibodies against melanoma antigens using murine antiidiotypic MAb vaccines. Murine antiidiotypic MAb alone, however, are not adequately immunogenic; these vaccines must be formulated with potent immune adjuvants. The experience with antiidiotypic MAb mimicking mCSP further suggests that murine MAb do not elicit help from T lymphocytes and that these molecules need to be presented on an appropriate carrier molecule, although this has not been definitively determined. Third, only a minority of patients responded immunologically, and titers induced against the tumor antigens have been low. Despite this, objective tumor responses have been observed in occasional patients. Although this strategy of immunization is exciting and potentially powerful, it remains to be determined whether this form of vaccine can be optimized to induce consistently specific immune responses against tumor antigens and whether these immune responses will have beneficial therapeutic effects.

FUTURE DIRECTIONS

MAb with potent inflammatory effector functions can induce major tumor responses in patients with metastatic melanoma.

TABLE 6. SELECTED CLINICAL TRIALS USING ANTIIDIOTYPIC MONOCLONAL ANTIBODY (MAb) VACCINES IN PATIENTS WITH MELANOMA

Antiidiotypic Vaccine	Antigen	No. of Patients	Disease Status	Results	Reference
MF11-30 MAb	mCSP	25	Metastatic	6 minor responses	186
MF11-30 MAb	mCSP	37	Metastatic	Antimelanoma antibodies not detected; 1 CR	162
MK-23 MAb conjugated to KLH, BCG adjuvant	mCSP	25	Metastatic	14/23 developed antibodies to antigen-positive melanoma; 3 PRs	160
MELIMMUNE-1 + SAFm adjuvant	mCSP	34	NED	Antibodies to mCSP identified in a subset of patients	187
MELIMMUNE-2 + SAFm	mCSP	26	Metastatic	1 PR	188
BEC2 MAb (and BEC2 conjugated to KLH), BCG adjuvant	GD3 ganglioside	32	NED	7/32 developed anti-GD3 antibodies	189,190
1A7 + QS21 adjuvant	GD2 ganglioside	12	Metastatic	Purified serum contained anti-GD2 antibodies; 1 CR	165

BCG, bacille Calmette-Guérin; CR, complete response; KLH, keyhole limpet hemocyanin; mCSP, melanoma chondroitin sulfated proteoglycan; NED, no evidence of disease; SAFm, syntax adjuvant formulation.

R24, an MAb against GD3 ganglioside, is active against metastatic melanoma, and the response rate with R24 is similar to the response rates observed with single agent chemotherapy drugs and interferon-α. Efforts to improve the inflammatory effects of MAb by combining them with cytokines have been unsuccessful. A major barrier, however, has been the immunogenicity of MAb. Most of the MAb used in melanoma trials have been of mouse origin and, as a result, induce human antimouse antibodies in the patients. This limits the ability to treat patients over a prolonged period. It was hoped that chimeric MAb might prove less immunogenic, but experiences with chimeric 14.18 demonstrate that the presence of murine framework regions can be immunogenic. Fully humanized MAb, or CDR-grafted recombinant MAb, although more technically difficult to produce, offer the possibility of significantly lower immunogenicity.

Recombinant CDR-grafted MAb can also be engineered as antibody fragments (e.g. Fab, Fv). Because of their much smaller size, these fragments may be superior to complete immunoglobulin at targeting melanoma tumors. These fragments may improve the delivery of radionuclides or toxins to tumors.

MAb tested to date have targeted differentiation antigens on the surface of melanoma cells. An alternative (or complementary) strategy is to target antigens on tumor vasculature. Initial trials in other tumor systems are under way, and future MAb trials in melanoma might exploit the fact that melanoma tumors are devoid of cellular stroma and depend entirely on neovascularization for tumor support.

Antiidiotypics MAb are being used as surrogate antigens for active immunotherapy trials in three melanoma antigen systems. It is clear that antiidiotypic MAb can induce antibody responses against defined antigens, and ongoing trials will explore methods to optimize the immunogenicity of these antiidiotypic MAb, such as novel adjuvants and alternative routes of administration. If specific immune responses can be generated reproducibly against melanoma antigens, randomized phase 3 trials will be required to determine whether these vaccines can impact on the natural history of the disease.

Future approaches may also exploit the constant regions of the immunoglobulin molecule. Many biologically active proteins have half-lives in the range of minutes, which significantly compromises their usefulness. The pharmacokinetics of such molecules may be improved by conjugation to an immunoglobulin structure. Such a recombinant molecule may provide prolonged serum half-lives for such agents.

REFERENCES

1. Marsoni S, Hoth D, Simon R. Clinical drug development. An analysis of phase II trials 1970–1985. *Cancer Treat Res* 1987;71:71.
2. Balch CM, Houghton AN, Milton GW, et al. *Cutaneous melanoma*. Philadelphia: JB Lippincott Co, 1992.
3. Rosenberg S, Lotze M, Yang J, et al. Experience with the use of high-dose interleukin-2 in the treatment of 652 cancer patients. *Ann Surg* 1989;210:474–484.
4. Comis RL. DTIC (NSC-45388) in malignant melanoma: a perspective. *Cancer Treat Res* 1976;64:1123.
5. Kirkwood JM, Ernstoff M. Therapeutic options with recombinant interferons. Lessons drawn from studies of human melanoma. *Semin Oncol* 1986;13:48.
6. Creagan ET, Ahman DL, Frytak S, et al. Recombinant leukocyte A interferon (rIFN-alpha A) in the treatment of disseminated malignant melanoma. Analysis of complete and long-term responding patients. Cancer 1986;58:2576.
7. Legha SS, Ring S, Bedikian A, et al. Treatment of metastatic melanoma with combined chemotherapy containing cisplatin, vinblastine and dacarbazine (CVD) and biotherapy using interleukin-2 and interferon-alpha. *Ann Oncol* 1996;7:827–835.
8. Houghton AN, Eisinger M, Albino AP, et al. Surface antigens of melanocytes and melanomas. Markers of melanocyte differentiation and melanoma subsets. *J Exp Med* 1982;156:1755–1766.
9. Lloyd KO. Human tumor antigens. Detection and characterization with mouse monoclonal antibodies. In: Herberman RB, ed. *Basic and clinical tumor immunology*. Boston: Martinus Nijhoff, 1983:159–214.
10. Reisfeld RA, Ferrone S. *Melanoma antigens and antibodies*. New York, Plenum Press, 1982.
11. Hellstrom KE, Hellstrom I. Monoclonal anti-melanoma antibodies and their possible clinical use. In: Baldwin BW, Byers VS, eds. *Monoclonal antibodies for tumor detection and drug targeting*. New York: Academic Press, 1985:17–51.
12. Houghton AN, Cordon-Cardo C, Eisinger M. Differentiation antigens of melanocytes and melanoma. *Int Rev Exp Pathol* 1986;28: 217–247.
13. Herlyn M, Koprowski H. Melanoma antigens: immunological and biological characterization and clinical significance. *Ann Rev Immunol* 1988;6:283–308.
14. Carrel SJ, Accolla RS, Carmagnola RL, et al. Common human melanoma-associated antigen(s) detected by monoclonal antibodies. *Cancer Res* 1980;40:2523–2528.
15. Hybridoma Workshop. Proceedings of the Natural Cancer Institute Workshop on monoclonal antibodies to human melanoma antigens. *Hybridoma* 1982;1:379–482.
16. Woodbury RG, Brown JP, Yeh MY, et al. Identification of a cell surface protein, p97, in human melanomas and certain other neoplasms. *Proc Natl Acad Sci U S A* 1980;77:2183–2186.
17. Brown JP, Wright P, Hart GG, et al. Protein antigens of normal and malignant tumor cells identified by immunoprecipitation with monoclonal antibodies. *J Biol Chem* 1980;255:4980–4983.
18. Brown JP, Nishiyama K, Hellstrom I, et al. Structural characterization of human melanoma-associated antigen p97 using monoclonal antibodies. *J Immunol* 1981;127:539–546.
19. Dippold WG, Lloyd KO, Li L, et al. Cell surface antigens of human malignant melanoma. Definition of six antigenic systems with mouse monoclonal antibodies. *Proc Natl Acad Sci U S A* 1980; 77:6114–6118.
20. Real FX, Houghton AN, Albino AP, et al. Surface antigens of melanomas and melanocytes defined by mouse monoclonal antibodies: antigen expression in cultured cells and tissues. *Cancer Res* 1985; 45:4401.
21. Khosravi MJ, Dent PB, Liao S-K. Structural characterization and biosynthesis of gp97, a melanoma-associated oncofetal antigen defined by monoclonal antibody. *Int J Cancer* 1985;35:73–80.
22. Brown JP, Woodbury RG, Hart CG, et al. Quantitative analysis of melanoma-associated antigen p97 in normal and neoplastic tissues. *Proc Nat Acad Sci U S A* 1981;78:539–543.
23. Woodbury RG, Brown JP, Loop SM, et al. Analysis of normal and neoplastic human tissues for the tumor-associated protein p97. *Int J Cancer* 1981;27:145–149.
24. Garrigues HJ, Tilgen W, Hellstrom I. Detection of a human melanoma-associated antigen, p97, in histological sections of primary human melanomas. *Int J Cancer* 1982;29:511–515.
25. Sciot R, deVos R, Van Eyken P, et al. In situ localization of melanotransferrin (melanoma-associated antigen p97) in human liver. A light and electron-microscopic immunohistochemical study. *Liver* 1989;9:110–119.
26. Morgan ACJ, Galloway DR, Reisfeld RA. Production and characterization of monoclonal antibody to a melanoma specific glycoprotein. *Hybridoma* 1981;1:27–36.
27. Bumol TF, Reisfeld RA. Unique glycoprotein-proteoglycan complex

defined by monoclonal antibody on human melanoma cells. *Proc Natl Acad Sci U S A* 1982;79:1245–1249.

28. Natali PG, Imai K, Wilson BS, et al. Structural properties and tissue distribution of the antigen recognized by the monoclonal antibody 653.405 to human melanoma cells. *J Natl Cancer Inst* 1981;67: 591–601.

29. Imai K, Ng AK, Ferrone S. Characterization of monoclonal antibodies to human melanoma-associated antigens. *J Natl Cancer Inst* 1981;66:489–496.

30. Ross AH, Cossu G, Herlyn M, et al. Isolation and chemical characterization of a melanoma-associated proteoglycan antigen. *Arch Biochem Biophys* 1983;225:370–383.

31. Wilson BS, Ruverto G, Ferrone S. Immunochemical characterization of a human high molecular weight melanoma associated antigen identified with monoclonal antibodies. *Cancer Immunol Immunother* 1983;14:196–201.

32. Hellstrom I, Garrigues HJ, Cabasso L, et al. Studies of a high molecular weight human melanoma-associated antigen. *J Immunol* 1983;130:1467–1472.

33. Harper JR, Bumol TF, Reisfeld RA. Characterization of monoclonal antibody 155.8 and partial characterization of its proteoglycan antigen on human melanoma cells. *J Immunol* 1984;132:2096–2104.

34. Giacomini P, Natali P, Ferrone S. Analysis of the interaction between a human high molecular weight melanoma-associated antigen and the monoclonal antibodies to three district antigenic determinants. *J Immunol* 1985;135:696–702.

35. Morgan ACJ, Woodhouse C, Bartholomew R, et al. Human melanoma-associated antigens: analysis of antigenic heterogeneity by molecular, serologic, and flow cytometric approaches. *Mol Immunol* 1986;23:193–200.

36. Pluschke G, Vanek M, Evans A, et al. Molecular cloning of a human melanoma-associated chondroitin sulfate proteoglycan. *Proc Natl Acad Sci U S A* 1996;93:9710–9715.

37. Rettig WJ, Real FX, Spengler BA, et al. Human melanoma proteoglycan. Expression in hybrids controlled by intrinsic and extrinsic signals. *Science* 1986;231:1281–1284.

38. Garrigues HJ, Lark MW, Lara S, et al. The melanoma proteoglycan. Restricted expression on microspikes, a specific domain of the cell surface. *J Cell Biol* 1986;103:1699–1710.

39. Harper JR, Reisfeld RA. Inhibition of anchorage-independent growth of human melanoma cells by a monoclonal antibody to a chondroitin sulfate proteoglycan. *J Natl Cancer Inst* 1983;139:59–79.

40. Portoukalian J, Zwingelstein G, Dore J. Lipid composition of human malignant melanoma tumors at various levels of malignant growth. *Eur J Biochem* 1979;94:19–23.

41. Tsuchida T, Saxton RG, Morton DL, et al. Gangliosides of human melanoma. *J Natl Cancer Inst* 1987;78:45–54.

42. Pukel CS, Lloyd KO, Travassos LR, et al. G$_{D3}$, a prominent ganglioside of human melanoma. Detection and characterization by mouse monoclonal antibody. *J Exp Med* 1982;155:1133–1147.

43. Nudelman E, Hakomori S, Kannazi R, et al. Characterization of a human melanoma-associated ganglioside antigen defined by a monoclonal antibody. *J Biol Chem* 1982;257:12752–12756.

44. Saito M, Yu RK, Cheung NKV. Ganglioside GD2 specificity of monoclonal antibodies to human neuroblastoma cell. *Biochem Biophys Res Commun* 1985;127:1.

45. Mujoo K, Kipps TJ, Yang HM, et al. Functional properties and effect on growth suppression of human neuroblastoma tumors by isotype switch variants of monoclonal antiganglioside G$_{D2}$ antibody 14.18. *Cancer Res* 1989;49:2857–2861.

46. Thurin J, Thurin M, Kimoto Y, et al. Monoclonal antibody-defined correlations in melanoma between levels of G$_{D2}$ and G$_{D3}$ antigens and antibody-mediated cytotoxicity. *Cancer Res* 1987;47:1229–1233.

47. Yeh M-Y, Hellstrom I, Abe K, et al. A cell surface antigen which is present in the ganglioside fraction and shared by human melanomas. *Int J Cancer* 1982;29:269–275.

48. Tai T, Kawashima I, Furukawa K, et al. Monoclonal antibody R24 distinguishes between different N-acetyl- and N-glycolylneuraminic acid derivatives of gangliosides GD3. *Arch Biochem Biophys* 1988;260:51–55.

49. Chapman PB, Lonberg M, Houghton AN. Light chain variants of an IgG3 anti-GD3 monoclonal antibody and the relationship between avidity, effector functions, tumor targeting, and antitumor activity. *Cancer Res* 1990;50:1503–1509.

50. Urmacher C, Coron-Cardo C, Houghton AN. Tissue distribution of GD3 ganglioside detected by mouse monoclonal antibody R24. *Am J Dermatopathol* 1989;11:577–581.

51. Carubia JM, Yu RK, Macala LJ, et al. Gangliosides of normal and neoplastic human melanocytes. *Biochem Biophys Res Commun* 1984;120:500–504.

52. Albino AP, Houghton AN, Eisinger M, et al. Class II histocompatibility antigen expression in human melanocytes transformed by Harvey murine sarcoma virus (Ha-MSV) and Kirsten MSV retroviruses. *J Exp Med* 1986;164:1710–1722.

53. Thurin J, Thurin M, Elder DE, et al. GD2 ganglioside biosynthesis is a distinct biochemical event in human melanoma tumor progression. *FEBS Lett* 1982;107:357–361.

54. Sela B-A, Iliopoulos D, Guerry D, et al. Levels of disialogangliosides in sera of melanoma patients monitored by sensitive thin-layer chromatography and immunostaining. *J Natl Cancer Inst* 1989;81: 1489–1492.

55. Cheresh DA, Pytela R, Pierschbacher MD, et al. An Arg-Gly-Asp-directed receptor on the surface of human melanoma cells exists in a divalent cation-dependent functional complex with the disialoganglioside GD2. *J Cell Biol* 1986;105:1167–1173.

56. Cheresh DA, Spiro RC. Biosynthetic and functional properties of an Arg-Gly-Asp-directed receptor involved in human melanoma cell attachments to vitronectin, fibrinogen, and von Willebrand factor. *J Biol Chem* 1987;262:17703–17711.

57. Nishinaka Y, Ravindranath MH, Irie RF. Development of a human monoclonal antibody to ganglioside GM2 with potential for cancer treatment. *Cancer Res* 1996;56:5666–5671.

58. Natoli EJ, Livingston PO, Pukel CS, et al. A murine monoclonal antibody detecting N-glycolyl-GM2: characterization of cell reactivity. *Cancer Res* 1986;46:4116–4120.

59. Cheresh DA, Reisfeld RA, Varki AP. O-acetylation of disialoganglioside GD3 by human melanoma cells creates a unique antigen determinant. *Science* 1984;225:844–846.

60. Cheresh DA, Varki AP, Varki NM, et al. A monoclonal antibody recognizes an O-acetylated sialic acid in a human melanoma-associated ganglioside. *J Biol Chem* 1984;259:7453–7459.

61. Mattes MJ, Thomson TM, Old LJ, et al. A pigmentation-associated, differentiation antigen of human melanoma defined by a precipitating antibody of human serum. *Int J Cancer* 1983;32:717–721.

62. Hara I, Takechi Y, Houghton AN. Implicating a role for immune recognition of self in tumor rejection: passive immunization against the *brown* locus protein. *J Exp Med* 1995;182:1609–1614.

63. Weber LW, Bowne WB, Wolchok JD, et al. Tumor immunity and autoimmunity induced by immunization with homologous DNA. *J Clin Invest* 1998;102:1258–1264.

64. Knuth A, Dippold W, Houghton AN, et al. ADCC reactivity of human melanoma cells with monoclonal antibodies. *Proc Am Assoc Cancer Res* 1984;25:1005.

65. Schultz G, Bumol TF, Reisfeld RA. Monoclonal-directed effector cells selectively lyse human melanoma cells *in vitro* and *in vivo*. *Proc Natl Acad Sci U S A* 1983;80:5407–5411.

66. Hellstrom I, Brankovan V, Hellstrom KE. Strong anti-tumor activities of IgG3 antibodies to a human melanoma-associated ganglioside. *Proc Natl Acad Sci U S A* 1985;82:1499–1502.

67. Hellstrom KE, Hellstrom I, Goodman GE, et al. Antibody dependent cellular cytotoxicity to human melanoma antigens. In: Reisfeld RA, Sell S, eds. *Monoclonal antibodies and cancer therapy*. New York: Alan R. Liss, Inc. 1985:149–164.

68. Herberman RB, Morgan AC, Reisfeld RA, et al. Antibody-dependent cellular cytotoxicity (ADCC) against human melanoma by human effector cells in cooperation with mouse monoclonal antibodies. In: Reisfeld RA, Sell S, eds. *Monoclonal antibodies and cancer therapy*. New York: Alan R. Liss, Inc., 1985:193–203.

69. Cheresh DA, Honsik CJ, Stafileno LK, et al. Disialoganglioside GD3 on human melanoma serves as a relevant antigen for mono-

clonal antibody-mediated tumor lysis. *Proc Natl Acad Sci U S A* 1985;82:5155–5159.

70. Welt S, Carswell EA, Vogel C-W, et al. Immune and nonimmune effector functions of IgG3 mouse monoclonal antibody R24 detecting the disialoganglioside GD3 on the surface of melanoma cells. *Clin Immunol Immunopathol* 1987;45:214–229.

71. Schultz G, Staffileno LK, Reisfeld RA, et al. Eradication of established human melanoma tumors in nude mice by antibody-directed effector cells. *J Exp Med* 1985;161:1315–1325.

72. Ortaldo JR, Woodhouse C, Morgan AC, et al. Analysis of effector cells in human antibody-dependent cellular cytotoxicity with murine monoclonal antibodies. *J Immunol* 1987;138:3566–3572.

73. Hellstrom I, Garrigues U, Lavic E, et al. Antibody-mediated killing of human tumor cells by attached effector cells. *Cancer Res* 1988;48:624–627.

74. Munn DH, Cheung NKV. Interleukin-2 enhancement of monoclonal antibody-mediated cellular cytotoxicity against human melanoma. *Cancer Res* 1987;47:6600–6605.

75. Honsik CJ, Jung G, Reisfeld RA. Lymphokine-activated killer cells targeted by monoclonal antibodies to the disialogangliosides GD2 and GD3 specifically lyse human tumor cells of neuroectodermal origin. *Proc Natl Acad Sci U S A* 1986;83:7893–7897.

76. Kushner BH, Cheung N-K. GM-CSF enhances 3F8 monoclonal antibody-dependent cellular cytotoxicity against human melanoma and neuroblastoma. *Blood* 1989;73:1936–1941.

77. Panneerselvam M, Bredehorst R, Vogel CW. Resistance of human melanoma cells against the cytotoxic and complement-enhancing activities of doxorubicin. *Cancer Res* 1987;47:4601–4607.

78. Goodman GE, Yen YP, Cox TC, et al. The effect of monoclonal antibody MG-21 plus human complement on in vitro cloning of fresh human melanoma. *Proc Am Assoc Cancer Res* 1987;28:389.

79. Hellstrom I, Brown J, Hellstrom KE. Monoclonal antibodies to two determinants of melanoma-antigen p97 act synergistically in complement-dependent cytotoxicity. *J Immunol* 1983;127:157–160.

80. Houghton AN, Scheinberg DA. Monoclonal antibodies. Potential applications to the treatment of cancer. *Semin Oncol* 1986;13:165–179.

81. Cheung NK, Walter EI, Smith-Mensah WH, et al. Decay-accelerating factor protects human tumor cells from complement-mediated cytotoxicity *in vitro*. *J Clin Invest* 1988;81:1122–1128.

82. Panneerselvam M, Welt S, Old LJ, et al. A molecular mechanism of complement resistance of human melanoma cells. *J Immunol* 1986;136:2534–2541.

83. Coit D, Houghton AN, Cordon-Cardo C, et al. Isolated limb perfusion with monoclonal antibody R24 in patients with malignant melanoma. *Proc Am Soc Clin Oncol* 1988;7:248.

84. Dippold WG, Bernhard H, Meyer zum Bushenfelde K-H. Immunological response to intrathecal GD3-ganglioside antibody treatment in cerebrospinal fluid melanosis. In: Oettgen HF, ed. *Gangliosides and cancer*. Weinheim: VCH, 1989;241–247.

85. Irie RF, Morton DL. Regression of cutaneous metastatic melanoma by intralesional injection with human monoclonal antibody to ganglioside GD2. *Proc Natl Acad Sci U S A* 1986;83:8694–8698.

86. Oldham RK, Foon KA, Morgan AC, et al. Monoclonal antibody therapy of malignant melanoma: *in vivo* localization in cutaneous metastasis after intravenous administration. *J Clin Oncol* 1984;2:1235–1244.

87. Schroff RW, Morgan AC, Woodhouse C, et al. Monoclonal antibody therapy in malignant melanoma: factors effecting *in vivo* localization. *J Biol Response Mod* 1987;6:457–472.

88. Goodman GE, Beaumier P, Hellstrom I, et al. Pilot trial of murine monoclonal antibodies in patients with advanced melanoma. *J Clin Oncol* 1985;3:340.

89. Vadhan-Raj S, Cordon-Cardo C, Carswell EA, et al. Phase I trial of a mouse monoclonal antibody against GD3 ganglioside in patients with melanoma: induction of inflammatory responses at tumor sites. *J Clin Oncol* 1988;6:1636–1648.

90. Cheung N, Lazarus H, Miraldi F, et al. Ganglioside GD2 specific monoclonal antibody 3F8: a phase I study in patients with neuroblastoma and malignant melanoma [published erratum, appears in 1992 April 10(4):671]. *J Clin Oncol* 1987;5:1430–1440.

91. Barnhill RL, Fandrey K, Levy MA, et al. Angiogenesis and tumor progression of melanoma. Quantification of vascularity in melanocytic nevi and cutaneous malignant melanoma. *Lab Invest* 1992;67:331–337.

92. Lanzavecchia A, Abrignani S, Moldenhauer G, et al. Antibodies as antigens. The use of monoclonal antibodies to focus human T-cells against selected targets. *J Exp Med* 1988;167:345–352.

93. Lanzavecchia A. Exploiting the immune system's own strategies for immunotherapy. *Immunol Today* 1988;9:167–168.

94. Koprowski H, Herlyn D, Sears HF, et al. Human anti-idiotype in cancer patients. Is the modulation of the immune system beneficial for the patient? *Proc Natl Acad Sci U S A* 1984;81:216–219.

95. Lonberg M, Bajorin D, Cheung N-K, et al. Phase I trial of a combination of two mouse monoclonal antibodies anti-GD3 (R24) and anti-GD2 (3F8) in patients with melanoma and soft tissue sarcoma. *Proc Am Soc Clin Oncol* 1988;7:173.

96. Albertini M, Hank J, Schiller J, et al. Phase Ib trial of combined treatment with ch14.18 and R24 monoclonal antibodies and interleukin-2 for patients with melanoma or sarcoma. *Proc Am Soc Clin Oncol* 1998;17:437a.

97. Saleh MN, Khazaeli MD, Wheeler RH, et al. Phase I trial of the chimeric anti-GD2 monoclonal antibody ch14.18 in patients with malignant melanoma. *Hum Antibodies Hybridomas* 1992;3:19–23.

98. Albertini M, Hank J, Schiller J, et al. Phase Ib trial of chimeric anti-disialoganglioside antibody plus interleukin 2 for melanoma patients. *Clin Cancer Res* 1997;3:1277–1288.

99. Murray JL, Stuckey SE, Pillow JK, et al. Differential *in vitro* effects of recombinant alpha-interferon and recombinant gamma-interferon alone or in combination on the expression of melanoma-associated surface antigens. *J Biol Response Mod* 1988;7:152–161.

100. Murray JL, Zukiwski AA, Rosenblum MG. Enhanced tumor targeting of indium-111 labeled anti-melanoma monoclonal antibody 96.5 in nude mice receiving recombinant alpha interferon subspecies A (rIFN-αA). *Proc Am Assoc Cancer Res* 1989;30:1598.

101. Bajorin DF, Chapman PB, Dimaggio J, et al. Phase I evaluation of a combination of monoclonal antibody R24 and interleukin 2 in patients with metastatic melanoma. *Cancer Res* 1990;50:7490–7495.

102. Creekmore S, Urba W, Koop W, et al. Phase IB/II trial of R24 antibody and interleukin-2 (IL2) in melanoma. *Proc Am Soc Clin Oncol* 1992;11:345.

103. Minasian LM, Szatrowski TP, Rosenblum M, et al. Hemorrhagic tumor necrosis during a pilot trial of tumor necrosis factor-α and anti-GD3 ganglioside monoclonal antibody in patients with metastatic melanoma. *Blood* 1994;83:56–64.

104. Matsui M, Nakanishi T, Noguchi C, et al. Synergistic in vitro and in vivo anti-tumor effects of daunomycin- anti-96kDa melanoma-associated antigen monoclonal antibody CL 207 conjugate and recombinant gamma IFN. *J Immunol* 1988;141:1410–1417.

105. Luders G, Kohnlein W, Sorg C, et al. Selective toxicity of neocarzinostatin-monoclonal antibody conjugates to the antigen bearing human melanoma cell line *in vitro*. *Cancer Immunol Immunother* 1985;20:85–90.

106. Matsui M, Nakanishi T, Noguchi T, et al. Suppression of human melanoma growth in nude mice injected with anti-high molecular weight melanoma-associated antigen monoclonal antibody 225.285 conjugated to purothionin. *Jpn J Cancer Res* 1985;76:119–123.

107. Imai K, Nakanishi T, Noguchi T, et al. Selective *in vitro* toxicity of purothionin conjugated to the monoclonal antibody 225.285 to a human high molecular weight melanoma-associated antigen. *Cancer Immunol Immunother* 1983;15:206–209.

108. Vitetta ES, Thorpe PE. Immunotoxins. In: DeVita VT Jr, Hellman S, Rosenberg SA, eds. *Biologic therapy of cancer*. Philadelphia: JB Lippincott Co, 1991:482–495.

109. Casellas P, Brown JP, Gros O, et al. Human melanoma cells can be killed *in vitro* by an immunotoxin specific for melanoma-associated antigen p97. *Int J Cancer* 1982;30:437–443.

110. Sivam G, Pearson JW, Bohn W, et al. Immunotoxins to a human melanoma-associated antigen: comparison of gelonin with ricin and other A chain conjugates. *Cancer Res* 1987;47:3169–3173.

111. Byers VS, Pimm MV, Scannon PJ, et al. Inhibition of growth of

human tumor xenografts in athymic mice treated with ricin A chain-monoclonal antibody T9IT/36 conjugates. *Cancer Res* 1987;47: 5042–5246.

112. Mujoo K, Reisfeld RA, Rosenblum MG. Effect of 14G2a-gelonin immunotoxin on human melanoma cells. *Proc Am Assoc Cancer Res* 1989;30:1596.

113. Rosenblum MG, Zuckerman JE, Cheung LH. An antimelanoma immunotoxin composed of antibody ZME-018 and the plant toxin gelonin. *Proc Am Assoc Cancer Res* 1988;29:1700.

114. Godal A, Fodstad O, Morgan AC, et al. Human melanoma cell lines showing striking inherent differences in sensitivity to immunotoxins containing holotoxins. *J Natl Cancer Inst* 1986;77:1247–1253.

115. Morgan AC, Bordomaro J, Pearson JW, et al. Immunotoxins to a human melanoma-associated antigen. Resistance to pokeweed antiviral protein conjugates *in vitro*. *J Natl Cancer Inst* 1987;78:1101–1106.

116. Spitler LE, del Rio M, Khentigan A, et al. Therapy of patients with malignant melanoma using a monoclonal antimelanoma antibody-ricin A chain immunotoxin. *Cancer Res* 1987;47:1717–1723.

117. Von Wussow P, Spitler L, Block B, et al. Immunotherapy in patients with advanced malignant melanoma using a monoclonal antimelanoma antibody ricin A immunotoxin. *Eur J Cancer Clin Oncol* 1988;24:S69–S73.

118. Spitler L, Minor DR. Monoclonal antimelanoma ricin A chain immunotoxin therapy of melanoma in outpatients. *Proc Am Soc Oncol* 1989;8:1117.

119. Oratz R, Speyer J, Wernz J, et al. Immunotoxin and cyclophosphamide in malignant melanoma. *Proc Am Soc Clin Oncol* 1988;7:981.

120. LoBuglio AF, Khazaeli MB, Lee J, et al. Pharmacokinetics and immune response to Xomazyme-Mel in melanoma patients. *Antibody Immunoconj Radiopharm* 1988;1:305–310.

121. Hertler AA, Spitler LE, Frankel AE. Humoral immune response to a ricin A chain immunotoxin in patients with metastatic melanoma. *Cancer Drug Deliv* 1987;42:245–253.

122. Khazaeli MB, LoBuglio AF, Wheeler R, et al. The effects of immunosuppressive regimens on human immune response to murine monoclonal anti-melanoma antibody-ricin A chain. *Proc Am Soc Clin Oncol* 1988;29:418.

123. Beaumier P, Krohn K, Carrasquillo J, et al. Melanoma localization in nude mice with monoclonal Fab against p97. *J Nucl Med* 1985; 26:1172–1179.

124. Chan SM, Hoddwe PB, Maric N, et al. Comparison of gallium-67 versus indium-111 monoclonal antibody (96.5, ZME-018B) in detection of human melanoma in athymic mice. *J Nucl Med* 1987; 28:1441–1446.

125. Hwang KM, Fodstad O, Oldham RK, et al. Radiolocalization of xenografted human malignant melanoma by a monoclonal antibody (9.2.27) to a melanoma-associated antigen in nude mice. *Cancer Res* 1985;45:150–155.

126. Wahl RL, Wilson BS, Liebert M, et al. High dose, unlabeled, non-specific antibody pretreatment. Influence on specific antibody localization to human xenografts. *Cancer Immunol Immunother* 1987; 24:221–224.

127. Buchegger F, Mach JP, Leonard P, et al. Selective tumor localization of radiolabeled anti-human melanoma monoclonal antibody fragment demonstrated in the nude mouse model. *Cancer* 1986;58:655–662.

128. Welt S, Mattes MJ, Grando R, et al. Monoclonal antibody to an intracellular antigen images human melanoma transplants in *nu/nu* mice. *Proc Natl Acad Sci U S A* 1987;84:4200–4204.

129. Wahl RL, Liebert M, Wilson BS. The influence of monoclonal antibody dose on tumor uptake of radiolabeled antibody. *Cancer Immunol Immunother* 1987;24:221–224.

130. Fawwaz RA, Wang TST, Estabrook A, et al. Immunoreactivity and biodistribution of indium-111 labeled monoclonal antibody to a high molecular weight-melanoma associated antigen. *J Nucl Med* 1985;26:488–492.

131. Matzku S, Kirchgessner H, Schmid U, et al. Melanoma targeting with a cocktail of monoclonal antibodies to distinct determinants of the human HMW-MAA. *J Nucl Med* 1989;30:390–397.

132. Neuwelt EA, Specht HD, Barnett PA, et al. Increased delivery of tumor-specific monoclonal antibodies to brain after osmotic blood-brain barrier modification in patients with melanoma metastatic to the central nervous system. *Neurosurgery* 1987;20:885–895.

133. Press OW. Immunotoxins. *Biotherapy* 1991;3:65–76.

134. DelVecchio S, Reynolds JC, Carrasquillo JA, et al. Local distribution and concentration of intravenously injected ^{131}I-9.2.27 monoclonal antibody in human malignant melanoma. *Cancer Res* 1989;49: 2783–2789.

135. Carrasquillo JA, Bunn PA, Keenan AM, et al. Radioimmunodetection of cutaneous T-cell lymphoma with indium-111-labeled T101 monoclonal antibody. *N Engl J Med* 1986;315:673–680.

136. Siccardi AG, Buraggi GL, Callegaro L, et al. Multicenter study of immunoscintigraphy with radiolabeled monoclonal antibodies in patients with melanoma. *Cancer Res* 1986;46:4817–4822.

137. Halpern SE, Haindl W, Beauregard J, et al. Scintigraphy with In-111-labeled monoclonal anti-tumor antibodies. Kinetics, biodistribution and tumor detection. *Radiology* 1988;168:529–536.

138. Abrahms PG, Eary F, Schroff RW, et al. The use of a radiolabeled monoclonal antibody for guiding patient management in melanoma. *Antibody Immunoconj Radiopharm* 1988;1:283–289.

139. Murray JL, Rosenblum MG, Sobol RL, et al. Radioimmunoimaging in malignant melanoma with ^{111}In-labeled monoclonal antibody 96.5. *Cancer Res* 1985;45:2376–2381.

140. Rosenblum MG, Murray JL, Haynie TP, et al. Pharmacokinetics of ^{111}In-labeled anti-p97 monoclonal antibody in patients with metastatic malignant melanoma. *Cancer Res* 1985;45:2382–2386.

141. Kirkwood JM, Neumann RD, Zoghbi SS, et al. Scintigraphic detection of metastatic melanoma using indium-111/DTPA conjugated anti-gp240 antibody (ZME-018). *J Clin Oncol* 1987;5:1247–1255.

142. Murray JL, Rosenblum MG, Lamki L, et al. Clinical parameters related to optimal tumor localization of ^{111}In-labeled mouse anti-melanoma monoclonal antibody ZME0.8. *J Nucl Med* 1987;28: 25–33.

143. Carasquillo JA, Abrams PG, Schroff RW, et al. Effects of antibody dose on the imaging and biodistribution of ^{111}In-9.2.27 anti-melanoma monoclonal antibody. *J Nucl Med* 1988;29:39–47.

144. Lotze MT, Carrasquillo JA, Weinstein JN, et al. Monoclonal antibody imaging of human melanoma. Radioimmunodetection by subcutaneous or system injection. *Ann Surg* 1986;204:223–235.

145. Larson SM, Carasquillo JA, McGuggin RW, et al. Use of I-131 labeled murine Fab against a high molecular weight antigen of human melanomas: a preliminary experience. *Radiology* 1985;155: 487–492.

146. Gaulton GN, Sharpe AH, Chang DW, et al. Syngeneic monoclonal internal image anti-idiotopes as prophylactic vaccines. *J Immunol* 1986;137:2930–2936.

147. Ertl HCJ, Finberg RW. Sendai virus-specific T-cell clones. Induction of cytolytic T cells by an anti-idiotypic antibody directed against a helper T-cell clone. *Proc Natl Acad Sci U S A* 1984;81:2850–2854.

148. Kennedy RC, Melnick JL, Dreesman GR. Antibody to hepatitis B virus induced by injecting antibodies to the idiotype. *Science* 1984;223:930–931.

149. Sharpe AH, Gaulton GN, McDade KK, et al. Syngeneic monoclonal anti-idiotype can induce cellular immunity to reovirus. *J Exp Med* 1984;160:1195–1205.

150. Shearer MH, Lanford RL, Kennedy RC. Monoclonal anti-idiotypic antibodies induce humoral immune responses specific for Simian virus 40 large tumor antigen in mice. *J Immunol* 1990;145:932–939.

151. Reagan KJ. Modulation of immunity to rabies virus induced by anti-idiotypic antibodies. *Curr Top Microbiol Immunol* 1985;119:15–30.

152. Stein KE, Soderstrom T. Neonatal administration of idiotype or anti-idiotype primes for protection against Escherichia coli K13 infection in mice. *J Exp Med* 1984;160:1001–1011.

153. McNamara MK, Ward RE, Kohler H. Monoclonal idiotype vaccine against Streptococcus pneumoniae infection. *Science* 1984;226: 1325–1326.

154. Schreiber JR, Patawaran M, Tosi M, et al. Anti-idiotype-induced, lipopolysaccharide-specific antibody response to Pseudomonas aeruginosa. *J Immunol* 1990;144:1023–1029.

155. Monafo WJ, Greenspan NS, Cebra-Thomas JA, et al. Modulation of the murine immune response to Streptococcal group A carbohydrate

by immunization with monoclonal anti-idiotype. *J Immunol* 1987;139:2702–2707.

156. Sacks DL, Kirchoff LV, Hieny S, et al. Molecular mimicry of a carbohydrate epitope on a major surface glycoprotein of Trypanosoma cruzi by using anti-idiotypic antibodies. *J Immunol* 1985;135:4155–4159.

157. Gryzych JM, Capron M, Lambert PH, et al. An anti-idiotype vaccine against experimental schistosomiasis. *Nature* 1985;316:74–76.

158. Chapman PB, Houghton AN. Induction of IgG antibodies against GD3 in rabbits by an anti-idiotypic monoclonal antibody. *J Clin Invest* 1991;88:186–192.

159. Chapman PB, Houghton AN. Anti-idiotype vaccines. In: DeVita VT Jr, Hellman S, Rosenberg SA, eds. *Biologic therapy of cancer updates*. Vol 2 (5). Philadelphia: JB Lippincott Co, 1992:1–9.

160. Mittelman A, Chen ZJ, Yang H, et al. Human high molecular weight melanoma-associated antigen (HMW-MAA) mimicry by mouse anti-idiotypic monoclonal antibody MK2-23. Induction of humoral anti-HMW-MAA immunity and prolongation of survival in patients with stage IV melanoma. *Proc Natl Acad Sci U S A* 1992;89:466–470.

161. Kahn M, Hellstrom I, Estin CD, et al. Monoclonal anti-idiotypic antibodies related to the p97 human melanoma antigen. *Cancer Res* 1989;49:3157–3162.

162. Mittelman A, Chen ZJ, Kageshita T, et al. Active specific immunotherapy in patients with melanoma. A clinical trial with mouse anti-idiotypic monoclonal antibodies elicited with syngeneic anti-high-molecular-weight melanoma-associated antigen monoclonal antibodies. *J Clin Invest* 1990;86:2136–2144.

163. Saleh MN, Stapleton JD, Khazaeli MB, et al. Generation of a human anti-idiotypic antibody that mimics the GD2 antigen. *J Immunol* 1993;151:3390–3398.

164. Cheung N-KV, Canete A, Cheung IY, et al. Disialoganglioside GD2 anti-idiotypic monoclonal antibodies. *Int J Cancer* 1993;54:499–505.

165. Foon KA, Sen G, Hutchins L, et al. Antibody responses in melanoma patients immunized with an anti-idiotype antibody mimicking disialoganglioside GD2. *Clin Cancer Res* 1998;4:1117–1124.

166. Yamamoto S, Yamamoto T, Saxton RE, et al. Anti-idiotype monoclonal antibody carrying the internal image of ganglioside GM3. *J Natl Cancer Inst* 1990;82:1757–1760.

167. Raymond J, Kirkwood J, Vlock D, et al. A phase Ib trial of murine monoclonal antibody R24 (anti-GD3) in metastatic melanoma. *Proc Am Soc Clin Oncol* 1991;10:298.

168. Bajorin DF, Chapman PB, Wong GY, et al. Treatment with high dose mouse monoclonal (anti-GD3) antibody R24 in patients with metastatic melanoma. *Melanoma Res* 1992;2:355–362.

169. Dippold WG, Bernhard H, Dienes HP, et al. Treatment of patients with malignant melanoma by monoclonal ganglioside antibodies. *Eur J Cancer Clin Oncol* 1988;24[Suppl 2]:S65–S67.

170. Dippold W, Bernhard H, Meyer zum Buschenfelde KH. Immunological response to intrathecal and systemic treatment with ganglioside antibody R-24 in patients with malignant melanoma. *Eur J Cancer* 1994;30A:137–144.

171. Nasi M, Meyers M, Livingston P, et al. Anti-melanoma effects of R24, a monoclonal antibody against GD3. *Vaccine Res* 1997;7[Suppl 2]:S155–S162.

172. Saleh MN, Khazaeli MB, Wheeler RH, et al. Phase I trial of murine monoclonal anti-GD2 antibody 14G2a in metastatic melanoma. *Cancer Res* 1992;52:4342–4347.

173. Murray JL, Cunningham JE, Brewer H, et al. Phase I trial of mouse monoclonal antibody 14G2a administered by prolonged intravenous infusion in patients with neuroectodermal tumors. *J Clin Oncol* 1994;12:184–193.

174. Cheung N-KV, Lazarus H, Miraldi FD, et al. Reassessment of patient response to monoclonal antibody 3F8. *J Clin Oncol* 1992;4:671.

175. Lichtin A, Iliopoulos D, Guerry D, et al. Therapy of melanoma with an anti-melanoma ganglioside monoclonal antibody. A possible mechanism of a complete response. *Proc Am Soc Clin Oncol* 1988;7:247.

176. Goodman GE, Hellstrom I, Stevenson U, et al. Phase I trial of murine monoclonal antibody MG-22 and IL-2 in patients with disseminated melanoma. *Proc Am Soc Clin Oncol* 1992;1190:346.

177. Zukiwski AA, Itoh K, Benjamin R, et al. Pilot study of rIL-2 administered with a murine anti-melanoma antibody in patients with metastatic melanoma. *Proc Am Assoc Cancer Res* 1989;1448:365.

178. Caulfield J, Barna B, Murthy S, et al. Phase Ia-Ib trial of an anti-GD3 monoclonal antibody in combination with interferon-α in patients with malignant melanoma. *J Biol Res Mod* 1990;9:319–328.

179. Murray JL, Kleinerman ES, Jia SF, et al. Phase Ia/Ib trial of anti-GD2 chimeric monoclonal antibody 14.18 (ch14.18) and recombinant human granulocyte-macrophage colony-stimulating factor (rhGM-CSF) in metastatic melanoma. *J Immunother* 1996;19:206–217.

180. Felice AJ, Chachoua A, Oratz R, et al. A phase Ib trial of GM-CSF with murine monoclonal antibody R24 in patients with metastatic melanoma. *Proc Am Soc Clin Oncol* 1992;1188:346.

181. Minasian LM, Yao TJ, Steffens TA, et al. A phase I study of anti-GD3 ganglioside monoclonal antibody R24 and recombinant human macrophage-colony stimulating factor in patients with metastatic melanoma. *Cancer* 1995;75:2251–2257.

182. Murray JL, Rosenblum MG, Lamki L, et al. Enhancement of tumor uptake of ^{111}indium-labeled anti-melanoma monoclonal antibody 96.5 in melanoma patients receiving partially purified alpha interferon. *Proc Am Soc Clin Oncol* 1986;5:226.

183. Larson SM, Carasquillo JA, Krohn KA, et al. Localization of p97 specific Fab fragments in human melanoma as a basis for immunotherapy. *J Clin Invest* 1983;72:2101–2114.

184. Bigner DD, Brown M, Coleman RE, et al. Phase I studies of treatment of malignant gliomas and neoplastic meningitis with 131I-radiolabeled monoclonal antibodies anti-tenascin 81C6 and anti-chondroitin proteoglycan sulfate Mel-14 F (ab′)2—a preliminary report. *J Neuro-Oncol* 1995;24:109–122.

185. Laske DW, Muraszko KM, Oldfield EH, et al. Intraventricular immunotoxin therapy for leptomeningeal neoplasia. *Neurosurgery* 1997;41:1039–1049(discussion 1049–1051).

186. Kageshita T, Chen ZJ, Kim J-W, et al. Murine anti-idiotypic monoclonal antibodies to syngeneic antihuman high molecular weight-melanoma associated antigen monoclonal antibodies: development, characterization and clinical applications. *Pigment Cell Res Suppl* 1988;1:185–191.

187. Livingston PO, Adluri S, Raychaudhuri S, et al. A phase I trial of the immunological adjuvant SAFm in melanoma patients vaccinated with the anti-idiotype antibody MELIMMUNE-1. *Vaccine Res* 1994;12(14):1275–1280.

188. Quan WDY Jr, Dean GE, Stevenson L, et al. Phase I/II trial of anti-idiotype antibody MelImmune™ temurtide in metastatic melanoma. *Proc Am Assoc Cancer Res* 1993;34:476.

189. Yao T-J, Meyers M, Livingston PO, et al. Immunization of melanoma patients with BEC2-Keyhole limpet hemocyanin plus BCG intradermally followed by intravenous booster immunizations with BEC2 to induce anti-GD3 ganglioside antibodies. *Clin Cancer Res* 1999;5:77–81.

190. McCaffery M, Yao T-J, Williams L, et al. Enhanced immunogenicity of BEC2 anti-idiotypic monoclonal antibody that mimics GD3 ganglioside when combined with adjuvant. *Clin Cancer Res* 1996;2:679–686.

15.4

MONOCLONAL ANTIBODIES: CLINICAL APPLICATIONS

Breast Cancer and Other Adenocarcinomas

MARGARET VON MEHREN
LOUIS M. WEINER

The primary impetus behind the development of therapeutic and diagnostic strategies using monoclonal antibodies (MAb) has been the specific targeting properties of these molecules. The development of hybridoma technology (1) ushered in a new era in antibody therapy. It allowed the production of significant amounts of MAb for evaluation as oncologic therapeutic agents. Since the early 1990s, the ability to alter antibody structures and binding capabilities through protein engineering has further allowed the development of effective cancer therapies. An increasing number of antibodies are available for both diagnostic purposes and for therapy. This chapter focuses on antibody-based therapeutic agents and strategies for the treatment of solid tumors, with a primary focus on breast cancer. The fundamentals of therapeutic antibody structures and their limitations are discussed. The diagnostic utility of antibodies in pathology and radiology are reviewed. Targets on adenocarcinomas and therapeutic antibodies are discussed.

BASICS OF ANTIBODIES

The structures of antibody-based therapeutic agents have expanded with the development of recombinant engineering technology (Fig. 1). Most therapeutic antibodies are IgG molecules, which contain two heavy chains with covalent linkages to two smaller light chains (see Fig. 1). Within each of these chains are constant and variable domains. The specificity of the antibody-binding site is conferred by these variable domains, as is the strength (affinity) with which the antibody binds to its target. The advent of phage display library techniques has also allowed for rapid screening and production of useful antibodies (2). Additionally, site-directed mutagenesis techniques and chain-shuffling have allowed for the production of antibodies with greater binding capacity for a particular antigen, which may allow for greater retention of antibodies at tumor sites (3).

Enzymatic digestion and recombinant engineering techniques have led to the production and testing of smaller antibody-based structures (4), which are better able to reach tumor targets, but also are cleared more rapidly via renal excretion (5) (Fig. 2). Enzymatic digestion of the Fc portion of the antibody molecule produces Fab or $F(ab')_2$ fragments (6,7). Recombinant technology has facilitated the production of single-chain Fv (scFv) fragments, which contain the variable domains of both the light and heavy chains, connected by a short amino acid link. A bivalent form of an scFv can be constructed by adding carboxy terminal cystine residues to scFv, followed by chemical conjugation of two scFv, yielding a covalently linked structure $(scFv')_2$. These smaller structures overcome some of the limitations of larger antibody structures, as discussed in the section Limitations to Antibodies, and therefore are ideal candidates for imaging. Other antibody fragments have also been developed, but have had limited clinical applications to date and therefore are not reviewed here.

The ability to alter protein structures allows for the production of antibodies with altered constant or variable domains, or with additional moieties. Initially, antibodies were derived by immunizing an animal, usually a mouse, with a human antigen, followed by the production of large quantities of antibodies by hybridomas obtained by the fusion of murine splenocytes with myeloma cell lines (1). The antigenicity of such murine antibodies limits some therapeutic applications in humans. The variable domains of an antibody can now be cloned into human constant domain regions, markedly decreasing the antigenicity of the antibody (8). This allows for repeated administration of these agents without inducing an immune response that rapidly clears the infused antibodies. Antibodies also can be modified by adding additional protein structures. For example, immunomodulatory compounds that can activate the immune system, such as superantigens (9), immunotoxin (10), or cytokines (11) have been produced as chemical conjugates or fusion proteins. Radioactive elements have long been conjugated to antibodies, allowing for targeted

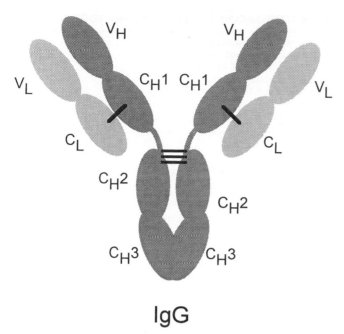

V_H V_H

V_L C_H1 C_H1 V_L

C_L C_L

C_H2 C_H2

C_H3 C_H3

IgG

FIGURE 1. Schematic diagram of an immunoglobulin G (IgG) molecule. There are two heavy chains consisting of one variable chain (V_H) and three constant domains (C_H1–3) linked by three interchain disulfide bonds. Linked to the heavy variable and first constant domain is the light chain, which also contains a variable and constant chain. The antigen-binding site is contained within the variable chains.

radiation. Similar approaches to target chemotherapeutic agents have been attempted, particularly with enzymes to activate prodrugs (12), thus targeting the tumor site for drug activation. Another pretargeting strategy uses antitumor antibodies fused to streptavidin (13–15). Then a biotinylated compound such as a cytokine, drug, or radioactive compound can be selectively accumulated at antibody-pretargeted tumor sites due to the high-affinity interaction between streptavidin and biotin. This approach may limit the toxicity associated with cytokines, chemotherapeutic agents, and radiation.

Another advance has been the development of bispecific antibodies (BsAb), which consist of two antibodies with specificity for distinct antigens (16). These constructs have been synthesized by covalently linking two MAb (17) or MAbFv (18) by the production of hybrid hybridomas (19), or by engineering recombinant bispecific molecules (20). This allows for the targeting of two different tumor antigens found on tumor cells or the simultaneous engagement of a tumor-associated antigen and a cytotoxic trigger molecule on effector cells. The rationale for the first approach is the hypothesis that the binding of two different antigens on tumor cells enhances targeting selectivity or may interrupt normal cellular metabolism by interfering with the function of either or both ligands (21). The second approach allows for targeting of an immune effector cell directly to a tumor cell, enhancing the immune response against the tumor. The majority of BsAb are of the latter type. A third strategy has been to combine a tumor-targeting antibody and an antibody with specificity for a thera-

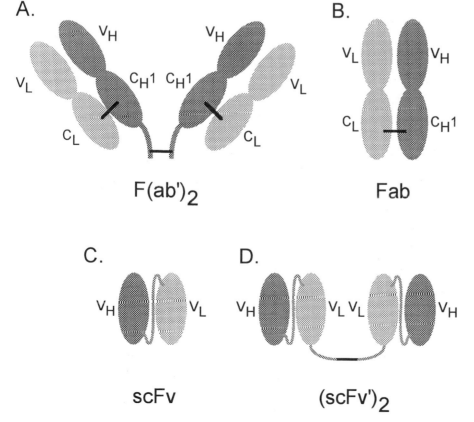

A.

V_H V_H

V_L C_H1 C_H1 V_L

C_L C_L

$F(ab')_2$

B.

V_L V_H

C_L C_H1

Fab

C.

V_H V_L

scFv

D.

V_H V_L V_L V_H

$(scFv')_2$

FIGURE 2. Schematic representations of smaller antibody structures. Diagrams **(A)** and **(B)** represent structures that are produced by enzymatic digestion of an immunoglobulin G molecule, whereas structures **(C)** and **(D)** are derived by recombinant engineering. These structures have mono- **(B and C)** or bivalent **(A and D)** antigen-binding site(s). A bivalent binding site is produced in an (scFv')$_2$ by adding a cysteine-containing linker to the carboxy terminus of the V_L chain of an scFv to allow two scFv to bond via a disulfide bond.

peutic agent to specifically target the drug or radiotherapeutic compound at tumor. Many of these molecules still are undergoing preclinical testing, while others have reached clinical trials and are discussed later in this chapter.

MECHANISMS OF TUMOR KILLING BY ANTIBODIES

Antibodies may direct antitumor effects by inducing apoptosis (22), interfering with ligand-receptor interactions (23), or by preventing the expression of proteins that are critical to the neoplastic phenotype. Antibodies have been developed to target receptors whose ligands are growth factors, such as the epidermal growth factor receptor. The antibody thus inhibits natural ligands that stimulate cell growth of the cell from binding to targeted tumor cells. Alternatively, antibodies may induce an antiidiotype network (24), complement-mediated cytotoxicity (25), or antibody-dependent cellular cytotoxicity (ADCC) (26). An antiidiotypic network results from the recognition of the antibody, called *Ab1*, by the host immune system. The antigenic binding site within the variable regions of the antibody is seen as foreign. When an antibody, termed *Ab2*, is formed against this binding site, it recapitulates the three-dimensional structure of the antigen targeted by Ab1. This chain of events can keep occurring, thus perpetuating the immune response against the primary antigen (27,28). Some classes of immunoglobulins (Ig) can activate complement or natural killer (NK) cells. The first component of the complement cascade, C1, is capable of binding the Fc portion of IgM and IgG molecules. C1 activation triggers the classical complement cascade, leading to the recruitment of phagocytic cells and death of the antibody-bound cells. This process occurs more efficiently with IgM molecules, but can also occur if IgG molecules are clustered on the cell surface. Cells coated by IgG1 or IgG3 isotype antibodies can also activate effector cells via the binding of the terminal Fc portion of the antibody to Fc receptors, found on NK cells, neutrophils, mononuclear phagocytes, some T cells, and eosinophils. ADCC occurs with the release of cytoplasmic granules containing perforins and granzymes from these effector cells. Some BsAb have been developed to facilitate ADCC by targeting a tumor antigen and an Fc receptor on immune effector cells and are discussed in the section Bispecific Antibody Therapy.

LIMITATIONS TO ANTIBODIES

Initial clinical trials with MAb led to some striking examples of antitumor effects (29), but the majority has served to illustrate the obstacles to successful therapy (Table 1). Most of the MAb used in clinical trials have been derived from mice, and patients exposed to them have developed human antimouse antibody (HAMA) responses, thus limiting the number of treatments patients can receive (30). Some tumor antigens are shed or secreted. Antibodies targeting these antigens bind their target in the circulation, limiting the amount of unbound antibody available to bind to tumor (31). Barriers impede antibody distribution within tumors, such as (a) disor-

TABLE 1. OBSTACLES TO EFFECTIVE ANTIBODY THERAPY

Immunogenicity of xenogeneic antibodies
Shedding of antigen into circulation
Disordered vasculature in tumors
Increased hydrostatic pressure in tumors
Heterogeneity of antigen on tumor surface
Limited numbers of effector cells at tumor
Immunosuppressive tumor microenvironment

dered vasculature, (b) increased hydrostatic pressure within tumors, and (c) heterogeneity of antigen distribution within tumors (32). Due to these barriers, the length of time for an IgG molecule to travel 1 mm and 1 cm in a tumor has been estimated to be 2 days and 7 to 8 months, respectively. Estimates for a smaller molecule, such as an Fab fragment, are 1 day or 2 months to travel 1 mm or 1 cm, respectively. If antibodies do reach their targets, there is little evidence that they efficiently mediate *in vivo* antibody-dependent cytotoxicity. For this to occur, sufficient numbers of effector cells, such as macrophages, NK cells, or cytotoxic T cells, must be present in the tumor (33). Finally, many tumors are known to secrete compounds that down-regulate the immune response (34,35), or have decreased effector cells as a consequence of hypoxia (36). Despite these impediments, preclinical and clinical data with improved antibody-based molecules continue to demonstrate an emerging role for antibody-based therapy as a component of the oncologic armamentarium.

TARGETS FOR ANTIBODY THERAPY

Any structure on the surface of a cancer cell can be a target for binding by an antibody. An optimal antigenic target for a therapeutic antibody is unique to tumor cells or is significantly overexpressed on tumor cells relative to normal cells. The antigen selected should not be shed into the circulation, because it binds to antibody before the therapeutic vehicle can reach tumor sites. The targeted protein should not be internalized when bound by the antibody if the antibodies are to mediate ADCC and complement-mediated cytotoxicity. However, an internalized antigen is desirable as a target for immunotoxins or radiolabeled antibodies. The following describes antigens found on adenocarcinomas, particularly on breast cancers.

HER-2/*neu* (c-erbB-2)

The *neu* proto-oncogene encodes for a receptor tyrosine kinase. It is part of the Heregulin (HER) family, consisting of epidermal growth factor receptor, HER-2/*neu*, HER-3 and HER-4 (37). HER-2/*neu* was discovered by detecting a murine humoral response to a 185-kd protein after inoculation of mice with rat tumors stimulated by *in utero* nitrosoethylurea injections (38). The human homologue was discovered due to its similarity to HER-2/*neu* (39–41). The protein receptor, when transfected into fibroblasts, transformed the phenotype of these cells (42,43). The endogenous ligand is unknown. However, HER-2/*neu* has been shown to mediate intracellular signals when dimerized with HER-3 and HER-4, or when bound with heregulin (44,45). Unlike the normal cellular homologue, which is not oncogenic, HER-2/*neu* contains a point mutation in the transmembrane portion of the molecule (46,47). Inserting truncated forms of HER-2/*neu* or overexpressing protein in the cell results in a transformed phenotype (48). In human tissues, HER-2/*neu* is detected in secretory epithelial tissues and the basal layer of skin (49,50). HER-2/*neu* also is overexpressed in approximately 30% of adenocarcinomas (51–55) of the lung, gastrointestinal tract, breast, and ovary. It is also found in comedo, large cell, and ductal carcinoma *in situ* (56). HER-2/*neu* has become a target for antibody-based therapies because of its role in oncogenesis and its relative overexpression in particular tumor types compared with normal host tissues.

Epidermal Growth Factor Receptor

Epidermal growth factor receptor (EGFR) is a 170-kd transmembrane glycoprotein that is overexpressed in many carcinomas, including 40% of breast cancers and many human gliomas (57). This receptor has a number of ligands, including epidermal growth factor (EGF) and transforming growth factor (TGF). Overexpression of EGFR and its ligands has been found in breast carcinoma cell lines and human carcinomas, providing evidence for the existence of an autocrine growth loop (58–60).

The most common mutant form of the receptor, EGFRvIII, has a deletion of exons 2 to 7 resulting in a truncated extracellular domain. The variant receptor is not found on normal tissues, but has been found on gliomas (61), non–small-cell lung cancer (62), and ovarian and breast cancer (63). Transfection with this mutant form results in transformation of fibroblasts (64), likely due to the constitutive activation of the c-Jun N-terminal kinase pathway (65). Evidence also exists for increased activation of phosphatidylinositol 3-kinase, which when blocked results in the loss of anchorage-independent growth and morphologic reversion of transformed cells (66). This mutant form is associated with drug resistance due to decreased apoptosis (67). When this receptor is bound, it leads to receptor internalization (68).

Carcinoembryonic Antigen

Carcinoembryonic antigen (CEA) is an 18-kd glycoprotein present on endodermally derived neoplasms and in the digestive organs of the human fetus (69,70). CEA is a member of the immunoglobulin superfamily located on chromosome 19 and is thought to be involved with intercellular interactions (71). CEA is thought to be an adhesion molecule, and may allow tumor cells to attach to normal cells in the metastatic process (72). Targeting CEA therefore may be important in the prevention of metastases. CEA is reported to be expressed in 68% to 88% of breast adenocarcinomas (73), the majority of colorectal adenocarcinomas, and in lung and gastric adenocarcinomas.

Carbohydrate Targets

Carbohydrate and mucin molecules are found on cell surfaces. Lewis-Y (Le^y) is a carbohydrate antigen found on the surface of many carcinomas, including breast (74), lung (75,76), ovary

(77), gastric (78), colorectal (79), and prostate. Its presence has been correlated with apoptosis in both normal and malignant cells (80). In colon cancer, its expression may correlate with lymph node metastasis (81). Mucin molecules, also termed *polymorphic epithelial mucins*, are found on most carcinoma cells and differ from those found on normal cell surfaces as a result of incomplete glycosylation (82). The carbohydrate side chains are shorter, thus exposing the core peptide and glycopeptide determinants (83). The core amino acid sequence of these mucins has a sequence of 20 amino acids that are repeated. Many antimucin antibodies recognize an immunodominant epitope within this repeated sequence (84,85). Patients with breast and pancreatic carcinoma have been reported to develop specific cytotoxic T-cell responses against the mucin core (86), suggesting that these carbohydrate antigens may be good targets for antiidiotypic antibody therapy. One mucin antigen, MUC-1, is shed into the serum of patients with breast and ovarian cancer (87) and may not be the ideal antibody target. Another glycoprotein, termed *gp72*, has been found on colorectal, gastric, and ovarian cancer (88). Several antibodies have also been developed against human milk-fat globules found on normal and malignant breast epithelium (89).

Ep-CAM (EGP-2 or GA 733-2)

A series of murine antibodies, identified by immunizing mice with cell lines from gastrointestinal cancers, have been found to recognize closely related tumor-associated epitopes. These antibodies detect a 38-kd surface glycoprotein variously referred to as *Ep-CAM*, *EGP-2*, or *GA733-2*. The normal distribution of Ep-CAM is on the basolateral surface of nonsquamous epithelium of the lower respiratory tract, lower gastrointestinal tract, tubules of the kidney, surface epithelium of the ovary, exocrine and endocrine pancreas, hair follicles, secretory tubules of sweat glands, bile ducts, and thymic epithelium. Ep-CAM expression also is associated with various cancers such as those derived from the colon, rectum, pancreas, lung, and breast. Although the antigen is abundantly expressed, it is not shed in the circulation (90). Ep-CAM has been shown to have homology to proteins involved with cell-to-cell, as well as cell-to-matrix interactions. Cells transfected with this gene demonstrate enhanced *in vitro* intercellular adhesion (91).

Transferrin Receptor

The transferrin receptor is comprised of two identical transmembrane subunits that are linked by disulfide bonds and is constitutively expressed on all cells. Its expression is controlled both by posttranscriptional iron response elements on messenger RNA and at the transcriptional level. When the receptor complexes with a ligand, it is rapidly internalized via endocytosis. The ligand is altered in the acidic pH of the endosome and becomes unbound in the endosome cytosol. The endosome is then recycled within minutes (92). The rapid internalization and regeneration on the cell surface makes this receptor ideal for targeting drugs, toxins, or radioisotopes conjugated to antibodies. Transferrin receptors are expressed on breast carcinoma cells (93).

In summary, these proteins and glycoproteins provide targets for antibody therapies. Some of these proteins are found on normal cells, but are overexpressed on tumor cells, such as EGFR and HER-2. They have been shown *in vitro* to transform cells. Some targets are utilized due to changes in the target associated with malignant cells only, as seen with the carbohydrate antigens. Others have been targeted because of rapid internalization of ligands bound to them, such as the transferrin receptor. This provides a means to deliver toxins or chemotherapeutic agents specifically into targeted cells.

ANTIBODIES AS DIAGNOSTIC TOOLS

The specific binding properties of antibodies has led to their extensive use in the diagnosis of cancers. They are mainstays in the pathologic diagnosis of malignancy, allowing for discrimination of histologically similar cancers. For example, CEA is expressed by most adenocarcinomas, not only by those of the gastrointestinal tract (94,95). D-14 MAb, directed against a specific epitope of CEA, has been shown to be specific for colon cancers, but not for ovarian adenocarcinomas (96). Cytokeratin-7 is used to distinguish ovarian cancers from colon cancers (97). Antibodies to detect estrogen (ER) and progesterone (PR) receptors are used to identify breast cancer primary lesions, although one or both receptors can be found on other cancers (98–100).

Immunochemistry has also been used to provide prognostic information about the cancer being evaluated. This is particularly true in breast cancers, in which routine evaluation for prognostic factors influences therapeutic decisions. ER and PR are evaluated to determine if the patient is eligible for hormonal therapy, but the presence of PR positivity also has prognostic value, as patients with hormone receptor–negative tumors have poorer outcomes (101,102). The presence of PR is the most reliable predictor of survival in endometrial carcinoma (103). Mutations in p53 result in a longer protein half-life that can be detected by immunohistochemistry. p53 Expression in breast cancer is associated with a poorer prognosis (104) and is inversely correlated with response to chemotherapy (105). Ki-67, a marker of cell proliferation, has prognostic relevance in breast (106) and non–small-cell lung cancers (107). Expression of Ki-67 in colon cancer is only associated with metastatic disease (108). High levels of HER-2/*neu* expression have also been correlated with a poorer prognosis in breast cancer (109,110), non–small cell lung cancer (111), and in FIGO III and IV ovarian cancer (112). In breast cancer patients, overexpression is associated with poor response to chemotherapy (113); it is also assessed to determine a patient's candidacy for treatment with trastuzumab (Herceptin), as will be discussed.

The use of antibodies in radiologic diagnostic procedures offers promise, but to date has not been shown to be significantly superior to other available modalities. Antibodies labeled with radioactive agents can be systemically administered to detect disease (114). The distribution of radiolabels can be measured using gamma counters, single-photon emission computed tomography, or radioactive probes (115). The foremost examples of this technology are the OncoScint CR/OV scan, used to detect CEA-expressing tumors, and ProstaScint, used to detect prostate-specific membrane antigen in men with adenocarcinoma of the prostate (116). Studies evaluating CEA and human milk fat globulin antibodies have been done in breast cancer patients at presentation as well as at disease recurrence (117–119). The antibodies detected lesions, including primary cancers smaller than 1 cm in size, but had 90% to 63% sensitivity in detecting lymph node metastases. The pancarcinoma antibody NR-LU-10 has also undergone evaluation for staging of small-cell lung cancer (120) and in a variety of adenocarcinomas (121). Compared with standard radiographic techniques, the technetium-99m-labeled antibody was able to detect 88% of known lesions, but missed some lesions smaller than 2 cm in size. The antibody can detect metastatic bone disease in patients with positive bone marrow biopsies (122).

Another approach used for diagnosis is pretargeted immunoscintigraphy utilizing a biotinylated antibody, followed by avidin and, subsequently, indium-111 (^{111}In)–labeled biotin. This approach has been evaluated in ovarian cancer (123), medullary thyroid cancer (124), pituitary adenomas (125), other endocrine tumors (126), and lung cancer (127). A higher rate of detection of endocrine tumors occurred using the pretargeted strategy compared with standard radiographic techniques.

More recently, radiolabeled antibodies have been applied to radioimmunoguided surgery (RIGS), improving the completeness of surgical resections by detecting occult disease because micrometastatic disease may be missed by radiographic studies or standard surgical exploration (128,129). An initial problem with this strategy has been the length of time required between the administration of the antibody until surgery was performed to allow background radioactivity to clear from the body. $F(ab')_2$ or Fab', which clear more rapidly from the circulation due to their smaller sizes, may address this problem. RIGS has been used primarily in patients with colorectal carcinoma, but has also been evaluated in breast and pancreatic carcinomas (130). Because cancers have variable antigen expression, a cocktail of radiolabeled antibodies may lead to increased sensitivity of RIGS (131). At the present time, no studies have compared these techniques to determine if one approach is superior to the others.

MONOCLONAL ANTIBODY THERAPY IN BREAST AND OTHER ADENOCARCINOMAS

Breast cancer has been the focus of considerable research, particularly since the early 1990s. New chemotherapeutic agents have clearly impacted on survival in the metastatic disease setting, with some suggestion of improved disease-free survival in the adjuvant setting as well. The strides in breast cancer therapy have not been limited to standard therapeutic agents. RhuMAb HER-2 antibody therapy has clearly resulted in responses in metastatic disease, as well as improved response and duration of disease-free progression when combined with chemotherapy. Antibody therapy in other adenocarcinomas has also been evaluated. Antibody 17-1A, which recognizes Ep-CAM, has been

TABLE 2. 17-1A CLINICAL TRIALS

Phase	Dose/Schedule	Disease	No. of Patients	Responses	References
1	25–200 mg i.v.	Met GI	4	1 MR	Sears (152)
1	15–1,000 mg i.v.	Met GI	20	3 CR	Sears (153)
1	200 mg i.v.[a]	Met GI	22	None	Verrill (154)
1	400 mg i.v.	Met GI	25	NR	Khazaeli (155)
1	400 mg i.v.	Met GI	20	NR	Lobuglio (156)
1	400 mg i.v. with FAM chemotherapy	Pancreas	16 (eight patients 17-1A only)	2 PR (chemotherapy and 17-1A)	Paul (157)
1	400 mg i.v.	Pancreas	25	4	Sindelar (158)
2	200–850 mg i.v.	Colorectal	20	1 CR	Sears (159)
2	500 mg i.v. t.i.w. × 8 wk	Pancreas	28	1 PR	Weiner (160)
2	GM-CSF d 1–10 with 400 mg i.v. d 3	Colorectal	20	2 CR	Ragnhammar (161)
2	IFN-γ d 1–15 i.v. with 400 mg i.v. d 5,7,9,12	Met colorectal	15	None	Saleh (162)
2	IFN-γ d 1–4 i.v. with 150 mg i.v. d 2–4	Colorectal	19	None	Weiner (163)
2	IFN-γ d 1–4 i.v. with 150 mg i.v. d 2–4	Pancreas	30	1 CR	Tempero (164)
3	500 mg i.v. × 1, then 100 mg i.v. q4wk × 4	Dukes' C colorectal	189	Improved DFS and OS	Reithmuller (165)

CR, complete response; DFS, disease-free survival; FAM, 5-fluorouracil, adriamycin, mitomycin; GI, gastrointestinal; GM-CSF, granulocyte-macrophage colony-stimulating factor; IFN-γ, interferon-γ; Met, metastatic; NR, not reported; OS, overall survival; PR, partial response.
[a]Antibody was mixed with leukopheresed mononuclear cells preinfusion.

extensively tested with studies, suggesting benefit in the adjuvant therapy of colon cancer.

HER-2/*neu* (c-erbB-2)

HER-2/*neu* (c-erbB-2), a member of the EGFR family, has been targeted for antibody therapy as it is overexpressed on approximately 25% of breast cancers. RhuMAb HER-2 (132), also known as *trastuzumab* (Herceptin), is a humanized antibody derived from 4D5, a murine monoclonal antibody, which recognizes an epitope on the extracellular domain of HER-2/*neu*. In a phase 2 trial in women with metastatic breast cancer, there was an objective response rate of 11.6%, with responses seen in the liver, mediastinum, lymph nodes, and chest wall. Patients received ten or more treatments with the antibody, and none developed an antibody response against RhuMAb HER-2. In a second phase 2 study, 222 women with metastatic breast cancer were treated with 2 mg per kg of RhuMAb HER-2 weekly, with an objective response rate of 16% (133). The median response duration was 9.1 months, with a median overall survival of 13 months, both of which are superior to outcomes reported for second-line chemotherapy in metastatic disease. In each of these trials, approximately 30% of the patients had stable disease lasting more than 5 months. Intriguingly, preclinical studies have demonstrated decreased expression of vascular endothelial cell growth factor and vascular permeability factor with 4D5 therapy, suggesting that an antiangiogenesis mechanism may account for some of the clinical impact of this antibody (134). RhuMAb HER-2 continues to be evaluated clinically in diverse adenocarcinoma types.

The results of a large randomized phase 3 trial comparing cytotoxic chemotherapy alone or with RhuMAb HER-2 have been reported in abstract form (135). Patients receiving initial therapy for metastatic breast cancer were treated with doxorubicin or epirubicin and cyclophosphamide, or with paclitaxel if they had received an anthracycline in the adjuvant setting. Patients were randomized to receive this chemotherapy alone or in combination with weekly antibody therapy. Response rates

for combination therapy with an anthracycline regimen increased from 43% to 52% with the addition of RhuMAb HER-2. Using paclitaxel, response rates increased from 16% to 42% with the addition of RhuMAb HER-2. Myocardial dysfunction was observed with increased frequency in patients receiving doxorubicin or epirubicin when RhuMAb HER 2 was added. Therefore, RhuMAb HER-2 is not recommended in combination with anthracyclines. Based on these clinical trial results, RhuMAb HER-2 has been approved by the U.S. Food and Drug Administration for the treatment of women with metastatic breast cancer with HER-2/*neu* overexpression given either alone or in combination with paclitaxel. RhuMAb HER-2 is being evaluated in combination with other chemotherapeutic drugs and in other adenocarcinomas that overexpress HER-2/*neu*.

Ep-CAM (EGP-2 and GA 733-2)

The 17-1A antibody, which recognizes Ep-CAM, has undergone extensive clinical testing, with some studies suggesting efficacy in colorectal carcinomas (Table 2). Initial trials used a murine antibody, with more recent trials using a human chimeric construct suppressing the development of HAMA responses. The chimeric antibody results in greater human peripheral mononuclear cell–mediated ADCC compared with the original murine MAb (136). Initial human studies with the chimeric antibody revealed a prolonged half-life compared with the murine antibody, no HAMA development, and radiolocalization to known sites of disease (137). Clinical trials have also incorporated cytokines because of *in vitro* data that suggest increased apoptosis when 17-1A is used in conjunction with interferon-γ (IFN-γ) (138). There is also *in vitro* evidence of increased ADCC with IFN-γ (139), granulocyte-macrophage colony-stimulating factor (GM-CSF) (140,141), the combination of GM-CSF and interleukin-2 (IL-2) (142), interleukin-4 (IL-4) (143), and interleukin-8 (IL-8) (144). The therapeutic use of this antibody has also been shown to induce potentially effective antiidiotypic antibodies (145–147); concomitant therapy with GM-CSF increased the induction of the antiidiotypic response (148) as well as increased infiltration of macrophages, CD4+ and CD8+ T cells within tumors (149). Induction of T cells against antiidiotypic epitopes has also been evaluated by proliferation assays, IFN-γ production, and delayed-type hypersensitivity reactions (150). Five of ten patients with antiidiotypic antibodies were also found to have induction of EP-CAM antigen–specific T cells. T cells were isolated from these samples and four patients demonstrated a proliferative response when stimulated with an antiidiotypic antibody *in vitro*. These four patients were reported to have clinical responses as well, in contrast to the six patients without evidence of T cells against antiidiotypic epitopes.

Initial phase 1 studies with 17-1A yielded promising results. Several studies demonstrated responses in patients with metastatic cancers of the gastrointestinal tract with only one intravenous dose of antibody. One patient received an intrahepatic infusion of autologous mononuclear cells mixed with 17-1A with regression of hepatic metastases. Antibody therapy was well tolerated with mild nausea, vomiting, or diarrhea. Phase 2 studies in colon and pancreatic cancers were less encouraging. Repeat dose injections and combinations with cytokines to enhance effector cell number and activity did not result in significant response rates, although *in vitro* assays of patient effector cells revealed increased activity with cytokine therapy. Repeat dose schedules with higher doses were theorized to induce tolerance to the murine antibody; however, this maneuver had no significant impact on the induction of HAMA. Evidence did exist of induction of antiidiotypic antibodies, with some trials showing a correlation with response. The overall lack of efficacy seen in these studies may have resulted from the large tumor burden or the associated immunosuppression seen in these patients with metastatic disease.

The initial study evaluating 17-1A in the adjuvant setting suggested the possibility of efficacy. A phase 3 clinical trial of patients with lymph-node positive colorectal cancer randomized patients to observation or therapy with 17-1A. The surgical approach was standardized and agreed to by all participating surgeons. All patients were followed postoperatively in a similar manner, irrespective of treatment. One hundred and eighty-nine patients were randomized, with 166 patients evaluated for overall survival and disease-free survival. Therapy with 17-1A was well tolerated except for malaise, low-grade fevers and chills, and mild gastrointestinal discomfort. Four episodes of anaphylactic reactions were treated without sequelae. At 5 years of follow-up, the death rate was 36% in the 17-1A group in contrast to 51% in the observation group, and the calculated recurrence rate was 48.7% versus 66.5% (165). At 7 years the death rates were 43% (17-1A) and 63% (controls), and the calculated recurrence rates were 52% and 68%, respectively, demonstrating a continued benefit in patients who received 17-1A (151). Treatment with 17-1A was associated with a decreased incidence of metastatic disease, but did not alter the incidence of local failure. This shift in failure pattern was thought to represent the ability of 17-1A to eradicate isolated metastatic cancer cells, but not bulkier disease. Alternatively, altered vasculature due to surgery and scar tissue may have limited antibody diffusion to tumor cells at the primary site. Another factor potentially accounting for the apparent lack of efficacy of 17-1A on local con-

trol is that 11 patients in the observation group received pre- or postoperative radiation therapy alone or in combination with chemotherapy. This trial has been criticized because of the higher rates of recurrence and death in the control arm than would be anticipated. Irrespective of these criticisms, this study is intriguing in demonstrating an effect of antibody-based therapy in the adjuvant setting of colorectal cancer. Current clinical trials are designed to confirm these results in stage II colon cancers and to test the value of adding 17-1A to standard chemotherapy in patients with stage III disease. Therapy with antibodies alone is likely not to be effective in all patients due to the antigenic heterogeneity of cancer cells. Combining standard adjuvant therapy with 17-1A would introduce therapies that have different mechanisms of action, are cell-cycle dependent and independent, and allow for death of cancer cells irrespective of antigen expression patterns.

Epidermal Growth Factor Receptor

EGFR is overexpressed on many cancers. The receptor and its ligands EGF and tumor necrosis factor–α (TNF-α) act in an autocrine loop to stimulate the growth of breast cancer cells. *In vitro*, some anti-EGFR antibodies have been shown to inhibit the binding of the receptor ligands (166,167). Antibodies that block the binding of EGFR ligands limit receptor activation by tyrosine kinases and inhibit growth of normal fibroblasts (168) as well as tumor cells in culture (169). Also, combining anti-EGFR antibodies with cisplatin leads to a significant decrease in the concentration that inhibits 50% of cisplatin (170), and cures of established tumors are seen when anti-EGFR antibodies are combined with cisplatin (171) or doxorubicin (172). *In vitro* and *in vivo* studies have also suggested that anti-EGFR antibodies may lead to terminal differentiation of squamous cell carcinoma cells, with accumulation of cells in G0-G1 phases of the cell cycle and expression of cell surface markers such as involucrin and cytokeratin-10 (173).

The anti-EGFR antibody MAb 225 blocks *in vitro* phosphorylation of the EGFR and induces receptor internalization as occurs with binding of the natural ligand (174). However, receptor processing is slower with antibody engagement than with natural ligand engagement (175). Smaller bivalent F(ab')₂ and univalent Fab' forms of this antibody also inhibit growth and decrease receptor phosphorylation, although the bivalent form is superior to the monovalent form (176). Because the smaller fragments lead to tumor regressions, the efficacy of antibody therapy is not dependent on ADCC, as these smaller fragments lack the Fc portion of the antibody required for ADCC. Rather, the efficacy of this antibody is due to its ability to inhibit binding of the natural ligand, limit receptor phosphorylation and thus downstream signals, and induce receptor internalization.

The chimeric form of MAb225, C225, has been evaluated *in vitro* and *in vivo* in hormone-sensitive and hormone-refractory prostate cancer (177). EGF is a strong chemoattractant for prostate cancer. Blocking the EGFR receptor with C225 *in vitro* results in decreased migration of prostate cancer cells in a dose-dependent manner due to decreased phosphorylation of the EGFR (178). This antibody has also been shown to lead to cell cycle arrest and decreased proliferation of prostate cancer cells (179,180). The binding of C225 to the EGFR results in multi-

ple events, leading to a decrease in proliferation and possibly decreased metastatic potential in prostate cancer. It has also been shown to inhibit the expression of vascular endothelial cell growth factor and vascular permeability factor, both involved in the induction of angiogenesis (134).

C225 has been tested in phase 1 studies in recurrent head and neck cancer in combination with cisplatin. Four out of seven patients demonstrated responses, three of whom had failed prior cisplatin therapy (181). C225 is currently undergoing phase 1 testing in combination with paclitaxel in women with stage IV breast cancer. ICR62, a rat monoclonal IgG, has been shown *in vitro* to block binding of the ligands of EGFR, inhibit growth of tumor cell lines that overexpress EGFR, and to cause differentiation of malignant cells to a normal phenotype. This antibody was evaluated in a phase 1 trial of patients with squamous head and neck and lung cancer. Evidence existed of localization of antibody to tumor sites at dosages of 40 to 100 mg and development of antirat antibodies (182). Another anti-EGFR antibody, RG 83853, has been used to treat patients with non–small cell lung cancer and head and neck cancer in a phase 1 setting. In this study, patients received up to 600 mg per m^2 by continuous infusion over 5 days without significant toxicity (183). Saturation of at least 50% of the EGFR at dosages of 200 mg per m^2 or more occurred. EGFR-expressing tumor cells demonstrate increased sensitivity to chemotherapy (184) and to radiation therapy (185) in the presence of EGF. In two of five patients with pre- and posttherapy biopsies of tumor, there was evidence for increased tyrosine kinase activity of EGFR, which provided rationale for combined modality therapy.

Carbohydrate Antigens

Carbohydrate antigens classically are described as poor immunogens and have not been used extensively as immunologic targets. However, by demonstrating the immunogenicity of such antigens as Le^y and the carcinoma-associated mucin epitopes Tf (β-D-Gal-(1-3)-α-GalNAc), Tn (*N*-acetyl-D-galactosamine-α-O-Ser/Thr), sialyl-Tn (dAcNeuα2-6(GalNAc-*O*-Ser/Thr), and MUC-1, these antigens have proved useful as targets for cancer therapy.

Lewis Antigens

Le^y antigen, which is expressed on 75% of breast adenocarcinomas, is recognized by ABL 364 (186). In a study treating breast cancer patients with bone metastases, patients were randomized to receive antibody therapy or albumin infusions. The number of metastatic cells selectively decreased in patients treated with the antibody and not albumin, especially those whose bone marrow samples contained a large percentage of malignant cells at baseline. Reduction in the number of malignant cells in patients with less bone marrow involvement was not demonstrable, likely due to a sampling error.

Le^x, also known as *CD15*, has been used as a target on granulocytes as well as breast cancer cells (187). FC-2.15, which recognizes Le^x, was used to treat 11 patients with advanced malignancies. One patient with metastatic breast cancer demonstrated a partial response (188). All patients demonstrated a transient neutropenia that developed within 1 hour of initiating the antibody infusion and resolved within 1 hour of ending the infusion. One patient's course was complicated by the development of *Pseudomonas* bacteremia.

Other Le^y and Le^x antibodies have been developed. B1, anti-Le^y and B3, which identifies Le^y, di-Le^x and tri-Le^x antigens, have been shown to have minimal reactivity with normal tissues (189). The antibodies BR64 and BR96 recognize Le^y, with limited reactivity to normal tissues except for the gastric mucosa, although BR64 also binds capillaries of the myocardium (190). These antibodies are internalized and therefore of interest as carriers of toxins; conjugates with doxorubicin and ricin have been evaluated and are described later.

MUC-1

Breast epithelial mucins are large, highly glycosylated molecules. Most antibodies derived against these mucins recognize the core structure MUC-1 (31). Five antibodies, Mc5, BrE-1, BrE-2, BrE-3, and Mc1, recognize an immunodominant 8-amino–acid sequence of the tandem repeat sequence of MUC-1. Immunohistochemistry assays of these antibodies demonstrate different distribution of antibody binding in both normal and malignant tissues, likely due to differences in glycosylation of mucin. These antibodies were developed for radioimmunotherapy and are described more fully in the section Radioimmunotherapy.

hCTMO1 recognizes the tetrameric epitope RPAP of MUC-1 (191). *In vitro* experiments have demonstrated that it is rapidly internalized, with a high degree of tumor-selective retention in *in vivo* tumor models. There is also evidence of tumor inhibition with an idarubicin conjugate, whereas idarubicin alone had no activity. To date, this antibody has only been tested as an imaging agent (192). ^{111}In-labeled antibody was evaluated in 31 patients with ovarian cancer with circulating MUC-1 (193). This study demonstrated persistent uptake of antibody 6 days after a single intravenous injection within tumor, with a greater percentage within tumor than in normal tissues or blood. Because this is a humanized antibody, a clearing step of unlabeled antibody has been given before the labeled antibody to allow for enhanced imaging (194). C595 is a murine IgG_3 that also recognizes RPAP. This antibody was used to immunize mice to develop an antiidiotypic antibody against the MUC-1 epitope RPAP, termed *MAb 911*. This antibody helps evaluate the potential for inducing tumor immunity to MUC-1 (195).

A number of mucins have been identified in pancreatic cancers (196), with the target of PAM4 found on malignant cells of the pancreas but not on the normal glandular tissue. Preclinical trials using a radiolabeled antibody have revealed growth delays even with large tumors (197). H23 recognizes MUC-1H23, which is overexpressed on 91% of human breast cancers but only 2% of normal breast tissue samples (198). The selectivity of this agent for malignant tissues is promising.

Other Mucin Antigens

Sialyl Tn tumor antigen is found on most adenocarcinomas, and a series of MAb have been found that recognize this antigen: B72.3, MAb B195.3R11, TKH2, B239.1, and CC49

(199). This antigen recognized by B72.3 and CC49 is also known as *tumor-associated glycoprotein-72* (TAG-72) (200). Human milk fat globule has also served as an antibody target (201), with therapeutic trials using radiolabled antibodies as described in the section Radioimmunotherapy.

Transferrin Receptor

The transferrin receptor TfR is another receptor on cancer cells that binds a growth-stimulatory ligand. Iron has been shown to be necessary for growth of malignant cells. Cells deprived of iron undergo growth arrest and apoptosis (202). Therefore, targeting the TfR found on most carcinomas, sarcomas, as well as some lymphomas and leukemias could have broad therapeutic applicability. 42/6, a murine IgA antitransferrin antibody, does not induce clinical responses, but decreases serum TfRs and increases serum iron and transferrin, suggesting blockade of iron uptake (203). Therapy with 42/6 was complicated by the induction of antibody responses against the murine antibody. This approach warrants further evaluation using a chimeric antibody that is administerable for protracted lengths of time. This target has also been used in immunotoxin constructs (204).

Carcinoembryonic Antigen

Although adenocarcinomas commonly express CEA, this has not been a common target in antibody-based therapies. It has been evaluated as a diagnostic antibody for RIGS and nuclear medicine scans, as previously discussed. Antiidiotypic antibody therapy has been evaluated and is reviewed in the section Antibodies as Vaccines.

BISPECIFIC ANTIBODY THERAPY

BsAb are constructed with two distinct binding sites. BsAb may be whole IgG molecules or constructed of smaller antibody fragments. Smaller BsAb are being constructed to optimize penetration into tumor tissues (205–207). The specificities of the two antibody-binding sites may be for distinct tumor-associated antigens. For example, BsAb with varied specificity for mucin, three different glycoproteins, transferrin receptor, and HER-2/*neu* were screened for direct tumor growth inhibition (208). Binding of the two different sites on tumor cells was hypothesized to alter normal cellular signaling pathways. Growth of the breast cancer cell line SKBR3 was best inhibited using a BsAb with specificities for HER-2/*neu* and the transferrin receptor. When combined with the iron chelator deferoxamine, enhanced growth inhibition is achieved with lower doses of antibody and deferoxamine than when either one is used alone. BsAb also have been made with specificity for tumor antigens and for therapeutic agents such as drugs, or radioactive elements.

Extensive work has been done in the construction, evaluation, and *in vivo* testing of BsAb that target tumor-associated antigens and effector cells. These antibodies have targeted either elements of the T-cell receptor complex or Fcγ receptors found on monocytes, macrophages, neutrophils, and NK cells. The receptors that are targeted may function as activation trig-

TABLE 3. BISPECIFIC ANTIBODIES IN CLINICAL TRI

Effector Cell Target	Tumor Target
CD64/FcγRI	
MDX-210	HER-2
MDX-H210	HER-2
MDX-447	EGFR
CD16/FcγRIII	
2B1	HER-2
CD3/T-cell receptor	
BIS-1	Ep-CAM
M26.1	EGFR
OC/TR	Folate-binding protein

EGFR, epidermal growth factor receptor; HER, Heregulin.

gers for the effector cell on binding of the antibody. BsAb promote the conjugation of effector T cells, NK cells, or macrophages (MØ) to malignant cell targets. When T-cell receptors are bound, the T cell is activated, leading to the production of IFN-γ and TNF-α, which may be responsible for the bystander effect observed in animal models in which cytotoxicity is not restricted to cells bound by antibody. Binding of T-cell receptors by these antibodies triggers cytotoxicity irrespective of the antigen specificity of the T cell (209,210) and is not dependent on major histocompatibility complex expression, which is often downregulated on malignant cells (211). The addition of IL-2 further activates these T cells. However, combinations of antibodies targeting three receptors on T cells results in profound T-cell activation that cannot be further manipulated by IL-2. This property may allow BsAb-promoted T-cell activation *in vivo* at tumor sites without the added systemic toxicities of IL-2 therapy (212).

Many of the BsAb-targeting T-cell receptors have been developed for lymphomas and leukemias. Table 3 provides a list of those BsAbs in clinical trials for solid tumors. One example of a clinically tested BsAb for solid tumors is OC/TR, which recognizes CD3 and the folate-binding protein on ovarian cancer cells (213). Patients with residual disease at the time of second-look surgery received autologous T-lymphocytes labeled with the BsAb via intraperitoneal administration daily for up to 9 days over 2 weeks with IL-2. Some patients underwent exploratory surgery after two cycles of therapy. Clinical responses lasted up to 12 months in duration. The significance of the responses is difficult to interpret, as patients with negative second-look surgeries are known to have prolonged disease-free survival (214). Another example is BIS-1, which recognizes CD3 and EGP-2, which has been evaluated in patients with lung cancer manifesting as malignant ascites or pleural effusions (215). Patients received therapy with preactivated T lymphocytes with BIS-1 injected directly into the pleural or peritoneal space. Limited toxicity occurred, in contrast with significant toxicity seen with intravenous administration of a F(ab')$_2$ of BIS-1 given with subcutaneous IL-2.

Two BsAb with specificity for FcγR have been characterized and are undergoing clinical trials. MDX-210 is the fusion of the F(ab')$_2$ of two murine MAb, which recognize FcγRI and the extracellular domain of HER-2/*neu* (216). The binding site on FcγRI is distinct from that for the Fc portion of immunoglobulins, allowing for binding to the Fc receptor *in vivo* even if it is

occupied by an Ig molecule, and for ADCC, phagocytosis, superoxide generation, and enzyme release. *In vitro* assays of PMNs and monocytes show an upregulation of FcγRI in response to granulocyte colony-stimulating factor (G-CSF) (217), and IFN-γ (218). The FcαRI receptor, CD89, has also been evaluated as a target for bispecific antibodies (219). The FcαRI receptor binds IgA and can lead to antibody-dependent cell cytotoxicity dependent on the presence of neutrophils, rather than complement. *In vitro*, BsAb targeting CD89 and either c-erbB-2 or *Candida albicans* have led to effective killing of cancer cells and phagocytosis of fungi in the presence of neutrophils. The toxic effects were enhanced in the presence of G-CSF.

In a phase 1 trial, patients with advanced breast and ovarian cancer overexpressing HER-2/*neu* were given one dose of MDX-210 antibody (216). Most patients developed fever and mild hypotension. One-third of patients were noted to have increases in transaminases for 48 to 72 hours after therapy. Transient monocytopenia was seen with increased TNF-α levels 1 to 3 hours after the initial infusion, followed by IL-6 and G-CSF increases. Biopsies demonstrated mononuclear cell infiltrates and antibody localization 48 hours after infusion. Ten patients were evaluated for clinical responses. One patient with breast cancer experienced a tumor flare and erythema after injection and a subsequent decrease in the size of subcutaneous metastases and axillary adenopathy; no change was seen in lymphangitic lung disease. Another patient with ovarian cancer had a 50% reduction in cervical lymph nodes, but progression of intraabdominal disease was suggested by the development of intestinal obstruction. In a separate phase 1 study, MDX-210 combined with G-CSF was well tolerated, with evidence *in vitro* of enhanced cytotoxicity in the presence of neutrophils and antibody (220). MDX-H210, a humanized form of the antibody, is currently in phase 2 trials in combination with GM-CSF for patients with renal cell carcinoma, prostate cancer, and colorectal cancer. An early report of these studies described responses in renal cell and prostate cancer (221). This antibody has also been evaluated with IFN-α with evidence of immunologic and clinical activity (222). MDX-447 combines anti-FcRI and anti-EGFR specificities. In 36 patients with renal cell, head and neck, bladder, ovarian, prostate, or skin cancer, nine patients treated with MDX-447 had stabilization of their disease for 3 to 6 months (220).

Preclinical data have demonstrated the ability of BsAb that bind tumor and FcγRIII to redirect lysis by large granular lymphocytes in the presence of competing human immunoglobulin (223,224). We have evaluated 2B1, which recognizes HER-2/*neu* and FcγRIII (225). In a phase 1 study, patients with HER-2/*neu* overexpressing tumors were treated with six infusions of antibody over 8 days (226). Immune activation was demonstrated by increases in circulating TNF-α, IL-6, IL-8, and, to a lesser extent, GM-CSF and INF-α. This group of patients developed antibody responses against the intracellular domain of HER-2/*neu* (227). These results suggest that BsAb-promoted cytolysis leads to processing of HER-2/*neu* via FcγRIII, leading to antigen presentation and immunization *in vivo* against HER-2/*neu*.

BsAb can also target a tumor-associated antigen and a chemotherapeutic agent (228–231) or radionuclide (232). An anti-

TAG-72 antibody has been combined with an antimethotrexate antibody, with *in vitro* data demonstrating targeting to and cytotoxicity of antigen-positive cells. In preclinical murine models, a bispecific targeting CEA and the vinca alkaloids vinblastine and vindesine demonstrate accumulation of drug at tumor sites, changes in drug biodistribution, and evidence of chemotherapeutic effect in tumor pathology. Similarly, a BsAb recognizing CEA and boron-10 can selectively concentrate boron in CEA-expressing tumors *in vivo*. Another construct targeting EGFR and doxorubicin also demonstrates altered biodistribution of the chemotherapeutic agent; of particular interest is evidence for decreased uptake in the myocardium compared with control animals not receiving the BsAb. This approach has not been tested in human clinical trials.

BsAb are also being evaluated in the preclinical setting in vaccine strategies (233). Tumor cells exposed to cytokines to upregulate major histocompatibility receptors and adhesion molecules were incubated with a BsAb that binds tumor and CD28, a costimulatory molecule on T cells. CD28, when bound, reverses T-cell anergy. When used as a vaccine *in vivo*, cytotoxic T-cell responses were induced, with cures of established tumors and inhibition of tumor rechallenges.

RADIOIMMUNOTHERAPY

Antibodies can also be used to deliver radioactive compounds to cells, leading to tumor cell death (234,235). Some preclinical studies suggest radioimmunotherapy can also decrease vascular permeability (236). Approaches using standard- and high-dose radiation therapy requiring bone marrow or stem cell transplant support have been evaluated with some efficacy. Antibodies, however, have limited capacity to penetrate into tumor tissues (32) and may therefore have limited therapeutic efficacy in large, bulky, solid tumors. Also, because tumor antigens are often found on normal host tissues, toxicity to normal organs has not been eliminated. Antibodies are cleared via the kidney or alternatively via the reticuloendothelial system, putting these organs at risk for injury from radiation. Last, the radionuclides distribute systemically, and therefore all tissues are exposed to radiation, particularly the bone marrow, which is quite sensitive to the effects of radiation. Some studies have used radiolabeled antibodies given by intraperitoneal injection in the setting of malignant ascites. However, this approach does not limit systemic absorption or toxicities (237–240). The following is an overview of antibodies targeting solid tumors that have been tested in clinical trials.

DeNardo and colleagues have developed a humanized antiadenocarcinoma antibody, chimeric L6 (ChL6) (241). It has been chelated with various radioisotopes, including Iodine-131 (^{131}I), and evaluated clinically (242,243). In chemotherapy-refractory metastatic breast cancer patients, ChL6 radioimmunotherapy has a 50% response rate; however, due to myelosuppression, doses of radiation could not be escalated above 60 to 70 mCi per m^2. More recent studies have escalated doses to 150 mCi per m^2, followed by autologous stem-cell transplantation. The clinical course of only three patients has been reported. These patients were given 200 mg of unconjugated antibody before ^{131}I-ChL6

treatment to block binding by normal vascular endothelium and Lugol's solution to block the uptake of radioactive iodine by the thyroid. One patient was able to receive three cycles of therapy with the addition of cyclosporin to inhibit the formation of HAMA, with an improvement in her performance status, a decline in her tumor markers, and 9-months' relief of bone pain. In a subsequent study, patients received up to four doses monthly of ^{131}I at doses of 20 to 70 μCi per m^2. Four of ten patients had partial responses lasting up to 5 months with an overall survival of 2.3 to 9.0 months (244). Further preclinical work is being done with a chimeric antibody conjugated to yttrium-90 (^{90}Y). This radiolabeled antibody and paclitaxel in a murine model have synergistic activity using human breast cancer xenografts (245).

The pancarcinoma antibody NR-LU-10 has been extensively evaluated for radioimmunotherapy. To limit normal host toxicity, radiolabeled NR-LU-10 was mixed with a collagen-based gel and injected intratumorally in a murine model, with improved tumor retention (246). Clinical trials have been done with rhenium-186 (^{186}Re)–labeled NR-LU-10 in ovarian cancer patients treated by intraperitoneal injection (238–240). Initial studies designed to estimate radiation doses to normal organs revealed dose-limiting hematologic toxicity at calculated bone marrow doses greater than 100 rad. A subsequent study treated patients with 25 to 150 mCi of ^{186}Re-NR-LU-10. Two patients at the highest dose experienced myelosuppression. Other clinically significant toxicities were fever and rash, but no significant gastrointestinal toxicity was found. Seven patients with minimal residual disease underwent repeat surgical exploration after therapy. Four of these patients had a decrease in residual disease. Another phase 1 study treated 15 refractory metastatic epithelial carcinoma patients with ^{186}Re-NR-LU-10 (247). Dose-limiting myelosuppression occurred at 120 mCi per m^2. This antibody has undergone clinical testing using a streptavidin-biotin pretargeting approach.

Mucin is an attractive target for radioimmunotherapy. Preclinical studies have demonstrated efficacy of ^{131}Iodine-Mc5 with no significant loss of MUC-1 expression in residual malignant tissue (248). ^{67}Copper-labeled MAb C595, another anti-MUC-1 antibody, is able to target transitional cell carcinoma and is being developed for intravesicular administration (249). BrE-3 has been investigated in the clinical setting (250). The initial phase 1 study done with the murine antibody conjugated to ^{90}Y demonstrated tolerable toxicity with doses of 6.25 to 9.25 MCi per m^2; however five of six treated patients developed HAMA after one dose of antibody (251). In a second phase 1 study escalating doses of 90Y-BrE-3 were used to treat heavily pretreated metastatic breast cancer patients. ^{90}Y conjugated to the antibody via MX-DPTA dissociates from the antibody and becomes incorporated into bone, resulting in a higher radiation dose to the bone marrow tissue than to other tissues. To minimize hematologic toxicity, patients were reinfused with autologous stem cells or bone marrow and treated with G-CSF after 1.5 mg per m^2 BrE-3 labeled with 15 MCi per m^2 or 20 MCi per m^2 ^{90}Y. Patients at both dose levels developed grade 4 thrombocytopenia, whereas grade 4 neutropenia was only seen at the higher dose level. Four patients had partial responses, with responses in lymph nodes, skin, and bone marrow. Another

patient experienced transient palliation of bone disease, but no objective response. Further dose escalation is planned with this compound. A humanized construct of this antibody has been developed and evaluated as an imaging agent for advanced breast cancer (252). This study demonstrated a longer biologic half-life than the murine construct. The decreased antigenicity of the antibody allows repeated administration in therapeutic trials, allowing for dose fractionation mimicking conventional radiation therapy. However, the longer half-life may increase the nonspecific deposition of radioactivity.

Methods of decreasing toxicity from nonspecific radiation are being developed. Preclinical studies suggest combining IFN-α with radioimmunotherapy may decrease bone marrow toxicity (253). Antibodies directed against the chelating agent used to conjugate the radionuclide to an antitumor antibody decrease the radiation dose to blood and normal tissues, with a relative increase in radiation delivery to tumor (254). A similar approach has been used to clear biotinylated, radiolabeled antibodies. Unbound biotinylated antibodies can be cleared rapidly from the circulation by streptavidin, which has a high affinity for biotin (255). Pretargeting offers another approach to limit nonspecific delivery of radiation. In this strategy, an antiantibody conjugated to streptavidin is systemically administered. After unbound antibody has cleared from normal organ reservoirs, a biotinylated radioactive element is subsequently administered. This radionuclide thus selectively binds to the tumorbound streptavidin. This approach need not be limited to radiotherapy, and indeed there are preclinical data using this approach to target cytokines to tumor sites (256). This approach has been tested in various disease settings. The biotinylated antibody Mov18 was injected intraperitoneally to 15 patients with known intraabdominal ovarian cancer (257). ^{111}In-streptavidin was given 3 to 5 days later followed by laparotomy 1 to 8 days later. Radioactivity in resected malignant and normal tissues demonstrated favorable ratios of radioactivity in tumor compared with normal organs. Using a murine NR-LU-10 antibody-streptavidin conjugate, biotinylated ^{90}Y was tested in the phase 2 setting in colon cancer and prostate cancer. Although there was some clinical activity in these patients, diarrhea was dose limiting due to expression in the gastrointestinal tract of the Le^y antigen recognized by NR-LU-10 (258).

Another approach to radioimmunotherapy is to combine it with other forms of therapy. Monoclonal antibody ^{125}Iodine-A33, specific for an epithelial antigen found in 90% of colorectal cancers (259), has demonstrated preliminary evidence of increased activity when combined with chemotherapy without added bowel or bone marrow toxicity at a dose of 350 mCi per m^2 (260). Some patients who achieved CEA response or stable disease were subsequently treated with carmustine, vincristine, 5-fluorouracil, and streptozocin, with 50% responding; a phase 1 study using the unlabeled antibody weekly with chemotherapy is being conducted to define the interaction between radioimmunotherapy and chemotherapy.

IMMUNOTOXINS

An immunotoxin (IT) is an engineered drug that consists of a targeting monoclonal antibody linked to a protein toxin (261). ITs were originally constructed using chemical cross-linking agents that couple the toxin to the antibody, resulting in a large protein structure with a molecular mass of 175 kd or more. More recently, IT have been cloned and expressed in bacterial expression systems as single-chain IT-fusion proteins linking the variable region of the antibody to the toxin (262), allowing for enhanced tumor penetration. The antibody component binds to the target on the malignant cell, is internalized, and the toxin or drug incapacitates the cell. Multiple compounds have been developed targeting various antigens linked to several different toxins.

The toxins used most commonly have been ricin, diphtheria toxin (DT), and *Pseudomonas* exotoxin (PE). Ricin and DT contain two chains, A and B. In ricin, the A chain is responsible for the toxic effects via *N*-glycosidase activity, which inactivates the 60S ribosomal subunit (263). The A chain of DT and domain 3 of PE have adenosine diphosphate ribosylation activity, which inactivates ribosomal elongation factor-2 and inhibits protein translation (264,265). The B chains and domains 1 and 2 of PE are required for intact toxin binding to the cell surface and translocation to the correct cytoplasmic compartment. Recombinant ITs engineered with specific intracellular translocation sequences can target the appropriate intracellular compartment where the toxin is active (266–269). This strategy has not always been successful due to poor internalization of the IT or inappropriate intracellular translocation of the toxin. Variations on this basic theme substitute chemotherapy agents or cytokines for the toxic moiety (270). More recently, two novel ribosome-inactivating proteins, ocymoidine and pyramidatine, have been evaluated. The ITs have activity both *in vitro* and *in vivo* (271).

Preclinical data and human clinical trials have identified challenges to the successful clinical use of ITs. Selecting an epitope on the antigen of interest closer to the cell surface appears to aid in improved internalization (272–274). Some ITs also have been found to have limited *in vivo* stability due to rapid clearance by the liver. Strategies have been developed to limit the recognition of the glycosylated proteins by the reticuloendothelial system (261,275,276), reduction of the proteins by glutathione (277), and complex formation with α_2-macroglobulin (278). Treatment with IT has been associated with unanticipated toxicities (279–282). The development of humoral responses directed against the toxin has limited the ability to administer repeated doses of drug. Common toxicities include fever, anorexia, malaise, arthralgias, and myalgias. A vascular leak syndrome characterized by weight gain, edema, dyspnea, and hypoalbuminemia has been seen in numerous studies with varying agents. The syndrome is hypothesized to be due to endothelial damage secondary to high concentrations of toxin (283); others have demonstrated binding of the immunotoxin to Fc receptors on monocytes releasing vasoactive compounds (282). Also observed were neurologic toxicities, including sensorimotor neuropathies associated with axonal loss and demyelination (281). Cases of rhabdomyolysis and acrocyanosis, manifested as reversible distal digital skin necrosis, have also been reported (284).

One IT that has been developed is based on BR96 (285), a murine IgG3 monoclonal antibody, which recognizes the Le^y antigen. It is rapidly internalized into lysosomes and endosomes by tumor cells and mediates antibody- and complement-dependent cytotoxicity, growth inhibition, and cell death. When this IT binds to cells bearing the Le^y antigen, protein synthesis is inhibited in a manner dependent on the number of Le^y surface receptors (286). Initial screens of the antibody revealed that it bound to a myriad of neoplasms and to a limited number of normal tissues, including the esophagus, stomach, intestines, and acinar cells of the pancreas. This normal tissue-binding pattern accounts for the gastrointestinal toxicity observed with this agent. BR96 has been conjugated to PE40 (287) (BR96 scFv-PE40) and to doxorubicin (BR96 IgG-DOX) (288). Preclinical studies of BR96 scFv-PE40 in murine and rat xenograft models using the human breast carcinoma cell line H3396 (289) and MCF-7 (290) demonstrated elimination of tumors in a dose- and schedule-dependent manner. Large tumors were cured when treated with 0.625 mg per kg intravenously every 4 days for a total of five doses. Preclinical toxicology studies revealed hepatotoxicity and vascular leak syndrome, which could be abrogated by premedicating with steroids (291).

The intracellular target of the toxin can also be targeted. Early IT with PE were found to be inactive when the antibody moiety was ligated to the carboxy terminus of PE. Analysis revealed that the amino acids, REDLK, at the end of the molecule are critical for the cytotoxicity of the molecule. These critical amino acids were changed to a similar sequence, KDEL, known to retain proteins in the lumen of the endoplasmic reticulum where protein synthesis occurs. Constructs combining an scFv directed against the IL-2 receptor and PE, PE-KDEL, or PE-(KDEL)$_3$ were compared. The KDEL modification enhanced *in vitro* cytotoxicity and *in vivo* antitumor effects by two- to threefold as compared with unmodified toxins (292).

More recently, ribonucleases (RNases) have been evaluated as candidate toxins (293,294). RNase from eosinophils (295,296), and pancreatic tissue (297) has been found to be cytotoxic to mammalian cells and to prolong survival in animal tumor models. Rybak and colleagues initially have evaluated bovine pancreatic ribonuclease A, and more recently angiogenin, a human protein with homology to pancreatic RNase. Angiogenin has been linked to an antitransferrin antibody (CH2.5-Ang). CH2.5-Ang supernatants selectively inhibit protein synthesis of cells from the leukemia cell line K562 by 50% after a 24-hour incubation. Adding excess parental antibody to the supernatant could block this toxicity. These observations suggest CH2.5-Ang is effective only when it is internalized into cells. Angiogenin is an attractive toxin to use as it is of human origin and should not be as immunogenic as catalytic toxins derived from prokaryotes.

Preclinical studies suggest limited toxicity when ITs are given intrathecally. LMB-7 is an IT constructed from a scFv that recognizes Le^y antigen linked to a component of the PE. Preclinical studies using a rat model demonstrated efficacy of intrathecal therapy with LMB-7 (298). After intrathecal seeding of A431 tumor, animals were treated with 10 µg of LMB-7 intrathecally on days 3, 5, and 7. Untreated animals died in 10 days. Twelve of 20 treated animals lived for more than 170 days. Nine of these animals demonstrated no histologic evidence of tumor at autopsy. An ongoing phase 1 clinical trial is determining the maximum tolerated dose of the LMB-7 for carcinomatous meningitis in patients with B3 expressing tumors.

CYTOKINE THERAPY WITH ANTIBODY THERAPY

Cytokines can expand or mitigate an immune response. The ability of certain cytokines to increase numbers of effector cells and activate these cells makes them ideal candidates to combine with antibody therapy. Increasing the number of activated cells at tumor sites may promote *in situ* ADCC. Commonly used cytokines include GM-CSF, due to its ability to activate macrophages and monocytes, and IL-2, due to its role in activating NK cells. IL-2 therapy has been shown to enhance ADCC (299,300). GM-CSF has also been examined in this context (301). Cytokine therapy can also increase the expression of some tumor antigens. Increased expression of some tumor antigens has been observed with IFNs (302,303); this provided the rationale for combining antibodies targeting CEA and TAG-72 with IFN-α and IFN-γ (304). TNF-α up regulates EGFR and in conjunction with an anti-EGFR antibody in a phase 1/2 clinical trial of patients with unresectable pancreatic cancer demonstrated enhanced growth inhibition, with increased doses of antibody and one complete remission lasting for 3 years (305). Cytokine therapy also upregulates major histocompatibility receptors, leading to enhanced cell surface antigen presentation (306,307).

MoAb L6, the original murine antibody from which ChL6 was developed, has been used to treat patients in conjunction with IL-2 (308). Sixteen patients were accrued to cohorts with escalating doses of IL-2, 2.0 to 4.5×10^6 U per day, given days 15 to 18, 22 to 25, and 29 to 32. All patients received 200 mg per m^2 of antibody on days 1 to 7. A patient with breast cancer had a mixed response with improvement in subcutaneous nodules, but developed a malignant pleural effusion. A colon cancer patient had a partial response lasting 12 weeks.

As described earlier, the antibody 17-1A has also been tested clinically with several cytokines. Three clinical trials in advanced colorectal cancer and pancreatic cancer were undertaken combining the antibody with IFN-γ because of *in vitro* data suggesting increased ADCC and apoptosis with combination therapy (138). The combination was not clinically effective (162,163). When 17-1A was combined with GM-CSF, clinical responses as well as increased induction of antiidiotypic antibodies were reported in one trial (309).

To increase antigen expression, IFN-α has been combined with the radiolabeled TAG-72 antibody CC49 (310). Patients were randomized to receive 3×10^6 U IFN-α subcutaneously daily for 14 days, or no interferon followed by ^{131}I-labeled CC49. Patients receiving the IFN were found to have significant increases in their TAG-72 antigen expression by tumors and improved localization of CC49 MAb. In a phase 3 breast cancer study, IFN-α increased the tumor uptake of radiolabeled CC49 and prolonged the circulation time of the radiolabeled antibody compared with patients receiving no cytokine therapy (311).

Another approach is the creation of fusion proteins containing an antibody linked to a cytokine. IFN-α has been conjugated to the humanized BrE-3 and Mc5. In murine models, there was enhanced efficacy of the conjugated antibody compared with IFN-α alone, or an irrelevant IgG conjugated with IFN-α. Upregulation of antigen recognized by BrE-3 was also observed (312).

MONOCLONAL ANTIBODY THERAPY IN CONJUNCTION WITH CHEMOTHERAPY

Combination therapy with MAb and chemotherapy has been approached in various ways. One strategy to minimize toxicity from chemotherapy has been to exploit the specificity of antibodies to target an enzyme to tumor, followed by the administration of a chemotherapeutic prodrug. The drug is then converted to its active form only at tumor sites. The enzymes used have been endogenous alkaline phosphatase and β-glucuronidase, as well as the bacterial enzymes β-lactamase and carboxypeptidase G2 (CPG2). The prodrugs for etoposide, mitomycin-c, and phenol mustards are substrates for alkaline phosphatase. β-Glucuronidase converts the prodrug of doxorubicin to its pharmacologically active form. Doxorubicin, mustard, and vinca alkaloid prodrugs can be converted by β-lactamase. CPG2 only activates the mustard-alkaloid prodrug. These bacterially derived enzymes are antigenic and thus may have limited therapeutic utility. β-Lactamase-conjugated Fab specific for CEA and TAG-72 target breast and ovarian cancer lines and activate the prodrug of doxorubicin, with *in vivo* efficacy in preclinical models (313). The tumor growth suppression seen with the antibody and prodrug was equal to using free doxorubicin; however, the maximum tolerated dose of doxorubicin increased using the prodrug strategy due to decreased systemic-free drug. Similarly, the use of a BsAb with specificities for a tumor antigen and a chemotherapeutic agent can lead to specific tumor retention of drug, as described in the section Bispecific Antibody Therapy.

Conjugation of chemotherapeutic agents to antibodies has been tested preclinically (314) and clinically (BR96-DOX). Initial phase 1 studies identified a dose-limiting toxicity of hematemesis secondary to an exudative gastritis (315), which could be ameliorated by premedicating with corticosteroids, 5-hydroxy-tryptoamine-3 antagonists, and infusing the antibody over 24 hours (316). The maximally tolerated dose was 700 mg per m^2, delivering 21 mg per m^2 of doxorubicin every 3 weeks. Two partial responses were observed in breast and gastric cancer. A randomized phase 2 study compared BR96-DOX, 21 mg per m^2 doxorubicin to single agent doxorubicin 60 mg per m^2, with patients crossing over to the alternate arm with disease progression or stable disease after four cycles (317). The toxicities of the immunoconjugate were gastrointestinal with limited hematologic toxicity, suggesting specific targeting of drug due to Le^y in the gut. The response rates were 7% for the immunoconjugate and 44% for doxorubicin. The decreased activity of the immunoconjugate may be due to the large antigen pool in the gastrointestinal tract limiting targeted delivery of antibody to tumor sites. Other constructs targeting HER-2/*neu* are under development (318).

Another means to combine drug and antibody therapy is to use agents that act intracellularly on overexpressed receptors on malignant cells. One such approach combined the anti-EGFR antibody C225 with inhibitors of type 1 cyclic adenosine monophosphate-dependent protein kinase (PKAI), 8-chloro-cAMP (319). PKAI overexpression has been demonstrated after transformation with TGF-α (320). Its overexpression has also been correlated with poor prognosis in breast cancers. *In vivo* models of combined therapy revealed prolonged survival of tumor-bearing animals with evidence of decreased production of autocrine growth factors by the malignant cells. The decrease in autocrine factors resulted in decreased tumor growth and a decrease in angiogenesis. There was no evidence of toxicity due to the antibody or PKAI. C225 was also combined with an antisense oligonucleotide that targets the expression of the regulator subunit of PKAI (321). Combined treatment of EGFR-expressing renal cell lines leads to loss of colony formation *in vitro* as well as growth inhibition and apoptosis. Tumor xenografts regressed with combination therapy. This exciting new therapeutic concept is an area for continuing drug development.

Last, the combined use of standard chemotherapy and antibody therapy is being increasingly explored, particularly in view of the effectiveness of RhuMAb HER-2 and paclitaxel therapy. Based on preclinical data in animal models, a phase 2 study has been completed in metastatic breast cancer, which overexpresses HER-2/*neu* combining RhuMAb HER-2 with cisplatin chemotherapy (322). Patients received an intravenous loading dose of 250 mg of antibody followed by 100 mg intravenously each week for 9 weeks. Treatment was combined with intravenous cisplatin 75 mg per m^2 days 1, 29, and 57. There were nine partial responses in 37 assessable patients with median response duration of 5.3 months. Another nine patients exhibited minor responses or stable disease. There were no unanticipated toxicities and pharmacokinetic studies revealed no change in antibody clearance with cisplatin. At the present time, the mechanisms underlying the efficacy of combination therapy are not understood at a cellular level. Studies are ongoing evaluating RhuMAb HER-2 with paclitaxel or docetaxel (Taxotere) in women with metastatic breast cancer and gemcitabine in patients with pancreatic cancer. RhuMAb HER-2 is also being combined with carboplatin and paclitaxel in patients with newly diagnosed metastatic breast cancer. If increased efficacy is seen with platinum-based combination therapy, other HER-2/*neu* overexpressing tumors, such as non–small cell or ovarian cancer, may benefit from this therapeutic approach. Similar encouraging results have been observed using the antiepidermal growth factor antibody C225 with cisplatin in head and neck cancer. *In vitro* studies continue to evaluate other antibody and chemotherapy combinations (323).

ANTIBODIES AS VACCINES

Based on the idiotypic network put forth by Lindenmann and Jerne, various investigators have created antiidiotypic antibodies to serve as vaccines (324–328). One such vaccine was derived by immunizing goats with the MAb 17-1A (325). Thirty patients with advanced colorectal cancer were immunized intradermally with 0.5 to 4.0 mg of the antibody weeks 0, 1, 2, and 5 with 11 patients subsequently receiving a booster dose between 1.5 to 11 months thereafter. All patients developed an antiidiotypic cascade of antibodies. Six patients had partial responses and seven patients had stable disease.

Response was not correlated with the dose of vaccine the patient received. However, only four of the patients with response or stabilization of their disease solely received vaccine. All others had received concurrent chemotherapy, making it unclear whether the clinical responses were due to vaccine, chemotherapy, or combination therapy.

An antiidiotypic antibody, created using an antibody directed against gp72 (324), has been used to treat patients with advanced colorectal cancer (329) and rectal cancer patients in an adjuvant setting (330). The antibody 105AD7 was produced by fusion of plasma cells from patients treated with an anti-gp72 antibody 791T/36 with EL41, a mouse/human heterohybrid. The 105AD7 hybridoma was found to produce a human IgG1 that bound to the binding site of the 791T/36 antibody. In 13 patients with metastatic colorectal cancer treated with the vaccine, survival was 12 months as compared to 4 months for patients in a contemporary control cohort; the significance of this increase in survival is unknown as this was not a prospectively randomized study. *In vitro* immunologic correlates demonstrated evidence of cellular responses as indicated by lymphocyte proliferation to gp72-expressing tumor cells and IL-2 production. In the adjuvant setting, six patients were vaccinated preoperatively. Three of these six patients subsequently demonstrated increased killing of autologous tumor cells by peripheral lymphocytes and by lymphocytes from draining lymph nodes; the killing observed by peripheral lymphocytes was increased as compared with baseline blood samples suggesting an immunologic impact of the vaccination. Evidence also existed of increased nonspecific killing of autologous tumor cells by NK cells.

Foon and his colleagues have evaluated an antiidiotypic vaccine strategy for CEA-expressing tumors. The antiidiotypic antibody 3H1 was derived from a murine antibody that targets a highly restricted epitope of CEA, which is not found on normal adult tissues or hematopoietic cells. Patients with advanced colorectal cancer treated with 3H1 injections developed both humoral and cellular responses against CEA (331). This response was not abrogated by concurrent chemotherapy (332). A phase 2 randomized study is ongoing evaluating 3H1 plus GM-CSF, or alum-precipitated 3H1 antibody with GM-CSF in patients with stage II or stage III colorectal cancer. This is the first trial evaluating an antibody as a vaccine in the adjuvant setting. Antiidiotypic antibodies against gp72 have also been developed (333), and 105AD7 has been tested in patients with advanced colorectal cancer (334). Patients were found to have a cellular, but not a humoral response to the immunization. Compared with contemporaneous controls, vaccinated patients survived a median of 12 months compared with nontreated patients who survived 4 months. In a follow-up study, the immunologic responses and progression-free survival were superior in patients who received a 100-μg versus 200-μg dose of vaccine (335).

Another antigen evaluated for immunization is the human milk-fat globule in women with breast cancer. Preclinical studies of 11D10, an antiidiotypic antibody derived against BrE-1, have been performed in cynomolgus monkeys (336). Immunization of the animals led to the production of both a cellular and humoral response. This vaccine strategy has been used in a limited number of breast cancer patients, both in the adjuvant and metastatic setting with evidence of cellular and humoral responses in both patient populations (337). Objective responses have not been observed in the metastatic setting.

The impact of antiidiotypic vaccines remains to be clarified. Most of the vaccines use nonhuman antibodies for the vaccine, which may help stimulate an immune response against the antibody. However, as has been seen with intravenously administered antibodies, multiple administrations of the antiidiotype vaccine may be limited by the immune response against the constant regions of the antibody (e.g., HAMA response). Also, although *in vitro* data supporting the induction immune responses have been demonstrated, there is not clear evidence for the induction of clinically meaningful responses. Clinical trials with various antibodies have demonstrated antiidiotypic cascades after therapy (338). There are also examples of antibodies with specificity for the tumor antigen that are being used as vaccines (339–340). The infused antibody may allow for *in vivo* immunization, and the induction of these antiidiotypic antibodies may serve to amplify the antigenic stimulus to the immune system. Ovarian and breast cancer patients receiving high-dose chemotherapy followed by stem-cell transplantation were immunized with Theratope STn-KLH, an antibody directed against the MUC-I epitope. Eleven of 26 patients developed STn specific T-cell responses (341). It remains to be determined if such responses are components of therapeutic responses.

NEW APPROACHES

Antibody therapy has been evaluated with chemotherapy and cytokines for many years. Various toxins added on to the antibody, such as radioactive elements, toxins, or cytokines, have also been evaluated. However, antibodies have been evaluated as potential enhancers of external beam radiation therapy only since the 1990s. One report of the anti-EGFR antibody C225 with radiation therapy in head and neck cancer has demonstrated the safety of the combination and superior outcomes compared to the published response rates for radiation therapy alone in patients with locally advanced head and neck cancer (342).

Gene therapy strategies have evaluated constructs that transcribe antibody or antibody fragments, also termed *intrabodies*. The delivery and production of an antibody within a cell can bind to oncogenic proteins and downregulate their expression. For example, HER-2/*neu* has been targeted in this fashion (343,344). Transfection with the gene for an anti-HER-2/*neu* scFv construct containing the endoplasmic reticulum-directed leader sequence led to decreased cell surface expression of the protein, loss of anchorage-independent growth in agar, and death of transfected malignant cells. This was not observed when the HER-2/*neu* overexpressing cells were transfected with a scFv gene that localized to the cytosol, demonstrating the importance of binding the protein before it reaches the cell surface. This same approach in HER-2/*neu* expressing prostate (345), breast (346), and lung (347) cancer cell lines led to cell death. The mechanism of this cell death

was shown to be apoptosis (348). In an ovarian cancer *in vivo* model, malignant ascites was treated with intraperitoneal injections of adenovirus complexed to the scFv plasmid DNA. The malignant cells were subsequently shown to have minimal cell surface expression of HER-2/*neu*. Thirty percent of animals treated with the scFv plasmid and cisplatin survived, whereas none survived when either was given as a single agent (349). This approach is intriguing, but like many gene therapy approaches is limited by the difficulty of delivering the gene into enough cells of interest.

Single chain fragments may provide a means to target genes to malignant cells by systemic administration. The sequence for a high-affinity scFv specific for CEA has been incorporated into the envelope protein of a retrovirus that contains the herpes simplex thymidine kinase (TK) gene (350). TK is a "suicide" gene, as cells that contain it die when exposed to ganciclovir. This approach allows for targeted delivery of the suicide gene to CEA-expressing cancer cells, specifically due to the binding of the scFv to cell surface CEA. *In vitro* there is evidence for efficient targeting and production of the kinase in CEA expressing cells.

New delivery systems are being evaluated for toxic therapies that incorporate antibodies. One example is the addition of antibodies to a lipid-encapsulated drug to specifically target the drug to the disease site. Another is the use of a gel in the delivery of a radioactive antibody for the treatment of liver metastases (351). Such an approach in a mouse model enhanced radioactive tumor retention, limited host toxicity, and allowed for the delivery of a higher dose to tumor site with improved therapeutic outcome.

CONCLUSIONS

We are in an era of tremendous growth and development in the field of antibody-based therapeutics. Clinical trials have documented the efficacy of some antibodies in the metastatic disease setting as single agents or in combination with chemotherapy. Our challenge is to continue to understand the mechanisms by which these antibodies achieve therapeutic efficacy and to use this information to seek new therapeutic targets and agents. Novel targets, such as receptors and proteins associated with drug resistance, may allow for killing of cells that are insensitive to the normal oncologic drug armamentarium (352). The increased ability to engineer antibody-based proteins assures an abundant supply of new therapeutic agents. These agents likely have the ability to target therapeutic agents such as cytotoxic drugs or radioactive compounds. Alternatively, cytokines that modify the tumor microenvironment can be targeted to the tumor, increasing immune responses at tumor sites. Strategies to optimize a particular type of immune response can be developed and used in conjunction with vaccines, allowing for the development of cellular antitumor responses. With the demonstration of clinical responses in the metastatic setting, the evaluation of effective antibodies in the settings of smaller bulk disease, such as in the posttransplant period or in the adjuvant disease setting, is anticipated with great interest.

REFERENCES

1. Kohler G, Milstein C. Continuous clusters of fused cells secreting antibody of predefined specificity. *Nature* 1975;256:495–497.
2. Marks C, Marks JD. Phage libraries—a new route to clinically useful antibodies. *N Engl J Med* 1996;33(5):730–733.
3. Osbourn JK, Field A, Wilton J, et al. Generation of a panel of related human scFv antibodies with high affinities for human CEA. *Immunotechnology* 1996;2:181–196.
4. Adams GP. Improving the tumor specificity and retention of antibody-based molecules. *In Vivo* 1998;12:11–22.
5. Adams GP, McCartney JE, Tai MS, et al. Highly specific in vivo tumor targeting by monovalent and divalent forms of 741F8 anti-c-erbB-2 single chain Fv. *Cancer Res* 1993;53:4026–4034.
6. Porter RR. Separation of fractions of Rabbit gamma-globulin containing the antibody and antigenic combining sites. *Nature* 1958;182:670–671.
7. Nisonoff A, Wissler FC, Lipman LN. Properties of the major component of a peptic digest of rabbit antibody. *Science* 1960;132: 1770–1771.
8. Winter G, Harris WJ. Humanized antibodies. *Trends Pharmacol* 1993;15:139–143.
9. Giantonio BJ, Alpaugh RK, Schultz J, et al. Superantigen-based immunotherapy: a phase I trial of PNU-2 14565, a monoclonal antibody-staphylococcal enterotoxin A recombinant fusion protein, in advanced pancreatic and colorectal cancer. *J Clin Oncol* 1997;15: 1994–2007.
10. Wawryzynczak EJ. Systemic immunotoxin therapy of cancer: advances and approaches. *Br J Cancer* 1991;64:624–630.
11. Kim YS, Maslinski W, Zheng XX, Schachter AD, Strom TB. Immunoglobulin-cytokine fusion molecules: the new generation of immunomodulating agents. *Transplant Proc* 1998;30:4031–4036.
12. Blakey DC, Burke PJ, Davies DH, et al. Antibody-directed enzyme prodrug therapy (ADEPT) for treatment of major solid tumour disease. *Biochem Soc Transactions* 1995;23:1047–1050.
13. Goodwin DA, Meares CF, McCall MJ, et al. Pretargeted immunoscintigraphy of murine tumors with indium-11-labeled bifunctional haptens. *J Nucl Med* 1988;29:226–234.
14. Paganelli G, Riva P, Deleide G, et al. In vivo labeling of biotinylated antibodies by radioactive avidin: a strategy to increase tumor radiolocalization. *Int J Cancer* 1988;2:121–125.
15. Axworthy DB, Beaumier PL, Bottino BJ, et al. Preclinical optimization of pretargeted radioimmunotherapy components: high efficiency curative ^{90}Y delivery to mouse tumor xenografts. *Tumor Targeting* 1993;2:156–157.
16. de Palazzo IG, Gercel-Taylor C, Kitson J, Weiner LM. Potentiation of tumor lysis by a bispecific antibody that binds to CA 19-9 antigen and the Fcγ receptor expressed by human large granular lymphocytes. *Cancer Res* 1990;50:7123–7128.
17. Segal DM, Wunderlich JM. Targeting of cytotoxic cells with heterocrosslinked antibodies. *Cancer Invest* 1988;6:83–92.
18. DeSilva BS, Wilson GS. Solid phase synthesis of bifunctional antibodies. *J Immunol Methods* 1995;188:9–19.
19. Staertz UD, Bevan MJ. Hybrid hybridoma producing a bispecific monoclonal antibody that can focus effector T-cell activity. *Proc Natl Acad Sci U S A* 1986;83:1453–1457.
20. Carter P, Ridgway J, Zhu Z. Toward the production of bispecific antibody fragments for clinical applications. *J Hematother* 1995;4:43–70.
21. Ring DB, Hsieh-Ma ST, Shi T, Reeder J. Antigen forks: bispecific reagents that inhibit cell growth by binding selected pairs of tumor antigens. *Cancer Immunol Immunother* 1994;39:41–48.
22. Trauth BC, Klas C, Peters AM, et al. Monoclonal antibody-mediated tumor regression by induction of apoptosis. *Science* 1989;245: 301–310.
23. Waidman TA. Monoclonal antibodies in diagnosis and therapy. *Science* 1991;252:387–394.
24. O'Connell MJ, Chen ZJ, Yang H, et al. Active specific immunotherapy with anti-idiotypic antibodies in patients with solid tumors. *Semin Surg Oncol* 1989;5:441–447.
25. Houghton AN, Mintzer D, Cordon-Cardo C, et al. Mouse monoclonal IgG3 antibody detecting GD3 ganglioside: a phase I trial in patients with malignant melanoma. *Proc Natl Acad Sci U S A* 1985;82:1242–1246.
26. Steplewski Z, Lubeck MD, Koprowski H. Human macrophages armed with murine immunoglobulin G2a antibodies to tumors destroy human cancer cells. *Science* 1983;221:865–867.
27. Lindenmann J. Speculations on Ids and homebodies. *Ann Immunol* 1973;124:171–184.
28. Jerne NK. Towards a network theory of the immune system. *Ann Immunol* 1974;125:373–389.
29. Miller RA, Maloney DG, Warnke R, Levy R. Treatment of B-cell lymphoma with monoclonal anti-idiotype antibody. *N Engl J Med* 1982;306:517–522.
30. Khazaeli MB, Conry RM, LoBuglio AF. Human immune response to monoclonal antibodies. *J Immunother* 1994;15:42–52.
31. Peterson JA, Couto JR, Taylor MR, Ceriani RL. Selection of tumor-specific epitopes on target antigens for radioimmunotherapy of breast cancer. *Cancer Res* 1995;55:5847–5851.
32. Jam RK, Baxter LT. Mechanisms of heterogeneous distribution of monoclonal antibodies and other macromolecules in tumors: significance of elevated interstitial pressure. *Cancer Res* 1988;48:7022–7032.
33. Badger CC, Anasetti C, Davis J, Bernstein ID. Treatment of malignancy with unmodified antibody. *Pathol Immunopathol Res* 1987;6:419–434.
34. Holland G, Zlotnik A. Interleukin-10 and cancer. *Cancer Invest* 1993;11:751–758.
35. Nørgaard P, Hougaard S, Poulsen HS, Thomsen M. Transforming growth factor β and cancer. *Cancer Treat Rev* 1995;21:367–403.
36. Lee J, Fenton BM, Koch CJ, Frelinger JG, Lord EM. Interleukin-2 expression by tumor cells alters both the immune response and the tumor microenvironment. *Cancer Res* 1998;58:1748–1785.
37. Lupu R, Cardillo M, Harris L, et al. Interaction between erbB-receptors and Heregulin in breast cancer tumor progression and drug resistance. *Semin Cancer Biol* 1995;6:135–145.
38. Schubert D, Heinemann S, Carlisle W, et al. Clonal cell lines from the rat central nervous system. *Nature* 1974;249:224–227.
39. King CR, Kraus MH, Aaronson SA. Amplification of a novel c-erbB-related gene in a human mammary carcinoma. *Science* 1985;229:974–976.
40. Coussens L, Yang-Feng TL, Liao YC, et al. Tyrosine kinase receptor with extensive homology to EGF receptor shares chromosomal location with neu oncogene. *Science* 1985;230:1132–1139.
41. Yamamoto T, Ikawa S, Akiyama T, et al. Similarity of protein encoded by the human c-erbB-2 gene to epidermal growth factor receptor. *Nature* 1986;319:230–237.
42. DiFiore PP, Pierce JH, Kraus MH, et al. erbB-2 is a potent oncogene when over-expressed in NIH/3T3 cells. *Science* 1989;237:178–182.
43. Hudziak RM, Schlessinger J, Ullrich A. Increased expression of the putative growth factor receptor p185 HER2 causes transformation and tumorigenesis of NIH/3T3 cells. *Proc Natl Acad Sci U S A* 1987;84:7159–7163.
44. Wallasch C, Weiss FU, Neiderfellner G, et al. Heregulin-dependent regulation of HER2/neu oncogene is signaling by heterodimerization with HER3. *Embo J* 1995;14:4267–4275.
45. Plowman GD, Green JM, Culouscou JM, et al. Heregulin induces tyrosine phosphorylation of HER2IP18OerbB4. *Nature* 1993;366: 473–475.
46. Schechter AL, Stern DF, Vaidyanathan L, et al. The neu-oncogene: an erbB related gene encoding a 185,000 MW tumor antigen. *Nature* 1984;312:513–516.
47. Bargmann CI, Hung M-C, Weinberg RA. Multiple independent activations of the neu oncogene by a point mutation altering the transmembrane domain of p185. *Cell* 1986;45:649–657.
48. Scott GK, Robles R, Park JW, et al. A truncated intracellular HER2/neu receptor produced by alternative RNA processing affects growth of human carcinoma cells. *Mol Cell Biol* 1993;13:2247–2257.
49. Press MF, Cordon-Cardo C, Slamon DJ. Expression of the HER-2/neu proto-oncogene in normal human and fetal tissues. *Oncogene* 1990;5:953–962.
50. Cohen JA, Weiner DB, More KF, et al. Expression pattern of the neu (NGL) gene-encoded growth factor receptor protein (p185^{neu}) in normal and transformed epithelial tissues. *Oncogene* 1989;4:81–88.
51. McGuire HC Jr, Greene MI. The neu (c-erbB-2) oncogene. *Semin*

Oncol 1989;16:148–155.

52. Tahara E. Growth factors and oncogenes in human gastrointestinal carcinomas. *J Cancer Res Clin Oncol* 1990;116:121–131.

53. Schneider PM, Hung MC, Chiocca SM. Differential expression of the c-erbB-2 gene in human small cell and non-small cell lung cancer. *Cancer Res* 1989;49:4968–4971.

54. Haldane JS, Hird V, Hughes CM. c-erbB-2 oncogene in ovarian cancer. *J Pathol* 1990;162:231–237.

55. Frankel AE, Ring DB, Tringale F. Tissue distribution of breast cancer-associated antigens defined by monoclonal antibodies. *J Biol Res Mod* 1985;4:273–286.

56. Klijn JGM, Berns PMJJ, Schmitz PIM, Foekens JA. The clinical significance of epidermal growth factor receptor (EGFR) in human breast cancer: a review of 5,232 patients. *Endocr Rev* 1992;13:3–17.

57. Wong AJ, Bigner SH, Bigner DD, Kinzler KW, Hamilton SR, Vogelstein B. Increased expression of the epidermal growth factor receptor gene in malignant gliomas is invariably associated with gene amplification. *Proc Natl Acad Sci U S A* 1987;84:6899–6903.

58. Salmon DS, Kim N, Saeki T, Ciardiello F. Transforming growth factor-α: an oncodevelopmental growth factor. *Cancer Cells* 1990;2: 389–397.

59. Barrett-Lee PJ, Travers MT, Lugmani Y, Coombs RC. Transcripts for transforming growth factors in human breast cancer: clinical correlates. *Br J Cancer* 1990;61:612–617.

60. Lundy J, Scuss A, Stanick D, et al. Expression of neu protein, EGF and TGFα in breast cancer. *Am J Pathol* 1991;138:1527–1534.

61. Ekstrand AJ, Sugawa N, James CD, Collins VP. Amplified and rearranged epidermal growth factor receptor genes in human glioblastomas reveal deletions of sequences encoding portions of the N- and/or C-terminal tails. *Proc Natl Acad Sci U S A* 1992;89:4309–4313.

62. Garcia de Palazzo I, Adams GP, Sundareshan P, et al. Expression of mutated epidermal growth factor receptor by non-small cell lung carcinomas. *Cancer Res* 1993;53:3217–3220.

63. Wikstrand CJ, Hale LP, Batra SK, et al. Monoclonal antibodies against EGFRvIII are tumor specific and react with breast and lung carcinomas and malignant gliomas. *Cancer Res* 1995;55:3140–3148.

64. Moscatello DK, Montgomery RB, Sundareshan P, McDanel H, Wong AJ. Transformational and altered signal transduction by a naturally occurring mutant EGF receptor. *Oncogene* 1996;13:85–96.

65. Antonyak MA, Moscatello DK, Wong AJ. Constitutive activation of c-Jun N-terminal kinase by a mutant epidermal growth factor receptor. *J Biol Chem* 1998;273:2817–2822.

66. Moscatello DK, Holgado-Madruga M, Emlet DR, Montgomery RB, Wong AJ. Constitutive activation of phosphatidylinositol 3-kinase by a naturally occurring mutant epidermal growth factor receptor. *J Biol Chem* 1998;273:200–206.

67. Nagane M, Levitzki A, Gazit A, Cavenee WK, Huang HJ. Drug resistance of human glioblastoma cells conferred by a tumor-specific mutant epidermal growth factor receptor through modulation of Bcl-XL and caspase-3-like proteases. *Proc Natl Acad Sci U S A* 1998;95:5724–5729.

68. Reist CJ, Garg PK, Aiston KL, Bigner DD, Zalutsky MR. Radioiodination of internalizing antibodies using N-succinimidyl 5-iodo-3-pyridinecarboxylate. *Cancer Res* 1996;56:4970–4977.

69. Gold O, Freedman SO. Demonstration of tumor specific antigens in human colonic carcinomata by immunological tolerance and absorption techniques. *J Exp Med* 1965;121:439–462.

70. Zimmerman W, Weber B, Ortlieb B, et al. Chromosomal localization of the carcinoembryonic antigen gene family and differential expression in various tissues. *Cancer Res* 1988;48:2443–2550.

71. Thompson J, Zimmerman W. The carcinoembryonic antigen gene family: structure, expression, and evolution. *Tumour Biol* 1988;9: 63–83.

72. Benchinol S, Fuks A, Jothy S, et al. Carcinoembryonic antigen, a human tumor marker functions as an intercellular adhesion molecule. *Cell* 1989;57:327–334.

73. Kuhajda FP, Offutt LE, Mendelsohn G. The distribution of carcinoembryonic antigen in breast carcinoma. Diagnostic and prognostic implications. *Cancer* 1983;52:1257–1264.

74. Kitamura K, Stockert E, Garin-Chesa P, et al. Specificity analysis of Ley antibodies generated against synthetic and natural Ley determi-

nants. *Proc Natl Acad Sci U S A* 1994;91:12957–12961.

75. Leoni F, Colnaghi MI, Canevari S, et al. Glycolipids carrying Leγ are preferentially expressed on small-cell lung cancer cells as detected by the monoclonal antibody MluC1. *Int J Cancer* 1992;51:225–231.

76. Anger B, Lloyd KO, Oettgen HF, Old U. Mouse monoclonal IgM antibody against human lung cancer cell line SK-LC-3 with specificity for h(O) blood group antigen. *Hybridoma* 1982;1:139–147.

77. Yin BWT, Finstad CL, Kitamura K, et al. Serological and immunochemical analysis of lewis y (Ley) blood group antigen expression in epithelial ovarian cancer. *Int J Cancer* 1996;65:406–412.

78. Blaszczyk-Thurin M, Thurin J, Hindsgaul O, Karlsson K-A, Steplewski Z, Koprowski H. Y and blood group B type 2 glycolipid antigens accumulate in a human gastric carcinoma cell line as detected by monoclonal antibody. *J Biol Chem* 1987;262:372–379.

79. Brown A, Ellis LO, Embleton MJ, et al. Immunohistochemical localization of Y hapten and the structurally related H type-2 blood-group antigen on large-bowel tumours and normal tissues. *Int J Cancer* 1984;33:727–736.

80. Hiraishi K, Suzuki K, Hakomori S, Adachi M. Ley antigen expression is correlated with apoptosis (programmed cell death). *Glycobiology* 1993;3:381–390.

81. Aoki R, Tanaka S, Hruma K, et al. MUC-1 expression as a predictor of the curative endoscopic treatment of submucosally invasive colorectal carcinoma. *Dis Colon Rectum* 1998;41:1262–1272.

82. Hanisch FG, Uhlenbruek G, Egge H, Peter-Katalinic J. A B72.3 second-generation monoclonal antibody (CC49) defines the mucin-carried carbohydrate epitope Galβ$(1\rightarrow3)$[NeuAcα$(2\rightarrow6)$]. *Biol Chem* 1989;370:21–26.

83. Springer GF. T and Tn, general carcinoma autoantigens. *Science* 1984; 224:1198–1206.

84. Petrakou E, Murray A, Price MR. Epitope mapping of anti-MUC 1 mucin protein core monoclonal antibodies. *Tumour Biol* 1998;19:21–29.

85. Kennedy RC. The impact of idiotope-based strategies on cancer immunity. *Immunol Allergy Clin North Am* 1991;11:425–444.

86. Jerome KR, Barnd DL, Bendt KM, et al. Cytotoxic T-lymphocytes derived from patients with breast cancer adenocarcinoma recognize an epitope present on the protein core of a mucin molecule preferentially expressed by malignant cells. *Cancer Res* 1991;51:2908–2916.

87. MacLean GD, Reddish MA, Longenecker BM. Prognostic significance of preimmunotherapy serum CA27.29 (MUC-1) mucin level after active specific immunotherapy of metastatic adenocarcinoma patients. *J Immunother* 1997;20:70–78.

88. Austin EB, Robins RA, Baldwin RW, Durrant LG. Induction of delayed hypersensitivity to human tumor cells with a human monoclonal anti-idiotypic antibody. *J Natl Cancer Inst* 1991;83: 1245–1248.

89. Peterson JA, Zava DT, Duwe AK, Blank EW, Battifora H, Ceriani RL. Biochemical and histological characterization of antigens preferentially expressed on the surface and cytoplasm of breast carcinoma cells identified by monoclonal antibodies against the human milk fat globule. *Hybridoma* 1990;9:221–235.

90. Moldenhauer G, Momburg F, Moller P, et al. Epithelium-specific surface glycoprotein of M_r 34,000 is a widely distributed human carcinoma marker. *Br J Cancer* 1987;56:714–721.

91. Litvinov SV, Velders MP, Bakker HAM, et al. Ep-CAM: a human epithelial antigen is a homophilic cell-cell adhesion molecule. *J Cell Biol* 1994;125:437–446.

92. Cook JD, Skikne BS, Baynes RD. Serum transferrin receptor. *Annu Rev Med* 1993;44:63–74.

93. Elliott RL, Elliott MC, Wang F, Head JF. Breast carcinoma and the role of iron metabolism. A cytochemical, tissue culture, and ultrastructural study. *Ann N Y Acad Sci* 1993;698:159–166.

94. Wittekind C. Carcinoembryonic antigen family members as diagnostic tools in immunohistopathology. *Tumour Biol* 1995;16:42–47.

95. Zamechek N, Kipchik HZ. Proceedings: the interdependence of clinical investigation and methodological development in the early evolution of assays for carcinoembryonic antigen. *Cancer Res* 1974;34:2131–2136.

96. Pavelic ZP, Pavelic L, Pavelic K, Peacock JS. Utility of anti-carcinoembryonic antigen monoclonal antibodies for differentiating ovarian adenocarcinomas from gastrointestinal metastasis to the ovary.

Gynecol Oncol 1991;40:112–117.

97. Ramaekers F, van Niekerk C, Poels L, et al. Use of monoclonal antibodies to keratin 7 in the differential diagnosis of adenocarcinomas. *Am J Pathol* 1990;136:641–655.

98. Colomer A, Martinez-Mas JV, Matias-Guim X, et al. Sex-steroid hormone receptors in human medullary thyroid carcinoma. *Mod Pathol* 1996;9:68–72.

99. Tonn JC, Ott MM, Paulus W, Meixensberger J, Roosen K. Progesterone receptors in tissue fragment spheroids of human meningiomas. *Acta Neurochir Suppl* 1996;65:105–107.

100. Khalid H, Shibata S, Kishikawa M, Yasunaga A, Iseki M, Hiura T. Immunohistochemical analysis of progesterone receptor and Ki-67 labeling index in astrocytic tumors. *Cancer* 1997;80:2133–2140.

101. McGuire WL. Estrogen receptor versus nuclear grade as prognostic factors in axillary node negative breast cancer. *J Clin Oncol* 1988;7:1071–1072.

102. Alexieva-Figusch J, Van Putten WLJ, Blankstein MA, Blonk-Van der Wijst J, Klijn JGM. The prognostic value and relationships of patient characteristics, estrogen and progestin receptors, and site of relapse in primary breast cancer. *Cancer* 1988;61:758–768.

103. Fukuda K, Mon M, Uichiyama M, Iwai K, Iwasaka T, Suymori H. Prognostic significance of progesterone receptor immunohistochemistry in endometrial carcinoma. *Gynecol Oncol* 1998;69:220–225.

104. Beck T, Weller EE, Weikel W, Brumm C, Wilkens C, Knapstein PG. Usefulness of immunohistochemical staining of p53 in the prognosis of breast carcinomas: correlations with established prognosis parameters and with the proliferation marker, MIB-1. *Gynecol Oncol* 1995;57:96–104.

105. Elledge RM, Gray R, Mansour E, et al. Accumulation of p53 protein as a possible predictor of response to adjuvant chemotherapy with cyclophosphamide, methotrexate, fluorouracil, and prednisone in breast cancer. *J Natl Cancer Inst* 1992;84:1109–1114.

106. Wintzer H-O, Zipfel I, Schulte-Montirg J, Hellerich U, von Kleist S. Ki-67 immunostaining in human breast tumors and its relationship to prognosis. *Cancer* 1991;67:421–428.

107. Simory J, Pujol J-L, Padal M, Ursule E, Michel F-B, Pujol H. In situ evaluation of growth fraction determined by monoclonal antibody ki-67 and ploidy in surgically resected non-small cell lung cancers. *Cancer Res* 1990;50:4382–4387.

108. Kyzer S, Gordon PH. Determination of proliferative activity in colorectal carcinoma using monoclonal antibody Ki-67. *Dis Colon Rectum* 1997;40:322–325.

109. Tandon AK, Clark GM, Chamness GC, et al. HER-2/neu oncogene protein and prognosis in breast cancer. *J Clin Oncol* 1989;7:1120–1128.

110. Tikannen S, Helm H, Isola J, Joensuu H. Prognostic significance of HER-2 oncoprotein expression in breast cancer: a 30-year follow up. *J Clin Oncol* 1992;10:1044–1048.

111. Giatromanolaki A, Koukourakis M, O'Byrne K, et al. Non-small cell lung cancer: c-erbB-2 overexpression correlates with low angiogenesis and poor prognosis. *Anticancer Res* 1996;16:3819–3826.

112. Tanner B, Kreutz E, Weikel W, et al. Prognostic significance of c-crbB-2 mRNA in ovarian carcinoma. *Gynecol Oncol* 1996;62:268–277.

113. Paik S, Hazan R, Fisher ER, et al. Pathologic findings from the National Surgical Adjuvant Breast and Bowel project: prognostic significance of c-erbB-2 protein overexpression in primary breast cancer. *J Clin Oncol* 1990;8:103–112.

114. Wong JY, Chu DZ, Yamauchi D, et al. Dose escalation trial of indium-111-labeled anti-carcinoembryonic antigen chimeric monoclonal antibody (chimeric T84.66) in presurgical colorectal cancer patients. *J Nucl Med* 1998;39:2097–2104.

115. Digvi CR. Status of radiolabeled monoclonal antibodies for diagnosis and therapy of cancer. *Oncology* 1996;10:939–950.

116. Textei JH Jr, Neal CE. The role of monoclonal antibody in the management of prostate adenocarcinoma. *J Urol* 1998;160:2393–2395.

117. Kairemo KJ. Immunolymphoscintigraphy with 99mTc-labeled monoclonal antibody (BW 431/26) reacting with carcinoembryonic antigen in breast cancer. *Cancer Res* 1990;50:949–954.

118. Rosner D, Nabi H, Wild L, Ortman-Nabi J, Hreshchyshyn MM. Diagnosis of breast carcinoma with radiolabeled monoclonal antibodies (MoAbs) to carcinoembryonic antigen (CEA) and human milk fat globulin (HMFG). *Cancer Invest* 1995;23:573–582.

119. Goldenberg DM, Wegencr W. Studies of breast cancer imaging with radiolabeled antibodies to carcinoembryonic antigen. Immunomedics Breast Cancer Study Group. *Acta Med Austriaca* 1997;24:55–59.

120. Balaban EP, Walker BS, Cox JV, et al. Detection and staging of small cell lung cancer with a technetium-labeled monoclonal antibody. A comparison with standard staging systems. *Clin Nucl Med* 1992;17:439–445.

121. Breitz HB, Tyler A, Bjorn MJ, Lesley T, Weiden PL. Clinical experience with Tc-99m nofetumomab merpentan (Verluma) radioimmunoscintigraphy. *Clin Nucl Med* 1997;22:615–620.

122. Balaban EP, Walker BS, Cox JV, et al. Radionuclide imaging of bone marrow metastases with a Tc-99 labeled monoclonal antibody to small cell lung cancer. *Clin Nucl Med* 1991;16:732–736.

123. Casalini P, Luison E, Menard S, et al. Tumor pretargeting: role of avidin/streptavidin on monoclonal antibody internalization. *J Nucl Med* 1997;38:1378–1381.

124. Magnani P, Paganelli G, Songini C, et al. Pretargeted immunoscintigraphy in patients with medullary thyroid carcinoma. *Br J Cancer* 1996;74:825–831.

125. Colobo P, Siccardi AG, Paganelli G, et al. Three-step immunoscintigraphy with anti-chromogranin A monoclonal antibody in tumours of the pituitary region. *Eur J Endocrinol* 1996;135:216-221.

126. Siccardi AG, Paganelli G, Pontiroli AE, et al. *In vivo* imaging of chromogranin A-positive endocrine tumours by three-step monoclonal antibody targeting. *Eur J Nucl Med* 1996;23:1455–1459.

127. Dosio F, Magnani P, Paganelli G, Samuel A, Chiesa G, Fazio F. Three-step tumor targeting in lung cancer immunoscintigraphy. *J Nucl Biol Med* 1993;37:228–232.

128. Bertsch DJ, Burak WE Jr, Young DC, Arnold MW, Martin LW. Radioimmunoguided surgery for colorectal cancer. *Ann Surg Oncol* 1996;3:310–316.

129. Nieroda CA, Mojzisik C, Hinkle G, Thurston MO, Martin LW Jr. Radioimmunoguided surgery (RIGS) in recurrent colorectal cancer. *Cancer Detect Prev* 1991;15:225–229.

130. Aftab F, Stodt HS, Tesori A, et al. Radioimmunoguided surgery and colorectal cancer. *Eur J Surg Oncol* 1996;22:381–396.

131. De Nardi P, Stella M, Magnani P, et al. Combination of monoclonal antibodies for radioimmunoguided surgery. *Int J Colorectal Dis* 1997;12:24–28.

132. Basegla J, Tripathy D, Mendelsohn J, et al. Phase II study of weekly intravenous recombinant humanized anti-p185^{HER2} monoclonal antibody in patients with HER2/*neu*-overexpressing metastatic breast cancer. *J Clin Oncol* 1996;14:737–744.

133. Cobleigh MA, Vogel CL, Tripathy D, et al. Efficacy and safety of Herceptin^{TM} (Humanized anti-HER2 antibody) as a single agent in 222 women with HER2 overexpression who relapsed following chemotherapy for metastatic breast cancer. *Proc Am Soc Clin Oncol* 1998;17:A376.

134. Petit AM, Rak J, Hung MC, et al. Neutralizing antibodies against epidermal growth factor and ErbB-2/neu receptor tyrosine kinases down-regulate vascular endothelial growth factor production by tumor cells *in vitro* and *in vivo*: angiogenic implications for signal transduction therapy in solid tumors. *Am J Pathol* 1997;151:1523–1530.

135. Slamon D, Shak S, Paton V, et al. Addition of Herceptin^{TM} (humanized anti-HER2 antibody) to first line chemotherapy for HER2 overexpressing metastatic breast cancer (HER2+/MBC) markedly increases anticancer activity: a randomized multinational controlled phase III trial. *Proc Am Soc Clin Oncol* 1998;17:A377.

136. Haga Y, Sivinski CL, Woo D, Tempero MA. Dose related comparison of antibody-dependent cellular cytotoxicity with chimeric and native murine monoclonal antibody 17-1A. Improved cytolysis of pancreatic cancer cells with chimeric 17-1A. *Int J Pancreatol* 1994;15:43–50.

137. Meredith RF, LoBuglio AF, Plott WE, et al. Pharmacokinetics, immune response, and biodistribution of iodine-131-labeled chimeric mouse/human IgG1 17-1A monoclonal antibody. *J Nucl Med* 1991;32:1162–1168.

138. Takarnuku K, Baba K, Arinaga S, Li J, Mon M, Akihoshi T. Apoptosis in antibody-dependent monocyte-mediated cytotoxicity with monoclonal antibody 17-1A against human colorectal carcinoma cells: enhancement with interferon gamma. *Cancer Immunol Immunother* 1996;43:220–225.

139. Reali E, Guiliani AL, Spisani S, et al. Interferon-gamma enhances monoclonal antibody 17-1A-dependent neutrophil cytotoxicity toward colorectal carcinoma cell line SW11-16. *Clin Immunol Immunopathol* 1994;71:105–112.

140. Ragnhammar P, Masucci G, Frodin JE, Hjelm AL, Mellstedt H. Cytotoxic functions of blood mononuclear cells in patients with colorectal carcinoma treated with mAb 17-1A and granulocyte/macrophage-colony-stimulating factor. *Cancer Immunol Immunother* 1992;35:158–164.

141. Ragnhammar P, Magnusson I, Masucci G, Mellstedt H. The therapeutic use of the unconjugated monoclonal antibodies (MAb) 17-1A in combination with GM-CSF in the treatment of colorectal carcinoma (CRC). *Med Oncol Tumor Pharmacother* 1993;10:61–70.

142. Masucci G, Ragnhammar P, Wersall P, Mellstedt H. Granulocyte-monocyte colony-stimulating-factor augments the interleukin-2-induced cytotoxic activity of human lymphocytes in the absence and presence of mouse or chimeric monoclonal antibodies (mAb 17-1 A). *Cancer Immunol Immunother* 1990;31:231–235.

143. Wersall P, Massucci G, Mellstedt H. Interleukin-4 augments the cytotoxic capacity of lymphocytes and monocytes in antibody-dependent cellular cytotoxicity. *Cancer Immunol Immunother* 1991; 33:45–49.

144. Reali E, Spisani S, Gavili R, Lanza F, Moretti S, Traniello S. IL-8 enhances antibody-dependent cellular cytotoxicity in human neutrophils. *Immunol Cell Biol* 1995;73:234–238.

145. Frodin JE, Faxas ME, Hagstrom B, et al. Induction of anti-idiotypic (ab2) and anti-idiotypic (ab3) antibodies in patients treated with the mouse monoclonal antibody 17-1A (ab1). Relation to the clinical outcome—an important antitumoral effector function? *Hybridoma* 1991;10:421–431.

146. Hanzawa Y, Tsujisaki M, Tokuchi S, et al. Detection of xenogeneic anti-idiotypic antibodies specific to murine monoclonal antibody 17-1A in patients with gastrointestinal cancer. *Tumour Biol* 1992;13:226–236.

147. Fagerberg J, Frodin JE, Wigzell H, Mellstedt H. Induction of an immune network cascade in cancer patients treated with monoclonal antibodies (ab1). I. May induction of ab-1 reactive T cells and anti-anti-idiotypic antibodies (ab3) lead to tumor regression after mAb therapy? *Cancer Immunol Immunother* 1993;37:264–270.

148. Ragnhammar P, Fagerberg J, Frodin J-E, et al. Granulocyte monocyte colony stimulating factor augments the induction of antibodies, especially anti-idiotypic antibodies to therapeutic monoclonal antibodies. *Cancer Immunol Immunother* 1993;37:264–270.

149. Shetye J, Ragnhammar P, Liljefors M, et al. Immunopathology of metastases in patients of colorectal carcinoma treated with monoclonal antibody 17-1A and granulocyte macrophage colony-stimulating factor. *Clin Cancer Res* 1998;4:1921–1929.

150. Fagerberg J, Frodin JE, Ragnhammar P, Steinitz M, Wigzell H, Mellstedt H. Induction of an immune network cascade in cancer patients treated with monoclonal antibodies (ab1). II. Is induction of anti-idiotype reactive T cells (T3) of importance for tumor response to mAb therapy? *Cancer Immunol Immunother* 1994;38:149–159.

151. Reithmuller G, Holz B, Schlirnok G, et al. Monoclonal antibody therapy for resected Dukes' C colorectal cancer: seven-year outcome of a multicenter randomized trial. *J Clin Oncol* 1988;16:1788–1794.

152. Sears HF, Atkinson B, Mattis J, et al. Phase I clinical trial of monoclonal antibody in treatment of gastrointestinal tumors. *Lancet* 1982;2:762–765.

153. Sears HF, Herlyn D, Steplewski Z, Koprowski H. Effects of monoclonal antibody immunotherapy on patients with gastrointestinal adenocarcinoma. *J Biol Res Mod* 1984;3:138–150.

154. Verrill H, Goldberg M, Rosenbaum R, et al. Clinical trial of Wistar Institute 17-1A monoclonal antibody in patients with advanced gastrointestinal adenocarcinoma: a preliminary report. *Hybridoma* 1986;1[Suppl 5]:175–183.

155. Khazaeli MB, Saleh MN, Wheeler RH, et al. Phase I trial of multiple large doses of murine monoclonal antibody CO 17-1 A. II; Pharmacokinetics and immune response. *J Natl Cancer Inst* 1988;80:937–942.

156. Lobuglio AF, Saleh M, Peterson L, et al. Phase I clinical trial of CO17-1A monoclonal antibody. *Hybridoma* 1986;1[5 Suppl]:117–123.

157. Paul AR, Engstrom PF, Weiner LM, Steplewski Z, Koprowski H. Treatment of advanced measurable or valuable pancreatic carcinoma with 17-1A murine monoclonal antibody alone or in combination with 5-fluorouracil, Adriamycin, and mitomycin (FAM). *Hybridoma* 1986;1[5 Suppl]:171–174.

158. Sindclar WF, Maher MM, Herlyn D, Sears HF, Steplewski Z, Koprowski H. Trial of therapy with monoclonal antibody 17-1A in pancreatic carcinoma: preliminary results. *Hybridoma* 1986;1[5 Suppl]:125–132.

159. Sears HF, Herlyn D, Steplewski Z, Koprowski H. Phase II clinical trial of a murine monoclonal antibody cytotoxic for gastrointestinal adenocarcinoma. *Cancer Res* 1985;45:5910–5913.

160. Weiner LM, Harvey E, Padavic-Shaller K, et al. Phase II multicenter evaluation of prolonged murine monoclonal antibody 17-1A therapy in pancreatic carcinoma. *J Immunother* 1993;13:110–116.

161. Ragnhammar P, Fragerberg J, Frodin J-E, et al. Effect of the monoclonal antibody 17-1A and granulocyte monocyte colony stimulating factor in patients with carcinoma. Long lasting complete remissions can be induced. *Int J Cancer* 1993;53:751–758.

162. Saleh MN, LoBuglio AF, Wheeler RH, et al. A phase II trial of murine monoclonal antibody 17-1A and interferon-γ: clinical and immunological data. *Cancer Immunol Immunother* 1990;32:185–190.

163. Weiner LM, Moldofsky PJ, Gatenby RA, et al. Antibody delivery and effector cell activation in a phase II trial of recombinant gamma interferon and the murine monoclonal antibody CO17-1A in advanced colorectal adenocarcinoma. *Cancer Res* 1988;45: 2568–2571.

164. Tempero MA, Sivinski C, Steplewski Z, Hsarvey E, Klassen E, Kay HD. Phase II trial of interferon gamma and monoclonal antibody 17-1A in pancreatic cancer: biologic and clinical effects. *J Clin Oncol* 1990;8:2019–2026.

165. Reithmuller G, Schneider-Gadicke E, Schlimok G, et al. Randomized trial of monoclonal antibody for adjuvant therapy of resected Dukes' C colorectal carcinoma. *Lancet* 1994;343:1177–1183.

166. Modjtahedi H, Komurasaki T, Toyoda H, Dean C. Anti-EGFR monoclonal antibodies which act as EGF, TGF alpha, HB-EGF, and BTC antagonists block the binding of epiregulin to EGFR-expressing tumours. *Int J Cancer* 1998;75:310–316.

167. Teramoto T, Onda M, Tokunaga A, Asano G. Inhibitory effect of an anti-epidermal growth factor receptor antibody on human gastric cancer. *Cancer* 1996;77:1639–1645.

168. Sato JD, Kawamoto T, Le AD, et al. Biologic effect *in vitro* of monoclonal antibodies to human EGF receptors. *Mol Biol Med* 1983; 1:511–529.

169. Artega CL, Corondo E, Osbore CK. Blockade of the epidermal growth factor receptor inhibits transforming growth factor alpha-induced but not estrogen-induced growth of hormone-dependent human breast cancer. *Mol Endocrinol* 1988;2:1064–1069.

170. Hoffman T, Hafner D, Ballo H, Haas I, Bier H. Antitumor activity of anti-epidermal growth factor receptor monoclonal antibodies and cisplatin in ten human head and neck squamous cell carcinoma lines. *Anticancer Res* 1997;17:4419–4425.

171. Fan Z, Baselga J, Masui H, Mendelsohn J. Antitumor effect of anti-epidermal growth factor receptor monoclonal antibodies plus cis-diaminedichloroplatinum on well established A431 cell xenografts. *Cancer Res* 1993;53:4637–4642.

172. Baselga J, Norton L, Masui H, et al. Antitumor effects of doxorubicin in combination with anti-epidermal growth factor receptor monoclonal antibodies. *J Natl Cancer Inst* 1993;85:1327–1333.

173. Modjtahedi H, Eccles S, Sandle J, Box G, Titley J, Dean C. Differentiation or immune destruction: two pathways for therapy of squamous cell carcinomas with antibodies to the epidermal growth factor receptor. *Cancer Res* 1994;54:1695–1701.

174. Sunada H, Magun G, Mendelsohn J, et al. Monoclonal antibody against the EGF receptor is internalized without stimulating receptor

phosphorylation. *Proc Natl Acad Sci U S A* 1986;83:3825–3928.

175. Sunada H, Yu P, Peacock JS, et al. Modulation of tyrosine serine and threonine phosphorylation and intracellular processing of the epidermal growth factor receptor by anti-receptor monoclonal antibody. *J Cell Physiol* 1990;142:284–292.

176. Fan Z, Masui M, Altas I, Mendelsohn J. Blockade of the epidermal growth factor receptor function by bivalent and monovalent fragments of 225 anti-epidermal growth factor receptor monoclonal antibodies. *Cancer Res* 1993;53:4322–4328.

177. Prewett M, Rockwell RF, Giorgio NA, Mendelsohn J, Scher HI, Goldstein NI. The biologic effects of C225, a chimeric monoclonal antibody to the EGFR, on human prostate carcinoma. *J Immunother* 1996;19:419–427.

178. Zolfaghari A, Djakiew D. Inhibition of chemomigration of a human prostatic carcinoma cell (TSU-pr1) line by inhibition of epidermal growth factor receptor function. *Prostate* 1996;28:232–238.

179. Peng D, Fan Z, Lu Y, DeBlasio T, Scher H, Mendelsohn J. Anti-epidermal growth factor receptor monoclonal antibody 225 up-regulates p27KIP1 and induces G1 arrest in prostatic cancer cell line DU145. *Cancer Res* 1996;56:3666–3669.

180. Wu X, Rubin M, Fan Z, et al. Involvement of p27KIP1 in G1 arrest mediated by an anti-epidermal growth factor receptor monoclonal antibody. *Oncogene* 1996;12:1397–1403.

181. Mendelsohn J, Shin DM, Donato N, et al. A phase I study of chimerized anti-epidermal growth factor receptor (EGFr) monoclonal antibody, C225, in combination with cisplatin (CDDP) in patient (PTS) with recurrent head and neck squamous cell carcinoma (SCC). *Proc Am Assoc Clin Oncol* 1999;18:A1502.

182. Modjtahedi H, Hickish T, Nicolson M, et al. Phase I trial and tumour localization of the anti-EGFR monoclonal antibody ICR62 in head and neck or lung cancer. *Br J Cancer* 1996;73:228–235.

183. Perez-Soler R, Donato NJ, Shin DM, et al. Tumor epidermal growth factor receptor studies in patients with non-small cell lung cancer or head and neck cancer treated with monoclonal antibody RG83852. *J Clin Oncol* 1994;12:730–739.

184. Christen RD, Horn DK, Porter DC, et al. Epidermal growth factor regulates the *in vitro* sensitivity of human ovarian carcinoma cells to cisplatin. *J Clin Invest* 1990;86:1632–1640.

185. Kwok TT, Sutherland RM. Differences in EGF related radio-sensitization of human squamous carcinoma cells with high and low numbers of EGF receptors. *Br J Cancer* 1991;64:251–254.

186. Hellstrom I, Garrigues HJ, Garrigues U, et al. Highly tumor-reactive, internalizing, mouse monoclonal antibodies to Le(Y)-related cell surface antigens. *Cancer Res* 1990;50:2183–2190.

187. Ball ED, Guyre PM, Mills L, Fisher J, Dinces NB, Fanger MW. Initial trial of bispecific antibody-mediated immunotherapy of CD-IS bearing tumors: cytotoxicity of human tumor cells using a bispecific antibody comprised of anti-CD 15 (MoAb PM81) and anti-CD64/Fc gamma RI (MoAb 32). *J Hematother* 1992;1:85–94.

188. Mordoh J, Silva C, Albarellos M, Bravo AI, Kairiyama C. Phase I clinical trial in cancer patients of a new monoclonal antibody FC-2.15 reacting with tumor proliferating cells. *J Immunother* 1995;17:151–160.

189. Pastan I, Lovelace ET, Gallo MG, Rutherford AV, Magnani JL, Willingham MC. Characterization of monoclonal antibodies B1 and B3 that react with mucinous adenocarcinomas. *Cancer Res* 1991;51:3781–3787.

190. Hellstrom I, Garrigues HJ, Garrigues U, Hellstrom KB. Highly tumor reactive, internalizing, mouse monoclonal antibodies to Ley-related cell surface antigens. *Cancer Res* 1990;50:2183–2190.

191. Pietersz GA, Wenjun L, Krauer K, Baker T, Wreschner D, McKenzie IFC. Comparison of the biological properties of two anti-mucin-1 antibodies prepared for imaging and therapy. *Cancer Immunol Immunother* 1997;44:323–328.

192. van Hof AC, Molthoff CF, Davies Q, et al. Biodistribution of (111) indium-labeled engineered human antibody CTM01 in ovarian cancer patients: influence of protein dose. *Cancer Res* 1996;56:5179–5185.

193. van Hof AC, Moithoff CF, Davies Q, et al. Biodistribution of (111) indium-labeled engineered human antibody CTM01 in ovarian cancer patients. *Cancer Res* 1996;56:5179–5185.

194. Prinssen HM, Molthoff CF, Verheijen RH, et al. Biodistribution of 111In-labelled engineered human antibody CTM01 (hCTM01) in

195. Bashford JA, Robins RA, Price MR. Development of an anti-idiotypic antibody reactive with an antibody defining the epitope RPAP in the MUC-l epithelial mucin core. *Int J Cancer* 1993;54:778–783.

196. Gold DV, Lew K, Maliniak R, Hernandez M, Cardillo T. Characterization of monoclonal antibody PAM4 reactive with a pancreatic cancer mucin. *Int J Cancer* 1994;57:204–210.

197. Gold DV, Cardillo T, Vardi Y, Blumenthal R. Radioimmunotherapy of experimental pancreatic cancer with 131I-labeled monoclonal antibody PAM4. *Int J Cancer* 1997;71:660–667.

198. Fiorentini S, Matczak E, Gallo RC, Reitz MS, Keydar I, Watkins BA. Humanization of an antibody recognizing a breast cancer epitope by CDR-grafting. *Immunotechnology* 1997;3:45–59.

199. Zhang S, Walberg LA, Ogata S, et al. Immune sera and monoclonal antibodies define two configurations for the Sialyl Tn tumor antigen. *Cancer Res* 1995;55:3364–3368.

200. O'Boyle KP, Goya V, Zuckier LS, Chun S, Bhargava K. Expression of human tumor mucin-associated carbohydrate epitopes, including sialylated Tn, and localization of murine monoclonal antibodies cc49 and B72.3 is a syngeneic rat colon carcinoma model. *J Immunother* 1994;16:251–261.

201. Couto JR, Blank EW, Peterson JA, Ceriani RL. Anti-BA46 monoclonal antibody Mc3: humanization using a novel positional consensus and *in vivo* and *in vitro* characterization. *Cancer Res* 1995;55:1717–1722.

202. Elliot RL, Elliot MC, Wang F, Head JF. Breast carcinoma and the role of iron metabolism. *Ann N Y Acad Sci* 1993;698:159–163.

203. Brooks D, Taylor C, Dos Santos B, et al. Phase Ia trial of murine immunoglobulin A antitransferrin receptor antibody 42/6. *Clin Cancer Res* 1995;1:1259–1265.

204. Batra JK, Fitzgerald DJ, Chaudhary VK, Pastan I. Single-chain immunotoxins directed as the human transferrin receptor containing *Pseudomonas* exotoxin A or diphtheria toxin: anti-TRF(Fv)-PE40 and DT3888-anti-TFR(Fv). *Mol Cell Biol* 1991;11:2200–2205.

205. Mack M, Riethmuller G, Kuffer P. A small bispecific antibody construct expressed as a functional single-chain molecule with high tumor cell cytotoxicity. *Proc Natl Acad Sci U S A* 1995;92:7021–7025.

206. Negri DR, Tosi E, Valota O, et al. *In vitro* and *in vivo* stability and anti-tumour efficacy of an anti-EGFR/anti-CD3 F(ab')2 bispecific monoclonal antibody. *Br J Cancer* 1995;72:928–933.

207. McCall AM, Adams GP, Amoroso AR, et al. Isolation and characterization of an anti-CD 16 single chain Fv fragment and construction of an anti-HER2/neu/anti-CD 16 bispecific scFv that triggers CD 16-dependent tumor cytolysis. *Mol Immunol* 1999(in press).

208. Ring DB, Hsieh-Ma ST, Shi T, Redder J. Antigen forks: bispecific reagents that inhibit cell growth by binding selected pairs of tumor antigens. *Cancer Immunol Immunother* 1994;39:41–48.

209. Staertz UD, Kanagawa O, Bevan MI. Hybrid antibodies can target sites for attack by T-cells. *Nature* 1985;314:628–631.

210. Perez P, Hoffman RW, Shaw S, et al. Specific targeting of cytotoxic T-cells by anti-T3 linked to anti-target cell antibody. *Nature* 1985;316:354–356.

211. Pantel K, Schlimok G, Kutter D, et al. Frequent down-regulation of major histocompatibility class I antigen expression on individual micrometastatic carcinoma cells. *Cancer Res* 1991;51:4712–4715.

212. Kroesen B-I, Bakker A, Van Lier RAW, The HT, de Leij L. Bispecific antibody-mediated target cell-specific costimulation of resting T cells via CD5 and CD28. *Cancer Res* 1995;55:4409–4415.

213. Bolhuis RLH, Lamers CHJ, Goey SH, et al. Adoptive immunotherapy of ovarian carcinoma with BS MAb-targeted lymphocytes: a multicenter study. *Int J Cancer* 1992;7:78–81.

214. Rutledge F, Burs B. Chemotherapy for advanced ovarian cancer. *Am J Obstet Gynecol* 1966;96:761–772.

215. Kroesen BJ, Nieken J, Sleijfer DT, et al. Approaches to lung cancer treatment using CD3 x EGP-2-directed bispecific monoclonal antibody BIS-1. *Cancer Immunol Immunother* 1997;45:203–206.

216. Valone FH, Kaufman PA, Guyre PM, et al. Phase Ia/Ib trial of bispecific antibody MDX-210 in patients with advanced breast or ovarian cancer that overexpresses the proto-oncogene HER-2/neu. *J Clin Oncol* 1995;13:2281–2292.

217. Stockmeyer B, Valerius T, Repp R, et al. Preclinical studies with FcγR bispecific antibodies and granulocyte colony-stimulating factor primed neutrophils as effector cells against HER-2/neu overexpressing breast cancer. *Cancer Res* 1997;57:696–701.

218. Shen L, Guyre PM, Anderson CL, et al. Heteroantibody-mediated cytotoxicity: antibody to the high-affinity Fc receptor for IgG mediates cytotoxicity by human monocytes which is enhanced by interferon-gamma and is not blocked by human IgG. *J Immunol* 1986;137:3378–3382.

219. Valerius T, Stockmeyer B, van Spriel AB, et al. FcalphaRl (CD89) as a novel trigger molecule for bispecific antibody therapy. *Blood* 1997;90:4485–4492.

220. Repp R, Valerius T, Wiekand G, et al. G-CSF-stimulated PMN in immunotherapy of breast cancer with a bispecific antibody to Fc gamma RI and HER-2/neu (MDX-210). *J Hematother* 1995;4:415–421.

221. Curnow RT. Clinical experience with CD64-directed immunotherapy. An overview. *Cancer Immunol Immunother* 1997;45:210–215.

222. Kaufman PA, Guyre PM, Barth RJ, et al. Phase I trial of interferon gamma (IFNγ) and MDX-210 (anti-HER-2/neu x anti-FcγRI) in patients (pts) with metastatic carcinomas that overexpress HER-2/neu: preliminary findings. *Proc Am Soc Clin Oncol* 1997;16:A1542.

223. de Palazzo IG, Gercel-Taylor C, Kitson J, Weiner LM. Potentiation of tumor lysis by a bispecific antibody that binds to CA 19-9 antigen and the Fcγ receptor expressed by human by large granular lymphocytes. *Cancer Res* 1990;50:7123–7128.

224. Ferrini S, Prigione I, Miotti S, et al. Bispecific monoclonal antibodies directed to CD16 and to a tumor-associated antigen induce target cell lysis by resting NK cells and a subset of NK clones. *Int J Cancer* 1990;48:227–233.

225. Weiner LM, Holmes M, Richeson A, et al. Binding and cytotoxicity characteristics of the bispecific murine monoclonal antibody 2B1. *J Immunol* 1993;151:2877–2886.

226. Weiner LM, Clark JI, Davey M, et al. Phase I trial of 2B1, a bispecific monoclonal antibody targeting c-erbB-2 and FcγRIII. *Cancer Res* 1995;55:4586–4593.

227. Gralow J, Weiner L, Ring D, et al. HER-2/neu specific immunity can be induced by therapy with 2B1, a bispecific monoclonal antibody binding to HER-2/neu and CD1 6. *Proc Am Soc Clin Oncol* 1995;14:A1807.

228. Pimm MV, Robins RA, Embleton E, et al. A bispecific monoclonal antibody against methotrexate and a human tumour associated antigen augments cytotoxicity of methotrexate-carrier conjugate. *Br J Cancer* 1990;61:508–513.

229. Corvalan JR, Smith W, Gore VA, Brandon DR. Specific *in vitro* and *in vivo* drug localization to tumour cells using a hybrid-hybrid monoclonal antibody recognizing both carcinoembryonic antigen (CEA) and vinca alkaloids. *Cancer Immunol Immunother* 1987;24:133–137.

230. Corvalan JR, Smith W, Gore VA, Brandon DR, Ryde PJ. Increased therapeutic effect of vinca alkaloids targeted to tumour by a hybrid-hybrid monoclonal antibody. *Cancer Immunother Immunol* 1987;24:138–143.

231. Morelli D, Menard S, Pozzi B, Balsari A, Colnaghi MI. Effect of a bifunctional monoclonal antibody directed against a tumor marker and doxorubicin on the growth of epidermoid vulvar carcinoma grafted in athymic mice. *Cell Biophys* 1994;24-25:119–126.

232. Primus FJ, Pak RH, Richard-Dickson KJ, et al. Bispecific antibody mediated targeting of nido-carboranes to human colon carcinoma cells. *Bioconjug Chem* 1996;1:532–535.

233. Guo YJ, Che XY, Shen F, et al. Effective tumor vaccines generated by in vitro modification of tumor cells with cytokines and bispecific monoclonal antibodies. *Nat Med* 1997;3:451–455.

234. Smellie WB, Dean CJ, Sacks NPM, et al. Radioimmunotherapy of breast cancer xenografts with monoclonal antibody ICR12 against c-erbB-2 p185: comparison of iodogen and N-succinimidyl 1-methyl-3-(tri-n-butylstannyl) benzoate radioiodination methods. *Cancer Res* 1995;55:5842–5846.

235. Juweid M, Sharkey RM, Behr T, et al. Targeting and initial radioimmunotherapy of medullary thyroid carcinoma with ^{131}I-labeled monoclonal antibodies to carcinoembryonic antigen. *Cancer Res* 1995;55:5946–5951.

236. Blumenthal RD, Sharkey RM, Kashi R, Sides K, Stein R, Goldenberg DM. Changes in tumor vascular permeability in response to experimental radioimmunotherapy: a comparative study of 11 xenografts. *Tumor Biol* 1997;18:367–377.

237. Buckman R, DeAngelis C, Shaw P, et al. Intraperitoneal therapy of malignant ascites associated with carcinoma of the ovary and breast using radioiodinated monoclonal antibody 2G3. *Gynecol Oncol* 1992;47:102–109.

238. Breitz HB, Durham JS, Fisher DR, Weiden PL. Radiation-absorbed dose estimates to normal organs following intraperitoneal 186Re-labeled monoclonal antibody: methods and results. *Cancer Res* 1995;55:5817–5822.

239. Breitz HB, Durham JS, Fisher DR, et al. Pharmacokinetics and normal organ dosimetry following intraperitoneal rhenium-186-labeled monoclonal antibody. *J Nucl Med* 1995;36:754–761.

240. Jacobs AJ, Fer M, Su FM, et al. A phase I trial of a rhenium 186-labeled monoclonal antibody administered intraperitoneally in ovarian carcinoma: toxicity and clinical responses. *Obstet Gynecol* 1993;82:586–593.

241. Adams GP, DeNardo GP, Amin A, et al. Comparison of the pharmacokinetics in mice and the biologic activity of murine L-6 and human-mouse chimeric Ch L-6 antibody. *Antibody Immunoconjugate Radiopharmaceuticals* 1992;5:81–95.

242. DeNardo SJ, Mirick GR, Kroger LA, et al. The biologic window for ChL6 radioimmunotherapy. *Cancer* 1994;73:1023–1032.

243. Richman CR, DeNardo SJ, O'Grady LF, DeNardo GL. Radioimmunotherapy for breast cancer using escalating fractionated doses of ^{131}I-labeled chimeric L6 antibody with peripheral blood progenitor cell transfusions. *Cancer Res* 1995;55:5916–5920.

244. Denardo SJ, O'Grady LF, Richman CR, et al. Radioimmunotherapy for advanced breast cancer using I-131-ChL6 Antibody. *Anticancer Res* 1997;17:1745–1752.

245. Denardo SJ, Kukis DL, Kroger LA, et al. Synergy of Taxol and radioimmunotherapy with yttrium-90-labeled chimeric L6 antibody: efficacy and toxicity in breast cancer xenografts. *Proc Natl Acad Sci U S A* 1997;94:4000–4004.

246. Ning S, Trisler K, Brown DM, et al. Intratumoral radioimmunotherapy of a human colon cancer xenograft using a sustained-release gel. *Radiother Oncol* 1996;39:179–189.

247. Breitz HB, Weiden PL, Vanderheyden JL, et al. Clinical experience with rhenium-186-labeled monoclonal antibodies for radioimmunotherapy: results of phase I trials. *J Nucl Med* 1992;33:1099–1109.

248. Peterson JA, Blank EW, Cerrani RL. Effects of multiple repeated dose of immunotherapy on target antigen expression (breast MUC-l mucin) in breast carcinomas. *Cancer Res* 1977;57:1103–1108.

249. Hughes OD, Bishop MC, Perkins AC, et al. Preclinical evaluation of copper-67 labeled anti-MUC1 mucin antibody C595 for therapeutic use in bladder cancer. *Eur J Nucl Med* 1997;24:439–443.

250. Schrier DM, Stemmer SM, Johnson T, et al. High dose ^{90}Y mx-diethylenetriaminepentaacetic acid (DPTA)-BrE-3 and autologous hematopoietic stem cell support (AHSCS) for the treatment of advanced breast cancer: a phase I trial. *Cancer Res* 1995;55: 5921–5924.

251. DeNardo SJ, Kramer EL, O'Donnell RT, et al. Radioimmunotherapy for breast cancer using indium-111/yttrium-90 brE-3: results of a phase I clinical trial. *J Nucl Med* 1997;38:1180–1185.

252. Kramer EL, Liebes L, Wasserheit C, et al. Initial evaluation of radiolabeled MX-DTPA humanized BrE-3 antibody in patients with advanced breast cancer. *Clin Cancer Res* 1998;4:1679–1688.

253. Thomas GE, Esteban JM, Raubitschek A, Wong JY. Gamma-Interferon administration after [90]yttrium radiolabeled antibody therapy: survival and hematopoietic toxicity studies. *Int J Radiat Oncol Biol Phys* 1995;31:529–534.

254. Casey JL, King DJ, Pedley RB, et al. Clearance of yttrium-90-labeled anti-tumour antibodies with antibodies raised against 12N4 DOTA macrocycle. *Br J Cancer* 1998;78:1307–1312.

255. Marshall D, Pedlwy RB, Boden JA, Boden R, Begent RH. Clearance of circulating radio-antibodies using streptavidin or second antibodies in a xenograft model. *Br J Cancer* 1994;69:502–507.

256. Moro M, Pelagi M, Fulci G, et al. Tumor cell targeting with anti-

body-avidin complexes and biotinylated tumor necrosis factor alpha. *Cancer Res* 1997;57:1992–1928.

257. Paganelli G, Belloni C, Magnani P, et al. Two-step tumour targeting in ovarian cancer patients using biotinylated monoclonal antibodies and radioactive streptavidin. *Eur J Nucl Med* 1992; 19:322–329.

258. Cheng JD, Knox SJ, Tempero M, et al. Phase II trial of NR-LU-10 pretargeted delivery of ^{90}yttrium in patients with metastatic colon cancer. *Proc Am Soc Clin Oncol* 1999;18:A1679.

259. Ji H, Moritz RL, Reid GE, et al. Electrophoretic analysis of the novel antigen for the gastrointestinal-specific monoclonal antibody, a33. *Electrophoresis* 1997;18:614–621.

260. Welt S, Scott AM, Divgi CR, et al. Phase I/II study of iodine 125-labeled monoclonal antibody A33 in patients with advanced colon cancer. *J Clin Oncol* 1996;14:1787–1797.

261. Wawrzynczak EJ, Davies AJS. Strategies in antibody therapy of cancer. *Clin Exp Immunol* 1990;82:189–193.

262. Siegall CB. Single-chain fusion toxins for the treatment of breast cancer: antitumor activity of BR96 sFv-PE40 and Heregulin-PE40. *Recent Results Cancer Res* 1995;140:51–60.

263. Endo Y, Mitsui K, Motizuki M, et al. The mechanism of action of ricin and related toxic lectins on eukaryotic ribosomes. *J Biol Chem* 1987;262:5908–5912.

264. Murphy JR, vanderSpek JC. Targeting diphtheria toxin to growth factor receptors. *Semin Cancer Biol* 1995;6:259–265.

265. Hwang J, Fitzgerald DJ, Adhya S, et al. Functional domains of *Pseudomonas* exotoxin identifies by deletion analysis of the gene expressed in *E. coli. Cell* 1987;48:129–136.

266. Colombatti M, Greenfield L, Youle RJ. Cloned fragment of diphtheria toxin linked to T cell-specific antibody identifies regions of B chain active in cell entry. *J Biol Chem* 1986;261:3030–3035.

267. Johnson VG, Wilson D, Greenfield L, et al. The role of the diphtheria toxin receptor in cytosol translocation. *J Biol Chem* 1988;263: 1295–1300.

268. Kihara A, Pastan I. Cytotoxic activity of chimeric toxins containing the epidermal growth factor-like domain of Heregulins fused to PE38 KDEL, a truncated recombinant form of *Pseudomonas* exotoxin. *Cancer Res* 1995;55:71–77.

269. Kreitman RJ, Pun RK, Pastan I. Increased antitumor activity of circularly permuted interleukin 4-toxin in mice with interleukin 4 receptor-bearing human carcinoma. *Cancer Res* 1995;55:3357–3363.

270. Ozello L, De Rosa CM, Blank EW, et al. The use of natural interferon alpha conjugated to a monoclonal antibody anti mammary epithelial mucin (Mc5) for the treatment of human breast cancer xenografts. *Breast Cancer Res Treat* 1993;25:265–276.

271. Di Massimo AM, Di Loreto M, Pacilli A, et al. Immunoconjugates made of an anti-EGF receptor monoclonal antibody and type 1 ribosome-inactivating proteins from *Saponaria ocymoides* or *Vaccinia pyramidata. Br J Cancer* 1997;75:822–828.

272. May RD, Finkelman FD, Wheeler HT, et al. Evaluation of ricin A chain-containing immunotoxins directed against different epitopes on the δ–chain of cell surface associated IgD on murine B cells. *J Immunol* 1990;144:3637–3642.

273. Press OW, Martin PJ, Thorpe PE, Vitetta ES. Ricin A chain-containing immunotoxins directed against different epitopes on the CD2 molecule differ in their ability to kill normal and malignant T cells. *J Immunol* 1988;141:4410–4417.

274. Till M, May RD, Uhr JW, et al. An assay that predicts the ability of monoclonal antibodies to form potent ricin A chain-containing immunotoxins. *Cancer Res* 1988;48:1119–1123.

275. Thorpe PB, Wallace PM, Knowles PP, et al. Improved antitumor effects of immunotoxins prepared with deglycosylated ricin A-chain and hindered disulfide linkages. *Cancer Res* 1988;48:6396–6403.

276. Wawrynczak EJ, Cumbe AJ, Henry RV, Parnell GD. Comparative biochemical cytotoxicity and pharmacokinetic properties of immunotoxins made with native ricin A chain, ricin A$_1$ chain and recombinant A chain. *Int J Cancer* 1991;47:130–135.

277. Cumbers AJ, Westwood JH, Henry RV, et al. Structural features of the antibody-A chain linkage that influences the activity and stability of ricin A chain immunotoxins. *Bioconjugate Chem* 1992;3:397–401.

278. Ghetie M-A, Uhr JW, Vitetta ES. Covalent binding of human α_2-macroglobulin to deglycosylated ricin A chain and its immunotoxins. *Cancer Res* 1991;51:1482–1487.

279. Chaudhary VK, Jinno Y, Gallo MG, et al. Mutagenesis of *Pseudomonas* exotoxin in identification of sequences responsible for animal toxicity. *J Biol Chem* 1990;265:16306–16310.

280. Bookman MA, Godfrey C, Padavic H, et al. Antitransferrin receptor immunotoxin therapy: phase I intraperitoneal trial. *Proc Am Soc Clin Oncol* 1990;9:A187.

281. Gould BJ, Borowitz MJ, Graves ES, et al. Phase I study of an anti-breast cancer immunotoxin by continuous infusion: report of a targeted toxic effect not predicted by animal studies. *J Natl Cancer Inst* 1989;81:775–781.

282. Weiner LM, O'Dwyer J, Kitson J, et al. Phase I evaluation of an anti-breast carcinoma monoclonal antibody 260F9-recombinant ricin A chain immunoconjugate. *Cancer Res* 1989;49:4062–4067.

283. Frankel AE, Tagge EP, Willingham MC. Clinical trials of targeted toxins. *Semin Cancer Biol* 1995;6:307–317.

284. Stone MJ, Sarscille EA, Fay JW, et al. A phase I study of bolus versus continuous infusion of the anti-CD 19 immunotoxin IgG-HD37-dgA, in patients with B-cell lymphoma. *Blood* 1996;88:1188–1197.

285. Hellström I, Garrigues HJ, Garrigues U, Hellström KE. Highly tumor-reactive internalizing, mouse monoclonal antibodies to Ley-related cell surface antigens. *Cancer Res* 1990;50:2183–2190.

286. Friedman PN, McAndrew SJM, Gawlak SL, et al. BR96 sFv-PE40, a potent single-chain immunotoxin that selectively kills carcinoma cells. *Cancer Res* 1993;53:334–339.

287. Siegall CB, Chace D, Mixan B, et al. *In vitro* and *in vivo* characterization of BR96 sFv-PE40. *J Immunol* 1994;152:2377–2384.

288. Trail PA, Willner D, Lasch SJ, et al. Cure of xenografted human carcinomas by BR96-doxorubicin immunoconjugates. *Science* 1993; 261:212–215.

289. Siegall CB, Chace D, Mixan B, et al. *In vitro* and *in vivo* characterization of BR96 sFv-PE40. *J Immunol* 1994;152:2377–2384.

290. Friedman PN, Chace DF, Trail PA, Siegall CB. Antitumor activity of the single-chain immunotoxin BR96 sFv-PE40 against established breast and lung tumor xenografts. *J Immunol* 1993;150:3054–3061.

291. Siegall CB, Ligitt D, Chace D, et al. Prevention of immunotoxin-mediated vascular leak syndrome in rats with retention of antitumor activity. *Proc Natl Acad Sci U S A* 1994;91:9514–9518.

292. Seetharam S, Chaudhary VK, Pastan I. Increased cytotoxic activity of *Pseudomonas* exotoxin and two chimeric toxins ending in KDEL. *J Biol Chem* 1991;266:17376–17381.

293. Rybak SM, Saxena SK, Ackerman LJ, Youle RJ. Cytotoxic potential of ribonuclease and ribonuclease hybrid proteins. *J Biol Chem* 1991;266:21202–21207.

294. Rybak SM, Hoogenboom HR, Meady MH, et al. Humanization of immunotoxins. *Proc Natl Acad Sci U S A* 1992;89:3165–3169.

295. Slifman NR, Loegering DA, McKean DJ, Gleich GJ. Ribonuclease activity associated with human eosinophil-derived neurotoxin and eosinophilic cationic protein. *J Immunol* 1986;137:2913–2917.

296. Gullberg U, Widegren B, Arnason U, et al. The cytotoxic eosinophil cationic protein (ECP) has ribonuclease activity. *Biochem Biophys Res Commun* 1986;139:1239–1242.

297. Roth J. Ribonuclease activity and cancer: a review. *Cancer Res* 1963;23:657–666.

298. Pastan IH, Archer GE, McLendon RE, et al. Intrathecal administration of single-chain immunotoxin, LMB-7 [B3(Fv)-PE38], produces cures of carcinomatous meningitis in a rat model. *Proc Natl Acad Sci U S A* 1995;92:2765–2769.

299. Munn DH, Cheung N-KV. Interleukin-2 enhancement of monoclonal antibody-mediated cellular toxicity against human melanoma. *Cancer Res* 1987;47:6600–6605.

300. Hank JA, Robinson RR, Surfus J, et al. Augmentation of antibody dependent cell mediated cytotoxicity following *in vivo* therapy with recombinant interleukin 2. *Cancer Res* 1990;50:5234–5239.

301. Saleh MN, Khazaeli MB, Wheeler RH, et al. Phase II trial of murine monoclonal antibody D612 combined with recombinant human monocyte colony-stimulating factor (rhM-CSF) in patients with metastatic gastrointestinal cancer. *Cancer Res* 1995;55:4339–4346.

302. Shimada S, Ogawa M, Schlom J, Greiner JW. Comparison of the interferon-gamma-mediated regulation of tumor-associated antigens expressed by human gastric carcinoma cells. *In Vivo* 1993;7:1–8.

303. Guadagni F, Roselli M, Nieroda C, Dansky-Ullmann G, Schlom J, Greiner JW. Biological response modifiers as adjuvants in monoclonal antibody-based treatment. *In Vivo* 1993;7:591–599.

304. Macey DJ, Grant EJ, Kasi L, et al. Effect of α-interferon on pharmacokinetics, biodistribution, toxicity, and efficacy of ^{131}I-labeled monoclonal antibody CC49 in breast cancer: a phase II trial. *Clin Cancer Res* 1997;3:1547–1555.

305. Schmiegel W, Schmielau J, Henne-Bruns D, et al. Cytokine-mediated enhancement of epidermal growth factor receptor expression provides an immunological approach to the therapy of pancreatic cancer. *Proc Natl Acad Sci U S A* 1997;94:12622–12626.

306. Raval A, Pun N, Rath PC, Saxena RK. Cytokine regulation of expression of class I MHC antigens. *Exp Mol Med* 1998;30:1–13.

307. Andalib AR, Lawry J, Ali SA, et al. Cytokine modulation of antigen expression in human melanoma cell lines derived from primary and metastatic tumour tissues. *Melanoma Res* 1997;7:32–42.

308. Zeigler LD, Palazzolo P, Cunningham J, et al. Phase I trial of murine monoclonal antibody L6 in combination with subcutaneous interleukin-2 in patients with advanced carcinoma of the breast, colorectum, and lung. *J Clin Oncol* 1992;10:1470–1478.

309. Rafnhammar P, Fagerberg J, Frodin JE, Wersall P, Hansson LO, Mellstedt H. Granulocyte/macrophage-colony stimulating factor augments the induction of antibodies, especially anti-idiotypic antibodies, to therapeutic monoclonal antibodies. *Cancer Immunol Immunother* 1995;40:367–375.

310. Murray JL, Macey DJ, Grant LJ, et al. Enhanced TAG-72 expression and tumor uptake of radiolabeled monoclonal antibody CC49 in metastatic breast cancer patients following alpha-interferon treatment. *Cancer Res* 1995;55:5925–5928.

311. Macey DJ, Grant EJ, Kasi L, et al. Effect of recombinant alpha-interferon on pharmacokinetics, biodistribution, toxicity, and efficacy of ^{131}I-labeled monoclonal antibody CC49 in breast cancer: a phase II trial. *Clin Cancer Res* 1997;3:1547–1555.

312. Ozzello L, Blank LW, De Rosa CM, et al. Conjugation of interferon alpha to humanized monoclonal antibody (HuBrE-3vl) enhances the selective localization and antitumor effects of interferon in breast cancer xenografts. *Breast Cancer Res Treat* 1998;48:135–147.

313. Meyers DL, Law KL, Payne JK, et al. Site-specific prodrug activation by antibody-beta-lactamase conjugates: preclinical investigation of the efficacy and toxicity of doxorubicin delivered by antibody directed catalysis. *Bioconjug Chem* 1995;6:440–446.

314. Affleck K, Embleton MJ. Monoclonal antibody targeting of methotrexate (MTX) against MTX-resistant tumour cell lines. *Br J Cancer* 1992;65:838–844.

315. Saleh M, LoBuglio A, Sugarman S, et al. Gastrointestinal effects of chimeric BR96-doxorubicin (DOX) conjugate. *Proc Am Assoc Cancer Res* 1995;36:A287.

316. Slichenmyer WJ, Saleh MN, Bookman MA, et al. Phase I studies of BR96 doxorubicin in patients with advanced solid tumors that express the Lewis Y antigen. *Anticancer Treat*, Sixth International Congress, A6-9, 1996.

317. Tolcher AW, Sugarman S, Gelman KA, et al. Randomized phase II study of BR96-doxorubicin conjugate in patients with metastatic breast cancer. *J Clin Oncol* 1999;17:478–484.

318. King CR, Kaspryk PG, Fischer PH, et al. Preclinical testing of an anti-erbB-2 recombinant toxin. *Breast Cancer Res Treat* 1996;38: 19–25.

319. Ciardiello F, Damiano V, Bianco R, et al. Antitumor activity of combined blockade of epidermal growth factor and protein kinase A. *J Natl Cancer Inst* 1996;88:1770–1776.

320. Ciardiello F, Tortora G. Interactions between the epidermal growth factor receptor and type I protein kinase A: biological significance and therapeutic implications. *Clin Cancer Res* 1998;4:821–828.

321. Ciardiello F, Capto R, Bianco R, et al. Cooperative inhibition of renal cancer growth by anti-epidermal growth factor receptor antibody and protein kinase A antisense oligonucleotide. *J Natl Cancer Inst* 1998;90:1087–1094.

322. Pegram MD, Lipton A, Hayes DF, et al. Phase II study of receptor-enhanced chemosensitivity using recombinant humanized anti-p185HER2/neu monoclonal antibody plus cisplatin in patients with HER2/neu-overexpressing metastatic breast cancer refractory to chemotherapy treatment. *J Clin Oncol* 1998;16:2659–2671.

323. Ballare C, Portela P, Schiaffi J, Yomha R, Mordoh J. Reactivity of monoclonal antibody FC-2.15 against drug resistant breast cancer cells. Additive cytotoxicity of Adriamycin and Taxol with FC-2.15. *Breast Cancer Res Treat* 1998;47:163–170.

324. Austin EB, Robins RA, Durrant LG, Price MR, Baldwin RW. Human monoclonal anti-idiotypic antibody to the tumour-associated antibody 791T/36. *Immunology* 1989;67:525–530.

325. Herlyn D, Wettendorff M, Schmoll E, et al. Anti-idiotype immunization of cancer patients: modulation of the immune response. *Proc Natl Acad Sci U S A* 1987;84:8055–8059.

326. Munn RK, Hutchins L, Garrison J, et al. Immune responses in patients with breast cancer treated with an anti-idiotype antibody that mimics the human milk fat globule (HMFG) antigen. *Proc Am Soc Clin Oncol* 1998;17:A1648.

327. Binzh H. Allo-antibodies: a de novo product. *J Immunol* 1973;111:1108–1111.

328. Jerne NK. Towards a network theory of the immune system. *Ann Immunol* (Paris) 1974;125:373–389.

329. Denton GW, Durrant LG, Hardcastle JD, Austin EB, Sewell HF, Robins RA. Clinical outcome of colorectal cancer patients treated with human monoclonal anti-idiotypic antibody. *Int J Cancer* 1994;57:10–14.

330. Durrant LG, Buckley TJ, Denton GW, Hardcastle JD, Sewell HF, Robins RA. Enhanced cell-mediated tumor killing in patients immunized with human monoclonal anti-idiotypic antibody 1 05AD7. *Cancer Res* 1994;54:4837–4840.

331. Foon KA, Chakraborty M, John WJ, Sherratt A, Kohler H, Bhattacharya-Chatterjee M. Immune response to the carcinoembryonic antigen in patients treated with an anti-idiotype antibody vaccine. *J Clin Invest* 1995;96:334–342.

332. Foon KA, John WJ, Chakraborty M, et al. Clinical and immune responses in surgically resected colorectal cancer (CRC) patients treated with an anti-idiotype (ID) monoclonal antibody that mimics carcinoembryonic antigen (CEA) with or without 5-fluorouracil (5-FU). *Proc Am Soc Clin Oncol* 1998;17:A1678.

333. Durrant LG, Doran M, Austin EB, Robins RA. Induction of cellular immune responses by a murine monoclonal anti-idiotypic antibody recognizing the 791Tgp72 antigen expressed on colorectal, gastric and ovarian human tumours. *Int J Cancer* 1995;61:62–66.

334. Pimm MV, Robins RA, Embleton MJ, et al. Clinical outcome of colorectal cancer patients treated with human monoclonal anti-idiotypic antibody. *Int J Cancer* 1994;57:10–14.

335. Durrant LG, Buckley DJ, Spendlove I, Robins RA. Low doses of 105AD7 cancer vaccine preferentially stimulate anti-tumor T-cell immunity. *Hybridoma* 1997;16:23–26.

336. Chakraborty M, Mukerjee S, Foon KA, Kohler H, Ceriani RL, Bhattacharya-Chatterjee M. Induction of human breast cancer-specific antibody responses in cynomolgus monkeys by a murine monoclonal anti-idiotype antibody. *Cancer Res* 1995;55:1525–1530.

337. Clark JI, Alpaugh RK, von Mehren M, et al. Induction of multiple anti-c-erbB-2 specificities accompanies a classical idiotypic cascade following 2B1 bispecific monoclonal antibody treatment. *Cancer Immunol Immunother* 1997;44:265–272.

338. Madiyalakan R, Yang R, Schultes BC, Baum RP, Noujaim AA. OVAREX MAb-B43, 13: IFN-gamma could improve the ovarian tumor cell sensitivity to CA 125-specific allogeneic cytotoxic T cells. *Hybridoma* 1997;16:41–45.

339. Livingston P. Ganglioside vaccines with emphasis on GM2. *Semin Oncol* 1998;25:636–645.

340. MacLean GD, Reddish MA, Koganty RR, Longenecker BM. Antibodies against mucin-associated sialyl-Tn epitopes correlate with survival of metastatic adenocarcinoma patients undergoing active specific immunotherapy with synthetic STn vaccine. *J Immunother* 1996;19:59–68.

341. Sandmaier BM, Oparin DV, Holmberg LA, Reddish MA, MacLean GD, Longenecker BM. Evidence of a cellular immune response against sialyl-Tn in breast and ovarian cancer patients after high-dose

chemotherapy, stem cell rescue, and immunization with Theratope STn-KLH cancer vaccine. *J Immunother* 1999;22:54–66.

342. Ezekiel MP, Bonner JA, Robert F, et al. Phase I trial of anti-epidermal growth factor receptor (Anti-EGFr) antibody in combination with either once-daily or twice-daily irradiation for locally advanced head and neck malignancies. *Proc Am Soc Clin Oncol* 1999;18:A1501.

343. Deshane J, Loechel F, Conry RM, Siegal GP, King CR, Curiel DT. Intracellular single-chain antibody directed against erbB2 down-regulates cell surface erbB2 and exhibits a selective anti-proliferative effect in erbB2 overexpressing cancer cell lines. *Gene Ther* 1994;1:332–337.

344. Deshane J, Cabrera G, Grim JE, et al. Targeted eradication of ovarian cancer mediated by intracellular expression of anti-erbB-2 single-chain antibody. *Gynecol Oncol* 1995;59:8–14.

345. Kim M, Wright M, Deshane J, et al. A novel gene therapy strategy for elimination of prostate carcinoma cells form human bone marrow. *Hum Gene Ther* 1997;8:157–170.

346. Wright M, Grim J, Deshane J, et al. An intracellular anti-erbB-2 single chain antibody is specifically cytotoxic to human breast carcinoma cells overexpressing erbB-2. *Gene Ther* 1997;4:317–322.

347. Grim H, Deshane J, Feng M, Lieber A, Kay M, Curiel DT. ErbB-2 knockout employing an intracellular single-chain antibody (sFv) accomplishes specific toxicity in erbB-2-expressing lung cancer cells. *Am J Res Cell Mol Biol* 1996;15:348–354.

348. Deshane J, Grim J, Loechel S, Siegal GP, Alvarez RD. Intracellular antibody against erbB-2 mediates targeted tumor cell eradication by apoptosis. *Cancer Gene Ther* 1996;3:89–98.

349. Barnes M, Vanderkwaak T, Wang MW, et al. *In vivo* efficacy of an anti-erbB-2 intracellular single chain antibody with cisplatin (CPPD) against a murine model of carcinoma of the ovary. *Proc Am Assoc Cancer Res* 1997;38:A1544.

350. Konishi H, Ochiya T, Chester KA, et al. Targeting strategy for gene delivery to carcinoembryonic antigen-producing cancer cells by retrovirus displaying a single-chain variable fragment antibody. *Hum Gene Ther* 1998;9:235–248.

351. Ning S, Trisler K, Brown DM, et al. Intratumoral radioimmunotherapy of a human colon cancer xenograft using a sustained-release gel. *Radiother Oncol* 1996;39:179–189.

352. Heike Y, Hamada H, Inamura N, Sone S, Ogura T, Tsuruo T. Monoclonal anti-P-glycoprotein antibody-killing of multidrug-resistant tumor cells by human mononuclear cells. *Jpn J Cancer Res* 1990;81:1155–1161.

15.5

MONOCLONAL ANTIBODIES: CLINICAL APPLICATIONS

Monoclonal Antibodies Directed Against Growth Factor Receptors

JOSE BASELGA
JOHN MENDELSOHN

Since the 1980s, monoclonal antibodies (MAb) have attracted considerable interest as potential agents in the treatment of human cancer. Potential uses of MAb in the therapy of cancer include activating the immune and inflammatory systems or carrying cytotoxic agents to specific target sites. An alternative approach is to use MAb to block or interfere with the physiologic function of a receptor; in this case, the antigen is a molecule with known biologic activity that acts in signal transduction when activated by a particular ligand.

Human tumors express high levels of growth factors and their receptors, and many types of malignant cells appear to exhibit autocrine- or paracrine-stimulated growth. MAb directed at growth factor receptors provide a selective strategy to interfere with receptor function and hence inhibit tumor growth. Because most studies have been conducted with MAb directed against the erbB tyrosine kinase receptors (also known as *type I receptor tyrosine kinases*), this review focuses on these receptors as targets for antibody therapy.

The erbB receptor family is comprised of four homolog receptors: erbB1 (also known as *epidermal growth factor receptor* [EGF-R] or *HER1*), erbB2 (also known as *HER2/neu/p185HER2*), erbB3 (HER3), and erbB4 (HER4). These receptors are composed of an extracellular binding domain, a transmembrane lipophilic segment, and an intracellular protein

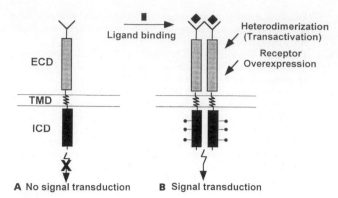

FIGURE 1. A: The erbB receptors are composed of an extracellular binding domain, a transmembrane lipophilic segment, and an intracellular protein tyrosine kinase domain with a regulatory carboxyl terminal segment. Monomeric receptors are inactive. B: Dimerization triggers receptor activation. In addition to ligand binding, mechanisms that promote the formation of dimers include receptor overexpression and transactivation (heterodimerization) (136). After receptor dimerization, activation of the intrinsic protein tyrosine kinase and tyrosine autophosphorylation occurs. These events lead to activation of a cascade of biochemical and physiologic responses that are involved in the mitogenic signal transduction of cells.

tyrosine kinase domain with a regulatory carboxyl terminal segment (Fig. 1) (1). erbB3, however, is different from the other members in that it has a deficient tyrosine kinase domain (2).

The rationale to target erbB receptors with MAb is compelling: These receptors are frequently overexpressed in human tumors; their overexpression typically confers a more aggressive clinical behavior; and MAb directed at these receptors inhibit tumor growth in laboratory model systems. Although an alternative approach would be to target the growth factors, the targeting of the receptors is preferred because of the multiplicity of ligands for a given receptor and the lack of known ligands for some of the family members.

Monoclonal Antibodies Against the Epidermal Growth Factor Receptor

Research with MAb against the EGF-R is presented in some detail as an example of the approach that can be taken in the exploration of receptor blockade as therapy for cancer.

Epidermal Growth Factor Receptor and Its Ligands

At least six different ligands, known as *EGF-like ligands*, activate the EGF-R (also known as *erbB1* or *HER1*) (3). These ligands include EGF, transforming growth factor–α (TGF-α), amphiregulin, heparin-binding EGF, betacellulin, and epiregulin. Some of the EGF-like ligands elicit differential biologic responses *in vitro*, suggesting that they may have unique physiologic roles (2–4).

The EGF-R with which these ligands interact is a 170-kd glycoprotein in the plasma membrane (see Fig. 1) (5). After binding of ligand, EGF-Rs form homodimers, an event believed to activate the intrinsic tyrosine kinase, resulting in transautophosphorylation of tyrosine residues, primarily in the carboxy

terminal segments (5). Phosphorylation on serine and threonine residues is mediated by secondary activation of protein kinase C or other kinases (5). In addition to the formation of erbB1/erbB1 homodimers, EGF-like ligands can also induce erbB1/erbB2 heterodimers, and erbB1/erbB3 and erbB1/erbB4 heterodimers can also be occasionally detected (2,3,6).

Epidermal Growth Factor Receptor and Human Malignancy

Many types of epithelial malignancies display increased EGF-Rs on their cell surface membranes. Examples include cancer of the breast, lung, glioblastoma, head and neck, and bladder (7). Gene amplification is not a commonly reported finding in these tumors with the exception of the glioblastomas. Furthermore, in the case of glioblastomas, mutant EGF-Rs have been described. Increased EGF-R expression correlates with a poorer clinical outcome in malignancies of the bladder, breast, and lung (7). The level of increased expression can reach an order of magnitude or greater. Increased receptor content is often associated with increased production of TGF-α by the same tumor cells (8). This establishes conditions conducive to receptor activation by an autocrine stimulatory pathway.

Laboratory Studies with Antiepidermal Growth Factor Receptor Monoclonal Antibodies

The concept of EGF-R blockade by specific MAb as a novel form of cancer therapy was founded in the overexpression of EGF-R on tumor cells relative to normal cells and in potential qualitative differences in the response to disrupted receptor function in cancer cells versus normal cells. This concept was tested using a panel of MAb against the EGF-R. Two MAb, 225 immunoglobulin G1 (IgG1) and 528 immunoglobulin G2a (IgG2a), were found to bind to the receptor with affinity comparable with the natural ligand (K_d = 2 nM), compete with EGF binding, and block activation of receptor tyrosine kinase by EGF or TGF-α (9–11). It is likely that these MAb do not react with the actual EGF binding site, but near enough it to prevent EGF from binding because they react with a human-specific sequence and do not recognize EGF-R on rodent cells. MAb 225 produces antibody-mediated receptor dimerization, resulting in receptor downregulation, and this effect appears to be important for its growth inhibitory capacity (12). MAb 225 and 528 can block EGF- and TGF-α–induced stimulation of growth rate of a variety of human cells that express EGF-R and ligand (9,10,13,14). The interruption of the EGF-R ligand autocrine pathway by MAb 225 affects cell cycle progression, resulting in a G1 phase arrest that is accompanied by elevated levels of p27KIP1 inhibitor of cyclin-dependent kinases (15,16). In cells in which the EGF-R ligands act as survival factors rather than growth-promoting factors, such as in colon adenocarcinoma DiFi cells, these antibodies cause an irreversible G1 arrest followed by apoptosis (17).

In vivo effects of these MAb were assayed against tumor xenografts with A431 vulvar squamous carcinoma cells or MDA-MD-468 breast carcinoma cells, which express extremely high levels of EGF-Rs (18). Administration of 225 or 528 MAb intraperitoneally, beginning concurrent with tumor cell implantation subcutaneously, caused a dose-dependent inhibition of tumor growth. The response to MAb treatment of well established (~ 0.5 cm diameter) xenografts varied with the cell line, but generally tumors were not eliminated. Based on antitumor activity, murine MAb 225 was selected for clinical development. A chimeric human:murine version of MAb 225 (C225) was produced to obviate the immune response produced in humans by repetitive exposure to murine MAb 225 (19). The chimeric antibody C225 binds to the EGF-R with higher affinity (kd = 0.39 nM) than the murine MAb and is capable of inducing complete regressions of well-established xenografts of tumors overexpressing the EGF-R. An interesting finding is that C225 has greater antitumor efficacy *in vivo* than in cell culture inhibitory studies. As possible mechanisms for this enhanced *in vivo* antitumor effect, C225 has been shown to downregulate vascular endothelial growth factor production and suppress angiogenesis (20). In addition, C225 may elicit an immune or inflammatory response mediated by the Fc portion of the MAb.

Other laboratories have produced anti–EGF-R MAb with inhibitory activity against cells bearing EGF-Rs. 425 is an IgG2a MAb that inhibits the proliferation of A431 cells and colorectal SW948 adenocarcinoma cells in culture and in xenografts (21). Iodine-131–labeled F(ab')2 fragments of this MAb detected xenografts that overexpress the EGF-R (22). MAb 108 against the high-affinity EGF-R inhibited human oral epidermoid carcinoma cell growth in culture and in xenografts (23).

LABORATORY STUDIES OF CHEMOTHERAPEUTIC AGENTS IN COMBINATION WITH ANTIEPIDERMAL GROWTH FACTOR RECEPTOR MONOCLONAL ANTIBODIES

A 1988 study reported synergistic cytotoxicity against human tumor xenografts when anti–EGF-R MAb 108 was combined with cisplatinum therapy against K562 squamous carcinoma cells (23). These observations stimulated us to explore the hypothesis that chemotherapy and growth factor blockade may work through common mechanisms to increase tumor cell kill, especially in the case of well-established xenografts, which are generally not completely eliminated by treatment with the anti–EGF-R MAb. Subsequent studies confirmed and extended the initial observation. In cultures of A431 or MDA-468 cells, doxorubicin in combination with MAb 528 or 225 (but not with control antibody) produced an additive inhibition of growth. In mice bearing well-established A431 tumor xenografts, doxorubicin alone, or MAb 528 (or 225) did not eliminate the tumors. In contrast, the combination of doxorubicin and MAb 528 resulted in a major antitumor effect with cure in all of the animals (24). In MDA-468 xenografts, the combined treatment with MAb 528 and doxorubicin also resulted in a major antitumor activity.

Further studies have been conducted against A431 cell xenografts with the chemotherapeutic agent cisplatin in combination with MAb 528 or 225. The results of these experiments show again a marked synergistic effect with disappearance of

well-established tumor xenografts, whereas the administration of cisplatin or MAb alone were not inhibitory (25). MAb 225 also enhances the antitumor activity of the paclitaxel in the MDA-468 breast cancer xenograft model (7).

What are the mechanisms underlying the enhancement of the activity of different classes of chemotherapeutic agents when given in combination with anti–EGF-R MAb? We favor an interpretation of our findings that implicates checkpoint regulation of the cell cycle as the activator of cell death (14). When cells are functioning properly, deprivation from the signaling pathways activated by essential growth factors activate the G_1 checkpoint, known as the *restriction point*, and the cells arrest in G1. Likewise, cells damaged by chemotherapy arrest typically in G2-M to repair alterations in DNA, tubulin, or other molecules. Malignant cells appear to be able to disobey checkpoints in some situations without jeopardizing cell survival. This was seen when MAb 225 was added to most tumor cell cultures, which resulted in incomplete G1 arrest. In contrast, cultures of nontransformed cells were completely arrested in G1 phase. We hypothesize that when tumor cells simultaneously disobey two checkpoint signals (activated by MAb 225 and chemotherapy), this becomes intolerable and results in cell death. Another way of conceptualizing this is to consider that in the face of chemotherapeutic damage, which signals the cell to pause for repair, the requirement for a growth factor for cell cycle traversal is converted to requirement of the growth factor for cell survival. Thus, malignant epithelial cells damaged by chemotherapy now act like DiFi cells, and when deprived of EGF-R kinase activity, they can no longer survive. Ample precedent exists for growth factors acting as survival factors in hematopoietic cell lines, in cultures of nerve cells, and in epithelial cells driven to proliferate by constitutive expression of myc (26,27). A corollary to this hypothesis is the prediction that nonmalignant epithelial cells, which obey the checkpoint signals, may be less susceptible to cytotoxicity from this combination therapy.

A newer approach to enhance the activity of anti–EGF-R MAb is the combination with inhibitors of related growth factor receptors, such as erbB2 (28), or with inhibitors that act on downstream signaling molecules, such as farnesyltransferase inhibitors (29), or with combined blockade of EGF-R and protein kinase A (30). Furthermore, anti–EGF-R antibodies may augment the activity of radiation therapy, as suggested by the observation that MAb 225 blocks the ability of the ligand EGF to enhance growth and radioresistance of breast cancer cells (31) and can potentiate the radiosensitivity of cultured cells (32,33).

Clinical Trials with Antiepidermal Growth Factor Receptor Monoclonal Antibodies

In an initial phase 1 single-dose study, indium-111–labeled murine MAb 225 was found to be safe, and satisfactory tumor localization was achieved (34). All patients produced human antimouse antibodies, however, which would have precluded the administration of multiple doses of antibody. To obviate the immune response, the chimeric human:murine version of MAb 225 (C225) was produced (19). An initial series of phase 1 trials with C225 have been recently completed in a total of 52 patients

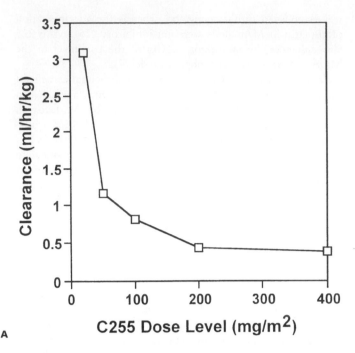

A

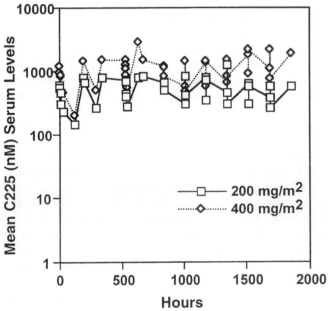

B

FIGURE 2. A: C225 clearance in relationship to the different dose levels. Data from the three phase 1 studies have been pooled and the average value obtained is presented in the graph. Clearance decreased with increasing C225 doses until reaching the 200 mg per m² dose level. Clearance values derived from study CP02–9503 indicated that little, if any, difference in drug clearance occurred between the 200 and 400 mg per m² dose levels (*p* = .179, t-test). **B:** Mean serum levels of circulating C225 in study CP02–9503 in dose levels 200 and 400 mg per m² shown on a semilogarithmic plot scale. Mean serum levels of C225 were sustained above approximately 200 nM throughout treatments at dose levels 200 and 400 mg per m². (doxo, doxorubicin; TAX, paclitaxel.) (From Baselga J, Pfister D, Cooper MR, et al. Phase I studies of antiepidermal growth factor receptor chimeric antibody C225 alone and in combination with cisplatin. *J Clin Oncol* 2000 (in press), with permission.)

with advanced, EGF-R–overexpressing tumors (35–37). In the first study, patients received a single intravenous dose of C225 at dose levels of 5, 20, 50, and 100 mg per m². In the second study, four weekly doses of 5, 20, 50, and 100 mg per m² were exam-

ined. In the third study of this series, cisplatin was added at a dose of 100 mg per m² on day 1 (cisplatin was later decreased to a dose of 60 mg per m²), and weekly C225 was continued at the dose levels of 5, 20, 50, 100, 200, or 400 mg per m². A critical issue in these trials was to define the optimal dose and schedule at which complete and sustained receptor saturation was achieved. In cell culture, murine MAb 225 levels at 20 times the receptor-binding affinity resulted in receptor saturation and maximal inhibition of growth (9,10). In nude mouse models, saturating MAb 225 levels in the serum produced optimal anti-tumor activity against the xenografts (18). These observations served to define initially the optimal biologic dose of C225 as the lowest dose that would continuously maintain serum concentrations of the antibody above 30 nM. Although this criterion was met in these trials with the 100 mg per m² weekly dose, consideration was given to the idea that the concentration of the antibody required for EGF-R saturation in preclinical models might not directly correlate with what is required in humans. Indeed, EGF-R is widely expressed in normal tissues, providing additional competing antibody-binding sites that would have to be completely saturated in addition to the tumor cells as well. Hence, it was specifically hypothesized that the systemic clearance of C225 would depend on the antibody binding to EGF-Rs in a large number of tissues (38). If this were the case, then complete saturation of EGF-R binding should be accompanied by saturation of the antibody systemic clearance. A dose-dependent antibody clearance within the 20 to 100 mg per m² dose range was observed, however, indicating that the process was not yet saturated (Fig. 2A). Therefore, further escalation of the dose of C225 was conducted in a study that combined cisplatin and antibody. In that study, no apparent effect of cisplatin on C225 clearance was observed. Furthermore, at the 200 and 400 mg per m² dose levels, complete saturation of drug clearance was achieved (see Fig. 2A), and this dose range was selected for phase 1 trials (35–37). Mean circulating C225 levels were sustained above 200 nM beyond the initial dose for patients treated with multiple doses at 200 and 400 mg per m² (Fig. 2B).

The difference between the optimal biologic dose projected from preclinical models and the higher C225 dose required to achieve saturation of drug clearance in patients could not have been predicted from studies with human xenografts in nude mice because of the lack of MAb 225 or C225 binding to the murine receptor. This observation emphasizes the need of developing reliable biologic markers in trials that evaluate agents that act on the EGF-R (39–41). The pharmacokinetic findings with C225 are in agreement with a prior phase 1 single-dose clinical trial with a different murine anti–EGF-R MAb, RG 83852, in patients with non–small-cell lung cancer or head and neck tumors (39). In that study, dose-dependent pharmacokinetics were observed with higher antibody doses that resulted in reduced plasma clearance, suggesting saturation of extravascular clearance mechanisms at higher antibody doses. In addition, tumor EGF-R saturation assessed in biopsied tumor samples by immunohistochemistry and EGF-R tyrosine kinase assays showed receptor saturation of equal to or more than 50% at doses equal to or more than 200 mg per m² (39). Overall, the results from these studies support the hypothesis that saturation of antibody binding to the EGF-R in humans occur only when complete saturation of drug clearance (i.e., zero order kinetics) is achieved.

C225 was well tolerated in these phase 1 trials, and the dose schedule that saturates the body clearance mechanisms was achieved before reaching the maximal tolerated dose (35–37). Although these trials were not designed to analyze clinical response, C225 given as a single agent did induce frequent stabilization of tumors. This was observed at all the C225 dose levels, although patients at higher dose levels had a higher tumor stabilization rate. Tumor regressions were demonstrated in two patients with head and neck tumors treated with C225 at doses of 200 mg per m^2 and 400 mg per m^2 in combination with cisplatin (36,37). A series of phase 2 studies of C225 given alone or in combination with several chemotherapeutic agents in head and neck cancer, prostate, renal cell, and breast cancer are ongoing. The most extensive studies with C225 have been on patients with advanced head and neck cancer. A phase 1/2 trial involving 15 patients with surgically unresectable disease combining radiation with MAb C225 treatment demonstrated a complete response in 13 patients and partial responses in the remaining two patients (42). The expected complete response rate was less than 50%. Based on these promising results, a randomized phase 3 trial comparing radiation with and without C225 is under way. A phase 2 trial of cisplatin plus C225 is ongoing. The results for six evaluable patients include three partial responses and one complete response. Two responders had previously failed regimens that included cisplatin (43). A phase 3 trial of cisplatin with or without C225 is planned.

In another phase 1 trial, the rat anti–EGF-R MAb ICR62 was evaluated in 20 patients with head and neck or lung cancer (44). This antibody effectively blocks the binding of EGF, TGF-α, and heparin-binding EGF to the EGF-R; inhibits the growth *in vitro* of tumor cell lines that overexpress the EGF-R; and eradicates such tumors when grown as xenografts in athymic mice. Groups of three patients were treated with 2.5 mg, 10 mg, 20 mg, or 40 mg of ICR62, and a further eight patients received 100 mg. In that trial, no serious toxicity was observed. Antibody ICR62 could be detected in the sera of patients treated with 40 mg or 100 mg of ICR62. Four patients showed human antirat antibodies. In four patients receiving doses of ICR62 at 40 mg or more, biopsies were obtained from metastatic lesions and showed the localization of MAb ICR62 to the membranes of tumor cells; this appeared to be more prominent at the higher dose of 100 mg (44).

Low-molecular-weight inhibitors of EGF-R also have been produced. These generally act intracellularly by blocking the activation of the tyrosine kinase portion of the receptor molecule (45). A number of these kinase inhibitors have been reported in preclinical studies, demonstrating efficacy in blocking the activation of the EGF-R kinase and inhibiting the growth of xenografts (46–48). Phase 1 trials of these receptor kinase inhibitors have been initiated.

MONOCLONAL ANTIBODIES AGAINST THE HER2 RECEPTOR

HER2 Receptor

The HER2 receptor (also known as *neu, erbB-2*, and *p185* ^{HER2} *receptor*), is a 185-kd tyrosine kinase receptor that belongs to the erbB receptor family and has partial homology to the EGF-R (49–51). The two other members of the erbB receptor family are erbB3 (HER3) and erbB4 (HER4).

Unlike the EGF-R (erbB1), a ligand for HER2 (erbB2) has not been identified. In spite of sequence homology between HER2 and the EGF-R, EGF-like ligands bind to the EGF-R but not to HER2 (3). A second class of ligands of erbB receptors, collectively termed *neuregulins* (also known as *neu differentiation factors* or *heregulins*), bind directly to erbB3 and erbB4, but not to HER2 or to the EGF-R (52). HER2, however, is the preferred heterodimerization partner within the family (53). HER2 is frequently transactivated by EGF-like ligands (see the section on Epidermal Growth Factor Receptor and Its Ligand), resulting from the formation of erbB1/HER2 heterodimers (2,3). In an analogous way, neuregulins can induce the formation of HER2/erbB3 and HER2/erbB4 heterodimers (54–57). This heterodimerization between HER2 and the other receptors of the family allows the participation of HER2 in signal transduction, even in the absence of a cognate ligand. The heterodimers between HER2 and the other members of the family (erbB1, erbB3, and erbB4) show relatively high ligand affinity and potent signaling activity and are synergistic for cell transformation (6,53,58–60). In one report, a transmembrane protein that contains two EGF-like domains, ASGP2, has been shown to interact with the extracellular domain of HER2 and potentiate signaling through the erbB receptor network (61).

HER2 has been shown to be overexpressed, most commonly by gene amplification, in an array of human carcinomas including, but not limited to, breast, ovarian, gastric, colon, and non–small-cell lung carcinoma (62). The most comprehensive studies have been conducted in breast cancer showing that HER2 is overexpressed in 25% to 30% of human breast cancers and predicts for a worse prognosis in patients with primary disease (63,64). In addition, several other lines of evidence support a direct role for HER2 in the pathogenesis and clinical aggressiveness of HER2 overexpressing tumors: The introduction of HER2 into nonneoplastic cells causes their malignant transformation (65,66); transgenic mice expressing HER2 develop mammary tumors (67), and MAb directed at the HER2 receptor inhibit the growth of tumors and transformed cells that express high levels of this receptor (62,68–71).

A distinct feature of the HER2 receptor when compared with other members of the erbB family is that the extracellular portion of the receptor can be cleaved and released into the media. This process is regulated and (72) of unknown importance, although high levels of extracellular HER2 in the serum of patients with breast cancer has been associated with a more aggressive clinical behavior and decreased sensitivity to conventional anticancer agents.

Laboratory Studies with Anti-HER2 Monoclonal Antibodies

Several groups have produced antibodies directed against the rat neu receptor (68,69) and the HER2 receptor on human cells (73–78). Genentech produced a series of murine MAb that inhibit the proliferation of monolayer cultures of breast and ovarian tumor cells overexpressing HER2 (70,73,79). In their extensive studies, a clear relationship between the level of HER2

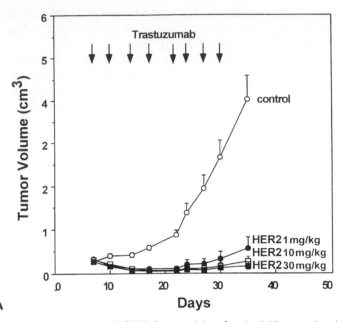

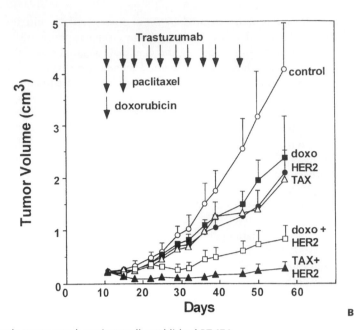

FIGURE 3. A: Activity of anti-erbB2 monoclonal antibody trastuzumab against well-established BT-474 tumor xenografts in athymic mice (80). Trastuzumab was given intraperitoneally twice a week for 4 weeks at doses of 1 mg per kg, 10 mg per kg, and 30 mg per kg. The control group was treated with a nonspecific rhu monoclonal antibody IgG at a dose of 30 mg per kg. Trastuzumab at doses equal to or greater than 1 mg per kg markedly suppressed the growth of BT-474 xenografts. **B:** Antitumor activity of trastuzumab in combination with paclitaxel or doxorubicin against well-established BT-474 tumor xenografts in athymic mice (137). The control group was treated with the control rhu monoclonal antibody IgG at a dose of 0.3 mg per kg twice weekly intraperitoneally. Trastuzumab was given intraperitoneally twice a week for 5 weeks at a dose of 0.3 mg per kg. Paclitaxel was given intravenously at a dose of 10 mg per kg on days 1 and 4. Doxorubicin was administered intraperitoneally at a dose of 10 mg per kg of body weight on day 1. Doxorubicin or paclitaxel, given each in combination with the control antibody, resulted in a modest antitumor activity. Trastuzumab also resulted in a modest inhibition of growth. The combined treatment with trastuzumab plus paclitaxel or doxorubicin resulted in a marked enhancement of the antitumor effects compared with either chemotherapeutic agent alone. Greater inhibition of tumor growth occurred in the group of animals treated with paclitaxel and trastuzumab. Results are given as mean tumor volume + SE. Arrows show days on which treatment was administered. (doxo, doxorubicin; HER2, trastuzumab; Tax, paclitaxel.)

proto-oncogene expression and sensitivity to the growth inhibitory effects of the antibodies were observed. One of the most potent growth inhibitory anti-HER2 MAb, 4D5, which is directed against the extracellular domain of HER2, was selected for further clinical development (72,73,79). As discussed previously, murine antibodies are limited clinically because they are immunogenic. To attempt to circumvent the antiglobulin response, a "humanized" antibody was constructed. The resulting recombinant humanized anti-erbB2 MAb, trastuzumab (Herceptin), has a higher binding affinity for erbB2 ($K_d = 0.1$ nM) than the murine 4D5 and has a marked growth inhibitory effect against cultured breast cancer cells overexpressing erbB2 (80). Furthermore, trastuzumab is much more efficient in supporting antibody-dependent cellular cytotoxicity against human tumor cell lines in the presence of human peripheral mononuclear cells, which can increase its antitumor activity (55,80,81).

In the first report using trastuzumab against human tumor xenografts, a single dose of antibody-inhibited tumor growth by 50% (82). Subsequently, we confirmed the *in vivo* antitumor activity of trastuzumab against human breast cancer BT-474 xenografts that overexpress erbB2 (83). Repeated administrations of the antibody given at doses equal to or greater than 1

mg per kg resulted in strong growth suppression and eradication of tumors in a significant proportion of animals. In our animal model, doses of 1 mg per kg given twice a week resulted in maximal inhibition of growth (Fig. 3A). This dose level is similar to the one being administered in the clinical trials in patients with advanced breast cancer (2 mg per kg × weekly).

In contrast with anti-EGF-R, MAb that mainly act by preventing ligand binding, the mechanism of action of antibodies directed against HER2, is not well understood. In fact, unlike MAb C225, binding of trastuzumab to its receptor activates the HER2 tyrosine kinase, resulting in autophosphorylation (84). Several possible mechanisms exist, however, by which anti-HER2 MAb could exert their tumor-inhibitory effects. Treatment of cancer cells overexpressing HER2 with MAb 4D5, trastuzumab, and other growth-inhibitory antibodies results in a marked downregulation of HER2 expression (79,84,85). Antibody-induced downregulation of erbB2 has been shown to induce reversion of the transformed phenotype in HER2-transformed cells (68). A relationship between receptor degradation and antitumor effects of anti-erbB2 MAb is supported by a study using a large battery of anti-HER2 antibodies (78). In that study, stimulation of erbB2 receptor phosphorylation was found to be uncoupled from the growth inhibitory effects of the antibodies (78). Another property of trastuzumab is its partial ability to disrupt the formation of erbB2/erbB3 and erbB2/erbB4 heterodimers, but a relationship between this effect and growth inhibition is not established (78,86). Possible additional *in vivo* mechanisms of action involve the observation that trastuzumab is a potent inducer of antibody-dependent cellular cytotoxicity (81) and has antiangiogenic activity with downregulation of vascular endothelial growth factor and other angiogenic factors (20). In addition to MAb, a variety of research approaches exist to target erbB2-overexpressing cells, including immunoconjugates, vaccines, tyrosine kinase inhibitors, antisense, and transcriptional downregulators.

Laboratory Studies of Chemotherapeutic Agents in Combination with Anti-HER2 Monoclonal Antibodies

As in the case of anti–EGF-R MAb, a way to optimize the efficacy of anti-HER2 MAb is to administer them in combination with chemotherapy. Hancock et al. showed that an anti-HER2 antibody, TAb 250, markedly enhanced the antitumor effects of cisplatin (74). Using the same antibody, Arteaga has shown enhanced etoposide-induced cytotoxicity against human breast carcinoma cells and postulated that erbB2 antibodies may alter the sensitivity of topoisomerase II toward etoposide (87). Studies by Slamon with MAb 4D5 or trastuzumab and chemotherapeutic agents have demonstrated that 4D5 promotes sensitivity to cisplatin in cisplatin-resistant ovarian carcinoma cell lines (88,89). Searching for mechanisms, it has been shown that anti-HER2 MAb interfere with repair of DNA damage owing to cisplatin, which could promote drug cytotoxicity against target cells (88,90).

Because paclitaxel and doxorubicin are two of the most active chemotherapeutic agents for the treatment of breast cancer (91), we hypothesized that finding enhanced antitumor activity of these drugs when combined with anti-HER2 MAb would have distinct clinical implications (83). Hence, a series of experiments with trastuzumab in combination with paclitaxel or doxorubicin was conducted. In cultured cells overexpressing HER2, an additive cytotoxic effect was observed with cotreatment combining trastuzumab plus paclitaxel. In our BT-474 tumor xenograft mouse model, doses of trastuzumab that modestly inhibit growth of well-established tumors effectively enhance the tumoricidal effects of paclitaxel and results in a striking rate of tumor eradication (Fig. 3B).

Trastuzumab enhanced the antitumor effects of doxorubicin as well, albeit to a lesser degree than was observed with paclitaxel (see Fig. 3B). Animals treated with trastuzumab alone or with trastuzumab plus chemotherapy had a significantly higher complete tumor regression rate than control animals. The highest complete tumor eradication rate was observed in those animals treated with trastuzumab plus paclitaxel (83). In addition to our data, a number of studies have shown that therapies leading to HER2 receptor downregulation or inhibition of its phosphorylation may enhance sensitivity to a variety of chemotherapeutic agents (92–94).

The simplest explanation for the enhanced activity of paclitaxel and trastuzumab is that it is the result of the summation of effects of two anticancer drugs that act on different targets; trastuzumab acts on the HER2 receptor signaling pathway and paclitaxel acts on tubulin. The magnitude of the enhanced antitumor activity with the combination, however, may be well beyond a simple summation of effects (83). It has been shown that overexpression of HER2 activates the cyclin-dependent kinase inhibitor p21, which inhibits $p34^{cdc2}$ kinase. $p34^{cdc2}$ kinase activation is required for paclitaxel-induced apoptosis, and overexpression of HER2 blocks paclitaxel-induced apoptosis by inhibiting $p34^{cdc2}$ activation (95). This finding provides a mechanistic link between erbB2 overexpression and paclitaxel sensitivity. Therefore, it is possible that trastuzumab, by downregulating HER2, may prevent or inhibit p21 activation and, as a result, increase paclitaxel-induced apoptosis because of the presence of activated $p34^{cdc2}$ kinase.

Clinical Trials with Anti-HER2 Monoclonal Antibodies

The first phase 2 study of multiple-dose intravenous administration of trastuzumab was conducted in patients with metastatic breast carcinoma overexpressing HER2 (96). The study included 46 patients that in general had extensive metastatic disease and had received prior chemotherapy. Based on prior phase 1 clinical trials, patients received a loading dose of 250 mg trastuzumab on day 0 and, beginning on day 7, 100 mg weekly for a total of 10 doses. More than 90% of the examined population had trastuzumab trough serum levels above the targeted 10 µg per mL level. Suboptimal serum concentrations, however, were found in those patients with high circulating levels of tumor-shed HER2 extracellular domain. Antibodies against trastuzumab were not detected in any patients. Trastuzumab was remarkably well tolerated. Out of a total of 768 administrations of trastuzumab, only 11 events occurred that were considered to be related to the use of the antibody. Among 43 evaluable patients, five had tumor responses (one complete remission and four partial remissions) for an overall response rate of 11.6% (Table 1). No responses were seen in patients with high serum levels of shed HER2 extracellular domain. Because elevated levels of shed HER2 ectodomain were associated with lack of response to trastuzumab and the shedding event is a regulated process, the results of laboratory studies examining a combined therapeutic approach with inhibitors of HER2 shedding and trastuzumab deserve consideration (72). Another important observation of this trial was that 37% of patients achieved minimal responses or stable disease (96). The median time to progression in patients with minor or stable disease was 5.1 months. The unusually long durations of minimal responses and stable disease seen in this trial suggested that stable disease may be an authentic reflection of the biologic action of the drug. This trial provided the first clinical evidence that anti–growth factor receptor–directed strategies were useful in the treatment of human cancer (96).

In a follow-up pivotal study (97), 222 women with HER2+ metastatic breast cancer and two prior chemotherapy regimens were enrolled in an open label, phase 2 trial of trastuzumab

TABLE 1. TRASTUZUMAB ACTIVITY: SINGLE-AGENT BREAST CANCER STUDIES

	Proof of Concept Phase 2 (%)	Pivotal Phase 2 (%)	Current Phase 2 (%)
No. of patients (intent-to-treat)	46	222	112
Prior CT regimens meta-static disease (median)	Yes (3)	Yes (2)	No
Complete response	1	8	6
Partial response	4	26	20
Response rate	11	14	23
95% CI	4–24	11–21	15–31
Median duration of response (mo)	6.6	9.1	8.0
Median survival (mo)	14	13	N/A
Reference	93	94	95

CI, confidence interval; CT, chemotherapy; N/A, not available.
Note: First-line therapy trial (patients without prior chemotherapy).

(loading dose, 4 mg per kg and weekly dose, 2 mg per kg). The overall response rate as determined by an independent Response Evaluation Committee was 14% (95% confidence interval, 10% to 20%) with a 2% complete response rate and a 12% partial response rate. Response Evaluation Committee–determined median duration of response was 8.5 months and estimated median survival is 13 months. Cardiac dysfunction was observed in ten patients, six of them symptomatic, including one death due to a ventricular arrhythmia; all had prior anthracycline chemotherapy or had a cardiac history.

A more recent study has analyzed the activity of trastuzumab in patients with metastatic breast cancer overexpressing HER2 as first-line therapy of breast cancer (98). A total of 114 women have been entered in this study. Patients were randomized to receive the conventional trastuzumab dose (loading dose, 4 mg per kg and weekly dose, 2 mg per kg) or a higher dose regimen (loading dose, 8 mg per kg and weekly dose, 4 mg per kg). Mean age in this study was 57 years, 26% had a metastatic-free interval of less than 12 months, and 86% had visceral disease. Of 112 evaluable patients, six complete remissions and 20 partial remissions have been observed for an overall response rate of 23% (95% confidence interval, 15% to 31%). The response rate in the group of patients with the higher level of HER2 overexpression (3+) (n = 85) was 31%. No differences existed in response between the two dose levels, and the median duration of response was 8 months.

In summary, trastuzumab is active as a single agent in women with HER2+ metastatic breast cancer and induces durable objective tumor responses as first-line therapy in previously treated patients. We conclude that trastuzumab is safe and effective for the therapy of patients with HER2+ metastatic breast cancer.

Clinical Trials with Anti-HER2 Monoclonal Antibodies and Chemotherapy

Based on the preclinical synergism, a phase 2 study of antibody and cisplatin was conducted in parallel to the first single-agent phase 2 trial (99). The study included patients with extensively pretreated advanced breast cancer with HER2 overexpression and disease progression during standard chemotherapy. The dose and schedule of trastuzumab administration was identical as in the single-agent phase 2 trial, and cisplatin (75 mg per m^2) was given every 4 weeks. Of 37 patients assessable for response, nine (24.3%) achieved a partial response, nine (24.3%) achieved a minor response or stable disease, and disease progression occurred in 19 (51.3%). The median response duration was 5.3 months (range, 1.6–18). No evidence exists that trastuzumab enhanced the toxicity of cisplatin. Mean pharmacokinetic parameters of trastuzumab were unaltered by coadministration of cisplatin. The presence of high serum levels of HER2 extracellular domain, however, was inversely related with the serum half-life of trastuzumab. The 24% response rate observed with the combination is greater than the reported response rate with cisplatin alone in patients who were previously treated for their metastatic disease (0% to 7%) and further supports the laboratory data showing marked enhancement of the antitumor effects of cisplatin when combined with trastuzumab.

The mentioned preclinical data showing marked antitumor effects when anthracyclines, and especially taxol, were combined with trastuzumab led to the design of a phase 3 multicenter clinical trial of chemotherapy (doxorubicin based or paclitaxel based) plus trastuzumab versus chemotherapy alone in patients with advanced breast cancers overexpressing HER2 (100). A total of 469 female patients with no prior chemotherapy for their metastatic breast cancer were included in the trial. The patients received doxorubicin-cyclophosphamide (AC) (n = 281) or paclitaxel (n = 188) as first chemotherapeutic regimen if they had not received prior adjuvant doxorubicin or paclitaxel if previously exposed to doxorubicin. The schedules of chemotherapy were: AC, doxorubicin (60 mg per m^2) (or epirubicin, 75 mg per m^2) plus cyclophosphamide (600 mg per m^2) or paclitaxel (175 mg per m^2) in a 3-hour infusion. All chemotherapeutic agents were given every 3 weeks for six cycles. One-half of the patients (stratified by the chemotherapeutic regimens) were randomized to additionally receive trastuzumab (4 mg per kg loading, then 2 mg per kg intravenously weekly). An independent Review Evaluation Committee–determined time to disease progression and response rates show a significant augmentation of the chemotherapy effect by trastuzumab without increase in overall severe adverse events. A syndrome of myocardial dysfunction similar to that observed with anthracyclines was reported more commonly with AC plus trastuzumab (16%, grade 3/4) than with AC alone (3%), paclitaxel alone (1%), or paclitaxel plus trastuzumab (2%). The benefits of adding trastuzumab to the chemotherapeutic regimens used are summarized in Table 2. Trastuzumab significantly increased time to progression and response rate and duration. The time to disease progression was 4.6 months with chemotherapy alone and increased to 7.6 months with combined therapy (p = .001). The increase in time to disease progression was particularly positive in the paclitaxel plus trastuzumab arm when compared with trastuzumab alone. The overall response rate was 32% with chemotherapy alone and 49% with combined therapy (p = .0002). The augmentation of response rate was more pronounced in the paclitaxel arm than in the AC arm (see Table 2). Of interest, the 1-year survival was 78% in patients treated with trastuzumab

TABLE 2. TRASTUZUMAB IN COMBINATION WITH CHEMOTHERAPY

	No. Patients	Median TTP (Mo) (*p* Value)	Response Rate (%) (*p* Value)	Median DR (Mo) (*p* Value)
H + AC	143	8.1 (.0003)	52 (.1038)	9.1 (.0025)
AC	138	6.1	43	6.5
H + P	92	6.9 (.0001)	42 (<.0001)	11.0 (.0001)
P	96	3.0	16	4.4
H + CT	235	7.6	49	9.3
CT	234	4.6 (.0001)	32 (.0002)	5.9 (.0001)

AC, doxorubicin + cyclophosphamide; CT, chemotherapy; DR, duration of response; H, Herceptin; P, paclitaxel; TTP, time to progression.

and chemotherapy versus 67% in patients treated with chemotherapy alone (*p* = .008) (97).

The results of these clinical trials have shown that trastuzumab is effective for the treatment of patients with HER2+ metastatic breast cancer. To further establish the role of trastuzumab in the therapy of patients with breast cancer, a series of clinical trials are under way or are in the planning process. The areas that appear to be of major interest for further development of trastuzumab are:

1. Studies of trastuzumab in combination with other active agents and regimens
2. Combination studies with hormonal therapy
3. New schedules with taxanes (± platinum)
4. Adjuvant and neoadjuvant studies

In addition, because HER2 is also overexpressed in other common malignancies, such as colon and non–small-cell lung cancer, studies are also being planned with trastuzumab alone or with conventional chemotherapeutic agents.

NOVEL ANTIBODY-BASED STRATEGIES DIRECTED AGAINST erbB RECEPTORS

In addition to antibodies that are directed against the extracellular domains of EGF-R or HER-2, recombinant antibody technology has been proved as a useful tool in designing and producing novel antibody-based molecules (101). These novel antibody-based molecules include intracellular antibodies, bispecific antibodies, and antireceptor antibody fusion molecules. Another therapeutic strategy involving antigrowth factor receptor MAb is the use of the receptor-mediated endocytosis pathway for gene delivery. Some of these antigrowth factor receptor strategies are entering clinical trials.

Intracellular Antibody

The intracellular antibody strategy is based on the delivery of a single-chain antibody construct containing the variable domains of heavy and light chains of the antibody (scFv) into target cells via a vehicle such as recombinant virus (102). When functionally expressed in target cells, the scFv antibody can bind to the targeted molecules and prevent their transit and delivery through the endoplasmic reticulum. This results in the func-

tional inactivation of the targeted molecules and, therefore, can be applied to selectively "knock out" some specific oncoproteins, potentially creating a new form of anticancer therapy. Research has been carried out on scFv antibodies directed against EGF-Rs and HER-2. Expression in the endoplasmic reticulum of the anti-HER-2 scFv antibody resulted in a profound downregulation of cell surface HER-2. This was accompanied by marked inhibition of proliferation in HER-2–overexpressing cell lines, and even killing of targeted tumors cells via apoptosis in some cases (102). Anti-HER-2 scFv can also reverse the phenotype of NIH3T3 cells transformed by HER-2 (103). Similar experiments with intracellular expression of an scFv antibody derived from anti–EGF-R MAb R1 also led to growth inhibition of cells expressing EGF-Rs (104).

Bispecific Antibody

Considerable progress has been made in the production of bispecific MAb (BsMAb) with dual specificity for cancer-associated antigens and for cells and molecules that can trigger cytotoxicity, such as leukocyte surface receptors or chemotherapeutic drugs. BsMAb have been produced by chemically cross-linking two individual F(ab') fragments by fusion of two parental hybridomas into a hybrid-hybridoma and screening for BsMAb expression or trough molecular construction of BsMAb fusion antibody using recombinant antibody technology (105).

Several BsMAb that bind to HER-2 or EGF-Rs have been made, and targeted lysis of tumor cells by BsMAb has been achieved. Some studies used BsMAb directed to the EGF-R coupled with reactivity to CD3 or doxorubicin; other studies used BsMAb directed to HER-2 coupled with reactivity to CD3, CD64 (FcγRI), CD43 (FcγRII), or CD16 (FcγRIII) (101). The results of these studies indicate that the BsMAb can significantly enhance the specific cytotoxicities of T cells, natural killer cells, or polymorphonuclear leukocyte cells on targeted tumor cell lines. 2B1, a hybrid-hybridoma BsMAb consisting of MAb 520C9 to HER-2 and MAb 3G8 to CD16 and MDX210, another BsMAb consisting of chemically cross-linked F(ab') fragments of MAb 520C9 to HER-2 and MAb H22 to CD64, have undergone phase 1 evaluation. No untoward toxicities were observed (106,107). As an alternative approach, the natural ligands for receptors may also be used for construction and expression of such fusion proteins (108).

Antireceptor Antibody Fusion Molecules

Genetically engineered fusion proteins coupling MAb with cytokines or toxins provide an approach that combines the specific targeting ability of antibodies with the multifunctional cytotoxicities of cytokines or toxins. This approach can be achieved via the fusion of genes encoding toxins or cytokines to the genes encoding for MAb with expression in a bacterial vector (109). With advances in recombinant DNA technology, scFv antibodies have been used as recognition domains. This novel form of fusion protein is superior to the conventional chemical conjugates of MAb with toxins, in that antibody single-chain fusion proteins are much smaller than the original conjugate and have superior properties in their penetration into large tumors. Also, the fusion proteins are easier to produce and purify and are more stable and consistent in activity. Research on the activity of antibody-cytokine or antibody-toxin fusion proteins has been carried out in cancer cells overexpressing EGF-Rs or HER2. These include anti–EGF-R MAb fusion proteins containing interleukin-2 (IL-2) (110) or lymphotoxin (111) and anti-HER2 receptor MAb fusion proteins containing B7-2 (CD80) (112).

The recombinant immune toxins scFv(225)-ETA and scFv(FRP5)-ETA contain a single-chain antibody against the EGF-R (225) or HER2 (FRP5), respectively, in fusion with a truncated gene encoding for the exotoxin (ETA) of *Pseudomonas aeruginosa* (109). The scFv(225)-ETA has been shown to specifically inhibit the growth of cultured cells expressing high levels of EGF-Rs, and scFv(FRP5)-ETA inhibited the growth of cultured cells, as well as xenografted tumor cells expressing HER2 (113). Another experimental capacity of these immunotoxins is the ability to purge, *ex vivo*, hematopoietic progenitor cells contaminated with mammary carcinoma cells because CD34+ hematopoietic progenitor cells do not express EGF-Rs or HER2 (114). Because some tumor cells express EGF-Rs and HER2 and the two receptors may synergize in cellular transformation, a bivalent scFv2(FRP5/225)-ETA fusion protein (a fusion containing HER2–specific and EGF-R–specific MAb domains fused to ETA) or, alternatively, a bivalent scFv2(FRP5)-TGF-α–ETA (a fusion immunotoxin containing HER2–specific MAb domain and TGF-α fused to ETA), were also constructed and expressed (115,116). In these studies, they were found to be more potent than the corresponding monovalent toxins in killing human tumor cells coexpressing HER2 and EGF-R *in vitro* and in xenografts.

MONOCLONAL ANTIBODIES AGAINST OTHER RECEPTORS

Monoclonal Antibodies Against the Receptor for Transferrin

The transferrin receptor is displayed on the cell surface when cells proliferate, and transferrin appears to be an essential ingredient of the culture medium for cells grown under serum-free conditions (117). In many cases, evidence exists that the transferrin receptor is expressed in higher numbers on tumor cells than in normal tissues (118). These properties suggest that the transferrin receptor may be a fruitful target for novel forms of anticancer therapies.

Antitransferrin receptor antibodies have shown antitumor activity in experimental murine and human xenograft models (119,120). 42/6 is a murine IgA monoclonal antihuman transferrin receptor MAb previously shown to have *in vitro* antitumor activity (119,121). 42/6, given as a 24-hour infusion, has been tested in an initial phase 1 clinical trial in patients with refractory malignancies (122). This represented the first clinical trial with an IgA mouse MAb, and antibody concentrations capable of inhibiting malignant cell growth were obtained without toxicity.

As with anti-erbB MAb, preclinical evidence exists that supports an enhanced antitumor activity when combined with other anticancer agents. Antitransferrin MAb enhance the antitumor effects of cyclophosphamide (Trowbridge, *unpublished observations*), desferroxamine (123), anti–IL-6 antibodies (124), and retinoid acid (125).

Monoclonal Antibodies Against the Interleukin-2 Receptor

The IL-2 receptor is a multisubunit complex containing two ligand-binding sites, IL-2 receptor α (p55 or Tac protein) and IL-2 receptor β (p75). In addition 22-, 35-, 75- (non–IL-2 binding), and 95- to 105-kd peptides, as well as class I major histocompatibility complex, intercellular adhesion molecule-I, and two tyrosine kinases are associated with the two IL-2–binding polypeptides (126). The distinct mature T-cell form of acute leukemia, termed *adult T-cell leukemia* (ATL), is a malignant proliferation of T cells that express IL-2 receptors, including the Tac peptide. Receptor expression is activated by the tax protein of human T leukemia virus-1, the primary etiologic agent in ATL. An early clinical trial evaluated the efficacy of anti-Tac MAb in patients with ATL. None of the 16 patients demonstrated any toxicity, one patient had a mixed response and another patient had a partial response, and four developed complete remissions lasting from 1 to more than 8 months (126–128). In one of these cases studied in great detail, there was a decline to normal in the number of Tac-expressing cells, paralleled by an elimination of circulating malignant cells characterized as cells bearing human T leukemia virus-1 integrated into their DNA and cells with a clonal T-cell receptor rearrangement. A bispecific humanized anti-IL receptor αβ has also been produced and may be more efficacious than anti-Tac or MAb, or both, directed at IL-2 receptor α and β, respectively (129).

To limit the immunogenicity, humanized anti-Tac MAb have been produced (130). In addition, to enhance their effector function, anti-Tac antibodies have been armed with immunotoxins or with α- and β-emitting radionuclides. Anti–IL-2 receptor antibodies linked to a deglycosylated ricin-A toxin have shown promising activity in patients with refractory Hodgkin's lymphoma (131). In a clinical trial with 90Y-anti-Tac, 11 of 17 patients with ATL underwent a remission (132).

A new class of receptor-active cytotoxic fusion protein, DAB$_{389}$IL-2, composed of the binding domain of diphtheria toxin and the receptor-binding domain of IL-2, has also been shown to be active in cutaneous T-cell lymphoma and in other non-Hodgkin's lymphomas (133). Five complete and eight partial remissions occurred in 35 patients with cutaneous T-cell lymphoma and one complete remission and two partial remissions out of 17 patients with non-Hodgkin's lymphomas. The median time to response was 2 months, and the duration of response was 2 to 39+ months. No responses were documented in patients with Hodgkin's disease. A randomized trial assessed the safety and efficacy of $DAB_{389}IL-2$ at two dose levels (134). Based on these studies, $DAB_{389}IL-2$ has undergone accelerated Food and Drug Administration approval for treatment of patients with persistent or recurrent cutaneous T-cell lymphoma that express the IL-2 receptor.

Antibodies Against Interleukin-6 Receptor

IL-6, also known as *B-cell stimulatory factor-2*, was originally described as a *T-cell product*, which enhances immunoglobulin synthesis by B cells. It has been shown that IL-6 stimulates the growth of multiple myeloma (135) and hematopoietic stem cells (136). Studies with anti–IL-6 antibody have demonstrated growth inhibition of freshly isolated human myeloma cells in culture (135). Because these cells produce IL-6 and express its receptor, these studies provide direct evidence that an autocrine growth regulatory pathway is active in the oncogenesis of human myelomas.

In patients with advanced multiple myeloma, an excess of production of IL-6 occurs *in vivo*, and elevated serum levels are associated with plasmablastic proliferative activity and short survival. These data provided the rationale to perform a clinical trial with a murine anti–IL-6 MAb to neutralize the activity of this putatively deleterious factor in these patients (137). Ten patients with extramedullary involvement were treated with anti–IL-6 MAb. Among seven patients receiving the anti–IL-6 MAb for more than 1 week, three had objective antiproliferative effects marked by a significant reduction of the myeloma cell labeling index within the bone marrow. One of these three patients achieved a 30% regression of tumor mass. None of the patients studied, however, achieved remission or improved outcome as judged by standard clinical criteria. Of major interest, objective antiproliferative effects were associated with complete inhibition of C-reactive protein synthesis and low daily IL-6 production *in vivo*. On the other hand, the lack of effect in four patients was associated with a higher IL-6 production and inability of the MAb to neutralize it. The generation of human antibodies to Fc fragment of the murine anti–IL-6 MAb observed in one patient was associated with dramatic progression (137).

Because the production of human antibodies against the MAb may limit their clinical applicability, a murine antibody, PM 1 MAb, which binds to the human IL-6 receptor and inhibits IL-6, has been humanized (138). The humanized PM1 MAb is equivalent to the murine PM1 MAb in terms of antigen binding and growth inhibition against multiple myeloma cells. This or other humanized anti–IL-6 receptor–humanized MAb could be useful agents in the treatment of patients with myeloma.

SUMMARY

A large body of preclinical evidence exists that demonstrates that targeting the EGF-R (erbB1) or HER2 (erbB2) by MAb is a successful approach to suppress malignant growth in *in vitro* and *in vivo* model systems. Furthermore, extensive studies have shown that these compounds markedly enhance the cytotoxicity of common chemotherapeutic agents. The clinical trials that build on these laboratory studies have confirmed the activity of antigrowth factor receptor MAb as anticancer agents and their ability to augment the benefits of standard chemotherapy.

The success of this hypothesis-based development of novel anticancer drugs is best represented by the approval of the anti-HER2 MAb trastuzumab for use as a single agent or in combination with paclitaxel for the treatment of patients with metastatic breast cancer whose tumors overexpress HER2 and who have received one or more chemotherapy regimens for their metastatic disease. The anti EGF-R MAb C225 is also being evaluated in phase 3 trials given in combination with radiotherapy or chemotherapeutic drugs. Hence, after almost two decades of intensive research in the field, the original hypothesis that targeting of receptors for growth factors may become a useful strategy in the treatment of cancer has proved to be right (9,18). In the years to come, it is anticipated that we will further define the indications and optimal regimens of these new antireceptor strategies.

REFERENCES

1. van der Geer P, Hunter T, Lindberg RA. Receptor protein-tyrosine kinases and their signal transduction pathways. *Annu Rev Cell Biol* 1994;10:251–337.
2. Pinkas-Kramarski R, Soussan L, Waterman H, et al. Diversification of Neu differentiation factor and epidermal growth factor signaling by combinatorial receptor interactions. *EMBO J* 1996;15(10): 2452–2467.
3. Pinkas-Kramarski R, Alroy I, Yarden Y. ErbB receptors and EGF-like ligands: cell lineage determination through combinatorial signaling. *J Mammary Gland Biol Neoplasia* 1997;2(2):97–108.
4. Alroy I, Yarden Y. The ErbB signaling network in embryogenesis and oncogenesis: signal diversification through combinatorial ligand-receptor interactions. *FEBS Lett* 1997;410(1):83–86.
5. Carpenter G. Receptors for epidermal growth factor and other polypeptide mitogens. *Annu Rev Biochem* 1987;56:881–914.
6. Lewis GD, Lofgren JA, McMurtrey AE, et al. Growth regulation of human breast and ovarian tumor cells by heregulin: evidence for the requirement of ErbB2 as a critical component in mediating heregulin responsiveness. *Cancer Res* 1996;56(6):1457–1465.
7. Baselga J, Mendelsohn J. Receptor blockade with monoclonal antibodies as anti-cancer therapy. *Pharmacol Ther* 1994;64(1):127–154.
8. Derynck R, Goeddel DV, Ullrich A, et al. Synthesis of messenger RNAs for transforming growth factors alpha and beta and the epidermal growth factor receptor by human tumors. *Cancer Res* 1987;47: 702–712.
9. Kawamoto T, Sato JD, Le A, Polikoff J, Sato GH, Mendelsohn J. Growth stimulation of A431 cells by EGF: identification of high affinity receptors for epidermal growth factor by an anti-receptor monoclonal antibody. *Proc Natl Acad Sci U S A* 1983;80:1337–1341.
10. Sato JD, Kawamoto T, Le AD, Mendelsohn J, Polikoff J, Sato GH. Biological effect *in vitro* of monoclonal antibodies to human EGF receptors. *Mol Biol Med* 1983;1:511–529.
11. Gill GN, Kawamoto T, Cochet C, et al. Monoclonal anti-epidermal

growth factor receptor antibodies which are inhibitors of epidermal growth factor binding and antagonists of epidermal growth factor-stimulated tyrosine protein kinase activity. *J Biol Chem* 1984;259: 7755–7760.

12. Fan Z, Lu Y, Wu X, Mendelsohn J. Antibody-induced epidermal growth factor dimerization mediates inhibition of autocrine proliferation of A431 squamous carcinoma cells. *J Biol Chem* 1994;269: 27595–27602.

13. Mendelsohn J, Baselga J. Antibodies to growth factors and receptors. In: DeVita AP Jr, Rosenberg SA, eds. *Biologic therapy of cancer,* 2nd ed. Philadelphia: JB Lippincott Co, 1994:607–623.

14. Mendelsohn J. Epidermal growth factor receptor inhibition by a monoclonal antibody as anticancer therapy. *Clin Cancer Res* 1997;3:2703–2707.

15. Wu X, Rubin M, DeBlasio T, Soos T, Koff A, Mendelsohn J. Involvement of p27kip1 in G1 arrest mediated by an anti-epidermal growth factor receptor monoclonal antibody. *Oncogene* 1996;12: 1397–1403.

16. Peng D, Fan Z, Lu Y, DeBlasio T, Scher H, Mendelsohn J. Anti-epidermal growth factor receptor monoclonal antibody 225 up-regulates p27KIP1 and induces G1 arrest in prostatic cancer cell line DU145. *Cancer Res* 1996;56(16):3666–3669.

17. Wu X, Fan Z, Masui H, Rosen N, Mendelsohn J. Apoptosis induced by an anti-epidermal growth factor receptor monoclonal antibody in a human colorectal carcinoma cell line and its delay by insulin. *J Clin Invest* 1995;95(4):1897–1905.

18. Masui H, Kawamoto T, Sato JD, Wolf B, Sato GH, Mendelsohn J. Growth inhibition of human tumor cells in athymic mice by anti-EGF receptor monoclonal antibodies. *Cancer Res* 1984;44:1002–1007.

19. Goldstein NI, Prewett M, Zuklys K, Rockwell P, Mendelsohn J. Biological efficacy of a chimeric antibody to the epidermal growth factor receptor in a human tumor xenograft model. *Clin Cancer Res* 1995;1(11):1311–1318.

20. Petit AM, Rak J, Hung MC, et al. Neutralizing antibodies against epidermal growth factor and ErbB-2/neu receptor tyrosine kinases down-regulate vascular endothelial growth factor production by tumor cells *in vitro* and *in vivo*: angiogenic implications for signal transduction therapy of solid tumors. *Am J Pathol* 1997;151(6): 1523–1530.

21. Rodeck U, Herlyn M, Herlyn D, et al. Tumor growth modulation by a monoclonal antibody to the epidermal growth factor receptor: immunologically mediated and effector cell–independent effects. *Cancer Res* 1987;47:3692–3696.

22. Takahaski H, Herlyn D, Atkinson B, et al. Radioimmunodetection of human glioma xenografts by monoclonal antibody to epidermal growth factor receptor. *Cancer Res* 1987;47:3847–3850.

23. Aboud-Pirak E, Hurwitz E, Pirak ME, Bellot F, Schlessinger J, Sela M. Efficacy of antibodies to epidermal growth factor receptor against KB carcinoma *in vitro* and in nude mice. *J Natl Cancer Inst* 1988;80:1605–1611.

24. Baselga J, Norton L, Masui H, et al. Anti-tumor effects of doxorubicin in combination with anti-epidermal growth factor receptor monoclonal antibodies. *J Natl Cancer Inst* 1993;85:1327–1333.

25. Fan Z, Baselga J, Masui H, Mendelsohn J. Antitumor effect of anti-EGF receptor monoclonal antibodies plus cis-Diaminedichloroplatinum (cis-DDP) on well established A431 cell xenografts. *Cancer Res* 1993;53(19):4637–4642.

26. Meikrantz W, Schelegel R. Apoptosis and the cell cycle. *J Cell Biochem* 1995;58:160–174.

27. Evan GI, Wyllie AH, Gilbert CS, et al. Induction of apoptosis in fibroblasts by c-myc protein. *Cell* 1992;69:119–128.

28. Ye D, Mendelsohn J, Fan Z. Augmentation of a humanized anti-HER2 mAb 4D5 induced growth inhibition by a human-mouse chimeric anti-EGF receptor mAb C225. *Oncogene* 1999;18:731–738.

29. Sepp-Lorenzino L, Bos M, Ma Z, et al. Farnesyl: protein transferase inhibitors (FTIs) block tyrosine kinase signal transduction and act in concert with an anti-EGF receptor antibody to inhibit cancer cell growth. *Proc Am Assoc Cancer Res* 1996;37:A421(abst).

30. Ciardiello F, Damiano V, Bianco R, et al. Antitumor activity of combined blockade of epidermal growth factor receptor and protein kinase A. *J Natl Cancer Inst* 1996;88(23):1770–1776.

31. Wollman R, Yahalom J, Maxy R, Pinto J, Fuks Z. Effect of epidermal growth factor on the growth and radiation sensitivity of human breast cancer cells *in vitro*. *Int J Radiat Oncol Biol Phys* 1994;30(1):91–98.

32. Huang S, Harari PM. Effects of anti-epidermal growth factor receptor (EGFR) antibody 225 on proliferation, apoptosis and radiosensitivity in human squamous cell carcinomas of the head and neck. *Proc Am Assoc Cancer Res* 1998;39:64(abst).

33. Balaban N, Moni J, Shannon M, Dang L, Mutphy E, Goldkorn T. The effect of ionizing radiation on signal transduction: antibodies to EGF receptor sensitize A431 cells to radiation. *Biochem Biophys Acta* 1996;1314:147–156.

34. Divgi CR, Welt C, Kris M, et al. Phase I and imaging trial of indium-111 labeled anti-EGF receptor monoclonal antibody 225 in patients with squamous cell lung carcinoma. *J Natl Cancer Inst* 1991;83:97–104.

35. Bos M, Mendelsohn J, Bowden D, et al. Phase I studies of anti-epidermal growth factor receptor (EGFR) chimeric monoclonal antibody C225 in patients with EGFR overexpressing tumors. *Proc Am Soc Clin Oncol* 1996;15:443(abst).

36. Falcey J, Pfister D, Cohen R, et al. A study of anti-epidermal growth factor receptor monoclonal antibody C225 and cisplatin in patients with head and neck to lung carcinomas (Meeting Abstract). *Proc Am Soc Clin Oncol* 1997;16:A1364.

37. Baselga J, Pfister D, Cooper MR, et al. Phase I studies of anti-epidermal growth factor receptor chimeric antibody C225 alone and in combination with cisplatin. *J Clin Oncol* 2000 (in press).

38. Real FX, Rettig WJ, Chesa PG, Melamed MR, Old LJ, Mendelsohn J. Expression of epidermal growth factor receptor in human cultured cells and tissues: relationship to cell lineage and stage of differentiation. *Cancer Res* 1986;46:4726–4731.

39. Perez-Soler R, Donato NJ, Shin DM, et al. Tumor epidermal growth factor receptor studies in patients with non-small-cell lung cancer or head and neck cancer treated with monoclonal antibody RG 83852. *J Clin Oncol* 1994;12(4):730–739.

40. Perez-Soler R, Shin DM, Donato N, et al. Tumor studies in patients with head & neck cancers treated with humanized anti-epidermal growth factor antibody C225 in combination with cisplatin. *Proc Am Soc Clin Oncol* 1998;17:A1514.

41. Baselga J, Cañadas MA, Codony J, et al. Activated epidermal growth factor receptor: studies in head and neck tumors and tumor cell lines after exposure to ligand and receptor tyrosine kinase inhibitors. *Proc Am Soc Clin Oncol* 1999(abst).

42. Ezekiel MP, Robert F, Meredith RF, et al. Phase I study if anti-epidermal growth factor receptor (EGFR) antibody C225 in combination with irradiation in patients with advanced squamous cell carcinoma of the head and neck. *Proc Am Soc Clin Oncol* 1998;17:395(abst).

43. Mendelsohn J, Shin DN, Donato F, et al. A phase I study of chimerized anti-epidermal growth factor receptor (EGFr) monoclonal antibody, C225, in combination with cisplatin in patients with recurrent head and neck squamous cell carcinoma (SCC). *Proc Am Soc Clin Oncol* 1999;18(abst).

44. Modjtahedi H, Hickish T, Nicolson M, et al. Phase I trial and tumour localization of the anti-EGFR monoclonal antibody ICR62 in head and neck or lung cancer. *Br J Cancer* 1996;73(2):228–235.

45. Levitzki A, Gazit A. Tyrosine kinase inhibition: an approach to drug development. *Science* 1995;267:1782–1785.

46. Klohs WD, Fry DW, Kraker AJ. Inhibitors of tyrosine kinase. *Curr Opin Oncol* 1997;9(6):562–568.

47. Panek RL, Lu GH, Klutchko SR, et al. *In vitro* pharmacological characterization of PD166285, a new nanomolar potent and broadly active protein tyrosine kinase inhibitor. *J Pharmacol Exp Ther* 1997;283:1433–1444.

48. Moyer JD, Barbacci ES, Iwata KT, et al. Induction of apoptosis and cell cycle arrest by CP-358,774, an inhibitor of epidermal growth factor receptor tyrosine kinase. *Cancer Res* 1997;57:4838–4848.

49. Coussens L, Yang-Feng TL, Liao YC, et al. Tyrosine kinase receptor with extensive homology to EGF receptor shares chromosomal location with neu oncogene. *Science* 1985;230:1132–1139.

50. Akiyama T, Sudo C, Ogawara H, Toyoshima K, Yamamoto T. The product of the human c-erbB2 gene: a 185,000 dalton glycoprotein with tyrosine kinase activity. *Science* 1986;232:1644–1646.

51. Stern DF, Hefferman PA, Weinberg RA. p185, a product of the neu proto-oncogene, is a receptor-like protein associated with tyrosine kinase activity. *Mol Cell Biol* 1986;6:1729–1740.

52. Tzahar ELG, Karunagaran D, Yi L, et al. ErbB-3 and ErbB-4 function as the respective low and high affinity receptors of all Neu differentiation factor/heregulin isoforms. *J Biol Chem* 1994;269:25226–25233.

53. Graus-Porta D, Beerly R, Daly JM, Hynes N. ErbB2, the preferred heterodimerization partner of all ErbB receptors, is a mediator of lateral signaling. *EMBO J* 1997;16:1647–1655.

54. Pinkas-Kramarski R, Shelly M, Guarino BC, et al. ErbB tyrosine kinases and the two neuregulin families constitute a ligand-receptor network. *Mol Cell Biol* 1998;18(10):6090–6101.

55. Baly DL, Wirth CM, Allison DA, Hotaling TE, Fox JA. Development and characterization of a rhuMAb HER2 antibody assay for clinical evaluation of cytotoxic potency. *Proc Am Assoc Cancer Res* 1997;38:181A(abst).

56. Burden S, Yarden Y. Neuregulins and their receptors: a versatile signaling module in organogenesis and oncogenesis. *Neuron* 1997;18(6):847–855.

57. Taetle R, Rhyner K, Castagnola J, To D, Mendelsohn J. Role of transferrin, Fe, and transferrin receptors in myeloid leukemia cell growth. Studies with an antitransferrin receptor monoclonal antibody. *J Clin Invest* 1985;75(3):1061–1067.

58. Tzahar E, Waterman H, Chen X, et al. A hierarchical network of interceptor interactions determines signal transduction by Neu differentiation factor/neuregulin and epidermal growth factor. *Mol Cell Biol* 1996;16(10):5276–5287.

59. Kokai Y, Myers JN, Wada T, et al. Synergistic interaction of p185c-neu and the EGF receptor leads to transformation in rodent fibroblasts. *Cell* 1989;58:287–292.

60. Zhang K, Sun J, Liu N, et al. Transformation of NIH 3T3 cells by HER3 or HER4 receptors requires the presence of HER1 or HER2. *J Biol Chem* 1996;271(7):3884–3890.

61. Carraway KL, Rossi EA, Komatsu M, et al. An intramembrane modulator of the ErbB2 receptor tyrosine kinase that potentiates neuregulin signaling. *J Biol Chem* 1999;274(9):5263–5266.

62. Hynes NE, Stern DF. The biology of erB-2/neu/HER-2 and its role in cancer. *Biochem Biophys Acta* 1994;1198:165–184.

63. Slamon DJ, Clark GM, Wong SG, Levin WJ, Ullrich A, McGuire WL. Human breast cancer: correlation of relapse and survival with amplification of the HER-2/neu oncogene. *Science* 1987;235:177–182.

64. Slamon DJ, Godolphin W, Jones LA, et al. Studies of the HER-2/neu proto-oncogene in human breast and ovarian cancer. *Science* 1989;244:707–712.

65. DiFiore PP, Pierce JH, Fleming TP, et al. Overexpression of the human EGF receptor confers an EGF-dependent transformed phenotype to NIH 3T3 cells. *Cell* 1987;51:1063–1070.

66. Hudziak RM, Schlessinger J, Ullrich A. Increased expression of the putative growth factor receptor p185HER2 causes transformation and tumorigenesis of NIH3T3 cell. *Proc Natl Acad Sci U S A* 1987;84:7159–7163.

67. Guy CT, Webster MA, Schaller M, Parsons TJ, Cardiff RD, Muller WJ. Expression of the neu proto-oncogene in the mammary epithelium of transgenic mice induces metastatic disease. *Proc Natl Acad Sci U S A* 1992;89(22):10578–10582.

68. Drebin JA, Link VC, Stern DF, Weinberg RA, Greene MI. Down-modulation of an oncogene protein product and reversion of the transformed phenotype by monoclonal antibodies. *Cell* 1985;41:695–706.

69. Drebin JA, Link VC, Weinberg RA, Greene MI. Inhibition of tumor growth by a monoclonal antibody reactive with an oncogene-encoded tumor antigen. *Proc Natl Acad Sci U S A* 1986;83:9129–9133.

70. Lewis GD, Figari I, Fendly B, et al. Differential responses of human tumor cell lines to anti-p185HER2 monoclonal antibodies. *Cancer Immunol Immunother* 1993;37(4):255–263.

71. Shepard HM, Lewis GD, Sarup JC, et al. Monoclonal antibody therapy of human cancer: taking the HER2 proto-oncogene to the clinic. *J Clin Immunol* 1991;11(3):117–127.

72. Codony-Servat J, Albanell J, Lopez-Talavera JC, Arribas J, Baselga J. Cleavage of the HER2 ectodomain is a pervanadate activable process that is inhibited by the tissue inhibitor of metalloproteases TIMP-1 in breast cancer cells. *Cancer Res* 1999;59:1196–1201.

73. Fendly BM, Winget M, Hudziak RM, Lipari MT, Napier MA, Ullrich A. Characterization of murine monoclonal antibodies reactive to either the human epidermal growth factor receptor or HER2/neu gene product. *Cancer Res* 1990;50:1550–1558.

74. Hancock MC, Langton BC, Chan T, et al. A monoclonal antibody against the c-erbB-2 protein enhances the cytotoxicity of cis-diaminedichloroplatinum against human breast and ovarian tumor cell lines. *Cancer Res* 1991;51:4575–4580.

75. Kasprzyk PG, Song SU, DiFiore PP, King CR. Therapy of an animal model of human gastric cancer using a combination of anti-erbB-2 monoclonal antibodies. *Cancer Res* 1992;52:2771–2776.

76. McKenzie SJ, Marks PJ, Lam T, et al. Generation and characterization of monoclonal antibodies specific for the human neu oncogene product, p185. *Oncogene* 1989;4:543–548.

77. Stancovski I, Hurwitz E, Leitner D, Ullrich A, Yarden Y, Sela M. Mechanistic aspects of the opposing effects of monoclonal antibodies to the erbB-2 receptor on tumor growth. *Proc Natl Acad Sci U S A* 1991;88:8691–8695.

78. Klapper LN, Vaisman N, Hurwitz E, Pinkas-Kramarski R, Yarden Y, Sela M. A subclass of tumor-inhibitory monoclonal antibodies to ErbB-2/HER2 blocks crosstalk with growth factor receptors. *Oncogene* 1997;14(17):2099–2109.

79. Hudziak RM, Lewis GD, Winget M, Fendly BM, Shepard HM, Ullrich A. p185HER2 monoclonal antibody has antiproliferative effects *in vitro* and sensitizes human breast tumor cells to tumor necrosis factor. *Mol Cell Biol* 1989;9(3):1165–1172.

80. Carter P, Presta L, Gorman CM, et al. Humanization of an anti-p185HER2 antibody for human cancer therapy. *Proc Natl Acad Sci U S A* 1992;89:4285–4289.

81. Pegram MD, Baly D, Wirth C, et al. Antibody dependent cell-mediated cytotoxicity in breast cancer patients in Phase III clinical trials of a humanized anti-HER2 antibody (meeting abstract). *Proc Am Assoc Cancer Res* 1997;38:A4044.

82. Tokuda Y, Ohnishi Y, Shimamura K, et al. In vitro and in vivo anti-tumour effects of a humanized monoclonal antibody against c-erbB-2 product. *Br J Cancer* 1996;73(11):1362–1365.

83. Baselga J, Norton L, Albanell J, Kim YM, Mendelsohn J. Recombinant humanized anti-HER2 antibody (Herceptin) enhances the antitumor activity of paclitaxel and doxorubicin against HER2/neu overexpressing human breast cancer xenografts. *Cancer Res* 1998;58(13):2825–2831.

84. Kumar R, Shepard HM, Mendelsohn J. Regulation of phosphorylation of the c-erbB-2/HER2 gene product by a monoclonal antibody and serum growth factor(s) in human mammary carcinoma cells. *Mol Cell Biol* 1991;11:979–986.

85. Sarup JC, Johnson RM, King KL, et al. Characterization of an anti-p185HER2 monoclonal antibody that stimulates receptor function and inhibits tumor cell growth. *Growth Reg* 1991;1(2):72–82.

86. Reese D, Arboleda J, Twaddell T, Akita R, Sliwkowski M, Slamon D. Effects of the 4D5 antibody on HER2/neu heterodimerization with other class I receptors in human breast cancer cells (Meeting abstract). *Proc Am Assoc Cancer Res* 1996;37:A353.

87. Arteaga CL, Carty-Dugger T, Winnier AR. Antibodies against p185HER2 enhance etoposide induced cytotoxicity against human breast carcinoma cells. *Proc Am Soc Clin Oncol* 1993;12:103.

88. Pietras RJ, Fendly BM, Chazin VR, Pegram MD, Howell SD, Slamon DJ. Antibody to HER-2/neu receptor blocks DNA repair after cisplatin in human breast and ovarian cancer cells. *Oncogene* 1994;9:1829–1838.

89. Pietras RJ, Pegram MD, Finn RS, Maneval DA, Slamon DJ. Remission of human breast cancer xenografts on therapy with humanized monoclonal antibody to HER-2 receptor and DNA-reactive drugs. *Oncogene* 1998;17:2235–2249.

90. Arteaga CL, Winnier AR, Poirier MC, et al. p185c-erbB-2 signal enhances cisplatin-induced cytotoxicity in human breast carcinoma

cells: association between an oncogenic receptor tyrosine kinase and drug-induced DNA repair. *Cancer Res* 1994;54(14):3758–3765.

91. Seidman AD. Chemotherapy for advanced breast cancer: a current perspective. *Semin Oncol* 1996;23(1)[Suppl 2]:55–59.

92. Ueno NT, Yu D, Hung MC. Chemosensitization of HER-2/neu-overexpressing human breast cancer cells to paclitaxel (Taxol) by adenovirus type 5 E1A. *Oncogene* 1997;15:953–960.

93. Tsai C-M, Levitzki A, Wu L-H, et al. Enhancement of chemosensitivity by tyrphostin AG825 in high-p185neu expressing non-small cell lung cancer cells. *Cancer Res* 1996;56:1068–1074.

94. Zhang L, Hung MC. Sensitization of HER-2/neu-overexpressing non-small cell lung cancer cells to chemotherapeutic drugs by tyrosine kinase inhibitor emodin. *Oncogene* 1996;12(3):57157–57160.

95. Yu D, Jing T, Liu B, et al. Overexpression of ErbB2 blocks taxol-induced apoptosis by upregulation of p21cip1, which inhibits p34cdc2 kinase. *Mol Cell* 1998;2:581–591.

96. Baselga J, Tripathy D, Mendelsohn J, et al. Phase II study of weekly intravenous recombinant humanized anti-p185HER2 monoclonal antibody in patients with HER2/neu-overexpressing metastatic breast cancer. *J Clin Oncol* 1996;14:737–744.

97. Cobleigh MA, Vogel CL, Tripathy D, et al. Efficacy and safety of Herceptin™ (humanized anti-HER2 antibody) as a single agent in 222 women with HER2 overexpression who relapsed following chemotherapy for metastatic breast cancer. *Proc Am Soc Clin Oncol* 1998;17:376A.

98. Vogel CL, Cobleigh MA, Tripathy D, et al. Efficacy and safety of herceptin (trastuzumab humanized anti-HER2 antibody) as a single agent in first line treatment of HER2 overexpressing metastatic breast cancer (HER2+/MBC) (Meeting abstract). *Breast Cancer Res Treat* 1998;50(3):23A.

99. Pegram MD, Lipton A, Hayes DF, et al. Phase II study of receptor-enhanced chemosensitivity using recombinant humanized anti-p185HER2/neu monoclonal antibody plus cisplatin in patients with HER2/neu-overexpressing metastatic breast cancer refractory to chemotherapy treatment. *J Clin Oncol* 1998;16(8):2659–2571.

100. Slamon D, Leyland-Jones B, Shak S, et al. Addition of Herceptin™ (humanized anti-HER2 antibody) to first line chemotherapy for HER2 overexpressing metastatic breast cancer (HER2+/MBC) markedly increases anticancer activity: a randomized, multinational controlled phase III trial. *Proc Am Soc Clin Oncol* 1998;377A.

101. Fan Z, Mendelsohn J. Therapeutic application of anti-growth factor receptor antibodies. *Curr Opin Oncol* 1998;10(1):67–73.

102. Deshane J, Grim J, Loechel S, Siegal GP, Alvarez RD, Curiel DT. Intracellular antibody against erbB-2 mediates targeted tumor cell eradication by apoptosis. *Cancer Gene Ther* 1996;3:89–98.

103. Beerli RR, Wels W, Hynes NE. Intracellular expression of single chain antibodies reverts ErbB-2 transformation. *J Biol Chem* 1994;269(39):23931–23936.

104. Jannot CB, Beerli RR, Mason S, Gullick WJ, Hynes NE. Intracellular expression of a single-chain antibody directed to the EGFR leads to growth inhibition of tumor cells. *Oncogene* 1994;13(2):275–282.

105. Featherstone C. Bispecific antibodies: the new magical bullets. *Lancet* 1996;348:536.

106. Weiner LM, Clark JI, Davey M, et al. Phase I trial of 2B1, a bispecific monoclonal antibody targeting c-erbB-2 and Fc gamma RIII. *Cancer Res* 1995;55(20):4586–4593.

107. Deo YM, Graziano RF, Repp R, van de Winkel JG. Clinical significance of IgG Fc receptors and Fc gamma R-directed immunotherapies. *Immunol Today* 1997;18(3):127–135.

108. Goldstein J, Graziano RF, Sundarapandiyan K, Somasundaram C, Deo YM. Cytolytic and cytostatic properties of an anti-human Fc gammaRI (CD64) x epidermal growth factor bispecific fusion protein. *J Immunol* 1997;158(2):872–879.

109. Wels W, Groner B, Hynes NE. Intervention in receptor tyrosine kinase-mediated pathways: recombinant antibody fusion proteins targeted to ErbB2. *Curr Top Microbiol Immunol* 1996;213:113–128.

110. Becker JC, Varki N, Gillies SD, Furukawa K, Reisfeld RA. An antibody-interleukin 2 fusion protein overcomes tumor heterogeneity by induction of a cellular immune response. *Proc Natl Acad Sci U S A* 1996;93(15):7826–7831.

111. Reisfeld RA, Gillies SD, Mendelsohn J, Varki NM, Becker JC. Involvement of B lymphocytes in the growth inhibition of human pulmonary melanoma metastases in athymic nu/nu mice by an antibody-lymphotoxin fusion protein. *Cancer Res* 1996;56(8):1707–1712.

112. Gerstmayer B, Hoffmann M, Altenschmidt U, Wels W. Costimulation of T-cell proliferation by a chimeric B7-antibody fusion protein. *Cancer Immunol Immunother* 1997;45(3-4):156–158.

113. Maurer-Gebhard M, Schmidt M, Azemar M, et al. Systemic treatment with a recombinant erbB-2 receptor-specific tumor toxin efficiently reduces pulmonary metastases in mice injected with genetically modified carcinoma cells. *Cancer Res* 1998;58(12):2661–2666.

114. Spyridonidis A, Schmidt M, Bernhardt W, et al. Purging of mammary carcinoma cells during *ex vivo* culture of CD34+ hematopoietic progenitor cells with recombinant immunotoxins. *Blood* 1998;91(5):1820–1827.

115. Schmidt M, Wels W. Targeted inhibition of tumour cell growth by a bispecific single-chain toxin containing an antibody domain and TGF alpha. *Br J Cancer* 1996;74(6):853–862.

116. Schmidt M, Hynes NE, Groner B, Wels W. A bivalent single-chain antibody-toxin specific for ErbB-2 and the EGF receptor. *Int J Cancer* 1996;65(4):538–546.

117. Barnes D, Sato G. Serum-free cell culture: a unifying approach. *Cell* 1980;22(3):649–655.

118. Trowbridge IS. Transferrin receptor as a potential therapeutic target. *Prog Allergy* 1988;45:121–146.

119. White S, Taetle R, Seligman PA, Rutherford M, Trowbridge I. Combinations of antitransferrin receptor monoclonal antibodies inhibit tumor cell growth *in vitro* and *in vivo*: evidence for synergistic antiproliferative effects. *Cancer Res* 1990;50:6295–6301.

120. Sauvage CA, Mendelsohn JC, Lesley JF, Trowbridge IS. Effects of monoclonal antibodies that block transferrin receptor function on the *in vivo* growth of a syngeneic murine leukemia. *Cancer Res* 1987;47(4):747–753.

121. Trowbridge IS, Lopez F. Monoclonal antibody to transferrin receptor blocks transferrin binding and inhibits human tumor cell growth *in vitro*. *Proc Natl Acad Sci U S A* 1982;79:1175–1179.

122. Brooks D, Taylor C, Dos Santos B, et al. Phase Ia trial of murine immunoglobulin A antitransferrin receptor antibody 42/6. *Clin Cancer Res* 1995;1(11):1259–1265.

123. Kemp JD, Smith KM, Kanner LJ, Gomez F, Thorson JA, Naumann PW. Synergistic inhibition of lymphoid tumor growth *in vitro* by combined treatment with the iron chelator deferoxamine and an immunoglobulin G monoclonal antibody against the transferrin receptor. *Blood* 1983;76(5):991–995.

124. Taetle R, Dos Santos B, Ohsugi Y, et al. Effects of combined antigrowth factor receptor treatment on *in vitro* growth of multiple myeloma. *J Natl Cancer Inst* 1994;86(6):450–455.

125. Taetle R, Dos Santos B, Akamatsu K, Koishihara Y, Ohsugi Y. Effects of all-trans retinoic acid and antireceptor antibodies on growth and programmed cell death of human myeloma cells. *Clin Cancer Res* 1996;2(2):253–259.

126. Waldmann TA, Tsudo M. The role of the multichain IL-2 receptor complex in the control of normal and malignant T-cell proliferation. *Prog Clin Biol Res* 1988;262:283–293.

127. Waldmann TA, Goldman CK, Bongiovanni KF, et al. Therapy of patients with human T-cell lymphotrophic virus I-induced adult T-cell leukemia with anti-Tac, a monoclonal antibody to the receptor for interleukin-2. *Blood* 1989;72(5):1805–1816.

128. Waldmann TA, Grant A, Tendler C, et al. Lymphokine receptor-directed therapy: a model of immune intervention. *J Clin Immunol* 1990;10(6S):19–28.

129. Pilson RS, Levin W, Desai B, et al. Bispecific humanized anti-IL-2 receptor alpha beta antibodies inhibitory for both IL-2- and IL-15-mediated proliferation. *J Immunol* 1997;159(3):1543–1556.

130. Junghans RP, Waldmann TA, Landolfi NF, Avdalovic NM, Schneider WP, Queen C. Anti-Tac-H, a humanized antibody to the interleukin 2 receptor with new features for immunotherapy in malignant and immune disorders. *Cancer Res* 1990;50(5):1495–1502.

131. Engert A, Diehl V, Schnell R, et al. A phase-I study of an anti-CD25 ricin A-chain immunotoxin (RFT5-SMPT-dgA) in patients with refractory Hodgkin's lymphoma. *Blood* 1997;89:403–410.

132. Waldmann TA, White JD, Carrasquillo JA, et al. Radioimmunotherapy of interleukin-2R alpha-expressing adult T-cell leukemia with Yttrium-90-labeled anti-Tac. *Blood* 1995;86:4063–4075.

133. LeMaistre CF, Saleh MN, Kuzel TM, et al. Phase I trial of a ligand fusion-protein (DAB389IL-2) in lymphomas expressing the receptor for interleukin-2. *Blood* 1998;91(2):399–405.

134. Duvic M, Kuzel T, Olseon E, et al. Quality of life is significantly improved in CTCL patients who responded to DAB389IL-2 (Ontak) fusion protein (meeting abstract). *Proc Am Soc Hematol* 1998;92[Suppl 1]:A2572.

135. Kawano M, Hirano T, Matsuda T, et al. Autocrine generation and requirement of BSF-2/IL-6 for human multiple myelomas. *Nature* 1988;332(6159):83–85.

136. Hirano T, Taga T, Matsuda T, et al. Interleukin 6 and its receptor in the immune response and hematopoiesis. *Int J Cell Cloning* 1990;[Suppl 1]:155–166 (discussion 166–167).

137. Bataille R, Barlogie B, Lu ZY, et al. Biologic effects of anti-interleukin-6 murine monoclonal antibody in advanced multiple myeloma. *Blood* 1995;86(2):685–691.

138. Sato K, Tsuchiya M, Saldanha J, et al. Humanization of a mouse anti-human interleukin-6 receptor antibody comparing two methods for selecting human framework regions. *Mol Immunol* 1993;31(5):371–381.

139. Weiss FA, Daub H, Ullrich A. Novel mechanisms of RTK signal generation. *Curr Opin Genet Dev* 1997;7:80–86.

140. Baselga J, Norton L, Coplan K, Shalaby R, Mendelsohn J. Antitumor activity of paclitaxel in combination with anti-growth factor receptor monoclonal antibodies in breast cancer xenografts. *Proc Am Assoc Cancer Res* 1994;35:A2262.

SECTION

IV

PRINCIPLES AND PRACTICE
OF CANCER VACCINES

16.1

CANCER VACCINES: CANCER ANTIGENS

Shared Tumor-Specific Antigens

THIERRY BOON
BENOÎT J. VAN DEN EYNDE

DISCOVERY OF THE *MAGE* GENES

The elucidation of antigens recognized by T lymphocytes on human tumor cells began with an analysis of metastatic melanoma. This is because the *in vitro* culture of metastatic melanoma has a much higher rate of success (approximately 50%) than that of nonmetastatic melanoma and other tumor types. A clonal cell line named MZ2-MEL was obtained from a melanoma patient with visceral metastasis. Lethally irradiated MZ2-MEL cells were used to stimulate autologous* peripheral blood lymphocytes in the presence of a small amount of interleukin-2 (20 U per mL).

The responder cells were restimulated weekly with irradiated melanoma cells. The lymphocytes of these autologous mixed lymphocyte tumor cell cultures were tested for their ability to lyse the MZ2-MEL cells in chromium-release assays (1). Significant and specific lytic activity was observed after 3 weeks. The responder lymphocyte populations were restimulated in limiting dilution conditions (one to 20 cells per well) so as to obtain cytolytic T lymphocyte (CTL) clones (i.e., long-term cultures of CTL derived from a single CTL). More than 50 CD8+ CTL clones directed against the MZ2-MEL cells were obtained in the course of several experiments. Most of these clones showed a high level of lytic activity on the autologous melanoma cells (e.g., 20% of lysis at a 1:1 effector to target ratio) (Fig. 1). Moreover, their specificity was remarkably strict: they did not lyse K562, which are natural killer target cells, nor did they lyse autologous Epstein-Barr virus–transformed B (EBV-B) cells or fibroblasts.†

---

*From the same patient.

†For a proper understanding of the difficulty of the field, it is worth mentioning that even the "best" CTL clones (i.e., those that multiply five/fold or more during a stimulation cycle of 7 days) and that show specific lysis, often lose their proliferative or lytic activity for reasons which, to this day, are not understood. Hence, the considerable importance of preparing many frozen stocks for each clone as soon as possible. Even so, the difficulty in sharing CTL clones between laboratories has remained a significant impediment to progress.

The CTL clones directed against the MZ2-MEL cells were used to select resistant tumor cell variants *in vitro* (2). Approximately 10 million MZ2-MEL cells were mixed with a number of CTL of a given clone. In many instances, a few surviving melanoma cells were observed after a few days. These cells were allowed to multiply before being submitted to another selection step with the same CTL clone. Thus, resistant melanoma cells were obtained. These were named *antigen-loss variants* under the presumption that their survival was due to their having lost the expression of the gene coding for the antigen recognized by the CTL. This presumption was based on previous findings from mouse tumor antigens and was confirmed later, when the genes coding for the antigens were identified. However, such *in vitro* selection procedures could also produce "presentation-loss variants" (i.e., cells that have lost the presenting HLA molecule or a component of the antigen-processing pathway). An important observation was that each antigen-loss variant obtained with one anti-MZ2-MEL CTL clone had usually kept its sensitivity to lysis by most of the other CTL clones directed against the same tumor (see Fig. 1). This led to the conclusion that the MZ2-MEL tumor carried not one but several (more than five) antigens that were recognized by autologous CTL. This observation, which has been extended to several other tumors, may have quite an important bearing on the prospects of immunotherapy; first, because immunization against several antigens borne by the same tumor may provide a more effective attack of the tumor cells by the CTL, and second, because the occurrence of antigen-loss variants leading to tumor escape ought to be much reduced under these circumstances.

We and our colleagues then set out to identify the gene coding for the antigen recognized by one of the anti-MZ2-MEL CTL clones (3). Our approach was to prepare a library of cosmids each carrying approximately 50 kilobases (kb) of DNA of the tumor cell line. This library was then transfected into an antigen-loss variant selected with the CTL clone. This CTL clone had been shown to produce tumor necrosis factor (TNF) only when presented with its target antigen: Pools of approxi-

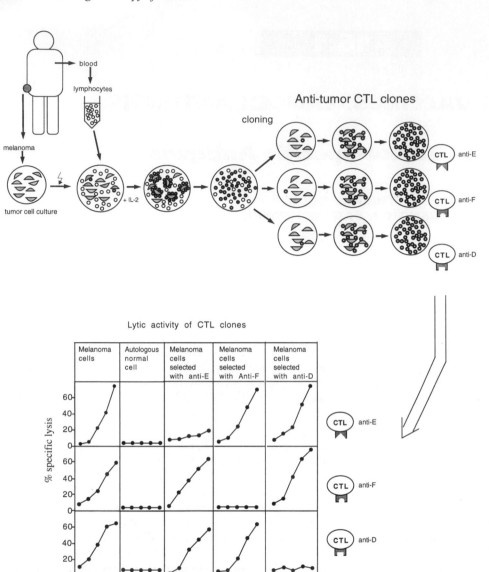

Lytic activity of CTL clones

FIGURE 1. Schematic drawing of the mixed lymphocyte tumor culture (MLTC) used to obtain anti-tumor cytolytic T lymphocyte (CTL) clones **(top)**, and lytic activity of three CTL clones tested against autologous melanoma cells, normal control cells (fibroblasts), and melanoma cells selected *in vitro* for resistance to each of the three CTL clones **(bottom)**. These antigen-loss variants are resistant to one CTL clone but still sensitive to the two others, indicating that the three CTL clones recognize three distinct antigens. Lysis was assessed by measuring the release of ^{51}chromium from target cells after 4 hours of incubation with the lymphocytes at the indicated effector to target ratios. (IL-2, interleukin-2.) (From Van den Eynde B, Hainaut M, Hérin A, et al. Presence on a human melanoma of multiple antigens recognized by autologous CTL. *Int J Cancer* 1989;44:634–640, with permission.)

mately 30 transfectants were mixed with the CTL, and the TNF released in the supernatant was measured. A few positive microcultures were obtained. Duplicates of the microcultures were then subcloned so that the antigen-bearing transfectant cells could be identified (4).

Thanks to a most useful property of the cosmids, it was possible to retrieve from the transfectant the cosmid that carried the gene responsible for the expression of the antigen. This led to the identification of a gene that was named *MAGE*, which contains three exons and codes for a protein of 309 amino acids (3). Previous work on mouse tumors had demonstrated that there are two main genetic mechanisms producing tumor-specific antigens. The first is the acquisition of point mutations by genes with ubiquitous expression (5). The mutation produces an amino-acid change enabling a peptide that is usually 9 or 10 amino acids long to bind to a class I major histocompatibility complex molecule, whereas the normal peptide cannot bind. In other cases the amino-acid change confers a new epitope to a peptide that was already capable of binding to a major histocompatibility complex molecule but was not recognized by T lymphocytes because of central or peripheral natural tolerance. The second major mechanism that generates tumor-specific antigens is the activation in the tumor cell of a gene that is silent in normal cells (6). This produces a tumor-specific protein, which can be degraded into tumor-specific antigenic peptides (Fig. 2).

The sequence of the *MAGE* gene (now called *MAGE-A1*) located in the MZ2-MEL tumor proved to be identical to that of the gene located in normal cells of the same patient. But the *MAGE-A1* gene was expressed in the MZ2-MEL tumor cell line and also in a frozen tumor sample, indicating that it was not an artefact of cell culture. The expression of the *MAGE* gene was then tested by reverse transcriptase–polymerase chain reaction on a large set of samples of normal tissues: no expression whatsoever was observed except in testis, where expression seemed to

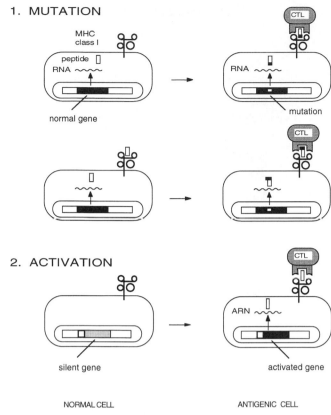

FIGURE 2. Main mechanisms of expression of tumor antigens. The peptide recognized by cytolytic T lymphocyte (CTL) on tumor cells can result either from a mutation **(1)** in a gene that is also expressed in normal cells or from the activation of a gene **(2)** that is normally silent. In the first mechanism, the nonmutated peptide may either be incapable of binding to the major histocompatibility complex (MHC) molecule, in which case the mutation is said to create an aggretope, or the nonmutated peptide may bind to the MHC but fail to be recognized by the immune system because of natural tolerance, in which case the mutation is said to create an epitope.

be of similar intensity as in the tumor (Fig. 3). The *MAGE-A1* gene was expressed in a large proportion of the melanoma samples. Remarkably, it was also expressed in many other types of tumor, such as bladder carcinoma, head and neck carcinoma, and lung carcinoma. For other types of tumor, such as renal carcinoma, colon carcinoma, and leukemia, expression was either infrequent or absent.

To identify the antigenic peptide recognized by the CTL clone used for the cloning of *MAGE-A1*, various regions of the coding sequence were transfected into target cells. When a small region was thus selected, a set of overlapping nonameric peptides encoded by the gene were tested for their ability to sensitize target cells to lysis by the CTL. This led to the identification of peptide EADPTGHSY, which is presented by the HLA-A1 molecule (7).

The only normal cells that express MAGE-A1 are male germ-line cells (8). As these cells do not express HLA class I molecules, they cannot present MAGE antigens (9). Therefore, these antigens appear to be strictly tumor-specific. And because they are shared by many tumors of various histologic types, they are referred to as *shared tumor-specific antigens.*

EXPRESSION OF MAGE-A1

	RT-PCR
MZ2 melanoma	+++
Liver	−
Muscle	−
Skin	−
Lung	−
Brain	−
Kidney	−
Breast	−
Uterus	−
Colon	−
Thymocytes	−
Lymphocytes	−
Testis	++

FIGURE 3. Expression of gene *MAGE-A1* in normal tissues. The expression of *MAGE-A1* was measured by reverse transcriptase-polymerase chain reaction (RT-PCR) using specific primers on RNA extracted from the indicated tissues. (+, positive; − negative.)

RECENT APPROACHES

Although successful for the identification of the first *MAGE* gene, the aforementioned approach was time consuming and difficult to repeat for the identification of other tumor antigens. Therefore, using MAGE-A1 as a model, we and our colleagues (10,11) searched for alternative transfection approaches. We observed that the well-known COS cells, which are monkey cells transfected with the SV40 large T antigen, strongly stimulated the anti-MAGE-A1 CTL when they were first transfected with both the MAGE-A1 and the HLA-A1 complementary DNAs (cDNAs). This showed that COS cells were capable of processing peptides encoded by transfected genes and of presenting them on transfected HLA. This opened the way for a cloning strategy based on cDNA libraries, which are substantially smaller than genomic cosmid libraries. Additionally, the COS can be transfected transiently rather than stably, thereby allowing the transfected cells to be tested as soon as 1 or 2 days after the transfection (10). The library is divided into 1,000 to 2,000 pools of 100 cDNAs each. DNA is extracted from each pool and transfected together with DNA from the gene encoding the HLA-presenting molecule. The CTL are then added to the transfected cells, and the TNF production is measured after an overnight incubation. When a positive cDNA pool is identified, it can be subcloned to identify the positive cDNA clone. The first antigen thus identified was tyrosinase, which is a melanocyte differentiation antigen (11). Many other antigens were subsequently identified by this approach, including two other antigens of melanoma MZ2-MEL, which are encoded by two new genes that were named BAGE and GAGE. Like the *MAGE* genes, these genes are totally silent in normal tissues except testis, but are expressed in many tumors (see below) (12,13). Despite their identical expression profile, these genes do not show any sequence homology to the *MAGE* genes, but rather belong to distinct gene families. The peptides were identified and presented by two HLA-C molecules, namely HLA-Cw16 and HLA-Cw6.

Once it became clear that the expression profiles of the *MAGE*, *BAGE*, and *GAGE* genes were so remarkably similar, it was reasonable to start looking for other genes that had the same expression pattern. The cDNA subtraction technique based on polymerase chain reaction, and known as *representative differential analysis*, was used to search for genes expressed in tumors but not in normal tissues (14,15). By applying this approach to several tumors, previously identified *MAGE* genes were retrieved several times, indicating that the number of gene families with *MAGE*-type expression is probably not very large (16). But a few new genes were discovered, including *MAGE-C1*, a new member of the *MAGE* family, and *LAGE-1*, which are also expressed only in testis and in tumors (17,18).

A completely different approach, which was used by Pfreundschuh and colleagues, relies on the use of the sera of cancer patients to screen expression libraries (19,20). It is called *SEREX* (for *serological analysis of recombinant expression libraries with autologous serum*). A cDNA library prepared in bacteriophage lambda is expressed in bacteria, transferred on filters, and screened directly with the serum of the patient (20). Quite unexpectedly, the first antigens found to be recognized by the patient's sera included intracellular proteins such as MAGE and tyrosinase, which had originally been identified as T-cell antigens. Apparently, these proteins are shed in the course of the necrosis of some cancer cells, thereby becoming immunogenic for B cells and CD4 T cells. The first new tumor-specific gene found by SEREX was *SSX-2* (21). *SSX-2* has a MAGE-type expression profile [i.e., it is silent in normal tissues except testis and is activated in a high proportion of tumors (50% of melanomas)]. Two other MAGE-type genes were then found by SEREX, namely *NY-ESO-1* and *SCP1* (22,23). *NY-ESO-1*, which is closely related to *LAGE-1*, was subsequently found to encode peptides that are recognized by antimelanoma CTL, indicating that it can stimulate both an antibody response and a CTL response in cancer patients (24).

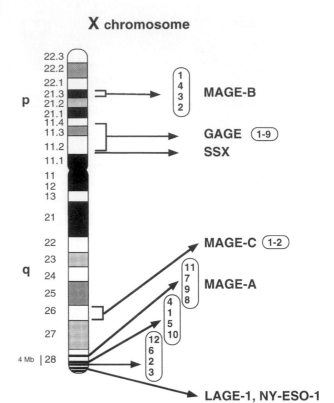

FIGURE 4. Localization of MAGE-type genes on chromosome X.

It is likely that other antigens discovered by SEREX will also prove to encode T-cell epitopes.

MAGE-TYPE GENE FAMILIES

After the identification of gene *MAGE-A1*, it became clear that it belonged to a multigenic family. Other members of the family were then identified using *MAGE-A1* as a probe to screen recombinant libraries. A first group of 12 *MAGE-A* genes was identified, all located in a cluster at the end of the long arm of chromosome X (Fig. 4, Table 1) (25). Like *MAGE-A1*, the other

TABLE 1. MAGE-TYPE GENES

Family Name	Number of Members	Chromosomal Location	Method of Identification	References
MAGE-A	12	Xq28	CTL/hybridization	25
MAGE-B	4	Xp21.3	Sequencing/hybridization	28
MAGE-C	2	Xq26-27	RDA	17
BAGE	≥2	Not on X	CTL	12
GAGE	9	Xp11.2-3	CTL/hybridization	13,31
LAGE-1, NY-ESO-1	2	Xq28	RDA/SEREX	18,22
SSX	10	Xp11.2	SEREX/hybridization	21
SCP1	—	1p13	SEREX	23

CTL, cytolytic T lymphocyte; RDA, representative differential analysis; SEREX, serological analysis of recombinant expression libraries with autologous serum.

MAGE-A genes have their entire coding sequence located in the last exon, which shows 64% to 85% identity with that of *MAGE-A1*. Because of the presence of a premature termination codon, the predicted MAGE-A5 protein is much shorter than the others. *MAGE-A7* is never expressed and appears to correspond to a pseudogene. Figure 5 shows an alignment of the remaining predicted protein sequences, which have 57% to 77% identity with MAGE-A1. At least seven of the MAGE-A genes code for T-cell epitopes that are presented by various HLA molecules.

Another cluster of *MAGE* genes was then identified by chance in the course of sequencing cosmids covering the Xp21.3 region, which is on the other arm of chromosome X (see Fig. 4) (26). This cluster contains four homologous genes, which were given the *MAGE-B* title (27) (see Table 1). Their coding region shows 45% to 63% identity with the *MAGE-A* genes (14% to 47% at the amino acid level). Remarkably, despite this homology, the *MAGE-B* genes were not detected by hybridization with probes derived from *MAGE-A* genes. As opposed to the MAGE-A proteins, which are acidic [isoelectric point (pI), 4.0 to 4.6] the MAGE-B proteins have a pI of 9.0 to 10.7 due to a higher content of basic residues.

Last, two additional *MAGE* genes were isolated by the representative differential analysis approach and located on a third cluster on chromosome Xq26, which was named *MAGE-C* (28). The 5' end of the coding region of *MAGE-C1* is composed almost exclusively of numerous short repetitive sequences. As a result, the predicted MAGE-C1 protein is much longer than the other MAGE proteins (1,142 amino acids). After this repetitive region, the C-terminal segment of the MAGE-C1 protein is 44% to 55% or 39% to 44% identical to the corresponding parts of the MAGE-A and B proteins, respectively.

The function of the MAGE proteins is not known. Their sequences show significant homology to a mouse protein, necdin, which is expressed in the nuclei of postmitotic neurons and may control cell growth during brain development (29). Mouse genes homologous to human *MAGE-A* and *MAGE-B* genes have been isolated. Some of them are expressed in blastocysts and embryonal stem cells, suggesting a function of the MAGE proteins in embryonic development (30). The analysis of MAGE knockout mice, which are currently being prepared, could shed some light on the function of MAGE.

The *GAGE* gene family is also clustered on chromosome X at position Xp11.2-p11.4. In addition to the six members initially described (13), two new *GAGE* genes have been uncovered (31). Each of these eight genes encodes at least one T-cell epitope that is presented either by HLA-Cw6 or HLA-A29. A ninth *GAGE* gene isolated from a prostate carcinoma line was initially named *PAGE-1* (32). It shows several insertions and deletions compared to the GAGE sequences, some of which can be explained by splicing differences (31). Given the high homology to the other *GAGE* genes, this *PAGE-1* gene clearly belongs to the same gene family and should be renamed *GAGE-9*. On the other hand, a related but distant family of genes was retrieved from the analysis of sequence databases, and these genes were also called *PAGE-1, -2,* and *-3* (33). As opposed to the *GAGE* genes, the latter *PAGE-1* gene is expressed in normal somatic tissues of the reproductive tract, including prostate and uterus. The antigenic peptides recognized by GAGE-specific CTL are absent from the PAGE-1 protein sequence. *PAGE-1* was mapped on chromosome X at the same locus as the *GAGE* family (33).

The proteins encoded by genes *LAGE-1* and *NY-ESO-1* share 84% identity (18). This homology and the location of both genes on the same locus on chromosome Xq28 clearly indicate that they belong to a single gene family (18,22). Two major transcripts of *LAGE-1* result from alternative splicing and code for two proteins that differ at their carboxy-terminus (18).

The first members of the *SSX* gene family were initially identified as the fusion partners on chromosome X of the t(X;18) chromosomal translocation that is present in the majority of human synovial sarcomas (34). The fusion partner on chromosome 18 is *SYT*, a gene coding for a putative transcription factor. As a result of the translocation, a hybrid transcript SYT-SSX1 or SYT-SSX2 is produced, which codes for a chimeric protein. Gene *SSX2* was picked up by the SEREX approach, indicating that it can induce antibody responses in melanoma patients (21,35). A study of the expression of *SSX2* then showed that it is activated in 50% of melanomas and in a few other tumor types (21). Unlike synovial sarcoma, this activation does not involve chromosomal translocation.

The only MAGE-type genes that are not located on chromosome X are *BAGE* and *SCP1* (see Table 1). The exact chromosomal localization of the *BAGE* family, which contains at least two different genes, is not known. *SCP1* has been mapped to chromosome 1. It codes for the major component of the synaptonemal complex, which is formed between homologous chromosomes during the prophase of the first meiotic division (36). This gene is expressed exclusively in sperm cells during this meiotic prophase. It was retrieved from a testis cDNA library by SEREX using serum from a female patient with renal cancer (23). This gene is activated in several tumor types, mainly glioma (40%) and breast cancer (27%).

Although not qualifying *sensu stricto* as a MAGE-type gene because of its expression in the retina, the *RAGE* gene is silent in all the other tissues tested, including the testis. It has been mapped to chromosome 14 (B. J. Van den Eynde, *unpublished results*). Different transcripts can be generated by alternative splicing, and *RAGE-1* has been found to encode a T-cell epitope recognized by CTL directed against renal cell carcinoma. It is expressed in 14% of sarcomas but only 2% of renal carcinomas (37).

EXPRESSION OF MAGE-TYPE GENES

The common feature of the MAGE-type genes is their pattern of expression: they are silent in normal tissues except in testis and expressed in a variety of tumors. Table 2 shows the frequency of expression of the MAGE-type genes known to encode T-cell epitopes, measured by reverse transcriptase-polymerase chain reaction in a large collection of tumor samples of different histologic types. Expression is frequently observed in melanomas and in carcinomas of the lung, head and neck, bladder, and esophagus. Expression is absent or infrequent in

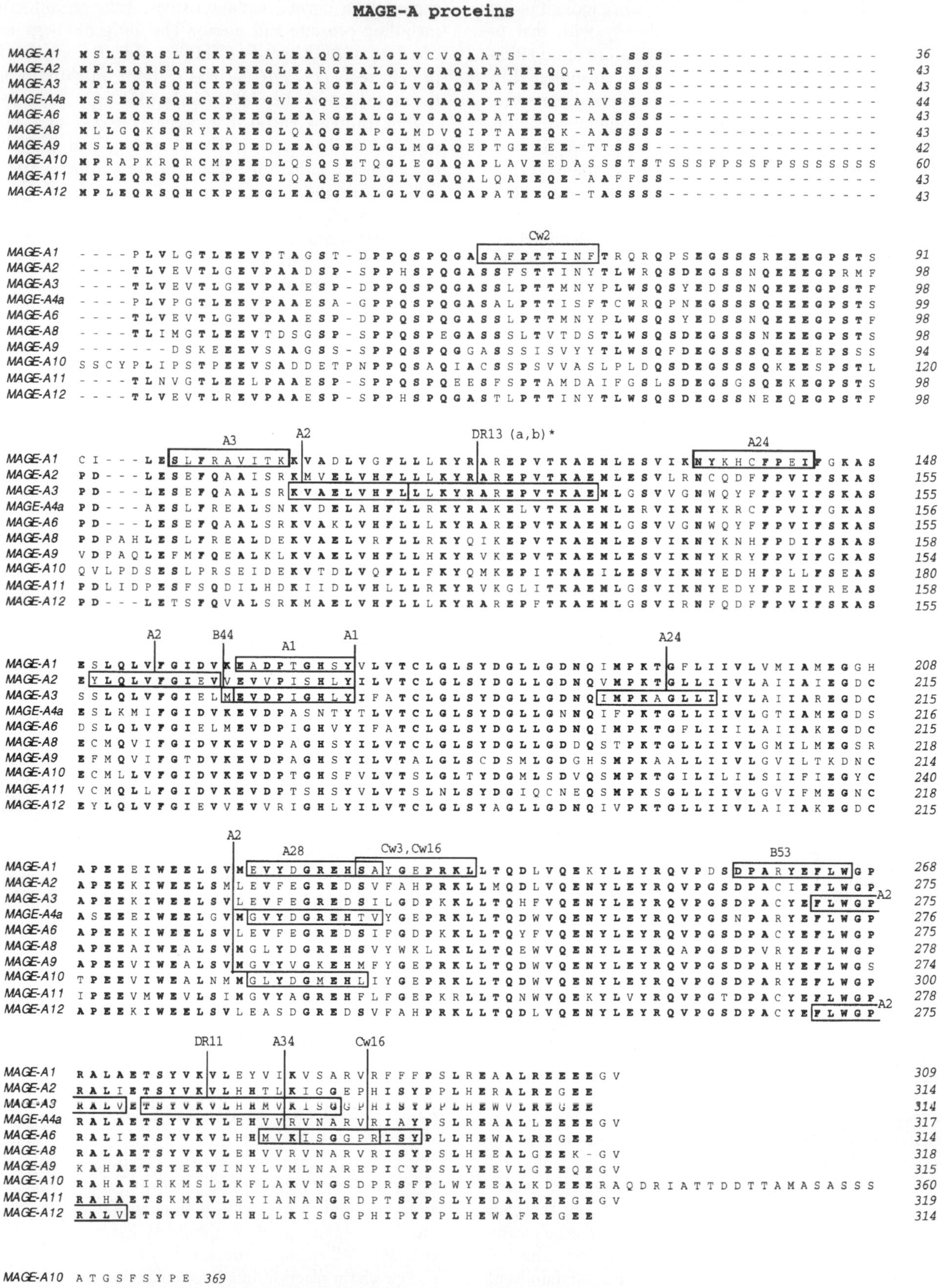

MAGE-A proteins

```
                                                                                                    Cw2
MAGE-A1    M S L E Q R S L H C K P E E A L E A Q Q E A L G L V C V Q A A T S - - - - - - - - - S S S - - - - - - - - - - - - - - -                                          36
MAGE-A2    M P L E Q R S Q H C K P E E G L E A R G E A L G L V G A Q A P A T E E Q Q - T A S S S S - - - - - - - - - - - - - - - -                                          43
MAGE-A3    M P L E Q R S Q H C K P E E G L E A R G E A L G L V G A Q A P A T E E Q E - A A S S S S - - - - - - - - - - - - - - - -                                          43
MAGE-A4a   M S S E Q K S Q H C K P E E G V E A Q E A L G L V G A Q A P T T E E Q E A A V S S S S - - - - - - - - - - - - - - - - -                                          44
MAGE-A6    M P L E Q R S Q H C K P E E G L E A R G E A L G L V G A Q A P A T E E Q E - A A S S S S - - - - - - - - - - - - - - - -                                          43
MAGE-A8    M L L G Q K S Q R Y K A E E G L Q A Q G E A P G L M D V Q I P T A E E Q K - A A S S S S - - - - - - - - - - - - - - - -                                          43
MAGE-A9    M S L E Q R S P H C K P D E D L E A Q G E A L G L M G A Q E P T G E E E E - T T S S S - - - - - - - - - - - - - - - - -                                          42
MAGE-A10   M P R A P K R Q R C M P E E D L Q S Q S E T Q G L E G A Q A P L A V E E D A S S S T S T S S S F P S S F P S S S S S S S                                          60
MAGE-A11   M P L E Q R S Q H C K P E E G L Q A Q E E D L G L V G A Q A L Q A E E Q E - A A F F S S - - - - - - - - - - - - - - - -                                          43
MAGE-A12   M P L E Q R S Q H C K P E E G L E A Q G E A L G L V G A Q A P A T E E Q E - T A S S S S - - - - - - - - - - - - - - - -                                          43


                                                                            Cw2
MAGE-A1    - - - - P L V L G T L E E V P T A G S T - D P P Q S P Q G A S A F P T T I N F T R Q R Q P S E G S S S R E E E G P S T S                                          91
MAGE-A2    - - - - T L V E V T L G E V P A A D S P - S P P H S P Q G A S S F S T T I N Y T L W R Q S D E G S S N Q E E E G P R M F                                          98
MAGE-A3    - - - - T L V E V T L G E V P A A E S P - D P P Q S P Q G A S S L P T T M N Y P L W S Q S Y E D S S N Q E E E G P S T F                                          98
MAGE-A4a   - - - - P L V P G T L E E V P A A E S A - G P P Q S P Q G A S A L P T T I S F T C W R Q P N E G S S S Q E E E G P S T S                                          99
MAGE-A6    - - - - T L V E V T L G E V P A A E S P - D P P Q S P Q G A S S L P T T M N Y P L W S Q S Y E D S S N Q E E E G P S T F                                          98
MAGE-A8    - - - - T L I M G T L E E V T D S G S P - S P P Q S P E G A S S S L T V T D S T L W S Q S D E G S S S N E E E G P S T S                                          98
MAGE-A9    - - - - - - - D S K E E E V S A A G S S - S P P Q S P Q G G A S S S I S V Y Y T L W S Q F D E G S S S Q E E E E P S S S                                          94
MAGE-A10   S S C Y P L I P S T P E E V S A D D E T P N P P Q S A Q I A C S S P S V V A S L P L D Q S D E G S S S Q K E E S P S T L                                          120
MAGE-A11   - - - - T L N V G T L E E L P A A E S P - S P P Q S P Q E E S F S P T A M D A I F G S L S D E G S G S Q E K E G P S T S                                          98
MAGE-A12   - - - - T L V E V T L R E V P A A E S P - S P P H S P Q G A S T L P T T I N Y T L W S Q S D E G S S N E E Q E G P S T F                                          98


                        A3              A2                        DR13 (a,b)*                              A24
MAGE-A1    C I - - - L E S L F R A V I T K K V A D L V G F L L L K Y R A R E P V T K A E M L E S V I K N Y K H C F P E I F G K A S                                          148
MAGE-A2    P D - - - L E S E F Q A A I S R K M V E L V H F L L L K Y R A R E P V T K A E M L E S V L R N C Q D F F P V I F S K A S                                          155
MAGE-A3    P D - - - L E S E F Q A A L S R K V A E L V H F L L L K Y R A R E P V T K A E M L G S V V G N W Q Y F F P V I F S K A S                                          155
MAGE-A4a   P D - - - A E S L F R E A L S N K V D E L A H F L L R K Y R A K E L V T K A E M L E R V I K N Y K R C F P V I F G K A S                                          156
MAGE-A6    P D - - - L E S E F Q A A L S R K V A K L V H F L L L K Y R A R E P V T K A E M L G S V V G N W Q Y F F P V I F S K A S                                          155
MAGE-A8    P D P A H L E S L F R E A L D E K V A E L V R F L L R K Y Q I K E P V T K A E M L E S V I K N Y K N H F P D I F S K A S                                          158
MAGE-A9    V D P A Q L E F M F Q E A L K L K V A E L V H F L L H K Y V K E P V T K A E M L E S V I K N Y K R Y F P V I F G K A S                                          154
MAGE-A10   Q V L P D S E S L P R S E I D E K V T D L V Q F L L F K Y Q M K E P I T K A E I L E S V I K N Y E D H F P L L F S E A S                                          180
MAGE-A11   P D L I D P E S F S Q D I L H D K I I D L V H L L L R K Y R V K G L I T K A E M L G S V I K N Y E D Y F P E I F R E A S                                          158
MAGE-A12   P D - - - L E T S F Q V A L S R K M A E L V H F L L L K Y R A R E P F T K A E M L G S V I R N F Q D F F P V I F S K A S                                          155


                  A2        B44        A1               A1                                                               A24
MAGE-A1    E S L Q L V F G I D V K E A D P T G H S Y V L V T C L G L S Y D G L L G D N Q I M P K T G F L I I V L V M I A M E G G H                                          208
MAGE-A2    Y L Q L V F G I E V V E V V P I S H L Y V L V T C L G L S Y D G L L G D N Q V M P K T G L L I I A I E G D C                                          215
MAGE-A3    S S L Q L V F G I E L M E V D P I G H L Y I F A T C L G L S Y D G L L G D N Q I M P K A G L L I I V L A I I A R E G D C                                          215
MAGE-A4a   E S L K M I F G I D V K E V D P A S N T Y T L V T C L G L S Y D G L L G N N Q I F P K T G L L I I V L G T I A M E G D S                                          216
MAGE-A6    D S L Q L V F G I E L M E V D P I G H V Y I F A T C L G L S Y D G L L G D N Q I M P K T G F L I I I L A I I A K E G D C                                          215
MAGE-A8    E C M Q V I F G I D V K E V D P A G H S Y I L V T C L G L S Y D G L L G D D Q S T P K T G L L I I M E G S R                                          218
MAGE-A9    E F M Q V I F G T D V K E V D P A G H S Y I L V T A L G L S C D S M L G D G H S M P K A A L L I I V L G V I L T K D N C                                          214
MAGE-A10   E C M L L V F G I D V K E V D P T G H S F V L V T S L G L T Y D G M L S D V Q S M P K T G I L I L I L S I I F I E G Y C                                          240
MAGE-A11   V C M Q L L F G I D V K E V D P T S H S Y V L V T S L N L S Y D G I Q C N E Q S M P K S G L L I I V L G V I F M E G N C                                          218
MAGE-A12   E Y L Q L V F G I E V V E V V R I G H L Y I L V T C L G L S Y A G L L G D N Q I V P K T G L L I I V L A I I A K E G D C                                          215


                                A2              A28          Cw3,Cw16                                              B53
MAGE-A1    A P E E E I W E E L S V M E V Y D G R E H S A Y G E P R K L L T Q D L V Q E K Y L E Y R Q V P D S D P A R Y E F L W G P                                          268
MAGE-A2    A P E E K I W E E L S M L E V F E G R E D S V F A H P R K L L M Q D L V Q E N Y L E Y R Q V P G S D P A C I E F L W G P                                          275
MAGE-A3    A P E E K I W E E L S V L E V F E G R E D S I L G D P K K L L T Q H F V Q E N Y L E Y R Q V P G S D P A C Y E F L W G P                                          275
MAGE-A4a   A S E E E I W E E L G V M G V Y D G R E H T V G E P R K L L T Q D W V Q E N Y L E Y R Q V P G S N P A R Y E F L W G P                                          276
MAGE-A6    A P E E K I W E E L S V L E V F E G R E D S I F G D P K K L L Q Y F V Q E N Y L E Y R Q V P G S D P A C Y E F L W G P                                          275
MAGE-A8    A P E E A I W E A L S V M G L Y D G R E H S V Y W K L R K L L T Q E W V Q E N Y L E Y R Q A P G S D P V R Y E F L W G P                                          278
MAGE-A9    A P E E V I W E A L S V M G V Y V G R E H S Y Y G E P R K L L T Q D W V Q E N Y L E Y R Q V P G S D P A H Y E F L W G S                                          274
MAGE-A10   T P E E V I W E A L N M M G L Y D G M E H L I Y G E P R K L L I Y G E P R K L L T Q D V Q E N Y L E Y R Q V P G S D P A R Y E F L W G P                                          300
MAGE-A11   I P E E V M W E V L S I M G V Y A G R E H F L F G E P K R L L T Q N W V Q E K Y L V Y R Q V P G T D P A C Y E F L W G P                                          278
MAGE-A12   A P E E K I W E E L S V L E A S D G R E D S V F A H P R K L L T Q D L V Q E N Y L E Y R Q V P G S D P A C Y E F L W G P                                          275


                    DR11            A34          Cw16
MAGE-A1    R A L A E T S Y V K V L E Y V I K V S A R V R F F F P S L R E A A L R E E E E G V                                          309
MAGE-A2    R A L I E T S Y V K V L H H T L K I G G E P H I S Y P P H E R A L R E G E E                                          314
MAGE-A3    R A L V E T S Y V K V L H H M V K I S G G P H I S Y P P L H E W V L R E G E E                                          314
MAGE-A4a   R A L A E T S Y V K V L E H V V R V N A R V R I A Y P S L R E A A L L E E E E G V                                          317
MAGE-A6    R A L I E T S Y V K V L H H M V K I S G G P R I S Y P P L L H E W A L R E G E E                                          314
MAGE-A8    R A L A E T S Y V K V L E H V V R V N A R V R I S Y P S L H E E A L G E E K - G V                                          318
MAGE-A9    K A H A E T S Y E K V I N Y L V M L N A R E P I C Y P S L Y E E V L G E E Q E G V                                          315
MAGE-A10   R A H A E I R K M S L L K F L A K V N G S D P R S F P L W Y E E A L K D E E E R A Q D R I A T T D D T T A M A S A S S S                                          360
MAGE-A11   R A H A E T S K M K V L E Y I A N A N G R D P T S Y P S L Y E D A L R E E G E G V                                          319
MAGE-A12   R A L V E T S Y V K V L H H L L K I S G G P H I P Y P P L H E W A F R E G E E                                          314
```

MAGE-A10   A T G S F S Y P E   *369*

FIGURE 5. Alignment of the predicted MAGE-A protein sequences. The antigenic peptides recognized by T lymphocytes are indicated with boxes, and the presenting HLA molecules are mentioned. *DR13 (a,b): Two DR13 peptides were found: AELVHFLLLKYRAR and LLKYRAREPVTKAE.

TABLE 2. EXPRESSION IN TUMOR SAMPLES OF MAGE-TYPE GENES ENCODING T-CELL ANTIGENS

Histologic Type	Percentages of Tumors Expressing:											
	MAGE-A1	MAGE-A2	MAGE-A3	MAGE-A4	MAGE-A6	MAGE-A10	MAGE-A12	BAGE	GAGE-1,2,7	GAGE-3-6,8	LAGE-1	NY-ESO-1
Melanoma												
Primary lesions	25	52	55	18	59	21	34	12	29	41	33	17
Metastases	46	70	74	28	72	47	62	31	41	50	41	35
Lung carcinoma												
Squamous cell carcinoma	44	42	48	59	53	50	28	9	39	42	27	17
Adenocarcinoma	49	47	44	35	49	40	33	13	36	45	44	40
Head and neck squamous cell carcinoma	31	38	51	53	58	35	27	6	26	28	35	24
Bladder carcinoma												
Superficial (<T2)	14	11	16	23	19	33	10	3	3	3		
Infiltrating (≥T2)	32	43	57	45	57	33	34	26	25	35	47	47
Esophageal carcinoma												
Squamous cell carcinoma	53	53	63	74	68	40	26	6	44	44	20	10
Adenocarcinoma	20	40	20	20	20		40	0	20	20	20	20
Prostate carcinoma	18	18	18	0	23	10	5	0	15		27	33
Sarcoma	8	15	8	15	15	7	8	0	17		24	35
Breast carcinoma	19	9	13	6	15	0	16	12	10		23	23
Colorectal carcinoma	0	13	17	11	22	0	11	0	0		0	0
Renal cell carcinoma	5	0	0	2	0	0	0	0	0		0	0
Leukemia and lymphoma	0	0	0	1	0	0	0	0	0	4	0	0
Myeloma												
Stages I–II	0	0	0	0	0	0	0	0	0	0	0	0
Stage III	30	19	31	12	33	7	15	15	44	44	52	30

Note: Expression was measured by reverse transcriptase-polymerase chain reaction on total RNA using primers specific for each gene.
From Brasseur F, Brussels Branch of the Ludwig Institute for Cancer Research, with permission.

renal carcinoma and leukemia. This picture is consistent for all the MAGE-type genes, even those from different families. Also consistently observed is a higher frequency of expression in metastatic versus primary melanoma, and in infiltrating versus superficial bladder carcinoma. This coordinated expression suggests that a common mechanism controls the activation of MAGE-type genes. Transfection studies of the MAGE-A1 promoter have shown that it can exert transcriptional activity in cells that do not express the gene, suggesting that the transcription factors capable of activating *MAGE-A1* are ubiquitous (38). Transcriptional control of *MAGE* genes therefore does not involve specific transcription factors. Indeed, it was found later to rely on the methylation of the promoter. The MAGE-A1 promoter contains binding sites for transcription factors of the Ets family, which are essential for its activity (38). These sites contain CpG dinucleotides, which are methylated in cells that do not express the gene, thereby preventing the binding of the Ets factor (39). Treatment of tumor cells or fibroblasts with the demethylating agent 5'-aza-2'-deoxycytidine activates gene *MAGE-A1* (40). This is also true for most MAGE-type genes. A global demethylation of the genome is often observed in tumor cells and is correlated with tumor progression. It is also correlated with *MAGE-A1* expression, which therefore appears to be a random consequence of this genome-wide demethylation (39). This provides an explanation for the higher frequency of MAGE expression in

advanced cancers. It also explains the expression of MAGE-type genes in male germ cells, which also have reduced levels of methylated DNA (41).

Among the *MAGE* genes not listed in Table 2, *MAGE-B2* is expressed in 45% of non–small-cell lung cancers and in 22% of melanomas, whereas *MAGE-C1* is expressed in 46% of melanomas and 18% of bladder cancers (17,27).

OTHER MECHANISMS PRODUCING SHARED TUMOR-SPECIFIC ANTIGENS

Two antigens that have been characterized on human melanoma also represent specific shared antigens, but their presence on tumor cells results from different genetic mechanisms. The first one is due to the activation of a cryptic promoter located in an intron of the gene coding for *N*-acetylglucosaminyltransferase V, an enzyme involved in protein glycosylation (42). An abnormal transcript is produced, containing the 5'-end of this intron and the following exon. This transcript is totally absent from normal cells but is present in approximately 50% of melanomas. The peptide recognized by the CTL is encoded by the intronic part of this transcript and is therefore strictly tumor specific. The reason why this cryptic promoter is active in melanoma and not in normal cells is unknown. The second antigen results from an incomplete splicing of the transcript of *TRP2*, a gene encoding a

TABLE 3. SHARED TUMOR-SPECIFIC ANTIGENS

Gene	HLA Restriction	Peptide	Position	Method of Stimulation of the CTL	References
MAGE-A1	A1	EADPTGHSY	161–169	Autologous tumor cells	7
	A24	NYKHCFPEI	135–143	Peptide	57
	A28	EVYDGREHSA	222–231	ALVAC-dendritic cells	49
	A3	SLFRAVITK	96–104	ALVAC-dendritic cells	49
	B53	DPARYEFLW	258–266	ALVAC-dendritic cells	49
	Cw2	SAFPTTINF	62–70	ALVAC-dendritic cells	49
	Cw16/Cw 3	SAYGEPRKL	230–238	Autologous tumor cells/ALVAC-dendritic cells[a]	45,49
MAGE-A2	A2	YLQLVFGIEV	157–166	Peptide	61
MAGE-A3	A1	EVDPIGHLY	168–176	Autologous tumor cells	62
	A2	FLWGPRALV	271–279	Peptide	46
	A2	KVAELVHFL	112–120	Peptide	61
	A24	IMPKAGLLI	195–203	Peptide	63
	B44	MEVDPIGHLY	167–176	Peptide	49
	DR11	TSYVKVLHHMVKISG	281–295	Peptide	64
	DR13	AELVHFLLLKYRAR	114–127	Protein	50
	DR13	LLKYRAREPVTKAE	121–134	Protein	50
MAGE-A4	A2	GVYDGREHTV	230–239	Adeno-dendritic cells[b]	Duffour[c]
MAGE-A6	A34	MVKISGGPR	290–298	Autologous tumor cells	65
	Cw16	ISGGPRISY	293–301	Autologous tumor cells	van der Bruggen[d]
MAGE-A10	A2	GLYDGMEHL	254–262	Autologous tumor cells	66
MAGE-A12	A2	FLWGPRALV	271–279	Peptide	46
BAGE	Cw16	AARAVFLAL	2–10	Autologous tumor cells	12
GAGE-1,2,8	Cw6	YRPRPRRY	9–16	Autologous tumor cells	13
GAGE-3 to 7	A29	YYWPRPRRY	10–18	Autologous tumor cells	31
NY-ESO-1	A2	QLSLLMWITQC[e]	155–165	Autologous tumor cells	24
	A31	ASGPGGGAPR	53–62	Autologous tumor cells	67
	A31	LAAQERRVPR	Alt.ORF	Autologous tumor cells	67
GnTV[f]	A2	VLPDVFIRC	38–64	Autologous tumor cells	42
TRP2-INT2[g]	A68011	EVISCKLIKR	Intron 2	Autologous tumor cells	43

Alt.ORF, alternative open reading frame; CTL, cytolytic T lymphocyte; GnTV, N-acetylglucosaminyl transferase V.
[a]ALVAC recombinant viruses carrying the entire gene were used to infect dendritic cells.
[b]Recombinant adenovirus carrying the entire gene was used to infect dendritic cells.
[c]Duffour M-T, Chaux P, Lurquin C, et al. A MAGE-A4 peptide presented by HLA-A2 is recognized by cytolytic T lymphocytes. *Eur J Immunol* 1999;29:3329–3337.
[d]van der Bruggen, unpublished results.
[e] The shortest effective peptide still has to be defined.
[f]Aberrant transcript of GnTV that is found only in melanomas.
[g]Incompletely spliced transcript found only in melanomas.

melanocytic protein (43). Again, the peptide recognized by the CTL is encoded by the retained intronic sequence. This incompletely spliced form of the message was not found in normal melanocytes, but was observed in approximately 50% of melanomas.

ANTIGENIC PEPTIDES

Antigenic Peptides Identified with Cytolytic T Lymphocytes

The complete characterization of the CTL–defined tumor antigens required the identification of the antigenic peptides actually presented to the T cells by the HLA molecules. This was achieved on the basis of the sequence of the genes that had been found to sensitize transfected cells to the CTL. A number of truncated genes were produced and tested in transfection experiments to delineate the region encoding the peptide. The predicted protein sequence of the relevant region was then searched for peptides bearing anchor residues for the presenting HLA molecule based on the published consensus binding motifs (44).

Synthetic peptides were then used to pulse target cells, which were then tested for recognition by the CTL. A comprehensive list of the peptides currently identified is provided in Table 3.

Antigenic Peptides Identified by Reverse Immunology

It seemed certain that genes like *MAGE-A1*, which was identified with a CTL clone restricted by HLA-A1, were also coding for many other antigenic peptides that could bind to various HLA class I molecules and be recognized by other CTL clones. This prediction was borne out when a CTL directed against a MAGE-A1 antigen presented by HLA-Cw16 was isolated by autologous stimulation with MZ2-MEL cells (45). Clearly, many antigenic peptides encoded by MAGE-type genes and binding to various HLA molecules remained to be defined. In addition, a wealth of MAGE-type gene sequences were obtained by DNA hybridization with probes of known MAGE-type genes, by enrichment for genes that are specifically expressed in tumors, and by the SEREX method. For all these new genes, the encoded epitopes remained to be discovered. Therefore, an effort was made to identify a number of these antigenic peptides by a reverse approach—that is, starting from the gene sequence rather than from an antitumor CTL clone.

A first approach was based on the results of Rammensee and others who demonstrated that the peptides binding to the product of a given HLA allele have consensus residues (i.e., preferred residues located at the anchoring points of the peptide in the groove of the HLA molecule) (44). The putative protein sequence encoded by a gene was screened for the presence of peptides bearing the consensus residues. The binding affinity of these peptides for the HLA molecule was then evaluated directly. The good binders were then mixed *in vitro* with blood lymphocytes from noncancerous donors to stimulate the putative CTL precursors present in these populations. This approach was applied with success to the identification of a MAGE-A3.A2 and a MAGE-A3.B44 epitope (46,47). However, it has many drawbacks. First, the search is limited to peptides corresponding to consensus motifs and such motifs are not available for all the HLA alleles. Moreover, some effective peptides proved to be different from the consensus peptides. Secondly, in a number of cases it proved difficult to obtain CTL directed against the peptide or, more seriously, when CTL that recognized cells pulsed with the peptide were obtained, they very often proved incapable of lysing cells that expressed the relevant gene and HLA allele, presumably because the peptide was not processed. As a result, the number of infertile attempts to identify peptides has vastly outnumbered the successful attempts. Moreover, for the MAGE-A3.A2 antigenic peptide, it became clear that, even though some tumor cells expressing MAGE-A3 and HLA-A2 are well lysed by the CTL clone, most such tumor cells are not. This suggested that only those cells expressing high levels of MAGE-A3 and HLA-A2 could be recognized, presumably because the MAGE-A3.A2 peptide is poorly processed. One reason for this poor processing appears to be the presence of internal cleavage sites for the proteasome within the MAGE-A3.A2 peptide (48).

These difficulties led us to try a different approach involving T-lymphocyte stimulation by dendritic cells infected with an ALVAC virus containing the MAGE-A1 sequence. After repeated stimulation with dendritic cells, CTL and CTL clones of noncancerous donors were obtained against five new MAGE-A1 epitopes (49). It seems likely that this method will be applicable generally. All the peptides thus identified appear to be well processed, as one would expect, because they must be processed by the presenting dendritic cells.

Because of the availability of highly purified MAGE-A3 protein produced in *Escherichia coli*, it has been possible to pulse dendritic cells with the protein and use these cells to stimulate CD4+ T lymphocytes of noncancerous donors. T-cell clones that recognize EBV-B cells pulsed with MAGE-A3 protein were obtained (50). Using sets of overlapping MAGE-A3 peptides, peptide MAGE-A3$_{121-134}$ was found to be recognized by the CD4+ clone on the DR13 molecule. Two other CD4 T-cell clones directed against this region of the MAGE-A3 protein were obtained from two other individuals. It should be noted that many CD4+ T-cell clones obtained in these stimulations turned out to recognize contaminants in the MAGE-A3 protein

preparation. MAGE-A3 protein prepared with a baculovirus construct ought to be very useful to screen out these T-cell clones conveniently. CD4+ T cells stimulated with the *E. coli* protein could be tested against the baculovirus protein, which ought to contain a completely different set of impurities. Immunization of patients against class II–presented tumor-specific antigens as well as class I–presented antigens may be of crucial importance for the obtention of T cells that can be stimulated and amplified on the tumor site.

THERAPEUTIC IMMUNIZATION

Eligible Patients

The proportion of metastatic melanoma patients who carry a known MAGE-type antigen is high (see Table 2). Less high but nevertheless considerable figures apply to other types of tumors, such as lung cancer, head and neck, and bladder cancer. It now appears quite certain that relatively large proteins, such as the *MAGE* proteins, contain at least one peptide that can be presented by any given HLA allele. It is therefore reasonable to embark on clinical trials of immunization with proteins or recombinant viruses carrying entire MAGE-type gene sequences without limiting the eligible patients to those who express an HLA allele corresponding to a known HLA-peptide combination for this gene.

For immunization trials involving peptides, the situation is quite different. Here the eligible patients are only those whose tumor expresses the relevant MAGE-type gene and also carry the appropriate HLA allele. With the exception of HLA-A2, an allele present in approximately 50% of the white population, this considerably restricts the number of eligible patients.

Modes of Immunization

Even though the extrapolation of animal observations to the human situation is not always straightforward, the careful study of a preclinical model may help to define general guidelines allowing a more rational design of human trials. The best model system for the human shared tumor-specific antigens is the antigen encoded by mouse gene *P1A*. This gene was cloned by the cosmid approach mentioned in the section Discovery of the *MAGE* Genes as the gene responsible for the expression of the antigen recognized by CTL directed against mouse tumor P815 (6). Like the MAGE-type genes, this gene is silent in normal tissues except in testis and is expressed in several mouse tumors, including mastocytomas, lymphomas, and sarcomas. A peptide derived from the P1A protein is presented to CTL by class I molecule H-2 L^d. When mice are injected with 1 million living cells transfected with P1A and with B7.1, they reject those cells, develop a strong CTL response against P1A, and are protected against a challenge injection of P1A-positive tumor cells P815 (51). Given the expression of P1A in testis, we have looked for autoimmune reactions in male mice immunized against P1A. We did not observe any sign of inflammation in their testes, nor did we record any reduction in their fertility (52). This is presumably related to the immune privilege of the testes, combined to the fact that P1A-positive testis cells are spermatogonia, which do not express class I molecules. Because MAGE-type genes also appear to be expressed in class I–negative male germ cells, this observation suggests that human beings can also be immunized safely against shared tumor-specific antigens. We also used this preclinical model to test different modes of immunization that are acceptable for human use and to compare the CTL responses induced. Three protocols appeared to give good responses in most animals. One is the injection of peptide with a QS21-based adjuvant and with interleukin-12 (IL-12) locally (53). A second is the injection of mononuclear cells pulsed with the peptide and injected with IL-12 (54), and a third is the injection of a recombinant adenovirus containing a P1A mini-gene, followed by boost injections of peptide plus adjuvant (55 and G. Warnier, personal communication, 1997).

Clinical Trials

A trial involving immunization of metastatic melanoma patients with a MAGE-A3 peptide binding to HLA-A1 has been completed (56). The patients had measurable disease, and the severity of the disease ranged from regional cutaneous (in transit) to visceral metastases. Patients with brain metastasis were excluded. The immunization schedule involved three monthly subcutaneous and intradermal injections of 100 μg or 300 μg of peptide without adjuvant. No significant difference was observed in the results obtained with either of the two doses of peptide. The locations of the injections were distant from the tumor sites.

Of the 39 patients who entered the treatment, 14 were removed after one or two injections because of disease progression. No significant toxicity was observed in any patient. Tumor regressions were observed in 7 out of the 25 patients who completed the treatment. Among the 17 patients who had no visceral metastases, six displayed tumor regressions. Two of these regressions were complete and long lasting (more than 4 and 2 years, respectively). Among the eight patients with visceral metastases, one showed complete regression of several lung metastases and of a mediastinal lymph node. This patient relapsed 6 months later and died approximately 2 years after that.

No convincing evidence for an anti-MAGE-A3 CTL response could be obtained even in those patients who showed tumor regression. The response was analyzed only in the blood. It may well be that CTL responses were obtained but that the CTL were confined to the tumor sites or lymph nodes.

In some instances, the onset of regression was not observed until a few months after the third injection. In most instances, the regressions that became complete took several months to reach this stage. This pattern of response would fit well with the notion that only a weak anti-MAGE CTL response was produced. Remarkably, patients with a partial or complete response could relapse at new sites in the absence of relapse at the sites that had regressed. This was particularly striking for the patient with lung metastases who cleared five lung metastases and relapsed in cutaneous sites, in lymph nodes, and in adrenals, but never in the lung. Thus, it appears that the immune response could clear up a tumor site completely without affecting small metastases present at that time. MAGE-A3 expression was retained in those tumor sites that did not regress in the course of mixed responses or that relapsed after complete responses. Thus,

neither the lack of a complete response nor the event of a relapse can be assigned solely to the selection of antigen-loss variants. We were not able to evaluate the antigen-presentation capability of these tumors, and it may well be that, as widely reported in the literature (57,58), many of them had a defect in the HLA molecule, β-2 microglobulin, transporter associated with antigen processing, or another component of the antigen-presentation machinery.

Finally, it seems that persistence in the injections may be an important component in obtaining regressions and preventing relapse. One of the patients recorded as nonregressing in this trial later received a large number of injections of MAGE-A3.A1 and MAGE-A1.A1 peptides. After several months of this treatment, most of approximately 50 cutaneous and subcutaneous metastases started to regress. At that point, two large cutaneous metastases were irradiated. A few months later, all of the metastases had disappeared.

Another trial involved the injection of advanced melanoma patients with autologous dendritic cells pulsed with MAGE-A3– and MAGE-A1–encoded peptides presented by HLA-A1. No significant toxicity was observed. A partial tumor response was observed in one of the six patients who received the treatment (56). Strong delayed-type hypersensitivity responses against the peptide-pulsed dendritic cells were observed in the responding patient and in one of the nonresponding patients.

Whereas the clinical trials reported here provide some hope that effective therapeutic vaccination may be achievable, they represent only a first step in a long series of trials aimed at finding effective ways of triggering T-cell responses and of monitoring them. It is particularly important to assess to what extent the failures can be attributed to defects in the antigen presentation of the tumor cells.

ACKNOWLEDGMENTS

We thank Drs. Francis Brasseur, Pascal Chaux, Olivier De Backer, Marie-Thérèse Duffour, Sophie Lucas, Pierre van der Bruggen, and Guy Warnier for communicating unpublished results. The editorial assistance of Saïda Khaoulali and Simon Mapp is gratefully acknowledged.

REFERENCES

1. Hérin M, Lemoine C, Weynants P, et al. Production of stable cytolytic T-cell clones directed against autologous human melanoma. *Int J Cancer* 1987;39:390–396.
2. Van den Eynde B, Hainaut P, Hérin M, et al. Presence on a human melanoma of multiple antigens recognized by autologous CTL. *Int J Cancer* 1989;44:634–640.
3. van der Bruggen P, Traversari C, Chomez P, et al. A gene encoding an antigen recognized by cytolytic T lymphocytes on a human melanoma. *Science* 1991;254:1643–1647.
4. Traversari C, van der Bruggen P, Van den Eynde B, et al. Transfection and expression of a gene coding for a human melanoma antigen recognized by autologous cytolytic T lymphocytes. *Immunogenetics* 1992;35:145–152.
5. Boon T. Toward a genetic analysis of tumor rejection antigens. *Adv Cancer Res* 1992;58:177–210.

6. Van den Eynde B, Lethé B, Van Pel A, De Plaen E, Boon T. The gene coding for a major tumor rejection antigen of tumor P815 is identical to the normal gene of syngeneic DBA/2 mice. *J Exp Med* 1991;173:1373–1384.

7. Traversari C, van der Bruggen P, Luescher IF, et al. A nonapeptide encoded by human gene MAGE-1 is recognized on HLA-A1 by cytolytic T lymphocytes directed against tumor antigen MZ2-E. *J Exp Med* 1992;176:1453–1457.

8. Takahashi K, Shichijo S, Noguchi M, Hirohata M, Itoh K. Identification of MAGE-1 and MAGE-4 proteins in spermatogonia and primary spermatocytes of testis. *Cancer Res* 1995;55:3478–3482.

9. Fiszer D, Kurpisz M. Major histocompatibility complex expression on human, male germ cells: a review. *Am J Reprod Immunol* 1998;40:172–176.

10. De Plaen E, Lurquin C, Lethé B, et al. Identification of genes coding for tumor antigens recognized by cytolytic T lymphocytes. *Methods* 1997;12:125–142.

11. Brichard V, Van Pel A, Wölfel T, et al. The tyrosinase gene codes for an antigen recognized by autologous cytolytic T lymphocytes on HLA-A2 melanomas. *J Exp Med* 1993;178:489–495.

12. Boël P, Wildmann C, Sensi M-L, et al. BAGE, a new gene encoding an antigen recognized on human melanomas by cytolytic T lymphocytes. *Immunity* 1995;2:167–175.

13. Van den Eynde B, Peeters O, De Backer O, Gaugler B, Lucas S, Boon T. A new family of genes coding for an antigen recognized by autologous cytolytic T lymphocytes on a human melanoma. *J Exp Med* 1995;182:689–698.

14. Lisitsyn N, Lisitsyn N, Wigler M. Cloning the differences between two complex genomes. *Science* 1993;259:946–951.

15. Hubank M, Schatz DG. Identifying differences in mRNA expression by representational difference analysis of cDNA. *Nucleic Acids Res* 1994;22:5640–5648.

16. De Smet C, Martelange V, Lucas S, Brasseur F, Lurquin C, Boon T. Identification of human testis-specific transcripts and analysis of their expression in tumor cells. *Biochem Biophys Res Commun* 1997;241:653–657.

17. Lucas S, De Smet C, Arden KC, et al. Identification of a new MAGE gene with tumor-specific expression by representational difference analysis. *Cancer Res* 1998;58:743–752.

18. Lethé B, Lucas S, Michaux L, et al. LAGE-1 a new gene with tumor specificity. *Int J Cancer* 1998;76:903–908.

19. Old LJ, Chen Y-T. New paths in human cancer serology. *J Exp Med* 1998;187:1163–1167.

20. Sahin U, Tureci O, Schmitt H, et al. Human neoplasms elicit multiple specific immune responses in the autologous host. *Proc Natl Acad Sci U S A* 1995;92:11810–11813.

21. Türeci Ö, Sahin U, Schobert I, et al. The SSX-2 gene, which is involved in the t(X;18) translocation of synovial sarcomas, codes for the human tumor antigen HOM-MEL-40. *Cancer Res* 1996;56:4766–4772.

22. Chen Y-T, Scanlan MJ, Sahin U, et al. A testicular antigen aberrantly expressed in human cancers detected by autologous antibody screening. *Proc Natl Acad Sci U S A* 1997;94:1914–1918.

23. Türeci Ö, Sahin U, Zwick C, Koslowski M, Seitz G, Pfreundschuh M. Identification of a meiosis-specific protein as a member of the class of cancer/testis antigens. *Proc Natl Acad Sci U S A* 1998;95:5211–5216.

24. Jäger E, Chen Y-T, Drijfhout JW, et al. Simultaneous humoral and cellular immune response against cancer-testis antigen NY-ESO-1: definition of human histocompatibility leukocyte antigen (HLA)-A2-binding peptide epitopes. *J Exp Med* 1998;187:265–270.

25. De Plaen E, Arden K, Traversari C, et al. Structure, chromosomal localization and expression of twelve genes of the MAGE family. *Immunogenetics* 1994;40:360–369.

26. Muscatelli F, Walker AP, De Plaen E, Stafford AN, Monaco AP. Isolation and characterization of a new MAGE gene family in the Xp21.3 region. *Proc Natl Acad Sci U S A* 1995;92:4987–4991.

27. Lucas S, De Plaen E, Boon T. MAGE-B5, MAGE-B6, MAGE-C2 and MAGE-C3: four new members of the MAGE family with tumor-specific expression. Int J Cancer 2000 (in press).

28. Lurquin C, De Smet C, Brasseur F, et al. Two members of the human MAGEB gene family located in Xp.21.3 are expressed in tumors of various histological origins. *Genomics* 1997;46:397–408.

29. Aizawa T, Maruyama K, Kondo H, Yoshikawa K. Expression of necdin, an embryonal carcinoma-derived nuclear protein, in developing mouse brain. *Dev Brain Res* 1992;63:265–274.

30. De Plaen E, De Backer O, Arnaud D, et al. A new family of mouse genes homologous to the human *MAGE* genes. *Genomics* 1999;55:176–184.

31. De Backer O, Arden KC, Boretti M, et al. Characterization of the GAGE genes that are expressed in various human cancers and in normal testis. Cancer Res 1999;59:3157–3165.

32. Chen ME, Lin S-H, Chung LWK, Sikes RA. Isolation and characterization of *PAGE-1* and *GAGE-7*. *J Biol Chem* 1998;273:17618–17625.

33. Brinkmann U, Vasmatzis G, Lee B, Yerushalmi N, Essand M, Pastan I. *PAGE-1*, an X chromosome-linked *GAGE*-like gene that is expressed in normal and neoplastic prostate, testis, and uterus. *Proc Natl Acad Sci U S A* 1998;95:10757–10762.

34. Clark J, Rocques PJ, Crew AJ, et al. Identification of novel genes, SYT and SSX, involved in the t(X;18) (p11.2;q11.2) translocation found in human synovial sarcoma. *Nat Genet* 1994;7:502–508.

35. Gure AO, Türeci Ö, Sahin U, et al. SSX: a multigene family with several members transcribed in normal testis and human cancer. *Int J Cancer* 1997;72:965–971.

36. Meuwissen RL, Meerts I, Hoovers JM, Leschot NJ, Heyting C. Human synaptonemal complex protein 1 (SCP1): isolation and characterization of the cDNA and chromosomal localization of the gene. *Genomics* 1997;39:377–384.

37. Gaugler B, Brouwenstijn N, Vantomme V, et al. A new gene coding for an antigen recognized by autologous cytolytic T lymphocytes on a human renal carcinoma. *Immunogenetics* 1996;44:323–330.

38. De Smet C, Courtois SJ, Faraoni I, et al. Involvement of two Ets binding sites in the transcriptional activation of the MAGE1 gene. *Immunogenetics* 1995;42:282–290.

39. De Smet C, De Backer O, Faraoni I, Lurquin C, Brasseur F, Boon T. The activation of human gene MAGE-1 in tumor cells is correlated with genome-wide demethylation. *Proc Natl Acad Sci U S A* 1996;93:7149–7153.

40. Weber J, Salgaller M, Samid D, et al. Expression of the MAGE1 tumor antigen is upregulated by the demethylating agent 5-aza-2'-deoxycytidine. *Cancer Res* 1994;54:1766–1771.

41. del Mazo J, Prantera G, Miguel T, Ferraro M. DNA methylation changes during mouse spermatogenesis. *Chromosome Res* 1994;2:147–152.

42. Guilloux Y, Lucas S, Brichard VG, et al. A peptide recognized by human cytolytic T lymphocytes on HLA-A2 melanomas is encoded by an intron sequence of the N-acetylglucosaminyltransferase V gene. *J Exp Med* 1996;183:1173–1183.

43. Lupetti R, Pisarra P, Verrecchia A, et al. Translation of a retained intron in tyrosinase-related protein (TRP)-2 mRNA generates a new cytotoxic T lymphocyte (CTL)-defined and shared human melanoma antigen not expressed in normal cells of the melanocytic lineage. *J Exp Med* 1998;188:1005–1016.

44. Rammensee H-G, Friede T, Stevanovic S. MHC ligands and peptide motifs: first listing. *Immunogenetics* 1995;41:178–228.

45. van der Bruggen P, Szikora J-P, Boël P, et al. Autologous cytolytic T lymphocytes recognize a MAGE-1 nonapeptide on melanomas expressing HLA-Cw*1601. *Eur J Immunol* 1994;24:2134–2140.

46. van der Bruggen P, Bastin J, Gajewski T, et al. A peptide encoded by human gene MAGE-3 and presented by HLA-A2 induces cytolytic T lymphocytes that recognize tumor cells expressing MAGE-3. *Eur J Immunol* 1994;24:3038–3043.

47. Herman J, van der Bruggen P, Luescher I, et al. A peptide encoded by the human gene MAGE-3 and presented by HLA-B44 induces cytolytic T lymphocytes that recognize tumor cells expressing MAGE-3. *Immunogenetics* 1996;43:377–383.

48. Valmori D, Gileadi U, Servis C, et al. Modulation of proteasomal activity required for the generation of a cytotoxic T lymphocyte-defined peptide derived from the tumor antigen MAGE-3. *J Exp Med* 1999;189:895–906.

49. Chaux P, Luiten R, Demotte N, et al. Identification of five MAGE-A1 epitopes recognized by cytolytic T lymphocytes obtained by in

vitro stimulation with dendritic cells transduced with MAGE-A1. J Immunol 1999;163:2928–2936.

50. Chaux P, Vantomme V, Stroobant V, et al. Identification of MAGE-3 epitopes presented by HLA-DR molecules to CD4(+) T lymphocytes. *J Exp Med* 1999;189:767–778.

51. Brändle D, Bilsborough J, Rülicke T, Uyttenhove C, Boon T, Van den Eynde BJ. The shared tumor-specific antigen encoded by mouse gene *P1A* is a target not only for cytolytic T lymphocytes but also for tumor rejection. *Eur J Immunol* 1998;28:4010–4019.

52. Uyttenhove C, Godfraind C, Lethé B, et al. The expression of mouse gene *P1A* in testis does not prevent safe induction of cytolytic T cells against a P1A-encoded tumor antigen. *Int J Cancer* 1997;70: 349–356.

53. Silla S, Fallarino F, Boon T, Uyttenhove C. Enhancement by IL-12 of CTL response of mice immunized with tumor-specific peptides in an adjuvant containing QS21 and MPL. *Eur Cytokine Netw* 1999 (*in press*).

54. Fallarino F, Uyttenhove C, Boon T, Gajewski TF. Improved efficacy of dendritic cell vaccines and successful immunization with tumor antigen peptide-pulsed peripheral blood mononuclear cells by coadministration of recombinant murine interleukin-12. *Int J Cancer* 1999;80:324–333.

55. Warnier G, Duffour M-T, Uyttenhove C, et al. Induction of a cytolytic T cell response in mice with a recombinant adenovirus coding for tumor antigen P815A. *Int J Cancer* 1996;67:303–310.

56. Marchand M, van Baren N, Weynants P, et al. Tumor regressions observed in patients with metastatic melanoma treated with an antigenic peptide encoded by gene *MAGE-3* and presented by HLA-A1. *Int J Cancer* 1999;80:219–230.

57. Ferrone S, Marincola FM. Loss of HLA class I antigens by melanoma cells: molecular mechanisms, functional significance and clinical relevance. *Immunol Today* 1995;16:487–494.

58. Garrido F, Ruiz-Cabello F, Cabrera T, et al. Implications for immunosurveillance of altered HLA class I phenotypes in human tumours. *Immunol Today* 1997;18:89–96.

59. Nestle FO, Alijagic S, Gilliet M, et al. Vaccination of melanoma patients with peptide- or tumor lysate-pulsed dendritic cells. *Nat Med* 1998;4:328–332.

60. Fujie T, Tahara K, Tanaka F, Mori M, Takesako K, Akiyoshi T. A *MAGE-1*-encoded HLA-A24-binding synthetic peptide induces specific anti-tumor cytotoxic T lymphocytes. *Int J Cancer* 1999;80: 169–172.

61. Kawashima I, Hudson S, Tsai V, et al. The multi-epitope approach for immunotherapy for cancer: identification of several CTL epitopes from various tumor-associated antigens expressed on solid epithelial tumors. *Hum Immunol* 1998;59:1–14.

62. Gaugler B, Van den Eynde B, van der Bruggen P, et al. Human gene MAGE-3 codes for an antigen recognized on a melanoma by autologous cytolytic T lymphocytes. *J Exp Med* 1994;179:921–930.

63. Tanaka F, Fujie T, Tahara K, Mori M, et al. Induction of antitumor cytotoxic T lymphocytes with a MAGE-3-encoded synthetic peptide presented by human leukocytes antigen-A24. *Cancer Res* 1997;57: 4465–4468.

64. Manici S, Sturniolo T, Imro MA, et al. Melanoma cells present a MAGE-3 epitope to CD4(+) cytotoxic T cells in association with histocompatibility leukocyte antigen DR11. *J Exp Med* 1999;189: 871–876.

65. Zorn E, Hercend T. A MAGE-6-encoded peptide is recognized by expanded lymphocytes infiltrating a spontaneously regressing human primary melanoma lesion. *Eur J Immunol* 1999;29:602–607.

66. Huang L-Q, Brasseur F, Serrano A, et al. Cytolytic T lymphocytes recognize an antigen encoded by *MAGE-A10* on a human melanoma. *J Immunol* 1999 (*in press*).

67. Wang R-F, Johnston SL, Zeng G, Topalian SL, Schwartzentruber DJ, Rosenberg SA. A breast and melanoma-shared tumor antigen: T cell responses to antigenic peptides translated from different open reading frames. *J Immunol* 1998;161:3596–3606.

16.2

CANCER VACCINES: CANCER ANTIGENS

Differentiation Antigens

PAUL F. ROBBINS

Studies carried out in the 1980s demonstrated that tumor-infiltrating lymphocytes (TILs) could recognize tumors in a class I major histocompatibility complex (MHC)–restricted manner. These extensive experiments carried out using TIL derived from melanoma patients indicated that human T cells could recognize widely shared tumor antigens. Additionally, *in vitro* stimulation of peripheral blood mononuclear cells (PBMCs) with autologous as well as allogeneic MHC-matched tumor cell lines

was found to result in the generation of tumor-reactive T cells. Further studies demonstrated that these T cells could, in many cases, recognize MHC-matched normal melanocyte-cultured cell lines, but not a variety of syngeneic or allogenic MHC-matched normal cell lines. These findings indicated that melanocyte differentiation gene products were recognized by some melanoma-reactive T cells. The subsequent cloning of the genes that encode these products directly demonstrated that T cells recognized melanocyte differentiation antigens in a conventional class I and class II restricted manner.

The majority of tumor antigens have been identified using a genetic approach. After the generation of a complementary DNA (cDNA) library from tumor-cell messenger RNA (mRNA) in a eukaryotic expression vector, pools of cDNA containing between 50 and 200 individual cDNA clones have been produced and cotransfected with a construct encoding the appropriate class I MHC gene into highly transfectable cell lines (Fig. 1). In a variation of this method, cDNA library pools have been transfected into cells that stably express the appropriate class I product. Cells transfected with the cDNA pools were then assayed for their ability to stimulate cytokine release from tumor-reactive T cells, and single clones were identified by subcloning from a positive pool.

The peptide epitopes derived from these antigens have primarily been identified through the use of HLA peptide-binding motifs. These motifs have been derived by comparing MHC-binding peptides that have been identified in a variety of antigens and by sequencing peptides that have been eluted from class I MHC molecules. The results of this analysis indicate that peptides that bind to a particular HLA allele contain a limited number of amino acids at particular positions that are termed *anchor residues*. These residues interact with amino acids in the MHC-binding pocket, providing the free energy for this interaction. Consensus sequences have been identified for a large number of class I molecules (1), allowing the generation of algorithms that can be used to predict potential class I MHC-binding peptides (2).

Another method that has been used to identify tumor antigens involves the elution of peptides from tumor-cell surface MHC molecules. Peptides are then fractionated using reversed phase high-performance liquid chromatography columns and are used to sensitize target cells for T-cell recognition (Fig. 2). After further fractionation of positive pools, individual peptides found in positive subpools that have been sequenced using a triple-quadrupole mass spectrometer have then been synthesized and tested for their ability to sensitize targets for recognition by specific T cells. The antigen from which the positive peptide is derived is then identified through the use of database searches.

Using these methods, a variety of melanocyte differentiation antigens have been isolated (Table 1). A number of homologues of these genes have now also been identified in the mouse, and therapeutic protocols have been established using some of these antigens in mouse model systems, providing a basis for future human clinical trials. Ongoing clinical trials are evaluating the efficacy of specific tumor antigen immunization using peptides that have been identified from these antigens, either administered singly or as mixtures of peptides in adjuvant. Recombinant viral constructs encoding these antigens, including vaccinia, fowlpox, and adenovirus, have been administered to cancer patients. Some studies have demonstrated that modified peptides that possess optimal anchor residues resulting in increased binding to MHC class I alleles are also more immunogenic. These studies, which are beginning to provide some insight into the nature of antitumor immune responses, should hopefully lead to the development of effective cancer vaccines that are capable of mediating tumor regression in the majority of cancer patients.

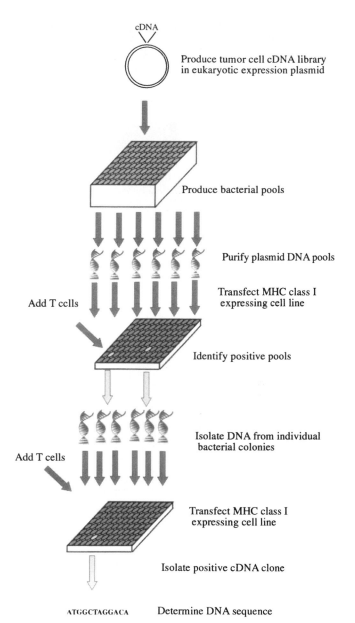

FIGURE 1. Genetic approach to the identification of tumor antigens. (cDNA, complementary DNA; MHC, major histocompatibility complex.)

MART-1

The observation that normal, cultured melanocytes were recognized by melanoma-reactive T cells suggested that tissue-specific antigens might serve as the targets of tumor-reactive T cells (3). The first member of this family to be isolated, termed *MART-1* (4) or *Melan-A* (5), was identified after the screening of a cDNA library with HLA-A2–restricted TILs or cytolytic T-lymphocyte (CTL) clones, respectively. High levels of expression of the MART-1 gene product were found in retinal tissues, which have been shown to contain melanocytes, and in normal skin melanocytes. This gene, which encodes 108 amino acid proteins of unknown function, contains a hydrophobic region between amino acids 27 and 47 and may represent a melanosomal membrane protein (6).

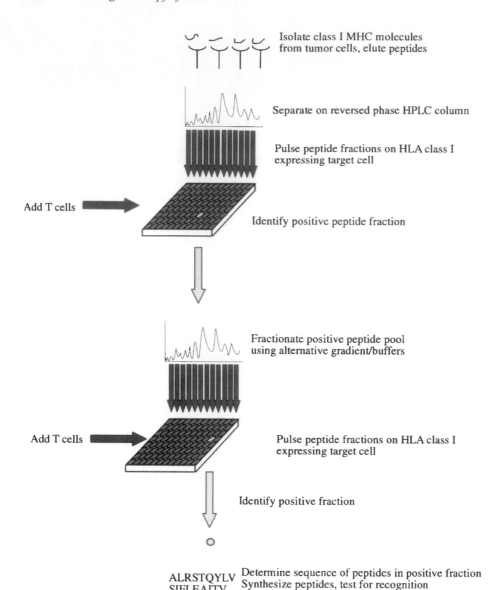

Isolate class I MHC molecules from tumor cells, elute peptides

Separate on reversed phase HPLC column

Pulse peptide fractions on HLA class I expressing target cell

Add T cells

Identify positive peptide fraction

Fractionate positive peptide pool using alternative gradient/buffers

Add T cells

Pulse peptide fractions on HLA class I expressing target cell

Identify positive fraction

ALRSTQYLV
SIFLEAITV
MLAVQSTRV

Determine sequence of peptides in positive fraction Synthesize peptides, test for recognition

FIGURE 2. Biochemical approach to the identification of tumor antigens. (HPLC, high-performance liquid chromatography; MHC, major histocompatibility complex.)

Identification of the T-cell epitopes from the MART-1 protein was initially carried out by synthesizing 23 peptides that were identified in this protein through the use of the HLA-A2–binding motif. The HLA-A2–expressing mutant cell line T2, which possesses a defect in antigen processing that facilitates the exogenous loading of high levels of peptides, was then pulsed individually with these peptides (7). In this study, ten out of ten MART-1 reactive TILs and the MART-1–reactive T-cell clone A42 reacted with target cells that had been pulsed with a single nonamer peptide, AAGIGILTV (MART-1:27–35), as well as decamer peptides that contain one additional amino acid at the amino (EAAGIGILTV) (MART-1:26–35) and carboxy (AAGIGILTVI) (MART-1:27–36) terminus of the MART-1:27–35 peptide. The A42 clone appeared to recognize targets pulsed at a minimum, with 1 nm of the MART-1:27–35 peptide, whereas 100 nm of the MART-1:26–35 peptide was required to sensitize targets for recognition by this T-cell clone. In contrast, TILs recognized targets pulsed with 1 nm of

either the MART-1:27–35 or the MART-1:26–35 peptides to a similar degree. This appears to represent a dominant T-cell epitope in HLA-A2 expressing in melanoma patients. In another study, 22 out of 30 HLA-A2–restricted TILs were found to recognize this peptide (8). Although it has been reported that HLA-A2–restricted, MART-1–reactive T cells recognize a partially overlapping peptide [ILTVILGVL (9)], the majority of MART-1–reactive T cells do not appear to react with this peptide [(10) and Y. Kawakami, personal communication, 1995]. Melanoma-reactive T cells have also been found to recognize two MART-1 peptides, AEEAAGIGILT and AEE-AAGIGIL, that partially overlap with the HLA-A2 peptide in the context of HLA-B45 (11).

A study has been carried out to examine the response of T cells generated from tumor-infiltrated lymph nodes (TILN) by stimulation with interleukin-2 (IL-2) to the MART-1:26–35 and MART-1:27–35 peptides, as well as several variants of these peptides (10). In contrast to previous results (7), targets pulsed

TABLE 1. DEFINED EPITOPES OF MELANOCYTE DIFFERENTIATION ANTIGENS

Gene	HLA Allele	Peptide Epitope	References
MART-1	A2	AAGIGILTV	7
MART-1	A2	EAAGIGILTV	7
MART-1	A2	AAGIGILTVA	7
MART-1	B45	AEEAAGIGILT	11
MART-1	B45	AEEAAGIGIL	11
gp100	A2	KTWGQYWQV	24
gp100	A2	ITDQVPFSV	24
gp100	A2	YLEPGPVTA	24
gp100	A2	LLDGTATLRL	24
gp100	A2	VLYRYGFSV	24
gp100	A2	RLMKQDFSV	28
gp100	A2	RLPRIFCSC	28
gp100	A3	SLIYRRRLMK	24
gp100	A3	ALLAVGATK	79
gp100	A24	VYFFLPDHL (intron)	30
gp100	Cw8	SNDGPTLI	31
Tyrosinase	A2	MLLAVLYCL	34
Tyrosinase	A2	YMDGTMSQV	34
Tyrosinase	A24	AFLPWHRLF	37
Tyrosinase	A1	KCDICTDEY	40
Tyrosinase	A1	SSDYVIPIGTY	28
TRP-1	A31	MSLQRQFLR	51
TRP-2	A31	LLPGGRPYR	61
TRP-2	A2	SVYDFFVWL	62
TRP-2	A68	EVISCKLIKR (intron)	65
TRP-2	Cw8	ANDPIFVVL	31
MC1R	A2	TILLGIFFL	66
MC1R	A2	FLALIICNA	66
MC1R	A2	AIIDPLIYA	66

with the MART-1:26–35 peptide were recognized at a five- to tenfold lower concentration than those pulsed with the MART-1:27–35 peptide. Several variants containing substitutions at positions 1, 2, or 3 of the MART-1:26–35 peptide with enhanced binding to HLA-A2 were also examined for their ability to be recognized by MART-1–reactive T cells. A variant containing a substitution of leucine for alanine at position 2 of the MART-1:26–35 peptide was recognized at a ten- to 1,000-fold lower concentration than the native peptide by T-cell clones as well as TILN, whereas more variable recognition of the other variants was observed. This peptide could also induce *in vitro* responses from the PBMC of melanoma patients more efficiently than the unmodified parental peptide. In another study, a peptide containing a substitution of alanine for the glutamic acid residue at position 1 of the MART-1:26–35 peptide was found to possess a higher affinity for HLA-A2, and was recognized more efficiently by eight out of ten MART-1–reactive CTL clones than was the unmodified peptide (12). This result was consistent with previous observations, indicating that the presence of a charged amino acid may be detrimental to the binding of peptides to HLA-A2 (13). In addition, a peptide containing a substitution of leucine for alanine at position 1 of the MART-1:27–35 nonamer peptide was significantly more efficient at generating tumor-reactive T cells *in vitro* than the parental MART-1:27–35 peptide (14).

Additional experiments to explore the immunogenicity of MART-1 peptide variants have been carried out in HLA-A2 transgenic mice (15). The mouse homologue of MART-1 is nearly identical to the human sequence, containing only a single substitution of isoleucine for threonine at position 34 of the human peptide. In agreement with the results of *in vitro* sensitizations that were carried out with human PBMC (12), the MART1:26–35 peptides containing substitutions of leucine for alanine at position 2 were significantly more immunogenic in HLA-A2 transgenic mice than the native MART-1 peptide. Moreover, the T cells generated with the modified peptide appeared to recognize melanoma cells expressing the naturally processed MART-1 epitope. These results provide additional support for the use of modified MART-1 peptides in clinical vaccine trials.

Responses to MART-1 appear to be immunodominant in HLA-A2 individuals, and responses can readily be elicited in HLA-A2+ normal, as well as melanoma patients. One possible explanation for these findings is that the MART-1 peptide represents an epitope mimic. In one study, evidence was obtained indicating that MART-1–reactive T cells reacted with peptides derived from a variety of sources, including viral proteins (16). Thus, T cells reactive with exogenous antigens, such as viral epitopes, may cross-react with the MART-1 epitope, thereby leading to the relatively high precursor frequency of T cells reactive with this epitope. Evidence has also been obtained suggesting that some self-antigens may serve as partial agonists or antagonists of MART-1–reactive T cells and thus may limit antitumor responses of these T cells (17).

Some data have indicated that T cells reactive with MART-1 may be present in individuals with vitiligo, an autoimmune disease that results from the destruction of normal skin melanocytes (18). In this study, T cells isolated from vitiligo patients were examined for their ability to recognize the MART-1 antigen using a class I MHC tetramer bound to the modified MART-1:26–35 peptide containing a substitution of leucine for alanine at position 2. The PBMC isolated from seven out of nine vitiligo patients appeared to contain between 0.1% and 0.5% of CD8+ T cells reactive with this peptide, whereas five out of six normal controls contained less than 0.05% MART-1–reactive CD8+ T cells. Many of the MART-1–reactive T cells obtained from vitiligo patients also expressed high levels of the skin-homing receptor cutaneous lymphocyte-associated antigen (CLA), a form of the P-selectin–binding glycoprotein 1 (19). A relatively high frequency of MART-1–reactive T cells was observed in one of the six normal HLA-A2+ individuals, but these cells did not appear to express CLA. These results suggest that expression of accessory molecules, such as the CLA homing receptor, may play a role in the maintenance of tolerance to normal tissue antigens.

gp100

The gene encoding a second melanocyte differentiation antigen, termed *Pmel17* or *gp100*, was initially isolated from melanocytes (20). Expression of this gene appeared to be correlated with melanin content, and subsequent studies demonstrated that gp100 is a melanosomal matrix protein that is directly involved with the synthesis of melanin (21). A number of monoclonal antibodies that are diagnostic for melanoma also have been shown to react

TABLE 2. RESPONSES OF HLA-A2 RESTRICTED TUMOR-INFILTRATING LYMPHOCYTES (TILS) TO EPITOPES FROM MART-1 AND GP100

Peptide	TIL Response												
	771	1,200	822	1,520	620	660	697	1,143	1,495	907	1,318	1,088	1,383
MART-1	−	−	−	−	++	++	++	++	++	++	++	++	+
G9-154	++	++	−	+	+	+	−	−	++	−	++	−	−
G9-209	++	−	+	++	++	−	+	−	−	−	−	++	−
G9-280	++	−	−	−	+	++	−	++	−	+	−	−	+
G10-457	−	+	−	−	−	−	−	−	−	−	−	−	−
G10-476	−	−	−	−	−	+	−	−	−	++	−	−	−
G9-619	−	−	−	−	−	−	−	−	−	−	−	−	+
G9-639	−	+	−	−	−	−	−	−	−	−	−	−	−

++, >500 pg/mL; +, 100–500 pg/mL; −, <100 pg/mL of interferon-γ secretion by TILs after stimulation with T2 cells that had been pulsed with the indicated peptides. From Kawakami Y, Dang N, Wang X, et al. Recognition of shared melanoma antigens in association with major HLA-A alleles by tumor infiltrating lymphocytes from 123 patients with melanoma. *J Immunother* (*in press*), with permission.

with gp100 (22). Screening a cDNA-expression library with a melanoma-reactive CTL also resulted in the isolation of a gene that was nearly identical to the previous gp100 isolates (23). Differential splicing and sequence polymorphisms appear to account for the differences between these sequences.

Identification of the T epitopes in gp100 was carried out by synthesizing 169 peptides from this protein that conformed to the HLA-A2 binding motif. The screening of candidate peptides from gp100 with four TILs resulted in the initial identification of three nonomer peptides, gp100:154–162, 209–217, and 280–288; and two decamer peptides, gp100:457–466 and 476–485 as peptide epitopes (24). Approximately 20% of HLA-A2–restricted, melanoma-reactive TILs reacted with each of the three peptide epitopes gp100:154–162, 209–217, and 280–288 (8) (Table 2). There appeared to be a significant correlation between the ability of TILs to recognize gp100 and patient responses to adoptive immunotherapy, whereas there was no significant correlation between MART-1 responses and patient responses to therapy. These observations indicate that gp100 may represent a significant tumor rejection antigen.

The gp100:280–288 peptide was also identified by testing HLA-A2–binding peptides that had been isolated from melanoma cells and fractionated by high-performance liquid chromatography. These peptides were tested for their ability to sensitize target cells for recognition by melanoma-reactive CTL lines that had been derived by stimulation of PBMC with autologous melanoma cells (25). Five out of the five lines that were tested in this study reacted with the gp100:280–288 peptide. It is not clear why, in contrast to the results obtained with TILs, responses to this epitope appeared to be so dominant. It is, however, possible that the source of cells plays a role in influencing the specificity of T cells.

Attempts were then made to enhance the immunogenicity of peptides from gp100 by substituting optimal for nonoptimal anchor residues. When the threonine at position 2 of the gp100:209–217 peptide was replaced with either a leucine or methionine residue, the HLA-A2–binding affinity was increased by a factor of 52 and nine, respectively (26). Tumor-reactive T cells could be elicited more reliably and after fewer *in vitro* stimulations when the modified peptide-containing methionine at position 2 (gp100:209–217 2M) was used than when the native

gp100:209–217 peptide was used. Clinical trials involving immunization with the gp100:209–217 2M peptide in Freund's incomplete adjuvant have demonstrated that this peptide is more immunogenic than the native peptide (27). In addition, patient response rate appeared to be increased when the modified peptide was administered in conjunction with IL-2.

Melanoma-reactive T cells have been shown to recognize additional gp100 epitopes. One peptide, gp100:619–627, has been found to be recognized by an HLA-A2–restricted CTL clone, but not bulk melanoma reactive HLA-A2–restricted TIL lines (28). This epitope contains the optimal anchor residues at positions 2 and 9, and this peptide has been shown to bind to HLA-A2 with a higher affinity than previously described gp100 epitopes (29). A second gp100 epitope, gp100:639–647, contains two cysteine residues, one at position 7 and one at the C-terminal anchor position (28). To explore the nature of the naturally processed epitopes, peptides were synthesized in which the cysteine residues were replaced with α-aminobutyric acid, an amino acid that contains a side chain similar in size to the cysteine side chain that cannot form disulfide bonds. Replacement of the cysteines at either position, individually, or at both positions with α-aminobutyric acid appeared to significantly enhance T-cell recognition, thus indicating that the formation of disulfide bonds, either with a second cysteine residue or another sulfhydryl compound, may inhibit binding of the peptide to class I. Although interactions with amino acids in the HLA-A2–binding pocket may prevent modification of cysteine residue side chains in this peptide, it is possible that cysteine residues present in the natural epitope may contain unknown modifications that interfere with disulfide bond formation.

The antigenic epitope recognized by an HLA-A24–restricted CTL clone has been found to be encoded by sequences within an intron of gp100 (30). The screening of a melanoma cDNA library with this T-cell clone resulted in the isolation of an insert that had retained a sequence corresponding to the fourth intron of the gp100 gene. Translation of this product in the normal gp100 open-reading frame resulted in the addition of 35 amino acids not found in the normal gp100 protein, which were followed by a stop codon, resulting in premature termination of translation. The T-cell epitope was encoded entirely within the intron region and conformed to the HLA-A24 consensus-binding motif. This appears to represent an aberrant transcript that is expressed at relatively low levels in melanomas. Expression of this product does not appear to be related to cellular transformation, however, because T cells that recognized this epitope also responded to an HLA-A24–expressing melanocyte cell line.

An epitope of gp100 that is recognized in the context of HLA-Cw8 has been identified (31). An octamer peptide, gp100:71–78, appeared to represent the optimal epitope, although significant recognition of nonamer and decamer peptides containing either one or two additional amino acids at the amino-terminal end of the octamer were also well recognized. This represented a predominant specificity in melanoma patient 15,392, because the majority of clones obtained from tumor-invaded lymph node cells that were isolated from this patient appeared to recognize this epitope. Additionally, this epitope appeared to be capable of rapidly generating tumor-reactive T cells using PBMC from this patient, although responses of additional HLA-Cw8–expressing patients were not examined in this report.

TYROSINASE

Tyrosinase represents a critical enzyme involved in the first steps of melanin synthesis. The gene encoding this product was first isolated in 1987 (32). Subsequently, two HLA-A2–restricted, melanoma-reactive T-cell clones were shown to recognize tyrosinase transfectants (33). These T-cell clones were found to recognize two distinct epitopes of tyrosinase, one beginning with the amino-terminal methionine of the tyrosinase signal sequence (MLLAVLYCL, tyr:1–9) and a second beginning with amino acid residue 368 (YMNGTMSQV, tyr:368–376) (34). The processed tyr:368–376 peptide that is expressed in association with HLA-A2 has been shown to be posttranslationally modified, containing a substitution of an aspartic acid for an asparagine residue at the third position (35). This modification, which was found at an asparagine residue that is part of an *N*-linked glycosylation site, may result from the activity of a mammalian enzyme that is responsible for the removal of *N*-linked oligosaccharide side chains from glycopeptides (36).

Additional studies have demonstrated T-cell recognition of tyrosinase in the context of the HLA-A24 (37,38), HLA-B44 (39), and HLA-A1 (40) class I restriction elements. Five out of six HLA-A1–restricted CTL lines isolated from melanoma patients appeared to recognize the tyrosinase nonamer KCDICTDEY and the overlapping dodecamer DAEKCDICTDEY (40). Modified peptides containing a substitution of either serine or alanine for cysteine at position 2 of the nonamer, as well as peptides containing these substitutions at the corresponding residue in the dodecamer, were recognized at concentrations that were 100- to 1,000-fold lower than the unmodified peptide. These results are similar to those found with the gp100:639–647 epitope, as discussed in the gp100 section. The status of the downstream cysteine residue was less clear, however, because some peptides containing modifications at this position were less stimulatory than the parental peptide.

A CD4+ melanoma-reactive TIL has been shown to recognize the nonmutated tyrosinase gene product after screening transfectants expressing candidate melanoma antigens (41) and two peptide epitopes of tyrosinase that are recognized in the context of HLA-DRB1*0401 have been identified (42). Although it is not clear what role class II–restricted T cells play in tumor regression, cytokine production in the tumor microenvironment by CD4+ cells may be involved in the activation of tumor-reactive CD8+ T cells. Some studies suggest that CD4+ T cells play an important role in activating antigen-presenting cells to facilitate efficient stimulation of naïve CD8+ T cells (43–45). The recruitment of inflammatory cells, such as neutrophils, by tumor-reactive CD4+ T cells may also play a role in tumor rejection (46).

TRP-1

The gp75 protein, which is recognized by immunoglobulin G antibodies in the serum of a patient with melanoma (47), represents one of the most abundant intracellular glycoproteins in melanocyte-lineage cells. The gene encoding gp75, *TRP-1*, was initially shown to represent the human homologue of the mouse brown-locus gene, a mouse-coat color gene (48). More recently, the gp75 protein has been found to possess DHI-2-carboxylic acid oxidase activity, demonstrating that this represents an enzyme involved in the synthesis of melanin (49).

Melanoma-reactive T cells have been shown to recognize an epitope of gp75 in the context of HLA-A31 (50). The gp75 epitope recognized by HLA-A31–restricted melanoma-reactive T cells was not encoded by the normal TRP-1 open reading frame (ORF). An alternative ORF consisting of only 24 amino acids and beginning at an AUG codon that is downstream from the normal TRP-1–initiation codon was found to encode the T-cell epitope recognized by this T cell (51). The amino terminus of the alternative ORF appeared to correspond with the amino terminus of the optimal T-cell epitope. This epitope also conformed to the HLA-A31 consensus motif that consists of a hydrophobic residue at position 2 and a positively charged residue at the carboxy terminus of the peptide.

A number of examples of T-cell epitopes that are encoded by alternative ORF have been described. A peptide derived from an alternative ORF of *NY-ESO-1*, a gene that encodes a cancer testis antigen, has been shown to be recognized by tumor-reactive T cells (52). Additionally, T-cell epitopes encoded by alternative ORF of a normal self-protein (53) and as a retroviral gene product (54) have been identified. These observations indicate that the translation of alternative ORF represents a general mechanism for generating T-cell epitopes.

Attempts have also been made to determine whether T-cell epitopes from TRP-1 and TRP-2 (described in the following section) that are recognized in the context of HLA-A31 are also recognized in the context of additional class I alleles. Both the TRP-1 and TRP-2 peptides were found to bind to HLA-A3, -A11, -A31, -A33, and -A68. T cells recognized the TRP-2 peptide in the context of HLA-A31 and -A33 (55). These HLA types appear to possess similar binding motifs and fit into what has been termed the *HLA-A3–like supertype* (56). Future studies should reveal whether it is possible to elicit response to these peptides in patients that express additional members of the HLA-A3 class I supertype.

Studies carried out in the B16 mouse melanoma tumor model have demonstrated that protective immunity can be generated by immunization with a vaccinia virus construct encoding mouse TRP-1 (57). The induction of protective immunity was found to be dependent on class II-restricted, but not class I-restricted, T cells. This protection may have resulted from the generation of antibodies directed against the TRP-1 protein. Alternatively, CD4+ T cells may recognize B16 antigens that are processed and presented by host antigen-presenting cells, resulting in the activation of nonspecific cells that mediate tumor destruction. In addition, immunization with this viral recombinant was found to induce vitiligo. A correlation between the development of vitiligo and responses to adoptive immunotherapy has been previously noted (58). This observation provides further evidence that responses directed against melanocyte differentiation antigens may be involved with tumor regression.

TRP-2

The TRP-2 gene product is approximately 40% identical at the amino acid level to *TRP-1*, and represents another melanosomal enzyme involved in the synthesis of melanin (59,60). The *TRP-2* gene was also found to encode an antigen that was recognized in the context of HLA-A31 (61). The T-cell epitope was encoded by the normal ORF of *TRP-2* and conformed to the consensus HLA-A31–binding motif. Results of one study also demonstrate T-cell recognition of a TRP-2 epitope in the context of HLA-Cw8 (31).

In an attempt to identify HLA-A2–restricted TRP-2 epitopes, peptides from this protein that fit the HLA-A2–binding motif were initially tested for binding to this class I molecule using a standard competitive inhibition assay (62). Twenty-one peptides were identified that inhibited the binding of a standard peptide at a concentration of 2 μM or below. These peptides were then used to carry out *in vitro* stimulations of peripheral blood lymphocytes from HLA-A2 melanoma patients. One of the peptides that was tested, SVYDFFVWL (TRP2:180–188), elicited CTL from patient peripheral blood lymphocytes that recognized T2 cells pulsed with this peptide as well as HLA-A2+ and TRP-2+ melanomas. The sequence of the human and corresponding mouse peptides are identical, and this peptide has been shown to represent an immunodominant epitope that is recognized by T cells reactive with the murine melanoma B16 in the context of H-2K^b (63,64). Adoptive transfer of CTL lines generated by stimulation with this peptide was shown to be effective at mediating the regression of established B16 lung metastases. In this model system, CTL lines that were generated using low concentrations of this peptide (10^{-9}M) were more efficient than CTL generated using a relatively high concentration (10^{-5}M) of peptide. Therapeutic strategies can therefore be evaluated in a mouse model system using the identical epitope recognized by human tumor-reactive T cells.

Melanoma-reactive T cells have also been shown to recognize an epitope that is encoded by a retained intron sequence from the *TRP-2* gene (65). The screening of an autologous melanoma cDNA library using an HLA-A68 restricted, melanoma-reactive T-cell clone resulted in the isolation of a partial cDNA clone containing the second intron of the *TRP-2* gene as well as a portion of the fourth intron of this gene. Extension of the normal *TRP-2* ORF through the region of the second intron resulted in the generation of a truncated protein of 227 amino acids, 39 of which are encoded by the intron sequence. The T-cell epitope was encoded entirely within the region derived from the second intron. Transcripts containing the second intron were either undetectable or were expressed at low levels in melanocytes, whereas this transcript was readily detected in melanomas that expressed TRP-2, as assessed by reverse transcriptase-polymerase chain reaction. As expected, T cells specific for the intron TRP-2 epitope failed to recognize melanocytes expressing HLA-A68. Previously, T cells that recognized a gp100 epitope encoded within the fourth intron of gp100 in the context of HLA-A24 had been found to react with melanoma cells and with normal melanocytes expressing this class I allele (30). Consistent with this observation, comparable levels of a gp100 gene transcript containing the fourth intron of this gene were found in melanocytes and melanomas (65). These findings indicate that epitopes derived from introns can represent both tumor-specific as well as normal-differentiation antigens and raise the question of whether these types of antigens differ in terms of their ability to generate therapeutic antitumor responses.

Some studies have also been carried out to evaluate the melanocortin-1 receptor (MC1R) as a candidate melanoma antigen (66). This protein, which is a member of a family of G-protein–coupled receptors that bind melanocyte-stimulating hormone, appears to be primarily expressed in cells of the melanocyte lineage. Peptides from MC1R that fit the HLA-A2–binding motif were synthesized and tested for their ability to bind to purified HLA-A2. When the 12 peptides with the highest affinities were tested for their ability to elicit CTL, three peptides were found to elicit peptide-specific T cells in the majority of normal donors tested. The CTL lines generated with each of the three peptides also appeared to recognize 8 out of 13 HLA-A2+, MC1R+ melanomas, and expression of the MC1R molecule correlated with recognition by specific T cells. These CTL lines failed to recognize melanomas that expressed only the HLA-A2 or MC1R molecules. This molecule thus represents another potential target for immunotherapy.

CLINICAL OBSERVATIONS

Several observations suggest that melanocyte-differentiation antigens may represent important tumor-regression antigens. Although TILs that induced tumor regression after adoptive transfer into autologous patients has been shown to recognize gp100 and MART-1, clinical responses to TIL therapy were significantly correlated with recognition of gp100 but not MART-1 in HLA-A2 patients (Table 3) (8). Vitiligo has also been observed in approximately 30% of the melanoma patients who responded to IL-2–based therapy in the Surgery Branch, National Cancer Institute, but was never seen in renal cancer patients after therapy (58). The destruction of normal skin mel-

TABLE 3. CORRELATION BETWEEN CLINICAL RESPONSE TO TUMOR-INFILTRATING LYMPHOCYTE (TIL) THERAPY AND ANTIGEN RESPONSIVENESS

Antigen Recognition	TILs																				
	771	1,200	822	620	660	697	1,143	1,495	907	1,088	1,318	1,383	1,104	1,074	1,235	1,287	1,363	1,381	1,399	1,138	1,374
	PR	PR	NR	PR	PR	PR	PR	PR	NR	NR	NR	PR	NR	NR	NR	NR	NR	NR	NR	PR	NR
gp100	++	++	+	++	++	+	++	++	++	++	++	+	–	–	–	–	–	–	–	–	–
MART-1	–	–	–	++	++	++	++	++	++	++	++	+	++	+	++	++	++	++	+	–	–
Tyrosinase	–	–	–	–	–	–	–	–	–	–	–	–	–	–	–	–	–	–	–	+	+
TRP-1	–	–	–	–	–	–	–	–	–	–	–	–	–	–	–	–	–	–	–	–	–
TRP-2	–	–	–	–	–	–	–	–	–	–	–	–	–	–	–	–	–	–	–	–	–

NR, no response; PR, partial response; ++, >500 pg/mL; +, >100 pg/mL but <500 pg/mL; –, <100 pg/mL of interferon-γ secretion in more than two experiments.
Note: Correlation between recognition of gp100 and clinical responses: $p = 0.024$ using Fisher's exact test. Correlation between recognition of MART-1 and clinical responses: $p = 0.611$.
From Kawakami Y, Dang N, Wang X, et al. Recognition of shared melanoma antigens in association with major HLA-A alleles by tumor infiltrating lymphocytes from 123 patients with melanoma. *J Immunother* (*in press*), with permission.

anocytes, which leads to the development of vitiligo, presumably results from the stimulation of T cells that recognize shared melanocyte-differentiation antigens, such as gp100, in these patients. The fact that clinical responses appear to correlate with the development of vitiligo suggests that immune responses to melanocyte-lineage antigens may play some role in the *in vivo* regression of tumors seen after treatment with immunotherapy.

Clinical trials are being carried out to evaluate the effect of immunization with specific peptides from these antigens and recombinant viral constructs encoding tumor antigens in combination with a variety of cytokines. The efficacy of immunization with modified peptides and the adoptive transfer of tumor-reactive T-cell clones are also being evaluated in patient clinical trials. The development of assays that facilitate the monitoring of patient responses represents an important aspect of these trials. Limiting dilution assays (67,68) and measurements of the ability of T cells to generate immune responses after *in vitro* stimulation have been used to monitor patient responses. The enzyme-linked immunospot assay has also been used to directly enumerate tumor-reactive T cells (69).

Complexes of class I MHC tetramers bound to specific peptides have been used for determining the frequency of peptide-specific T cells, in bulk populations of T cells, and for the direct isolation of antigen-reactive cells (70,71). The precursor frequency of T cells reactive with the MART-1:26–35 peptide has been estimated to be between 1 in 50 and 1 in 500 in tumor-infiltrated lymph nodes, whereas the frequency of T cells reactive with a peptide epitope from tyrosinase was below the limit of detection (<0.05%) (72). Another approach to monitoring involves the identification of T-cell receptors' subfamilies or clonotypes that are expressed by tumor-reactive T cells (73,74). Analysis of the expression of specific T-cell receptors in tumor sites and peripheral blood should allow monitoring of lymphocyte trafficking after immunization or adoptive transfer.

A number of peptides from MART-1, gp100, and tyrosinase are being evaluated in clinical trials. In one trial, the MART-1 peptide and two HLA-A2 binding tyrosinase peptides were administered intradermally in a soluble form to melanoma patients (75). Delayed-type hypersensitivity responses directed against the tyrosinase signal peptides were observed in some patients, but significant tumor regressions were not observed in this trial. The ability to induce tumor-reactive T cells after *in vitro* stimulation of PBMC with peptides appeared to be modestly enhanced after the immunization of HLA-A2 patients with the MART-1 and gp100:209–217 peptides in Freund's incomplete adjuvant (76,77). Significant clinical responses, however, were only observed in small numbers of patients in these trials.

The modified gp100:209–217 2M peptide has been used to immunize HLA-A2 melanoma patients in one phase 1 clinical trial (27). The responses of PBMC from 10 out of 11 immunized patients after one *in vitro* stimulation with the gp100:209–217 2M peptide were significantly enhanced by this immunization protocol. The precursor frequency of T cells reactive with the gp100:209–217 peptide was estimated to be between 1 in 3,000 and 1 in 6,000 in immunized patients, whereas the preimmunization frequency of peptide-reactive T cells was estimated to be less than 1 in 30,000. Analysis of the responses of an additional 19 patients that were immunized with the gp100:209–217 2M peptide, along with high-dose IL-2, indicated that only 3 out of the 19 patients treated with this regimen developed enhanced-peptide reactivity. Although none of the patients that had received the gp100:209–217 2M peptide alone in adjuvant demonstrated a clinical response, 8 of the 19 patients treated with the gp100:209–217 2M peptide plus IL-2 demonstrated objective cancer regressions. This represents a higher response rate than was seen in previous clinical trials carried out with IL-2 alone, which ranged between 15% and 20%.

It is not clear why decreased peptide reactivity was observed in patients that were treated with the combination of the gp100:209–217 2M plus IL-2. Patients that had been initially immunized with peptide plus IL-2 responded when subsequent immunizations were carried out with peptide alone, indicating that the IL-2 did not lead to a general inability to detect memory T cells. The diminished responses did not simply result from enhanced migration of T cells from the peripheral blood to lymph nodes or other tissues following the administration of IL-2, because patients that had first been immunized with peptide alone appeared to develop reactivity after immunization with the peptide plus IL-2.

Clinical trials have also been carried out with recombinant viral vaccines that encode melanoma antigens. Only a small number of patients that had been immunized with adenoviral or vaccinia, constructs encoding gp100, and MART-1 demonstrated clinical responses. *In vitro* responses to these antigens were not enhanced in immunized patients. One possible explanation for these findings is the observation that high titers of neutralizing antibodies directed against these viruses, presumably resulting from smallpox vaccination and environmental exposure to adenovirus, may have had a negative impact on these responses (78).

These studies have provided the basis for a number of ongoing as well as future clinical trials. One clinical trial that has been initiated in the Surgery Branch of the National Cancer Institute involves the immunization of melanoma patients with peptides derived from MART-1, tyrosinase, and gp100 in an attempt to prevent the recurrence of tumors that have lost the expression of one of these antigens. Recombinant viral constructs have now been generated that encode gp100 epitopes that have been modified to enhance their immunogenicity, as described above, either in the context of full-length genes or as minigenes. Another strategy that is now being evaluated in clinical trials is the adoptive transfer of highly reactive, melanoma-specific T-cell clones. The identification of additional shared antigens recognized by CD4+ tumor-reactive T cells may also lead to the development of peptide and protein vaccines that can be utilized as immunogens either alone or in combination with class I antigens. Hopefully, some of these approaches, used either alone or in combination, may lead to the development of cancer vaccines that result in long-term cures in the majority of patients.

REFERENCES

1. Rammensee HG, Friede T, Stevanoviic S. MHC ligands and peptide motifs: first listing. *Immunogenetics* 1995;41:178–228.
2. Parker KC, Shields M, DiBrino M, Brooks A, Coligan JE. Peptide binding to MHC class I molecules: implications for antigenic peptide prediction. *Immunol Res* 1995;14:34–57.
3. Anichini A, Maccalli C, Mortarini R, et al. Melanoma cells and normal melanocytes share antigens recognized by HLA-A2 restricted cytotoxic T cell clones from melanoma patients. *J Exp Med* 1993;177:989–998.
4. Kawakami Y, Eliyahu S, Delgado CH, et al. Cloning of the gene coding for a shared human melanoma antigen recognized by autologous T cells infiltrating into tumor. *Proc Natl Acad Sci U S A* 1994;91:3515–3519.
5. Coulie PG, Brichard V, Van Pel A, et al. A new gene coding for a differentiation antigen recognized by autologous cytolytic T lymphocytes on HLA-A2 melanomas. *J Exp Med* 1994;180:35–42.
6. Kawakami Y, Battles JK, Kobayashi T, et al. Production of recombinant MART-1 proteins and specific antiMART-1 polyclonal and monoclonal antibodies: use in the characterization of the human melanoma antigen MART-1. *J Immunol Methods* 1997;202:13–25.
7. Kawakami Y, Eliyahu S, Sakaguchi K, et al. Identification of the immunodominant peptides of the MART-1 human melanoma antigen recognized by the majority of HLA-A2 restricted tumor infiltrating lymphocytes. *J Exp Med* 1994;180:347–352.
8. Kawakami Y, Dang N, Wang X, et al. Recognition of shared melanoma antigens in association with major HLA-A alleles by tumor infiltrating lymphocytes from 123 patients with melanoma. *J Immunother* (in press).
9. Castelli C, Storkus WJ, Maeurer MJ, et al. Mass spectrometric identification of a naturally processed melanoma peptide recognized by CD8+ cytotoxic T lymphocytes. *J Exp Med* 1995;181:363–368.
10. Valmori D, Fonteneau JF, Lizana CM, et al. Enhanced generation of specific tumor-reactive CTL in vitro by selected Melan-A/MART-1 immunodominant peptide analogues. *J Immunol* 1998;160:1750–1758.
11. Schneider J, Brichard V, Boon T, Meyer zum Buschenfelde KH, Wolfel T. Overlapping peptides of melanocyte differentiation antigen Melan-A/MART-1 recognized by autologous cytolytic T lymphocytes in association with HLA-B45.1 and HLA-A2. *Int J Cancer* 1998;75:451–458.
12. Valmori D, Gervois N, Rimoldi D, et al. Diversity of the fine specificity displayed by HLA-A*0201-restricted CTL specific for the immunodominant Melan-A/MART-1 antigenic peptide. *J Immunol* 1998;161:6956–6962.
13. Ruppert J, Sidney J, Celis E, Kubo RT, Grey HM, Sette A. Prominent role of secondary anchor residues in peptide binding to HLA-A2. 1 molecules. *Cell* 1993;74:929–937.
14. Rivoltini L, Squarcina P, Loftus DJ, et al. A superagonist variant of peptide MART 1/Melan A27-35 elicits anti-melanoma CD8+ T cells with enhanced functional characteristics: implication for more effective immunotherapy. *Cancer Res* 1999;59:301–306.
15. Men Y, Miconnet L, Valmori D, Rimoldi D, Cerottini JC, Romero P. Assessment of immunogenicity of human melan-A peptide analogues in HLA-A*0201/Kb transgenic mice. *J Immunol* 1999;162:3566–3573.
16. Loftus DJ, Castelli C, Clay TM, et al. Identification of epitope mimics recognized by CTL reactive to the melanoma/melanocyte-derived peptide MART-1(27-35). *J Exp Med* 1996;184:647–657.
17. Loftus DJ, Squarcina P, Nielsen MB, et al. Peptides derived from self-proteins as partial agonists and antagonists of human CD8+ T-cell clones reactive to melanoma/melanocyte epitope MART 1(27-35). *Cancer Res* 1998;58:2433–2439.
18. Ogg GS, Rod Dunbar P, Romero P, Chen JL, Cerundolo V. High frequency of skin-homing melanocyte-specific cytotoxic T lymphocytes in autoimmune vitiligo. *J Exp Med* 1998;188:1203–1208.
19. Fuhibrigge RC, Kieffer JD, Armerding D, Kupper TS. Cutaneous lymphocyte antigen is a specialized form of PSGL-1 expressed on skin-homing T cells. *Nature* 1997;389:978–981.
20. Kwon BS, Chintamaneni C, Kozak CA, et al. A melanocyte-specific gene, Pmel 17, maps near the silver coat color locus on mouse chromosome 10 and is in a syntenic region on human chromosome 12. *Proc Natl Acad Sci U S A* 1991;88:9228–9232.
21. Lee ZH, Hou L, Moellmann G, et al. Characterization and subcellular localization of human Pmel 17/silver, a 110-kDa (pre)melanosomal membrane protein associated with 5,6-dihydroxyindole-2-carboxylic acid (DHICA) converting activity. *J Invest Dermatol* 1996;106:605–610.
22. Adema GJ, de Boer AJ, van't Hullenaar R, et al. Melanocyte lineage specific antigens recognized by monoclonal antibodies NKI-beteb, HMB-50, and HMB-45 are encoded by a single cDNA. *Am J Pathol* 1993;143:1579–1585.
23. Kawakami Y, Eliyahu S, Delgado CH, et al. Identification of a human melanoma antigen recognized by tumor infiltrating lymphocytes associated with in vivo tumor rejection. *Proc Natl Acad Sci U S A* 1994;91:6458–6462.
24. Kawakami Y, Eliyahu S, Jennings C, et al. Recognition of multiple epitopes in the human melanoma antigen gp100 associated with in vivo tumor regression. *J Immunol* 1995;154:3961–3968.
25. Cox AL, Skipper J, Chen Y, et al. Identification of a peptide recognized by five melanoma-specific human cytotoxic T cell lines. *Science* 1994;264:716–719.

26. Parkhurst MR, Salgaller M, Southwood S, et al. Improved induction of melanoma reactive CTL with peptides from the melanoma antigen gp100 modified at HLA-A0201 binding residues. *J Immunol* 1996;157:2539–2548.

27. Rosenberg SA, Yang JC, Schwartzentruber DJ, et al. Immunologic and therapeutic evaluation of a synthetic peptide vaccine for the treatment of patients with metastatic melanoma [see comments]. *Nat Med* 1998;4:321–327.

28. Kawakami Y, Robbins PF, Wang X, et al. Identification of new melanoma epitopes on melanosomal proteins recognized by tumor infiltrating lymphocytes restricted by HLA-Al, -A2 and -A3 alleles. *J Immunol* 1998;161:6985–6992.

29. Tsai V, Southwood S, Sidney J, et al. Identification of subdominant CTL epitopes of the GP 100 melanoma-associated tumor antigen by primary *in vitro* immunization with peptide-pulsed dendritic cells. *J Immunol* 1997;158:1796–1802.

30. Robbins PF, El-Gamil M, Li YF, Fitzgerald EB, Kawakami Y, Rosenberg SA. The intronic region of an incompletely spliced gp100 gene transcript encodes an epitope recognized by melanoma-reactive tumor-infiltrating lymphocytes. *J Immunol* 1997;159:303–308.

31. Castelli C, Tarsini P, Mazzocchi A, et al. Novel HLA-Cw8-restricted T cell epitopes derived from tyrosinase-related protein-2 and gp100 melanoma antigens [In Process Citation]. *J Immunol* 1999;162:1739–1748.

32. Kwon BS, Haq AK, Pomerantz SH, Halaban R. Isolation and sequence of a cDNA clone for human tyrosinase that maps at the mouse c-albino locus. *Proc Natl Acad Sci U S A* 1987;84:7473–7477.

33. Brichard V, Van Pel A, Wolfel T, et al. The tyrosinase gene codes for an antigen recognized by autologous cytolytic T lymphocytes on HLA-A2 melanomas. *J Exp Med* 1993;178:489–495.

34. Wolfel T, Van Pel A, Brichard V, et al. Two tyrosinase nonapeptides recognized on HLA-A2 melanomas by autologous cytolytic T lymphocytes. *Eur J Immunol* 1994;24:759–764.

35. Skipper JC, Hendrickson RC, Gulden PH, et al. An HLA-A2-restricted tyrosinase antigen on melanoma cells results from post-translational modification and suggests a novel pathway for processing of membrane proteins. *J Exp Med* 1996;183:527–534.

36. Suzuki T, Seko A, Kitajima K, Inoue Y, Inoue S. Identification of peptide: N-glycanase activity in mammalian-derived cultured cells. *Biochem Biophys Res Commun* 1993;194:1124–1130.

37. Kang XQ, Kawakami Y, Sakaguchi K, El-Gamil M, et al. Identification of a tyrosinase epitope recognized by HLA-A24 restricted tumor-infiltrating lymphocytes. *J Immunol* 1995;155:1343–1348.

38. Robbins PF, El-Gamil M, Kawakami Y, Stevens E, Yannelli J, Rosenberg SA. Recognition of tyrosinase by tumor infiltrating lymphocytes from a patient responding to immunotherapy. *Cancer Res* 1994;54:3124–3126.

39. Brichard VG, Herman J, Van Pel A, Wildmann C, Gaugler B, Wolfel T, Boon T, Lethe B. A tyrosinase nonapeptide presented by HLA-B44 is recognized on a human melanoma by autologous cytolytic T lymphocytes. *Eur J Immunol* 1996;26:224–230.

40. Kittlesen DJ, Thompson LW, Gulden PH, et al. Human melanoma patients recognize an HLA-A1-restricted CTL epitope from tyrosinase containing two cysteine residues: implications for tumor vaccine development. *J Immunol* 1998;160:2099–2106.

41. Topalian SL, Rivoltini L, Mancini M, et al. Human CD4+ T cells specifically recognize a shared melanoma-associated antigen encoded by the tyrosinase gene. *Proc Natl Acad Sci U S A* 1994;91: 9461–9465.

42. Topalian SL, Gonzales MI, Parkhurst M, et al. Melanoma-specific CD4+ T cells recognize nonmutated HLA-DR-restricted tyrosinase epitopes. *J Exp Med* 1996;183:1965–1971.

43. Schoenberger SP, Toes RE, van der Voort EL, Offringa R, Melief CJ. T-cell help for cytotoxic T lymphocytes is mediated by CD40-CD40L interactions. *Nature* 1998;393:413–414.

44. Bennett SR, Carbone FR, Karamalis F, Miller JF, Heath WR. Induction of a CD8+ cytotoxic T lymphocyte response by cross-priming requires cognate CD4+ T cell help. *J Exp Med* 1997;186:65–70.

45. Bennett SR, Carbone FR, Karamalis F, Flavell RA, Miller JF, Heath WR. Help for cytotoxic-T-cell responses is mediated by Cd40 signaling. *Nature* 1998;393:478–480.

46. Cavallo F, Giovarelli M, Gulino A, et al. Role of neutrophils and CD4+ T lymphocytes in the primary and memory response to nonimmunogenic murine mammary adenocarcinoma made immunogenic by IL-2 gene. *J Immunol* 1992;149:3627–3635.

47. Mattes MJ, Thomson TM, Old LJ, Lloyd KO. A pigmentation-associated, differentiation antigen of human melanoma defined by a precipitating antibody in human serum. *Int J Cancer* 1983;32:717–721.

48. Vijayasyradhi S, Bouchard BB, Houghton AN. The melanoma antigen gp75 is the human homologue of mouse b (brown) locus gene. *J Exp Med* 1990;171:1375–1380.

49. Jimenez-Cervantes C, Solano F, Kobayashi T, et al. A new enzymatic function in the melanogenic pathway. *J Biol Chem* 1994;269:17993–18001.

50. Wang R-F, Robbins PF, Kawakami Y, Kang X-Q, Rosenberg SA. Identification of a gene encoding a melanoma tumor antigen recognized by HLA-A31-restricted tumor-infiltrating lymphocytes. *J Exp Med* 1995;181:799–804.

51. Wang RF, Parkhurst MR, Kawakami Y, Robbins PF, Rosenberg SA. Utilization of an alternative open reading frame of a normal gene in generating a novel human cancer antigen. *J Exp Med* 1996;183: 1131–1140.

52. Wang R-F, Johnston SL, Zeng G, Topalian SL, Schwartzentruber DJ, Rosenberg SA. A breast and melanoma-shared tumor antigen: T cell responses to antigenic peptides translated from different open reading frames. *J Immunol* 1998;161:3596–3606.

53. Malarkannan S, Afkarian M, Shastri N. A rare cryptic translation product is presented by Kb major histocompatibility complex class I molecule to alloreactive T cells. *J Exp Med* 1995;182:1739–1750.

54. Mayrand SM, Schwarz DA, Green WR. An alternative translational reading frame encodes an immunodominant retroviral CTL determinant expressed by an immunodeficiency-causing retrovirus. *J Immunol* 1998;160:39–50.

55. Wang RF, Johnston SL, Southwood S, Sette A, Rosenberg SA. Recognition of an antigenic peptide derived from tyrosinase-related protein-2 by CTL in the context of HLA-A31 and -A33. *J Immunol* 1998;160:890–897.

56. Sidney J, Grey HM, Southwood S, et al. Definition of an HLA-A3-like supermotif demonstrates the overlapping peptide-binding repertoires of common HLA molecules. *Hum Immunol* 1996;45:79–93.

57. Overwijk WW, Lee DS, Surman DR, et al. Vaccination with a recombinant vaccinia virus encoding a "self" antigen induces autoimmune vitiligo and tumor cell destruction in mice: requirement for CD4(+) T lymphocytes. *Proc Natl Acad Sci U S A* 1999;96:2982–2987.

58. Rosenberg SA, White DE. Vitiligo in patients with melanoma: normal tissue antigens can be target for cancer immunotherapy. *J Immunother* 1996;19:81–84.

59. Tsukamoto K, Jackson IJ, Urabe K, Montague PM, Hearing VJ. A second tyrosinase-related protein, TRP-2, is a melanogenic enzyme termed DOPAchrome tautomerase. *Embo J* 1992;11:519–526.

60. Yokoyama K, Suzuki H, Yasumoto K, Tomita Y, Shibahara S. Molecular cloning and functional analysis of a cDNA coding for human DOPAchrome tautomerase/tyrosinase-related protein 2. *Biochem Biophys Acta* 1994;1217:317–321.

61. Wang RF, Appella E, Kawakami Y, Kang X, Rosenberg SA. Identification of TRP-2 as a human tumor antigen recognized by cytotoxic T lymphocytes. *J Exp Med* 1996;184:2207–2216.

62. Parkhurst MR, Fitzgerald EB, Southwood S, Sette A, Rosenberg SA, Kawakami Y. Identification of a shared HLA-A*0201 restricted T cell epitope from the melanoma antigen tyrosinase related protein 2 (TRP-2). *Cancer Res* 1998;58: 4895–4901.

63. Bloom MB, Perry-Lalley D, Robbins PF, et al. Identification of tyrosinase-related protein 2 as a tumor rejection antigen for the B16 melanoma. *J Exp Med* 1997;185:453–459.

64. Zeh HJ III, Perry-Lalley D, Dudley ME, Rosenberg SA, Yang JC. High avidity CTLs for two self-antigens demonstrate superior *in vitro* and *in vivo* antitumor efficacy. *J Immunol* 1999;162:989–994.

65. Lupetti R, Pisarra P, Verrecchia A, et al. Translation of a retained intron in tyrosinase-related protein (TRP) 2 mRNA generates a new cytotoxic T lymphocyte (CTL)-defined and shared human melanoma antigen not expressed in normal cells of the melanocytic lineage. *J Exp Med* 1998;188:1005–1016.

66. Salazar-Onfray F, Nakazawa T, Chhajlani V, et al. Synthetic peptides derived from the melanocyte-stimulating hormone receptor MC1R can stimulate HLA-A2-restricted cytotoxic T lymphocytes that recognize naturally processed peptides on human melanoma cells. *Cancer Res* 1997;57:4348–4355.

67. Coulie PG, Somville M, Lehmann F, et al. Precursor frequency analysis of human cytolytic T lymphocytes directed against autologous melanoma cells. *Int J Cancer* 1992;50:289–297.

68. Mazzocchi A, Belli F, Mascheroni L, Vegetti C, Parmiani G, Anichini A. Frequency of cytotoxic T lymphocyte precursors (CTLp) interacting with autologous tumor via the T-cell receptor: limiting dilution analysis of specific CTLp in peripheral blood and tumor-invaded lymph nodes of melanoma patients. *Int J Cancer* 1994;58:330–339.

69. Scheibenbogen C, Lee KH, Stevanovic S, et al. Analysis of the T cell response to tumor and viral peptide antigens by an IFNgamma-ELISPOT assay. *Int J Cancer* 1997;71:932–936.

70. Altman JD, Moss PAH, Goulder PJR, et al. Phenotypic analysis of antigen-specific T lymphocytes. *Science* 1996;274:94–96.

71. Dunbar PR, Ogg GS, Chen J, Rust N, van der Bruggen P, Cerundolo V. Direct isolation, phenotyping and cloning of low-frequency antigen-specific cytotoxic T lymphocytes from peripheral blood. *Curr Biol* 1998;8:413–416.

72. Romero P, Dunbar PR, Valmori D, et al. *Ex vivo* staining of metastatic lymph nodes by class I major histocompatibility complex tetramers reveals high numbers of antigen-experienced tumor-specific cytolytic T lymphocytes. *J Exp Med* 1998;188:1641–1650.

73. Sensi M, Farina C, Maccalli C, Anichini A, Berd D, Parmiani G. Intralesional selection of T cell clonotypes in the immune response to melanoma antigens occurring during vaccination. *J Immunother* 1998;21:198–204.

74. McKee MD, Clay TM, Rosenberg SA, Nishimura MI. Quantitation of T-cell receptor frequencies by competitive PCR: generation and evaluation of novel TCR subfamily and clone specific competitors. *J Immunother* 1999;22:93–102.

75. Jaeger E, Bernhard H, Romero P, et al. Generation of cytotoxic T-cell responses with synthetic melanoma-associated peptides *in vivo*: implications for tumor vaccines with melanoma-associated antigens. *Int J Cancer* 1996;66:162–169.

76. Salgaller ML, Marincola FM, Cormier JN, Rosenberg SA. Immunization against epitopes in the human melanoma antigen gp100 following patient immunization with synthetic peptides. *Cancer Res* 1996;56:4749–4757.

77. Cormier JN, Salgaller ML, Prevette T, et al. Enhancement of cellular immunity in melanoma patients immunized with a peptide from MART-1/Melan A [see comments]. *Cancer J Sci Am* 1997;3:37–44.

78. Rosenberg SA, Zhai Y, Yang JC, et al. Immunizing patients with metastatic melanoma using recombinant adenoviruses encoding MART-1 or gp100 melanoma antigens. *J Natl Cancer Inst* 1998;90:1894–1900.

79. Skipper JC, Kittlesen DJ, Hendrickson RC, et al. Shared epitopes for HLA-A3-restricted melanoma-reactive human CTL include a naturally processed epitope from Pmel-17/gp100. *J Immunol* 1996;157:5027–5033.

16.3

CANCER VACCINES: CANCER ANTIGENS

Viral Antigens

SJOERD H. VAN DER BURG
RIENK OFFRINGA
CORNELIS J. M. MELIEF

Viruses are recognized as a major etiologic factor in human cancer. Estimates of the frequency of virus-induced cancer worldwide as a proportion of all cancers are in the order of 15% to 20% (1,2). The tumor viruses involved in human cancers are Epstein-Barr virus (EBV), human T-cell lymphotropic virus type I (HTLV-I), human herpesvirus type 8 (HHV-8), hepatitis B and C viruses (HBV and HCV, respectively) and human papillomavirus (HPV) types 16 and 18 (and other less prevalent oncogenic-HPV types). The pathways by which these tumor viruses induce cancer are often long and characterized by pre-malignant stages. Malignant transformation by these viruses involves the expression of at least some viral genes in the premalignant lesions and in the ultimate cancers, providing target antigens for the immune system.

Immunocompromised individuals, such as transplant patients and human immunodeficiency virus 1 (HIV-1)–infected subjects display an increased risk to most types of virus-induced cancer (3,4). This indicates that the host immune response plays an important role in the prevention of virus-induced cancers. To persistently infect human cells and induce transformation, some viruses interfere with cell-cycle control or prevent or delay apoptosis, whereas others have coevolved with the host's immune system and developed ways to slow down host defenses or even hide themselves from it.

To treat or prevent the outgrowth of these virus-associated tumors by immunotherapy (e.g., by adoptive cell therapy or by prophylactic or therapeutic vaccination) one has to consider the following four questions:

1. Which cells are primarily infected?
2. Which antigens are expressed during different stages of viral infection or tumorigenesis?
3. Which types of immune response play a role in the normal defense against these viruses?
4. How does the virus or the arising tumor evade the immune response?

This chapter globally describes the human tumor viruses, the immune response against them, and the evasive actions of these viruses. HPV is dealt with in somewhat more detail as an example of a human tumor virus. We describe the kinetics of HPV infection and pinpoint the HPV-derived specific antigens that might be suitable targets for immunoprophylaxis and T-cell immunotherapy at different disease stages.

IMMUNITY AGAINST TUMOR VIRUSES AND THEIR SUBSEQUENT EVASIVE ACTIONS

The viral life cycle, the host immune response to the virus, and other host factors together determine the natural outcome of infection with oncogenic viruses. Ideally, the increased knowledge of the natural history of infection with these viruses, the viral antigens that are expressed at each stage of disease, and the immune response against them should allow the development of prophylactic vaccines providing long-lasting immunity or therapeutic vaccines to treat minimal residual disease. We broadly review the human tumor viruses and then focus on vaccination against HPV-16 as a detailed example for the other tumor viruses.

Epstein-Barr Virus

More than 95% of the world's population are infected with EBV. Primary infection occurs through the throat where the virus replicates in the epithelial cells and infects circulating B cells. Productive infection by EBV involves the expression of more than 80 virus lytic-cycle genes and formation of infectious virus particles in the epithelium of the throat. EBV infection of the epithelium is characterized by lack of an inflammatory response, which can, in part, be explained by the production of the viral homologue of human interleukin-10 (IL-10) (5) that inhibits full deployment of a type 1 T-cell response and decreases the magnitude of CD8 cytolytic T lymphocyte (CTL) responses generated by limiting the production of IL-2 and interferon-γ (IFN-γ). When EBV is transmitted to B cells, the virus enters a latent stage in which a limited set of latency-associated genes is expressed.

After infection, the virus persists for the lifetime of the infected individual, and it rarely causes disease in the immunocompetent host. Detailed studies on the immune response to EBV have firmly established that EBV-infected B-cell growth is under control of CTL-recognizing peptide epitopes in the latent proteins Epstein Barr (virus) nuclear antigen 2-6 (EBNA2-6), latent membrane protein-1, and latent membrane protein-2a (6–8). Furthermore, CD4+ T-helper (Th) cells specific for the major envelope protein gp340 as well as EBNA2-specific CD4+ major histocompatibility complex (MHC) class-II–restricted CTL have been described (9). EBV-infected cells evade the immune response by controlling the expression of latency-associated genes (10) and thus the available targets for T-cell recognition.

In immunocompromised individuals, expression of all nuclear- and late-membrane proteins is found in EBV-infected B cells (Table 1). Due to the loss of immunologic control of viral infection, these patients are often faced with immunoblastic lymphoma. However, the broad expression of EBV proteins makes it possible to treat, for example, immunodeficient patients after bone-marrow transplantation with adoptive transfer of donor-derived virus-specific T cells (10,11). In contrast, EBV-associated Hodgkin's lymphoma (HL), nasopharyngeal carcinoma, and Burkitt's lymphoma (BL) are found in patients with an intact immune system. The first two cancers express a restricted number of antigens (see Table 1). It is difficult to explain how HL and nasopharyngeal carcinoma escape from immunosurveillance, but downregulation of surface HLA class I, as noted in HL, might facilitate escape from virus-specific CTL (10). Furthermore, local inhibitory factors might play a role (12). BL cells are poorly immunogenic, the likely result of exclusive EBNA-1 protein expression. This protein is needed to maintain the virus episome in dividing cells (13). *In vivo*, the EBNA-1 protein does not elicit CTL responses. EBNA-1 consists of an N-terminal part that is followed by a polymorphic Gly-Ala co-repeat unit and a conserved C-terminal region. This Gly-Ala repeat-unit blocks processing of the protein by the proteasome and thus presentation of EBNA-1 peptides at the cell surface and subsequent recognition of the peptides by CTL (14). Recognition of EBNA-1–derived peptides potentially generated by proteolytic enzymes other than the proteasome is further impaired by defects that have been found in the transporter-associated proteins (TAPs) (15) or allele-specific downregulation of HLA–class-I molecules (16). In addition, the cell surface of BL cells expresses no adhesion molecules (17).

The EBV-derived protein expression in immunoblastic lymphoma, HL, and nasopharyngeal carcinoma leads to the conclusion that these diseases might be treated by the use of EBV-specific, CD8+ or CD4+ T cells, or both, directed at the available antigens. Treatment of disease might be achieved by adoptive transfer of T cells or therapeutic vaccination aimed at the activation of EBV-specific T cells. T-cell based immunotherapy for the treatment of BL seems not feasible.

Human T-Cell Lymphotropic Virus Type I

HTLV-I is a retrovirus and the etiologic agent of adult T-cell leukemia (ATL), a condition in which the CD4+ T cells are

TABLE 1. ANTIGEN EXPRESSION AND IMMUNITY AGAINST TUMOR-ASSOCIATED VIRUSES

Virus	Disease	Antigen Expression	T-Cell Reactivity/Immune Evasion
EBV	Burkitt's lymphoma	EBNA-1	No gly-ala repeat at N-terminus of protein prohibits antigen processing by proteasome. Lack of costimulatory molecules at surface infected cells. TAP defects inhibit transport of peptides to ER and subsequent expression at cell surface. HLA class I downregulation.
	Hodgkin's lymphoma Nasopharyngeal carcinoma T-cell lymphoma	EBNA-1 LMP-1, LMP-2a, LMP-2b	CTL activity toward LMP1 and LMP2a and LMP2b. Possible escape due to local expression of inhibitory factors and/or HLA class I downregulation.
	Immunoblastic lymphoma in immunocompromised individuals	EBNA-1, 2, 3 EBNA leader protein LMP1, LMP2a, LMP2b	All proteins (except EBNA-1) provide target epitopes for CTL.
HTLV-1	Adult T-cell leukemia	Gag, envelope, reverse-transcriptase, integrase, protease, tax, rex	CTL activity against envelope, gag and tax has been found. Other proteins probably provide T-cell epitopes as is noted for HIV-1. Latent infection and mutation of T-cell epitopes provide temporary escape. TGF-β production by ATL inhibits induction of CTL response. Infection of CD4+ T cells results in loss of T-helper cell function.
HHV-8	Kaposi's sarcoma Primary effusion lymphoma	HHV-8 shows sequence similarity to two other oncogenic γ-herpes viruses: Herpesvirus of Saimiri and EBV; similarly early and late antigens will probably be expressed.	No T-cell antigens have been identified yet. The mechanisms of how HHV-8 infected cells evade host immune responses are not yet known.
HBV	Hepatocellular carcinoma in HBsAg positive patients	Pre-S, HBsAg, HBeAg, HBcAg, HBxAg, polymerase	CTL have been found against epitopes in the surface, core, and polymerase antigens. T-helper cells strongly reacted against the core antigens (HBe and HBc) in patients with acute hepatitis.
	Hepatocellular carcinoma in HBsAg-negative patients	HBxAg (HBeAg and HBcAg are deleted in numerous tumors)	Deletion or mutation of T-cell epitopes weakens the response, allowing *HBV* virus– or HBV-containing tumors to persist.
HCV	Hepatocellular carcinoma	Core, envelope 1, and envelope 2, nonstructural proteins: NS2, NS3, NS4, and NS5	CTL and T-helper cells react to all proteins.
HPV	Cervical intraepithelial neoplasia	E1, E2, E4, E5, E6, E7, L1, and L2	CTLs have been found to react against E2 and E7. T-helper cells have been found against E7. Tumor escape by HLA class I and/or TAP downregulation.
	Cervical carcinoma	E6 and E7	Possible escape by E7-mediated impairment of IFN-γ response.

ATL, adult T-cell leukemia; CTL, cytolytic T lymphocyte; EBNA, Epstein Barr (virus) nuclear antigen; EBV, Epstein-Barr virus; ER, endoplasmic reticulum; HBcAg, hepatitis B core antigen; HBeAg, hepatitis B early antigen; HBsAg, hepatitis B surface antigen; HBxAg, hepatitis B X antigen; HBV, hepatitis B virus; HCV, hepatitis C virus; HHV, human herpesvirus; HIV-1, human immunodeficiency virus 1; HPV, human papillomavirus; HTLV-1, human T-cell lymphoma/leukemia virus type 1; IFN, interferon; LMP, latent membrane protein; pre-S, pre-surface; TAP, transporter-associated protein; TGF-β, transforming growth factor–β.

mainly affected (18). Breast-feeding, sexual intercourse, blood transfusions, and needle sharing transmit HTLV vertically and horizontally. In addition to genes common to all retroviruses, the HTLV genome carries a region that is related to the T-cell immortalizing phenotype of the virus and codes for two transacting regulatory proteins, tax and rex (19,20) (see Table 1).

HTLV-I–specific CTL directed against env, gag, and tax have been observed in 57% of asymptomatic HTLV-I carriers (21), and these CTL appear to control viral replication (22,23). At an early stage of viral gene expression, tax and rex proteins are predominantly produced (24). Therefore, these antigens are attractive targets for the immune system (25) and may be used as target antigens for prophylactic vaccination. Besides HTLV-I–specific T-cell responses, HTLV-I–neutralizing antibodies that inhibit cell fusion have been reported (26).

ATL develops in a small proportion of HTLV-I–infected people (1 per 1,000) (27). HTLV tax induces the expression of IL-2 and IL-2 receptor genes in infected T cells, therefore providing an autocrine loop for T-cell proliferation (28,29). During progression, ATL cells no longer produce IL-2, but they continue to express the IL-2 receptor. Widespread infection of CD4+ T cells might result in a loss of T-cell help during the CTL-mediated response and form a plausible reason for the escape of HTLV-I from the immune system and the subsequent development of ATL. Furthermore, HTLV-I–induced immunosuppression is indicated by the fact that most ATL patients are susceptible to various opportunistic infections by bacteria, fungi, protozoa, and viruses (18), which are normally under control of T-cell mediated immunity. HTLV-I infection of CD4+ T cells impairs T-cell function by decreasing the surface expression of the T-cell receptor/CD3 complex and diminishing helper function (30). Indeed, only 18% of ATL patients show an HTLV-I–specific CTL response (21), suggesting that the capacity to induce HTLV-I–specific CTL is decreased. The positive and negative regulation by tax and rex regulatory molecules result in transient expression of HTLV-I and allows a temporal escape from the immune system (24). HTLV tax transactivates various cellular molecules, including transforming growth factor–β (TGF-β) and IL-6 (31,32), and ATL cells constitutively produce IL-10 (33). Although both IL-6 and IL-10 might decrease the inflammatory response, TGF-β might inhibit the induction of a T-cell response. TGF-βs are highly immunosuppressive, and they inhibit the proliferation and effector functions of T cells, B cells, natural killer cells, and macrophages (34).

Conventional therapy by combination chemotherapy or treatment of ATL patients with radioactively labeled anti-IL-2 receptor antibodies results in partial or complete remissions in approximately 50% of treated patients (35). Alternative therapies for the treatment of ATL patients, such as the adoptive transfer of CD8+ HTLV-I tax-specific CTL, seems more attractive but only when the negative effects of tumor-produced cytokines are circumvented (36). Immunotherapy of established disease, therefore, appears a tough task. Prophylaxis of tumors by vaccination against HTLV-I (e.g., by induction of neutralizing antibodies against intact envelope components) in endemic regions seems more attractive.

Human Herpesvirus Type 8

In 1994, HHV-8 has been identified as an etiologic agent in Kaposi's sarcoma (KS) and primary effusion lymphomas (37,38). HHV-8 is sexually transmitted and may infect 10% of the general population. In HIV and acquired immunodeficiency syndrome patients, a higher fraction of the population is affected (39,40).

Antibodies directed against HHV-8 are detected in HIV patients and in some blood donors (41,42). The presence of antibodies to HHV-8 in HIV-1–infected patients is a predictor for the development of KS, showing that antibodies do not mediate full protection against HHV-8. Although no cell-mediated T-cell responses against HHV-8 have been described at present, several studies indicate a prominent role for the T-cell

mediated control of HHV-8. Detection of HHV-8 in peripheral blood mononuclear cells increases with immunosuppression, as shown by the correlation with a reduced number of CD4+ T cells (43). Furthermore, HHV-8 produces the chemokine homologue vMIP-II that displaces the CC chemokines MIP-1α and monocyte chemotactic protein 1 from their receptors (44,45). Chemokines are potent leukocyte chemoattractants that are involved in the recruitment of immune cells to sites of inflammation and infection. Production of viral homologues by HHV-8 prevents a local inflammatory response and thus protects the virus from immune-mediated clearance. It is not known how HHV-8 transforms cells into tumor cells, but some of the open reading frames (ORFs) of HHV-8 encode homologues that are important for transformation such as ORF72, the D-type cyclin homologue (46), and ORF16, a bcl-2 homologue (47,48). Additionally, the HHV-8 K2 gene encodes a functional IL-6 homologue. Human IL-6 inhibits apoptosis in myeloma cell lines (49) and viral IL-6 might play the same role. Furthermore, the HHV-8 K9 gene encodes a homologue of the viral interferon regulatory factor (vIRF). vIRF inhibits IFN-β inducibility of p21$^{waf1/cip1}$ and thus indirectly prevents p53-induced cell cycle arrest (50). The oncogenic potential of vIRF is demonstrated by the fact that expression of vIRF fully transforms NIH3T3 cells (50). The ORF of HHV-8 K13 shows a significant homology to the ORFs present in three other γ-herpesviruses encoding viral inhibitors that interfere with apoptosis signaled through death receptors (51). These inhibitors, called *vFLIP*, inhibit the recruitment and activation of the ICE-like protease FLICE by FAS/CD95 and might protect HHV-8–infected cells against apoptosis, leading to a higher virus production and persistence of HHV-8. At present, it is not known which antigens are expressed at which stage of disease, but based on the sequence similarity of HHV-8 to two other oncogenic γ-herpesviruses, herpesvirus of Saimiri and EBV, early and late antigens are probably expressed (see Table 1).

Hepatitis B Virus

HBV is a noncytopathic, enveloped virus with a circular double-stranded DNA genome. HBV causes acute and chronic necroinflammatory liver disease. Approximately 5% of the world's population is infected by HBV. More than 95% of adults acutely infected with HBV are able to clear all viral antigens and develop antiviral antibodies (52,53). During the acute phase of the disease, the T-cell response to HBV in these patients is vigorous, polyclonal, and multispecific (53). Sterilizing immunity, however, frequently fails to occur, as traces of HBV surface antigen and activated HBV-specific CTL can be detected in HBV surface–antigen-negative patients that have recovered years ago (54). The antibody response to HBV probably prevents viral spread, whereas the CTLs control HBV replication (53,55). Some HLA class-II alleles are associated with clearance of HBV infection (56), and patients that clear HBV show a concomitant HBV-specific CD4+ T-cell response that is absent in patients who do not (57). In addition to killing of infected hepatocytes, CTLs downregulate the expression and replication of HBV in surrounding liver tissue (58). Cytokines secreted by CTLs, such as IFN-γ and tumor necrosis factor α

(TNF-α), play an important role. TNF-α mediates the accelerated degradation of cytoplasmic HBV messenger RNA (mRNA) and IFN-γ plays a role in the upregulation of MHC class I expression, proteasomal cleavage of antigens, and expression of a variety of cellular antiviral proteins. Furthermore, IFN-γ is a powerful activator of macrophages. Activated hepatic macrophages have been shown to persistently abolish HBV gene expression and replication from the hepatocytes, possibly by the secretion of TNF-α and IFN-α/β (59).

The dominant cause of viral persistence seems to be a weak antiviral response to the viral antigens. Indeed, a relatively narrow and weak T-cell response is correlated with high viral load in patients with chronic hepatitis (53,57). Viral evasion by mutations in CTL or Th epitopes can contribute to viral persistence, as might the infection of immunologically privileged sites. Obviously, vaccination-induced upgrading of the natural T-cell response against the envelope, nucleocapsid, and polymerase antigens (60) into a vigorous HBV-specific immune response may result in control of HBV infection and prevent the development of hepatocellular carcinoma (HCC).

HCC is a common complication of chronic HBV infection. Most HCC tumors contain clonally integrated HBV DNA. Indeed the HBV-X gene product and preS2/S can transactivate cellular genes that are involved in cellular growth control and inhibit p53 gene function (61–64). Like other retroviruses, HBV integration can only take place in dividing cells, and an active immune response, resulting in an enhanced hepatocellular turnover, has been implicated as mediator of hepatocarcinogenesis in chronic HBV infection (65). No evidence of a rise in hepatocellular cancer incidence was found in HIV-1 seropositive subjects, which suggests that the development of HCC might be dependent on a chronic and weak immune response to HBV (4).

Numerous tumors contain viral RNAs encoding the HBV-X, -S, and -C genes, whereas in other tumors these genes are disrupted and only HBV-X is expressed (66). CTLs recognizing surface and core antigens that are encoded by HBV-S and HBV-C have been found, suggesting that tumors expressing these antigens might be treated by immunotherapy (see Table 1). Considering the decreased immune status of tumor-bearing patients (2,67) and the routes tumor cells follow to resist T-cell immunity (36,68,69), adoptive transfer of *in vitro*-expanded HBV-specific T cells might be feasible, provided that the primary tumor has been resected. CTLs directed at the transactivating gene X have not been reported, suggesting that treatment of tumors expressing only HBV-X may be much harder. Prevention of HBV infection and incidence of HCC might decrease by prophylactic vaccination with HBV antigens, as was shown by vaccination-induced reduction of HBV-related HCC in children (70,71).

Hepatitis C Virus

HCV is a small, enveloped RNA virus that encodes a single polyprotein of approximately 3,000 amino acids. At the 5' end, a highly conserved region encoding the core protein is located, which is followed by five less-conserved nonstructural regions and a hyper-variable region encoding the envelope. *In vivo* replication of HCV takes place predominantly in the liver. Most patients with acute infection are asymptomatic, nevertheless

50% to 70% of the infected individuals progress to chronic liver disease (72). Viremia may be lifelong, although clearance of HCV-RNA may occur transiently. In 20% of these patients, symptomatic cirrhosis develops after one or more decades, which then might slowly evolve to hepatocellular cancer (73).

The immune response necessary to elicit protective immunity against HCV is presently unknown. Humoral responses to multiple HCV antigens are present, but the antibody titer of the response does not correlate with course of disease. Moreover, high-titer antibodies have been associated with disease transmission and persistent viremia (74,75). In addition to antibodies, lymphocytes are observed within the hepatic parenchyma of individuals infected with HCV. Both HCV-specific CD4+ and CD8+ T cells exist, and these responses appear to be directed at many HCV epitopes (76–81). All HCV-derived proteins are a target for CD4+ Th cells, but CD4+ T cells specific for HCV core are associated with a benign course of infection (81). In view of the HIV-like high RNA replication rates and poor proofreading ability of HCV, which leads to frequent transcription errors, a Th response directed at the conserved core protein might be better able to maintain the humoral and CTL response. Furthermore, current data on HCV suggest that in the case of HBV, HCV infection of immunologically privileged sites or weakening of T-cell–mediated immune responses might allow the virus to persist. Continuous priming of the CTL response by persistent virus, long after clinical recovery, might wear out the T-cell response. Moreover, HCV proteins containing epitopes that elicit neutralizing antibodies mutate frequently and appear to permit the virus to escape.

A role for T cells in the pathogenesis of liver injury is indicated by the fact that HCV-specific CTL produces cytokines, including IFN-γ, TNF-α, granulocyte-macrophage colony-stimulating factor, IL-8, and IL-10 in an antigen- and class I–restricted manner (80). The release of these proinflammatory cytokines by CTL on recognition of their cognate target may contribute to the pathogenesis of liver injury. Direct liver damage of noninfected hepatocytes might also occur by molecular mimicry between an HCV-derived CTL epitope and a cytochrome p450-derived peptide (82) and it can be envisaged that this type of CTL epitope might also play a role in HBV infection and the development of HCC. The nature of HCV replication makes it unlikely that HCV integrates in the host genome, and HCV-positive tumors, therefore, express all HCV proteins (see Table 1). If protection from HCV infection turns out to be T-cell mediated, the conserved antigens of HCV are attractive immunotherapeutic targets to treat HCV-associated HCC.

HUMAN PAPILLOMAVIRUS TYPE 16

HPVs of the high-risk types (e.g., HPV-16, -18, -31, -33, and -45) are responsible for cancer. The HPV genomes can be divided into three regions: a long control region (LCR) and an early (E) and a late (L) region. The L genes encode structural proteins, the E region codes mainly for regulatory proteins engaged in genome persistence, DNA replication, and activation of the lytic cycle (83). Virus gene expression is controlled by viral- and cellular-derived transcription factors such as Brn3a (84) or the epithelial factor Epoc1/Skn-1a (85) that regulates papillomavirus transcription in a differentiation-dependent fashion in the suprabasal cells of the cervical epithelium. The E1 and E2 genes regulate viral replication. Furthermore, E2 and E5 regulate transcription. The E2 protein controls the expression of the E6- and E7-oncoproteins by binding to sites close to the TATA box within their common promoter (86). E5 enhances the transcription of the immediate early genes (87,88). The E5 protein of HPV shows only weak transforming activity in NIH3T3 cells by *in vitro* transfection experiments. Indeed, the E5 ORF is frequently deleted in cervical cancers (89). The early genes E6 and E7 interfere with cell cycle control. The E6 protein of the high-risk HPV types specifically binds to p53 and targets its rapid degradation through the ubiquitin pathway (90). p53 Is involved in initiation of apoptosis, and loss of this protein results in the prevention of apoptosis. HPV-16 viruses, with an E6 protein that displays variation in areas likely to be important for protein-protein interaction with p53, reportedly are more prevalent in invasive cervical carcinoma than are prototype viruses (91). The E7 protein of high-risk types binds to pRB, which normally prevents cells from entering the cell cycle by inactivating E2F, a protein needed for cell cycle entry (92). E7 expression results in the failure of infected cells to withdraw from the cell cycle and differentiate. In addition, HPV-16 E7 can bind to another identified cellular partner, the human homologue hTID56 of the *Drosophila* tumor-suppressor protein TID56 (93). The combined actions of E6 and E7 create an environment conducive to viral replication. Finally, E4 expression correlates exactly with the start of viral DNA replication (94) suggesting a role for the E4 protein in DNA replication, but the exact role of E4 remains unclear.

Kinetics of Human Papillomavirus Infection and Development of Human Papillomavirus-Induced Cervical Carcinoma

Papillomaviruses infect basal keratinocytes, and the differentiation of these cells allows HPV to replicate and assemble new virions. These new viruses are released when the superficial cells flake off (95). After infection of the basal epithelial cells, the immediate HPV early genes E1, E2, E5, E6, and E7 are expressed. As the infected basal cell migrates through the differentiating layers of the epidermis, HPV late gene expression is initiated. Expression of the nonstructural early protein E4 precedes the expression of the L1 and L2 capsid proteins for one or two cell layers (94). In the most superficial epithelial layers, L1 and L2 are expressed. Here, the new HPV virions are assembled and released.

Low-risk HPV types (e.g., HPV-6 and -11) cause benign warts, whereas the high-risk types are responsible for cancer in more than 99% of cases. In some cases, HPV of the high-risk types persist and the viral genome is linearized and integrated. Malignant transformation occurs when the E2 region is disrupted. Loss of E2-protein expression leads to elevated expression of the E6 and E7 oncoproteins and in abortion of the productive infection cycle. Prolonged and elevated expression of the E6 and E7 oncoproteins is tightly associated with HPV-induced dysplasia and transformation into cervical carcinoma (83). This sets the stage for a transformation process involving progression from precursor lesions, termed *cervical intraepithe-*

lial neoplasia (CIN), and potentially evolving to monoclonal cervical carcinoma. Indeed, in a high proportion of CIN III lesions, and in all tumors, the E2 gene was disrupted although no detectable E2 transcripts were found (96,97). The precursor lesions (CIN I to III) are classified on the basis of a progressive increase in cellular atypia and tissue architecture. CIN I lesions spontaneously regress in 60% of cases and are mostly associated with infection of low-risk HPV types 6 and 11. Approximately 10% of CIN I lesions progress to CIN II or CIN III (severe dysplasia and carcinoma *in situ*). With progression to high-grade CIN, the chance of spontaneous regression diminishes, but the chance of developing cervical carcinoma and the incidence of high-risk HPV types increases (98–101). A strong relationship was found between persistence of oncogenic HPV types and progression of premalignant cervical lesions. In contrast, the absence of progression was often found to be associated with HPV clearance or fluctuation. HPV-16 can be found in 30% to 70% of CIN III lesions, the majority of which progress to cervical carcinoma in the absence of treatment (83,102).

Immunity to Human Papillomavirus

In most women, infection with genital HPV is a transient phenomenon. Natural HPV infection at the genitomucosal surfaces is poorly immunogenic. Premalignant HPV infections are restricted to the epithelium, limiting contact with immune-effector cells and antigen-presenting cells (APCs). Moreover, HPV is a nonlytic virus that exploits the normal differentiation of the keratinocytes for viral replication and production. Viral particles are shed from the upper layers of the epithelium and, as a consequence, HPV infection produces little or no local inflammation. Involvement of the immune system in the defense against HPV infection was suggested by (a) an increased incidence of HPV-induced epithelial lesions in immunosuppressed patients (3); (b) association of particular HLA alleles with increased susceptibility to, or protection from, HPV infection and cervical neoplasia (103,104); (c) seemingly spontaneous regressions of CIN lesions and clearance of concomitant HPV infections (105); and (d) downregulation of MHC class I or TAPs, or both, in the majority of cervical cancers (106).

More direct proof of natural HPV-directed immunity has accumulated since the mid-1990s. The existence of natural HPV-16 E7-specific CTL immunity, and homing of these CTLs to the site of premalignant and malignant lesions, has been shown in the blood, lymph nodes, or tumor material of patients with HPV-16 or -18 DNA–positive lesions (107–111). In a non-intervention follow-up study, HPV-16 E7-specific CTLs, as well as Th cells, were found only in the blood of patients with a persistent HPV infection or with progressive cervical lesions (112,113). This agrees with the idea that the cells of the basal layer that are most likely to contact immune cells express only a limited repertoire of viral gene products. Antigen expression is probably too low to induce a protective immune response, and T cells are only triggered on viral persistence and progression of HPV-infected lesions when the expression of the E6 and E7 protein is increased and the normal epithelial organization is disrupted and thus accessible for antigen-presenting cells.

In addition to T-cell responses, antibodies to the early genes E2, E4, E6, and E7 have been described (114–117). These antibodies do not appear to have any antiviral effect once HPV infection has been established but merely reflect progression of disease. E2- and E4-specific antibodies have been found at the time of replication, whereas E6- and E7-specific antibodies were found in tumor-bearing patients when E1 and E2 expression is disrupted and the antigen burden of the E6 and E7 oncoproteins is increased. Furthermore, HPV capsid-specific antibodies of the immunoglobulin G (IgG) class have been found. These antibodies seem to be insufficient in mediating a protective response because the presence of capsid-specific IgG antibodies is associated with and predictive for persistent HPV-16 infection and the development of high-grade CIN (118).

A Th type 1 cytokine profile of the HPV-specific immune response seems in favor of the host. IgG2 (Th type 1) reactivity against HPV-16 E7 in CIN patients is associated with viral clearance, whereas an increase in HPV-16 E7-specific IgG1 antibodies (Th type 2) is found in cervical cancer patients, indicating a possible shift from a Th type 1 to Th type 2 response (119). Indeed, IL-2 production by peripheral blood lymphocytes in response to stimulation with soluble antigen was reported to be reduced in HPV-infected individuals with high-grade lesions or carcinoma (120,121). In contrast, production of IL-4 and IL-10 was found to be elevated in HPV-infected patients with high-grade disease (121). Moreover, high expression of the Th type 1 cytokine IFN-γ correlated with good prognosis in cervical cancer, whereas an abnormally elevated concentration of the Th type 2 cytokine IL-6 was associated with poor prognosis (122).

Persistence of oncogenic HPV types might be achieved by multiple pathways. Lack of a local inflammatory response and low antigen expression of viral antigens in the basal layer of the epithelium can be just enough to avoid induction of protective immunity. Whether the viral genome is involved in downregulation of APC function, particularly of Langerhans' cells in the skin, remains unclear at present. HPV-16 E7 seems to impair the IFN-γ response of infected cells (123). Furthermore, high-risk HPV harbor glucocorticoid responsive elements within the LCR (124), and exposure of infected cells to glucocorticoids could have multiple effects. Glucocorticoids were found to substantially enhance immortalization of HPV-16 but not of HPV-11–infected cells *in vitro* (125). Exposure of transgenic mice expressing HPV-16 oncogenes under the human keratin-14 promotor to estrogen, which enhances the action of glucocorticoids, is known to induce cancer in these transgenic mice (126). Alternatively, hydrocortisone and progesterone were found to downregulate human HLA class I molecule expression at the surface of HPV-positive cells (127) leading to reduced presentation of peptide antigen to T cells. Downregulation of HLA class-I molecules or TAP expression has also been noted in cervical carcinoma cells (106).

Antigens Accessible for Prophylactic Vaccination Against Human Papillomavirus-16

Approximately 50% of young, sexually active women are infected at one time or another with HPV types that have the potential to progress to malignancy (128). An early termination of viral infection might not only protect the host from subsequent reinfection of newly assembled virus or the potential formation of premalignant lesions, but may also limit the spread of the virus in the population and thus the incidence of HPV infection. Prophylactic vaccination aimed at the suppression of HPV infection at the port of entry, thus, is preferred. Generation of local antibody responses against the capsid antigens L1 and L2 could block the interaction between the infectious virion and its cellular receptor and prevent infection of the cervical epithelium. Moreover, these antibodies might facilitate the degradation of virions through antibody-mediated uptake by macrophages. It is, however, not formally proven that such antibodies are capable of preventing virus transmission by flaked-off virus-infected epithelial cells. L1-specific antibodies of the IgG class were found in the majority of patients with persistent infections and histologically confirmed high-grade lesions, suggesting that these antibodies are insufficient for the control of established HPV infections (118). More relevant than L1- or L2-specific IgG antibodies might be mucosal IgA responses with the capacity to neutralize virions. Cervical mucous antibodies of the IgA type that reacted with HPV-16 capsid proteins were found particularly in patients who displayed low-grade lesions (CIN I) (129).

In addition to mucosal L1- or L2-specific antibodies of the IgG and IgA type, a cell-mediated immune response against the early gene products E1, E2, E5, E6, and E7 might protect against HPV-16. The L1, L2, and E4 proteins are unlikely to be suitable CTL targets, as these proteins are expressed in the late phase of infection when the cells are already dying as part of their differentiation program. Furthermore, the manifestation of E6 and E7 proteins is low as a result of E2 expression. The E1 and E2 proteins constitute a replication complex necessary for the maintenance of the episomal genome and thus should be expressed in all cells that contain episomal HPV. Therefore, the E1 and E2 proteins are attractive targets for CTL as well as for supportive Th type 1 responses (see Table 1). Prophylactic vaccines must include L1, L2, and, preferably, E2 antigens of multiple oncogenic HPV types to make an impact in the reduction of cancer and high-grade cervical lesions. Luckily, each of the types of HPV is highly conserved globally, and the viral genomes are not ostensibly prone to mutation. Phase 1, phase 2, and phase 3 efficacy trials of prophylactic vaccination with virus-like particles composed of HPV-16/18 L1 with or without L2 and other viral proteins are currently under way and should answer the question whether reduction of viral burden or disease, or both, induced by these high-risk HPV types is feasible.

Antigens Accessible for Therapeutic Treatment of Human Papillomavirus-16 Positive Lesions

Constitutive expression of E6 and E7 is needed for maintenance of the transformed state of cervical carcinoma cells. The E6 and E7 proteins thus form attractive targets for the treatment of disease characterized by the presence of transformed cells. E7-specific CTLs have been found in high-grade lesions, and the frequency of these CTLs was higher in tumors and tumor-draining lymph nodes than in the blood of these patients (107). This shows that HPV-specific CTLs can home to the sites of disease. However, this also indicates that these CTLs are not sufficiently effective to accomplish tumor regression. Furthermore, HPV-16 E7-specific Th responses, as well as E7-specific CTLs, seem to develop as a consequence of increased viral antigen burden resulting from tumor growth, and, therefore, their induction is probably too late to have any effect on established tumor (112,113). Active immune intervention aiming at E6 and E7 in premalignant or minimal residual disease after cancer surgery may provide adequate and effective immunity. Therapeutic treatment should result in the elimination of residual cancer, the regression of existing lesions, or prevention of progression from low-grade into high-grade disease. Two approaches can be followed: therapeutic vaccination or adoptive immunotherapy, or both.

Many animal studies have shown that vaccination with various formulations of E7-derived peptides, E7 protein, dendritic cells pulsed with peptide or protein, virus-like particle–containing E7, or recombinant viruses expressing E7 protein, elicit E7-specific CD8+ CTL capable of protecting animals from a tumor challenge (130–134). Moreover, therapeutic intravenous vaccination with dendritic cells, pulsed with either an E7-derived CTL epitope or with unfractionated acid-eluted peptides from an HPV-16+ tumor, resulted in tumor regression and long-term immunity (135,136). Of note, the time span allowed between onset of tumors and start of treatment for therapy to be effective was limited in these murine tumor models relative to the situation found in cervical cancer patients. Instead of therapeutic vaccination, adoptive transfer of antigen-specific Th cells and CTL might be a practical way to control advanced disease. Indeed, established virus-induced or p53-overexpressing tumors of considerable size can be eradicated in murine models when treated with adoptively transferred CTL (137,138) or injection of E7-specific CTL directly into an HPV-16+ tumor (139). In humans, CTL were shown to control persistent viral infection or exert antitumor reactivity as illustrated by the therapeutic activity of *ex vivo* expanded autologous cytomegalovirus or EBV-specific T cells in bone marrow transplant patients (11,140), or the infusion of expanded tumor-infiltrating lymphocytes in patients with malignant melanoma (141).

We are currently not aware of any trials that conduct the adoptive transfer of HPV-specific T cells in patients with HPV-induced tumors. Possibly this is due to the fact that good protocols needed for the expansion of HPV-specific memory T cells are still lacking. Additionally, the restricted repertoire of viral gene products in basal cells, the limited contact of immune cells with HPV-infected epithelium, and downregulation of epithelial APC function probably impede vigorous priming of HPV-specific T cells. This is confirmed by the fact that the majority of T-cell responses were found in patients in later stages of disease when antigen burden is high and the structure of cervical epithelium is altered (112,113).

Instead of expanding existing HPV-specific T cells *ex vivo*, priming of autologous naïve T cells to react to HPV may be considered. Priming of CTLs able to react against HPV-16–positive tumor cells is feasible (142,143), but *in vitro* induction of antigen-specific CTLs is quite laborious and, except for melanoma antigens, the success rate and reproducibility are low. *In vitro* generation of antigen-specific Th cells seems more success-

ful and reproducible (144). Previously, it was shown in an animal model that murine leukemia virus-specific Th cells were needed for the induction of CTL-mediated protection against challenge with the aggressive virus-induced RMA tumor (145). Dissection of the cellular interactions involved in the generation of effective CTL responses revealed that Th cells and CTLs must recognize antigen on the same APC (146,147). Recognition of APCs by Th cells induces APC maturation through CD40L-CD40 cognate interactions (148–150). This is associated with IL-12 production by the APC, with upregulation of MHC class I and class II molecules, and costimulatory molecules that convert the APC into a CTL-priming state. Thus, in essence, adoptive transfer of HPV-specific Th cells, which can recognize their antigen captured by local APC, results in maturation of the APC and potentiates priming of HPV-specific CTL. Furthermore, antigen-specific Th cells are able to activate macrophages and eosinophils that produce both superoxide and nitric oxide, resulting in MHC-independent antitumor activity (151). We have identified E7-derived peptides that were able to prime and expand HLA-DR–restricted E7-specific Th cells from the blood of healthy blood donors in a time span of 3 to 4 weeks (S. H. van der Burg, *in preparation*). Such T cells, if prepared under good manufacturing practice conditions, could be used for immunotherapy by adoptive transfer, possibly resulting in a more efficient local activation of effector cells. In general, the importance of exploiting the full therapeutic potential of tumor-specific CD4+ Th cells, orchestrating several effector functions that can cooperate in an effective antitumor response, should be stressed here (152).

Stage of Patients and Efficacy of Therapeutic Treatment

The stage of disease might have a profound outcome on the efficacy of treatment. Late-stage cancer patients display impaired immunity as shown by loss of CTL responses to influenza or diminished proliferative Th responses against *Mycobacterium tuberculosis* or tetanus toxin (153). Furthermore, cervical tumor cells tend to lose MHC class I expression or downregulate peptide transport into the endoplasmic reticulum, or both, resulting in loss of recognition by the immune system. Several groups have vaccinated HPV-16–infected late-stage cervical carcinoma patients with E7-derived CTL epitopes and Th peptide formulations, E6 and/or E7 proteins, or recombinant vaccinia virus expressing E6 and E7. Only a few of the patients reacted to the vaccine and displayed E7-specific CTL responses (110,153,154) or Th peptide-specific responses (153,155). In general, these vaccines were shown to be safe, but due to the small groups and, more important, the impaired immunity of late-stage cancer patients, it was difficult to evaluate the full potential of these vaccines.

Based on these experiences, new trials should include patients with less advanced stages of disease, and HPV-specific Th epitopes should be included in these vaccines. Therapeutic vaccination or adoptive transfer of HPV-specific T cells in addition to the standard treatment of HPV-16–infected patients with severe dysplasia or noninvasive tumor might shed a light on a potential beneficial effect of HPV-specific CTL and Th cells in the elimination or control of residual disease.

Cost-Effectiveness of Treatment Modalities

Apart from the feasibility of prophylactic vaccination, one should remember that of the 30% to 50% of the sexually active population that is infected with HPV, only a small percentage (less than 1%) progress to full-blown invasive cancer. This can be compared to other viruses such as EBV and HBV (155). Thus, cancer induction by these viruses is an accident of an otherwise uneventful virus-host relationship. Furthermore, the generation of long-term high-titer neutralizing antibodies at the mucosal surfaces may be hard to achieve and may not be enough to fully control disease. Additionally, substantial numbers of HPV-specific Th cells and CTLs should be maintained over prolonged periods. Both probably require regular boosts and antibody, and HPV-specific T-cell levels need to be high for many years. It requires many years of patience to observe a reduction of cervical carcinoma after vaccination, but prophylactic vaccination inducing both humoral and cellular immunity might limit the spread of virus in populations at risk.

Assuming that T cells play an important role in the control of HPV infections, immunotherapy of people with severe dysplasia or noninvasive carcinoma as adjuvant therapy to the standard treatment limits the number of individuals that should be treated (less than 1% of infected subjects). Adoptive transfer of HPV-specific T cells enhances the costs due to the necessity for cytokines and specialized personnel for T- and dendritic-cell culturing and antigen preparation, which are needed to obtain clinical-grade HPV-specific T cells at sufficient numbers (if possible).

Therapeutic vaccination might lower the costs dramatically if no cell culture is needed. Ideally prophylactic and therapeutic vaccines are identical and may be composed of recombinant proteins or viruses (vaccinia or adenovirus) expressing HPV antigens. Because this kind of active immunotherapy depends heavily on an intact immune system, it is only possible in immunocompetent patients.

REFERENCES

1. Masucci MG. Viral immunopathology of human tumors. *Curr Opin Immunol* 1993;5(5):693.
2. zur Hausen H. Viruses in human cancers. *Science* 1991;254 (5035):1167.
3. Benton C, Shahidullah H, Hunter JAA. Human papillomavirus in the immunosuppressed. *Papillomavirus Rep* 1992;3:23.
4. Beral V, Newton R. Overview of the epidemiology of immunodeficiency-associated cancers. *J Cancer Inst Monogr* 1998;23:1.
5. Liu Y, de Waal Malefyt R, Briere F, et al. The EBV IL-10 homologue is a selective agonist with impaired binding to the IL-10 receptor. *J Immunol* 1997;158(2):604.
6. Khanna R, Burrows SR, Kurilla MG, et al. Localization of Epstein-Barr virus cytotoxic T cell epitopes using recombinant vaccinia: implications for vaccine development. *J Exp Med* 1992;176(1):169.
7. Murray RJ, Kurilla MG, Brooks JM, et al. Identification of target antigens for the human cytotoxic T cell response to Epstein-Barr virus (EBV): implications for the immune control of EBV-positive malignancies. *J Exp Med* 1992;176(1):157.
8. Nazaruk RA, Rochford R, Hobbs MV, Cannon MJ. Functional diversity of the CD8(+) T-cell response to Epstein-Barr virus (EBV): implications for the pathogenesis of EBV-associated lymphoproliferative disorders. *Blood* 1998;91(10):3875.
9. Khanna R, Burrows SR, Thomson SA, et al. Class I processing-defective Burkitt's lymphoma cells are recognized efficiently by CD4+ EBV-specific CTLs. *J Immunol* 1997;158(8):3619.
10. Rooney CM, Smith CA, Heslop HE. Control of virus-induced lymphoproliferation: Epstein-Barr virus-induced lymphoproliferation and host immunity. *Mol Med Today* 1997;3(1):24.
11. Heslop HE, Ng CY, Li C, Smith CA, et al. Long-term restoration of immunity against Epstein-Barr virus infection by adoptive transfer of gene-modified virus-specific T lymphocytes. *Nat Med* 1996; 2(5):551.
12. Frisan T, Sjoberg J, Dolcetti R, et al. Local suppression of Epstein-Barr virus (EBV)-specific cytotoxicity in biopsies of EBV-positive Hodgkin's disease. *Blood* 1995;86(4):1493.
13. Yates JL, Warren N, Sugden B. Stable replication of plasmids derived from Epstein-Barr virus in various mammalian cells. *Nature* 1985;313(6005):812.
14. Levitskaya J, Coram M, Levitsky V, et al. Inhibition of antigen processing by the internal repeat region of the Epstein-Barr virus nuclear antigen-1. *Nature* 1995;375(6533):685.
15. Khanna R, Burrows SR, Argaet V, Moss DJ. Endoplasmic reticulum signal sequence facilitated transport of peptide epitopes restores immunogenicity of an antigen processing defective tumour cell line. *J Immunol* 1994;6(4):639.
16. Masucci MG, Zhang QJ, Gavioli R, et al. Immune escape by Epstein-Barr virus (EBV) carrying Burkitt's lymphoma: *in vitro* reconstitution of sensitivity to EBV-specific cytotoxic T cells. *Int Immunol* 1992;4(11):1283.
17. Brooks LA, Lear AL, Young LS, Rickinson AB. Transcripts from the Epstein-Barr virus BamHI A fragment are detectable in all three forms of virus latency. *J Virol* 1993;67(6):3182.
18. Uchiyama T. Human T cell leukemia virus type I (HTLV-I) and human diseases. *Annu Rev Immunol* 1997;15:15.
19. Seiki M, Hattori S, Hirayama Y, Yoshida M. Human adult T-cell leukemia virus: complete nucleotide sequence of the provirus genome integrated in leukemia cell DNA. *Proc Natl Acad Sci U S A* 1983; 80(12):3618.
20. Sodroski JG, Rosen CA, Haseltine WA. Transacting transcriptional activation of the long terminal repeat of human T lymphotropic viruses in infected cells. *Science* 1984;225(4660):381.
21. Kannagi M, Matsushita S, Shida H, Harada S. Cytotoxic T cell response and expression of the target antigen in HTLV-I infection. *Leukemia* 1994;8[Suppl 1]:S54.
22. Kannagi M, Harada S, Maruyama I, et al. Predominant recognition of human T cell leukemia virus type I (HTLV-I) pX gene products by human CD8+ cytotoxic T cells directed against HTLV-I-infected cells. *Int Immunol* 1991;3(8):761.
23. Jacobson S, Reuben JS, Streilein RD, Palker TJ. Induction of CD4+, human T lymphotropic virus type-1-specific cytotoxic T lymphocytes from patients with HAM/TSP. Recognition of an immunogenic region of the gp46 envelope glycoprotein of human T lymphotropic virus type-1. *J Immunol* 1991;146(4):1155.
24. Yoshida M, Suzuki T, Hirai H, Fujisawa J. Regulation of HTLV-I gene expression and its roles in ATL development. In: Takatsuki K, ed. *Adult T-cell leukemia*. Oxford, UK: Oxford University Press, 1994:28.
25. van Baalen CA, Pontesilli O, Huisman RC, et al. Human immunodeficiency virus type 1 Rev- and Tat-specific cytotoxic T lymphocyte frequencies inversely correlate with rapid progression to AIDS. *J Gen Virol* 1997;78(8):1913.
26. Kuroki M, Nakamura M, Itoyama Y, et al. Identification of new epitopes recognized by human monoclonal antibodies with neutralizing and antibody-dependent cellular cytotoxicity activities specific for human T cell leukemia virus type 1. *J Immunol* 1992;149(3):940.
27. Tajima K. The 4th nation-wide study of adult T-cell leukemia/lymphoma (ATL) in Japan: estimates of risk of ATL and its geographical and clinical features. The T- and B-cell Malignancy Study Group. *Int J Cancer* 1990;45(2):237.
28. Uchiyama T, Hori T, Tsudo M, et al. Interleukin-2 receptor (Tac antigen) expressed on adult T cell leukemia cells. *J Clin Invest* 1985; 76(2):446.

29. Arima N, Daitoku Y, Ohgaki S, et al. Autocrine growth of interleukin 2-producing leukemic cells in a patient with adult T cell leukemia. *Blood* 1986;68(3):779.

30. Inatsuki A, Yasukawa M, Kobayashi Y. Functional alterations of herpes simplex virus-specific CD4+ multifunctional T cell clones following infection with human T lymphotropic virus type I. *J Immunol* 1989;143(4):1327.

31. Noma T, Nakakubo H, Sugita M, Kumagai S, Maeda M, Shimizu A, Honjo T. Expression of different combinations of interleukins by human T cell leukemic cell lines that are clonally related. *J Exp Med* 1989;169(5):1853.

32. Kim SJ, Kehrl JH, Burton J, Tendler CL, et al. Transactivation of the transforming growth factor beta 1 (TGF-beta 1) gene by human T lymphotropic virus type 1 tax: a potential mechanism for the increased production of TGF-beta 1 in adult T cell leukemia. *J Exp Med* 1990;172(1):121.

33. Mori N, Prager D. Interleukin-10 gene expression and adult T-cell leukemia. *Leuk Lymphoma* 1998;29(3-4):239.

34. Taipale J, Saharinen J, Keski-Oja J. Extracellular matrix-associated transforming growth factor-beta: role in cancer cell growth and invasion. *Adv Cancer Res* 1998;75:87.

35. Waldmann TA. The promiscuous IL-2/IL-15 receptor: a target for immunotherapy of HTLV-I-associated disorders. *J Acquir Immune Defic Syndr Hum Retrovirol* 1996;13[Suppl 1]:S179.

36. Chouaib S, Asselin-Paturel C, Mami-Chouaib F, Caignard A, Blay JY. The host-tumor immune conflict: from immunosuppression to resistance and destruction. *Immunol Today* 1997;18(10):493.

37. Chang Y, Cesarman E, Pessin MS, et al. Identification of herpesvirus-like DNA sequences in AIDS-associated Kaposi's sarcoma. *Science* 1994;266(5192):1865.

38. Weiss RA, Whitby D, Talbot S, Kellam P, Boshoff C. Human herpesvirus type 8 and Kaposi's sarcoma. *J Natl Cancer Inst Monogr* 1998;23:51.

39. Kedes DH, Operskalski E, Busch M, Kohn R, Flood J, Ganem D. The seroepidemiology of human herpesvirus 8 (Kaposi's sarcoma-associated herpesvirus): distribution of infection in KS risk groups and evidence for sexual transmission. *Nat Med* 1996;2(8):918.

40. Gao SJ, Kingsley L, Li M, et al. KSHV antibodies among Americans, Italians and Ugandans with and without Kaposi's sarcoma. *Nat Med* 1996;2(8):925.

41. Rezza G, Lennette ET, Giuliani M, et al. Prevalence and determinants of anti-lytic and anti-latent antibodies to human herpesvirus-8 among Italian individuals at risk of sexually and parenterally transmitted infections. *Int J Cancer* 1998;77(3):361.

42. Lin SF, Sun R, Heston L, et al. Identification, expression, and immunogenicity of Kaposi's sarcoma-associated herpesvirus-encoded small viral capsid antigen. *J Virol* 1997;71(4):3069.

43. Whitby D, Howard MR, Tenant-Flowers M, et al. Detection of Kaposi's sarcoma associated herpesvirus in peripheral blood of HIV-infected individuals and progression to Kaposi's sarcoma. *Lancet* 1995;346(8978):799.

44. Kiedal TN, Rosenkilde MM, Coulin F, et al. A broad-spectrum chemokine antagonist encoded by Kaposi's sarcoma-associated herpesvirus. *Science* 1997;277(5332):1656.

45. Boshoff C, Endo V, Collins PD, et al. Angiogenic and mV-inhibitory functions of KSHV-encoded chemokines. *Science* 1997;278 (5336):290.

46. Godden-Kent D, Talbot SJ, Boshoff C, et al. The cyclin encoded by Kaposi's sarcoma-associated herpesvirus stimulates cdk6 to phosphorylate the retinoblastoma protein and histone H1. *J Virol* 1997;71(6):4193.

47. Neipel F, Albrecht JC, Fleckenstein B. Cell-homologous genes in the Kaposi's sarcoma-associated rhadinovirus human herpesvirus 8: determinants of its pathogenicity? *J Virol* 1997;71(6):4187.

48. Sand R, Sato T, Bohenzky RA, Russo JJ, Chang V. Kaposi's sarcoma-associated herpesvirus encodes a functional bcl-2 homologue. *Nat Med* 1997;3(3):293.

49. Lichtenstein A, Tu V, Fady C, Vescio R, Berenson J. Interleukin-6 inhibits apoptosis of malignant plasma cells. *Cell Immunol* 1995; 162(2):248.

50. Gao SJ, Boshoff C, Jayachandra S, Weiss RA, Chang V, Moore PS. KSHV ORF K9 (vIRF) is an oncogene which inhibits the interferon signaling pathway. *Oncogene* 1997;15(16):1979.

51. Thome M, Schneider P, Hofmann K, et al. Viral FLICE-inhibitory proteins (FLIPs) prevent apoptosis induced by death receptors. *Nature* 1997;386(6624):517.

52. Chisari FV, Ferrari C. Hepatitis B virus immunopathogenesis. *Annu Rev Immunol* 1995;13:29.

53. Chisari FV, Ferrari C. Hepatitis B virus immunopathology. *Springer Semin Immunopathol* 1995;17(2-3):261.

54. Rehermann B, Ferrari C, Pasquinelli C, Chisari FV. The hepatitis B virus persists for decades after patients' recovery from acute viral hepatitis despite active maintenance of a cytotoxic T-lymphocyte response. *Nat Med* 1996;2(10):1104.

55. Rehermann B, Fowler P, Sidney J, et al. The cytotoxic T lymphocyte response to multiple hepatitis B virus polymerase epitopes during and after acute viral hepatitis. *J Exp Med* 1995;181(3):1047.

56. Thursz MR, Kwiatkowski D, Allsopp CE, Greenwood BM, Thomas HC, Hill AV. Association between an MHC class II allele and clearance of hepatitis B virus in the Gambia (see comments). *N Engl J Med* 1995;332(16):1065.

57. Ferrari C, Bertoletti A, Penna A, et al. Identification of immunodominant T cell epitopes of the hepatitis B virus nucleocapsid antigen. *J Clin Invest* 1991;88(1):214.

58. Guidotti LG, Ishikawa T, Hobbs MV, Matzke B, Schreiber R, Chisari FV. Intracellular inactivation of the hepatitis B virus by cytotoxic T lymphocytes. *Immunity* 1996;4,(1):25.

59. Guidotti LG, Chisari FV. To kill or to cure: options in host defense against viral infection. *Curr Opin Immunol* 1996;8(4):478.

60. Cerny A, Ferrari C, Chisari FV. The class I-restricted cytotoxic T lymphocyte response to predetermined epitopes in the hepatitis B and C viruses. *Curr Top Microbiol Immunol* 1994;189:169.

61. Matsubara K, Tokino T. Integration of hepatitis B virus DNA and its implications for hepatocarcinogenesis. *Mol Biol Med* 1990;7(3):243.

62. Maguire HF, Hoeffler JP, Siddiqui A. HBV X protein alters the DNA binding specificity of CREB and ATF-2 by protein-protein interactions. *Science* 1991;252(5007):842.

63. Natoli G, Avantaggiati ML, Chirillo P, et al. Induction of the DNA-binding activity of c-jun/c-fos heterodimers by the hepatitis B virus transactivator pX. *Mol Cell Biol* 1994;14(2):989.

64. Wang XW, Forrester K, Yeh H, Feitelson MA, Gu JR, Harris CC. Hepatitis B virus X protein inhibits p53 sequence-specific DNA binding, transcriptional activity, and association with transcription factor ERCC3. *Proc Natl Acad Sci U S A* 1994;91(6):2230.

65. Nakamoto V, Guidotti LG, Kuhlen CV, Fowler P, Chisari FV. Immune pathogenesis of hepatocellular carcinoma. *J Exp Med* 1998;188(2):341.

66. Paterlini P, Poussin K, Kew M, Franco D, Brechot C. Selective accumulation of the X transcript of hepatitis B virus in patients negative for hepatitis B surface antigen with hepatocellular carcinoma. *Hepatology* 1995;21(2):313.

67. Ioannides CG, Whiteside TL. T cell recognition of human tumors: implications for molecular immunotherapy of cancer. *Clin Immunol Immunopathol* 1993;66(2):91.

68. Tada T, Ohzeki S, Utsumi K, et al. Transforming growth factor-beta-induced inhibition of T cell function. Susceptibility difference in T cells of various phenotypes and functions and its relevance to immunosuppression in the tumor-bearing state. *J Immunol* 1991;146(3):1077.

69. Jaffe ML, Arai H, Nabel GJ. Mechanisms of tumor-induced immunosuppression: evidence for contact-dependent T cell suppression by monocytes. *Mol Med* 1996;2(6):692.

70. Chen HL, Chang MH, Ni VH, et al. Seroepidemiology of hepatitis B virus infection in children: Ten years of mass vaccination in Taiwan. *JAMA* 1996;276(11):906.

71. Chang MH. Hepatocellular carcinoma in children. *Chung Hua Min Kuo Hsiao Erh Ko I Hsueh Hui Tsa Chih* 1998;39(6):366.

72. Alter MJ, Margolis HS, Krawczynski K, et al. The natural history of community-acquired hepatitis C in the United States. The Sentinel Counties Chronic non-A, non-B Hepatitis Study Team. *N Engl J Med* 1992;327(27):1899.

73. Saito I, Miyamura T, Ohbayashi A, et al. Hepatitis C virus infection is associated with the development of hepatocellular carcinoma. *Proc Natl Acad Sci U S A* 1990;87(17):6547.

74. Alter HJ, Purcell RH, Shih JW, et al. Detection of antibody to hepatitis C virus in prospectively followed transfusion recipients with acute and chronic non-A, non-B hepatitis. *N Engl J Med* 1989; 321(22):1494.

75. Bortolotti F, Tagger A, Cadrobbi P, et al. Antibodies to hepatitis C virus in community-acquired acute non-A, non-B hepatitis. *J Hepatol* 1991;12(2):176.

76. Cerny A, McHutchison JG, Pasquinelli C, et al. Cytotoxic T lymphocyte response to hepatitis C virus-derived peptides containing the HLA A2.1 binding motif. *J Clin Invest* 1995;95(2):521.

77. Battegay M, Fikes J, Di Bisceglie AM, et al. Patients with chronic hepatitis C have circulating cytotoxic T cells which recognize hepatitis C virus-encoded peptides binding to HLA-A2.1 molecules. *J Virol* 1995;69(4):2462.

78. Koziel MJ, Dudley D, Afdhal N, et al. Hepatitis C virus (HCV)-specific cytotoxic T lymphocytes recognize epitopes in the core and envelope proteins of HCV. *J Virol* 1993;67(12):7522.

79. Koziel MJ, Dudley D, Wong JT, et al. Intrahepatic cytotoxic T lymphocytes specific for hepatitis C virus in persons with chronic hepatitis. *J Immunol* 1992;149(10):3339.

80. Koziel MJ, Dudley D, Afdhal N, et al. HLA class I-restricted cytotoxic T lymphocytes specific for hepatitis C virus. Identification of multiple epitopes and characterization of patterns of cytokine release. *J Clin Invest* 1995;96(5):2311.

81. Botarelli P, Brunetto MR, Minutello MA, et al. T-lymphocyte response to hepatitis C virus in different clinical courses of infection. *Gastroenterology* 1993;104(2):580.

82. Kammer AR, van der Burg SH, Grabscheid B, et al. Molecular mimicry of human cytochrome P450 by hepatitis C virus at the level of cytotoxic T cell recognition. 1999 (submitted).

83. zur Hausen H. Papillomavirus infections—a major cause of human cancers. *Biochimica et Biophysica Acta* 1996;1288:F55.

84. Ndisdang D, Morris PJ, Chapman C, Ho L, Singer A, Latchman DS. The HPV-activating cellular transcription factor Brn-3a is overexpressed in CIN3 cervical lesions. *J Clin Invest* 1998;101:1687.

85. Vukawa K, Butz K, Vasui T, Kikutani H, Hoppe-Seyler F. Regulation of human papillomavirus transcription by the differentiation-dependent epithelial factor Epoc-1/skn-1a. *J Virol* 1996;70(1):10.

86. Cripe TP, Haugen TH, Turk JP, et al. Transcriptional regulation of the human papillomavirus-16 E6-E7 promoter by a keratinocyte-dependent enhancer, and by viral E2 trans-activator and repressor gene products: implications for cervical carcinogenesis. *EMBO J* 1987;6(12):3745.

87. Crusius K, Auvinen E, Steuer B, Gaissert H, Alonso A. The human papillomavirus type 16 E5-protein modulates ligand-dependent activation of the EGF receptor family in the human epithelial cell line HaCaT. *Exp Cell Res* 1998;241(1):76.

88. Venuti A, Salani D, Poggiali F, Manni V, Bagnato A. The E5 oncoprotein of human papillomavirus type 16 enhances endothelin-1-induced keratinocyte growth. *Virology* 1998;248(1):1.

89. Schwarz E, Freese UK, Gissmann L, et al. Structure and transcription of human papillomavirus sequences in cervical carcinoma cells. *Nature* 1985;314(6006):111.

90. Scheffner M, Werness BA, Huibregtse JM, Levine AJ, Howley PM. The E6 oncoprotein encoded by human papillomavirus types 16 and 18 promotes the degradation of p53. *Cell* 1990;63(6):1129.

91. Zehbe I, Wilander E, Delius H, Tommasino M. Human papillomavirus 16 E6 variants are more prevalent in invasive cervical carcinoma than the prototype. *Cancer Res* 1998;58:829.

92. Dyson N, Howley PM, Munger K, Harlow E. The human papilloma virus-16 E7 oncoprotein is able to bind to the retinoblastoma gene product. *Science* 1989;243(4893):934.

93. Stanley M. Papillomavirus: biology and clinical implications for immunotherapy. *Mol Med Today* 1997;3(6):239.

94. Doorbar J, Foo C, Coleman N, et al. Characterization of events during the late stages of HPV16 infection in vivo using high-affinity synthetic Fabs to E4. *Virology* 1997;238(1):40.

95. Stanley MA. Virus-keratinocyte interactions in the infectious cycle. In: Stern PL, Stanley MA, eds. *Human papillomaviruses and cervical cancer: biology and immunology.* Oxford: Oxford University Press, 1994:116.

96. Vernon SD, Unger ER, Miller DL, Lee DR, Reeves WC. Association of human papillomavirus type 16 integration in the E2 gene with poor disease-free survival from cervical cancer. *Int J Cancer* 1997;74:50.

97. Daniel B, Rangarajan A, Mukherjee G, Vallikad E, Krishna S. The link between integration and expression of human papillomavirus type 16 genomes and cellular changes in the evolution of cervical intraepithelial neoplastic lesions. *J Gen Virol* 1997;78:1095.

98. Lorincz AT, Temple GF, Kurman RJ, Jenson AB, Lancaster WD. Oncogenic association of specific human papillomavirus types with cervical neoplasia. *J Natl Cancer Inst* 1987;79(4):671.

99. Downey GP, Bavin PJ, Deery AR, et al. Relation between human papillomavirus type 16 and potential for progression of minor-grade cervical disease. *Lancet* 1994;344(8920):432.

100. Londesborough P, Ho L, Terry G, Cuzick J, Wheeler C, Singer A. Human papillomavirus genotype as a predictor of persistence and development of high-grade lesions in women with minor cervical abnormalities. *Int J Cancer* 1996;69:364.

101. Pirami L, Giache V, Becciolini A. Analysis of HPV16, 18, 31, and 35 DNA in pre-invasive and invasive lesions of the uterine cervix. *J Clin Pathol* 1997;50(7):600.

102. Bosch FX, Manos MM, Munoz N, et al. Prevalence of human papillomavirus in cervical cancer: a worldwide perspective. International biological study on cervical cancer (IBSCC) Study Group. *J Natl Cancer Inst* 1995;87(11):796.

103. Stern PL. Immunity to human papillomavirus-associated cervical neoplasia. *Adv Cancer Res* 1996;69:175.

104. Krul EJT, Schipper RF, Schreuder GMT, Fleuren GJ, Kenter GG, Melief CJM. HLA and susceptibility to cervical neoplasia. *Hum Immunol* 1999;60 (*in press*).

105. Aiba S, Rokugo M, Tagami H. Immunohistologic analysis of the phenomenon of spontaneous regression of numerous flat warts. *Cancer* 1986;58(6):1246.

106. Keating PJ, Cromme FV, Duggan-Keen M, et al. Frequency of down-regulation of individual HLA-A and -B alleles in cervical carcinomas in relation to TAP-1 expression. *Br J Cancer* 1995;72(2):405.

107. Evans EM, Man S, Evans AS, Borysiewicz LK. Infiltration of cervical cancer tissue with human papillomavirus-specific cytotoxic T-lymphocytes. *Cancer Res* 1997;57:2943.

108. Nimako M, Fiander A, Wilkinson GWG, Borysiewicz LK, Man S. Human papillomavirus-specific cytotoxic T lymphocytes in patients with cervical intraepithelial neoplasia grade III. *Cancer Res* 1997; 57:4855.

109. Nakagawa M, Stites DP, Farhat S, et al. Cytotoxic T lymphocyte responses to E6 and E7 proteins of human papillomavirus type 16: relationship to cervical intraepithelial neoplasia. *J Infect Dis* 1997; 175:927.

110. Borysiewicz LK, Fiander A, Nimako M, et al. A recombinant vaccinia virus encoding human papillomavirus types 16 and 18, E6 and E7 proteins as immunotherapy for cervical cancer. *Lancet* 1996; 347:1523.

111. Ressing ME, van Driel WJ, Celis E, et al. Occasional memory cytotoxic T-cell responses of patients with human papillomavirus type 16-positive cervical lesions against a human leukocyte antigen-A*0201-restricted E7-encoded epitope. *Cancer Res* 1996;56:582.

112. Bontkes HJ, de Gruiji TD, van den Muysenberg AJC, et al. Human papillomavirus type 16 E6 and E7 specific cytotoxic T lymphocyte responses are associated with persistent viral infection in patients with cervical intraepithelial neoplasia. *17th International Papillomavirus Conference*, Charleston, South Carolina, USA. 1999.

113. de Gruiji T, Bontkes HJ, Walboomers JMM, et al. Differential T helper cell responses to human papillomavirus type 16 E7 related to viral clearance or persistence in patients with cervical neoplasia: a longitudinal study. *Cancer Res* 1998;58:1700.

114. Kochel HG, Monazahian M, Sievert K, et al. Occurrence of antibodies to L1, L2, E4 and E7 gene products of human papillomavirus

types 6b, 16 and 18 among cervical cancer patients and controls. *Int J Cancer* 1991;48(5):682.

115. Muller M, Viscidi RP, Ulken V, et al. Antibodies to the E4, E6, and E7 proteins of human papillomavirus (HPV) type 16 in patients with HPV-associated diseases and in the normal population. *J Invest Dermatol* 1995;104(1):138.

116. Kanda T, Onda T, Zanma S, et al. Independent association of antibodies against human papillomavirus type 16 E1/E4 and E7 proteins with cervical cancer. *Virology* 1992;190(2):724.

117. Di Lonardo A, Marcante ML, Poggiali F, Venuti A. HPV 16 E7 antibody levels in cervical cancer patients: before and after treatment. *J Med Virol* 1998;54(3):192.

118. de Gruijl TD, Bontkes HJ, Walboomers JM, et al. Immunoglobulin G responses against human papillomavirus type 16 virus-like particles in a prospective nonintervention cohort study of women with cervical intraepithelial neoplasia. *J Natl Cancer Inst* 1997;89(9):630.

119. de Gruijl TD, Bontkes HJ, Walboomers JM, et al. Analysis of IgG reactivity against human papillomavirus type-16 E/ in patients with cervical intraepithelial neoplasia indicates an association with clearance of viral infection: results of a prospective study. *Int J Cancer* 1996;68(6):731.

120. Tsukui T, Hildesheim A, Schiffman MH, et al. Interleukin 2 production in vitro by peripheral lymphocytes in response to human papillomavirus-derived peptides: correlation with cervical pathology. *Cancer Res* 1996;56(17):3967.

121. Clerici M, Merola M, Ferrario E, et al. Cytokine production patterns in cervical intraepithelial neoplasia: association with human papillomavirus infection. *J Natl Cancer Inst* 1997;89(3):245.

122. Tartour E, Gey A, Sastre-Garau X, Lombard Surin I, Mosseri V, Fridman WH. Prognostic value of intratumoral interferon gamma messenger RNA expression in invasive cervical carcinomas. *J Natl Cancer Inst* 1998;90(4):287.

123. Perea SE, Massimi P, Banks L. Human papillomavirus type 16 (HPV-16) E7 impairs the interferon regulatory factor-1 (IRF-1) activation. *17th International Papillomavirus Conference*, Charleston, South Carolina, USA. 1999.

124. Gloss B, Bernard HU, Seedorf K, Klock G. The upstream regulatory region of the human papilloma virus-16 contains an E2 protein-independent enhancer which is specific for cervical carcinoma cells and regulated by glucocorticoid hormones. *EMBO J* 1987; 6(12):3735.

125. Pater MM, Hughes GA, Hyslop DE, Nakshatri H, Pater A. Glucocorticoid-dependent oncogenic transformation by type 16 but not type 11 human papilloma virus DNA. *Nature* 1988;335(6193):832.

126. Arbeit JM, Howley PM, Hanahan D. Chronic estrogen-induced cervical and vaginal squamous carcinogenesis in human papillomavirus type 16 transgenic mice. *Proc Natl Acad Sci U S A* 1996;93:2930.

127. Bartholomew JS, Glenville S, Sarkar S, et al. Integration of high-risk human papillomavirus DNA is linked to the down-regulation of class I human leukocyte antigens by steroid hormones in cervical tumor cells. *Cancer Res* 1997;57:937.

128. Galloway DA. Is vaccination against human papillomavirus a possibility? *Lancet* 1998;351:22.

129. Wang Z, Hansson BG, Forslund O, et al. Cervical mucus antibodies against human papillomavirus type 16, 18, and 33 capsids in relation to presence of viral DNA. *J Clin Microbiol* 1996;34(12):3056.

130. Feltkamp MC, Smits HL, Vierboom MP, et al. Vaccination with cytotoxic T lymphocyte epitope-containing peptide protects against a tumor induced by human papillomavirus type 16-transformed cells. *Eur J Immunol* 1993;23(9):2242.

131. De Bruijn ML, Schuurhuis DH, Vierboom MP, et al. Immunization with human papillomavirus type 16 (HPV16) oncoprotein-loaded dendritic cells as well as protein in adjuvant induces MHC class I restricted protection to HPV16-induced tumor cells. *Cancer Res* 1998;58(4):724.

132. Greenstone HL, Nieland JD, de Visser KE, et al. Chimeric papillomavirus virus-like particles elicit antitumor immunity against the E7 oncoprotein in an HPV16 tumor model. *Proc Natl Acad Sci U S A* 1998;95(4):1800.

133. Meneguzzi G, Cerni C, Kieny MP, Lathe R. Immunization against human papillomavirus type 16 tumor cells with recombinant vaccinia viruses expressing E6 and E7. *Virology* 1991;181(1):62.

134. Toes REM, Hoeben RC, van der Voort EIH, et al. Protective antitumor immunity induced by vaccination with recombinant adenoviruses encoding multiple tumor-associated cytotoxic T lymphocyte epitopes in a string-of-bead fashion. *Proc Natl Acad Sci U S A* 1997;94:14660.

135. Mayordomo JI, Zorina T, Storkus WJ, et al. Bone marrow-derived dendritic cells pulsed with synthetic tumour peptides elicit protective and therapeutic antitumor immunity. *Nat Med* 1995;1(12):1297.

136. Zitvogel L, Mayordomo JI, Tjandrawan T, et al. Therapy of murine tumors with tumor peptide-pulsed dendritic cells: dependence on T cells, B7 costimulation, and T helper cell 1-associated cytokines. *J Exp Med* 1996;183(1):87.

137. Kast WM, Offringa R, Peters PJ, et al. Eradication of adenovirus E1-induced tumors by E1A-specific cytotoxic T lymphocytes. *Cell* 1989;59(4):603.

138. Vierboom MP, Nijman HW, Offringa R, et al. Tumor eradication by wild-type p53-specific cytotoxic T lymphocytes. *J Exp Med* 1997;186(5):695.

139. Feltkamp MC, Vreugdenhil GR, Vierboom MP, et al. Cytotoxic T lymphocytes raised against a subdominant epitope offered as a synthetic peptide eradicate human papillomavirus type 16-induced tumors. *Eur J Immunol* 1995;25(9):2638.

140. Walter EA, Greenberg PD, Gilbert MJ, et al. Reconstitution of cellular immunity against cytomegalovirus in recipients of allogeneic bone marrow by transfer of T-cell clones from the donor. *N Engl J Med* 1995;333(16):1038.

141. Rosenberg SA, Packard BS, Aebersold PM, et al. Use of tumor-infiltrating lymphocytes and interleukin-2 in the immunotherapy of patients with metastatic melanoma. A preliminary report. *N Engl J Med* 1988;319(25):1676.

142. Alexander M, Salgaller ML, Celis E, et al. Generation of tumor-specific cytolytic T lymphocytes from peripheral blood of cervical cancer patients by in vitro stimulation with a synthetic human papillomavirus type 16 E7 epitope. *Am J Obstet Gynecol* 1996; 175:1586.

143. Ressing ME, Sette A, Brandt RMP, et al. Human CTL epitopes encoded by human papillomavirus type 16 E6 and E7 identified through *in vivo* and *in vitro* immunogenicity studies of HLA-A*0201 binding peptides. *J Immunol* 1995;154:5934.

144. van der Burg SH, Kwappenberg KM, Geluk A, et al. Identification of a conserved universal Th epitope in HIV-1 reverse transcriptase that is processed and presented to HIV-specific CD4+ T cells by at least four unrelated HLA-DR molecules. *J Immunol* 1999; 162(1):152.

145. Ossendorp F, Mengede E, Camps M, Filius R, Melief CJM. Specific T helper cell requirement for optimal induction of cytotoxic T lymphocytes against major histocompatibility complex class II negative tumors. *J Exp Med* 1998;187(5):1.

146. Keene JA, Forman J. Helper activity is required for the *in vivo* generation of cytotoxic T lymphocytes. *J Exp Med* 1982;155(3):768.

147. Bennett SR, Carbone FR, Karamalis F, Miller JF, Heath WR. Induction of a CD8+ cytotoxic T lymphocyte response by cross-priming requires cognate CD4+ T cell help. *J Exp Med* 1997;186(1):65.

148. Bennett SRM, Carbone FR, Karamalis F, Flavell RA, Miller JFAP, Heath WR. Help for cytotoxic-T-cell responses is mediated by CD40 signaling. *Nature* 1998;393(6684):478.

149. Schoenberger SF, Toes RE, van der Voort EI, Offringa R, Melief CJ. T-cell help for cytotoxic T lymphocytes is mediated by CD40-CD40L interactions. *Nature* 1998;393(6684):480.

150. Ridge JP, Di Rosa F, Matzinger P. A conditioned dendritic cell can be a temporal bridge between a CD4+ T-helper and a T-killer cell. *Nature* 1998;393(6684):474.

151. Hung K, Hayashi R, Lafond-Walker A, Lowenstein C, Pardoll D, Levitsky H. The central role of CD4(+) T cells in the antitumor immune response. *J Exp Med* 1998;188(12):2357.

152. Toes REM, Ossendorp F, Offringa R, Melief CJM. CD4 T cells and their role in antitumor immune responses. *J Exp Med* 1999;185(5):753.

153. Ressing ME, van Driel WJ, Brandt RMP, et al. Detection of immune responses to helper peptide, but not to viral CTL epitopes, following peptide vaccination of immunocompromised patients with recurrent cervical carcinoma. 1999 (submitted).

154. Steller MA, Gurski KJ, Murakami M, et al. Cell-mediated immuno- logical responses in cervical and vaginal cancer patients immunized with a lipidated epitope of human papillomavirus type 16 E7. *Clin Cancer Res* 1998;4(9):2103.

155. Tindle RW. Human papillomavirus vaccines for cervical cancer. *Curr Opin Immunol* 1998;8:643.

16.4

CANCER VACCINES: CANCER ANTIGENS

Oncogenes and Mutations

JAY A. BERZOFSKY
LEE J. HELMAN
DAVID P. CARBONE

Two of the important criteria for a good tumor antigen are (a) unique expression in the tumor cell that allows the immune system to distinguish cancer cells from normal cells and (b) essentialness of the function of the protein for malignant transformation, preventing the tumor from escaping the immune response by suppressing expression of the antigen without losing its malignant phenotype. Mutations that occur in oncogenes and tumor suppressor genes often fulfill both of these criteria, because the mutation is unique to the tumor and also results in a function that contributes to the malignant phenotype. For these reasons, mutant oncogene and tumor suppressor gene products, such as mutant ras or mutant p53, have been widely studied as potential tumor antigens against which to target immunotherapeutic vaccines. Of a similar nature, but not a mutation in the strict sense, are the fusion proteins created by chromosomal translocations. These are formed when a chromosomal translocation juxtaposes the 5' portion of one gene with the 3' portion of another to create a new gene and a novel gene product not present in normal cells. Several of these, such as those that occur in several leukemias and sarcomas (see Novel Fusion Proteins Created by Chromosomal Translocations), result in novel transcription factors that cause aberrant transcription of genes that lead to the malignant phenotype. Thus, they meet the criterion that they are causal and hence essential for the malignant transformation. Furthermore, the junction or breakpoint at which the two sequences join may create a neoantigenic determinant that is not present in either of the parent proteins from which the fusion was derived. Any epitope that spans this breakpoint junction is unique to the tumor. Thus, these fusion proteins meet the same criteria as missense mutations in oncogenes and in effect create novel oncogenes. All of these types of tumor-unique antigens are discussed in this chapter. Also discussed are certain oncoprotein/receptors that are overexpressed in the tumor, albeit not unique to the tumor, such as HER-2/*neu*. These may serve as tumor markers, because, if the level of expression in normal cells is too low to be detected by the immune system, only the tumor cells that overexpress these proteins may be detected.

One key aspect of most of these oncogene product or mutant protein potential tumor antigens, other than receptors or receptor-like proteins such as HER-2/*neu*, is that they are not cell-surface proteins and thus are not accessible to antibodies. Indeed, many of these are predominantly nuclear proteins. Such internal proteins were not originally considered candidate tumor antigens because of the inaccessibility to antibodies. However, the key discovery from basic immunology, that the T-cell immune system is designed to detect internal proteins that are not necessarily ever expressed intact on the cell surface (1,2), has opened the door to exploiting these unique tumor markers as potential vaccine targets. In particular, class I major histocompatibility complex (MHC)–encoded molecules such as HLA-A, -B, and -C in humans or H-2K, D, or L in mice, appear to have evolved to provide surveillance of all proteins synthesized in a cell and displaying fragments of these for recognition by CD8+ T lymphocytes, such as cytotoxic T lymphocytes (CTLs). A portion of all protein molecules made in the cell is degraded by proteasomes in the cytosol and short peptide fragments of these are actively transported from the

TABLE 1. POTENTIAL TUMOR-SPECIFIC ANTIGENS DISCUSSED

Tumor Antigen	Major Histocompatibility Complex Class	Tumor Type
Mutant Proteins		
ras	I and II	Wide variety of tumors
p53	I	Wide variety of tumors
p16	I	Wide variety of tumors
β-Catenin	I	Melanoma
Triosephosphate isomerase	II	Melanoma
CDC 27	II	Melanoma
Fusion proteins		
BCR-ABL	I and II	Leukemia
TEL-AML-1	I	Leukemia
EWS-FLI-1	I (and II?)	Sarcoma
PAX-3-FKHR	I (and II?)	Sarcoma
EWS-ATF1	I (and II?)	Sarcoma
EWS-WT1	I (and II?)	Sarcoma
SSX-SYT	I (and II?)	Sarcoma
Overexpressed oncoproteins		
HER-2/*neu*	I	Variety of tumors

cytosol to the endoplasmic reticulum by a heterodimer complex called the *transporter of antigenic peptides.* In the endoplasmic reticulum, these peptides bind to newly synthesized class I MHC molecules that then carry them out to the cell surface and display them within their peptide-binding groove, for recognition by CD8+ T cells. The T-cell receptors are specific for the complex of a particular peptide bound to a particular MHC molecule, accounting for the phenomenon of genetic restriction of T cells that has played so critical a role in immunology that its discovery led to the award of a Nobel prize (3). T cells with receptors that could recognize fragments of normal cell proteins presented by the host's own MHC molecules are most often deleted in the thymus, by a process called *negative selection,* or are tolerized by other mechanisms of peripheral self-tolerance. Thus, the T cells would be expected to react primarily to any protein that is not present in normal cells, such as viral proteins made in virally infected cells or mutant or otherwise abnormal proteins expressed in tumor cells. The surveillance provided by the class-I MHC molecule thus declares these abnormal cells to the immune system and facilitates their elimination.

If these unique tumor antigen markers exist and can be presented by MHC molecules, why are not all tumors harboring them deleted by the immune system before they reach a clinical stage? The answer probably lies in the fact that most tumor cells are not effective antigen-presenting cells (APCs), lacking the critical costimulatory molecules, such as CD80 and CD86, or intercellular adhesion molecule-1 (ICAM-1) and leukocyte function-associated antigen-3 (LFA 3), that contribute to activating T cells. Thus, they may never initiate an immune response and so avoid detection. These accessory molecules are needed only for the afferent limb of the immune response and its induction, however, not for the efferent limb or effector phase. Thus, if a vaccine that allows the relevant tumor antigens to be presented on professional APCs, such as dendritic cells (4,5), which express these accessory or costimulatory molecules at high levels, can induce CTLs specific for the tumor antigens presented on the patient's class I MHC molecules, these

CTLs should be able to recognize the tumor cells and destroy them. Only the expression of the antigen presented by the MHC molecules is necessary for the tumor cells to function as targets of the CTLs. Therefore, lack of immunogenicity of the tumor does not imply that it is not amenable to specific immunotherapy.

A review of the progress in developing these mutant proteins, fusion proteins, and other oncogene products as tumor antigen targets of vaccines for the immunotherapy of cancer, both in animal models and in human clinical trials, is covered in this chapter. The potential tumor antigens discussed are listed in Table 1. Other reviews of tumor antigens, including some in these categories, have been published (6,7).

MUTANT ras

Mutant ras protein constitutes a potentially valuable tumor antigen because ras mutations are present in approximately 15% of cancers, including, for example, approximately 90% of adenocarcinoma of the pancreas and almost 50% of colorectal adenocarcinomas, approximately 30% of lung adenocarcinomas, and approximately 50% of thyroid tumors as well as 30% of myeloid leukemias (8), but are not present in normal cells. Furthermore, they fulfill the second criterion mentioned in the first paragraph of this chapter, in that they contribute directly to malignant transformation, and thus their expression cannot be suppressed to escape immune detection without loss of the malignant state. ras Is a key molecule in the signal transduction pathway for cell activation. Another advantage of ras mutations is that the vast majority occurs at one of three codons, 12, 13, and 61, and thus they are limited in variety. For example, in one large study of colorectal cancer (9), 80.8% of the Ki-ras mutations occurred at codon 12, which is a glycine in the wild-type protein. Most of the remainder were codon-13 mutations. Of the codon-12 mutations, Asp was the most common (30.6% of codon-12 mutations), followed by Val (23.4%). Other common but less frequent codon-12 mutations were to cysteine, alanine, and serine. Of the codon 13 mutations, the vast majority was from Gly to Asp. Thus, a few mutant sequences might provide a vaccine for a large number of different cancers. Meta-analysis of a number of epidemiologic studies indicates that mutations in ras may have an adverse impact on prognosis in colorectal cancer (9). In this study, ras 12-Val stood out as the only mutation that by itself conveyed an increased risk of recurrence and death (p = 0.007 and 0.004, respectively). Thus, mutant ras-bearing tumors may be important targets also because they are present in more aggressive cancers.

Animal Models of Mutant ras

To obtain proof of principle that mutant ras could serve as a tumor antigen for immunotherapy of cancer, several groups developed mouse models. Both CD4[+] and CD8[+] T-cell responses were obtained.

CD4[+] T Cells

Peace et al. (10) from the group of Cheever pioneered the use of ras as a tumor antigen in murine models (7). First to be detected were CD4[+] T-cells from C57BL/6 (H-2[b]) mice specific for the codon-12 Arg mutation presented by the class II MHC molecule I-A[b]. T cells raised by immunization with a synthetic peptide spanning residues 5 to 16 responded not only to the immunizing peptide but also to the intact mutant ras p21 protein. Additionally, C3H/HeN (H-2[k]) mice immunized with peptide spanning residues 54 to 66, containing the Leu mutation at codon 61, responded to this mutant peptide. In both cases, the wild-type peptide was not recognized, indicating that the T cells could distinguish the single point mutation from the wild-type sequence, an essential requirement if a vaccine is to be tumor specific. Furthermore, immunization with the intact 61 Leu mutant p21 ras protein was able to elicit CD4[+] T cells from C3H/HeN mice specific for the 61 Leu-containing synthetic peptide (11), indicating that the flanking sequences in the native mutant protein did not interfere with immunogenicity of the epitope.

Abrams et al. (12) were able to raise CD4[+] T cells from BALB/c mice immunized with a peptide spanning residues 5 to 17 and containing the codon-12 Val mutation. These cells were phenotyped as Th1 by their cytokine production [including interleukin-2 (IL-2), interferon-γ (IFN-γ), and tumor necrosis factor] and by their ability to lyse target cells in a class II MHC–restricted fashion. The restriction element was mapped using monoclonal antibodies and transfected L cells to the hybrid molecule containing the A[b]β chain and the Eα chain. Importantly, these T cells, CD4[+] not CD8[+], could lyse A20 B lymphoma cells transfected with the mutant K-ras oncogene with the 12 Val mutation. Abrams et al. (13) then went on to identify an overlapping epitope in the same mutant sequence presented by the H-2K[d] class-I molecule. These CD8[+] CTLs recognized the ras 4-12 peptide containing the 12-Val mutation, but not the corresponding wild-type peptide. They also lysed the A20 lymphoma transduced with the corresponding mutant ras oncogene. Thus, the same mutant peptide can serve to induce both

CD4[+] and CD8[+] CTLs specific for closely overlapping epitopes in mutant ras, which might function together to reject tumor cells. Furthermore, Th1 cells specific for this site might provide help for the induction or maintenance of the CD8[+] CTLs.

CD8[+] T Cells

Murine CD8[+] CTLs specific for mutant ras peptides were first described by Skipper and Stauss (14). C57BL/10 mice immunized with recombinant vaccinia viruses expressing either N-ras with the mutation of Gln to Lys at codon 61 or wild-type N-ras produced CTLs that recognized the same segment 60 to 67 of ras but did not cross-react, so that the ones immunized with the mutant sequence recognized only that and not the wild-type and vice versa. They also recognized targets expressing the whole mutant or wild-type ras, respectively, expressed either by transfection or infection with recombinant vaccinia virus. However, they did not lyse normal cells expressing the normal endogenous levels of ras. These were just the characteristics that one would like to obtain for immunotherapy (i.e., specificity for the mutation and ability to lyse cells expressing mutant ras but not normal cells). Peace et al. (15) carried out binding assays for overlapping ras peptides spanning the Gln to Leu mutation at codon 61 to determine which bound with highest affinity to the murine class I MHC molecule H-2K[b], and identified the nonamer 59 to 67 as the best binder. They used this for induction of a primary *in vitro* CTL response from naive C57BL/6 spleen cells, and raised a CTL line that they showed recognized this peptide presented by H-2K[b], as well as a B6-fibroblast line transformed by transfection with the c-Ha-ras 61-Leu gene. These CTLs were specific for the mutation, as they did not recognize untransfected fibroblasts or cells incubated with the wild-type sequence peptide. Thus, CTLs could be raised that were mutation-specific and killed tumor cells expressing the mutant ras gene. To test whether soluble ras protein could elicit CTLs that could protect an animal from a tumor expressing the ras mutation, Fenton et al. (16) immunized BALB/c mice with 5-μg soluble recombinant-ras protein expressing the 12-Arg mutation intraperitoneally and were able to elicit mutation-specific CD8[+] CTLs as well as protection in nine of ten mice against challenge with tumor cells expressing the Arg-12 mutation. The protected animals were disease free for more than 6 months after tumor challenge. The protection was specific in that no protection was observed after challenge with tumor cells expressing the Val-12 mutation instead of Arg 12, and no protection against the Arg-12 tumors was seen after immunization with the wild-type ras protein. Thus, ras mutation-specific CTLs could be induced that protected mice *in vivo* against a tumor expressing the corresponding mutation in ras. These results are promising for the immunotherapy of human tumors expressing mutant ras.

Human T-Cell Responses to Mutant ras Epitopes

Human CD4[+] T Cells

Jung and Schluesener (17) first identified human CD4[+] T cells specific for mutant ras by *in vitro* stimulation of peripheral blood mononuclear cells (PBMCs) from normal healthy blood donors with a mutant peptide corresponding to residues 5 to 16 of ras containing the mutation of Gly to Val at codon 12. These were found to be restricted by the class II MHC molecule HLA-DR1. Importantly, they did not respond to the corresponding wild-type ras peptide with Gly 12. Gedde-Dahl et al. (18) similarly were able to induce human primary *in vitro* T-cell responses to mutant ras peptides corresponding to residues 1 to 25, including T-cell lines specific for ras-12-Arg and ras-12-Lys restricted by HLA-DR and ones specific for ras-12-Val restricted by HLA-DQ. Gedde-Dahl et al. (19) also identified HLA-DQ8–restricted memory T cells from a patient with follicular thyroid carcinoma specific for the ras-61 Gln to Leu mutation that did not cross-react with the corresponding wild-type ras. Inability to detect this ras mutation in tumor biopsies was puzzling, but taken to suggest the possibility that tumor cells expressing this mutation had arisen and been cleared by the immune system, as this response was not seen in healthy, nontumor-bearing patients. Since these 1992 studies, this group of Thorsby and Gaudernack has continued to be perhaps the most productive in pursuing the induction of human T cells against mutant ras for the therapy of cancer. Gedde-Dahl et al. (20) went on to show that overlapping epitopes spanning the ras-61-Leu mutation were presented by HLA-DQ8 and by HLA-DQ4 to several T-cell clones with different T-cell receptors from this same patient, suggesting some promiscuity of presentation. Similarly, in a study by Fossum et al. (21), the same group went on to show that the segment spanning residues 9 to 16 of the mutant ras with codon 12 Arg was a promiscuous epitope presented by at least three distinct human class II HLA molecules, HLA-DR2, -DQ7, and -DP3. This result suggested that a broad segment of the HLA-diverse population might be able to respond to mutant-ras peptides. Fossum et al. (22,23) also found that HLA-DQ7 presented two overlapping epitope peptides containing the ras-13-Asp mutation to independent T-cell clones with distinct T-cell receptors from a colon cancer patient. In an analysis of 251 colon cancer patients, 26 of whom had ras-13-Asp mutations, they did not find a decreased frequency of HLA-DQ7 among those with ras-13-Asp mutations, as might have been expected if this HLA allele were protective, but fewer ras-13-Asp–expressing tumors were classified in advanced Dukes' stages when DQ7 was present (p <0.025, among 26 patients studied), suggesting a modifying effect of this HLA molecule. Cheever's group (24) also examined pancreatic and colon cancer patients for the presence of CD4+ T-cell proliferative responses to mutant ras-12-Asp, the most common of the ras mutations, and found responses in 7 of 16 (44%) of the pancreatic cancer patients, and 2 of 25 (8%) of the colon cancer patients, but not in any of 11 normal individuals, suggesting natural immune responses to mutant ras can be generated by the tumor. It should also be noted that Chicz et al. (25) identified a ras peptide naturally processed and able to be eluted from HLA-DR8 molecules, indicating that endogenous ras can be processed and presented by class II MHC molecules in human cells. Cheever's group also demonstrated serum antibodies to mutant ras-12-Asp p21 protein in 51 of 160 colon cancer patients (32%), compared to 1 of 40 (2.5%) normal individuals, consistent with the induction of antibodies to ras by the presence of the tumor (26). Most of the antibodies were directed to the unmutated portions of the molecule, espe-cially the carboxyl terminus, although some was directed to the mutant epitope. Thus, the breaking of tolerance to ras by the presence of the tumor could be due to level of expression, increased apoptosis of tumor cells and resulting antigen presentation, or the induction of T-helper cells specific for the mutant epitope, providing help for autoimmune B cells.

Based on these promising studies, Gjertsen et al. (27,28) carried out a human clinical trial of vaccine immunotherapy in pancreatic cancer patients. They immunized five patients with pancreatic cancer and ras mutations (three patients with 12 Asp, one each with 12 Val and 12 Arg) with 1 to 4 x 10⁹ leukaphere-sed, autologous PBMCs pulsed overnight with 25 µmol of the ras 5 to 21 peptide corresponding to the mutation with Val, Arg, or Asp at codon 12 in their tumor. None of the patients had T-cell proliferative responses to the peptide before vaccination, and two developed transient responses after immunization, one specific for ras-12-Val uniquely and the other responsive to ras-12-Asp (but cross-reactive with wild-type ras-12-Gly). No adverse effects of the vaccination were detected, even in the patient who developed T cells cross-reactive with wild-type ras. No complete or partial tumor response was seen to the therapy, but the two responding patients survived longer (9 and 12 months) than the nonresponding patients (3.5, 4.5, and 5 months, respectively). Whether this intriguing observation in the small group of patients reflects a result of the therapy, a greater ability of healthier patients to mount an immune response, or a mere coincidence cannot be determined.

Human CD8+ T-Cell Responses

In the case of CD8+ T-cell responses primarily measured as CTLs, Fossum et al. (23) first described CD8+ T cells isolated from the blood of a colon cancer patient specific for mutant ras-13-Asp. Importantly, these cells were shown to kill a human tumor cell line, HCT116, which expresses the ras-13-Asp mutation and shares both HLA-A2 and -B12 with the patient (29), if the tumor cells were treated with IFN-γ. The lytic activity could be blocked by anti-CD8 and by anti-HLA-B12, mapping the restriction element, and proving for the first time that a human tumor cell could process and present endogenous mutant p21-ras in association with a human class I MHC molecule on the tumor cell (29).

Elsas et al. (30) identified a peptide containing the ras-61-Leu mutation as the C-terminal anchor residue that bound to HLA-A2.1 and were able to raise primary *in vitro* CTL responses to this peptide in PBMCs of normal healthy HLA-A2.1–positive individuals by stimulation with T2 cells deficient in the transporter of antigenic peptides that were loaded homogeneously with the mutant ras peptide bound to HLA-A2.1. The wild-type peptide, with Gln at the C-terminus, which is not a functional anchor residue, bound much more weakly to HLA-A2.1 than the mutant peptide and was not recognized by the CTLs. However, the CTLs in this case did not lyse melanoma cells transfected with the mutant ras gene, perhaps because their avidity was too low. Similarly, Juretic et al. (31) were able to raise *in vitro* CTLs against ras-61-Leu peptides presented by HLA-A2.1 from PBMCs of healthy individuals, but none of these killed tumor cells expressing the specific mutation.

Peptide	Sequence	Relative Affinity	Origin
WT	YKLVVVGAGGVGKSALT	±	Ras wild-type
PR5	--------V--------	Not tested	Ras mutants
PR6	--------D--------	±	
PR7	--------A--------	±	
PR18	--------C--------	+++	
PR24	--------R--------	±	
PR54	KLVVVGAGDVGKSALTI	+++	
WT V10	KLVVVGAGGV	±	Ras wild-type
PR5 V10	-------V--	±	Ras mutants
PR6 V10	-------D--	+++	
	-------A--	+++	
	-------C--	+	
	--------D-	±	
P18-I10	RGPGRAFVTI	+++	Human immunodeficiency virus envelope protein
FMP	GILGFVFTL	+++++	Influenza matrix protein

FIGURE 1. Mutations in ras peptides affect binding to HLA-A2.1 as well as extracellular processing. Peptides shown from ras residues 4 to 20 or 5 to 14, with or without mutations at codon 12 or 13, were tested along with control peptides for binding to the most common human class I major histocompatibility complex molecule, HLA-A2.1, in a T2 cell–binding assay. The assay, described by Nijman et al. (34), takes advantage of the fact that T2 cells lack the transporter of antigenic peptides, and so do not load endogenous peptides to newly synthesized class I molecules. The few empty class I molecules that reach the cell surface are unstable and rapidly lost unless they bind a peptide, which stabilizes the conformation. Thus, in the presence of a peptide that can bind to HLA-A2.1, the steady-state level of HLA-A2.1 on the surface of the T2 cells increases and can be measured by fluorescence-activated cell sorter scan. The relative affinity is determined from the relative concentration required to induce a 50% increase in HLA-A2.1 expression. Some of the ras peptides bind better as decapeptides, such as ras-12-Asp and ras-12-Ala, whereas some bind better as 17-mers, such as ras-12-Cys and ras-13-Asp. However, most of the mutant ras sequences in one form or the other bind better than the wild-type peptide. The differences in binding between the longer and shorter peptides depend in part on the need for proteolysis of the longer peptides and the sensitivity to proteolysis of the shorter peptides, both of which appear to be influenced by the mutation at codon 12 or 13. The 17-mers were designed to include all possible 9-mers containing the point mutation. Note: Nine- and ten-residue peptides were tested in the presence of protease inhibitor 1, 10-phenanthrolene. (HIV, human immunodeficiency virus; NT, not tested; +, positive; +++, strongly positive; ±, marginally positive.) (Based on results described in Smith MC, Pendleton CD, Maher VE, Kelley MJ, Carbone DP, Berzofsky JA. Oncogenic mutations in ras create HLA-A2.1 binding peptides but affect their extracellular processing. *Internat Immunol* 1997;9:1085–1093, with permission.)

On the other hand, Gjertsen et al. (32) were able to raise CD8+ CTLs (as well as CD4+ T cells) specific for ras-12-Val from a pancreatic cancer patient whom they immunized with a mutant ras-17-mer peptide containing this mutation. In this case, they were able to raise an autologous pancreatic tumor cell line and show that these tumor cells were killed by the ras-12-Val–specific CD8+ CTLs (as well as by the CD4+ CTLs) from the patient. Using tumor cell lines matched for either HLA-B35 or for the ras-12-Val mutation, or both, they showed that the CTLs were specific for the mutant peptide endogenously presented by HLA-B35 on the tumor cells. Thus, mutant ras in these pancreatic tumors is endogenously processed and presented to autologous CTLs by the tumor's class I MHC molecules. The most common human class I MHC molecule is HLA-A2.1, present in almost one-half of most populations. Smith et al. (33) found that the ras peptides spanning residues 5 to 14 contained an HLA-A2.1–binding sequence motif and, using a binding assay with T2 cells described by Nijman et al. (34), they found that most of the ras-12 and ras-13 mutant peptides bound to HLA-A2.1 with higher affinity than the wild-type ras-12-Gly, 13-Gly peptide (Fig. 1). This preferential binding may favor generation of responses specific for the mutant sequence in the tumor that do not cross-react with the wild-type sequence present in normal cells. The mutations were also found to have some effect on the processing of the peptides by extracellular serum or cell-surface proteases, making the 10-mers more effective in some cases and longer (17-mer) peptides more effective in other cases (33) (see Fig. 1). In a phase 1 trial just being completed, we immunized cancer patients with autologous PBMCs pulsed with synthetic 17-mer peptides, with the mutation in the center, containing all possible nonapeptides spanning the mutation present in the patient's tumor. We were able to raise mutant ras-specific CTLs against ras-13-Asp, ras-12-val, and ras-12-Cys, especially in patients bearing HLA-A2.1, but did not have tumor specimens to test the ability of the CTLs to lyse tumors (Carbone et al., manuscript in preparation). In a phase 1 phase 2 trial, Khleif et al. (35) and Abrams et al. (36) immunized patients with mutant ras-13-mer peptides containing codon-12 Asp, Cys, or Val mutations. They were able to raise both class II, HLA-DQ–restricted CD4+ T cells and class-I HLA-A2.1–restricted CD8+ T cells specific for the ras-12-Val mutant peptide from one patient, as well as a CD4+ T-cell line specific for ras-12-Cys, and a CD8+ T-cell line specific for ras-12-Asp from other patients. In this case also, the CD8+ CTLs specific for ras-

12-Val could lyse a nonautologous SW480 colon carcinoma cell line expressing both HLA-A2.1 and the mutant ras-12-Val if the tumor cells were treated with IFN-γ. Thus, at least three independent studies demonstrate that human CD8+ CTLs from cancer patients, in two of the cases immunized with mutant ras peptides, can kill human tumor cells naturally, endogenously expressing the corresponding mutant ras. In one of these cases, the tumor was autologous. These studies provide unequivocal proof that human tumor cells naturally process and present p21 ras in such a way as to present mutant peptides in association with human class I HLA molecules on their surface, and can be recognized and destroyed by human CTLs specific for these mutations. Moreover, the most common mutations at ras codon-12 and -13 can be presented by the most common class I MHC molecule, HLA-A2.1, more effectively than the wild-type peptide, as well as by at least one other human class-I molecule, HLA-B35, making these peptides potentially widely recognized as candidate tumor antigens despite the HLA diversity of the population. These results are promising for the ultimate development of mutant ras-based cancer immunotherapy.

MUTANT AND WILD-TYPE p53

p53 Is a nuclear phosphoprotein located on chromosome 17p with specific DNA binding and transcriptional activation capabilities. p53 Is frequently abnormal in human cancer, with mutation rates of more than 50% of non–small-cell lung cancer and colon cancer, and more than 90% in certain tumors such as small-cell lung cancer (37). Compared to the relatively limited number of missense mutations commonly found in activated ras, mutations in p53 are of all types: missense, nonsense, splicing, and large deletions. Approximately 80% of all somatic mutations in p53 are single amino acid substitutions, but again unlike ras, these missense mutations occur throughout the open reading frame (ORF), though they tend to be concentrated in the central region, approximately codons 140 to 300 or exons 5 to 8. For most tumor suppressor genes, mutation is usually associated with decreased or absent expression. Missense mutations in p53, however, are associated with significantly prolonged protein half-life, and thus greatly increased steady-state protein levels (38), usually by orders of magnitude. The overexpressed protein can be detected by immunohistochemistry, whereas the p53 in normal cells is usually below the detection threshold, forming the basis for a simple "screening" immunohistochemical test of clinical material for the presence of p53 mutations. Positive immunostaining shows approximately a 66% correlation with the presence of a mutation (39). The locations of missense mutations in p53 are similar between different tumor types, but there may be a preference for mutations between codon 150 to 160 in non–small cell lung cancer, and codon 175 mutations are common in colon cancer but are uncommon in lung cancer. The significance of these differences is unclear.

p53 As an Immunologic Target

Because it is so frequently mutated in cancer, when mutant p53 is usually highly overexpressed, p53 protein represents an excellent candidate as an immunotherapeutic target. Additionally,

missense mutant p53 is thought to have a dominant transforming function, resulting in selection pressure to maintain expression throughout tumor evolution. It is also clear that p53 can be recognized by the immune system. Antibodies to p53 have been observed in lung cancer patients, and their presence is highly correlated with the presence of a p53 mutation in the tumor (40). In addition, in small-cell lung cancer, an association has been observed between the presence of antibodies to any tumor cell protein (not just p53) and improved survival. Antibodies to p53 may also precede the development of clinical cancer (41), and their titer varies with disease status, suggesting that continuous antigen stimulation is required (42).

Because p53 is a nuclear protein, however, it is unlikely that the antibodies themselves could have therapeutic effect, and it is more likely that T cell responses directed toward short-peptide epitopes in the p53 protein would be the response of interest for therapy. Antibody responses usually require T-cell "help" so the presence of antibody responses suggested that T cells could indeed recognize p53 protein epitopes. In fact, immunization with anti-p53 antibodies can induce an "antiidiotype network" response and result in effective tumor protection (43,44).

The most tumor-selective potential epitopes would be the peptides containing the somatic mutation itself. If it could be recognized by CTLs, this mutant epitope would be absolutely restricted to tumor cells and not present in normal cells. Animal studies have demonstrated the induction of effective CTL responses against the mutant p53 protein. Using peptides that spanned the mutation site in human-mutant p53 coated on murine APCs to immunize animals, it is possible to show the development of p53-specific CTLs. Some of these CTLs recognized the mutant-peptide sequence and not the corresponding wild-type one (45). Specific responses to mutant epitopes were also observed to mutant p53 in the carcinogen-induced mouse tumor MethA (46). It is remarkable that a CTL response can be generated in such animals that are selective for the presence of a single amino acid substitution in the p53 protein. This underscores the specificity achievable when a finely tuned biologic process, such as the cellular immune system, is evoked, as opposed to the lack of specificity observed for standard chemotherapeutic agents. This CTL response provided tumor protection in control mice against subsequent challenge with tumor cells bearing specific mutation (46–54). It has also been possible to treat established tumors by immunization with peptide-pulsed dendritic cells (53,54) (Fig. 2) or peptide, plus IL-12 (51). Tumor size either stopped increasing and remained stable throughout the course of immunization (compared to tumors in control animals that grew rapidly) (see Fig. 2), or actually decreased. Enhancement of the immunogenicity of a mutant p53 epitope was also observed after transduction of the costimulatory molecule B7 via recombinant adenovirus (55). Improved effectiveness of peptide immunization has also been reported if the immunization is done together with IL-12 (51), or with IL-12 and peptide-pulsed dendritic cells (52,53). This underscores the fact that appropriate antigens may be present in the tumor but not recognized without therapeutic manipulation of cytokines, costimulatory molecules, or APCs.

Although there are a few hotspots for mutations in p53 (such as codons 175, 248, and 273), these make up only a small fraction of the mutations observed. This complicates mutation-spe-

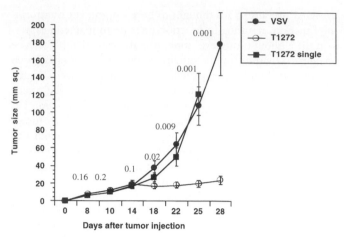

FIGURE 2. Ability of immunization with mutant p53-pulsed dendritic cells to inhibit growth of established tumors in mice (54). Groups of 5 BALB/c mice were injected subcutaneously with 2×10^5 D459 fibrosarcoma cells expressing mutant human p53 gene T1272, with mutation of Cys to Tyr at position 135 creating a neoantigenic determinant with a new H-2K^d–binding motif not present in the wild-type p53 (45). Immunizations were begun at day 8, when the tumors were palpable (2 to 4 mm diameter), and were given on day 8 only (T1272 single) or on days 8, 14, 18, and 22 [T1272 and ventricular stomatitis (VSV) peptide]. The immunogen consisted of 1 to 2×10^5 syngeneic dendritic cells generated from bone marrow of normal BALB/c mice and pulsed for 2 hours with either T1272 mutant p53 peptide or control VSV-8 peptide. Average tumor size (mm^2) and SEM are given. *p* Values for differences between the group immunized multiply with T1272 peptide-pulsed dendritic cells and the group immunized with the VSV peptide-pulsed dendritic cells are indicated by the numbers above the points. No significant difference occurred between the group immunized only once with T1272 and the control group. Similar results were obtained in three independent experiments. (From Gabrilovich DI, et al. Dendritic cells in antitumor immune responses. II. Dendritic cells grown from bone marrow precursors, but not mature DC from tumor-bearing mice, are effective antigen carriers in the therapy of established tumors. *Cell Immunol* 1996;170:111–119, with permission from Academic Press.)

cific immunotargeting, as each patient is likely to have a different mutation, each requiring a different peptide vaccine. Mutant-specific epitope targeting may, however, not be necessary, as several authors have demonstrated efficient recognition of wild-type p53 sequences in murine models (46,53,56–59) or human cells *in vitro* (60). This occurs in spite of the fact that every normal cell in normal individuals expresses a low level of structurally identical p53 protein. The typical massive overexpression of the mutant protein may allow sufficient tumor-normal discrimination to be of clinical utility. The antibodies that develop in cancer patients recognize sequences in either the amino or carboxy terminal regions of p53, and not in the central DNA-binding region of the molecule, where most of the somatic mutations occur (61). Consequently, these antibodies recognize both mutant and wild-type p53 *in vitro*, in spite of the fact that individuals might be expected to be tolerant to these epitopes. These antibodies are found much less commonly, if at all, in patients without cancer or cancer patients whose tumors do not have missense mutations in p53. It is possible that anti-p53 antibodies are induced due to the resulting overproduction of the mutant protein, a conformational change associated with the mutation, or induction of T-cell help by the mutant epitope to break tolerance. The major practical advantage of targeting a wild-type

epitope is that a single vaccine preparation can be used to target a wide variety of tumors producing different mutated p53 proteins, and these sequences can be selected to match the peptide-binding preferences of large classes of patients with common MHC antigens.

Many studies have shown the ability to kill murine tumors with T cells specific for wild-type–p53 epitopes (46,53,62,63). Adoptively transferred wild-type p53-specific T cells can also eradicate established tumors in mice (57). HLA-A2-restricted, wild-type, p53-specific T cells can be developed in A2-transgenic mice that exhibit antitumor effects in human-tumor nude mouse xenografts (64,65). One study used the intact wild-type p53 gene–transduced dendritic cells to induce specific immunologic and tumor responses in animal tumors expressing a variety of mutant p53 proteins (66).

Anti-p53 Cellular Immune Responses in Cancer Patients

Cellular immune responses specific for p53 have also been observed in humans. Induction of the humoral response described in the previous section requires antigen presentation on APCs and T-helper cells, so detection of these antibodies implies a T-cell response to the same antigen. CD4+ T cells (those which produce cytokines and proliferate in response to antigen) that respond to p53 peptides have been reported in breast cancer patients (67). All of the patients with detectable T-helper cell responses also had antibodies against p53, demonstrating the existence of a combined cellular and humoral response in these patients. CTLs have also been isolated that are specific for either wild-type or mutant-p53 epitopes. Kast and Melief showed *in vitro* induction of human CTLs to both normal and mutant p53 epitopes (60). Low levels of CTL precursors recognizing wild-type p53 epitopes have even been identified in the peripheral blood of individuals with no apparent cancer (68). It is unclear what the clinical significance of these responses is and whether they are *in vitro* primary responses (artifacts) or true recall responses. In breast cancer patients, significant CTL responses specific for the mutant p53 in a cancer patient's tumor have been observed (69). In most cases, these CTLs recognized mutant, but not the corresponding wild-type p53 sequences. The role of these CTLs in affecting the clinical course of the cancer is unclear, but the majority of patients in this study with these responses were apparently cured of their disease with surgery alone. Wild-type p53-specific T cells stimulated *in vitro* from a normal donor have been shown to be able to kill human squamous cell carcinoma cells naturally overexpressing mutant p53 (70,71). Therefore, p53 protein can behave as an antigenic target for CTLs during the natural process of tumorigenesis without external immunization or other immunotherapy.

Induction of Epitope-Specific Immunity to p53 in Cancer

For defined target antigens, induction of epitope-specific immunity in animals has been typically accomplished using synthetic peptides (72–75). The use of peptides as immunogens is complicated by their weak inherent immunogenicity and variable chemical and physical properties, so a variety of strategies have been used to enhance the efficacy of peptide-based vaccines (75–86). The chemical and physical problems of protein or peptide-based vaccines can be avoided by the use of genetic vaccines, purified-plasmid DNA-expression vectors encoding the entire cloned ORF of proteins introduced into living animals. These DNA-vaccine vectors may generate substantial humoral and cellular immunity with little or no toxicity (87–91). We have shown the induction of T-cell epitope-specific (mutant p53) cellular immune responses and antitumor effects after introduction of a "genetic epitope" vaccine consisting of an expression cassette containing only an oligonucleotide coding for the desired epitope (48). In this study, we used a particle gun, which atraumatically delivers microscopic gold particles coated with the plasmid DNA into the shaved skin of living animals. A plasmid vector containing the adenovirus-E3 leader sequence, which facilitates transport of the mutant-p53 epitope into the endoplasmic reticulum, was constructed and used to show the importance of this transport for optimal CTL induction and tumor-protective immunity. The use of epitope-mini-gene genetic vaccines may thus have significant potential for the induction of responses against identified T-cell epitopes in tumors.

When the p53 gene was expressed in a recombinant poxvirus vector and used to immunize animals, protection from lethal tumor challenge was observed (56). The wild-type p53 was just as effective as the mutant p53 in this system. Studies with animals bearing pre-existing tumors (a more clinically relevant situation) have not yet been reported using recombinant viral immunization.

Human Clinical Trials of p53 Vaccines

Human clinical trials have been conducted that aim to induce CTLs in cancer patients using a custom p53-derived peptide corresponding to the mutant-p53 sequence in the particular patient's tumor. In one such trial, DNA from each patient's tumor was evaluated for mutations in p53 and if a mutation was found that altered the predicted protein sequence, a customized synthetic peptide was constructed and used to immunize the patient (Carbone et al., manuscript in preparation). Frequent T-cell immunologic responses to the peptide were observed, including both CTL and cytokine responses. Results showed that the T cells could distinguish between the mutant-p53 sequence, to which they responded, and the corresponding homologous wild-type p53 sequence, to which they did not, avoiding any potential for autoimmunity. Future studies are planned to use dendritic cells as antigen carriers and might be able to use peptides derived from normal p53 protein sequences or the intact p53 protein. A cocktail of p53 peptides is also possible, analogous to multivalent pneumococcal vaccines, particularly if wild-type sequences are used.

The use of a complex vaccine containing more than a single peptide epitope may have advantages. One study observed that the mutant site in human p53 was found statistically significantly less frequently in sites that matched the patient's MHC class I consensus sequence (92). Another study found that mutation of arginine to histidine at the hotspot codon 273 in

human p53 altered the processing of the surrounding sequence and eliminated presentation of an epitope effectively presented in the absence of mutation (93).

Therefore, there is ample evidence that both wild-type and mutant-p53 sequences can be the specific targets of CTL recognition and can kill tumors overexpressing p53. The optimal immunization technique and the ability of such CTLs to effect clinically significant improvements in the outcome for human cancer patients remains uncertain. These issues are under clinical evaluation at this time.

OTHER MUTATIONS AS TUMOR ANTIGENS

In addition to known oncogenes and tumor suppressor genes that are commonly mutated, sporadic mutations in other proteins can create novel tumor antigens. These have often been identified when searches are made for tumor antigens in tumors by methods that do not assume the nature of the tumor antigenic protein in advance. Perhaps the first of these discovered is the tum⁻P91A antigen in mutated P815-mastocytoma cells characterized by Thierry Boon's group in a novel cloning strategy that they developed (94). The point mutation in the novel antigen was shown to be an Arg-to-His mutation that created a sequence with strong binding to H-2L^d and allowed the induction of class I MHC H-2L^d–restricted CTLs. Another similar tumor antigen was also identified by Boon's group in a mutant P815 tumor, in this case a point mutation in the P198 antigen and not homologous to any other protein in the data banks (95). This mutation of Ala to Thr did not create a new binding site, as both the mutant and wild-type sequences bound to H-2K^d, but created a new epitope recognized by CTLs.

Using a different approach, acid elution of peptides from MHC molecules on tumor cells, Mandelboim et al. (96) identified a tumor antigen from the Lewis lung carcinoma. This was found to represent a point-mutated epitope from the connexin-37 protein presented by H-2K^b.

When a cloning approach similar to that pioneered by Boon's group in mice was applied to a human melanoma using tumor infiltrating lymphocytes as the source of CTLs to define the antigen, an interesting mutation in β-catenin was discovered by Robbins et al. (97) that created a novel tumor antigen. The mutation, from Ser to Phe, created a neoantigen determinant by introducing Phe, which could serve as the C-terminal anchor residue for binding to HLA-A24, whereas the wild-type peptide did not bind. Thus, strikingly, the mutant peptide was found to sensitize targets for lysis at a million-fold lower concentration than the wild-type peptide (97) (Fig. 3). Because β-catenin is involved in cell adhesion through its interaction with cadherins, it is possible that the mutation contributed to the malignant phenotype of tumor cells and provided a possible target for attack by the immune system.

Similarly, mutations have been found in other known critical proteins that might function as tumor antigens. P16Ink4a is a cyclin-dependent kinase inhibitor responsible for keeping the tumor suppressor Rb in its cell-cycle suppressive state. Mutations in p16 are frequently observed in a variety of cancers, and human CTLs have been identified from a patient

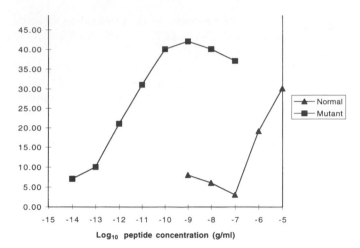

FIGURE 3. Mutation in the β-catenin gene creates a neoantigenic determinant that sensitizes targets at a million-fold lower concentration than the wild-type peptide. Mutant and wild-type peptides were titrated for sensitization of Epstein-Barr virus–transformed lymphoblasts for lysis by tumor-infiltrating lymphocytes from the patient in whose tumor the mutation was discovered. (Reprinted from Robbins PF, El-Gamil M, Li YF, et al. A mutated beta-catenin gene encodes a melanoma-specific antigen recognized by tumor infiltrating lymphocytes. *J Exp Med* 1996;183:1185–1192 by copyright permission of The Rockefeller University Press.)

with melanoma that specifically recognize the mutant protein (98).

Mutations have also been found to create tumor antigens presented by class II molecules. A new technique has been developed that allows screening of a complementary DNA (cDNA) library in which the genes are fused to the invariant chain of class II molecules to target them to the class II processing pathway and transfected to a cell in which the appropriate class II molecule and other necessary genes have also been transfected (99). This approach has allowed the identification of novel mutant tumor antigens in melanoma, including a mutant form of CDC27 presented by HLA-DR4 and a mutated triosephosphate isomerase presented by HLA-DR1 (99). Of interest is the fact that both mutations, like the β-catenin mutation presented by a class I HLA molecule, were found to be C to T mutations, consistent with a possible role of UV light in inducing the mutation (99). Similarly, another novel melanoma antigen presented by HLA-DR1 and recognized by CD4+ T cells was identified as a fusion protein created by a chromosomal rearrangement (100). All three melanoma tumor antigens so far identified, as presented by class II HLA molecules, are unique to the tumor, in contrast to many melanoma antigens presented by class I molecules that were parts of normal melanocyte proteins (83,101,102).

Thus, sporadic tumor-unique antigens can often be point mutations that occur in a variety of proteins and may or may not contribute to the malignant phenotype. In some cases, these novel tumor antigens are sufficiently immunogenic as to cause spontaneous regression of the tumor by immunologic rejection. Alternatively, it may be possible to boost the immunogenicity with custom vaccines containing these mutations or expand CTLs from tumor-infiltrating lymphocytes, preferably ones with high avidity (85,103–106) for adoptive immunotherapy.

NOVEL FUSION PROTEINS CREATED BY CHROMOSOMAL TRANSLOCATIONS

The use of translocation-specific fusion proteins as targets for CTL therapy is attractive for several reasons. First, they meet the criteria articulated earlier in this chapter—namely, that they would be expected to be uniquely expressed in tumor cells, and they are either presumed or proven to be causally related to the oncogenic process. Thus, loss of fusion protein expression to escape immune recognition would not permit maintenance of the transformed state. Second, because the expression of these tumor-specific fusion proteins are shared by most, if not all patients with a specific tumor, developing a successful vaccination strategy would be expected to be applicable to many patients whose tumors harbor the same translocation. There has been a growing interest in targeting tumor-specific, translocation fusion proteins for immunotherapeutic approaches. This section reviews work undertaken to determine the possibility of targeting tumor-specific, translocation-generated fusion proteins as targets for therapy.

Examples of Fusion Proteins Targeted for Immunotherapy

Cataloging the extensive list of tumor-specific translocations—and, hence, potential tumor-specific antigens that have been identified to date—is beyond the scope of this review. However, this chapter presents multiple examples of both preclinical and clinical models that attempt to generate tumor-specific CTL responses targeted at specific fusion proteins generated by the tumor-specific translocations. Several examples are discussed in detail in the following sections.

BCR-ABL

Among the best-studied fusion proteins is the BCR-ABL fusion protein generated by the t(9;22)(q34;q11), historically known as the *Philadelphia chromosome of chronic myelogenous leukemia* (CML) patients. The BCR-ABL fusion protein is present in more than 95% of patients with CML and in approximately 10% of children with acute lymphocytic leukemia (ALL) and 25% of adults with ALL (107). This translocation results in the fusion of exon 2 of the C-ABL tyrosine kinase on chromosome 9 with either exon 2 or exon 3 of the BCR gene on chromosome 22 at the amino-terminal region. If the fusion is from exon 2 of BCR, it is referred to as *b2a2*, and if the fusion is from exon 3 of BCR, it is referred to as *b3a2* (Fig. 4A). In either case, the ORF of BCR and ABL are fused in-frame to encode a 210-kd protein that includes 1,004 amino acids derived from C-ABL and either 902 or 927 amino acids derived from BCR (108). The resultant fusion has been shown to encode a protein with enhanced tyrosine kinase activity when compared to the normal C-ABL–encoded cytosolic tyrosine kinase activity (109–111). Furthermore, the p210[b2a2] and the p210[b3a2] have been shown to have transforming activity in fibroblasts and lymphoid cells, and thus are believed to play a critical role in leukemogenesis (112).

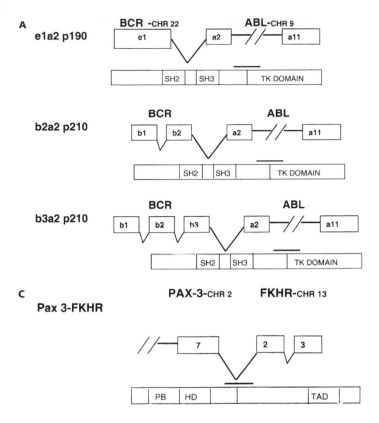

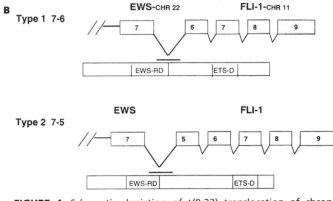

FIGURE 4. Schematic depiction of t(9;22) translocation of chronic myelogenous leukemia **(A)**, t(11;22) translocation of Ewing's sarcoma/peripheral primitive neuroepitheliomas **(B)**, and t(2;13) translocation of alveolar rhabdomyosarcoma **(C)**. Upper panel in each pair shows genomic organization. Lower panel is schematic of chimeric protein. The horizontal line represents the fusion region and a potential immunogenic peptide spanning the breakpoint. The vertical line centered below the horizontal line indicates the fusion breakpoint junction. Some critical regions of the fusion protein are indicated (not to scale). In the case of BCR-ABL, the fusion alters the target protein specificity of a tyrosine kinase, creating an oncogenic effect. In the case of EWS-FLI-1 and PAX-3-FKHR, the fusions bring together the activation domain of one parent molecule with the nucleotide-binding domain of the other parent molecule, creating an aberrant transcription factor that is transforming. (ETS-D, ETS DNA-binding domain of FLI-1; EWS-RD, EWS regulatory domain; HD, homeodomain of PAX-3; PB, paired box of PAX-3; SH2, SRC-homology-2 domain of BCR; SH3, SRC homology-3 domain of BCR; TAD, transactivating domain of FKHR; TK, tyrosine kinase domain of ABL.)

Approximately 40% of patients with BCR-ABL–positive CMLs have the b2a2 fusion, 40% have the b3a2 fusion, and 20% contain both fusions due to alternative splicing (113,114). In approximately 10% of children and 25% of adults with ALL, the same region of C-ABL is translocated to a region of BCR upstream of exon 2, called *e1*, yielding a p190^{e1a2} BCR-ABL fusion protein with similar function to the p210 fusion protein (115,116).

Chen et al. from the group of Cheever were the first to report the use of a p210^{b3a2} fusion 12-mer peptide to immunize mice and generate MHC class II–restricted CD4$^+$ T-cell clones that specifically recognized the fusion peptide that contained six amino acids from BCR and five amino acids from ABL (117). tenBosch et al. (118) have gone on to demonstrate that a similar b3a2 17-mer peptide spanning the breakpoint region was capable of eliciting an *in vitro* CD4$^+$ T cell class II–restricted response. Furthermore, a DR4-restricted response was demonstrated against allogeneic p210^{b3a2}-expressing leukemic blasts from a patient in blast crisis (118). This response required the expression of both DR4 and p210 in the same cell. These data strongly suggest that the p210^{b3a2} oncoprotein is endogenously processed through the HLA class II pathway and presented on the surface of leukemic blast cells and thus fully capable of serving as a target for tumor-specific CD4 cells. Subsequently, Chen et al. (119) demonstrated the ability to elicit CD8$^+$, H-2K^d–restricted CTLs using a breakpoint B392 peptide in mice. Despite lytic activity against syngeneic cells pulsed with the vaccinating peptide, however, the CTL clones did not lyse either syngeneic murine leuke-

mia cells expressing the identical p210^{b3a2} or human K562 cells expressing p210^{b3a2} transfected with mouse H-2K^d (119).

Greco et al. (120) showed that a nonamer peptide spanning the b3a2 fusion region was capable of binding HLA-A3. Subsequent studies using peptide-pulsed antigen-presenting cell (APC) *in vitro* immunizations led to specific CTL responses (120). Likewise, Bocchia et al. (121) found that 9-mer and 11-mer b3a2 spanning peptides were able to elicit an HLA-A3–restricted CTL response *in vitro* using peptide-pulsed APC vaccination approaches. The CTLs generated were shown to be capable of lysing autologous or HLA-A3–matched allogeneic peptide-pulsed targets. These investigators also used a 25-mer spanning the b3a2 breakpoint to show that this peptide could elicit HLA class II (DR11)–restricted peptide-induced CD4 proliferation (121).

TEL(ETV6)-AML-1

The TEL-AML-1 fusion protein seen in approximately 25% of childhood ALL is generated by a reciprocal t(12;21)(p13;q22) translocation (122,123). This translocation results most commonly in the in-frame fusion of exon 5 of TEL on chromosome 12, with exon 2 of AML-1 on chromosome 21. The resultant fusion protein generates a novel transcription factor combining helix-loop-helix TEL with the DNA-binding domain of the AML-1/CBFβ transcription factor.

The Lemonnier/Langlade-Demoyen group has tested a series of peptides spanning this translocation breakpoint for evidence of binding to HLA-A2.1 (124). This group identified a non-apeptide spanning the translocation breakpoint that bound HLA-A2.1. They subsequently demonstrated that this nonamer could elicit a primary CTL response in peripheral blood lymphocytes from healthy donors. Furthermore, these CTLs were shown to specifically lyse HLA-A2.1–positive tumor cells that expressed endogenous TEL-AML-1 fusion protein. These investigators were also able to identify CTLs specific for this fusion peptide at high frequency in the bone marrow of a patient with TEL-AML-1-positive ALL. These CTLs were capable of lysing HLA-matched ALL tumor cells bearing the TEL-AML-1 translocation (124), making this a promising tumor antigen.

EWS-FLI-1

The EWS-FLI-1 fusion protein is generated by a reciprocal t(11;22)(q24;q12) translocation that is the hallmark of Ewing's sarcoma (ES)/peripheral primitive neuroepitheliomas (PPNET). The EWS-FLI-1 fusion is present in approximately 85% of such tumors (125,126). The translocation results in the fusion, most commonly, of exon 7 of the EWS gene on chromosome 22, with either exon 5 or exon 6 of the FLI-1 gene on chromosome 11. If the fusion is from exon 7 of EWS to exon 6 of FLI-1, it is referred to as the *type I* or *7 to 6 fusion*. If the fusion is from exon 7 of EWS to exon 5 of FLI-1, it is referred to as the *type II* or *7 to 5 fusion* (Fig. 4B). Either fusion results in an apparently enhanced nuclear transcription factor with transactivation domains derived from EWS and DNA-binding activity encoded by the ETS transcription family member, FLI-1. Studies have demonstrated both the transforming activity of EWS-FLI-1 in fibroblasts, as well as the critical role of EWS-FLI-1 in maintaining the transformed phenotype in ES cells (127,128). Of interest is the finding that there may be prognostic differences between the type I and type II fusion-positive ES tumors (129).

In an attempt to generate CTL responses aimed at the EWS-FLI-1 fusion protein, 15- to 18-mer peptides spanning the type I or type II breakpoints were synthesized and analyzed for potential binding motifs for MHC class I and class II molecules. Based on predictions for a variety of class I and -II human-binding motifs as well as mouse class I binding motifs, we went on to develop an *in vitro* model using peptide-pulsed mouse APCs. In these studies, intravenously administered peptide-pulsed APCs generated CD8[+] CTLs capable of lysing peptide-pulsed targets *in vitro*. The cytolytic activity was shown to be class I H-2K^d–restricted, using mouse L-cell transfectants as targets. In these mouse experiments, the 18-mer peptides were incubated with APCs in the presence of serum that presumably contains proteolytic activity capable of generating smaller peptide fragments able to bind MHC class I molecules. Minimal epitope mapping identified a 9-mer overlapping the translocation breakpoint (130,131, and *unpublished data*).

We are currently attempting to generate an *in vivo* model using mouse tumor cells transfected with an EWS-FLI-1 cDNA. Although these data clearly demonstrate that peptides spanning the EWS-FLI-1 fusion protein can generate specific CD8[+] CTLs, it remains to be determined whether such peptides are processed similarly in ES tumor cells and, thus, are

capable of acting as targets for CTLs in patients bearing ES/PPNET tumors.

PAX-3-FKHR

PAX-3-FKHR is generated by the reciprocal t(2;13)(q35;q14) translocation and is present in approximately 80% of alveolar rhabdomyosarcomas. PAX-3 is a transcription factor that plays an important role in embryonic development, including skeletal muscle differentiation (132,133). PAX genes contain both paired box (PB) and paired-type homeodomain (HD) DNA-binding domains. FKHR is a member of the forkhead family of transcription factors that contain a conserved DNA-binding motif related to the homeotic gene *forkhead*. The PAX-3-FKHR fusion protein contains the PB and HD DNA-binding domains of PAX-3 at the amino-terminal end, fused to the carboxy-terminal end of FKHR, which retains its putative transactivation domain (Fig. 4C). Thus it appears that the DNA-binding specificity is encoded by PAX-3, whereas the transactivation domain is contributed by FKHR. The PAX-3-FKHR fusion has been demonstrated to transform chicken embryo fibroblasts (134).

Synthetic 18-mer peptides spanning the PAX-3-FKHR breakpoint were synthesized and pulsed onto the surface of murine splenocytes (containing APCs) or onto purified mouse dendritic cells using a 2-hour incubation in the presence of serum. Intravenous infusion of such peptide-pulsed, irradiated APCs led to the generation of CTLs specific for the peptide within 21 days, as assayed by chromium-release studies. Of further note, these CTLs also lysed mouse CT26 adenocarcinoma cells that had been transfected with the full-length PAX-3-FKHR cDNA (130,131). This finding demonstrates that the full-length fusion protein can be endogenously processed in CT26 tumor cells and presented in the context of class I HLA on the surface of the cell. The CTL activity was found to be H-2L^d–restricted. Minimal epitope mapping identified a 10-mer overlapping the breakpoint. Most recently, this same 10-mer was noted to bind a human HLA molecule (unpublished observations of the authors).

Based on the *in vitro* activity, we went on to study the activity of this approach using an *in vivo* model of CT26 cells transfected with the PAX-3-FKHR cDNA. Immunization using the same peptide-pulsed APCs in mice was shown to be specifically protective of PAX-3-FKHR expressing CT26 cells in tumor-challenge studies, and adoptive transfer of bulk-immunized splenocytes was shown to lead to tumor reduction in a micrometastatic model (130).

We have begun a clinical study to determine whether immunization of patients bearing either EWS-FLI-1– or PAX-3-FKHR–expressing tumors with peptide-pulsed APCs can lead to the generation of tumor-specific CTL activity.

Several other sarcomas have been shown to have tumor-specific translocations generating fusion transcription factors. Some of these currently under investigation in our laboratories include the EWS-ATF1 fusion protein generated by the t(12;22)(q13;q12) seen in clear cell sarcoma, the EWS-WT1 fusion protein generated by the t(11;22)(p13;q12) in desmoplastic small round cell tumor, and the SSX-SYT fusion protein generated by the t(x;18)(p11.2;q11.2) in synovial sarcoma (135,136).

As the efforts to develop CTL responses targeting tumor-specific translocations continue, several critical questions remain to be answered. Most important, the presence of these fusion peptides on the surface of tumor cells bound to MHC molecules must be formally proven. Although the generation of tumor-specific CTL responses would not be expected to affect normal cells, it is possible that CTLs recognizing epitopes contained within normal proteins also could be generated, with the possibility of developing autoimmune phenomena. We hope that ultimately the use of immunotherapy directed against tumor-specific fusion proteins may be used after more standard cytoreductive therapy to improve the outcome in patients with these tumors.

OTHER ONCOGENES AS TARGETS OF IMMUNOTHERAPY

When overexpressed, even nonmutated oncogene products may serve as tumor antigens. An oncogene that has received extensive scrutiny is known as HER-2/*neu*. HER-2/*neu* is a cell-surface receptor that was originally identified as a dominant oncogene from a rat neuroblastoma cell line. It has subsequently been shown to be amplified or overexpressed in many human solid tumors, particularly adenocarcinomas of the breast, lung, ovary, and pancreas. It is overexpressed in 20% to 30% of the cases, and in these cases it represents a potentially useful tumor-associated target antigen. Immunotherapeutic targeting of HER-2/*neu* has been reviewed in detail elsewhere (7). Antibodies to Her-2/*neu* have been found in 44% to 55% of breast cancer patients and are correlated with overexpression, compared to 4% to 5% of normal individuals, suggesting that overexpression in the tumor can break self-tolerance to this unmutated oncogene product (7,137). The fact that these were IgG antibodies also suggests the existence of T-cell help. Indeed, CD4[+] T-proliferative responses were observed in PBMCs of three of seven patients studied to HER-2/*neu* proteins and selected synthetic peptides from the HER-2/*neu* sequence (7,137,138). Additionally, human CTLs have been isolated that recognize HER-2/*neu* epitopes on human breast and ovarian cancer (7,138–142), as well as non–small-cell lung cancer (143), pancreatic cancer (144), prostate cancer (145), and gastric cancer (146). At least some of these human CTLs can kill a breast cancer cell line expressing HER-2/*neu* as well as HLA-A2.1 (7,138). In contrast, one study immunizing patients with HER-2/*neu* peptide 369–377 that binds to HLA-A2.1 found that CTLs could be induced that recognized peptide-pulsed target cells, but these CTLs failed to kill HLA-A2.1–positive human tumor cells, even after treatment with IFN-γ to upregulate class I HLA expression (147). Effective immunotherapy against animal model tumors expressing HER-2/*neu* has been demonstrated using nanoparticle/protein immunization (148), or this protein pulsed onto dendritic cells (149). In a novel approach to break tolerance, it was shown that HER-2/*neu* peptides could break tolerance and induce CD4[+] T-cell responses and antibodies to rat HER-2/*neu* in rats that were not able to be immunized with the intact rat HER-2/*neu* protein (7,150). A human phase 1 study is currently being conducted by Dr. Mary Disis at the University of Washington.

CONCLUSIONS

A number of oncogene products, mutant oncogene products, other mutant proteins, and fusion proteins created by tumor-specific chromosomal translocations have been identified in tumors that have the properties necessary to serve as tumor antigens. Oncogene products and tumor-specific fusion proteins have the advantage that they contribute to the malignant phenotype and thus cannot be lost under immune selective pressure without loss of this phenotype. Mutations and the breakpoint regions of fusion proteins also have the advantage of being unique to the tumor, allowing the immune system to distinguish the cancer cells from normal cells. This allows immunotherapeutic approaches to fully exploit the hallmark of the immune system, namely its exquisite specificity. Even in cases in which the oncogene product is not mutated, such as HER-2/*neu*, or in which the immune system recognizes a nonmutated epitope of an oncogene or tumor-suppressor gene product, such as p53, overexpression of this product can sometimes allow immune recognition of the tumor without autoimmune responses against normal cells expressing much lower levels of these proteins.

A number of examples have been given in this chapter that are promising tumor antigens for active or passive immunotherapy. These have been studied in both animal and human models. In many cases, human T cells recognizing these mutant or fusion epitopes specifically have been identified, and in some of these cases, the T cells have been shown to kill human tumor cells expressing the antigen. Currently, a number of clinical studies are ongoing that are designed to determine the clinical utility of these approaches. As this field is rapidly advancing, additional new tumor antigens of this type are likely to be identified. Concurrent rapid advances in new techniques to increase immunogenicity hold promise for producing more potent antitumor immune responses that have clinical benefit (85,86,151–155). Thus, the field is poised at the threshold of a new and promising era in the immunotherapy of cancer.

REFERENCES

1. Townsend A, Bodmer H. Antigen recognition by class I-restricted T lymphocytes. *Annu Rev Immunol* 1989;7:601–624.
2. Germain RN, Margulies DH. The biochemistry and cell biology of antigen processing and presentation. *Annu Rev Immunol* 1993;11:403–450.
3. Zinkernagel RM, Doherty PC. MHC-restricted cytotoxic T cells: studies on the biological role of polymorphic major transplantation antigens determining T-cell restriction-specificity, function, and responsiveness. *Adv Immunol* 1979;27:51–177.
4. Steinman R. The dendritic cell system and its role in immunogenicity. *Annu Rev Immunol* 1991;9:271–296.
5. Banchereau J, Steinman RM. Dendritic cells and the control of immunity. *Nature* 1998;392:245–252.
6. Henderson RA, Finn OJ. Human tumor antigens are ready to fly. *Adv Immunol* 1996;62:217–256.
7. Cheever MA, Disis ML, Bernhard H, et al. Immunity to oncogenic proteins. *Immunol Rev* 1995;145:33–59.
8. Bos JL. *ras* oncogenes in human cancer: a review. *Cancer Res* 1989;49:4682–4689.
9. Andreyev HJN, Norman AR, Cunningham D, Oates JR, Clarke PA. Kirsten ras mutations in patients with colorectal cancer: the multicenter "RASCAL" study. *J Natl Cancer Inst* 1998;90:675–684.

10. Peace DJ, Chen W, Nelson H, Cheever MA. T cell recognition of transforming proteins encoded by mutated ras proto-oncogenes. *J Immunol* 1991;146:2059–2065.

11. Peace DJ, Smith JW, Disis ML, Chen W, Cheever MA. Induction of T cells specific for the mutated segment of oncogenic P21ras protein by immunization *in vivo* with the oncogenic protein. *J Immunol* 1993;14:110–114.

12. Abrams SI, Dobrzanski MJ, Wells DT, et al. Peptide-specific activation of cytolytic CD4+ T lymphocytes against tumor cells bearing mutated epitopes of K-ras p21. *Eur J Immunol* 1995;25:2588–2597.

13. Abrams SI, Stanziale SF, Lunin SD, Zaremba S, Schlom J. Identification of overlapping epitopes in mutant ras oncogene peptides that activate CD4+ and CD8+ T cell responses. *Eur J Immunol* 1996;26:435–443.

14. Skipper J, Stauss HJ. Identification of two cytotoxic T lymphocyte-recognized epitopes in the ras protein. *J Exp Med* 1993;177:1493–1498.

15. Peace DJ, Smith JW, Chen W, et al. Lysis of Ras oncogene-transformed cells by specific cytotoxic T lymphocytes elicited by primary *in vitro* immunization with mutated Ras peptide. *J Exp Med* 1994;179:473–479.

16. Fenton RG, Taub DD, Kwak LW, Smith MR, Longo DL. Cytotoxic T-cell response and in vivo protection against tumor cells harboring activated ras proto-oncogenes. *J Natl Cancer Inst* 1993;85:1294–1302.

17. Jung S, Schluesener HJ. Human T lymphocytes recognize a peptide of single point-mutated, oncogenic ras proteins. *J Exp Med* 1991;173:273–276.

18. Gedde-Dahl III T, Eriksen JA, Thorsby E, Gaudernack G. T-cell responses against products of oncogenes: generation and characterization of human T-cell clones specific for p21 ras-derived synthetic peptides. *Hum Immunol* 1992;33:266–274.

19. Gedde-Dahl III T, Spurkland A, Eriksen JA, Thorsby E, Gaudernack G. Memory T cells of a patient with follicular thyroid carcinoma recognize peptides derived from mutated p21 ras (Gln Leu61). *Int Immunol* 1992;4:1331–1337.

20. Gedde-Dahl III T, Spurkland A, Fossum B, Wittinghofer A, Thorsby E, Gaudernack G. T cell epitopes encompassing the mutational hot spot position 61 of p21 ras. Promiscuity in peptide binding to HLA. *Eur J Immunol* 1994;24:410–414.

21. Fossum B, Gedde-Dahl T III, Hansen T, Eriksen JA, Thorsby E, Gaudernack G. Overlapping epitopes encompassing a point mutation (12 Gly → Arg) in p21 ras can be recognized by HLA-DR, -DP and -DQ restricted T cells . *Eur J Immunol* 1993;23:2687–2691.

22. Fossum B, Breivik J, Meling GI, et al. A K-ras 13gly asp mutation is recognized by HLA-DQ7 restricted t cells in a patient with colorectal cancer. Modifying effect of DQ7 on established cancers harboring this mutation? *Int J Cancer* 1994;58:506–511.

23. Fossum B, Gedde-Dahl T III, Breivik J, et al. p21-ras-peptide-specific T-cell responses in a patient with colorectal cancer. CD4+ and CD8+ T cells recognize a peptide corresponding to a common mutation (13Gly→Asp). *Int J Cancer* 1994;56:40–45.

24. Qin H, Chen W, Takahashi M, et al. CD4+ T-cell immunity to mutated ras protein in pancreatic and colon cancer patients. *Cancer Res* 1995;55:2984–2987.

25. Chicz RM, Urban RG, Gorga JC, Vignali DAA, Lane WS, Strominger JL. Specificity and promiscuity among naturally processed peptides bound to HLA-DR alleles. *J Exp Med* 1993;178:27–47.

26. Takahashi M, Chen W, Byrd DR, et al. Antibody to ras proteins in patients with colon cancer. *Clin Cancer Res* 1995;1:1071–1077.

27. Gjertsen MK, Bakka A, Breivik J, et al. Vaccination with mutant ras peptides and induction of T-cell responsiveness in pancreatic carcinoma patients carrying the corresponding RAS mutation. *Lancet* 1995;346:1399–1400.

28. Gjertsen MK, Bakka A, Breivik J, et al. *Ex vivo* ras peptide vaccination in patients with advanced pancreatic cancer: results of a phase I/II study. *Int J Cancer* 1996;65:450–453.

29. Fossum B, Olsen AC, Thorsby E, Gaudernack G. CD8+ T cells from a patient with colon carcinoma, specific for a mutant p21-Ras derived peptide (GLY13 ASP), are cytotoxic towards a carcinoma cell line harboring the same mutation. *Cancer Immunol Immunother* 1995;40:165–172.

30. Elsas AV, Nijman HW, Van der minne CE, et al. Induction and characterization of cytotoxic T-lymphocytes recognizing a mutated p21RAS peptide presented by HLA-A*0201. *Int J Cancer* 1995;61:389–396.

31. Juretic A, Jürgens-Göbel J, Schaefer C, et al. Cytotoxic t-lymphocyte responses against mutated p21 ras peptides: an analysis of specific t-cell-receptor gene usage. *Int J Cancer* 1996;68:471–478.

32. Gjertsen MK, Bjorheim J, Saeterdal I, Myklebust J, Gaudernack G. Cytotoxic CD4+ and CD8+ T lymphocytes, generated by mutant p21-ras (12VAL) peptide vaccination of a patient, recognize 12VAL-dependent nested epitopes present within the vaccine peptide and kill autologous tumour cells carrying this mutation. *Int J Cancer* 1997;72:784–790.

33. Smith MC, Pendleton CD, Maher VE, Kelley MJ, Carbone DP, Berzofsky JA. Oncogenic mutations in ras create HLA-A2.1 binding peptides but affect their extracellular processing. *Internat Immunol* 1997;9:1085–1093.

34. Nijman HW, Houbiers JGA, Vierboom MPM, et al. Identification of peptide sequences that potentially trigger HLA-A2.1-restricted cytotoxic T lymphocytes. *Eur J Immunol* 1993;23:1215–1219.

35. Khleif SN, Abrams SI, Hamilton JM, et al. A phase I vaccine trial with peptides reflecting ras oncogene mutations of solid tumors. *J Immunother* 1999; 22(2):155–165.

36. Abrams SI, Khleif SN, Bergmann-Leitner ES, et al. Generation of stable CD4+ and CD8+ T cell lines from patients immunized with ras oncogene-derived peptides reflecting codon 12 mutations. *Cell Immunol* 1997;182:137–151.

37. Chiba I, Takahashi T, Nau MM, et al. Mutations in the p53 gene are frequent in primary, resected non-small cell lung cancer. *Oncogene* 1990;5:1603–1610.

38. Bodner SM, Minna J, Jensen SM, et al. Expression of mutant p53 proteins in lung cancer correlates with the class of p53 gene mutation. *Oncogene* 1992;7:743–749.

39. Carbone DP, Mitsudomi T, Chiba I, et al. p53 immunostaining positivity is associated with reduced survival and is imperfectly correlated with gene mutations in resected non-small cell lung cancer. *Chest* 1994;106:S377–S381.

40. Winter SF, Minna JD, Johnson BE, Takahashi T, Gazdar AF, Carbone DP. Development of antibodies against p53 in lung cancer patients appears to be dependent on the type of p53 mutation. *Cancer Res* 1992;52:4168–4174.

41. Lubin R, Zalcman G, Bouchet L, et al. Serum p53 antibodies as early markers of lung cancer. *Nat Med* 1995;1:701–702.

42. Zalcman G, Schlichtholz B, Tredaniel J, et al. Monitoring of p53 autoantibodies in lung cancer during therapy: relationship to response to treatment. *Clin Cancer Res* 1998;4:1359–1366.

43. Erez-Alon N, Herkel J, Wolkowicz R, et al. Immunity to p53 induced by an idiotypic network of anti-p53 antibodies: generation of sequence-specific anti-DNA antibodies and protection from tumor metastasis. *Cancer Res* 1998;58:5447–5452.

44. Ruiz PJ, Wolkowicz R, Waisman A, et al. Idiotypic immunization induces immunity to mutated p53 and tumor rejection. *Nat Med* 1998;4:710–712.

45. Yanuck M, Carbone DP, Pendleton CD, et al. A mutant p53 tumor suppressor protein is a target for peptide-induced CD8+ cytotoxic T cells. *Cancer Res* 1993;53:3257–3261.

46. Noguchi Y, Chen Y T, Old LJ. A mouse mutant p53 product recognized by CD4+ and CD8+ T cells. *Proc Natl Acad Sci U S A* 1994;91:3171–3175.

47. Ciernik IF, Berzofsky JA, Carbone DP. Mutant oncopeptide immunization induces CTL specifically lysing tumor cells endogenously expressing the corresponding intact mutant p53. *Hybridoma* 1995;14:139–142.

48. Ciernik IF, Berzofsky JA, Carbone DP. Induction of cytotoxic T lymphocytes and anti-tumor immunity with DNA vaccines expressing single T cell epitopes. *J Immunol* 1996;156:2369–2375.

49. Ciernik IF, Berzofsky JA, Carbone DP. Human lung cancer cells endogenously expressing mutant p53 process and present the mutant epitope, and are lysed by mutant-specific CTL. *Clin Cancer Res* 1996;2:877–882.

50. Ciernik IF, Krayenbuhl BH, Carbone DP. Puncture-mediated gene transfer to the skin. *Hum Gene Ther* 1996;7:893–899.

51. Noguchi Y, Richards EC, Chen Y-T, Old LJ. Influence of interleukin 12 on p53 peptide vaccination against established Meth A sarcoma. *Proc Natl Acad Sci U S A* 1995;92:2219–2223.

52. Gabrilovich DI, Cunningham HT, Carbone DP. IL-12 and mutant P53 peptide-pulsed dendritic cells for the specific immunotherapy of cancer. *J Immunother Emphasis Tumor Immunol* 1996;19:414–418.

53. Mayordomo JI, Loftus DJ, Sakamoto H, et al. Therapy of murine tumors with p53 wild-type and mutant sequence peptide-based vaccines. *J Exp Med* 1996;183:1357–1365.

54. Gabrilovich DI, Nadaf S, Corak J, Berzofsky JA, Carbone DP. Dendritic cells in anti-tumor immune responses. II. Dendritic cells grown from bone marrow precursors, but not mature DC from tumor-bearing mice are effective antigen carriers in the therapy of established tumors. *Cell Immunol* 1996;170:111–119.

55. Lee CT, Ciernik IF, Wu S, et al. Increased immunogenicity of tumors bearing mutant p53 and P1A epitopes after transduction of B7-1 via recombinant adenovirus. *Cancer Gene Ther* 1996;3:238–244.

56. Roth J, Dittmer D, Rea D, Tartaglia J, Paoletti E, Levine AJ. p53 as a target for cancer vaccines: recombinant canarypox virus vectors expressing p53 protect mice against lethal tumor cell challenge. *Proc Nat Acad Sci U S A* 1996;93:4781–4786.

57. Vierboom MPM, Nijman HW, Offringa R, et al. Tumor eradication by wild-type p53-specific cytotoxic T lymphocytes. *J Exp Med* 1997;186:695–704.

58. Theobald M, Biggs J, Dittmer D, Levine AJ, Sherman LA. Targeting p53 as a general tumor antigen. *Proc Natl Acad Sci U S A* 1995;92: 11993–11997.

59. Theobald M, Biggs J, Hernández J, Lustgarten J, Labadie C, Sherman LA. Tolerance to p53 by A2.1-restricted cytotoxic T lymphocytes. *J Exp Med* 1997;185:833–841.

60. Houbiers JGA, Nijman HW, van der Burg SH, et al. *In vitro* induction of human cytotoxic T lymphocyte responses against peptides of mutant and wild-type p53. *Eur J Immunol* 1993;23:2072–2077.

61. Schlichtholz B, Tredaniel J, Lubin R, Zalcman G, Hirsch A, Soussi T. Analysis of p53 antibodies in sera of patients with lung carcinoma define immunodominant regions in the p53 protein. *Br J Cancer* 1994;69:809–816.

62. Stuber G, Leder GH, Storkus WT, et al. Identification of wild-type and mutant p53 peptides binding to HLA-A2 assessed by a peptide loading-deficient cell line assay and a novel major histocompatibility complex class I peptide binding assay. *Eur J Immunol* 1994;24: 765–768.

63. Lacabanne V, Viguier M, Guillet JG, Choppin J. A wild-type p53 cytotoxic T cell epitope is presented by mouse hepatocarcinoma cells. *Eur J Immunol* 1996;26:2635–2639.

64. McCarty TM, Liu X, Sun JY, Peralta EA, Diamond DJ, Ellenhorn JD. Targeting p53 for adoptive T-cell immunotherapy. *Cancer Res* 1998;58:2601–2605.

65. McCarty TM, Yu Z, Liu X, Diamond DJ, Ellenhorn JD. An HLA-restricted, p53 specific immune response from HLA transgenic p53 knockout mice. *Ann Surg* 1998;5:93–99.

66. Ishida T, Stipanov M, Chada S, Gabrilovich DI, Carbone DP. Dendritic cells transduced with wild type p53 gene elicit potent antitumor immune responses. *J Clin Exp Immunol* 1999; 117(2):244–251.

67. Tilkin AF, Lubin R, Soussi T, et al. Primary proliferative T cell response to wild-type p53 protein in patients with breast cancer. *Eur J Immunol* 1995;25:1765–1769.

68. Ropke M, Regner M, Claesson MH. T cell-mediated cytotoxicity against p53-protein derived peptides in bulk and limiting dilution cultures of healthy donors. *Scand J Immunol* 1995;42:98–103.

69. Gabrilovich DI, Nadaf S, Cunningham T, et al. Cytotoxic T-lymphocytes (CTL) specific for mutant p53-peptides in peripheral blood of patients with cancer: support for specific immune intervention. *9th International Congress of Immunol* 1995;A3964(abst).

70. Ropke M, Hald J, Guldberg P, et al. Spontaneous human squamous cell carcinomas are killed by a human cytotoxic T lymphocyte clone recognizing a wild-type p53-derived peptide. *Proc Natl Acad Sci U S A* 1996;93:14704–14707.

71. DeLeo A. Killing of human squamous cell carcinomas with wild-type specific T cells. *International Dendritic Cell Meeting* 1998;(abst).

72. Ishioka GY, Colon S, Miles C, Grey HM, Chesnut RW. Induction of class I MHC-restricted, peptide-specific cytolytic T lymphocytes by peptide priming *in vivo*. *J Immunol* 1989;143:1094–1100.

73. Carbone FR, Bevan MJ. Induction of ovalbumin-specific cytotoxic T cells by in vivo peptide immunization. *J Exp Med* 1989;169:603–612.

74. Shirai M, Pendleton CD, Ahlers J, Takeshita T, Newman M, Berzofsky JA. Helper-CTL determinant linkage required for priming of anti-HIV CD8⁺ CTL *in vivo* with peptide vaccine constructs. *J Immunol* 1994;152:549–556.

75. Takahashi H, Nakagawa Y, Yokomuro K, Berzofsky JA. Induction of CD8⁺ CTL by immunization with syngeneic irradiated HIV-1 envelope derived peptide-pulsed dendritic cells. *Int Immunol* 1993;5:849–857.

76. Deres K, Schild H, Wiesmüller KH, Jung G, Rammensee HG. *In vivo* priming of virus-specific cytotoxic T lymphocytes with synthetic lipopeptide vaccine. *Nature* 1989;342:561–564.

77. Gupta RK, Relyveld EH, Lindblad EB, Bizzini B, Ben-Efraim S, Gupta CK. Adjuvants—a balance between toxicity and adjuvanticity. *Vaccine* 1993;11:293–306.

78. Romero P, Cerottini JC, Luescher I. Efficient *in vivo* induction of CTL by cell-associated covalent H-2K^d-peptide complexes. *J Immunol Methods* 1994;171:73–84.

79. Berzofsky JA. Epitope selection and design of synthetic vaccines: molecular approaches to enhancing immunogenicity and crossreactivity of engineered vaccines. *Ann N Y Acad Sci* 1993;690:256–264.

80. Ahlers JD, Takeshita T, Pendleton CD, Berzofsky JA. Enhanced immunogenicity of HIV-1 vaccine construct by modification of the native peptide sequence. *Proc Natl Acad Sci U S A* 1997;94:10856–10861.

81. Sarobe P, Pendleton CD, Akatsuka T, et al. Enhanced *in vitro* potency and *in vivo* immunogenicity of a CTL epitope from hepatitis C virus core protein following amino acid replacement at secondary HLA-A2.1 binding positions. *J Clin Invest* 1998;102:1239–1248.

82. Parkhurst MR, Salgaller ML, Southwood S, et al. Improved induction of melanoma-reactive CTL with peptides from the melanoma antigen gp100 modified at HLA-A*0201-binding residues. *J Immunol* 1996;157:2539–2548.

83. Rosenberg SA, Yang JC, Schwartzentruber DJ, et al. Immunologic and therapeutic evaluation of a synthetic peptide vaccine for the treatment of patients with metastatic melanoma. *Nat Med* 1998;4:321–327.

84. Ahlers JD, Dunlop N, Alling DW, Nara PL, Berzofsky JA. Cytokine-in-adjuvant steering of the immune response phenotype to HIV-1 vaccine constructs: GM-CSF and TNFα synergize with IL-12 to enhance induction of CTL. *J Immunol* 1997;158:3947–3958.

85. Oscherwitz J, Gotch FM, Cease KB, Berzofsky JA. New insights and approaches regarding B and T cell epitopes in HIV vaccine design. *AIDS* 1999;13[Suppl A]:S163–174.

86. Soengas MS, Alarcon RM, Yoshida H, et al. Apaf-1 and caspase-9 in p53-dependent apoptosis and tumor inhibition. *Science* 1999;284: 156–159.

87. Tang D, DeVit M, Johnston SA. Genetic immunization is a simple method for eliciting an immune response. *Nature* 1992;356:152–154.

88. Ulmer JB, Donnelly JJ, Parker SE, et al. Heterologous protection against influenza by injection of DNA encoding a viral protein. *Science* 1993;259:1745–1749.

89. Eisenbraun MD, Heydenburg Fuller D, Haynes JR. Examination of parameters effecting the election of humoral immune response by particle bombardment-mediated genetic immunization. *DNA Cell Biol* 1993;12:791–797.

90. Wang B, Ugen KE, Srikantan V, et al. Gene inoculation generates immune response against human immunodeficiency virus type 1. *Proc Natl Acad Sci U S A* 1993;90:4156–4160.

91. Fynan EF, Webster RG, Fuller DH, Haynes JR, Santoro JC, Robinson HL. DNA vaccines: protective immunization by parental, mucosal and gene-gun inoculation. *Proc Natl Acad Sci U S A* 1993;90:11478–11482.

92. Wiedenfeld EA, Fernandez-Viña M, Berzofsky JA, Carbone DP. Evidence for selection against human lung cancers bearing p53 missense mutations which occur within the HLA A*0201 peptide consensus motif. *Cancer Res* 1994;54:1175–1177.

93. Theobald M, Ruppert T, Kuckelkorn U, et al. The sequence alter-

ation associated with mutational hotspot in p53 protects cells from lysis by cytotoxic T lymphocytes specific for a flanking peptide epitope. *J Exp Med* 1998;188:1017–1028.

94. Lurquin C, Van Pel A, Mariamé B, et al. Structure of the gene of tum-transplantation antigen P91A: the mutated exon encodes a peptide recognized with L^d by cytolytic T cells. *Cell* 1989;58:293–303.

95. Sibille C, Chomez P, Wildmann C, et al. Structure of the gene of tum-transplantation antigen P198: a point mutation generates a new antigenic peptide. *J Exp Med* 1990;172:35–45.

96. Mandelboim O, Berke G, Fridkin M, Feldman M, Eisenstein M, Eisenbach L. CTL induction by a tumour-associated antigen octapeptide derived from a murine lung carcinoma. *Nature* 1994;369:67–71.

97. Robbins PF, El-Gamil M, Li YF, et al. A mutated β-catenin gene encodes a melanoma-specific antigen recognized by tumor infiltrating lymphocytes. *J Exp Med* 1996;183:1185–1192.

98. Wolfel T, Hauer M, Schneider J, et al. p16INK4a-insensitive CDK4 mutant targeted by cytolytic T lymphocytes in a human melanoma. *Science* 1995;269:1281–1284.

99. Wang R-F, Wang X, Atwood AC, Topalian SL, Rosenberg SA. Cloning genes encoding MHC class II-restricted antigens: mutated CDC27 as a tumor antigen. *Science* 1999;284:1351–1354.

100. Wang R-F, Wang X, Rosenberg SA. Identification of a novel major histocompatibility complex class II-restricted tumor antigen resulting from a chromosomal rearrangement recognized by CD4 T cells. *J Exp Med* 1999;189:1659–1667.

101. Kawakami Y, Eliyahu S, Delgado CH, et al. Identification of a human melanoma antigen recognized by tumor-infiltrating lymphocytes associated with *in vivo* tumor rejection. *Proc Natl Acad Sci U S A* 1994;91:6458–6462.

102. Rosenberg SA. Cancer vaccines based on the identification of genes encoding cancer regression antigens. *Immunol Today* 1997;18:175–182.

103. Alexander-Miller MA, Leggatt GR, Berzofsky JA. Selective expansion of high or low avidity cytotoxic T lymphocytes and efficacy for adoptive immunotherapy. *Proc Natl Acad Sci U S A* 1996;93:4102–4107.

104. Gallimore A, Dumrese T, Hengartner H, Zinkernagel RM, Rammensee HG. Protective immunity does not correlate with the hierarchy of virus-specific cytotoxic T cell responses to naturally processed peptides. *J Exp Med* 1998;187:1647–1657.

105. Zeh III HJ, Perry-Lalley D, Dudley ME, Rosenberg SA, Yang JC. High avidity CTLs for two self-antigens demonstrate superior in vitro and in vivo antitumor efficacy. *J Immunol* 1999;162:989–994.

106. Yee C, Savage PA, Lee PP, Davis MM, Greenberg PD. Isolation of high avidity melanoma-reactive CTL from heterogeneous populations using peptide-MHC tetramers. *J Immunol* 1999;162:2227–2234.

107. Kurzrock R, Gutterman J, Talpaz M. The molecular genetics of Philadelphia chromosome positive leukemias. *N Engl J Med* 1988;319:990–998.

108. Shtivelman E, Lifshitz B, Gale R, Canaani E. Fused transcripts of abl and bcr genes in chronic myelogenous leukemia. *Nature* 1985;315:550.

109. Cheever M, Chen W, Disis M, Takahashi M, Peace D. T-cell immunity to oncogenic proteins including mutated RAS and chimeric BCR-ABL. *Ann N Y Acad Sci* 1993;690:101–112.

110. Konopka J, Witte O. Detection of c-abl tyrosine kinase activity *in vitro* permits direct comparison of normal and altered abl gene products. *Mol Cell Biol* 1985;5:3116.

111. Daley G, vanEtten R, Baltimore D. Induction of chronic myelogenous leukemia in mice by the p210 bcr/abl gene of the Philadelphia chromosome. *Science* 1990;247:824–830.

112. Daley G, Baltimore D. Transformation of an interleukin-3 dependent cell line by the chronic myelogenous leukemia-specific p210 bcr/abl protein. *Proc Natl Acad Sci U S A* 1988;85:9312–9316.

113. Lange W, Snyder D, Castro R, Rossi J, Blume K. Detection by enzymatic amplification of BCR-ABL mRNA in peripheral blood and bone marrow cells of patients with chronic myelogenous leukemia. *Blood* 1989;73:1735.

114. Lee M, LeMaistre A, Kantarjian H, et al. Detection of two alternative bcr/abl mRNA junctions and minimal residual disease in Philadelphia chromosome positive chronic myelogenous leukemia by polymerase chain reaction. *Blood* 1989;73:2165.

115. Clark S, McLaughlin J, Crist W, Champlin R, Witte O. Unique forms of the abl tyrosine kinase distinguish Ph1-positive CML from Ph1-positive ALL. *Science* 1987;235:85–88.

116. Kurzrock R, Shtalrid M, Romero P, et al. A novel c-abl protein product in Philadelphia-positive acute lymphoblastic leukemia. *Nature* 1987;325:631–635.

117. Chen W, Peace DJ, Rovira DK, You S-G, Cheever MA. T-cell immunity to the joining region of p210BCR-ABL protein. *Proc Natl Acad Sci U S A* 1992;89:1468–1472.

118. tenBosch G, Joosten A, Kessler J, Melief C, Leeksma O. Recognition of BCR-ABL positive leukemic blasts by human CD4⁺ T cells elicited by primary *in vitro* immunization with a BCR-ABL breakpoint peptide. *Blood* 1996;88:3522–3527.

119. Chen W, Qin H, Reese V, Cheever M. CTL specific for BCR-ABL joining region segment peptides fail to lyse leukemia cells expressing P210 BCR-ABL protein. *J Immunother* 1999;4:257–268.

120. Greco G, Fruci D, Accapezzato D, et al. Two bcr-abl junction peptides bind HLA-A3 molecules and allow specific induction of human cytotoxic T lymphocytes. *Leukemia* 1996;10:693–699.

121. Bocchia M, Korontsvit T, Xu Q, et al. Specific human cellular immunity to bcr-abl oncogene-derived peptides. *Blood* 1996;87:3587–3592.

122. Shurtleff S, Buijs A, Behm F, et al. TEL/AML1 fusion resulting from a cryptic t(12;21) is the most common genetic lesion in pediatric ALL and defines a subgroup of patients with an excellent prognosis. *Leukemia* 1995;9:1985–1989.

123. Raynaud S, Cave M, Baens C, et al. The 12;21 translocation involving TEL and deletion of the other TEL allele: two frequently associated alterations found in childhood acute lymphoblastic leukemia. *Blood* 1996;87:2891–2897.

124. Yotnda P, Garcia F, Peuchmaur M, et al. Cytotoxic T cell response against the chimeric ETV6-AML1 protein in childhood acute lymphoblastic leukemia. *J Clin Invest* 1998;102:455–462.

125. Whang-Peng J, Triche T, Knutsen T, Miser J, Douglass E, Israel M. Chromosome translocation in peripheral neuroepithelioma. *New Engl J Med* 1984;311:584–585.

126. Turc-Carel C, Aurias A, Mugneret F, et al. Chromosomes in Ewing's sarcoma: an evaluation of 85 cases and remarkable consistency of t(11;22)(q24;q12). *Cancer Genet Cytogenet* 1988;32:229–238.

127. Lessnick SL, Braun BS, Denny CT, May WA. Multiple domains mediate transformation by the Ewing's sarcoma EWS/FLI-1 fusion gene. *Oncogene* 1995;10:423–431.

128. May WA, Lessnick SL, Braun BS, et al. The Ewing's sarcoma EWS/FLI-1 fusion gene encodes a more potent transcriptional activator and is a more powerful transforming gene than FLI-1. *Mol Cell Biol* 1993;13:7393–7398.

129. deAlava E, Kawai A, Healey J, et al. EWS-FLI1 fusion transcript structure is an independent determinant of prognosis in Ewing's sarcoma. *J Clin Oncol* 1998;16:1–9.

130. Goletz T, Zhan S, Pendleton C, Helman L, Berzofsky J. Cytotoxic T cell responses against the EWS/FLI-1 Ewing's sarcoma fusion protein and the PAX3/FKHR alveolar rhabdomyosarcoma fusion protein. *Proc Am Assoc Clin Res* 1996;3243.

131. Goletz T, Mackall C, Berzofsky J, Helman L. Molecular alterations in pediatric sarcomas: potential targets for immunotherapy. *Sarcoma* 1998;2:77–87.

132. Chalepakis G, Jones F, Edelman G, Gruss P. Pax-3 contains domains for transcription activation and transcription inhibition. *Proc Natl Acad Sci U S A* 1994;91:12745–12749.

133. Barr F, Nauta L, Davis R, Schafer B, Nycum L, Biegel J. *In vivo* amplification of the PAX3-FKHR and PAX7-FKHR fusion genes in alveolar rhabdomyosarcoma. *Hum Mol Genet* 1996;5:15–21.

134. Scheidler S, Fredericks Ward FR, Barr F, Vogt P. The hybrid PAX3-FKHR fusion protein of alveolar rhabdomyosarcoma transforms fibroblasts in culture. *Proc Natl Acad Sci U S A* 1996;93:9805–9809.

135. Goletz TJ, Mackall CL, Berzofsky JA, Helman LJ. Molecular alterations in pediatric sarcomas: potential targets for immunotherapy. *Sarcoma* 1998;2:77–87.

136. Maher VE, Worley BS, Contois D, et al. Mutant oncogene and tumor suppressor gene products and fusion proteins created by chromosomal translocations as targets for cancer vaccines. In: Kast WM, ed. *Peptide-based cancer vaccines*. Austin: Landes Bioscience, 1999.

137. Disis ML, Calenoff E, McLaughlin G, et al. Existent T-cell and antibody immunity to HER-2/neu protein in patients with breast cancer. *Cancer Res* 1994;54:16–20.

138. Disis ML, Smith JW, Murphy AE, Chen W, Cheever MA. *In vitro* generation of human cytolytic T-cells specific for peptides derived from the HER-2/neu proto-oncogene protein. *Cancer Res* 1994;54:1071–1076.

139. Linehan DC, Goedegebuure PS, Peoples GE, Rogers SO, Eberlein TJ. Tumor-specific and HLA-A2-restricted cytolysis by tumor-associated lymphocytes in human metastatic breast cancer. *J Immunol* 1995;155:4486–4491.

140. Peoples GE, Goedegebuure PS, Smith R, Linehan DC, Yoshino I, Eberlein TJ. Breast and ovarian cancer-specific cytotoxic T lymphocytes recognize the same HER2/neu-derived peptide. *Proc Natl Acad Sci U S A* 1995;92:432–436.

141. Yoshino I, Goedegebuure PS, Peoples GE, et al. HER2/neu-derived peptides are shared antigens among human non-small cell lung cancer and ovarian cancer. *Nature* 1994;54:3387–3390.

142. Fisk B, Chesack B, Pollack MS, Wharton JT, Ioannides CG. Oligopeptide induction of a cytotoxic T lymphocyte response to HER-2/neu proto-oncogene in vitro. *Proc Am Assoc Cancer Res* 1994;35:498.

143. Peoples GE, Smith RC, Linehan DC, Yoshino I, Goedegebuure PS, Eberlein TJ. Shared T cell epitopes in epithelial tumors. *Cell Immunol* 1995;164:279–286.

144. Peiper M, Goedegebuure PS, Linehan DC, Ganguly E, Douville CC, Eberlein TJ. The HER2/neu-derived peptide p654-662 is a tumor-associated antigen in human pancreatic cancer recognized by cytotoxic T lymphocytes. *Eur J Immunol* 1997;27:1115–1123.

145. Zhang S, Zhang HS, Reuter VE, Slovin SF, Scher HI, Livingston PO. Expression of potential target antigens for immunotherapy on primary and metastatic prostate cancers. *Clin Cancer Res* 1998;4:295–302.

146. Kono K, Rongcun Y, Charo J, et al. Identification of HER2/neu-derived peptide epitopes recognized by gastric cancer-specific cytotoxic T lymphocytes. *Int J Cancer* 1998;78:202–208.

147. Zaks TZ, Rosenberg SA. Immunization with a peptide epitope (p369-377) from HER-2/neu leads to peptide-specific cytotoxic T lymphocytes that fail to recognize HER-2/neu tumors. *Cancer Res* 1998;4902–4908.

148. Gu XG, Schmitt M, Hiasa A, et al. A novel hydrophobized polysaccharide/oncoprotein complex vaccine induces *in vitro* and *in vivo* cellular and humoral immune responses against HER2/expressing murine sarcomas. *Cancer Res* 1998;58:3385–3390.

149. Wang L, Ikeda H, Ikuta Y, et al. Bone marrow-derived dendritic cells incorporate and process hydrophobized polysaccharide/oncoprotein complex as antigen presenting cells. *Int J Oncol* 1999;14:695–701.

150. Disis ML, Gralow JR, Bernhard H, Hand SL, Rubin WD, Cheever MA. Peptide-based, but not whole protein, vaccines elicit immunity to HER-2/neu, oncogenic self-protein. *J Immunol* 1996;156:3151–3158.

151. Berzofsky JA, Berkower IJ. Immunogenicity and antigen structure. In: Paul WE, ed. *Fundamental immunology.* 4th ed. Philadelphia: Lippincott–Raven, 1999:651–699.

152. Berzofsky JA, Berkower IJ. Novel approaches to peptide and engineered protein vaccines for HIV using defined epitopes: advances in 1994–95. *AIDS* 1995;9[Suppl A]:S143–S157.

153. Irvine KR, Rao JB, Rosenberg SA, Restifo NP. Cytokine enhancement of DNA immunization leads to effective treatment of established pulmonary metastases. *J Immunol* 1996;156:238–245.

154. Chamberlain RS, Carroll MW, Bronte V, et al. Costimulation enhances the active immunotherapy effect of recombinant anticancer vaccines. *Cancer Res* 1996;56:2832–2836.

155. Hodge JW, McLaughlin JP, Abrams SI, Shupert WL, Schlom J, Kantor JA. Admixture of a recombinant vaccinia virus containing the gene for the costimulatory molecule B7 and a recombinant vaccinia virus containing a tumor-associated antigen gene results in enhanced specific T-cell responses and antitumor immunity. *Cancer Res* 1995;55:3598–3603.

16.5

CANCER VACCINES: CANCER ANTIGENS

Carbohydrate Antigens on Glycolipids and Glycoproteins

PHILIP O. LIVINGSTON
KENNETH O. LLOYD

BASIS FOR FOCUSING ON CANCER ANTIGENS THAT ARE CARBOHYDRATES

Carbohydrate antigens have been surprisingly potent targets for immune recognition and attack against cancer cells, both because of their abundance at the cell surface and because of their unexpected immunogenicity. Despite these and other obvious advantages to the use of carbohydrate antigens as targets for immune attack, there are also limitations.

Vaccines Against Bacterial Diseases

Of the many well-defined bacterial antigens studied as targets for vaccine therapy, carbohydrate antigens are the most effective

(1–3). Antibodies against capsular polysaccharides on *Neisseria meningitidis, Streptococcus pneumoniae,* and *Haemophilus influenzae* type B protect against subsequent bacterial challenge, and these vaccines are approved and widely available for human use.

Abundant Expression at the Cancer Cell Surface

Cancer cells may occasionally express as many as 10^6 copies of individual protein antigens at the cell surface, as has been reported for epidermal growth factor and HER-2/*neu* (4,5), but most protein antigens are expressed in far smaller numbers. The number of carbohydrate epitopes expressed at the cell surface, however, is often far greater. Thus, the median number of glycolipid molecules, such as gangliosides GM2 and GD2 on melanoma cells, is close to 10^7 and for sarcomas and neuroblastomas is more than 5×10^7 (6–8). The median number of GD3 molecules expressed on melanoma and sarcoma cells is also approximately 5×10^7. The number of copies of a given glycoprotein carbohydrate epitope on cancer cells is less well defined. However, each mucin molecule has 30 to 100 tandem repeats, each of which can express five to 15 carbohydrate epitopes. Some of these mucins (e.g., MUC1) have transmembrane domains and are integral membrane components, whereas others (e.g., MUC2 and MUC5AC) are shed and surround the tumor cell *in vivo*, though they are not actually membrane components. Because the surface of epithelial cancer cells is covered by a dense glycocalyx of various mucins, most epithelial cancer cells are probably covered by at least 100,000 mucin molecules (9,10). Consequently, the number of small carbohydrate epitopes, such as Thomsen-Friedenreich antigen (TF), Tn, or sialyl Tn (sTn), at or near the cell surface is probably well in excess of 10^7.

Effective Targets for Immune Attack

In our series of 110 patients immunized with melanoma cell or melanoma cell lysate vaccines mixed with various adjuvants (11) and in the series of patients immunized with allogeneic melanoma cell vaccines described by Tai et al. (12), gangliosides GM2 and GD2 were the only antigens recognized by multiple patients. Gangliosides are acidic glycosphingolipids overexpressed at the cell surface of melanomas, sarcomas, and other tumors of neuroectodermal origin. Gangliosides have also been shown to be effective targets for immunotherapy with monoclonal antibodies (MAb), with major responses seen in patients after treatment with MAb against GM2, GD2, and GD3 (13–19). The experience with mono or disaccharide epitopes TF, Tn, and sTn that are expressed on mucins in a great variety of epithelial cancers has been similar. Immunization with Tn and TF protects mice from subsequent challenge with cancer cells expressing these antigens (20,21), and the presence of antibodies against TF and sTn in cancer patients has been increased by vaccination (22–24). Patients with increased antibodies against GM2 and sTn have been shown to have a more favorable prognosis (22,25). Hence, active and passive immunotherapy trials have identified carbohydrate epitopes on glycolipids and glycoproteins as uniquely effective targets for cancer immunotherapy.

The chemical structure of these carbohydrate antigens is demonstrated in Figure 1.

Limitations

The general inability of carbohydrate vaccines to induce T-cell immunity against carbohydrate epitopes and the probable inability of a strictly antibody response to alter the course of well-established cancers is a limitation that results from selecting carbohydrate antigens as targets for cancer immunotherapy. Carbohydrates are considered T lymphocyte–independent antigens. Whether this is invariably true is unclear at this time. Although T lymphocytes with $\gamma\delta$ receptors can recognize nonpeptide antigens (26) and T lymphocytes with standard $\alpha\beta$ receptors can recognize carbohydrate substituents on peptides (27), it has not been possible to use this knowledge to construct vaccines capable of inducing T-lymphocyte immunity against carbohydrate cancer antigens. This may be in part because it is not known to which amino acids on which peptides any given carbohydrate epitope is linked, and whether the resulting glycopeptide sequences bind to HLA molecules. In any case, skin tests for delayed-type hypersensitivity, cytokine release assays, and cytotoxic T-lymphocyte responses have not been convincingly demonstrated against human cancer antigens or cells after immunization with antibody-inducing carbohydrate antigen vaccines.

Advantages

A number of advantages exist to using cell-surface carbohydrate antigens as targets for immunotherapy of cancer with vaccines, especially in the adjuvant setting. These include

- They are the most abundant antigens at the tumor-cell surface.
- They are immunogenic in terms of antibody response after vaccination with properly constructed conjugate vaccines.
- Antibodies induced against carbohydrate antigens are ideally suited for tumor eradication in the adjuvant setting where the targets are micrometastases and circulating tumor cells.
- Carbohydrates are uniquely effective targets for active and passive immunotherapy of cancer.
- It is possible to purify or synthesize these carbohydrate antigens in sufficient quantities for vaccine construction.
- Carbohydrates play key roles in intracellular interactions as targets for selectins and adhesins, which may be crucial, not discretionary, to tumor-cell survival and the metastatic process. Vaccine-induced antibodies may be capable of interfering with these processes.

BIOLOGIC ROLES OF CELL SURFACE CARBOHYDRATES

The great majority of the molecules of the mammalian plasma membrane are glycosylated such that glycan structures form a dense forest covering the cell surface. These glycan chains are found on glycolipids and integral membrane glycoproteins and

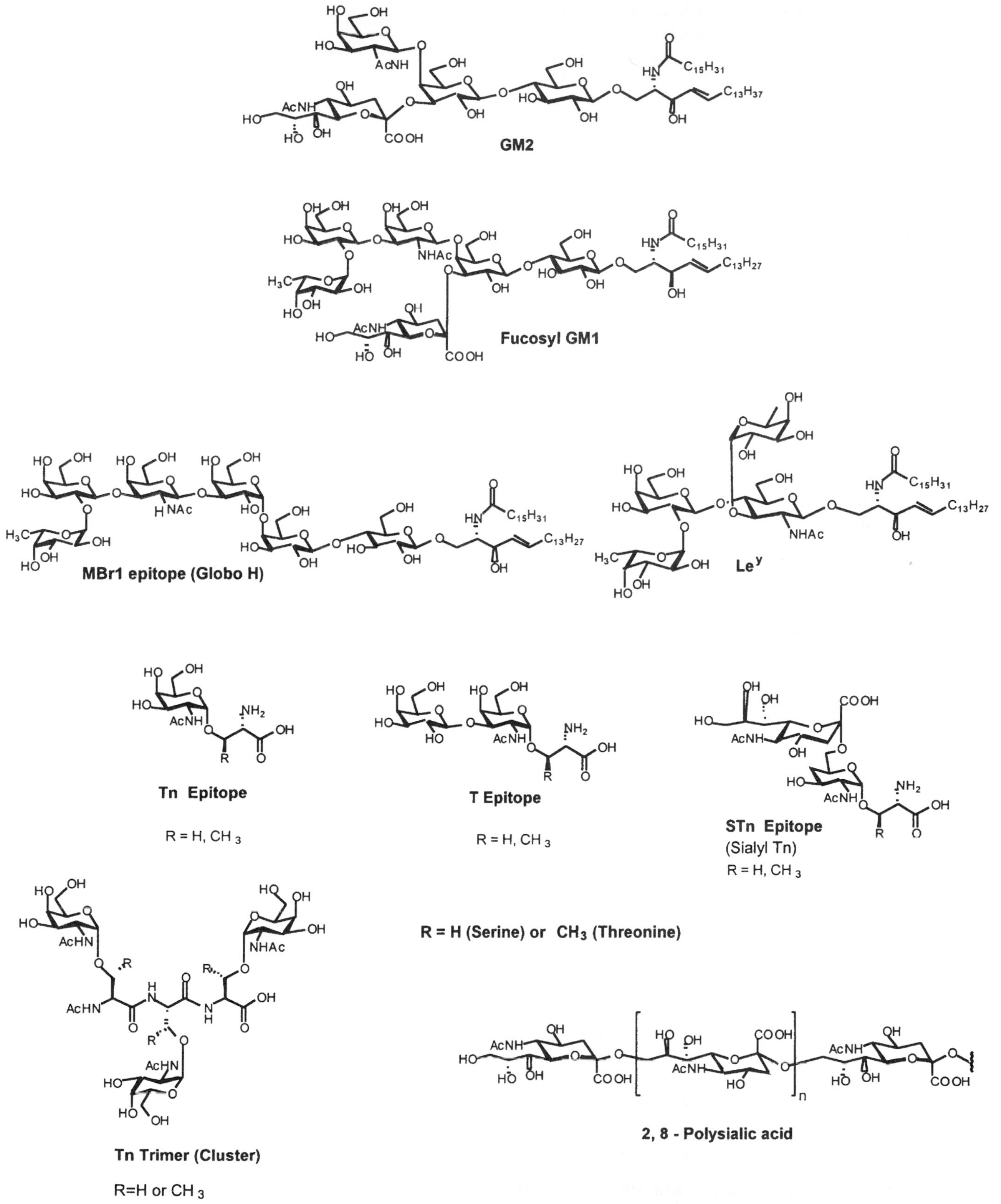

FIGURE 1. Structures of some of the defined carbohydrate tumor antigens used as targets in clinical tumor vaccine trials.

on more specialized glycoproteins such as mucins and proteoglycans. To some extent, these carbohydrates serve structural, protective, and stabilizing roles, but it is becoming increasingly recognized that they can have information-bearing functions in cell-cell recognition and adhesion (28–32). Much of this work has centered on carbohydrates as the ligands for selectins, sialoadhesins, and other cell-surface lectins. The E, L, and P selectins are involved in the interaction of endothelial cells, leukocytes, and platelets, respectively, with other cells. All three proteins recognize sialylated or sulfated Le^x (or Le^a)-bearing ligands, although in the context of different carriers (28,32). Sialoadhesins are more widely expressed and recognize α-2,6- and α-2,3-linked sialic acid–containing structures (33). Other carbohydrate structures have been implicated in such normal cell functions as embryogenesis, neural cell adhesion, and sperm adhesion. A large body of circumstantial evidence also links glycosylation to the biology of tumor cells. All tumors studied have changes in the expression of carbohydrate structures that are characteristic of the tissue of origin of the tumor. As a general rule, tumors of neural-crest origin (e.g., melanoma, sarcoma, and neuroblastoma) exhibit overexpression of gangliosides (sialylated glycolipids), whereas epithelial cancers (carcinomas) have altered fucosylated structures and mucin-core structures (TF, Tn, sTn) as their characteristic antigens. Although the precise role that these structures play in the aberrant behavior of tumor cells is unclear, numerous studies have shown a relationship between the expression of certain carbohydrate specificities (including Le^y, Le^b, sTn, and Tn blood group antigens) and metastatic potential and patient survival (34,35). The authors suggest that these effects be mediated through the influence of carbohydrate structures on the metastatic spread of tumor cells. Another glycosylation change frequently found on tumor cells—that is, a higher proportion of branched complex structures on Asn-linked chains of their glycoprotein—has also been correlated with metastatic properties in experimental systems (36). In contrast to the emerging picture of the role of oligosaccharides on glycoproteins, there is much less information on the role of cell-surface glycolipids. Evidence is accumulating that glycolipids may also play important roles in cell/cell interactions, cell proliferation, and tumor metastasis (37,38).

BASIS FOR CANCER VACCINES THAT INDUCE ONLY ANTIBODIES

Antibodies prevent infections with viral or bacterial pathogens by preventing their spread through the bloodstream and by eliminating early tissue invasion. They are also ideally suited for eliminating circulating tumor cells and micrometastasis.

Evidence in Experimental Animals

The basis for vaccines that induce only antibodies is well documented in experimental animals (39). Experiments involving administration of MAb 3F8 against the ganglioside GD2 have been particularly informative (40). Administration of 3F8 before, 2 days after, or 4 days after intravenous tumor challenge

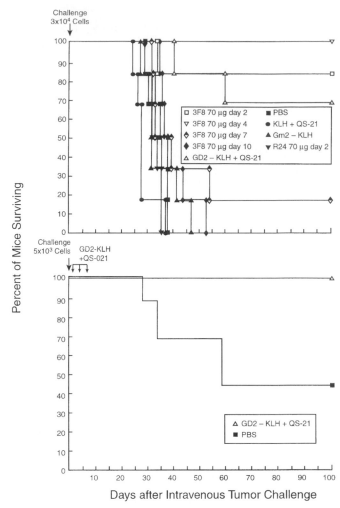

FIGURE 2. Prevention of EL4 lymphoma recurrence by immunotherapy with monoclonal antibody 3F8 or vaccination with GD2-KLH plus QS-21 after intravenous challenge. In the top panel, immunizations were administered on days -14, -7, and 1. (KLH, keyhole limpet hemocyanin.)

with EL4 lymphoma (which expresses GD2) results in complete protection (cure) of most mice. Vaccinations with GD2-KLH initiated either before the challenge or immediately after the challenge has the same effect (Fig. 2). This timing may be comparable to antibody induction in the adjuvant setting, after surgical resection of the primary malignancy or lymph node metastasis, because in both cases the targets are circulating tumor cells and micrometastases. Administration of 3F8 7 days or longer after intravenous tumor challenge had little impact on tumor progression.

The adjuvant setting in the clinic has been more closely modeled by injecting EL4-lymphoma cells into the footpad on day 1, amputating the visible tumor and foot on day 17, and then treating with 3F8 or initiating a series of vaccinations with GD2-KLH plus immunologic adjuvant QS-21. All untreated mice died or were in obvious distress and were euthanized by day 50. All mice treated with 3F8 or vaccine survived at least 60 days, and 60% and 40%, respectively, were tumor free when they were sacrificed at day 100.

Evidence in Patients

Evidence that naturally acquired or passively administered anti-bodies are associated with a more favorable prognosis exists in cancer patients.

1. Patients with resected melanoma having natural antibodies against GM2 ganglioside had an 80% to 90% 5-year survival compared to the expected 40% rate in studies at two different medical centers (25,41,42).

2. Patients with small-cell lung cancer and naturally acquired antibodies against small-cell lung cancer had a prolonged survival compared to antibody-negative patients (43).

3. Paraneoplastic syndromes in cancer patients have been associated with high titers of natural antibodies against onconeural antigens expressed on neurons and certain malignant cells. The antibodies were apparently induced by tumor growth and have been associated with autoimmune neurologic disorders and with delayed tumor progression and prolonged survival (44,45).

4. Patients with resected Dukes' C colon cancer who were treated with monoclonal antibody (MAb) 17-1A in the adjuvant setting had a significantly prolonged disease-free and overall survival compared to randomized controls. This is the only randomized clinical trial of MAb therapy conducted in the adjuvant setting reported to date (46).

Mechanism of Action

The effect of all commonly used vaccines against infectious agents is thought to be primarily a consequence of antibody induction. Based on studies of bacterial infections, the mechanism of protection against tumors by antibodies probably includes complement-mediated attack and lysis, antibody-dependent cell-mediated cytotoxicity (ADCC), and Fc-mediated opsonization, with cell-surface tumor antigens as targets. Some antibodies may have direct effects, such as by inhibiting tumor-cell attachment or inhibiting growth hormone receptors, but in general the interaction of antibody and antigen is without consequence unless Fc-mediated secondary effector mechanisms are activated. Binding of antibody to antigen results in a functional change in the Fc portion of the antibody and activation of several effector mechanisms. For cancer carbohydrate antigens, immunoglobulin M (IgM) bound to antigen is the most active complement activator in the intravascular space and IgG1 and IgG3 are the most important complement activators extravascularly. Complement activation at the cell surface mediates inflammatory reactions, opsonization for phagocytosis, clearance of antigen or antibody complexes from the circulation, and membrane-attack complex-mediated lysis. Opsonization for ingestion and destruction by phagocytosis can occur through complement activation but also can occur directly as a consequence of Fc receptors on phagocytic cells. Fc receptors on cell-surface–bound IgG1 and IgG3 are the primary targets for ADCC of tumor cells. FcδRI (CD64), FcδRII (CD32), and FcδRIII (CD16) receptors on a range of effector cells, including especially natural killer cells but also cells of myeloid lineage, react with tumor cell–bound antibody, resulting in activation of inherent cytotoxic mechanisms in these effector cells.

TABLE 1. CARBOHYDRATE TARGETS FOR VACCINE CONSTRUCTION

Tumor	Antigens
Melanoma	GM2, GD2, GD3
Neuroblastoma	GM2, GD2, GD3, polysialic acid
Sarcoma	GM2, GD2, GD3
B-cell lymphoma	GM2, GD2
Small-cell lung cancer	GM2, fucosyl GM1, polysialic acid, globo H, sialyl Le^a
Breast	GM2, globo H, Le^y, TF
Prostate	GM2, Tn, sTn, TF, Le^y
Colon	GM2, Tn, sTn, TF, sialyl Le^a, Le^y
Ovary	GM2, globo H, sTn, TF, Le^y
Stomach	GM2, Le^y, Le^a, sialyl Le^a

Note: Antigens present on at least 50% of cancer cells in at least 60% of biopsy specimens.

SELECTION OF CARBOHYDRATE ANTIGENS FOR VACCINE CONSTRUCTION

Carbohydrate antigens expressed at the cancer-cell surface have generally been identified first by antibodies, usually murine MAb. Immunohistochemistry with MAb of known specificity is the most widely used procedure for defining the distribution of carbohydrate antigens on cancers and normal tissues. This is performed on frozen sections when glycolipids are the target to prevent glycolipid loss during paraffin imbedding. Results with immunohistochemistry have been confirmed in the case of glycolipid antigens by extraction and thin-layer chromatography. This is possible because glycolipids can be extracted from biopsy specimens using chloroform and methanol, and because cancer biopsy specimens of neuroectoderm origin contain predominantly tumor cells. The identity of these glycolipids can be confirmed by immunostaining of thin-layer chromatography plates. GM2, GD2, and GD3 ganglioside-expression on melanomas, sarcomas, and neuroblastomas have been defined in this way (6,7,47). This approach is not applicable to carbohydrate antigens on glycoproteins because glycoproteins are difficult to fractionate and to isolate, and because these antigens are characteristic of epithelial cancers in which tumor cells frequently constitute only 10% to 20% of the biopsy specimen, the remainder being normal connective tissue or stroma. Using panels of MAb against carbohydrate antigens, we have screened a variety of malignant and normal tissues by immunohistochemistry (48,49). In general, ganglioside antigens have a different distribution on various malignancies than the other carbohydrate antigens. Melanomas, sarcomas, and neuroblastomas express GM2, GD2, and GD3 but none of the other antigens, whereas the epithelial cancers express a broad range of carbohydrate antigens but rarely express GD2 or GD3. The carbohydrate antigens expressed on 50% or more of tumor cells in 60% or more of biopsy specimens of various types of cancers are listed in Table 1.

Each of these antigens are also expressed on some normal tissues. GM2, GD2, and GD3 are all expressed in the brain, especially GD2, which is also expressed on some peripheral nerves and, unexpectedly, a subpopulation of B lymphocytes in the

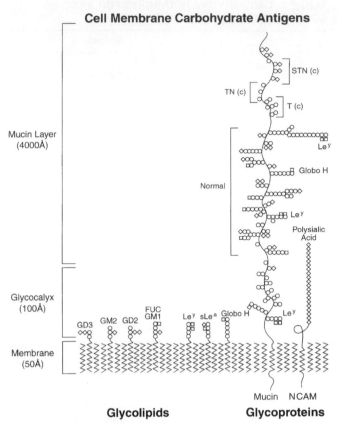

FIGURE 3. Comparison of the cell surface profiles of clinically relevant carbohydrate antigens expressed at the cancer cell surface as glycolipids or glycoproteins. Note the log scale. (NCAM, neural cell adhesion molecule; □, fucose; ○, glucose, galactose, N-acetylgalactosamine or N-acetylglucosamine; ◇, sialic acid.)

spleen and lymph nodes. Also unexpectedly, GM2 as defined by MAb 696 is expressed at the secretory borders of most epithelial tissues. GD2 and GD3 are also expressed at low levels in connective tissues of multiple organs, and GD3 is known to be expressed on some human T lymphocytes (50). Fucosyl GM1 is expressed on occasional cells in the islets of Langerhans and in some sensory neurons in the dorsal root ganglia. Polysialic acid is expressed significantly in brain and some bronchial epithelial cells. Globo H, Le^y, TF, Tn, and sTn were expressed at the secretory borders of a variety of epithelial tissues. Le^x and sialyl Le^x were expressed at the secretory border of many epithelial tissues but also on polymorphonuclear leukocytes, and sTn was found on Leydig cells of the testis.

The broad expression of most of these carbohydrate antigens on normal tissues raises concern for their suitability as targets for immunotherapy. However, there is sufficient experience from clinical trials with MAb against GD2, GD3, Le^x, sTn, and with vaccine-induced antibody responses against GM2, GD2, GD3, TF, Tn, sTn, globo H, and Le^y to draw conclusions about the consequences of antigen distribution on various normal tissues (11,13–19,22–24,51–53). Expression of gangliosides in the brain and expression of many of these antigens at the secretory borders of epithelial tissues has induced neither

immunologic tolerance nor autoimmunity once antibodies were present, suggesting that they are sequestered from the immune system. The known expression of Le^x and sialyl Le^x on polymorphonucleocytes and the granulocytopenia seen after treatment of patients with MAb FC-2.15 (later found to recognize Le^x) (52) excludes these two carbohydrates as candidates for vaccine construction, and so they have been omitted from Table 1. The expression of fucosyl GM1 on subpopulations of cells in the islets of Langerhans and the dorsal-root ganglia was initially of concern, but no evidence of autoimmunity has been detected in nine patients vaccinated with fucosyl GM1 who produced high titers of IgM and IgG antibodies against fucosyl GM1 (54). Administration of high doses of some, but not other, IgG MAb against GD2 has been associated with peripheral neuropathy in melanoma patients (18,19). High, but not lower, doses of anti-Le^y MAb-BR96 conjugated to doxorubicin has resulted in vomiting, hematemesis, and amylase elevations in some patients (55), whereas BR55, a second MAb against Le^y studied by the same investigators, resulted in no such toxicity. With regard to vaccines, ongoing trials with vaccines against GD2, fucosyl GM1, and Le^y have addressed these questions more directly (54,56,57). Moderate to high titers of IgM and IgG antibodies have been induced and have not been associated with any evidence of autoimmunity or other adverse clinical effects. Consequently, Table 1, which lists the carbohydrate antigens expressed at the cell surface of each of the common solid tumors, serves as a guide as single antigen or polyvalent antigen vaccine trials are planned.

Carbohydrate epitopes on tumor cells can be expressed on glycolipids with the carbohydrate epitopes covalently attached to ceramide that is anchored in the lipid membrane by hydrophobic forces or on glycoproteins linked to proteins. This is illustrated in Figure 3. The carbohydrate epitopes of gangliosides are expressed exclusively as glycolipids. Carbohydrate epitopes of Tn, sTn, and TF are only known to be expressed O-linked to the hydroxy moiety of the many serines and threonines characteristic of mucins. Le^y and globo H are known to be expressed both on glycolipids and glycoproteins (especially on mucins). A clear dichotomy exists between the close association of glycolipid carbohydrate epitopes with the lipid bilayer of the cell membrane and the considerable distance between many glycoprotein epitopes and the cell membrane.

DISTINCTIONS BETWEEN GLYCOLIPIDS AND GLYCOPROTEINS AS TARGETS FOR IMMUNE ATTACK

While analyzing the serologic responses in a series of vaccine trials in cancer patients immunized with various carbohydrate antigens, we noted that while sera in most of the trials were readily able to react with the tumor cell surface as detected by flow cytometry, only responses against glycolipid antigens were able to mediate complement-dependent cytotoxicity (CDC). The results of studies with immunized patient sera and with MAb against these same antigens are summarized in Table 2.

TABLE 2. COMPLEMENT-DEPENDENT CYTOTOXICITY (CDC) IS MEDIATED BY ANTIBODIES AGAINST ANTIGENIC EPITOPES ON GLYCOLIPIDS BUT NOT AGAINST EPITOPES ON MUCINS

| | Target Antigens on MCF7 or LSC Cells | | | | | | |
| | Glycolipids | | | Glycoproteins | | | |
	GM2	Globo H	Le^y	TF	Tn	sTn^a	MUC1
Murine MAb	696	MBr1	S193	4911.8	13239.1	Cc49	HMFG2
Class/subclass	IgM	IgM	IgG3	IgM	IgM	IgG1	IgG
% positive cells (FACS)	4+^{b}	4+	4+	4+	4+	4+	4+
% lysis (CDC)	2+^{c}	4+	4+	0	0	0	0
Immune patient serum	Pt1^d	Pt2	Pt3	Pt4	Pt5	Pt6	Pt7
Class/subclass	IgM	IgM	IgM	IgM	IgM	IgM	IgM
% positive cells (FACS)	2+	3+	2+	4+	3+	4+	2+
% lysis (CDC)	2+	3+	2+	0	0	0	0

FACS, flow cytometry; IgM, immunoglobulin M; MAb, monoclonal antibody; Pt, patient; TF, Thomsen-Friedenreich antigen; sTn, sialyl Tn.
^{a}Target cells LSC colon cancer cell line in place of MCF7 breast cancer cell line.
^{b}4+, >85%, 3+, 50% to 85%; 2+, 30% to 50%; 1+, 10% to 30% positive cells by FACS.
^{c}4+, >85%; 3+, 50% to 85%, 2+, 30% to 50%; 1+, 10% to 30% lysis by chromium release assay.
^{d}Each patient was immunized with the antigen shown above conjugated to keyhole limpet hemocyanin plus QS-21. These results are representative of all results obtained with immune sera from these trials.

Although MUC1 is a mucin peptide backbone and not a carbohydrate, it is included in Table 2 to demonstrate that the inability to mediate CDC is not unique to Tn, sTn, and TF but rather includes many, if not all, antigenic epitopes on mucins. Antibodies of the IgG1 and IgG3 subclasses and IgM antibodies (all of which are induced by these vaccines) are known to be able to mediate complement activation. It is likely that cell-surface reactivity demonstrated by flow cytometry results in complement activation, and that most of the complement and Fc-mediated effector mechanisms are activated by these antibodies. Complement activation by antibody binding to sites on cell-surface proteins that are distant from the cell surface may not be capable of mediating CDC. Even antibodies of lower titer that recognize glycolipid antigens that are intimately associated with the cell membrane have no difficulty lysing the same cells.

SUMMARY

Antibodies induced against tumor antigens are ideally suited for tumor eradication in the adjuvant setting where the targets are micrometastases and circulating tumor cells. Carbohydrate antigens have proved to be surprisingly potent targets for antibody recognition and attack against cancer cells, both because of their unexpected immunogenicity and because of their abundance at the cancer cell surface. Carbohydrates play key roles in intracellular interactions as targets for selectins and adhesins, which may be crucial, not discretionary, to tumor cell survival and the metastatic process. Vaccine-induced antibodies may be capable of interfering with these processes directly and are clearly capable of inducing complement-mediated inflammation and lysis and ADCC and of mediating opsonization, inflammation, and tumor cell death by other Fc-mediated mechanisms. Passively administered MAb and vaccine-induced antibodies can protect

against growth of previously administered cancer cells in a variety of preclinical models for treatment in the adjuvant setting. Strong circumstantial evidence exists that antibodies against tumor antigens, especially against carbohydrate tumor antigens, can protect against tumor recurrence in humans. Carbohydrate antigens are expressed at the tumor cell surface as glycolipids or as glycoproteins (frequently on mucins). Carbohydrate epitopes on glycolipids appear to be uniquely potent at inducing complement-mediated cell lysis, probably as a consequence of their close association with the cell membrane. However, antibodies against both glycolipids and glycoproteins can activate complement- and other Fc-mediated effector mechanisms, and have been associated with prevention of tumor recurrence in preclinical models and in cancer patients.

REFERENCES

1. Flexner S. The results of the serum treatment in thirteen hundred cases of epidemic meningitis. *J Exp Med* 1913;17:553.
2. Heidelberger M, Avery OT. The soluble specific substance of pneumococcus. *J Exp Med* 1923;38:73–79.
3. Kayhty H, Peltola H, Karanko V. The protective level of serum antibodies to the capsular polysaccharide of *Haemophilus influenzae* type B. *J Infec Dis* 1983;147:1100.
4. Davidson NE, Gelmann EP, Lippman ME, Dickson RB. Epidermal growth factor gene expression in estrogen-positive and negative human breast cancer cell lines. *Mol End* 1987;1:216–223.
5. Lewis GD, Figari I, Fendly B, et al. Differential responses of human tumor cell lines to anti p185 HER2 monoclonal antibodies. *Cancer Immunol Immunother* 1993;37: 255–263.
6. Hamilton WB, Helling F, Lloyd KO, Livingston PO. Ganglioside expression on human malignant melanoma assessed by quantitative immune thin layer chromatography. *Int J Cancer* 1993;53: 566–573.
7. Hamilton WB, Helling F, Livingston PO. Ganglioside expression on sarcoma and small-cell lung carcinoma compared to tumors of neuroectodermal origin. *Proc Am Assoc Clin Res* 1993;34:491.
8. Helling F, Livingston PO. Ganglioside conjugate vaccines. In: *Mol*

Chem Neuropathol 1994; 21:299–309.

9. Gendler SJ. Molecular cloning and expression of human tumor associated polymorphic epithelial mucin. *J Biol Chem* 1990;265: 15286–15293.

10. Carrato C, Balague C, De Bolos C, et al. Differential apomucin expression in normal and neoplastic human gastrointestinal tissues. *Gastroenterology* 1994;107:160–172.

11. Livingston P. Approaches to augmenting the immunogenicity of melanoma gangliosides: from whole melanoma cells to ganglioside-KLH conjugate vaccines. *Immunol Rev* 1995;145:147–166.

12. Tai T, Cahan LD, Tsuchida T, Saxton RE, Irie RF, Morton DL. Immunogenicity of melanoma-associated gangliosides in cancer patients. *Int J Cancer* 1985;35:607.

13. Irie RF, Matsuki T, Morton DL. Human monoclonal antibody to ganglioside GM2 for melanoma treatment. *Lancet* 1989;1(8641): 786–787.

14. Irie RF, Morton DL. Regression of cutaneous metastatic melanoma by intralesional injection with human monoclonal antibody to ganglioside GD2. *Proc Natl Acad Sci U S A* 1986;83:8694–8698.

15. Houghton AN, Mintzer D, Cordon-Cardo C, et al. Mouse monoclonal antibody IgG3 antibody detecting GD3 ganglioside: a phase I trial in patients with malignant melanoma. *Proc Natl Acad Sci U S A* 1985;82:1242–1246.

16. Dippold WG, Bernhard H, Peter Dienes H, Meyer zum Buschenfelde K-H. Treatment of patients with malignant melanoma by monoclonal ganglioside antibodies. *Eur J Cancer Clin Oncol* 1988;24: S65–S67.

17. Raymond J, Kirkwood J, Vlock D, et al. A phase 1B trial of murine monoclonal antibody R24 (anti-GD3) in metastatic melanoma (abstract). *Proc Am Soc Clin Oncol* 1988;7:A958.

18. Cheung N-K V, Lazarus H, Miraldi FD, et al. Ganglioside GD2 specific monoclonal antibody 3F8: a phase I study in patients with neuroblastoma and malignant melanoma. *J Clin Oncol* 1987;5:1430–1440.

19. Saleh MN, Khazaeli MB, Wheeler RH, et al. Phase I trial of the murine monoclonal anti-GD2 antibody 14G9a in metastatic melanoma. *Cancer Res* 1992;52:4342.

20. Fung PYS, Madej M, Koganty RR, Longenecker BM. Active specific immunotherapy of a murine mammary adenocarcinoma using a synthetic tumor-associated glycoconjugate. *Cancer Res* 1990;50: 4308–4314.

21. Singhal A, Fohn M, Hakomori S-I. Induction of a-N-acetylgalactosamine-O-serine/threonine (Tn) antigen-mediated cellular immune response for active immunotherapy in mice. *Cancer Res* 1991;51: 1406–1411.

22. MacLean GD, Reddish MA, Koganty RR, Longenecker BM. Antibodies against mucin-associated sialyl-Tn epitopes correlate with survival of metastatic adenocarcinoma patients undergoing active specific immunotherapy with synthetic sTn vaccine. *J Immunol* 1996;9:59–68.

23. Springer GF. T and Tn, general carcinoma autoantigens. *Science* 1984;224:1198–1206.

24. Adluri S, Helling F, Calves MJ, Lloyd KO, Livingston PO. Immunogenicity of synthetic TF- and sTn-KLH conjugates in colorectal carcinoma patients. *Cancer Immunol Immunother* 1995;41:185–192.

25. Livingston PO, Wong GY, Adluri S, et al. Improved survival in stage II melanoma patients with GM2 antibodies: a randomized trial of adjuvant vaccination with GM2 ganglioside. *J Clin Oncol* 1994;12: 1036–1044.

26. Kaufmann SHE. Gamma/delta and other unconcentianal T lymphocytes: what do they see and what do they do? *Proc Natl Acad Sci U S A* 1996;93:2272–2279.

27. Haurum JS, Arsequell G, Lellouch AC, et al. Recognition of carbohydrate by major histocompatibility complex class I-restricted, glycopeptide-specific cytotoxic T lymphocytes. *J Exp Med* 1994;180: 739–744.

28. Varki A. Biological roles of oligosaccharides: all of the theories are correct. *Glycobiology* 1993;3:97–130.

29. Kobata A. Structures and functions of the sugar chains of glycoproteins. *Eur J Biochem* 1992;209:483–501.

30. Hart GW. Glycosylation. *Curr Opin Cell Biol* 1992;4:1017–1023.

31. Ashwell G, Harford J. Carbohydrate-specific receptors of the liver. *Annu Rev Biochem* 1982;51:531–554.

32. Rosen SD, Bertozzi CR. The selectins and their ligands. *Curr Opin Cell Biol* 1994;6:663–673.

33. Kelm S, Schauer R, Crocker PR. The sialoadhesins—a family of sialic acid-dependent cellular recognition molecules within the immunoglobulin superfamily. *Glycoconj J* 1996;13:913–926.

34. Miyake M, Taki T, Hitomi S, Hakomori S-I. Correlation of expression of H/Le^y/Le^b antigens with survival in patients with carcinoma of the lung. *N Engl J Med* 1992;327:14–18.

35. Ghazizadeh M, Ogawa H, Sasaki Y, Araki T, Aihara K. Mucin carbohydrate antigens (T, Tn, and sialyl-Tn) in human ovarian carcinomas: relationship with histopathology and prognosis. *Hum Pathol* 1977;960–966.

36. Kobata A. A retrospective and prospective view of glycopathology. *Glycoconj J* 1998;15:323–331.

37. Hakomori S-I. Tumor malignancy defined by aberrant glycosylation and sphingo(glyco)lipid metabolism. *Cancer Res* 1996;56:5309–5318.

38. Nakano J, Raj BKM, Asagami C, Lloyd KO. Human melanoma cell lines deficient in G$_{D3}$ ganglioside expression exhibit altered growth and tumorigenic characteristics. *J Invest Dermatol* 1996; 107:543–548.

39. Livingston PO. The case for melanoma vaccines that induce antibodies. In: Kirkwood JM, ed. *Molecular diagnosis, prevention and treatment of melanoma*. New York: Marcel Dekker, Inc. 1998:139–157.

40. Zhang H, Zhang S, Cheung NK, Ragupathi G, Livingston PO. Antibodies can eradicate cancer micrometastases. *Cancer Res* 1998;58:2844–2849.

41. Livingston PO, Ritter G, Srivastava P, et al. Characterization of IgG and IgM antibodies induced in melanoma patients by immunization with purified GM2 ganglioside. *Cancer Res* 1989;49:7045–7050.

42. Jones PC, Sze LL, Liu PY, Morton DL, Irie RF. Prolonged survival for melanoma patients with elevated IgM antibody to oncofetal antigen. *J Natl Cancer Inst* 1981;66:249–254.

43. Winter SF, Sekido Y, Minna JD, et al. Antibodies against autologous tumor cell proteins in patients with small-cell lung cancer: association with improved survival. *J Natl Cancer Inst* 1993;85(24): 2012–2018.

44. Darnell RB. Onconeural antigens and the paraneoplastic neurologic disorders: at the intersection of cancer, immunity, and the brain. *Proc Natl Acad Sci U S A* 1996;93:4529–4536.

45. Dalmau J, Graus F, Cheung N-KV, et al. Major histocompatibility proteins, Anti-Hu antibodies, and paraneoplastic encephalomyelitis in neuroblastoma and small cell lung cancer. *Cancer* 1995;75: 99–109.

46. Riethmuller G, Schneider-Gadicke E, Schlimok G, et al, and the German Cancer Aid 17-1A Study Group. Randomized trial of monoclonal antibody for adjuvant therapy of resected Dukes' C colorectal carcinoma. *Lancet* 1994;343:1177–1183.

47. Tsuchida T, Saxton RE, Kmorton DL. Gangliosides of human melanoma. *J Natl Cancer Inst* 1987;78:45–54.

48. Zhang S, Cordon-Cardo C, Zhang HS, et al. Selection of carbohydrate tumor antigens as targets for immune attack using immunohistochemistry: I. focus on gangliosides. *Int J Cancer* 1997;73:42–49.

49. Zhang S, Zhang HS, Cordon-Cardo C, Reuter VI, Lloyd KO, Livingston PO. Selection of carbohydrate tumor antigens as targets for immune attack using immunohistochemistry: II. blood group-related antigens. *Int J Cancer* 1997;73:50–56.

50. Merritt WD, Taylor BJ, Der-Minassian V, Reaman GH. Coexpression of GD$_3$ ganglioside with CD45RO in resting and activated human T lymphocytes. *Cell Immunol* 1996;173:131–148.

51. Ragupathi G, Slovin S, Adluri S, Sames D, et al. A fully synthetic globo H carbohydrate vaccine induces a focused humoral response in prostate cancer patients: a proof of principle. *Angewandte Chemie* 1999;38(45):334–339.

52. Mordoh J, Silva C, Albarellos M, Bravo AI, Kairiyama C. Phase I clinical trial in cancer patients of a new monoclonal antibody FC-

2.15 reacting with tumor proliferating cells. *J Immunother* 1995;17: 151–180.

53. Capurro M, Bover L, Portela P, Livingston PO, Mordoh J. FC-2.15, a monoclonal antibody active against human breast cancer, specifically recognizes Lewis X hapten. *Cancer Immunol Immunother* 1998;45:334–339.

54. Dickler MN, Ragupathi G, Liu NX, et al. Immunogenicity of the fucosyl-GM1-keyhole limpet hemocyanin (KLH) conjugate vaccine in patients with small cell lung cancer. *Clin Cancer Res* 1999;5:2773–2779.

55. Giantonio BJ, Gilewski T, Bookman MA, et al. A phase I study of weekly BR96-doxorubicin in patients with advanced carcinoma expressing the Lewis (Le^y) antigen. *Proc Am Soc Clin Oncol* 1996;15:53(abst).

56. Chapman PB, Meyers ML, Williams L, et al. Immunization of melanoma patient (pts) with a bivalent GM2/GD2 ganglioside conjugate vaccine. *Proc Assoc Cancer Res* 1998;39:2515.

57. Sabbatini P, Kudryashov V, Ragupathi G. Immunization of ovarian cancer patients with a synthetic LewisY–protein conjugate: clinical and serological. *Int J Cancer* (in press).

16.6

CANCER VACCINES: CANCER ANTIGENS

Glycoprotein Antigens

OLIVERA J. FINN

The term *tumor antigen* has been given a new and much more precise definition as a result of important developments in immunology in the 1990s, particularly in the area of antigen presentation and antigen recognition. For something to be a tumor antigen it must be recognized by specific immune effector cells or antibodies on tumor cells, but not on normal cells. If a tumor is recognized by CD8+ cytotoxic T lymphocytes (CTLs), in the greatest majority of cases it can be assumed that the tumor antigen is a small peptide (eight, nine, or ten amino acids long) that has been processed from a larger protein from tumor cells and presented in the peptide-binding cleft of major histocompatibility complex (MHC) class I molecules on the surface of the tumor cell. If the antigen is recognized by CD4+ T cells, it can be assumed that it is a slightly longer peptide (on an average 12 to 18 amino acids), most likely derived from a larger protein expressed or secreted by tumor cells and processed and presented in MHC class II molecules. Tumor-specific antibodies recognize either small linear peptides or conformational peptide- or nonpeptide-epitopes that are carried on proteins made by normal and tumor cells. Often, antibodies recognize tumor-specific carbohydrate epitopes on proteins that are otherwise identical in normal cells and tumor cells.

Because tumor specificity resides in small epitopes, the term *tumor antigen* must be dissociated from whole molecules and specifically applied to their much smaller fragments. Having reserved the tumor-antigen definition for small peptides, it may not be immediately obvious why we have chosen in this chapter to maintain the older definition "glycoprotein tumor antigens," which refers to the whole molecules. The glycoproteins that are discussed in this chapter are, by and large, products of normal genes that encode proteins whose amino-acid sequences are identical in normal and tumor cells. Thus, as whole proteins they do not warrant the tumor antigen designation. However, the fact that these proteins are glycosylated during their normal biosynthesis, combined with the fact that most tumor cells exhibit defects in the ability to correctly glycosylate proteins (1), creates a situation in which the repertoire of peptides derived from two differentially glycosylated but otherwise identical amino-acid sequences can be different between normal cells and tumor cells. Furthermore, antigen-presenting cells (APCs) appear to process the glycoproteins from tumor cells differently than the same molecules from normal cells, producing a tumor-specific repertoire of peptides. Some of the peptides in this new repertoire are apparently capable of stimulating a tumor-specific immune response.

Differential glycosylation affects the processed peptide repertoire not only qualitatively but also quantitatively. Aberrantly glycosylated proteins may be easier to process than their fully glycosylated normal counterparts, resulting in many more peptides derived from the same glycoprotein on the surface of tumor cells as compared to normal cells. Even though these peptides are not different in sequence from peptides presented on normal cells, their increased density of expression on the cell surface can reach the threshold level necessary for immune recognition. Whereas low levels of peptide MHCs might be ignored on normal cells, their higher density on APCs and on tumor cells can lead to effector-cell activation.

Altered glycosylation of normal cellular proteins is associated with altered immunogenicity not only in cancer but also in many inflammatory and autoimmune diseases that are accompanied by changes in *N*- or *O*-linked glycosylation of normal cellular proteins, some of which become targets of the autoimmune response (2).

ALTERED GLYCOSYLATION OF GLYCOPROTEINS IN CANCER AND RELATIONSHIP TO IMMUNOGENICITY

All glycoproteins are divided into two groups, those that carry predominantly *N*-linked and those that carry predominantly *O*-linked carbohydrate chains. Proteins are modified with *N*-linked glycans in the endoplasmic reticulum (ER) and the Golgi in a well-ordered process orchestrated by specific glycosyltransferases and glycosidases (3). *O*-glycans are added to proteins in the Golgi. The process of protein glycosylation involves a complex regulation of large families of enzymes that are tightly controlled at many levels, including gene expression, enzyme activity, presence or absence of specific cofactors, and correct trafficking of the protein substrate. All of these processes can differ or change, depending on the cell and tissue type and state of differentiation.

Transformation of a cell from a normal to a malignant phenotype can be accompanied by a dramatic change in its protein glycosylation (1). When hybridoma technology began to be used to identify tumor antigens, it was immediately noticed that many monoclonal antibodies raised against various types of tumors recognized carbohydrate epitopes that were either a novel form made by the tumor cell or more often a truncated form of the carbohydrate chain made in normal cells. A lot of work over many years on the *N*- and *O*-linked glycosylation pathways in tumor cells suggests that tumor cells lose control over the balance of their glycosyltransferases, upregulating some of them while simultaneously downregulating others (4). Another common change in tumors is truncation of the carbohydrate chains through increased action of capping glycosyltransferases. These changes have defined a whole group of carbohydrate tumor antigens, such as T or Tn, resulting from carbohydrate chain truncation and an unusual terminal oligosaccharide sequence Lewis$^{x/a}$, resulting from an inappropriate upregulation of a glycosyltransferase. Purified or synthetic versions of these carbohydrates, when coupled to carrier proteins, can be used to induce an antibody response against tumor cells.

For the purpose of this chapter, the importance of carbohydrate tumor antigens is that they are markers of glycoproteins that are aberrantly glycosylated in tumor cells. To a tumor immunologist, their presence raises the possibility that there might be changes in how the whole glycoprotein is handled and presented to the immune system by either the tumor cells or by APCs that take up glycoproteins secreted or shed from tumor cells.

ABERRANT GLYCOSYLATION IN TUMOR CELLS MAY DETERMINE ABERRANT PROCESSING AND PRESENTATION OF TUMOR GLYCOPROTEINS

MHC class I molecules are primarily responsible for presenting peptides derived from endogenously synthesized proteins made and degraded by the proteasomes in the cytosol (5,6). All cellular proteins are made in the cytosol. Those that need to be further processed or are destined to the cell surface or secretion are translocated to the ER where they must be folded correctly, *N*-glycosylated if glycoproteins, transported to the Golgi, further glycosylated with *N*- and/or *O*-linked glycans, and finally trafficked to the cell surface. Parallel with this process is the continuous process of protein degradation that also takes place in the cytosol and is carried out by a large multicatalytic protease complex called the *proteasome*. Proteasomes generate small peptides that are transported to the ER through the transporters associated with antigen processing-1 and -2 (TAP-1 and TAP-2) molecules where they bind newly synthesized MHC class I molecules. MHC class I peptide complexes are then transported to the cell surface where they can be recognized by CD8$^+$ T cells.

It is easy to imagine how the repertoire of the peptides presented on the surface of a cell would depend on the processing of proteins inside the cell. As Figure 1 illustrates, a normal cellular glycoprotein that finds itself in the cytosol is degraded predictably and consistently to a certain number of peptides, thus providing an expected repertoire of class I–restricted peptides on the cell surface (top left panel). Lack of an immune response to this normal peptide repertoire is maintained through numerous mechanisms of peripheral tolerance. If malignant transformation results in a profound difference in glycosylation or other posttranslational modifications of this same glycoprotein, proteasomes may handle it differently, resulting in the appearance of certain peptide fragments not otherwise generated from the normal glycoprotein (top right panel). These new peptides carried to the cell surface in class I molecules are not subject to the established tolerance mechanisms specific for the normal peptides and may now elicit a class I–restricted T-cell response. This response is then, by definition, a tumor-specific response.

Proteins destined to be presented to CD4$^+$ T cells are also degraded into peptide fragments, but this is accomplished by the action of vesicular proteases in specialized vesicles. This pathway is used for the processing of internalized antigens, either cell-surface molecules or soluble proteins taken up from the outside of the cell by endocytosis (6). Endocytosed proteins become enclosed into vesicles called *endosomes*, which travel into the interior of a cell where they meet with vesicles carrying MHC class II molecules. The repertoire of peptides generated by this process from glycoproteins derived from normal cells versus tumor cells can also be very different. As Figure 1 shows, endocytosed normal cell-surface glycoproteins result in a predictable, and most likely tolerated, peptide repertoire (lower left

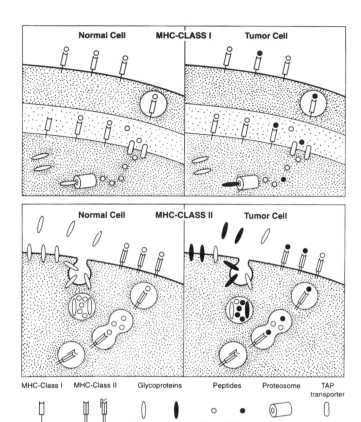

FIGURE 1. Normal pathways of antigen processing and presentation can yield tumor-specific peptides. Upper left panel illustrates the process by which a normal glycoprotein (indicated in white) made by a normal cell is processed in the cytosol by proteasomes into a normal peptide repertoire. These peptides are transported into the endoplasmic reticulum by transporters associated with antigen-processing molecules where they bind to nascent major histocompatibility complex (MHC) class I chains. They are then transported to the cell surface where the normal repertoire (*white circles only*) is not reacted against by CD8⁺ T cells. The upper right panel illustrates what happens if the same glycoprotein is changed in a tumor cell to a tumor-specific form (indicated in black). Processing of this modified glycoprotein results in a different peptide repertoire (*white and black circles*) on the surface of the tumor cell, which could be reacted against by CD8⁺ T cells.

Lower left panel illustrates the process by which a normal glycoprotein (indicated in white) is internalized from the cell surface or extracellular space into endocytic vesicles where it is degraded into normal peptides (all white). Fusion of these vesicles with vesicles containing MHC class II molecules loads the peptide fragments into MHC class II for presentation on the surface. The peptide repertoire is normal and not reacted against by T cells. Lower right panel represents uptake and processing of the same glycoprotein made in tumor cells (indicated in black). Processing of this tumor form of the glycoprotein results in a different MHC class II–presented peptide repertoire (*white and black circles*) on the surface of tumor cells, which could be reacted against by CD4⁺ T cells.

panel), whereas modified tumor glycoproteins can be processed to present new class II–restricted epitopes (lower right panel).

The same phenomenon described in Figure 1 for normal and tumor cells is operational at the level of APCs. Normal glycoproteins that are shed from surfaces of normal cells and picked up by APCs are processed into an expected repertoire of self-peptides that are not recognized by T cells. Any change in the glycoproteins shed from a malignant cell may be reflected in how it is handled by APCs. For example, if a certain glycopro-

tein is overexpressed by tumor cells compared to normal cells, it might be considered a potential tumor antigen. But the effect might be just the opposite if overexpression is accompanied by a loss or a change in its glycosylation. The result of this change may be a protein that cannot be efficiently internalized by specialized receptors on APCs. If not taken up and presented by APCs, this highly expressed tumor protein can remain hidden from the immune system. On the other hand, a specific change in glycosylation that puts a different sugar on, or truncates a sugar chain and reveals otherwise concealed core sugars on the tumor glycoprotein, may make it a much better ligand for some of the receptors, thereby increasing its uptake by APCs and thus its potential immunogenicity. Additionally, new epitopes may be generated from the aberrantly glycosylated polypeptide if certain enzyme-sensitive sites have been exposed due to the lack of glycosylation.

All of these possibilities have been documented for one or another tumor glycoprotein and are highlighted in the following specific examples.

Melanoma Glycoproteins

The best known and most studied of melanoma glycoproteins are tyrosinase, glycoprotein 100 (gp100), and gp75. Their biochemical structure has been elucidated, and they have been confirmed as glycoproteins. The biochemical nature as glycoproteins of several other melanoma antigens, in particular MART1/Melan-A, has not yet been confirmed.

Tyrosinase

Tyrosinase is a part of the melanin biosynthesis pathway and catalyzes the synthesis of the melanin precursor dihydroxyphenylalanine. That this glycoprotein, a normal tissue differentiation antigen, is recognized as a tumor antigen was first shown by the reactivity of melanoma-specific CTLs with a COS-7 cell cotransfected with both a complementary DNA (cDNA) library derived from a melanoma tumor and a plasmid-encoding HLA-A2 (7). It was subsequently shown that it contains multiple antigenic peptides restricted by a number of human HLA class I and class II molecules. Most of these peptides are derived from the normal tyrosinase sequence.

Tyrosinase-specific T cells have only been detected in melanoma patients, suggesting that *in vivo* the immune system is faced with different processing and presentation of this antigen when it is derived from melanomas rather than from normal melanocytes. *In vitro*, using optimal priming conditions, which most likely activate APCs as well as present high density of antigen, tyrosinase-specific CTLs have also been generated (8). One example of antigenicity being dependent on posttranslational modifications is the naturally occurring HLA-A2.1–associated peptide YMDGTMSQV that was identified by mass spectrometry from peptides extracted from purified HLA-A2.1 molecules expressed by melanoma cells. The peptide corresponded to residues 368 to 376 of tyrosinase except that it contained aspartic acid (D) instead of asparagine (N) predicted by the tyrosinase gene sequence (9). The peptide with aspartic acid sensitized target cells for CTL lysis at a 100 fold lower concentration than the asparagine-containing peptide. It was determined that the naturally processed peptide arose as a result of a posttranslational modification that converts a glycosylated asparagine to aspartic acid by enzymatic deamidation through the action of peptide:*N*-glycanase. This is a clear example of how changes in the posttranslational modification of glycoproteins in tumor cells may lead to the generation of new peptide epitopes that could be relevant to tumor rejection. One can also postulate that aberrant glycosylation in some tumors might instead leave the asparagine unglycosylated, which would result in a completely different peptide being presented in HLA class I, with a completely different, in this case inferior, potential as a CTL target.

Tyrosinase is also processed into peptides that can be presented by class II MHC molecules and recognized by CD4+ T cells (10,11). These class II–restricted peptides have been identified by *in vitro* stimulation with either autologous Epstein-Barr virus–immortalized B cells loaded with lysates of COS-7 cells transfected with tyrosinase cDNA or with autologous APCs infected with vaccinia virus encoding tyrosinase. Neither of these preparations that have been used to identify the epitopes mimics the tyrosinase glycoprotein synthesized by melanomas. This makes it difficult to predict with certainty that the tumor-derived glycoprotein would be processed and presented exactly the same way as the recombinant molecule. For any of these peptides derived from normal tissue differentiation antigens to become serious candidates for vaccines, issues of their tumor-specific processing and presentation should be fully resolved.

Glycoprotein 100

gp100 Is a lineage-specific antigen that is expressed in melanomas but not in other tumor-cell types or normal cells, with the exception of melanocytes and pigmented cells in the retina. It was defined as a melanoma-specific T-cell antigen when it was first demonstrated that transfection of this gene into target cells could reconstitute the epitope recognized by CD8+ HLA-A2.1–restricted tumor-infiltrating lymphocytes (TILs) (12,13). The antigenic peptide YLEPGPVTA responsible for this specificity was identified through mass spectrometric isolation of a naturally processed peptide eluted from HLA-A2.1 molecules on a melanoma cell line (14). Many other HLA-A2–restricted gp100-derived peptides have been reported to date, and TILs containing a strong anti-gp100 activity have been shown to be effective in adoptive immunotherapy of melanoma, making these peptides promising candidates for inclusion into a melanoma vaccine preparation. Importantly, there are reports that peptides derived from gp100 have also been eluted from HLA class II antigens on melanomas and found to be able to stimulate CD4+ T cells (15).

Glycoprotein 75

Similar to gp100 and tyrosinase, gp75 is expressed in human melanocytic cells and melanoma tumors. It was first identified using serum immunoglobulin G antibodies from a melanoma patient (16,17) and later found to encode a shared melanoma antigen recognized by HLA-A31–restricted TILs (18). Unlike the other melanoma differentiation antigens, however, the peptide MSLQRQFLR recognized by the TILs was not derived from the normal gp75 protein but from an alternative open reading frame that directs the translation of a small 24 amino acid protein. Alternative translation of otherwise normal cellular genes, in addition to alternative posttranslational modification and processing, is another way by which new tumor-specific antigens may be derived.

MART-1/MelanA

MART-1/MelanA was first defined by melanoma-specific HLA-A2.1–restricted CTLs (19,20). It is a transmembrane protein whose expression parallels that of tyrosinase. Several other peptide epitopes contained in this glycoprotein sequence have been identified as CTL targets. Although considerable information exists about the gene structure and antigenicity of this protein, little is known about its biochemical nature, including whether it is a glycoprotein. Monoclonal antibodies have been generated that react with this protein, and they are going to be useful in deciphering its primary structure and posttranslational modifications (21). Already, it is obvious that the precipitated protein is larger (23 kd) than its predicted molecular weight (13 kd) from the gene sequence. It is not clear yet if this additional weight is a result of glycosylation or other posttranslational modifications. Regardless of the precise modification of the primary structure, however, the chance that a tumor may modify this protein differently than a normal cell provides an opportunity for the immune system to see it as a tumor-specific antigen.

GLYCOPROTEINS FROM EPITHELIAL TUMORS

Among the best known epithelial cell glycoproteins, which are also classified as tumor antigens, are carcinoembryonic antigen (CEA), CO17-1A, prostate-specific antigen (PSA), HER-2/*neu*, and MUC1. All of them have been first identified by antibodies and later shown to also contain T-cell epitopes.

Carcinoembryonic Antigen

The CEA glycoprotein belongs to a family of cell-surface glycoproteins extensively explored to date for potential application in diagnosis and treatment of cancer (22,23). It is expressed primarily on colon, breast, and lung adenocarcinomas, but it is assumed that most tumor cells of epithelial origin express some low level of this antigen. It is also expressed on normal epithelia, primarily colon, and to a lesser extent other normal epithelial as well as endothelial cells. Its expression on epithelial tumors is characterized by drastically different levels of expression and differences in posttranslational modification of the protein (24). For a long time it was not clear if this difference between CEA expression on normal cells and tumor cells would have any consequence on its immunogenicity. Although low titers of CEA antibodies were found occasionally in cancer patients, it was difficult to show T-cell reactivity. Using advances in recombinant expression vector technology as well as antigen presentation, numerous peptide epitopes have been identified that can stimulate human CTLs. CEA has also been tested in phase 1 and 2 clinical trials as a vaccine against colon cancer (25). All of the immunization protocols, both *in vitro* and *in vivo*, have used some form of recombinant CEA. Having the tumor form of the molecule would appear more likely to generate immune responses against epitopes presented on tumor cells. However, published data suggests that quantitative rather than qualitative differences in CEA expression on tumor cells may be important in the tumor-specific effector phase of an immune response, whereby low levels of CEA on normal tissues are ignored by the immune system, whereas high levels on tumors specifically target those cells for killing by CTLs.

CO17-1A

CO17-1A is another human colorectal cancer antigen with a promising role in cancer immunotherapy. This 40-kd glycoprotein is expressed on gastrointestinal cancers and treatment with an anti-17-1A antibody has been shown in a randomized phase 2 trial with 189 patients and a placebo control to significantly prolong survival of colon cancer patients over a median follow-up of 5 to 7 years (26,27).

Prostate-Specific Antigen

PSA is present in the circulation of prostate cancer patients at elevated levels and has been used for diagnosis of prostate cancer (28). It is a glycoprotein of 33-kd molecular weight, and it is a member of the serine protease family with trypsin-like and chymotrypsin-like protease activity (29). PSA can also be found in milk of lactating women and in amniotic fluid, and its production by normal breast can be stimulated by oral contraceptives (30,31). PSA expression has been documented in various other tumors in addition to prostate, most frequently in breast, and some tumors of the skin, ovary, and salivary gland. A lot of interest in this molecule as a possible immunogen exists, but only limited information is available to date about its antigenicity to human T and B cells. No differences have been observed between the PSA glycoprotein expressed on tumors versus normal tissues. Two studies report generation of human CTLs against PSA. One defines two HLA-A2–binding peptides designated PSA-1 (amino acids 141 to 150) and PSA-3 (amino acids 154 to 163) that stimulate human CTLs that can kill HLA-A2+ PSA+ tumor cells (32). The other uses a longer PSA peptide of 30 amino acids to show an additional HLA-A2– and -A3–restricted CTL activity (33). These results encourage further study of PSA as a possible prostate tumor-specific antigen.

It is important to mention that other prostate glycoproteins have begun to be explored for use in prostate tumor immunotherapy. These are prostatic acid phosphatase (34) and prostate-specific membrane antigen (35). Both have been shown to induce an immune response, but this response is directed against normal as well as malignant prostate cells. Breaking of tolerance to these antigens and induction of autoimmune prostatitis is considered to be one possible approach to prostate tumor therapy.

Also promising are molecules that are being identified by representational differential analysis as genes that are upregulated during prostate cancer progression. An interesting cell-surface glycoprotein, prostate stem cell antigen, has been reported (36). It encodes a 123-aa protein with an amino-terminal signal sequence, carboxy-terminal glycosylphosphatidylinositol anchoring sequence, and multiple *N*-glycosylation sites. It is of interest to attempt to target this molecule by the immune system.

The technique of cDNA library subtraction in conjunction with a high-throughput screening has identified additional genes that were shown by reverse transcriptase-polymerase chain reaction, Northern blot, and real-time polymerase chain reaction to be overexpressed in prostate tissues or prostate tumors, or both (37). The proteins have not yet been identified, but potentially one or all of these new gene products could be explored for cancer diagnosis and immunotherapy.

HER-2/*neu*

Another category of cell surface glycoproteins that have been studied by tumor immunologists as candidate tumor-rejection antigens are various cell surface growth-factor receptors that are aberrantly expressed on tumor cells and provide autocrine growth signals. The best described to date is HER-2/*neu*, a proto-oncogene product with homology to the epidermal growth factor receptor. It is expressed in breast, ovarian, and several other types of epithelial tumors, but primarily explored in the setting of breast cancer immunotherapy. Anti-HER-2/*neu* antibodies are thought to mimic the natural ligands of this molecule, several of which have been described elsewhere (38). It has been shown that treatment with one such anti-HER-2/*neu* antibody known by the name of *trastuzumab* (Herceptin) has some therapeutic effects in metastatic breast cancer (39). On tumors, HER-2/*neu* is characterized by an increased rather than mutated expression. Like many antigens discussed in this chapter, it is also weakly expressed on normal tissues (40). The normal expression apparently fails to induce tolerance, as both antibodies (41) and T cells specific for this molecule can be found in cancer patients (42,43). This encourages further manipulations of this antigen or its gene to be used as an anti-cancer vaccine (41). Several clinical trials based on this immunogen are in progress.

Although HER-2/*neu* is touted primarily as a breast cancer antigen, there are reports of a successful elicitation of HER-2–specific T-cell responses in other malignancies, such as gastric cancer (44) and renal and colon cancer (45).

MUC1 Mucin

One of the first epithelial tumor antigens to be shown to be a target of human T-cell immunity is a mucin-like glycoprotein MUC1 (46–48). MUC1 is the only integral membrane glycoprotein among a large number of other mucins that are expressed at high levels on the surface of epithelial cell tumors, primarily breast, pancreas, colon, ovary, and lung adenocarcinomas (49). Expression of these molecules on normal tissues is usually at a much lower level and characterized by a different repertoire of immune epitopes (50). Some of the epitopes are exquisitely tumor specific (51). MUC1 is a high-molecular-weight glycoprotein extensively *O*-glycosylated on serines and threonines that are

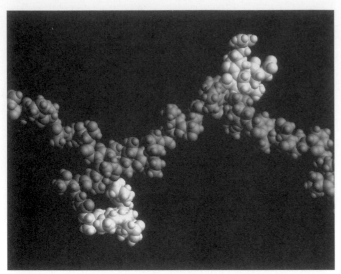

FIGURE 2. Three-dimensional structure of the tumor form of the MUC1 glycoprotein. Inability of tumor cell to glycosylate the polypeptide core leads to a formation of new knob-like epitopes (indicated in white) that are recognized by tumor-specific antibodies and T cells.

found in tandemly repeated 20 amino acid–long segments. The carbohydrate chains on the tumor-produced mucin are shorter than those on mucin produced by normal cells. An indication also exists that in tumor mucin not all the potential glycosylation sites are used. This results in the unmasking on tumor mucin of cryptic protein-core epitopes that serve as tumor-specific antigens. The same epitopes are concealed in normal mucin by complete glycosylation. In the latest International Workshop on Monoclonal Antibodies against MUC1 (52), it was observed that antibodies that recognize MUC1 only when expressed on human epithelial adenocarcinomas but not on the corresponding normal tissue were all specific for the same epitope on the tandem repeats. The amino-acid sequence of the tandem repeat is GVTS**AP-DTRP**APGSTAPPAH. The tumor-specific epitope includes amino acids APDRTP, highlighted in bold type in the preceding sequence. The nuclear magnetic resonance data revealed that the PDTRP sequence forms the tip of a protruding knob exposed to solvent and forming a stable type II β-turn (Fig. 2) (53). The formation of these "knobs" is a result of underglycosylation of serine and threonine residues just preceding and just after the knob sequence. Normal MUC1 with completely and extensively glycosylated serine and threonine residues does not form the knob-like epitopes. Differences in glycosylation between MUC1 in normal cells and MUC1 in tumor cells thus create profound changes in the 3-D structure of the native molecule, which in turn affects direct recognition, processing, and presentation of peptide epitopes derived from this molecule. The knobs are immunogenic, and antibodies against them have been detected in cancer patients (54,55). There appears to be a correlation between the presence of the antibody and increased disease-free survival (56). There are also T-cell responses against the knobs and against processed peptides presented by HLA molecules.

In patients *in vivo*, anti-MUC1 immune responses are characterized by low titer of immunoglobulin M antibodies and low frequency of MHC unrestricted CTLs. MUC1-specific T-helper cells

had not been identified *in vivo*, but they have been generated by *in vitro* priming (57), suggesting that helper-cell unresponsiveness was not due to a deletion of MUC1-specific CD4+ T cells. It was determined that the glycosylated soluble form of MUC1 that is cleaved off of the tumor cell surface and made available for APCs to take up, process, and present to T-helper cells is in fact not processed by the APCs. This hampers the development of both class I (58) and class II (59) restricted T-cell responses. When the antigen is supplied in a synthetic or a recombinant form as unglycosylated polypeptide, vigorous CTL and T-helper cell responses are generated that also react with the MUC1+ tumor cells.

The inability of APCs to present the form of MUC1 available *in vivo* explains in great part the inability of this potentially good tumor-cell target to serve in its native state as a tumor-rejection antigen. On the other hand, it appears that if the unglycosylated form is used as a vaccine to prime the T-cell responses, this problem might be solved. A synthetic MUC1 peptide, at least 100 amino acids long and composed of five or more tandem repeats, has been successfully used to prime T-helper and CTL responses in primates (60) and in several ongoing phase 1 clinical trials in patients with metastatic colon, breast, and pancreatic cancer (61) and in early diagnosed and/or resected pancreatic cancer (Finn et al., unpublished data, 1999).

Several other investigators around the world are testing MUC1 peptide-based vaccine approaches. One peptide vaccine strategy is designed to facilitate presentation of the peptides by both MHC class I and class II molecules. This is accomplished by conjugating a similarly long MUC1 peptide to mannans (polymannose) that then targets this conjugate to the mannose receptors on APCs. Patients were immunized subcutaneously eight times over a 13-week period, and antibody delayed-type hypersensitivity and CTL responses were monitored (62). This treatment resulted in the development of antibody responses of the immunoglobulin G isotype, T-helper cell responses and, in a small number of patients, a CTL response. These results collectively suggest that MUC1 peptide vaccines may serve as a powerful method to enhance or induce T-cell responses to class I and class II MUC1 epitopes.

Other MUC1-based immunogens that are also being tested in phase 1 clinical trials have included the whole protein, short peptides derived from its amino-acid sequence, or carbohydrate moieties mimicking those exposed on the tumor MUC1 due to its aberrant glycosylation (63–65). These antigenic preparations have been expressed in bacterial or viral vectors as fusion proteins, expressed in or pulsed onto several cell types, or used with different adjuvants. Some success has been seen in eliciting immune responses to these various immunogens as well.

MUC1 is an excellent example of how changes in a normal glycoprotein caused by the inability of tumor cells to glycosylate it fully can make this glycoprotein immunogenic. Clever design of vaccine approaches that take advantage of these changes can lead to development of immune responses that are tumor specific.

NEWLY EMERGING AND POTENTIALLY PROMISING TUMOR GLYCOPROTEINS

Even though many tumor-associated antigens are fully characterized and their immunogenicity is being explored, continuous developments of new techniques of antigen discovery prompt further searches for new and perhaps better candidates for tumor antigen–based immunotherapies. The road to discovery of new antigens has two parts, one that is biochemical or genetic and traveled a little faster, yielding at its destination numerous potential candidates. It is at that point in the journey that the road turns unpaved and the travel a lot slower. The destination is to determine antigenicity, immunogenicity, and modes of delivery of these antigens to the immune system. Several tumor glycoproteins are taking the later part of the road for the first time. One of them is the secreted glycoprotein Mammaglobin, a product of a mammary-specific member of the uteroglobin gene family overexpressed in breast cancer (66). Another interesting tumor glycoprotein is designated 90K (67,68). It is not so much a tumor antigen as it is a stimulator of APCs and may facilitate presentation of other tumor antigens. Human A33-antigen is a 43-kd glycoprotein with characteristics similar to the members of CEA family. It is a novel palmitoylated cell surface, *N*-linked glycoprotein expressed on normal human colonic and small-bowel epithelium and on more than 95% of primary and metastatic colon cancer cells (69,70).

Many more candidate molecules are being identified through a screening strategy using patients' humoral responses to screen cDNA expression libraries derived from human tumors. This is known as *SEREX technology* (*s*erological analysis of *r*ecombinant *ex*pression libraries with autologous serum) (71). The candidates obtained by this approach are already numerous (72–74) (see Chapter 16.7), but they are for now mostly recombinant unmodified proteins that require extensive study until their biochemical characterization is completed. None of them are yet confirmed glycoproteins and for that reason are not described in this chapter.

An important lesson that has been learned from working with the "old" tumor glycoproteins, and that should be applied to the "new" antigens, is that posttranslational modifications of these proteins differ between normal cells and tumor cells and between different tumor types. This may determine whether these molecules are presented to the immune system and how they are presented to the immune system. In testing their immunogenicity and antigenicity, it is important to use the form of antigen found on a tumor cell of interest that is known to be processed by APCs and that can generate an immune response that is likely to react with tumor cells and not with normal tissues.

REFERENCES

1. Kim YJ, Varki A. Perspectives on the significance of altered glycosylation of glycoproteins in cancer. *Glycoconj J* 1997;14:569–576.
2. Brockhausen I, Schutzbach J, Kuhns W. Glycoproteins and their relationship to human disease. *Acta Anat* 1998;161:36–78.
3. Brockhausen I, Schachter H. Glycosyltransferases involved in N- and O-glycan biosynthesis. In: Gabius HJ, Gabius S, eds. *Glycosciences: status and perspectives*. Weinheim: Chapman and Hall, 1997;79–113.
4. Corfield AP, Myerscough N, Gough M, Brockhausen I, Schauer R, Paraskeva C. Glycosylation patterns of murins in colonic disease. *Biochem Soc Trans* 1995;23:840–845.
5. Lehner PJ, Cresswell P. Processing and delivery of peptides presented by MHC class I molecules. *Curr Opin Immunol* 1996;8:59–67.
6. Germain RN, Castellino F, Han RE, Romagnoli P, Sadegh Nasseri S, Zhong GM. Processing and presentation of endocytically acquired protein antigens by MHC class I and class II molecules. *Immunol Rev* 1996;151:5–30.
7. Brichard V, Van Pel A, Wolfel T, et al. The tyrosinase gene codes for an antigen recognized by autologous cytolytic T lymphocytes on HLA-A2 melanoma. *J Exp Med* 1993;178:489–495.
8. Visseren MJW, van Elsas A, van der Vort EIH, et al. CTL specific for tyrosinase autoantigen can be induced from healthy donor blood to lyse melanoma cells. *J Immunol* 1995;154:3991–3998.
9. Skiper JC, Hendrickson RC, Gulden PH, et al. An HLA-A2-restricted tyrosinase antigen on melanoma cells results from post-translational modification and suggests a novel pathway for processing of membrane proteins. *J Exp Med* 1996;183:527–534.
10. Topalian SL, Rivoltini L, Mancini M, et al. Human CD4$^+$ T cells specifically recognize a shared melanoma-associated antigen encoded by the tyrosinase gene. *Proc Natl Acad Sci U S A* 1994;91:9461–9465.
11. Cassian Y, Gilbert M, Riddell SR, et al. Isolation of tyrosinase-specific CD8$^+$ and CD4$^+$ T cell clones from peripheral blood of melanoma patients following *in vitro* stimulation with recombinant vaccinia virus. *J Immunol* 1996;157:4079–4086.
12. Bakker ABH, Schreurs MWJ, de Boer AJ, et al. Melanocyte lineage-specific antigen gp100 is recognized by melanoma-derived tumor-infiltrating lymphocytes. *J Exp Med* 1994;179:1005–1009.
13. Kawakami Y, Eliyahu S, Jennings C, et al. Recognition of multiple epitopes in the human melanoma antigen gp100 by tumor-infiltrating T lymphocytes associated with *in vivo* tumor regression. *J Immunol* 1995;154:3961–3968.
14. Cox AL, Skipper J, Chen Y, et al. Identification of a peptide recognized by five melanoma-specific human cytotoxic T cell lines. *Science* 1994;264:716–719.
15. Li K, Adibzadeh M, Halder T, et al. Tumor-specific MHC-class-restricted responses after *in vitro* sensitization to synthetic peptides corresponding to gp100 and Annexin II eluted from melanoma cells. *Cancer Immunol Immunother* 1998;47:32–38.
16. Mattes MJ, Thomson TM, Old LJ, Lloyd KO. A pigmentation-associated, differentiation antigen of human melanoma defined by a precipitating antibody in human serum. *Int J Cancer* 1983;32:717–721.
17. Vijayasyradhi S, Bouchard BB, Houghton AN. The melanoma antigen gp75 is the human homologue to mouse b (BROWN) locus gene. *J Exp Med* 1990;171:1375–1380.
18. Wang R-F, Robbins PF, Kawakami Y, Kang X-Q, Rosenberg SA. Identification of a gene encoding a melanoma tumor antigen recognized by HLA-A31-restricted tumor-infiltrating lymphocytes. *J Exp Med* 1995;181:799–804.
19. Kawakami Y, Eliyahu S, Sakaguchi K, et al. Identification of the immunodominant epitope of the MART-1 human melanoma antigen recognized by the majority of HLA-A2-restricted tumor infiltrating lymphocytes. *J Exp Med* 1994;180:347–352.
20. Coulie PG, Brichard V, Van Pel A, et al. A new gene coding for a differentiation antigen recognized by autologous cytolytic lymphocytes on HLA-A2 melanomas. *J Exp Med* 1994;180:35–42.
21. Chen Y-T, Stockert E, Jungbluth A, et al. Serological analysis of Melan-A(MART-1), a melanocyte-specific protein homogenously expressed in human melanomas. *Proc Natl Acad Sci U S A* 1996;93:5915–5919.
22. Shively J, Beatty J. CEA related antigens: molecular, biological and clinical significance. *CRC Crit Rev Oncol Hematol* 1985;2:355–399.
23. Thomson J, Grunert F, Ziemerman W. CEA gene family: molecular biology and clinical perspective. *J Clin Lab Anal* 1991;5:344–366.
24. Majuri ML, Hakkarainen M, Paavonen T, Renkonen R. Carcinoembryonic antigen is expressed on endothelial cells. A putative mediator of tumor cell extravasation and metastasis. *APMIS* 1994;102:432–438.
25. Schlom J. Carcinoembryonic antigen (CEA) peptides and vaccines for carcinoma. In: Kast M, ed. *Peptide-based cancer vaccines. Bioscience* 1999;(submitted).
26. Riethmuller G, Schneider-Gadicke E, Schlimok G, et al., and the German Cancer Aid 17-1A Study Group. Randomized trial of monoclonal antibody for adjuvant therapy of resected Dukes' C colorectal carcinoma. *Lancet* 1994;343:1177–1183.

27. Riethmuller G, Holz E, Schlimok G, et al. Monoclonal antibody therapy for resected Dukes' C colorectal cancer: seven-year outcome of a multicenter randomized trial. *J Clin Oncol* 1998;16:1788–1794.

28. Wang MC, Papsider LD, Kuriyama M, Valenzuela LA, Murphy GP, Chu TM. Prostate antigen: a new potential marker for prostatic cancer. *Prostate* 1981;2:89–96.

29. Wat WWK, Lee P-J, M'Timkulu T, Chan W-P, Loor R. Human prostate-specific antigen: structural and functional similarity with serine proteases. *Proc Natl Acad Sci U S A* 1986;83:3166–3170.

30. Yu H, Diamandis EP. Prostate specific antigen in milk of lactating women. *Clin Chem* 1995;41:54–58.

31. Yu H, Diamandis EP. Prostate specific antigen immunoreactivity in amniotic fluid. *Clin Chem* 1995;41:204–210.

32. Correale P, Walmsly K, Nieroda C, et al. *In vitro* generation of human cytotoxic T lymphocytes specific for peptides derived from prostate-specific antigen. *J Natl Cancer Inst* 1997;89:293–299

33. Correale P, Walmsley K, Zaremba S, Zhu M, Schlom J, Tsang KY. Generation of human cytolytic T lymphocyte lines directed against prostate-specific antigen (PSA employing a PSA oligoepitope peptide. *J Immunol* 1998;161:3186–3194.

34. Fong L, Ruegg CL, Brockstedt D, Engleman EG, Laus R. Induction of tissue-specific autoimmune prostatitis with prostatic acid phosphatase immunization. *J Immunol* 1997;159:3113–3117.

35. Tyoa BA, Simmons VA, Radge H, et al. Evaluation of phase I/II clinical trials in prostate cancer with dendritic cells and PSMA peptides. *Prostate* 1998;36:39–44.

36. Reiter RE, Gu Z, Watabe T, et al. Prostate stem cell antigen: a cell surface marker overexpressed in prostate cancer. *Proc Natl Acad Sci U S A* 1998;95:1735–1740.

37. Xu J, Stolk JH, Zhang X, Silva SJ, Houghton RL, Reed SG. Identification of differentially expressed genes in human prostate tumor using subtraction and microarray. *Cancer Res* 2000 (*in press*).

38. Peles E, Bacus S, Koski R, et al. Isolation of the HER2/neu stimulatory ligand: a 44 kd glycoprotein that induces differentiation of mammary tumor cells. *Cell* 1992;69:205–216.

39. Pegram MD, Lipton A, Hayes DF, et al. Phase II study of receptor-enhanced chemosensitivity using recombinant humanized anti-p185HER2/neu monoclonal antibody plus cisplatin in patients with HER2/neu-overexpressing metastatic breast cancer refractory to chemotherapy treatment. *J Clin Oncol* 1998;16:2659–2671.

40. Press M, Cordon-Cardo C, Slamon D. Expression of HER-2/neu proto-oncogene in normal human adult and fetal tissues. *Oncogene* 1990;5:953–962.

41. Disis ML, Cheever MA. HER-2/neu oncogenic protein: issues in vaccine development. *Crit Rev Immunol* 1998;18:37–45.

42. Fisk B, Blevins TL, Wharton JT, Ioannides CG. Identification of an immunodominant peptide of HER-2/neu proto-oncogene recognized by ovarian tumor-specific cytotoxic T lymphocyte lines. *J Exp Med* 1995;181:2109–2117.

43. Disis ML, Grabstein KH, Sleath P, Cheever MA. Generation of immunity to the HER-2/neu oncogenic protein in patients with breast and ovarian cancer using a peptide-based vaccine. *Clin Cancer Res* 1999;5:1289–1298.

44. Kono K, Rongcun Y, Charo J, et al. Identification of HER2/neu-derived peptide epitopes recognized by gastric cancer-specific cytotoxic lymphocytes. *Int J Cancer* 1998;78:202–208.

45. Brossart P, Stuhler G, Flad T, et al. Her-2/neu-derived peptides are tumor-associated antigens expressed by human renal cell and colon carcinoma lines and are recognized by *in vitro* induced specific cytotoxic T lymphocytes. *Cancer Res* 1998;58:732–736.

46. Barnd DL, Lan M, Metzgar RS, Finn OJ. Specific, MHC-unrestricted recognition of tumor-associated mucins by human cytotoxic T cells. *Proc Natl Acad Sci U S A* 1998;86:7159–7163.

47. Jerome KR, Barnd DL, Bendt KM, et al. Cytotoxic T lymphocytes derived from patients with breast adenocarcinoma recognize an epitope present on the protein core of a mucin molecule preferentially expressed by malignant cells. *Cancer Res* 1991;51:2908–2916.

48. Finn OJ, Jerome K, Henderson RA, et al. MUC-1 epithelial tumor mucin-based immunity and cancer vaccines. *Immunol Rev* 1995;145:61–89.

49. Zotter S, Hageman PC, Lossnitzer A, Mooi WJ, Hilgers J. Tissue and tumor distribution of human polymorphic epithelial mucin. *Cancer Rev* 1988;11:55–101.

50. Burchell J, Durbin H, Taylor-Papdimitriou J. Complexity of expression of antigenic determinants recognized by monoclonal antibodies HMFG-1 and HMFG-2, in normal and malignant mammary epithelial cells. *J Immunol* 1983;131:508–511.

51. Girling A, Bartkov AJ, Gendler S, Gillet C, Taylor PJ. A core protein of the polymorphic epithelial mucin detected by the monoclonal antibody SM-3 is selectively exposed in a range of primary carcinomas. *Int J Cancer* 1989;43:1072–1075.

52. Rye PD, Price MR. ISOBM TD-4 International Workshop on Monoclonal Antibodies against MUC1. *Tumor Biol* 1998;19[Suppl 1]:1–152.

53. Fontenot JS, Mariappan S, Catasti V, Domenech N, Finn OJ, Gupta G. Structure of a tumor associated antigen containing a tandemly repeated immunodominant epitope. *J Biomol Struct Dyn* 1994;13:245–260.

54. Rughetti A, Turchi V, Ghetti CA, et al. Human B-cell immune response to the polymorphic epithelial mucin. *Cancer Res* 1993;53:2457–2459.

55. Kotera Y, Fontenot JD, Pecher G, Metzgar RS, Finn OJ. Humoral immunity against a tandem repeat epitope of human mucin MUC-1 in sera from breast, pancreatic and colon cancer patients. *Cancer Res* 1994;54:2856–2860.

56. Von Mensdorff-Pouilly S, Gourevitch MM, Kenemans P, et al. Humoral immune response to polymorphic epithelial mucin (MUC1) in patients with benign and malignant breast tumors. *Eur J Cancer* 1996;32A:1325–1331.

57. Hiltbold EH, Ciborowski P, Finn OJ. Naturally processed class II epitope from the tumor antigen MUC1 primes human CD4+ T cells. *Cancer Res* 1998;58:5066–5070.

58. Hiltbold EM, Alter MD, Ciborowski P, Finn OJ. Efficiency of processing and presentation of class I-restricted MUC1 epitopes and CTL function correlate with the glycosylation state of the soluble protein taken up by dendritic cells. *J Cell Immunol* 1999;194:143–149.

59. Hiltbold EM, Vlad AM, Ciborowski P, Watkins SC, Finn OJ. Mechanism of T cell tolerance to glycosylated antigen MUC1 is a block in intracellular sorting and processing by dendritic cells. 1999 (submitted).

60. Barrat-Boyes SM, Vlad A, Finn OJ. Immunization of chimpanzees with tumor antigen MUC1 mucin tandem repeat peptide elicits both helper and cytotoxic T cell responses. *Clin Cancer Res* 1999;5:1918–1924.

61. Goydos JS, Elder E, Whiteside TL, Finn OJ, Lotze MT. A phase I clinical trial of a synthetic mucin peptide vaccine. *J Surg Res* 1996;63:289–304.

62. Karanikas V, Hwang LA, Pearson J, et al. Antibody and T cell responses of patients with adenocarcinoma immunized with mannan-MUC1 fusion protein. *J Clin Invest* 1997;100:2783–2792.

63. Longenecker BM, Reddish M, Koganty R, MacLean GD. Immune responses of mice and breast cancer patients following immunization with synthetic sialyl-Tn conjugated to KLH plus detox adjuvant. *Ann N Y Acad Sci* 1993;690:276–283.

64. Longenecker BM, Reddish M, Koganty R, MacLean GD. Specificity of the IgG response in mice and human breast cancer patients following immunization against synthetic sialyl-Tn, an epitope with possible functional significance in metastasis. In: Ceriani RL, ed. *Antigen and antibody molecular engineering in breast cancer diagnosis*. New York: Plenum Publishing, 1994:105–124.

65. MacLean DG, Redidsh M, Koganty R, et al. Immunization of breast cancer patients using a synthetic sialyl-Tn glycoconjugate plus Detox adjuvant. *Cancer Immunol Immunother* 1993;36:215–221.

66. Watson AM, Fleming T. Mammaglobin, a mammary-specific member of the uteroglobin gene family, is overexpressed in breast cancer. *Cancer Res* 1996;56:860–865.

67. Powel TJ, Schreck R, McCall M, et al. A tumor-derived protein which provides T-cell costimulation through accessory cell activation. *J Immunother* 1995;17:209–221.

68. Tinari N, D'egidio M, Iacobelli S, et al. Identification of the tumor antigen 90K domains recognized by monoclonal antibodies SP2 and L3 and preparation and characterization of novel anti-90K monoclonal antibodies. *Biochem Biophys Res Commun* 1997;232: 367–372.

69. Heath JK, White SJ, Johnstone CN, et al. The human A33 antigen is a transmembrane glycoprotein and a novel member of the immunoglobulin superfamily. *Proc Natl Acad Sci* 1997;94:469–474.

70. Ritter G, Cohen LS, Nice EC, et al. Characterization of posttranslational modifications of human A33 antigen, a novel palmitoylated surface glycoprotein of human gastrointestinal epithelium. *Biochem Biophys Res Commun* 1997;236:682–686.

71. Sahin U, Tureci O, Schmitt H, et al. Human neoplasms elicit multiple specific immune responses in the autologous host. *Proc Natl Acad Sci U S A* 1995;92:11810–11813.

72. Jager E, Chen Y-T, Drijfhout JW, et al. Simultaneous humoral and cellular immune responses against cancer-testis antigen NY-ESO-1: definition of human histocompatibility leukocyte antigen (HLA)-A2-binding peptide epitopes. *J Exp Med* 1998;187:265–270.

73. Chen Y-T, Gure AO, Tsang S, Stockert E, Jager E, Knuth A, Old LJ. Identification of multiple cancer/testis antigens by allogeneic antibody screening of melanoma cell line library. *Proc Natl Acad Sci U S A* 1998;95:6919–6923.

74. Scanlan MJ, Chen Y-T, Williamson B, et al. Characterization of human colon cancer antigens recognized by autologous antibodies. *Int J Cancer* 1998;76:652–658.

16.7

CANCER VACCINES: CANCER ANTIGENS

Identification of Human Tumor Antigens by Serological Expression Cloning

YAO-TSENG CHEN
MATTHEW J. SCANLAN
YUICHI OBATA
LLOYD J. OLD

The search for antibodies that distinguish cancer cells from normal cells is one of the longest uninterrupted inquiries in cancer research (1). The history of this pursuit can be divided into four phases. The first, dominated by immunologists such as Witebsky and Hirszfeld, dealt mainly with the analysis of heteroimmune serum obtained from rabbits and other animals immunized with human cancer (2). The challenge, generally unmet, was to remove antibodies reactive with normal tissue antigens; a variety of absorption techniques were devised to accomplish this. Complement fixation and, later, agar gel immunoprecipitation provided the primary systems to analyze the heteroimmune sera. Although little of enduring value came from this vast effort, two useful antigens were identified—alpha fetoprotein, a serum marker for hepatoma and germ-cell tumors (3); and carcinoembryonic antigen, a serum marker for colon and other epithelial cancers (4). The second phase in this odyssey was initiated by the work of Peter Gorer, a scientist best known for his discovery of the mouse histocompatibility locus. Gorer also had an intense interest in tumor antigens, and he introduced the approaches and test systems involving cytotoxic alloantibodies prepared in inbred mice that led to the serological dissection of normal and malignant lymphoid cells and the discovery of cell surface "differentiation antigens" such as TL, Ly1, Lyt2 (CD8), Thy-1, and PCA (5), and endogenous retroviral-coded antigens such as Gross cell surface antigen, G_{IX}, and ML (6). The emergence of hybridoma technology (7) transformed the field of serology and opened the floodgates for identifying new cell-surface antigens in mice and humans and for analyzing the antigenic phenotype of human cancer. Although there was great hope that monoclonal antibodies (MAb) would uncover tumor-specific antigens in humans, this has not proven to be the case. Rather, experience has shown that even the most restricted tumor antigen generally turns out to be a restricted normal differentiation antigen (8). In addition to the use of polyclonal and MAb of heterologous and allogeneic origin in the search for tumor-specific antigens, there has been a sustained effort to determine whether the autologous host recognizes cancer cells.

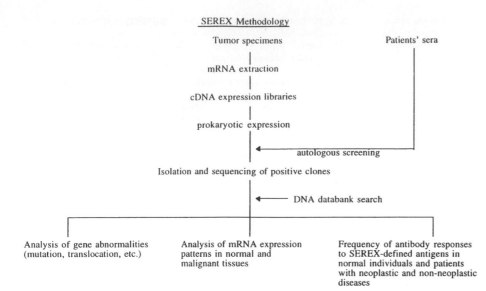

FIGURE 1. Serological expression cloning (SEREX) approach to defining human tumor antigens. (cDNA, complementary DNA; mRNA, messenger RNA.)

To establish as rigorous and unambiguous a serological test system as possible for this purpose, an approach called *autologous typing* was developed (9), initiating what can be seen as the third phase in human cancer serology. The intention of autologous typing was to restrict the analysis to autologous reagents—tumor cells, serum, and normal cells such as fibroblasts and lymphocytes from the same patient—to eliminate the contribution of alloantigens in the reactions observed and to establish tumor specificity by absorption with autologous normal cells. With the exception of leukemia cells (10), cultured tumor-cell lines were required for autologous typing, and this limited analysis to tumor types that could be adapted to growth *in vitro* with some regularity [i.e., melanoma (11,12), renal cancer (13), and brain cancer (14)]. The conclusion coming from the autologous typing of a large series of patients is that a small fraction of patients do develop autologous antibody with specificity for cell-surface antigens of the tumor. With few exceptions (15–18), however, molecular characterization of the antigen was generally beyond reach, primarily because the antibodies were not of sufficient titer to monitor biochemical purification or cloning.

This limitation in autologous typing has been overcome by a new approach introduced by Michael Pfreundschuh and his colleagues Ugur Sahin and Özlem Türeci at the University of Saarland (19,20). They called their approach *SEREX*, for *se*rological analysis of *re*combinant cDNA *ex*pression libraries of human tumors with autologous serum. In their initial application of the method, tumor antigens, such as MAGE and tyrosinase that had originally been defined as T-cell–recognized epitopes, were detected by autologous antibody. SEREX analysis has identified a series of provocative cancer antigens that have relevance to the etiology, diagnosis, and therapy of cancer. What is so encouraging about SEREX is that it provides a way to analyze the humoral immune response to intracellular cancer antigens, a generally impenetrable forest for cancer serologists in the past. The development of the SEREX technique has inaugurated the fourth phase in cancer serology, bringing with it the prospect of providing a comprehensive view of the immune recognition of human cancer.

SEREX: THE TECHNIQUE AND STEPS INVOLVED IN THE ANALYSIS OF SEREX-DEFINED ANTIGENS

SEREX was developed to combine serological analysis with antigen cloning techniques to identify human tumor antigens eliciting high-titer immunoglobulin G (IgG) antibodies. The SEREX technique is shown schematically in Figure 1. Although the concept behind SEREX is straightforward, a number of technical challenges needed resolution. One of the most crucial involved eliminating antibodies in human sera that react with bacterial or phage components. This step, usually done by repeated absorption of the diluted serum with bacterial and phage lysates, is absolutely essential because such contaminating antibodies would completely obscure the detection of other classes of antibodies. The second challenge is the presence of B cells in tumors, sometimes in quite large numbers. These B cells give rise to IgG complementary DNA (cDNA), which is expressed and detected in SEREX. The frequency of such IgG clones varies in each library but can represent substantial percentages of the clones. When present in high numbers, these clones have to be distinguished before the human serum screening step, and Türeci et al. (21) have devised a prescreening procedure that serves this purpose quite effectively. The third challenge, at least initially, was the suspicion that the majority of antibodies detected in SEREX would be autoantibodies with little or no relevance to cancer. Although known autoantigens do constitute a fraction of the SEREX antigens identified to date, such antigens have not been overrepresented. Part of the reason may be attributed to the initial decision of Pfreundschuh and his colleagues to exclude IgM from the analysis (by using secondary antibodies specific to IgG) and to focus on high-titered IgG antibodies (by performing the immunoscreening at serum dilution of 1:100 to 1:1,000).

After the initial selection of antibody-reactive clones in SEREX analysis, subsequent steps in SEREX analysis are directed to answering the following questions:

1. Why is the antigen immunogenic?
2. What role, if any, does the antigen have in the malignant process?
3. Is the immune response to the antigen cancer related?

To address these issues, the first step is to sequence the clone to determine its relationship to known genes or motifs and to search for structural or functional modifications in the gene (e.g., mutations, translocations, and gene amplification). The messenger RNA (mRNA) expression pattern of the gene in panels of normal tissues and malignancies by reverse transcriptase-polymerase chain reaction (RT-PCR) and Northern analysis represents the next step to determine whether the gene has a restricted or nonrestricted pattern of expression. This expression pattern of the gene product is then extended to the protein level by generating polyclonal or MAb from animals immunized with recombinant SEREX-defined proteins and using them for biochemical characterization of the cellular protein and for immunohistochemical analysis. If not previously known, chromosomal mapping of the SEREX-defined gene is another important aspect of characterizing SEREX antigens. In evaluating the importance of SEREX-defined antigen in the context of cancer, the serological screening of sera from normal individuals, cancer patients, and patients with nonneoplastic diseases is of critical importance. These surveys of antibody responses to SEREX-defined antigens define whether the immune response is cancer restricted or whether the antigen is recognized by humans in a non-cancer–restricted fashion. To initiate such serological surveys, a small panel of sera from normal individuals and patients with cancer are screened against the SEREX-defined bacteriophage clone, a process called *petit serology*. SEREX isolates showing a cancer-restricted seroreactivity can then be tested in larger-scale serological surveys (grand serology) using purified recombinant protein as the antigenic target in enzyme-linked immunoassay (ELISA).

At this stage in the development of SEREX, few SEREX-defined antigens have been through this battery of steps in SEREX analysis. However, it is already known that the vast majority of SEREX-defined antigens appear to show universal or near universal mRNA expressions in normal tissues. Examples of differentially expressed SEREX genes have been found, but these are uncommon. Also, mutations and other structural modifications are rare, but more extensive sequencing should be carried out to exclude structural changes in the coding genes. What is encouraging is that SEREX has identified a number of gene products that have known or suspected relevance to cancer development (e.g., oncogenes and suppressor genes) and other products that have potential as targets for cancer vaccine. Additionally, the finding of SEREX-defined gene products that appear to be recognized by the humoral immune system of subsets of cancer patients but not normal individuals further emphasizes the potential of SEREX. The fact that a number of these genes are widely expressed in normal tissues indicates that cancer-specific recognition can occur

TABLE 1. VARIATIONS IN SEREX METHODOLOGY

cDNA library source
  Allogeneic tumor
  Testis
  Tumor cell lines
Vector system
  Filamentous phage and other prokaryotic expression systems
  Baculovirus and other eukaryotic expression systems
Antibody source
  Allogeneic sera from cancer patients
  Sera from cancer patients after cancer vaccination
  IgM and other Ig subclasses
  Oligoclonal or monoclonal human antibody
  Recombinant clonal IgG
Combined approaches of SEREX with other cloning methods
  RDA/SEREX, SAGE/SEREX, differential display/SEREX

cDNA, complementary DNA; Ig, immunoglobulin; RDA, representational difference analysis; SAGE, serial analysis of gene expression; SEREX, serological expression cloning.

in the absence of cancer-specific expression. The basis for this cancer-specific immunogenicity is one of the central challenges that need resolving.

MODIFICATIONS IN THE SEREX TECHNIQUE

Although SEREX analysis was initially developed to analyze the autologous humoral response to cancer—that is, tumor and serum from the same patient—a number of modifications on the original SEREX design have been introduced or are being considered (Table 1). The first variation, developed to discover new antigens belonging to the cancer-testis (CT) category—that is, antigens with restricted expression in normal testis and in cancer (see below)—involves the screening of sera from cancer patients on allogeneic testicular cDNA libraries, either unsubtracted or after subtraction with cDNA derived from nontesticular normal tissue. This approach has led to the recognition of several CT antigens, including new members of the SSX family (22), SCP-1 (23), and HOM-TES-85/CT8 (24). Another modification involves established tumor cell lines rather than fresh tumor as the source of cDNA for SEREX analysis. Although one of the great advantages of SEREX is that it circumvents the requirement for cultured tumor cells, cell lines can be a useful alternative target source of cDNA. This is illustrated by the analysis of SK-MEL-37, an established melanoma cell line that was chosen for SEREX because it expressed most, if not all, of the known CT antigens (25). A cDNA library from SK-MEL-37 was screened with allogeneic sera from a patient having high titers of antibody to two CT antigens, NY-ESO-1 and MAGE-1. This screening resulted in the isolation of the two known CT antigens, NY-ESO-1 and MAGE-4, and the discovery of a new member of the CT family, CT7. The use of cell lines for SEREX may be particularly useful in the case of tumors in which tumor specimens are difficult to obtain (e.g., small-cell lung cancer). A third modification involves a combination of representational difference analysis (RDA) (26) and SEREX. This approach is not SEREX-based cloning in the strictest sense, but rather uses

TABLE 2. SEREX ANALYSIS OF HUMAN CANCER

cDNA Source	Serum Source	No. Positive Clones	No. Genes (Known/Unknown)	Examples of Genes	References
Melanoma	Autologous	40	10	MAGE-1, tyrosinase, SSX2	Sahin et al. (19)
Testis	Allogeneic melanoma	8	8 (7/1)	SSX2, SSX3	Güre et al. (22)
Melanoma cell line	Allogeneic melanoma	61	16 (10/6)	CT7, KOC, MAGE-4	Chen et al. (25)
Esophageal cancer	Autologous	13	8 (5/3)	NY-ESO-1, U1snRNP	Chen et al. (28)
Colon cancer[a]	Autologous	234	48 (31/17)	p53, galectin-4, PDZ-73	Scanlan et al. (29,45)
Gastric cancer[a]	Autologous	297	135(87/48)	E-cadherin/gene Y, AKT1	Obata et al. (33)
Renal cancer	Autologous	7	5	Carbonic anhydrase XII	Sahin et al. (19)
Testis	Allogeneic renal cancer	5	3	SCP1	Sahin et al. (23)
Renal cancer[a]	Autologous	169	65 (36/29)	LKB/STK11, *bcr*, LUCA15, g21	Scanlan et al. (33)
Lung cancer	Autologous	35	19 (10/9)	eIF-4 gamma, amplified genes	Brass et al. (30,31)
Lung cancer	Autologous	20	12 (5/7)	Aldolase A, NY-LU-12/g16	Güre et al. (32)
Breast cancer	Autologous	38	16 (13/3)	NY-ESO-1, SSX2, *ING1*	Jäger et al. (35)
Breast cancer	Allogeneic	23	9 (9/0)	NY-ESO-1	Jäger et al. (35)
Testis	Allogeneic breast cancer	28	10 (8/2)	SSX2, *ING1*	Jäger et al. (35)
Breast cancer[a]	Autologous	86	48 (26/22)	CDC10, Notch/int3-like, helicase-like	Scanlan et al. (36)
Breast cancer[a]	Autologous	94	55 (34/21)	SSX2, hsp105	Obata et al. (37)
Hodgkin's disease	Autologous	14	4	Galectin-9, restin	Türeci et al. (21)
Prostate cancer	Autologous	19	18 (10/8)	Replication licensing factor β unit	Chen et al. (38)
Prostate cancer	Autologous	56	30 (17/13)	eIF-4 gamma, NFκB p105	Obata et al. (39)
Astrocytoma	Autologous	48	5	Tegt	Sahin et al. (19)
CML	Autologous	8	8(6/2)	clone no. 4 (CT gene?)	Ling et al. (40)
Bladder cancer line	Allogeneic hepatoma	1	1	p62/KOC3	Zhang et al. (43)
Testis	Allogeneic seminoma	9	6(4/2)	CT8, hook-1 protein	Sahin et al. (23)

cDNA, complementary DNA; CML, chronic myeloid leukemia; CT, cancer-testis; Tegt, testis-enhanced gene transcript.
[a]Multiple libraries screened: four colon cancers, five gastric cancers, four breast cancers, and four renal cancers (including one autologous renal cancer cell line).

SEREX-based serology to identify seroreactivity to the products of genes cloned by the RDA approach. An example of this was the cloning of CT10 (27). CT10, a gene sharing homology to CT7 and members of the MAGE family, was initially cloned by RDA as a gene abundantly expressed in SK-MEL-37 but not in normal skin. After initial RDA cloning, the cDNA was subcloned into the same expression vector used for SEREX, and the resulting phage clone was tested against a panel of absorbed serum samples from tumor patients. In this manner, the immunogenicity of RDA-identified gene products can be analyzed and documented.

In addition to extending the antigenic targets for SEREX analysis beyond the autologous tumor (e.g., testis, tumor-cell lines, and RDA) different sources of antibodies other than autologous and allogeneic sera are being explored. Human oligoclonal or MAb generated from B cells (directly after isolation or after expansion *in vitro*) from peripheral blood, tumor, or draining lymph nodes of cancer patients are promising sources that need investigation. Additional serological probes could come from cDNA cloning of IgG sequences expressed by tumor-infiltrating B cells of cancer patients.

SEREX-DEFINED ANTIGENS BY TUMOR TYPE

SEREX has been applied to a range of tumor types, including melanoma (19,22,25), esophageal cancer (28), colon cancer (29), lung cancer (30–32), renal cancer (23,33), gastric cancer (34), breast cancer (35–37), astrocytoma (19), prostate cancer (38,39), seminoma (24), and hematologic malignancies, including Hodgkin's lymphoma (19) and leukemia (40). These SEREX

studies and examples of the clones isolated are summarized in relation to individual tumor types in Table 2.

Melanoma

Several SEREX studies have focused on melanoma tumor specimens, melanoma cell lines, and sera from melanoma patients (19,22,25). In their initial analysis, Sahin et al. (19) screened a melanoma library of 1.0×10^6 clones and isolated 40 positive clones representing ten different gene products. These included tyrosinase and two CT antigens, MAGE-1 and HOM-MEL-40/SSX2. To extend the search for CT antigens recognized by melanoma patient sera, a testicular cDNA library was screened by Güre et al. (22). This resulted in the isolation of eight gene products, including six universally expressed genes and two members of the SSX family, SSX2 and a new member SSX3. Southern blot analysis confirmed SSX as a multigene family, and subsequent PCR-based cDNA cloning led to the identification of two additional SSX members, SSX4 and SSX5, both transcribed in testis and in malignancy (scc below).

To further extend this search for CT antigens, a cDNA library was constructed from SK-MEL-37, a melanoma cell line expressing multiple CT antigens, and the library was screened with an allogeneic melanoma patient serum known to have antibodies to two CT antigens, NY-ESO-1 and MAGE-1 (25). Sixty-one positive clones were identified, including four CT antigen genes: MAGE-4a, NY-ESO-1, LAGE-1 [a gene closely related to NY-ESO-1 (28,41)], and a new CT antigen CT7. Additionally, the most abundantly represented clones in this screening, 33 of 61 positive clones, were derived from three closely related genes. One of these three genes, called *KOC* (*K*H domain-containing gene *o*verexpressed in *c*an*c*cr), had been previously identified as a gene overexpressed in pancreatic cancer (42). These three genes were designated KOC1 (the original KOC gene), KOC2, and KOC3, of which KOC3 was most abundantly expressed (30 of 33 isolated clones). Northern blot analysis of KOC3 expression showed variable levels of mRNA expression in melanoma cell lines and no detectable mRNA in any normal tissue examined. Subsequently, KOC3 was also cloned from a bladder cancer line by antibody screening using serum from a hepatocellular carcinoma patient (43) (see below).

Esophageal Cancer

An esophageal cancer cDNA library derived from a squamous cell carcinoma has been analyzed (28). Thirteen positive clones were identified, derived from eight different genes, designated NY-ESO-1 through NY-ESO-8. Among these, NY-ESO-1 showed a characteristic cancer-testis expression pattern, and NY-ESO-5 appeared to be preferentially expressed in squamous epithelium. Other genes were found to be universally expressed, including two genes coding for autoimmune antigens in the U1 small nuclear ribonucleoprotein family.

Colon Cancer

SEREX analysis of four colon cancer cDNA libraries has been carried out by Scanlan et al. (29). A total of 234 immunoreactive cDNA clones encoding 48 different antigens were identified. Sequence analysis revealed 17 novel genes and 31 known genes coding for a vast array of cellular components. A large proportion of the antigens were nuclear proteins, such as transcription factors, mRNA splicing factors, and DNA-binding proteins, and a smaller percentage represented metabolic enzymes, molecular chaperones, signaling molecules, cytoskeletal proteins, and membrane-associated proteins. In addition to these common cellular constituents, however, several of the colon cancer antigens stood out as having a known or suspected etiologic association with human cancer; the most obvious example of this being the isolation of a mutated version of p53 tumor-suppressor gene (NY-CO-13). RT-PCR analysis and Northern blotting showed that transcripts encoding 3 of the 48 antigens were differentially expressed, whereas the other 45 genes were universally expressed. NY-CO-27 is identical to the S-type lectin galectin-4 (44), and is expressed primarily in normal colon and small intestine. The other two differentially expressed antigens, NY-CO-37 and NY-CO-38, are related isoforms encoded by a previously unknown gene that maps to chromosome 11p15.4-p15.1 (45). These two antigens are members of a group of differentially expressed isoforms that are characterized by a variable number of PDZ domains, the presence or absence of a PEST protein degradation motif, a large coiled-coil domain, and the existence of a putative C-terminal module that may function as a binding site for PDZ domains (indicating that it may form homomeric or heteromeric protein complexes). In general, PDZ domains function as scaffolding sites for the organization of signal transduction complexes, cell junctions, and cytoskeletal-plasma membrane linkages (46). A yeast 2-hybrid screen of proteins that interact with the Coxsackie and adenovirus receptor identified NY-CO-38 (or a related isoform) as an interacting protein (R. Finberg, *personal communication*, 1999). One of the NY-CO-38 isoforms is expressed in some normal tissues but is not found in normal colon. In contrast, this isoform is expressed in colon cancer, and this aberrant expression of a normally expressed isoform in cancer may be the basis for its immunogenicity in cancer patients (see below).

Gastric Cancer

SEREX analysis of five cases of gastric carcinoma derived from tumors of various histologic types and grades has been carried out by Obata et al. (34). The screening of each cDNA library with autologous serum was continued until approximately 50 positive clones were isolated from each library. In total, 297 positive clones were obtained, representing 135 distinct genes, 87 of which were previously known. Of the 135 gene products, 21 were identified in two or more gastric cancer libraries and 24 were identified in SEREX analysis of other tumor types. No CT antigens were isolated, consistent with the low frequency of CT gene expression in gastrointestinal cancer (28,47).

Of the genes isolated, two showed possible etiologic significance for gastric cancer. One was derived from a fusion gene product between E-cadherin (E-Cad) and a novel gene designated as *GeneY*. E-Cad is an adhesion molecule involved in the regulation of various cellular functions, including normal differentiation and tumor invasion (48). Mutations in E-Cad have been identified in gastric and other cancers and inherited mutations have been related to familial gastric cancer (49,50). Nine independent cDNA clones encompassing the fusion gene were isolated and the combined sequencing data indicated that the 5' end of E-Cad was fused to the 3' end of GeneY. RT-PCR using a 5' primer derived from E-Cad and a 3' primer derived from GeneY showed that the amplification product was restricted to the tumor and was not detected in autologous nonneoplastic tissue or allogeneic normal or tumor tissues. This finding indicates a somatic translocation event involving E-Cad and GeneY in the cancer, an event possibly contributing to the cancer's origin or progression. Although this translocational event was not found in five other cases of gastric cancer in this small series or reported in the literature, a larger panel of gastric cancer specimens should be evaluated to assess the frequency and significance of this genetic alteration.

A second gene, recognized by the serum of a different gastric cancer patient and also related to gastric carcinogenesis, is the AKT1 (PKB) oncogene. AKT1 gene is thought to promote cell survival by modulating antiapoptotic signals, and AKT1 gene amplification has been reported in a primary gastric cancer (51). AKT1 expression was elevated in five of eight gastric cancers, and one of the five patients with amplified AKT1 expression had an anti-AKT1 antibody response. Overexpression of this gene presumably forms the basis for its immunogenicity in cancer patients.

Renal Cancer

In the initial study by Sahin et al., five different antigens were isolated from a single renal cell carcinoma cDNA library screened with autologous serum (19). Of these, HOM-RCC-

3.1.3 is a type I integral-membrane protein (40 kd) representing a novel tumor-associated carbonic anhydrase (CA XII). The coding gene for CA XII maps to chromosome 15q22 (52). CA XII is expressed in normal kidney, small intestine, and renal cancer. In 10% of the renal cancer examined, RCC-3.1.3 mRNA was expressed at a much higher level than in adjacent normal kidney tissue (19,52).

In a subsequent study by Sahin et al. (24), serum from a patient with renal cancer was used to screen a testicular library subtracted with a range of normal tissues. The aim of the screening was to uncover new members of the CT family. Five positive clones representing three genes were isolated, one encoding synaptonemal complex protein 1 (SCP1), a protein involved in chromosome reduction during meiosis. The expression of SCP1 is normally restricted to germ cells and was not previously known to be expressed in cancer. However, Sahin et al. found SCP1 mRNA and protein expression in a subset of malignant gliomas, breast cancers, renal cancers, and ovarian cancers. Thus, SCP1 belongs to the CT antigen category.

Four additional cases of renal cancer were analyzed in SEREX by Scanlan et al. (33) using autologous patient sera. These studies yielded a total of 169 clones representing 65 different gene products. Sequence analysis showed that 36 were coded by known genes and 29 were novel gene products. Four of the antigens, NY-REN-9, -10, -19, and -26, have a known association with human cancer. NY-REN-9 (LUCA-15) and NY-REN-10 (gene 21) map to the p21.3 locus on chromosome 3, a region presumably containing tumor suppressor gene(s), which is often deleted in small-cell and non–small-cell lung cancer (53) and renal cancer (53,54). REN-19 is identical to LKB/STK11 serine-threonine kinase. Defects in the LKB/STK11 gene are responsible for Peutz-Jeghers syndrome, a disease characterized in part by an increased risk of gastrointestinal cancer (55). Somatic mutations in the LKB1/STK11 gene have also been reported in cases of colon cancer (56), breast cancer (57), and gastric cancer (58). NY-REN-26 is encoded by the *bcr* gene involved in the [t(9:22)] *bcr/abl* translocation associated with chronic myelogenous leukemia (59). No evidence of gene mutation was detected in the cDNA sequences of clones defining NY-REN-9, -10, -19, or -26. In addition to these four genes, two others, NY-REN-33 and NY-REN-65, are related to less well-characterized potential tumor suppressor genes. NY-REN-33 is identical to a possible tumor suppressor, SNC6 (GenBank U28918), which maps to 22q13.1, a region known to be deleted in cases of breast cancer (60). NY-REN-65 maps to 11q12 and is a possible human homologue of the rat HREV107 tumor suppressor gene (GenBank X92814).

With regard to tissue mRNA expression, transcripts encoding all 65 antigens are expressed in a range of normal tissues as determined by expressed sequence tag analysis, RT-PCR, and/or Northern blotting. However, three antigens, NY-REN-3, NY-REN-21, and NY-REN-43, have a differential mRNA expression pattern. NY-REN-3 is identical to NY-CO-38 (described above), belonging to a family of differentially expressed isoforms with PDZ domains. Both NY-REN-21 and NY-REN-43 transcripts are expressed at higher levels in testis than in other normal tissues. NY-REN-21 represents a possible human homologue of mouse zinc finger protein-38 (61), a DNA-binding protein thought to be involved in meiosis, and NY-REN-43

cDNA encodes a putative protein containing a ring-zinc finger domain and a polyserine domain.

Lung Cancer

Two SEREX studies of lung cancer have been reported (30–32). Brass et al. (30,31) derived 35 positive clones representing 19 genes from the autologous screening of a squamous cell carcinoma cDNA library. Six clones coded for eIF-4 gamma, an eukaryotic translation initiation factor, which maps to chromosome 3q26.1-3q26.3, a region that is amplified in 30% of squamous lung cancer (62). By comparative PCR analysis, the authors showed that eIF-4 gamma and eight other genes were amplified in the tumor of origin, including DnaJ heat shock protein and Jk-recombinant signal binding protein, two genes also found in the SEREX analysis of renal cancer (NY-REN-14, NY-REN-30) (29). Three of the amplified genes were located on chromosome 3, and two of these mapped to the 3q region. The authors suggested that immune recognition is a consequence of amplified gene expression, and that amplified eIF-4 gamma may be important in the development of squamous cell carcinoma.

In a separate study, Güre et al. (32) analyzed a moderately differentiated adenocarcinoma of the lung with autologous serum and isolated 20 positive clones representing 12 genes. One of these was aldolase A, a gene known to be expressed at high levels in most lung cancer (63,64). Aldolase A has been subsequently isolated in SEREX analysis of breast cancer (35), indicating a possible linkage of aldolase A overexpression to adenocarcinomas of various tissue origin. Another SEREX-defined gene of special interest, NY-LU-12, maps to the tumor suppressor gene locus on chromosome 3p21.3, as do NY-REN-9 and NY-REN-10 from renal cancer (see above). NY-LU-12 encodes a nuclear zinc finger protein with two RNA-binding domains. To date, no mutations have been found in the NY-LU-12, NY-REN-9, or NY-REN-10 coding genes. What is the basis for the immunogenicity of these 3p antigens? Further sequencing is necessary to exclude the possibility of mutation as the immune stimulus. Another possibility is that loss or downregulated expression of a gene product such as allelic 3p deletion can result in an immune response, just as gain or overexpression can be an immunogenic event.

In addition to the published studies, Güre and Chen (*unpublished data*) have screened three additional non–small-cell lung cancers. These three screenings yielded only eight positive clones from a total of more than 2×10^6 bacteriophages, and the clones represented two known genes and two unknown genes, all of them widely expressed in normal tissues. Low-yield SEREX screening is, in fact, not uncommonly encountered, most likely reflecting low tumor immunogenicity or low host immune reactivity, or both. Such essentially negative studies should be recognized because they are unlikely to be published and are therefore underrepresented in the literature.

Breast Cancer

A number of studies targeting breast cancer are ongoing within the SEREX efforts coordinated by the Ludwig Institute for Cancer Research (see below).

Jäger et al. (35) screened one breast cancer library with two separate serum sources—autologous serum and a pool of seven allogeneic sera from breast cancer patients. Additionally, a testicular library was also screened with the autologous serum. These analyses led to the isolation of 89 clones derived from 30 different genes, 27 known and three unknown. Among the known genes were two encoding CT antigens, NY-ESO-1 and SSX2, and these were prominently represented, constituting 31 (14 NY-ESO-1, 17 SSX2) of the 89 positive clones. In addition to these two genes, a candidate breast tumor suppressor gene, *ING1*, was isolated from both the breast cancer library and the testicular library. *ING1* was initially identified in the cloning of genes preferentially expressed in a normal breast epithelial cell line but not in breast cancer lines; transfection of a breast cancer cell line with the *ING1* gene was shown to lead to growth inhibition (65). No mutation has been found in the SEREX-defined *ING1* gene from the breast cancer specimen. By analyzing cDNA clones obtained by hybridization screening of the testicular library, however, three splice variants of *ING1* (variants A, B, and C) were identified. These three variants differed in their 5' sequences, encoding putative products with different amino terminal sequences. By RT-PCR analysis, only variant A showed universal expression in all tissues examined. Variants B and C were expressed in a tissue-specific fashion, whereas variant C showed expression almost exclusively in the testis. Among tumor cell lines, variant C was silent in six breast cell lines tested, and variant B, although not expressed in normal breast, was weakly expressed in four of six breast cancer cell lines tested. As discussed above in relation to NY-CO-37/38, perturbation in the tumor expression of *ING1* splice variants may account for immune recognition in the human host.

Scanlan and Gout (36) have screened four breast cancer cDNA libraries with autologous sera, yielding 53 different genes, half of them known genes and half of them novel. Of the novel gene products, three may be of etiologic significance for cancer: LONY-BR-23, which is structurally related to members of the CDC 10 family of cell-cycle regulators; LONY-BR-49, which is similar to Notch/int3; and LONY-BR-53, which shows homology to SNF2/RAD54 helicase.

Obata et al. (37) have performed autologous SEREX screenings of two breast cancers and isolated 94 reactive clones. These clones represented 55 different genes, 34 known and 21 unknown. Eighteen (33%) of the 55 were also identified by previous SEREX analysis of other breast cancers or other cancers. Among the gene products identified in these two screenings were the CT antigen SSX2, heat shock protein hsp105 (nine clones), and guanylate binding protein isoform II (five clones).

Hodgkin's Disease

A case of Hodgkin's disease was analyzed in the initial SEREX study of Sahin et al. (19). Of 1.0×10^6 clones screened, 14 positive clones were identified, representing four genes. Of most interest was HOM-HD-21, which encodes a new member of the galactoside-binding protein family, designated galectin-9 by Türeci et al. (21). This gene contains two lectin domains with galactoside binding capacity, and its expression was found to be restricted to peripheral blood leukocytes and to lymphoid tis-

sues. Serum reactivity to galactin-9 has been found to be restricted to patients with Hodgkin's disease, supporting a close association of galectin-9 with the disease. Another clone identified in this initial SEREX screening was a splice variant of the intermediate filament protein restin. Unlike seroreactivity to galectin-9, antibody to the restin splice variant was frequently found in normal individuals, as well as in patients with Hodgkin's disease (19).

Prostate Cancer

SEREX analysis of prostate cancer with autologous sera is being carried out by Chen et al. (38) and by Obata et al. (39). Chen et al. isolated 19 positive clones derived from 18 genes (ten known and eight unknown), including genes encoding DNA replication licensing factor β subunit, acid finger protein, and scaffold attachment factor. Obata et al. isolated 56 positive clones, representing 30 different genes, 17 known and 13 unknown. Among the known gene products were cIF-4 gamma and NFκB p105. The known and unknown genes derived from these studies of prostate cancer were found to be widely expressed in normal tissues.

Other Tumor Types

SEREX analysis of astrocytoma (19), chronic myeloid leukemia (40), hepatocellular carcinoma (43), and seminoma (24) have also been initiated.

In the study of astrocytoma by Sahin et al. (19), 48 positive clones were isolated representing five gene products. One of the genes was Tegt (testis-enhanced gene transcript), a gene developmentally regulated in the testis (66). Tegt was found to be overexpressed in 8 of 12 astrocytomas, but not in other cancers.

SEREX analysis of a cDNA library from a case of chronic myeloid leukemia with autologous serum identified eight positive clones, corresponding to six known and two unknown genes (40). One of the two unknown genes, referred to as *clone #4*, was shown to be expressed exclusively in testis, and not in the normal tissues tested (bone marrow, brain, lung, small intestine, muscle, or spleen), suggesting that it is a new member of the CT family.

Zhang et al. (43) have carried out an analysis of T24 bladder cancer cell line with serum from a patient with hepatocellular carcinoma. The KOC3 gene, previously identified as SEREX-defined antigen in melanoma, was isolated (see above). This indicates that KOC-related gene products are overexpressed in more than one tumor type and are often immunogenic.

In one study, Sahin et al. (24) screened a cDNA library enriched for testis-specific transcripts with serum from a seminoma patient. Nine clones were isolated, derived from four known and two unknown genes. The known genes included human hook-1 protein and a mitotic protein. One of the two unknown genes, HOM-TES-85, was found to encode a new CT antigen, and this gene was designated CT8. Sequence analysis revealed that CT8 gene product is a leucine zipper protein. Of interest, the leucine zipper region of the CT8 protein shows an atypical amphipathy, a feature that has only been observed in the N-myc proto-oncogene (24).

TABLE 3. CATEGORIES OF SEREX-DEFINED HUMAN TUMOR ANTIGENS

Antigen Category	Examples	Serum Source for Initial Isolation
Cancer-testis	NY-ESO-1	Esophageal cancer
	SSX	Melanoma
	CT7	Melanoma
Mutational	p53	Colon cancer
Differentiation	Tyrosinase	Melanoma
	Galectin-4	Colon cancer
Amplified/over-expressed	Carbonic anhydrase XII	Renal cancer
	KOC3	Melanoma, hepatoma
	eIF-4 gamma	Lung cancer
	HER-2/*neu*	Breast cancer
Splice variant	Restin	Hodgkin's disease
	NY-CO-37/38	Colon cancer
Retroviral	HERV-K10	Renal cancer

HERV, human endogenous retrovirus; KOC, *KH* domain-containing gene overexpressed in cancer.

CLASSIFICATION OF SEREX-DEFINED ANTIGENS

Given the large number of gene products identified by SEREX, it would be useful to develop a classification system that could organize them into meaningful categories. The challenge is to decide on which characteristic or characteristics of the antigen should be chosen to form the basis for categorization. As unknown genes are responsible for approximately 30% of the SEREX sequences and the number of SEREX-defined antigens continue to increase at a rapid rate, it is clearly premature to attempt a comprehensive classification at this time. However, antigens with related characteristics can readily be identified at this point. For instance, antigens can be grouped according to their cellular location, and it is particularly striking that so many of the SEREX-defined antigens are nuclear proteins (e.g., enzymes and factors involved in DNA replication, transcriptional control, RNA elongation, DNA repair, including zinc finger proteins, RNA helicases, proteins related to the mitotic apparatus, and chromosome condensation proteins). Although it is tempting to conclude that the immune responses to these

nuclear antigens are nonspecific and are related to the high cell turnover and necrosis associated with cancer, it would be premature to exclude the possibility that immunogenicity is a consequence of specific structural changes in these proteins or their expression patterns.

Another way to group the antigens would be by functional characteristics, and a broad array of functionally related proteins can be found among SEREX-defined antigens, including metabolic enzymes (e.g., lactic dehydrogenase, aldolases, pyridoxal kinase, adenylosuccinate lyase, glyceraldehyde-3-phosphate dehydrogenase), transcriptional and translational factors (e.g., zinc finger proteins, translation initiation factors), structural proteins (e.g., histone proteins, keratin, restin, and lamin), and stress proteins (e.g., heat shock proteins). In the context of tumor biology and tumor immunity, however, antigens of greatest interest would be those having a known relation to cancer or showing cancer-restricted expression or cancer-restricted immunogenicity. These would be tumor antigens of most importance for diagnostic or therapeutic applications (e.g., vaccine use). A number of SEREX antigens with these cancer-related characteristics have been identified and can be classified into one of the following six categories (Table 3).

Cancer-Testis Antigens

CT antigens share the following characteristics:

1. Predominant mRNA expression in testis, but generally not in other normal somatic tissues.
2. Gene activation and mRNA expression in a variable proportion of a wide range of human tumor types.
3. Existence of multigene families.
4. Frequent mapping of coding genes to chromosome X.

Table 4 summarizes the CT antigens identified to date. Of these, MAGE, BAGE, and GAGE were initially identified as cytotoxic T lymphocyte (CTL)–recognized antigens (47,67), and SSX, NY-ESO-1, SCP1, CT7, and CT8 were discovered by SEREX analysis. MAGE-C1, a gene identical to CT7, was independently cloned by representational difference analysis (RDA) using testicular cDNA after subtraction hybridization with other

TABLE 4. CHARACTERISTICS OF HUMAN CANCER/TESTIS ANTIGENS

Gene/Gene Family	No. of Genes	Chromosome	CTL Recognition	Ab Recognition	References
MAGE	16	Xq28/Xp21	+	I	19, 67, 85
BAGE	Unknown[a]	Unknown	+	Unknown	67
GAGE	6	Xp21-pter	+	Unknown	67
SSX	5	Xp11	Unknown	+	22, 67, 85
NY-ESO-1	2	Xq28	+	+	28, 41, 85, 86
SCP1	Unknown[a]	1p13	Unknown	+	23
CT7/MAGE-C1	1	Xq26	Unknown	+	25, 68
CT8	Unknown	Unknown	Unknown	+	24
CT9	1	1p	Unknown	Unknown	69
CT10	1	Xq27	Unknown	+[b]	28

CT, cancer-testis; CTL, cytologic T lymphocyte.
[a]Southern blot analysis suggests a multigene family for both BAGE and SCP1.
[b]CT10 recognition by human serum has been shown by enzyme-linked immunoassay.

normal tissue cDNAs (68). Similar RDA approaches have also led to the identification of LAGE-1 (42), a second gene in the NY-ESO-1 family, and CT10 (27). Both LAGE-1 and CT10 have subsequently been found to be recognized by antibodies in patient sera, confirming that they are immunogenic. CT9 was identified through mRNA-expression analysis of known or suspected testis-specific genes in tumors (69), but has not been shown to elicit an antibody response in humans.

Of the MAGE family, MAGE-1, first defined by CTL epitope cloning (47,67), was also isolated by SEREX from a case of melanoma (19). MAGE-4a, another member of the MAGE family, though not as yet been shown to elicit a CTL response, has been isolated from melanoma and ovarian cancer by SEREX (25). Other members of the MAGE family (e.g., MAGE-3 and MAGE-6), although shown to be CTL targets (47,67,70), have not been identified by SEREX.

SSX2, also known as *HOM-MEL-40*, was isolated from melanoma by SEREX (19). SSX2 was originally recognized as a gene mapping to chromosome X that was involved in the t(X;18) translocation invariably associated with synovial sarcoma (71). Additional members of the SSX family have been cloned (71, 22), and the five members of the SSX family have been shown to be transcribed in testis. Of these, only SSX1, -2, and -4 show significant expression in cancers. Expression pattern analysis revealed expression of SSX1, -2, and -4 in a proportion of malignancies of various origins, whereas SSX5 is only rarely expressed (~1% of the tumors examined), and SSX3 is silent in all tumors examined. This pattern of discordant expression of SSX genes and other CT genes mapped to chromosome X suggests the existence of gene-specific mechanisms for activation of CT antigens, in addition to other general mechanisms of gene activation, such as global demethylation (72).

NY-ESO-1 was isolated from an esophageal squamous cell carcinoma by SEREX and has been shown to be expressed in 20% to 40% of several common tumor types, including breast cancer, lung cancer, prostate cancer, bladder cancer, head and neck cancer, and melanoma. A highly homologous gene (84% amino acid identity), LAGE-1, has been found by RDA by Lethè et al. (42). Both NY-ESO-1 and LAGE-1 appear to be expressed in tumors in similar frequencies, and both are recognized by patients' sera (25).

SCP1 is a synaptonemal complex protein involved in chromosome reduction in meiosis (73) and was detected in a subtractive testicular library with serum from a patient with renal cancer (23). SCP1 has the distinction of being the only CT antigen with a defined function. The finding of a meiotic protein aberrantly expressed in a somatic neoplastic cell raises the provocative question of its role in the chromosomal aneuploidy of cancer.

CT7 was isolated by allogeneic screening of melanoma cell line SK-MEL-37 with a melanoma patient serum. This gene encodes a protein of 1,142 amino acid residues, with a carboxyl terminus highly homologous to the MAGE-10 gene over an ~210 amino acid stretch (57% identity, 75% homology, including conserved substitutions). Sequences N-terminal to this segment, however, show no homology to the MAGE family, having instead a striking repetitive pattern, with a core of ten almost exact repeats of 35 amino acids. This gene has also been isolated

by Lucas et al. (68) using the RDA approach and has been designated MAGE-C1.

CT8 was isolated by Sahin et al. (24) by SEREX analysis of a subtracted testicular library with serum from a seminoma patient. It encodes a 36-kd protein with a leucine zipper motif, characteristic of proteins involved in DNA binding and gene transcription.

CT9 (69) is the bromo domain, testis-specific gene product BRDT (74). BRDT is a putative nuclear protein of 947 amino acids (108 kd) containing two copies of the bromo domain, a motif associated with transcriptional regulation. BRDT was identified as a CT antigen during the screening of previously defined testis-specific genes for expression in malignancies. Unlike other CT antigens that are expressed in a wide range of tumors, CT9 appears to show preferential expression in lung cancer.

CT10 was isolated from melanoma using RDA by Güre et al. (27). It is structurally closely related to CT7 but lacks the repetitive sequences of CT7. It maps to chromosome Xq27 in close proximity to CT7 and MAGE genes. ELISA analysis of 100 melanoma patient sera against recombinant CT10 protein revealed seroreactivity in two cases, demonstrating the immunogenicity of CT10.

Mutational Antigens

A mutated p53, identified during a SEREX analysis of a colon cancer (29), carried a single-base substitution (TAT to TGT). Another example in this category is the translocation involving E-Cad, detected in the SEREX analysis of gastric cancer (34). These findings illustrate the capacity of SEREX to identify products of mutated genes. As discussed above, three genes coding for products identified by SEREX are clustered in chromosome 3p21, a region long known to be a hot spot of genetic aberrations in many cancer types and postulated to harbor tumor suppressor genes (53,54). Two of the three genes, NY-REN-9 and NY-REN-10, were derived from renal carcinoma and correspond to LUCA-15 and gene 21, respectively (33). The third gene, NY-LU-12, isolated from lung cancer, was identical to gene 16, which maps to the telomeric breakpoint of a small-cell lung cancer line NCI-H740 (32). Although no mutation has been detected to date in these three genes, mutations may have been missed: wild-type rather than the mutated allele of the 3p genes might have been isolated in SEREX because the antibody elicited by the mutated 3p product cross-reacts with the wild-type product.

Differentiation Antigens

The classic example of a differentiation antigen recognized by SEREX is the melanocyte-specific protein tyrosinase (19). Another example is NY-CO-27, a gene identical to galectin-4, that was isolated during a SEREX analysis of colon cancer (29). Normal tissue expression of galectin-4 is restricted to normal colon and small intestine. Because galectin-4 is localized to the leading edge of lamellipodia, it is thought to have a role in cell adhesion (44).

A number of other genes isolated by SEREX could also be classified as differentiation antigens because they show a differential pattern of gene expression in normal tissues. For instance, CT antigens, because of their restricted expression in normal testis, represent a special category of differentiation antigens. As many of these other SEREX-defined genes with differential expression are either amplified, overexpressed, or show aberrant splice variants in cancer, however, they are discussed under these categories of tumor antigens.

Amplified or Overexpressed Antigens

Overexpression of normal gene products in cancer may be a major underlying mechanism for the immunogenicity of cancer antigens in cancer patients. Examples of amplified or overexpressed SEREX-defined antigens include carbonic anhydrase XII in renal cancer (52), galectin-9/HOM-HD-21 in Hodgkin's disease (21), eIF-4 gamma (30) in lung cancer, aldolase A in lung cancer (32) and breast cancer (35), KOC family genes in melanoma (25), hepatoma (41), and AKT1 (37) and HER-2/*neu* (36) in breast cancer. Several mechanisms can account for amplified expression of gene products in cancer, including gene amplification (e.g., eIF-4 gamma), increased steady-state mRNA (e.g., KOC3), and increased protein stability (e.g., p53) (75). The frequency of gene amplification in SEREX-defined genes has been examined by Brass et al. (31), and 9 of 14 genes detected in a SEREX analysis of lung cancer were shown to be amplified by quantitative PCR, including three genes from chromosome 3, at least two of which were from a region known to be amplified in squamous cell carcinoma.

Splice Variant Antigens

Another category of SEREX-defined antigens are splice variants of genes that are differentially expressed in normal tissues. In the initial SEREX study by Sahin et al. (19), a splice variant of the intermediate filament protein restin was isolated from Hodgkin's lymphoma and was found to react with sera from both cancer patients and normal donors. In the SEREX analysis of colon cancer (29), two of the isolated antigens NY-CO-37 and NY-CO-38 represent differentially expressed isoforms of a previously unknown gene containing PDZ protein-protein interaction domains (45). In total, five splice variants of NY-CO-38 have been defined [PDZ-37, PDZ-45 (NY-CO-37), PDZ-54, PDZ-59, and PDZ-73 (NY-CO-38)], and their expression patterns in normal and malignant tissues have been characterized. One of these variants, PDZ-54, is normally expressed in normal kidney and brain but not in normal colon. However, PDZ-54 is expressed in all cases of colon cancer tested.

Viral Antigens

Human endogenous retrovirus (HERV)–related sequences have been shown to represent at least 1% of the human genome, and their gene products have been linked to the development of autoimmune and neoplastic diseases, including systemic lupus erythematosus (76), rheumatoid arthritis (77), and germ cell tumors (78). Of these sequences, HERV-K exists in 25 to 30 copies per haploid human genome, and HERV-K–encoded env and gag proteins are expressed consistently in germ cell tumors, leading to high-titer antibodies in 60% to 85% of patients with these tumors (78,79). Although HERV-K has not been shown to be expressed in renal tissue, the env protein of this retroviral sequence, HERV-

K10, was isolated from renal cancer by SEREX (19) and represents the sole example of a SEREX-identified viral antigen to date.

BASIS FOR THE IMMUNOGENICITY OF SEREX-DEFINED ANTIGENS

In the case of the great majority of SEREX-defined antigens, it is unclear why they elicit a humoral immune response. The important point would be to distinguish antigens that have no direct relevance to cancer (e.g., antigens detected by preexisting autoantibodies or antibodies elicited by antigens related to necrotic tumor products) from antigens that have some casual relation to cancer etiology or cancer phenotype. Past studies have demonstrated a high frequency of autoantibodies to known normal tissue autoantigens in cancer patients (80), and it would not be surprising that a significant proportion of the currently defined SEREX antigens are autoantigens of this kind. However, the importance of these antigens in the context of cancer antigens should not be dismissed without understanding the reason for their immunogenicity in cancer patients. For instance, mutational events in the tumor may elicit antibodies that cross-react with the corresponding nonmutated counterparts in normal cells. Under these circumstances, the immunogenic stimulus for the antibody response in cancer patients is in fact a mutated or altered gene product, but, because the resulting antibody cross-reacts with the wild-type protein, the wild-type gene (from admixed normal cells or nonmutated alleles) might be isolated in SEREX. Unless the mutated gene is identified, such antibodies would be classified as conventional autoantibodies. This scenario has been recognized as a major problem in interpreting the fact that mutations have been detected so rarely in SEREX-defined genes (29). Sequencing of repeated isolates of the gene from the cancer, microdissected cancer cells, or cell lines derived from the cancer would be one way to address this critical issue. Given the large number of SEREX-defined antigens, however, this clearly represents a daunting task.

With regard to SEREX antigens with obvious or suspected cancer relatedness, immunogenicity can be ascribed to one of several mechanisms: gene activation or depression, mutation, amplification, mRNA overexpression, or expression of abnormal splice variants. The immune response to CT antigens is clearly related to anomalous expression of gene products in cancer that are normally only expressed in primitive germ cells. CT antigen expression in cancer has been ascribed to abnormal demethylation (72), although other mechanisms may well be involved. Anomalous antigen expression also appears to be the basis for certain paraneoplastic syndromes affecting the central nervous system. These syndromes are believed to result from autoimmune recognition of neural antigens aberrantly expressed by nonneural cancers, and specific autoantibodies are often found to be associated with specific tumor types (81). For example, in paraneoplastic cerebellar degeneration, a syndrome seen in patients with breast and ovarian cancers, autoantibodies have been found to react with neuronal antigens, including CDR34, an antigen strongly expressed in Purkinje cells of the cerebellum (82). The experimental precedent for immunogenicity due to anomalous activation of a gene in cancer comes from the study of the TL system of antigens in the mouse (83). In some mouse

TABLE 5. SEROEPIDEMIOLOGICAL ANALYSIS OF SEVEN SEREX-DEFINED ANTIGENS FROM COLON AND RENAL CANCER WITH A CANCER-RESTRICTED RECOGNITION PATTERN

Clone Number	Gene	Serum Source (No. Positive/Total No. Tested)					
		Normal Sera	Colon Cancer	Renal Cancer	Lung Cancer	Breast Cancer	Esophageal Cancer
NY-CO-8	Leucine zipper protein	0/26	8/29	5/31	2/29	0/10	0/15
NY-CO-9	Histone deacetylase	0/26	5/29	1/31	1/29	0/10	0/15
NY-CO-13	p53	0/26	6/29	0/13	1/29	0/10	2/15
NY-CO-38[a]	PDZ-73	0/26	7/37	8/32	0/29	1/26	0/15
NY-REN-21	Zfp38 homolog	0/22	3/16	3/32	2/21	0/16	0/15
NY-REN-31	Syntaxin	0/19	0/16	5/32	2/21	0/16	1/15
NY-REN-60	Tre oncogene-related	0/19	0/16	7/32	0/21	0/16	0/15

SEREX, serological expression cloning.
[a]Same as NY-REN-3.

strains (TL+ strains), TL is a normal alloantigen whose expression is limited to thymocytes. In other strains (TL– strains), no normal cell types express TL. However, leukemias arising in TL– as well as TL+ strains can express TL, and a strong humoral immunity against TL can be elicited in TL– mice.

With regard to mutations as a basis for immunogenicity, p53 can be considered the prime example among SEREX-defined antigens. However, it is unclear whether mutation or accumulation of high levels of p53 in cells harboring p53 mutations represents the initial antigenic stimulus leading to the development of p53 antibodies. Nevertheless, what is clear is that the resulting p53 antibodies recognize wild-type p53 sequences rather than showing specificity for mutated sequences (84).

Amplified expression appears to be one of the most frequent reasons for immunogenicity of antigens isolated by SEREX, and many examples of antibodies to overexpressed gene products in cancer have been detected in SEREX analysis. Thus, the immune system appears poised to respond to quantitative as well as qualitative changes in antigen expression in cancer cells. Until the basis for amplification or overexpression has been understood and the specificity established, however, the relation between antigen overexpression and antibody response can only be regarded as a strong correlation rather than a causal relationship.

Finally, another stimulus for an immune response has been postulated to be splice variants of genes, which are differentially expressed in normal tissues but aberrantly expressed in cancer. For example, PDZ-54, one of five splice variants of NY-CO-38 normally expressed in kidney, brain, but not colon, was found to be expressed in colon cancer (see above). Thus, tolerance may not extend to normal splice variants that are aberrantly expressed in a cancer, but this idea remains to be formally demonstrated.

SEROEPIDEMIOLOGY OF SEREX-DEFINED ANTIGENS

Serology plays a central role in three phases of SEREX analysis.

1. In the initial identification of reactive clones

2. In screening small panels of sera from normal individuals and cancer patients for antibody (petit serology)
3. In large-scale surveys of human sera (grand serology)

Petit serology, using the isolate as target antigen, provides some indication of cancer-specific recognition of the antigen, whereas grand serology, using recombinant protein as target antigen, establishes the seroreactivity pattern of humans with or without cancer on a larger scale. Although only a small percentage of SEREX-defined antigens has been subjected to petit or grand serology, there is a growing list of antigens that show a promising degree of cancer-specific recognition in petit serology. For instance, in the SEREX analysis of four colon cancers by Scanlan et al. (29), 6 of 48 antigens isolated in the study showed a cancer-restricted recognition pattern in tests with 16 normal sera and 29 colon cancer sera. In a SEREX analysis of four renal cancers by Scanlan et al. (33), 12 of the 65 antigens isolated in the study showed a cancer-restricted recognition pattern in tests with 19 normal serum and 32 renal cancer patients. As a rule, the highest reactivity frequency with these antigens is 20% to 25% of patients, and there is a distinctive seroreactivity pattern with each of the antigens. As a consequence, the combined use of the six restricted antigens in the colon cancer panel detected 69% of sera from colon cancer patients, and the 12 restricted antigens in the renal cancer panel detected 72% of sera from renal cancer patients. Reactivity is not restricted to patients with the corresponding cancer type; sera from patients with other forms of cancer (e.g., lung or breast cancers) recognize a proportion of the antigens derived from colon and renal cancer. Table 5 shows an updated seroepidemiologic survey by Scanlan et al. (29,33, and *unpublished data*) of seven SEREX-defined antigens showing a cancer-restricted recognition pattern identified in our analysis of colon and renal cancer.

Petit serology, although useful to identify antigens worthy of future study, is laborious and has several limitations:

1. It requires large amounts of sera.
2. Sera must be preabsorbed to remove *Escherichia coli* or phage reactivity.
3. Only small numbers of sera can be tested at one time.

For this reason, ELISA tests with recombinant protein (grand serology) offers a number of advantages (e.g., does not require preabsorbed sera, requires small amounts of sera, a large number of sera can be tested, and the analysis is quantitative). However, some degree of sensitivity (~1 log) is sacrificed in grand serology as compared to petit serology. NY-ESO-1 is the first SEREX-defined antigen to be analyzed in grand serology (85). No reactivity was found with 70 sera from normal individuals. Antibody to NY-ESO-1 was found in ~10% of sera from unselected patients with melanoma and ovarian cancer. To investigate the relation between NY-ESO-1 expression in the tumor and antibody response, a series of 62 melanoma patients were tested, 15 with NY-ESO-1+ tumors and 47 with NY-ESO-1– tumors. The conclusions were clear—NY-ESO-1 antibody was only found in patients with NY-ESO-1+ tumors, and up to 50% of patients with advanced NY-ESO-1+ tumors formed NY-ESO-1 antibody.

SEREX-defined antigens showing cancer-restricted seroreactivity offer a range of opportunities for cancer diagnosis and disease monitoring. To explore these applications, the current approach using ELISA technology and recombinant SEREX-defined antigens provides a satisfactory methodology. In the future, however, protein chip technology holds great promise for miniaturized, rapid, and large-scale screening of human sera for antibodies against SEREX-defined antigens.

T-CELL RECOGNITION OF SEREX-DEFINED ANTIGENS

The detection of tyrosinase and MAGE-1 by SEREX, two tumor antigens initially recognized by epitope cloning as targets for CD8 T cells, established the critical principle that the analysis of humoral immunity to tumor antigens has the potential for identifying CD8 T-cell recognized antigens. In addition, because production of IgG antibodies is known to require CD4 T-cell help, SEREX analysis can be viewed as a way to define the CD4 T-cell repertoire against human tumor antigens. A number of laboratories are developing approaches for defining the peptide targets for CD8+ and CD4+ T-cell recognition of SEREX-defined antigens. NY-ESO-1, one of the first antigens isolated by SEREX, provides a model for defining the T-cell recognized peptides of a tumor protein initially identified by antibody (86). In the case of CD8 T cells, an HLA-A2+ melanoma patient with high-titered NY-ESO-1 antibody was also found to have strong CTL reactivity against the autologous NY-ESO-1+ melanoma. To investigate the possibility that NY-ESO-1 was the target for the CD8 recognition in this patient, COS cells were cotransfected with HLA-A2 and the NY-ESO-1 coding gene, and these transfectants were found to be lysed by CTLs from the patient with high-titered NY-ESO-1 antibody. Additionally, the reactivity of these CTLs cotyped with NY-ESO-1 expression in a panel of HLA-A2+ melanoma. To identify the NY-ESO-1 peptide epitopes recognized by the CTLs, a series of overlapping peptides were synthesized on the basis of known HLA-A2 peptide-binding motifs, and three of these peptides were found to be specifically recognized. Subsequent studies with CTLs from other HLA-A2+ patients with

NY-ESO-1+ tumors and NY-ESO-1 antibody showed recognition of these HLA-A2 restricted peptides. For the identification of CD4-recognized NY-ESO-1 peptides, a similar general strategy was followed (87). CD4 T cells from two patients with NY-ESO-1+ melanoma and NY-ESO-1 antibody recognized NY-ESO-1 target cells pulsed with NY-ESO-1 protein in a HLA–DRB4 0101-0103–restricted fashion in enzyme-linked immunospot (ELISPOT) analysis. Overlapping NY-ESO-1 peptides were synthesized, and three of these were recognized by CD4 T cells in ELISPOT and proliferation assays using peptide-pulsed target cells.

Because the definition of targets for T-cell recognition is a far more complex and laborious task than defining antibody targets, current technologies place a limit on the number of antigens that can be analyzed from the T-cell perspective. In our opinion, SEREX-defined antigens eliciting high-titered antibodies with a cancer-restricted pattern in a substantial number of patients constitute the most promising targets for T-cell analysis. Newer techniques involving efficient transfection of coding genes with viral or nonviral vectors, better methods for long-term propagation and stabilization of specifically reactive CD8 and CD4 T cells, and new approaches to identify and expand low-frequency–specific T-cell populations should facilitate T-cell analysis of SEREX-defined antigens.

CANCER IMMUNOME

The past decade has seen enormous strides in our understanding of the immune response to human cancer. In major part, this has been due to the development of methodologies capable of defining the antigenic targets on cancer cells that elicit an immune response (19,67,88). The cloning of T-cell recognized epitopes by Boon et al. (67) and Kawakami and Rosenberg et al. (88) has provided a growing list of tumor peptides that allows detailed monitoring of CD8 T-cell responses to these antigens in cancer patients and offers promising targets for cancer vaccine development. SEREX technology, because it is generally applicable to all tumor types and is less technically demanding than T-cell epitope cloning, holds promise for greatly extending the understanding of the immune response to cancer. In fact, identifying the complete repertoire of immunogenic gene products in human cancer—what is becoming known as the cancer immunome—is now an achievable goal for tumor immunology. To this end, a SEREX collaborative group was established in 1996 by the Ludwig Institute for Cancer Research, involving investigators at the University of Saarland (Homburg, Germany); Ludwig Institute Branches in New York, Melbourne, and London (University College); Aichi Cancer Center (Japan); Krankenhaus Nordwest (Frankfurt, Germany); and Moscow State University (Russia). A SEREX database has been organized by Victor Jongeneel (Director of Information Technology, Ludwig Institute for Cancer Research, http://www.licr.org/SEREX) and more than 500 SEREX-identified antigens have been deposited at last count (February 2000). Even at this early stage of SEREX analysis, repeated isolation of the same gene is being seen, indicating the limited range of immunogenic cancer antigens and the feasibility of defining the cancer immunome.

REFERENCES

1. Oettgen HF, Old LJ. The history of cancer immunotherapy. In: DeVita VT Jr, Hellman S, Rosenberg SA, eds. *Biologic therapy of cancer.* Philadelphia: JB Lippincott Co, 1991:87–119.
2. Day EA. *The immunochemistry of cancer.* Springfield, IL: Charles C. Thomas Publisher, 1965.
3. Abelev GI, Perova SD, Khramkova NI, Postnikova ZA, Irlin IS. Production of embryonal alpha-globulin by transplantable mouse hepatomas. *Transplantation* 1963;1:174–180.
4. Gold P, Freeman SO. Specific carcinoembryonic antigens of the human digestive system. *J Exp Med* 1965;122:467–468.
5. Boyse EA, Old LJ. Some aspects of normal and abnormal cell surface genetics. *Annu Rev Genet* 1969;3:269–290.
6. Old LJ, Stockert E. Immunogenetics of cell surface antigens of mouse leukemia. *Annu Rev Genet* 1977;11:127–160.
7. Köhler G, Milstein C. Continuous cultures of fused cells secreting antibody of predefined specificity. *Nature* 1975;236:495–497.
8. Rettig WJ, Old LJ. Immunogenetics of human cell surface differentiation. *Annu Rev Immunol* 1989;7:481–511.
9. Old LJ. Cancer immunology: the search for specificity—G.H.A. Lowes Memorial Lecture. *Cancer Res* 1981;41:361–375.
10. Garrett TJ, Takahashi T, Clarkson BD, Old LJ. Detection of antibody to autologous human leukemia cells by immune adherence assay. *Proc Natl Acad Sci U S A* 1977;74:4587–4590.
11. Carey TE, Takahashi T, Resnick LA, Oettgen HF, Old LJ. Cell surface antigens of human malignant melanoma. I. Mixed hemadsorption assays for humoral immunity to cultured autologous melanoma cells. *Proc Natl Acad Sci U S A* 1976;73:3278–3282.
12. Shiku H, Takahashi T, Oettgen HF, Old LJ. Cell surface antigens of human malignant melanoma. II. Serological typing with immune adherence assays and definition of two new surface antigens. *J Exp Med* 1976;144:873–881.
13. Ueda R, Shiku H, Pfreundschuh M, et al. Cell surface antigens of human renal cancer defined by autologous typing. *J Exp Med* 1979;150:564–579.
14. Pfreundschuh M, Shiku H, Takahashi T, et al. Serological analysis of cell surface antigens of malignant human brain tumors. *Proc Natl Acad Sci U S A* 1978;75:5122–5126.
15. Carey TE, Lloyd KO, Takahashi T, Travassos L, Old LJ. Solubilization and partial characterization of the AU cell surface antigen of human malignant melanoma. *Proc Natl Acad Sci U S A* 1976;73:3278–3282.
16. Watanabe T, Pukel CS, Takeyama H, et al. Human melanoma antigen AH is an autoimmunogenic ganglioside related to GD2. *J Exp Med* 1982;156:1884–1894.
17. Real FX, Mattes MJ, Houghton AN, Oettgen HF, Lloyd KO, Old LJ. Class 1 (unique) antigens of melanoma: identification of a 90,000 dalton cell surface glycoprotein by autologous antibody. *J Exp Med* 1984;160:1219–1233.
18. Mattes MJ, Thomson TM, Old LJ, Lloyd KO. A pigmentation-associated differentiation antigen of human melanoma defined by a precipitating antibody in human serum. *Int J Cancer* 1983;32:717–721.
19. Sahin U, Türeci Ö, Schmitt H, et al. Human neoplasms elicit multiple specific immune responses in the autologous host. *Proc Natl Acad Sci U S A* 1995;92:11810–11813.
20. Sahin U, Türeci Ö, Pfreundschuh M. Serological identification of human tumor antigens. *Curr Opin Immunol* 1997;9:709–716.
21. Türeci Ö, Schmitt H, Fadle N, Pfreundschuh M, Sahin U. Molecular definition of a novel human galactin which is immunogenic in patients with Hodgkin's disease. *J Biol Chem* 1997;272:6416–6422.
22. Güre AO, Türeci Ö, Sahin U, et al. SSX, a multigene family with several members transcribed in normal testis and human cancer. *Int J Cancer* 1997;72:965–971.
23. Türeci Ö, Dahin U, Zwick C, Koslowski M, Seitz G, Pfreundschuh M. Identification of a meiosis-specific protein as a new member of the class of cancer/testis antigens. *Proc Natl Acad Sci U S A* 1998;95:5211–5216.
24. Sahin U, Türeci Ö, Eberle T, et al. A novel tumor-specific leucine zipper protein which shares features with the n-myc oncoprotein and

25. elicits immune responses in tumor-bearing patients. 2000 (submitted).
25. Chen YT, Güre AO, Tsang S, et al. Identification of multiple cancer/testis antigens by allogeneic antibody screening of a melanoma cell line library. *Proc Natl Acad Sci U S A* 1998;95:6919–6923.
26. O'Neill MJ, Sinclair AH. Isolation of rare transcripts by representational difference analysis. *Nucleic Acids Res* 1997;25:2681–2682.
27. Güre A, Stockert E, Arden KC, et al. CT10: a new cancer-testis (CT) antigen homologous to CT7 and the MAGE family, identified by representational difference analysis. *Int J Cancer* 2000;85:726–732.
28. Chen YT, Scanlan M, Sahin U, et al. A testicular antigen aberrantly expressed in human cancers detected by autologous antibody screening. *Proc Natl Acad Sci U S A* 1997;94:1914–1918.
29. Scanlan MJ, Chen YT, Williamson B, et al. Characterization of human colon cancer antigens recognized by autologous antibodies. *Int J Cancer* 1998;76:652–658.
30. Brass N, Heckel D, Sahin U, Pfreundschuh M, Sybrecht GW, Meese EU. Translation initiation factor eIF-4 gamma is encoded by an amplified gene and induces an immune response in squamous cell lung carcinoma. *Hum Mol Genet* 1997;6:33–39.
31. Brass N, Racz A, Bauer C, Heckel D, Sybrecht GW, Meese EU. Role of amplified genes in the production of autoantibodies. *Blood* 1999;93:2158–2166.
32. Güre AO, Altorki NK, Stockert E, Scanlan MJ, Old LJ, Chen YT. Human lung cancer antigens recognized by autologous antibodies: definition of a novel cDNA derived from the tumor suppressor gene locus on chromosome 3p21. *Cancer Res* 1998;58:1034–1041.
33. Scanlan MJ, Gordan JD, Williamson B, et al. Antigens recognized by autologous antibody in patients with renal cell carcinoma. *Int J Cancer* 1999;83:456–464.
34. Obata Y, Sakamoto J, Hamajima N, et al. In preparation.
35. Jäger D, Stockert E, Scanlan MJ, et al. Cancer-testis antigens and ING1 tumor suppressor gene product are breast cancer antigens: characterization of tissue specific ING1 transcripts and a homolog gene. *Cancer Res* 1999;59:6197–6204.
36. Scanlan MJ, Gout I, Mackay A, Chen YT, O'Hare M, Old LJ. In preparation.
37. Obata Y, Miura S, Iwase T, et al. In preparation.
38. Chen YT, Güre AO, Scanlan MJ, Jäger E, Knuth A, Old LJ. In preparation.
39. Obata Y, Kinukawa T, Chen YT, Old LJ, Takahashi T, Tamaki H. In preparation.
40. Ling M, Wen YJ, Lim SH. Prevalence of antibodies against proteins derived from chronic myeloid leukemia. *Blood* 1998;92:4764–4770.
41. Lethé B, Lucas S, Michaux L, et al. LAGE-1: a new gene with tumor specificity. *Int J Cancer* 1998;76:903–908.
42. Müller-Pillasch F, Lacher U, Wallrapp C, et al. Cloning of a gene highly overexpressed in cancer coding for a novel KH-domain containing protein. *Oncogene* 1997;14:2729–2733.
43. Zhang JY, Chan EKL, Peng XX, Tan EM. A novel cytoplasmic protein with RNA-binding motifs is an autoantigen in human hepatocellular carcinoma. *J Exp Med* 1999;189:1101–1110.
44. Huflejt ME, Jordan ET, Gitt MA, Barondes SH, Leffler H. Strikingly different localization of galectin-3 and galectin-4 in human colon adenocarcinoma T84 cells: galectin-4 is localized at sites of cell adhesion. *J Biol Chem* 1997;272:14294–14303.
45. Scanlan MJ, Williamson B, Jungbluth A, et al. Isoforms of the human PDZ-73 protein exhibit differential tissue expression. *Biochem Biophys Acta* 1999;1445:39–52.
46. Ponting CP, Phillips C, Davies KE, Blake DJ. PDZ domains: targeting signaling molecules to sub-membranous sites. *Bioessays* 1997;19:469–479.
47. Van den Eynde BJ, van der Bruggen P. T cell defined tumor antigens. *Curr Opin Immunol* 1997;9:684–693.
48. Geiger B, Ayalon O. Cadherins. *Annu Rev Cell Biol* 1992;8:307–332.
49. Takeichi M. Cadherins in cancer: implications for invasion and metastasis. *Curr Opin Cell Biol* 1993;5:806–811.
50. Guilford P, Hopkins J, Harraway J, et al. E-cadherin germline mutations in familial gastric cancer. *Nature* 1998;392:402–405.
51. Staal SP. Molecular cloning of the akt oncogene and its human

homologues AKT1 and AKT2: amplification of AKT1 in a primary human gastric adenocarcinoma. *Proc Natl Acad Sci U S A* 1987;84: 5034–5037.

52. Türeci Ö, Sahin U, Vollmar E, et al. Human carbonic anhydrase XII: cDNA cloning, expression, and chromosomal localization of a carbonic anhydrase gene that is overexpressed in some renal cell cancers. *Proc Natl Acad Sci U S A* 1998;95:7608–7613.

53. Kok K, Naylor SL, Buys CH. Deletions of the short arm of chromosome 3 in solid tumors and the search for tumor suppressor genes. *Adv Cancer Res* 1997;71:27–92.

54. van den Berg A, Hulsbeek MF, de Jong D, et al. Major role for a 3p21 region and lack of involvement of the t(3;8) breakpoint region in the development of renal cell carcinoma suggested by loss of heterozygosity analysis. *Genes Chrom Cancer* 1996;15:64–72.

55. Jenne DE, Reimann H, Nezu J, et al. Peutz-Jeghers syndrome is caused by mutations in a novel serine threonine kinase. *Nat Genet* 1998;18:38–43.

56. Dong SM, Kim KM, Kim SY, et al. Frequent somatic mutations in serine/threonine kinase 11/Peutz-Jeghers syndrome gene in left-sided colon cancer. *Cancer Res* 1998;58:3787–3790.

57. Bignell GR, Barfoot R, Seal S, Collins N, Warren W, Stratton MR. Low frequency of somatic mutations in the LKB1/Peutz-Jeghers syndrome gene in sporadic breast cancer. *Cancer Res* 1998;58:1384–1386.

58. Park WS, Moon YW, Yang YM, et al. Mutations of the STK11 gene in sporadic gastric carcinoma. *Int J Oncol* 1998;13:601–604.

59. Hariharan IK, Adams JM. cDNA sequence for human bcr, the gene that translocates to the abl oncogene in chronic myeloid leukaemia. *EMBO J* 1987;6:115–119.

60. Iida A, Kurose K, Isobe R, et al. Mapping of a new target region of allelic loss to a 2-cM interval at 22q13.1 in primary breast cancer. *Genes Chromosomes Cancer* 1998;21:108–112.

61. Chowdhury K, Goulding M, Walther C, Imai K, Fickenscher H. The ubiquitous transactivator Zfp-38 is unregulated during spermatogenesis with differential transcription. *Mech Develop* 1992;39:129–142.

62. Brass N, Ukena I, Remberger K, Mack U, Sybrecht GW, Meese EU. DNA amplification on chromosome 3q26.1-q26.3 in squamous cell carcinoma of the lung detected by reverse chromosome painting. *Eur J Cancer* 1996;32:1205–1208.

63. Ojila T, Imaizumi M, Abe T, Kato K. Immunochemical and immunohistochemical studies on three aldolase isozymes in human lung cancer. Cancer 1991;67:2153–2158.

64. Asaka M, Kimura T, Meguro T, et al. Alteration of aldolase isozymes in serum and tissues of patients with cancer and other diseases. *J Clin Lab Anal* 1994;8:144–148.

65. Garkavtsev I, Kazarov A, Gudkov A, Riabowol K. Suppression of the novel growth inhibitor p33ING1 promotes neoplastic transformation. *Nat Genet* 1996;14:415–420.

66. Walter L, Marynen P, Szpirer J, Levan G, Gunther E. Identification of a novel conserved human gene, TEGT. *Genomics* 1995;28:301–304.

67. Boon T, van der Bruggen P. Human tumor antigens recognized by T lymphocytes. *J Exp Med* 1996;183:725–729.

68. Lucas S, De Smet C, Arden KC, et al. Identification of a new MAGE gene with tumor-specific expression by representational difference analysis. *Cancer Res* 1998;58:743–752.

69. Scanlan MJ, Altorki NK, Güre AO, et al. Expression of cancer-testis antigens in lung cancer: definition of bromodomain testis-specific gene (BRDT) as a new CT gene CT9. *Cancer Lett* 2000 (*in press*).

70. Zorn E, Hercend T. A MAGE-6-encoded peptide is recognized by expanded lymphocytes infiltrating a spontaneously regressing human primary melanoma lesion. *Eur J Immunol* 1999;29:602–607.

71. Crew AJ, Clark J, Fisher C, et al. Fusion of SYT to two genes, SSX1 and SSX2, encoding proteins with homology to the Kruppel-associated box in human synovial sarcoma. *EMBO J* 1994;14:2333–2340.

72. DeSmet C, DeBacker O, Faraoni I, et al. The activation of human gene MAGE-1 in tumor cells is correlated with genome-wide demethylation. *Proc Natl Acad Sci U S A* 1996;93:7149–7153.

73. Meuwissen RJL, Meerts I, Hoovers JMN, Leschot NJ, Heyting C. Human synaptonemal protein 1 (SCP1): isolation and characterization of the cDNA and chromosomal localization of the gene. *Genomics* 1997;39:377–384.

74. Jones MH, Numata M, Shimane M. Identification and characterization of BRDT: a testis-specific gene related to the bromodomain genes RING3 and Drosophila fsh. *Genomics* 1997;45:529–534.

75. Reich NC, Oren M, Levine AJ. Two distinct mechanisms regulate the levels of a cellular tumor antigen, p53. *Mol Cell Biol* 1983;3: 2143–2150.

76. Herrmann M, Hagenhofer M, Kalden JR. Retrovirus and systemic lupus erythematosus. *Immunol Rev* 1996;152:145–156.

77. Walchner M, Leib-Mosch C, Messer G, Germaier H, Plewig G, Kind P. Endogenous retroviral sequences in the pathogenesis of systemic autoimmune disease. *Arch Dermatol* 1997;133:767–771.

78. Herbst H, Sauter M, Mueller-Lantzsch N. Expression of human endogenous retrovirus K elements in germ cell and trophoblastic tumors. *Am J Pathol* 1996;149:1727–1735.

79. Boller K, Janssen O, Schuldes H, Tonjes RR, Kurth R. Characterization of the antibody response specific for the human endogenous retrovirus HTDV/HERV-K. *J Virol* 1997;71:4581–4588.

80. Burek CL, Rose NR, eds. *Autoantibodies.* New York: Raven Press, 1995:207–230.

81. Posner JB. Paraneoplastic syndromes: a brief review. *Ann N Y Acad Sci U S A* 1997;835:83–90.

82. Dropcho EJ, Chen YT, Posner JB, Old LJ. Cloning of a brain protein identified by autoantibodies from a patient with paraneoplastic cerebellar degeneration. *Proc Natl Acad Sci U S A* 1987;84: 4552–4556.

83. Chen YT, Obata Y, Stockert E, Takahashi T, Old LJ. *Tla* region genes and their products. *Immunol Res* 1987;6:30–45.

84. Schlichtholz B, Legros Y, Gillet D, et al. The immune response to p53 in breast cancer patients is directed against immunodominant epitopes unrelated to the mutational hot spot. *Cancer Res* 1992;52: 6380–6384.

85. Stockert E, Jäger E, Chen YT, Gout I, Knuth A, Old LJ. A survey of the humoral immune response of cancer patients to a panel of human tumor antigens. *J Exp Med* 1998;187:1349–1354.

86. Jäger E, Chen YT, Drijfout JW, et al. Simultaneous humoral and cellular immune response against cancer-testis antigen NY-ESO-1: definition of HLA-A2-binding peptide epitopes. *J Exp Med* 1998;187: 265–270.

87. Jäger E, Jäger D, Karbach J, et al. Identification of NY-ESO-1 epitopes presented by HLA-DRB4 0101-0103 and recognized by CD4⁺ T lymphocyte of patients with NY-ESO-1 expressing melanoma. *J Exp Med* 2000 (*in press*).

88. Kawakami Y, Rosenberg SA. Human tumor antigens recognized by T cells. *Immunol Res* 1997;16:313–339.

CANCER VACCINES: BASIC PRINCIPLES

General Concepts and Preclinical Studies

NICHOLAS P. RESTIFO

What are the basic principles of the design of cancer vaccines? Because a number of efficacious tumor vaccines are not available to draw "principles" from, the answer to this question, at least in the clinic, is far from definitive. It is only in experimental animals where enough progress has been made that patterns of efficacy begin to emerge. Thus, the general concepts and "principles" of cancer vaccination described in this chapter are largely derived from work in laboratory animals, especially from preclinical mouse models.

Human clinical trials using experimental cancer vaccines are being performed at an accelerating pace. These trials have confirmed some early findings obtained from animal studies while refuting others. Most important, findings in human clinical trials are an engine for hypotheses about how cancer vaccines work. Once generated, these hypotheses can be explored in experimental animals (1). It is through the interplay of *in vivo* and *in vitro* data from experimental animals and human clinical trials that a set of general immunologic principles is emerging, which may guide the immunotherapist in the successful vaccination against cancer (Table 1).

Vaccines are traditionally thought of as preventing infectious diseases, but they may have new uses in the treatment of malignancies. In the case of cancer, it is clear that the immune system can recognize and destroy even large quantities of established tumor. Evidence for this immune-mediated destruction comes primarily from clinical trials using interleukin-2 (IL-2), which is a U.S. Food and Drug Administration–approved treatment for melanoma and renal cell carcinoma (2). New immunotherapies based on vaccines designed to treat cancer have been used in the clinic. These therapeutic vaccines have been clearly demonstrated to elicit antitumor immune responses. In a number of cases, these vaccines have also been reported to mediate the destruction of established cancer (3–5).

Although the notion of vaccines designed to prevent cancer may be appealing, a variety of practical and theoretical problems arise in creating such a prophylactic vaccine. One problem has to do with predicting which patients will develop cancer, although an increased knowledge of genetic and environmental factors that contribute to carcinogenesis may enhance our ability to make these kinds of predictions. In addition to these practical considerations, theoretical reasons exist as to why prophylactic vaccination against defined antigens may be problematic. For example, the difficulty in predicting which of a myriad of mutations may occur in any one of a large number of genes makes vaccination against mutated tumor antigens unlikely to be successful. Similarly, vaccination against unmutated "self" antigens may be subject to chronic immunologic toleration or may produce untoward side effects resulting from the destruction of normal tissues that express the same antigen.

The only true preventive cancer vaccines that are under serious consideration are really variants of vaccines designed to prevent infectious diseases (6,7). For example, vaccines that prevent human papilloma virus or hepatitis infections should also prevent cervical cancer and liver cancer, respectively. Most cancers affecting individuals in developed cancers, however, have not been associated with viruses. Thus, prophylactic vaccines for cancer are likely to be the exception rather than the rule. Most research in the field of cancer vaccines is devoted to vaccines designed to activate the immune system to destroy established cancer cells. These vaccines are the primary focus of this chapter.

Seven Principles to Consider When Designing an Anticancer Vaccine

We attempt to enunciate a few of the basic immunologic principles that may be useful in the design of anticancer vaccines, whether these vaccines are based on irradiated or gene-modified tumor cells or synthetic or recombinant forms of a tumor antigen. Some general principles follow:

Human Cancers Are Poorly Immunogenic

Every cancer that kills a person is a cancer that has not been destroyed by the immune system. The reason for this apparent lack of immunogenicity may be that cancer antigens are generally not presented to the immune system in a microenvironment that favors the activation of immune cells. Although no

TABLE 1. SEVEN PRINCIPLES TO CONSIDER WHEN DESIGNING AN ANTICANCER VACCINE

Human cancers are poorly immunogenic.
The vaccine must express an appropriate tumor antigen target.
Immunizations most effective in generating reactive T cells are the most therapeutically effective.
Dendritic cells mediate vaccine function.
Vaccination can be enhanced with cytokines, chemokines, and costimulatory molecules.
The immunogen chosen must be effective in the treatment of established disease.
Optimal dose, boosting, and route of the immunization are determined by basic immunologic principles.

single known mechanism can explain poor tumor immunogenicity in all experimental models studied, the molecular bases can be separated conceptually into two distinct groupings. The first concerns mechanisms of poor immune activation shared by normal cells in the body, whereas the second has to do with the inherent genetic instability of cancer cells (Table 2). This instability leads to a great deal of heterogeneity among tumor cells, making the immune destruction of all tumor cells in the body an extremely difficult task (8).

Tumor Microenvironment May Inhibit Immune Activation

Like most normal cells in the body, tumor cells generally do not express costimulatory molecules, such as B7-1 (CD80) and B7-2 (CD86). In the absence of costimulation, T cells tend to become anergic. For self-antigens, this may protect against autoreactivity. B7-1 and B7-2 are expressed on professional antigen-presenting cells (APCs) and on a variety of other tissues after exposure to inflammatory cytokines (9). Transfection of tumor cells with both isoforms has been used successfully to trigger their immune-mediated rejection of experimental mouse tumors, which have some inherent immunogenicity (10,11). This strategy, however, is insufficient for nonimmunogenic tumors, a category into which most, if not all, human tumors would fall (11).

Another mechanism that may explain why patients with cancer usually do not reject their tumors involves the lack of inflammation at the tumor site. Important differences exist between the site of a tumor deposit and a site of infection. Tumors produce few, if any, immunologic "danger signals" to stimulate the immune response (12,13). In contrast, at a site of infection, the innate immune response is triggered because of tissue destruction. Inflammatory cells, such as monocytes, macrophages, and dendritic cells (DCs), are activated as a result of

TABLE 2. WHY TUMOR CELLS ARE POORLY IMMUNOGENIC

Lack of expression of costimulatory molecules (B7-1/CD80, B7-2/CD86, and CD40L)
Production of immunoinhibitory substances (transforming growth factor–β and interleukin-10)
Poor antigen processing and presentation (loss or poor expression of B2m, major histocompatibility class I, TAP, and LMP)
Variability in the expression of antigen by tumors

this tissue destruction, and because of components of the infectious agents themselves, such as lipopolysaccharide, nonmethylated CpG sequences, and double-stranded RNA, each of which are components of invading microbes that are not shared by normal host cells or growing cancer cells. In the absence of these "danger signals," the immune system may not be fully activated (14).

Induction of Tolerance by Tumor Cells

Despite cancer cells' expression of clearly immunogenic molecules, the host does not always mount an effective immune response to these antigens. A number of groups have conducted experiments in which highly immunogenic foreign antigens, such as the hemagglutinin protein from influenza (15), the β-galactosidase (β-gal) enzyme from *Escherichia coli* (16), and the ovalbumin protein from the chicken are expressed in tumor cells (17). The results are fairly uniform: tumors tend to grow progressively, retaining their lethality despite the expression of a foreign and highly immunogenic protein by the tumor cell.

Alternative immune mechanisms, designated *tolerance* and *ignorance*, have been used to explain why the immune system fails to recognize such tumors. *Tolerance* generally refers to the lack of a destructive immune reaction to a given antigen. In the tumor context, an active state of tolerance may be distinguished in which the immune system undergoes a functional and phenotypic change after encounter with antigen from ignorance, a passive process where immune cells do not have any contact with the antigen that alters their phenotype or function (18–21). Both mechanisms likely play a role in the immune system's unresponsiveness to tumor cells.

Tumors Produce Immunoinhibitory Factors

Tumor cells may ectopically use normal immunosuppressive mechanisms, such as the production of transforming growth factor–β, normally produced by certain immune and other somatic cells, but potentially antiproliferative for cytotoxic T lymphocytes (CTL), natural killer cells, and lymphokine-activated T cells (22–25). Another example, IL-10, produced by activated T cells, B cells, monocytes, and keratinocytes, may be produced by certain solid tumors and may interfere with macrophage-mediated antigen presentation and other immune functions.

Hahne et al. reported in 1996 that expression of Fas ligand (FasL/CD95L) by melanoma cells was responsible for their escape from immune recognition (26). Because FasL was reportedly expressed in areas of immune privilege, such as the eye and testis, it was reasoned that expression of FasL by melanoma cells indicated that the tumor bed was also an "immune privileged" site. In our own study, however, we found no FasL expressed by a panel of 26 human melanoma lines we tested (27–29). Thus, our data do not support a role for FasL expression in the escape of melanoma cells from immune destruction.

Tumor as a "Moving Target"

Tumor cells can be a moving target when it comes to immune recognition. The field of chemotherapy has produced a number of well-known examples of tumor escape from treatment, including the induction of the expression of the multidrug resistance gene. As recombinant and synthetic vaccines become more effective, the selective pressure on the loss of particular target antigens may increase. Indeed, some evidence exists that tumor cells may preferentially lose the gp100 tumor antigen as a result of treatment with the gp100 209-217 (2M) peptide plus IL-2 (FM Marincola, *unpublished*, 1999 and 30,31).

Tumors have unstable genomes, which leads them to be heterogeneous for the expression of tumor-associated antigens. Further, their unstable genomes may enable them to escape immune recognition because they lose or mutate key elements of the antigen-processing machinery, such as the TAP transporters, β_2-microglobulin, or the major histocompatibility complex (MHC) class I α chain molecules (32–37). Other mechanisms underlying the poor immunogenicity of tumors includes the downregulation of two interferon-γ–inducible proteasomal components, called *LMP2* and *LMP7*, in certain human tumors (32). The proteasome is a large multicatalytic complex involved in the degradation of many of the peptides that later find their way into the MHC class I pathway.

Not All Tumor-Associated Antigens Are Suitable Targets for Vaccine Development

How does one go about choosing an antigen appropriate for use in the design of a cancer vaccine? Some workers have picked target antigens because they are frequently mutated in tumors, as in the case of p53 (38) or Ras (39–42), at the site of joining a translocation, such as bcr-abl (43), or are aberrantly glycosylated and thus the subject of recognition by antibodies, as is the case for MUC1 (44–46) and carcinoembryonic antigen (47,48).

What Fraction of Potential Tumor Antigens Can Actually Be Found on the Tumor Cell Surface?

A simple estimate of the number of possible epitopes in expressed proteins to the number of expressed MHC molecules clearly reveals that only a fraction of all antigenic peptides are presented by MHC on the cell surface. Estimates place the total number of MHC/peptide complexes on the cell surface at between 10^5 and 10^6 molecules per cell (49). T lymphocytes, however, may be able to recognize a single peptide on the surface of a target cell (50–52). Nevertheless, many of these MHC/peptide complexes presented on the cell surface are redundant, and some "self," particularly stable, complexes may be present in quantities of hundreds or even thousands of copies per cell (53,54), making the total number of different complexes significantly lower than the total number of MHC class I molecules per cell. Consequently, a tumor with excellent MHC expression and antigen-processing capacity is likely to express a maximum of approximately 10,000 different MHC/peptide complexes on its surface.

On the other side of the ledger, how many possible tumor-derived antigenic peptides are expressed by a tumor? An individual tumor cell may express approximately 20,000 of an estimated 100,000 genes in the genome. Each encoded protein contains dozens of epitopes that could bind to any given

MHC molecule. For example, a total of ten different epitopes derived from the 661 amino acid–long gp100 molecule have been shown to be presented by the HLA-A*0201 molecule. These ten were chosen, however, from a list of actual binders that exceeded 50 different potential binders in the primary open reading frame of the molecule. Peptides derived from alternative open reading frames can also load MHC molecules, further increasing the number of potential epitopes encoded by the tumor genome (55,56).

A conservative estimate of the total number of peptides that are actually able to bind to any given MHC molecule may thus be greater than a million. Furthermore, each MHC molecule is codominantly expressed, so a tumor may express six different "classical" MHC class I molecules. Thus, using conservative estimates, millions of potential binders exist competing for tens of thousands of MHC molecules.

It is then clear that not every peptide that can be generated is presented in an MHC class I–restricted fashion. Peptides can be created or destroyed by a large number of specificities in the proteolytic machinery. Furthermore, after their creation, peptides must traffic to the appropriate compartment for binding to MHC class I (the endoplasmic reticulum) or class II (the compartment for peptide loading).

Based on the numbers presented above, we estimate that the chances that any given peptide will be presented on the tumor cell surface are approximately 1%, although this number is an estimate. Because not every good MHC-binding tumor-derived peptide is actually presented on the tumor cell surface, it is possible to make a CTL that can kill peptide-pulsed targets but not actual tumors (43,57).

Identifying Tumor Antigens Recognized by T Lymphocytes

The molecular identification of the antigens present on cancers that are recognized by the immune system is central to the development of recombinant and synthetic vaccines. Because of the difficulty in predicting what peptides are present on the cell surface, one of the most successful approaches to identifying tumor-associated antigens suitable for the development of cancer vaccines starts with the antitumor immune response. The specificity of this response is then used to identify tumor-associated antigens (58). One approach has been to start the cloning process using T cells with antitumor reactivity to screen complementary DNA libraries made from melanoma cell lines. In many cases, the antitumor T cells were derived from cultures of tumor-infiltrating lymphocytes that had been adoptively transferred to patients with cancer. Our group focused on the T-cell reactivities that were associated with objective regressions of metastatic melanoma lesions after their adoptive transfer (59).

Complementary DNA libraries of expressed melanoma genes were screened by transfecting these genes along with the gene for the restricting MHC molecule into an antigen-negative cell line, which is then admixed with T lymphocytes that have antitumor activity. If the T cells recognize the transfected cell line, they lyse it and release cytokines, such as granulocyte-macrophage colony-stimulating factor, tumor necrosis factor–α, and interferon-γ, any of which can be measured. The process of cloning genes encoding tumor antigens is under constant improvement and has become considerably faster and more streamlined (60–62).

Targeting "Self" Antigens

Many of the tumor antigens that have been identified are tissue differentiation antigens in melanocytes and include gp100 (63–69), MART-1/MelanA (70–74), tyrosinase (65,75–78), and tyrosinase-related protein-1/gp75 (79) and -2 (62,80,81). These antigens are involved in the synthesis of melanin and give melanocytes and deposits of melanoma tumor their dark pigment.

The fact that differentiation antigens are nonmutated in most tumors has two important implications. First, expression of these tissue differentiation enzymes are shared by the great majority of melanoma nodules from the great majority of patients, and thus an "off-the-shelf" vaccine strategy targeting these antigens is possible (a strategy that targets a mutated antigen may have to be individualized for every mutation). Second, the nonmutated nature of these antigens suggests that immunotherapies that target these antigens could elicit autoreactivity. One consequence of this "autoreactivity" may be vitiligo, the patchy and permanent loss of pigment from the skin and hair thought to result from the autoimmune destruction of pigment cells. Vitiligo has been correlated with objective shrinkage of deposits of metastatic melanoma in patients receiving high-dose IL-2, a cytokine known to activate and expand T lymphocytes (2,82).

Thus, evidence exists that vitiligo can be coupled with tumor regression, and that adoptive transfer of antitumor T cells recognizing differentiation antigens is associated with objective shrinkage of melanoma deposits. Although the focus of this review is on melanocyte differentiation antigens, two other groups of antigens should be mentioned. Those in the first category are expressed by a diversity of tumor histologies, but are not expressed by normal tissues (other than testis). Cloned in large part by Boon and colleagues, these antigens are encoded by genes with family names like *MAGE, BAGE, GAGE, RAGE,* and *LAGE* (83–85). *NY-ESO-1* also falls into this group and is expressed in a significant proportion of human melanoma cells, as well as other tumor histologies, including breast, ovary, bladder, prostate, and liver (60,86–89).

Are Mutated Tumor Antigens Better Targets for Immune Recognition?

Tumor protection experiments using experimental animals have shown that protective responses are generally tumor specific, leading to the conclusion that, at least in mice, tumor rejection antigens are often unique (90). These antigens are thought to be the result of mutations in the genome. Human tumors also express mutated antigens that can be processed and presented for recognition by T cells. Neoantigens produced as a result of mutation often are found to originate in ubiquitously expressed proteins. Examples include epitopes from beta-catenin (91), CDK4 (92), MUM1 (93), FLICE (caspase-8) (94), HLA-A2 (95) and, most recently, a mutant gene from a bladder carcinoma that is recorded in databases under the name *KIAA0205*, whose function is unknown

(94,96). Some of these antigens are also oncogenic, including the mutations described for beta-catenin and CDK4.

Mutated antigens may not lend themselves easily to off-the-shelf vaccines consisting of purely recombinant and synthetic components because each neoantigen for each patient must be checked for sequence, and that sequence must be verified to be present on the surface of a tumor cell. Some workers, however, have asserted that mutated tumor antigens are superior targets for vaccine design because immune cells are not tolerated to these antigens (97). Recent work, especially by Levitsky's and Sherman's groups, has shown that even the most immunogenic "foreign" antigen, such as the hemagglutinin antigen from the influenza A virus, can be tolerating when expressed peripherally (i.e., outside the thymus) in normal cells (98) or in tumor cells (15). Thus, mutated or otherwise "foreign" antigens may also induce peripheral tolerance when expressed by tumor cells.

Immunizations Most Effective in Generating Reactive T Cells Are the Most Therapeutically Effective

The principle that T cells were critically important in the immune response was derived originally in mice with methylcholanthrene-induced tumors. A large body of work in which T-cell subsets were depleted using antibodies or gene knockout mice revealed that CD8$^+$ and CD4$^+$ T cells could play a role in the antitumor immune response.

Role of CD8$^+$ T Cytotoxic Cells in Antitumor Immunity

It has long been known that elements of the cellular immune response are capable of specifically recognizing and destroying tumor cells. Classic studies showed that mice immunized with irradiated methylcholanthrene-induced sarcoma cells were fully protected against a subsequent challenge with that same tumor, but not with other tumors (99). This protection was dependent on CD8$^+$ T lymphocytes, whereas CD4$^+$ T lymphocytes often played little if any role. Furthermore, adoptive transfer of pure populations of CD8$^+$ T lymphocytes was shown to mediate tumor regression in mice (100–102). Thus, many efforts to develop therapeutic anticancer vaccines have focused on CD8$^+$ T lymphocytes, and the molecular targets of these cells have been identified in human and mouse systems (1,103).

"Mini-gene" constructs have been created to favor immune responses against the heterologously inserted target antigen. These viruses are constructed to encode immunodominant epitopes (i.e., the fragments of antigens that are presented by MHC molecules) from cancer antigens alone or in combination with endoplasmic reticulum insertion signal sequences that can bypass the TAP transporters, in some cases profoundly enhancing the function of virus-based vaccines in animal models (17,104,105).

The use of synthetic peptide vaccines that have been altered to increase their ability to bind MHC class I molecules is a promising new avenue to augment CD8$^+$ T-cell function. Crystal structures of peptide MHC complexes, together with mass sequencing of peptides eluted from class I molecules, have revealed that peptides bind to their restricting class I molecules in large part by "anchor" residues. These residues can be modified to increase the peptide-MHC interaction without compromising the interaction of this complex with the T-cell receptor (106,107).

Role of CD4⁺ T "Helper" Cells in Antitumor Immunity

Compared with the comprehensive studies using CD8⁺ T cells in tumor models, relatively little is known about how CD4⁺ T cells influence antitumor immunity. Early work demonstrated that disseminated murine leukemia could be eradicated by a combination of cyclophosphamide and adoptively transferred cells, then known as *Lyt1⁺2⁻ cells*, a phenotype later shown to be L3T4⁺, Lyt2⁻ cells, now designated *CD4⁺ T cells* (108,109). The most dramatic examples of the power of CD4⁺ T cells in the immune response to "self" proteins can be found in murine models of autoimmune diseases, such as experimental allergic encephalomyelitis, systemic lupus erythematosus, and diabetes. In these models, disease can often be transferred to naïve mice with purified, "self" reactive CD4⁺ splenocytes or specific CD4⁺ T lymphocyte clones (110–115). These studies and others suggest that the full activation of autoreactive CD4⁺ T cells may be a key element missing from many current clinical cancer vaccine trials.

We understand how CD4⁺ T lymphocytes help initiate and maintain the antitumor immune response (116,117). CD4⁺ T cells regulate antigen-specific immune responses by regulating the functions of other components of the immune system, including B lymphocytes and CD8⁺ T lymphocytes (118,119). Conversely, CD4⁺ T cells can be preferentially activated by B cells under some conditions (120). In the experimental B16 tumor system, B lymphocytes, under the control of CD4⁺ T cells, play an important role in inducing autoimmunity and antitumor immunity (121–126). CD4⁺ T lymphocytes also appear to attract and activate other non–antigen-specific components of the immune system, including eosinophils and macrophages (127).

CD4⁺ T cells have recently been shown to alter the function of DCs, as well as other APCs (128,129). This activation occurs, in part, through the interaction of CD40 on the APC surface with its ligand (gp39), which is expressed on the surfaces of activated CD4⁺ T cells (129,130). Engagement of CD40 prompts the APC to secrete proinflammatory cytokines, such as interferon-γ and IL-2, and attract a host of other cells to the site of immune reactivity (128,129).

One potentially important experimental thrust in the use of adoptively transferred T cells may be the intentional addition of "helper" CD4⁺ T cells to adoptively transferred CD8⁺ T cells. In studies using T cells specific for cytomegalovirus, Greenberg and his colleagues have reported that the cytotoxic activity of adoptively transferred CD8⁺ clones declined in patients deficient in helper CD4⁺ T cells specific for cytomegalovirus (131). These results suggested that CD4⁺ T-cell function is needed for the persistence of transferred CD8⁺ T cells. Attempts to identify the molecular targets of antitumor CD4⁺ T cells have already been successful (132–137). Thus, work focuses on efforts to harness the potential capabilities of antitumor CD4⁺ T cells.

Dendritic Cells Mediate Vaccine Function

The initiation of T-cell immunity is largely the result of a specialized subset of APCs, called *dendritic cells* (138,139). DCs activate T-cell responses because they are able to capture, process, and present antigens in the context of MHC molecules to T lymphocytes. Signaling through the interaction of T-cell receptor and peptide/MHC, however, is insufficient to activate a T cell. In this light, DCs also have another more specialized function: they are capable of costimulating T cells. The importance of costimulation comes from understanding the "two signal" hypothesis of T-cell activation, first proposed by Bretscher and Cohn (140). Although the first signal delivered through the T-cell receptor is necessary, it is not sufficient to activate the T cell. It is known that T cells receive a large number of second signals through the interaction of what are generally integral membrane glycoproteins on the surfaces of T cells and APCs (141). These signals are mediated through the interactions of intracellular adhesion molecules and through the lymphocyte function–associated antigens.

The interaction of the B7 molecules B7.1 (CD80) and B7.2 (CD86) with their ligands on the surface of T cells, known as *CD28* and *CTLA4*, are critical to the provision of a "second signal" (142,143). Whether B7 family molecules trigger the activation or inhibition is dependent on their interaction with molecules on the T cell: engagement of CD28 is associated with proliferation and differentiation, whereas an encounter with CTLA-4 may trigger functional unresponsiveness (144,145). Blocking CTLA-4 engagement has been reported to enhance immune responses to tumor cells (146). Activating T cells by DCs is thus accomplished by presenting antigen/MHC complexes in the context of a variety of other activating signals.

Optimizing Vaccine Function in Dendritic Cells

One line of evidence illustrating the importance of DC in anticancer vaccines comes from studies using recombinant viral vectors encoding tumor-associated antigens. Poxvirus-based immunogens are one class of candidate vectors that has been explored extensively. Poxvirus-specific promoters placed upstream of a heterologous sequence can determine the timing and quantity of antigen production. In a mouse model system, we explored the capacity of recombinant vaccinia virus promoters to mediate tumor regression and the elicitation of T cell responses (147). The recombinant poxviruses mediating the highest expression of β-gal under the control of an "early" promoter (i.e., a promoter operating before viral DNA replication) expressed approximately 30-fold less β-gal than the best construct using a "late" promotor (i.e., active after viral DNA replication in permissive tissue culture cells). Only the recombinant vaccinia virus using early promoters prolonged the survival of mice bearing established tumor expressing the model antigen, β-gal. When a variety of cells were infected with the panel of viruses *in vitro*, DCs were found to express β-gal only under the control of the early promoters. Moreover, in a functional assay, DCs infected *in vitro* with recombinants using late promoters did not activate β-gal–specific CTLs, whereas the CTL responses were powerful and specific when early promoters were used. These data suggested that promoter strength was not the most critical quality of a recombinant poxvirus-based vaccine. Rather, the success of recombinant poxviruses in the immunotherapy of established cancer may require the use of early promoters capable of driving the production of the heterologous protein in infected DCs and other "professional" APCs.

In another study using cutaneous DNA bombardment (the so-called gene-gun), substantial expression of an encoded model antigen was found in the epidermal layer (148). In addition, a low but detectable level of expression was also found in DCs and in draining lymph nodes. Under these conditions, it was clear that two possible modes of DC antigen presentation to naive CD8$^+$ T cells might exist: (a) presentation directly by gene-transfected DC trafficking to local lymph nodes, and (b) cross-presentation by untransfected DCs of antigen released from or associated with transfected epidermal cells. When the relative contributions of these distinct modes of antigen presentation to priming of CD8$^+$ T cells was evaluated, however, the predominant pathway for T-cell activation was the presentation of directly transfected DCs, indicating that augmenting direct DC gene expression may enhance the function of gene-gun–based DNA-based immunization (148).

Vaccine Efficacy May Depend on the "Super-Activation" of Dendritic Cells

DCs can undergo maturation or "super activation" through the activity of tumor necrosis factor–α and other macrophage-derived cytokines, as well as through the engagement of CD40 by CD40L on the surfaces of activated T cells. On activation, DCs can effectively activate naïve T cells. Other key noncytokine immunomodulators include molecules vital to costimulation. One of these, CD40 and its ligand, which, like other members of the tumor necrosis factor family, naturally forms homotrimers, has been shown to be important in B-cell activation, the production of type 1 cytokines by T helper cells, and the generation of cytotoxic memory responses. We and others have found that the addition of CD40L trimer to DNA vaccination can significantly increase antitumor efficacy (149). Another molecule, called *FLT3 ligand*, can induce the apparent growth and differentiation of functional DCs and has been reported to have antitumor effects (150,151). The role, if any, of FLT 3 ligand in the augmentation of the function of recombinant and synthetic anticancer vaccines is the subject of a great deal of investigation in experimental mouse models.

Vaccination Can Be Enhanced with Cytokines, Chemokines, and Costimulatory Molecules

A number of immunomodulatory molecules can augment immunization. One group of these molecules, called *cytokines*, are substances that generally act locally on immune cells and usually have a limited half-life in circulation. Cytokines can be produced by and have activity on cells outside of those with specialized immune function cells. These effects may blur the distinction between cytokines and other classes of soluble intercellular signals, such as hormones and growth factors.

The ILs are a subset of cytokines that are produced by leukocytes and have activity on leukocytes, although they have direct and indirect effects on a wide range of cells. Cytokines and, in particular, the ILs, have powerful effects on the activation and proliferation of T cells. Cytokines that are chemoattractant are called *chemokines*. Chemokines induce the activation and directional migration in a variety of immune cells (152–158). Chemokines are produced locally in the tissues, often as a result of the presence of pathogens, and act on leukocytes through a family of at least a dozen receptors. They function as regulatory molecules in leukocyte maturation, traffic and homing of lymphocytes, and the development of lymphoid tissues.

Cytokines, Chemokines, and Costimulatory Molecules as Molecularly Defined Adjuvants

From the vaccinologist's point of view, cytokines, chemokines, and costimulatory molecules can be used as molecularly defined adjuvants, significantly improving vaccine-induced immune responses. They can be administered systemically as protein or their genes can be inserted into recombinant vaccines (159–162). Mouse models have been used to evaluate large panels of molecularly defined adjuvant antitumor activity elicited by a vaccine. We have found that gene-gun delivery of a model antigen was protective by itself but was only therapeutic when codelivered with IL-2, IL-6, IL-7, or, especially, IL-12 (160). Other useful cytokine adjuvants include granulocyte-macrophage colony-stimulating factor, a cytokine thought to play an important role in the recruitment and maturation of DCs (163–165). Studies using vaccinia virus–based immunogens have revealed that IL-2 and IL-12 (151–161) are extremely potent in their ability to increase the efficacy of cancer vaccines. In addition, the costimulatory molecules B7-1, B7-2, and CD40L also have a beneficial effect on vaccination (149,161,162,166).

Importantly, not all of the findings in murine models were confirmed in human clinical trials. When patients with metastatic melanoma were immunized with a modified immunodominant peptide derived from gp100, no increase in efficacy as measured by objective clinical response was observed using granulocyte-macrophage colony-stimulating factor or IL-12. Only IL-2 was found to have a beneficial effect as an adjuvant for peptide immunization.

Bacterial DNA sequences, called *immunostimulatory sequences*, have been reported to be potent adjuvants. Nonmethylated palindromic DNA sequences containing CpG-oligodinucleotides can activate an "innate" immune response by activating monocytes, natural killer cells, DCs, and B cells in an antigen-independent manner (167–170). Indeed, methylation of the CpG-oligodinucleotides reportedly abrogates the immunogenicity of the DNA vaccine. Thus, the use of large amounts of plasmid for immunization may not only overcome the low transfection efficiency *in vivo*, but may also serve as an adjuvant driving a Th1-response (171,172).

Not All Immunogens Are Created Equal

Early attempts at developing cancer vaccines were based on the use of tumor cells that were irradiated; admixed with a number of adjuvants, including *Corynebacterium parvum* and bacille Calmette-Guérin; or infected with viruses to create "oncolysates." Since the 1990s, tumor cells have been gene-modified in an attempt to turn them into effective vaccines. Because cancer cells are notoriously poor immunogens, workers in a number of laboratories have attempted to remove tumor antigens from the tumor microenvironment with strategies, such as purifying heat shock proteins, which are thought to bind precursors of peptides destined for the MHC complex (173,174). Others have acid-eluted peptides to pulse them onto DCs (175,176). Yet another approach is transfecting DCs with tumor-derived RNA (177).

The use of recombinant and synthetic vaccines is predicated on the identification of tumor-associated antigens. A large number of recombinant vectors are available. A partial list of recombinant viral immunogens includes vaccinia, fowlpox, canarypox, adenovirus, influenza, polio, and Sindbis (178). Recombinant organisms include *Listeria, Salmonella,* and bacille Calmette-Guérin (179,180). In addition, "naked" nucleic acid–based vectors include the administration of DNA by intramuscular or intradermal injection or by gene-gun and, most recently, the administration of "self-replicating" nucleic acid–based immunogens (160,181).

Recombinant Virus-Based Vaccines

Recombinant virus-based cancer vaccines are created by inserting genes encoding tumor antigens into the viral genome. The safety of these recombinant viruses, always of paramount importance, can be insured in a number of ways. For example, some of the recombinant vaccines are comprised of viruses incapable of replicating in mammalian cells because of their host range (e.g., the avian poxviruses) (16), whereas others are highly attenuated (like certain influenza A viruses) (182) or the Wyeth and modified vaccinia virus Ankara strains of vaccinia virus (183), and still others are made safe by the removal of viral genes that are critical to viral replication and virulence, such as adenoviruses (184).

Vaccines based on live, attenuated, or killed viruses can be highly effective in preventing human viral diseases, such as polio, smallpox, and even influenza A. Recombinant viruses encoding tumor antigens, however, have an important shortcoming that is not shared by the viral vaccines from which they derive. Any immune response elicited by a viral vaccine is, at least potentially, virus-specific, and thus relevant to the immune response against the viral challenge. This is not the case for cancer vaccines where the only component of the immune response that can be tumor specific is the response elicited by the expression of the transgene(s) encoding the tumor antigen(s). Although viral elements might help boost immune reactivity through their activity as helper epitopes, they do not contribute any specificity of immune reactivity for tumors. The only exception to this generalization would be if a recombinant virus-based immunogen were used to vaccinate against a virally induced cancer (e.g., the use of recombinant human papillomavirus to treat cervical cancer).

Problem of Preexisting Immunity to Viral Immunogens

Although viral vaccines are potent inducers of antitumor immunity in animal models, the obstacle of preexisting immunity

remains an important problem in the translation of these strategies to the clinic. We have learned in the conduct of our own clinical trials that humans have high neutralizing titers to recombinant viral vaccines based on adenoviruses (185). These antibodies are likely owing to the ubiquitous environmental presence of adenoviruses and heterotypic immunity resulting from pandemic adenoviral infection, especially in children and in military recruits (186–188). Adenoviruses frequently are the causes of respiratory illness, conjunctivitis, and gastroenteritis (189,190). Our patients almost uniformly have been exposed to adenovirus because of its ubiquitous presence in the environment in each of our upper respiratory systems (185).

Vaccinia virus was widely used in the campaign to eradicate smallpox (191–193). Thus, anyone born in the United States before approximately 1970 (the majority of patients who currently have cancer) have already been immunized to vaccinia (194,195). Elsewhere in the world, immunization with vaccinia was continued well after the early 1970s (196). Indeed, most patients appear to be able to rapidly clear these viruses, making it difficult or impossible to effectively use cancer vaccines based on these viruses. One way of circumventing the problem of preexisting immunity is the use of viruses whose natural hosts are nonmammalian, such as the avian poxviruses (16).

Recombinant Vaccines Based on "Naked" Nucleic Acid

Reports dating from the early 1990s indicated the finding that the intramuscular injection of "naked" plasmid DNA (i.e., DNA without a viral coat) could result in an immune response (197). Like viral vaccines, the activity of DNA vaccines appears to be mediated through DCs and other "professional" APCs. Clear evidence exists for a predominant role for directly transfected DCs in antigen presentation to CD8$^+$ T cells after nucleic acid immunization (148).

In contrast to vaccines that use recombinant bacteria or viruses, naked nucleic acid vaccines consist only of DNA or RNA, which is taken up by cells and translated into protein. In case of gene-gun delivery, nucleic acid is precipitated onto an inert particle (generally gold beads) and forced into the cells with a helium blast. Transfected cells then express the antigen encoded on the plasmid, resulting in an immune response. Like live or attenuated viruses, DNA vaccines effectively engage MHC class I and II pathways, allowing for the induction of CD8$^+$ and CD4$^+$ T cells, whereas antigen present in soluble form, such as recombinant protein, generally induces only antibody responses.

DNA-based vaccines are relatively safe and easy to engineer and produce. In animal models, they are generally not as potent as recombinant viruses at eliciting immune responses capable of destroying tumors. Significant effort has been exerted to improve the efficacy of DNA vaccines. Important innovations in the design of these vectors include promoter optimization, enhancement of polyadenylation sequences, the removal of 5' and 3' untranslated regions from the inserted gene, and the use of intronic sequences to improve nuclear export.

Clinical trials using naked DNA vaccines encoding tumor antigens have begun. One of the first of these trials was launched in 1999 at the Surgery Branch, National Cancer Insti tute. It uses a plasmid encoding a modified form of the human gp100 melanoma antigen first alone, then in combination with IL-2, previously shown in murine study to enhance vaccination with plasmid (160).

Naked nucleic acid vaccines are potentially useful candidates as therapeutic vaccines for patients with cancer, but their clinical efficacy has not been demonstrated. One promising approach to the development of nucleic acid vaccines may be strategies designed to make them "self-replicating." Self-replication can be accomplished by using a gene encoding an RNA replicase polyprotein derived from alphaviruses, a family of viruses that includes Semliki Forest virus, Sindbis virus, and the Venezuelan equine encephalomyelitis virus. A gene encoding a tumor antigen can be added to such a construct under the control of viral promoter. Such constructs can elicit antigen-specific antibody and CD8$^+$ T-cell responses at doses as low as 0.1 µg (198). Although the self-replicating vectors do not mediate the production of substantially more model antigens than a conventional vaccine, the enhanced efficacy of the vector may be owing to its ability to induce caspase-dependent apoptotic death in transfected cells. Such death has been shown to facilitate the uptake of apoptotic cells by DCs, providing a potential mechanism for enhanced immunogenicity.

Synthetic Peptide Vaccines

Knowledge of the amino acid sequences of the epitopes presented by MHC molecules on the surfaces of tumor cells can be used to generate synthetic peptide immunogens for use as vaccines. When admixed with adjuvant, these peptide immunogens have been shown to enhance antitumor T-cell responses in cancer patients. A variety of adjuvants can be used, including oil-in-water–based adjuvants, like incomplete Freund's adjuvant, saponin-based adjuvants like QS-21, and others, like the monophosphoryl lipid A and trehalose dimycolate adjuvant system (199–205).

In a 1996 study, we used a synthetic peptide immunogen corresponding to an epitope from the gp100 melanoma antigen. When the second amino acid from the amino terminus was modified from a threonine to a methionine to create a peptide called *g209-2M*, binding to the HLA-A*0201 molecule could be increased ninefold in an *in vitro* competitive binding assay (106). *In vivo*, 91% of patients vaccinated with this peptide were successfully immunized on the basis of immunologic assays. Perhaps more important, when the T-cell growth and differentiation cytokine, IL-2, is added to the treatment regimen, 13 of 31 patients (42%) who were given IL-2 had objective clinical responses, and four additional patients had mixed or minor responses (see Table 2) (3). These results compare favorably and are significantly different than results from clinical trials using high-dose IL-2 alone where objective response rates generally fall between 15% and 17%.

Future directions in the development of synthetic peptide vaccines may include the use of modified peptides embedded into microspheres, a maneuver that can target antigen for uptake and MHC class I–restricted presentation by professional APCs. Other promising novel strategies developed in experimental animal systems use toxin-linked peptides

(206,207) and peptides linked to endoplasmic reticulum insertion signal sequences covalently attached to the amino terminus of a peptide immunogen (208). The enhanced hydrophobicity of the resultant peptide may be responsible for its increased immunogenicity, but the mechanism of action is not fully understood.

Optimal Dose, Boosting, and Route of the Immunization Is Determined by Basic Immunologic Principles

The immunotherapist faces a number of bewildering choices when administering an anticancer vaccine. In addition to the issues already described (choice of antigen, immunogen, and adjuvant), a number of additional questions immediately present themselves. What is the appropriate dose of the immunogen? What route is most effective? Is a boosting of the immune response required and, if so, how many times and at what intervals? Should the vaccine be administered monthly, weekly, or daily? Answering these questions requires an understanding of the immunophysiology of vaccination *in vivo*. *In vitro* work with human cells is of limited benefit, whereas work in human subjects must necessarily be limited in its scope. Too many questions exist that must be answered in what are ultimately a limited number of clinical trials, each of which is based on a relatively small number of patients. Thus, in practice, questions regarding dose, route, and boosting are generally addressed in mouse models.

Evidence from animal models suggests that increasing the dose of immunogen beyond certain limits can hinder, or even abrogate, an immune response against that antigen. This has been shown to be the case after infection with high doses of a virus called *lymphocytic choriomeningitis virus*, as well as after administration of large amounts of peptide antigen (209–212). On the other hand, this observation may not be generalizable to all viruses or all immunogens based on synthetic peptide immunogens. For example, in early clinical studies using patients with melanoma, a similar state of immune unresponsiveness has not been observed at immunizing doses as high as 10 mg (213). It may be difficult to administer doses of viruses or peptides to humans that are equivalent to the large doses given to mice.

Based on the idea that more antigen is better, most viral and DNA vaccines are geared towards maximum expression and use the strongest available promoters. In our own preclinical trials using immunogens based on vaccinia viruses, as well as DNA given by blasts with the gene-gun, efficacy improves as the dose of immunogen increases (104,160).

It has long been known that boosting an immune response can increase its intensity. We now understand, however, that the efficacy of synthetic and recombinant anticancer vaccines can be enhanced with prime/boost regimens that use two different vectors. When primary and booster treatment regimens using a single vector (i.e., homologous boosting) are compared with regimens that used two different vectors (i.e., heterologous boosting), the heterologous boosting regimens generally result in significantly more potent antigen-specific CTL responses than are seen in animals who receive homologous boosting (214,215).

Using the optimal route of administration of any given immunogen can significantly improve the efficacy of an immunization strategy. Indeed, the administration of a synthetic peptide immunogen by the intraperitoneal route can lead to toleration, whereas administration of the same peptide immunogen subcutaneously leads to activation (210). For poxviral vectors, the intravenous route of immunization is optimal in mice (216). For any given immunogen, we surmise that the optimal route of immunization is likely to be dictated by the route that leads to the presence of the antigen on the maximal number of activated DCs, perhaps with the least amount of antigen presentation by normal, immunologically quiescent cells.

CONCLUSION

In this chapter, we have attempted to describe the basic immunologic principles that may be useful in the design of anticancer vaccines. These principles are derived in large part from a deeper understanding of immune function that has resulted from a "reductionistic" approach characterized by understanding the interactions between the immune system and tumor cells on a molecular level (217). We have described the weak immunogenicity of human tumors, perhaps owing to their lack of expression of important immune activating signals *in vivo*. Specifically, tumors may lack expression of appropriate costimulatory molecules, tumor antigens, and MHC molecules, and they may directly suppress immune function through the expression of suppressive molecules, such as transforming growth factor–β and IL-10.

Nevertheless, tumor-associated antigens can be identified, making possible the design of recombinant and synthetic vaccines for cancer. Potential targets include the products of mutations in tumor cells, as well as normal (nonmutated) differentiation antigens. To achieve direct recognition of the tumor cell, target antigen must be presented on the tumor cell surface. Work with these antigens in animal models and preliminarily in human clinical trials has shown that immunizations that are most effective in generating reactive T cells are the most therapeutically effective. T lymphocytes provide the specificity of recognition of the cellular immune response. Independent and collaborative roles for the CD8+ and CD4+ T-cell subsets are being elucidated. The activation of T cells by cancer vaccines is likely to be effected largely by DCs. Thus, the function of promoters for recombinant vaccines must be optimized in these "professional" APCs. Further adjuvants might best be designed to "super-activate" DCs.

A variety of immunogens can be used as cancer vaccines, including physically altered or gene-modified tumor cells. In the case of recombinant and synthetic vaccines, a number of different classes of immunogens are available, including peptides and proteins, naked nucleic acids, and recombinant viruses or organisms. The immunotherapist can add cytokines, chemokines, and costimulatory molecules to a vaccination to enhance its efficacy. To get the best response from a cancer vaccine, considerable evidence exists that more antigen is usually better, although some evidence exists to the contrary. The vaccine should be administered by a route that places it in contact with a maximal number of DCs, and heterologous boosting is usually better than homologous boosting. Finally, it is likely that mutable tumor cells are capable of altering their phenotype in a way that can result in their escape from immune recognition, but it is also abundantly clear that the immune system can recognize and destroy even large deposits of solid tumors in patients with cancer.

REFERENCES

1. Restifo NP, Rosenberg SA. Developing recombinant and synthetic vaccines for the treatment of melanoma. *Curr Opin Oncol* 1999;11:50.
2. Rosenberg SA. Keynote address: perspectives on the use of interleukin-2 in cancer treatment. *Cancer J Sci Am* 1997;3[Suppl 1]:S2–S6.
3. Rosenberg SA, Yang JC, Schwartzentruber DJ, et al. Immunologic and therapeutic evaluation of a synthetic peptide vaccine for the treatment of patients with metastatic melanoma. *Nat Med* 1998;4:321.
4. Nestle FO, Alijagic S, Gilliet M, et al. Vaccination of melanoma patients with peptide- or tumor lysate-pulsed dendritic cells. *Nat Med* 1998;4:328.
5. Jaeger E, Bernhard H, Romero P, et al. Generation of cytotoxic T-cell responses with synthetic melanoma-associated peptides *in vivo*: implications for tumor vaccines with melanoma-associated antigens. *Int J Cancer* 1996;66:162.
6. Lowy DR, Schiller JT. Papillomaviruses: prophylactic vaccine prospects. *Biochim Biophys Acta* 1999;1423:M1.
7. Lowy DR, Schiller JT. Papillomaviruses and cervical cancer: pathogenesis and vaccine development. *J Natl Cancer Inst Monogr* 1998;23:27–30.
8. Kageshita T, Kawakami Y, Hirai S, Ono T. Differential expression of MART-1 in primary and metastatic melanoma lesions. *J Immunother* 1997;20:460.
9. Liebowitz DN, Lee KP, June CH. Costimulatory approaches to adoptive immunotherapy. *Curr Opin Oncol* 1998;10:533.
10. La Motte RN, Sharpe AH, Bluestone JA, Mokyr MB. Importance of B7-1-expressing host antigen-presenting cells for the eradication of B7-2 transfected P815 tumor cells. *J Immunol* 1998;161:6552.
11. Chen L, McGowan P, Ashe S, et al. Tumor immunogenicity determines the effect of B7 costimulation on T cell-mediated tumor immunity. *J Exp Med* 1994;179:523.
12. Fuchs EJ, Matzinger P. Is cancer dangerous to the immune system? *Semin Immunol* 1996;8:271.
13. Matzinger P. An innate sense of danger. *Semin Immunol* 1998; 10:399.
14. Matzinger P. Tolerance, danger, and the extended family. *Annu Rev Immunol* 1994;12:991–1045.
15. Staveley-O'Carroll K, Sotomayor E, Montgomery J, et al. Induction of antigen-specific T cell anergy: an early event in the course of tumor progression. *Proc Natl Acad Sci U S A* 1998;95:1178.
16. Wang M, Bronte V, Chen PW, et al. Active immunotherapy of cancer with a nonreplicating recombinant fowlpox virus encoding a model tumor-associated antigen. *J Immunol* 1995;154:4685.
17. McCabe BJ, Irvine KR, Nishimura MI, et al. Minimal determinant expressed by a recombinant vaccinia virus elicits therapeutic antitumor cytolytic T lymphocyte responses. *Cancer Res* 1995;55:1741.
18. Ochsenbein AF, Klenerman P, Karrer U, et al. Immune surveillance against a solid tumor fails because of immunological ignorance. *Proc Natl Acad Sci U S A* 1999;96:2233.
19. Chen L. Overcoming T cell ignorance by providing costimulation. Implications for the immune response against cancer. *Adv Exp Med Biol* 1998;451:159–165.
20. Chen L. Immunological ignorance of silent antigens as an explanation of tumor evasion. *Immunol Today* 1998;19:27.

21. Melero I, Bach N, Chen L. Costimulation, tolerance and ignorance of cytolytic T lymphocytes in immune responses to tumor antigens. *Life Sci* 1997;60:2035.

22. Stearns ME, Garcia FU, Fudge K, Rhim J, Wang M. Role of interleukin-10 and transforming growth factor beta1 in the angiogenesis and metastasis of human prostate primary tumor lines from orthotopic implants in severe combined immunodeficiency mice. *Clin Cancer Res* 1999;5:711.

23. Shim KS, Kim KH, Han WS, Park EB. Elevated serum levels of transforming growth factor-beta1 in patients with colorectal carcinoma: its association with tumor progression and its significant decrease after curative surgical resection. *Cancer* 1999;85:554.

24. Lahn M, Fisch P, Kohler G, et al. Pro-inflammatory and T cell inhibitory cytokines are secreted at high levels in tumor cell cultures of human renal cell carcinoma. *Eur Urol* 1999;35:70.

25. Kim IY, Ahn HJ, Zelner DJ, et al. Loss of expression of transforming growth factor beta type I and type II receptors correlates with tumor grade in human prostate cancer tissues. *Clin Cancer Res* 1996;2:1255.

26. Hahne M, Rimoldi D, Schroter M, et al. Melanoma cell expression of Fas(Apo-1/CD95) ligand: implications for tumor immune escape. *Science* 1996;274:1363.

27. Chappell DB, Restifo NP. T cell-tumor cell: a fatal interaction? *Cancer Immunol Immunother* 1998;47:65.

28. Chappell DB. Human melanoma cells do not express Fas (Apo-1/CD95) ligand. *Cancer Res* 1999;59:59.

29. Zaks TZ, Chappell DB, Rosenberg SA, Restifo NP. Fas-mediated suicide of tumor-reactive T cells following activation by specific tumor: selective rescue by caspase inhibition. *J Immunol* 1999;162:3273.

30. Cormier JN, Hijazi YM, Abati A, et al. Heterogeneous expression of melanoma-associated antigens and HLA-A2 in metastatic melanoma *in vivo*. *Int J Cancer* 1998;75:517.

31. Cormier JN, Abati A, Fetsch P, et al. Comparative analysis of the *in vivo* expression of tyrosinase, MART-1/Melan-A, and gp100 in metastatic melanoma lesions: implications for immunotherapy. *J Immunother* 1998;21:27.

32. Restifo NP, Esquivel F, Kawakami Y, et al. Identification of human cancers deficient in antigen processing. *J Exp Med* 1993;177:265.

33. Restifo NP, Kawakami Y, Marincola F, et al. Molecular mechanisms used by tumors to escape immune recognition: immunogenetherapy and the cell biology of major histocompatibility complex class I. *J Immunother* 1993;14:182.

34. Restifo NP, Marincola FM, Kawakami Y, Taubenberger J, Yannelli JR, Rosenberg SA. Loss of functional beta 2-microglobulin in metastatic melanomas from five patients receiving immunotherapy. *J Natl Cancer Inst* 1996;88:100.

35. Marincola FM, Shamamian P, Simonis TB, et al. Locus-specific analysis of human leukocyte antigen class I expression in melanoma cell lines. *J Immunother Emphasis Tumor Immunol* 1994;16:13.

36. Rivoltini L, Barracchini KC, Viggiano V, et al. Quantitative correlation between HLA class I allele expression and recognition of melanoma cells by antigen-specific cytotoxic T lymphocytes. *Cancer Res* 1995;55:3149.

37. Cormier JN, Panelli MC, Hackett JA, et al. Natural variation of the expression of HLA and endogenous antigen modulates CTL recognition in an *in vitro* melanoma model. *Int J Cancer* 1999;80:781.

38. Yanuck M, Carbone DP, Pendleton CD, et al. A mutant p53 tumor suppressor protein is a target for peptide-induced CD8+ cytotoxic T-cells. *Cancer Res* 1993;53:3257.

39. Smith MC, Pendleton CD, Maher VE, Kelley MJ, Carbone DP, Berzofsky JA. Oncogenic mutations in ras create HLA-A2.1 binding peptides but affect their extracellular antigen processing. *Int Immunol* 1997;9:1085.

40. Peace DJ, Smith JW, Chen W, et al. Lysis of ras oncogene-transformed cells by specific cytotoxic T lymphocytes elicited by primary *in vitro* immunization with mutated ras peptide. *J Exp Med* 1994;179:473.

41. Khleif SN, Abrams SI, Hamilton JM, et al. A phase I vaccine trial with peptides reflecting ras oncogene mutations of solid tumors. *J Immunother* 1999;22:155.

42. Abrams SI, Hand PH, Tsang KY, Schlom J. Mutant ras epitopes as targets for cancer vaccines. *Semin Oncol* 1996;23:118.

43. Chen W, Qin H, Reese VA, Cheever MA. CTLs specific for bcr-abl joining region segment peptides fail to lyse leukemia cells expressing p210 bcr-abl protein. *J Immunother* 1998;21:257.

44. Goydos JS, Elder E, Whiteside TL, Finn OJ, Lotze MT. A phase I trial of a synthetic mucin peptide vaccine. Induction of specific immune reactivity in patients with adenocarcinoma. *J Surg Res* 1996;63:298.

45. Hiltbold EM, Ciborowski P, Finn OJ. Naturally processed class II epitope from the tumor antigen MUC1 primes human CD4+ T cells. *Cancer Res* 1998;58:5066.

46. Magarian-Blander J, Ciborowski P, Hsia S, Watkins SC, Finn OJ. Intercellular and intracellular events following the MHC-unrestricted TCR recognition of a tumor-specific peptide epitope on the epithelial antigen MUC1. *J Immunol* 1998;160:3111.

47. Kass E, Schlom J, Thompson J, Guadagni F, Graziano P, Greiner JW. Induction of protective host immunity to carcinoembryonic antigen (CEA), a self-antigen in CEA transgenic mice, by immunizing with a recombinant vaccinia-CEA virus. *Cancer Res* 1999;59:676.

48. Tsang KY, Zaremba S, Nieroda CA, Zhu MZ, Hamilton JM, Schlom J. Generation of human cytotoxic T cells specific for human carcinoembryonic antigen epitopes from patients immunized with recombinant vaccinia-CEA vaccine. *J Natl Cancer Inst* 1995;87:982.

49. Meunier L, Vian L, Lagoueyte C, et al. Quantification of CD1a, HLA-DR, and HLA class I expression on viable human Langerhans cells and keratinocytes. *Cytometry* 1996;26:260.

50. Sykulev Y, Joo M, Vturina I, Tsomides TJ, Eisen HN. Evidence that a single peptide-MHC complex on a target cell can elicit a cytolytic T cell response. *Immunity* 1996;4:565.

51. Kageyama S, Tsomides TJ, Sykulev Y, Eisen HN. Variations in the number of peptide-MHC class I complexes required to activate cytotoxic T cell responses. *J Immunol* 1995;154:567.

52. Christinck ER, Luscher MA, Barber BH, Williams DB. Peptide binding to class I MHC on living cells and quantitation of complexes required for CTL lysis. *Nature* 1991;352:67.

53. Hunt DF, Henderson RA, Shabanowitz J, et al. Characterization of peptides bound to the class I MHC molecule HLA-A2.1 by mass spectrometry. *Science* 1992;255:1261.

54. Hunt DF, Michel H, Dickinson TA, et al. Peptides presented to the immune system by the murine class II major histocompatibility complex molecule I-Ad. *Science* 1992;256:1817.

55. Wang RF, Johnston SL, Zeng G, Topalian SL, Schwartzentruber DJ, Rosenberg SA. A breast and melanoma-shared tumor antigen: T cell responses to antigenic peptides translated from different open reading frames. *J Immunol* 1998;161:3598.

56. Wang RF, Parkhurst MR, Kawakami Y, Robbins PF, Rosenberg SA. Utilization of an alternative open reading frame of a normal gene in generating a novel human cancer antigen. *J Exp Med* 1996;183:1131.

57. Zaks TZ, Rosenberg SA. Immunization with a peptide epitope (p369-377) from HER-2/neu leads to peptide-specific cytotoxic T lymphocytes that fail to recognize HER- 2/neu+ tumors. *Cancer Res* 1998;58:4902.

58. Kawakami Y, Robbins PF, Wang RF, Parkhurst M, Kang X, Rosenberg SA. The use of melanosomal proteins in the immunotherapy of melanoma. *J Immunother* 1998;21:237.

59. Rosenberg SA. A new era for cancer immunotherapy based on the genes that encode cancer antigens. *Immunity* 1999;10:281.

60. Wang RF, Johnston SL, Zeng G, Topalian SL, Schwartzentruber DJ, Rosenberg SA. A breast and melanoma-shared tumor antigen: T cell responses to antigenic peptides translated from different open reading frames. *J Immunol* 1998;161:3598.

61. Wang RF, Wang X, Johnston SL, Zeng G, Robbins PF, Rosenberg SA. Development of a retrovirus-based complementary DNA expression system for the cloning of tumor antigens. *Cancer Res* 1998;58:3519.

62. Wang RF, Johnston SL, Southwood S, Sette A, Rosenberg SA. Recognition of an antigenic peptide derived from tyrosinase-related pro-

tein-2 by CTL in the context of HLA-A31 and -A33. *J Immunol* 1998;160:890.

63. Kawakami Y, Eliyahu S, Delgado CH, et al. Identification of a human melanoma antigen recognized by tumor-infiltrating lymphocytes associated with *in vivo* tumor rejection. *Proc Natl Acad Sci U S A* 1994;91:6458.

64. Kawakami Y, Eliyahu S, Jennings C, et al. Recognition of multiple epitopes in the human melanoma antigen gp100 by tumor-infiltrating T lymphocytes associated with *in vivo* tumor regression. *J Immunol* 1995;154:3961.

65. Kawakami Y, Robbins PF, Wang X, et al. Identification of new melanoma epitopes on melanosomal proteins recognized by tumor infiltrating T lymphocytes restricted by HLA-A1, -A2, and -A3 alleles. *J Immunol* 1998;161:6985.

66. Bakker AB, Schreurs MW, de Boer AJ, et al. Melanocyte lineage-specific antigen gp100 is recognized by melanoma-derived tumor-infiltrating lymphocytes. *J Exp Med* 1994;179:1005.

67. Skipper J, Kittlesen DJ, Hendrickson RC, et al. Shared epitopes for HLA-A3 restricted melanoma reactive human CTL include a naturally processed epitope from Pmel-17/gp100. *J Immunol* 1996;157:5027.

68. Cox A, Skipper J, Celm Y, et al. Identification of a peptide recognized by five melanoma-specific human cytotoxic T cell lines. *Science* 1994;264:716.

69. Robbins PF, El-Gamil M, Li YF, Fitzgerald EB, Kawakami Y, Rosenberg SA. The intronic region of an incompletely spliced gp100 gene transcript encodes an epitope recognized by melanoma-reactive tumor-infiltrating lymphocytes. *J Immunol* 1997;159:303.

70. Kawakami Y, Eliyahu S, Delgado CH, et al. Cloning of the gene coding for a shared human melanoma antigen recognized by autologous T cells infiltrating into tumor. *Proc Natl Acad Sci U S A* 1994;91:3515.

71. Kawakami Y, Eliyahu S, Sakaguchi K, et al. Identification of the immunodominant peptides of the MART-1 human melanoma antigen recognized by the majority of HLA-A2-restricted tumor infiltrating lymphocytes. *J Exp Med* 1994;180:347.

72. Schneider J, Brichard VG, Boon T, Buschenfelde K, Wolfel T. Overlapping peptides of melanocyte differentiation antigen MELAN-A/MART-1 recognized by autologous cytolytic T lymphocytes in association with HLA-B45.1 and HLA-A2.1. *Int J Cancer* 1998;75(3):451–458.

73. Valmori D, Gervois N, Rimoldi D, et al. Diversity of the fine specificity displayed by HLA-A*0201-restricted CTL specific for the immunodominant Melan-A/MART-1 antigenic peptide. *J Immunol* 1998;161:6956.

74. Romero P, Gervois N, Schneider J, et al. Cytolytic T lymphocyte recognition of the immunodominant HLA-A*0201-restricted Melan-A/MART-1 antigenic peptide in melanoma. *J Immunol* 1997;159:2366.

75. Wolfel T, van Pel A, Brichard VG, et al. Two tyrosinase nonapeptides recognized on HLA-A2 melanomas by autologous cytolytic T lymphocytes. *Eur J Immunol* 1994;24:759.

76. Kittlesen DJ, Thompson LW, Gulden PH, et al. Human melanoma patients recognize an HLA-A1-restricted CTL epitope from tyrosinase containing two cysteine residues: implications for vaccine development. *J Immunol* 1998;160:2099.

77. Brichard VG, Herman J, van Pel A, et al. A tyrosinase nonapeptide presented by HLA-B44 is recognized on a human melanoma by autologous cytolytic T lymphocytes. *Eur J Immunol* 1996;26:224.

78. Kang X-Q, Kawakami Y, Sakaguchi K, et al. Identification of a tyrosinase epitope recognized by HLA-A24 restricted tumor-infiltrating lymphocytes. *J Immunol* 1995;155:1343.

79. Wang RF, Parkhurst MR, Kawakami Y, Robbins PF, Rosenberg SA. Utilization of an alternative open reading frame of a normal gene in generating a novel human cancer antigen. *J Exp Med* 1996;183:1131.

80. Wang RF, Appella E, Kawakami Y, Kang X, Rosenberg SA. Identification of TRP-2 as a human tumor antigen recognized by cytotoxic T lymphocytes. *J Exp Med* 1996;184:2207.

81. Parkhurst MR, Fitzgerald EB, Southwood S, Sette A, Rosenberg SA, Kawakami Y. Identification of a shared HLA-A*0201-restricted T-cell epitope from the melanoma antigen tyrosinase-related protein 2 (TRP2). *Cancer Res* 1998;58:4895.

82. Rosenberg SA, Yang JC, White DE, Steinberg SM. Durability of complete responses in patients with metastatic cancer treated with high-dose interleukin-2: identification of the antigens mediating response. *Ann Surg* 1998;228:307.

83. De Plaen E, De Backer O, Arnaud D, et al. A new family of mouse genes homologous to the human MAGE genes. *Genomics* 1999;55:176.

84. van Baren N, Chambost H, Ferrant A, et al. PRAME, a gene encoding an antigen recognized on a human melanoma by cytolytic T cells, is expressed in acute leukaemia cells. *Br J Haematol* 1998;102:1376.

85. Lethe B, Lucas S, Michaux L, et al. LAGE-1, a new gene with tumor specificity. *Int J Cancer* 1998;76(6):903.

86. Jager E, Chen YT, Drijfhout JW, et al. Simultaneous humoral and cellular immune response against cancer-testis antigen NY-ESO-1: definition of human histocompatibility leukocyte antigen (HLA)-A2-binding peptide epitopes. *J Exp Med* 1998;187:265.

87. Stockert E, Jager E, Chen YT, et al. A survey of the humoral immune response of cancer patients to a panel of human tumor antigens. *J Exp Med* 1998;187(8):1349.

88. Chen YT, Scanlan MJ, Sahin U, et al. A testicular antigen aberrantly expressed in human cancers detected by autologous antibody screening. *Proc Natl Acad Sci U S A* 1997;94(5):1914.

89. Boon T, Old LJ. Cancer tumor antigens. *Curr Opin Immunol* 1997;9(5):681.

90. Srivastava PK. Do human cancers express shared protective antigens? or the necessity of remembrance of things past. *Semin Immunol* 1996;8:295.

91. Robbins PF, El-Gamil M, Li YF, et al. A mutated beta-catenin gene encodes a melanoma-specific antigen recognized by tumor infiltrating lymphocytes. *J Exp Med* 1996;183:1185.

92. Wolfel T, Hauer M, Schneider J, et al. A p16INK4a-insensitive CDK4 mutant targeted by cytolytic T lymphocytes in a human melanoma. *Science* 1995;269:1281.

93. Coulie PG, Lehmann F, Lethe B, et al. A mutated intron sequence codes for an antigenic peptide recognized by cytolytic T lymphocytes on a human melanoma. *Proc Natl Acad Sci U S A* 1995;92:7976.

94. Mandruzzato S, Brasseur F, Andry G, Boon T, van der Bruggen P. A CASP-8 mutation recognized by cytolytic T lymphocytes on a human head and neck carcinoma. *J Exp Med* 1997;186(5):785.

95. Brandle D, Brasseur F, Weynants P, Boon T, van den Eynde B. A mutated HLA-A2 molecule recognized by autologous cytotoxic T lymphocytes on a human renal cell carcinoma. *J Exp Med* 1996;183:2501.

96. Gueguen M, Patard JJ, Gaugler B, et al. An antigen recognized by autologous CTLs on a human bladder carcinoma. *J Immunol* 1998;160(12):6188.

97. Blachere NE, Srivastava PK. Heat shock protein-based cancer vaccines and related thoughts on immunogenicity of human tumors. *Semin Cancer Biol* 1995;6:349.

98. Lo D, Freedman J, Hesse S, Palmiter RD, Brinster RL, Sherman LA. Peripheral tolerance to an islet cell-specific hemagglutinin transgene affects both CD4+ and CD8+ T cells. *Eur J Immunol* 1992;22:1013.

99. Prehn RT, Main JM. Immunity to methylcholanthrene-induced sarcomas. *J Natl Cancer Inst* 1957;18:769–774.

100. Barth RJJ, Bock SN, Mule JJ, Rosenberg SA. Unique murine tumor-associated antigens identified by tumor infiltrating lymphocytes. *J Immunol* 1990;144:1531.

101. Melief CJ, Kast WM. T-cell immunotherapy of tumors by adoptive transfer of cytotoxic T lymphocytes and by vaccination with minimal essential epitopes. *Immunol Rev* 1995;145:167–177.

102. Yee C, Riddell SR, Greenberg PD. Prospects for adoptive T cell therapy. *Curr Opin Immunol* 1997;9:702.

103. De Smet C, Lurquin C, De Plaen E, et al. Genes coding for melanoma antigens recognized by cytolytic T lymphocytes. *Eye* 1997;11(Pt 2):243.

104. Restifo NP, Bacik I, Irvine KR, et al. Antigen processing *in vivo* and the elicitation of primary CTL responses. *J Immunol* 1995;154:4414.

105. Irvine KR, McCabe BJ, Rosenberg SA, Restifo NP. Synthetic oligonucleotide expressed by a recombinant vaccinia virus elicits therapeutic CTL. *J Immunol* 1995;154:4651.

106. Parkhurst MR, Salgaller ML, Southwood S, et al. Improved induction of melanoma-reactive CTL with peptides from the melanoma antigen gp100 modified at HLA-A*0201-binding residues. *J Immunol* 1996;157:2539.

107. Lu L, McCaslin D, Starzl TE, Thomson AW. Bone marrow-derived dendritic cell progenitors (NLDC 145+, MHC class II+, B7-1dim, B7-2-) induce alloantigen-specific hyporesponsiveness in murine T lymphocytes. *Transplantation* 1995;60:1539.

108. Greenberg PD, Cheever MA, Fefer A. Eradication of disseminated murine leukemia by chemoimmunotherapy with cyclophosphamide and adoptively transferred immune syngeneic Lyt-1+2- lymphocytes. *J Exp Med* 1981;154:952.

109. Greenberg PD, Kern DE, Cheever MA. Therapy of disseminated murine leukemia with cyclophosphamide and immune Lyt-1+,2- T cells. Tumor eradication does not require participation of cytotoxic T cells. *J Exp Med* 1985;161:1122.

110. McDevitt HO, Wakeland EK. Autoimmunity. *Curr Opin Immunol* 1998;10:647.

111. McDevitt HO. The role of MHC class II molecules in susceptibility and resistance to autoimmunity. *Curr Opin Immunol* 1998;10:677.

112. McDevitt H, Singer S, Tisch R. The role of MHC class II genes in susceptibility and resistance to type I diabetes mellitus in the NOD mouse. *Horm Metab Res* 1996;28:287.

113. Goodnow CC. Balancing immunity, autoimmunity, and self-tolerance. *Ann N Y Acad Sci* 1997;815:55–66.

114. Kumar V, Sercarz E. Induction or protection from experimental autoimmune encephalomyelitis depends on the cytokine secretion profile of TCR peptide-specific regulatory CD4 T cells. *J Immunol* 1998;161:6585.

115. Kumar V, Stellrecht K, Sercarz E. Inactivation of T cell receptor peptide-specific CD4 regulatory T cells induces chronic experimental autoimmune encephalomyelitis (EAE). *J Exp Med* 1996;184:1609.

116. Toes RE, Ossendorp F, Offringa R, Melief CJ. CD4 T cells and their role in antitumor immune responses. *J Exp Med* 1999;189:753.

117. Ossendorp F, Mengede E, Camps M, Filius R, Melief CJ. Specific T helper cell requirement for optimal induction of cytotoxic T lymphocytes against major histocompatibility complex class II negative tumors. *J Exp Med* 1998;187:693.

118. Toes RM, Schoenberger SP, van der Voort EH, Offringa R, Melief CJ. CD40-CD40Ligand interactions and their role in cytotoxic T lymphocyte priming and anti-tumor immunity. *Semin Immunol* 1998;10:443.

119. Cornall RJ, Goodnow CC. B cell antigen receptor signaling in the balance of tolerance and immunity. *Novartis Found Symp* 1998;215:21–30.

120. Macaulay AE, DeKruyff RH, Goodnow CC, Umetsu DT. Antigen-specific B cells preferentially induce CD4+ T cells to produce IL-4. *J Immunol* 1997;158:4171.

121. Overwijk WW, Lee DS, Surman DR, et al. Vaccination with a recombinant vaccinia virus encoding a "self" antigen induces autoimmune vitiligo and tumor cell destruction in mice: requirement for CD4(+) T lymphocytes. *Proc Natl Acad Sci U S A* 1999;96:2982.

122. Pardoll DM. Inducing autoimmune disease to treat cancer. *Proc Natl Acad Sci U S A* 1999;96:5340.

123. Weber LW, Bowne WB, Wolchok JD, et al. Tumor immunity and autoimmunity induced by immunization with homologous DNA. *J Clin Invest* 1998;102:1258.

124. Clynes R, Takechi Y, Moroi Y, Houghton A, Ravetch JV. Fc receptors are required in passive and active immunity to melanoma. *Proc Natl Acad Sci U S A* 1998;95:652.

125. Hara I, Takechi Y, Houghton AN. Implicating a role for immune recognition of self in tumor rejection: passive immunization against the brown locus protein. *J Exp Med* 1995;182:1609.

126. Hirschowitz EA, Leonard S, Song W, et al. Adenovirus-mediated expression of melanoma antigen gp75 as immunotherapy for metastatic melanoma. *Gene Ther* 1998;5:975.

127. Hung K, Hayashi R, Lafond-Walker A, Lowenstein C, Pardoll D, Levitsky H. The central role of CD4(+) T cells in the antitumor immune response. *J Exp Med* 1998;188:2357.

128. Ridge JP, Di Rosa F, Matzinger P. A conditioned dendritic cell can be a temporal bridge between a CD4+ T-helper and a T-killer cell. *Nature* 1998;393:474.

129. Schoenberger SP, Toes RE, van der Voort EI, Offringa R, Melief CJ. T-cell help for cytotoxic T lymphocytes is mediated by CD40-CD40L interactions. *Nature* 1998;393:480.

130. Balasa B, Krahl T, Patstone G, et al. CD40 ligand-CD40 interactions are necessary for the initiation of insulitis and diabetes in non-obese diabetic mice. *J Immunol* 1997;159:4620.

131. Walter EA, Greenberg PD, Gilbert MJ, et al. Reconstitution of cellular immunity against cytomegalovirus in recipients of allogeneic bone marrow by transfer of T-cell clones from the donor [see comments]. *N Engl J Med* 1995;333:1038.

132. Wang RF, Wang X, Atwood AC, Topalian SL, Rosenberg SA. Cloning genes encoding MHC class II-restricted antigens: mutated CDC27 as a tumor antigen. *Science* 1999;284:1351.

133. Wang RF, Wang X, Rosenberg SA. Identification of a novel major histocompatibility complex class II-restricted tumor antigen resulting from a chromosomal rearrangement recognized by CD4(+) T cells. *J Exp Med* 1999;189:1659.

134. Topalian SL, Gonzales MI, Parkhurst M, et al. Melanoma-specific CD4+ T cells recognize nonmutated HLA-DR-restricted tyrosinase epitopes. *J Exp Med* 1996;183:1965.

135. Pieper R, Christian RE, Gonzales MI, et al. Biochemical identification of a mutated human melanoma antigen recognized by CD4(+) T cells. *J Exp Med* 1999;189:757.

136. Chaux P, Vantomme V, Stroobant V, et al. Identification of MAGE-3 epitopes presented by HLA-DR molecules to CD4(+) T lymphocytes. *J Exp Med* 1999;189:767.

137. Manici S, Sturniolo T, Imro MA, et al. Melanoma cells present a MAGE-3 epitope to CD4(+) cytotoxic T cells in association with histocompatibility leukocyte antigen DR11. *J Exp Med* 1999; 189:871.

138. Banchereau J, Steinman RM. Dendritic cells and the control of immunity. *Nature* 1998;392:245.

139. Steinman RM, Witmer MD. Lymphoid dendritic cells are potent stimulators of the primary mixed leukocyte reaction in mice. *Proc Natl Acad Sci U S A* 1978;75:5132.

140. Bretscher P, Cohn M. A theory of self-nonself discrimination. *Science* 1970;169:1042.

141. Brown MJ, Shaw S. T-cell activation: interplay at the interface. *Curr Biol* 1999;9:R26.

142. Bluestone JA. Cell fate in the immune system: decisions, decisions, decisions. *Immunol Rev* 1998;165:5–12.

143. Schwartz RH. T cell clonal anergy. *Curr Opin Immunol* 1997;9:351.

144. Van Parijs L, Abbas AK. Homeostasis and self-tolerance in the immune system: turning lymphocytes off. *Science* 1998;280:243.

145. Walunas TL, Bluestone JA. CTLA-4 regulates tolerance induction and T cell differentiation in vivo. *J Immunol* 1998;160:3855.

146. Leach DR, Krummel MF, Allison JP. Enhancement of antitumor immunity by CTLA-4 blockade. *Science* 1996;271:1734.

147. Bronte V, Carroll MW, Goletz TJ, et al. Antigen expression by dendritic cells correlates with the therapeutic effectiveness of a model recombinant poxvirus tumor vaccine. *Proc Natl Acad Sci U S A* 1997;94:3183.

148. Porgador A, Irvine KR, Iwasaki A, Barber BH, Restifo NP, Germain RN. Predominant role for directly transfected dendritic cells in antigen presentation to CD8+ T cells after gene gun immunization. *J Exp Med* 1998;188:1075.

149. Gurunathan S, Irvine KR, Wu CY, et al. CD40 ligand/trimer DNA enhances both humoral and cellular immune responses and induces protective immunity to infectious and tumor challenge. *J Immunol* 1998;161:4563.

150. Esche C, Subbotin VM, Maliszewski C, Lotze MT, Shurin MR. FLT3 ligand administration inhibits tumor growth in murine melanoma and lymphoma. *Cancer Res* 1998;58(3):380.

151. Shurin MR, Pandharipande PP, Zorina TD, et al. FLT3 ligand induces the generation of functionally active dendritic cells in mice. *Cell Immunol* 1997;179:174.

152. Mantovani A. The chemokine system: redundancy for robust outputs. *Immunol Today* 1999;20:254.

153. Sallusto F, Lanzavecchia A. Mobilizing dendritic cells for tolerance, priming, and chronic inflammation. *J Exp Med* 1999;189:611.

154. Sallusto F, Lanzavecchia A, Mackay CR. Chemokines and chemokine receptors in T-cell priming and Th1/Th2-mediated responses. *Immunol Today* 1998;19:568.

155. Ward SG, Bacon K, Westwick J. Chemokines and T lymphocytes: more than an attraction. *Immunity* 1998;9:1.

156. Nelson PJ, Krensky AM. Chemokines, lymphocytes and viruses: what goes around, comes around. *Curr Opin Immunol* 1998;10:265.

157. Baggiolini M. Chemokines and leukocyte traffic. *Nature* 1998;392:565.

158. Luster AD. Chemokines—chemotactic cytokines that mediate inflammation. *N Engl J Med* 1998;338:436.

159. Bronte V, Tsung K, Rao JB, et al. IL-2 enhances the function of recombinant poxvirus-based vaccines in the treatment of established pulmonary metastases. *J Immunol* 1995;154:5282.

160. Irvine KR, Rao JB, Rosenberg SA, Restifo NP. Cytokine enhancement of DNA immunization leads to effective treatment of established pulmonary metastases. *J Immunol* 1996;156:238.

161. Rao JB, Chamberlain RS, Bronte V, et al. IL-12 is an effective adjuvant to recombinant vaccinia virus-based tumor vaccines: enhancement by simultaneous B7-1 expression. *J Immunol* 1996;156:3357.

162. Carroll MW, Overwijk WW, Surman DR, Tsung K, Moss B, Restifo NP. Construction and characterization of a triple-recombinant vaccinia virus encoding B7-1, interleukin 12, and a model tumor antigen. *J Natl Cancer Inst* 1998;90:1881.

163. Dranoff G, Jaffee E, Lazenby A, et al. Vaccination with irradiated tumor cells engineered to secrete murine granulocyte-macrophage colony-stimulating factor stimulates potent, specific, and long-lasting anti-tumor immunity. *Proc Natl Acad Sci U S A* 1993;90:3539.

164. Simons JW, Jaffee EM, Weber CE, et al. Bioactivity of autologous irradiated renal cell carcinoma vaccines generated by ex vivo granulocyte-macrophage colony-stimulating factor gene transfer. *Cancer Res* 1997;57:1537.

165. Witmer-Pack MD, Olivier W, Valinsky J, Schuler G, Steinman RM. Granulocyte/macrophage colony-stimulating factor is essential for the viability and function of cultured murine epidermal Langerhans cells. *J Exp Med* 1987;166:1484.

166. Chamberlain RS, Carroll MW, Bronte V, et al. Costimulation enhances the active immunotherapy effect of recombinant anticancer vaccines. *Cancer Res* 1996;56:2832.

167. Wloch MK, Pasquini S, Ertl HC, Pisetsky DS. The influence of DNA sequence on the immunostimulatory properties of plasmid DNA vectors. *Hum Gene Ther* 1998;9:1439.

168. Klinman DM. Therapeutic applications of CpG-containing oligodeoxynucleotides. *Antisense Nucleic Acid Drug Dev* 1998;8:181.

169. Krieg AM, Yi AK, Schorr J, Davis HL. The role of CpG dinucleotides in DNA vaccines. *Trends Microbiol* 1998;6:23.

170. Lipford GB, Bauer M, Blank C, Reiter R, Wagner H, Heeg K. CpG-containing synthetic oligonucleotides promote B and cytotoxic T cell responses to protein antigen: a new class of vaccine adjuvants. *Eur J Immunol* 1997;27:2340.

171. Kovarik J, Bozzotti P, Love-Homan L, et al. CpG oligodeoxynucleotides can circumvent the Th2 polarization of neonatal responses to vaccines but may fail to fully redirect Th2 responses established by neonatal priming. *J Immunol* 1999;162:1611.

172. Brazolot MC, Weeratna R, Krieg AM, Siegrist CA, Davis HL. CpG DNA can induce strong Th1 humoral and cell-mediated immune responses against hepatitis B surface antigen in young mice. *Proc Natl Acad Sci U S A* 1998;95:15553.

173. Blachere NE, Li Z, Chandawarkar RY, et al. Heat shock protein-peptide complexes, reconstituted in vitro, elicit peptide-specific cyto-toxic T lymphocyte response and tumor immunity. *J Exp Med* 1997;186:1315.

174. Tamura Y, Peng P, Liu K, Daou M, Srivastava PK. Immunotherapy of tumors with autologous tumor-derived heat shock protein preparations. *Science* 1997;278:117.

175. Celluzzi CM, Mayordomo JI, Storkus WJ, Lotze MT, Falo LDJ. Peptide-pulsed dendritic cells induce antigen-specific CTL-mediated protective tumor immunity. *J Exp Med* 1996;183:283.

176. Zitvogel L, Mayordomo JI, Tjandrawan T, et al. Therapy of murine tumors with tumor peptide-pulsed dendritic cells: dependence on T cells, B7 costimulation, and T helper cell 1-associated cytokines. *J Exp Med* 1996;183:87.

177. Ashley DM, Faiola B, Nair S, Hale LP, Bigner DD, Gilboa E. Bone marrow-generated dendritic cells pulsed with tumor extracts or tumor RNA induce antitumor immunity against central nervous system tumors. *J Exp Med* 1997;186:1177.

178. Restifo NP. The new vaccines: building viruses that elicit antitumor immunity. *Curr Opin Immunol* 1996;8:658.

179. Paterson Y. Rational approaches to immune regulation. *Immunol Res* 1998;17:191.

180. Paterson Y, Ikonomidis G. Recombinant Listeria monocytogenes cancer vaccines. *Curr Opin Immunol* 1996;8:664.

181. Polo JM, Dubensky TWJ. DNA vaccines with a kick. *Nat Biotechnol* 1998;16:517.

182. Restifo NP, Surman DR, Zheng H, Palese P, Rosenberg SA, Garcia-Sastre A. Transfectant influenza A viruses are effective recombinant immunogens in the treatment of experimental cancer. *Virology* 1998;249:89.

183. Carroll MW, Overwijk WW, Chamberlain RS, Rosenberg SA, Moss B, Restifo NP. Highly attenuated modified vaccinia virus Ankara (MVA) as an effective recombinant vector: a murine tumor model. *Vaccine* 1997;15:387.

184. Chen PW, Wang M, Bronte V, Zhai Y, Rosenberg SA, Restifo NP. Therapeutic antitumor response after immunization with a recombinant adenovirus encoding a model tumor-associated antigen. *J Immunol* 1996;156:224.

185. Rosenberg SA, Zhai Y, Yang JC, et al. Immunizing patients with metastatic melanoma using recombinant adenoviruses encoding MART-1 or gp100 melanoma antigens. *J Natl Cancer Inst* 1998;90:1894.

186. Schowalter DB, Himeda CL, Winther BL, Wilson CB, Kay MA. Implication of interfering antibody formation and apoptosis as two different mechanisms leading to variable duration of adenovirus-mediated transgene expression in immune-competent mice. *J Virol* 1999;73:4755.

187. Gurwith MJ, Horwith GS, Impellizzeri CA, Davis AR, Lubeck MD, Hung PP. Current use and future directions of adenovirus vaccine. *Semin Respir Infect* 1989;4:299.

188. Barraza EM, Ludwig SL, Gaydos JC, Brundage JF. Reemergence of adenovirus type 4 acute respiratory disease in military trainees: report of an outbreak during a lapse in vaccination. *J Infect Dis* 1999;179:1531.

189. Wood DJ. Adenovirus gastroenteritis. *Br Med J (Clin Res Ed)* 1988;296:229.

190. Zahradnik JM. Adenovirus pneumonia. *Semin Respir Infect* 1987;2:104.

191. Wehrle PF. A reality in our time—certification of the global eradication of smallpox. *J Infect Dis* 1980;142:636.

192. Deria A. The world's last endemic case of smallpox: surveillance and containment measures. *Bull World Health Organ* 1980;58:279.

193. Wehrle PF. Smallpox eradication. A global appraisal. *JAMA* 1978;240:1977.

194. Koplan JP, Hicks JW. Smallpox and vaccinia in the United States—1972. *J Infect Dis* 1974;129:224.

195. Gregorio L. The smallpox legacy: a history of pediatric immunizations. *Pharos* 1996;59:7.

196. Fenner F. Risks and benefits of vaccinia vaccine use in the worldwide smallpox eradication campaign. *Res Virol* 1989;140:465.

197. Liu MA. Vaccine developments. *Nat Med* 1998;4:515.

198. Ying H. Cancer therapy using a self-replicating RNA vaccine. *Nat Med* 1999;5:823–827.

199. Adluri S, Gilewski T, Zhang S, Ramnath V, Ragupathi G, Livingston P. Specificity analysis of sera from breast cancer patients vaccinated with MUC1-KLH plus QS-21. *Br J Cancer* 1999;79:1806.

200. McNeal MM, Rae MN, Ward RL. Effects of different adjuvants on rotavirus antibody responses and protection in mice following intramuscular immunization with inactivated rotavirus [In Process Citation]. *Vaccine* 1999;17:1573.

201. Sasaki S, Sumino K, Hamajima K, et al. Induction of systemic and mucosal immune responses to human immunodeficiency virus type 1 by a DNA vaccine formulated with QS-21 saponin adjuvant via intramuscular and intranasal routes. *J Virol* 1998;72:4931.

202. Kensil CR, Wu JY, Anderson CA, Wheeler DA, Amsden J. QS-21 and QS-7: purified saponin adjuvants. *Dev Biol Stand* 1998;92:41.

203. Romieu R, Baratin M, Kayibanda M, Guillet JG, Viguier M. IFN-gamma-secreting Th cells regulate both the frequency and avidity of epitope-specific CD8+ T lymphocytes induced by peptide immunization: an *ex vivo* analysis. *Int Immunol* 1998;10:1273.

204. Deeb BJ, DiGiacomo RF, Kunz LL, Stewart JL. Comparison of Freund's and Ribi adjuvants for inducing antibodies to the synthetic antigen (TG)-AL in rabbits. *J Immunol Methods* 1992;152:105.

205. Fitzgerald TJ. Syphilis vaccine: up-regulation of immunogenicity by cyclophosphamide, Ribi adjuvant, and indomethacin confers significant protection against challenge infection in rabbits. *Vaccine* 1991;9:266.

206. Goletz TJ, Klimpel KR, Arora N, Leppla SH, Keith JM, Berzofsky JA. Targeting HIV proteins to the major histocompatibility complex class I processing pathway with a novel gp120-anthrax toxin fusion protein. *Proc Natl Acad Sci U S A* 1997;94:12059.

207. Goletz TJ, Klimpel KR, Leppla SH, Keith JM, Berzofsky JA. Delivery of antigens to the MHC class I pathway using bacterial toxins. *Hum Immunol* 1997;54:129.

208. Minev B, McFarland BJ, Spiess PJ, Rosenberg SA, Restifo NP. Insertion signal sequence fused to a minimal peptide elicits specific CD8+ T cell responses and prolongs survival of thymoma-bearing mice. *Cancer Res* 1994;54(15):4155.

209. Zinkernagel RM, Hengartner H. Virally induced immunosuppression. *Curr Opin Immunol* 1992;4:408.

210. Aichele P, Brduscha-Riem K, Zinkernagel RM, Hengartner H, Pircher H. T cell priming versus T cell tolerance induced by synthetic peptides. *J Exp Med* 1995;182:261.

211. Toes RE, van der Voort EI, Schoenberger SP, et al. Enhancement of tumor outgrowth through CTL tolerization after peptide vaccination is avoided by peptide presentation on dendritic cells. *J Immunol* 1998;160:4449.

212. Toes RE, Blom RJ, Offringa R, Kast WM, Melief CJ. Enhanced tumor outgrowth after peptide vaccination. Functional deletion of tumor-specific CTL induced by peptide vaccination can lead to the inability to reject tumors. *J Immunol* 1996;156:3911.

213. Cormier JN, Salgaller ML, Prevette T, et al. Enhancement of cellular immunity in melanoma patients immunized with a peptide from MART-1/Melan A. *Cancer J Sci Am* 1997;3:37.

214. Hodge JW, McLaughlin JP, Kantor JA, Schlom J. Diversified prime and boost protocols using recombinant vaccinia virus and recombinant non-replicating avian pox virus to enhance T-cell immunity and antitumor responses. *Vaccine* 1997;15:759.

215. Irvine KR, Chamberlain RS, Shulman EP, Surman DR, Rosenberg SA, Restifo NP. Enhancing efficacy of recombinant anticancer vaccines with prime/boost regimens that use two different vectors. *J Natl Cancer Inst* 1997;89:1595.

216. Irvine KR, Chamberlain RS, Shulman EP, Rosenberg SA, Restifo NP. Route of immunization and the therapeutic impact of recombinant anticancer vaccines. *J Natl Cancer Inst* 1997;89:390.

217. Restifo NP. Cancer vaccines '98: a reductionistic approach. *Mol Med Today* 1998;4:327.

17.2

CANCER VACCINES: BASIC PRINCIPLES

Immune Adjuvants

MICHAEL L. SALGALLER

The general principle of adjuvants is to promote, expedite, or lengthen the immune response to a given vaccine. The development of vaccines directed against human cancer has been facilitated by concurrent progress in the arena of adjuvants. Adjuvants aid immunotherapy by enhancing reactivity to tumors. This is true regardless of the immunogenicity of the tumor, although the most use would be found with those cancers of poor immunogenicity. For the purpose of this chapter, we usually do not discriminate between the establishment of immunogenicity *in vitro* versus *in vivo*. Some of the agents described herein have established themselves in the laboratory or in animal models, whereas others have shown promise in human clinical trials. For the purpose of this review, it is also of less importance whether the primary treatment uses defined

TABLE 1. TYPES OF IMMUNOMODULATORY ADJUVANTS

Category	Example
Gel-type	Alum (aluminum hydroxide)
	Calcium phosphate
Synthetic	Nonionic block copolymers
	Muramyl peptides and peptide analogues
Emulsifier-based or oil emulsion	Saponins
	Freund's incomplete adjuvant
	MF59
Particulate	Immunostimulatory complexes
	Liposomes and liposomal complexes
Bacterial	Bacillus Calmette-Guérin
	Oligodeoxynucleotides
	Monophosphoryl lipid A
Immunogenic proteins and peptides	Keyhole limpet hemocyanin
	Pan-DR epitopes
Cytokines and growth factors	Interleukin-2
	Interleukin-4
	Interleukin-12
	Interferon-α and -γ
	Granulocyte-macrophage colony-stimulating factor
Haptens	Dinitrophenyl
	Trinitrophenyl

(epitopes associated with tumor rejection) or undefined immune targets (whole cells or lysates). Using intact tumor cells as immunogens has achieved protective immunity (protection against a subsequent challenge with tumor cells) in murine experiments. Most human cancers, however, are markedly less immunogenic, thereby validating the need for additional stimulation (1). Augmenting the response to weak immunogens is not the only reason for including an adjuvant. They can also: (a) increase vaccine potency with immunocompromised subjects, (b) bolster CD8$^+$ T-cell–mediated immunity without diminishing humoral responses, (c) potentially decrease the vaccine titer needed, and (d) potentially decrease the number of booster vaccinations required (2).

Adjuvants possess diverse mechanisms of action (2–4), the discussion of which is beyond the scope of this summary. Initially, immunization with an adjuvant increases the durability, concentration at site of introduction, and stability of the antigen. After this, an adjuvant can enhance antigen uptake by antigen-presenting cells, even targeting certain cells of interest, such as macrophages or dendritic cells (DCs). It is important that the adjuvant not hinder antigen processing and presentation to immune cells that are major histocompatibility (MHC) class I–, class II–, or non–MHC-restricted. Lastly, potent adjuvants stimulate T- and B-cell responses via cytokine secretion after immunostimulation, thereby attracting and activating cell subsets. Certainly, many adjuvants mediate effects during more than one step of this process.

This chapter emphasizes those adjuvants under intense investigation as opposed to more classic agents, such as *Corynebacteria parvum*, whose clinical development is being deemphasized at this juncture. The list of adjuvants discussed in this chapter is outlined in Table 1.

GEL-TYPE ADJUVANT

Alum

The most common adjuvants in human clinical trials are aluminum hydroxide (alum) and aluminum phosphate (5). As of 1996, alum remained the only adjuvant licensed for human use in the United States (3). The principal function of alum adjuvants is to enhance humoral immune responses. The extensive surface area of aluminum salts—in particular, the hydroxide and phosphate variants—possess a large absorptive capacity for immunogens (6). Early studies showed stimulation primarily of Th2-type responses, as reflected by the interleukin-4 (IL-4), immunoglobulin 1 (IgG1), and immunoglobulin E (IgE) production they elicited. Most alum-based adjuvants involve the admixing of antigen with preformed aluminum salts, a process known as *aluminum absorption*. Owing to their biochemical characteristics, such as charge and surface area, alum-based adjuvants can be difficult to reproducibly produce. Yet these formulations possess an extensive and excellent safety record with human testing. As a result, alum is a component of several licensed human vaccines for diseases, including hepatitis B, diphtheria, and rabies (7). A novel class of adjuvant combining alum with gamma-inulin (Algammulin) is under development. The inulin component is a polysaccharide and is nontoxic and nonpyogenic in humans (8). Algammulin produced high titers of antibody against infectious agents, such as *meningococci*, after injection of the adjuvant and immunogen into mice (9). It elicits the Th1 and Th2 immune pathway. Lastly, immunization of mice with Algammulin and the E7 protein of human papillomavirus-16 (HPV-16) produces tumor regression in a 14-day tumor protection experiment (10). Future studies will determine how effective it is for augmenting cell-mediated antitumor activity in human subjects.

SYNTHETIC ADJUVANTS

Nonionic Block Copolymers

Block copolymers are similar to saponin-based adjuvants in that they use a noninfectious, chemically defined formulation (11). Nonionic block copolymers are surfactants manufactured with propylene oxide and ethylene oxide (12). The adjuvant activity of a particular copolymer is directly related to its ability to bind protein antigen and capacity to stimulate complement and macrophages. In an *in vitro* system, a copolymer consisting of a central core of hydrophobic polyoxypropylene [POP; $(C_3H_6O_n)$] between two side blocks of hydrophobic polyoxyethylene [POE; $(C_2H_4O_n)$] demonstrated increased presentation of exogenous ovalbumin (OVA) via MHC class I and II pathways (13). Animal studies used mice immunized with a crude oil-in-water emulsion of block copolymer admixed with OVA or the gp120 protein derived from human immunodeficiency virus. MHC class I–restricted cytotoxic T lymphocyte (CTL) were induced that could recognize targets exogenously pulsed with the OVA253-276 synthetic peptide. Vibrant cytolytic activity was noted as long as 4 months after a single treatment (11). A later derivation of this compound, termed *CRL1005*, was used in subsequent studies and had a slightly greater molecular weight. The CRL1005 copolymer elicited high titers of IgG_1 and IgG_{2b}. Its construction overcame a major deficiency of smaller block copolymers—poor solubility in aqueous solution that necessitated their use in oil-based formulations. The ability to administer CRL1005 in aqueous solution lessened the risk of systemic toxicity and localized reactivity at the site of injection. It aggregated into particles in aqueous solution, thus making it compatible with protein-based vaccines and enhancing its ability to act as a carrier moiety (14).

Muramyl Dipeptides and Tripeptides

Muramyl dipeptide (MDP) and tripeptide (MTP) are minimal components derived from the cell walls of bacterial peptioglycan that retain adjuvant activity (15). Their adverse effects, primarily vasculitis and nephrotoxicity, were initially demonstrated in early animal experiments (16). By loading MDP and MTP into liposomal microcarriers (17) or modifying them into analogues of the parent compound, such adverse effects were mitigated without affecting adjuvant potency (18). One derivative, glucosaminyl-MDP, displayed greater antitumor activity than MDP in a Meth A fibrosarcoma murine model. Glucosaminyl-MDP induced activated macrophages to produce IL-1, IL-6, and tumor necrosis factor–α (TNF-α) (19). When encapsulated into liposomes, the derivative MTP-phosphatidylserine (MTP-PE) demonstrated promise as a potent adjuvant in an interferon-γ (IFN-γ)–based therapy regimen for bladder cancer in athymic nude mice (17). The results of a randomized trial for osteosarcoma (20) and mammary carcinoma (21) in dogs, however, showed no survival advantage using adjuvant therapy with liposome-encapsulated MTP-PE compared with treatment with cisplatin or a placebo (empty liposomes), respectively. A 1989 phase 1 trial of liposomal MTP-PE in patients with renal cell carcinoma (RCC) (22) found no objective tumor regression. These disappointing results have greatly diminished the interest in MDP and its derivatives as a vaccine adjuvant, and, to our knowledge, no current clinical pronouncements have reached the literature.

OIL/EMULSIFIER-BASED SURFACE ACTIVE AGENTS

Saponins

A crude saponin mixture, known as *Quil-A*, was initially shown to produce primarily a Th1 response. That is, it stimulated T cells and generated large titers of IL-2 and IFN-γ (23). Experiments with a more purified form showed it also upregulated Th2 responses, evoking strong humoral activity, including IgG1 and IgG2a production (24,25). It enhanced IL-10 production after immunization in mice. Human preclinical studies with Quil-A have targeted the HPV-16 protein after the demonstration that more than 90% of cervical cancer cells contain HPV genetic material integrated into the host genome (26). The E7 protein derived from HPV-16 is required for maintenance of the transformed state. Furthermore, the HPV-16–derived protein can serve as a tumor-rejection antigen (27–29), and peptides contained within it are immunogenic *in vitro* (30). Fernando et al. (31) vaccinated mice with various adjuvants and E7 protein. When admixed with Quil-A, the vaccine elicited Th1 responses, primarily CTL activity against an E7+-transfected EL4 murine thymoma cell line. E7 protein plus Quil-A also produced the most durable CTL activity. Quil-A, complete Freund's adjuvant (CFA), and Algammulin all produced similar titers of IgG1. Quil-A plus E7 protein could not generate Th1-type immunity in immunized animals with a preexisting Th2-type response to E7. These data indicate that saponin adjuvants may be contraindicated in those patients with a preexisting Th2-type response to the immunogen.

More recently, experiments were conducted with highly purified saponins, such as QS-21, and, to a lesser extent, QS-7. C57BL/6 mice were vaccinated with soluble native or denatured OVA in a form containing various amounts of QS-21. OVA-restricted CTL responses were detected in splenocytes only from mice given antigen, including adjuvant. The antigen was effectively delivered to draining lymph nodes and spleen where, after a single vaccination, naïve lymph node cells were induced to proliferate and secrete IL-2 and IFN-γ. CD8+ T cells specifically recognized the OVA258-276 epitope, demonstrating the ability of QS-21 to evoke MHC class I–restricted, antigen-specific CTL after vaccination with soluble protein (32).

Human studies with QS-21 began in the 1990s, the majority of which were conducted at Memorial Sloan-Kettering Cancer Center. Such studies combined several adjuvants, among them QS-21, with gangliosides that are overexpressed in melanoma, including GM2, GD2, and GD3 (33). In addition, clinical trials were performed or are being planned that combine QS-21 with neutral glycolipids (Lewis[y] and Globo H), and glycoproteins (Tn and sialylated Tn antigens) (34). Investigators sought to improve their preexisting GM2/bacillus Calmette-Guérin (BCG) vaccine (35,36), which produced transient IgM and infrequent IgG titers. Indeed, the features of the antibody response included: (a) high IgM titers after initial administration, (b) swift secondary IgM production after booster administration, (c) prolonged IgM antibody titers as long as 10 weeks after booster administration, and (d) uniform IgG antibody production. The anti-GM2 humoral immunity displayed several hallmarks of a T-cell–dependent response, such as the prolonged induction of IgG1 and IgG3 antibodies (37). In addition, when coupled to the carrier keyhole limpet hemocyanin (KLH), a long-lasting, high-titer, anti-KLH antibody response was seen. The regimen was well tolerated with no severe side effects. After this, investigators began treating advanced melanoma patients with 1A7, an antiidiotypic antibody that mimicked the disialoganglioside GD2. After four weekly vaccinations with 1A7/QS-21, immune sera from all 12 subjects had detectable anti-antiidiotype responses. The hyperimmune sera specifically recognized tumor cells expressing GD2. One complete response (CR) and six instances of stable disease were achieved (38). Based on these results, a randomized phase 3 adjuvant trial with KLH/GM2 plus QS-21 was initiated in stage 2 and 3 melanoma patients by the Eastern Cooperative Oncology Group, the Southwest Oncology Group, the North Central Cancer Treatment Group, Cancer and Leukemia Group B,

Memorial Sloan-Kettering Cancer Center, and M. D. Anderson Cancer Center (39).

Incomplete Freund's Adjuvant

Incomplete Freund's Adjuvant (IFA) is composed of mineral oil and the emulsifier Arlacel A. It is the less toxic counterpart of CFA that includes *Mycobacterium tuberculosis*. Notwithstanding its long history of use in humans with only moderate toxicity, it has not been approved for commercial use (40). Despite its tendency to cause sterile abscesses and cysts, as well as carcinogenicity in mice, IFA does not appear to increase mortality, tumors, or autoimmunity in human recipients (7).

IFA has been included in tumor-associated peptide-based immunotherapeutics for patients with cervical cancer (41) and melanoma (42,43). In each instance, peptide epitopes were admixed with IFA before vaccination. In the melanoma study, 13 of 31 patients (42%) showed objective clinical responses (43). All melanoma patients received IL-2 in addition to IFA/gp100, however, making it difficult to assess the contribution of IFA to the observed effects. Enhanced T-cell reactivity *in vitro* could be demonstrated after treatment (44,45). Once again, though, it was not possible to separate the individual contributions made by IFA and IL-2 to the increased CTL and cytokine secretion observed in patient immune cells posttreatment versus pretreatment.

MF59

A number of submicron particulate adjuvants are under development as potential adjuvants for cancer treatment. MF59, a squalene-water emulsion, was planned as a delivery vehicle for the synthetic muramyl peptide MTP-PE. Early in its development, MF59 demonstrated an immunostimulatory capacity approaching that of the Freund's adjuvants, but without the concomitant toxicity (46). In fact, it was observed that the MTP-PE portion of the MF59-MTP-PE complex was responsible for the induction of major side effects. Further, the MTP-PE segment was inessential to evoke antibody reactivity. As a result, MF59 emulsion has been studied as a stand-alone intramuscular adjuvant. It has been further refined to reduce the size of the emulsion droplets from 1–2 μm to 200–300. This has resulted in a substantial increase in adjuvant activity, possibly owing to enhanced uptake of the smaller droplets by macrophages (7). A recombinant form of herpes simplex virus (HSV) type 2 (gD2) was complexed with MF59 and injected into Balb/C mice. Humoral responses of mice given MF59 were compared with animals injected with gD2 encapsulated into microparticles (47). The MF59 induced greater levels of serum IL-4 and IL-5 cytokines, implying a more Th2-type response. The microparticles induced more serum IFN-γ and IgG2a production, suggesting more of a Th1-type response. MF59 was again combined with gD2 in a 1998 report investigating how the immune system processes this adjuvant (48). MF59/gD2 was labeled with a fluorescent dye and injected intramuscularly into BALB/c mice. Only 3 hours after injection, a small portion of the MF59 could be detected in the subcapsular sinus of draining lymph nodes. At 48 hours, a majority of the MF59 was found within DEC-205[+], MHC class II[+] antigen-presenting cells. This observation strongly indicated that the vaccine was efficiently taken up by DCs. During this time, intracellular MF59 was also abundant in the paracortical (T cell) region of lymph nodes. This report indicates that MF59 interacts with DCs and later migrates to the draining lymph nodes, the site of efficient antigen presentation to naïve T cells (48).

MF59 has received its most extensive testing, more than 8,000 patients in several studies, combined with recombinant gp120 protein from human immunodeficiency virus–1, cytomegalovirus, HSV (7), influenza, and other viruses. It maintains an impressive record of safety and potency in seronegative and seropositive subjects (40,47). When combined with HSV type 2 in a phase 1/2 clinical trial, MF59 elicited antibody levels equivalent to that obtained with alum. Strong helper T-cell responses were induced as well (49). Safety and efficacy studies using MF59 as an adjuvant with cancer immunotherapy are planned.

PARTICULATE ADJUVANTS

Immune-Stimulating Complexes

Immune-stimulating complexes are hydrophobically bonded micelles that are produced naturally after the admixture of cholesterol, lipid, and saponins (50). Immune-stimulating complexes form a particle of repeating units icosahedral in shape, approximately 30 to 40 nm in diameter (51). They were developed to enhance immunogenicity by: (a) physical presentation in the form of particles with multimeric formation of surface antigens, (b) guiding vaccine antigens to antigen-presenting cells and to the appropriate intracellular processing pathway, and (c) immune modulation (52). The saponin portion is derived from aqueous extracts of bark from the South American tree *Quillaja saponaria*. Although the extract is complex, the adjuvant activity is associated with the saponin component (53). During their creation, they may be combined with other moieties, such as hydrophobic glycoproteins or hydrophilic/amphipathic proteins (54). The ability to modify the chemical structure of immune-stimulating complexes greatly broadened their applicability.

Liposomes

The use of liposomes for targeted immunogen delivery has several favorable characteristics: (a) low cost, (b) low toxicity, (c) is itself a nonimmunogenic carrier, (d) stable, (e) biodegradable, and (f) can act synergistically with other agents (55). In the last decade, technical improvements simplified their construction and facilitated large-scale preparation. By using this improvement involving dehydration and rehydration, small vesicles are produced (~100 nm), which have the ability to hold onto most of the loaded solute (55,56). Positively charged multilamellar vehicles are actively phagocytized by macrophages, beginning the cascade of events that culminate in the induction of CTLs (57–59). Negatively charged liposomes encapsulating OVA markedly bolstered IFN-γ production in mice vaccinated only once without boosting.

For a humoral antitumor approach, immunoliposomes are manufactured via linkage of antibody to a hydrophobic moiety stably integrated in the lipid bilayer (60). The antibody can be covalently or noncovalently attached to the hydrophobic region. Noncovalent linkages (e.g., to streptavidin or avidin), however, impart a strong binding constant to the molecule. The drawback of this approach is the potential immunogenicity of bulky side chains. It is largely for this reason that covalent coupling chemistry was developed (61). Complexing with lipid also promoted the monoclonal antibody stability in the circulation, increasing the terminal plasma half-life in rats fivefold as compared with its native form. In addition, the ability to detect the anti-HER2/neu immunoliposomes in the plasma 10 hours after vaccination indicated insignificant leakage or disassociation (60). Biodistribution and tumor localization studies further confirmed confidence in this adjuvant. The ability of immunoliposomes to treat established tumor xenografts was demonstrated in several nude mouse model reports (61,62). In another active treatment report, Zhou et al. (63) prolonged the survival of mice bearing an OVA-expressing tumor by immunization with OVA encapsulated in liposomes. Antitumor efficacy was ascribed to CTLs because cytolytic activity, not specific antibody, was detected.

The capacity of cytokines to enhance and regulate antitumor immunity made them attractive candidates to be combined with a liposomal delivery system. Owing to the superior efficacy of negatively charged liposomes, the charge and hydrophobicity of the cytokine had to be considered. Highly hydrophobic cytokines, such as IL-2, demonstrate incorporation rates of more than 80% (64). IL-2 was one of the first cytokines to demonstrate adjuvant activity in murine experiments, so it was not unexpected that it was the first to be tested as a vaccine adjuvant in concert with liposomes. Guinea pigs with established HSV-2 infections were given overlapping vaccinations with IL-2 liposomes and a soluble form of HSV-2 glycoprotein. Animals treated with both vaccinations showed a 70% decrease in disease recurrence compared with a 30% decrease for those animals given either agent alone. Soluble IL-2 was not beneficial. Importantly, it was demonstrated that a substantial clearance of the liposomal complex to regional lymph nodes occurred (65). In a similar study, male CD-1 mice received two injections intramuscularly with several tetanus toxoid-containing liposome formulations with or without IL-2/liposome complex. Secondary humoral immunity, as evidenced by IgG$_1$ secretion, was maximal when IL-2 was complexed with liposome-entrapped toxoid. IL-2 plus liposome-entrapped toxoid additionally augmented IgG$_{2a}$ and IgG$_{2b}$ titers, indicating concurrent induction of Th1 and Th2 cells (66). IL-1α, IL-7, TNF-α, and IFN-γ have also been efficiently incorporated into liposomes, and their adjuvant activity has been demonstrated in *in vivo* animal studies (64).

BACTERIAL PRODUCTS AND DERIVATIVES

Bacillus Calmette-Guérin

BCG is a modified form of the *Tubercle bacillus*. It is most often used alone or admixed with tumor cells or lysates. It causes an inflammatory reaction at the site of administration, resulting in the recruitment and activation of macrophages, production of chemokines, and secretion of immunomodulators, such as IFN-γ, IL-2, and TNF-α. The putative mechanism of its antitumor activity is finally being elucidated. It is thought that it can induce antigen-specific effector cells, B and T lymphocytes, at the site of administration. Rapid proliferation and migration of specific immune effectors results in systemic response. It was established that BCG has profound effects on DCs, arguably the most efficient antigen-presenting cells in the body's arsenal. This is important because Langerhans' cells, a type of DC found primarily in the skin, is likely the first antigen-presenting cell to uptake antigen after intradermal or subcutaneous injection of BCG, its most common route of administration. Addition of BCG expedited homotypic adhesion of DCs. BCG increases expression of the DC maturation antigen CD83 and of the T-cell costimulator CD86 (B7-2) in a dose-dependent manner (67). BCG bacteria stimulates TNF-α gene transcription and TNF-α protein release from DCs also in a dose-dependent fashion. Furthermore, BCG augments the DC-derived production of IL-8, a potent chemokine of T cells and granulocytes, as well as the T-cell stimulatory potential of human DCs (68).

Since the 1970s, BCG administration has resulted in clinical regression of tumor. Morton et al. (69) injected BCG into the lesions of patients with cutaneous melanoma, resulting in tumor regression in five of eight subjects. In a study of 668 stage 2 melanoma patients, all those initially nonreactive to BCG became tuberculin-positive during treatment. The instances of disease-free and overall survival were statistically greater for those with negative skin reactivity before therapy (70). Over the years, BCG has been used in several studies as a postoperative adjuvant for those with high-risk primary metastatic lesions or lymph nodes (71–75). The number of patients varied from 30 to 327, and the duration of follow-up ranged from 1.8 to 6.0 years. None of these trials could demonstrate a significant impact of BCG on overall survival, disease-free survival, or recurrence. Berd and coworkers (76) treated 64 patients with melanoma, injecting a vaccine consisting of autologous, enzymatically dissociated, irradiated tumor mixed with BCG. Of 40 evaluable subjects, four partial responses (PRs) and one CR were achieved, with a median duration of 10 months. Delayed-type hypersensitivity (DTH) responses increased significantly during therapy, although any clinical correlation was not investigated.

Since the 1980s, BCG has remained the standard treatment for superficial bladder cancer (77–80) after transurethral resection owing to the 40% to 80% recurrence rate after surgery (81). The local cellular immune response in the bladder wall of patients receiving BCG has been studied. After a 6-week regimen, results showed a marker infiltration of T cells and mononuclear cells, mostly in suburothelial tissue. The ratio of Th:T suppressor cells in the bladder wall increased fourfold and remained detectable in biopsies for more than 1 year from treatment onset (82,83). No difference in lymphocyte infiltration pre- versus post-BCG treatment was observed in nonresponding subjects. The interaction of fibronectin on the extracellular matrix of the mycobacteria with tumor cells is thought to help prevent tumor cell motility (84).

BCG has been combined with mitomycin C to try to further reduce the rate of recurrence in patients with intermediate and high-risk papillary superficial bladder cancer *in situ* (85). Treatment benefit was not significantly different with regard to time to initial recurrence (p = .53), frequency of recurrence (p = .36), progression (p = .70), or survival (p = .16). In a large, retrospective study organized by the European Organization for Research and Treatment of Cancer (86), 344 patients with papillary superficial bladder cancer *in situ* were randomized after resection to receive six weekly instillations with BCG or four weekly instillations with mitomycin C. Investigators were not able to establish that BCG was more effective than mitomycin C as a treatment option in high-risk patients with regard to disease recurrence.

The potential clinical benefit of BCG adjuvant therapy with other cancer types has been more difficult to assess. A prospective randomized trial at the Cross Cancer Institute (87) reported no therapeutic benefit of BCG treatment for 253 patients with Dukes' stage B_2 and C colorectal cancer after curative surgery. These findings contrasted with a 1984 report from The Johns Hopkins University (88) that demonstrated a significant enhancement in time to recurrence and disease-free survival for patients with stage B_2, C, or D colon cancer receiving BCG. In 1999, Vermoken et al. (89) randomized 254 patients with stage II or III colon cancer to receive three weekly vaccinations of autologous tumor cells and BCG or no additional treatment. A significant improvement in recurrence-free disease (p = .011) was obtained in stage II patients given active specific immunotherapy. In the studies demonstrating no treatment benefit, BCG was administered orally after surgery. In those studies reporting clinical efficacy, active specific immunotherapy (BCG was admixed with autologous tumor cells) was used. And so, conclusions are difficult because of the different protocols used. Different conclusions were also reached in two large clinical trials investigating the role of BCG in the treatment of non-Hodgkin's lymphoma (16,90).

In a large study of BCG-based active specific immunotherapy and RCC, 120 cancer patients were randomized to two groups: control (receiving no treatment) or experimental (receiving three weekly intradermal injections of 10^7 autologous irradiated tumor cells mixed with 10^7 BCG) (91). Fifty patients were classified as stages I–II with the remaining 70 patients classified as stage III according to the tumor node metastasis staging system. Treatment commenced 4 weeks after surgery to permit the subject to recover from any immunosuppression brought on by surgery and anesthesia. No systemic toxicity was observed. One month after the final injection, 38 of 54 immunized and evaluable subjects demonstrated a significant DTH response to tumor but not normal cells. Positive DTH responses were durable, remaining positive at 12 months follow-up in 16 of 28 patients. No enhancement of disease-free or overall survival was observed with patients given tumor/BCG therapy. Further, the contribution of BCG to the induction of DTH responses could not be determined because no subjects were given autologous tumor without BCG.

Reports of BCG adjuvant therapy for prostate cancer are infrequent. In 1982, Guinan and coworkers (92) randomized 42 patients with advanced prostate cancer to receive conventional therapy (consisting of exogenous estrogens and/or orchiectomy or observation alone) with or without four monthly injections of BCG. Forty-four percent of subjects receiving BCG had grade I or II tumors, whereas 62% of control patients had low-grade disease. Performance status and alkaline phosphatase levels were not significantly different between groups. The BCG-treated patients demonstrated a mean survival of 38 weeks compared with 28 weeks in control patients (p <.05). The BCG-treated patients, however, had a significantly reduced rate of infections, and so investigators acknowledged that this, rather than BCG-mediated tumoricidal activity, might account for the enhanced survival.

Oligodeoxynucleotides

Several diverse groups of bacterial proteins, such as lipopolysaccharide (93,94) are capable of inducing immune cell activation or increasing immune function (95). Bacterial DNA—but not mammalian DNA—activated B-cell proliferation and antibody secretion, whereas mammalian DNA did not (96). It is postulated that lymphocyte activation by bacterial DNA represents an early immune defense system in humans capable of distinguishing bacterial from host genetic material (97). Investigations of bacterial DNA mitogenicity revealed that CpG dinucleotides were detected at a frequency of 1 per 16 dinucleotides; approximately 25% as common in vertebrates and with markedly hypomethylated cytosines (98). Methylation of bacterial CpG motifs abrogated mitogenicity as determined by proliferative assay (98). Pretreatment of CpG motifs with deoxyribonuclease totally abolished lymphocyte stimulation, indicating that the observed effects were not owing to other culture components (96). Antigen-restricted B-cell activation by bacteria DNA requires antigen binding, as well as costimulation. Indeed, CpG oligonucleotides were able to provide such costimulatory signals by the synergistic activation of antigen-specific Ig production in the mouse B-cell line CH12.LX, which contains an antigen receptor for binding sheep red blood cells (98).

The molecular mechanism responsible for the immunostimulatory effects of oligonucleotides remains largely unclear. CpG motifs stimulated nuclear factor-κB (NF-κB) by inducing a reactive oxygen intermediate–dependent pathway. After enhanced NF-κB activity, increased levels of IL-6, a cytokine produced in response to microbial infection, were detected (99). Plasmid DNA was ingested by bone marrow–derived macrophages, as well as the macrophage cell line RAW 263, whereas methylated CpG dinucleotides were not (100). Ingestion induced a signaling pathway leading to NF-κB activation, and inflammatory gene (TNF-α) induction was demonstrated as indicated by Northern blot and electromobility shift analysis. To assess whether such effects occurred *in vivo*, mice were injected with bacterial DNA or calf thymus DNA. Within 4 hours of treatment, only the mice receiving injections with bacterial DNA demonstrated an increase in serum IFN-γ titers. Splenic natural killer (NK) cells from mice immunized with bacterial DNA were also induced to secrete IFN-γ (101).

In animal studies, Weiner and associates (97) used the 38C13 B-cell lymphoma model in which the idiotype (Id) of the 38C13 surface IgM acts as a highly specific tumor-associated antigen (102). Mice were immunized with 50 μg KLH, along with oligodeoxynucleotides (ODN) or CFA. The ODN-containing CpG motifs induced the greatest amounts of anti-Id IgG2a (more effective than IgG1 at mediating antibody-dependent cellular cytotoxicity) and IgM as compared with ODN without such motifs. The absence of nonspecific IgM indicated that the humoral activity was directed against the idiotype of the 38C13 IgM. For *in vivo* survival experiments, mice received a single vaccination followed 2 weeks later by 38C13 cell administration. Mice given Id-KLH and CFA showed a median survival of 42 days with two animals remaining free of disease. Mice given Id-KLH and CpG ODN showed a median survival of 51 days with four animals remaining free of disease. In a subsequent study, the 38C13 model was again used to demonstrate the benefit of ODN and granulocyte-macrophage colony-stimulating factor (GM-CSF) combination therapy (103). CpG ODN and GM-CSF were additive in their ability to evoke anti-Id IgG after vaccination with Id-KLH. It was noteworthy that repeated vaccinations shifted the response from IgG1 to primarily IgG2a. In a 3-day tumor protection experiment, ODN plus GM-CSF resulted in 70% of mice remaining disease free—a superior finding compared with either agent by itself. Similar experiments demonstrated enhanced survival in mice treated with a combination of ODN plus IL-2 (104). Direct application of CgG ODN had no direct effect on tumor cell growth, and only minor treatment benefit was observed in the group immunized with CpG ODN alone. Therefore, it was most likely that the observed effects were owing to the CpG ODN–induced production of cytokines that caused greater susceptibility of the tumor cells to antibody-mediated cell cytotoxicity. Having established a relationship between ODN and B and NK cells, researchers went on to investigate the connection between ODN and human DCs. *In vitro*, treatment with CpG ODN induced the maturation of murine fetal skin DCs. That is, E-cadherin–mediated adhesion diminished, MHC class II was upregulated, and the cell surface expression of costimulatory molecules (CD40, CD80, CD86) increased. *In vivo*, CpG ODN injection augmented IL-12 production by DCs but had no effect on keratinocytes, indicating that, at least in murine skin, immunostimulatory DNA acted primarily on DCs (105). Lastly, the observation that subcutaneous injection of CpG ODN caused regional lymphadenopathy suggested that DCs activated by bacterial DNA could properly migrate to lymph nodes and, as per their normal function, stimulate DCs in lymphoid tissue.

Monophosphoryl Lipid A

Monophosphoryl lipid A (MPL) is produced after the acid hydrolysis of purified bacterial cell walls (16). This reaction produces a safe, immunogenic adjuvant. In the 1990s, MPL was shown to be nontoxic in mice and capable of increasing the extent of antibody responses to pneumococcal polysaccharides (106). In 1998, a vaccine construct consisting of a MUC-1–derived 24-MER synthetic peptide encapsulated with MPL in liposomes was tested in a mouse mammary adenocarcinoma model (107). Low-dose human MUC-1 peptide (5 µg) with MPL in liposomes given subcutaneously or intravenously generated enhanced survival and decreased the number of established lung metastases when administered three times before tumor

challenge. The protective antitumor activity correlated with a Th1-type immune response involving MUC-1–restricted T-cell proliferation and the specific production of IgG2a antibodies.

As an adjuvant in humans, MPL has most frequently been used as a component of DETOX. DETOX is an adjuvant made up of detoxified MPL from *Salmonella minnesota*, cell wall skeletons of *Mycobacterium phlei*, squalane oil, and emulsifier (108). Schultz et al. (109) immunized 19 patients with resected stage III melanoma using a polyvalent melanoma antigen vaccine (40 µg) admixed with DETOX three times weekly for 4 weeks in a dose-escalation trial. A nonrandomized control group of 35 patients were immunized using the vaccine admixed with alum. A significantly greater percentage of patients receiving DETOX developed antibody responses. The DTH responses were similar for the two groups. Nevertheless, median disease-free survival was significantly better for the group receiving alum, thereby showing little treatment benefit for DETOX. Similarly, only two durable responses out of 42 patients were reported in a study of active immunotherapy with ultraviolet B–irradiated autologous whole melanoma cells plus DETOX (110). A randomized phase 2 study of sialyl-Tn and DETOX for 23 patients with breast cancer also demonstrated enhanced humoral immunity but little clinical impact (111). In contrast, Mitchell et al. (112) achieved promising results from several phase 1, 2, and 3 studies of two mechanically disrupted melanoma cell lines (M-1 and M-2 cell lines, also known as *Melacine*) injected subcutaneously along with the adjuvant DETOX. In one phase 1/2 report (108), 25 subjects were given 200 antigenic units (2×10^7 tumor cell equivalents) along with 0.25 mL of DETOX (consisting of 250 µg of cell wall skeletons and 25 µg of MPL) subcutaneously on weeks 1, 2, 3, 4, and 6. Adverse events were minimal and without anaphylactic reactions. Nineteen percent (20 of 106 patients) had objective tumor regression of tumor masses, including five CR. The median duration of response was 46 months. A strong association existed between clinical response and an increase in CTL activity, although antibody production did not correlate with treatment outcome (108). In a phase 3 study in patients with resected stage III melanoma, melacine plus DETOX again showed therapeutic benefit (113). A 66% overall survival rate was attained with a median relapse-free survival time of 36 months. All subjects responded to or failed treatment by 4 months after treatment onset.

IMMUNOGENIC PROTEINS AND PEPTIDES

Keyhole Limpet Hemocyanin

KLH is a powerful immunostimulatory protein that is produced by the mollusk *Megathura crenulata*. Originally, the capacity of KLH to evoke IgM, IgG, and DTH responses in normal recipients inspired subsequent studies in cancer patients. In earlier cancer investigations, it was used primarily as a carrier molecule for those immunotherapeutic approaches using haptens. More recently, its role has expanded to include acting as a surrogate marker of immunologic memory, providing a nonspecific indication about the effectiveness of the vaccine in enhancing a recipient's tumor antigen-specific immune responses.

Moltro and coworkers showed that KLH augmented NK cell activity in patients with transitional cell carcinoma of the bladder. Most studies have shown that KLH primarily elicits a CD4⁺ T-cell response (82,83). Jurincic-Winkler et al. (114) confirmed that KLH administered intravesically enhanced local cellular immunity within the bladder wall of patients with superficial bladder carcinoma. Twelve patients underwent complete tumor resections immediately before six weekly treatments with 20 mg KLH in saline followed by monthly treatments for the balance of 1 year. Using immunohistochemistry, they noted a marked infiltration of immunocompetent cells into the bladder wall 6 weeks into treatment. The majority of the cell infiltrate into the submucosa were CD4⁺ T cells, but CD8⁺ T cells and B cells were also observed to a lesser extent. The immunophenotypic characteristics of the control group (recipients without malignant bladder disease or cystitis) was similar. HLA-DR–positive cells were found in bladder walls with the number of such cells increasing during treatment and persistent up to 9 months of follow-up. NK cells and macrophages were rare, confirming previous findings (115). Several studies with bladder cancer patients demonstrated that KLH given subcutaneously (116) or intravesically (114,117,118) produced a reduction in tumor burden without major side effects. Yet, no clinical responses were shown. Nestle et al. (119) vaccinated 16 melanoma patients with autologous DCs pulsed with melanoma-derived peptides or tumor lysates combined with KLH. All patients displayed a positive immune response to KLH as demonstrated by a KLH-restricted DTH response. It could then be implied that KLH helped evoke a more vibrant and durable Th-cell response—two patients still had positive DTH reactions more than 6 months after their final treatment. All groups received KLH. Thus, it remains to be conclusively established that KLH administration enhances tumor regression *in vivo*, despite its ability to augment immunity. It certainly is valid to state, however, that KLH acts as a neoantigen of great potency, permitting investigators to monitor the induction of specific immune reactivity (119).

Pan-DR Epitope

The numerous reasons for eliciting Th activity led to the development of artificial Th pan (HLA)-DR epitopes (PADRE). This group of nonnatural peptides has a polyalanine backbone and bind with intermediate or high affinity to nine of ten common HLA-DR specificities (120). The idea for this approach arose from research suggesting that bulk or charged side chains, oriented at angles away from the DR-peptide complex, are frequently recognized as immunodominant regions (121). PADRE peptides were more strongly immunostimulatory to peripheral blood mononuclear cells *in vitro* as compared with the tetanus toxoid peptides previously used to elicit Th cells (120). Several PADRE peptides of various lengths and forms (mono- and multimeric) have been studied. Some variants cross-react with particular murine MHC class II alleles, thereby establishing the ability of PADRE epitopes to provide T-cell help for MHC class I–restricted immune responses (122). From the murine experiments arose studies concerning human cancer and infectious disease. One of the types of cancers investigated involved those containing p53 mutations. p53 is a cellular regulatory molecule,

which is overexpressed in approximately 50% of all malignant cells (123,124). Moreover, its overexpression frequently is associated with poor prognosis. Yu and coworkers (125) immunized HLA-A2.1 transgenic mice with immunodominant p53 peptide epitopes (p53$_{149-157}$ and p53$_{264-272}$) in conjunction with PADRE peptides in IFA. CTL with strong affinity to the p53 peptides were elicited. CTL were cytolytic against the established breast carcinoma cell line MDA-MB231 (HLA-A2.1⁺ and overexpressing p53), but without concurrent lysis of human HLA-A2.1⁺ cells displaying normal p53 expression. The specific lytic activity confirmed earlier findings that showed vaccination with p53 peptides resulted in potent antitumor efficacy against murine tumors overexpressing mutated murine p53 (126). The precise contribution, however, of PADRE peptides in cancer vaccines targeting p53 or other gene products remains unclear.

CYTOKINES

Interleukin-2

IL-2 is produced principally by Th cells and induces the activation and proliferation of a variety of cells (127), including T cells, NK cells, macrophages, epidermal Langerhans' cells, and oligodendrocytes (4). IL-2 also enhances the secretion of cytokines, such as IFN-γ and TNF-α (128). Initial work using murine tumor models indicated that IL-2 could retard the development of 3-day liver and lung micrometastases in a dose-dependent fashion (129). A phase 1 clinical trial with IL-2 therapy alone was unsatisfactory, as none of 66 metastatic melanoma patients responded to treatment (130). The balance of escalated dose of IL-2 with minimal treatment-related mortality (>1.5%) and acceptable toxicity resulted in a 15% combined CR plus PR against several cancers, including melanoma, renal, colorectal, breast cancer, and non-Hodgkin's lymphoma (131). In a 1998 study, IL-2 adjuvant therapy was combined with immunodominant peptides from the gp100 melanoma-associated antigens and IFA. Based on *in vitro* immune monitoring analysis, 91% of patients were successfully immunized with these synthetic peptides. *In vivo*, 13 of 31 patients (42%) receiving the peptide vaccine plus IL-2 had objective cancer responses, and four additional patients demonstrated mixed or minor responses (43).

Some clinical benefit was observed in 29 patients with stage IV colorectal cancer who received 15 doses of IL-2 and IFN-α with only four partial responses (17%) (132). Even fewer clinical responders resulted from bolus IL-2 administration combined with the adoptive transfer of anti-CD3–stimulated T-killer cells (133). Also, capillary leak syndrome was observed in several of these reports.

The approach of combining IL-2 with lymphokine-activated killer (LAK) cells most commonly harvested from peripheral blood and activated *in vitro* was first studied in a clinical trial of 180 patients treated with IL-2 and LAK cells, which resulted in a CR plus PR rate of 35% and 21% for RCC and melanoma, respectively (134,135). Duration of response varied from 1 month to more than 5 years. Histologic analysis of subcutaneous melanoma lesions revealed widespread infiltration of lymphocytes, suggesting that the mechanism of action was enhancement of local immune reactivity (129). Another report concerned six melanoma patients who had failed previous treatment with chemotherapy and isolated perfusion. They were treated with 7 to 16×10^9 LAK cells plus bolus IL-2. All six responded to some degree with four PR, one CR, and one patient with stable disease (136). Blay et al. (137) gave a continuous infusion of IL-2 (20 to 28×10^6 units per m^2 per course) in combination with LAK cells (4.8 to 7.5×10^{10}) to 25 patients with metastatic RCC and achieved a 20% overall response rate. A larger follow-up phase 1/2 trial treated 68 evaluable RCC patients with a combination of IL-2, LAK, and IFN-α (138). Four (24%; three CR, one PR) and 19 responders (37%; 6 CR, 13 PR) were obtained in the phase 1 and 2 trials, respectively. No patient was administered only IL-2 and LAK, so it was not possible to assess if the IFN-α accounted for the enhanced clinical efficacy as compared with the previous report (137).

IL-2 has also been used as an adjuvant in tumor-infiltrating lymphocyte (TIL) studies. Abundant IL-2 receptors on the surface of TIL permitted *in vitro* expansion by culturing in the presence of IL-2 (129). After *in vitro* growth with IL-2 and autologous tumor, TIL demonstrated cytolytic activity against autologous and HLA-matched allogeneic tumors of murine, as well as human, origin (139–142). Most likely, the largest study on the therapeutic benefit of IL-2/TIL immunotherapy reported on a 5-year experience with 86 metastatic melanoma patients treated with autologous TIL and high-dose bolus IL-2 (720,000 IU per kg at 8-hour intervals) (143). Thirty-four percent of patients displayed a partial or complete clinical response, which compared favorably with the 17% overall response rate observed in melanoma or RCC patients receiving only high-dose IL-2 (135).

A combined regimen of TIL, IL-2, and IFN-α was used to treat 11 patients with metastatic RCC. IFN-α alone was given before radical nephrectomy, as well as in conjunction with IL-2 (6×10^6 U per m^2 per day IFN-α, 2×10^6 U per m^2 per day IL-2) during the weeks of TIL infusion. $0.14–16 \times 10^{10}$ TIL were infused, containing mostly (>80%) CD3$^+$ T cells and an average ratio of 2:1 CD8$^+$:CD4$^+$ lymphocytes. The treatment was fairly toxic. Reversible thyroid dysfunction, mild to moderate fever, chills, fatigue, diarrhea, and nausea occurred in at least nine of ten evaluable patients. In this and a second similar investigation, a 32% total response rate was observed (seven CR, three PR) with disease-free survival lasting more than 3 and one-half years (144).

Interleukin-4

IL-4 expression is limited to T cells, mast cells, basophils, and eosinophils, unlike several other cytokines that are expressed by various hematopoietic and nonhematopoietic cell lineages (145). Development of type II T-cell cytokine profiles is strongly affected by IL-4 (146), although the cell source during this process is uncertain (147). IL-4 augments the ontogeny of B lymphocytes by enhancing their activation, proliferation, and differentiation. It upregulates the expression of MHC class II antigens, human leukocyte function-associated antigen-1 (148). It increases CTL cytotoxicity (149) and stimulates lytic activity and expansion of TIL *in vitro* (150). IL-4 also has profound

effects on the generation of DCs from precursors of the monocytic lineage pathway (151–154), in part by downregulating CD14 expression (148). In conjunction with phase 1 clinical testing, IL-4 injections produced moderate eosinophilia in all 17 cancer patients (155). Systemic eosinophil degranulation was noted based on dose-dependent elevations in serum major basic protein and urine major basic protein. Blood samples from eight patients showed enhanced eosinophil survival that could be abrogated by antibodies to IL-3, IL-5, and GM-CSF. Cells previously activated before IL-4 exposure generally exhibited increased proliferation and biologic function. Yet, if already activated before IL-4 exposure, the same cell types could be similarly inhibited (156).

Earlier animal studies focused on the ability of IL-4 to demonstrate antitumor efficacy against a variety of tumors, including chemically induced fibrosarcoma, spontaneous adenocarcinoma, melanoma, and RCC (16). In 1998, Husain and coworkers (157) further expanded the potential clinical benefit of IL-4 by analyzing its activity in the treatment of glioblastoma. It had been previously determined that: (a) glioblastoma cells express IL-4 receptors with high affinity, and (b) a chimeric molecule consisting of IL-4 and *Pseudomonas* exotoxin was highly cytolytic in a dose-dependent fashion (158). Female athymic nude mice were implanted with the U251 human glioblastoma cell line by subcutaneous injection into the flank, generating tumors in less than 6 days. Animals given the IL-4/endotoxin chimeric protein intratumorally on alternate days for 3 to 4 days demonstrated a complete remission of small and large tumors without accompanying toxicity. A marked antitumor response was observed as well with intravenous and intraperitoneal administration of chimeric protein. A phase 1 clinical trial for the treatment of recurrent glioma using intratumoral vaccination with IL-4 toxin is planned.

By 1994, the safety and tolerability of recombinant human IL-4 (rhIL-4) was established in phase 2 and 3 studies in human subjects with several different cancers at doses as high as 5 μg per kg per day (159). A phase 2 clinical trial of rhIL-4 involved 36 patients with malignant melanoma and no previous systemic therapy for metastatic disease (156). Subjects received 5 μg per kg per day subcutaneous injections for 1 to 28 days succeeded by a 7-day rest period, then another cycle. Aggressive supportive care was implemented to try to prevent serious side effects that could force a dose reduction. Although 68% (23/36) of subjects developed at least one grade 3 or 4 toxicity distinct from elevated liver function tests (the most frequent side effect), all but three completed treatment. One durable CR (15+ months) and two cases of stable disease were achieved. The areas of tumor that were eliminated in the lone CR were a large cervical lymph node and several minute lung nodules. The estimated median survival was 6 months. Serum levels of IL-4 were not measured. Therefore, although the clinical responses were minimal, it remained unknown whether the IL-4 levels previously shown to display antitumorigenicity *in vitro* (160) had been reached *in vivo*. Some degree of therapeutic benefit was also observed in a phase 2 clinical trial of rhIL-4 for patients with recurrent or advanced non–small-cell lung cancer (101). Of the 63 subjects enrolled, eleven had stage IIIB disease and 53 had stage IV disease. Patients were randomized to receive low-dose (0.25 μg per kg) or high-dose (1.0 μg per kg) rhIL-4 injected subcutaneously three times per week. The regimen consisted of at least two cycles of 4 weeks' duration each or until disease progression or severe toxicity occurred. No grade IV toxicity developed in either group. No cardiac toxicity was observed. One patient per group discontinued treatment owing to toxicity. The most common side effects at both dosages were mild to moderate fever and rigors. One PR (1 of 41 patients; 2.5%) and eight cases of stable disease (8 of 41 patients; 20%) were achieved in the high-dose group. Only a single case (1 of 22 patients; 5%) of stable disease was achieved in the low-dose group. No significant difference existed between the dosage groups in median survival time or the percentage of subjects alive after 1 year. The promising percentage of subjects at the higher dose with decreased disease progression combined with the lack of dose-limiting toxicity has led to ongoing clinical testing using rhIL-4 at higher doses in patients with stage IV non–small-cell lung cancer.

Interleukin-12

IL-12, a heterodimeric cytokine first demonstrated as being secreted by phagocytic cells as part of the innate immune repertoire, has lately shown antitumor potency. It is produced by many kinds of immune cells, including macrophages, monocytes, B cells, granulocytes, keratinocytes, mast cells, and DCs. It induces the maturation and proliferation of preactivated T and NK cells and augments T- and NK-mediated cytolytic activity. IL-12 stimulates T and NK cells to make several cytokines, such as IFN-γ, TNF-α, IL-2, IL-3, IL-8, IL-10, and numerous colony-stimulating factors. It also directs the naïve Th cell towards a Th1 (effector cell) phenotype while at the same time promoting its expansion (161–163). IL-12 does not exert its antitumor effects directly (164,165), probably because only T cells, NK cells, and DCs express the cognate receptor. The effect of IL-12 on DCs has just been elucidated. DCs contain IL-12 receptors, and signaling via this receptor involves activating members of the NF-κB family for DNA binding (166). Recombinant IL-12 primes purified DCs exogenously pulsed with tumor peptides *in vitro* for potent sensitization *in vivo* (167,168).

Brunda and colleagues (169) administered systemic IL-12 five times per week for a total of 4 weeks to mice previously injected with B16F10 melanoma cells. Tumor growth was markedly diminished, even when treatment did not begin until day 28 when tumors were well established. Antitumorigenicity resulted largely from the contribution of CD8+ cells and not as much from CD4+ or NK cells. Studies involving antiangiogenic factors capable of cutting off a tumor's blood supply by preventing new vessel formation or by blocking those already formed suggested an additional role for IL-12 in tumor inhibition. Voest et al. (170) examined the effect of IL-12 in a model of basic fibroblast growth factor–induced corneal neovascularization in normal and immunodeficient mouse strains. In normal, T-cell–deficient and in T- and B-cell–deficient mice, IL-12 injection strongly abolished vessel formation. The effect could be reversed by concurrent administration of antiinterferon monoclonal antibodies, indicating that antiangiogenesis was mediated through this cytokine (170). But, in a previous study, injection of anti-NK cell monoclonal antibody, not anti-IFN-γ monoclonal antibody, abrogated the enhancement of IFN-γ–producing T cells (171). These findings imply that IL-12 may promote an antitumor effect via more than one pathway, including one distinct from that mediated via various immune effector cells. After the observation that tumors in IL-12–treated mice displayed a severely diminished system of blood vessels, it was established that IL-12 promoted production of an antiangiogenic protein, IPO-10, and became the basis of an IL-12–based phase 1 clinical trial for the treatment of kidney cancer (172).

A phase 1 dose-escalation study to assess safety, maximum tolerated dose, pharmacokinetics, and antitumor activity after intravenous injection of rhIL-12 was reported in 1997 (173). Patients received escalating doses (3 to 1,000 ng per kg per day) of rhIL-12 via bolus intravenous infusion. The regimen consisted of one injection followed by a 2-week rest period, and then once daily for 5 days every 3 weeks. Forty patients participated, including 20 with RCC, 12 with melanoma, and five with colon cancer. Routine toxicities included fever, chills, fatigue, nausea, vomiting, and headache. Common laboratory affects included anemia, neutropenia, lymphopenia, hyperglycemia, thrombocytopenia, and hypoalbuminemia. The dose-limiting toxicities included oral stomatitis and abnormal liver function tests. The elimination half-life was between 5.3 and 10.3 hours. One RCC patient achieved a partial tumor regression that was still ongoing after 2 years. One melanoma patient achieved a complete regression of small pleural-based nodules and cervical adenopathy lasting 4 weeks. None of the 14 patients injected at the maximum tolerated dose demonstrated a clinical response. Owing to the low number of patients per dose level and prior immunotherapy, it was not possible to assess the therapeutic benefit of rhIL-12. It should be mentioned that a phase II clinical trial for RCC had to be stopped when two patients died after IL-12 administration and several others experienced severe side effects. The initial investigation theorized that the subjects received multiple doses of IL-12 before the previous dose had time to clear from their systems (174). No such severe toxicities were observed in a phase 1/2 clinical trial of patients with breast cancer, melanoma, and head and neck cancer after direct intratumoral injection of autologous fibroblasts secreting IL-12 (175). Clinical benefit occurred, as shrinkage of the injected lesions and more than one-half the distal lesions was noted in three melanoma patients, two breast cancer patients, and one patient with head and neck cancer.

Interferon-α

IFN-α has been shown to be one of the more effective cytokine adjuvants in the treatment of melanoma and renal carcinoma. The proposed mechanisms of action included activation of intracellular signaling pathways that, in turn, modulate numerous cytokines including IL-1, IL-2, IL-6, IL-8, and TNF-α (176). In 1995, Doveil and associates (177) reported that IFN–α-2b treatment (3 MU intramuscularly three times a week) was well tolerated and increased 5-year survival from 36% to 62% in patients with stage IIIB melanoma (177). A 1996 report from the Eastern Cooperative Oncology group also underscored the potential clinical benefit of IFN-α-2b therapy in the treatment of melanoma (178). Two hundred fifty-two subjects were treated with maximum tolerated doses of 20 MU per m^2 per day intravenously for 1 month and 10 MU per m^2 three times per week subcutaneously for 48 weeks. A significant increase in relapse-free survival was achieved after periodic examination of tumor burden, as well as regional lymph node metastasis. Despite severe toxicity (67% of all patients demonstrated grade 3 toxicity and two patients died from lethal hepatic toxicity), 5-year survival rates increased from 37% to 46% (178). It should be noted, however, that using a different method of statistical analysis (two-sided instead of one-sided *p* test) and quality-of-life survival analysis (Q-TwiST), a reinvestigation of the data concluded that the improvement was significant only for those patients who considered toxicity to have a high relative value and relapse to have a low relative value (179). In 1998, a comprehensive summary of adjuvant IFN-α therapy for melanoma reported clinical benefit in several multicenter trials (180). High-dose IFN-α-2b treatment of patients with stage IIB and III melanoma received 20 MU per m^2 intravenously daily for 5 of 7 days per week for 4 weeks, followed by 10 MU per m^2 subcutaneously three times weekly for the remainder of 1 year. Statistically significant improvements in overall and recurrence-free survival (*p* = .47 and *p* = .004, respectively) were achieved (181). Severe toxicities prompted the study of low-dose IFN-α (e.g., 3 MU subcutaneously daily three times weekly for 36 months), but, thus far, durable responses have not been obtained.

Because IFN-α is important in priming tumor-specific lymphocytes and IL-2 enhanced lymphocyte expansion, immunotherapy using IFN-α and IL-2 was thought to have synergistic activity. This theory was substantiated in clinical trials of IFN-α and IL-2 in metastatic renal cancer, which achieved a 30% response rate. Combined IFN-α and IL-2 did not seem to significantly benefit patients with metastatic colorectal carcinoma, but this could reflect the failure to show treatment benefit when either cytokine was used singly (132). IFN-α adjuvant therapy has also been combined with other adoptive cellular immunotherapy. In one such study, renal carcinoma patients received IFN-α before nephrectomy. TIL were isolated from autologous tumor, cultivated in IL-2, and returned to the patient along with continuous *in vivo* IL-2 infusion. An overall response rate of 30% was achieved in this regimen. In addition, the responses appeared to be more durable than those observed with TNF-α and IL-2 combination therapy (144). IFN-α has also been used with melanoma patients who were nonresponders to previous treatment with an allogeneic melanoma vaccine (182). Forty percent of patients responded as measured by regression of tumor. Although this response rate is greater than the response to IFN-α or vaccine alone, the study design did not allow comparison of combination therapy with either single therapy. In 1998, Tonini and associates (183) used TNF-α and IL-2 in combination with chemotherapy [cyclophosphamide, methotrexate, and 5-fluorouracil (5-FU)] in a pilot study of ten patients with stage I and II breast carcinoma. The regimen was well tolerated, although transient leukopenia and fever were common. No clinical responses were reported.

The literature indicates that the potential clinical benefit of IFN-α as an adjuvant for cancer treatment is dependent on tumor type. When seven randomized trials for chronic myeloid leukemia were analyzed, it was evident that regimens using IFN-α produced a significant improvement of 5-year

overall survival rates (from 42% to 57%), as compared with standard chemotherapy treatments with drugs such as busulfan or hydroxyurea (184). Yet, for patients with advanced colorectal cancer, the addition of IFN-α-2b to standard therapies has not proved beneficial. When used as an adjuvant to single modulation chemotherapy [leucovorin (folinic acid) concurrently with 5-FU], IFN-α-2b (5 MU subcutaneously three times weekly) actually decreased overall survival rates and had more frequent toxicity and contraindications (including neutropenia, anemia, diarrhea, and flulike syndrome) as compared with the group given only leucovorin and 5-FU (185). In a subsequent report, the combination of IFN-α-2b with 5-FU did not provide any benefit over treatment solely with 5-FU (186). In summary, when used alone or in combination with other immunotherapeutic modalities, studies suggest that IFN-α has potential therapeutic benefit for certain cancer types, the durability and frequency of which await long-term follow-up (187).

Interferon-γ

IFN-γ mediates numerous biologic activities. It enhances the expression of MHC class I and II molecules and other surface molecules, such as tumor-associated antigens and IL-2 receptors. IFN-γ modulates lipid metabolism. It displays antiviral and antimicrobial activity (4). NK-produced IFN-γ plays a key role in acute inflammation. During antigen-specific immune response, it modulates antigen presentation, as well as lymphocyte differentiation, in a classic Th1-type reaction (188). It affects the nonspecific and specific arms of the immune system in a myriad of ways, including Ig synthesis by B cells and activation of CTL (4). Although it has been investigated for many years as an immune adjuvant in cancer patients, the number of clinical trials with IFN-γ have been much less frequent as those with IFN-α.

The several clinical trials using IFN-γ for the treatment of RCC achieved disparate results (189–193), which is not entirely surprising considering the disparate schedules and doses. Aulitzky et al. (192) performed a dose-escalation phase 1 study using 10, 100, and 500 μg of subcutaneus IFN-γ weekly for a total of three injections. Beta-2-microglobulin and neopterin served as biologic surrogate end points. Patients at the 100 μg dose demonstrated beta-2-microglobulin and neopterin levels comparable to those given 500 μg, yet without the toxicity levels resulting from the highest dosage. A subsequent phase 2 study with 100 μg of rhIL-4 reported a 30% response rate with a duration of from 6 to 24+ months (192). Ellhorst et al. (193) achieved a 15% response rate with a duration of from 2 to 18 months. In one of the largest multicenter studies, 202 RCC patients were evaluated after treatment with 60 μg per m^2 0 rhIL-4 subcutaneously once every 7 days until disease progression. During the initial year of treatment, subjects were analyzed for therapeutic benefit and adverse events every 57 days. Ninety-two percent of subjects experienced a drug-related adverse event, but only 14% had a grade 3 or 4 toxicity. Clinical responses were disappointing: only 6% of subjects were classified as responders. In addition, the median survival observed (13.4 months from treatment onset) was not an increase over that obtained in other studies. Bruntsch et al. (190) also obtained minimal clinical responses in a phase 2 study in metastatic RCC.

Granulocyte-Macrophage Colony-Stimulating Factor

GM-CSF is a glycoprotein that modulates the maturation, production, and function of the granulocyte and monocyte-macrophage subpopulations of human white blood cells (194,195). It is produced by monocytes, B lymphocytes, neutrophils, eosinophils, mast cells, keratinocytes, fibroblasts, endothelial cells, osteoblasts, and various epithelial cell types. Constitutive expression by resting cells is low, but after stimulation, such as infection by microbes or microbial products, secretion is greatly enhanced (196). GM-CSF has pronounced effects on the immune system, including:

1. Upregulating MHC class II expression
2. Modulating other hematopoietic growth factors
3. Eliciting localized inflammatory responses at the site of antigen deposition
4. Stimulating myeloid precursors in bone marrow
5. Promoting DC migration and development (197–200)

As far as the effect on DCs is concerned, GM-CSF potentiates several *in vitro* effects that would suggest it being advantageous as an adjuvant in immunotherapeutics. The addition of GM-CSF to peripheral blood DCs has been shown to prolong cell viability beyond 30 days of culture. Such long-lived DCs remain immunostimulatory, as evidenced by their ability to provoke T-cell proliferation in autologous and allogeneic-mixed leukocyte reactions. Total cell number, however, does not increase over time, implying the inability of GM-CSF to induce DC division and proliferation (201).

Clinical trials of GM-CSF as an adjuvant began in earnest after a 1994 report by the American Society of Clinical Oncology recommended further research for adult and pediatric cancers (202). In a 1996 study of GM-CSF's *in vivo* immunomodulatory properties (203), 12 patients with small-cell lung cancer were given a single 2.5, 5.0, or 10.0 μg per kg injection of the cytokine 3 days before ACO (cyclophosphamide, doxorubicin, and vincristine) chemotherapy. After chemotherapy, patients received supportive therapy with recombinant human GM-CSF 5 μg per kg daily for 8 days. GM-CSF enhanced the MHC class II expression on monocytes, confirming earlier *in vitro* findings (204). GM-CSF demonstrated a minor effect on adhesion molecules: only CD44 (a molecule important for the binding of leukocytes to bone marrow stroma and lymphoid organs) levels were markedly induced. An increase in IL-1 receptor α plasma and soluble IL-2 receptor levels were detected as well. To assess whether such immunomodulation could translate into therapeutic benefit, Samanci et al. (205) treated 18 colorectal carcinoma patients with recombinant human carcinoembryonic antigen with or without 80 μg per day of GM-CSF subcutaneously on days 1–4. The regimen was repeated six times over a term of 9 months. The recombinant human carcinoembryonic antigen–specific proliferative activity and IFN-γ secretion levels were higher in the nine GM-CSF recipients compared with the non–GM-CSF group. A smaller percentage of GM-CSF recipients also demonstrated IL-4 secretion via enzyme-linked immunospot assay indicative of a type II response. Those given GM-CSF had an increased humoral response as well, as evidenced by nine out of nine patients developing increasingly higher IgG antibodies against recombinant human carcinoembryonic antigen after each cytokine injection, whereas only three out of nine patients not given GM-CSF displayed no antibodies whatsoever. No evidence of clinical benefit for any subject was indicated.

Two reports involving GM-CSF adjuvant therapy for metastatic prostate cancer (206,207) and RCC (208) also showed no treatment benefit. In the first report, a phase 2 trial was performed to determine the efficacy of infusions of DCs exogenously pulsed with two HLA-A2–restricted peptides derived from prostate-specific membrane antigen. Each subject received six infusions of DCs and prostate-specific membrane antigen peptide-1 and prostate-specific membrane antigen peptide-2 peptides (LLHETDSAV and ALFDIESKV, respectively) every 6 weeks. GM-CSF was self-administered by subcutaneous injection at a dose of 75 μg per m^2 per day for 7 days with each of six infusion cycles. Most reported side effects (local reactions at the injection sites, pain, fever, and fatigue) were of mild severity, although 11 patients with such symptoms requested discontinuation of GM-CSF. DTH responses against a panel of highly immunogenic recall antigens improved in five control patients and only three patients receiving GM-CSF. One CR plus eight PRs were obtained among 44 subjects who were given adjuvant therapy compared with 2 CRs plus 17 PRs among 51 subjects who did not receive GM-CSF (209). Thus, no *in vitro* or *in vivo* treatment benefit was observed in this prostate cancer vaccine study. In the second report, 24 patients with metastatic RCC were given 10 μg per kg of GM-CSF per day using a 14-days-on/14-days-off regimen. Toxicity, including nausea, vomiting, fever, pain, skin reactions, fatigue, myalgia, and hyperleukocytosis, often required dose modifications. Three patients demonstrated a slowing in the progress of their cancer, but 21 of 24 subjects died from their respective illnesses. Because 17 of 24 patients had received prior immunotherapy, it is possible that a more definitive assessment of GM-CSF activity could be conducted using untreated patients.

Finally, supportive adjuvant GM-CSF therapy has also been used to try to mitigate the side effects of chemotherapy and increase the maximum tolerated dose. As with its use as an antitumor agent, the results with GM-CSF were mixed. Stoger et al. (210) found that posttreatment administration of GM-CSF allowed for dose intensification of epidoxorubicin and cyclophosphamide in a randomized phase 2/3 study in patients with advanced breast cancer. The ability of GM-CSF to enhance hematologic recovery in a chemotherapy setting was demonstrated in phase 1/2 studies of advanced sarcomas (211,212). In a phase 2 study of patients with squamous cell carcinoma of the head and neck, however, GM-CSF adjuvant therapy did not improve antitumor activity for patients receiving cisplatin and 5-FU (213).

HAPTENS

A hapten is a small moiety that is unable to elicit an immune response by itself unless it is linked to a larger moiety, such as a protein, peptide, or lipid (214). In 1965, Weigle and colleagues (215) initially established that haptens could:

1. Enhance immunogenicity to the hapten-protein (in this instance, thyroglobulin) complex
2. Concurrently increase immunogenicity to the carrier protein itself
3. Induce an immune response to the normal "self-protein," which manifested itself with the development of autoimmunity.

Since then, class I–restricted T-cell responses have been generated against haptenized proteins. Once more, immune responses can be demonstrated against the hapten-carrier complex, as well as to the unmodified carrier. The most commonly used haptens are dinitrophenyl (DNP) and trinitrophenyl.

In the first human clinical trial using a haptenized vaccine, 24 metastatic melanoma patients were immunized with autologous, irradiated tumor cells conjugated to DNP (216). Fourteen subjects (60%) demonstrated intense inflammatory responses using physical examination and immunohistochemistry. Tumor biopsies revealed T-cell and DC infiltration. In a follow-up report, 20 of 46 subjects identically vaccinated developed inflammatory reactions, consisting of erythema, warmth, and tenderness at the site of tumor nodules. Five patients achieved a PR, including one durable response still evident 16 months after the initial immunization. The 2-year overall and disease-free survivals attained, 85% and 59%, respectively, were significantly better than those of participants given the unmodified vaccine (217). Later, Berd et al. (218) showed that melanoma patients vaccinated with DNP-modified autologous tumor cells acquire a hapten-restricted T-cell response, as evidenced by DTH and HLA-specific proliferation and IFN-γ production *in vitro*. The combination of DNP- and melanoma-specific immunity seems to enhance clinically relevant antitumor activity: results of two phase 2 trials attained a median relapse-free survival duration (24–37 months) and rate (45%) superior to those attained with high-dose IFN in an Eastern Cooperative Oncology Group trial (214).

CONCLUSION

The extensive body of research that has accumulated in the field of adjuvants does not paint a clear picture. Some adjuvants are efficacious only in animal tumor model systems, whereas others have shown clinical benefit only with certain human tumors. Many of the most promising agents will soon enter large, multi-center clinical trials in which their use can truly be affirmed or denied. Yet, unless a cohort group is established for each trial in which patients are given all vaccine components save the adjuvant, it will continue to be difficult to gauge their contribution. The added complexity and cost of including such cohort groups certainly contributes to why so few adjuvant-inclusive trials have been performed this way. The reality of medicine today is that cost and ease of manufacture will be increasingly important factors in future adjuvant development (40). In addition, an adjuvant should be stable and readily mass-produced so that it

could potentially be used worldwide. It should elicit a wide range of immune events to overcome potential problems with tumor-escape mechanisms, such as downregulation of MHC expression (219,220). Ideally, it should be immunostimulatory and safe by several routes of administration. Several candidate adjuvants with many of these parameters are in ongoing phase 1, 2, and 3 clinical trials. Within a few years, it will be possible to draw firm conclusions about the validity of their approach towards enhancing antitumor immunity.

REFERENCES

1. Berd D. Cancer vaccines: reborn or just recycled? *Semin Oncol* 1998;25:605–610.
2. Vogel FR. Adjuvants in perspective. *Dev Biol Stand* 1998;92:241–248.
3. Kwak LW, Longo DL. Modern vaccine adjuvants. In: Chabner BA, Longo DL, eds. *Cancer chemotherapy and biotherapy*. Philadelphia: Lippincott–Raven Publishers, 1996:749–763.
4. Rosenberg SA. Principles of cancer management: biologic therapy. In: DeVita Jr VT, Hellman S, Rosenberg SA, eds. *Cancer: principles and practice of oncology*. Philadelphia: Lippincott–Raven Publishers, 1997:349–373.
5. Gupta RK, Siber GR. Adjuvants for human vaccines—current status, problems and future prospects. *Vaccine* 1995;13:1263–1276.
6. Edsall G. Application of immunological principles to immunization practices. *Med Clin North Am* 1965;49:1729–1743.
7. McElrath MJ. Selection of potent immunological adjuvants for vaccine construction. *Semin Cancer Biol* 1995;6:375–385.
8. Cooper PD. Vaccine adjuvants based on gamma inulin. *Pharm Biotechnol* 1995;6:559–580.
9. Gonzalez S, Nazabal C, Vina L, Caballero E. Influence of several adjuvants on the immune response against a recombinant meningococcal high molecular weight antigen. *Dev Biol Stand* 1998;92:269–276.
10. Fernando GJ, Stewart TJ, Tindle RW, Frazer IH. Th2-type CD4+ cells neither enhance nor suppress antitumor CTL activity in a mouse tumor model. *J Immunol* 1998;161:2421–2427.
11. Raychaudhuri S, Tonks M, Carbone F, Ryskamp T, Morrow WJ, Hanna N. Induction of antigen-specific class I-restricted cytotoxic T cells by soluble proteins *in vivo*. *Proc Natl Acad Sci U S A* 1992; 89:8308–8312.
12. Newman MJ, Todd CW, Balusubramanian M. Design and development of adjuvant-active nonionic block copolymers. *J Pharm Sci* 1998;87:1357–1362.
13. Ke Y, McGraw CL, Hunter RL, Kapp JA. Nonionic triblock copolymers facilitate delivery of exogenous proteins into the MHC class I and class II processing pathways. *Cell Immunol* 1997;176:113–121.
14. Todd CW, Pozzi LA, Guarnaccia JR, et al. Development of an adjuvant-active nonionic block copolymer for use in oil-free subunit vaccine formulations. *Vaccine* 1997;15:564–570.
15. Ellouz F, Adam A, Ciorbaru R, Lederer E. Minimal structural requirements for adjuvant activity of bacterial peptidoglycan derivatives. *Biochem Biophys Res Commun* 1974;59:1317–1325.
16. Akporiaye ET, Hersh EM. Immune adjuvants. In: DeVita Jr VT, Hellman S, Rosenberg SA, eds. *Biologic therapy of cancer*. Philadelphia: Lippincott–Raven Publishers, 1995:635–647.
17. Dinney CP, Tanguay S, Bucana CD, Eve BY, Fidler IJ. Intravesical liposomal muramyl tripeptide phosphatidylethanolamine treatment of human bladder carcinoma growing in nude mice. *J Interferon Cytokine Res* 1995;15:585–592.
18. Allison AC. The mode of action of immunological adjuvants. *Dev Biol Stand* 1998;92:3–11.
19. Shimizu T, Iwamoto Y, Yanagihara Y, Ikeda K, Achiwa K. Combined effects of synthetic lipid A analogs or bacterial lipopolysaccharide with glucosaminylmuramyl dipeptide on antitumor activity against Meth A fibrosarcoma in mice. *Int J Immunopharmacol* 1992;14: 1415–1420.

20. Kurzman ID, MacEwen EG, Rosenthal RC, et al. Adjuvant therapy for osteosarcoma in dogs: results of randomized clinical trials using combined liposome-encapsulated muramyl tripeptide and cisplatin. *Clin Cancer Res* 1995;1:1595–1601.

21. Teske E, Rutteman GR, Ingh TS, van Noort R, Misdorp W. Liposome-encapsulated muramyl tripeptide phosphatidylethanolamine (L-MTP-PE): a randomized clinical trial in dogs with mammary carcinoma. *Anticancer Res* 1998;18:1015–1019.

22. Murray JL, Kleinerman ES, Cunningham JE, et al. Phase I trial of liposomal muramyl tripeptide phosphatidylethanolamine in cancer patients. *J Clin Oncol* 1989;7:1915–1925.

23. Fossum C, Bergstrom M, Lovgren K, Watson DL, Morein B. Effect of iscoms and their adjuvant moiety (matrix) on the initial proliferation and IL-2 responses: comparison of spleen cells from mice inoculated with iscoms and/or matrix. *Cell Immunol* 1990;129:414–425.

24. Kensil CR, Patel U, Lennick M, Marcotte R. Separation and characterization of saponins with adjuvant activity from Quillaja saponaria Molina cortex. *J Immunol* 991;146:431–437.

25. Maloy KJ, Donachie AM, Mowat AM. Induction of Th1 and Th2 CD4+ T cell responses by oral or parenteral immunization with ISCOMS. *Eur J Immunol* 1995;25:2835–2841.

26. Messina JP, Gilkeson GS, Pisetsky DS. Stimulation of *in vitro* murine lymphocyte proliferation by bacterial DNA. *J Immunol* 1991;147:1759–1764.

27. Feltkamp MCW, Smits HL, Vierboom MPM, et al. Vaccination with cytotoxic T lymphocyte epitope-containing peptide protects against a tumor induced by human papillomavirus type 16-transformed cells. *Eur J Immunol* 1993;23:2242–2249.

28. Chen L, Ashe S, Brady WA, et al. Costimulation of antitumor immunity by the B7 counterreceptor for the T lymphocyte molecules CD28 and CTLA-4. *Cell* 1992;71:1093–1102.

29. Hariharan K, Braslawsky G, Barnett RS, et al. Tumor regression in mice following vaccination with human papillomavirus E7 recombinant protein in PROVAX. *Int J Oncol* 1998;12:1229–1235.

30. Alexander M, Salgaller ML, Celis E, et al. Generation of tumor-specific cytolytic T lymphocytes from peripheral blood of cervical cancer patients by *in vitro* stimulation with a synthetic human papillomavirus type 16 E7 epitope. *Am J Obstet Gynecol* 1996;175:1586–1593.

31. Fernando GJ, Stewart TJ, Tindle RW, Frazer IH. Vaccine-induced Th1-type responses are dominant over Th2-type responses in the short term whereas pre-existing Th2 responses are dominant in the longer term. *Scand J Immunol* 1998;47:459–465.

32. Newman MJ, Wu JY, Gardner BH, et al. Saponin adjuvant induction of ovalbumin-specific CD8+ cytotoxic T lymphocyte responses. *J Immunol* 1992;148:2357–2362.

33. Hamilton WB, Helling F, Lloyd KO, Livingston PO. Ganglioside expression on human malignant melanoma assessed by quantitative immune thin-layer chromatography. *Int J Cancer* 1993;53:566–573.

34. Livingston PO. Augmenting the immunogenicity of carbohydrate tumor antigens. *Semin Cancer Biol* 1995;6:357–366.

35. Wolchok JD, Livingston PO, Houghton AN. Vaccines and other adjuvant therapies for melanoma. *Hematol Oncol Clin North Am* 1998;12:835–848.

36. McCaffrey M, Yao T-J, Williams L, Livingston PO, Houghton AN, Chapman PB. Immunization of melanoma patients with BEC2 anti-idiotypic monoclonal antibody that mimics GD3 ganglioside: enhanced immunogenicity when combined with adjuvant. *Clin Cancer Res* 1996;2:679–686.

37. Helling F, Zhang S, Shang A, et al. GM2-KLH conjugate vaccine: increased immunogenicity in melanoma patients after administration with immunological adjuvant QS-21. *Cancer Res* 1995;55:2783–2788.

38. Foon KA, Sen G, Hutchins L, et al. Antibody responses in melanoma patients immunized with an anti-idiotype antibody mimicking disialoganglioside GD2. *Clin Cancer Res* 1998;4:1117–1124.

39. Livingston P. Ganglioside vaccines with emphasis on GM2. *Semin Oncol* 1998;25:636–645.

40. O'Hagan DT. Recent advances in vaccine adjuvants for systemic and mucosal administration. *J Pharm Pharmacol* 1998;50:1–10.

41. Zaks TZ, Rosenberg SA. Immunization with a peptide epitope (p369–377) from HER-2/neu leads to peptide-specific cytotoxic T lymphocytes that fail to recognize HER-2/ncu+ tumors. *Cancer Res* 1998;58:4902–4908.

42. Kawakami Y, Robbins PF, Wang RF, Parkhurst M, Kang X, Rosenberg SA. The use of melanosomal proteins in the immunotherapy of melanoma. *J Immunother* 1998;21:237–246.

43. Rosenberg SA, Yang JC, Schwartzentruber DJ, et al. Immunologic and therapeutic evaluation of a synthetic peptide vaccine for the treatment of patients with metastatic melanoma. *Nat Med* 1998;4:321–327.

44. Salgaller ML, Marincola FM, Cormier JN, Rosenberg SA. Immunization against epitopes in the human melanoma antigen gp100 following patient immunization with synthetic peptides. *Cancer Res* 1996;56:4749–4757.

45. Cormier JN, Salgaller ML, Prevette T, et al. Enhancement of cellular immunity in melanoma patients immunized with a peptide from MART-1/Melan A. *Cancer J Sci Am* 1997;3.37–44.

46. O'Hagan DT, Ott GS, van Nest G. Recent advances in vaccine adjuvants: the development of MF59 emulsion and polymeric microparticles. *Mol Med Today* 1997;3:69–75.

47. Minutello M, Senatore F, Cecchinelli G, et al. Safety and immunogenicity of an inactivated subunit influenza virus vaccine combined with MF59 adjuvant emulsion in elderly subjects, immunized for three consecutive influenza seasons. *Vaccine* 1999;17:99–104.

48. Dupuis M, Murphy TJ, Higgins D, et al. Dendritic cells internalize vaccine adjuvant after intramuscular injection. *Cell Immunol* 1998;186:18–27.

49. Langenberg AG, Burke RL, Adair SF, et al. A recombinant glycoprotein vaccine for herpes simplex virus type 2: safety and immunogenicity. *Ann Intern Med* 1995;122:889–898.

50. Smith RE, Donachie AM, Mowat AM. Immune stimulating complexes as mucosal vaccines. *Immunol Cell Biol* 1998;76:263–269.

51. Sjolander A, Cox JC, Barr IG. ISCOMs: an adjuvant with multiple functions. *J Leukoc Biol* 1998;64:713–723.

52. Morein B, Bengtsson KL. Functional aspects of iscoms. *Immunol Cell Biol* 1998;76:295–299.

53. Kensil CR, Wu JY, Anderson CA, Wheeler DA, Amsden J. QS-21 and QS-7: purified saponin adjuvants. *Dev Biol Stand* 1998;92:41–47.

54. Deliyannis G, Jackson DC, Dyer W, et al. Immunopotentiation of humoral and cellular responses to inactivated influenza vaccines by two different adjuvants with potential for human use. *Vaccine* 1998;16:2058–2068.

55. Gregoriadis G. The immunological adjuvant and vaccine carrier properties of liposomes. *J Drug Target* 1994;2:351–356.

56. Gregoriadis G. Immunological adjuvants: a role for liposomes. *Immunol Today* 1990;11:89–97.

57. Nakanishi T, Kunisawa J, Hayashi A, et al. Positively charged liposome functions as an efficient immunoadjuvant in inducing immune responses to soluble proteins. *Biochem Biophys Res Commun* 1997;240:793–797.

58. Reddy R, Nair S, Brynestad K, Rouse BT. Liposomes as antigen delivery systems in viral immunity. *Semin Immunol* 1992;4:91–96.

59. Reddy R, Zhou F, Nair S, Huang L, Rouse BT. *In vivo* cytotoxic T lymphocyte induction with soluble proteins administered in liposomes. *J Immunol* 1992;148:1585–1589.

60. Park JW, Hong K, Kirpotin DB, Papahadjopoulos D, Benz CC. Immunoliposomes for cancer treatment. In: *Advances in pharmacology.* San Diego: Academic Press, 1997:399–435.

61. Park JW, Hong K, Carter P, et al. Development of anti-p185HER2 immunoliposomes for cancer therapy. *Proc Natl Acad Sci U S A* 1995;92:1327–1331.

62. Huang SK, Lee KD, Hong K, Friend DS, Papahadjopoulos D. Microscopic localization of sterically stabilized liposomes in colon carcinoma-bearing mice. *Cancer Res* 1992;52:5135–5143.

63. Zhou F, Rouse BT, Huang L. Prolonged survival of thymoma-bearing mice after vaccination with a soluble protein antigen entrapped in liposomes: a model study. *Cancer Res* 1992;52:6287–6291.

64. Lachman LB, Ozpolat B, Rao XM. Cytokine-containing liposomes as vaccine adjuvants. *Eur Cytokine Netw* 1996;7:693–698.

65. Ho RJ, Burke RL, Merigan TC. Liposome-formulated interleukin-2 as an adjuvant of recombinant HSV glycoprotein gD for the treatment of recurrent genital HSV-2 in guinea-pigs. *Vaccine* 1992;10:209–213.

66. Gursel M, Gregoriadis G. The immunological co-adjuvant action of liposomal interleukin-2: the role of mode of localization of the cytokine and antigen in the vesicles. *J Drug Target* 1998;5:93–98.

67. Thurnher M, Ramoner R, Gastl G, et al. Bacillus Calmette-Guerin mycobacteria stimulate human blood dendritic cells. *Int J Cancer* 1997;70:128–134.

68. Ramoner R, Rieser C, Herold M, et al. Activation of human dendritic cells by bacillus Calmette-Guerin. *J Urol* 1998;159:1488–1492.

69. Morton DL, Eilber FR, Malmgren RA, Wood WC. Immunological factors which influence response to immunotherapy in malignant melanoma. *Surgery* 1970;68:158–164.

70. Cascinelli N, Rumke P, MacKie R, Morabito A, Bufalino R. The significance of conversion of skin reactivity to efficacy of bacillus Calmette-Guerin (BCG) vaccinations given immediately after radical surgery in stage II melanoma patients. *Cancer Immunol Immunother* 1989;28:282–286.

71. Czarnetzki BM, Macher E, Suciu S, Thomas D, Steerenberg PA, Rumke P. Long-term adjuvant immunotherapy in stage I high risk malignant melanoma, comparing two BCG preparations versus non-treatment in a randomized multicentre study (EORTC Protocol 18781). *Eur J Cancer* 1993;29A:1237–1242.

72. Sterchi JM, Wells HB, Case LD, et al. A randomized trial of adjuvant chemotherapy and immunotherapy in Stage I and Stage II cutaneous melanoma. An interim report. *Cancer* 1985;55:707–712.

73. Fisher RI, Terry WD, Hodes RJ, et al. Adjuvant immunotherapy or chemotherapy for malignant melanoma. Preliminary report of the National Cancer Institute randomized clinical trial. *Surg Clin North Am* 1981;61:1267–1277.

74. Brocker EB, Suter L, Czarnetzki BM, Macher E. BCG immunotherapy in stage I melanoma patients. Does it influence prognosis determined by HLA-DR expression in high-risk primary tumors? *Cancer Immunol Immunother* 1986;23:155–157.

75. Aranha GV, McKhann CF, Grage TB, Gunnarsson A, Simmons RL. Adjuvant immunotherapy of malignant melanoma. *Cancer* 1979;43:1297–1303.

76. Berd D, Maguire Jr HC, McCue P, Mastrangelo MJ. Treatment of metastatic melanoma with an autologous tumor-cell vaccine: clinical and immunologic results in 64 patients. *J Clin Oncol* 1990;8:1858–1867.

77. Morales A, Eidinger D, Bruce AW. Intracavitary Bacillus Calmette-Guerin in the treatment of superficial bladder tumors. *J Urol* 1976;116:180–183.

78. Brosman SA. Experience with bacillus Calmette-Guerin in patients with superficial bladder carcinoma. *J Urol* 1982;128:27–30.

79. Nseyo UO, Lamm DL. Immunotherapy of bladder cancer. *Semin Surg Oncol* 1997;13:342–349.

80. Rubben H, Lutzeyer W, Fischer N, Deutz F, Lagrange W, Giani G. Natural history and treatment of low and high risk superficial bladder tumors. *J Urol* 1988;139:283–285.

81. Torti FM, Lum BL. The biology and treatment of superficial bladder cancer. *J Clin Oncol* 1984;2:505–531.

82. Bohle A, Gerdes J, Ulmer AJ, Hofstetter AG, Flad HD. Effects of local bacillus Calmette-Guerin therapy in patients with bladder carcinoma on immunocompetent cells of the bladder wall. *J Urol* 1990;144:53–58.

83. Boccafoschi C, Montefiore F, Pavesi M, et al. Immunophenotypic characterization of the bladder mucosa infiltrating lymphocytes after intravesical BCG treatment for superficial bladder carcinoma. *Eur Urol* 1992;21:304–308.

84. Garden RJ, Liu BC, Redwood SM, Weiss RE, Droller MJ. Bacillus Calmette-Guerin abrogates *in vitro* invasion and motility of human bladder tumor cells via fibronectin interaction. *J Urol* 1992;148:900–905.

85. Witjes JA, Caris CT, Mungan NA, Debruyne FM, Witjes WP. Results of a randomized phase III trial of sequential intravesical therapy with mitomycin C and bacillus Calmette-Guerin versus mitomycin C alone in patients with superficial bladder cancer. *J Urol* 1998;160:1668–1671.

86. Witjes JA, Meijden AP, Sylvester LC, Debruyne FM, van Aubel A, Witjes WP. Long-term follow-up of an EORTC randomized prospective trial comparing intravesical bacille Calmette-Guerin-RIVM and mitomycin C in superficial bladder cancer. EORTC GU Group and the Dutch South East Cooperative Urological Group. European Organization for Research and Treatment of Cancer Genito-Urinary Tract Cancer Collaborative Group. *Urology* 1998;52:403–410.

87. Abdi EA, Hanson J, Harbora DE, Young DG, McPherson TA. Adjuvant chemoimmuno- and immunotherapy in Dukes' stage B2 and C colorectal carcinoma: a 7-year follow-up analysis. *J Surg Oncol* 1989;40:205–213.

88. Hoover HCJ, Brandhorst JS, Peters LC, et al. Adjuvant active specific immunotherapy for human colorectal cancer: 6.5-year median follow-up of a phase III prospectively randomized trial. *J Clin Oncol* 1993;11:390–399.

89. Vermorken JB, Claessen AM, van Tinteren H, et al. Active specific immunotherapy for stage II and stage III human colon cancer: a randomized trial. *Lancet* 1999;353:345–350.

90. Jones SE, Grozea PN, Miller TP, et al. Chemotherapy with cyclophosphamide, doxorubicin, vincristine, and prednisone alone or with levamisole or with levamisole plus BCG for malignant lymphoma: a Southwest Oncology Group Study. *J Clin Oncol* 1985;3:1318–1324.

91. Galligioni E, Quaia M, Merlo A, et al. Adjuvant immunotherapy treatment of renal carcinoma patients with autologous tumor cells and bacillus Calmette-Guerin. *Cancer* 1996;77:2560–2566.

92. Guinan P, Toronchi E, Shaw M, Crispin R, Sharifi R. Bacillus Calmette-Guerin (BCG) adjuvant therapy in stage D prostate cancer. *Urology* 1982;20:401–403.

93. De Smedt T, Pajak B, Muraille E, et al. Regulation of dendritic cell numbers and maturation by lipopolysaccharide *in vivo*. *J Exp Med* 1996;184:1413–1424.

94. Rescigno M, Martino M, Sutherland CL, Gold MR, Ricciardi-Castagnoli P. Dendritic cell survival and maturation are regulated by different signaling pathways. *J Exp Med* 1998;188:2175–2180.

95. Hennemann B, Beckmann G, Eichelmann A, Rehm A, Andreesen R. Phase I trial of adoptive immunotherapy of cancer patients using monocyte-derived macrophages activated with interferon gamma and lipopolysaccharide. *Cancer Immunol Immunother* 1998;45:250–256.

96. Messina JP, Gilkeson GS, Pisetsky DS. Stimulation of *in vitro* murine lymphocyte proliferation by bacterial DNA. *J Immunol* 1991;147:1759–1764.

97. Weiner GJ, Liu HM, Wooldridge JE, Dahle CE, Krieg AM. Immunostimulatory oligodeoxynucleotides containing the CpG motif are effective as immune adjuvants in tumor antigen immunization. *Proc Natl Acad Sci U S A* 1997;94:10833–10837.

98. Krieg AM, Yi AK, Matson S, et al. CpG motifs in bacterial DNA trigger direct B-cell activation. *Nature* 1995;374:546–549.

99. Yi AK, Klinman DM, Martin TL, Matson S, Krieg AM. Rapid immune activation by CpG motifs in bacterial DNA. Systemic induction of IL-6 transcription through an antioxidant-sensitive pathway. *J Immunol* 1996;157:5394–5402.

100. Stacey KJ, Sweet MJ, Hume DA. Macrophages ingest and are activated by bacterial DNA. *J Immunol* 1996;157:2116–2122.

101. Cowdery JS, Chace JH, Yi AK, Krieg AM. Bacterial DNA induces NK cells to produce IFN-gamma *in vivo* and increases the toxicity of lipopolysaccharides. *J Immunol* 1996;156:4570–4575.

102. Bergman Y, Haimovich J. Characterization of a carcinogen-induced murine B lymphocyte cell line of C3H/eB origin. *Eur J Immunol* 1977;7:413–417.

103. Liu HM, Newbrough SE, Bhatia SK, Dahle CE, Krieg AM, Weiner GJ. Immunostimulatory CpG oligodeoxynucleotides enhance the immune response to vaccine strategies involving granulocyte-macrophage colony-stimulating factor. *Blood* 1998;92:3730–3736.

104. Wooldridge JE, Ballas Z, Krieg AM, Weiner GJ. Immunostimulatory oligodeoxynucleotides containing CpG motifs enhance the efficacy of monoclonal antibody therapy of lymphoma. *Blood* 1997;89:2994–2998.

105. Jakob T, Walker PS, Krieg AM, Udey MC, Vogel JC. Activation of cutaneous dendritic cells by CpG-containing oligodeoxynucleotides: a role for dendritic cells in the augmentation of Th1 responses by immunostimulatory DNA. *J Immunol* 1998;161:3042–3049.

106. Baker PJ, Hiernaux JR, Fauntleroy MB, et al. Ability of monophosphoryl lipid A to augment the antibody response of young mice. *Infect Immun* 1988;56:3064–3066.

107. Samuel J, Budzynski WA, Reddish MA, et al. Immunogenicity and antitumor activity of a liposomal MUC1 peptide-based vaccine. *Int J Cancer* 1998;75:295–302.

108. Mitchell MS, Harel W, Kempf RA, et al. Active-specific immunotherapy for melanoma. *J Clin Oncol* 1990;8:856–869.

109. Schultz N, Oratz R, Chen D, Zeleniuch-Jacquotte A, Abeles G, Bystryn JC. Effect of DETOX as an adjuvant for melanoma vaccine. *Vaccine* 1995;13:503–508.

110. Eton O, Kharkevitch DD, Gianan MA, et al. Active immunotherapy with ultraviolet B-irradiated autologous whole melanoma cells plus DETOX in patients with metastatic melanoma. *Clin Cancer Res* 1998;4:619–627.

111. Miles DW, Towlson KE, Graham R, et al. A randomized phase II study of sialyl-Tn and DETOX-B adjuvant with or without cyclophosphamide pretreatment for the active specific immunotherapy of breast cancer. *Br J Cancer* 1996;74:1292–1296.

112. Morton DL, Barth A. Vaccine therapy for malignant melanoma. *CA Cancer J Clin* 1996;46:225–244.

113. Mitchell MS. Perspective on allogeneic melanoma lysates in active specific immunotherapy. *Semin Oncol* 1998;25:623–635.

114. Jurincic-Winkler C, Metz KA, Beuth J, Engelmann U, Klippel KF. Immunohistological findings in patients with superficial bladder carcinoma after intravesical instillation of keyhole limpet haemocyanin. *Br J Urol* 1995;76:702–707.

115. el-Demiry MI, Smith G, Ritchie AW, et al. Local immune responses after intravesical BCG treatment for carcinoma in situ. *Br J Urol* 1987;60:543–548.

116. el-Demiry MI, Smith G, Ritchie AW, et al. Local immune responses after intravesical BCG treatment for carcinoma in situ. *Br J Urol* 1987;60:543–548.

117. Jurincic CD, Engelmann U, Gasch J, Klippel KF. Immunotherapy in bladder cancer with keyhole-limpet hemocyanin: a randomized study. *J Urol* 1988;139:723–726.

118. Flamm J, Bucher A, Holtl W, Albrecht W. Recurrent superficial transitional cell carcinoma of the bladder: adjuvant topical chemotherapy versus immunotherapy. A prospective randomized trial. *J Urol* 1990;144:260–263.

119. Nestle FO, Alijagic S, Gilliet M, et al. Vaccination of melanoma patients with peptide- or tumor lysate-pulsed dendritic cells. *Nat Med* 1998;4:328–332.

120. Alexander J, Sidney J, Southwood S, et al. Development of high potency universal DR-restricted helper epitopes by modification of high affinity DR-blocking peptides. *Immunity* 1994;1:751–761.

121. Alexander J, Fikes J, Hoffman S, et al. The optimization of helper T lymphocyte (HTL) function in vaccine development. *Immunol Res* 1998;18:79–92.

122. Del Guercio MF, Alexander J, Kubo RT, et al. Potent immunogenic short linear peptide constructs composed of B cell epitopes and Pan DR T helper epitopes (PADRE) for antibody responses *in vivo*. *Vaccine* 1997;15:441–448.

123. Theobald M, Biggs J, Dittmer D, Levine AJ, Sherman LA. Targeting p53 as a general tumor antigen. *Proc Natl Acad Sci U S A* 1995;92: 11993–11997.

124. Yanuck M, Carbone DP, Pendleton CD, et al. A mutant p53 tumor suppressor protein is a target for peptide-induced CD8+ cytotoxic T-cells. *Cancer Res* 1993;53:3257–3261.

125. Yu Z, Liu X, McCarty TM, Diamond DJ, Ellenhorn JD. The use of transgenic mice to generate high affinity p53 specific cytolytic T cells. *J Surg Res* 1997;69:337–343.

126. Mayordomo JI, Loftus DJ, Sakamoto H, et al. Therapy of murine tumors with p53 wild-type and mutant sequence peptide-based vaccines. *J Exp Med* 1996;183:1357–1365.

127. Smith KA. Interleukin-2: inception, impact, and implications. *Science* 1988;240:1169–1176.

128. Maas RA, Dullens HF, Den Otter W. Interleukin-2 in cancer treatment: disappointing or (still) promising? *Cancer Immunol Immunother* 1993;36:141–148.

129. Rosenberg SA. The immunotherapy and gene therapy of cancer. *J Clin Oncol* 1992;10:180–199.

130. Rosenberg SA. Immunotherapy and gene therapy of cancer. In: *Origins of human cancer: a comprehensive review*. Plainview, NY: Cold Spring Harbor Laboratory Press, 1991:865–883.

131. Rosenberg SA, Lotze MT, Yang JC, et al. Experience with the use of high-dose interleukin-2 in the treatment of 652 cancer patients. *Ann Surg* 1989;210:474–484; discussion 484–485.

132. Chang AE, Cameron MJ, Sondak VK, Geiger JD, Vander Woude DL. A phase II trial of interleukin-2 and interferon-alpha in the treatment of metastatic colorectal carcinoma. *J Immunother Emphasis Tumor Immunol* 1996;18:253–262.

133. Curti BD, Ochoa AC, Urba WJ, et al. Influence of interleukin-2 regimens on circulating populations of lymphocytes after adoptive transfer of anti-CD3-stimulated T cells: results from a phase I trial in cancer patients. *J Immunother Emphasis Tumor Immunol* 1996;19:296–308.

134. Rosenberg SA, Lotze MT, Muul LM, et al. A progress report on the treatment of 157 patients with advanced cancer using lymphokine-activated killer cells and interleukin-2 or high-dose interleukin-2 alone. *N Engl J Med* 1987;316:889–897.

135. Rosenberg SA, Yang JC, Topalian SL, et al. Treatment of 283 consecutive patients with metastatic melanoma or renal cell cancer using high-dose bolus interleukin 2. *JAMA* 1994;271:907–913.

136. Belli F, Arienti F, Rivoltini L, et al. Treatment of recurrent in transit metastases from cutaneous melanoma by isolation perfusion in extracorporeal circulation with interleukin-2 and lymphokine activated killer cells. A pilot study. *Melanoma Res* 1992;2:263–271.

137. Blay JY, Favrot MC, Negrier S, et al. Correlation between clinical response to interleukin 2 therapy and sustained production of tumor necrosis factor. *Cancer Res* 1990;50:2371–2374.

138. Gratama JW, Schmitz PI, Goey SH, Lamers CHJ, Stoter G, Bolhuis RLH. Modulation of immune parameters in patients with metastatic renal-cell cancer receiving combination immunotherapy (IL-2, IFN-alpha and autologous IL-2-activated lymphocytes). *Int J Cancer* 1996;65:152–160.

139. Topalian SL, Solomon D, Rosenberg SA. Tumor-specific cytolysis by lymphocytes infiltrating human melanomas. *J Immunol* 1989;142: 3714–3725.

140. Rosenberg SA, Spiess P, Lafreniere R. A new approach to the adoptive immunotherapy of cancer with tumor-infiltrating lymphocytes. *Science* 1986;233:1318–1321.

141. Topalian SL, Solomon D, Avis FP, et al. Immunotherapy of patients with advanced cancer using tumor-infiltrating lymphocytes and recombinant interleukin-2: a pilot study. *J Clin Oncol* 1988;6:839–853.

142. Barth RJ Jr, Bock SN, Mule JJ, Rosenberg SA. Unique murine tumor-associated antigens identified by tumor infiltrating lymphocytes. *J Immunol* 1990;144:1531–1537.

143. Rosenberg SA, Yannelli JR, Yang JC, et al. Treatment of patients with metastatic melanoma with autologous tumor-infiltrating lymphocytes and interleukin 2. *J Natl Cancer Inst* 1994;86:1159–1166.

144. Belldegrun A, Pierce W, Kaboo R, et al. Interferon-alpha primed tumor-infiltrating lymphocytes combined with interleukin-2 and interferon-alpha as therapy for metastatic renal cell carcinoma. *J Urol* 1993;150:1384–1390.

145. Kelso A. Cytokines: principles and prospects. *Immunol Cell Biol* 1998;76:300–317.

146. Swain SL, Weinberg AD, English M, Huston G. IL-4 directs the development of Th2-like helper effectors. *J Immunol* 1990;145:3796–3806.

147. Brewer JM, Alexander J. Cytokines and the mechanisms of action of vaccine adjuvants. *Cytokines Cell Mol Ther* 1997;3:233–246.

148. Chomarat P, Banchereau J. An update on interleukin-4 and its receptor. *Eur Cytokine Netw* 1997;8:333–344.

149. Widmer MB, Grabstein KH. Regulation of cytolytic T-lymphocyte generation by B-cell stimulatory factor. *Nature* 1987;326:795–799.

150. Kawakami Y, Rosenberg SA, Lotze MT. Interleukin-4 promotes the growth of tumor-infiltrating lymphocytes cytotoxic for human autologous melanoma. *J Exp Med* 1988;168:2183–2191.

151. Bender A, Sapp M, Schuler G, Steinman RM, Bhardwaj N. Improved methods for the generation of dendritic cells from nonproliferating progenitors in human blood. *J Immunol Methods* 1996;196:121–135.

152. Lardon F, Snoeck HW, Berneman ZN, et al. Generation of dendritic cells from bone marrow progenitors using GM-CSF, TNF-alpha, and additional cytokines: antagonistic effects of IL-4 and IFN-gamma and selective involvement of TNF-alpha receptor-1. *J Immunol* 1997;91:553–559.

153. Romani N, Reider D, Heuer M, et al. Generation of mature dendritic cells from human blood. An improved method with special regard to clinical applicability. *J Immunol Meth* 1996;196:137–151.

154. Tjoa B, Erickson S, Barren R III, et al. *In vitro* propagated dendritic

cells from prostate cancer patients as a component of prostate cancer immunotherapy. *Prostate* 1995;27:63–69.

155. Sosman JA, Bartemes K, Offord KP, et al. Evidence for eosinophil activation in cancer patients receiving recombinant interleukin-4: effects of interleukin-4 alone and following interleukin-2 administration. *Clin Cancer Res* 1995;1:805–812.

156. Whitehead RP, Unger JM, Goodwin JW, et al. Phase II trial of recombinant human interleukin-4 in patients with disseminated malignant melanoma: a Southwest Oncology Group study. *J Immunother* 1998;21:440–446.

157. Husain SR, Behari N, Kreitman RJ, Pastan I, Puri RK. Complete regression of established human glioblastoma tumor xenograft by interleukin-4 toxin therapy. *Cancer Res* 1998;58:3649–3653.

158. Puri RK, Leland P, Kreitman RJ, Pastan I. Human neurological cancer cells express interleukin-4 (IL-4) receptors which are targets for the toxic effects of IL4-Pseudomonas exotoxin chimeric protein. *Int J Cancer* 1994;58:574–581.

159. Leach MW, Rybak ME, Rosenblum IY. Safety evaluation of recombinant human interleukin-4. II. Clinical studies. *Clin Immunol Immunopathol* 1997;83:12–14.

160. Defrance T, Vanbervliet B, Aubry JP, et al. B cell growth-promoting activity of recombinant human interleukin 4. *J Immunol* 1987;139:1135–1141.

161. Trinchieri G. Interleukin 12: a proinflammatory cytokine with immunoregulatory functions that bridge innate resistance and antigen-specific adaptive immunity. *Ann Rev Immunol* 1995;13:251–276.

162. Wang M, Chen PW, Bronte V, Rosenberg SA, Restifo NP. Antitumor activity of cytotoxic T lymphocytes elicited with recombinant and synthetic forms of a model tumor-associated antigen. *J Immunother Emphasis Tumor Immunol* 1995;18:139–146.

163. Scott P. IL-12: initiation cytokine for cell-mediated immunity [comment]. *Science* 1993;260:496–497.

164. Tahara H, Zeh HJ III, Storkus WJ, et al. Fibroblasts genetically engineered to secrete interleukin 12 can suppress tumor growth and induce antitumor immunity to a murine melanoma *in vivo*. *Cancer Res* 1994;54:182–189.

165. Hiscox S, Hallett MB, Puntis MC, Jiang WG. Inhibition of cancer cell motility and invasion by interleukin-12. *Clin Exp Metastasis* 1995;13:396–404.

166. Grohmann U, Belladonna ML, Bianchi R, et al. IL-12 acts directly on DC to promote nuclear localization of NF-kappaB and primes DC for IL-12 production. *Immunity* 1998;9:315–323.

167. Bianchi R, Grohmann U, Belladonna ML, et al. IL-12 is both required and sufficient for initiating T cell reactivity to a class I-restricted tumor peptide (P815AB) following transfer of P815AB-pulsed dendritic cells. *J Immunol* 1996;157:1589–1597.

168. Grohmann U, Fioretti MC, Bianchi R, et al. Dendritic cells, interleukin 12, and CD4+ lymphocytes in the initiation of class I-restricted reactivity to a tumor/self peptide. *Crit Rev Immunol* 1998;18:87–98.

169. Brunda MJ, Luistro L, Warrier RR, et al. Antitumor and antimetastatic activity of interleukin 12 against murine tumors. *J Exp Med* 1993;178:1223–1230.

170. Voest EE, Kenyon BM, O'Reilly MS, Truitt G, D'Amato RJ, Folkman J. Inhibition of angiogenesis *in vivo* by interleukin 12. *J Natl Cancer Inst* 1995;87:581–586.

171. McKnight AJ, Zimmer GJ, Fogelman I, Wolf SF, Abbas AK. Effects of IL-12 on helper T cell-dependent immune responses *in vivo*. *J Immunol* 1994;152:2172–2179.

172. Baringa M. Designing therapies that target tumor blood vessels. *Science* 1997;275:482–484.

173. Atkins MB, Robertson MJ, Gordon M, et al. Phase I evaluation of intravenous recombinant human interleukin 12 in patients with advanced malignancies. *Clin Cancer Res* 1997;3:409–417.

174. Cohen J. IL-12 deaths: explanation and a puzzle. *Science* 1995;270:908.

175. Lotze MT, Hellerstedt B, Stolinski L, et al. The role of interleukin-2, interleukin-12, and dendritic cells in cancer therapy. *Cancer J Sci Am* 1997;3[Suppl 1]:S109–S114.

176. Taylor JL, Grossberg SE. The effects of interferon-α on the production and action of other cytokines. *Semin Oncol* 1998;25:23–29.

177. Doveil GC, Fierro MT, Novelli M, et al. Adjuvant therapy of stage IIIb melanoma with interferon alfa-2b: clinical and immunological relevance. *Dermatology* 1995;191:234–239.

178. Kirkwood JM, Strawderman MH, Ernstoff MS, Smith TJ, Borden EC, Blum RH. Interferon alfa-2b adjuvant therapy of high-risk resected cutaneous melanoma: the Eastern Cooperative Oncology Group trial EST 1684. *J Clin Oncol* 1996;14:7–17.

179. Cole BF, Gelber RD, Kirkwood JM, Goldhirsch A, Barylak E, Borden E. Quality-of-life-adjusted survival analysis of interferon alfa-2b adjuvant treatment of high-risk resected cutaneous melanoma: an Eastern Cooperative Oncology Group study. *J Clin Oncol* 1996;14:2666–2673.

180. Agarwala SS, Kirkwood JM. Adjuvant interferon treatment for melanoma. *Hematol Oncol Clin North Am* 1998;12:823–833.

181. Kirkwood JM. Systemic adjuvant treatment of high-risk melanoma: the role of interferon alfa-2b and other immunotherapies. *Eur J Cancer* 1998;34[Suppl 3]:S12–S17.

182. Mitchell MS, Jakowatz J, Harel W, et al. Increased effectiveness of interferon alfa-2b following active specific immunotherapy for melanoma. *J Clin Oncol* 1994;12:402–411.

183. Tonini G, Nunziata C, Prete SP, et al. Adjuvant treatment of breast cancer: a pilot immunochemotherapy study with CMF, interleukin-2 and interferon alpha. *Cancer Immunol Immunother* 1998;47:157–166.

184. Delannoy A, Kluin-Nelemans JC, Louwagie A, et al. Interferon alfa versus chemotherapy for chronic myeloid leukemia: a meta-analysis of seven randomized trials. *J Natl Cancer Inst* 1997;89:1616–1620.

185. Kosmidis PA, Tsavaris N, Skarlos D, et al. Fluorouracil and leucovorin with or without interferon alfa-2b in advanced colorectal cancer: analysis of a prospective randomized phase III trial. Hellenic Cooperative. *J Clin Oncol* 1996;14:2682–2687.

186. Greco FA, Figlin R, York M, et al. Phase III randomized study to compare interferon alfa-2a in combination with fluorouracil versus fluorouracil alone in patients with advanced colorectal cancer. *J Clin Oncol* 1996;14:2674–2681.

187. Salgaller ML, Lodge PA. Use of cellular and cytokine adjuvants in the immunotherapy of cancer. *J Surg Oncol* 1998;68:122–138.

188. Billiau A, Heremans H, Vermeire K, Matthys P. Immunomodulatory properties of interferon-gamma. An update. *Ann N Y Acad Sci* 1998;856:22–32.

189. Richtsmeier WJ, Koch WM, McGuire WP, Poole ME, Chang EH. Phase I-II study of advanced head and neck squamous cell carcinoma patients treated with recombinant human interferon gamma. *Arch Otolaryngol Head Neck Surg* 1990;116:1271–1277.

190. Bruntsch U, de Mulder PH, ten Bokkel H, et al. Phase II study of recombinant human interferon-gamma in metastatic renal cell carcinoma. *J Biol Response Mod* 1990;9:335–338.

191. Boue F, Pastran Z, Spielmann M, et al. A phase I trial with recombinant interferon gamma (Roussel UCLAF) in advanced cancer patients. *Cancer Immunol Immunother* 1990;32:67–70.

192. Aulitzky WE, Lerche J, Thews A, et al. Low-dose gamma-interferon therapy is ineffective in renal cell carcinoma patients with large tumour burden. *Eur J Cancer* 1994;30A:940–945.

193. Ellerhorst JA, Kilbourn RG, Amato RJ, Zukiwski AA, Jones E, Logothetis CJ. Phase II trial of low dose gamma-interferon in metastatic renal cell carcinoma. *J Urol* 1994;152:841–845.

194. Metcalf D. The granulocyte-macrophage colony-stimulating factors. *Science* 1985;229:16–22.

195. Clark SC, Kamen R. The human hematopoietic colony-stimulating factors. *Science* 1987;236:1229–1237.

196. Tarr PE. Granulocyte-macrophage colony-stimulating factor and the immune system. *Med Oncol* 1996;13:133–140.

197. Inaba K, Inaba M, Romani N, et al. Generation of large numbers of dendritic cells from mouse bone marrow cultures supplemented with granulocyte/macrophage colony-stimulating factor. *J Exp Med* 1992;176:1693–1702.

198. Szabolcs P, Moore MA, Young JW. Expansion of immunostimulatory dendritic cells among the myeloid progeny of human CD34+ bone marrow precursors cultured with c-*kit* ligand, granulocyte-macrophage colony-stimulating factor, and TNF-alpha. *J Immunol* 1995;154:5851–5861.

199. Jones T, Stern A, Lin R. Potential role of granulocyte-macrophage colony-stimulating factor as vaccine adjuvant. *Eur J Clin Microbiol Infect Dis* 1994;13[Suppl 2]:S47–S53.

200. Pardoll DM. Paracrine cytokine adjuvants in cancer immunotherapy. *Annu Rev Immunol* 1995;13:399–415.
201. Markowicz S, Engleman EG. Granulocyte-macrophage colony-stimulating factor promotes differentiation and survival of human peripheral blood dendritic cells *in vitro. J Clin Invest* 1990;85:955–961.
202. American Society of Clinical Oncology. American Society of Clinical Oncology recommendations for the use of hematopoietic colony-stimulating factors: evidence-based, clinical practice guidelines. *J Clin Oncol* 1994;12:2471–2508.
203. Aman MJ, Stockdreher K, Thews A, et al. Regulation of immunomodulatory functions by granulocyte-macrophage colony-stimulating factor and granulocyte colony-stimulating factor *in vivo. Ann Hematol* 1996;73:231–238.
204. Willman CL, Stewart CC, Miller V, Yi TL, Tomasi TB. Regulation of MHC class II gene expression in macrophages by hematopoietic colony-stimulating factors (CSF). Induction by granulocyte/macrophage CSF and inhibition by CSF-1. *J Exp Med* 1989;170:1559–1567.
205. Samanci A, Yi Q, Fagerberg J, et al. Pharmacological administration of granulocyte/macrophage-colony-stimulating factor is of significant importance for the induction of a strong humoral and cellular response in patients immunized with recombinant carcinoembryonic antigen. *Cancer Immunol Immunother* 1998;47:131–142.
206. Murphy GP, Tjoa BA, Simmons SJ, et al. Infusion of dendritic cells pulsed with HLA-A2-specific prostate-specific membrane antigen peptides: a phase II prostate cancer vaccine trial involving patients with hormone-refractory metastatic disease. *Prostate* 1999;38:73–78.
207. Murphy GP, Tjoa BA, Simmons SJ, et al. Phase II prostate cancer vaccine trial: report of a study involving 37 patients with disease recurrence following primary treatment. *Prostate* 1999;39:54–59.
208. Rini BI, Stadler WM, Spielberger RT, Ratain MJ, Vogelzang NJ. Granulocyte-macrophage–colony stimulating factor in metastatic renal cell carcinoma: a phase II trial. *Cancer* 1998;82:1352–1358.
209. Simmons SJ, Tjoa BA, Elgamal A, et al. GM-CSF as a systemic adjuvant in a phase II prostate cancer vaccine trial. 1999 (*in press*).
210. Stoger H, Samonigg H, Krainer M, et al. Dose intensification of epidoxorubicin and cyclophosphamide in metastatic breast cancer: a randomized study with two schedules of granulocyte-macrophage colony stimulating factor. *Eur J Cancer* 1998;34:482–488.
211. Leyvraz S, Bacchi M, Cerny T, et al. Phase I multicenter study of combined high-dose ifosfamide and doxorubicin in the treatment of advanced sarcomas. Swiss Group for Clinical Research (SAKK). *Ann Oncol* 1998;9:877–884.
212. Buesa JM, Lopez-Pousa A, Martin J, et al. Phase II trial of first-line high-dose ifosfamide in advanced soft tissue sarcomas of the adult: a study of the Spanish Group for Research on Sarcomas (GEIS). *Ann Oncol* 1998;9:871–876.
213. Merlano M, Benasso M, Numico GM, et al. 5-Fluorouracil dose intensification and granulocyte-macrophage colony-stimulating factor in cisplatin-based chemotherapy for relapsed squamous cell carcinoma of the head and neck: a phase II study. *Am J Clin Oncol* 1998;21:313–316.
214. Berd D, Kairys J, Dunton C, Mastrangelo MJ, Sato T, Maguire HC Jr. Autologous, hapten-modified vaccine as a treatment for human cancers. *Semin Oncol* 1998;25:646–653.
215. Weigle WO. The production of thyroiditis and antibody following injection of unaltered thyroglobulin without adjuvant into rabbits previously stimulated with altered thyroglobulin. *J Exp Med* 1965;122:1049–1062.
216. Berd D, Murphy G, Maguire HC Jr, Mastrangelo MJ. Immunization with haptenized, autologous tumor cells induces inflammation of human melanoma metastases. *Cancer Res* 1991;51:2731–2734.
217. Berd D, Maguire HC Jr, Mastrangelo MJ. Treatment of human melanoma with a hapten-modified autologous vaccine. *Ann N Y Acad Sci* 1993;690:147–152.
218. Sato T, Maguire HC Jr, Mastrangelo MJ, Berd D. Human immune response to DNP-modified autologous cells after treatment with a DNP-conjugated melanoma vaccine. *Clin Immunol Immunopathol* 1995;74:35–43.
219. Bodmer WF, Browning MJ, Krausa P, Rowan A, Bicknell DC, Bodmer JG. Tumor escape from immune response by variation in HLA expression and other mechanisms. *Ann N Y Acad Sci* 1993;690:42–49.
220. Khanna R. Tumour surveillance: missing peptides and MHC molecules. *Immunol Cell Biol* 1998;76:20–26.

17.3

CANCER VACCINES: BASIC PRINCIPLES

Mechanisms of Immune Escape and Immune Tolerance

FRANCESCO M. MARINCOLA

A remarkable breakthrough in the understanding of human tumor immunology is the demonstration that the host immune system can mount humoral and cellular responses against antigens expressed by autologous cancer cells (1–3). Serologic analysis of recombinant complementary DNA–expression libraries has identified humoral immune responses directed against autologous cancer-specific proteins. The antitumor role of these antibodies, however, remains unclear because the proteins that they recognize are expressed in the intracellular compartment where immunoglobulins cannot reach them (3). Cellular immune responses are directed toward intracellular proteins because T cells recognize molecules that have been cleaved into short peptides and presented on target cell surfaces in association with major histocompatibility complex (MHC) class I molecules (called *human leukocyte antigens* or *HLA* in humans) (4). Because tumor antigens consist in large part of intracellular proteins, it is generally assumed that cellular immune responses are the prevalent immunologic defense of the organism against tumors (5). Indeed, most experimental models support a predominant role of the cellular rather than humoral arm of the immune response in cancer (6). Thus, T-cell–based immune interactions with tumor cells have been more extensively studied.

Among human tumors, malignant melanoma has been the most comprehensively studied because of the ease with which tumor-associated antigen (TAA)–specific T cells can be expanded by *in vitro* incubation of tumor-infiltrating lymphocytes (TILs) (7) with T-cell growth factors, such as interleukin-2 (IL-2) (8,9). The availability of tumor-specific TILs has led to the identification of several cytotoxic T lymphocyte (CTL)–defined melanoma-associated antigens (MAAs). MAAs fall into distinct categories according to various genetic and physiologic properties. Some MAAs are tissue specific because they are expressed by melanoma cells and normal melanocytes (10). These MAAs are called *tumor differentiation antigens* (TDAs). Other MAAs consist of proteins that are not expressed in normal adult tissues except for the testes (10). In addition, these antigens are expressed by tumors other than melanoma and are called *tumor-specific antigens* (TSAs) or *cancer-testis antigens*. The remaining MAAs are products of genes overexpressed in comparison with normal tissues (oncogenes) or of aberrant transcription of intronic sequences, mutated genes, or alternate open reading frames (10). Characterization of antigen-specific TILs has demonstrated that cellular immune responses are most commonly directed toward nonmutated TDAs or TSAs.

It was previously believed that the immune system could control tumor growth by recognizing foreign "new" molecules expressed by tumor cells (11,12). Proteins selectively expressed by tumors are not included in the repertoire of molecules determining negative selection of T cells in the thymus. Therefore, T cells recognizing "neoantigens" are not eliminated, and tumor cells are killed as they originate on the basis of self/nonself discrimination. Accordingly, most cancer cells were thought to have a "nonself" identity and to be eliminated by a vigorous immune reaction. Occasionally, however, under immune selection, tumor cells lacking neoantigens could survive, replicate, and produce clinically detectable tumors. This theory, referred to as *immune surveillance*, postulates a predominant role of escape mechanisms adopted by cancer cells to offset a brisk immune response against them. Immune surveillance is, however, questioned by the modern understanding of the immune biology of melanoma. Obviously, self/nonself discrimination does not apply broadly to tumor immunology because most identifiable immune responses against cancer are directed against self-molecules (1–3) and tolerance of self is the expected default reaction of the host toward them. Yet, the immune system is not totally unaware of cancer cells, as evidenced by the ease with which TAA-specific TILs can be generated from tumors (13–16). Thus, an indolent, rather than absent, immune response appears to govern the overall balance of tumor/host interactions. This guarantees a relatively pacific coexistence of effector and target cells, as evil and good seen from a distance seem to peacefully coexist in the society. The TAA-specificity of TILs observed *ex vivo* is likely to constitute an exaggeration of the immune reaction existing naturally at tumor site. If a cell suspension from a tumor is expanded *in vitro* without the addition of T-cell growth factors, tumor cells or fibroblasts (or both) take over the culture. TILs expand and tumor cells die only when cytokines stimulating T-cell proliferation are provided, unless resistant tumor cells arise (17). Because *in vivo* such growth factors are not provided, T cells that can kill tumor targets *in vitro* can coexist with the same cells *in vivo*. This view of tumor/host interaction (opposite to the immune/surveillance theory) suggests that tumor growth most often does not represent an escape from an effective immune response, rather an insensitivity to an insufficient immune response. When tumor rejection exceptionally occurs, the balance between tumor cell growth and destruction by T cells is overturned by immune stimulatory conditions similar, perhaps, to those causing autoimmunity. Thus, the term *immune escape* might be misleading because, in most cases, there is nothing to escape from. Therefore, for the rest of the chapter we refer to *tumor escape* when an immune response of sufficient magnitude to cause immune regression is postulated. In this case, the presence of tumor masses is attributed to countermeasures adopted by tumor cells or other cells, or both, within the tumor microenvironment to offset such response. We instead refer to *tumor tolerance* when an absent or insufficient immune response is postulated independently from the ability of tumor cells to escape it.

Expression of shared CTL-defined MAAs in a large percentage of patients with melanoma has stimulated enthusiasm for their use in clinical trials of active specific immunization. Thus, large amounts of information have been accrued on immune and clinical responses in these trials (18–22). These studies have shown that immunization with MAAs induces detectable MAA-specific CTL responses (19,22,23) but does not yield the clinical responses predicted by murine models. In mice, established immunogenic tumors can be cured by innumerable immune treatments. Furthermore, growth of poorly immunogenic tumors can be controlled or prevented in protection experiments in which animals are immunized before implantation of tumor cells. The exciting results obtained in mice are, however, invariably tempered by follow-up clinical studies, which, as noted long ago (24), regularly fail to yield similar results. Protection experiments illustrate the need for immune T cells to face small cell burdens for successful control of tumor growth. Bulky tumors may exhaust the host immune competence by altering its metabolism or producing immune suppression (25). Large cell populations may tolerize immune-reactive CTLs because of lack of costimulation (26) or by overwhelming the immune reaction. It is also possible that the greater number of cell divisions in larger lesions may statistically increase chances for the development of tumor cell variants resistant to treatment. Human treatments deal with the polymorphic nature of the human immune systems and tumors. Furthermore, the extreme heterogeneity of cancer cells has to be faced. Therefore, tumor escape mechanisms may play a bigger role in human disease than in prefabricated oligoclonal murine models. Thus, a pessimistic interpretation of the discrepant results observed between preclinical and clinical studies is the higher likelihood of human tumors to escape immune recognition.

MULTIPLE WAYS TO TUMOR TOLERANCE

Immune escape and *immune tolerance* are general terms that include a variety of mechanisms (Table 1). Inadequate immune responses in patients with cancer and other chronic illness have been attributed to decreased T-cell receptor (TCR) signaling capacity (25,27). No convincing evidence exists, however, that cancer patients are immune compromised. Flu-specific CTL reactivity is not different between patients with melanoma and healthy controls (28). Furthermore, MAA-specific CTL reactivity is easier to induce in patients with melanoma than in non–tumor-bearing individuals (28,29). Clonal deletion or exhaustion (30–35), replicative senescence (36,37), circulating immune-suppressive cytokines (25), soluble HLA molecules (38,39), and epitope mimicry (40) have been implicated in the induction of systemic, epitope-specific immune tolerance. Because MAA-specific T cells, however, can be activated and expanded *in vivo* by antigen-specific vaccines (19,22,23), deletion of tumor-reactive clones may not play in human cancers the role it plays in some preclinical models (30,33,36,37,41). We believe that the natural history of tumor growth and its response to immune manipulation is predominantly influenced by local factors. The ease with which MAA-specific CTLs can be detected among peripheral blood mononuclear cells and TILs suggests that the host immune system is sensitized against MAAs. The observation of "mixed responses" also suggests local factors as major modulators of tumor behavior. A mixed response is a relatively frequent (although the actual frequency has never been documented) phenomenon characterized by different behavior of synchronous metastases in response to T-cell–based immunotherapy. Although some metastases decrease in size or disappear, others grow unaffected by therapy. As a patient's immune response at a single time point is a constant, mixed responses reflect the major role played by the interactions between tumor and immune cells at each tumor site. Thus, we focus on local factors that could account for immune escape or peripheral tolerance of tumors, or both.

METHODOLOGIC CONSIDERATIONS

Although the clinical results of TAA-specific vaccinations have been disappointing, the use of well-defined immunogens represents an unprecedented human model to test hypotheses suggested by preclinical studies. Epitope-specific vaccines allow for analyses of immune responses confined to a single TAA/HLA allele combination targeted by the vaccination (42). This simplification might be incredibly important considering the com-

TABLE 1. MULTIPLE WAYS TO TUMOR TOLERANCE

I. Systemic mechanisms
  A. Immune suppression
    1. Cancer cachexia
    2. Alteration in T-cell receptor signal transduction (ζ-chain downregulation)
    3. Circulating immune-suppressive cytokines (transforming growth factor–β, interleukin-10, etc.)
  B. Systemic tolerance
    1. Clonal exhaustion
    2. Replicative senescence
    3. Fas/Fas ligand-induced apoptosis
    4. Soluble HLA
    5. Epitope mimicry
II. Local mechanisms
  A. Lack of localization
  B. Inadequate immunogenicity of tumor cells
    1. Lack of danger signal
    2. Insufficient epitope density
  C. Escape mechanisms
    1. Tumor-associated antigen loss or downregulation
    2. Abnormalities in antigen processing
    3. HLA loss or downregulation
  D. Peripheral tolerance
    1. Fas/Fas ligand-induced apoptosis
    2. Soluble HLA
    3. Paracrine secretion of immune suppressive cytokines by tumor cells (transforming growth factor-β, interleukin-10, etc.)
    4. Epitope mimicry

plexity of the algorithm governing tumor/host interactions. The difficulty of correlating laboratory findings with clinical outcome is the primary obstacle to the assessment of the role of immune escape or tolerance, or both, in cancer progression. Tumor/host interactions *in situ* have traditionally been studied in excised surgical specimens with immunohistochemistry (IHC) to estimate protein expression, DNA amplification to identify genetic abnormalities, and messenger RNA amplification for the assessment of gene expression. Fixed material, however, is not suitable for the assessment of T-cell function. Freshly isolated tumor cells or lymphocytes are suboptimal for accurate functional studies because of their extensive contamination by various cell types and the altered conditions of cells recently subjected to enzymatic or mechanical treatment. Expansion of TIL/tumor cell pairs from excised tumors has provided elegant models for the characterization *in vitro* of CTL/tumor interactions at a given time point (43). Although it is not clear whether cultured cells are representatives of *in vivo* conditions, experiments performed with cell lines establish important principles of T-cell/epitope interaction, which allow formulation of hypotheses to be tested *in vivo*. Analysis of reagents obtained from excised specimens, however, yields static information about a disease characterized by extreme genetic instability (44). As the natural course of the removed tumor cannot be followed prospectively to take the excised lesion as representative of other lesions left *in vivo*, homogeneity among metastases must be assumed. Even synchronous metastases, however, are quite heterogeneous (i.e., in the expression of MAA and HLA molecules) (45). This limitation could be overcome by serial analysis of identical tumor samples through fine needle aspiration (FNA) biopsies, which provide the opportunity to evaluate dynamically the expression of relevant markers (46,47). Because of the limited amount of material obtainable, however, FNA suffers from its own limitations. FNA could be combined with other techniques, allowing analysis of limited materials. Distinct populations of cells could be sorted by microdissection (48,49) or epitope/HLA tetramers (50,51), and their status of activation could be tested using accurate and sensitive methodologies, such as Taqman-based real-time polymerase chain reaction (52) or intracellular fluorescence-activated cell sorter analysis (53). This theoretically allows evaluation of the status of activation of CTLs *in vivo*. Collection of complementary DNA libraries from FNA of metastases could profile patterns of expression of thousands of genes in a single experiment (54). This information, combined with knowledge of the natural history of the lesion left *in situ*, might yield clinical material for correlation of laboratory findings with clinical outcome and identification of the algorithm necessary for tumor regression.

T-CELL LOCALIZATION AT TUMOR SITE

CTLs kill their victims by direct contact. Thus, localization of TAA-specific CTLs at tumor site is expected for their effector function. Adoptive transfer of indium-111–labeled TILs has shown that their localization is necessary for a clinical response to occur (55). In some cases, TILs home within the tumor and no regression is observed, suggesting that other factors within the tumor microenvironment may influence the status of CTL activation or the sensitivity of tumor cells to CTLs.

T Cells as "Lazy" Soldiers

Paradoxically, TILs can routinely be expanded *ex vivo* from growing melanoma metastases and shown to be able to effectively kill tumor cells in *in vitro* assays. Thus, TIL/tumor cell interactions observed *in vitro* do not explain *in vivo* phenomena. The discrepancy may reflect lack of sufficient stimulation *in vivo*, as the expansion *ex vivo* of TILs requires incubation not only with tumor cells but also with IL-2. Indeed, the requirements necessary to induce and sustain a CTL response in target organs are higher than that necessary for the execution of effector responses by the same CTL (26,56,57). Matzinger's "danger model" (26,58) proposes an explanation for the coexistence of effector and target cells in tissues without the development of tumor rejection, suggesting that the default interaction between tumor cells and host immune systems is absent or minimal. This model, in antithesis with self/nonself discrimination, suggests that immune responses start when tissue distress (danger) is detected. T cells require two types of stimulation to become activated, to stay activated, or both: (a) a "first signal" (signal one) provided by specific antigen/TCR interaction and (b) a "second signal" (signal two) bearer of the environmental conditions in which the immune interaction is occurring (59,60). The second message can be provided by cytokines ("help") or by costimulatory molecules expressed by specialized antigen-presenting cells (APCs) (61) in condition of tissue distress. Cancer cells do not constitutively express costimulatory molecules and do not secrete immune-stimulatory cytokines. Furthermore, by

offering only signal one, tumors might induce tolerance because the interaction of antigen-specific T cells with signal one in the absence of signal two causes their deletion (26). Thus, the majority of tumors do not "escape" immune recognition but simply survive in a favorable environment. In particular circumstances, however, the host immune response is awakened, resulting in spontaneous or therapeutically provoked regression of disease. The nature of the extra stimulation operating in such circumstances is unknown.

CTL requirements for induction of IL-2 or other cytokines promoting their activation and proliferation are relatively high (57), and "help" from HLA class II–restricted CD4+ T cells may be required (5,62–65). Tumors, particularly melanoma, express HLA class II molecules (66) and their expression in metastases correlates with response to T-cell–based therapy (67). Furthermore, HLA class II–associated MAAs have been identified (65,68), and evidence exists that malignant cells can present endogenous antigens in the context of HLA class II (69–72). Thus, it is possible that tumor cells could cross-prime effector and helper T cells; however, this possibility is difficult to accept considering the difficulties in identifying MAA-specific, HLA class II–restricted CD4+ T cells in tumor specimens. Furthermore, tumor cells do not provide signal two necessary for T-cell activation, and it is likely that APCs are required for activation of TAA-specific CTLs. It is assumed that TAAs shed by cancer cells are incorporated into lysosomes by APCs cleaved into peptides and presented on their surface bound to HLA class II molecules (5). Interactions with HLA class II–restricted helper T cells would cause release of cytokines capable of recruiting, expanding, and activating TAA-specific CTLs *in situ*. No direct evidence exists in humans, however, that APCs present TAAs shed by tumor cells *in vivo*. In murine models, APCs can present endocytosed antigens in association with MHC class I and class II molecules, and, if an adequate amount of antigen is provided, APCs induce concomitant activation of CD8+ and CD4+ T cells (73,74). High doses of antigen are necessary for efficient cross-presentation. If the amount of antigen incorporated by APCs is not sufficient, no CD4+ T-cell activation occurs, and tolerance is induced. Whether the efficiency of TAA incorporation by APCs in the tumor microenvironment is adequate for cross-presentation to helper and CTL populations or inadequate, leading to tumor tolerance, is not known. Tumor cells die without causing inflammation probably through an apoptotic pathway. Human CD14 (abundantly present on the surface of phagocytes) mediates phagocytosis of apoptotic cells (75) without induction of inflammatory processes. Thus, macrophages infiltrating tumors act as scavengers for senescent cancer cells, which remain "unnoticed" by the immune system. If, however, activated dendritic cells (DCs) incorporate and present antigen to CD8+ T cells, a powerful CTL response is induced (76). Viral models suggest that APCs activated by the viral infection can efficiently present antigens to CD8+ T cells (77). It is possible, therefore, that an activating step is required in tumors to turn macrophages into efficient APCs (78).

The primary interaction between tumor and T cells leads to expansion of APC-activated TAA-specific helper T cells, which, although unable to kill tumor cells, are capable of producing cytokines for the proliferation of TAA-specific, HLA class I–

TABLE 2. HYPOTHESIZED BEHAVIOR OF TUMOR-ASSOCIATED ANTIGEN EXPRESSION DURING DISEASE PROGRESSION

Type of Tumor-Associated Antigen	Expression			
	Relationship with Oncogenesis	Relative to Normal	Expected Expression with Disease Progression	Expected Effect on HLA Class I Expression
Tumor differentiation antigens	None	Decreased	Gradual loss	Less powerful
Tumor-specific antigens	Associated	Increased	Increased	Powerful
Oncogenes	Causative	Increased	Stable	Powerful

restricted CTLs. The difficulty encountered in identifying TAA-specific CD4$^+$ helper cells suggests that tumors may escape immune recognition simply because of the low chances of productive encounters among the various cell populations. It is possible, however, that non–TAA-specific CD4$^+$ helper cells are all that are needed for induction of TAA-specific CD8$^+$ T-cell responses. Environmental immunogens coincidentally expressed at the tumor site might suddenly stimulate proliferation of CD4$^+$ T cells. These helper cells would in turn promote proliferation and activation of dormant TAA-specific CD8$^+$ T cells (58). The coincidental nature of such events could offer a rationale for rare and serendipitous spontaneous tumor regressions. CD4$^+$ T cells can also directly activate and mature APCs through CD40/CD40L interactions (79). In this case, no close contact between CD8 and CD4 T cells is necessary. The activated APC then acts as a temporal bridge between a helper and a killer cell (79) and can activate more than one DC, which, in turn, could activate more than one CTL, leading to exponential expansion of the immune response. In this case, the presence of a helper epitope in the tumor microenvironment could be all that is required to initiate effective anticancer responses. Yet, most commonly, tumors might not express such helper molecules.

Tumor Cells as Inadequate Targets

Expression of MHC class I molecules is necessary for tumor recognition by CTLs (15,80,81). The molecular basis of this phenomenon has been well characterized by crystallographic resolution of peptide/HLA class I (82) and peptide/HLA class I/TCR complexes (83). Thus, complete loss of expression of TAA or HLA has, as undisputed consequence, loss of recognition by TAA-specific CTLs. It is, however, still controversial whether decreased expression of TAA or HLA, or both, affects significantly tumor/host interactions *in vivo*. An extensive description of TAA and HLA loss or downregulation has recently been prepared and we refer the reader to this review (10). Here we limit the discussion to the salient points with particular attention to the functional implications.

Loss or Decreased Expression of Tumor-Associated Antigens

Alterations in TAA expression were originally identified in murine tumor models as a cause of tumor escape (84–88). In humans, TAA expression is quite heterogeneous. TSAs are variably expressed in tumors (89) in correlation with a genome-wide demethylation process associated with tumor progression

(90–92). Treatment with demethylating agents, such as 5-Aza-2'-deoxycytidine, can induce expression of TSAs and sensitize cell lines to lysis by TAA-specific CTLs (90,93,94). The ability of demethylating agents to restore recognition of tumor cells by CTLs has not been exploited in clinical grounds because of the widespread effects that these agents have on normal cells (90,93). TDAs are more commonly expressed than TSAs. Earlier studies detected MART-1/MelanA messenger RNA in all cell lines and melanoma lesions tested (95). These studies, however, might have underestimated the heterogeneity of TDA protein expression. Idiopathic hemochromatosis (IHC) analysis with monoclonal antibody specific for gp100/Pmel17, MART-1/MelanA, and tyrosinase revealed that their expression is not as ubiquitous as suggested by molecular methods (46,96–105). Furthermore, contrary to TSAs, the frequency of TDA expression decreases with disease progression (45,106–109), probably because TSAs are not related to neoplastic transformation (Table 2). In particular, gp100/Pmel17 is less frequently expressed than MART-1/MelanA, which is less frequently expressed than tyrosinase (45,102,108–110).

Approximately 25% of synchronous metastases of patients with melanoma display significant differences in the percent of tumor cells expressing a given TAA (45,108,109). In addition, IHC of metastatic lesions has shown heterogeneity not only in percentage of tumor cells expressing a TAA but also in the level of TAA expression by demonstrating differences in intensity of staining (45,102,106). These findings have been corroborated in cell lines by analysis of TDAs by fluorescence-activated cell sorter analysis (111) and by quantitative real-time polymerase chain reaction (108). *In vitro* studies have also shown a correlation between the variability of expression of TAAs and recognition of tumor cells by CTLs (46,111–113). Variation in the level of TAA expression may explain the coexistence of TAA specific TILs in tissues expressing the target TAA. It is possible that productive engagements between TCRs and HLA class I antigen/peptide complexes proceed to a point of balance between avidity for and availability of epitope, which might correspond clinically to a temporary shrinkage of the tumor. At this point, T cells fail to destroy the remaining malignant cells efficiently, and the size of metastases is determined predominantly by the rate of growth of the remaining cancer cells. Yet, MAA-specific CTLs roam the tumor mass because TAAs shed by dying cancer cells may be presented by intratumoral APCs, which, with their superior antigen-presenting capability, can perpetuate the presence of TILs within the tumor.

Decreased expression of MAA or HLA class I molecules, or both, has been noted in residual tumors after immunotherapy

TABLE 3. ABERRANT HLA CLASS I PHENOTYPES

Phenotype	Mechanism
Loss of Expression	
Loss of all HLA class I alleles	Mutations in the β_2m gene
Selective loss of one HLA haplotype	Loss of large genomic unit
Selective allelic loss	Mutation in heavy chain gene
Downregulation	
Locus specific downregulation	Locus linked variability in transcriptional regulation
Allele downregulation	Unknown

(45,108,109,114). In 1999, an analysis of pooled metastases from HLA-A*0201 melanoma patients showed a significant increase in frequency of gp100-negative lesions (29% of 155 lesions) after immunization against this TDA compared with metastases analyzed before immunization (18% of 175 lesions) (108). Another study has shown a reduced expression of the ErbB-2 protooncogene in HLA-A2–expressing breast cancer lesions compared with HLA-A2–negative lesions (115). Because this antigen has a well-defined HLA-A2–associated epitope, this finding suggests that lesions expressing HLA alleles other than HLA-A2 may experience reduced immune pressure against this TAA.

Loss or Decreased Expression of HLAs

Altered MHC class I antigen expression in tumors was also first observed in murine tumor models (116–123) and shown to be a factor determining tumor escape from immune response (124–133). Surface expression of HLA molecules on human tumor cells has also been extensively studied, mostly with monoclonal antibody–recognizing monomorphic determinants of the HLA class I heavy chain (10). In 1999, however, monoclonal antibodies recognizing determinants restricted to the gene products of HLA-A and HLA-B loci or polymorphic determinant–defining HLA class I alleles were used to analyze malignant cells (10). HLA class I loss or downregulation has been described in several human tumors, including melanoma and carcinomas of the bladder, breast, cervix, colon, head and neck, kidney, lung, pancreas, prostate, and stomach (10,134,135). The frequency of HLA class I antigen loss and downregulation in various tumor types is presently controversial and has been discussed elsewhere (10).

Characterization of the molecular basis of altered HLA class I expression could be performed by the study of tumor cell lines. Several phenotypes have been identified and classified differently by various authors (134,135). They include: (a) total HLA class I loss, (b) selective loss of an HLA haplotype, (c) selective loss of one HLA allele, and (d) locus-specific or allele-specific downregulation (Table 3). Total HLA class I loss in tumor cells is caused by mutations in the β_2m gene, which results in loss of functional β_2m expression necessary for the stability of the peptide/HLA complex (136–140). Loss of β_2m expression has been observed by IHC staining of HLA class I-negative tumor specimens (141,142). Abnormalities ranging from point mutations to large deletions within the

β_2m gene are responsible in the majority of cases for altered translation of the protein product. These mutation occur most often within a "hot spot" in cell lines with a high mutation rate (44,138,139,143,144). Because two identical β_2m genes exist in the human genome, both genes need to be knocked out before HLA class I expression is totally lost. This may account for the relative rarity with which this phenotype is detected and its occurrence in the later stages of tumor progression. β_2m loss and identification of the same molecular abnormalities identified in cell lines have also been described *in situ* in the tumor lesions from which the cell lines were derived (137,139,145–147). Selective loss of an HLA class I allele has been documented by IHC staining of malignant lesions and by analysis of cell lines (148–150). Loss of an HLA class I heavy chain gene owing to loss of an HLA class I haplotype has been described in malignant melanoma (151), pancreatic (152), cervical (150), and colon carcinoma (*unpublished data*, 1999). This loss is most often caused by a large genomic deletion of the region encoding for HLA class II, III, and I genes (134,135,151). This relatively common mechanism leads to a 50% reduction in the ability of cells to express antigens in association with HLA molecules and is not reversible by treatment with interferon-γ (IFN-γ). This defect arises through mechanisms of defective chromosomal segregation, nondisjunction, or mitotic recombination that cause loss of variable portions of genomic DNA in the short arm of chromosome 6. In the 1990s, allelic loss was characterized in a melanoma and in cervical cell lines (149,150). In the melanoma cell, the loss of the HLA allele is caused by a defect in HLA-A*0201 premessenger RNA splicing (153).

Locus-specific abnormalities affect more commonly the HLA-B and -C loci and can be reversed in vitro by incubation of cell lines with IFN-γ (151,154). The systemic administration of IFN-γ, however, does not achieve a tissue concentration sufficient to achieve the same effect *in vivo* (155). It is likely that a common pathway is responsible for HLA class I locus-specific downregulation in tumor cells, as most HLA class I alleles within the same locus are simultaneously downregulated or upregulated (154). Although a correlation was described between HLA-B downregulation and elevated c-myc expression (156–159), it is unlikely related to the oncogenic process because HLA-B molecules are downregulated with the same frequency in normal cells (151) and in tumor cells not overexpressing c-myc (160,161). The selective downregulation of HLA class I alleles has been less extensively studied. Marked variation in the level of HLA-A2 was identified in clones isolated from a bulk melanoma cell line (149) and confirmed by an analysis in 1999 of a large panel of melanoma cell lines (111). The mechanism(s) underlying the variability of allelic expression noted in cell lines has not been investigated. Furthermore, it is not known whether the naturally occurring variation in HLA class I allele expression noted in cell lines corresponds to similar variability *in vivo*.

Little is known about the expression of nonclassical MHC molecules, such as HLA-E or -G. HLA-G expression has been reported on lymphoma (162) and melanoma (163) cell lines. Furthermore, a higher level of HLA-G expression was found in metastatic melanoma lesions than in normal skin (163). No conclusive information is available about the expression of HLA-E by solid tumor cells.

Defects in HLA Class I–Dependent Antigen Processing

Correct assembly of HLA class I molecules and efficient presentation of antigenic peptides depends on the generation of peptides by the proteasome complex and transport of these peptides into the endoplasmic reticulum, where they are assembled with HLA class I heavy chains and β_2m. Tumor cells may alter expression of components of the HLA class I antigen-processing pathway, leading to abnormal processing and presentation of TAAs. Several studies have demonstrated defective expression of the proteasome subunits LMP2 and LMP7 or the transporter subunits TAP1 and TAP2, or both, in cell lines derived from various tumor types (10). These defects have been shown to cause defective processing and presentation of antigenic peptides to CTLs (164–168). Synchronous loss of LMP and TAP observed in tumor cell lines and restoration of their expression by incubation in IFN-γ suggest that mechanisms of gene regulation are defective in these cells (164,168–170). Analysis of tissue specimen expression has identified examples of TAP1 downregulation in head and neck, breast, lung, colon, and cervical carcinomas and in melanomas (10), and noted more frequent losses in metastatic than primary lesions. The role of TAA processing defects in tumor immunology is, however, not clear, as these defects may not cause detectable loss of HLA class I expression because peptides may be generated by alternative proteasome complexes (171) and supplied through TAP-independent mechanisms (172).

Functional Significance of Tumor-Associated Antigens or HLA Loss or Downregulation, or Both

The majority of studies correlating HLA class I expression by tumor cells with their recognition by TAA-specific CTLs has evaluated this relationship in terms of an all-or-none phenomenon. The effect of variability in the surface expression of a specific TAA/HLA epitope on the recognition of tumor cells by cognate CTLs has been investigated only to a limited extent. The scanty information on this topic is likely to reflect at least in part the general assumption that as few as 1–5 peptide/MHC class I complexes on a target cell are sufficient for its recognition by CTLs (173–176). As a consequence, one may be inclined to dismiss the possibility that downregulation of the restricting HLA class I allele or associated TAA, or both, may provide tumor cells with an escape mechanism from CTL recognition. Intracellular peptides, however, compete with thousands of other peptides for a specific HLA class I allele (177). Therefore, not all possible endogenous epitopes can be presented with a density sufficient for recognition by CTLs (178), especially when the restricting HLA class I allele is downregulated. Furthermore, it has been proposed that high-avidity TCR/ligand interactions in the context of self-recognition are eliminated during thymic selection (179). As a consequence, TCR activation may require a threshold of self-epitope density higher than

1–5 HLA/peptide complexes (174,175). Studies in 1999 have shown that the level of HLA class I allele expression may vary considerably among tumor cells (111). Furthermore, level of TAA expression is an independent cofactor determining recognition by CTLs (111). Because of the highly competitive characteristics of MHC/peptide binding (180,181), variations in MHC molecule expression may significantly affect recognition of antigenic peptides by MHC-restricted CTLs. This variability may be particularly important for poorly immunogenic human tumors in which a combination of low expression of TAAs, low affinity of the TAA-derived peptide for HLA class I allele, and HLA class I allele downregulation may switch on and off TAA-specific CTLs. When HLA class I allele availability is sufficient to present one or more TAA-derived peptides on the cell surface, a target cell could be lysed through serial TCR engagement as an all-or-none phenomenon (182,183). If a cell population rather than a single cell is considered, a proportional relationship is expected to exist between epitope density and extent of CTL-mediated lysis of target cells. A normal distribution predicts that in borderline conditions the epitope density is on some cells below and on others above the threshold level required for recognition of targets by CTLs. Furthermore, the statistical probability of productive encounters between TCRs and epitopes increases with their density. These mechanism(s) account for the statistically significant relationship found between the level of the restricting HLA class I allele and extent of CTL-mediated lysis when the TAA-derived peptide recognized by CTLs is not a limiting variable.

As suggested by the "missing self" hypothesis, HLA class I downregulation on cells renders cells more susceptible to NK cell–mediated lysis (184). NK cell function is inhibited by the interaction of two distinct families of NK cell inhibitory receptors with HLA class I molecules (185). The first family of receptors, referred to as *killer inhibitory receptors*, includes molecules with two (p50, p58) or three (p70) immunoglobulinlike domains in their extracellular region and interacts with specific HLA-A, -B, and -C alleles. The second family of inhibitory receptors includes heterodimers composed of a CD94 glycoprotein and a NKG2 protein specific for the nonclassical HLA-E. The expression of HLA-E is of particular interest because it depends on binding of peptides derived from the signal sequence of most HLA-A, -B, -C, and -G molecules, therefore acting as a gauge for the overall expression HLA class I molecules (186–188). NK cells monitor HLA class I expression on target cells through these inhibitory receptors and eliminate those with low expression. Increased susceptibility of tumor cells with HLA class I downregulation to NK cell–mediated lysis has been demonstrated in several studies (134,184,189–192), although examples of tumor cell lines resistant to NK cell lysis despite HLA class I downregulation have been identified (Ferrone S. *unpublished data*, 1997;191,193). HLA-G has also been implicated as an inhibitor of NK cell activity and to protect melanoma cells from NK cell lysis (163). It is not clear what NK receptor interacts with HLA-G (194–199). Inhibitory receptors are expressed also on T cells (200,201), and the presence of killer-inhibitory receptors on TAA-specific CTL clones may have important implications for recognition of tumor cells with altered HLA class I (202). The frequency of expression of inhibitory receptors in TAA-specific CTLs, however, is not known.

It is unknown whether TAA or HLA class I expression, or both, gradually decreasing along with advancing stage of disease (203–209) reflects the progressive dedifferentiation of tumor cells or is the result of immune selection (205,208–210). Several *in vivo* observations suggest that MAA loss may lead to tumor escape from host immune recognition. Reports about loss of HLA or MAA owing to a particular treatment have been, however, anecdotal (45,47,109,114,166,202,211). Some larger studies have suggested MAA loss in relation to the specificity of the expected immune response (108,115), whereas others did not (111). Thus, circumstantial but not conclusive evidence exists that TAAs during progression of disease is owing to immune selection. Still, independent from its cause, loss, or downregulation of TAA or HLA, or both, MAA loss makes tumor cells unsuitable targets for HLA class I–restricted CTLs. Considering the extreme stringency of the human TCR repertoire for unique epitope/HLA allele combinations (212,213), it could be predicted that the HLA phenotype may influence the chance of a patient to respond to T cell–based immunotherapy. Conversely, loss of particular TAAs might be noted more frequently in patients with an HLA phenotype associated with a strong immune response toward that TAA. An extensive analysis of HLA phenotypes in patients undergoing T-cell–based immunotherapy, however, failed to demonstrate any association between HLA phenotype and disease stage or response to therapy, or both (214). The inability to identify a relationship between a particular HLA phenotype and clinical correlates remains an unsolved question going beyond the domains of tumor immunology (215).

TUMOR MICROENVIRONMENT IS A MESSY BATTLEFIELD

Immune Regulatory Cytokines

Within the environment where tumor cells live, immunologic mediators, particularly cytokines (216), may control host defenses. Cytokines can modulate interactions between CTLs and tumor cells by interfering with production and function of other cytokines or by altering the expression of adhesion or costimulatory molecules on various cell types (217–220). Intracellular adhesion molecule-1, which reinforces CTL/tumor interactions, can be induced or enhanced in normal and malignant cells *in vitro* and *in vivo* by tumor necrosis factor-α (TNF-α) (221–225), IFN-γ (224,226), and IL-10 (227). Furthermore, TNF-α and IFN-γ have been implicated in the shedding of soluble intracellular adhesion molecule-1 by malignant cells, which may inhibit CTL and NK lytic function (228). The effect of adhesion molecule expression on the cytotoxic activity of CTL and NK cells, however, remains controversial (218–220,229–231). Cytokines can also induce maturation and differentiation of APCs (232), or, like IL-10, have direct depressing effects on T-cell function (25). These include suppression of IL-2, IFN-γ, and granulocyte-macrophage colony-stimulating factor production by T helper cells (233,234) and inhibition of T-cell proliferation (235). IL-10 has also been described as a growth

factor for human melanoma cells (227). IL-10 is produced by immune cells (233), but it can also be secreted by melanoma cells and has been found in tissues from patients with metastatic melanoma (236). Furthermore, elevated serum levels of IL-10 were found in patients with metastatic melanoma, suggesting that this cytokine may have a systemic immune-suppressive effect (237).

Wojtowicz-Praga suggested a predominant role of transforming growth factor–β (TGF-β) as a cause of "tumor-induced immune suppression" (25). *In situ* expression of various isoforms of TGF (TGF-β1, -β2, and -β3) is common in tumors and correlates with progression of melanoma (238–240) and other skin tumors (241). The expression of TGF-β *in situ* is possibly owing to paracrine secretion by tumor cells, which can secrete cytokines *in vitro* (242,243). TGF isoforms have similar biologic effects acting as inhibitors or stimulators of cell replication (240,244,245). In murine models, TGF-β modulates melanoma growth by inducing immunosuppression of the host (246,247). It is not clear, however, whether the immunosuppressive effects of TGF-β produced by tumor cells are limited to the tumor microenvironment or affect the entire host immune system. In patients with melanoma, a correlation exists between plasma levels of TGF-β and disease progression (25). This association, however, may simply reflect the higher tumor burden in patients with progressive disease. *In vitro* TGF-β is also a powerful inhibitor of NK (248) and CTL function (246). TGF-β and IL-10 have been shown to act synergistically to induce immune privilege in the eye by inducing downregulation of Th1 immune responses (249). It is not known, however, whether IL-10 produced by melanoma cells plays a similar role by turning tumors into immune-privileged sites. In 1997 and 1998, different expression of lymphoattractant C-X-C chemokines was proposed as a relevant variable for the recruitment of T cells at the site of pathology (250–253). Evidence that these chemokines may play a significant role in cancer, however, is not available. Cytokines secreted by normal cells or tumor cells, or both, can also facilitate tumor growth. One example is IL-6, which can have a direct effect on tumor growth and progression (254). In addition, some cytokines can act as stimulus for induction of angiogenesis factors required for the supply of blood to tumor cells.

Interactions between the vascular endothelium and tumor cells may also affect the outcome of the antitumor immune response. Swelling, tenderness, and other inflammatory signs precede the disappearance of tumor masses and characterize tumor regression. This extraordinary behavior is difficult to consider the sole effect of CTL-mediated lysis of tumor cells because lysis induces apoptosis, which, per se, is not inflammatory. Alternatively, by selectively recognizing a target tissue, CTLs may trigger *in situ* an inflammatory cascade by producing TNF-α, IFN-γ, and other cytokines. Some tumors might be more sensitive than others to these inflammatory signals. This may explain why tumors respond with similar frequency to different biologic agents (CTLs, bacille Calmette-Guérin, IL-2, IFN, etc.). In all cases, the therapeutic agent might trigger inflammation, but tumor response would depend on the sensitivity of the tumor to the cytotoxic substances produced by the inflammatory process or the ability of the tumor environment to sustain an inflammatory process. This hypothesis could also explain why melanoma and renal cell cancer, two tumors that are characterized by different immunogenic potential (in melanoma, it is easy to derive MAA-specific CTLs, and multiple MAAs have been identified, the contrary for renal cell cancer), overall have similar sensitivity to biologic manipulation (255,256). It is possible that, although immunologically different, these tumor types have the same frequency of lesions sensitive to inflammation. TNF-α could play a significant role by exercising antitumor effects by a direct induction of apoptosis after contact of T cell with the target cell (257) or by indirect effects on tumor vasculature (258). As TNF-α is one of the cytokines secreted by activated CTLs, it is reasonable to postulate that factors modulating its antitumor effects could play a significant role in determining the sensitivity of a tumor to T-cell attack. In 1998, Wu et al. have shown that melanoma cell lines produce a cytokine called *endothelial monocyte-activating polypeptide II,* which increases sensitivity of endothelial cells to TNF-α (259). Melanoma cell lines secreting higher amounts of endothelial monocyte-activating polypeptide II are more sensitive *in vivo* to the antineoplastic effects of TNF-α. The expression of endothelial monocyte-activating polypeptide II in various tumor types, however, is not known, nor has this parameter been correlated with clinical outcome.

Surface Expression of Apoptotic Signals

Fas ligand (FasL) has been reported to be expressed in a high percentage of melanoma lines and melanoma lesions and to be detectable in sera of patients with melanoma (260). These findings suggested a novel mechanism of tumor escape whereby, through interaction with Fas on the surface of TILs, FasL could counter attack CTLs and extinguish anti-TAA CTLs. This model was accepted originally with enthusiasm because it provides a mechanism for the rarity of tumor regressions in spite of the presence of TAA-specific CTLs in malignant lesions. Furthermore, several studies described the detection of FasL in a number of other tumor types, including glioblastoma (261); astrocytoma (262); and lung (263), colon (264,265), and esophageal carcinoma (266). On scrutiny, however, it was realized that this model is not supported by the available experimental data. TILs and CTLs can be expanded *ex vivo* by repeated exposure to freshly isolated tumor cells or cell lines. In addition, Rivoltini et al. reported that TILs are insensitive to FasL (267) and, in murine models, the implantation of FasL-transduced tumors does not abrogate antitumor immune responses (268,269). In 1997 and 1998, an analysis of a large panel of melanoma cell lines found no evidence of FasL in melanoma (265,270). These studies were carried out on extensive control populations and with multiple methods, including real-time polymerase chain reaction, flow cytometry, and functional assays. One study included cell lines established from melanoma metastases, which had not responded to active specific immunotherapy with MAA-derived peptides (108). The conflicting information in the literature is likely to reflect the limited specificity of the anti-FasL antibodies used in IHC and flow cytometry and the contamination of tumor cells with other types of cells in studies, which have used real-time polymerase chain

reaction. Thus, the available information indicates that the expression of FasL in malignant lesions is minimal and its role in inducing immune escape limited as recognized by the same group, which had originally proposed this theory (271). Alternatively, tumor tolerance may be explained by Fas/FasL interactions between activated CTLs expressing FasL (272). Therefore, CTLs may not be able to efficiently attack tumor targets because on engagement of the TCR with the appropriate epitope they become activated and express FasL. Fas/FasL interactions occurring within the same T cell (suicide) or between closely proliferating activated T cells could cause their apoptotic death. Such effect would be specific for areas within the tumor microenvironment rich in activated T cells.

Soluble HLA

Soluble HLA (sHLA) class I molecules have been implicated in the induction of peripheral tolerance (39). Multiple mechanisms have been described that could induce secretion of sHLA molecules from cells, including alternative splicing of messenger RNA, proteolytic cleavage of membrane-bound HLA molecules, or secretion of unloaded heavy chains. sHLA molecules have been identified in serum, urine, and other body fluids (273,274). Among solid organs, the liver seems to contain the highest amount of sHLA, a curious finding considering the resistance of transplanted livers to rejection compared with other transplanted organs (275,276). Possibly, sHLA molecules could tolerize the host immune system by inducing apoptosis of alloreactive CTLs (38). Although sHLA have been implicated in the modulation of immune responses during rejection of HLA-mismatched organs, little evidence exists that these molecules could interfere with TAA-specific CTL function (39,277). Only a few studies have measured levels of sHLA molecules in cancer patients (278,279) and no studies assessing the effect of sHLA on TAA-specific T cells have been reported. Thus, the relevance of sHLA in the induction of tumor tolerance still needs evaluation.

Downregulation of Cytotoxic T-Lymphocyte Activity by Tumor-Associated Antigen Epitope Mimics

Among various factors that can shape TCR repertoire after birth are repeated encounters with degenerate epitopes from endogenous or exogenous sources. This phenomenon is called *molecular mimicry* (280–282). Molecular mimicry interactions between environmental pathogens or self-antigens and TAA-CTL reactions have also been described (283). A database search for peptides structurally similar to the MART-1 immunodominant epitope MART-1$_{27-35}$ identified multiple mimicry sequences occurring in proteins of viral, bacterial, and human (self) proteins. Some of these mimicry peptides could react with MART-1–specific CTLs. Although an individual TCR can engage different (though biochemically related) peptide sequences, the result of the various TCR/epitope interactions can yield remarkably different outcomes on a particular T cell, ranging from fully agonistic to totally antagonistic reactions (284). In 1998, Loftus et al. identified partial agonists of

MART-1$_{27-35}$, which could partially tolerize MART-1–specific CTLs (40). These experiments suggested that encounters with partial agonist or antagonist peptides may hamper CTL responses to their natural ligands and, in the case of TAA-specific CTLs, be responsible for impaired antitumor responses. Most of the MART-1$_{27-35}$ analogues so far identified are peptide sequences from proteins produced by human pathogens or expressed by human normal tissues. Therefore, it could be postulated that such analogue peptides could be commonly present in the organism and be responsible for decreased function of TAA-specific CTLs. Evidence is lacking, however, that these analogue peptides are present in the systemic circulation or in the tumor microenvironment in concentrations sufficient to cause the effects described *in vitro*. Thus, future work should demonstrate a tissue distribution of weak agonist or antagonist epitope mimics compatible with induction of tumor tolerance.

GETTING TO THE END OF THE WAR

For the immunotherapist, cancer is a fratricidal war that leads most often to the demise of the society in which it occurs. Like in most civil wars, the fight is complicated by a (sub)conscious repulsion of brothers to kill brothers (tolerance) and by the ease in which differences can be concealed by similarities (escape mechanisms). Contrary to regular wars, the end of a civil war is rarely achieved by force, as it is difficult to overpower a concealed enemy. This war is more likely ended by understanding its causes and the reasons extending it. Sorting the evil from good might depend on subtleties more likely to be appreciated by the patience of a diplomat than the power of a general. Thus, it is likely that the defeat of cancer will be achieved by crafters of smarter bombs rather than more powerful ones.

The identification of MAAs and their respective CTL epitopes has raised interest in peptide-based vaccinations (2), as clinical studies have shown that MAA-specific vaccines can powerfully enhance TAA-specific CTL reactivity (19,22,23). Systemic CTL responses to the vaccines, however, most often do not correspond to clinical regression, leaving investigators with the paradoxical observation of identifiable CTL reactivity that is not capable of destroying the targeted tissues. Among the questions raised by this paradox stands the enigma of whether tumors resist immunotherapy because the immune response elicited is insufficient (26) or because tumor cells rapidly adapt to immune pressure by switching into less immunogenic phenotypes (10). As discussed, animal models support either point of view and this dichotomy is far from solved in humans. It is possible that a balance between subliminal immune responses and fading immunogenicity of tumors governs the fine equilibrium, allowing tumor survival in the immune competent host. Epitope-specific vaccinations for the immunotherapy of melanoma, although disappointing in their clinical results, have given us the unique opportunity of comparing systemic T-cell responses with localization and status of activation of the same T cells in the target organ. At the same time, accurate analyses of the molecules targeted by the vaccination (TAA/HLA complex) can be performed. Prospective analyses of large cohorts of patients undergoing these "immunologically simplified" treatments will allow, in the near future, an expedited understanding of the issues raised in this chapter.

REFERENCES

1. Boon T, Coulie PG, Van den Eynde B. Tumor antigens recognized by T cells. *Immunol Today* 1997;18:267–268.
2. Rosenberg SA. Cancer vaccines based on the identification of genes encoding cancer regression antigens. *Immunol Today* 1997;18:175–182.
3. Old LJ, Chen YT. New paths in human cancer serology. *J Exp Med* 1998;187:1163–1167.
4. Germain RN. The ins and outs of antigen processing and presentation. *Nature* 1996;322:687–689.
5. Yewdell JW, Bennink JR. The binary logic of antigen processing and presentation to T cells. *Cell* 1990;62:203–206.
6. Restifo NP, Wunderlich JR. Principles of tumor immunity: biology of cellular immune responses. In: DeVita VT, Hellman S, Rosenberg SA, eds. *Biologic therapy of cancer*, 1st ed. Philadelphia: JB Lippincott Co, 1996:3–21.
7. Rosenberg SA, Spiess P, Lafreniere R. A new approach to the adoptive immunotherapy of cancer with tumor-infiltrating lymphocytes. *Science* 1986;233:1318–1321.
8. Taniguchi T, Matsui H, Fujita T, et al. Structure and expression of a cloned cDNA for human interleukin-2. *Nature* 1983;302:305–310.
9. Knuth A, Danowski B, Oettgen HF, et al. T-cell-mediated cytotoxicity against autologous malignant melanoma: analysis with interleukin 2-dependent T-cell cultures. *Proc Natl Acad Sci U S A* 1984;81:3511–3515.
10. Marincola FM, Jaffe EM, Hicklin DJ, et al. Escape of human solid tumors from T cell recognition: molecular mechanisms and functional significance. *Adv Immunol* 2000;74:181–273.
11. Thomas L. *Cellular and humoral aspects of the hypersensitive state*, 1st ed. New York: Hoeber, 1959.
12. Burnet FM. The concept of immunological surveillance. *Prog Exp Tumor Res* 1970;13:1–27.
13. Topalian SL, Solomon D, Rosenberg SA. Tumor-specific cytolysis by lymphocytes infiltrating human melanomas. *J Immunol* 1989;142:3714–3725.
14. Topalian SL, Rosenberg SA. Tumor-infiltrating lymphocytes: evidence for specific immune reactions against growing cancers in mice and humans. *Important Adv Oncol* 1990;19–41.
15. Wolfel T, Klehmann E, Muller C, Schutt KH, et al. Lysis of human melanoma cells by autologous cytolytic T cell clones. Identification of human histocompatibility leukocyte antigen A2 as a restriction element for three different antigens. *J Exp Med* 1989;170:797–810.
16. Kawakami Y, Zakut R, Topalian SL, et al. Shared human melanoma antigens. Recognition by tumor-infiltrating lymphocytes in HLA-A2.1-transfected melanomas. *J Immunol* 1992;148:638–643.
17. Topalian SL, Kasid A, Rosenberg SA. Immunoselection of a human melanoma resistant to specific lysis by autologous tumor-infiltrating lymphocytes. Possible mechanisms for immunotherapeutic failures. *J Immunol* 1990;144:4487–4495.
18. Marchand M, Weynants P, Rankin E, et al. Tumor regression responses in melanoma patients treated with a peptide encoded by gene MAGE-3. *Int J Cancer* 1995;63:883–885.
19. Cormier JN, Salgaller ML, Prevette T, et al. Enhancement of cellular immunity in melanoma patients immunized with a peptide from MART-1/Melan A [see comments]. *Cancer J Sci Am* 1997;3:37–44.
20. McRae BL, Vanderlugt CL, Dal Canto MC, et al. Functional evidence for epitope spreading in the relapsing pathology of experimental autoimmune encephalomyelitis. *J Exp Med* 1995;182:75–85.
21. Nestle FO, Alijagic S, Gilliet M, et al. Vaccination of melanoma patients with peptide- or tumor lysate-pulsed dendritic cells. *Nat Med* 1998;4:328–332.
22. Rosenberg SA, Yang JC, Schwartzentruber DJ, et al. Immunologic and therapeutic evaluation of a synthetic tumor associated peptide vaccine for the treatment of patients with metastatic melanoma. *Nat Med* 1998;4:321–327.

23. Salgaller ML, Marincola FM, Cormier JN, et al. Immunization against epitopes in the human melanoma antigen gp100 following patient immunization with synthetic peptides. *Cancer Res* 1996;56: 4749–4757.

24. Sell S. Tumor immunity: relevance of animal models to man. *Hum Pathol* 1978;9:63–69.

25. Wojtowicz-Praga S. Reversal of tumor-induced immunosuppression: a new approach to cancer therapy [see comments]. *J Immunother* 1997;20:165–177.

26. Matzinger P. An innate sense of danger. *Semin Immunol* 1998; 10:399–415.

27. Zea AH, Curti BD, Longo DL, et al. Alterations in T cell receptor and signal transduction molecules in melanoma patients. *Clin Cancer Res* 1995;1:1327–1335.

28. Marincola FM, Rivoltini L, Salgaller ML, et al. Differential anti-MART-1/MelanA CTL activity in peripheral blood of HLA-A2 melanoma patients in comparison to healthy donors: evidence for *in vivo* priming by tumor cells. *J Immunother* 1996;19:266–277.

29. D'Souza S, Rimoldi D, Lienard D, et al. Circulating Melan-A/Mart-1 specific cytolytic T lymphocyte precursors in HLA-A2+ melanoma patients have a memory phenotype. *Int J Cancer* 1998;78:699–706.

30. Lauritzsen GF, Hofgaard PO, Schenck K, et al. Clonal deletion of thymocytes as a tumor escape mechanism. *Int J Cancer* 1998;78: 216–222.

31. Toes RE, Blom RJ, Offringa R, et al. Enhanced tumor outgrowth after peptide vaccination. Functional deletion of tumor-specific CTL induced by peptide vaccination can lead to the inability to reject tumors. *J Immunol* 1996;156:3911–3918.

32. Van Parijs L, Abbas AK. Homeostasis and self-tolerance in the immune system: turning lymphocytes off. *Science* 1998;280: 243–248.

33. Moskophidis D, Lechner F, Pircher HP, et al. Virus persistence in acutely infected immunocompetent mice by exhaustion of antiviral cytotoxic effector T cells. *Nature* 1993;362:758–761.

34. Alexander-Miller MA, Leggatt GR, Sarin A, et al. Role of antigen, CD8, and cytotoxic T lymphocyte (CTL) avidity in high dose antigen induction of apoptosis of effector CTL. *J Exp Med* 1996;184:485–492.

35. Toes RE, Schoenberger SP, van der Voort EI, et al. Activation or frustration of anti-tumor responses by T-cell-based immune modulation. *Semin Immunol* 1997;9:323–327.

36. Effros RB, Pawelec G. Replicative senescence of T cells: does the Hayflick Limit lead to immune exhaustion? *Immunol Today* 1997;18:450–454.

37. Effros RB, Allsopp R, Chiu CP, et al. Shortened telomeres in the expanded CD28-CD8+ cell subset in HIV disease implicate replicative senescence in HIV pathogenesis. *AIDS* 1996;10:F17–F22.

38. Zavazava N, Kronke M. Soluble HLA class I molecules induce apoptosis in alloreactive cytotoxic T lymphocytes. *Nat Med* 1996;2: 1005–1010.

39. Zavazava N. Soluble HLA class I molecules: biological significance and clinical implications. *Mol Med Today* 1998;4:116–121.

40. Loftus DJ, Squarcina P, Nielsen MB, et al. Peptides derived from self-proteins as partial agonists and antagonists of human CD8+ T-cell clones reactive to melanoma/melanocyte epitope MART1(27-35). *Cancer Res* 1998;58:2433–2439.

41. Toes RE, Offringa R, Blom RJ, et al. Peptide vaccination can lead to enhanced tumor growth through specific T-cell tolerance induction. *Proc Natl Acad Sci U S A* 1996;93:7855–7860.

42. Salgaller ML. Monitoring of cancer patients undergoing active or passive immunotherapy. *J Immunother* 1997;20:1–14.

43. Pandolfi F, Boyle LA, Trentin L, et al. Expression of HLA-A2 antigen in human melanoma cell lines and its role in T-cell recognition. *Cancer Res* 1991;51:3164–3170.

44. Lengauer C, Kinzler KW, Vogelstein B. Genetic instabilities in human cancers. *Nature* 1998;396:643–649.

45. Cormier JN, Hijazi YM, Abati A, et al. Heterogeneous expression of melanoma-associated antigens (MAA) and HLA-A2 in metastatic melanoma *in vivo*. *Int J Cancer* 1998;75:517–524.

46. Marincola FM, Hijazi YM, Fetsch P, et al. Analysis of expression of the melanoma associated antigens MART-1 and gp100 in metastatic melanoma cell lines and in in situ lesions. *J Immunother* 1996; 19:192–205.

47. Lee K-H, Panelli MC, Kim CJ, et al. Functional dissociation between local and systemic immune response following peptide vaccination. *J Immunol* 1998;161:4183–4194.

48. Bonner RF, Emmert-Buck M, Cole K, et al. Laser capture microdissection: molecular analysis of tissue. *Science* 1997;278:1481–1483.

49. Peterson LA, Brown MR, Carlisle AJ, et al. An improved method for construction of directionally cloned cDNA libraries from microdissected cells. *Cancer Res* 1998;58:5326–5328.

50. Altman JD, Moss PH, Goulder PR, et al. Phenotypic analysis of antigen-specific T lymphocytes. *Science* 1996;274:94–96.

51. Romero P, Dunbar PR, Valmori D, et al. *Ex vivo* staining of metastatic lymph nodes by class I major histocompatibility complex tetramers reveals high numbers of antigen-experienced tumor-specific cytolytic T lymphocytes. *J Exp Med* 1998;188:1641–1650.

52. Kruse N, Pette M, Toyka K, et al. Quantification of cytokine mRNA expression by RT PCR in samples of previously frozen blood. *J Immunol Methods* 1997;210:195–203.

53. Kern F, Surel IP, Brock C, et al. T-cell epitope mapping by flow cytometry. *Nat Med* 1998;4:975–978.

54. Duggan DJ, Bittner M, Chen Y, et al. Expression profiling using cDNA microarrays. *Nat Genet* 1999;21:10–14.

55. Pockaj BA, Sherry RM, Wei JP, et al. Localization of [111]indium-labeled tumor infiltrating lymphocytes to tumor in patients receiving adoptive immunotherapy. Augmentation with cyclophosphamide and correlation with response. *Cancer* 1994;73:1731–1737.

56. Valitutti S, Muller S, Dessing M, et al. Different responses are elicited in cytotoxic T lymphocytes by different levels of T cell receptor occupancy. *J Exp Med* 1996;183:1917–1921.

57. Gervois N, Guilloux Y, Diez E, et al. Suboptimal activation of melanoma infiltrating lymphocytes (TIL) due to low avidity of TCR/MHC-tumor peptide interactions. *J Exp Med* 1996;183:2403–2407.

58. Fuchs EJ, Matzinger P. Is cancer dangerous to the immune system? *Semin Immunol* 1996;8:271–280.

59. Schwartz RH. A cell culture model for T lymphocyte clonal anergy. *Science* 1990;248:1349–1356.

60. Matzinger P. Tolerance, danger, and the extended family. *Annu Rev Immunol* 1994;12:991–1045.

61. Jenkins MK, Schwartz RH. Antigen presentation by chemically modified splenocytes induces antigen-specific T cell unresponsiveness *in vitro* and *in vivo*. *J Exp Med* 1987;165:302–319.

62. Kalams SA, Walker BD. The critical need for CD4 help in maintaining effective cytotoxic T lymphocyte responses. *J Exp Med* 1998;188:2199–2204.

63. Zajac AJ, Blattman JN, Murali-Krishna K, et al. Viral immune evasion due to persistence of activated T cells without effector function. *J Exp Med* 1998;188:2205–2213.

64. Hung K, Hayashi R, Lafond-Walker A, et al. The central role of CD4+ T cells in the antitumor immune response. *J Exp Med* 1998;188:2357–2368.

65. Toes RE, Ossendorp F, Offringa R, et al. CD4 T cells and their role in antitumor immune responses. *J Exp Med* 1999;189:(5)753–756.

66. Pellegrino MA, Natali PG, Ng AK, et al. Unorthodox expression of IA-like antigens on human tumor cells of nonlymphoid origin: immunological properties, structural profile and clinical relevance. In: Nakamura RM, Dito WR, Tucker ES, eds. *Immunologic analysis. Recent progress in diagnostic laboratory immunology*, 1st ed. New York: Mason, 1982:159–173.

67. Rubin JT, Elwood LJ, Rosenberg SA, et al. Immunohistochemical correlates of response to recombinant interleukin-2 based immunotherapy in humans. *Cancer Res* 1989;49:7086–7092.

68. Topalian SL, Rivoltini L, Mancini M, et al. Human CD4+ T cells specifically recognize a shared melanoma-associated antigen encoded by the tyrosinase gene. *Proc Natl Acad Sci U S A* 1994;91:9461–9465.

69. Brady MS, Eckels DD, Ree SY, et al. MHC class II-mediated antigen presentation by melanoma cells [see comments]. *J Immunother Emphasis Tumor Immunol* 1996;19:387–397.

70. Armstrong TD, Clements VK, Ostrand-Rosenberg S. MHC class II-transfected tumor cells directly present antigen to tumor-specific CD4+ T lymphocytes. *J Immunol* 1998;160:661–666.

71. Akporiaye ET, Panelli MC. Functional class II antigen presentation pathway in metastatic melanoma cell lines. *J Immunother* 1996; 19:398.

72. Panelli MC, Wang E, Shen S, et al. Interferon gamma (IFN-gamma) gene transfer of an EMT6 tumor that is poorly responsive to IFN-gamma stimulation: increase in tumor immunogenicity is accompanied by induction of a mouse class II transactivator and class II MHC. *Cancer Immunol Immunother* 1996;42:99–107.

73. Kurts C, Heath WR, Carbone FR, et al. Cross-presentation of self antigens to CD8+ T cells: the balance between tolerance and autoimmunity. *Novartis Found Symp* 1998;215:172–181.

74. Kurts C, Kosaka H, Carbone FR, et al. Class I-restricted cross-presentation of exogenous self-antigens leads to deletion of autoreactive CD8(+) T cells. *J Exp Med* 1997;186:239–245.

75. Devitt A, Moffatt OD, Raykundalia C, et al. Human CD14 mediates recognition and phagocytosis of apoptotic cells. *Nature* 1998;392:505–509.

76. Albert ML, Sauter B, Bhardwaj N. Dendritic cells acquire antigen from apoptotic cells and induce class I-restricted CTLs. *Nature* 1998;392:86–89.

77. Bhardwaj N, Bender A, Gonzalez N, et al. Influenza virus-infected dendritic cells stimulate strong proliferative and cytolytic responses from human CD8+ T cells. *J Clin Invest* 1994;94:797–807.

78. Sallusto F, Lanzavecchia A. Efficient presentation of soluble antigen by cultured human dendritic cells is maintained by granulocyte/macrophage colony-stimulating factor plus interleukin 4 and downregulated by tumor necrosis factor alpha. *J Exp Med* 1994; 179:1109–1118.

79. Ridge JP, Di Rosa F, Matzinger P. A conditioned dendritic cell can be a temporal bridge between a CD4+ T-helper and a T-killer cell. *Nature* 1998;393:474–478.

80. Crowley NJ, Darrow TL, Quinn-Allen MA, et al. MHC-restricted recognition of autologous melanoma by tumor-specific cytotoxic T cells. Evidence for restriction by a dominant HLA-A allele. *J Immunol* 1991;146:1692–1699.

81. Rosenberg SA, Packard BS, Aebersold PM, et al. Use of tumor-infiltrating lymphocytes and interleukin-2 in the immunotherapy of patients with metastatic melanoma. *N Engl J Med* 1988;319: 1676–1680.

82. Bjorkman PJ, Saper MA, Samraoui B, et al. Structure of the human class I histocompatibility antigen, HLA-A2. *Nature* 1987; 329:506–512.

83. Garboczi DN, Ghosh P, Utz U, et al. Structure of the complex between human T-cell receptor, viral peptide and HLA-A2. *Nature* 1996;384:134–141.

84. Biddison WE, Palmer JC. Development of tumor cell resistance to syngeneic cell-mediated cytotoxicity during growth of ascitic mastocytoma P815Y. *Proc Natl Acad Sci U S A* 1977;74:329–333.

85. Uyttenhove C, Maryanski J, Boon T. Escape of mouse mastocytoma P815 after nearly complete rejection is due to antigen-loss variants rather than immunosuppression. *J Exp Med* 1983;157: 1040–1052.

86. Lethe B, Van den Eynde B, Van Pel A, et al. Mouse tumor rejection antigens P815A and P815B: two epitopes carried by a single peptide. *Eur J Immunol* 1992;22:2283–2288.

87. Van den Eynde B, Lethe B, Van Pel A, et al. The gene coding for a major tumor rejection antigen of tumor P815 is identical to the normal gene of syngeneic DBA/2 mice. *J Exp Med* 1991;173: 1373–1384.

88. Boon T, De Plaen E, Lurquin C, et al. Identification of tumour rejection antigens recognized by T lymphocytes. *Cancer Surv* 1992;13: 23–37.

89. van der Bruggen P, Traversari C, Chomez P, et al. A gene encoding an antigen recognized by cytolytic T lymphocytes on a human melanoma. *Science* 1991;254:1643–1647.

90. De Smet C, De Backer O, Faraoni I, et al. The activation of human gene MAGE-1 in tumor cells is correlated with genome-wide demethylation. *Proc Natl Acad Sci U S A* 1996;93:7149–7153.

91. Bedford MT, van Helden PD. Hypomethylation of DNA in pathological conditions of the human prostate. *Cancer Res* 1987;47: 5274–5276.

92. Liteplo RG, Kerbel RS. Reduced levels of DNA 5-methylcytosine in metastatic variants of the human melanoma cell line MeWo. *Cancer Res* 1987;47:2264–2267.

93. Weber J, Salgaller M, Samid D, et al. Expression of the MAGE-1 tumor antigen is up-regulated by the demethylating agent 5-aza-2'-deoxycytidine. *Cancer Res* 1994;54:1766–1771.

94. Lee L, Wang RF, Wang X, et al. NY-ESO-1 may be a potential target for lung cancer immunotherapy. *Cancer J Sci Am* 1999;5:20–25.

95. Coulie PG, Brichard V, Van Pel A, et al. A new gene coding for a differentiation antigen recognized by autologous cytolytic T lymphocytes on HLA-A2 melanomas. *J Exp Med* 1994;180:35–42.

96. Vennegoor C, Hageman P, Van Nouhuijs, et al. A monoclonal antibody specific for cells of the melanocyte lineage. *Am J Pathol* 1988;130:179–192.

97. Vennegoor C, Calafat J, Hageman P, et al. Biochemical characterization and cellular localization of a formalin-resistant melanoma-associated antigen reacting with monoclonal antibody NKI/C-3. *Int J Cancer* 1985;35:287–295.

98. Kawakami Y, Eliyahu S, Delgado CH, et al. Identification of a human melanoma antigen recognized by tumor-infiltrating lymphocytes associated with *in vivo* tumor rejection. *Proc Natl Acad Sci U S A* 1994;91:6458–6462.

99. Kang X, Kawakami Y, el-Gamil M, et al. Identification of a tyrosinase epitope recognized by HLA-A24-restricted, tumor-infiltrating lymphocytes. *J Immunol* 1995;155:1343–1348.

100. Wolfel T, Van Pel A, Brichard V, et al. Two tyrosinase nonapeptides recognized on HLA-A2 melanomas by autologous cytolytic T lymphocytes. *Eur J Immunol* 1994;24:759–764.

101. Brichard VG, Herman J, Van Pel A, et al. A tyrosinase nonapeptide presented by HLA-B44 is recognized on a human melanoma by autologous cytolytic T lymphocytes. *Eur J Immunol* 1996;26: 224–230.

102. Chen Y-T, Stockert E, Tsang S, et al. Immunophenotyping of melanomas for tyrosinase: implications for vaccine development. *Proc Natl Acad Sci U S A* 1995;92:8125–8129.

103. Kawakami Y, Battles JK, Kobayashi T, et al. Production of recombinant MART-1 proteins and specific antiMART-1 polyclonal and monoclonal antibodies: use in the characterization of the human melanoma antigen MART-1. *J Immunol Methods* 1997;202:13–25.

104. Scott-Coombes DM, Whawell SA, Vipond MN, et al. Fibrinolytic activity of ascites caused by alcoholic cirrhosis and peritoneal malignancy. *Gut* 1993;34:1120–1122.

105. Busam KJ, Iversen K, Coplan KA, et al. Immunoreactivity for A103, an antibody to melan-A (Mart-1), in adrenocortical and other steroid tumors. *Am J Surg Pathol* 1998;22:57–63.

106. de Vries TJ, Fourkour A, Wobbes T, et al. Heterogeneous expression of immunotherapy candidate proteins gp100, MART-1, and tyrosinase in human melanoma cell lines and in human melanocytic lesions. *Cancer Res* 1997;57:3223–3229.

107. Busam KJ, Chen YT, Old LJ, et al. Expression of melan-A (MART1) in benign melanocytic nevi and primary cutaneous malignant melanoma. *Am J Surg Pathol* 1998;22:976–982.

108. Riker A, Kammula US, Panelli MC, et al. Immune selection following antigen specific immunotherapy of melanoma. *Surgery* 1999; 126:112–120.

109. Scheibenbogen C, Weyers I, Ruiter D, et al. Expression of gp100 in melanoma metastases resected before or after treatment with IFN alpha and IL-2. *J Immunol* 1996;19:375–380.

110. Cormier JN, Abati A, Fetsch P, et al. Comparative analysis of the *in vivo* expression of tyrosinase, MART-1/Melan-A, and gp100 in metastatic melanoma lesions: implications for immunotherapy. *J Immunother* 1998;21:27–31.

111. Cormier JN, Panelli MC, Hackett JA, et al. Natural variation of the expression of HLA and endogenous antigen modulates CTL

recognition in an *in vitro* melanoma model. *Int J Cancer* 1999;80: 781–790.

112. Yoshino I, Peoples GE, Goedegebuure PS, et al. Association of HER2/neu expression with sensitivity to tumor-specific CTL in human ovarian cancer. *J Immunol* 1994;152:2393–2400.

113. Caux C, Massacrier C, Dezutter-Dambuyant C, et al. Human dendritic Langerhans cells generated *in vitro* from CD34+ progenitors can prime naive CD4+ T cells and process soluble antigen. *J Immunol* 1995;155:5427–5435.

114. Jager E, Ringhoffer M, Karbach J, et al. Inverse relationship of melanocyte differentiation antigen expression in melanoma tissues and CD8+ cytotoxic-T-cell responses: evidence for immunoselection of antigen-loss variants *in vivo. Int J Cancer* 1996;66:470–476.

115. Nistico P, Moulese M, Mammi C, et al. Low frequency of ErbB-2 proto-oncogene overexpression in human leukocyte antigen A2 positive breast cancer patients. *J Natl Cancer Inst* 1997;89:319–321.

116. Cikes M. Variations in expression of surface antigens on cultured cells. *Ann N Y Acad Sci* 1971;177:190–200.

117. Cikes M, Friberg SJ. Expression of H-2 and Moloney leukemia virus-determined cell-surface antigens in synchronized cultures of a mouse cell line. *Proc Natl Acad Sci U S A* 1971;68:566–569.

118. Haywood GR, McKhann CF. Antigenic specificities on murine sarcoma cells. Reciprocal relationship between normal transplantation antigens (H-2) and tumor-specific immunogenicity. *J Exp Med* 1971;33:1171–1187.

119. Kersey JH, Yunis EJ, Todaro GJ, et al. HL-A antigens of human tumor-derived cell lines and viral transformed fibroblasts in culture. *Proc Soc Exp Biol Med* 1973;143:453–456.

120. Seigler HF, Kremer WB, Metzgar RS, et al. HL-A antigenic loss in malignant transformation. *J Natl Cancer Inst* 1971;46:577–584.

121. Garrido F, Festenstein H, Schirrmacher V. Further evidence for depression of H-2 and Ia-like specificities of foreign haplotypes in mouse tumour cell lines. *Nature* 1976;261:705–707.

122. Garrido F, Perez M, Torres MD. Absence of four H-2d antigenic specificities in an H-2d sarcoma. *J Immunogenet* 1979;6:83–86.

123. Wolf JE, Faanes RB, Choi YS. Antigenic changes of DBA/2J mastocytoma cells when grown in the BALB/c mouse. *J Natl Cancer Inst* 1977;58:1407–1412.

124. Hui K, Grosveld F, Festenstein H. Rejection of transplantable AKR leukaemia cells following MHC DNA-mediated cell transformation. *Nature* 1984;311:750–752.

125. Hui KM, Sim BC, Foo TT, et al. Promotion of tumor growth by transfecting antisense DNA to suppress endogenous H-2Kk MHC gene expression in AKR mouse thymoma. *Cell Immunol* 1991; 136:80–94.

126. Wallich R, Bulbuc N, Hammerling GJ, et al. Abrogation of metastatic properties of tumour cells by de novo expression of H-2K antigens following H-2 gene transfection. *Nature* 1985;315:301–305.

127. Bahler DW, Frelinger JG, Harwell LW, et al. Reduced tumorigenicity of a spontaneous mouse lung carcinoma following H-2 gene transfection. *Proc Natl Acad Sci U S A* 1987;84:4562–4566.

128. Porgador A, Feldman M, Eisenbach L. H-2Kb transfection of B16 melanoma cells results in reduced tumourigenicity and metastatic competence. *J Immunogenet* 1989;16:291–303.

129. Plaksin D, Gelber C, Feldman M, et al. Reversal of the metastatic phenotype in Lewis lung carcinoma cells after transfection with syngeneic H-2Kb gene. *Proc Natl Acad Sci U S A* 1988;85: 4463–4467.

130. Tanaka K, Isselbacher KJ, Khoury G, et al. Reversal of oncogenesis by the expression of a major histocompatibility complex class I gene. *Science* 1985;228:26–30.

131. Eisenbach L, Segal S, Feldman M. MHC imbalance and metastatic spread in Lewis lung carcinoma clones. *Int J Cancer* 1983;32: 113–120.

132. Eisenbach L, Hollander N, Greenfeld L, et al. The differential expression of H-2K versus H-2D antigens, distinguishing high-metastatic from low-metastatic clones, is correlated with the immunogenic properties of the tumor cells. *Int J Cancer* 1984;34: 567–573.

133. De Baetselier P, Katzav S, Gorelik E, et al. Differential expression of H-2 gene products in tumour cells is associated with their metastatogenic properties. *Nature* 1980;288:179–181.

134. Ferrone S, Marincola FM. Loss of HLA class I antigens by melanoma cells: molecular mechanisms, functional significance and clinical relevance. *Immunol Today* 1995;16:487–494.

135. Garrido F, Ruiz-Cabello F, Cabrera T, et al. Implications for immunosurveillance of altered HLA class I phenotypes in human tumours. *Immunol Today* 1997;18:89–95.

136. D'Urso CM, Wang ZG, Cao Y, et al. Lack of HLA class I antigen expression by cultured melanoma cells FO-1 due to a defect in B2m gene expression. *J Clin Invest* 1991;87:284–292.

137. Wang Z, Cao Y, Albino AP, et al. Lack of HLA class I antigen expression by melanoma cells SK-MEL-33 caused by a reading frameshift in beta 2-microglobulin messenger RNA. *J Clin Invest* 1993;91: 684–692.

138. Bicknell DC, Rowan A, Bodmer WF. Beta 2-microglobulin gene mutations: a study of established colorectal cell lines and fresh tumors. *Proc Natl Acad Sci U S A* 1994;91:4751–4756.

139. Hicklin DJ, Wang Z, Arienti F, et al. beta2-Microglobulin mutations, HLA class I antigen loss, and tumor progression in melanoma. *J Clin Invest* 1998;101:2720–2729.

140. Wang Z, Seliger B, Mike N, et al. Molecular analysis of the HLA-A2 antigen loss by melanoma cells SK-MEL-29.1.22 and SK-MEL-29.1.29. *Cancer Res* 1998;58:2149–2157.

141. Ruiter DJ, Bergman W, Welvaart K, et al. Immunohistochemical analysis of malignant melanomas and nevocellular nevi with monoclonal antibodies to distinct monomorphic determinants of HLA antigens. *Cancer Res* 1984;44:3930–3935.

142. Cabrera T, Concha A, Ruiz-Cabello F, et al. Loss of HLA heavy chain and beta 2-microglobulin in HLA negative tumours. *Scand J Immunol* 1991;34:147–152.

143. Chen HL, Gabrilovich D, Tampe R, et al. A functionally defective allele of TAP1 results in loss of MHC class I antigen presentation in a human lung cancer. *Nat Genet* 1996;13:210–213.

144. Branch P, Bicknell DC, Rowan A, et al. Immune surveillance in colorectal carcinoma. *Nat Genet* 1995;9:231–232.

145. Wang Z, Arienti F, Parmiani G, et al. Induction and functional characterization of beta-2-microglobulin (beta2-mu)-free HLA class I heavy chains expressed by beta2-mu-deficient human FO-1 melanoma cells. *Eur J Immunol* 1998;28:2817–2826.

146. Bicknell DC, Kaklamanis L, Hampson R, et al. Selection for beta 2-microglobulin mutation in mismatch repair-defective colorectal carcinomas. *Curr Biol* 1996;6:1695–1697.

147. Benitez R, Godelaine D, Lopez-Nevot MA, et al. Mutations of the b2-microglobulin gene result in a lack of HLA class I molecules on melanoma cells of two patients immunized with MAGE peptides. *Tissue Antigens* 1998;52:520–529.

148. Browning MJ, Krausa P, Rowan A, et al. Tissue typing the HLA-A locus from genomic DNA by sequence-specific PCR: comparison of HLA genotype and surface expression on colorectal tumor cell lines. *Proc Natl Acad Sci U S A* 1993;90:2842–2845.

149. Rivoltini L, Baracchini KC, Viggiano V, et al. Quantitative correlation between HLA Class I allele expression and recognition of melanoma cells by antigen specific cytotoxic T lymphocytes. *Cancer Res* 1995;55:3149–3157.

150. Koopman LA, Mulder A, Corver WE, et al. HLA class I phenotype and genotype alterations in cervical carcinomas and derivative cell lines. *Tissue Antigens* 1998;51:623–636.

151. Marincola FM, Shamamian P, Alexander RB, et al. Loss of HLA haplotype and B locus down-regulation in melanoma cell lines. *J Immunol* 1994;153:1225–1237.

152. Torres MJ, Ruiz-Cabello F, Skoudy A, et al. Loss of an HLA haplotype in pancreas cancer tissue and its corresponding tumor derived cell line. *Tissue Antigens* 1996;47:372–381.

153. Wang Z, Marincola FM, Mazzocchi A, et al. Selective HLA-A2 antigen loss by melanoma cells 624MEL28: molecular analysis and functional implications. 1999 (submitted).

154. Marincola FM, Shamamian P, Simonis TB, et al. Locus-specific anal-

ysis of human leukocyte antigen class I expression in melanoma cell lines. *J Immunother* 1994;16:13–23.

155. Kim CJ, Taubenberger JK, Simonis TB, et al. Combination therapy with Interferon-gamma and Interleukin-2 for the treatment of metastatic melanoma. *J Immunother* 1996;19:50–58.

156. Versteeg R, Noordermeer IA, Kruse-Wolters M, et al. c-myc downregulates class I HLA expression in human melanomas. *EMBO J* 1988;7:1023–1029.

157. Versteeg R, Peltenburg LT, Plomp AC, et al. High expression of the c-myc oncogene renders melanoma cells prone to lysis by natural killer cells. *J Immunol* 1989;143:4331–4337.

158. Versteeg R, Kruse-Wolters KM, Plomp AC, et al. Suppression of class I human histocompatibility leukocyte antigen by c-myc is locus specific. *J Exp Med* 1989;170:621–635.

159. Peltenburg LT, Schrier PI. Transcriptional suppression of HLA-B expression by c-Myc is mediated through the core promoter elements. *Immunogenetics* 1994;40:54–61.

160. Redondo M, Ruiz-Cabello F, Concha A, et al. Altered HLA class I expression in non-small cell lung cancer is independent of c-myc activation. *Cancer Res* 1991;51:2463–2468.

161. Feltner DE, Cooper M, Weber J, et al. Expression of class I histocompatibility antigens in neuroectodermal tumors is independent of the expression of a transfected neuroblastoma myc gene. *J Immunol* 1989;143:4292–4299.

162. Amiot L, Onno M, Renard I, et al. HLA-G transcription studies during the different stages of normal and malignant hematopoiesis. *Tissue Antigens* 1996;48:609–614.

163. Paul P, Rouas-Freiss N, Khalil-Daher I, et al. HLA-G expression in melanoma: a way for tumor cells to escape from immunosurveillance. *Proc Natl Acad Sci U S A* 1998;95:4510–4515.

164. Restifo NP, Esquivel F, Kawakami Y, et al. Identification of human cancers deficient in antigen processing. *J Exp Med* 1993;177:265–272.

165. Sanda MG, Restifo NP, Walsh JC, et al. Molecular characterization of defective antigen processing in human prostate cancer. *J Natl Cancer Inst* 1995;87:280–285.

166. Maeurer MJ, Gollin SM, Martin D, et al. Tumor escape from immune recognition: lethal recurrent melanoma in a patient associated with downregulation of the peptide transporter protein TAP-1 and loss of expression of the immunodominant MART-1/Melan-A antigen. *J Clin Invest* 1996;98:1633–1641.

167. Rowe M, Khanna R, Jacob CA, et al. Restoration of endogenous antigen processing in Burkitt's lymphoma cells by Epstein-Barr virus latent membrane protein-1: coordinate up-regulation of peptide transporter and HLA-class I antigen expression. *Eur J Immunol* 1995;25:1374–1384.

168. White RL. Excess risk of colon cancer associated with a polymorphism of the APC gene? *Cancer Res* 1998;58:4038–4039.

169. Johnsen A, France J, Sy MS, et al. Down-regulation of the transporter for antigen presentation, proteasome subunits, and class I major histocompatibility complex in tumor cell lines. *Cancer Res* 1998;58:3660–3667.

170. Seliger B, Hohne A, Knuth A, et al. Reduced membrane major histocompatibility complex class I density and stability in a subset of human renal cell carcinomas with low TAP and LMP expression. *Clin Cancer Res* 1996;2:1427–1433.

171. York IA, Rock KL. Antigen processing and presentation by the class I major histocompatibility complex. *Annu Rev Immunol* 1996;14:369–396.

172. Wei ML, Cresswell P. HLA-A2 molecules in an antigen-processing mutant cell contain signal sequence-derived peptides. *Nature* 1992;356:443–446.

173. Christinck ER, Luscher MA, Barber BH, et al. Peptide binding to class I MHC on living cells and quantitation of complexes required for CTL lysis. *Nature* 1991;352:67–70.

174. Sykulev Y, Joo M, Vturina I, Tsomides TJ, et al. Evidence that a single peptide-MHC complex on a target cell can elicit a cytolytic T cell response. *Immunity* 1996;4:565–571.

175. Brower RC, England R, Takeshita T, et al. Minimal requirements for peptide mediated activation of CD8+ CTL. *Mol Immunol* 1994;31:1285–1293.

176. Porgador A, Yewdell JW, Deng Y, et al. Localization, quantitation, and in situ detection of specific peptide-MHC class I complexes using a monoclonal antibody. *Immunity* 1997;6:715–726.

177. Hunt DF, Henderson RA, Shabanowitz J, et al. Characterization of peptides bound to the class I MHC molecule HLA-A2.1 by mass spectrometry. *Science* 1992;255:1261–1263.

178. Carbone FR, Moore MW, Sheil JM, et al. Induction of cytotoxic T lymphocytes by primary in vitro stimulation with peptides. *J Exp Med* 1988;167:1767–1779.

179. Chen Y, Sidney J, Southwood S, et al. Naturally processed peptides longer than nine amino acid residues bind to the class I MHC molecule HLA-A2.1 with high affinity and in different conformations. *J Immunol* 1994;152:2874–2881.

180. Foa R, Guarini A, Gansbacher B. IL2 treatment for cancer: from biology to gene therapy. *Br J Cancer* 1992;66:992–998.

181. Schild H, Rotzschke O, Kalbacher H, et al. Limit of T cell tolerance to self proteins by peptide presentation. *Science* 1990;247:1587–1589.

182. Viola A, Lanzavecchia A. T cell activation determined by T cell receptor number and tunable thresholds. *Science* 1996;273:104–106.

183. Valitutti S, Muller S, Cella M, et al. Serial triggering of many T-cell receptors by a few peptide-MHC complexes. *Nature* 1995;375:148–151.

184. Ljunggren HG, Karre K. Host resistance directed selectively against H-2-deficient lymphoma variants. Analysis of the mechanism. *J Exp Med* 1985;162:1745–1759.

185. Lopez-Botet M, Moretta L, Strominger J. NK-cell receptors and recognition of MHC class I molecules. *Immunol Today* 1996;17:212–214.

186. Braud VM, Allan DS, O'Callaghan CA, et al. HLA-E binds to natural killer cell receptors CD94/NKG2A, B and C. *Nature* 1998;391:795–799.

187. Braud V, Jones EY, McMichael A. The human major histocompatibility complex class Ib molecule HLA-E binds signal sequence-derived peptides with primary anchor residues at positions 2 and 9. *Eur J Immunol* 1997;27:1164–1169.

188. Lanier LL. Follow the leader: NK cell receptors for classical and non-classical MHC class I. *Cell* 1998;92:705–707.

189. Maio M, Altomonte M, Tatake R, et al. Reduction in susceptibility to natural killer cell-mediated lysis of human FO-1 melanoma cells after induction of HLA class I antigen expression by transfection with B2m gene. *J Clin Invest* 1991;88:282–289.

190. Schrier PI, Peltenburg LT. Relationship between myc oncogene activation and MHC class I expression. *Adv Cancer Res* 1993;60:181–246.

191. Porgador A, Mandelboim O, Restifo NP, et al. Natural killer cell lines kill autologous beta-2-microglobulin-deficient melanoma cells: implications for cancer immunotherapy. *Proc Natl Acad Sci U S A* 1997;94:13140–13145.

192. Pende D, Accame L, Pareti L, et al. The susceptibility to natural killer cell-mediated lysis of HLA class I-positive melanomas reflects the expression of insufficient amounts of different HLA class I alleles. *Eur J Immunol* 1998;28:2384–2394.

193. Pena J, Alonso C, Solana R, et al. Natural killer susceptibility is independent of HLA class I antigen expression on cell lines obtained from human solid tumors. *Eur J Immunol* 1990;20:2445–2448.

194. Pazmany L, Mandelboim O, Vales-Gomez M, et al. Protection from natural killer cell-mediated lysis by HLA-G expression on target cells. *Science* 1996;274:792–795.

195. Munz C, Holmes N, King A, et al. Human histocompatibility leukocyte antigen (HLA)-G molecules inhibit NKAT3 expressing natural killer cells. *J Exp Med* 1997;185:385–391.

196. Pende D, Sivori S, Accame L, et al. HLA-G recognition by human natural killer cells. Involvement of CD94 both as inhibitory and as activating receptor complex. *Eur J Immunol* 1997;27:1875–1880.

197. Perez-Villar JJ, Melero I, Navarro F, et al. The CD94/NKG2-A inhibitory receptor complex is involved in natural killer cell-mediated recognition of cells expressing HLA-G1. *J Immunol* 1997;158:5736–5743.

198. Mandelboim O, Pazmany L, Davis DM, et al. Multiple receptors for HLA-G on human natural killer cells. *Proc Natl Acad Sci U S A* 1997;94:14666–14670.

199. Allan DS, Colonna M, Lanier LL, et al. Tetrameric complexes of HLA-G bind to peripheral blood myelomonocytic cells. *J Exp Med* 1999;189:1149–1156.

200. Moretta A, Biassoni R, Bottino C, et al. Major histocompatibility complex class I-specific receptors on human natural killer and T lymphocytes. *Immunol Rev* 1997;155:105–177.

201. Lanier LL, Phillips JH. Inhibitory MHC class I receptors on NK cells and T cells. *Immunol Today* 1996;17:86–91.

202. Ikeda H, Lethe B, Lehmann F, et al. Characterization of an antigen that is recognized on a melanoma showing partial HLA loss by CTL expressing an NK inhibitory receptor. *Immunity* 1997;6:199–208.

203. Cromme FV, van Bommel PF, Walboomers JM, et al. Differences in MHC and TAP-1 expression in cervical cancer lymph node metastases as compared with the primary tumours. *Br J Cancer* 1994;69:1176–1181.

204. Hilders CG, Munoz IM, Nooyen Y, et al. Altered HLA expression by metastatic cervical carcinoma cells as a factor in impaired immune surveillance. *Gynecol Oncol* 1995;57:366–375.

205. Kageshita T, Hirai S, Ono T, et al. Downregulation of HLA class I antigen processing molecules in malignant melanoma. Association with disease progression. *Am J Pathol* 1999;154:745–754.

206. van Driel WJ, Tjiong MY, Hilders CG, et al. Association of allele-specific HLA expression and histopathologic progression of cervical carcinoma. *Gynecol Oncol* 1996;62:33–41.

207. Hilders CG, Houbiers JG, Krul EJ, et al. The expression of histocompatibility-related leukocyte antigens in the pathway to cervical carcinoma. *Am J Clin Pathol* 1994;101:5–12.

208. Ottesen SS, Kieler J, Christensen B. Changes in HLA A, B, C expression during "spontaneous" transformation of human urothelial cells *in vivo*. *Eur J Cancer Clin Oncol* 1987;23:991–995.

209. Tomita Y, Matsumoto Y, Nishiyama T, et al. Reduction of major histocompatibility complex class I antigens on invasive and high-grade transitional cell carcinoma. *J Pathol* 1990;162:157–164.

210. Tomita Y, Nishiyama T, Fujiwara M, et al. Immunohistochemical detection of major histocompatibility complex antigens and quantitative analysis of tumour-infiltrating mononuclear cells in renal cell cancer. *Br J Cancer* 1990;62:354–359.

211. Lehmann F, Marchand M, Hainaut P, et al. Differences in the antigens recognized by cytolytic T cells on two successive metastases of a melanoma patient are consistent with immune selection. *Eur J Immunol* 1995;25:340–347.

212. Bettinotti M, Kim CJ, Lee K-H, et al. Stringent allele/epitope requirements for MART-1/Melan A immunodominance: implications for peptide-based immunotherapy. *J Immunol* 1998;161:877–889.

213. Kim CJ, Parkinson DR, Marincola FM. Immunodominance across the HLA polymorphism: implications for cancer immunotherapy. *J Immunother* 1997;21:1–16.

214. Marincola FM, Shamamian P, Rivoltini L, et al. HLA associations in the anti-tumor response against malignant melanoma. *J Immunother* 1996;18:242–252.

215. Kaufman J, Volk H, Wallny HJ. A "minimal essential MHC" and an "unrecognized MHC": two extremes in selection for polymorphism. *Immunol Rev* 1995;143:63–88.

216. Chouaib S, Asselin-Paturel C, Mami-Chouaib F, et al. The host-tumor immune conflict: from immunosuppression to resistance and destruction. *Immunol Today* 1997;18:493–497.

217. Yoong KF, McNab G, Hubscher SG, et al. Vascular adhesion protein-1 and ICAM-1 support the adhesion of tumor-infiltrating lymphocytes to tumor endothelium in human hepatocellular carcinoma. *J Immunol* 1998;160:3978–3988.

218. Vanky F, Wang P, Patarroyo M, et al. Expression of the adhesion molecule ICAM-1 and major histocompatibility complex class I antigens on human tumor cells is required for their interaction with autologous lymphocytes *in vitro*. *Cancer Immunol Immunother* 1990;31:19–27.

219. Cao X, Chen G, He L, et al. Involvement of MHC class I molecule and ICAM-1 in the enhancement of adhesion and cytotoxic susceptibility to immune effector cells of tumor cells transfected with the interleukin (IL)-2, IL-4 or IL-6 gene. *J Cancer Res Clin Oncol* 1997;123:602–608.

220. Lefor AT, Fabian DF. Enhanced cytolytic activity of tumor infiltrating lymphocytes (TILs) derived from an ICAM-1 transfected tumor in a murine model. *J Surg Res* 1998;75:49–53.

221. Budinsky AC, Brodowicz T, Wiltschke C, et al. Decreased expression of ICAM-1 and its induction by tumor necrosis factor on breast-cancer cells *in vitro*. *Int J Cancer* 1997;71:1086–1090.

222. Krunkosky TM, Fischer BM, Akley NJ, et al. Tumor necrosis factor alpha (TNF alpha)-induced ICAM-1 surface expression in airway epithelial cells *in vitro*: possible signal transduction mechanisms. *Ann N Y Acad Sci* 1996;796:30–37.

223. Kilgore KS, Shen JP, Miller BF, et al. Enhancement by the complement membrane attack complex of tumor necrosis factor-alpha-induced endothelial cell expression of E-selectin and ICAM-1. *J Immunol* 1995;155:1434–1441.

224. Mortarini R, Belli F, Parmiani G, et al. Cytokine-mediated modulation of HLA-class II, ICAM-1, LFA-3 and tumor-associated antigen profile of melanoma cells. Comparison with anti-proliferative activity by rIL1-beta, rTNF-alpha, rIFN-gamma, rIL4 and their combinations. *Int J Cancer* 1990;45:334–341.

225. Krutmann J, Kock A, Schauer E, et al. Tumor necrosis factor beta and ultraviolet radiation are potent regulators of human keratinocyte ICAM-1 expression. *J Invest Dermatol* 1990;95:127–131.

226. Kitsuki H, Katano M, Ikubo A, et al. Induction of inflammatory cytokines in effusion cavity by OK-432 injection therapy for patients with malignant effusion: role of interferon-gamma in enhancement of surface expression of ICAM-1 on tumor cells *in vivo*. *Clin Immunol Immunopathol* 1996;78:283–290.

227. Yue FY, Dummer R, Geertsen R, et al. Interleukin-10 is a growth factor for human melanoma cells and down-regulates HLA class-I, HLA class-II and ICAM-1 molecules. *Int J Cancer* 1997;71:630–637.

228. Becker JC, Dummer R, Hartmann AA, et al. Shedding of ICAM-1 from human melanoma cell lines induced by IFN-gamma and tumor necrosis factor-alpha. Functional consequences on cell-mediated cytotoxicity. *J Immunol* 1991;147:4398–4401.

229. Gwin JL, Gercel-Taylor C, Taylor DD, Eisenberg B. Role of LFA-3, ICAM-1, and MHC class I on the sensitivity of human tumor cells to LAK cells. *J Surg Res* 1996;60:129–136.

230. Webb DS, Mostowski HS, Gerrard TL. Cytokine-induced enhancement of ICAM-1 expression results in increased vulnerability of tumor cells to monocyte-mediated lysis. *J Immunol* 1991;146:3682–3686.

231. Akella R, Hall RE. Expression of the adhesion molecules ICAM-1 and ICAM-2 on tumor cell lines does not correlate with their susceptibility to natural killer cell-mediated cytolysis: evidence for additional ligands for effector cell beta integrins. *Eur J Immunol* 1992;22:1069–1074.

232. Gabrilovich DI, Chen HL, Girgis KR, et al. Production of vascular endothelial growth factor by human tumors inhibits the functional maturation of dendritic cells. *Nat Med* 1996;2:1096–1103.

233. Fiorentino DF, Bond MW, Mosmann TR. Two types of mouse T helper cell. IV. Th2 clones secrete a factor that inhibits cytokine production by Th1 clones. *J Exp Med* 1989;170:2081–2095.

234. Vieira P, de Waal-Malefyt R, Dang MN, et al. Isolation and expression of human cytokine synthesis inhibitory factor cDNA clones: homology to Epstein-Barr virus open reading frame BCRFI. *Proc Natl Acad Sci U S A* 1991;88:1172–1176.

235. Taga K, Tosato G. IL-10 inhibits human T cell proliferation and IL-2 production. *J Immunol* 1992;148:1143–1148.

236. Dummer W, Bastian BC, Ernst N, et al. Interleukin-10 production in malignant melanoma: preferential detection of IL-10-secreting tumor cells in metastatic lesions. *Int J Cancer* 1996;66:607–610.

237. Dummer W, Becker JC, Schwaaf A, et al. Elevated serum levels of interleukin-10 in patients with metastatic malignant melanoma. *Melanoma Res* 1995;5:67–68.

238. Van Belle P, Rodeck U, Nuamah I, et al. Melanoma-associated expression of transforming growth factor-beta isoforms. *Am J Pathol* 1996;148:1887–1894.

239. Schmid P, Itin P, Rufli T. In situ analysis of transforming factor-beta s (TGF-beta 1, TGF-beta 2, TGF-beta 3), and TGF-beta type II receptor expression in malignant melanoma. *Carcinogenesis* 1995;16:1499–1503.

240. Moretti S, Pinzi C, Berti E, et al. In situ expression of transforming growth factor beta is associated with melanoma progression and correlates with Ki67, HLA-DR and beta 3 integrin expression. *Melanoma Res* 1997;7:313–321.

241. Schmid P, Itin P, Rufli T. In situ analysis of transforming factors-beta (TGF-beta 1, TGF-beta 2, TGF-beta 3) and TGF-beta type II receptor expression in basal cell carcinomas. *Br J Dermatol* 1996;134:1044–1051.

242. Rodeck U, Melber K, Kath R, et al. Constitutive expression of multiple growth factor genes by melanoma cells but not normal melanocytes. *J Invest Dermatol* 1991;97:20–26.

243. Gorsch SM, Memoli VA, Stukel TA, et al. Immunohistochemical staining for transforming growth factor beta 1 associates with disease progression in human breast cancer. *Cancer Res* 1992;52:6949–6952.

244. Sporn MB, Roberts AB. Transforming growth factor-beta: recent progress and new challenges. *J Cell Biol* 1992;119:1017–1021.

245. Wakefield LM, Letterio JJ, Geiser AG, et al. Transforming growth factor-beta s in mammary tumorigenesis: promoters or antipromoters? *Prog Clin Biol Res* 1995;391:133–148.

246. Wojtowicz-Praga S, Verma UN, Wakefield L, et al. Modulation of B16 melanoma growth and metastasis by anti-transforming growth factor beta antibody and interleukin-2. *J Immunother* 1996;19:169–175.

247. Park JA, Wang E, Kurt RA, et al. Expression of an antisense transforming growth factor-beta1 transgene reduces tumorigenicity of EMT6 mammary tumor cells. *Cancer Gene Ther* 1997;4:42–50.

248. Bellone G, Aste-Amezaga M, Trinchieri G, et al. Regulation of NK cell functions by TGF-beta 1. *J Immunol* 1995;155:1066–1073.

249. D'Orazio TJ, Niederkorn JY. A novel role for TGF-beta and IL-10 in the induction of immune privilege. *J Immunol* 1998;160:2089–2098.

250. Tensen CP, Vermeer MH, van der Stoop PM, et al. Epidermal interferon-gamma inducible protein-10 (IP-10) and monokine induced by gamma-interferon (Mig) but not IL-8 mRNA expression is associated with epidermotropism in cutaneous T cell lymphomas. *J Invest Dermatol* 1998;111:222–226.

251. Piali L, Weber C, LaRosa G, et al. The chemokine receptor CXCR3 mediates rapid and shear-resistant adhesion-induction of effector T lymphocytes by the chemokines IP10 and Mig. *Eur J Immunol* 1998;28:961–972.

252. Sgadari C, Farber JM, Angiolillo AL, et al. Mig, the monokine induced by interferon-gamma, promotes tumor necrosis *in vivo*. *Blood* 1997;89:2635–2643.

253. Farber JM. Mig and IP-10: CXC chemokines that target lymphocytes. *J Leukoc Biol* 1997;61:246–257.

254. Klein B, Zhang XG, Jourdan M, et al. Paracrine rather than autocrine regulation of myeloma-cell growth and differentiation by interleukin-6. *Blood* 1989;73:517–526.

255. Rosenberg SA, Lotze MT, Yang JC, et al. Experience with the use of high-dose interleukin-2 in the treatment of 652 cancer patients. *Ann Surg* 1989;210:474–484.

256. Rosenberg SA, Yang JC, Topalian SL, et al. Treatment of 283 consecutive patients with metastatic melanoma or renal cell cancer using high-dose bolus interleukin 2. *JAMA* 1994;271:907–913.

257. Wang CY, Mayo MW, Baldwin ASJ. TNF- and cancer therapy-induced apoptosis: potentiation by inhibition of NF-kappaB. *Science* 1996;274:784–787.

258. Nawroth P, Handley D, Matsueda G, et al. Tumor necrosis factor/cachectin-induced intravascular fibrin formation in meth A fibrosarcomas. *J Exp Med* 1988;168:637–647.

259. Wu PC, Alexander HR, Huang J, et al. *In vivo* sensititivy of human melanoma to tumor necrosis factor (TNF)-alpha is determined by tumor production of the novel cytokine endothelial-monocyte activating polypeptide II (EMAII). *Cancer Res* 1999;59:205–212.

260. Hahne M, Rimoldi D, Schroter M, et al. Melanoma cell expression of Fas (Apo-1/CD95) ligand: implications for tumor immune escape. *Science* 1996;274:1363–1366.

261. Gratas C, Tohma Y, Van Meir EG, et al. Fas ligand expression in glioblastoma cell lines and primary astrocytic brain tumors. *Brain Pathol* 1997;7:863–869.

262. Saas P, Walker PR, Hahne M, et al. Fas ligand expression by astrocytoma *in vivo*: maintaining immune privilege in the brain? *J Clin Invest* 1997;99:1173–1178.

263. Niehans GA, Brunner T, Frizelle SP, et al. Human lung carcinomas express Fas ligand. *Cancer Res* 1997;57:1007–1012.

264. O'Connell J, O'Sullivan GC, Collins JK, et al. The Fas counterattack: Fas-mediated T cell killing by colon cancer cells expressing Fas ligand. *J Exp Med* 1996;184:1075–1082.

265. Shiraki K, Tsuji N, Shioda T, et al. Expression of Fas ligand in liver metastases of human colonic adenocarcinomas. *Proc Natl Acad Sci U S A* 1997;94:6420–6425.

266. Bennett MW, O'Connell J, O'Sullivan GC, et al. The Fas counterattack *in vivo*: apoptotic depletion of tumor-infiltrating lymphocytes associated with Fas ligand expression by human esophageal carcinoma. *J Immunol* 1998;160:5669–5675.

267. Rivoltini L, Radrizzani M, Accornero P, et al. Human melanoma-reactive CD4+ and CD8+ CTL clones resist Fas ligand-induced apoptosis and use Fas/Fas ligand-independent mechanisms for tumor killing. *J Immunol* 1998;161:1220–1230.

268. Arai H, Gordon D, Nabel EG, et al. Gene transfer of Fas ligand induces tumor regression *in vivo*. *Proc Natl Acad Sci U S A* 1997;94:13862–13867.

269. Seino K, Kayagaki N, Okumura K, et al. Antitumor effect of locally produced CD95 ligand. *Nat Med* 1997;3:165–170.

270. Chappell DB, Zaks TZ, Rosenberg SA, et al. Human melanoma cells do not express Fas (Apo-1/Cd95) ligand. *Cancer Res* 1999;59:59–62.

271. Rimoldi D, Muehlethaler K, Romero P, et al. Limited involvement of the Fas/FasL pathway in melanoma-induced apoptosis of tumor-specific T cells. *Proc Cancer Vacc Week* 1998;1:382.

272. Zaks TZ, Chappell DB, Rosenberg SA, et al. Fas-mediated suicide of tumor-reactive T cells following activation by specific tumor: selective rescue by Caspase inhibition. *J Immunol* 1999;162:3273–3279.

273. Allison JP, Pellegrino MA, Ferrone S, et al. Biologic and chemical characterization of HLA antigens in human serum. *J Immunol* 1977;118:1004–1009.

274. Zavazava N, Muller-Ruchholtz W. Quantitative and biochemical characterization of soluble HLA class I antigens shed by cultured human cells. *Hum Immunol* 1994;40:174–178.

275. Davies H, Kamada N, Roser B. Liver allografts and the induction of donor-specific unresponsiveness. In: Calne RY, ed. *Transplantation immunology clinical and experimental*, 1st ed. Oxford: Oxford University Press, 1984:222–253.

276. Kamada N, Davies HS, Wight D, et al. Liver transplantation in the rat. Biochemical and histological evidence of complete tolerance induction in non-rejector strains. *Transplantation* 1983;35:304–311.

277. Puppo F, Indiveri F, Scudeletti M, et al. Soluble HLA antigens: new roles and uses. *Immunol Today* 1997;18:154–155.

278. Westhoff U, Fox C, Otto FJ. Soluble HLA class I antigens in plasma of patients with malignant melanoma. *Anticancer Res* 1998;18:3789–3792.

279. Shimura T, Hagihara M, Yamamoto K, et al. Quantification of serum-soluble HLA class I antigens in patients with gastric cancer. *Hum Immunol* 1994;40:183–186.

280. Wucherpfennig KW, Strominger JL. Molecular mimicry in T cell-mediated autoimmunity: viral peptides activate human T cell clones specific for myelin basic protein. *Cell* 1995;80:695–705.

281. Bevan MJ. In thymic selection, peptide diversity gives and takes away. *Immunity* 1997;7:175–178.
282. Matsushita S, Kohsaka H, Nishimura Y. Evidence for self and nonself peptide partial agonists that prolong clonal survival of mature T cells *in vitro*. *J Immunol* 1997;158:5685–5691.
283. Loftus DJ, Castelli C, Clay TM, et al. Identification of epitope

mimics recognized by CTL reactive to the melanoma/melano-cyte-derived peptide MART-1(27-35). *J Exp Med* 1996;184:647–657.
284. Lyons DS, Lieberman SA, Hampl J, et al. A TCR binds to antagonist ligands with lower affinities and faster dissociation rates than to agonists. *Immunity* 1996;5:53–61.

17.4

CANCER VACCINES: BASIC PRINCIPLES

Principles of Immune Monitoring in Cancer Vaccine Trials

MARIO SZNOL
FRANCESCO M. MARINCOLA

Cancer vaccines are designed to induce or enhance antigen-specific immune responses against cancer cells. On entering clinical trials, selection of an optimum dose and schedule for a vaccine and decisions regarding subsequent clinical development are based in large part on laboratory studies that monitor and measure the vaccine-induced immune response. The laboratory correlative studies also have the potential to provide further insight into host tumor biology and support alternate methods of administration or combination with other agents that may result in more effective immunization strategies.

A major challenge in monitoring cancer vaccine trials is determining which parameters to measure *in vivo*. Cancer vaccines are capable of inducing complex and diverse immune responses, and the quantitative and qualitative aspects of effective antitumor immune responses are not completely understood. Furthermore, patient and tumor-related factors may influence the response to the vaccine, as well as the capacity of the immune response to produce tumor regression. The complex interactions and feedback mechanisms that occur *in vivo* when modulating an immunologic response also complicate the establishment of a direct dose effect. Major advances in molecular biology, immunology, and the biology of cancer have provided the scientific basis to discover and understand some of the basic principles that govern the interactions between the host immune system and cancer cells. In particular, the identification of tumor antigens recognized by T cells and their T-cell epitopes

have given the unprecedented opportunity to characterize and follow the development of cancer-specific immune responses *in vivo*, including the interactions between molecularly defined T-cell responses and the relevant antigen in the target tissue (1,2).

GENERAL PRINCIPLES

To fully assess and understand the effects of a cancer vaccine in the initial clinical trials, the laboratory studies are generally focused on:

1. Monitoring the method of vaccination, including the parameters of vaccine administration, biologic properties, and local or systemic effects that lead to effective immune responses, as predicted from preclinical data.
2. Measuring the immune response to the vaccine, based on the best available understanding of the type, quality, and magnitude of immune response necessary to mediate antitumor effects.
3. Assessment of patient and tumor-related factors known or suspected to influence the development and evolution of an effective antitumor immune response *in vivo*.

Several general principles of monitoring cancer vaccine trials can be proposed that may be applicable regardless of the vaccine or immunization approach. The immunologic concepts that underlie the selection and interpretation of the assays are fully covered in other chapters and reviews (3).

Selecting Relevant End Points for Immune Monitoring

Depending on the antigen form and source, relevant immune responses may include CD4$^+$ helper, CD8$^+$ cytotoxic T lymphocyte (CTL), and antibody responses. It is essential, but often neglected, to demonstrate that the vaccine induces an immune response that recognizes the antigens as naturally processed and presented by tumor cells or host professional antigen-presenting cells (APCs) because antitumor efficacy could not occur otherwise. Furthermore, assessment of the magnitude and quality of the immune response is likely to be important in determining the potential efficacy of the vaccine in subsequent studies. For example, the number of tumor antigen–specific cells (4), their avidity for the antigen (5), the cytokines they produce (6), and their ability to traffic to tumor may be critical for mediating antitumor effects (7,8). Similarly, for antibody responses, the titer, epitope or number of epitopes recognized, class and isotype, and affinity for the antigen as expressed by tumor may influence antitumor efficacy (9). Monitoring of immune responses against tumor antigens not targeted directly by the vaccine may also be relevant to the outcome, as destruction of tumor cells by vaccine-induced effectors may lead to the release of other abundant antigenic molecules in the tumor milieu, and to inflammatory reactions that facilitate the presentation and development of immune responses to the antigenic molecules. The latter phenomenon, which results in broadening the specificity of the host immune response, is referred to as *epitope spreading*.

Issues Related to Selection of Tissue and Timing for Sampling

The immune response to a vaccine can be assessed at the vaccine site, draining lymph nodes, peripheral blood, and the tumor. Theoretically, the tumor is the most relevant tissue because lymphocytes or antibodies must reach the tumor to mediate antitumor effects (except, perhaps, in the situation where the immune response is eliminating circulating malignant cells before implantation). Furthermore, examination of the tumor prevaccination can confirm that the relevant antigen and the major histocompatibility complex (MHC) molecules associated with the presentation of antigen to T cells are expressed. Postvaccination sampling of tumor specimens can provide important information on immune selection, such as the development of antigen loss variants as a result of an effective immune response. For practical purposes, in most circumstances, it is only possible to monitor the relevant antigen-specific response in draining lymph nodes or peripheral blood. The limited data obtained from the latter sites are still considered useful because they verify the ability of the vaccine to produce a systemic immune response, although without the more relevant information on the ability of vaccine-elicited T cells to localize, function, and sustain an immune reaction within tumor.

Another consideration that has scientific and practical implications is the timing of tissue sampling after vaccine administra-

tion. Substantial *in vitro* and clinical data support the observation that antibody- and cell-mediated responses to vaccines evolve over time *in vivo*; therefore, the ability to detect the response in any particular site may vary as a function of the time from immunization. Clear data regarding optimal timing of sampling are not available from animal or human trials, particularly for T-lymphocyte responses to cancer vaccines.

Selecting Assays to Monitor the Parameters of Effective Immunization

Where possible and applicable, monitoring the parameters of effective antigen presentation aids in the interpretation of the clinical trial. Several examples are relevant. If the gene for the antigen is delivered by a viral, plasmid DNA or other vector, consideration should be given to confirming the extent and duration of gene expression *in vivo* and comparing the results to effective parameters in the animal models. For cytokine-transduced tumor cells, the levels of cytokine produced by the tumor cells in the vaccine (or gene expression) should be similar to that required for effective immunization and antitumor activity in preclinical experiments (10). Furthermore, the vaccine site can be biopsied and examined histologically to determine whether the local inflammatory response conducive to antigen presentation is similar in quality and magnitude to that observed with analogous vaccines in the animal models (10,11). Measurement of immune responses against non–tumor-related antigens in the vaccine may provide important information on the duration of expression of the relevant tumor antigen *in vivo* and the possibility of successful immunization with future application of the same vaccine construct. For example, vaccinia and adenovirus constructs induce potent neutralizing antivirus immune responses. Therefore, in subsequent use of the same viral construct, the infection is cleared rapidly, and the antigen gene insert is not expressed sufficiently to stimulate an effective immune response (12,13).

Determination of Assay Performance Characteristics

The usefulness of data generated during the monitoring of a cancer vaccine trial is highly dependent on the quality of the assays and the availability of sufficient numbers of samples to conduct valid analyses. Assays used for immune monitoring should be validated by showing that they are reproducable and specific, and sufficiently sensitive to detect relevant immune responses. If possible, the immune studies should be defined and prioritized prospectively, and levels of response worthy of further study should be clearly stated.

Appropriate controls are essential to the interpretation of any outcome in laboratory monitoring of cancer vaccine trials. Simple measurement of prevaccination versus postvaccination immune responses must be demonstrated to be specific for the immunizing preparation and, where applicable, to a tumor antigen and not a bystander component of the vaccine. For example, in allogeneic or autologous tumor cell vaccines, enzymes used in the preparation and dissociation of tumor samples and components of culture media can be immunogenic and responsible for positive delayed-type hypersensitivity (DTH) responses or an apparent increase in a T-lymphocyte response postvaccination (14). The results can be interpreted correctly only if appropriate controls are included.

Inclusion of positive and negative controls for *in vivo* immunization and *in vitro* testing can aid in identifying nonspecific effects of the vaccine, as well as potential problems in the patient population being studied, the immunization method, or the assay itself. For example, measurement of immune responses to influenza antigens is commonly included as a positive *in vitro* control because most patients have been immunized to influenza and have strong baseline immune responses that can be readily detected *in vitro* (15). No agreement exists on a standard positive control antigen that reliably induces primary immune responses *in vivo* in most individuals.

Correlation of Laboratory Studies to Clinical Outcome

A common objective of monitoring in early clinical studies is to correlate immune response to clinical outcome. Although this provides some useful information in the context of a single-arm trial, a responder-to-nonresponder analysis, which generally shows that responders fare better than nonresponders, often leads to the incorrect conclusion that treatment and the induced immune response produced clinical benefit. Often, immune responders simply represent a better prognostic group of patients who are therefore better able to generate immune responses to the vaccine. Placement of a control immunogenic antigen together with the cancer antigen may allow more accurate correlation between induced response to the cancer antigen and clinical outcome.

Monitoring of Patient-Related Factors

Induction of an immune response in a patient may depend on several patient-related factors, including prior treatment with cytotoxic agents, type of disease, stage of disease, performance status, and other variables. Some animal studies suggest that growing tumors may induce conditions that affect overall immune status, ability to respond to new antigens, or the type of immune response to an antigen. Several investigators have reported generalized or specific defects in T-cell signaling in animal models and patients with advanced cancer (16–18). Defects in maturation of professional APCs have been reported in animals and patients owing to tumor overproduction of vascular endothelial growth factor and other cytokines (19,20). Clearly, it would be desirable to determine the immune competence of a patient before immunization to interpret the results of vaccination, and, perhaps, to select patient populations that are most appropriate to test the vaccine. No reliable tests for immune competence and the ability to respond to new antigens have been developed. Many investigators perform recall-antigen DTH tests or measure CD4/CD8 ratios or lymphocyte responsiveness to mitogens, viral antigens, or alloantigens. The significance of the results from these studies to overall immune status, ability to respond to immunization, and clinical outcome has not been fully defined.

MHC phenotyping has become an important aspect of patient selection for vaccine trials and monitoring of immune response to the vaccine (21). Patients selected for treatment with a particular MHC-restricted peptide antigen must be shown to express that MHC molecule. Such a requirement may not be present when the immunizing preparation is a whole protein or derived from whole tumor cells because the antigens are taken up and processed by host APCs, and the appropriate epitopes are bound to the patient's own MHC molecules. Because of the higher level of difficulty in measuring and characterizing immune responses to proteins or whole tumor cells, monitoring in the latter trials has, in certain settings, been directed to specific MHC-restricted epitopic determinants of the proteins contained in the immunizing preparation (12,22,23). Precise determination of the MHC phenotype has become increasingly important after demonstration that even one amino acid variant within the MHC molecule may totally alter the ability of an antigen to function as immunogen in a particular patient (24). Knowledge of each patient's MHC phenotype also enables investigators to characterize and identify possible shared antigens recognized by the induced T-lymphocyte response within the context of vaccines composed of proteins or whole cells. Methods for identifying antigens recognized by tumor-specific T lymphocytes are described in another chapter.

Monitoring of Tumor-Related Factors

Events that occur in tumors are the most relevant to the clinical outcome of any anticancer therapeutic approach. Indeed, clinical and preclinical data suggest the possibility of a dissociation between immune responses detected in peripheral blood versus tumor (25). Assessment of the tumor can also be used to guide selection of appropriate patients for treatment with a vaccine or can provide data to explain the biologic basis for treatment failures and successes, which may lead to improved vaccine approaches. Obtaining sufficient tumor tissue for these studies in most patients can be quite difficult, particularly when tumors are not in easily accessible sites. Furthermore, assays conducted on tumor are expensive and labor intensive, and interpretation of the results is complicated by heterogeneity within and between tumor specimens. Compared with full biopsies, fine-needle aspirates of tumors (which, in many cases, can be performed with relative ease and minimal morbidity) can provide sufficient tissue for some correlative studies, give information on antigen expression, and be used to establish lymphocyte cultures and tumor cell lines for *in vitro* immune assays (26). Nevertheless, even fine-needle aspirates can be used only in a subset of patients with minimal morbidity.

Perhaps the primary reason to examine tumor tissue within the context of a vaccine trial is to assess the extent to which tumors express the antigen in the vaccine and, where appropriate, the restricting MHC molecule. This is because lack of appropriate antigen presentation by the tumor precludes therapeutic efficacy (27,28). Indeed, *in vitro* data suggest that CTL recognition of tumor cell lines can vary depending on the level, as opposed to just the presence or absence, of antigen and MHC expression (29). It is possible to measure relative expression of the protein antigen and the restricting MHC molecule for the relevant peptide epitope with various techniques, such as immunohistochemistry or polymerase chain reaction (PCR) (30,31), but techniques are not available to accurately assess the number of MHC complexes containing the relevant peptide on the surface of the cell. In the future, it may be possible to raise antibodies that are specific for a single peptide/MHC complex, which can therefore be used to more accurately determine tumor antigen presentation.

A number of other tumor-related factors have been identified that may determine responsiveness to a vaccine, including expression by tumor of immunosuppressive molecules, such as Fas ligand that binds to death receptors on T cells, or the lack of expression of certain adhesion molecules on tumor vasculature that allow penetration by T cells (7). In some settings, interactions between tumor-related products may influence the developing immune response. For example, the combined expression of transforming growth factor–β and Fas ligand by tumor has been shown to markedly inhibit the activation, function, and survival of infiltrating T cells, whereas expression of Fas ligand alone promoted tumor regression (32). Defects in certain tumor cell signaling pathways can also affect immune recognition. For example, disruption of the interferon-γ (IFN-γ) signaling pathway in tumors was associated with resistance to lymphocyte-mediated control of growth in animal models (33). Because of the many factors that appear to impact on the antitumor immune response, newer technologies, such as gene chip arrays that can measure expression of many genes simultaneously within a sample of tumor tissue, may be necessary to fully characterize the tumor phenotype before immunization (34).

Theoretically, lymphocytes, antibodies, or both must reach the tumor to mediate antitumor effects. Tumor can be examined histologically for lymphocytic infiltration and presence of other immune effector cells, as well as the induction of apoptosis in tumor cells and induced changes in tumor vasculature. The interpretation of histologic findings is subject to variations in sampling, observer bias, or error. Therefore, assessment of the slides should be blinded with regard to the treatment received and the time of tissue sampling (pre versus post), and overall conclusions should be based on examination of multiple samples from multiple patients. In addition to visual examination, infiltrating lymphocytes can be assessed directly by staining or PCR measurement of gene expression or indirectly through subsequent *in vitro* culture; the latter may be necessary to expand infiltrating lymphocytes to sufficient numbers for functional studies. Lymphocytes are generally examined for surface expression of markers that determine identity, activation state, ability to home within target organs, and antigen specificity and function (avidity, cytokine production, and cytotoxicity). The data generated by these laboratory assays can confirm that activated antigen-specific T lymphocytes were produced as a result of immunization and reached the tumor site. These types of analyses, although extremely important, cannot be performed routinely. It should be emphasized, however, that the collection of clinically relevant material might be all that is necessary. The availability of an "off the shelf" clinically relevant library of tissue specimens allows eventual selection of the most interesting samples for further study and interpretation of clinical results.

SPECIAL ISSUES CONCERNING THE MONITORING OF VACCINES DERIVED FROM AUTOLOGOUS OR ALLOGENEIC TUMOR

A large number of vaccines are derived from autologous or allogeneic tumors in which the specific tumor antigens are not known. For autologous tumor vaccines, an assumption is made that the more relevant antitumor immune responses are generated to unknown unique antigens. Vaccines derived from allogeneic sources of tumor are presumably inducing immune responses to shared tumor antigens, which may or may not be known. In either case, if the tumors are likely to contain known or putative shared defined tumor antigens, it may be possible to monitor the overall immunogenicity of the vaccine by measuring immune responses to the defined shared antigens. Monitoring of immune responses to defined antigens is discussed in the next section.

If the antigens contained in the vaccine are not known, then other monitoring approaches must be considered. The major goal is to determine whether immune responses are induced to antigens expressed by the vaccine preparation. T-lymphocyte and serologic responses can be measured, but instead of a defined antigen, established autologous or HLA-matched allogeneic cell lines from the vaccine preparation are used as targets for *in vitro* assays. Another measure of immune response to the vaccine preparation is development of DTH reaction to a skin test, consisting of the whole or some fraction of the vaccine (35). Appropriate controls should be included because enzymes used in the preparation and dissociation of tumor samples and components of culture media can be immunogenic and can be responsible for positive DTH responses or an apparent increase in a T-lymphocyte response postvaccination.

Vaccine efficacy can also be monitored by assessing and comparing local or tumor site–specific biologic effects to those that correlated with effective immunization in animal models (10,11,36). Even before the administration of autologous or allogeneic tumor cells transfected with a cytokine gene, production of cytokine by the cells (i.e., measurement of cytokine production per number of cells per unit of time) should be demonstrated to be in the same range as that required for increasing immunogenicity in the animal models. After placement of the vaccine, a biopsy of the site some days later can be examined histologically for infiltration by T lymphocytes, plasma cells, dendritic cells, eosinophils, or other populations, providing some indication that the local effects of the vaccine in humans mimic those conducive to antigen presentation observed in animals. Ultimately, the vaccine is expected to induce an inflammatory response in the tumor. Tumor biopsies can provide an indication of effective immunization if the postvaccine sample shows an increase in the inflammatory infiltrate, which again can be correlated to findings in the preclinical models. T lymphocytes isolated from biopsy sites can be phenotyped for expression of cell surface markers by immunohistochemistry and possibly expanded *in vitro* culture to examine functional properties, such as ability to recognize cell lines from the immunizing preparation. With the inclusion of appropriate controls, the sum of the data could provide convincing evidence of effective immunization against tumor antigens, even if the tumor antigens are not defined.

TABLE 1. VARIOUS ASSAYS USED FOR MONITORING OF EPITOPE-SPECIFIC CD8⁺ T-CELL RESPONSES

	Main Characteristic	Sensitivity	Comments
Direct Assays			
HLA tetramers	Requires only engagement of TCR with epitope/MHC complex	1:5,000	Does not yield information about the ability of T cells to respond to stimulation
Intracellular cytokine expression	Requires engagement of TCR with epitope/MHC complex and activation of T cell	1:5,000	Does not identify epitope-specific T cells incapable of responding to the stimulatory conditions applied by the assay
Enzyme-linked immunospot	—	1:10,000	—
Reverse transcriptase polymerase chain reaction	—	1:50,000	—
Indirect Assays			
In vitro sensitization	Requires engagement of TCR with epitope/MHC complex, activation and proliferation of T cell	Undetermined (probably higher than all other assays)	Does not identify epitope-specific T cells incapable of proliferation in response to the stimulatory conditions applied by the assay
Limiting dilution assay	—	1:10,000 to 1:50,000	—
Proliferation assay	—	Undetermined	Nonspecific, does not correlate with antigen-specific reactivity, practically obsolete

MHC, major histocompatibility complex; TCR, T-cell receptor.

MEASURING T-LYMPHOCYTE RESPONSES TO CANCER VACCINES

Many cancer vaccines in development are designed to induce T-lymphocyte responses against tumor antigens based on the prevalent role of T cells in mediating tumor regression in preclinical animal models. Parallel with clinical evaluation of the vaccines, several assays were adapted or developed for measuring the vaccine-induced T-lymphocyte responses (Table 1). Although each has advantages and disadvantages, none can measure the full spectrum of possible lymphocyte responses. Furthermore, no clear correlations at this time exist between a measured immune response and antitumor activity. For these reasons, the assays must be considered research techniques rather than fully validated instruments that can be routinely used to guide the development of cancer vaccines in the clinic. Selection of the particular assay and the target for measuring the response depends on the form and source of vaccine, its antigen contents, and the expected immune response. Monitoring becomes increasingly more directed as the antigen in the vaccine becomes more defined and restricted. Broad monitoring of immune responses must be considered even in studies of well-defined single antigens because tumor lysis by a specific immune response may promote more effective and broader presentation of tumor antigens *in vivo*.

The immunology of CD4⁺ and CD8⁺ lymphocyte responses on which the monitoring studies are based is described in another chapter. Both cell types may play a role in mediating antitumor responses. In general, cellular responses to antigen recognition include cell activation, changes in expression of surface markers, proliferation, cytokine production, and antigen-specific lysis of target cells. CD4⁺ cells are primarily nonlytic and produce cytokines, whereas CD8⁺ lymphocytes can produce cytokines and lyse tumor cells. CD4⁺ cells are capable of differentiating along separate pathways, leading to different patterns of cytokine production, which may affect their ability to promote versus inhibit an effective antitumor response. CD4⁺ cells with immune-suppressive properties have also been reported.

The significance of CD4⁺ T-cell responses in tumor immunology has been reviewed (37). For CD4⁺ and CD8⁺ immune responses, the magnitude of response (the frequency of antigen-specific T cells), as well as the avidity of the T cells for their respective peptide/MHC complex, may be important factors in determining whether immunization results in tumor regression.

The subsequent sections focus primarily on assessment of CD8⁺ T-cell responses. Few shared CD4⁺ antigen epitopes of tumor antigens have been identified, and the majority of CD4⁺ tumor antigen–specific responses that have been well characterized in humans have been against unique mutations in cellular proteins (38,39). Nevertheless, assessment of CD4⁺ responses is appropriate for vaccines containing long peptides, proteins, or cells.

Assays in Bulk Cultures of Lymphocytes

Immunization against various antigens in animal models and humans has been shown to produce expansion of antigen-specific T-cell precursors in peripheral blood. When the antigen-specific T cells reach a threshold percentage of the overall peripheral blood mononuclear cell (PBMC) population, it becomes possible to detect proliferation and cytokine production in response to or cytotoxicity against target cells bearing the antigen of interest. In some cases (i.e., infection with or immunization against some viral antigens), a large expansion of antigen-specific precursors in peripheral blood occurs, and reactivity against the target antigen can be detected without further expansion of the specific T-cell precursors. With lower numbers of precursors in peripheral blood, detection of T-cell reactivity against a specific antigen in bulk cultures requires expansion of the precursors *in vitro*. Bulk PBMCs or sorted subpopulations from PBMCs (i.e., CD8⁺ T cells) are exposed to the antigen in combination with interleukin-2 (IL-2) in repeated cycles of approximately 7 days. The conditions of *in vitro* expansion vary depending on the particular assay and may include one or more of the following in various concentrations depending on the optimal conditions established for the assay: IL-7, IL-6, IL-12, other cytokines, antibodies activating CD28, irradiated feeder cells, and activated mature dendritic cells. The higher the baseline number of precursors in fresh peripheral blood, the fewer the number of *in vitro* sensitization cycles required to expand the precursors to a level where proliferation, cytotoxicity, or cytokine production in response to the relevant target antigen can be demonstrated in the bulk culture (Fig.1).

Although lymphocytes can produce several cytokines (IFN-γ, granulocyte-macrophage colony-stimulating factor, IL-2, tumor necrosis factor, IL-4, IL-10), assays for detection of antigen-specific cells in bulk cultures, particularly for CD8⁺ CTLs, are often designed to measure production of IFN-γ. The choice of IFN-γ is based in part on preclinical studies of adoptively transferred CTLs to treat murine tumors, which demonstrated a correlation between IFN-γ production by CTLs (but not cytotoxicity) and *in vivo* antitumor effects (6). CTL cytotoxicity for target cells generally correlates with IFN-γ production, but the two functions may be dissociated, partly because the different functions of T cells can require different levels of activation (40). Proliferative assays are usually conducted by measuring the incorporation of tritiated thymidine, which is added over the last 24 hours of an *in vitro* culture of PBMCs with antigen and IL-2. The proliferative assays are used less commonly because they provide minimal information on function of the antigen-specific cells.

Assays for lysis or cytokine production are conducted against target cells expressing the relevant antigen and MHC restriction element. If a generic target cell is used, antigen is placed on the target by pulsing with the appropriate peptide or transfecting the cell with the gene coding for the antigen. Autologous tumor cell lines, or, more commonly, allogeneic tumor cells that contain the antigen and the appropriate MHC restriction element matched to the patient, are also used as targets. The assays are conducted at various ratios of T cells:targets for periods ranging from 4 to 24 hours. Cytokine production is generally measured in the supernatant after a 24-hour incubation using commercially available kits. Lysis is measured by release of a chromium-51 or other label from the target cell, usually over a 4-hour period. To determine the specificity of response, cytotoxicity or cytokine-release assays are conducted in parallel against target cells alone (without peptide) or pulsed with irrelevant peptide, antigen-positive cells mismatched at the MHC restriction element, or antigen-negative MHC-matched cells. In certain circumstances, a blocking antibody against the MHC restriction element is added to verify that recognition is through a receptor-peptide-MHC interaction. For lytic assays, unlabeled antigen-negative target cells can be added to determine if any of the observed lysis is caused by non–antigen-specific killer cells. After correction for background release, the percent of target cells lysed at each effector:target ratio is plotted. Various publications present the data as lytic units, defined as the number of effector cells necessary to give *x*% lysis (usually 33%) of *x* target cells (usually 2,500), divided into 1×10^7 effector cells.

The sensitivity of a cytokine release or lytic assay depends on many variables, including the effector:target ratio, amount of antigen/MHC expressed by the target, the avidity of the T cell, and its capacity for specific lysis or cytokine production. Even such factors as the solubility of the peptide may affect the outcome of the *in vitro* assays. For example, a poorly solu-

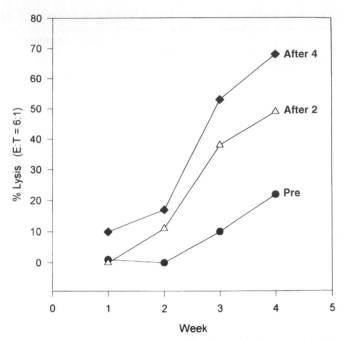

FIGURE 1. *In vitro* sensitization assay for the evaluation of MART-1–specific immune reactivity in peripheral blood mononuclear cells of a patient who received MART-1 (27–35) peptide vaccine in incomplete Freund's adjuvant. Peripheral blood mononuclear cultures were stimulated *in vitro* repetitively with the MART-1 (27–35) peptide and tested after each restimulation for their ability to lyse cancer cells in a cytotoxicity assay. Immune-reactive cells specific to the vaccine and able to kill cancer cells were developed more efficiently after four vaccinations than after two vaccinations and before vaccination. (E:T, effector:target.) [Data from this trial are reported in Cormier JN, Salgaller ML, Prevette T, et al. Enhancement of cellular immunity in melanoma patients immunized with a peptide from MART-1/Melan A (see comments). *Cancer J Sci Am* 1997;3:37.]

ble peptide may give falsely low CTL read-out when pulsed on target cells *in vitro*. A reasonable estimate of the sensitivity of a typical cytotoxicity or cytokine release assay has been provided by spiking PBMCs with increasing numbers of cloned high-avidity CTLs recognizing their respective peptide antigen loaded on target cells or expressed by tumor (41). (M. Nishimura, *personal communication*, 1999). Under the prescribed experimental conditions, the cloned cells must comprise approximately 0.2% to 1.0% of the bulk PBMC population to detect IFN-γ production above background in a standard 24-hour cytokine release assay or cytotoxicity against tumor or peptide-pulsed target cells. Thus, unless immunization results in specific precursor frequencies in peripheral blood or other sampled tissue of approximately 1% (for these particular peptides and assays), detecting the antigen-specific cells requires some *in vitro* expansion. Indeed, successful immunization to the MART-1 melanoma peptide, among the first to be studied in the clinic, was demonstrated by showing detection of CTLs with fewer *in vitro* stimulations postimmunization compared with preimmunization (42,43). (see Fig. 1). For peptides capable of inducing potent immune responses, such as the modified gp100:209-217 (210M) melanoma peptide, production of IFN-γ above background against a peptide-pulsed target cell rarely can be detected directly out of peripheral blood and,

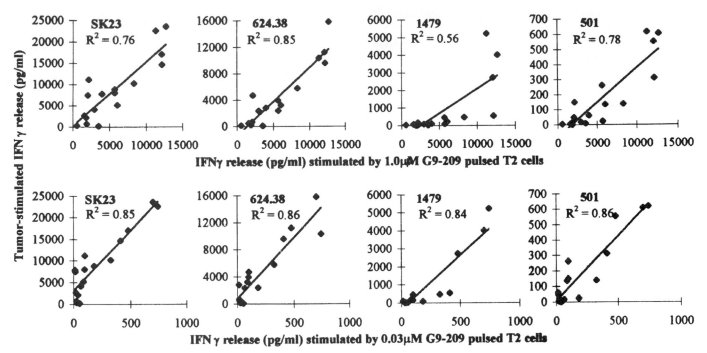

FIGURE 2. Recognition of tumor by vaccine-specific T-cell clones derived from a patient vaccinated with gp100-209-2M in incomplete Freund's adjuvant. Recognition of tumor highly correlates with recognition of antigen-pulsed T2 cells. Interferon-γ (IFN-γ) secretion by individual clones for each indicated tumor is plotted as tumor-stimulated release (*y axis*) versus peptide-pulsed T2 cell–stimulated release (*x axis*). The trendline for the population of clones is shown with the regression coefficient indicated (R^2 value). Top graphs: T2 pulsed with 1.0 μm gp100-209 peptide. Bottom graphs: T2 pulsed with 0.03 mm gp100-209 peptide. SK23, 624.38, 1479, and 501 are gp100 and HLA-A*0201–expressing cell lines. [Adapted from Dudley ME, Nishimura MI, Holt AKC, Rosenberg SA. Anti-tumor immunization with a minimal peptide epitope (G90209-2M) leads to a functionally heterogeneous CTL response. *J Immunother* 1999;22(4):288.]

in most cases, is detected after a single 7- to 11-day *in vitro* sensitization with peptide and IL-2 (44,45).

Characterization of CTL responses in bulk culture can be expanded to examine production of other relevant cytokines and to estimate the avidity of the CTL for the antigen target. For the latter, detection of CTL activity at low effector:target ratios or recognition of peptide-pulsed target cells at low concentrations of peptide suggests that CTLs have high avidity for the antigen-MHC complex. In patients immunized with the modified gp100:209-217 (210M) peptide, Dudley et al. have shown that the avidity of CTLs in bulk culture, as measured by IFN-γ production against peptide-pulsed target cells, correlates with their capacity to recognize tumor cell lines *in vitro* (46) (Fig. 2). Further characterization of the CTL response in bulk culture can be accomplished by cloning and analyzing antigen-specific T cells. The latter analysis in patients immunized with the modified gp100:209-217 (210M) peptide revealed the diversity of the T-cell response (47). Many of the clones recognized only target cells pulsed with the modified peptide or with the native peptide, but not antigen-positive tumor containing the appropriate MHC restriction element HLA-A*0201. Furthermore, analysis of T-cell receptor (TCR) alpha and beta chain usage among these and other antigen-specific clones has demonstrated the broad variability in TCRs that are capable of recognizing a particular peptide-MHC complex (48).

Enzyme-Linked Immunospot Assays

The enzyme-linked immunospot (ELISPOT) assay was developed to increase the quantitative capacity of monitoring T-cell responses (49–51). Plates are coated with antibody to a specific cytokine, most commonly IFN-γ. Target cells pulsed with peptide or target tumor cells are placed onto the plate on which the lymphocytes are added to form a layer one cell thick. The conditions of the assay can be varied. For example, lymphocytes may be sorted to select CD4+ or CD8+ cells before plating, or, if unsorted populations are used, blocking antibodies can be added to decrease background and increase detection specificity (i.e., adding anti-MHC class II antibodies to the plates to block nonspecific CD4+ cell responses and, therefore, increase the specificity for detecting MHC class I–restricted responses) (52). Plates are incubated for approximately 24 to 48 hours in most settings. In each spot that a lymphocyte specific for the target antigen is located, IFN-γ is produced and captured by the bound IFN-γ antibodies on the plate. A second antibody to IFN-γ is added and, after washing, is visualized with a process that forms a colored spot at the site of the second IFN-γ antibody. The spots are counted, each representing a T cell specific for the antigen target. The total number of spots in plates loaded with the relevant target minus the spots formed in the plates with a nonrelevant target divided by the number of PBMCs per plate represents the frequency of antigen-specific T cells. Spots can be read manually or with special instruments.

ELISPOT assays can be used to detect CD4⁺ or CD8⁺ responses. Theoretically, depending on the number of plates used and the extent of background, an ELISPOT assay could allow detection of antigen-specific T cells directly from peripheral blood without any *in vitro* culture and expansion. Similar to the bulk culture techniques, the development of a spot (and, therefore, the assay results) can be affected by several variables, including the amount of antigen/MHC complex presented by the target, the avidity of the T cells for the antigen/MHC complex, their ability to produce the particular cytokine, the length of time required to activate the antigen-specific cells (incubation time), and the sensitivity of detecting the second antibody in the colorimetric reaction.

The published experience using the ELISPOT assay to monitor T-cell responses to cancer antigens is still limited (52–55). Pass et al. reported results of ELISPOT assays conducted in patients immunized with peptides derived from the melanocyte protein gp100. 10^4 or 10^5 PBMCs were plated with 10^5 target cells, either T2 cells pulsed with peptide or MHC-matched antigen-positive tumor cells. In general, an 8- to 12-day *in vitro* sensitization with peptide and IL-2 was necessary to detect reactivity above background in the ELISPOT assay. After the *in vitro* sensitization, peptide-reactive CTLs could be detected in most patients immunized with the gp100:209-217 (210M) modified peptide or the native gp100:209-217 peptide and in approximately 20% of patients immunized with the gp100:280-288 (288V) peptide. The frequency of CTLs after the 8- to 12-day *in vitro* sensitization was in the range of 0.1% to 1.0%. When tumor was used as the target in the ELISPOT assay, reactive CTLs at a frequency of 0.1% to 1.0% were demonstrated in several patients immunized with the modified gp100 peptide.

Reynolds et al. used the ELISPOT assay in monitoring immune responses in 22 consecutive patients receiving a melanoma vaccine composed of shed antigens of cultured melanoma cell lines (52). The ELISPOT assay was used to measure directly from peripheral blood pre- and postimmunization PBMC reactivity to a large number of HLA-A*0201–binding peptides derived from several antigens known to be expressed by melanoma. The ELISPOT assay was modified by adding anti–MHC class II antibodies (to block CD4⁺ responses), and the number of peptide-specific T cells were determined by first subtracting the number of spots in wells containing an anti-CD8⁺ antibody (which would block peptide-specific CTL responses) and further subtracting the number of spots in wells with control non-melanoma peptide. A value of 5 out of 500,000 PBMCs was considered positive in the assay. Frequencies of peptide-specific CTLs pre- or postvaccination ranged from 1 in 100,000 to as high as approximately 1 in 5,000 although most were less than 1 in 25,000. Substantial heterogeneity was found in positive CTL responses between peptides and between patients. The ability of the CTL to recognize HLA-A*0201 antigen–positive melanoma cell lines was not reported.

Intracellular Cytokine Production

Techniques have been developed to quantify antigen-specific T cells by sorting on the basis of intracellular cytokine production

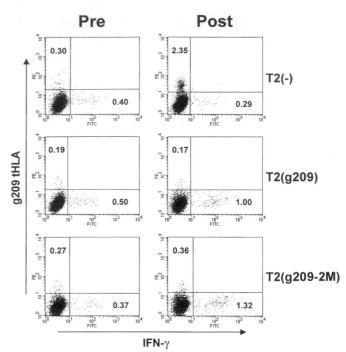

FIGURE 3. Fluorescene-activated cell sorter analysis for intracellular interferon-γ (IFN-γ) expression in pre- and postvaccination peripheral blood mononuclear cells from a patient vaccinated with gp100-209-2M in incomplete Freund's adjuvant. Peripheral blood mononuclear cells were stimulated with unpulsed T2 cells [T2(-)] pulsed with g209 [T2(g209)] or g2092M [T2(g209-2M)] peptides (1 μm). CD3⁺/CD8⁺ cells were gated for analysis, and numbers indicate the percentage of cells in the quadrants over the total gated cells. g209 tHLA staining decreased on stimulation because of downregulation of T-cell receptor as previously noted analyzing epitope-specific clonal populations. [Adapted from Lee K-H, Wang E, Nielsen M-B, et al. Enhanced T-cell response to peptide-based vaccination against melanoma correlates with increased vaccine-specific T-cell frequency and susceptibility to stimulation but does not lead to tumor regression. 1999 (submitted).]

in response to recognition of specific antigen (56,57). T-cell membrane permeability is increased using chemical means, which allows penetration and binding by antibodies specific to the cytokine of interest, usually IFN-γ. Multicolor flow cytometry can then be used to quantify and subset the activated T cells among a bulk PBMC population. The technique has not been fully developed or used extensively in monitoring of cancer vaccine trials and is limited in overall sensitivity by the sensitivity of flow cytometry (Fig. 3) (58,41).

Limiting Dilution Assays

The limiting dilution assay (LDA) is designed to yield an estimate of T-cell precursor frequency in the circulation and is therefore a relatively quantitative assay. Furthermore, as expansion of T cells is integral to the conduct of this assay, it has the capacity for increased sensitivity compared with assays such as ELISPOT and intracellular cytokine and tetramer analysis, which are often used to enumerate the number of antigen-specific T cells directly from peripheral blood without expansion. Nevertheless, the capabilities of the tetramer technology (described in the section Tetramer Assays) may ultimately surpass the sensitivity of the LDA in certain settings.

LDA is based on the principle that the number of *in vitro* PBMC cultures from which an antigen-specific T-cell population can be expanded is proportional to the frequency of the precursors in fresh PBMCs. In making serial dilutions of the initial PBMC population and plating replicate cultures at each dilution, the number of cultures containing the antigen-specific lymphocytes should decrease. The number of "negative" cultures per dilution of the starting lymphocyte population can be plotted, and statistical methods can be used to determine the frequency of the target antigen–specific lymphocytes in the undiluted lymphocyte population obtained from peripheral blood (59).

Each culture per dilution is set up by adding feeder cells (usually irradiated PBMCs) and then adding the antigen of interest (a peptide in many cases) or a tumor target. A parallel series of control cultures are established with irrelevant targets. The lymphocytes are added at a predetermined effector:target ratio along with IL-2. The *in vitro* stimulation with antigen and IL-2 may be repeated at set intervals. After a sufficient period for the antigen-specific lymphocytes to proliferate, labeled target cells containing the antigen are added to the cultures, and the end point of interest is measured (usually cytotoxicity or cytokine production for detection of CTLs). In some circumstances, cold antigen-negative target cells are added with the labeled relevant targets to negate nonspecific effector cell activity generated by IL-2. Positive cultures are scored when the values are higher than the mean plus three standard deviations.

The results of the LDA depend on several variables, including the type of cellular response that is assayed, the target cells, the frequency of the antigen-specific cells in the starting population, the ability of those cells to expand in culture, the number of cultures established per dilution, and the number of dilutions that are examined. Overall, the sensitivity of LDA appears to be superior to other assays that use a functional end point for detection of antigen-specific lymphocytes with a range of 1 in 30,000 to 1 in 100,000, although some investigators report sensitivity to 1 in 10^6. Even under the most favorable circumstances, measurement of lymphocyte responses with the LDA is labor intensive and not practical for routine monitoring of cancer vaccine trials. Furthermore, comparison of the LDA with the tetramer assays (discussed in the section Tetramer Assays) for detection of T-cell responses in the setting of a viral infection suggests that LDA detects only a fraction (approximately 1.0% to 20%) of T lymphocytes that express a TCR capable of recognizing the antigen of interest.

The LDA has been used to monitor several cancer vaccine studies, including trials of allogeneic melanoma cell lines or lysates (60,61), poxvirus vectors containing the carcinoembryonic antigen gene (using an HLA-A2–restricted carcinoembryonic antigen peptide as the *in vitro* target) (22), and peptides derived from MUC-1 and gp100 (62). Although precursor frequencies of CTLs against the immunogen or the selected target increased in some patients for most of the studies, postvaccination CTL frequencies were generally still quite low. Patients treated with the modified gp100:209-217 (210M) peptide, however, were found to have T cells specific for the native gp100 peptide in the range of 0.1% to 0.01% of

the bulk PBMC population (S.A. Rosenberg, *personal communication*, 1998).

Tetramer Assays

Theoretically, the most sensitive and specific assay for antigen-specific T cells would permit identification and enumeration of all cells in a population that contained a TCR that bound to a particular peptide-MHC complex. The lymphocyte TCR binds to a single peptide-MHC complex with relatively low affinity followed by rapid dissociation. Single peptide-MHC complexes are therefore poor reagents for use in cell-sorting analyses of T cells. When two to four MHC molecules are linked and the peptide antigen is allowed to bind to the MHC molecules, the dissociation rate of the peptide-MHC complex from the lymphocyte TCR is diminished substantially, allowing for identification and sorting of lymphocytes using a fluorescence-activated cell sorter instrument (63). The sensitivity of peptide-MHC tetramers to detect antigen-specific CTLs is predicted to be greater than the standard limiting dilution assays because the tetramers detect T cells based primarily on the binding properties of the TCR, whereas detection of T cells by LDA depends inherently on the ability of a T cell to proliferate and perform a function, such as cytotoxicity or cytokine release in response to its antigen. The increased sensitivity conferred by tetramer binding is offset partially by the limited sensitivity of the fluorescence-activated cell sorter instrument, which can only reliably detect approximately 1 in 10,000 cells (0.01% to 0.02%). Furthermore, production of high-quality pure peptide-MHC tetramer reagents can be difficult, requiring relatively pure peptide and a refolding of the recombinant-produced heavy chain and beta-2-microglobulin in the presence of peptide. Nevertheless, the peptide-MHC tetramers appear to provide more reliable quantization of antigen-specific T cells than other techniques, and, in certain settings, may allow analysis of CTL responses directly on peripheral blood or tissue. Furthermore, once the antigen-specific cells are sorted, they can be analyzed for functional properties in bulk or after additional cloning.

In animal and human studies of viral infections, tetramers have detected remarkable peripheral blood expansion of CD8$^+$ cells specific for a viral peptide epitope, in some cases comprising 5% to 10% of the total CD8$^+$ lymphocyte population (64–68). The published experience with tetramers to monitor CTL responses to cancer antigens remains limited (69,70). Tetramers have been generated for the melanocyte HLA-A201–restricted peptide epitopes MART-1/Melan-A:27-35 and 26-35 (27L), gp100:209-217, and its 210M modification gp100:154-162 and tyrosinase:368-376 (370D), all of which are in clinical trials for patients with metastatic melanoma. Ogg et al. used the MART-1/Melan-A:26-35 (27L) tetramers to study the frequency of CTLs specific for MART-1 in the PBMCs of HLA-A201 individuals diagnosed with vitiligo compared with a normal HLA-A201 cohort. Individuals with vitiligo had higher frequencies of MART-1–specific CTLs in the range of 0.01% to 0.50% of all CD8$^+$ lymphocytes. The majority of tetramer-positive CD8$^+$ lymphocytes also expressed the skin homing receptor cutaneous lymphocyte antigen. *In vitro* expansion of PBMCs with the corresponding MART-1/Melan-A peptide and cytokines produced greater expansion of tetramer-positive lymphocytes in the vitiligo cohort compared with the control cohort, confirming the observations made directly from peripheral blood. Expanded tetramer-positive cells were also shown to have cytolytic activity against HLA-A201 MART-1–positive melanoma cell lines. Using similar techniques, Romero et al. demonstrated higher frequencies of MART-1/Melan-A CTL in CD8⁺ lymphocytes obtained from melanoma-involved, resected regional lymph nodes when compared with CD8⁺ lymphocytes from tumor-involved lymph nodes in patients with other cancers. The tyrosinase peptide tetramer detected antigen-specific CTLs at low frequencies and only in some patients, although higher frequencies could be detected in two of three PBMCs cultured *in vitro* for 2 to 3 weeks in IL-2 and IL-7.

Lee et al. used tetramers to tyrosinase (as above) MART1:27-35, and gp100:154-162 peptides to stain PBMCs from 11 nonvaccinated melanoma patients (71). In four patients, MART-1–specific CTLs were detected at a frequency of 0.014% to 0.160%, whereas tyrosinase-specific CTLs were detected in two separate patients (0.19% and 2.2%). Tetramer-positive cells were characterized for expression of multiple surface markers, as well as cytolytic activity, cytokine production, and expression of the activation marker CD69 in response to peptide-pulsed target cells. CTLs in two of the patients expressed an unusual phenotype with characteristics of naïve and memory cells. In contrast to control populations of cytomegalovirus or Epstein-Barr virus peptide–specific CTLs from the same patients or normal donors, MART-1– and tyrosinase tetramer–positive CTLs isolated directly from peripheral blood were unable to kill or upregulate CD69 expression in response to peptide-pulsed target cells. *In vitro* exposure of CTLs to IL-2 for 48 hours did not restore lytic activity. Furthermore, the CTLs were unable to produce IFN-γ or tumor necrosis factor in response to phorbol ester and a calcium ionophore. The results illustrate the potential of the tetramer assay to identify and characterize function of specific populations of tumor antigen–specific CTLs and compare them within the same patient to CTLs recognizing nontumor antigens. The investigators were also able to demonstrate a decline in the tyrosinase tetramer–positive CTLs over time in response to chemotherapy.

The gp100:209-217 and 209-217 (210M) tetramers have been used to measure PBMC frequencies of CTLs specific to the gp100:209-217 epitope in patients immunized with the 210M modification of this peptide (58). Samples are generally obtained 3 weeks after the second q3w immunization with peptide administered in incomplete Freund's adjuvant. Whereas up to a one-log increase in CTL frequency could be detected postimmunization directly from peripheral blood in some patients, the absolute number of antigen-specific cells was only 1.0% to 1.5% of PBMCs in patients with the best response. When PBMCs were expanded *in vitro* with peptide and IL-2 for several days, however, the tetramer assay showed a marked expansion in the gp100-specific CTLs only in the postimmunization PBMCs.

Molecular Techniques for Monitoring T-Lymphocyte Responses

Direct monitoring of specific T-cell populations using molecular approaches may improve sensitivity and allow examination of small samples of tissue. One potential approach is to monitor the genes used to code for the TCR of the CTL that recognizes a particular peptide-MHC complex. The TCR is composed of an alpha and beta chain, each of which is formed by recombination of DNA sequences from two and three gene families, respectively, within the respective gene locus. Various combinations of TCR alpha and beta chains can form a binding site for a specific peptide/MHC complex. This marked plasticity of the potential T-cell response within and between patients (before the stimulation of an immune response) precludes determining the genes that will be preferentially used to form the TCRs that bind to the peptide-MHC complex. Once a CTL clone specific for a peptide-MHC complex is available, however, the fate of cells expressing the particular genes coding for the TCR alpha and beta chain and a CDR3 region of specific length (the area that forms the specific antigen-binding region) can be monitored *in vitro* or *in vivo*. A competitive reverse transcriptase PCR assay has been described that can quantitatively assess the absolute number and percent of message for a particular gene of the TCR alpha or beta gene family (72). The assay was reported as being capable of detecting one copy per 100,000 of the message of interest. A second PCR technique estimates the percent of cells within a population that express a particular gene of the TCR beta gene family and a specific length (number of amino acids) of the CDR3 region (the area that makes contact with the peptide-MHC complex) (73). The techniques have substantial value in dissecting the evolution of immune responses to specific antigens in animal models (74,75). For clinical trials, the techniques appear to be most useful in following adoptive transfer of specific CTL clones *in vivo* or for tracking expansion and localization of a subpopulation of CTLs once an immune response has been induced (76,77).

Rather than following the fate of specific clones of T cells, investigators have developed molecular methods to estimate the presence or changes in frequency of T cells in peripheral blood or tumor that have the characteristics of activation in response to antigen recognition. After activation of a T cell, RNA message for several cytokines and other activation-induced genes increases within 2 to 4 hours. Quantitative reverse transcriptase PCRs can measure the absolute amount of messenger RNA (mRNA) for a particular gene and the increase in message related to T-cell activation. Investigators at the Surgery Branch of the National Cancer Institute have used the quantitative reverse transcriptase PCR techniques to detect evidence of immunization to a peptide vaccine directly from peripheral blood. A sample of PBMCs is exposed to peptide antigen for a short period, and quantitative PCR for various genes is performed at several time points after the completion of peptide incubation (78) (Fig. 4). Among several genes, IFN-γ has been most sensitive for detecting activation of MHC class I–restricted CD8 T cells when normalized to mRNA copies of the CD8 gene. The sensitivity of the assay, determined by adding titrated

Principle of the Technique

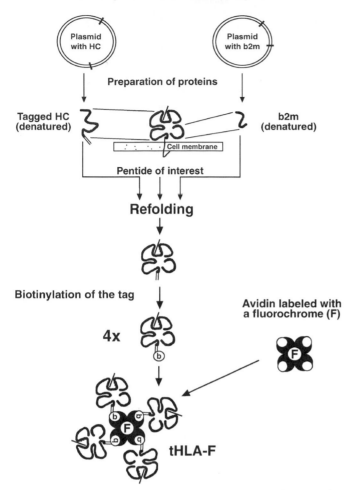

FIGURE 4. Preparation of soluble major histocompatibility complex/peptide complexes for staining of epitope-specific T cells. Both major histocompatibility complex heavy chains tagged with a biotinylation sequence (HC) and beta-2-microglobulin (b2m) are produced in bacteria. Purified molecules are then reconstituted in the presence of a relevant peptide into a trimer, including HC, b2m, and peptide (refolding step). The biotinylation is then performed, and then avidin is added to the biotinylated complexes. Because avidin is a tetravalent molecule, tetramers with four HC/b2m/peptide complexes are obtained.

amounts of cloned CTLs to PBMCs, can be in the range of one activated antigen-specific cell among 50,000 PBMCs. In preliminary studies of patients immunized with the gp100:209-217 (210M) peptide, the sensitivity of the quantitative PCR directly from peripheral blood is still below that of bulk *in vitro* culture of PBMCs, because the latter method allows expansion of the antigen-specific CTLs, and the signal can be amplified by secretion of the target cytokine. Nevertheless, the sensitivity of PCR may be sufficient for the purpose of detecting clinically relevant immune responses, and the technique is substantially less labor intensive. Use of PCR in combination with limiting dilution techniques may provide quantitative estimates of specific T-cell precursors in peripheral blood. It may also be possible to assess the avidity of the T-cell response by varying the concentration of peptide used to stimulate the T cells.

In Vivo Biologic Measures of T-Lymphocyte Responses

Regardless of the source of antigen or method of immunization, induction of an effective T-lymphocyte response against tumor should result in tumor infiltration by T cells and other inflammatory effector cells drawn to the site by the antigen-specific T-cell response. Therefore, a direct method of monitoring vaccine efficacy is to obtain pre- and postimmunization samples of tumor and assess the tumor inflammatory response. The issues related to monitoring of responses within tumor and interpretation of the results have been discussed in the section Monitoring of Tumor-Related Factors.

Optimally, monitoring of T-cell responses within tumor in response to a particular cancer vaccine would include assessment of the change in number of tumor antigen–specific cells, their activation state, and functional properties. Techniques capable of monitoring all aspects of the T-cell response, however, are not available, and the serial tumor biopsies necessary for these laboratory studies and full histologic examination are difficult to obtain, particularly in patients who have poorly accessible metastatic disease. To address these concerns, investigators at the Surgery Branch of the National Cancer Institute have adapted quantitative PCR techniques (Taq-man) to serially measure absolute amounts of RNA message for genes expressed within samples of tumor obtained by fine-needle aspirates (Fig. 5). Although not able to ascribe changes to a particular group of antigen-specific T cells, the technique can theoretically provide important information on changes in overall amount of T-cell infiltrate and the activation state and function of those cells. More important, the technique has the capacity to quantitatively measure biologic functions that are activated as part of a presumed common pathway for antigen-specific, T-cell–mediated antitumor response (i.e., amount of IFN-γ produced within the tumor as a result of infiltration and activation of tumor antigen–specific T cells).

Preliminary experiments were conducted retrospectively on cohorts of patients that had received a melanoma peptide vaccine from gp100 [gp100:209-217 (210M)] on Surgery Branch immunotherapy protocols and undergone serial fine-needle aspirates of melanoma lesions (78). Copies of mRNA for IFN-γ were normalized to CD8 messenger RNA, and copies of gp100 messenger RNA were normalized to beta-actin mRNA. In eight of nine patients, posttreatment tumor samples revealed at least a twofold increase in copies of IFN-γ message. Furthermore, the increase in IFN-γ message was correlated strongly to prevaccination tumor expression of gp100. The increase in tumor IFN-γ mRNA was not observed in a cohort of control patients that were treated on other immunotherapy protocols but had no evidence of CTL response against the native gp100:209-217 peptide epitope, as measured in peripheral blood by standard bulk culture techniques. Of substantial interest was the observation that none of the sampled lesions had shown evidence of objective response, suggesting that the immune response was insufficient to mediate tumor regression. The PCR assay is being expanded to measure RNA message for other relevant genes, such as IL-2. If confirmed in larger groups of patients and in prospective trials, the technique will offer a simple and rapid indication of effective

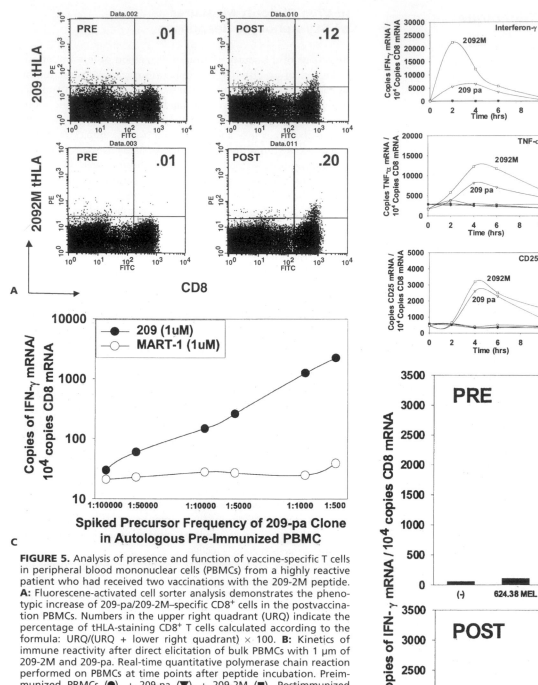

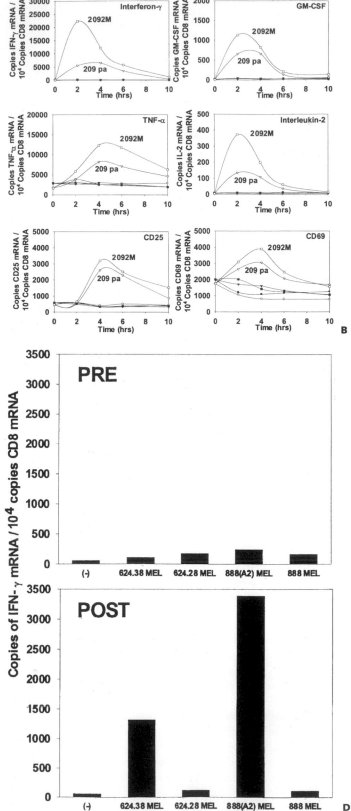

FIGURE 5. Analysis of presence and function of vaccine-specific T cells in peripheral blood mononuclear cells (PBMCs) from a highly reactive patient who had received two vaccinations with the 209-2M peptide. **A:** Fluorescene-activated cell sorter analysis demonstrates the phenotypic increase of 209-pa/209-2M–specific CD8+ cells in the postvaccination PBMCs. Numbers in the upper right quadrant (URQ) indicate the percentage of tHLA-staining CD8+ T cells calculated according to the formula: URQ/(URQ + lower right quadrant) × 100. **B:** Kinetics of immune reactivity after direct elicitation of bulk PBMCs with 1 μm of 209-2M and 209-pa. Real-time quantitative polymerase chain reaction performed on PBMCs at time points after peptide incubation. Preimmunized PBMCs (●), + 209-pa (▼), + 209-2M (■), Postimmunized PBMCs (○) +209-pa (▽) +209-2M (□). **C:** Sensitivity of direct molecular assay; 209-pa–reactive T-cell clone was spiked into preimmunized PBMCs. Elicitation of 209-pa reactivity [interferon-γ (IFN-γ) messenger RNA (mRNA)] could be seen at a spiked dilution of 1 clone in 50,000 PBMCs. Negative control was performed with exposure to irrelevant peptide, MART 27-35. **D:** Direct reactivity (IFN-γ mRNA production) of pre- and postimmunized PBMCs to HLA-A2+/gp100 + melanomas, 624.38 Mel and 888 Mel (A2+), and HLA-A2-/gp100 + melanomas 624.28 Mel and 888 Mel. (GM-CSF, granulocyte-macrophage colony-stimulating factor.) [Adapted from Kammula U, Lee K-H, Riker AI, et al. Evidence of effective immunization by serial gene expression analysis of tumors. 1999 (submitted).]

immunization against a tumor antigen because it assesses the integration of events necessary for tumor response (i.e., T-cell activation, migration into tumor, and production of cytokines by the T-cell infiltrate).

Because tumor sampling is not possible in many patients, an alternative to measure effective immunization *in vivo* has been the DTH. The tumor antigen is administered by intradermal injection, and, 24 to 72 hours later, the local inflammatory response, as determined by the diameter of induration, is measured. The reaction is considered positive if induration measures at least 5 mm. The DTH reaction is mediated by an antigen-specific T-cell response. Therefore, a positive DTH test indicates a T-cell response to the antigen placed at the site. The specificity of the reaction is ascertained by placing appropriate controls and further confirmed by biopsy of the site and functional characterization of the T-cell infiltrate (see below).

DTH testing as a monitoring tool has been used primarily for cell-based vaccines (35,79,80). Typically, the cell line used for vaccination is placed intradermally without adjuvant in successively higher concentrations. For autologous tumor cell vaccines, the best available controls are autologous non–tumor-derived cells that have been prepared using procedures identical to those used in generation of the tumor cell line used for immunization (i.e., normal tissue adjacent to the tumor, peripheral blood lymphocyte, or Epstein-Barr virus–transformed autologous lymphoblastoid cell lines). Comparison of pre- versus postimmunization DTH responses is often insufficient to determine whether the immune response is directed to a tumor-related antigen, because tumor cells may be exposed to highly immunogenic enzymes and fetal calf serum in the preparation procedure (14). Tumor cells that are dissociated mechanically without the use of enzymes and are stored without exposure to foreign proteins, however, may be appropriate for comparison of pre- versus postimmunization DTH responses, although controls are still necessary to increase the certainty that the DTH response is a direct result of immunization. To avoid investigator bias, the skin test results should be read by an independent observer unaware of which site contains the antigen versus the control. In allogeneic cell–based vaccines, skin-test reactivity to tumor antigens is difficult to differentiate from the more likely responses to allogeneic antigens in the vaccine. DTH tests have been performed in studies of defined antigens using the antigen alone or pulsed on dendritic cells, and, in some studies, DTH tests were performed with tumor lysates pulsed on dendritic cells (81).

PRINCIPLES OF MEASURING ANTIBODY RESPONSES TO CANCER VACCINES

Depending on the type of cancer vaccine, the method of delivery, and the antigens used for immunization, antibody responses may be elicited in patients. For some vaccines, immunization is intended solely to induce antibody responses to the cancer antigen. Reliable techniques for measuring antibody responses have been available for many years. Studies often use a combination of Western blot and enzyme-linked

immunosorbent assay to determine presence or absence of antibody to the antigen and the titer, respectively (82–86). The time course of response in serum is usually determined, as well as the immunoglobulin M (IgM) and IgG component and the subclass of the IgG response. The antibody response is sometimes further characterized to assess complement fixation in the presence of the antigen target and ability to mediate antibody-dependent cellular cytotoxicity. As with vaccines that induce cell-mediated responses, it is critical to demonstrate that the antibody response recognizes tumor cells because the conformation or composition of purified antigen may be quite different than that found on tumor. Although not a common feature of vaccine trials, obtaining tumor tissue to demonstrate saturation of antibody binding sites after immunization may provide useful information.

SUMMARY

Substantial progress has been made in the development and application of techniques to immune monitoring of cancer vaccine studies. Ongoing studies dissecting the type, quality, magnitude, and targets of effective antitumor immune responses in more sophisticated and predictive preclinical models will lead to even more rapid progress and focus in the development of immune-monitoring assays for early clinical trials. Current assays are able to detect evidence of T-cell responses and antibody responses to immunization with reasonable sensitivity and specificity; however, full characterization of the complex immune response *in vivo* is still beyond the resources and technical capabilities of most investigators. New molecular techniques that assess expression of many genes within tumor before and after treatment offer great hope for more fully characterizing the events necessary for tumor regression, and, most important, reasons for failure and means to improve the efficacy of cancer vaccines in future trials.

REFERENCES

1. Rosenberg SA. A new era for cancer immunotherapy based on the genes that encode cancer antigens. *Immunity* 1999;10:281–287.
2. Boon T, Coulie PG, Van den Eynde B. Tumor antigens recognized by T cells. *Immunol Today* 1997;18:267–268.
3. Salgaller ML. Monitoring of cancer patients undergoing active or passive immunotherapy. *J Immunother* 1997;20:1–14.
4. Speiser DE, Miranda R, Zakarian A, et al. Self antigens expressed by solid tumors do not efficiently stimulate naive or activated T cells: implications for immunotherapy. *J Exp Med* 1997;186:645–653.
5. Zeh HJ III, Perry-Lalley D, Dudley ME, Rosenberg SA, Yang JC. High avidity CTLs for two self-antigens demonstrate superior *in vitro* and *in vivo* antitumor efficacy. *J Immunol* 1999;162:989–994.
6. Barth RJ Jr, Mulé JJ, Spiess PJ, Rosenberg SA. Interferon gamma and tumor necrosis factor have a role in tumor regressions mediated by murine CD8+ tumor-infiltrating lymphocytes. *J Exp Med* 1991;173:647–658.
7. Ganss R, Hanahan D. Tumor microenvironment can restrict the effectiveness of activated antitumor lymphocytes. *Cancer Res* 1998;58:4673–4681.
8. Pockaj BA, Sherry RM, Wei JP, et al. Localization of [111]indium-labeled tumor infiltrating lymphocytes to tumor in patients receiving

adoptive immunotherapy. Augmentation with cyclophosphamide and correlation with response. *Cancer* 1994;73:1731–1737.

9. Zhang H, Zhang S, Cheung NK, Ragupathi G, Livingston PO. Antibodies against GD2 ganglioside can eradicate syngeneic cancer micrometastases. *Cancer Res* 1998;58:2844–2849.

10. Soiffer R, Lynch T, Mihm M, et al. Vaccination with irradiated autologous melanoma cells engineered to secrete human granulo-cyte-macrophage colony-stimulating factor generates potent antitu-mor immunity in patients with metastatic melanoma. *Proc Natl Acad Sci U S A* 1998;95:13141–13146.

11. Simons JW, Jaffee EM, Weber CE, et al. Bioactivity of autologous irradiated renal cell carcinoma vaccines generated by ex vivo granulo-cyte-macrophage colony-stimulating factor gene transfer. *Cancer Res* 1997;57:1537–1546.

12. Rosenberg SA, Zhai Y, Yang JC, et al. Immunizing patients with metastatic melanoma using recombinant adenoviruses encoding MART-1 or gp100 melanoma antigens. *J Natl Cancer Inst* 1998; 90:1894–1900.

13. Hodge JW, McLaughlin JP, Kantor JA, Schlom J. Diversified prime and boost protocols using recombinant vaccinia virus and recombi-nant non-replicating avian pox virus to enhance T-cell immunity and antitumor responses. *Vaccine* 1997;15:759–768.

14. Berd D, Mastrangelo MJ. Active immunotherapy of human mela-noma exploiting the immunopotentiating effects of cyclophospha-mide. *Cancer Invest* 1988;6:337–349.

15. Marincola FM, Rivoltini L, Salgaller ML, Player M, Rosenberg SA. Differential anti-MART-1/MelanA CTL activity in peripheral blood of HLA-A2 melanoma patients in comparison to healthy donors: evidence of *in vivo* priming by tumor cells. *J Immunother Emphasis Tumor Immunol* 1996;19:266–277.

16. Mizoguchi H, O'Shea JJ, Longo DL, Loeffler CM, McVicar DW, Ochoa AC. Alterations in signal transduction molecules in T lym-phocytes from tumor-bearing mice [see comments]. *Science* 1992; 258:1795–1798.

17. Correa MR, Ochoa AC, Ghosh P, Mizoguchi H, Harvey L, Longo DL. Sequential development of structural and functional alterations in T cells from tumor-bearing mice. *J Immunol* 1997;158:5292–5296.

18. Kolenko V, Wang Q, Riedy MC, et al. Tumor-induced suppression of T lymphocyte proliferation coincides with inhibition of Jak3 expression and IL-2 receptor signaling: role of soluble products from human renal cell carcinomas. *J Immunol* 1997;159:3057–3067.

19. Gabrilovich D, Ishida T, Oyama T, et al. Vascular endothelial growth factor inhibits the development of dendritic cells and dramatically affects the differentiation of multiple hematopoietic lineages *in vivo*. *Blood* 1998;92:4150–4166.

20. Gabrilovich DI, Chen HL, Girgis KR, et al. Production of vascular endothelial growth factor by human tumors inhibits the functional maturation of dendritic cells [published erratum appears in *Nat Med* 1996;2(11):1267]. *Nat Med* 1996;2:1096–1103.

21. Kim CJ, Parkinson DR, Marincola F. Immunodominance across HLA polymorphism: implications for cancer immunotherapy. *J Immunother* 1998;21:1–16.

22. Marshall JL, Hawkins MJ, Tsang KY, et al. Phase I study in cancer patients of a replication-defective avipox recombinant vaccine that expresses human carcinoembryonic antigen. *J Clin Oncol* 1999;17: 332–337.

23. Tsang KY, Zaremba S, Nieroda CA, Zhu MZ, Hamilton JM, Schlom J. Generation of human cytotoxic T cells specific for human carcinoembryonic antigen epitopes from patients immunized with recombinant vaccinia-CEA vaccine [see comments]. *J Natl Cancer Inst* 1995;87:982–990.

24. Bettinotti MP, Kim CJ, Lee KH, et al. Stringent allele/epitope require-ments for MART-1/Melan A immunodominance: implications for peptide-based immunotherapy. *J Immunol* 1998;161:877–889.

25. Lee KH, Panelli MC, Kim CJ, et al. Functional dissociation between local and systemic immune response during anti-melanoma peptide vaccination. *J Immunol* 1998;161:4183–4194.

26. Panelli M, Riker A, Kammula U, et al. Expansion of tumor/T cell pairs from fine needle aspirates (FNA) of melanoma metastases. *J Immunol* 2000;164:495–504.

27. Ferrone S, Marincola FM. Loss of HLA class I antigens by mela-noma cells: molecular mechanisms, functional significance and clini-cal relevance. *Immunol Today* 1995;16:487–494.

28. Marincola FM, Jaffe EM, Hicklin DJ, Ferrone S. Escape of human tumor from T cell recognition: molecular mechanisms and func-tional significance. *Adv Immunol* 2000;74:181–273.

29. Cormier JN, Panelli MC, Hackett JA, et al. Natural variation of the expression of HLA and endogenous antigen modulates CTL recogni-tion in an *in vitro* melanoma model. *Int J Cancer* 1999;80:781–790.

30. Cormier JN, Hijazi YM, Abati A, et al. Heterogeneous expression of melanoma-associated antigens and HLA-A2 in metastatic melanoma in vivo. *Int J Cancer* 1998;75:517–524.

31. Cormier JN, Abati A, Fetsch P, et al. Comparative analysis of the in vivo expression of tyrosinase, MART-1/Melan-A, and gp100 in met-astatic melanoma lesions: implications for immunotherapy. *J Immu-nother* 1998;21:27–31.

32. Chen JJ, Sun Y, Nabel GJ. Regulation of the proinflammatory effects of Fas ligand (CD95L). *Science* 1998;282:1714–1717.

33. Kaplan DH, Shankaran V, Dighe AS, et al. Demonstration of an interferon gamma-dependent tumor surveillance system in immuno-competent mice. *Proc Natl Acad Sci U S A* 1998;95:7556–7561.

34. Duggan DJ, Bittner M, Chen Y, Meltzer P, Trent JM. Expression profiling using cDNA microarrays. *Nat Genet* 1999;21:10–14.

35. Berd D, Maguire HC Jr, Schuchter LM, et al. Autologous hapten-modified melanoma vaccine as postsurgical adjuvant treatment after resection of nodal metastases. *J Clin Oncol* 1997;15:2359–2370.

36. Berd D, Murphy G, Maguire HC Jr, Mastrangelo MJ. Immuniza-tion with haptenized, autologous tumor cells induces inflammation of human melanoma metastases. *Cancer Res* 1991;51:2731–2734.

37. Hung K, Hayashi R, Lafond-Walker A, Lowenstein C, Pardoll D, Lev-itsky H. The central role of CD4(+) T cells in the antitumor immune response [In Process Citation]. *J Exp Med* 1998;188:2357–2368.

38. Wang RF, Wang X, Rosenberg SA. Identification of a novel major histocompatibility complex class II-restricted tumor antigen result-ing from a chromosomal rearrangement recognized by CD4(+) T cells [In Process Citation]. *J Exp Med* 1999;189:1659–1668.

39. Pardoll DM, Topalian SL. The role of CD4+ T cell responses in anti-tumor immunity. *Curr Opin Immunol* 1998;10:588–594.

40. Valitutti S, Muller S, Dessing M, Lanzavecchia A. Different responses are elicited in cytotoxic T lymphocytes by different levels of T cell receptor occupancy. *J Exp Med* 1996;183:1917–1921.

41. Labarriere N, Pandolfino MC, Raingeard D, et al. Frequency and rela-tive fraction of tumor antigen-specific T cells among lymphocytes from melanoma-invaded lymph nodes. *Int J Cancer* 1998;78:209–215.

42. Jager E, Ringhoffer M, Arand M, et al. Cytolytic T cell reactivity against melanoma-associated differentiation antigens in peripheral blood of melanoma patients and healthy individuals. *Melanoma Res* 1996;6:419–425.

43. Cormier JN, Salgaller ML, Prevette T, et al. Enhancement of cellular immunity in melanoma patients immunized with a peptide from MART-1/Melan A [see comments]. *Cancer J Sci Am* 1997;3:37–44.

44. Salgaller ML, Marincola FM, Cormier JN, Rosenberg SA. Immuni-zation against epitopes in the human melanoma antigen gp100 fol-lowing patient immunization with synthetic peptides. *Cancer Res* 1996;56:4749–4757.

45. Rosenberg SA, Yang JC, Schwartzentruber DJ, et al. Immunologic and therapeutic evaluation of a synthetic peptide vaccine for the treatment of patients with metastatic melanoma [see comments]. *Nat Med* 1998;4:321–327.

46. Dudley ME, Nishimura MI, Holt AKC, Rosenberg SA. Anti-tumor immunization with a minimal peptide epitope (G90209-2M) leads to a functionally heterogeneous CTL response. *J Immunother* 1999;22(4):288–298.

47. Clay TM, Custer MC, McKee MD, et al. Changes in the fine speci-ficity of gp100(209-217)-reactive T cells in patients following vacci-nation with a peptide modified at an HLA-A2.1 anchor residue. *J Immunol* 1999;162:1749–1755.

48. Shilyansky J, Nishimura MI, Yannelli JR, et al. T-cell receptor usage by melanoma-specific clonal and highly oligoclonal tumor-infiltrat-ing lymphocyte lines. *Proc Natl Acad Sci U S A* 1994;91:2829–2833.

49. Scheibenbogen C, Lee KH, Mayer S, et al. A sensitive ELISPOT assay for detection of CD8+ T lymphocytes specific for HLA class I-binding peptide epitopes derived from influenza proteins in the blood of healthy donors and melanoma patients [In Process Citation]. *Clin Cancer Res* 1997;3:221–226.

50. Schmittel A, Keilholz U, Scheibenbogen C. Evaluation of the interferon-gamma ELISPOT-assay for quantification of peptide specific T lymphocytes from peripheral blood. *J Immunol Methods* 1997;210:167–174.

51. Herr W, Schneider J, Lohse AW, Meyer zum Buschenfelde KH, Wolfel T. Detection and quantification of blood-derived CD8+ T lymphocytes secreting tumor necrosis factor alpha in response to HLA-A2.1-binding melanoma and viral peptide antigens. *J Immunol Methods* 1996;191:131–142.

52. Reynolds SR, Celis E, Sette A, et al. HLA-independent heterogeneity of CD8+ T cell responses to MAGE-3, Melan-A/MART-1, gp100, tyrosinase, MC1R, and TRP-2 in vaccine-treated melanoma patients [In Process Citation]. *J Immunol* 1998;161:6970–6976.

53. Pass HA, Schwarz SL, Wunderlich JR, Rosenberg SA. Immunization of patients with melanoma peptide vaccines: immunologic assessment using the ELISPOT assay [see comments]. *Cancer J Sci Am* 1998;4:316 323.

54. Schmittel A, Keilholz U, Max R, Thiel E, Scheibenbogen C. Induction of tyrosinase-reactive T cells by treatment with dacarbazine, cisplatin, interferon-alpha +/- interleukin-2 in patients with metastatic melanoma. *Int J Cancer* 1999;80:39–43.

55. Schmittel A, Keilholz U, Thiel E, Scheibenbogen C. Quantification of tumor-specific T lymphocytes with ELISPOT assay. *J Immunother* 1999 (in press).

56. Gallimore A, Glithero A, Godkin A, et al. Induction and exhaustion of lymphocytic choriomeningitis virus-specific cytotoxic T lymphocytes visualized using soluble tetrameric major histocompatibility complex class I-peptide complexes. *J Exp Med* 1998;187:1383–1393.

57. Murali-Krishna K, Altman JD, Suresh M, et al. Counting antigen-specific CD8 T cells: a reevaluation of bystander activation during viral infection. *Immunity* 1998;8:177–187.

58. Lee K-H, Wang E, Nielsen M-B, et al. Enhanced T cell response to peptide-based vaccination against melanoma correlates with increased vaccine-specific T cell frequency and susceptibility to stimulation but does not lead to tumor regression. 1999 (submitted).

59. Coulie PG, Somville M, Lehmann F, et al. Precursor frequency analysis of human cytolytic T lymphocytes directed against autologous melanoma cells. *Int J Cancer* 1992;50:289–297.

60. Mitchell MS, Harel W, Kempf RA, et al. Active-specific immunotherapy for melanoma. *J Clin Oncol* 1990;8:856–869.

61. Mitchell MS, Harel W, Kan-Mitchell J, et al. Active specific immunotherapy of melanoma with allogeneic cell lysates. Rationale, results, and possible mechanisms of action. *Ann N Y Acad Sci* 1993;690:153–166.

62. Goydos JS, Elder E, Whiteside TL, Finn OJ, Lotze MT. A phase I trial of a synthetic mucin peptide vaccine. Induction of specific immune reactivity in patients with adenocarcinoma. *J Surg Res* 1996;63:298–304.

63. Altman JD, Moss PAH, Goulder PJR, et al. Phenotypic analysis of antigen-specific T lymphocytes [published erratum appears in *Science* 1998;280(5371):1821]. *Science* 1996;274:94–96.

64. Bieganowska K, Hollsberg P, Buckle GJ, et al. Direct analysis of viral-specific CD8+ T cells with soluble HLA-A2/Tax11-19 tetramer complexes in patients with human T cell lymphotropic virus-associated myelopathy. *J Immunol* 1999;162:1765–1771.

65. Tan LC, Gudgeon N, Annels NE, et al. A re-evaluation of the frequency of CD8+ T cells specific for EBV in healthy virus carriers. *J Immunol* 1999;162:1827–1835.

66. Murali-Krishna K, Altman JD, Suresh M, Sourdive D, Zajac A, Ahmed R. *In vivo* dynamics of anti-viral CD8 T cell responses to different epitopes. An evaluation of bystander activation in primary and secondary responses to viral infection [In Process Citation]. *Adv Exp Med Biol* 1998;452:123–142.

67. Butz E, Bevan MJ. Dynamics of the CD8+ T cell response during acute LCMV infection. *Adv Exp Med Biol* 1998;452:111–122.

68. Butz EA, Bevan MJ. Massive expansion of antigen-specific CD8+ T cells during an acute virus infection. *Immunity* 1998;8:167–175.

69. Ogg GS, Rod Dunbar P, Romero P, Chen JL, Cerundolo V. High frequency of skin-homing melanocyte-specific cytotoxic T lymphocytes in autoimmune vitiligo. *J Exp Med* 1998;188:1203–1208.

70. Romero P, Dunbar PR, Valmori D, et al. Ex vivo staining of metastatic lymph nodes by class I major histocompatibility complex tetramers reveals high numbers of antigen-experienced tumor-specific cytolytic T lymphocytes. *J Exp Med* 1998;188:1641–1650.

71. Lee PL, Yee C, Savage PA, et al. Characterization of circulating T cells specific for tumor-associated antigens in melanoma patients. *Nat Med* 1999;5:677–685.

72. McKee MD, Clay TM, Rosenberg SA, Nishimura MI. Quantitation of T-cell receptor frequencies by competitive PCR: generation and evaluation of novel TCR subfamily and clone specific competitors. *J Immunother* 1999;22:93–102.

73. Pannetier C, Even J, Kourilsky P. T-cell repertoire diversity and clonal expansions in normal and clinical samples. *Immunol Today* 1995;16:176–181.

74. Bousso P, Casrouge A, Altman JD, et al. Individual variations in the murine T cell response to a specific peptide reflect variability in naive repertoires. *Immunity* 1998;9:169–178.

75. Fernandez NC, Levraud JP, Haddada H, Perricaudet M, Kourilsky P. High frequency of specific CD8+ T cells in the tumor and blood is associated with efficient local IL-12 gene therapy of cancer. *J Immunol* 1999;162:609–617.

76. Hishii M, Andrews D, Boyle LA, et al. *In vivo* accumulation of the same anti-melanoma T cell clone in two different metastatic sites. *Proc Natl Acad Sci U S A* 1997;94:1378–1383.

77. Maccalli C, Farina C, Sensi M, Parmiani G, Anichini A. TCR beta-chain variable region-driven selection and massive expansion of HLA-class I-restricted antitumor CTL lines from HLA-A*0201+ melanoma patients. *J Immunol* 1997;158:5902–5913.

78. Kammula U, Lee K-H, Riker AI, et al. Evidence of effective immunization by serial gene expression analysis of tumors. 1999(submitted).

79. Berd D, Maguire HC Jr, McCue P, Mastrangelo MJ. Treatment of metastatic melanoma with an autologous tumor-cell vaccine: clinical and immunologic results in 64 patients. *J Clin Oncol* 1990;8:1858–1867.

80. Bystryn JC, Oratz R, Roses D, Harris M, Henn M, Lew R. Relationship between immune response to melanoma vaccine immunization and clinical outcome in stage II malignant melanoma. *Cancer* 1992;69:1157–1164.

81. Nestle FO, Alijagic S, Gilliet M, et al. Vaccination of melanoma patients with peptide- or tumor lysate-pulsed dendritic cells [see comments]. *Nat Med* 1998;4:328–332.

82. Livingston PO, Natoli EJ, Calves MJ, Stockert E, Oettgen HF, Old LJ. Vaccines containing purified GM2 ganglioside elicit GM2 antibodies in melanoma patients. *Proc Natl Acad Sci U S A* 1987;84:2911–2915.

83. Kitamura K, Livingston PO, Fortunato SR, et al. Serological response patterns of melanoma patients immunized with a GM2 ganglioside conjugate vaccine. *Proc Natl Acad Sci U S A* 1995;92:2805–2809.

84. Helling F, Zhang S, Shang A, et al. GM2-KLH conjugate vaccine: increased immunogenicity in melanoma patients after administration with immunological adjuvant QS-21. *Cancer Res* 1995;55:2783–2788.

85. MacLean GD, Reddish M, Koganty RR, et al. Immunization of breast cancer patients using a synthetic sialyl-Tn glycoconjugate plus Detox adjuvant. *Cancer Immunol Immunother* 1993;36:215–222.

86. Longenecker BM, Reddish M, Koganty R, MacLean GD. Specificity of the IgG response in mice and human breast cancer patients following immunization against synthetic sialyl-Tn, an epitope with possible functional significance in metastasis. *Adv Exp Med Biol* 1994;353:105–124.

CANCER VACCINES: CLINICAL APPLICATIONS

Whole Cell and Lysate Vaccines

MUTHUKUMARAN SIVANANDHAM
CHRISTOS I. STAVROPOULOS
MARC K. WALLACK

The concept of host immunity against tumor was developed by Ehrlich (1) nearly one century ago and was later reinforced in the early 1900s by several laboratories that studied transplantable tumor cell lines in mice. In 1910, Cantamin (2) demonstrated the development of protective immunity against transplantable tumor in mice immunized with the same irradiated tumor cells. Furthermore, in 1935, Besredka and Gross (3) showed that some animals inoculated with tumor cell homogenate experienced tumor regression, as well as protection to tumor reinoculation challenges. These studies, however, were inconclusive because the distinction between immunity against histocompatibility antigens and tumor antigens was not entirely understood.

After the development of inbred mouse strains with stringent criteria, tumor-specific immunity was clearly demonstrated in murine tumor models. In 1943, Gross (4) showed that C3H inbred mice immunized with methylcholanthrene-induced sarcoma were protected against the same tumor, whereas the nonimmunized inbred mice experienced tumor development. Subsequently, in 1954, Foley (5) and Donaldson (6) also demonstrated the induction of specific protective immunity in mice against sarcoma and Ehrlich's ascites tumor, respectively.

Because these experimental tumor models suggested that tumors could indeed generate host immunity, a search for tumor-specific antibodies was initiated using serologic techniques. Antisera prepared against murine tumor tissue were formerly studied in an immunodiffusion approach; the resultant precipitation reaction indicated the presence of antibodies in the sera reacting to tumor antigens (7). Based on this evidence, antisera for human cancers were prepared in various animals and then tested for reactivity to human cancer. For example, human tumor tissue was used to develop antisera in horses, which was then shown to lyse tumor cells from that particular human tumor (8). The specificity of these antisera to tumor was demonstrated by preventing tumor cell lysis with antisera absorbed in tumor while retaining tumor cell lysis with antisera absorbed in normal tissues (8). These humoral responses to tumor antigens encouraged investigators to identify tumor-specific antigens.

TUMOR-ASSOCIATED ANTIGENS

Several tumor-associated antigens (TAAs) were initially defined in mouse tumors based on components from oncogenic viruses, such as polyoma virus, SV-40, and Friend leukemia virus. These antigens, however, could not be identified on human tumor cells. After the development of monoclonal antibody technology, several TAAs identified previously were confirmed unequivocally and many new TAAs were detected on human tumor cells.

These TAAs are unique to individual tumor or shared between tumors of the same histiotype. The unique tumor antigens are characterized by restricted expression on autochthonous human tumor cells. They are derived from mutated cellular gene products, such as p53, ras, cyclin-dependent kinase, and p21, often secondary to chemical or radiation-induced carcinogenesis. These unique antigens are not detected in normal tissue of the same histologic type. The shared tumor antigens, such as common acute lymphocytic leukemia antigen, carcinoembryonic antigen, fetal-associated antigen, gp100 (melanocyte lineage antigens), MUC-1 (mucin glycoprotein), prostate-specific antigen, carcinoma antigen–125, and GD3 and GM2 (glycolipid antigens of tumors originated from neuro crest), are normal cellular antigens that are overexpressed in tumor. These antigens also include the neonatal antigens (fetal-associated antigen and carcinoembryonic antigen) that are overexpressed on cancer cells of different origin. In addition, antigens of oncogenic viruses, such as human T-cell leukemia virus, Epstein-Barr virus, human papilloma virus, and hepatitis B virus, are expressed on leukemia/lymphoma, cervical cancer, nasopharyngeal cancer, and liver cancer, respectively.

Although TAAs were shown to induce host antibody responses, immunologists remained puzzled for many years thereafter in search of TAAs that can induce T-cell responses. Boon (9) performed elegant work in identifying cytolytic T lymphocyte (CTL)–recognizing tumor antigens using variants of p815 plasmacytoma tumor cell lines. They extended this undertaking to identify human TAAs that can induce a CTL response. Consequently, the CTL-inducing melanoma antigen encoding gene–1 (MAGE-1) antigen was recognized using a melanoma-specific CTL clone that had HLA-A1 restriction properties. Subsequently, several other CTL-inducing cytoplasmic tumor antigens, such as MAGE-3, MART-1, and gp100, were identified for human cancers from numerous laboratories (10,11). Some antibody-inducing antigens, such as carcinoembryonic antigen, gp100, and NY-ESO-1, have also been shown to contain peptide epitopes that induce CTLs (11,12). Moreover, these antigens were expressed on a majority of tumor cells of the same histiotype and could thus stimulate antigen-specific CTLs in most patients, provided that an HLA compatibility exists. In addition to the above-described antigens, several novel tumor antigens that induce antibody responses were identified using serologic analysis of recombinant expression libraries (13). These antigens are also shared between tumor cell lines.

The heterogeneity in the expression of TAAs has been documented in several types of tumor (14,15) and clearly plays a role in the escape of tumor cells from immune surveillance (16). Therefore, the development of tumor cell lysate vaccines (TCLVs) or whole tumor cell vaccines (WCVs) should embody a polyvalent antigen approach. This method incorporates two or more cell lines of the same tumor histiotype and thus offsets any potentially lost antigens.

TCLVs and WCVs from autologous tumor cells target unique antigens and shared antigens as vaccine components. TCLVs and WCVs derived from allogeneic tumor cell targets, however, only shared antigens as vaccine components and rarely contain unique antigens. Unlike cancer vaccines derived from purified proteins, glycoproteins, glycolipids, carbohydrates, and synthetic peptides, TCLVs and WCVs derived from allogeneic tumor cells have several advantages. Most important, the polyvalent nature of TCLVs and WCVs covers most of the identified TAAs, such that an immunization with these vaccines neutralizes the tumor's escape mechanisms from host immune surveillance. Other advantages include the ease in preparing, storing, and transporting the actual vaccine. Notwithstanding, TCLVs and WCVs prepared from autologous or allogeneic tumor cells have demonstrated induction of cellular and humoral immune responses in cancer patients (17–20).

Expression of shared tumor antigens and the induction of host immune responses by these antigens form the basis for using TCLVs and WCVs in the active specific immunotherapy of cancer patients. Clinical trials with TCLVs and WCVs have been shown to increase the survival of patients, and, in some cases, even induce clinical remission. The clinical application of WCVs and TCLVs is detailed in this chapter. Because Chapter 18.2 discusses cancer vaccines using gene-modified tumor cells, this review does not consider this subject matter.

PREPARING TUMOR CELL LYSATE VACCINES AND WHOLE TUMOR CELL VACCINES

Autologous or allogeneic tumor cells are the major components of TCLVs and WCVs. Chemical or biologic adjuvants are often used as additional vaccine components, although a few clinical trials have used tumor vaccines without any adjuvants.

Selection of tumor tissue or cells is a critical step in the preparation of a tumor vaccine. Tumor tissue isolated from different sites on a patient is the most appropriate method of preparing autologous TCLVs and WCVs. Several autologous TCLVs and WCVs have been used in clinical trials of cancer patients. The major advantage to these vaccines is that they do not contain any allogeneic tissue–specific antigens that induce undesired immune responses when administered. Nevertheless, several reasons exist as to why it is difficult to use autologous tumor tissue or cells in the preparation of TCLVs and WCVs. First, the patient's own tumor cells are not usually available during early stage of disease. Second, several arduous steps are involved in the preparation and standardization of TCLVs and WCVs, such that batch-to-batch consistency would be difficult to maintain. This is particularly true of TCLVs made from different cell lines and in various laboratories. For example, one laboratory reported that 60% of autologous colon WCVs were contaminated with normal microflora (21).

To avoid such problems, several investigators have decided to use allogeneic tumor cells for the preparation of TCLVs (19,22–26) and WCVs (27–35). When selecting an appropriate allogeneic tumor cell line, it should be screened for the highest expression of TAAs that can induce humoral or cellular responses, or both. Moreover, the expression of HLA class I and class II antigens on these tumor cells should be analyzed and correspond to a profile consistent with most patients. Morton et al. (26) illustrated this point by preparing a second-generation whole-cell melanoma vaccine using three melanoma cell lines that express high levels of six melanoma antigens and cover more than 95% of melanoma patients' HLA type.

Similar characterization was applied to tumor cell lines that were used in the preparation of our laboratory's melanoma vaccine (17). In light of studies reporting TAA expression heterogeneity on different tumor cell lines despite identical histiotype (14,15), cell lines inclusive of all shared TAAs and HLAs are to be selected for preparing TCLVs and WCVs. We and others have used fluorescent-activated cell sorter aided immunofluorescence assays to characterize the expression of TAAs and measure the density of TAAs on tumor cells. Furthermore, we have used reverse transcriptase polymerase chain reaction to characterize the cytoplasmic peptide antigens of the tumor cells. More than one cell line (17,26,35), and, in some cases, even seven cell lines (24) are used to prepare TCLVs or WCVs to incorporate as many TAAs as possible. These cell lines should be subjected to rigorous quality control inquiries, such as optimal tissue culture conditions, karyotyping, and freedom from bacterial or viral (including human immunodeficiency virus) contamination. These screening methods establish the stability and sterility of a tumor cell line and can then render it appropriate for use in the preparation of TCLVs. Finally, a manufacturer's working cell bank should be instituted for all cell lines used in vaccine preparation.

This cell bank system would allow one to expand the production of these vaccines to an industrial level without sacrificing quality.

Although some clinical trials with TCLVs and WCVs have used plain tumor cell lysates without any adjuvants (36,37), the majority have indeed used adjuvants. They include bacterial (19,21,26,29), viral (24,25,38), chemical (39,40), and cytokine (41,42) adjuvants. Haptens, such as dinitrophenyl, and enzymes, including neuraminidase, have also been used to modify tumor cell vaccines (20).

Bacterial adjuvants, such as bacille Calmette-Guérin (BCG) and *Corynebacterium parvum*, have been used as cancer vaccine adjuvants. BCG is the most commonly used bacterial adjuvant in preparing TCLVs and WCVs (19,26,31). These ancillary components are mixed with the tumor vaccine before injection or given separately, even at an entirely different site.

Several pathogenic and nonpathogenic viruses have also been used as adjuvants in the preparation of cell lysate and whole cell vaccines. Nonpathogenic viruses, including influenza and vaccinia, have demonstrated tumor cell lytic activity (25,38,43). Other nonlytic viruses used as adjuvants are the budding viruses, including Newcastle disease virus (NDV), RNA C-type virus, and vesicular stomatitis virus (23,24,44,45).

In our laboratory's TCLV preparation, vaccinia virus was used as a vaccine adjuvant for multiple reasons. It can modify membrane-associated tumor antigens using neuraminidase, as well as reexpress tumor antigens (46). Moreover, it can enhance expression of antigen chaperone heat-shock proteins (47,48) and nonspecifically help the induction of tumor-specific CTLs (49). Most importantly, it was documented to be safe in the mass immunizations against smallpox. Killed pathogenic viruses, such as influenza virus and vesicular stomatitis virus, have also been used as adjuvants in tumor cell vaccines.

Carefully tailored synthetic products, such as detoxified endotoxin (DETOX) and QS21, are yet another group of adjuvants that have been used in tumor cell vaccines (42). The DETOX adjuvant contains bacterial cell wall skeleton derived from *Mycobacterium phlei,* monophosphoryl lipid–A from the *Salmonella minnesota* squalane, egg phosphatidyl choline, and α-tocopherol. Chemical adjuvants to cancer vaccines include muramy dipeptide, cholesteryl hemisuccinate, and monophosphoryl lipid–A. Moreover, the cytokines interferon-α (INF-α), INF-γ, granulocyte-macrophage colony-stimulating factor, interleukin-2 (IL-2), and IL-12 have been studied as adjuvants in cancer vaccine therapy.

WCVs contain autologous or allogeneic tumor cells, γ-irradiated with 50 to 200 Gy, and adjuvants that are added before or after irradiation. The irradiation itself is often performed before freezing or just before injection. Until that point, these cells are maintained in appropriate medium and then frozen at a controlled rate. The frozen tumor cells are ultimately stored in the vapor phase immersed in liquid nitrogen. Before injecting patients, they must be thawed quickly and washed.

TCLVs contain mechanically lysed autologous or allogeneic tumor cells. Similarly, adjuvants are added before or after cell lysis. The tumor cell lysates are then reconstituted in a buffer and stored at –70°C until use. Alternately, tumor cell lysates can be freeze-dried and stored at refrigeration temperatures if anti-genic quality is maintained. Dried tumor cell lysates are reconstituted with a diluent just before injection.

All final TCLVs and WCVs should be subjected to quality control screening, such as freedom from bacterial, fungal, mycoplasma, and other human pathogenic viral (cytomegalovirus, Epstein-Barr virus, hepatitis B virus, human papillomavirus, human immunodeficiency syndrome, and human T-cell leukemia virus) contamination. Likewise, the antigenic quality of TCLVs should also be tested by measuring representative tumor antigens.

CLINICAL TRIALS WITH WHOLE CELL AND CELL LYSATE VACCINES

Almost all tumor vaccine studies have initially tested their vaccine approach in a "feasibility clinical trial" in which a small number of advanced-stage patients are treated with one dose of vaccine. The prototype trial to test vaccination against tumors was attempted by Leyden and Blumenthal (50) in 1902; however, details of this trial are not documented. Later, in 1909, Coca and Gilman (51) reported a feasibility clinical trial using autologous TCLVs for the treatment of fourteen patients with early and advanced stages of carcinomas, including buccal cavity, bladder, breast, cervix, cheek, pelvic, neck, and rectum, and one of Hodgkin's lymphoma. Although problems with vaccine sterility were addressed in this trial, a standard had not been established for the preparation of these vaccines. Patients were injected subcutaneously with 10 to 25 g of tumor lysates. Sterilization of the vaccine was performed by chemical treatments that would have altered the nature of tumor antigens. Furthermore, only some patients received a booster injection 3 weeks after the first vaccine injection, whereas others received just one injection. The follow-up of patients was likewise not uniform. Despite these problems, four patients with carcinomas displayed softening and disappearance of some tumor mass, three patients with inoperable cancers showed stable growth, and seven patients were disease-free for 6 months.

Finney et al. (52) performed immunotherapy studies in nine patients with melanoma, sarcoma, or carcinoma to evaluate the induction of tumor-specific antibodies. They used intratumoral injection of autologous tumor tissue lysates mixed with Freund's adjuvant. The first three vaccine injections were given to patients on alternative days. An additional vaccine injection was given 2 to 4 weeks after the peak antibody response in these patients' sera. All nine patients immunized with this vaccine showed increased titers of antibodies in their postimmune sera when compared with their preimmune sera. All patients exhibited uniform erythema, swelling, edema, and tenderness at the tumor site 15 to 25 days after initial injection, which then persisted for 2 to 7 days thereafter. Moreover, to document humoral antitumor cytotoxicity, purified immunoglobulins from these patients' sera were injected into tumor nodules. Sixty-three percent of injected tumor nodules were rendered nonpalpable in 10 days, suggesting the specificity of antibodies to tumor. This study clearly demonstrated the induction of tumor-specific cytotoxic antibodies by tumor cell lysate vaccination.

Czajkowski et al. (53) used intact, irradiated autologous tumor cells modified with bisdiazobenzidine and rabbit γ-globulin in 14 patients with squamous cell carcinoma of cervix and skin, adenocarcinoma of the breast, ovary, pancreas, colon, and prostate, melanoma, hepatoma, or chronic lymphocytic leukemia. Patients received a vaccine injection every 2 to 3 weeks for a total of 4 to 11 injections. One patient with squamous cell carcinoma and another with adenocarcinoma of the breast lived tumor free for 4 years longer than the expected survival. Four patients also revealed stabilization or slowed progression of tumor. Sera from 13 patients contained a high titer of antibodies that were reactive to melanoma antigens from their own melanoma cells.

McCune et al. (30) performed a phase 1 clinical trial using autologous tumor cells mixed with *C. parvum* in 15 patients with renal, melanoma, breast, lung, or colon cancer. Patients were treated with irradiated 10^6 to 10^8 tumor cells weekly for a minimum of three injections. Minimal toxicity was noted, such as fever, chills, tiredness, and pain at the site of injection. Only one patient had actual regression of tumor, whereas seven patients had stable disease that lasted for 1–13 months; seven other patients, however, did experience disease progression.

Wallack et al. (54) studied viral oncolysate vaccines in 29 patients with different types of advanced-stage cancers, including colon, melanoma, breast, thyroid, ovarian, cervical, and gastric carcinoma; hypernephroma; hepatoma; and fibrosarcoma. Patients were immunized intradermally with vaccinia virus–modified autologous tumor cell lysate vaccines. The majority of patients who participated in this trial had melanoma (9 of 29 patients) or colon carcinoma (10 of 29 patients). None of the patients experienced untoward responses during the trial. It was concluded that vaccinia oncolysate vaccine treatment is safe and produces only minimal side effects, such as fever, chills, malaise, headache, nausea, and inflammation with minimal pain at the injection site. Nine of the 29 patients experienced controlled tumor growth. Three of the nine patients who showed lack of progression of disease were melanoma patients, perhaps owing to the highly immunogenic nature of melanoma.

Pattillo (27) conducted an active specific immunotherapy (ASI) trial using autologous and allogeneic tumor cell–derived antigens mixed with BCG for patients with melanoma and cervical, ovarian, and breast cancers. Patients with advanced stages of cancer were treated with this vaccine preparation. Clinical responses included regression, as well as stabilization of tumor growth. Imperato et al. (55) conducted a similar immunotherapy study for a patient with advanced-stage ovarian carcinoma. This patient was primed with two intradermal injections of BCG followed by immunization with 2×10^8 autologous tumor cells. The patient also received a booster vaccine containing the same amount of tumor cells mixed with BCG. Only a partial clinical response was noted.

To avoid problems with the isolation of tumor cells from patients for the preparation of TCLVs or WCVs, several investigators studied ASI via intratumoral injection of adjuvants. Biologic adjuvants, such as vaccinia virus and BCG, were used in this approach. Hunter-Craig et al. (56) and Roenigk Jr et al. (57) used intratumoral injection of vaccinia virus for patients with melanoma. Their studies yielded some clinical responses, including regression of tumor and increased survival. Morton

(58) also studied intratumoral injection of BCG for patients with melanoma and sarcoma and demonstrated tumor regression in some patients.

All of these aforementioned clinical studies were preliminary trials that tested the feasibility of their respective vaccine approach. None of the described vaccines produced significant toxicity. Collectively, these trials demonstrated minimal clinical responses. Possible reasons include a lack of standardized vaccine production and the fact that multiple kinds of cancers with variable immunogenic properties were studied concurrently. Accordingly, cancer vaccine preparation adopted standardized techniques and approaches, including standard amounts of antigen(s) and adjuvant(s). These changes have assured vaccine quality for future clinical trials.

Several clinical trials have put to use whole cell vaccines or cell lysate vaccines prepared under these new standards. Patients in these trials generally fall into one of the following categories: (a) minimal disease (early stage of disease) or (b) free of tumor via surgery but with advanced stage of disease. Most important, these clinical trials studied patients with only one distinct type of cancer. Testing methods were also organized incorporating phase 1 through phase 3 clinical protocols (summarized in Tables 1 and 2).

WHOLE CELL VACCINE

Breast Cancer

Although the immunogenic nature of breast cancer is controversial (59,60), a few studies have evaluated the use of cell vaccine therapy. Anderson et al. (61) treated breast cancer patients with an autologous tumor cell vaccine after radical mastectomy but were not able to demonstrate any clinical benefit. Giuliano et al. (62) used allogeneic breast cancer cells with BCG in stage II breast cancer patients, and they, too, did not show any significant clinical response.

Colorectal Cancer

Hoover and his coworkers (63) initiated a pilot ASI study in five patients with colorectal cancer. They initially demonstrated ASI using tumor cells mixed with BCG to induce antitumor responses in guinea pig hepatocarcinoma models. The clinical trial had patients treated intradermally with irradiated autologous colon cancer cells mixed with BCG. Patients experienced minimal toxicity. After the preliminary trial, they performed a prospective randomized clinical trial to determine the efficacy of ASI with this type of vaccine (64). Their objective was to test vaccine efficacy in terms of increased disease-free interval (DFI) and overall survival (OS) of patients with lymph node metastases (stage B2 and B3 colon cancer or stage C1 and C2 rectal cancer). Ninety-eight patients were randomized between vaccine (treatment) and observation (control) groups. Autologous tumor cells from patients' tumor tissues were prepared using standardized procedures. Patients were then immunized intradermally with 10 million viable, irradiated tumor cells mixed with 10 million viable BCG organisms. The first vaccine injection was performed approximately 4 weeks after surgical removal of tumor. Three consecutive weekly vaccines then followed, the third vaccine consisting of irra-

TABLE 1. CLINICAL TRIALS PERFORMED WITH WHOLE CELL VACCINES

Cancer	Vaccine Therapy	Patient Characteristics (n)	Responses	Reference
Breast cancer	Irra. auto. tumor cells; i.d.	Stage II (131)	No clinical benefit	61
	randomized trial; irra. allo. tumor cells + BCG and CT		No clinical benefit	62
Colorectal cancer	Randomized trial; auto. tumor cell + BCG; i.d.	B2 and B1 colon C1 and C2 rectal (98)	No significant difference in DFI or OS; patients with positive DTH showed improved survival	64
	Phase 2 trial; NDV-modified irra. auto. tumor cells	Advanced stage (48)	Survival rate at 2-yr time point was 97.9%	66
Colon cancer	Randomized trial; auto. tumor cell + BCG; i.d.	Stages II and III (254)	Significant DFI in all patients with stage II disease at median follow-up of 5.3 yrs	21
Glioblastoma	Randomized trial; irra. auto. tumor cells	Grades III and IV (62)	No survival difference	67
	Phase 1 trial; irra. auto. tumor cells + BCG	Advanced stage (19)	One patient showed response	33
Gynecologic cancer	Irra. allo. tumor cells + BCG and CT	Advanced or recurrent ovarian cancer (10)	A better DFI and OS with vaccine compared with matched controls	68
Leukemia	Irra. allo. tumor cells. BCG and *Corynebacterium parvum*, i.d.; CT and radiation therapy	All stages (100)	33% DFI in all patients; 43% DFI in patients <15 yrs of age	34
	Irra. allo. tumor cells mixed with BCG	Patients with AML in remission (8)	6/8 DFI for 1 yr	69
	Randomized trial; irra. and nonirra. allo. tumor cells mixed with BCG, s.c.; CT	Patients with AML in remission or with disease (100)	Significantly longer survival with immunotherapy	70
Lung cancer	Irra. allo. tumor cells + BCG, i.d.	Stages I and II (13)	No significant DFI	71
	Irra. auto. tumor cells mixed with BCG, i.d.	Stages I–IV (18)	13/18 positive to DTH. Seven of these 13 had relapse	72
Melanoma	Phase 2, irra. allo. tumor cells with BCG, i.d. CY, cimetidine, or indomethacin	Stages III and IV (136)	Significant survival when compared with controls; significant IgM type antibody to melanoma	74
	Phase 2, irra. allo. tumor cells mixed with BCG, i.d.	Stage III (30)	33.3% DFI at 20-mo interval	75
	Phase 2, irra. auto. melanoma modified with DNP, i.d. Initially sensitized with DNFB, i.v., plus CY.	Stage III (62); stage IV (15)	At 5-yr point, DFI 45% and OS 58% for stage III; at 5-yr point, OS of stage IV >50 yrs, 71% and >50 yrs, 41%	76
Renal cancer	Irra. auto. tumor cells and *C. Parvum*, s.c.;	All stages (14)	Four patients had CR; one had stable disease	77
	Irra. auto. tumor cells mixed with BCG, i.d. and i.l., plus hormonal therapy	Stages I–III (24)	At 3-yr point, DFI 54% and OS 65% on vaccine + hormone vs. DFI 34% and OS 52% on hormone	78
	Irra. auto./allo. cells mixed with *Candida* antigens	Stages III and IV (35)	No significant improvement in survival	32
Sarcoma	Irra. auto. tumor cells, i.d.	All stages (12)	No clinical response	79
	Irra. allo. tumor cells mixed with BCG, i.d., plus RT	Stages I–III (18)	11/18 were disease free	80

allo., vaccine derived from allogeneic tumor cells; auto., vaccine derived from autologous tumor cells; BCG, bacillus Calmette-Guérin; CT, chemotherapy; CR, complete response; CY, cyclophosphamide; DFI, disease-free interval; DNFB, dinitroflurobenzene; DNP, dinitrophenyl; irra., irradiated; DTH, delayed-type hypersensitivity; IgM, immunoglobulin M; NDV, Newcastle disease virus; OS, overall survival; RT, radiotherapy.

diated tumor cells only. Patients were monitored at 3-month intervals for the first 2 years, every 4–6 months for the next 3 years, and once a year after 5 years. Data from 80 eligible patients were analyzed with a median follow-up of 83 months for patients with colon cancer and 57 months for patients with rectal cancer. When compared with the controls, patients treated with the vaccine did not show a significant DFI or OS. Patients with colon cancer, however, did reveal an increased survival trend with vaccine therapy when compared with controls. Moreover, the induction of immunity by this ASI was determined by a delayed-type cutaneous hypersensitivity (DTH) response.

The Eastern Cooperative Oncology Group subsequently sponsored another randomized trial in patients with Dukes' B2, B3, or C stage colorectal cancer (65). Four hundred and twelve patients were randomized between the observation and vaccine groups; the latter group was immunized intradermally with irradiated autologous tumor cells mixed with BCG. Survival analysis of patients in this trial did not yield any significant treatment differences with respect to OS or DFI. A subset analysis of patients with DTH response greater than 5 mm, however, did indeed demonstrate improved survival with respect to vaccine therapy. These results suggested that an additional immunization would be required to induce enhanced immunity against colon cancer.

Accordingly, a third prospective randomized vaccine trial was performed in patients with stage II and III colon cancer (21). Three months after the third injection, patients received a booster vaccine containing 10 million irradiated tumor cells. Median follow-up was 5.3 years. The results of this trial showed a significant DFI with vaccine therapy when compared with controls, as well as a trend toward improved OS in the treatment

TABLE 2. CLINICAL TRIALS PERFORMED WITH CELL LYSATE VACCINES

Cancer	Vaccine Therapy	Patient Characteristics (n)	Responses	Reference
Breast cancer	Auto./allo. tumor cells lysate; i.d.	Stages I and II (5)	At 5 yrs, 83% stage I survived, 53% stage II survived	37
Colon cancer	Phase 1 allo. lysate with Freund's adjuvant; i.d.	Dukes' B2, C, and D (28)	At 21 mos, 82% OS; DTH response in all patients	82
Gynecologic cancer	Allo. ovarian tumor cells modified with influenza; i.p. and intrapleural	Advanced or ovarian cancer (40)	9/40 PR	83
Leukemia	Allo. cell lysate modified with fowl plaque virus + CT	Patients in remission (27)	No significant improvement in survival	85
Melanoma	Vaccinia virus–augmented allo. cell lysate, i.d. Phase 1	Stages I and II (48)	24/48 NED	87
	Phase 2	Stage III (39)	21/39 NED	88
	Phase 3	Stage III (217)	No significant DFI or OS	38
	Allo./auto. cells modified with VSV, i.d.	Stages II–IV (24)	1/24 SR	23
	Allo. cells modified with vaccinia, i.d., some with CY phase 2	Early stage (62)	A significant survival with vaccine	91
	Allo. cells lysate modified with influenza A, i.m. and s.c., plus BCG + CT Phase 1	Stage III (13)	6/13 PR	90
	Phase 2	Stages II and III (32)	28/32 DFS at 3 yr	91
	Allo. cell lysate mixed with DETOX + CY Phase 1/2	Stages III and IV (109)	5 CR, 17 PR	42
	Phase 3	Stages II and III	In progress	42
	Phase 3	Stage IV (56)	No significant difference	42
	Allo. tumor lysate	Stages I and II (190)	Stage I did not show significant OS; stage II showed significant survival	36
Renal cancer	Auto./allo. cell lysate mixed with BCG, i.d.	Stage IV (30)	7% CR, 7% PR, 37% SD	92
Lung cancer	Allo. cell lysate, s.c.	Advanced stage (8)	Two had increased survival	93
Sarcoma	Allo. cells lysate modified with influenza A, s.c., plus CT	All stages (19)	4/19 CR, 9/19 PR	94
	Auto. tumor cell lysate	All stages (15)	Seven survived disease free	79

allo., vaccine derived from allogeneic tumor cells; auto., vaccine derived from autologous tumor cells; BCG, bacillus Calmette-Guérin; CR, complete response; CT, chemotherapy; CY, cyclophosphamide; DETOX, detoxified endotoxin; DFI, disease-free interval; DFS, disease-free survival; DTH, delayed-type hypersensitivity; NED, no evidence of disease; OS, overall survival; PR, partial response; SD, stable deisease; SR, serologic response; VSV, vesicular stomatitis virus.

group. Subset analysis of stage III disease did not produce significant DFI or OS in patients treated with vaccine when compared with appropriate controls. A significant DFI, however, occurred in the vaccine-treated group of patients with stage II disease when compared with controls, as well as a trend toward improved survival. Clearly, this data confirms that vaccine therapy was indeed effective in patients with stage II disease but not stage III disease.

In another series, a phase 2 clinical trial using 10^7 autologous colon tumor cells modified with NDV was performed in 48 patients with colorectal cancer (66). Patients were immunized intradermally at 2-week intervals for three injections. The survival rate at 2 years was 97.9% with the vaccine when compared with historical controls (73.8%). These results, however, should be verified in a randomized trial.

Glioblastoma

Bloom et al. (67) investigated the use of ASI for patients with glioblastoma multiforme using irradiated autologous tumor cells in a randomized prospective trial. Sixty-two patients randomized into two groups with grade III or IV glioblastoma were initially treated with radical surgery and postoperative radiation. One group with 27 patients received a subcutaneous injection of crude irradiated autologous tumor cell suspension. Only nine

patients received three vaccine injections, one patient received two injections of vaccine, and 17 patients received only one vaccine injection within 2 hours after surgery. Thirty-five patients comprised the control group. No standards were followed regarding vaccine quality or quantity per patient, or both. Moreover, no adjuvant was used with this vaccine. Results were analyzed at a 30-month follow-up time point during which all 27 vaccine-treated patients had expired. No survival difference existed between the vaccine-treated group and the control group. Marked skin reactions at the vaccine injected sites, however, were observed in two of six patients who received only one vaccine injection and four of four patients who received three vaccine injections.

In 1983, Mahaley et al. (33) conducted a phase 1 clinical trial using cells from two allogeneic glioblastoma tumor lines with BCG adjuvant for patients with gliomas. Nineteen patients were immunized with this vaccine. Sera from these patients were analyzed for the presence of antibodies binding to glioblastoma cell lines. Only one of the patient's serum contained tumor-specific antibodies.

Gynecologic Cancers

Hudson et al. (68) performed ASI trials using irradiated allogeneic tumor cells mixed with BCG for patients with advanced or recurrent ovarian cancer having completed chemotherapy. At 24-month follow-up, DFI and OS of these patients were better than the matched controls of chemotherapy alone.

Leukemia

The feasibility of ASI trials in patients with leukemia were based on preliminary studies using murine models. The first tumor cell vaccine therapy for patients with leukemia was performed by Mathe et al. (34). This trial used irradiated, pooled allogeneic tumor cells isolated from leukemia patients. Patients were immunized intradermally with 4×10^7 irradiated leukemia cells every week for 3 months and then once every 3 months. Patients also received intradermal immunizations with adjuvants such as BCG, *C. parvum*, and polyinosinic-polycytidylic acid at 20 different sites on every fourth and seventh day thereafter. At 5-years follow-up, 33% of all patients who received immunotherapy survived disease free. Moreover, 43% of patients younger than 15 years of age survived disease free with immunotherapy. It is difficult to draw conclusions about the efficacy of this vaccine because patients in this trial received chemotherapy and radiotherapy, both of which could have suppressed host immunity.

Freeman et al. (69) studied ASI for patients with acute myeloid leukemia (AML). Eight patients who showed complete remission with chemotherapy were immunized with 10^9 irradiated allogeneic tumor cells with BCG as an adjuvant at weekly intervals. Six of the eight patients survived without disease for more than 1 year. Because this trial was performed in only a few patients and without a chemotherapy-alone control, it is also difficult to conclude on the efficacy of this vaccine therapy.

A controlled ASI trial was conducted by Powles (70) in 100 patients with AML who were in remission or failed to achieve remission with chemotherapy. These patients were divided into five treatment groups:

1. Patients in remission receiving chemotherapy
2. Patients in remission receiving chemotherapy plus vaccine therapy with irradiated 10^9 allogeneic AML cells
3. Patients in remission receiving chemotherapy plus vaccine therapy with nonirradiated 10^9 allogeneic AML cells
4. Patients who failed to achieve remission receiving chemotherapy
5. Patients who failed to achieve remission receiving a combination of chemotherapy and vaccine therapy with irradiated 10^9 allogeneic AML cells. BCG was also used as a vaccine adjuvant.

Survival data showed that patients given the vaccine therapy survived significantly longer than those receiving chemotherapy alone. A prospective randomized trial is under way to confirm these findings.

Lung Cancer

The first vaccine therapy trial for patients with stages I and II non–small-cell lung cancer was performed by Perlin et al. (71) in 1980. This trial used 5×10^7 allogeneic irradiated tumor cells mixed with 3 to 5×10^8 BCG organisms as a vaccine. Patients

were administered the vaccine twice monthly for 24 months. Fifty-one patients were divided into three groups: (a) a control group of 18 patients who had lobectomy, (b) a nonspecific immunotherapy group of 13 patients who had BCG alone, and (c) a vaccine group of 13 patients. No statistically significant DFI differences were noted between the three groups. On the other hand, a remarkable and significant difference was found in the DFI of stage I patients treated with vaccine therapy alone when compared with matched controls. Another interesting finding concerns the lack of statistically significant differences observed between the nonspecific BCG therapy and the vaccine therapy. Regardless, the results would be inconclusive because the number of patients in each group was insufficient to yield meaningful statistical analysis.

Schulof et al. (72) performed a nonrandomized vaccine trial using 10^7 irradiated autologous tumor cells mixed with 10^7 BCG organisms as a vaccine for 20 patients with stages I to IV non–small-cell lung cancer. Vaccine therapy was initiated 1 to 3 months after surgery. Patients received three consecutive weekly vaccinations intradermally. Moreover, patients were tested before and after vaccine therapy for DTH responses to tumor cells alone and purified protein derivatives of BCG. DTH responses greater than 5 mm were scored as positive. Ten of 18 patients immunized with this vaccine experienced disease relapse with a median follow-up of 17 months. Thirteen patients showed a DTH response to purified protein derivatives before the initiation of the vaccine therapy. Only 5 of 18 patients showed a DTH response to tumor cells before vaccine therapy. Eight patients, however, converted to a positive DTH response after the vaccine therapy. Seven of the 13 patients who showed an initial positive DTH response had relapsed and two DTH negative patients survived without relapsing. Therefore, it was concluded that little correlation of patients' DTH response existed between their actual clinical responses.

Melanoma

Melanoma is perhaps the best-studied cancer in various tumor vaccine approaches. Reasons include the presence of melanoma-specific antibodies and T cells within the sera and peripheral blood lymphocytes (PBLs) of melanoma patients, respectively. Furthermore, reported spontaneous regression of melanoma provides sound evidence in favor of vaccine therapy for this highly immunogenic cancer.

After the demonstration of approximately 90% antibody response to tumor with intratumoral BCG injections, Morton (58) performed a preliminary clinical trial using allogeneic melanoma cells mixed with BCG. Only 35% of patients, however, developed high levels of antimelanoma antibodies. Hence, a new polyvalent allogeneic melanoma cell vaccine was constructed using three melanoma cell lines that contain high concentrations of six representative melanoma antigens (73). They conducted a clinical trial with this new vaccine using 24 million irradiated allogeneic melanoma cells mixed with BCG. This vaccine induced antimelanoma humoral responses that correlated with increased survival. A phase 2 clinical trial was subsequently performed using this vaccine for patients with stage III and IV melanoma (74). One hundred thirty-six melanoma patients were immunized (intradermally) as follows: every 2 weeks for 4 weeks, then monthly for 1 year, every 3 months for the following year (4 injections), and every 6 months thereafter. Only the first two vaccine injections contained irradiated melanoma cells mixed with BCG, whereas subsequent injections contained only irradiated melanoma cells. Some patients also received biologic-response modifiers, such as cimetidine, indomethacin, and cyclophosphamide. Minor toxicity, such as local erythema, induration, and ulceration at the injection sites, as well as mild fever with occasional myalgia, arthralgia, and chills, were again experienced. Patients were followed at 3-month intervals with pre- and postimmune sera analyses for the presence of antibodies to melanoma antigens. Furthermore, DTH responses against melanoma cells were also measured. Stage III and IV patients receiving vaccine therapy survived significantly longer than those patients treated with other methods. Moreover, those patients with a median survival of 30 months had a significantly higher immunoglobulin M (IgM) antibody response to melanoma antigens and a significantly higher DTH response (>10 mm) to melanoma cells. These results led to a phase 3 multicenter randomized clinical trial to elucidate the efficacy of this melanoma cell vaccine. Results of this trial are awaited.

A nonrandomized phase 2 melanoma vaccine trial was performed by Mordoh et al. (75) for patients with stage III melanoma. This trial used 5 million irradiated allogeneic melanoma cells mixed with 5 million BCG organisms. Thirty patients were immunized intradermally as follows: one vaccine injection every 3 weeks (four injections) every 2 months for the rest of the first year, every 3 months in the second year, and then once every 6 months until the fifth year. Patients received cyclophosphamide 3 days before each vaccination. DTH and antibody responses were analyzed. Twenty-four patients with the same stage of disease served as controls in this study. A significant DFI was noted at 20 months with 33.3% survival with vaccine therapy when compared with only 4.1% survival in the control group. Moreover, a large portion of patients who experienced the induction of antibody response also had positive DTH responses. The efficacy of this vaccine, nevertheless, needs to be confirmed in a randomized trial with a larger number of patients.

Berd et al. (76) used dinitrophenyl as a hapten to modify autologous melanoma cells and used it as a vaccine for patients with stage III or IV melanoma (palpable masses in two lymph node sites). A recent publication in 1997 of their nonrandomized trial reviews results from 62 patients with stage III melanoma and 15 patients with stage IV melanoma, all treated with this vaccine. Each dose of the vaccine contained 5 to 25 million autologous tumor cells. All patients were initially sensitized with 1% of dinitroflurobenzine in acetone corn oil on 2 consecutive days and intravenous cyclophosphamide (300 mg per kg) 2 days before the dinitroflurobenzine to reduce suppressor T-cell activity. These patients were subjected to two different vaccine schedules. In the first schedule, the dinitrophenyl-modified tumor cells were mixed with BCG and administered intradermally every 4 weeks for eight doses. Cyclophosphamide was given only for the first two doses. In the second schedule, six weekly vaccine injections were performed. Only the first three vaccines were modified with dinitrophenyl. Patients were then followed every 2 months for 2 years and tested for DTH

responses. With a median follow-up of 55 months, DFI of stage III patients treated with vaccine was 45% at 5 years, and OS was 58% at that point. In contrast, with a median follow-up of 73 months, OS of stage IV patients older than 50 years of age and younger than 50 years of age were 71% and 41%, respectively, at a 5-year time point. These survival rates were better than the survival rates of patients with no treatment. Moreover, a significant survival rate was detected in patients who showed a positive DTH response when compared with negative DTH responders; 71% versus 49% at 5 years. A phase 3 clinical trial with this vaccine is in progress.

Dillman et al. (41) conducted a clinical trial with cultured autologous melanoma cells for patients with metastatic melanoma. Fifty-seven patients were immunized subcutaneously with 10 million irradiated cultured autologous tumor cells 3 consecutive weeks and then once a month for 6 months. Adjuvants included BCG, INF-α, INF-γ, and granulocyte-macrophage colony-stimulating factor. DTH responses in 27 patients with no evidence of metastases were higher than those in 25 patients with metastases.

Renal Cancer

Similar to melanoma, renal cancer also demonstrated immunogenicity, such as spontaneous regression of metastases, tumor infiltration of lymphocytes, and *in vitro* demonstration of T-cell proliferation against renal tumor cells. McCune et al. (77) performed a vaccine trial for patients with renal carcinoma in 1981. They used 3 to 20×10^7 irradiated autologous renal cancer cells mixed with *C. parvum* at a concentration of 37.5 µg per 10^7 tumor cells. Fourteen patients were immunized weekly intracutaneously with this vaccine. The number of doses varied with the availability of tumor cells. Four patients had complete or partial responses, or both. One patient had stable disease for 27+ months. Patients who received vaccines with more than 20×10^7 tumor cells per dose had a higher rate of clinical response than those who received smaller doses. Nevertheless, the important conclusion from this study was that vaccine therapy could induce clinical responses in renal cancer patients.

Adler et al. (78) performed a randomized trial combining a renal cancer cell vaccine and hormonal therapy for patients with all stages of renal cell carcinoma. They used 3×10^6 irradiated autologous tumor cells mixed with BCG as a vaccine. The vaccine was given intradermally for 5 to 6 consecutive weeks, then monthly for 24 months or until recurrence. Patients were also immunized intralymphatically via endolymphatic instillation and lymphangiography. For this procedure, 80 to 100 million irradiated autologous tumor cells in 2 to 3 mL of saline was mixed with 0.1 mL of BCG and slowly injected into lymph vessels. At least one lymphatic immunization was performed in each patient (5 to 6 weeks after the intradermal immunization), as well as an additional two injections (excluding three patients). Patients received hormonal therapy with intramuscular primostat (200 mg per day) five times per week for 1 month, followed by vaccine twice per week for 2 months, and then weekly for 24 months. Forty-three patients with stage I to III renal cell carcinoma were randomized between the hormonal therapy alone (19 patients) and hormonal plus vaccine therapy with 24 patients.

Patients in the vaccine therapy group were evaluated for DTH responses against autologous tumor cells. Although DFI and OS with a median follow-up of 30 months were in favor of immunotherapy over hormonal therapy alone, their respective differences were not statistically significant. At a 3-year time point, DFI was 54% with vaccine therapy and 34% with hormonal therapy. Likewise, OS was 65% in the former and 52% in the latter. Both DFI and OS were also better in positive (i.e., >8 mm) rather than negative DTH responders in the immunotherapy group. These positive DTH responders also demonstrated a significantly higher DFI and OS when compared with hormone-treated controls. A lymphocyte migration inhibition test was also used to evaluate the induction of immunity in patients treated with this vaccine. Accordingly, a higher number of patients in the vaccine therapy group experienced positive lymphocyte migration inhibition to autologous tumor extract. These findings, collectively, strongly suggest that ASI induces clinical and immunologic responses in renal cancer patients.

Rauschmeier (32) conducted a renal cancer vaccine trial using irradiated autologous/allogeneic tumor cells for patients with advanced stage (III and IV) renal cancer patients. Thirty-five patients were treated with 2 million irradiated renal cancer cells mixed with Candida antigen. Two different testing modalities characterized this trial to address vaccine therapy efficacy. The first modality initiated the therapy immediately after surgery, whereas the second initiated the therapy when metastases were diagnosed. Moreover, two different schemas were tested in the vaccination protocol to determine the most effective method of immunization. In the first schema, two cycles of vaccines were given as follows: four weekly primary vaccine injections with booster vaccine injections at monthly intervals for 1 year or four injections, each 1 month apart after 1 year. In the latter protocol schema, the first booster injection was given 2 weeks after the primary vaccination and 24 consecutive months thereafter. Neither stage III or IV patients (median follow-up of 3 years) experienced a significant improvement in survival with vaccine therapy when compared with age-matched controls.

Sarcoma

Vaccine therapy for patients with sarcoma was initially studied in the early 1960s. Marcove et al. (79) performed a clinical trial with a γ-irradiated autologous tumor cell vaccine for 12 sarcoma patients but could not elicit any clinical responses. Townsend et al. (80) also performed a preliminary clinical trial in 15 patients with skeletal and soft tissue sarcomas. Their patients were immunized with 50 to 75 million irradiated tumor cells mixed with BCG. Nine of the 12 patients' postimmune sera yielded increased antisarcoma antibody titers. A positive DTH reaction to autologous tumor cells also developed in seven of 15 patients. Although no significant clinical responses were observed, some patients did experience prolonged survival. Subsequently, these investigators performed a clinical trial in 18 patients with stage I, II, and III skeletal and soft tissue sarcoma using irradiated allogeneic sarcoma tumor cells (10×10^7) mixed with BCG. The vaccine was injected intradermally in five separate sites. Patients received the vaccine weekly for 3 months and then biweekly for 2 years or until recurrence. Although 11 of 18

patients with localized soft tissue sarcoma who had received immunotherapy were free of disease, these results were not significant against appropriate controls.

TUMOR CELL LYSATE VACCINES

The preparation, storage, and transportation of WCVs are difficult because their use emphasizes the preservation of cell viability. Moreover, WCVs with irradiated autologous tumor cells are at risk of radioresistant viable tumor cells that can proliferate at the injection sites. Therefore, TCLVs derived from autologous tumors or allogeneic tumors have also been studied in various cancer patients, including breast, gynecologic, leukemia, lung, melanoma, and sarcoma. The following sections summarize the clinical application of TCLVs in these cancer patients.

Breast Cancer

Surgical adjuvant ASI trials for patients with breast cancer were performed by Humphrey et al. (81) using breast cancer tissue lysates as vaccines. The vaccine was prepared by homogenizing tumor tissues in 0.25 mol/L sucrose solution and removing the cell nucleus and debris by ultracentrifugation. Patients with stage I and II breast cancer were treated with this vaccine weekly for eight injections and then every 3 months for 1 year. The vaccine was administered in two portions, one intradermally and another subcutaneously. Survival results from 95 patients treated with this vaccine were reviewed by Lytle et al. (37). The 5-year survival rate was 83% for those with stage I disease and 53% for those with stage II disease. This data was then compared with survival rates of control patients who underwent standard adjuvant chemotherapy or radiotherapy in studies conducted by the American College of Surgeons and The National Surgical Adjuvant Breast and Bowel Project. At a 5-year interval, vaccine therapy patients with stage II breast cancer demonstrated a survival rate comparable to those of control American College of Surgeons and The National Surgical Adjuvant Breast and Bowel Project patients (53% vs. 51% vs. 59%, respectively). The authors, therefore, suggested that the addition of this adjuvant immunotherapy to other proven adjuvant modalities would further enhance the survival of breast cancer patients.

Colon Cancer

Hollinshead et al. (82) conducted a phase 1 clinical trial with vaccine therapy using allogeneic colon tumor lysate mixed with Freund's adjuvant in patients with colon adenocarcinoma. Twenty-eight patients with Dukes' B2, C, and D stages of colon cancer were treated intradermally for 3 consecutive months. With a median follow-up of 21 months, 82% of immunized patients survived with a mean survival rate of 21 months. A strong DTH response was also observed in these patients.

Gynecologic Cancers

Freedman et al. (83) reported the use of influenza-modified allogeneic ovarian cell lysate vaccines for patients with ovarian cancer. The vaccine was prepared from two cultured ovarian cell lines. Forty patients with advanced ovarian cancer were given intrapleural and intraperitoneal vaccine injections. All patients had previously received cisplatin and 31 patients received two or more systemic treatments. During the first month of vaccine therapy, 28 patients received a single injection, six received biweekly injections, and six received weekly injections. After the first month, all patients received a monthly booster vaccination. Observed clinical responses included complete or partial regression of ascites and stabilization of a pelvic mass.

Similarly, Freedman et al. (84) used influenza A virus–augmented vulva carcinoma cell lysate from an established squamous vulvar carcinoma cell line in combination with radiotherapy for patients with vulvar carcinoma. Sixteen patients were immunized intradermally weekly for 3 weeks and then biweekly for 2 years. The median DFI was 26+ months for the vaccine therapy patients, considerably longer when compared with controls (e.g., received either surgery alone or surgery plus radiotherapy).

Leukemia

Schuepbach and Sauter (85) performed a clinical trial with avian virus–augmented cell lysate vaccine therapy in combination with chemotherapy for AML patients in remission. The vaccine was prepared using fowl plague virus–infected formalin-treated allogeneic leukemia cells. Twenty-seven patients received the vaccine monthly along with chemotherapy. No significant improvement occurred in survival between those treated with the vaccine plus chemotherapy versus chemotherapy alone. Nevertheless, most patients did develop antiviral antibodies. This trial, however, did not measure antitumor immune responses. In addition, immunized patients may not have induced antitumor immunity because the viral oncolysate was initially treated with formaldehyde, which may have denatured tumor antigens. Chemotherapy may have suppressed host antitumor immunity as well.

Melanoma

Our laboratory has investigated the use of vaccinia virus–modified tumor cell lysate vaccines in various cancer patients. The preliminary clinical trial, described in the section Clinical Trial with Whole Cell and Cell Lysate Vaccines, did not yield significant toxicity with vaccine therapy. Because three of nine patients with melanoma experienced a lack of disease progression in that preliminary clinical trial, the ensuing trial was initiated exclusively for patients with melanoma (86). An allogeneic vaccinia vaccine virus–augmented melanoma cell lysate (VMO) vaccine was prepared from four established melanoma cell lines expressing the identified melanoma antigens. The objective of this preliminary trial was to determine the toxicity and feasibility of VMO therapy. The 12 patients with advanced-stage melanoma who received VMO experienced minimal toxicity, similar to that observed in the previous trial. Moreover, four of 12 patients had improved survival when matched to disease stage.

These encouraging results suggested that this therapy would be even more beneficial to patients with earlier stages of disease.

Advanced melanoma patients may be somewhat more immunosuppressed, and, thus, at a disadvantage. Subsequently, a phase 1 trial was designed using patients with stage I and II melanoma. The objective was to establish the most effective dose of VMO in terms of induction of antimelanoma serologic response (87). Forty-eight patients with melanoma were treated with VMO at six different dose levels (0.05 to 2.00 mg protein). Patients' serum at the highest dose produced the most antimelanoma activity, and, therefore, was chosen to be used in future trials. In addition, patients having a high antibody titer showed significant clinical responses, such as stabilization of tumor growth and increased disease-free survival.

After this trial, a phase 2 trial was performed in patients with high-risk stage I and II melanoma in a surgical adjuvant setting (88). Patients were treated with 2.0 mg of VMO, the most active dose established from the previous phase 1 trial. Again, toxicity was minimal. Statistical comparison of VMO-treated patients with 39 matched controls (patients treated with BCG or *C. parvum*) revealed a significant ($p = .04$) increase in the disease-free survival.

A phase 3 randomized, double-blinded, multiinstitutional trial followed the efficacy of the VMO vaccine in patients with high-risk stage III melanoma. The VMO vaccine was used with patients in the treatment group, and live vaccinia virus (V), a component of the VMO, was used in the control group. The objective of this trial was to evaluate the clinical efficacy of VMO versus V to increase the DFI and OS of stage III melanoma patients. The Institute of Mariuex (known as *Pasteur Mariuex and Connaught Laboratories*, Lyon, France) prepared one lot of VMO (#17) and one lot of V (#1) for this trial; 250 patients were accrued from 11 U.S. Medical Centers. Informed consent was obtained from all patients at the individual institutions. All patients registered in this study underwent a central pathology review of the preregistration biopsy and the subsequent wide excision and lymph node dissection. Furthermore, all patients registered in this study underwent a surgical review to confirm that the surgery was performed according to criteria specified in the protocol. Patients in group I (VMO) and group II (V) were treated weekly for 13 weeks and then biweekly for 39 weeks or until recurrence. A total of 33 injections were administered to the patients unless any patient was withdrawn from the study. All patients received a smallpox booster, supplied by Mariuex, at least 48 hours before the first injection of VMO or V. One mL of VMO or V was equally divided among 4 to 6 injections and administered at different sites near several nodal groups. Dates of recurrence documented radiographically or pathologically were used to determine the disease-free intervals.

The first interim survival analysis was performed with a mean follow-up time of 30.38 months after prerandomization surgery (38). Thirty-three patients were deemed ineligible and excluded from the trial. The toxicity of VMO or V was minimal. Data from this trial demonstrated that no significant difference was detected in DFI or OS between the VMO and the V arms. This analysis did show, however, that approximately a 10% difference was detected in the OS at a 4-year time point in favor of VMO-treated patients. Moreover, a retrospective subset analysis was performed to determine any groups of patients that did benefit from VMO treatment. Based on sex, age, positive node status, depth of invasion, and location of primary tumor, the following populations were identified as having improved survival on VMO: (a) males, (b) males younger than 57 years with 1 to 5 positive nodes, and (c) patients with clinical stage I but pathologic stage II disease. The final analysis of data with a median follow-up of 46.3 months revealed that the surgical adjuvant ASI with VMO did not increase the DFI or OS of patients with stage III melanoma (89). Notwithstanding, VMO continued to show survival advantages in a subset of males between the ages of 44 and 57 years with 1 to 5 positive nodes.

Other laboratories also reported the use of virus-augmented melanoma cell lysate vaccines for patients with melanoma. Sinkovics (25) used influenza A–modified allogeneic melanoma cell lysate in combination with BCG and chemotherapy for patients with stage III melanoma. In this 5-year follow-up study, no evidence of disease was observed in 36% (n = 30) of patients compared with 29% with chemotherapy and BCG alone. Cassel et al. (90) used a NDV-modified allogeneic melanoma cell lysate vaccine for patients with melanoma and observed clinical responses, such as complete remission and lack of progression of tumor, in 6 of 13 patients. Hershey et al. (91), in Australia, also reported an improved survival in patients treated with vaccinia melanoma cell lysate (VMCL) vaccine, a viral oncolysate similar to VMO but containing viral melanoma cell lysates from two allogeneic melanoma tumor cell lines.

Livingston et al. (23) used vesicular stomatitis virus–modified autologous or allogeneic melanoma cell lysate vaccine for melanoma patients. No clinical responses were observed in patients from this trial using this type of vaccine. Furthermore, they reported that most of these patients' sera contained only antibodies to fetal calf serum components rather than antibodies to melanoma antigens. This viral oncolysate vaccine was exposed to ultraviolet irradiation before its administration into patients. This procedure may have provided the minimal clinical responses observed in patients treated with this viral oncolysate vaccine.

Cassel et al. (24) and Hersey et al. (22) also performed independent phase 2 trials with cell lysate vaccines in early stage melanoma patients. They reported a significant increase in disease-free survival. The latter investigators also performed a phase 3 randomized trial with their VMCL vaccine to evaluate its efficacy in patients with stage 3 melanoma. An interim analysis of data from this trial showed survival advantage with VMCL when compared with observation controls. The survival with VMCL, however, has not reached statistical significance.

Mitchell et al. (19,42) performed phase 1 and 2 clinical trials with a melanoma cell lysate vaccine plus the adjuvant DETOX for advanced-stage melanoma patients. The phase 1 trial and the earlier part of the phase 2 trial used frozen melanoma cell lysate suspended in a buffer. The latter part of the phase 2 trial also used a lyophilized melanoma cell lysate vaccine. Some patients in the phase 2 trial also received cyclophosphamide. A review of the results from these trials of 109 patients, collectively, rendered five complete responses, 17 partial responses, and nine minor responses. Subsequently, a randomized clinical trial with a combination of vaccine mixed with DETOX and cyclophosphamide was performed in patients with resected stage II and III melanoma. The final analysis of data from this trial will be presented over the next few years. Results from this trial, however, would not clearly define the efficacy of this vaccine because patients in the observation arm received experimental therapies from other institutions.

Mitchell et al. (42) have also performed a phase 3 randomized clinical trial with the TCLV melacine, using the adjuvant DETOX and low-dose cyclophosphamide in patients with stage IV melanoma. The TCLV arm was compared with the control chemotherapy arm; however, the objective responses between these treatments were not statistically significant. The median survival of patients treated with TCLV is 9.4 versus 12.1 months with chemotherapy alone. The toxicity of TCLV therapy was far less than that observed with chemotherapy.

A tumor tissue lysate vaccine without any bacterial or viral adjuvants for patients with melanoma was studied by McGee et al. (36). This vaccine therapy was conducted in a nonrandomized clinical trial for 129 patients with stage I melanoma and 61 patients with stage II melanoma. Immunizations were given weekly for 8 weeks and then every 3 months for 24 months. The vaccine was administered in two portions, one intradermally and another subcutaneously. At 5-years follow-up, patients with stage I melanoma did not show any significant survival when compared with their historical controls. Patients with stage II melanoma, however, demonstrated a significant increase in survival rate when compared with historical controls (64% vs. 40%, respectively).

Renal Cancer

Neidhart et al. (92) studied ASI using TAAs derived from homogenized renal cancer tissues admixed with BCG or phytohemagglutinin in patients with stage IV renal carcinoma. Autologous and allogeneic tumor tissues were used in preparation of the cell lysate vaccine. Thirty patients were treated intradermally biweekly until disease progression. Seven percent, 7%, and 37% of patients had complete, partial, and stable disease, respectively.

Lung Cancer

Specific immunotherapy trials for patients with advanced lung cancer were conducted by Alth et al. (93). The vaccine was derived from six bronchogenic carcinoma cell lines of various histologic types. A group of eight patients with advanced stage bronchogenic carcinoma was immunized subcutaneously twice weekly throughout the study time. Two of the eight patients had longer survival with 19 and 22 months, respectively.

Sarcoma

Marcove et al. (79) reported a study with 15 patients with osteogenic sarcoma. These patients were treated with autologous tumor cell lysate containing tumor cell membranes. Fifteen patients were treated with this vaccine subcutaneously at 3-week intervals for 30 injections. Seven patients were free of disease and 46% of patients in the treatment group survived with good performance, whereas only 17% survived in the control group.

Greene et al. (94) used influenza virus–augmented cell lysate vaccines for patients with osteosarcoma. Toxicity was related to the influenza virus itself present in their TCLVs. Only a minimal clinical response was observed in patients treated with this type of TCLVs. Sinkovics (95) used influenza A virus–modified allogeneic sarcoma cell lysate in combination with BCG and chemotherapy for patients with metastatic sarcoma but observed complete response in four of 19 patients and partial response in nine of 19 patients.

IMMUNE RESPONSES IN PATIENTS TREATED WITH CANCER VACCINES

In addition to evaluating the antitumor efficacy of tumor vaccines in cancer patients, analyzing their induction of immune responsiveness is as equally important. Results of immune response data could further be used to demonstrate a correlation with the observed clinical response(s). Finally, the induction of humoral and cellular responses could be used to evaluate vaccine potency, as well as provide prognostic information.

In T-cell–immunocompromised patients and studies in CTL-depleted animal tumor models clearly suggest the importance of the cellular immune response. The CTL response arm is regarded as the most important aspect of antitumor immunity. The relative importance of cellular immune responses over antibody responses to tumors, however, has not been elucidated in humans. The following sections summarize studies that assessed *in vitro* cellular and humoral responses using PBLs and sera from vaccine-treated patients, respectively, as well as *in vivo* DTH responses in the same patients.

Antibody Response

Humoral immune responses in vaccine-treated patients were well documented in most of the above clinical trials (29,33,40,73,86). Tumor-reacting antibodies of IgG and IgM classes were observed in patients treated with TCLV or WCV using enzyme-linked immunosorbent assay (73,88). In a dose-response phase 1 trial with VMO vaccine, IgG and IgM antibody responses were found to be proportional to the increasing doses of VMO vaccine (86). Additionally, antibodies induced by allogeneic TCLVs and WCVs were found to be reacting to tumor-specific antigens (29) and HLA antigens, although some trials reported that the reactivity was directed to fetal calf serum components (23). The specificity of antibodies to tumor antigens was further characterized by Western blot analysis that revealed the recognition of different tumor antigens present in tumor cells of the same histiotype (17). These antibodies have demonstrated tumor cell lysis via antibody-dependent cellular cytotoxicity assays. Antibody responses correlated with patients' clinical responses; increased concentration of antibodies to melanoma antigens corresponded to increased survival of vaccine-treated patients (73).

Cellular Response

In addition to the induction of humoral immune responses, cellular immune responses have been demonstrated in patients treated with cancer vaccines (19,40). Vaccine-treated patients'

postimmune PBLs showed an enhanced proliferative response. Likewise, PBLs from vaccine-treated patients lysed proper tumor target cells in a 4-hour chromium-release assay (19,31,40), suggesting that these patients developed tumor-specific cytolytic cellular immunity. The induction of cytolytic cellular response by tumor vaccines was also confirmed by analyzing the frequency of tumor-specific precursor cytolytic T cells (CTLp) before and after tumor vaccine therapy using a microcytotoxicity assay. An increased amount of CTLp was detected in the postimmune PBLs when compared with the preimmune PBLs of patients immunized with vaccines. The increase in CTLp frequency also correlated to patients' increased survival time. In some studies with a peptide vaccine, patients' improved clinical status could not be demonstrated with an increase in the CTLp in their postimmune PBLs (96). One speculation is that all the CTLp in the circulation may be homed to the tumor site, which could have resulted in an undetectable level of CTLp in the PBLs. For this reason, CTLp analysis is performed from biopsies taken in regressing tumors. Alternately, CTLp analysis could be performed in the vaccine-injected sites. In fact, a 1998 study measured the CTLp in the vaccine-injected site and showed a higher preference of tumor antigen-specific CTLp when compared with a control site that was not presented with the same antigen (97).

The microcytotoxicity assay to determine the CTLp frequency is cumbersome to perform. The enzyme-linked immunospot assay simplifies the CTLp frequency analysis. Clinical trials have shown that the enzyme-linked immunospot assay can be used to measure CTLp in PBLs, and, thus, determine the induction of immunity in patients treated with a cancer vaccine (98). Moreover, a novel technique of staining antigen-specific T cells with a tetramer complex could further simplify the CTLp frequency analysis. This future staining method will undoubtedly be used to measure the induction of CTLp by cancer vaccines (99).

Enhancement of natural killer cell and lymphokine-activated killer cell responses can improve the antitumor potency of a given vaccine therapy. Hence, these responses have been analyzed in patients treated with TCLVs. Some tumor vaccine studies have shown an increase in the natural killer cell and lymphokine-activated killer cell responses, probably owing to the presence of adjuvants.

Helper T cells are known to augment the induction of tumor-specific CTL responses. Only a few helper T-cell–stimulating tumor antigens have been identified. The role of these antigens in the induction of tumor-specific CTLs and antibody responses has been the endeavor of many laboratories. Furthermore, the role of adjuvant vaccine components in the induction of antitumor responses (via stimulation of helper T cells) has been widely studied. In a virus-augmented tumor cell lysate–treated host, an increased immunoglobulin production was correlated with virus-stimulated T-cell helper activity (100). We (19) and others (101) have demonstrated that virus-specific helper T cells enhanced antimelanoma cytolytic activity in patients treated with vaccinia virus–augmented melanoma cell lysate vaccine.

In addition to the above *in vitro* assays, DTH responses have been used to measure *in vivo* induction of antitumor immunity by a vaccine. Many clinical trials performed this DTH test in patients undergoing the vaccine therapy (20,21,102). Although the nature of the DTH response to T cell, B cell, or other infiltrating mononuclear cells is not known, patients' DTH responses have correlated well to clinical responses. Ongoing problems include the lack of standard positive responses, although wheels of 5–10 mm have been considered positive in previous studies.

MECHANISM OF THE INDUCTION OF IMMUNITY BY A TUMOR CELL LYSATE VACCINE OR A WHOLE TUMOR CELL VACCINE

The mechanisms of the induction of helper T cell and antibody responses by a TCLV are not different than those of viral or bacterial antigen. Mechanisms for the induction of CTL responses by soluble antigens from a TCLV, however, are not clear. These antigens are known to be generally processed by endosomal pathways for class II major histocompatibility complex (MHC) binding only. Nevertheless, several reports suggested new pathways for processing soluble antigens through the MHC class I pathways for the stimulation of CTLs (103,104). Several studies demonstrated that tumor cell lysate–pulsed dendritic cells (DCs), efficient antigen processing and presenting cells, induced *in vitro* and *in vivo* CTL responses.

Although an intact whole tumor cell can present CTL-inducing peptide antigens in context with MHC, these cells are poor stimulators of CTL because of the absence of T-cell costimulatory factors, such as B7.1 and B7.1, on their membranes. Moreover, a study by Huang et al. (104) clearly showed in a murine tumor model that bone marrow–derived cells, perhaps of DC lineage, were essential for an effective immune response. These bone marrow–derived cells are rich in costimulatory factors and MHC molecules, and they are presumably involved in the processing of soluble antigen from the necrotic tumor cells and effectively priming CTLs. Hence, the suggested mechanism for induction of antitumor immune responses by TCLVs and WCVs is represented in Figure 1. Tumor antigens present in a lysate or WCV are captured by antigen processing and presenting cells by simple pinocytosis or by receptor-mediated uptake using Fc and mannose receptors. These cells then process these antigens into peptides, assembled with MHC class I and class II molecules, and transport them to the membrane. The helper and the cytolytic T cells specific for these antigens are then stimulated. Cytokines produced from helper T cells help in the proliferation and expansion of the T and B cells. Furthermore, tumor vaccines contain antigens that can stimulate B cells to produce antibodies; IgA, IgG, and IgM type antibodies, TAA-specific, have been produced by tumor vaccines. Because both arms of the immune system are induced by the TCLV and WCV, an effective and potent antitumor immune response can clearly be generated with cancer vaccines.

FUTURE OF THE WHOLE CELL AND CELL LYSATE VACCINES

Several areas of interest exist regarding the improvement of TCLVs and WCVs. The first one is to combine immunomodulating cytokines with cancer vaccines to augment their efficacy.

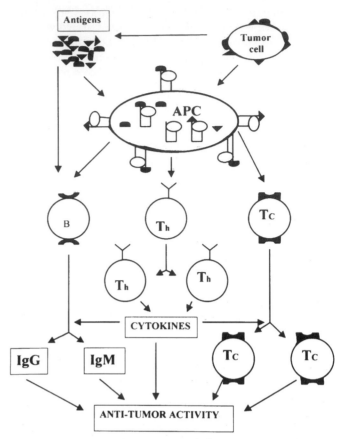

FIGURE 1. Mechanisms of the induction of antitumor responses by tumor cell lysate vaccines and whole cell vaccines. Tumor-associated antigens present in tumor cell lysate vaccines or whole cell vaccines are captured by antigen-processing cells (APC). These cells then process antigens into peptides assembled with major histocompatibility complex class I and class II molecules and transport them to the cell membrane. These peptide–major histocompatibility complexes stimulate helper T cells (Th) and cytolytic T cells (Tc) specific for these antigens. Simultaneously, cytokines produced from Th are used in the proliferation and expansion of Th and Tc. Furthermore, soluble tumor-associated antigens from tumor cell lysate vaccines and whole cell vaccines stimulate B cells to produce antibodies [immunoglobulin A (IgA), IgG, and IgM] using the cytokines from Th. Collectively, tumor-specific Tc cytotoxic cytokines form Th, and tumor-specific antibodies mount an effective antitumor response.

Several murine model experiments suggest that the addition of cytokines and chemotherapeutic drugs, including antiangiogenic factors or radiotherapy to cancer vaccine therapy, improve their efficacy. In fact, Mitchell et al. (42) and Dillman et al. (41) have used combinations of cytokines and cancer vaccines for patients with melanoma and demonstrated significant clinical responses. Immunomodulating cytokines, such as IL-2, IL-12, granulocyte-macrophage colony-stimulating factor and tumor necrosis factor, are candidates for such combination therapy. Cytokine gene–encoded bacterial and viral adjuvants can also be used to augment the efficacy of TCLVs. Our laboratory has studied the IL-2 gene–encoded recombinant vaccinia virus to augment the efficacy of a cell lysate vaccine in a murine colon cancer model. An enhanced antitumor effect was observed with a TCLV containing IL-2 gene–encoded vaccinia virus in comparison with a TCLV containing plain vaccinia virus (105). Antiviral immunity is a major problem, however, regarding repeated boosters with this approach. In addition, several

WCVs with cytokine gene–transduced tumor cells have been tested as potential vaccines in clinical trials; these are discussed in Chapter 18.2.

Finally, the use of DCs to augment TCLV therapy is being explored. DCs are the most potent antigen processing and presenting cells because they express surface markers (e.g., mannose receptors, Fc receptors, etc.) that are involved in capturing and retaining antigens. They also express a high level of HLA class I and class II antigens and T-cell costimulatory molecules CD80, CD86, intracellular adhesion molecule–1, and lymphocyte function-associated antigen-3 that are involved in the effective stimulation of cytotoxic and helper T cells. Moreover, DCs secrete immunomodulating cytokines, such as IL-12, IL-15, and INF-γ, which are involved in expanding the cellular response. DCs have demonstrated migration to lymph nodes, where they can effectively prime T cells.

DC-pulsed tumor cell lysates have demonstrated antitumor immunity in patients with melanoma (106). We have studied vaccinia virus–augmented tumor cell lysate vaccine–pulsed DCs in the ASI of mice with CC-36 colon tumor and demonstrated enhanced survival when compared with no treatment control (107). Melanoma patients immunized with unfractionated melanoma tumor cell lysate–pulsed DC therapies experienced the induction of melanoma-specific CTLs, as well as clinical responses. DC-aided TCLV therapies, hence, represent the next generation of cancer vaccines.

REFERENCES

1. Ehrlich P. Uber den jetzgen Stand der Karzinom-forschung. In: Himmelweit F, ed. *The collected papers of Paul Ehrlich—Vol. II. Immunology and cancer research*. London: Pergamon Press, 1957:559.
2. Cantamin MA. Immunization contre le cancer de la souris inoculec avec des tumeurs modifiees par les rayons. *Academie Des Sciences* 1910;150:128.
3. Besredka A, Gross L. Du role dela peau dans la sarcomatose de la souris. *Ann Inst Pasteur* 1935;55:402–416.
4. Gross L. Intradermal Immunization of C3H mice against sarcoma that originated in an animal of the same line. *Cancer Res* 1943;3:326–333.
5. Foley EJ. Antigenic properties of methylcholanthrene-induced tumors in mice of the strain of origin. *Cancer Res* 1953;13:835–837.
6. Donaldson DM, Mitchell JR. Immunization against Ehrlich's ascites carcinoma with x-irradiated tumor cells. *Proc Soc Exp Biol Med* 1959;101:204–207.
7. Old LJ, Benacerraf B, Clarke DA, et al. The role of endothelial system in the host reaction to neoplasia. *Cancer Res* 1961;2:1281–1301.
8. Bjorklund B, Lundbland, Bjorklund V. Antigenicity of pooled human malignant and normal tissues by cyto-immunological techniques. Presence of insoluble, heat-labile tumor antigens. *Int Arch Allergy Immunol* 1957;10:153–184.
9. Boon T. Antigenic tumor cell variant obtained with mutagens. *Adv Cancer Res* 1983;39:121–151.
10. Van-der-bruggen P, Traversari C, Chomez P, et al. A gene encoding an antigen recognized by cytolytic T lymphocytes on a human melanoma. *Science* 1991;254:1643–1647.
11. Rosenberg SA. A new era for cancer immunotherapy based on the genes that encode cancer antigens. *Immunity* 1999;10:281–287.
12. Tsang KY, Zhu M, Nieroda CA, et al. Phenotypic stability of a cytotoxic T-cell line directed against an immunodominant epitope of human carcinoembryonic antigen. *Clin Cancer Res* 1997;3:2439–2449.
13. Chen YT, Gure AO, Tsang S, et al. Identification of multiple cancer/testis antigens by allogeneic antibody screening of a melanoma cell line library. *Proc Natl Acad Sci U S A* 1998;95:6919–6923.
14. Natali PG, Giacomini P, Bigotti A, et al. Heterogeneity in the expression of HLA and tumor-associated antigens by surgically removed and cultured breast carcinoma cells. *Cancer Res* 1983;43:660–666.
15. Houghton AN, Davis LJ. Phenotypic heterogeneity of melanoma. In: Bagnara JT, ed. *Advances in pigment cell research*. New York: Alan R. Liss Inc. 1988:333–342.
16. Jager E, Ringhoffer M, Altmannsberger M, et al. Immunoselection *in vivo*: independent loss of MHC class I and melanocyte differentiation antigen expression in metastatic melanoma. *Int J Cancer* 1997;71:142–147.
17. Sivanandham M, Shaw P, Ditaranto K, et al. Active specific immunotherapy with vaccinia melanoma oncolysates for patients with melanoma—an overview. *Vaccine Res* 1996;5:215–232.
18. Hsuesh EC, Famatiga E, Gupta RK, et al. Enhancement of complement-dependent cytotoxicity by polyvalent melanoma cell vaccine (cancer vax): correlation with survival *Ann Surg Oncol* 1998;5(7):595–602.
19. Mitchell MS, Mitchell JK, Kempf RF, et al. Active specific immunotherapy for melanoma: a phase I trial of allogeneic lysates and a novel adjuvant. *Cancer Res* 1988;48:5883–5889.
20. Berd D, Danna V, Maguire HC, et al. Induction of cell-mediated immunity to autologous melanoma cells and regression of metastases after treatment with melanoma cell vaccine preceded by cyclophosphamide. *Cancer Res* 1986;46:2572–2577.
21. Vermorken JB, Claessen AME, Tinteren H, et al. Active specific immunotherapy for stage II and stage III human colon cancer: a randomized trial. *Lancet* 1999;353:345–350.
22. Hershey P, Edwards S, D'Alessandro D, et al. Phase II study of vaccinia melanoma cell lysate (VMCL) as an adjuvant to surgical treatment of stage II melanoma. II. Effect of cell mediated cytotoxicity and leukocyte dependent antibody activity: immunological effects of VMCL in melanoma patients. *Cancer Immunol Immunother* 1986;22:221–231.
23. Livingston PO, Albino AP, Chung TJ, et al. Serological responses of melanoma patients to vaccines prepared from VSV lysates of autologous and allogeneic cultured melanoma cells. *Cancer* 1985;55:713–720.
24. Cassel WA, Murray DR, Phillips HS. A phase II study on the post-surgical management of malignant melanoma with Newcastle disease virus oncolysate. *Cancer* 1983;52:856–862.
25. Sinkovics JG, Papadopoulos NE, Plager G. Viral oncolysate in immunotherapy of human tumors. In: Yohan DS, ed. *Advances in comparative leukemia research in leukemia and related disease*. New York: Elsevier Science, 1981:613–615.
26. Morton DL, Foshag LJ, Hoon DSB, et al. Prolongation of survival in metastatic malignant melanoma after active specific immunotherapy with a new polyvalent melanoma vaccine. *Ann Surg* 1992;216:463–482.
27. Patillo RA. Immunotherapy and chemotherapy of gynecologic cancers. *Am J Obstet Gynecol* 1976;124:808–817.
28. Kurth KH, Marquet R, Zwartendijk J, et al. Autologous anticancer antigen preparation for specific immunotherapy in advanced renal cell carcinoma. *Eur Urol* 1987;13:103–109.
29. Seigler HF, Wallack MK, Vervaert CE, et al. Melanoma patient antibody responses to melanoma tumor-associated antigens defined by murine monoclonal antibodies. *J Biol Response Mod* 1989;8:37–52.
30. McCune CS, Patterson WB, Henshaw EC. Active specific immunotherapy with tumor cells and corynebacterium parvum—a phase I study. *Cancer* 1979;43:1619–1623.
31. Perlin MCE, Oldham RK, Weese JL, et al. Carcinoma of the lung: immunotherapy with intradermal BCG and allogeneic tumor cells. *Int J Radiat Oncol Biol Phys* 1980;6:1033–1039.
32. Rauschmeier HA. Immunotherapy of metastatic renal cancer. *Semin Surg Oncol* 1988;4:169–173.
33. Mahaley Jr MS, Gillespie GY, Gillespie RP, et al. Immunobiology of primary intracranial tumors. Part 8: serological responses to active immunization of patients with anaplastic gliomas. *J Neurosurg* 1983;59:208–216.
34. Mathe G, Pouillart P, Schwarzenberg L, et al. Attempts at immunotherapy of 100 patients with acute lymphoid leukemia: some factors influencing results. *Natl Cancer Inst Monogr* 1972;35:361–371.
35. Reid JW, Perlin E, Oldham RK, et al. Immunotherapy of carcinoma of the lung with intradermal BCG and allogeneic tumor cells. In: Terry WD, Rosenberg SA, eds. *Immunotherapy of human cancer*. New York: Elsevier North Holland, 1982:147–152.

36. McGee JMC, Lytle GH, Malnar KF, et al. Melanoma tumor vaccine: five-year follow-up. *J Surg Oncol* 1991;47:233–238.

37. Lytle GH, McGee JM, Yamanashi WS, et al. Five-year survival in breast cancer treated with adjuvant immunotherapy. *Am J Surg* 1994;168:19–21.

38. Wallack MK, Sivanandham M, Balch C, et al. A phase III randomized, double-blind, multi-institutional trial of vaccinia melanoma oncolysate (VMO) active specific immunotherapy for patients with stage II (UICC) melanoma. *Cancer* 1995;75:34–42.

39. Eggers AE, Tarmin L, Gamboa ET. *In vivo* immunization against autologous glioblastoma-associated antigens. *Cancer Immunol Immunother* 1985;19:43–45.

40. Skornick YG, Rong GH, Sindelar WF, et al. Active immunotherapy of human solid tumor with autologous cells treated with cholesteryl hemisuccinate—a phase I study. *Cancer* 1986;58:650–654.

41. Dillman RO, Nayak SK, Barth NM, et al. Clinical experience with autologous tumor cell lines for patient-specific vaccine therapy of metastatic melanoma. *Society for Biological Therapy 12th Annual Meeting* 1997:25 (abstract).

42. Mitchell MS. Perspective on allogeneic melanoma lysates in active specific immunotherapy. *Semin Oncol* 1998;25:623–625.

43. Boone CW, Blackman K. Augmented immunogenicity of tumor cell homogenates infected with influenza virus. *Cancer Res* 1972;32:1018–1022.

44. Austin FC, Boone CW, Levin DL, et al. Breast cancer skin test antigens of increased sensitivity prepared from vesicular stomatitis virus-infected tumor cells. *Cancer* 1982;49:2034–2042.

45. Greenberger JS, Aaronson SA. *In vivo* inoculation of RNA C-type viruses inducing regression of experimental solid tumors. *J Natl Cancer Inst* 1973;51:1935–1938.

46. Berthier-Vergnes O, Portoukalian J, Leftheriotis E, et al. Induction of IgG antibodies directed to a M(r) 31,000 melanoma antigen in patients immunized with vaccinia virus melanoma oncolysates. *Cancer Res* 1994;54:2433–2439.

47. Sedger L, Ruby J. Heat shock response to vaccinia virus infection. *J Virol* 1994;68:4685–4689.

48. Jindal S, Young RA. Vaccinia virus infection induces a stress response that leads to association of Hsp 70 with viral proteins. *J Virol* 1992;66:5357–5362.

49. Shimizu Y, Asumi K, Masubuchi K, et al. Immunotherapy of tumor bearing mice utilizing virus help. *Cancer Immunol Immunother* 1988;27:223–227.

50. Leyden VE, Blumenthal. Vorlaufige mittheilungen uber einige ergebnisse der kresforschung auf der I. *Medizinischen klinik deutsche medizinische wochenschriff* 1902;28:637–638.

51. Coca AF, Gilman PK. The specific treatment of carcinoma. *Philippine J Sci* 1909;4:391–402.

52. Finney JW, Byers EH, Wilson RH. Studies in tumor auto-immunity. *Cancer Res* 1960;20:351–356.

53. Czajowski NP, Rosenblatt M, Wolf PL, et al. A new method of active immunization to autologous human tumour tissue. *Lancet* 1967;2:905–909.

54. Wallack MK. Specific active immunotherapy with vaccinia oncolysates. In: Crispen R, ed. *Tumor progression.* New York: Elsevier North Holland Inc., 1980:277–287.

55. Imperato S, Rossi R, Ermiglia G, et al. Active specific and non specific immunotherapy with immunological monitoring in late stage ovarian cancers. *Acta Eur Fertil* 1974;5:25–39.

56. Hunter-Craig I, Westbury G. Use of vaccinia virus in the treatment of metastatic melanoma. *Br Med J* 1970;2:512–515.

57. Roenigk HH Jr, Deodhar S, Jacques RS, et al. Immunotherapy of malignant melanoma with vaccinia virus. *Arch Dermatol* 1974;109:668–673.

58. Morton DL. Immunotherapy of human melanomas and sarcomas. *Natl Cancer Inst Monogr* 1972;35:375–378.

59. Wallack MK, Scoggin SD. Immunological evaluation of patients with breast cancer has no siginificant role in their management. In: Wise L, Johnson Jr H, eds. *Breast cancer: controversies in management.* New York: Futura Publishing, 1994:539–547.

60. Black MM, Zachrau RE. Immunological evaluation of patients with breast cancer has a significant role in their management. In: Wise L, Johnson Jr H, eds. *Breast cancer: controversies in management.* New York: Futura Publishing, 1994:539–547.

61. Anderson JM, Kelly F, Wood SE, et al. Stimulatory immunotherapy in mammary cancer. *Br J Surg* 1974;61:778–784.

62. Giuliano AE, Sparks FC, Patterson K, et al. Adjuvant chemo-immunotherapy in stage II carcinoma of the breast. *J Surg Oncol* 1986;31:255–259.

63. Hoover HC Jr, Surdyke M, Dangel RB, et al. Delayed cutaneous hypersensitivity to autologous tumor cells in colorectal cancer patients immunized with an autologous tumor cell: bacillus Calmette-Guerin vaccine. *Cancer Res* 1984;44:1671–1676.

64. Hoover HC Jr, Brandhorst JS, Peters LC, et al. Adjuvant active specific immunotherapy for human colorectal cancer: 6.5-year median follow-up of a phase III prospectively randomized trial. *J Clin Oncol* 1993;11:390–399.

65. Harris J, Ryan L, Adams G, et al. Survival and Relapse in Adjuvant Autologous Tumor Vaccine Therapy for Dukes B and C Colon Cancer. *Proc Am Soc Clin Oncol* 1994;13:294.

66. Ockert D, Schirrmacher V, Beck N, et al. Newcastle disease virus-infected intact autologous tumor cell vaccine for adjuvant active specific immunotherapy of resected colorectal carcinoma. *Clin Cancer Res* 1996;2:21–28.

67. Bloom HJG, Peckham MJ, Richardson AE, et al. Glioblastoma multiforme: a controlled trial to assess the value of specific active immunotherapy in patients treated by radical surgery and radiotherapy. *Eur J Cancer* 1973;27:253–267.

68. Hudson CN, McHardy JE, Curling OM, et al. Active specific immunotherapy for ovarian cancer. *Lancet* 1976;2:877–879.

69. Freeman CB, Harris R, Geary CG, et al. Active immunotherapy used alone for maintenance of patients with acute myeloid leukaemia. *Br Med J* 1973;4:571–573.

70. Powles RL. Imunologic maneuvers in the management of acute leukemia. *Med Clin North Am* 1976;60:463–472.

71. Perlin E, Weese JL, Heim W, et al. Immunotherapy of carcinoma of the lung with bcg and allogeneic tumor cells. In: Crispen RG, ed. *Neoplasm immunity: solid tumor therapy.* Chicago: Franklin Institute Press, 1977:9–21.

72. Schulof RS, Mai D, Nelson MA, et al. Active specific immunotherapy with an autologous tumor cell vaccine in patients with resected non-small-cell lung cancer. *Mol Biother* 1988;1:30–36.

73. Euhus DM, Gupta RK, Morton DL. Induction of antibodies to a tumor-associated antigen by immunization with a whole melanoma cell vaccine. *Cancer Immunol Immunother* 1989;29:247–254.

74. Morton DL, Foshag LJ, Hoon DS, et al. Prolongation of survival in metastatic melanoma after active specific immunotherapy with a new polyvalent melanoma vaccine. *Ann Surg* 1992;216:463–482.

75. Mordoh J, Kairiyama C, Bover L, et al. Allogeneic cells vaccine increases disease-free survival in stage III melanoma patients. A non-randomized phase II study. *Medicina (B Aires)* 1997;57:421–427.

76. Berd D, Maguire HC Jr, Schuchter LM, et al. Autologous hapten-modified melanoma vaccine as postsurgical adjuvant treatment after resection of nodal metastases. *J Clin Oncol* 1997;15:2359–2370.

77. McCune CS, Schapira DV, Henshaw EC. Specific immunotherapy of advanced renal carcinoma: evidence for the polyclonality of metastases. *Cancer* 1981;47:1984–1987.

78. Adler A, Gillon G, Lurie H, et al. Active specific immunotherapy of renal cell carcinoma patients: a prospective randomized study of hormono-immuno-versus hormonotherapy. Preliminary report of immunological and clinical aspects. *J Biol Res Mod* 1987;6:610–624.

79. Marcove RC, Southam CM, Levin A, et al. A clinical trial of autogenous vaccine in osteogenic sarcoma in patients under the age of twenty-five. In: Mathe G, Weiner R, eds. *Investigation and stimulation of immunity in cancer patients.* New York: Springer-Verlag, 1974:434–435.

80. Townsend CM Jr, Eilber FR, Morton DL. Skeletal and soft tissue sarcomas—treatment with adjuvant immunotherapy. *JAMA* 1976;236:2187–2189.

81. Humphrey LJ, Taschler-Collins S, Volenec FJ. Treatment of primary breast cancer with immunotherapy. *Am J Surg* 1984;148:649–652.

82. Hollinshead A, Elias EG, Arlen M, et al. Specific active immunotherapy in patients with adenocarcinoma of the colon utilizing tumor-associated antigens (TAA). A phase I clinical trial. *Cancer* 1985;56:480–489.

83. Freedman RS, Edwards CL, Bowen JM, et al. Viral oncolysates in patients with advanced ovarian cancer. *Gynecol Oncol* 1988;29:337–347.

84. Freedman RS, Bowen JM, Herson JH, et al. Immunotherapy for vulvar carcinoma with virus-modified homologous extracts. *Obstet Gynecol* 1983;62:707–714.

85. Schuepbach J, Sauter C. Inverse correlation of antiviral antibody titers and the remission length in patients treated with viral oncolysate: a possible new prognostic sign in acute myelogenous leukemia. *Cancer* 1981;48:1363–1367.

86. Wallack MK, Michaelides M. Serological response to human melanoma cell lines from patients with melanoma undergoing treatment with melanoma oncolysates. *Surgery* 1984;96:791–800.

87. Wallack MK, McNally KR, Leftheriotis S, et al. A Southeastern cancer study group phase I/II trial using vaccinia melanoma oncolysate. *Cancer* 1986;57:649–656.

88. Wallack MK, McNally KR, Leftheriotis S, et al. A Southeastern cancer study group phase I/II trial using vaccinia melanoma oncolysate. *Arch Surg* 1987;122:1460–1463.

89. Wallack MK, Sivanandham M, Balch CM, et al. Surgical adjuvant active specific immunotherapy for patients with stage III melanoma: the final analysis of data from a phase III, randomized, double-blind, multicenter vaccinia melanoma oncolysate trial. *J Am Coll Surg* 1998;187:69–77.

90. Cassel WA, Murras DR, Torbin AH, et al. Viral oncolysate in the management of malignant melanoma. I. Preparation of the oncolysate and measurement of immunologic responses. *Cancer* 1977;40:672–679.

91. Hershey P, Edwards A, Coates A, et al. Evidence with treatment with vaccinia melanoma cell lysate (VMCL) may improve survival of patients with stage II melanoma patients. *Cancer Immunol Immunother* 1987;25:257–265.

92. Neidhart JA, Murphy SG, Hennick LA, et al. Active specific immunotherapy of stage IV renal carcinoma with aggregated tumor antigen adjuvant. *Cancer* 1980;46:1128–1134.

93. Alth G, Denck H, Fischer M, et al. Aspects of the immunologic treatment of lung cancer. *Cancer Chemother Rep* [3] 1973;4:271–274.

94. Greene A, Pratt C, Webster R, et al. Immunotherapy of osteosarcoma patients with virus-modified tumor cells. *Ann N Y Acad Sci* 1976;2777:396–411.

95. Sinkovics J. Immunotherapy with viral oncolysates for sarcoma. *JAMA* 1977;237:869.

96. Rosenberg SA, Yang JC, Schwartzentruber DJ, et al. Immunologic and therapeutic evaluation of a synthetic peptide vaccine for the treatment of patients with metastatic melanoma. *Nat Med* 1998;4:321–327.

97. Chakraborty NG, Sporn JR, Tortora AF. Immunization with a tumor-cell-lysate-loaded autologous-antigen-presenting-cell-based vaccine in melanoma. *Cancer Immunol Immunother* 1998;47:58–64.

98. Pass HA, Schwarz SL, Wunderlich JR, Rosenberg SA. Immunization of patients with melanoma peptide vaccines: immunologic assessment using the ELISPOT assay. *Cancer J Sci Am* 1998;4:316–323.

99. Altman JD, Moss PAH, Goulder PJR, et al. Phenotypic analysis of antigen-specific T lymphocytes. *Science* 1996;274:94–96.

100. Shimizu Y, Asumi K, Masubuchi K, et al. Immunotherapy of tumor bearing mice utilizing virus help. *Cancer Immunol Immunother* 1988;27:223–227.

101. Ioannides CG, Platsoucas CD, Patenia R, et al. T-cell functions in ovarian cancer patients with viral oncolysates: I. Increased helper activity to immunoglobulins production. *Anticancer Res* 1990;10:645–654.

102. Barth A, Hoon DSB, Foshag LJ, et al. Polyvalent melanoma cell vaccine induces delayed-type hypersensitivity *in vitro* immune response. *Cancer Res* 1994;54:3342–3345.

103. Rock KL, Rothstein L, Gamble S, et al. Characterization of antigen-presenting cells that present exogenous antigens in association with Class I MHC molecules. *J Immunol* 1993;150:438–446.

104. Huang AY, Golumbek P, Ahmadzadeh M, et al. Role of bone marrow-derived cells in presenting MHC class I–restricted tumor antigens. *Science* 1994;264:961–965.

105. Sivanandham M, Scoggin SD, Sperry RG, Wallack MK. Therapeutic effect of oncolysate prepared with the interleukin-2 gene encoded vaccinia virus: study with the C-C36 murine colon hepatic metastases model. *Cancer Immunol Immunother* 1994;38:259–264.

106. Nestle FO, Alijagic S, Gilliet M, et al. Vaccination of melanoma patients with peptide—or tumor lysate-pulsed dendritic cells. *Nat Med* 1998;4:328–332.

107. Yang Y, Sivanandham M, Stavropoulous CI, Wahal A, Wallack MK. Dendritic cells pulsed with vaccinia virus-augmented colon tumor cell-lysate therapy increased survival of mice bearing CC36 colon tumor. *Surg Forum* 1999;L:291–292.

18.2

CANCER VACCINES: CLINICAL APPLICATIONS

Genetically Modified Tumor Vaccines

DREW M. PARDOLL
ELIZABETH M. JAFFEE

The concept of cancer vaccination, also referred to as *active immunotherapy,* is based on the notion that exposure of a cancer patient's immune system to tumor antigens expressed by their cancer in an "immunogenic" fashion activates therapeutically useful antitumor immunity. For a limited number of tumors, such as melanoma and virus-associated tumors, candidate immunodominant tumor–associated antigens have been identified, providing the basis for antigen-specific vaccines in the form of adjuvanted peptide, protein or recombinant DNA, or virus or bacterium. For the majority of cancers, however, we have essentially no information regarding the identity of the most relevant tumor-associated antigens. Therefore, cancer vaccines for these tumors necessitate the use of tumor cells as the source of antigens.

Earlier approaches to enhance the immunogenicity of tumor cells have involved mixing them with bacterial adjuvants, such as bacillus Calmette-Guérin or *Corynebacterium parvum* (1–4). With the cloning of gene-encoding immune system regulatory molecules, a new generation of cell-based cancer vaccine strategies has arisen through transduction of tumor cells with genes encoding immunologically active molecules. The evaluation of antitumor immunity induced by vaccination with genetically modified tumor cells has been extensively studied in preclinical (mostly murine) models, and results of early-stage clinical trials applying this vaccine approach have been reported in a number of centers. In general, the types of immunologically active genes that have been introduced into tumors can be divided into three categories: (a) major histocompatibility complex (MHC) genes, (b) genes encoding membrane-associated costimulatory molecules (i.e., B7), and (c) cytokine genes. Although it is impossible to completely review all of the published information on genetically modified tumor vaccines, this chapter summarizes general principles and concepts and highlights concordant themes derived from multiple studies in different tumor models.

CENTRAL ROLE OF THE ANTIGEN-PRESENTING CELL IN CANCER VACCINATION

One of the most important principles emerging from mechanistic studies of immunologic priming, as well as tolerance induction to tissue and tumor antigens, is that the response of the immune system to a particular antigen is largely determined by the characteristics of the antigen-presenting cell (APC), which presents that antigen to cognate T cells *in vivo*. Increasing evidence supports the idea that tolerance and activation of immune responses depends on antigen presentation by different subsets or differentiation states of bone marrow–derived APCs.

The original notion that most tumors arising *in vivo* are efficiently eliminated by immune surveillance (5,6) has been replaced by an increasing appreciation that tumors can induce tolerance to their tumor-associated antigens through pathways that reflect natural mechanisms of tolerance induction to self tissue antigens expressed in the periphery (7–12). The application of transgenic mouse models and bone marrow chimera approaches, which allow the distinction of *in vivo* antigen presentation by bone marrow–derived versus parenchymal or tumor cells, has demonstrated a critical role for the "cross tolerance" pathway in which tissue and tumor antigens are transferred to a specialized class of "tolerizing" bone marrow–derived APCs, which, in turn, present them to T cells in a tolerogenic fashion (13). Hence, therapeutic vaccines for cancer of any type must overcome this tolerant state of the immune system to activate clinically useful immune responses. Strategies to break tolerance with vaccination must not only provide a high density of

peptide-MHC complexes on APCs but also cause the activation of APCs to states in which they activate T cells most efficiently. APCs in this "activated" differentiation state are generally referred to as *dendritic cells* (DCs) (14). Taking into account the central role of the APC in vaccine efficacy, genetically modified vaccines seek to convert the tumor cell itself into an APC or to attract APC progenitors to the site of the vaccine, which can then differentiate *in situ* to DCs.

HISTORY OF GENETICALLY MODIFIED TUMOR VACCINES

The first studies demonstrating enhanced immunogenicity of genetically altered tumors were performed in the late 1960s, starting with Lindenmann and Klein (15), who showed that vaccination with influenza virus–infected tumor cell lysates generated enhanced systemic immune responses against a challenge with the original wild-type tumor cells. Furthermore, these early studies showed that nonvirally infected tumor cell lysates or tumor cell lysates mixed with the same virus are not immunogenic and cannot elicit a systemic immune response against challenge with the parental tumor cells. The process of introducing strong foreign antigens into tumors (by infection or gene transfer) to enhance their immunogenicity has been referred to as *xenogenization*. Because adequate immunization against the tumor required that the tumor cells be infected with the virus, Lindenman and Klein hypothesized that weak antigens derived from the tumor cells might become associated with or incorporated into the virus and subsequently become potent immunogens. Based on what we have learned since, the enhanced immune response generated by the virally infected tumor cells probably occurred as a consequence of the inflammatory responses induced by viral infection together with "bystander help." As described earlier, these inflammatory responses are critical to the *in situ* differentiation of bone marrow–derived progenitors into activated APCs that can present antigens in an immunogenic rather than tolerogenic fashion. Once this is achieved, CD4 T–cell responses against the strong foreign antigens can provide increased help for the amplification of weaker responses against the endogenous tumor antigens.

The next generation of genetically altered tumor cell vaccines involved the use of mutagenesis to generate immunogenic variants of nonimmunogenic tumor cells, which on immunization could generate enhanced immune responses against the original nonimmunogenic variants. As newer techniques of gene transfer have been developed, infection with virus and mutagenesis was replaced with specific gene transfer in an attempt to more carefully regulate the nature of the genetic alteration within the tumor. The first studies of genetic modification of tumors to enhance immunogenicity involved transfer of the influenza hemagglutinin (HA) gene into a murine colon tumor (16). This approach met with limited success because the majority of HA transfectants failed to be rejected or demonstrated increased immunogenicity. Based on the more recent appreciation of the capacity of tumors to tolerize immune responses specific for their antigens (see above), this result is not surprising in retrospect. Subcutaneous injection of clones selected to express

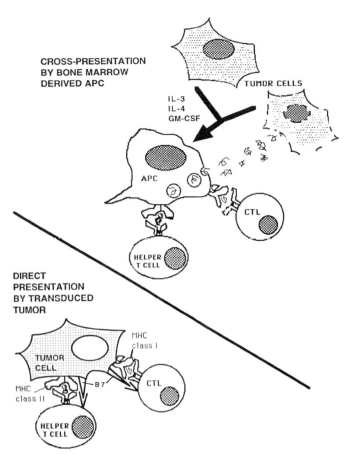

FIGURE 1. Potential mechanisms by which gene-transduced tumor cells may enhance the activation of tumor-specific T cells. Shown are examples of different classes of gene products that attract and activate antigen-presenting cells (APCs) for more efficient presentation of tumor antigens to T cells or allow for enhanced direct presentation of antigens by the transduced tumor cell. (GM-CSF, granulocyte-macrophage colony-stimulating factor; IL, interleukin; MHC, major histocompatibility complex.)

1. Enhancement of the presentation of antigens to T cells. This mechanism implies an increase in peptide-MHC density at the site of activation of T cells.

2. Enhancement of costimulation. This mechanism takes into account the fact that T cells require extra costimulatory signals in addition to engagement of the T-cell receptor to become efficiently activated. Costimulatory signals may be membrane-bound ligands, such as B7, that are critical for T-cell activation, or soluble mediators, such as cytokines.

3. Local elaboration of cytokines that attract and locally activate bone marrow–derived APCs, which process and present tumor antigens to T cells.

GENETIC MODIFICATION OF TUMORS WITH MAJOR HISTOCOMPATIBILITY GENES

Introduction of MHC genes into tumors was one of the first approaches for enhancing the immunogenicity of tumors by gene transfer. A number of studies in the 1980s suggested that increasing MHC class I expression by gene transfection typically results in decreased tumorigenic capacity in murine tumor models (17). The decreased tumorigenicity was felt to be caused by enhanced presentation of tumor-specific antigens to CD8+ cytotoxic T lymphocytes (CTLs) *in vivo*. Enhanced expression of self-MHC class I molecules, however, does not always increase the immunologic potency of a tumor, and, in certain circumstances, has been shown to inhibit natural killer (NK) cells, thereby resulting in paradoxically increased tumorigenicity (18). Tumor immunogenicity has also been enhanced by the transfer of allogeneic MHC class I genes (19,20). In certain cases, the rejection of tumors expressing allogeneic MHC class I molecules may result in enhanced systemic immune responses against subsequent challenge with the unmodified parental tumor. This represents an example of the general phenomenon of enhancing tumor vaccine potency by introducing genes encoding any foreign antigen, as in the case of viral infection or introduction of the viral genes. The mechanism by which tumors "xenogenized" with allo-MHC genes enhance systemic immune responses against challenge is likely identical to the original virus infected or foreign antigen–transduced tumor vaccines, namely bystander effects caused by the high frequency of allo-MHC–reactive T cells.

In some murine tumors, introduction of MHC class II genes into tumor cells decreases their immunogenicity and can result in generation of enhanced systemic immune responses against parental MHC class II–negative tumor (21). Further enhancement of vaccine potency has been achieved by cointroduction of MHC class II and B7 genes (22) (see next section). It was postulated that the expression of MHC class II molecules on tumor cells allowed for the presentation of MHC class II–restricted tumor-specific antigen CD4 helper T cells, which ultimately could provide enhanced *in vivo* help for action of cytotoxic T cells and possibly other CD4-dependent effector pathways. In one study, evidence was provided that MHC class II molecules introduced into tumors would preferentially present endogenous tumor antigens in the absence of expression of invariant chain (Ii), presumably because of the failure of Ii to block access

extremely high levels of HA, however, resulted in some immune response induction to the parental tumor akin to that which was achieved earlier with viral infection. The limited success of these approaches to introduce foreign genes encoding "strong" antigens into tumors to enhance their immunogenicity can be attributed to the inflammatory responses produced by the mechanical trauma of subcutaneous injection together with the bystander help effect, just as was produced with virally infected tumors.

PRECLINICAL EVALUATION OF GENETICALLY MODIFIED TUMOR VACCINES

Despite limited success, the xenogenization experiments described earlier encouraged increasing efforts aimed at directly altering the tumor cell's genetic material to enhance immune responses generated against endogenous tumor antigens. The enhancement of immune responses in the vaccine setting can be divided mechanistically into three categories (Fig. 1):

of peptides to the MHC class II groove in the endoplasmic reticulum (23). Because Ii is also important in the trafficking of MHC class II molecules to MIIC compartments in which proteases, a low pH environment, and H2M are necessary for efficient peptide loading of MHC class II molecules, the exact nature of antigens expressed by MHC class II molecules in Ii-negative tumors remains to be determined.

Genetic Modification with Genes Encoding B7 and Other Costimulatory Molecules

The original basis for the introduction of the B7 gene into tumors stems from the critical role of B7-CD28 interactions in costimulating T-cell activation. CD28 is well characterized as a critical costimulatory receptor for activation of CD4 and CD8 T cells (24). Cross-linking of CD28 has been shown to enhance the level of lymphokine production by CD4⁺ T cells subsequent to antigen recognition. This enhanced lymphokine production appears to be caused by enhanced transcription, as well as enhanced messenger RNA stability (25,26). Engagement of CD28 also decreases the number of T-cell receptors necessary to be engaged by peptide-MHC complexes for maximum T-cell stimulation (27). Blocking the interaction between B7 and CD28 not only decreases lymphokine production, but it can also result in a functional anergy to subsequent antigen stimulation (28). These important roles of the B7-CD28 interaction in T-cell activation made B7 a promising gene candidate to introduce into tumor cells to enhance their immunogenicity. Indeed, certain tumors are rejected in their syngeneic host subsequent to transfection with the B7 gene, and systemic immune responses capable of generating protection against challenges from the wild-type tumor at a distant site were noted (29–39). One study comparing vaccination with tumors expressing B7.1 versus B7.2 suggested that B7.1-transduced tumors elicited superior antitumor immunity to B7.2-transduced tumors (37). Subsequent analyses of B7-transduced tumor vaccines have suggested that the systemic immunity is only generated with immunogenic tumors and not with poor or nonimmunogenic tumors, such as B16-F10. In some cases, it was necessary to introduce an additional "strong" tumor antigen into the tumors to see the B7 effect (39).

The original postulated mechanism for enhanced immunogenicity of B7-transduced tumors was that expression of B7 by the tumor cell itself was converted into a more potent activating APC. This notion was further enhanced by the findings that the cointroduction of B7 and MHC class II genes synergized in enhancing T-cell dependent antitumor immunity (22). Other studies, however, have suggested a different mechanism for the B7 effect. B7 can represent a target antigen for killing by NK cells. Thus, B7-transduced tumors are efficiently killed *in vivo* by an NK-dependent mechanism. Hence, it is possible that enhanced immunogenicity of B7-transduced tumors results from enhanced antigen release to bone marrow–derived APCs mediated by increased killing of the B7-transduced tumor cells by NK cells (35). Evidence for this "cross-priming" pathway was derived through the application of bone marrow chimera experiments, which demonstrated that, although B7 expression could indeed confer some *de novo* capacity of tumor cells to directly present antigens to T cells, the majority of antigen presentation

with B7-transduced tumor vaccines was via bone marrow–derived APCs (36,38).

Expression of other cell membrane–bound costimulatory molecules in tumor cells has also been explored, although to a much lesser extent than B7. In particular, members of the tumor necrosis factor (TNF) family, including 4-1BBL, FasL, CD70, CD153, and CD154 genes, have been introduced into tumor cells (40,41). In one study, introduction of FasL into tumor cells induced local tumor regression rather than the expected protection from immunologic attack reported by previous investigators. This effect was shown to be caused by a FasL-Fas dependent activation of neutrophils with resultant local inflammatory destruction (40). In another study, tumor cells expressing CD70 and CD154 were able to induce antitumor immunity at higher frequency than nontransduced irradiated cells when tested in vaccination and therapy models (41). As signaling through the TNF–TNF receptor pathways between T cells and APCs can travel in both directions (and, in some cases, bidirectionally), it is possible that enhanced immunogenicity of tumor vaccines transduced with TNF (or corresponding TNF receptor) family members could work through costimulation of T cells by the transduced tumor or by providing a ligand for the activation of APCs or other inflammatory cells local to the environment of the tumor that are in the process of ingesting released tumor antigens. As agonist antibodies have been produced against a number of the TNF receptor family members, it remains to be determined whether *in vivo* treatment with agonist antibodies or transduction of the gene encoding the ligand will be most effective. In one study, the combination of B7-transduced tumors with agonist antibodies to 4-1BB resulted in synergistic enhancement of antitumor immunity (34).

Genetic Modification with Cytokine Genes

The most actively investigated approach to genetically modified tumor vaccination involves introduction of cytokine genes into tumors. This approach seeks to locally alter the immunologic environment of the tumor cell so as to enhance antigen presentation of tumor-specific antigens to the immune system or enhance the activation of tumor-specific lymphocytes. One of the most important concepts underlying the use of cytokine gene–transduced tumor cells is that the cytokine is produced at high concentrations local to the tumor. Systemic concentrations are generally quite low. Conversely, systematic administration of the cytokine such that blood concentrations are much higher than after injection of the corresponding genetically modified tumor fails to produce the same biologic effects. This paracrine physiology much more closely mimics the natural biology of cytokine action than does the systemic administration of recombinant cytokines. Furthermore, gene transduction allows for a sustained local cytokine release at the vaccine site. Thus, although coinjection of free cytokine at the vaccine site can produce similar effects as gene transfer, they are generally weaker (42).

Many cytokine genes have been introduced into tumor cells with varying effects on tumorigenicity and immunogenicity. When produced by tumors, some of these cytokines induce a local inflammatory response that results in elimination of the injected tumor. This local inflammatory response is often predominantly dependent on leukocytes or NK cells as opposed to classic T cells. These systems have been used to uncover *in vivo* effects of cytokines that result in activation of tumoricidal potential by various types of leukocytes. In addition to rejecting the genetically modified tumor cells, vaccinated animals may develop a T-cell–dependent systemic immunity, which, in some cases, can cure micrometastases established before treatment with the genetically altered tumor cells. In all cases in which systemic immunity against wild-type tumor challenge has been analyzed, it is mediated by T cells. Given the number of studies done with cytokine-transduced tumor cells, it is not surprising that variable results have been observed when different tumor systems are analyzed. Additional variables to the cytokines used include cell dose, level of cytokine expression, location of immunization and challenge sites, and vaccination schedule. Summarized in Table 1 and in following sections are results of murine studies using some of the more commonly analyzed cytokine genes.

Interleukin-2

In several murine tumor systems, injection of autologous tumor cells transfected with the interleukin-2 (IL-2) gene (43–51) leads to IL-2 secretion and MHC class I–restricted CTL activity against transduced and parental tumor. IL-2–transduced tumor vaccines are characterized by a predominantly lymphocytic infiltrate that includes NK cells. All IL-2–transduced tumors are rejected as long as secretion levels of the transductants are sufficiently high. Rejection is dependent on CD8$^+$ T cells and NK cells. Vaccination with IL-2–transduced tumors can also induce systemic antitumor immunity, although not as potently as other cytokine genes. In a number of IL-2 transduction studies that analyzed T-cell subsets, systemic immunity required CD8$^+$ but not CD4$^+$ cells, suggesting that IL-2 was truly bypassing the helper T-cell arm. In one case (47), CD4$^+$ and CD8$^+$ cells were required, indicating that IL-2 can also induce a local inflammatory response, leading to activation of helper and cytotoxic T cells. Cotransduction of tumors with the IL-2 and B7 genes has been reported to synergistically enhance vaccine potency, although the mechanism of synergy has not been specifically determined (52).

Interleukin-4

IL-4 has broad immunoregulatory properties, affecting MHC class II antigens and immunoglobulin isotype switching in B cells, T-cell growth and development, and the secretion or action of IL-1, IL-2, granulocyte colony-stimulating factor (G-CSF), macrophage colony-stimulating factor, and granulocyte-macrophage colony-stimulating factor (GM-CSF). The prominent acute inflammatory reaction and rejection of the transduced tumors occurs even in nude mice and is mediated primarily by macrophages and eosinophils. This contrasts with the predominantly lymphocytic infiltrates seen in IL-2–mediated tumor rejection and suggests an important role for the recruitment and enhancement of APCs in antitumor immune responses. In several murine tumor systems, IL-4 gene–transduced vaccines pro-

TABLE 1. BIOLOGIC ACTIVITIES OF COMMONLY INVESTIGATED CYTOKINE GENE–TRANSDUCED TUMOR VACCINES

Cytokine	*In Vivo* Effects of Cytokine Gene–Transduced Tumors
IL-2	Expression of high levels of IL-2 results in regression of transduced tumors. Transduced tumors are characterized by massive infiltrate of lymphocytic cells. In some tumor models, a systemic immune response is generated against challenge with parental tumor. Rejection of the IL-2–transduced tumor cells is dependent on CD8$^+$ and natural killer cells but not on CD4$^+$ cells, suggesting that helper T cells are rendered irrelevant in the rejection response. A correlation exists between increased levels of local IL-2 production and systemic, as well as local, antitumor responses.
IL-4	Expression of high levels of IL-4 results in regression of transduced tumors, characterized by massive infiltrate of macrophages and eosinophils. In some tumor models, a systemic immune response is generated against challenge with parental tumor that is greater than those generated by irradiated nontransduced tumor cells. Systemic antitumor responses are dependent on CD8$^+$ cells and partially on CD4$^+$ cells, suggesting enhanced presentation of tumor antigens by influxing macrophages to CD4$^+$ helper T cells is an important event in the ultimate stimulation of tumor-specific CD8$^+$ cytotoxic lymphocytes.
IFN-γ	Introduction of the IFN-γ gene into tumor cells generally induces or upregulates MHC class I and II gene products. In some tumors, IFN-γ expression results in rejection of transduced tumors and induction of systemic immunity. The effects of IFN-γ are quite tumor system dependent, and, in certain cases, the cotransduction of IFN-γ with other cytokine genes actually reveals an inhibitory effect of IFN-γ in the generation of systemic immune responses.
TNF	TNF-transduced tumor cells typically grow more slowly *in vitro* and are sometimes rejected when injected into syngeneic animals. It is unclear whether the rejection phenomenon is simply owing to the direct effects of TNF on the tumor cells or whether additional effects of TNF occur on inflammatory cells, such as macrophages. Immunization with TNF-transduced tumor cells does not generate enhanced systemic immunity relative to irradiated nontransduced tumor cells.
IL-7	Systemic antitumor immune responses have been reported with an MHC class II + myelocytoma line by immunization with tumor cells engineered to secrete IL-7. Immunity was independent of CD8$^+$ T cells, but dependent on CD4$^+$ T cells (presumably macrophages).
IL-12	IL-12–transduced tumors are vigorously rejected *in vivo* via NK and T-cell–dependent mechanisms. IL-12–transduced tumors variably induce systemic antitumor immunity.
GM-CSF	GM-CSF–transduced cells induce long-lived systemic antitumor immunity relative to irradiated nontransduced tumors in a number of different tumor models. Potency of GM-CSF's effect locally may relate to its unique ability in promoting the differentiation of hematopoietic precursors to dendritic cells. Immunity is dependent on CD4$^+$ and CD8$^+$ T cells, even when tumors are MHC class II-dependent. Effector mechanisms include activation of macrophages to produce reactive nitrogen and oxygen species, as well as recruitment of eosinophils to metastatic sites.

GM-CSF, granulocyte-macrophage colony-stimulating factor; IFN, interferon; IL, interleukin; MHC, major histocompatibility complex; NK, natural killer; TNF, tumor necrosis factor.

duce systemic antitumor immunity (53–56). In these cases, immune responses were systemic, tumor antigen–dependent and specific, IL-4 level–dependent, mediated by CD4$^+$ and CD8$^+$ T cells, and they exhibited immunologic memory. As determined by cellular depletion studies, T cells appear to be more critical than B cells, particularly for long-lasting systemic immunity.

Interferon-γ

Interferon-γ (IFN-γ) has direct antitumor properties, as well as several immunoregulatory properties. It induces MHC class I antigens on several tumor cells and class II antigens on macrophages and DCs. It also upregulates lymphotoxin, TNF-α, intracellular adhesion molecule–1, and lymphocyte function antigen-1. IFN-γ can stimulate CTL activity, NK and B cells, and the phagocytic activity of macrophages and monocytes by upregulating Fc receptors and increasing superoxide production.

Transduction of the IFN-γ gene into some murine tumors can induce specific and persistent antitumor immunity that is probably related to MHC class I expression on tumor cells and T-cell activation (57–59). In other murine models, MHC class I antigen induction and T-cell activity are not needed, and a strong nonspecific antitumor effect is seen.

Tumor Necrosis Factor–α

TNF-α has pleiotropic biologic properties, including the ability to cause hemorrhagic necrosis of established tumors, and the ability to induce multiple cytokines, including IL-6, IL-8, GM-CSF, and G-CSF. Systemic TNF-α shows antitumor effects in mice but minimal activity in humans, where severe dose-limiting toxicity arises at doses one-fortieth of those tolerated by mice on a milligram per kilogram basis. Responses in several human malignancies are reported with intralesional TNF-α injections, which permit high local concentrations. Transduction of the gene provides a technique for delivering similar levels of this active antitumor and immune modulatory agent directly to the tumor site. Gene transfer experiments in preclinical models have demonstrated considerable antitumor activity for TNF-α (60–62). This activity can be specific and long lasting; it is dependent on CD4$^+$ and CD8$^+$ cells, and its acute inflammatory infiltrate is composed primarily of macrophages. Relatively modest systemic vaccine effects have been observed, however, particularly with poorly immunogenic tumors.

Interleukin-7

Similar generation of antitumor immune responses has been reported by immunization with tumor cells engineered to secrete IL-7 (63). Of interest, the systemic immunity in one system of IL-7–transduced cells was independent of CD8$^+$ T cells but dependent on CD4$^+$ T cells. Furthermore, CR3$^+$ cells, presumably macrophages, were also required for tumor rejection. As the tumor used in this study was an MHC class II plus plasmacytoma line, it is possible that the antitumor response generated by CD4 cells was in response to MHC class II–restricted tumor antigens. The CD4 cells responding to MHC class II–restricted tumor-specific antigens may have subsequently

secreted cytokines, which acted as macrophage-activating factors, thereby recruiting tumoricidal macrophages responsible for the ultimate tumor destruction. In a study conducted in 1997, an IL-7–transduced alveolar cell carcinoma vaccine was shown to be much more potent when admixed with *ex vivo*–generated DCs (64).

Interleukin-12

Interest in IL-12–transduced tumor vaccines stems from its extremely potent biologic activity in activating innate immune responses, NK cells, and Th1-type T-cell responses (48,55,56,65–68). Systemic administration of IL-12 in mice generates potent antitumor responses, although increased sensitivity in humans led to prohibitive toxicity (akin to TNF), which has diminished enthusiasm for systemically administered IL-12 as a viable cancer therapy. IL-12–transduced tumors are potently rejected by NK and T-cell infiltrates similarly to IL-2 transductants. Although induction of systemic immunity has been reported, it is not as potent as with other cytokine transductants. Synergy between IL-12 and B7 gene transduction has been reported by a number of groups.

Granulocyte-Macrophage Colony-Stimulating Factor

Since the study by Dranoff et al. (69), which compared multiple cytokine, adhesion molecules, and costimulatory genes introduced into a number of different murine tumor lines, GM-CSF gene–transduced tumors have become the most actively studied genetically modified vaccines at the mechanistic level, as well as clinically. In the original study, each of the genes were introduced into the poorly immunogenic B16-F10 tumor using a replication-defective retroviral vector that produced consistent high levels of expression of each of the transgenes in the absence of selection, thereby eliminating variability caused by different levels of gene expression and resultant cytokine expression. Animals were vaccinated with irradiated transductants, followed by challenge with unirradiated wild-type B16-F10 cells at doses 3 to 4 logs higher than the minimal tumoricidal dose. Although a number of cytokine genes in this study, such as IL-4 and IL-6, induced some measure of systemic antitumor immunity, the most potent systemic antitumor immunity was produced by GM-CSF–transduced tumor cells. Subsequent studies in other tumor models have validated the potent systemic immunity induced by GM-CSF–transduced tumor vaccines (31,33,55,70–84).

In most, but not all, subsequent studies comparing vaccine potency of tumors transduced with various cytokine and costimulatory genes, GM-CSF–transduced tumor vaccines have proved to be the most potent, as long as a sufficiently high level of GM-CSF production is achieved. A careful analysis of immunity induction as a function of gene transduction and expression demonstrated a steep dose–response curve. Maximal systemic immunity was achieved with vaccines producing 40 ng per 10^6 cells or more per 24 hours (84). Once this dose response between GM-CSF production levels by the transduced vaccine and systemic immunity was established, it became apparent that previous studies, which failed to detect a significant vaccination effect by GM-CSF–transduced tumors, had not achieved high enough levels of GM-CSF expression by the vaccines.

Antitumor immunity induced by GM-CSF–transduced vaccines has been shown to depend on CD4$^+$ and CD8$^+$ T cells. In addition to the classic MHC class–I restricted CTLs, other effector arms mediated by CD4 cells have been shown to participate in the generation of maximal antitumor immunity. Th1 and Th2 effector arms have been delineated. The Th1 effector arm depends on IFN-γ and involves the activation of macrophages at sites of metastases to produce reactive nitrogen species (NO), as well as reactive oxygen species (superoxides). These effectors have been demonstrated to be critically based on the diminished antitumor responses of GM-CSF–transduced vaccines in NOS-2 (inducible nitric oxide synthase) and gp91 (subunit of the reduced nicotinamide adenine dinucleotide phosphate oxidase complex) knockout mice. Eosinophils appear to be important Th2 effectors that are dependent on the production of cytokines, such as IL-4 and IL-5, by tumor-specific CD4 cells (81). The presence of the eosinophils at delayed-type hypersensitivity (DTH) sites and in tumor metastases subsequent to vaccination with GM-CSF–transduced tumors is not only observed in mouse models, but also has been a consistent observation in clinical trials with different tumor types (see the section Clinical Experience with Granulocyte-Macrophage Colony-Stimulating Factor–Transduced Vaccines).

GM-CSF–transduced vaccines represent a prototypical example of paracrine cytokine adjuvants in which local production of a cytokine induces the differentiation of bone marrow–derived progenitors into activated APCs (Fig. 2). In particular, numerous *in vitro* studies have demonstrated that, at high enough doses, GM-CSF is an extremely potent differentiation factor for DCs. The three following findings all underscore the likely mechanism of action of these vaccines as working through the differentiation of bone marrow–derived progenitors into DCs *in situ* at the vaccine site followed by antigen uptake, processing, and traffic to draining lymph nodes:

1. Higher doses of GM-CSF lead to DC differentiation *in vitro*.
2. Maximal systemic immunity is only found with vaccines that produce high quantities of GM-CSF .
3. Increased DCs are found in lymph nodes draining GM-CSF–transduced vaccines.

Formal evidence that presentation of the tumor antigens to T cells is mediated by bone marrow–derived APCs for MHC class I– and MHC class II–restricted antigens has been obtained through direct analysis of infiltrating DCs, as well as bone marrow chimera models (82). Similar results have been demonstrated for IL-3–transduced tumor vaccines, which have a potency and mechanism of action similar to GM-CSF (85). Indeed, IL-3 and GM-CSF have similar biologic activities, and their receptors share common subunits. Recent evidence that GM-CSF and IL-3 induced the differentiation of different types of DCs capable of inducing different functional responses in T cells suggests that GM-CSF and IL-3–transduced tumor vaccines should be more carefully compared.

It is important to note that, although irradiated GM-CSF–transduced vaccines can induce potent T-cell–dependent immu-

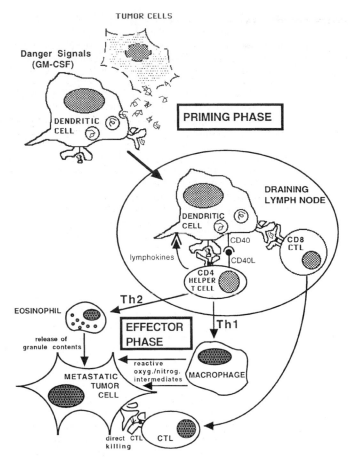

FIGURE 2. Summary of cellular and molecular components of the priming phase and effector phase of systemic antitumor immunity induced by granulocyte-macrophage colony-stimulating factor (GM-CSF) gene–modified vaccines. This diagram represents a synthesis of multiple studies into the mechanism of immunity generation by GM-CSF gene–modified tumor vaccines. At the site of vaccination, high concentrations of local GM-CSF secreted by the transduced tumors attract bone marrow–derived cells and induce their differentiation into early-stage dendritic cells capable of efficiently ingesting antigens released over a 2- to 4-day period by the dying tumor cells. These early-stage dendritic cells then begin to migrate to draining lymph nodes, during which time they process tumor antigens into the major histocompatibility complex (MHC) class I and II pathways. In the draining lymph nodes, dendritic cells present MHC class II–restricted peptides to CD4 cells, which further activates dendritic cell differentiation via CD40, CD40 ligand interactions, and other signals. Mature dendritic cells efficiently process and present ingested tumor antigens to MHC class I–restricted CD8 cells. In the effector stage, CD4-mediated and CD8-mediated antitumor responses collaborate to generate maximal killing at the site of metastases. CD8$^+$ T cells directly recognize peptide MHC complexes expressed on tumor cells in metastatic phosphides. CD4 cells recognize MHC class II–restricted tumor peptides that have been processed and presented by macrophages within the metastatic tumor mass. The CD4 cells produce Th1 cytokine, such as interferon-γ, which, in turn, activates the macrophages to produce tumoricidal products, such as nitric oxide and superoxides. Th2 CD4 cells produce cytokines, such as IL-4 and IL-5, which attract and activate the eosinophils, thereby inducing them to discharge their cytocidal granule contents. (CTL, cytotoxic T lymphocyte.)

nity against challenge at a distant site, nonirradiated GM-CSF–transduced tumors are not always rejected themselves. This is because GM-CSF induces differentiation of bone marrow–derived progenitors into potent APCs (e.g., DCs) but does not induce tumoricidal properties of bone marrow–derived cells nearly as much as other cytokines. In fact, rejection of nonirradiated tumor cells expressing GM-CSF at modest levels has been shown to preferentially induce differentiation of macrophages capable of suppressing immune responses *in vitro* (86). It has also been shown that IL-10 production by some tumor cells can interfere with *in situ* APC differentiation and subsequent generation of antitumor immunity. In one study, GM-CSF transduction failed to significantly enhance vaccine potency of an IL-10–producing B-cell lymphoma; however, cointroduction of the GM-CSF gene and an IL-10 antisense gene restored immunogenicity (76). These studies underscore the importance of careful attention to parameters, such as gene expression level, expression of interfering genes, and preparation of the transduced vaccines, in determining the ultimate potency of any genetically modified vaccine.

Other Cytokine Genes

Additional cytokines, such as G-CSF (87), macrophage chemotactic protein-1 (88), IL-6 (89), and IL-3 (85), have been shown in isolated reports to be associated with local inflammatory-mediated rejection of tumors engineered to secrete these cytokines locally. In the case of G-CSF, the local inflammatory infiltrate was characterized by large numbers of granulocytes. In the case of macrophage chemotactic protein-1, the local inflammatory infiltrate was characterized by large numbers of macrophages. In neither of these cases was a systemic immune response demonstrated. IL-3– and IL-6–transduced vaccines did produce systemic immunity dependent on CD4$^+$ and CD8$^+$ T cells.

Given the large number of potential immunologically active genes in the armamentarium and the technical difficulties in transducing human tumor cells to make vaccines, it is critical that they be compared for efficacy. Also, given that most mouse tumors show significant immunogenicity when simply irradiated, identification of genes that truly enhance a tumor's immunogenicity above that of irradiated wild-type cells is important.

VECTORS USED FOR TRANSDUCTION OF TUMORS

A variety of gene transfer vectors has been used to create genetically modified tumor vaccines. For the creation of autologous gene–modified tumor vaccines, high-efficiency gene transfer, as well as consistent high levels of gene expression in transduced cells, are critical parameters because numerous preclinical studies have verified the importance of levels of gene expression (particularly in the case of cytokine genes) in determining the potency of immunologic priming. In addition, primary human tumor explants are difficult to passage in culture for extended periods, thereby limiting the feasibility of drug-selecting transduced cells *in vitro*.

Initially, replication-defective retroviral vectors constituted the major gene transfer vehicle (69,90). The properties of retroviral vectors, however, are poorly suited for creating genetically modified tumor vaccines. Limitations in achievable virion titers (10^6 plaque-forming units per mL) limit efficiency of gene transfer, and retroviruses have severe limitations in the amount of foreign genetic material they can carry. Also, transduction requires replication of the target cell. Indeed, the major advantage of retroviral gene transfer systems, namely stable gene expression based on their ability to integrate into the host genome, is, in fact, unnecessary for genetically modified tumor vaccines, as the vaccine cells themselves are ultimately destroyed within the first week after immunization. For these reasons, other gene transfer systems have supplanted retroviruses for the production of genetically modified tumor vaccines.

Replication-defective adenoviral vectors (77,91) represent a more attractive gene transfer system that is being extensively used for tumor transduction *ex vivo*, as well as *in vivo*, because they can be produced at much higher titer (up to 10^{12} plaque-forming units per mL). The limited duration of expression of adenoviruses (which do not integrate into the host genome) does not represent a disadvantage for this particular application, as discussed earlier. Adenoviruses have another advantage in that their larger genome allows for the introduction of larger sized, as well as larger numbers, of inserted genes than is possible with conventional retroviruses. As more experience has developed with adenoviral vectors, a tremendous variability in transduction efficiency and gene expression levels have been observed for different tumors, even from within the same histologic category. Some of this variability in transduction efficiency is accounted for by the variable levels of expression of the primary adenoviral receptor, coxsackievirus and adenovirus receptor, to which the fiber protein binds in the initial adsorption step, and integrins, to which the penton protein binds to effect cell entry (92–94). Other unidentified factors additionally contribute to the variability of transduction and gene expression, which represents a major barrier to consistent transduction for purposes of autologous vaccine production.

A number of other viral and nonviral vectors, including herpesvirus amplicon vectors (49), adeno-associated virus vectors (95), avipox vectors (96), ballistically delivered gold particles (75), and liposomal DNA carriers (50), are being explored as gene transfer systems for *ex vivo* and *in vivo* transduction of tumors. In addition, replication-competent vectors, such as vaccinia virus, are also being used (71,73). The application of replication-competent viral vectors carries potential advantages and potential disadvantages. Advantages include the ability to locally expand the level of production of cytokine (or other costimulatory molecules) via multiple rounds of infection and replication at the injection site. Also, inflammatory or "danger" signals generated by local viral replication can potentially enhance the priming to tumor antigens released at the vaccine site. Potential disadvantages of cell vaccines transduced with replication-competent viral vectors include the potential danger of systemic infections by the virus after vaccine injection, as well as potential limitations in transgene expression by infected cells, resulting from the cytolytic properties of the particular virus. New generations of attenuated replication-competent viruses that are slow to lyse infected cells and present little danger from systemic infection may represent ideal vector systems that maintain the advantages but diminish the disadvantages of replication-competent viral vectors (52).

Replacement of Direct Tumor Transduction with Bystander Cells

Despite the continued improvement in vector delivery systems, rapid, efficient, and consistent transduction of autologous tumors

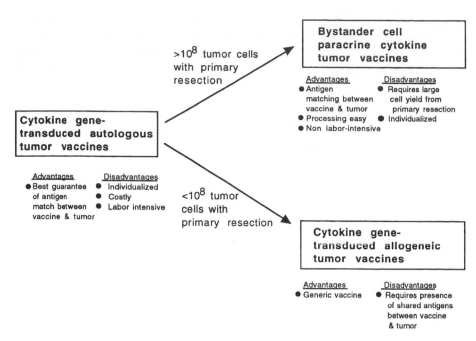

FIGURE 3. Clinical development of cytokine cancer vaccines. For some tumors (cancers of colon, kidney, ovary; leukemias, and lymphomas) from which large numbers of tumor cells can be obtained, vaccines are produced by admixture of patient cells with bystander cells that have been transduced with cytokine genes or with biopolymer microspheres containing cytokines. When autologous tumor is not available, patients can be immunized with allogeneic tumor cells (derived from cell lines of the same type as the patient's tumor) that have been transduced with cytokine genes. This strategy depends on the existence of appropriate antigens shared by the patient's tumor and the tumor cells in the vaccine.

continues to represent a major barrier to the broad application of genetically modified autologous tumor vaccines. For cytokine gene–transduced vaccines in which immune response induction depends on the paracrine biology of cytokine production local to the injected vaccine cells, increasing attention has been paid to the idea of replacing direct gene transfer into the tumor with admixture of bystander depots of cytokine. Indeed, a number of studies using bystander-transduced cells or cytokine-containing biodegradable polymer microspheres have demonstrated equivalent vaccine potency to directly transduced tumor cells (54,97). As discussed in the section Clinical Evaluation of Genetically Modified Vaccines, a number of clinical trials have used autologous or allogeneic fibroblast lines as the transduced cell admixed with nongenetically modified tumor cells. An MHC-negative K562 line transduced with the GM-CSF gene and selected to secrete extremely high levels of GM-CSF has been developed as a standardized bystander for human clinical trials (97).

The use of generic transduced bystander lines completely obviates the need for culture or transduction of autologous tumor cells, as long as enough cells can be harvested from the patient to produce the vaccine. Therefore, this approach is most suitable for the treatment of cancers in which a large number of relatively pure tumor cells can be collected through pheresis (in the case of hematologic tumors) or surgical excision of the tumor masses (Fig. 3). Examples of tumors that commonly fit these criteria include leukemia, lymphoma, multiple myeloma, colon cancer, renal cancer, and ovarian cancer.

Genetically Modified Allogeneic Vaccines

Even through the application of genetically modified bystander cells, the production of autologous tumor vaccines by necessity includes some degree of individualized cell processing. Two discoveries that have occurred since the early 1990s in the cancer immunology field provide a rationale for the development of generic genetically modified allogeneic cancer vaccines. First and foremost, the finding that some relevant immunologic targets are shared antigens (tissue specific or tumor associated) indicates that established cell lines of a particular tumor type may indeed contain "cross-reactive" antigens associated with that tumor type. Second, the finding that antigen presentation with cell-based vaccines occurs predominantly, if not exclusively, through the cross-priming pathway by host bone marrow–derived APCs indicates that matching of HLA alleles between the vaccine cells and the host is unnecessary. A number of preclinical models have verified that as long as immunorelevant antigens are shared between vaccine and challenge tumor, complete MHC mismatching between the vaccine and the host does not interfere with priming of host-restricted immune responses capable of recognizing the challenge tumor (98). As discussed in the section Clinical Evaluation of Genetically Modified Vaccines, genetically modified allogeneic vaccines are being actively investigated clinically in a number of cancer types (see Fig. 3).

IN VIVO INTRODUCTION OF CYTOKINE GENES INTO TUMOR CELLS

Interest exists in the use of viral and other gene delivery vehicles to introduce immunologically active genes into tumor deposits *in vivo* that cannot be easily surgically removed (68,79,99,100). Such approaches have two distinct goals, each of which would be most appropriately achieved by different genes. One goal is to increase the local production of cytokine within a metastatic tumor mass, so as to induce a tumoricidal inflammatory infiltrate. Lymphokine genes, such as IL-2 and IL-12, which induce strong NK and NK target responses, in addition to enhancing CD8 T-cell responses, would likely be the most potent for this purpose. In addition to destruction of the tumor itself, it would also be advantageous to enhance T-cell–dependent systemic immunity at the same time. Such an outcome might be best achieved through transfer of the GM-CSF gene, thereby enhancing local DC differentiation within the *in vivo*–transduced metastatic tumor mass. Thus, it is not surprising that some of the most potent antitumor effects generated by *in vivo* gene transfer approaches have used IL-2, IL-12, and GM-CSF. Using direct injection of recombinant replication-defective adenoviral vectors, Chen and colleagues have demonstrated that combined gene transfer of the herpes simplex virus thymidine kinase suicide gene, the GM-CSF gene, and the IL-2 gene resulted in the most potent antitumor responses in a murine model of liver metastases (100).

The first clinical evaluation of direct *in vivo* injection of genetic material into tumor masses used a gene encoding an allo-MHC antigen, HLA-B7 (101). As with the *ex vivo* gene transfer experiments with allogenic MHC genes, it is postulated that expression of a foreign HLA antigen by the tumor cells would generate a strong allogeneic immune response, resulting in the bystander stimulation of immunity against the bystander tumor antigens in the transduced mass. A DNA-liposome complex was used to accomplish the *in vivo* gene transfer. Five patients were treated with direct injections into accessible lymph nodes containing melanoma metastases. Analysis of needle biopsy specimens taken from the injected masses revealed that the HLA-B7 gene was expressed in 1% to 10% of the tumor cells near the injection site. No apparent toxicity was associated with this therapy and regression of the treated lesion, as well as several distant metastases, was observed in one patient. CTL precursor frequencies against the HLA-B7 alloantigen were detected, as well as an increase in bulk CTL activity against the autologous melanoma.

One of the great limitations of *in vivo* gene transfer for immunologic, as well as other purposes, is the relatively poor *in vivo* gene transfer efficiency of replication-defective viruses. Approaches that may improve *in vivo* gene transfer, resulting in enhanced immunologic effects, involve the development of targeted vectors, as well as the use of replication-competent recombinant viruses, which are capable of propagating a temporary infection and subsequent amplification within the injected or targeted tumor site. Along these lines, a number of groups are exploring the use of recombinant vaccinia to carry the GM-CSF gene into tumor masses *in vivo*.

Combination of Genetically Modified Tumor Vaccines and Adoptive Immunotherapy

A number of groups have explored combination strategies of vaccination with genetically modified vaccines, followed by *ex vivo* expansion of draining lymph node cells, followed by adoptive transfer back into the tumor-bearing animal (102,103). The rationale behind this approach is that the initial stages of activation and expansion of T cells specific for tumor antigens in the vaccine occurs in the draining lymph node subsequent to traffic of APCs from the vaccine site via afferent lymphatics. Studies using tumor vaccines transduced with allogeneic MHC genes, the IL-2 gene, and the GM-CSF gene have indeed indicated that prevaccination with certain genetically modified vaccines can enhance the ultimate number and potency of T cells cul-

tured *ex vivo* from draining lymph nodes. In one study, adoptive transfer of T cells grown from lymph nodes draining GM-CSF–transduced vaccines provided enhanced immunity relative to vaccination alone (103). These sorts of studies indeed highlight the potential value for approaches that combine multiple immunologic manipulations.

Amplification of Vaccine Potency Through Blockade of Immunologic Checkpoints

As more is learned about the molecular regulation of immune responses, additional strategies to block inhibitory pathways of T-cell activation, so called immunologic checkpoints, have been explored as approaches to amplify the potency of cancer vaccines. One of the most extensively studied examples has been the blockade of cytoxic T lymphocyte antigen-4 (CTLA-4) pathway. CTLA-4 binds B7 with roughly a tenfold higher affinity than CD28. Occupancy of CTLA-4 appears to directly counter the effects of CD28 on T-cell activation and lymphokine induction (104,105). The importance of the CTLA-4 pathway as an immunologic checkpoint *in vivo* is most dramatically exemplified in CTLA-4 knockout mice, which develop a severe lymphoproliferative disease with immunologically mediated organ destruction (106,107). If CTLA-4 could be transiently blocked *in vivo*, it might be possible to enhance vaccine potency while limiting the collateral damage seen in the constitutive genetic knockouts.

Indeed, anti–CTLA-4 infusions produced an enhanced antitumor effect in a number of murine cancer models without overt toxicity in the treated animals (108). The CTLA-4 blockade was found to be most effective when given together with a genetically modified cancer vaccine (109). In initial synergy studies, anti–CTLA-4 treatment was shown to synergize with a B7-transduced prostate cancer vaccine. Subsequently, a number of studies have demonstrated dramatic synergy between anti–CTLA-4 treatment with GM-CSF–transduced vaccines in treating established cancer in two poorly immunogenic tumor models—B16 melanoma (110) and breast cancer (111). In a third model of spontaneously arising prostate cancer in probasin-SV40 Tag transgenic mice (the TRAMP model), neither GM-CSF–transduced vaccines nor CTLA-4 blockade alone significantly affected the rate of spontaneous tumor outgrowth, whereas the combination significantly reduced the rate of tumor growth (112). Further evidence of potent synergy came from the findings that vaccination with B16-GM-CSF plus CTLA-4 blockade induced vitiligo in B6 mice, whereas vaccination with TRAMP-GM-CSF plus CTLA-4 blockade induced autoimmune prostatitis. A report regarding the role of the CD30 pathway as a later immunologic checkpoint in autoimmunity models (113) suggests that multiple opportunities may exist to combine tumor vaccination with blockade of immunologic checkpoints.

CLINICAL EVALUATION OF GENETICALLY MODIFIED TUMOR VACCINES

The majority of activity in the clinical evaluation of genetically modified tumor vaccines involves cytokine genes. Results of the early-stage clinical trials have been reported for vaccines transduced with IL-2 (114–117), IL-4 (118), IL-7 (119), IFN-γ (120), IL-12 (121), and GM-CSF (122–126). We have used different gene transfer approaches, including retroviruses, adenoviruses, lipofectant, and ballistically delivered gold particles. Although the majority of clinical trials have been performed in melanoma, genetically modified vaccines are also being evaluated in neuroblastoma, lung cancer, pancreatic cancer, prostate cancer, sarcoma, renal cancer, ovarian cancer, and hematologic malignancies. Autologous and allogeneic genetically modified vaccines have been tested, and, in some cases, tumor cells have been admixed with genetically modified autologous fibroblasts.

In addition to the cancer type and the particular cytokine gene transferred, four additional parameters that preclinical models predict would dramatically affect the outcome of vaccination are as follows:

1. Total number of tumor cells expressing antigen needed for generating an effective antitumor immune response: In all preclinical models in which vaccine cell number has been evaluated, increasing the number of vaccinating cells seems to increase the potency of systemic immunity. Importantly, widening the distribution of vaccine injections to involve more lymph node groups at the priming stage also enhances systemic immunity.

2. Expression level of cytokine required for generating an effective antitumor immune response: The importance of concentration of cytokine expression appears to depend on particular cytokines. In the case of IL-2 and IL-4, increasing amounts seem to correlate with increased systemic immunity. In the case of GM-CSF, maximal immunity plateaus at a secretion rate of 40 to 50 ng per 10^6 cells per 24 hours.

3. Route of administration of vaccine most effective at generating an effective antitumor immune response: It is difficult to completely analyze routes of injection in preclinical models because the dermis of rodents is too thin to place large numbers of cells. Studies using soluble GM-CSF to treat cutaneous leprosy, however, suggest that the dermal route of injection is superior. This may be owing to the presence of Langerhans' cells, which are induced by GM-CSF to differentiate into potent APCs. The optimal route of administration, however, may differ for different histologic types of tumors; therefore, this question should be adequately addressed in preclinical models and clinical trials.

4. Methods of pretreatment of reintroduced tumor cells: As described earlier, many of the gene products of the transduced tumor vaccines, particularly the cytokines, generate a local inflammatory response that eventually destroys the transduced tumor. This result is highly variable, however, and depends on levels of cytokine, tumor type, and cell dose. Also, for different cytokines, relative efficiency of elimination of the transduced tumor does not correlate with relative potency of the systemic immunity against distant sites of tumor—the only clinically relevant feature. For the ultimate use of genetically modified tumor vaccines in low tumor–burden patients, additional safeguards must be used. The most feasible and reliable method of inactivating the vaccine cells is radiation. For essentially all tumors, it is possible to find a window of γ irradiation dose that maintains metabolic activity and immunogenicity of the tumor for a few days while inhibiting replication.

Because variability exists in transduced genes, as well as these other critical parameters, it is difficult to derive much consistent information from the outcomes of the reported clinical trials, most of which have involved relatively small numbers of patients from diverse clinical settings; however, a few concordant themes, however, have emerged. First and foremost, the vaccines have not shown any significant systemic toxicity in any of the diverse clinical trials reported. Local inflammatory toxicities at the vaccine site have been reported in a number of trials, consistent with the bioactivity of locally secreted cytokines after injection of the transduced tumor cells. In a number of the studies, increased postvaccination proliferative and cytolytic responses from peripheral blood lymphocytes against the vaccine or autologous tumor cells have been reported. In the absence of information regarding which specific antigens are the targets of induced immune responses, it has been difficult to reliably measure increases in tumor antigen–specific T-cell precursor frequencies or activity. In some cases, increases in titers of serum antibodies reactive with tumor-associated antigens have been identified postvaccination. In the case of an IFN-γ–transduced autologous melanoma vaccine and a GM-CSF–transduced allogeneic prostate cancer vaccine trial, specific species appear to be selectively recognized on serum Western blots by postvaccine but not preimmune serum.

At the clinical level, anecdotal partial responses, mixed responses, and disease stabilization have been reported in a number of clinical trials, although the small patient numbers preclude any statistically significant evaluation of efficacy at this time.

The greatest clinical experience with cytokine gene–modified tumor vaccines has been with the IL-2 and GM-CSF genes.

Clinical Experience with Interleukin-2–Transduced Vaccines

A number of early-stage clinical trials using autologous and allogeneic vaccines have been performed using IL-2 gene transfer. A small trial in patients with metastatic renal cancer and melanoma used autologous untransduced tumor cells admixed with an immortalized fibroblast line stably transduced with the IL-2 gene introduced through cationic lipofection (116). Significant transient inflammatory responses developed at vaccine sites, as well as at DTH sites, where only irradiated tumor cells were injected. Infiltrates consisted of CD4+ and CD8+ T cells, which, on culture, demonstrated a suggestion of specific lytic activity against the autologous tumor cells. Clinical trials using directly IL-2–transduced tumor vaccines have been reported (115–117). Two of the vaccine trials involved patients with metastatic melanoma. Evidence of immune response induction was found in both cases; however, in neither case were responses against specific melanoma antigens assessed. In one of the trials, disease stabilization was noted in four of 12 patients treated, and mixed responses were observed in two of the 12 patients. Results of a clinical trial using an allogeneic neuroblastoma line transduced with the IL-2 gene were reported in children with relapsed stage IV neuroblastoma (117). As with other clinical IL-2–transduced vaccine trials, a strong lymphocytic infiltrate was observed at vaccine sites. One of the 12 children demonstrated more than a 90% tumor response (partial response), seven had stable disease, and four had progressive disease in response to vaccine administration as a single agent. The authors concluded that this outcome was indicative of immune response induction to shared antigens, but noted that these results were somewhat less dramatic than with their previous trials using autologous IL-2–transduced neuroblastoma vaccines. It is thus possible that allogeneic vaccination may miss the opportunity to activate responses against relevant unique tumor antigens.

Clinical Experience with Granulocyte-Macrophage Colony-Stimulating Factor–Transduced Vaccines

The results of autologous GM-CSF–transduced vaccine trials in melanoma and renal cell cancer have been reported. In both of the original clinical trials, retroviral vectors were used for gene transfer of cells cultured *ex vivo*. In the renal cancer trial, patients were randomly assigned to be vaccinated with autologous nontransduced tumor cells or with GM-CSF gene–transduced tumor cells (123). Evaluation on the GM-CSF gene transduction arm was only done in cases in which vaccine cells secreted equal or more than 40 ng per 10^6 cells per 24 hours of GM-CSF posttransduction (based on preclinical studies, which demonstrated that this level produced maximal systemic antitumor immunity). This has been the only clinical trial that evaluated genetically modified vaccines that directly compared transduced versus nontransduced vaccines. The results of the trial demonstrated that GM-CSF–transduced vaccines induced a strong infiltration of mononuclear cells (including cells expressing "DC-specific" markers) at the vaccine site relative to nontransduced vaccines. Evaluation of immune response generation indicated that, at the highest dose tier (4×10^7 cells per vaccine dose), a greater magnitude of DTH response to irradiated autologous nongenetically modified cells was detected. Biopsy analysis of the DTH site revealed a significant qualitative difference between patients receiving GM-CSF–transduced vaccines versus patients receiving nontransduced vaccines. In particular, patients receiving GM-CSF–transduced vaccines demonstrated significant eosinophil infiltration at DTH sites reminiscent of the Th2-dependent eosinophil infiltration observed at challenge sites in murine tumor models of GM-CSF–transduced vaccination. One of four patients receiving the highest dose of GM-CSF–transduced autologous vaccine cells achieved more than a 90% regression (partial response) in metastases that lasted 1 year. This patient mounted the greatest DTH response of all the patients in the trial.

In a similar trial using the same retroviral vector to introduce the GM-CSF gene into autologous melanoma cells, dramatic postvaccination responses were observed (124). Increases in melanoma-reactive serum antibody titers were detected, as well as DTH responses. Biopsy of cutaneous melanoma lesions postvaccination revealed strong infiltrates, which included eosinophils (largely perivascular), T cells, macrophages, and quite a large number of plasma cells. A number of the patients demonstrated near complete destruction of tumor cells on biopsy of cutaneous lesions. Although no classic partial responses or complete responses occurred in terms of regression of metastatic lesions, a number of the patients who demonstrated tumor destruction in biopsy specimens achieved long-term stabilization of disease.

Two new directions exist for GM-CSF gene–transduced vaccine development—the application of allogeneic vaccines and the treatment of patients with minimal residual disease. The rationale for the application of these vaccines in the minimal residual disease setting is twofold. First, preclinical evidence indicates that they are significantly more effective with minimal tumor burdens. Second, as multiple clinical trials have verified the lack of toxicity, essentially no risk appears to exist in the vaccination process itself. An allogeneic GM-CSF–transduced prostate vaccine is entering a phase 2 clinical trial and has used two well-characterized prostate-specific antigen (PSA) + prostate cancer lines, LNCAP and PC3 (125). This vaccine was tested in a phase 1/2 trial in patients with postradical prostatectomy with no clinical evidence of metastatic disease but with rising PSA levels. In this clinical trial, 15 of 21 (71%) patients demonstrated a statistically significant decrease in the rate of rise of PSA with approximately one-half of patients demonstrating PSA stabilization. Two patients showed a decrease in PSA levels of more than 50% of their maximal prevaccine levels. Serologic analysis suggested a correlation between the development of antibodies specific for certain protein species (as yet unidentified) in the vaccinating tumors and PSA response. In an allogeneic GM-CSF–transduced pancreatic cancer vaccine trial, patients postradical pancreaticoduodenectomy (Whipple procedure) were vaccinated with two pancreatic cancer cell lines transduced with the GM-CSF gene using the pc-DNA-3 plasmid followed by drug selection of lines secreting approximately 100 ng per 10^6 cells per 24 hours (122). A number of patients at the highest dose tier demonstrated positive DTH responses to autologous tumor postvaccination and some patients demonstrated recurrent inflammatory responses at old vaccine sites. Biopsy in these cases was characterized by a strong eosinophil component to the inflammatory infiltrate, further suggesting that the Th2 response originally identified in murine models may in fact translate to patients with a variety of cancer types.

CONCLUSION

Major advances in gene transfer technology together with the understanding of immune recognition and regulation have provided the basis for an expanding effort in the development of genetically modified tumor vaccines. Particularly with cytokine gene–transduced vaccines, the concept of paracrine cytokine adjuvants and their role in local activation of APCs has been established. Many decades may pass before the critical shared immunodominant antigens are identified for most cancers. Thus, clinical development of genetically modified vaccines plays a major role in human cancer immunotherapy as clinical and scientific tools. Carefully designed clinical studies together with appropriate immunologic evaluation of vaccinated patients are the critical steps to take to successfully define the most effective application of this approach in the treatment of cancer patients.

REFERENCES

1. Berd D, Maguire HCJ, Mastrangelo MJ. Induction of cell-mediated immunity to autologous melanoma cells and regression of metastases after treatment with a melanoma cell vaccine preceded by cyclophosphamide. *Cancer Res* 1986;46(5):2572–2577.

2. Livingston PO, Albino AP, Chung TJ, et al. Serological response of melanoma patients to vaccines prepared from VSV lysates of autologous and allogeneic cultured melanoma cells. *Cancer* 1985;55(4): 713–720.

3. Berd D, Maguire HCJ, McCue P, Mastrangelo MJ. Treatment of metastatic melanoma with an autologous tumor-cell vaccine: clinical and immunologic results in 64 patients. *J Clin Oncol* 1990;8(11): 1858–1867.

4. McCune CS, O'Donnell RW, Marquis DM, Sahasrabudhe DM. Renal cell carcinoma treated by vaccines for active specific immunotherapy: correlation of survival with skin testing by autologous tumor cells. *Cancer Immunol Immunother* 1990;32(1):62–66.

5. Lawrence HS. Discussion of cellular and humoral aspects of the hypersensitive states. New York: Hoeber-Harper, 1959:529–532.

6. Burnet FM. The concept of immunological surveillance. *Prog Exp Tumor Res* 1970;13(1):1–27.

7. Ohashi PS, Oehen S, Buerki K, et al. Ablation of "tolerance" and induction of diabetes by virus infection in viral antigen transgenic mice. *Cell* 1991;65(2):305–317.

8. Miller JF, Morahan G, Allison J. Extrathymic acquisition of tolerance by T lymphocytes. *Cold Spring Harb Symp Quant Biol* 1989;2(807):807–813.

9. Burkly LC, Lo D, Kanagawa O, Brinster RL, Flavell RA. T-cell tolerance by clonal anergy in transgenic mice with nonlymphoid expression of MHC class II I-E. *Nature* 1989;342(6249):564–566.

10. Staveley-O'Carroll K, Sotomayor E, Montgomery J, et al. Induction of antigen-specific T cell anergy: an early event in the course of tumor progression. *Proc Natl Acad Sci U S A* 1998;95(3): 1178–1183.

11. Wick M, Dubey P, Koeppen H, et al. Antigenic cancer cells grow progressively in immune hosts without evidence for T cell exhaustion or systemic anergy. *J Exp Med* 1997;186(2):229–238.

12. Speiser DE, Miranda R, Zakarian A, et al. Self antigens expressed by solid tumors do not efficiently stimulate naive or activated T cells: implications for immunotherapy. *J Exp Med* 1997;186(5):645–653.

13. Adler AJ, Marsh DW, Yochum GS, et al. CD4+ T cell tolerance to parenchymal self-antigens requires presentation by bone marrow-derived antigen-presenting cells. *J Exp Med* 1998;187:1555–1564.

14. Banchereau J, Steinman RM. Dendritic cells and the control of immunity. *Nature* 1998;392:245–252.

15. Lindenmann J, Klein PA. Viral oncolysis: increased immunogenicity of host cell antigen associated with influenza virus. *J Exp Med* 1967;126(1):93–108.

16. Fearon ER, Itaya T, Hunt B, Vogelstein B, Frost P. Induction in a murine tumor of immunogenic tumor variants by transfection with a foreign gene. *Cancer Res* 1988;48(11):2975–2980.

17. Wallich R, Bulbuc N, Hammerling GJ, Katzav S, Segal S, Feldman M. Abrogation of metastatic properties of tumour cells by de novo expression of H-2K antigens following H-2 gene transfection. *Nature* 1985;315(6017):301–305.

18. Karre K, Ljunggren HG, Piontek G, Kiessling R. Selective rejection of H-2-deficient lymphoma variants suggests alternative immune defense strategy. *Nature* 1986;319(6055):675–678.

19. Itaya T, Yamagiwa S, Okada F, et al. Xenogenization of a mouse lung carcinoma (3LL) by transfection with an allogeneic class I major histocompatibility complex gene (H-2Ld). *Cancer Res* 1987;47(12):3136–3140.

20. Plautz GE, Yang ZY, Wu BY, Gao X, Huang L, Nabel GJ. Immunotherapy of malignancy by *in vivo* gene transfer into tumors. *Proc Natl Acad Sci U S A* 1993;90(10):4645–4649.

21. Ostrand-Rosenberg S, Roby C, Clements VK, Cole GA. Tumor-specific immunity can be enhanced by transfection of tumor cells with syngeneic MHC-class-II genes or allogeneic MHC-class-I genes. *Int J Cancer Suppl* 1991;6:61–68.

22. Baskar S, Ostrand-Rosenberg S, Nabavi N, Nadler LM, Freeman GJ, Glimcher LH. Constitutive expression of B7 restores immunogenicity of tumor cells expressing truncated major histocompatibility class

23. II molecules. *Proc Natl Acad Sci U S A* 1993;90(12):5687–5690.

23. Armstrong TD, Clements VK, Ostrand-Rosenberg S. MHC class II-transfected tumor cells directly present antigen to tumor-specific CD4+ T lymphocytes. *J Immunol* 1998;160(2):661–666.

24. Linsley PS, Brady W, Grosmaire L, Aruffo A, Damle NK, Ledbetter JA. Binding of the B cell activation antigen B7 to CD28 costimulates T cell proliferation and interleukin-2 mRNA accumulation. *J Exp Med* 1991;173:721–730.

25. Lindsten T, June CH, Ledbetter JA, Stella G, Thompson CB. Regulation of lymphokine messenger RNA stability by a surface-mediated T cell activation pathway. *Science* 1989;244(4902):339–343.

26. Fraser JD, Irving BA, Crabtree GR, Weiss A. Regulation of interleukin-2 gene enhancer activity by the T cell accessory molecule CD28. *Science* 1991;251(4991):313–316.

27. Viola A, Hadjur C, Jeunet A, Julliard M. Electron paramagnetic resonance evidence of the generation of superoxide (O2.-) and hydroxyl (.OH) radicals by irradiation of a new photodynamic therapy photosensitizer, Victoria Blue BO. *J Photochem Photobiol B* 1996;32(1-2):49–58.

28. Harding FA, McArthur JG, Gross JA, Raulet DH, Allison JP. CD28-mediated signaling co-stimulates murine T cells and prevents induction of anergy in T-cell clones. *Nature* 1992;356(6370):607–609.

29. Townsend SE, Allison JP. Tumor rejection after direct costimulation of CD8+ T cells by B7-transfected melanoma cells [see comments]. *Science* 1993;259(5093):368–370.

30. Chen L, Ashe S, Brady WA, et al. Costimulation of antitumor immunity by the B7 counterreceptor for the T lymphocyte molecules CD28 and CTLA-4. *Cell* 1992;71(7):1093–1102.

31. Sumimoto H, Tani K, Nakazaki Y, et al. GM-CSF and B7-1 (CD80) co-stimulatory signals cooperate in the induction of effective antitumor immunity in syngeneic mice. *Int J Cancer* 1997;73(4):556–561.

32. Dummer R, Yue FY, Pavlovic J, et al. Immune stimulatory potential of B7.1 and B7.2 retrovirally transduced melanoma cells: suppression by interleukin 10. *Br J Cancer* 1998;77(9):1413–1419.

33. Nakazaki Y, Tani K, Lin ZT, et al. Vaccine effect of granulocyte-macrophage colony-stimulating factor or CD80 gene-transduced murine hematopoietic tumor cells and their cooperative enhancement of antitumor immunity. *Gene Ther* 1998;5(10):1355–1362.

34. Guinn BA, DeBenedette MA, Watts TH, Berinstein NL. 4-1BBL cooperated with B7-1 and B7-2 in converting a B cell lymphoma cell line into a long-lasting antitumor vaccine. *J Immunol* 1999;162, 8:5003–5010.

35. Wu TC, Huang AYC, Jaffee EM, Levitsky HI, Pardoll DM. A reassessment of the role of B7-1 expression in tumor rejection. *J Exp Med* 1995;182:1415–1421.

36. Cayeux S, Richter G, Noffz G, Dorken B, Blankenstein T. Influence of gene-modified (IL-7, IL-4 and B7) tumor cell vaccines on tumor antigen presentation. *J Immunol* 1997;158(6):2834–2841.

37. Gajewski TF, Fallarino F, Uyttenhove C, Boon T. Tumor rejection requires a CTLA4 ligand provided by the host or expressed on the tumor: superiority of B7-1 over B7-2 for active tumor immunization. *J Immunology* 1996;156(8):2909–2917.

38. Huang AY, Bruce AT, Pardoll DM, Levitsky HI. Does B7-1 expression confer antigen-presenting cell capacity to tumors *in vivo*? *J Exp Med* 1996;183(3):769–776.

39. Chen L, McGowan P, Ashe S, Johnston J, Li Y, Hellstrom KE. Tumor immunogenicity determines the effect of B7 costimulation on T cell-mediated tumor immunity. *J Exp Med* 1994;179(2):523–532.

40. Chen JJ, Sun Y, Nabel GJ. Regulation of the proinflammatory effects of Fas ligand (CD95L). *Science* 1998;282(5394):1714–1717.

41. Couderc B, Zitvogel L, Douin-Echinard V, et al. Enhancement of antitumor immunity by expression of CD70 (CD27 ligand) or CD154 (CD40 ligand) costimulatory molecules in tumor cells. *Cancer Gene Ther* 1998;5(3):163–175.

42. Kwak LW, Young HA, Pennington RW, Weeks SD. Vaccination with syngeneic, lymphoma-derived immunoglobulin idiotype combined with granulocyte/macrophage colony-stimulating factor primes mice for a protective T-cell response. *Proc Natl Acad Sci U S A* 1996; 93(20):10972–10977.

43. Fearon ER, Pardoll DM, Itaya T, et al. Interleukin-2 production by tumor cells bypasses T helper function in the generation of an antitumor response. *Cell* 1990;60(3):397–403.

44. Gansbacher B, Zier K, Daniels B, Cronin K, Bannerji R, Gilboa E. Interleukin 2 gene transfer into tumor cells abrogates tumorigenicity and induces protective immunity. *J Exp Med* 1990;172(4):1217–1224.

45. Bubenik J, Simova J, Jandlova T. Immunotherapy of cancer using local administration of lymphoid cells transformed by IL-2 cDNA and constitutively producing IL-2. *Immunol Lett* 1990;23(4):287–292.

46. Cavallo F, Giovarelli M, Gulino A, et al. Role of neutrophils and CD4+ T lymphocytes in the primary and memory response to non-immunogenic murine mammary adenocarcinoma made immunogenic by IL-2 gene. *J Immunol* 1992;149(11):3627–3635.

47. Bannerji R, Arroyo CD, Cordon CC, Gilboa E. The role of IL-2 secreted from genetically modified tumor cells in the establishment of antitumor immunity. *J Immunol* 1994;152(5):2324–2332.

48. Rodolfo M, Zilocchi C, Melani C, et al. Immunotherapy of experimental metastases by vaccination with interleukin gene-transduced adenocarcinoma cells sharing tumor-associated antigens: comparison between IL-12 and IL-2 gene-transduced tumor cell vaccines. *J Immunol* 1996;157(12):5536–5542.

49. D'Angelica M, Karpoff H, Halterman M, et al. *In vivo* interleukin-2 gene therapy of established tumors with herpes simplex amplicon vectors. *Cancer Immunol Immunother* 1999;47(5):265–271.

50. Koppenhagen FJ, Kupcu Z, Wallner G, et al. Sustained cytokine delivery for anticancer vaccination: liposomes as alternative for the gene-transfected tumor cells. *Clin Cancer Res* 1998;4(8):1881–1886.

51. de Vos S, Kohn DB, Cho SK, McBride WH, Said JW, Koeffler HP. Immunotherapy against murine leukemia. *Leukemia* 1998;12(3):401–405.

52. Sivanandham M, Shaw P, Bernik SF, Paloetti E, Wallack MK. Colon cancer cell vaccine prepared with replication-deficient vaccinia viruses encoding B7.1 and interleukin-2 induce antitumor response in syngeneic mice. *Cancer Immunol Immunother* 1998;46(5):261–267.

53. Tepper RI, Pattengale PK, Leder P. Murine interleukin-4 displays potent anti-tumor activity *in vivo*. *Cell* 1989;57(3):503–512.

54. Golumbek PT, Lazenby AJ, Levitsky HI, et al. Treatment of established renal cancer by tumor cells engineered to secrete interleukin-4. *Science* 1991;254(5032):713–716.

55. Stoppacciaro A, Paglia P, Lombardi L, Parmiani G, Baroni C, Colombo MP. Genetic modification of a carcinoma with the IL-4 gene increases the influx of dendritic cells relative to other cytokines. *Eur J Immunol* 1997;27(9):2375–2382.

56. Rodolfo M, Melani C, Zilocchi C, et al. IgG2a induced by interleukin (IL) 12-producing tumor cell vaccines but not IgG1 induced by IL-4 vaccine is associated with the eradication of experimental metastases. *Cancer Res* 1998;58(24):5812–5817.

57. Gansbacher B, Bannerji R, Daniels B. Retroviral vector-mediated gamma-interferon gene transfer into tumor cells generates potent and long lasting antitumor immunity. *Cancer Res* 1990;50:7820–7826.

58. Watanabe Y, Kuribayashi K, Miyatake S, et al. Exogenous expression of mouse interferon gamma cDNA in mouse neuroblastoma C1300 cells results in reduced tumorigenicity by augmented anti-tumor immunity. *Proc Natl Acad Sci U S A* 1989;86(23):9456–9460.

59. Restifo NP, Spiess PJ, Karp SE, Mule JJ, Rosenberg SA. A nonimmunogenic sarcoma transduced with the cDNA for interferon gamma elicits CD8+ T cells against the wild-type tumor: correlation with antigen presentation capability. *J Exp Med* 1992;175(6):1423–1431.

60. Asher M, Mule J, Kasid A. Murine tumor cells transduced with the gene for tumor necrosis factor-a. *J Immunol* 1991;146:3227–3229.

61. Karp SE, Farber A, Salo JC, et al. Cytokine secretion by genetically modified nonimmunogenic murine fibrosarcoma. Tumor inhibition by IL-2 but not tumor necrosis factor. *J Immunol* 1993;150(3):896–908.

62. Blankenstein T, Qin Z, Uberla K. Tumor suppression after tumor cell-targeted tumor necrosis factor via gene transfer. *J Exp Med* 1991;173:1047–1052.

63. Hock H, Dorsch M, Diamantstein T, Blankenstein T. Interleukin 7 induces CD4+ T cell-dependent tumor rejection. *J Exp Med* 1991;174(6):1291–1298.

64. Sharma S, Miller PW, Stolina M, et al. Multicomponent gene therapy vaccines for lung cancer: effective eradication of established murine tumors *in vivo* with interleukin-7/herpes simplex thymidine kinase-transduced autologous tumor and *ex vivo* activated dendritic cells. *Gene Ther* 1997;4(12):1361–1370.

65. Nanni P, Rossi I, De Giovanni C, et al. Interleukin 12 gene therapy of MHC-negative murine melanoma metastases. *Cancer Res* 1998;58(6):1225–1230.

66. Hallez S, Detremmerie O, Giannouli C, Thielemans K, Gajewski TF, Burny A, Leo O. Interleukin-12-secreting human papillomavirus type 16-transformed cells provide a potent cancer vaccine that generates E7-directed immunity. *Int J Cancer* 1999;81(3):428–437.

67. Popvic D, El-Shami KM, Vadai E, Feldman M, Tzehoval E, Eisenbach L. Antimetastatic vaccination against Lewis lung carcinoma with autologous tumor cells modified to express murine interleukin 12. *Clin Exp Metastasis* 1998;16(7):623–632.

68. Toda M, Martuza RL, Kojima H, Rabkin SD. In situ cancer vaccination: an IL-12 defective vector/replication-competent herpes simplex virus combination induces local and systemic antitumor activity. *J Immunol* 1998;160(9):4457–4464.

69. Dranoff G, Jaffee E, Lazenby A, et al. Vaccination with irradiated tumor cells engineered to secrete murine granulocyte-macrophage colony-stimulating factor stimulates potent, specific, and long-lasting antitumor immunity. *Proc Natl Acad Sci U S A* 1993;90(8):3539–3543.

70. Hsieh CL, Pang VF, Chen DS, Hwang LH. Regression of established mouse leukemia by GM-CSF-transduced tumor vaccine: implications for cytotoxic T lymphocyte responses and tumor burdens. *Hum Gene Ther* 1997;8(16):1843–1854.

71. McLaughlin JP, Abrams S, Kantor J, Dobrzanski MJ, Greenbaum J, Schlom J, Greiner JW. Immunization with a syngeneic tumor infected with recombinant vaccinia virus expressing granulocyte-macrophage colony-stimulating factor induces tumor regression and long-lasting systemic immunity. *J Immunother* 1997;20(6):449–459.

72. Herrlinger U, Kramm CM, Johnston KM, et al. Vaccination for experimental gliomas using GM-CSF-transduced glioma cells. *Cancer Gene Ther* 1997;4(6):345–352.

73. Qin H, Chatterjee SK. Cancer gene therapy using tumor cells infected with recombinant vaccinia virus expressing GM-CSF. *Hum Gene Ther* 1996;7(15):1853–1860.

74. Sampson JH, Archer GE, Ashley DM, et al. Subcutaneous vaccination with irradiated, cytokine-producing tumor cells stimulates CD8+ cell-mediated immunity against tumors located in the "immunologically privileged" central nervous system. *Proc Natl Acad Sci U S A* 1996;93(19):10399–10404.

75. Turner JG, Tan J, Crucian BE, et al. Broadened clinical utility of gene gun-mediated, granulocyte macrophage colony-stimulating factor cDNA-based tumor cell vaccines as demonstrated with a mouse myeloma model. *Hum Gene Ther* 1998;9(8):1121–1130.

76. Qin Z, Noffz G, Mohaupt M, Blankenstein T. Interleukin-10 prevents dendritic cell accumulation and vaccination with granulocyte-macrophage colony-stimulating factor gene-modified tumor cells. *J Immunol* 1997;159(2):770–776.

77. Nagai E, Ogawa T, Kielian T, Ikubo A, Suzuki T. Irradiated tumor cells adenovirally engineered to secrete granulocyte macrophage-colony stimulating factor establish antitumor immunity and eliminate pre-existing tumors in syngeneic mice. *Cancer Immunol Immunother* 1998;47(2):72–80.

78. Hogge GS, Burkholder JK, Culp J, et al. Development of human granulocyte macrophage colony-stimulating factor-transfected tumor cell vaccines for the treatment of spontaneous canine cancer. *Hum Gene Ther* 1998;9(13):1851–1861.

79. Bonnekoh B, Greenhalgh DA, Chen SH, et al. *Ex vivo* and *in vivo* adenovirus-mediated gene therapy strategies induce a systemic antitumor immune defense in the B16 melanoma model. *J Invest Dermatol* 1998;110(6):867–871.

80. Dunussi-Joannopoulos K, Dranoff G, Weinstein HJ, Ferrara JL, Bierer BE, Croop JM. Gene immunotherapy in murine acute myeloid leukemia: granulocyte-macrophage colony-stimulating factor tumor cell vaccines elicit more potent antitumor immunity compared with B7 family and other cytokine vaccines. *Blood* 1998;91(1):222–230.

81. Hung K, Hayashi R, Lafond-Walker A, Lowenstein C, Pardoll DM, Levitsky H. The central role of CD4+ T cells in the anti-tumor immune response. *J Exp Med* 1998;188:2357–2368.

82. Huang AY, Golumbek P, Ahmadzadeh M, Jaffee E, Pardoll D, Levitsky H. Role of bone marrow-derived cells in presenting MHC class I-restricted tumor antigens. *Science* 1994;264(5161):961–965.

83. Thompson RC, Pardoll DM, Jaffee EM, et al. Systemic and local paracrine cytokine therapies using transduced tumor cells are synergistic in treating intracranial tumors. *J Immunother Emphasis Tumor Immunol* 1996;19(6):405–413.

84. Jaffee EM, Pardoll DM. Considerations for the clinical development of cytokine gene-transduced tumor cell vaccines. *Methods* 1997;12(2):143–153.

85. Pulaski BA, McAdam AJ, Hutter EK, Biggar S, Lord EM, Frelinger JG. Interleukin 3 enhances development of tumor-reactive cytotoxic cells by a CD4-dependent mechanism. *Cancer Res* 1993;53(9): 2112–2117.

86. Bronte V, Chappell DB, Apolloni E, et al. Unopposed production of granulocyte-macrophage colony-stimulating factor by tumors inhibits CD8+ T cell responses by dysregulating antigen-presenting cell maturation. *J Immunol* 1999;162(10):5728–5737.

87. Colombo MP, Ferrari G, Stoppacciaro A, et al. Granulocyte colony-stimulating factor gene transfer suppresses tumorigenicity of a murine adenocarcinoma *in vivo*. *J Exp Med* 1991;173(4):889–897.

88. Rollins BJ, Sunday ME. Suppression of tumor formation *in vivo* by expression of the JE gene in malignant cells. *Mol Cell Biol* 1991;11(6):3125–3131.

89. Porgador A, Tzehoval E, Katz A, et al. Interleukin-6 gene transfection into Lewis lung carcinoma tumor cells suppresses the malignant phenotype and confers immunotherapeutic competence against parental metastatic cells. *Cancer Res* 1992;52(13):3679–3686.

90. Dranoff G, Mulligan RC. Gene transfer as cancer therapy. *Adv Immunol* 1995;58:417–454.

91. Dachs GU, Dougherty GJ, Stratford IJ, Chaplin DJ. Targeting gene therapy to cancer: a review. *Oncol Res* 1997;9(6-7):313–325.

92. Bergelson JM, Cunningham JA, Droguett G, et al. Isolation of a common receptor for Coxsackie B viruses and adenoviruses 2 and 5. *Science* 1997;275(5304):1320–1323.

93. Roelvink PW, Lizonova A, Lee JG, et al. The coxsackievirus-adenovirus receptor protein can function as a cellular attachment protein for adenovirus serotypes from subgroups A, C, D, E, and F. *J Virol* 1998;72(10):7909–7915.

94. Li Y, Pong RC, Bergelson JM, et al. Loss of adenoviral receptor expression in human bladder cancer cells: a potential impact on the efficacy of gene therapy. *Cancer Res* 1999;59(2):325–330.

95. Ferrari FK, Xiao X, McCarty D, Samulski RJ. New developments in the generation of Ad-free, high-titer rAAV gene therapy vectors. *Nat Med* 1997;3(11):1295–1297.

96. Pincus S, Tartaglia J, Paoletti E. Poxvirus-based vectors as vaccine candidates. *Biologicals* 1995;23(2):159–164.

97. Borrello I, Sotomayor EM, Cooke S, Levitsky HI. A universal granulocyte-macrophage colony-stimulating factor producing bystander cell line for use in the formulation of autologous tumor cell-based vaccines. *Hum Gene Ther* 1999;10:1983–1991.

98. Thomas MC, Greten TF, Pardoll DM, Jaffee EM. Enhanced tumor protection by GM-CSF expression at the site of an allogeneic vaccine. *Hum Gene Ther* 1998;9:835–843.

99. Caruso M, Pham-Nguyen K, Kwong YL, et al. Adenovirus-mediated interleukin-12 gene therapy for metastatic colon carcinoma. *Proc Natl Acad Sci U S A* 1996;93(21):11302–11306.

100. Chen SH, Shine HD, Goodman JC, Grossman RG, Woo SL. Gene therapy for brain tumors: regression of experimental gliomas by adenovirus-mediated gene transfer *in vivo*. *Proc Natl Acad Sci U S A* 1994;91(8):3054–3057.

101. Nabel GJ, Nabel EG, Yang ZY, et al. Direct gene transfer with DNA-liposome complexes in melanoma: expression, biologic activity, and lack of toxicity in humans. *Proc Natl Acad Sci U S A* 1993;90(23):11307–11311.

102. Lipshy KA, Kostuchenko PJ, Hamad GG, Bland CE, Barrett SK, Bear HD. Sensitizing T-lymphocytes for adoptive immunotherapy by vaccination with wild-type or cytokine gene-transduced melanoma. *Ann Surg Oncol* 1997;4(4):334–341.

103. Schmidt W, Schweighoffer T, Herbst E, et al. Cancer vaccines: the interleukin 2 dosage effect. *Proc Natl Acad Sci U S A* 1995;92(10):

4711–4714.

104. Villanueva MS, Fischer P, Feen K, Pamer EG. Efficiency of MHC class I antigen processing: a quantitative analysis. *Immunity* 1994;1(6):479–489.

105. Krummel MF, Allison JP. CTLLA-4 engagement inhibits IL-2 accumulation and cell cycle progression upon activation of resting T cells. *J Exp Med* 1996;183:2533–2540.

106. Waterhouse P, Penninger JM, Timms E, et al. Lymphoproliferative disorders with early lethality in mice deficient in CTLA-4. *Science* 1995;270(5238):985–988.

107. Tivol EA, Borriello F, Schweitzer AN, Lynch WP, Bluestone JA, Sharpe AH. Loss of CTLA-4 leads to massive lymphoproliferation and fatal multiorgan tissue destruction, revealing a critical negative regulatory role of CTLA-4. *Immunity* 1995;3(5):541–547.

108. Leach DR, Krummel MF, Allison JP. Enhancement of antitumor immunity by CTLA-4 blockade. *Science* 1996;271:1734–1736.

109. Kwon ED, Hurwitz AA, Foster BA, et al. Manipulation of T cell costimulatory and inhibitory signals for immunotherapy of prostate cancer. *Proc Natl Acad Sci U S A* 1997;94:8099–8103.

110. van Elsas A, Hurwitz AA, Allison JP. Combination immunotherapy of B16 melanoma using anti-cytoxic T lymphocyte-associated antigen 4 (CTLA-4) and granulocyte/macrophage colony-stimulating factor (GM-CSF)-producing vaccines induces rejection of subcutaneous and metastatic tumors accompanied by autoimmune depigmentation. *J Exp Med* 1999;190:355–366.

111. Hurwitz AA, Yu TF, Leach DR, Allison JP. CTLA-4 blockade synergizes with tumor-derived granulocyte-macrophage colony-stimulating factor for treatment of an experimental mammary carcinoma. *Proc Natl Acad Sci U S A* 1998;95(17):10067–10071.

112. Hurwitz A, Choi E, Fasso M, Allison JP. Combination vaccination and CTLA-4 blockade for spontaneous murine prostate cancer. *Cancer Res* 2000 (*in press*)

113. Kurts C, Carbone FR, Krummel MF, Koch KM, Miller JFAP, Heath WR. Signaling through CD30 protects against autoimmune diabetes mediated by CD8 cells. *Nature* 1999;398(6725):341–344.

114. Stingl G, Brocker EB, Mertelsmann R, et al. Phase I study to the immunotherapy of metastatic malignant melanoma by a cancer vaccine consisting of autologous cancer cells transfected with the human IL-2 gene. *J Mol Med* 1997;75(4):297–299.

115. Belli R, Arienti F, Sule-Suso J, et al. Active immunization of metastatic melanoma patients with interleukin-2-transduced allogeneic melanoma cells: evaluation of efficacy and tolerability. *Cancer Immunol Immunother* 1997;44(4):197–203.

116. Veelken H, Mackensen A, Lahn M, et al. A phase I clinical study of autologous tumor cells plus interleukin-2-gene-transfected allogeneic fibroblasts as a vaccine in patients with cancer. *Int J Cancer* 1997;70(3):269–277.

117. Bowman LC, Grossmann M, Rill D, et al. Interleukin-2 gene-modified allogeneic tumor cells for treatment of relapsed neuroblastoma. *Hum Gene Ther* 1998;9(9):1303–1311.

118. Suminami Y, Elder EM, Lotze MT, Whiteside TL. In situ interleukin-4 gene expression in cancer patients treated with genetically modified tumor vaccine. *J Immunother Emphasis Tumor Immunol* 1995;17(4):238–248.

119. Moller P, Sun Y, Dorbic T, et al. Vaccination with IL-7 gene-modified autologous melanoma cells can enhance the anti-melanoma lytic activity in peripheral blood of patients with a good clinical performance status: a clinical phase I study. *Br J Cancer* 1998;77(11):1907–1916.

120. Abdel-Wahab Z, Weltz C, Hester D, et al. A phase I clinical trial of immunotherapy with interferon-gamma gene-modified autologous melanoma cells: monitoring the humoral immune response. *Cancer* 1997;80(3):401–412.

121. Sun Y, Jurgovsky K, Moller P, et al. Vaccination with IL-12 gene-modified autologous melanoma cells: preclinical results and a first clinical phase I study. *Gene Ther* 1998;5(4):481–490.

122. Jaffee EM, Schutte M, Gossett J, et al. Development and characterization of a cytokine-secreting pancreatic adenocarcinoma vaccine from primary tumors for use in clinical trials. *Cancer J Sci Am* 1998;4(3):194–203.

123. Simons JW, Jaffee EM, Weber CE, et al. Bioactivity of autologous irradiated renal cell carcinoma vaccines generated by *ex vivo* granulocyte-macrophage colony-stimulating factor gene transfer. *Cancer Res* 1997;57(8):1537–1546.

124. Soiffer R, Lynch T, Mihm M, et al. Vaccination with irradiated autologous melanoma cells engineered to secrete human granulocyte-macrophage colony-stimulating factor generates potent antitumor immunity in patients with metastatic melanoma. *Proc Natl Acad*

Sci U S A 1998;95(22):13141–13146.

125. Simons JW, Mikhak B. *Ex vivo* gene therapy using cytokine-transduced tumor vaccines: molecular and clinical pharmacology. *Semin Oncol* 1998;25(6):661–676.

126. Mahvi DM, Shi FS, Yang NS, et al. Immunization by particle-mediated transfer of the GM-CSF gene into autologous tumor cells in melanoma or sarcoma patients: report of a Phase I/IB study. *Clin Cancer Res* (in press).

18.3

CANCER VACCINES: CLINICAL APPLICATIONS

Peptides and Protein Vaccines

STEVEN A. ROSENBERG

PEPTIDE PRESENTATION ON MAJOR HISTOCOMPATIBILITY COMPLEX MOLECULES

The T-cell receptor on lymphocytes with antitumor activity recognize a unique conformation on the tumor cell surface comprised of a peptide nestled in the groove of a surface major histocompatibility complex (MHC) molecule (1,2). CD8$^+$ T cells recognize peptides attached to class I molecules, and CD4 cells recognize peptides attached to class II molecules. Class I MHC molecules consist of a heavy chain of 45,000 d and a noncovalently attached beta-2-microglobulin of 12,000 d. There are three major HLA class I alleles called *HLA-A, -B*, and *-C*. Class II molecules are heterodimers consisting of an alpha and beta chain of approximately 30,000 d each, and the three class II alleles are called *HLA-DR, -DQ*, and *-DP*. X-ray diffraction crystallography has characterized the three-dimensional structure of class I and II molecules and their peptide-binding sites.

The cellular processes resulting in the binding of peptides to class I and II molecules are different. The great majority of class I–presented peptides result from the degradation of cytosolic proteins by a multi-unit structure in the cytoplasm called the *proteosome*. Cleaved peptides are transported into the lumen of the endoplasmic reticulum (ER) by the transporter associated with processing molecule, possibly protected from complete degradation by chaperone heat-shock proteins before entering the ER. The trimmed peptides are bound to the groove of the

assembled class I molecule in the ER, and the complex is transported to the cell surface.

Most peptides that are loaded onto class II molecules are derived from proteins that are endocytosed into the cell and are degraded in intracellular compartments in endosomal or lysosomal structures. The alpha and beta chains of class II molecules are assembled in the ER and are bound to a chaperone-like molecule called *invariant chain*. A stretch of the invariant chain called the *CLIP peptide* binds in the groove of the class II molecule to prevent premature peptide binding. A targeting sequence in the cytoplasmic tail of the invariant chain also appears to be responsible for transport of class II molecules from the ER to endosomal or lysosomal intracellular compartments where they can bind peptides and are then transported to the cell surface. Although the great majority of class I molecules are bound to peptides from endogenous cellular proteins and the great majority of class II peptides are derived from endogenous endocytosed proteins, there are examples of endogenous proteins entering the class II pathway and exogenous proteins entering the class I pathway.

Thus, a variety of steps can affect which peptides are found on the cell surface, including (a) the presence of endogenous and exogenous proteins, (b) the appropriate degradation of these proteins in intracellular compartments, (c) the ability of the degraded peptides to bind in the groove of the particular HLA class I or II molecules present in that patient, and (d) the successful transport of these molecules to the cell surface. Absence or dysfunction of any of these steps can lead to defective peptide presentation on the tumor cell surface.

The interaction of the three-dimensional structure of the peptide-binding groove of the class I and II molecules with the conformation of the associated peptide determines which peptides can bind to particular HLA molecules as well as the affinity of this interaction. Particular sites in the groove of HLA molecules (called *anchor sites*) play a major role in determining binding of the peptide to the MHC molecule. Other amino acid residues are more involved in interacting with the T-cell receptor, leading to recognition of this peptide and MHC complex. Analysis of known peptides recognized by T cells as well as the analysis of sequences of pooled peptides eluted from MHC molecules have helped to determine the characteristics of peptides associated with particular MHC molecules (3–5). The relatively uniform length of these peptides (e.g., eight to ten amino acids for most class I molecules and slightly longer peptides for class II molecules) has enabled the definition of these allele-specific motifs for most of the common class I and II specificities. An example of one such peptide-binding analysis derived from studies by Rammensee and colleagues (3) is shown in Table 1. Examples of the peptide ligands derived from pooled sequences and from known T-cell antigenic epitopes are shown. From these and other studies, it was determined that position 2 was an anchor residue favoring a leucine or methionine, and position 9 was a second anchor residue favoring binding of a valine or leucine to the HLA-A*0201 molecule. Other residues with a lesser degree of preferred binding to HLA-A2 were also found. Examples of predominant anchor-binding residues for HLA-A1, -A3, and -A24 are shown in Table 2. Knowledge of these allele-specific motifs has facilitated the identification of the immunogenic peptides of tumor antigens.

IDENTIFICATION OF IMMUNOGENIC PEPTIDES FROM TUMOR ANTIGENS

Three main techniques have been used to identify peptides derived from tumor antigens. The most common method has been the analysis of synthetic peptides based on the known amino acid sequence of tumor antigens detected by T cells. Most tumor antigens that have been characterized were identified by cloning the genes that encode proteins recognized by T cells with antitumor activity (see Chapter 16). The amino acid sequences of these proteins are analyzed, and peptides conforming to the allele-specific motifs of the particular HLA-restriction molecules used by these antigens can then be synthesized and pulsed onto antigen-presenting cells (APCs) and tested for recognition by the antitumor T cells. Estimates of the avidity of T cells for these peptide antigens were determined by pulsing differing concentrations of peptides to APCs and determining the minimal concentrations required for recognition. Algorithms developed to predict the peptides most likely to bind to individual MHC molecules have been useful in facilitating peptide identification (6). Alternatively, it has been possible to use exonuclease digestion to produce fragments that can narrow the areas within the amino acid sequence that contain the immunogenic peptides (7).

A second technique also dependent on the availability of T cells capable of recognizing tumor antigens, but that does not depend on knowing the identity of the antigen, uses the direct elution and identification of peptides from tumor cells. In this approach, class I or II molecules are purified from tumor cells by affinity chromatography, peptides are released from the MHC molecules by acid elution and are fractionated by high-performance liquid chromatography (HPLC) (8,9). These HPLC fractions are pulsed to APCs containing the appropriate MHC molecule, and T cells that recognize tumor antigens can be used to identify the fractions containing the immunogenic peptides. Further fractionation of the peptides by microcapillary HPLC with direct elution into a triple quadruple mass spectrometer can be used to further identify fractions containing immunogenic peptides. Automated Edman degradation or collision-activated dissociation analysis can then be used to identify the amino acid sequence of the peptides. Finally, the ability of these peptides to be recognized by antitumor T cells after pulsing onto APCs can confirm the identity of the appropriate tumor peptide. A peptide at amino acid positions 280 to 288 of the gp100 molecule was identified as a melanoma antigen using this technique (9).

A third approach to the identification of immunogenic tumor peptides uses what has been called *reverse immunology* and does not depend on the availability of T cells capable of recognizing tumor antigens. In this approach, candidate proteins thought to have a high probability of representing tumor antigens because of their overexpression or unique distribution on tumor cells are identified and their amino acid sequence analyzed for the presence of peptides with motifs capable of binding to HLA molecules. Based on these allele-specific motifs, multiple peptides are synthesized and *in vitro* sensitization techniques can be used to generate T cells capable of recognizing the particular peptide. The critical step of this process is the test of whether cloned T cells raised *in vitro* against this synthetic peptide can recognize tumor cells in an MHC-restricted fashion. Using this reverse immunology approach, immunogenic peptides derived from the melanocyte-stimulating hormone receptor as well as tyrosinase-related protein-2 (TRP-2) have been identified as human melanoma antigens restricted by HLA-A2 (10,11).

PEPTIDE VACCINES IN PATIENTS WITH MELANOMA

The majority of tumor antigens that have been described were derived from melanomas and thus initial experience with peptide vaccination has been in patients with metastatic melanoma. Peptides identified in the MAGE-1 and MAGE-3 tumor antigens (see Chapter 16.1) were used in pilot studies in melanoma patients whose tumors were shown to express MAGE-3 protein as evaluated by reverse transcriptase-polymerase chain reaction analysis. Marchand et al. reported on 12 patients with evaluable melanoma metastases who were treated with an HLA-A1–restricted peptide (EVDPIGHLY) injected at monthly intervals (12). The peptide was injected in saline at a dose of 100 or 300 mg divided between two sites subcutaneously, and 13 to 30 mg given intradermally. Of the 12 melanoma patients included in this study, six were withdrawn from treatment after one or two injections because of rapid progression of disease. Six remaining patients received at least three immunizations, and three of these patients

TABLE 1. PEPTIDE BINDING TO HLA-A*0201

Position

		1	2	3	4	5	6	7	8	9						Source
Anchor or auxiliary anchor residues	—	—	L	—	—	—	V	—	—	V	—	—	—	—	—	—
	—	—	M	—	—	—	—	—	—	L	—	—	—	—	—	—
Preferred residues	—	—	—	—	E	—	—	—	K	—	—	—	—	—	—	—
	—	—	—	—	K	—	—	—	—	—	—	—	—	—	—	—
Other residues	—	—	I	—	A	G	I	I	A	E	—	—	—	—	—	—
	—	—	L	—	Y	P	K	L	Y	S	—	—	—	—	—	—
	—	—	F	—	F	D	Y	T	H	—	—	—	—	—	—	—
	—	—	K	—	P	T	N	—	—	—	—	—	—	—	—	—
	—	—	M	—	M	—	G	—	—	—	—	—	—	—	—	—
	—	—	Y	—	S	—	F	—	—	—	—	—	—	—	—	—
	—	—	V	—	R	—	V	—	—	—	—	—	—	—	—	—
	—	—	—	—	—	H	—	—	—	—	—	—	—	—	—	—
Examples for ligands	—	S	L	L	P	A	I	V	E	L	—	—	—	—	—	Protein phosphatase 2A 389–397
	—	Y	L	L	P	A	I	V	H	I	—	—	—	—	—	ATP-dependent RNA helicase 148–156
	—	T	L	W	V	D	P	Y	E	V	—	—	—	—	—	B-cell translocation gene 1 protein 103–111
	—	S	X	P	S	G	G	X	G	V	—	—	—	—	—	Unknown
	—	G	X	V	P	F	X	V	S	V	—	—	—	—	—	Unknown
	—	S	X	X	V	R	A	X	E	V	—	—	—	—	—	Unknown
	—	K	X	N	E	P	V	X	X	X	—	—	—	—	—	Unknown
	—	A	L	W	G	F	F	P	V	X+	—	—	—	—	—	Unknown mouse protein
	—	L	L	D	V	P	T	A	A	V	—	—	—	—	—	IP-30 signal sequence 27–35
	L	L	L	D	V	P	T	A	A	V	—	—	—	—	—	IP-30 signal sequence 26–35
	L	L	L	D	V	P	T	A	A	V	Q	A	—	—	—	IP-30 signal sequence 26–37
	L	L	L	D	V	P	T	A	A	V	Q	—	—	—	—	IP-30 signal sequence 26–36
	—	V	L	F	R	G	G	P	R	G	L	L	A	V	A	SSR α signal sequence 12–25
	—	M	V	D	G	T	L	L	L	L	—	—	—	—	—	HLA-E signal sequence 1–9
	—	Y	M	N	G	T	M	S	Q	V+	—	—	—	—	—	Tyrosinase 369–377
	—	M	L	L	S	V	P	L	L	L	G	—	—	—	—	Calreticulin signal sequence 1–10
	—	S	L	L	G	L	L	V	E	V[a]	—	—	—	—	—	Unknown
	—	A	L	L	P	P	I	N	I	L[a]	—	—	—	—	—	Unknown
	—	T	L	I	K	I	Q	H	T	L[a]	—	—	—	—	—	Unknown
	—	A	L	I	V	G	X	N	D	D[a]	—	—	—	—	—	Unknown
	—	H	L	I	D	Y	L	V	T	S[a]	—	—	—	—	—	Carboxypeptidase M 91–99
	—	I	L	A	P	P	V	V	K	L	L	V[a]	F	P	—	Unknown
	—	A	L	F	P	Q	L	V	K	L[a]	—	—	—	—	—	Unknown
	—	G	I	L	G	F	V	F	T	L[a]	—	—	—	—	—	Influenza matrix protein 58–66
T-cell epitopes	—	I	L	K	E	P	V	H	G	V	—	—	—	—	—	HIV-1 RT 476–484
	—	I	L	G	F	V	F	T	L	T	V	—	—	—	—	Influenza matrix protein 59–68
	—	L	L	F	G	Y	P	V	Y	V	—	—	—	—	—	HTLV-1 tax 11–19
	—	G	L	S	P	T	V	W	L	S	V	—	—	—	—	Hepatitis BsAg 348–357
	—	W	L	S	L	L	V	P	F	V	—	—	—	—	—	Hepatitis BsAg 335–343
	—	F	L	P	S	D	F	F	P	S	V	—	—	—	—	Hepatitis B nucleocapsid 18–27
	—	C	L	G	G	L	L	T	M	V	—	—	—	—	—	EBC LMP2 426–434
	—	F	I	A	G	N	S	A	Y	E	Y	V	—	—	—	HCMV glycoprotein B 618–628
	—	K	L	G	E	F	Y	N	Q	M	M	—	—	—	—	Influenza B NP 85–94
	—	K	L	V	A	L	G	I	N	A	V	—	—	—	—	HCV-1 1406–1415
	—	D	L	M	G	Y	I	P	L	V	—	—	—	—	—	HCV core 132–140
	—	R	L	V	T	L	K	D	I	V	—	—	—	—	—	HPV 11 E7 4–12
	—	M	L	L	A	L	L	Y	C	L	—	—	—	—	—	Tyrosinase 1–9
	—	A	A	G	I	G	I	L	T	V	—	—	—	—	—	Melan A/MART-1
	—	Y	L	E	P	G	P	V	T	A	—	—	—	—	—	pmel 17/gp100
	—	I	L	D	G	T	A	T	L	R	L	—	—	—	—	pmel 17/gp100

ATP, adenosine triphosphate; BsAg, hepatitis B surface antigen; EBC, ; HCMV, human cytomegalovirus; HCV-1, hepatitis C virus type 1; HIV-1, human immunodeficiency virus 1; HPV, human papillomavirus; HTLV, human T-cell lymphoma/leukemia virus; RT, reverse transcriptase.
[a]Class I ligands allocated to A2 by motif. Also a T-cell epitope.
From Rammensee H, Friede R, Stevanovic S. MHC ligands and peptide motifs: first listing. *Immunogenetics* 1995;41:178, with permission.

were reported to have some clinical response to the immunizations. One patient had a mixed response but died 1 month after the third treatment. One patient had a partial response of multiple 1- to 3-mm cutaneous metastases, and an additional patient was reported to have a partial response of lung metastases. Also treated in this protocol were two melanoma patients who had no evaluable disease, one patient with non–small-cell lung cancer and one patient with bladder cancer. Neither of the two latter patients showed a clinical response. None of the patients in this study developed evidence of cytotoxic T lymphocyte (CTL) precursors

TABLE 2. PEPTIDE BINDING TO HLA-A MOLECULES

HLA-A1

	Position									
	1	2	3	4	5	6	7	8	9	10
Anchor or auxiliary anchor residues	—	T	D	P	—	—	L	—	Y	—
	—	S	E	—	—	—	—	—	—	—
Other preferred residues	—	L	—	G	G	G	—	—	—	—
	—	—	—	I	N	V	—	—	—	—
	—	—	—	—	Y	I	—	—	—	—

HLA-A3

	Position									
	1	2	3	4	5	6	7	8	9	10
Anchor or auxiliary anchor residues	—	L	F	—	—	I	I	—	K	K
	—	V	Y	—	—	M	L	—	Y	—
	—	M	—	—	—	Γ	M	—	F	—
	—	—	—	—	—	V	F	—	—	—
	—	—	—	—	—	L	—	—	—	—
Other preferred residues	I	—	—	—	I	T	—	Q	—	—
	—	—	—	—	P	—	—	S	—	—
	—	—	—	—	V	—	—	T	—	—
	—	—	—	—	K	—	—	K	—	—

HLA-A24

	Position									
	1	2	3	4	5	6	7	8	9	10
Anchor or auxiliary anchor residues	—	Y	—	—	I	F	—	—	I	—
	—	—	—	—	V	—	—	—	L	—
	—	—	—	—	—	—	—	—	F	—
Other preferred residues	—	—	N	D	—	—	Q	E	—	—
	—	—	E	P	—	—	N	K	—	—
	—	—	L	—	—	—	—	—	—	—
	—	—	M	—	—	—	—	—	—	—
	—	—	P	—	—	—	—	—	—	—
	—	—	G	—	—	—	—	—	—	—

From Rammensee H, Friede R, Stevanovic S. MHC ligands and peptide motifs: first listing. *Immunogenetics* 1995;41:178, with permission.

TABLE 3. HLA-A*0201-RESTRICTED CYTOKINE RELEASE BY PERIPHERAL BLOOD MONONUCLEAR CELL CULTURES SENSITIZED *IN VITRO* WITH MART-1:27–35

	IFN-γ Release (pg/5 $\times$ 10^5 effectors/24 hr)	
	Before Immunization	After Immunization
Patient Number	T2 + MART-1	T2 + MART-1
1	476	7,839
2	10	360
3	498	6,785
4	1,614	8,580
5	5,976	27,080
6	262	25,620
7	131	5,952
8	0	7,499
9	12	960
10	696	23,760
11	1,146	3,240
12	82	1,570
13	1,664	2,668
14	46	192
15	540	4,336
16	0	64
17	1,864	3,264
18	60	8,848

IFN-γ, interferon-γ.

Release of cytokine is expressed as the amount of IFN-γ (pg/mL) secreted by 5 $\times$ 10^5 effector cells/mL cytotoxic T lymphocyte co-cultured for 24 hours in the presence of 5 $\times$ 10^5 relevant (T2 + MART-1:$_{27-35}$) stimulators per milliliter. The assay was performed after three *in vitro* stimulations.

From Cormier JN, Salgaller ML, Prevette T, et al. Enhancement of cellular immunity in melanoma patients immunized with a peptide from MART-1/Melan A. *Cancer J Sci Am* 1997;3:37, with permission.

in the blood, including analysis of patients who appeared to show clinical evidence of tumor regression.

Chakraborty et al. treated 17 patients with melanoma, including 11 with metastatic disease using autologous APCs pulsed with a MAGE-1, HLA-A1–restricted peptide (EADPTGHSY) given intradermally monthly for 4 months (13). Thirteen of these patients completed all four immunizations, and one patient was reported to show a partial regression of a subcutaneous nodule. Monitoring of biologic response using conventional natural killer or CTL assays in these patients revealed no consistent differences between pre- and postimmunization peripheral blood lymphocytes. Nestle et al. reported four patients who received HLA-A1– and HLA-A3–restricted MAGE-3 peptides pulsed to APCs and two additional patients who received MAGE-3 peptides in conjunction with HLA-A2–restricted melanoma differentiation antigen peptides also pulsed on APCs (14). In the Nestle et al. study these cells were injected into lymph nodes, and one of these six patients was reported to have a partial response.

The predominant antigens recognized by tumor-infiltrating lymphocytes (TILs) obtained from patients with metastatic melanoma are the melanoma and melanocyte differentiation antigens (see Chapter 16.2). Pilot studies have been performed in the Surgery Branch, National Cancer Institute (NCI) immunizing restricted peptides from the MART-1 and gp100 melanoma antigens (15–17). In one study, 18 HLA-A*0201 patients with metastatic melanoma were immunized with the MART-1:27-35 peptide (AAGIGILTV) in incomplete Freund's adjuvant (IFA) subcutaneously every 3 weeks (15). Evidence of significant immunization to the MART-1 peptide as well as to MART-1–expressing tumors was obtained in most patients, although only one of these patients developed a partial response (ongoing at longer than 4 years). Lymphoid precursors reactive with the MART-1 peptide were detected using *in vitro* assays based on repeated *in vitro* sensitization with autologous peripheral blood mononuclear cells (PBMCs) pulsed with the MART-1:27-35 peptide. In 15 of these patients, postvaccination CTL cultures exhibited more than a threefold increase in specific release of interferon gamma compared with prevaccination samples (Table 3). No dose response was seen in patients receiving from 0.1 to 10 mg per injection. Because of the low precursor frequency both before and after immunization, it was necessary to perform three *in vitro* stimulations of PBMCs to detect the precursors seen in these patients. This increase in peptide reactivity after immunization was also reflected in increased recognition of MART-1–expressing melanomas (Table 4). Thus, it appeared that the normal nonmutated MART-1 peptide in IFA was capable of immunizing the majority of patients after immunization, although only one patient in this trial developed a partial response.

A similar study in the Surgery Branch, NCI evaluated the ability to immunize HLA-A2 metastatic melanoma patients

TABLE 4. HLA-A*0201–RESTRICTED RECOGNITION OF NATURALLY PROCESSED MART-1 ANTIGEN BY PERIPHERAL BLOOD MONONUCLEAR CELL (PBMC) CULTURES SENSITIZED *IN VITRO* WITH MART-1:27–35

| | IFN-γ Release (pg/5 × 10⁵ effectors/24 hr) | | | |
| | Before Immunization | | After Immunization | |
Patient Number	624.38 (HLA-A2⁺)	624.28 (HLA-A2⁻)	624.38 (HLA-A2⁺)	624.28 (HLA-A2⁻)
1	0	0	6,708	0
3	131	38	6,215	0
6	0	0	16,936	480
7	32	0	4,998	16
8	0	0	4,098	0
10	2,180	1,372	24,356	240
11	0	0	5,806	27
12	0	0	2,384	0
15	0	0	6,761	0
17	0	0	5,009	202
18	0	0	7,454	0

IFN-γ, interferon-γ.
IFN-γ release by PBMC cultures in the presence of the melanoma cell clones 624.38 (MART-1+ and HLA-A*0201+) and 624.28 (MART-1+ and HLA-A*0201–).
From Cormier JN, Salgaller ML, Prevette T, et al. Enhancement of cellular immunity in melanoma patients immunized with a peptide from MART-1/Melan A. *Cancer J Sci Am* 1997;3:37, with permission.

using one of three different immunodominant peptides from the gp100 antigen, gp100:209-217 (ITDQVPFSY), gp100:280-288 (YLEPGPVTA), or the gp100:154-162 peptide (KTWGQYWQV) (16). These peptides were injected in IFA at doses between 1 and 10 mg subcutaneously every 3 weeks. Of the 28 patients immunized with one of these peptides, one patient receiving the gp100:209-217 peptide had a complete response of cutaneous metastases that lasted 4 months. All of the patients receiving the gp100:209-217 or the gp100:280-288 peptide, but none receiving the gp100:154-162 peptide, showed evidence of *in vivo* immunization when multiple *in vitro* sensitizations to compare pre- and postvaccination PBMC samples were performed. Thus, these studies of the nonmutated MART-1 and gp100 peptides revealed that significant increases in circulating precursor levels could be induced by immunization, although clinical responses were rare.

Jager et al. reported on the treatment of patients with metastatic melanoma using combinations of peptides from the MART-1, tyrosinase, and gp100 tumor antigens (18,19). Patients in this trial received 100 μg of each peptide intrader-

mally weekly for 4 weeks. No clinical responses were seen in six treated patients. Several patients showed evidence of precursor development against the MART-1 and tyrosinase peptides, but no reactivity was seen against the gp100 peptides. In a subsequent study, these same investigators reported on three patients who received intradermal injections of these melanoma-associated peptides along with the daily systemic administration of granulocyte-macrophage colony-stimulating factor (GM-CSF) starting 3 days before immunization until 2 days after immunization (20). Delayed-type hypersensitivity responses were seen in each of the patients, and each of these three patients were reported to have experienced clinical regression of disease. There has, however, been no follow-up study of this approach since 1996, and thus the reproducibility of these findings remains to be determined.

A pilot trial has also been conducted using melanoma and melanocyte differentiation antigens from MART-1, gp100, and tyrosinase pulsed onto autologous dendritic cells from HLA-A*0201 patients with metastatic melanoma (14). These peptide-pulsed dendritic cells were injected directly into lymph nodes at weekly intervals, and clinical response was evaluated. Eight patients received immunization with autologous–dendritic cells pulsed with A2 peptides, including two patients who received dendritic cells pulsed with A1 and A2 peptides. One complete response and one partial response were seen in these eight patients, and several developed delayed-type hypersensitivity skin reactions to peptide.

MODIFICATION OF MELANOMA PEPTIDES TO INCREASE IMMUNOGENICITY

In contrast to most immunogenic viral peptides that have high binding affinity for their corresponding MHC molecules (21–23), most of the immunogenic melanoma and melanocyte differentiation antigen peptides have a modest or relatively low affinity for the HLA-A*0201 molecule (24,25). Of the four immunodominant HLA-A*0201–restricted peptides derived from the MART and gp100 antigens, three of the four peptides have a suboptimal amino acid residue at anchor position two and the other peptide has a suboptimal residue at anchor position nine (Table 5). It is likely that T-cell precursors capable of binding peptides with high affinity for HLA-A*0201 are deleted during lymphocyte maturation in the thymus and that only T cells with relatively weak recognition of peptides survive negative selection (26,27). Thus, although a correlation has been demonstrated between immunogenicity and peptide binding affinity to class I

TABLE 5. PEPTIDE BINDING TO HLA-A2

Anchor	2⁰	1⁰	2⁰	—	—	—	—	—	1⁰
	1	2	3	4	5	6	7	8	9
	—	Leu	—	—	—	—	—	—	Val
Preferred amino acids	—	Met	—	—	—	—	—	—	Leu
MART-1:27–35	Ala	Ala	Gly	Ile	Gly	Ile	Leu	Thr	Val
gp100:154–162	Lys	Thr	Try	Gly	Gln	Tyr	Try	Gln	Val
gp100:209–217	Ile	Thr	Asp	Gln	Val	Pro	Phe	Ser	Val
gp100:280–288	Tyr	Leu	Glu	Pro	Gly	Pro	Val	Thr	Ala

TABLE 6. INITIAL SCREENING OF MODIFIED gp100:209-217 PEPTIDES FOR RECOGNITION BY TIL AND CTL INDUCTION

G9$_{209}$ Peptide Modification	Sequence	HLA-A*0201 Binding Affinity[a] ID$_{50}$ (parent) ID$_{50}$ (mod) (pg/mL)	Recognition of TIL620[b] (1 µM peptide) IFN-γ	Patient 1 % specific lysis (40:1 E:T)	Patient 2 IFN-γ[d] (pg/mL)		Patient 3 IFN-γ[d] (pg/mL)	
Parent	ITDQVPFSV	1.0	2,672	6(0)[e]	—	2	—	346
2L	ILDQVPFSV	52	2,316	ND	145	—	46	—
2M	IMDQVPFSV	9.0	2,574	2(0)	—	555	—	438
2I	IIDQVPFSV	4.3	2,266	10(0)	—	4	—	19
1F	FTDQVPFSV	2.8	2,541	ND	6	—	41	—
1W	WTDQVPFSV	0.24	1,994	ND	0	—	0	—
1Y	YTDQVPFSV	2.0	2,382	ND	0	—	31	—
3W	ITWQVPFSV	5.0	113	ND	ND	—	ND	—
3F	ITFQVPFSV	2.6	562	ND	ND	—	ND	—
3Y	ITYQVPFSV	5.2	257	ND	ND	—	ND	—
3A	ITAQVPFSV	1.8	120	ND	ND	—	ND	—
3M	ITMQVPFSV	4.3	2,214	ND	ND	—	ND	—
3S	ITSQVPFSV	0.27	1,212	ND	ND	—	ND	—
2L3W	ILWQVPFSV	102	329	ND	0	—	8	—
2L3F	ILFQVPFSV	86	243	ND	ND	—	ND	—
2L3Y	ILYQVPFSV	35	120	ND	ND	—	ND	—
2L3A	ILAQVPFSV	15	163	ND	ND	—	ND	—
2L3M	ILMQVPFSV	23	564	ND	ND	—	ND	—
2L3S	ILSQVPFSV	8.6	464	ND	ND	—	ND	—
1W2L	WLDQVPFSV	15	2,359	ND	0	—	195	—
1F2L	FLDQVPFSV	79	2,688	85(0)	—	0	—	2
1Y2L	YLDQVPFSV	76	2,445	ND	2	—	103	—

CTL, cytotoxic T lymphocyte; IFN-γ, interferon-γ; ND, not done; TIL, tumor-infiltrating lymphocyte.

[a]Peptide binding affinity to HLA-A*0201 was evaluated by measuring the concentration of peptide necessary to inhibit the binding of a standard radiolabeled peptide by 50% (ID$_{50}$). The ratio (R) presented here indicates the relative HLA-A*0201 binding affinity of the modified peptide (mod) compared to the parent peptide (parent):R> indicates the modified peptide bound with greater affinity than the parent peptide. ID$_{50}$ (G9$_{209}$ parent) = 172 nM.

[b]IFN-γ release by TIL in the presence of T2 cells preincubated with 1 µM peptide. IFN-γ (T2 cells without exogenous peptide) = 454 pg/mL.

[c]Cytotoxicity or IFN-γ release by CTLs in the presence of T2 cells preincubated with 1 µM peptide.

[d]IFN-γ release by CTLs above the background of T2 cells without exogenous peptide.

[e]Values in parentheses indicate background percent cytolysis of T2 cells without exogenous peptide.

From Parkhurst MR, Salgaller ML, Southwood S, et al. Improved induction of melanoma-reactive CTL with peptides from the melanoma antigen gp100 modified at HLA-A*0201-binding residues. *J Immunol* 1996;157:2539, with permission.

MHC molecules for peptides derived from viral antigens, this appears not to be the case for the immunogenicity of peptides derived from nonmutated self determinants (21–24).

The relatively low binding affinity of the immunodominant self-peptides suggested that amino acid substitutions at anchor residues could increase binding affinity without interfering with peptide recognition and therefore increase the immunogenicity of the peptide (28,29). These modified peptides have been referred to as *heteroclytic peptides*. Parkhurst et al. studied a large number of synthetic peptides with one or two amino acid substitutions of the gp100:209-217 peptide designed to increase binding affinity to the HLA-A*0201 molecule (25). An example is shown in Table 6. The relative binding affinity of each synthetic peptide to HLA-A*0201 was evaluated based on the inhibition of binding of a standard radiolabeled peptide to the purified HLA-A*0201 molecule. The relative binding affinity of the leucine modification instead of threonine at the second position resulted in a peptide with a 52-fold higher binding affinity compared to the native peptide and yet was recognized as well as the native peptide by a specific TIL. CTLs induced by *in vitro* sensitization using the modified peptide exhibited superior recognition of the native peptide compared to CTLs raised with the native peptide. Similarly, a peptide with a modification of methionine at the second position was more effective than the

native peptide in inducing CTLs reactive with the native peptide *in vitro*.

On the basis of these *in vitro* studies, a pilot clinical protocol was performed in the Surgery Branch, NCI in which HLA-A*0201 patients with metastatic melanoma were immunized with the gp100:209-217 (210 M) modified peptide (M substituted for T at the second anchor position, amino acid 210) (17). Using a stringent *in vitro* assay comparing pre- and postimmunization samples after a single *in vitro* exposure to peptide, only two of eight patients immunized with the native peptide showed evidence of successful immunization compared to 10 of 11 patients immunized with the modified peptide. A detailed example of one such assay is shown in Table 7, and the results of the *in vitro* monitoring of all 11 patients who received the modified peptide is shown in Table 8. Increase in precursors was also seen against HLA-A*0201–matched tumors and not against HLA-A*0201–negative tumors (Table 9). Only mixed responses were seen in patients receiving the modified peptide alone in IFA; however, when interleukin 2 (IL-2) was administered along with the modified peptide in IFA, 42% of 31 patients showed an objective anticancer response (17). This 42% response rate appeared higher than the 17% response rate seen in studies of patients using IL-2 alone (30) or the 15% response rate in 62 melanoma patients receiving the same high-dose IL-2 concurrently at the same insti-

TABLE 7. SPECIFICITY OF REACTIVITY AGAINST gp209-217 PEPTIDE AND HLA-A2⁺ MELANOMAS

Number of Immunizations	In Vitro[a] Sensitization with Peptide	T2	T2(280)	T2(flu)	T2(209)	501 (A2+) (pg IFN-γ/mL)	SK23 (A2+)	624.28 (A2–)	888 (A2–)
None	209-2M	135	102	230	146	195	180	89	115
	209	118	90	238	84	148	231	162	261
	Flu	178	123	35,570[b]	124	290	284	172	282
2	209-2M	86	74	61	24,150	72,780	43,250	124	33
	209	86	62	165	9,890	25,710	19,480	104	98
	Flu	121	118	36,460	132	313	448	85	362

The "Stimulator" header spans the T2 through 888 columns.

IFN-γ, interferon-γ.
[a]Day 11 after culture with 1 µg/mL peptide; peripheral blood mononuclear cells were tested for IFN-γ release after culture with tumor or T2 cells pulsed with peptide.
[b]In this and subsequent tables, values greater than 100 pg IFN-γ mL and at least twice that of all controls are underlined.
From Rosenberg SA, Yang JC, Schwartzentruber DJ, et al. Immunologic and therapeutic evaluation of a synthetic vaccine for the treatment of patients with metastatic melanoma. *Nat Med* 1998;4:321, with permission.

tution but not with peptide immunization. A randomized trial is necessary to test whether immunization with the modified peptide can increase the responses seen when IL-2 is administered concurrently with peptide.

The mechanisms by which immunization with the modified peptide in IFA resulted in high circulating levels of cellular immunity against the native peptide as well as against melanoma cells is under intensive study. The emulsification of pep-

TABLE 8. REACTIVITY OF PERIPHERAL BLOOD MONONUCLEAR CELLS (PBMCS) FROM PATIENTS IMMUNIZED WITH 209-2M PEPTIDE IN INCOMPLETE FREUND'S ADJUVANT

Patient	Experiment	T2	T2(280)	T2(209)	T2(209-2M)	T2 (pg IFN-γ/mL)[b]	T2(280)	T2(209)	T2(209-2M)
1	1	21	22	12	20	42	37	6,897	57,060
2	1	58	56	66	50	54	48	1,851	4,012
	2	1	4	2	ND	30	22	>1,000	ND
3	1	33	26	33	35	46	53	56	54
	2	145	127	124	ND	49	36	46	ND
4	1	133	123	184	213	40	35	2,631	6,086
	2	50	36	41	43	45	52	1,618	3,751
	3	351	299	501	470	86	825	944	1,057
5	1	28	30	21	24	41	35	4,366	6,402
	2	154	156	152	142	128	129	295	323
	3	29	18	37	32	27	22	856	1,126
6	1	38	28	24	31	44	47	152	671
	2	154	166	210	153	128	72	662	887
	3	96	61	117	127	22	14	2,374	5,407
7	1	44	66	72	82	104	81	4,424	5,411
	2	10	8	13	16	197	224	1,293	1,583
	3	127	105	ND	120	61	67	1,244	ND
8	1	ND	ND	ND	ND	17	25	845	ND
	2	1,553	562	719	ND	79	78	2,326	ND
	3	ND	ND	ND	ND	43	ND	1,768	ND
9	1	345	337	355	ND	209	183	2,253	ND
	2	13	13	10	ND	229	262	1,550	ND
	3	1,434	816	513	ND	495	517	2,408	ND
10	1	247	283	413	ND	29	39	1,271	ND
	2	135	102	146	ND	86	74	24,150	ND
	3	117	147	150	ND	6	9	39,690	ND
11	1	53	53	56	ND	65	71	154	ND
	2	46	50	47	ND	29	39	63	ND
	3	ND	ND	ND	ND	87	83	205	ND

The "Before Immunization" header spans the T2, T2(280), T2(209) columns; "Assay Stimulator" spans T2(209-2M) and T2 (pg IFN-γ/mL)[b]; "After Immunization[a]" spans T2(280), T2(209), T2(209-2M).

IFN-γ, interferon-γ; ND, not done.
[a]Day 11 to 13 after culture with 209-2M peptide, PBMCs were tested for IFN-γ release after 24-hour incubation with peptide-pulsed T2 cells.
[b]Patient 1 after one immunization; all other patients after two immunizations.
From Rosenberg SA, Yang JC, Schwartzentruber DJ, et al. Immunologic and therapeutic evaluation of a synthetic vaccine for the treatment of patients with metastatic melanoma. *Nat Med* 1998;4:321, with permission.

TABLE 9. REACTIVITY AGAINST TUMOR CELLS OF PERIPHERAL BLOOD MONONUCLEAR CELLS (PBMCS) FROM PATIENTS BEFORE AND AFTER IMMUNIZATION WITH 209-2M PEPTIDE IN INCOMPLETE FREUND'S ADJUVANT

Patient	Number of Immunizations	Stimulator[a]						
		T2	T2 (280)	T2 (209) (pg IFN-γ/mL)	501-mel (A2+)	SK23-mel (A2+)	888-mel (A2–)	624.28-mel (A2–)
7	0	169	175	220	28	72	84	51
	2	209	243	2,555	1,211	2,037	98	60
8	0	528	691	729	70	640	933	806
	4	202	284	13,600	11,580	14,720	408	489
9	0	13	13	10	ND	ND	ND	ND
	4	229	590	3,987	676	889	291	235
10	0	117	147	150	19	90	39	42
	4	15	18	24,040	23,860	21,580	2	4
11	0	46	50	47	11	39	14	17
	4	29	30	106	5	43	4	10

IFN-γ, interferon-γ; ND, not done.

[a]PBMCs incubated with gp209-2M peptide for 13 days and then tested for reactivity to tumors and to T2 cells pulsed with 1 μM of the g209–217 peptide on the central gp280-288 peptide.

From Rosenberg SA, Yang JC, Schwartzentruber DJ, et al. Immunologic and therapeutic evaluation of a synthetic vaccine for the treatment of patients with metastatic melanoma. *Nat Med* 1998;4:321, with permission.

tide in adjuvant is thought to prolong the exposure of the immune system to antigen and to activate nonspecific inflammatory cells with recruitment of APCs to the site of immunization. Of particular interest was the decrease in circulating precursor cells when IL-2 was administered along with peptide, possibly due to redistribution of immune cells out of the circulation to sites of tumor (31).

Some studies have identified peptides from the MART-1 tumor antigen that appear to be more immunogenic *in vitro* than is the native MART-1:27-35 peptide (32,33). Modifications of this peptide with a methionine at the second position appear to be more immunogenic *in vitro* than the native nine-mer peptide, and modifications of the MART-1:26-35 ten-mer with a leucine or methionine in the second position appear to be more immunogenic than the native ten-mer peptide. Clinical trials evaluating the ability of modified MART peptides to immunize melanoma patients are under way.

IMMUNIZATION WITH PEPTIDES FROM THE ras ONCOGENE

Increasing efforts are being made to develop peptide immunization for patients with common epithelial tumors. Mutated oncogenes or tumor-suppressor genes are particularly attractive targets for these immunizations (see Chapter 16.4), because the malignant phenotype of the tumor often depends on the expression of these oncogene products, and thus antigen loss variants are unlikely to survive.

Mutations in the ras oncogene have been reported in from 20% to 90% of different human epithelial malignancies (34). Ninety percent of ras mutations occur at codon 12, in which a normal glycine residue is replaced by an aspartic acid, valine, or cysteine. These point mutations lead to the production of aberrant proteins that can affect early events in tumorigenesis. Gjertsen et al. (35) identified the exact ras mutations in five patients with adenocarcinoma of the pancreas using polymerase

chain reaction amplification and sequencing and immunized patients with up to 4×10^9 PBMCs pulsed with the synthetic mutated ras peptide (amino acid positions 5 to 21) infused intravenously with booster vaccinations on days 14 and 35 and then every 4 to 6 weeks. In this study, two of five patients were reported to exhibit a transient PBMC proliferative T-cell response to peptide on approximately day 40. One of these responses specifically recognized only the mutated peptide and the other recognized both the mutated and nonmutated peptides. In subsequent reports, specific anti-ras class II–restricted and class I–restricted T-cell responses were described (36). The position 12 valine mutation in one patient was shown to be HLA-B35–restricted and the exact nine amino-acid peptide with the sequence VVVGAVGVG was identified. Of particular interest was the ability of the class I–restricted cells to recognize tumors expressing this K-ras mutation. These studies were encouraging because they demonstrated that peptides arising from these individual point mutations could be presented on the surface of tumor cells and thus potentially serve as targets for immune attack.

Abrams et al. used a similar approach to immunize patients with adenocarcinomas of the colon, lung, or pancreas whose tumors contained point mutations in the K-ras gene at codon 12 (37). Mutant ras peptides, 13 amino acids in length, corresponding to the individual patient's mutation were synthesized and injected subcutaneously admixed with Detox adjuvant (a combination of cell-wall skeletons from *Mycobacterium phlei* and lipid-A from *Salmonella* prepared in oil and water emulsion). Each of the patients received three vaccinations of 0.1 to 1.0 mg peptide separated by 4 weeks. Immunologic responses in these patients were assessed by the generation of cell lines derived from lymphocyte populations incubated *in vitro* and sensitized with autologous APCs, the mutant ras peptides, and IL-2. T-cell lines derived from three of eight patients receiving these vaccinations were reported to recognize the mutated peptide with no detectable crossreactivity against normal ras sequences. A CD8+ T-cell line sensitized to a mutant-ras peptide

TABLE 10. PREVIOUS STUDIES IDENTIFYING HLA-A2–RESTRICTED EPITOPES FROM HER-2/*neu*

Source of CTLs	Method of Induction	Peptides Identified	Tumor Recognition	References
Ovarian TALs, including three derived clones	CD8$^+$ selection	p369(4/4 lines), P971(2/4 lines)	SKBR-3.A2, OVA-16 HER-2^{high}	40
Ovarian TILs and TALs, including nine clones	*In vitro* stimulation with autologous tumor followed by cloning	p369(2/9 clones), p971(1/9 clones)	Autologous and A2$^+$ HER-2$^+$ lines	41
HLA-A2.1 huCD8 transgenic mouse	*In vitro* peptide vaccination	p369, p773	Panel of A2$^+$ HER-2$^+$ lines	42
Donor PBLs	*In vitro* stimulation with pulsed autologous dendritic cells	p369, p654	A2$^+$ HER-2$^+$ breast (MB 231, MCF-7), colon (HCT 116), and RCC (A_498) tumor lines	62
Donor PBLs	*In vitro* stimulation with pulsed autologous dendritic cells	p369, p435, p9	Not shown for p369-reactive cells	59
Ovarian TALs	*In vitro* stimulation with autologous tumor	p971	Autologous	63
Donor PBLs	*In vitro* stimulation with pulsed autologous PBMCs	p968-981, p968-981 611 p971, p971, 9V	Autologous and allogeneic A2$^+$ HER-2$^+$ lines	64
Ovarian, breast, and NSCLC TILs	*In vitro* stimulation with autologous tumor, pulsed T2, or pulsed dendritic cells	p654	Autologous and allogenic A2$^+$ HER-2^{high} tumors from ovarian, breast, NSCLC, and pancreatic cancer	65–67
Donor PBLs	*In vitro* stimulation with pulsed autologous PBMCs	p48, p789	None shown	68

NSCLC, non–small-cell lung cancer; PBLs, peripheral blood leukocytes; PBMCs, peripheral blood mononuclear cells; TALs, tumor-associated lymphocytes; TILs, tumor-infiltrating lymphocytes.
From Zaks TZ, Rosenberg SA. Immunization with a peptide epitope (p369-377) from HER-2/neu leads to peptide-specific cytotoxic T lymphocytes that fail to recognize HER-2/neu+ tumors. *Cancer Res* 1998;58:4902, with permission.

also exhibited lysis of a tumor-cell line naturally expressing the same endogenous mutation.

Khleif et al. studied 139 tumors and identified 37 (26.6%) that carried K-ras mutations in position 12 of the ras gene (38). Fifteen patients were vaccinated with Detox adjuvant containing 0.1 to 5.0 mg of the specific mutated peptide found in their tumor. Immunologic data was available from 10 of the 11 patients that completed at least three vaccinations, and three of these ten generated either CD4$^+$ or CD8$^+$ T-cell responses to the specific mutant ras peptide used for immunization. A CD8$^+$ CTL line was capable of lysing an HLA-A2 matched tumor-cell line carrying the corresponding mutation.

No clinical antitumor effects were reported in any of the patients immunized with ras peptides.

IMMUNIZATION WITH PEPTIDES FROM THE HER-2/*neu* ONCOGENE

The HER-2/*neu* protein is a member of the tyrosine kinase family of growth factor receptors and is frequently amplified and overexpressed in adenocarcinomas of the breast, ovary, colorectum, and other histologies (39). The expression of HER-2/*neu* correlates with poor prognosis and appears to be involved in the tumorigenic and metastatic phenotype of these tumors.

HER-2/*neu* contains 1,255 amino acids, and multiple potential HLA-binding epitopes exist for most human MHC haplotypes. Several groups have identified peptides that appear to be recognized by human lymphocytes in an HLA-A2–restricted fashion (Table 10). Fisk et al. identified a nine-amino acid peptide (KIFGSLAFL) at amino acids 369 to 377 (referred to as *p369*) that was recognized by ovarian tumor–associated lymphocytes as well as tumor-reactive clones from four of four

patients (40). Independently, Kono et al. reported that two of nine clones derived from ovarian and breast TILs also recognized the p369 epitope (41). Lustgarten immunized HLA-A2.1 transgenic mice with this epitope; splenocytes from these immunized mice recognized HLA-A2$^+$ HER-2/*neu* overexpressing human tumor lines (42). Additionally, multiple other HLA-A2–binding peptides from HER-2/*neu* have been recognized by PBMCs from HLA-A2$^+$ patients with ovarian or breast cancer (see Table 10).

A variety of laboratory studies have also suggested the potential importance of immunologic reactions against HER-2/*neu* in immunotherapy. Disis et al. demonstrated that specific CD4$^+$ T-cell immunity against HER-2/*neu* could be generated in the rat by vaccination with immunogenic rat peptides but not by immunization with the intact protein (43). No evidence of autoimmunity was seen directed against organs that expressed low basal levels of the HER-2/*neu* protein.

Although several groups have shown that human T cells could be generated *in vitro* that were capable of reacting with HER-2/*neu* peptides, controversy exists concerning the ability of these cells to recognize processed HER-2/*neu* peptides on the surface of tumor cells. Zaks et al. raised highly avid T cells capable of recognizing the p369 peptide but could not detect reactivity against HER-2/*neu*–overexpressing human tumors (44). Four patients were then treated with the HER-2/*neu* p369 peptide administered subcutaneously in IFA every 3 weeks, and PBMCs collected before and after two and four immunizations were analyzed. Strong peptide reactivity was raised in the PBMCs of three of these four patients that could recognize peptide concentrations of 1 ng per mL, yet failed to react with a panel of HLA-A2$^+$ HER-2/*neu* overexpressing tumors or with HLA-A2$^+$ cells infected with recombinant *vaccinia virus* encoding the HER-2/*neu* protein. It thus appeared from these studies that the p369 peptide was not presented on the surface of tumors cells. Further work is necessary to clarify this point.

IMMUNIZATION WITH PEPTIDE VACCINES FROM HUMAN PAPILLOMAVIRUS–INDUCED TUMORS

Cancers known to be induced by viruses represent attractive candidates for the development of cancer vaccines because of the possible presence of foreign virally encoded epitopes presented on the tumor cell surface (see Chapter 16.3). Human papillomavirus (HPV) infection is strongly associated with the presence of cervical cancer; greater than 90% of cervical cancers harbor DNA encoding HPV (45). The HPV genotype 16 is detected in approximately 50% of squamous carcinomas of the cervix. The E6 and E7 genes of HPV16 encode nucleoproteins that are involved in the malignant transformation of cells and have been shown to inactivate the tumor-suppressor protein p53 and retinoblastoma, respectively (46). Continued expression of the E6 and E7 encoded proteins is essential for maintenance of the malignant phenotype. Studies by Ressing et al. using HLA-A*0201 Kb transgenic mice as well as *in vitro* sensitization of human PBMCs have identified a series of E6- and E7-binding peptides that appear to be immunogenic *in vitro* and are capable of giving rise to reactive T cells that recognize not only the peptide but an HLA-A*0201 HPV-positive cervical carcinoma cell line as well (47). Because HPV16 is foreign to both mice and humans, animal models have been particularly valuable in developing immunization protocols capable of preventing the growth of tumors expressing these viral proteins (48).

The HPV16-E7 peptide with amino acids 86 to 93 (TLGIVCPI) has been of particular interest because of its high binding to HLA-A*0201 as well as its ability to mediate the generation of antitumor lymphocytes *in vitro* (47). Clinical studies have been initiated attempting to raise specific CTLs against these peptides in humans (49).

PEPTIDE VACCINES DIRECTED AGAINST PROSTATE AND COLON CANCER–ASSOCIATED PROTEINS

Murine monoclonal antibodies have identified a variety of proteins, such as carcinoembryonic antigen (CEA) and prostate-specific antigen (PSA), that exhibit a high degree of selective expression on tumor cells and have been useful in monitoring cancer patients. Because of the selective expression of these proteins in unique organs or their overexpression in tumors, these proteins have been the subjects of study for the development of cancer vaccines. Prostate-specific membrane antigen (PSMA) is a protein found in the prostate gland and is recognized by monoclonal antibody 7E11.C5 (50,51). PSMA is present in seminal fluid, prostate epithelial cells, and low levels are found in normal male sera. By studying allele-specific motifs, two PSMA peptides called *PSMA-P1* (LLHETDSAV) and *PSMA-P2* (ALFDIESKV) were identified that exhibited

high binding to HLA-A*0201. Murphy et al. reported on 51 patients with advanced hormone-resistant prostate cancer treated in a phase 1 study with these two PSMA peptides (52). Thirty of these patients were HLA-A2$^+$. Patients received between 0.2 mg and 20.0 mg of either the PSMA-P1 or PSMA-P2 peptides given intravenously or autologous dendritic cells produced *in vitro* using GM-CSF and IL-4 given either alone or pulsed with the PSMA-P1 or PSMA-P2 peptides. Between 10^6 and 2×10^7 dendritic cells were administered at 6- to 8-week intervals for four or five doses. Many of the patients in this study had advanced disease, and 39 of the 51 patients were stage D2 patients. Some impairment of cellular immunity was seen in 39 of these 51 patients based on failure to develop a standard delayed-type hypersensitivity reaction to at least one standard test antigen. In this study, and in follow-up evaluations, an increase in PSMA peptide-specific cellular reactivity was reported in some patients who received dendritic cells plus peptide (53,54). Seven of these patients were reported to have a clinical response based largely on reduction of circulating PSA levels. In more recent studies, this group has added the systemic administration of GM-CSF to the peptide immunizations.

Study of the class I HLA-A*0201 binding motifs of PSA have identified several candidate peptides for use in immunization (55,56). A 30-mer oligopeptide called *PSA-OP* encompassed two HLA-A2 binding epitopes as well as an HLA-A3 binding epitope (57). *In vitro* stimulation for six to seven cycles with this PSA-OP lead to the generation of CTL lines capable of lysing target cells pulsed with these peptides as well as a PSA-positive prostate cancer cell line. The difficulty in generating prostate cancer lines has limited the ability to test T-cell reactivity against naturally processed peptides. The description of techniques to generate prostate cancer lines using transduction with E6- and E7-expressing retroviruses has provided additional lines of value in subsequent studies of PSA (58).

Attempts are under way to identify peptides that may be useful for immunization of patients with a variety of epithelial tumors. Kawashima et al. used peptide-specific motifs to identify several CEA peptides that could give rise to CTL precursors in an HLA-A2–restricted fashion (59). Tsang et al. immunized patients with a recombinant *vaccinia virus* encoding CEA and used these postimmunization PBMCs stimulated with candidate CEA peptides to identify a nine amino-acid peptide called *CAP-1* comprised of amino acids 571 to 579 (YLSGANLNL) (60). *In vitro* immunization with this CAP-1 peptide was capable of generating T-cell lines capable of recognizing the peptide as well as an HLA-A2 CEA expressing colon cancer line. Subsequent studies demonstrated that a substitution with aspartic acid of the asparagine at position six of this peptide led to a peptide that exhibited significantly increased immunogenicity *in vitro* (61). Clinical trials using these peptides for immunization are planned.

CONCLUDING COMMENTS

In preliminary studies, immunization of humans with peptides in adjuvant has been surprisingly effective in generating circulating lymphocytes with antipeptide and in some instances antitumor recognition. Except in rare cases, these antitumor immune responses have not been sufficient by themselves to mediate tumor regression, and additional manipulations to increase the avidity of the lymphocytes for tumor or to increase lymphocyte number and traffic are required. The modification of native peptides with amino acid substitutions to increase binding to MHC molecules, the systemic administration of cytokines such as IL-2, the use of improved adjuvants, and the simultaneous administration of multiple class I and class II peptides are approaches that may increase the therapeutic effectiveness of peptide immunization.

REFERENCES

1. Restifo NP, Wunderlich JR. Essentials of immunology. In: DeVita VT, Hellman S, Rosenberg SA, eds. *Cancer: principles & practice of oncology*, 5th ed. Philadelphia: Lippincott–Raven Publishers, 1997:47.
2. Unanue ER. Macrophages, antigen-presenting cells, and the phenomena of antigen handling and presentation. In: Paul WE, ed. *Fundamental immunology*, 2nd ed. New York: Raven Press, 1993:111.
3. Rammensee H, Friede R, Stevanovic S. MHC ligands and peptide motifs: first listing. *Immunogenetics* 1995;41:178.
4. Ruppert J, Sidney J, Celis E, Kubo RT, Grey HM, Sette A. Prominent role of secondary anchor residues in peptide binding to HLA-A2.1 molecules. *Cell* 1993;74:929.
5. Kubo R, Sette A, Grey H, et al. Definition of specific peptide motifs for four major HLA-A alleles. *J Immunol* 1994;152:3913.
6. Parker KC, Bednarek MA, Coligan JE. Scheme for ranking potential HLA-A2 binding peptides based on independent binding of individual peptide side-chains. *J Immunol* 1994;152:163.
7. Kang X-Q, Kawakami Y, Sakaguchi K. Identification of a tyrosinase epitope recognized by HLA-A24 restricted tumor-infiltrating lymphocytes. *J Immunol* 1995;155:1343.
8. Hunt DF, Henderson RA, Shabanowitz J, et al. Characterization of peptides bound to the Class I MHC molecule HLA-A2.1 by mass spectrometry. *Science* 1992;255:1261.
9. Cox AL, Skipper J, Chen Y, et al. Identification of a peptide recognized by five melanoma-specific human cytotoxic T cell lines. *Science* 1994;264:716.
10. Salazar-Onfray F, Nakazawa T, Chhajlani V, et al. Synthetic peptides derived from the melanocyte-stimulating hormone receptor MC1R can stimulate HLA-A2-restricted cytotoxic T lymphocytes that recognize naturally processed peptides on human melanoma cells. *Cancer Res* 1997;57:4348.
11. Parkhurst MR, Fitzgerald EB, Southwood S, Sette A, Rosenberg SA, Kawakami Y. Identification of a shared HLA-A*0201-restricted T-cell epitope from the melanoma antigen tyrosinase-related protein 2 (TRP2). *Cancer Res* 1998;58:4895.
12. Marchand M, Weynants P, Rankin E, et al. Tumor regression responses in melanoma patients treated with a peptide encoded by gene MAGE-3 [Letter]. *Int J Cancer* 1995;63:883.
13. Chakraborty NG, Sporn JR, Tortora AF, et al. Immunization with a tumor-cell-lysate-loaded autologous-antigen-presenting-cell-based vaccine in melanoma. *Cancer Immunol Immunother* 1998;47:58.
14. Nestle FO, Alijagic S, Gilliet M, et al. Vaccination of melanoma patients with peptide- or tumor lysate-pulsed dendritic cells. *Nat Med* 1998;4:328.
15. Cormier JN, Salgaller ML, Prevette T, et al. Enhancement of cellular immunity in melanoma patients immunized with a peptide from MART-1/Melan A. *Cancer J Sci Am* 1997;3:37.
16. Salgaller ML, Marincola FM, Cormier JN, Rosenberg SA. Immunization against epitopes in the human melanoma antigen gp100 following patient immunization with synthetic peptides. *Cancer Res* 1996;56:4749.
17. Rosenberg SA, Yang JC, Schwartzentruber DJ, et al. Immunologic and therapeutic evaluation of a synthetic vaccine for the treatment of patients with metastatic melanoma. *Nat Med* 1998;4:321.
18. Jager E, Bernhard H, Romero P, et al. Generation of cytotoxic T-cell responses with synthetic melanoma-associated peptides *in vivo*: implications for tumor vaccines with melanoma-associated antigens. *Int J Cancer* 1996;66:162.
19. Jager E, Ringhoffer M, Karbach J. Inverse relationship of melanocyte differentiation antigen expression in melanoma tissues and CD8+ cytotoxic-T-cell responses: evidence for immunoselection of antigen-loss variants *in vivo*. *Int J Cancer* 1996;66:470.
20. Jager E, Ringhoffer M, Dienes HP, et al. Granulocyte-macrophage-colony-stimulating factor enhances immune responses to melanoma-associated peptides *in vivo*. *Int J Cancer* 1996;67:54.
21. Sette A, Vitiello A, Reherman V, et al. The relationship between class I binding affinity and immunogenicity of potential cytotoxic T cell epitopes. *J Immunol* 1994;153:5586.
22. Lipford G, Bauer S, Wagner H, Heeg K. *In vivo* CTL induction with point-substituted ovalbumin peptides: immunotherapy correlates with peptide-induced MHC class I stability. *Vaccine* 1995;13:313.
23. Chen W, Khilko S, Fecondo J, Margulies D, McCluskey J. Determinant selection of major histocompatibility complex class I-restricted antigenic peptides is explained by class I-peptide affinity and is strongly influenced by nondominant anchor residues. *J Exp Med* 1994;180:1471.
24. Kawakami Y, Eliyahu S, Jennings C, et al. Recognition of multiple epitopes in the human melanoma antigen gp100 by tumor infiltrating T-lymphocytes associated with in vivo tumor regression. *J Immunol* 1995;154:3461.
25. Parkhurst MR, Salgaller ML, Southwood S, et al. Improved induction of melanoma-reactive CTL with peptides from the melanoma antigen gp100 modified at HLA-A*0201-binding residues. *J Immunol* 1996;157:2539.
26. Sercarz E, Lehmann P, Ametani A, Benichou G, Miller A, Moudgil K. Dominance and crypticity of T cell antigenic determinants. *Ann Rev Immunol* 1993;11:729.
27. Ohno S. How cytotoxic T cells manage to discriminate nonself from self at the nonapeptide level. *Proc Natl Acad Sci U S A* 1992;89:4643.
28. Lipford G, Bauer S, Wagner H, Heeg K. Peptide engineering allows cytotoxic T-cell vaccination against human papilloma virus tumour antigen, E6. *Immunol* 1995;84:298.
29. Pogue R, Eron J, Frelinger J, Matsui M. Amino-terminal alteration of the HLA-A* 0201-restricted human immunodeficiency virus pol peptide increases complex stability and in vitro immunogenicity. *Proc Natl Acad Sci U S A* 1995;92:8166.
30. Rosenberg SA, Yang JC, Topalian SL, et al. Treatment of 283 consecutive patients with metastatic melanoma or renal cell cancer using high-dose bolus interleukin-2. *JAMA* 1994;271:907.
31. Rosenberg SA, Yang JC, Schwartzentruber DJ, et al. Impact of cytokine administration on the generation of antitumor reactivity in patients with metastatic melanoma receiving a peptide vaccine. *J Immunol* 1999 (*in press*).
32. Valmori D, Fonteneau JF, Lizana CM. Enhanced generation of specific tumor-reactive CTL in vivo by selected Melan-A/MART-1 immunodominant peptide analogues. *J Immunol* 1998;160:1750.
33. Rivoltini L, Squarcina P, Loftus DJ, et al. A superagonist variant of peptide MART1/Melan A27-35 elicits anti-melanoma CD8+ T cells with enhance functional characteristics: implication for more effective immunotherapy. *Cancer Res* 1999;59:301.
34. Bos JL. ras oncogenes in human cancer: a review. *Cancer Res* 1989;49:4682.
35. Gjertsen MK, Bakka A, Breivik J, et al. Vaccination with mutant ras peptides and induction of T-cell responsiveness in pancreatic carcinoma patients carrying the corresponding ras mutation. *Lancet* 1995;346:1399.
36. Gjertsen MK, Bjorheim JSI, Myklebust J, Gaudernack G. Cytotoxic CD4+ and CD8+ T lymphocytes, generated by mutant p21-ras (12VAL) peptide vaccination of a patient, recognized 12VAL-dependent nested epitopes present within the vaccine peptide and kill autologous tumour cells carrying this mutation. *Int J Cancer* 1997;72:784.

37. Abrams SI, Khleif SN, Bergmann-Leitner ES, et al. Generation of stable CD4$^+$ and CD8$^+$ T cell lines from patients immunized with ras oncogene-derived peptides reflecting codon 12 mutations. *Cell Immunol* 1997;182:137.

38. Khleif SN, Abrams SI, Hamilton M, et al. A phase I vaccine trial with peptides reflecting ras oncogene mutations of solid tumors. *J Immunother* 1999;22:155.

39. Coussens L, Yang-Feng TL, Liao YC, et al. Tyrosinase kinase receptor with extensive homology to EGF receptor shares chromosomal location with neu oncogene. *Science* 1985;230:1132.

40. Fisk B, Blevins TL, Wharton JT, Ioannides CG. Identification of an immunodominant peptide of HER-2/neu proto-oncogene recognized by ovarian tumor-specific cytotoxic T lymphocytes lines. *J Exp Med* 1995;181:2109.

41. Kono K, Halapi E, Hising C. Mechanisms of escape from CD8$^+$ T-cell clones specific for the HER-2/neu proto-oncogene expressed in ovarian carcinomas: related and unrelated to decreased MHC class I expression. *Int J Cancer* 1997;70:112.

42. Lustgarten J, Theobald M, Labadie C, et al. Identification of Her-2/Neu CTL epitopes using double transgenic mice expressing HLA-A2.1 and human CD.8. *Hum Immunol* 1997;52:109.

43. Disis ML, Gralow JR, Bernhard H, Hand SL, Rubin WD, Cheever MA. Peptide-based, but not whole protein, vaccines elicit immunity to HER-2/neu, an oncogenic self-protein. *J Immunol* 1996;156:3151.

44. Zaks TZ, Rosenberg SA. Immunization with a peptide epitope (p369-377) from HER-2/neu leads to peptide-specific cytotoxic T lymphocytes that fail to recognize HER-2/neu+ tumors. *Cancer Res* 1998;58:4902.

45. Bosch FX, Manos MM, Munoz M, et al. Prevalence of human papillomavirus in cervical cancer: a world-wide perspective. International biological study on cervical cancer (BSCC) Study Group. *J Natl Cancer Inst* 1995;87:796.

46. Munger K, Scheffner M, Huibregts JM, Howley PM. Interactions of HPV E6 and E7 oncoproteins with tumour suppressor gene products. *Cancer Surv* 1992;12:197.

47. Ressing ME, Sette A, Brandt RM. Human CTL epitopes encoded by human papillomavirus type 16 E6 and E7 identified through *in vivo* and *in vitro* immunogenicity studies of HLA-A*0201-binding peptides. *J Immunol* 1995;154:5934.

48. Feltkamp MCW, Smits HL, Vierboom MPM, et al. Vaccination with cytotoxic T lymphocyte epitope-containing peptide protects against a tumor induced by human papillomavirus type 16-transformed cells. *Eur J Immunol* 1993;23:2242.

49. Steller MA, Gurski KJ, Murakami M, et al. Cell-mediated immunological responses in cervical and vaginal cancer patients immunized with a lipidated epitope of human papillomavirus type 16 E7. *Clinical Cancer Res* 1998;4:2103.

50. Horoszewicz JS, Kawinski E, Murphy GP. Monoclonal antibodies to a new antigenic marker in epithelial prostate cells and serum of prostatic cancer patients. *Anticancer Res* 1987;7.927.

51. Israeli RS, Powell CT, Corr JG, Fair WR, Heston WD. Molecular cloning of a complementary DNA encoding a prostate-specific membrane antigen. *Cancer Res* 1993;54:1807.

52. Murphy G, Tjoa B, Ragde H, Kenny G, Boynton A. Phase I clinical trial: T-cell therapy for prostate cancer using autologous dendritic cells pulsed with HLA-A0201-specific peptides from prostate-specific membrane antigen. *Prostate* 1996;29:371.

53. Tjoa BA, Erickson SJ, Bowes VA, et al. Follow-up evaluation of prostate cancer patients infused with autologous dendritic cells pulsed with PSMA peptides. *Prostate* 1997;32:272.

54. Salgaller ML, Lodge PA, McLean JG, et al. Report of immune monitoring of prostate cancer patients undergoing T-cell therapy using dendritic cells pulsed with HLA-A2-specific peptides from prostate-specific membrane antigen (PSMA). *Prostate* 1998;35:144.

55. Zue BH, Zhang Y, Sosman JA, Peace DJ. Induction of human cytotoxic T lymphocytes specific for prostate-specific antigen. *Prostate* 1997;2:73.

56. Alexander RB, Brady F, Leffell MS, Tsai V, Celis E. Specific T cell recognition of patients derived from prostate-specific antigen in patients with prostate cancer. *Urology* 1998;1:150.

57. Correale P, Walmsley K, Zaremba S, Zhu M, Schlom J, Tsang KY. Generation of human cytolytic T lymphocyte lines directed against prostate-specific antigen (PSA) employing a PSA oligoepitope peptide. *J Immunol* 1998;161:3186.

58. Bright RK, Vocke CD, Emmert-Buck MR, et al. Generation and genetic characterization of immortal human prostate epithelial cell lines derived from primary cancer specimens. *Cancer Res* 1997;57:995.

59. Kawashima I, Hudson SJ, Tsai V, et al. The multi-epitope approach for immunotherapy for cancer: identification of several CTL epitopes from various tumor-associated antigens expressed on solid epithelial tumors. *Hum Immunol* 1998;59:1.

60. Tsang KY, Zaremba S, Nieroda CA, et al. Generation of human cytotoxic T cells specific for human carcinoembryonic antigen epitopes from patients immunized with recombinant vaccinia-CEA vaccine. *J Natl Cancer Inst* 1995;87:982.

61. Zaremba S, Barzaga E, Zhu M, Soares N, Tsang KY, Schlom J. Identification of an enhancer agonist cytotoxic T lymphocyte peptide from human carcinoembryonic antigen. *Cancer Res* 1997;57:4570.

62. Brossart P, Stuhler G, Flad T, et al. HER-2/neu-derived peptides are tumor-associated antigens expressed by human renal cell and colon carcinoma lines and are recognized by in vitro induced specific cytotoxic T lymphocytes. *Cancer Res* 1998;58:732.

63. Ioannides CG, Fisk B, Fan D, Biddison WE, Wharton JT, O'Brian CA. T cells isolated from ovarian malignant ascites recognize a peptide derived from the HER-2/neu proto-oncogene. *Cell Immunol* 1993;151:225.

64. Fisk B, Chesak B, Pollack MS, Wharton JT, Ioannides CG. Oligopeptide induction of a cytotoxic T lymphocyte response to HER-2/neu proto-oncogene *in vitro*. *Cell Immunol* 1994;157:415.

65. Peoples GE, Goedegeburre PS, Smith R. Breast and ovarian cancer-specific cytotoxic T lymphocytes recognize the same HER-2/neu-derived peptide. *Proc Natl Acad Sci U S A* 1995;92:432.

66. Yoshino I, Goedegebuure PS, Peoples GE, et al. HER-2/neu-derived peptides are shared antigens among human non-small-cell lung cancer and ovarian cancer. *Cancer Res* 1994;54:3387.

67. Peiper M, Goedegeburre PS, Linehan DC, Ganguly E, Douville CC, Eberlein TJ. The HER-2/neu-derived peptide p654-662 is a tumor-associated antigen in human pancreatic cancer recognized by cytotoxic T lymphocytes. *Eur J Immunol* 1997;27:1115.

68. Disis ML, Smith JW, Murphy AE, Chen W, Cheever MA. *In vitro* generation of human cytolytic T-cells specific for peptides derived from the HER-2/neu proto-oncogene protein. *Cancer Res* 1994;54:1071.

18.4

CANCER VACCINES: CLINICAL APPLICATIONS

DNA Vaccines

STEPHEN A. WHITE
ROBERT M. CONRY

The term *DNA vaccination* designates a form of active immunization or immunotherapy in which antigen-specific humoral and cellular immune responses are induced by direct introduction of recombinant plasmids encoding immunogens. This process was first described in 1992 by Tang et al., who noted the elicitation of antibody responses against human growth hormone in mice after intramuscular injection of a growth hormone–expressing plasmid construct (1). Subsequently, Ulmer's group reported that inoculation of a DNA vector encoding influenza virus nucleoprotein (NP) into murine muscle generated NP-specific humoral and cytotoxic T lymphocyte (CTL) responses with resultant immunoprotection against intranasal challenge with influenza A virus (2). Since these initial reports, numerous investigators have used the direct injection of antigen-encoding plasmids to induce protective humoral and cellular immune responses against a broad range of microbial proteins and tumor-associated antigens (TAAs) in numerous animal species. Immune responses to DNA vaccines have been described after administration by needle injection into muscle, skin, spleen, and subcutaneous tissue, as well as by particle bombardment–mediated transfer into muscle, skin, and mucosa (3–6). Additionally, several groups have reported induction of immune responses by intranasal administration of lipid-encapsulated DNA vaccines (7,8) and by oral administration of attenuated *Salmonella* carriers transfected with antigen-encoding plasmids (9,10).

Some studies have demonstrated the ability of DNA vaccination to elicit meaningful immune responses in nonhuman primates. For example, Boyer et al. noted the generation of antigen-specific humoral and cellular immunity with resultant protection against challenge with human immunodeficiency virus 1 (HIV-1) in chimpanzees vaccinated with DNA constructs encoding HIV-1 *rev, env,* and *gag/pol* (11). This group has subsequently reported the boosting of anti-*env* antibodies and a decline in viral load in HIV-1–infected chimpanzees after immunization with an HIV-1–*env/rev* DNA vaccine (12). Liu's group has described the utilization of a DNA vaccine construct

encoding influenza virus hemagglutinin (HA) in African green monkeys to elicit HA-specific humoral immune responses equal or superior to those induced by commercially available whole inactivated influenza virus vaccines (13). These findings have generated considerable interest in the application of DNA vaccination to human disease.

DNA vaccination provides several advantages over protein or peptide vaccines. First, DNA vaccines possess greater chemical stability and are more easily sequenced and purified than proteins or peptides. Second, plasmid vaccines are inherently immunogenic and generally do not require coadministration of adjuvants. Third, DNA immunization generates antigen expression within the cytosol of transfected cells, permitting direct entry of antigen to intracellular major histocompatibility complex (MHC) class I processing pathways and facilitating the induction of CTL responses. In addition, intracellular synthesis with posttranslational modification generates antigenic proteins with native tertiary structure. Finally, in preclinical studies, DNA vaccines have elicited a broad range of antigen-specific immune responses, including antibodies, lymphoproliferation, CTL activation, and delayed-type hypersensitivity (DTH). Similarly, immunization with plasmid constructs provides certain advantages over recombinant viral vaccination. First, DNA vaccines are easier to construct, produce, and control for quality than viral recombinants. Second, recombinant viral vaccines frequently evoke vector-specific immune responses that preclude their use in multidose immunization schedules. Third, DNA vaccines carry less risk of insertional mutagenesis than viral vectors, particularly retroviral recombinants. Fourth, unlike adenoviral and vaccinia recombinants, DNA vaccines are not known to downregulate MHC class I gene expression in transfected cells (14). Finally, DNA vaccines do not confer a risk of recombinational events leading to the derivation of revertant or recombinant pathogenic viruses.

This chapter describes preclinical advances in DNA vaccination and reviews applications of this form of active immunotherapy in the prevention and treatment of human infectious disease and cancer.

CELLULAR MECHANISMS OF DNA VACCINATION

The cellular mechanisms responsible for T-lymphocyte activation after DNA vaccination have been partially elucidated. Antigen-specific induction of naïve T-helper cells and CTLs involves two discrete processes: antigen synthesis and MHC-restricted antigen presentation. The specific roles of bone marrow–derived antigen-presenting cells (APCs) and locally transfected nonhematopoietic cells (i.e., myocytes or keratinocytes) in these processes are discussed below.

Bone marrow-derived APCs appear to be the predominant cells involved in MHC-restricted antigen presentation after intramuscular or cutaneous DNA immunization. This contention is supported by several observations. Myocytes and keratinocytes lack cell surface costimulatory molecules (B7-1, B7-2) that promote T-cell adhesion and thereby facilitate antigen-specific T-cell induction. Antigen presentation in the absence of these ligands is thought to induce tolerance rather than immunity (15). Furthermore, *in vivo* expression of MHC class II molecules is generally limited to cells of hematopoietic origin. This fact, coupled with the efficient MHC class II–restricted induction of $CD4^+$ T cells after DNA immunization, suggests antigen presentation by bone marrow–derived APCs. In further support of this contention, several investigators have noted the preservation of immune responses to intramuscular DNA vaccination despite excision of the inoculated muscle within 1 minute of immunization (16,17). However, the most compelling evidence of antigen presentation by bone marrow–derived cells after DNA immunization is provided by studies of murine bone marrow transplant chimeras (18,19). In these studies, DNA vaccine–induced CTL responses after intramuscular immunization were restricted to MHC haplotypes expressed by cells of hematopoietic origin.

Two hypotheses have been proposed regarding the source of antigen for bone marrow–derived APC presentation: (a) direct transduction of these APCs at the inoculation site or draining nodes, and (b) antigen synthesis within transduced myocytes or keratinocytes with subsequent transfer to bone marrow–derived APCs. The former hypothesis is supported by several lines of evidence:

1. First, the efficacy of intravenous and intrasplenic DNA vaccination suggests a myocyte- and keratinocyte-independent mechanism of antigen expression sufficient for induction of immunity.
2. Second, the preservation of immune responses to intramuscular DNA immunization despite ablation of the inoculated muscle within minutes of vaccine administration argues for plasmid transduction and antigen synthesis at distant sites. Of note, the excision of inoculated skin within 24 hours of cutaneous DNA vaccination markedly diminishes antigen-specific CTL induction (16,20). This attenuation may reflect the importance of transfected keratinocytes in immunogen expression after DNA vaccination of skin. Alternatively, this finding could be attributable to the removal of transfected, cutaneous

dendritic (Langerhans') cells before their migration to regional lymph nodes.
3. Third, some studies have described the detection of plasmid DNA sequences by polymerase chain reaction (PCR) in lymph-node dendritic cells and in epidermal Langerhans' cells after intramuscular and cutaneous DNA vaccination, respectively (21).
4. Finally, the presence of green fluorescent protein (GFP) in rhodamine-positive lymph-node dendritic cells has been observed 24 hours after biolistic delivery of a GFP-encoding plasmid to rhodamine-stained murine epidermis (22). This finding suggests direct transfection of cutaneous dendritic cells with ensuing migration to regional lymph nodes. In a similar study, GFP expression was detectable in bone marrow–derived APCs in lymph nodes, peripheral blood, and the spleen after intramuscular inoculation of mice with a DNA construct encoding GFP (23). GFP signals display a diffuse pattern within the cytoplasm of positive cells consistent with intracellular synthesis, as opposed to a focal distribution that would suggest endocytic uptake of presynthesized GFP.

The second hypothesis regarding DNA vaccine immunogen expression, the synthesis of antigen within myocutaneous cells with subsequent transfer to bone marrow–derived APCs for presentation, is supported by the following observations.

1. First, numerous immunohistochemical studies have demonstrated the presence of plasmid-encoded antigens within myocytes and keratinocytes at sites of DNA immunization (24).
2. Second, some investigations have established the ability of bone marrow–derived APCs to endocytose, process, and present extracellular antigen in association with MHC class I molecules. For example, dendritic cell phagocytosis of apoptotic cells with subsequent stimulation of MHC class I restricted CTLs specific for phagocytosed antigens has been described (25).
3. Third, augmentation of antigen-specific humoral and CTL responses against human immunoglobulin G (IgG) has been reported after fusion of human IgG complementary DNA (cDNA) with cDNA encoding the APC-targeting ligand CTLA4 within a plasmid construct (26). This observation is highly suggestive of APC cross-priming with antigen presynthesized in myocytes, keratinocytes, or other cells after DNA immunization.
4. Finally, two reports have described the induction of antigen-specific CTL immunity after the transplantation of lipid-encapsulated myoblasts stably transduced with antigen-encoding plasmid (27,28). Of note, CTL responses in these studies were restricted to MHC haplotypes absent from transplanted myoblasts, further confirming the contention that antigen presentation after intramuscular DNA vaccination is a function of bone marrow–derived APCs, not myocytes.

ROLE OF CPG DINUCLEOTIDE MOTIFS IN DNA VACCINATION

One important advantage of DNA vaccines is the inherent adjuvanticity of the plasmid vector. This immunogenicity results from the presence of unmethylated CpG-dinucleotide motifs in the six-residue nucleotide sequence 5' Purine-Purine-CpG-Pyrimidine-Pyrimidine 3' (29). CpG dinucleotides occur with a frequency of 1 per 16 base pairs in bacterial DNA versus a frequency of 1 per 50 base pairs in vertebrate DNA (30). Additionally, the incidence of cytosine methylation is much lower in prokaryotic DNA (5%) than in eukaryotic DNA (70% to 90%) (31). Thus, unmethylated CpG motifs are much more common in bacterial DNA (and in DNA from certain nonbacterial species, including yeast, nematodes, mollusks, and insects) than in mammalian genomic DNA (32,33). These immunostimulatory sequences enhance cell-mediated immunity and promote the generation of T helper 1 (Th1) immune responses by inducing macrophages, B cells, and natural killer cells to secrete interferons, tumor necrosis factor alpha (TNF-α), interleukin-6 (IL-6), IL-12, and IL-18 (29,34–36). Unmethylated CpG motifs promote the maturation and activation of dendritic cells (37). The immunomodulatory effects of plasmid DNA can be abrogated by cytosine residue methylation (38), by reversal of the central dinucleotide within immunostimulatory sequences from CpG to GpC (38), or by the removal of CpG motifs (35). Conversely, in a single report, the addition of immunostimulatory sequences to the plasmid backbone of a DNA vaccine construct has been demonstrated to enhance antigen-specific humoral and cellular immune responses without alteration in the level of antigen synthesis (35).

The immunogenic properties of plasmid DNA and of synthetic oligodeoxynucleotides (ODNs) containing CpG motifs have prompted interest in their use as vaccine adjuvants. Several investigators have reported that coadministration of irrelevant plasmid DNA with DNA vaccines reduces the minimum dose of vaccine required for the elicitation of measurable immune responses (39–41). However, the use of immunostimulatory ODNs as DNA vaccine adjuvants may be precluded by an ODN dose–dependent reduction in vaccine antigen expression (42). Numerous murine studies have demonstrated augmentation of antigen-specific Th1 immune responses to protein vaccines [e.g., hepatitis B surface antigen (43,44), hen egg lysozyme (45), influenza NP (46), and B-cell lymphoma idiotype (47)] and inactivated viral vaccines [e.g., formalin-inactivated influenza virus (48)] by codelivery of CpG-rich synthetic ODNs.

Potential mechanisms whereby plasmid DNA produces Th1-biased immunostimulation have been elucidated. APC internalization of DNA into endosomes is sequence-independent (29). After DNA uptake, sequence-dependent activation of two separate signal transduction pathways has been described. First, acidification of double-stranded DNA containing immunostimulatory nucleotide sequences induces the generation of reactive oxygen species with resultant expression of specific cellular proto-oncogenes (e.g., c-myc) and cytokines (e.g., IL-12) (49). Second, CpG-rich DNA induces the phosphorylation-mediated activation of two members of the mitogen-activated protein kinase superfamily, leading to lymphokine gene expression (50). *In vitro* studies suggest that inhibitors of endosomal acidification (e.g., quinacrine and chloroquine) block the activation of B lymphocytes and mononuclear cells by DNA-containing immunostimulatory CpG motifs (49,50,51).

Krieg et al. have reported the existence of neutralizing oligonucleotide sequences, which, if present in DNA vaccine con-

structs, counteract the immunostimulatory sequences (52). These neutralizing motifs, initially described in adenoviral DNA, include CpG dinucleotides in direct repeats, the nucleotide sequence 5'CpCpG3', and the nucleotide sequence 5'CpGpG3'. Coadministration of synthetic ODNs containing neutralizing sequences with DNA vaccines containing immunostimulatory motifs markedly inhibits immune induction by the latter. Conversely, elimination of neutralizing sequences from the plasmid backbone of a DNA vaccine construct has been demonstrated to augment the elicitation of antigen-specific Th1 immunity.

Nucleotide sequences flanking immunostimulatory motifs within DNA vaccines may also influence the pattern of cytokine secretion elicited from immune effector cells. As noted above, CpG-rich DNA typically induces the production and release of IL-6, IL-12, and TNF-α. An 18-residue, CpG-rich nucleotide sequence derived from the murine IL-12 p40 gene has been identified that elicits IL-12 secretion without stimulation of IL-6 or TNF-α release (53).

In summary, unmethylated CpG dinucleotide motifs clearly explain many of the inherent adjuvant properties of bacterial plasmid DNA. Furthermore, synthetic ODNs containing CpG motifs appear to represent an important new class of adjuvant molecules to enhance immune responses to protein and inactivated viral vaccines. However, most plasmid DNA vectors contain many immunostimulatory CpG dinucleotide motifs by random chance. Thus, the clinical impact of engineering plasmid DNA vaccines based on the number and potency of CpG motifs remains to be determined.

MODULATION OF IMMUNE RESPONSES TO DNA VACCINATION

The magnitude and character of immune responses to DNA vaccination are influenced by multiple factors, including the site and mode of vaccine administration, the level of expression and cellular localization of the encoded antigen, and the concurrent use of genetic and chemical adjuvants. In preclinical DNA vaccination studies, manipulation of these and other variables has altered the level and orientation of vaccine-induced immunity.

The influence of the site and technique of vaccine administration on immune responses to DNA immunization has been extensively studied in animals. In general, needle inoculation of DNA vaccines into muscle preferentially elicits Th1 immune responses characterized by enhanced CTL immunity, IgG2a antibody production, and interferon-γ (INF-γ) release (54). Biolistic vaccine delivery into skin or muscle typically induces Th2 responses with increased IgG1 antibody production and IL-4 release (6,54). The orientation of immune responses to intradermal needle DNA immunization is variable, with both Th1 and Th2 responses reported (6,54,55). These differences in immune response patterns may be secondary to Th1-biased immunostimulation associated with the high doses of plasmid DNA generally used for needle immunization. In support of this contention, Barry and Johnston noted IgG1 (Th2) humoral responses to minute doses of an α-1 antitrypsin DNA vaccine administered to mice by gene-gun cutaneous inoculation, whereas biolistic delivery of high doses (50 μg) of this construct induced antigen-specific IgG2a (Th1) production (56). Conversely, in studies of a DNA vaccine encoding influenza virus hemagglutinin, Robinson's group reported dose-independent generation of Th1 antibody responses after needle injection and Th2 antibody responses after biolistic delivery (6).

Several groups have investigated the utilization of plasmid-encoded cytokines as molecular adjuvants for DNA vaccination. In general, coadministration of proinflammatory cytokine genes (e.g., IL-1, TNF-α, TCA3, and INF-γ) or Th1-associated cytokine genes (e.g., IL-2, IL-12, IL-15, and IL-18) with antigen-encoding DNA constructs induces enhanced CTL activity, lymphocyte proliferation, and DTH responses with variable effects on antibody production (57). For example, Xin's group noted increased IgG2a-antibody production, INF-γ secretion, CTL activity, and DTH as well as decreased IgG1 antibody production and IL-4 release after intranasal vaccination of mice with DNA constructs encoding HIV-1 antigens and IL-2 (58). Similarly, codelivery of the murine IL-12 gene with an HIV-1 DNA vaccine has been demonstrated to promote antigen-specific lymphoproliferation and CTL immunity and reduce antibody responses in mice (59). Conversely, coadministration of plasmids encoding Th2-associated cytokines (e.g., IL-4 and IL-10) with DNA vaccines typically augments overall antibody and IgG1 production, reduces IgG2a production, and diminishes CTL and DTH responses (57,60,61). Codelivery of the granulocyte-macrophage colony-stimulating factor gene with DNA constructs encoding antigens generally promotes antibody production, Th1 cytokine (e.g., IL-2) release, lymphoproliferative responses, CTL activity, and DTH (62–65). In two reports, enhanced antigen-specific humoral responses associated with the use of plasmid-encoded granulocyte-macrophage colony-stimulating factor entailed increases in both IgG1 and IgG2a antibody production (64,66).

The utilization of plasmid-encoded costimulatory molecules (e.g., CD80 and CD86) and APC ligands (e.g., CTLA4 and CD40 ligand) as molecular adjuvants for DNA immunization has been investigated. Codelivery of cDNA encoding an immunogen and CD86 (B7-2), either as separate plasmids or within a single bicistronic expression plasmid, is consistently associated with enhanced antigen-specific lymphoproliferative responses and CTL immunity (67,68). However, the effect of coadministration of the CD80 (B7-1) gene with DNA vaccines on T-cell responses is variable (53,67–69). Boyle's group has reported augmentation of humoral and cellular immune responses to a DNA vaccine encoding human IgG after fusion of the Ig gene to cDNA encoding the costimulatory molecule ligand CTLA4 (26). Another group used codelivery of a plasmid-encoding CD40 ligand, a stimulatory signal for CD40-bearing APCs, to enhance antigen-specific antibody and CTL responses to a DNA vaccine encoding β-galactosidase (70).

Several investigators have attempted to manipulate the cellular localization of antigens encoded by DNA vaccines and thereby influence the magnitude and character of resultant immune responses. In some reports, DNA constructs encoding antigens with secretory signals preferentially enhance antibody (especially IgG1) responses, whereas plasmids expressing nonsecreted immunogens promote CTL immunity and IgG2a humoral responses (71,72). Other groups have investigated the use of DNA constructs containing immunogen cDNA fused in frame with ubiquitin coding sequences (73–75). In these studies, antigen ubiquitinization is consistently associated with enhanced CTL immunity and abrogation of humoral responses, presumably reflecting antigen targeting for rapid proteosome-dependent degradation and subsequent MHC-restricted epitope presentation.

Other strategies for modulation of responses to DNA vaccination have been proposed and investigated. First, optimization of gene-expression regulatory elements (e.g., promoters) within plasmid constructs may upregulate antigen expression and thereby facilitate immune induction (76). Second, some studies have suggested that the sequential use of DNA vaccines and recombinant viral vaccines (e.g., fowlpox recombinants) may synergistically induce durable and protective immune responses (77–79). Third, several investigators have reported that fusion of antigen DNA sequences and cDNA encoding highly immunogenic proteins [e.g., fragment C of tetanus toxoid, hepatitis B surface antigen (HBsAg)] within DNA vaccine constructs promotes the generation of immunity against poorly immunogenic antigens (80,81). Finally, chemical adjuvants may modulate the magnitude and character of immune responses induced by DNA vaccination. For example, one report described enhanced antigen-specific IgG2a production, IL-2 and IFN-γ secretion, CTL immunity, and DTH responses to HIV-1 DNA vaccines encoding *env* and *rev* after coadministration of the anticancer immunomodulator Ubenimex into mouse muscle (82). Similar immune modulation was noted after intranasal or intramuscular administration of an HIV-1 *env* DNA vaccine with the saponin adjuvant QS-21 (83). Myolytic agents (e.g., bupivacaine and cardiotoxin), when inoculated into muscle several days before DNA vaccination, promote DNA uptake by myofiber cells and thereby increase the level of antigen synthesis within regional myocytes (84,85). However, the use of these agents as adjuvants in DNA immunization studies has not consistently augmented vaccine-induced immune responses (86).

RNA VACCINATION

To circumvent the risk of vaccine integration into host chromosomal DNA, our group and others have investigated the use of naked RNA constructs encoding antigenic proteins for immunization. We noted priming of an anti-carcinoembryonic antigen (CEA) antibody response in mice after multiple intramuscular injections of messenger RNA (mRNA) transcripts encoding CEA (87). Similarly, biolistic delivery of an mRNA construct encoding human α-1 antitrypsin into mouse epidermis elicited antigen-specific humoral immunity (88). Direct injection of mRNA transcripts is generally associated with a low level and brief duration of transgene expression, an advantageous characteristic for vaccines encoding transformation-associated oncoproteins (e.g., erb-B2). However, such limited antigen expression is frequently inadequate for the induction of immune responses.

To enhance the level and duration of transgene expression from naked RNA vaccine constructs, several investigators have incorporated antigen-encoding sequences into self-replicative vector RNA derived from alphavirus, including Sindbis virus and Semliki Forest virus. The alphavirus genome consists of a

TABLE 1. PRECLINICAL TRIALS OF DNA VACCINES ENCODING TUMOR ANTIGENS

Tumor Antigen	Associated Human Cancers	Animal Models	Route	Immune Responses	References
Her-2/*neu*	Breast, ovarian, gastric	Mouse	i.m.	Ab, TP	94,95
CEA	Adenocarcinoma	Mouse, rabbit, dog, primate	i.m., i.d., g.g., i.v., i.s.	Ab, LP, TP	4,40,69,96–98
HCG-β	Testicular, choriocarcinoma	Mouse	i.m.	Ab, LP, CTL, TP	99
HuD	Small-cell lung	Mouse	i.m.	Ab, TP	100
Ig idiotype	B-cell lymphoma	Mouse	i.m.	Ab, LP, TP	101–105
CD4	T-cell malignancies	Mouse	i.m.	Ab, CTL, TP	106
HTLV-1	ATLL	Rabbit, rat	i.m.	Ab, LP, TP	107
MAGE-1, MAGE-3	Melanoma, breast, NSCLC	Mouse	i.m.	TP	108
gp100	Melanoma	Mouse	i.m., i.d.	Ab, CTL, TP	109
MART-1	Melanoma	Mouse	i.m.	Ab	Unpublished observation
TRP-1	Melanoma	Mouse	g.g.	Ab, TP	110
Mutant p53	Widely expressed	Mouse	g.g.	CTL, TP	78
PSA	Prostate	Mouse	i.m.	Ab, LP, CTL	111

Ab, antibody; ATLL, adult T-cell leukemia/lymphoma; CEA, carcinoembryonic antigen; CTL, cytotoxic T lymphocyte; g.g., gene gun (skin); HCG-β, β subunit of human chorionic gonadotropin; HTLV-1, human T-cell lymphotrophic virus-1; Ig, immunoglobulin; i.s., intrasplenic; LP, lymphoproliferation; MART-1, melanoma antigen recognized by T cells-1; NSCLC, non–small-cell lung cancer; PSA, prostate-specific antigen; TP, tumor protection; TRP-1, tyrosinase-related protein-1.

positive-polarity, single-stranded RNA molecule containing coding regions for viral replicase and transcriptase and structural proteins, including basic capsid protein (89). After alphavirus infection of susceptible cells, this genomic RNA serves as a template for translation (by host ribosomal complexes) of viral proteins. Nascent viral transcriptase then uses genomic RNA to synthesize full-length minus-strand RNA, which provides a template for the production of multiple genome-length positive-polarity RNA molecules and subgenomic-positive strand transcripts encoding structural proteins. Our group and others have replaced structural genes from alphavirus genomic RNA with heterologous coding sequences to derive self-replicative, packaging-defective RNA species. We used Sindbis virus RNA to produce a self-replicative transcript encoding luciferase (90). Injection of this construct into mouse muscle generated markedly increased and prolonged reporter-gene expression relative to that obtained with nonreplicative transcripts. The efficiency of heterologous gene expression from alphavirus-based recombinant RNA may be further augmented by the retention within chimeric RNA of a translational enhancer located near the beginning of the open reading frame of basic capsid protein (91).

Several investigators have conducted murine vaccination studies using alphavirus-based constructs with heterologous antigen–encoding sequences. For example, intramuscular injection of recombinant Semliki Forest virus genomic RNA encoding influenza virus HA induced seroconversion against HA and protected against intranasal challenge with influenza virus (92). Other groups have attempted to combine the advantages of DNA vaccines (e.g., stability and ease of production) with the enhanced gene expression of alphavirus-based replicons by the production of plasmid constructs driving expression of self-replicative, antigen-encoding transcripts. Intramuscular injection of a DNA vaccine encoding a Sindbis virus–based replicon containing coding sequences for herpes simplex virus, glycoprotein B elicited, antigen-specific, humoral and cellular immune responses in mice (93). This was a highly efficient vector, requiring 100- to 1,000-fold lower doses of plasmid to induce immunity, as compared to a conventional DNA vaccine encoding the same antigen. This efficiency presumably reflects enhanced transgene expression due to cytoplasmic amplification of self-replicative RNA transcripts.

PRECLINICAL STUDIES OF ANTITUMOR DNA VACCINATION

Several investigators have reported the generation of antigen-specific humoral and cellular immune responses and the rejection of tumor transplants in animals vaccinated with DNA constructs encoding TAAs. Examples of these studies are provided in Table 1, and our preclinical experience with DNA vaccines encoding CEA is outlined in Table 2. In preparation for a phase

TABLE 2. PRECLINICAL EXPERIENCE WITH DNA VACCINES ENCODING CARCINOEMBRYONIC ANTIGEN

Species/Immune Response	Route of Administration					
	i.m.	i.m. (Biojector)	i.d.	i.v.	i.s.	g.g.
Mouse						
Ab	+	ND	+	ND	+	+
LP	+	ND	+	ND	ND	+
TP	+	ND	+	ND	+	–
Rabbit						
Ab	+	+	+	–	ND	ND
Dog						
Ab	+	+	+	±	ND	ND
LP	+	+	ND	ND	ND	ND
Primate						
Ab	+	ND	ND	ND	ND	+
LP	+	ND	ND	ND	ND	+
DTH	+	ND	ND	ND	ND	–

Ab, antibody; DTH, delayed-type hypersensitivity; g.g., gene gun (skin); i.s., intrasplenic; LP, lymphoproliferation; ND, not done; TP, tumor protection; +, immune response or protection against tumor challenge; –, absence of immune response or tumor protection.

1 trial of DNA vaccination against CEA in patients with colorectal carcinoma, we immunized a group of pig-tailed macaques with a single plasmid-encoding CEA and HBsAg by repetitive intramuscular injections (98). Lymphoproliferative and antibody responses to CEA and HBsAg were not consistently observed until 4 months after primary immunization, suggesting the need for a protracted immunization schedule in human trials of DNA vaccines.

We have investigated the efficacy of intrasplenic administration of a DNA vaccine encoding CEA (pCEA) (4). In this study, several groups, each containing 15 mice, were immunized with 50-µg doses of pCEA by intrasplenic or intramuscular injection. Six weeks later, sera were collected followed by subcutaneous challenge with syngeneic, CEA-expressing colon carcinoma cells. Intrasplenic administration of pCEA induced anti-CEA antibody responses at a frequency comparable to the intramuscular route. Anti-CEA IgG antibodies were observed in 73% (11 of 15) and 53% (8 of 15) of mice receiving 50-µg doses of pCEA by intrasplenic or intramuscular injection, respectively. Both intrasplenic and intramuscular administration of pCEA elicited CEA-specific IgG1, IgG2a, and IgG2b antibody responses, an isotype pattern consistent with the activation of T helper 1 cells. Additionally, partial immunoprotection against tumor challenge occurred with comparable frequency after either route of immunization. No anti-CEA antibodies or tumor-free survival occurred after intrasplenic or intramuscular injections of a control plasmid lacking CEA coding sequences.

Two antitumor DNA vaccine studies have reported induction of immune responses against tumor-associated self-antigens in animals. First, a DNA construct encoding the human small-cell carcinoma antigen HuD elicited anti-Hu humoral immunity in mice (100). Sera from vaccinated animals were reactive with murine neuron Hu antigens *in vitro*, but seroconversion was not associated with the development of neuropathologic changes. Additionally, immunization with plasmid-encoded human HuD conferred immunoprotection against challenge with syngeneic neuroblastoma cells constitutively expressing native mouse HuD. A second report described the induction of tyrosinase-related protein 1 (TRP-1)–specific autoantibodies with consequent coat depigmentation after the immunization of mice with a plasmid construct encoding homologous human TRP-1 (110). Vaccination with this construct also provided protection against challenge with a syngeneic melanoma cell line expressing native mouse TRP-1. Of note, immunization with a DNA vaccine encoding syngeneic murine TRP-1 produced neither seroconversion against TRP-1 nor tumor protection. Two additional murine studies have described the use of DNA vaccines to break tolerance to self-antigens. One group has noted the induction of anti-HBsAg antibodies in HBsAg-transgenic mice after intramuscular administration of a plasmid encoding HBsAg. Immune response to this vaccine was accompanied by loss of circulating antigen and complete disappearance of hepatitis B virus (HBV) mRNA in the liver (112). In another report, vaccination of mice with DNA encoding the human thyrotropin receptor induced a humoral response against this antigen and produced histologic evidence of murine thyroiditis (113). Collectively, these observations support the use of DNA vaccine constructs encoding TAA homologues

from other species to break tolerance to tumor-associated self-antigens in humans.

SAFETY CONSIDERATIONS IN DNA VACCINATION

Potential adverse effects associated with the use of DNA vaccines in the management of human cancer include the elicitation of anti-DNA autoantibodies with resultant induction or exacerbation of systemic autoimmune disease, integration of plasmid into host genomic DNA with consequent insertional mutagenesis, induction of deleterious host immune responses against plasmid-transfected tissues, and provocation of immune responses against host tissues expressing proteins homologous to vaccine-encoded antigens.

The risk of induction or acceleration of systemic autoimmune disease by DNA vaccines has been extensively evaluated in murine studies. For example, multiple intramuscular injections of a plasmid-DNA construct into normal mice was associated with a threefold increase in the number of splenic B cells secreting IgG with anti-DNA specificity and an associated modest increase in serum anti-DNA antibody levels (114). This serologic response was not accompanied by the development of proteinuria or other clinical findings suggestive of glomerulonephritis or systemic autoimmune disease. In subsequent studies, DNA vaccination of lupus-prone mice neither accelerated the development of anti-DNA antibodies nor altered the age of onset or severity of glomerulonephritis (114). Several investigators have reported the induction of anti-DNA antibodies in mice by the administration of bacterial DNA complexed to a charged carrier protein with adjuvant (115,116). Inoculation of *Escherichia coli* DNA complexed to methylated bovine serum albumin in complete Freund's adjuvant into the peritonei of lupus-prone mice accelerated the development of anti-DNA antibodies but appeared to attenuate the clinical manifestations of systemic lupus erythematosus (117). Inoculated mice displayed less proteinuria, less histologic evidence of glomerulonephritis, and a longer life span than controls. Moreover, administration of protein-complexed bacterial DNA in adjuvant to lupus-prone mice after the spontaneous development of DNA autoantibodies stabilized nephritis and prolonged survival (117). These murine studies collectively suggest that the use of DNA vaccines may result in the elicitation of anti-DNA antibodies but is unlikely to induce or accelerate systemic autoimmune disease. This contention is supported by reports describing the presence of anti-DNA antibodies in sera from normal human subjects that target nonconserved epitopes on bacterial DNA, presumably reflecting exposure to bacterial DNA in the setting of colonization or infection (118). These antibodies lack cross-reactivity with host DNA, and their detection does not correlate with the presence or subsequent development of autoimmune disease. Several phase 1 clinical trials of DNA vaccines have specifically looked for development of anti-DNA antibodies but none have been detected (119–122).

Potential mechanisms whereby a DNA vaccine could integrate into host chromosomal DNA include homologous recombination and random insertion. Integration by these means could be tumorigenic by virtue of host proto-oncogene activation or disruption of expression of a host tumor suppressor gene. Additionally, chromosomal integration of a DNA vaccine encoding a transformation-associated oncoprotein (e.g., erb-B2) could induce cellular transformation independent of the site of plasmid insertion. The risk of DNA vaccine integration to host genomic DNA by homologous recombination is low given the lack of sequence homology between bacterial and mammalian DNA, as well as the general absence of chromosomal replication and cell division in cells transfected with DNA vaccine reagents. Two lines of evidence suggest that the risk of insertional mutagenesis secondary to random plasmid integration is similarly small. First, widespread clinical use of live replicating DNA virus vaccines (e.g., vaccinia) has not been associated with tumorigenesis. Second, PCR-based studies of myocytes transfected with DNA vaccine constructs have suggested an absence of plasmid integration into host chromosomal DNA. In one of these investigations, inoculated mouse quadriceps were harvested at various time points after injection of a large dose of a DNA vaccine (123). After whole DNA extraction, high-molecular-weight host chromosomal DNA was separated from nonintegrated vaccine DNA by agarose gel electrophoresis. Isolated host genomic DNA was then evaluated for the presence of integrated plasmid by PCR using plasmid-specific primers. No plasmid integration was demonstrable at a sensitivity of 1.0 to 7.5 copies of integrated plasmid per 150,000 cell nuclei. Based on these observations, the authors of this study estimate that the risk of insertional mutagenesis of a given gene secondary to random DNA vaccine integration is at least three orders of magnitude lower than the rate of spontaneous mutation. Although the risk of host chromosomal integration appears to be low, some investigators have proposed the inclusion of apoptotic signals within DNA vaccine constructs intended for human use to circumvent any potential risk of plasmid-mediated oncogenesis (124).

A third theoretical adverse effect of DNA vaccination is the provocation of destructive immune responses against plasmid-transfected cells, which has not been reported in preclinical DNA immunization studies. Klinman's group noted no increase in serum antibodies reactive with myosin and no evidence of muscle inflammation following multiple intramuscular DNA immunizations of adult mice (114). Similarly, intradermal and epidermal delivery of DNA vaccines have not been associated with the development of dermatitis. Several phase 1 clinical trials of DNA vaccines have reported the absence of serologic or clinical evidence of myositis despite successful elicitation of immune responses to plasmid-encoded antigens (119–122). Absence of local immunologic sequelae may reflect the relative inefficiency of target-cell transduction by DNA vaccines. Immunohistochemical studies suggest that generally less than 1% of regional myocytes are transfected by intramuscular DNA vaccines (86). Thus, immune-mediated destruction of transfected cells would likely be a subclinical event.

The potential destruction of host tissues expressing proteins identical or homologous to plasmid-encoded antigens is of particular concern with the use of DNA vaccines encoding tumor-associated self-antigens. To investigate this possibility, we administered a DNA vaccine construct encoding human CEA to macaques, a primate species with low-level expression of human CEA homologues on intestinal mucosal cells and neutrophils (CD66) (98). In this study, we noted frequent anti-CEA immune responses among immunized animals without generation of autoimmune colitis or neutropenia. However, as noted in the section Preclinical Studies of Antitumor DNA Vaccination, immunization of mice with a DNA vaccine encoding human TRP-1–elicited antibodies that cross-reacted with the native mouse homologue resulting in autoimmune coat depigmentation (110). If immunologic tolerance to tumor-associated self-antigens can be broken in humans by DNA vaccines, the likelihood and clinical relevance of the resultant autoimmune toxicity depends on several factors, including the expression level and tissue distribution of the antigen as well as the magnitude and character of the vaccine-induced immune response.

CLINICAL TRIALS OF DNA VACCINES IN INFECTIOUS DISEASES

Since 1996, phase 1 clinical trials have been conducted with DNA vaccines directed against a variety of viral pathogens and malaria, an intracellular parasitic infection. These trials are summarized in Table 3. Only a few DNA vaccine clinical trials have reached phase 2, and no large-scale phase 3 trial has yet begun. Although the safety database is still accumulating, the data obtained from vaccinating approximately 400 human subjects indicate that plasmid DNA vaccination is safe and well tolerated. Clinical trials to date have reported minimal local toxicity consisting of occasional injection-site erythema or tenderness (135). No systemic toxicity has been reported, including no laboratory abnormalities (119,121,125,127–129). Specifically, no anti-DNA antibodies or muscle enzyme elevations have been reported (119,121,125).

One of the first DNA vaccine clinical trials to be reported involved immunization of 15 asymptomatic HIV-infected patients with a DNA plasmid containing HIV *env* and *rev* genes (119,120). Successive groups received three intramuscular injections of vaccine (30, 100, or 300 μg) at 10-week intervals in a dose-escalation trial. CD4/CD8-lymphocyte levels and plasma HIV concentration remained relatively unchanged throughout the study. Antibody against the *env* gene product (gp120) increased modestly in a minority of patients in the 100 μg and 300 μg groups, though no consistent effect on cellular responses to HIV was noted (57,119,120). Interpretation of humoral and cellular immune response data was hampered by significant preexisting immunity in these HIV-infected individuals.

In a second clinical trial, nine asymptomatic HIV-infected patients were immunized with one of three DNA constructs encoding the *nef, rev,* or *tat* regulatory genes of HIV-1 (125). Groups of three patients received 100-μg doses of a single DNA construct by intramuscular injection on days 0, 60, and 180. DNA vaccination induced antigen-specific lymphoproliferative and CTL responses. CTLs were MHC class I restricted and primarily CD8 positive (125). More recently, more than 80 HIV seronegative volunteers have been enrolled in clinical trials testing both *env/rev* and *gag/pol* DNA vaccines (121,126,127,130–

TABLE 3. CLINICAL TRIALS OF DNA VACCINES

Disease	Antigen	Application	Status	Immune Response	Institution	References
AIDS	HIV *env/rev*	Therapeutic	Complete	Ab, LP, CTL	Univ. of Pennsylvania	119,120
AIDS	HIV *nef/rev/tat*	Therapeutic	Complete	LP, CTL	Karolinska Institute, Sweden	125
AIDS	HIV *gag/pol*	Prophylactic	Active	LP	NIH AVEG	121,126,127
AIDS	HIV *env/rev*	Prophylactic	Active	NA	NIH	126,127
Hepatitis B	HBsAg	Prophylactic	Complete	Ab	Univ. of Wisconsin	Web site
Hepatitis B	HBsAg	Prophylactic	Active	NA	Univ. of Cincinnati	128
Herpesvirus	HSV antigen gd	Therapeutic	Active	NA	Univ. of Washington	128
Influenza	Hemagglutinin	Prophylactic	Complete	Ab	Johns Hopkins Univ.	128,129
Malaria	PfCSP	Prophylactic	Complete	CTL	Naval Medical Research Institute	130
Colon cancer	CEA/HBsAg	Therapeutic	Complete	Ab	Univ. of Alabama at Birmingham	122,131
CTCL	Idiotypic TCR	Therapeutic	Active	NA	Univ. of Pennsylvania	106,128
B-cell lymphoma	Idiotype	Therapeutic	Active	NA	Univ. of Southampton, Great Britain	Web site
Melanoma	gp100	Therapeutic	Active	NA	NIH	Web site
Melanoma	HLA-B7	Therapeutic	Complete	CTL, CR	Univ. of Michigan	132–134

Ab, antibody response; AVEG, AIDS Vaccine Evaluation Group; CEA, carcinoembryonic antigen; CTCL, cutaneous T-cell lymphoma; CTL, cytotoxic T lymphocyte; CR, clinical antitumor response; HBsAg, hepatitis B surface antigen; HIV, human immunodeficiency virus; HSV, herpes simplex virus; LP, lymphoproliferative response; NA, not available; NIH, National Institutes of Health; PfCSP, *Plasmodium falciparum* circumsporozoite protein; TCR, T-cell receptor; Web site, http://DNAvaccine.com.

135). One such trial evaluated intramuscular delivery of a DNA vaccine encoding HIV *gag/pol* at 0, 1, 2, and 6 months in 39 healthy subjects (121). The vaccine dose was escalated from 100 to 1,000 μg of DNA. Vaccine-induced lymphoproliferative responses to *gag* occurred. However, no antibody responses were observed to *gag* or *pol,* and only rare CTL responses were induced with plasmid DNA doses up to 1 mg. Knowledgeable sources have expressed doubt that the first generation HIV DNA vaccines, as currently designed, can induce significant CTL responses in uninfected human volunteers (127).

In the largest DNA vaccine trial reported to date, 219 healthy volunteers were randomized to receive up to three doses of a plasmid-encoding influenza hemagglutinin or placebo (129). Doses ranged from 1 to 500 μg of plasmid DNA administered intramuscularly. Virus-neutralizing and hemagglutination-inhibiting antibodies were observed in a minority of subjects. However, the immunogenicity of this first-generation vaccine appears to have been somewhat disappointing.

More encouraging results have emerged from the initial clinical trial of a DNA vaccine against malaria. Twenty healthy malaria-naive adults were randomized into four dosage groups to receive three intramuscular injections of 20, 100, 500, or 2,500 μg of plasmid DNA encoding the *Plasmodium falciparum* circumsporozoite protein (130). Vaccinees developed antigen-specific, CD8+ CTLs restricted by multiple HLA alleles. Immunization with either 500 or 2,500 μg of DNA induced significantly better CTL responses in comparison with either 20 or 100 μg of DNA. Furthermore, a significantly higher frequency of CTL response was induced with 2,500 μg of DNA in comparison to 500 μg of DNA after the second immunization. This trial represents the first demonstration in healthy naive humans of the induction of CD8+ CTLs by a DNA vaccine, providing a foundation for further human testing of this potentially revolutionary vaccine technology (130).

Encouraging results have also emerged from the first clinical trial of a DNA vaccine administered by cutaneous particle bombardment. Twelve healthy naive volunteers received a prime and

two boosts of a DNA vaccine encoding the surface antigen of HBV adhered to gold particles and delivered by the Dermal PowderJect System (PowderJect Pharmaceuticals, Madison, WI). Interim analysis showed that all 11 subjects completing the vaccination schedule seroconverted to antibody levels, which are accepted as conferring protection against HBV. Thus, early clinical trials of DNA vaccines against infectious pathogens have provided mixed results. Trials conducted in HIV-infected individuals have been difficult to interpret due to preexisting immunity; and trials of HIV and influenza DNA vaccines in healthy volunteers have been somewhat lackluster. However, DNA vaccine trials against malaria and HBV have provided unequivocal evidence for the induction of antigen-specific CTL and antibody responses, respectively.

CLINICAL TRIALS OF DNA VACCINES FOR CANCER THERAPY

Our group at the University of Alabama at Birmingham has completed a dose-escalation clinical trial of a dual-expression plasmid encoding CEA and HBsAg in 17 patients with metastatic colorectal carcinoma (122,131). This represents the first completed clinical trial of a DNA vaccine in patients with cancer. The HBsAg cDNA was included as a positive control for immune response to the DNA vaccine without relying on breaking immunologic tolerance to the tumor-associated self-antigen, CEA. Groups of three patients each received the DNA vaccine by intramuscular injection at 3-week intervals in a dose-escalation format as follows: group one, 100-μg single dose; group two, 300-μg single dose; group three, 1-mg single dose; group four, 300 μg × three doses; group five, 1 mg × three doses; and group six, 2 mg × three doses. No significant toxicity occurred, including no autoimmune toxicity (122). All five patients receiving repetitive 1- to 2-mg doses of the DNA vaccine seroconverted to antibodies against HBsAg, and three of these five patients achieved antibody levels that are accepted as

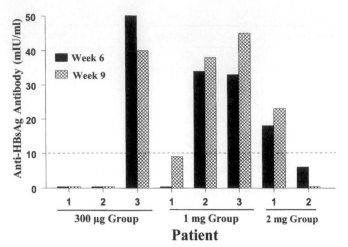

FIGURE 1. Antibody response to hepatitis B surface antigen (HBsAg) after intramuscular DNA vaccination. Colorectal carcinoma patients received three repetitive doses of a DNA vaccine encoding both carcinoembryonic antigen and HBsAg at 3-week intervals in a dose-escalation trial. Anti-HBsAg antibodies were quantitated by commercial enzyme-linked immunosorbent assay (Abbott Laboratories, Abbott Park, IL). Prevaccination values were zero for all patients, and the dashed line at 10 mIU per mL indicates the accepted threshold conferring protection against hepatitis B virus.

conferring protection against HBV (Fig. 1). Antibody responses to HBsAg occurred less frequently at lower doses and among patients receiving only a single vaccination. Notably, anti-HBsAg seroconversion was achieved within 9 weeks after primary immunization, a constraint imposed by vaccination of patients with limited life expectancy due to metastatic colorectal carcinoma. We have previously reported immunization of three pig-tailed macaques by intramuscular injection of the same DNA vaccine (98). Only one of three animals developed anti-HBsAg antibodies within 19 weeks after primary immunization, whereas all three seroconverted to protective levels of antibody by week 28. Thus, a more protracted vaccination schedule may increase the frequency of seroconversion to protective levels of anti-HBsAg antibodies, particularly when lower doses of DNA are used. No anti-CEA antibodies or lymphoproliferative response to CEA or HBsAg occurred. Analysis of CTL response to CEA and HBsAg is ongoing.

Additional phase 1 and phase 2 trials of DNA vaccines for cancer therapy are summarized in Table 3. A trial initiated in 1997 at the University of Pennsylvania is evaluating a DNA vaccine encoding the idiotypic T-cell receptor Vβ in patients with CTL (106,128). Similarly, a British trial initiated in 1998 is examining a DNA vaccine encoding a fusion protein consisting of fragment C of tetanus toxin and a tumor-derived single-chain idiotypic antibody-variable region in patients with B-cell lymphoma in first remission (80). Phase 1 and phase 2 trials of DNA vaccines are also ongoing in patients with prostate cancer, renal cell carcinoma, and melanoma (135).

The first clinical trial of a plasmid DNA vaccine in patients with melanoma was conducted at the University of Michigan in the early 1990s (132–134). In this trial, five HLA-B7–negative patients with metastatic melanoma and subcutaneous tumor nodules received intralesional injections of a plasmid DNA vaccine encoding a foreign human MHC class I gene, HLA-B7,

complexed with liposomes (134). This strategy was designed to enhance the immunogenicity of tumor cells through immune activation by the foreign MHC antigen. Recombinant HLA-B7 protein was demonstrated in tumor biopsy tissue from all five patients, and circulating tumor-specific CTLs were detected in three of five patients after vaccination. One patient demonstrated regression of injected nodules and regression at distant sites. No harmful side effects occurred. More recently, the Surgical Oncology Branch of the National Cancer Institute initiated a trial of a DNA vaccine encoding gp100 in patients with metastatic melanoma in late 1988. Approximately 24 patients have received 1 mg of plasmid DNA by intramuscular or intradermal needle injection every 4 weeks for four doses with or without systemic IL-2. One partial clinical response is ongoing, as is the analysis of immune response to gp100 immunodominant peptides (James Yang, *personal communication*, 1999).

Our group at the University of Alabama at Birmingham is conducting a phase 1 dose-escalation trial of a DNA vaccine encoding MART-1, melanoma antigen recognized by T cells-1, in patients with resected melanoma at significant risk for relapse. A separate DNA vaccine encoding HBsAg is administered into the contralateral deltoid as a positive control for immune response. Because this trial is in the adjuvant setting, we have selected a more protracted vaccination schedule consisting of DNA vaccine injections (100, 300, or 1,000 µg of each plasmid) every 6 weeks for four doses.

In summary, a trial in a small number of patients has demonstrated the ability of plasmid DNA complexed with liposomes to direct expression of a foreign MHC antigen within subcutaneous melanoma nodules with resultant tumor-specific immune responses. Our phase 1 trial in colorectal cancer has not yet demonstrated immune responses to the tumor-associated antigen. However, protective levels of anti-HBsAg antibodies were induced in the majority of patients receiving repetitive 1- to 2-mg doses of DNA vaccine. This information, together with the phase 1 malaria DNA vaccine trial (130), suggests enhanced frequency and magnitude of immune responses to DNA vaccines when 1.0- to 2.5-mg doses are used in humans. Furthermore, data from our group and others in nonhuman primate models suggest that a protracted vaccination schedule over 4 to 6 months may enhance the immune response to DNA vaccines. Otherwise, clinical trials of DNA vaccines have been initiated in a wide range of malignancies; whether this new technology represents hope or hype for patients with cancer remains to be seen.

CONCLUSION

Data obtained from first-generation clinical trials indicate that DNA vaccination is safe and well tolerated. DNA vaccine clinical trials have also unequivocally elicited antigen-specific CTL and antibody responses against malaria and HBV, respectively. Furthermore, humoral and cellular immune responses against TAAs have been induced in numerous preclinical models with resultant antitumor effects. This has led to the initiation of clinical DNA vaccine trials in six human malignancies. Second-generation clinical trials examine exciting augmentation strategies for preferential induction of Th1 and CTL immunity. The next half-decade promises to provide much insight into the clinical utility of this revolutionary vaccine technology in the fields of infectious disease and cancer.

REFERENCES

1. Tang DC, DeVit M, Johnston SA, et al. Genetic immunization is a simple method for eliciting an immune response. *Nature* 1992;356:152–154.
2. Ulmer JB, Donnelly JJ, Parker SE, et al. Heterologous protection against influenza by injection of DNA encoding a viral protein. *Science* 1993;259:1745–1749.
3. Fynan EF, Webster RG, Fuller DH, et al. DNA vaccines: protective immunizations by parental, mucosal, and gene gun inoculations. *Proc Natl Acad Sci U S A* 1993;90:11478–11482.
4. White SA, LoBuglio AF, Shaw DR, et al. Intrasplenic administration of a DNA vaccine encoding carcinoembryonic antigen (CEA) elicits CEA-specific antibody responses and tumor protection. *J Gene Med* 2000;2:1–6.
5. Gerloni M, Ballou WR, Billetta ZM. Immunity to plasmodium falciparum malaria sporozoites by somatic transgene immunization. *Nat Biotech* 1997;15:876–881.
6. Feltquate DM, Heaney S, Webster RG, et al. Different T helper cell types and antibody isotypes generated by saline and gene gun DNA immunization. *J Immunol* 1997;158:2278–2284.
7. Xin KQ, Hamajima K, Sasaki S, et al. Intranasal administration of human immunodeficiency virus type-1 (HIV-1) DNA vaccine with interleukin-2 expression plasmid enhances cell-mediated immunity against HIV-1. *Immunol* 1998;94:438–444.
8. Sasaki S, Hamajima K, Fukushima J, et al. Comparison of intranasal and intramuscular immunization against human immunodeficiency virus type 1 with a DNA-monophosphoryl lipid A adjuvant vaccine. *Infect Immun* 1998;66:823–826.
9. Toebe CS, Clements JD, Cardenas L, et al. Evaluation of immunogenicity of an oral Salmonella vaccine expressing recombinant Plasmodium berghei merozoite surface protein-1. *Am J Trop Med Hyg* 1997;56:192–199.
10. Paglia P, Medina E, Arioli I, et al. Gene transfer in dendritic cells induced by oral DNA vaccination with Salmonella typhimurium, results in protective immunity against a murine fibrosarcoma. *Blood* 1998;92:3172–3176.
11. Boyer JD, Ugen KE, Wang B, et al. Protection of chimpanzees from high-dose heterologous HIV-1 challenge by DNA vaccination. *Nat Med* 1997;3:526–532.
12. Boyer JD, Ugen KE, Chattergoon M, et al. DNA vaccination as anti-human immunodeficiency virus immunotherapy in infected chimpanzees. *J Infect Dis* 1997;176:1501–1509.
13. Liu MA, McClements W, Ulmer JB, et al. Immunization of non-human primates with DNA vaccines. *Vaccine* 1997;15:909–912.
14. Donnelly JJ, Ulmer JB, Liu MA. Protective efficacy of intramuscular immunization with naked DNA. *Ann N Y Acad Sci* 1995;772:40–46.
15. Harding FA, McArthur JG, Gross JA, et al. CD28-mediated signaling co-stimulates murine T cells and prevents induction of anergy in T-cell clones. *Nature* 1992;356:607–609.
16. Torres CA, Iwasaki A, Barber BH, et al. Differential dependence on target site tissue for gene gun and intramuscular DNA immunizations. *J Immunol* 1997;158:4529–4532.
17. Eartl HCJ, Xiang ZQ. Genetic immunization. *Viral Immunol* 1996;9:1–9.
18. Corr M, Lee DJ, Tighe H. Gene vaccination with naked plasmid DNA: mechanism of CTL priming. *J Exp Med* 1996;184:1555–1560.
19. Iwasaki A, Torres AT, Ohashi PS, et al. The dominant role of bone marrow-derived cells in CTL induction following plasmid DNA immunization at different sites. *J Immunol* 1997;159:11–14.
20. Klinman DM, Sechler JMG, Conover J, et al. Contribution of cells at the site of DNA vaccination to the generation of antigen-specific immunity and memory. *J Immunol* 1998;160:2388–2392.
21. Casares S, Inaba K, Brumeanu T-D, et al. Antigen presentation by dendritic cells after immunization with DNA encoding a major histocompatibility complex class II-restricted viral epitope. *J Exp Med* 1997;186:1481–1486.
22. Condon C, Watkins SC, Celluzzi CM, et al. DNA-based immunization by *in vivo* transfection of dendritic cells. *Nat Med* 1996;2:1122–1125.
23. Chattergoon MA, Robinson TM, Boyer JD, et al. Specific immune induction following DNA-based immunization through *in vivo* transfection and activation of macrophages/antigen-presenting cells. *J Immunol* 1998;160:5707–5718.
24. Wolff JA, Dowty ME, Jiao S, et al. Expression of naked plasmids by cultured myotubes and entry of plasmids into T-tubules and caveolae of mammalian skeletal muscle. *J Cell Sci* 1993;103:1249–1259.
25. Albert ML, Sauter B, Bhardwaj N. Dendritic cells acquire antigen from apoptotic cells and induce class I-restricted CTLs. *Nature* 1998;392:86–89.
26. Boyle JS, Brady JL, Lew AM. Enhanced responses to a DNA vaccine encoding a fusion antigen that is directed to sites of immune induction. *Nature* 1998;392:408–411.
27. Ulmer JB, Deck CM, Dewitt CM, et al. Generation of MHC class I-restricted cytotoxic T lymphocytes by expression of a viral protein in muscle cells: antigen presentation by non-muscle cells. *Immunol* 1996;89:59–67.
28. Fu TM, Ulmer JB, Caulfield MJ, et al. Priming of cytotoxic T lymphocytes by DNA vaccines: requirement for professional antigen presenting cells and evidence for antigen transfer from myocytes. *Mol Med* 1997;3:362–371.
29. Kreig AM, Yi AK, Matson S, et al. CpG motifs in bacterial DNA trigger direct B-cell activation. *Nature* 1995;374:546–549.
30. Bird AP. CpG islands as gene markers in the vertebrate nucleus. *Trends Genet* 1987;3:342–346.
31. Hergersberg M. Biological aspects of cytosine methylation in eukaryotic cells. *Experientia* 1991;47:1171–1185.
32. Sun S, Beard C, Jaenisch R, et al. Mitogenicity of DNA from different organisms for murine B cells. *J Immunol* 1997;159:119–125.
33. Sun S, Kishimoto H, Sprent J. DNA as an adjuvant: capacity of insect DNA and synthetic oligodeoxynucleotides to augment T cell responses to specific antigen. *J Exp Med* 1998;187:1145–1150.
34. Halpern MD, Kurlander RJ, Pisetsky DS. Bacterial DNA induces murine interferon-gamma production by stimulation of IL-12 and tumor necrosis factor-alpha. *Cell Immunol* 1996;167:72–78.
35. Sato Y, Roman M, Tighe H, et al. Immunostimulatory DNA sequences necessary for effective intradermal gene immunization. *Science* 1996;273:352–354.
36. Klinman DM, Yi A, Beaucage SL, et al. CpG motifs expressed by bacterial DNA rapidly induce lymphocytes to secrete IL-6, IL-12 and IFN-γ. *Proc Natl Acad Sci U S A* 1996;93:2879–2883.
37. Sparwasser T, Koch ES, Vabulas RM, et al. Bacterial DNA and immunostimulatory CpG oligonucleotides trigger maturation and activation of murine dendritic cells. *J Immunol* 1998;28:2045–2054.
38. Klinman DM, Yamshchikov G, Ishigatsubo Y. Contribution of CpG motifs to the immunogenicity of DNA vaccines. *J Immunol* 1977;158:3635–3639.
39. Yi AK, Chang M, Peckham DW, et al. CpG oligodeoxyribonucleotides rescue mature spleen B cells from spontaneous apoptosis and promote cell cycle entry. *J Immunol* 1998;160:5898–5906.
40. Conry RM, LoBuglio AF, Curiel DT. Polynucleotide-mediated immunization therapy of cancer. *Semin Oncol* 1996;23:135–147.
41. Porter KR, Kochel TJ, Wu SJ, et al. Protective efficacy of a dengue 2 DNA vaccine in mice and the effect of CpG immuno-stimulatory motifs on antibody responses. *Archives Virol* 1998;143:997–1003.
42. Weeratna R, Brazolot Millan CL, Kreig AM, et al. Reduction of antigen expression from DNA vaccines by coadministered oligodeoxynucleotides. *Antisense Nucleic Acid Drug Dev* 1998;8:351–356.
43. McCluskie MJ, Davis HL. CpG DNA is a potent enhancer of systemic and mucosal immune responses against hepatitis B surface

antigen with intranasal administration to mice. *J Immunol* 1998;161:4463–4466.

44. Davis HL, Weeranta R, Waldschmidt TJ, et al. CpG DNA is a potent enhancer of specific immunity in mice immunized with recombinant hepatitis B surface antigen. *J Immunol* 1998;160:870–876.

45. Chu RS, Targoni OS, Kreig AM, et al. CpG oligodeoxynucleotides act as adjuvants that switch on T helper 1 (Th1) immunity. *J Exp Med* 1997;186:1623–1631.

46. Donnelly JJ, Ulmer JB, Shiver JW, et al. DNA vaccines. *Pharmacol Ther* 1997;15:17–48.

47. Weiner GJ, Liu HM, Woolridge JE, et al. Immunostimulatory oligodeoxynucleotides containing the CpG motif are effective as immune adjuvants in tumor antigen immunization. *Proc Natl Acad Sci U S A* 1997;94:10833–10837.

48. Roman M, Martin-Orozco E, Goodman JS, et al. Immunostimulatory DNA sequences function as T helper-1-promoting adjuvants. *Nat Med* 1997;3:849–854.

49. Yi A-K, Tuetken R, Redford T, et al. CpG motifs in bacterial DNA activate leukocytes through the pH-dependent generation of reactive oxygen species. *J Immunol* 1998;160:4755–4761.

50. Yi AK, Kreig AM. Rapid induction of mitogen-activated protein kinases by immune stimulatory CpG DNA. *J Immunol* 1998;161:4493–4497.

51. Macfarlane DE, Manzel L. Antagonism of immunostimulatory CpG-oligodeoxynucleotides by quinacrine, chloroquine, and structurally related compounds. *J Immunol* 1998;160:1122–1131.

52. Krieg AM, Wu T, Weeratna R, et al. Sequence motifs in adenoviral DNA block immune activation by stimulatory CpG motifs. *Proc Natl Acad Sci U S A* 1998;95:12631–12636.

53. Lipford GB, Sparwasser T, Bauer M, et al. Immunostimulatory DNA: sequenced-dependent production of potentially harmful or useful cytokines. *Eur J Immunol* 1997;27:3420–3426.

54. Pertmer TM, Roberts TR, Haynes JR. Influenza virus nucleoprotein-specific immunoglobulin G subclass and cytokine responses elicited by DNA vaccination are dependent on the route of vector DNA delivery. *J Virol* 1996;70:6119–6125.

55. Raz E, Tighe H, Sato Y, et al. Preferential induction of a Th1 immune response and inhibition of specific IgE antibody formation by plasmid DNA immunization. *Proc Natl Acad Sci U S A* 1996;93:5141–5145.

56. Barry MA, Johnston SA. Biological features of genetic immunization. *Vaccine* 1997;15:788–791.

57. Cohen AD, Boyer JD, Weiner DB. Modulating the immune response to genetic immunization. *FASEB* 1998;12:1611–1626.

58. Xin KQ, Hamajima K, Sasaki S, et al. Intranasal administration of human immunodeficiency virus type-1 (HIV-1) DNA vaccine with interleukin-2 expression plasmid enhances cell-mediated immunity against HIV-1. *Immunol* 1998;94:438–444.

59. Kim JJ, Ayyavoo V, Bagarazzi ML, et al. *In vivo* engineering of a cellular immune response by coadministration of IL-12 expression vector with a DNA immunogen. *J Immunol* 1997;158:816–826.

60. Sin JI, Boyer JD, Ciccarelli RB, et al. *In vivo* modulation of vaccine-induced immune responses toward a Th1 phenotype increases potency and vaccine effectiveness in a herpes simplex virus type 2 mouse model. *J Virol* 1999;73:501–509.

61. Kim JJ, Trivedi NN, Nottingham LK, et al. Modulation of amplitude and direction of *in vivo* immune responses by co-administration of cytokine gene expression cassettes with DNA immunogens. *Eur J Immunol* 1998;28:1089–1103.

62. Lee SW, Cho JH, Sung YC. Optimal induction of hepatitis C virus envelope-specific immunity by bicistronic plasmid DNA inoculation with the granulocyte-macrophage colony-stimulating factor gene. *J Virol* 1998;72:8430–8436.

63. Sin JI, Kim JJ, Ugen KE, et al. Enhancement of protective humoral (Th2) and cell-mediated (Th1) immune responses against herpes simplex virus-2 through co-delivery of granulocyte-macrophage colony-stimulating factor expression cassettes. *Eur J Immunol* 1998;28:3530–3540.

64. Uchijima M, Yoshida A, Nagata T, et al. Development of Th1 and Th2 populations and the nature of immune responses to hepatitis

65. Okada E, Sasaki S, Ishii N, et al. Intranasal immunization of a DNA vaccine with IL-12- and granulocyte-macrophage colony-stimulating factor (GM-CSF)-expressing plasmids in liposomes induces strong mucosal and cell-mediated immune responses against HIV-1 antigens. *J Immunol* 1997;159:3638–3647.

66. Weiss WR, Ishii KJ, Hedstrom RC, et al. A plasmid encoding murine granulocyte-macrophage colony stimulating factor increases protection conferred by a malaria DNA vaccine. *J Immunol* 1998;161:2325–2332.

67. Kim JJ, Bagarazzi ML, Trivedi N, et al. Engineering of *in vivo* immune responses to DNA immunization via codelivery of costimulatory molecule genes. *Nat Biol* 1997;15:641–646.

68. Iwasaki A, Niclas-Stiernholm BJ, Chan AK, et al. Enhanced CTL responses mediated by plasmid DNA immunogens encoding costimulatory molecules and cytokines. *J Immunol* 1997;158:4591–4601.

69. Conry RM, Widera G, LoBuglio AF, et al. Selected strategies to augment polynucleotide immunization. *Gene Ther* 1996;3:67–74.

70. Mendoza RB, Cantwell MJ, Kipps TJ. Immunostimulatory effects of a plasmid expressing CD40 ligand (CD154) on gene immunization. *J Immunol* 1997;159:5777–5781.

71. Haddad D, Liljeqvist S, Stahl S, et al. Differential induction of immunoglobulin G subclasses by immunization with DNA vectors containing or lacking a signal sequence. *Immunol Lett* 1998;61:201–204.

72. Inchauspe G, Vitvitski L, Major ME, et al. Plasmid DNA expressing a secreted or a nonsecreted form of hepatitis C virus nucleocapsid: comparative studies of antibody and T-helper responses following genetic immunization. *DNA Cell Biol* 1997;16:185–195.

73. Wu Y, Kipps TJ. Deoxyribonucleic acid vaccines encoding antigens with rapid proteasome-dependent degradation are highly efficient inducers of cytolytic T lymphocytes. *J Immunol* 1997;159:6037–6043.

74. Rodriguez F, Zhang J, Whitton JL. DNA immunization: ubiquitization of a viral protein enhances cytotoxic T-lymphocyte induction and antiviral protection but abrogates antibody induction. *J Virol* 1997:8497–8503.

75. Ciernik IF, Berzofsky JA, Carbone DP. Induction of cytotoxic T lymphocytes and antitumor immunity with DNA vaccines expressing single T cell epitopes. *J Immunol* 1996;156:2369–2375.

76. Norman JA, Hobart P, Manthorpe M, et al. Development of improved vectors for DNA-based immunization and other gene therapy applications. *Vaccine* 1997;15:801–803.

77. Ramsay AJ, Leong KH, Ramshaw IA. DNA vaccination against virus infection and enhancement of antiviral immunity following consecutive immunization with DNA and viral vectors. *Immunol Cell Biol* 1997;75:382–388.

78. Kent SJ, Zhao A, Best SJ, et al. Enhanced T-cell immunogenicity and protective efficacy of a human immunodeficiency virus type 1 vaccine regimen consisting of consecutive priming with DNA and boosting with recombinant fowlpox virus. *J Virol* 1998;72:10180–10188.

79. Sedegah M, Jones TR, Kaur M, et al. Boosting with recombinant vaccinia increases immunogenicity and protective efficacy of malaria DNA vaccine. *Proc Natl Acad Sci U S A* 1998;95:7648–7653.

80. King CA, Spellerberg MB, Zhu D, et al. DNA vaccines with single-chain Fv fused to fragment C of tetanus toxin induce protective immunity against lymphoma and myeloma. *Nat Med* 1998;4:1281–1286.

81. Le Borgne S, Mancini M, Le Grand R, et al. *In vivo* induction of specific cytotoxic T lymphocytes in mice and rhesus macaques immunized with DNA vector encoding an HIV epitope fused with hepatitis B surface antigen. *Virology* 1998;240:304–315.

82. Sasaki S, Fukushima J, Hamajima K, et al. Adjuvant effect of Ubenimex on a DNA vaccine for HIV-1. *Clin Exp Immunol* 1998;111:30–35.

83. Sasaki S, Sumino K, Hamajima K, et al. Induction of systemic and mucosal immune responses to human immunodeficiency virus type 1 by a DNA vaccine formulated with QS-21 saponin adjuvant via intramuscular and intranasal routes. *J Virol* 1998:4931–4939.

virus DNA vaccines can be modulated by co-delivery of various cytokine genes. *J Immunol* 1998;160:1320–1329.

84. Wells DJ. Improved gene transfer by direct plasmid injection associated with regenerating muscle. *Biochem Soc* 1993;332:179–182.

85. Danko L, Fritz JD, Jiao S, et al. Pharmacological enhancement of *in vivo* foreign gene expression in muscle. *Science* 1993:179–182.

86. Fomsgaard A, Neilsen HV, Neilsen C, et al. Comparisons of DNA-mediated immunization procedures directed against surface glycoproteins of human immunodeficiency virus type-1 and hepatitis B virus. *APMIS* 1998;106:636–646.

87. Conry RM, LoBuglio AF, Wright M, et al. Characterization of a messenger RNA polynucleotide vaccine vector. *Cancer Res* 1994;55:1397–1400.

88. Qui P, Ziegelhoffer P, Sun J, et al. Gene gun delivery of mRNA *in situ* results in efficient transgene expression and genetic immunization. *Gene Ther* 1996;3:262–268.

89. Rice CM. Alphavirus-based expression systems. *Adv Exp Med Biol* 1996;397:31–40.

90. Johanning FW, Conry RM, LoBuglio AF, et al. A Sindbis virus mRNA polynucleotide vector achieves prolonged and high level heterologous gene expression *in vivo*. *Nucleic Acids Res* 1995;23:1495–1501.

91. Sjoberg JH, Suomalainen M, Garoff H. A significantly improved Semliki Forest virus expression based on translation enhancer segments from the viral capsid gene. *BioTech* 1994;12:1127–1131.

92. Dalemans W, Delers A, Delmelle C, et al. Protection against homologous influenza challenge by genetic immunization with SFV-RNA encoding Flu-HA. *Ann N Y Acad Sci* 1995;772:255–256.

93. Hariharan MJ, Driver DA, Townsend K, et al. DNA immunization against herpes simplex virus: enhanced efficacy using a Sindbis virus-based vector. *J Virol* 1998;72:950–958.

94. Concetti A, Amici A, Petrelli C, et al. Autoantibody to p185erB2/neu oncoprotein by vaccination with xenogenic DNA. *Cancer Immunol Immunother* 1996;43:307–315.

95. Chen Y, Hu D, Eling DJ, et al. DNA vaccines encoding full-length or truncated *neu* induce protective immunity against *neu*-expressing mammary tumors. *Cancer Res* 1998;58:1965–1971.

96. Conry RM, LoBuglio AF, Loechel F, et al. A carcinoembryonic antigen polynucleotide vaccine for human clinical use. *Gene Ther* 1995;2:33–38.

97. Smith BF, Baker HJ, Curiel DT, et al. Humoral and cellular immune responses of dogs immunized with a nucleic acid vaccine encoding human carcinoembryonic antigen. *Gene Ther* 1998;5:865–868.

98. Conry RM, White SA, Fultz PN, et al. Polynucleotide immunization of nonhuman primates against carcinoembryonic antigen. *Clin Cancer Res* 1998;4:2903–2912.

99. Geissler M, Wands G, Gesien A, et al. Genetic immunization with the free human chorionic gonadotropin β subunit elicits cytotoxic T lymphocyte responses and protects against tumor formation in mice. *Lab Invest* 1997;76:859–871.

100. Carpentier AF, Rosenfeld MR, Delattre JY, et al. DNA vaccination with HuD inhibits growth of a neuroblastoma in mice. *Clin Cancer Res* 1998;4:2819–2824.

101. Syrengelas AD, Chen TT, Levy R, et al. DNA immunization induces protective immunity against B-cell lymphoma. *Nat Med* 1996;2:1038–1041.

102. Hakim I, Levy S, Levy R. A nine-amino acid peptide from IL-1 beta augments antitumor immune responses induced by protein and DNA vaccines. *J Immunol* 1996;157:5503–5511.

103. Hawkins RE, Winter G, Hamblin TJ, et al. A genetic approach to idiotypic vaccination. *J Immunol* 1993;14:273–278.

104. Stevenson FK, Zhu D, King CA, et al. Idiotypic DNA vaccines against B-cell lymphoma. *Immunol Rev* 1995;145:211–228.

105. Spelerberg MB, Zhu D, Thomsett A, et al. DNA vaccines against lymphoma. *J Immunol* 1997;159:1885–1892.

106. Wang B, Godillot AP, Madaio MP, et al. Vaccination against pathogenic cells by DNA inoculation. *Curr Topics Microbiol Immunol* 1991;221:21–35.

107. Agadjanyan MG, Wang B, Nyland SB, et al. DNA plasmid based vaccination against the oncogenic human T cell leukemia virus type 1. *Curr Topics Microbiol Immunol* 1998;226:175–192.

108. Beuler H, Mulligan RC. Induction of antigen-specific tumor immunity by genetic and cellular vaccines against MAGE: enhanced tumor protection by coexpression of granulocyte-macrophage colony-stimulating factor and B7-1. *Mol Med* 1996;2:545–555.

109. Schreurs MWJ, de Boer AJ, Figdor CG, et al. Genetic vaccination against the melanocyte lineage-specific antigen gp100 induces cytotoxic T lymphocyte-mediated tumor protection. *Cancer Res* 1998;58:2509–2514.

110. Weber LW, Browne WB, Wolchok JD, et al. Tumor immunity and autoimmunity induced by immunization with homologous DNA. *J Clin Invest* 1998;102:1258–1264.

111. Kim JJ, Trivedi NN, Wilson DM, et al. Molecular and immunological analysis of genetic prostate specific antigen (PSA) vaccine. *Oncogene* 1998;17:3125–3135.

112. Davis HL, Brazolot Millan CL. DNA-based immunization against hepatitis B virus. *Springer Semin Immunopathol* 1997;19:195–209.

113. Costagliola S, Rodien P, Many MC, et al. Genetic immunization against the human thyrotropin receptor causes thyroiditis and allows production of monoclonal antibodies recognizing the native receptor. *J Immunol* 1998;160:1458–1465.

114. Mor G, Singla M, Steinberg AD, et al. Do DNA vaccines induce autoimmune disease? *Hum Gene Ther* 1997;8:293–300.

115. Stollar BD. The specificity and applications of antibodies to helical nucleic acids. *CRC Crit Rev Biochem* 1975;3:45–69.

116. Madaio MPS, Moller A, Nordheim BD, et al. Responsiveness of autoimmune and normal mice to nucleic acid antigens. *J Immunol* 1984;132:872–876.

117. Gilkeson GS, Ruiz P, Pippen MM, et al. Modulation of renal disease in autoimmune NZB/NZW mice by immunization with bacterial DNA. *J Exp Med* 1996;183:1389–1397.

118. Pisetsky DS, Reich C, Crowley SD, et al. Immunological properties of bacterial DNA. *Ann N Y Acad Sci* 1995;772:152–163.

119. MacGregor RR, Boyer JD, Ugen KE, et al. First human trial of a DNA-based vaccine for treatment of human immunodeficiency virus type 1 infection: safety and host response. *J Infect Dis* 1998;178:92–100.

120. Boyer JD, Chattergoon MA, Ugen KE, et al. Enhancement of cellular immune response in HIV-1 seropositive individuals: a DNA-based trial. *Clin Immunol* 1999;90:100–107.

121. Goepfert P, Mulligan M, Corey L, et al. AVEG 031: phase I evaluation of a gag-pol facilitated DNA vaccines for HIV-1 prevention. 12th World AIDS Conference, Geneva, June 1998(abst).

122. Conry RM, Strong TV, White SA, et al. Phase I trial of polynucleotide immunization to carcinoembryonic antigen in patients with metastatic colorectal cancer. *Cancer Gene Ther* 1997;4:S49(abst).

123. Nichols WW, Ledwith BJ, Manam SV, et al. Potential DNA vaccine integration into host cell genome. *Ann N Y Acad Sci* 1995;772:30–39.

124. Cohen IR, Steinman L. Exploring the potential of DNA vaccination. *Hosp Pract* 1997;32:169–171, 176–178.

125. Calarota S, Bratt G, Nordland S, et al. Cellular cytotoxic response induced by DNA vaccination in HIV-1-infected patients. *Lancet* 1998;351:1320–1325.

126. Kim JJ, Weiner DB. DNA gene vaccination for HIV. In: *Springer Seminars in Immunopathology*. New York: Springer-Verlag, 1997:175–194.

127. Gold D, Avrett S. HIV DNA vaccines move slowly into human trials. *IAVI Report* 1998;3:1–10.

128. Chattergoon M, Boyer J, Weiner DB. Genetic immunization: a new era in vaccines and immune therapeutics. *FASEB* 1997;11:753–763.

129. Clements-Mann ML, Eichelberger M, Boslego JW, et al. *Am Soc Virol Ann Meeting*. 1998;17:W31–W10.

130. Wang R, Doolan DL, Le TP, et al. Induction of antigen-specific cytotoxic T lymphocytes in humans by a malaria DNA vaccine. *Science* 1998;282:476–480.

131. Conry RM, LoBuglio AF, Curiel DT. Clinical protocol: phase Ia trial of a polynucleotide anti-tumor immunization to human carcinoembryonic antigen in patients with metastatic colorectal cancer. *Hum Gene Ther* 1996;7:755–772.

132. Nabel EG, Yang ZY, Muller D, et al. Safety and toxicity of catheter gene delivery to the pulmonary vasculature in a patient with metastatic melanoma. *Hum Gene Ther* 1994;5:1089–1094.

133. Nabel GJ, Nabel EG, Yang Z, et al. Molecular genetic interventions for cancer. *Cold Spr Harb Symp Quant Biol* 1994;59: 699–707.

134. Nabel GJ, Nabel EG, Yang ZY, et al. Direct gene transfer with DNA-liposome complexes in melanoma: expression, biologic activity and lack of toxicity in humans. *Proc Natl Acad Sci U S A* 1993;90:11307–11311.

135. Shroff KE, Smith LR, Baine Y, et al. Potential for plasmid DNAs as vaccines for the new millennium. *Pharm Sci Tech Today* 1999 (*in press*).

18.5

CANCER VACCINES: CLINICAL APPLICATIONS

Recombinant Poxvirus Vaccines

JEFFREY SCHLOM
DENNIS PANICALI

POXVIRUS FAMILY

Poxviruses are not strangers to the world of vaccines. In 1796, Edward Jenner administered the first vaccine containing a cowpox virus, which subsequently demonstrated resistance to smallpox (variola) infection. This milestone eventually led to the worldwide eradication of smallpox, a disease that had plagued humankind for thousands of years. To date, vaccinia virus has been administered to more than 1 billion people. The last endemic case of smallpox occurred in 1977 (1).

The *Poxviridae* family consists of two major genera of large DNA viruses that are being used in cancer vaccine development. The *Orthopoxvirus* group includes the replication-competent vaccinia virus, originally derived from cowpox, and the replication-defective modified vaccinia virus Ankara (MVA). The *Avipoxvirus* group consists of fowlpox and canarypox (ALVAC); both are replication-defective. Excellent review articles have been written on poxviruses and on the use of genetically engineered poxviruses (1–5).

POTENTIAL ADVANTAGES AND DISADVANTAGES OF RECOMBINANT POXVIRUS VACCINES

Recombinant poxviruses have been used in a wide range of vaccines in experimental and clinical studies. Most of these vaccines have been directed against viral antigens such as rabies and human immunodeficiency virus (HIV) (6–11). Thus, both rodent models and clinical studies have revealed many of the advantages and disadvantages of recombinant poxvirus vectors.

Vaccination with a live recombinant vaccinia (rV) virus allows expression of foreign antigens encoded by a transgene directly in various cells of the host, including professional antigen-presenting cells (APCs). This method of vaccination enables antigen processing and presentation of antigenic peptides along with host histocompatibility antigens and other necessary cofactors found on the APC. These foreign antigens are presented to the immune system with the large number of proteins produced by the vector itself, which likely is responsible for the significant inflammatory response to the poxvirus vector. In turn, this inflammatory process could lead to an environment of cytokine production and T-cell proliferation, which may act to further amplify the immune response to the foreign antigen. This process favors induction of a cell-mediated immune response and humoral responses to the foreign antigen. Because vaccinia actively replicates in the host, it can present high levels of antigen to the immune system over a period of 1 to 2 weeks, substantially increasing the potential for immune stimulation. The immune response to the vaccinia vector then eliminates the virus.

Thus, one of the main advantages of using rV viruses to develop cancer vaccines is that when a gene for a weakly immunogenic protein is inserted into rV and used as an immunogen, the expressed recombinant protein is much more immunogenic as a vaccine than the use of that protein with adjuvant (12–14).

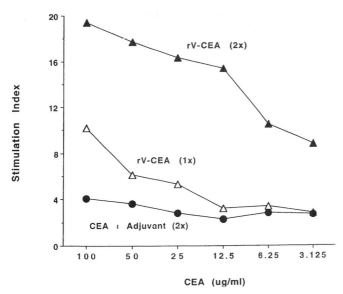

FIGURE 1. Carcinoembryonic antigen (CEA)–specific splenic CD4+ proliferative responses from CEA. Tg mice vaccinated with rV-CEA (1 to 2×) or CEA protein. CEA.Tg mice (H-2D) (2 to 3/group) were administered 10^7 plaque-forming units rV-CEA 1× (open triangles) or 2× (closed triangles) by tail scarification. Another group of CEA.Tg mice (4/group) was administered 100 µg CEA in 100 µL adjuvant (*RTBT* Superdetox) by tail scarification (solid circles). Fourteen days later, mice were sacrificed, splenic T cells were isolated, and the proliferative responses to soluble CEA were measured by a T-cell lymphoproliferative assay. The assay included splenic T cells, isolated and purified from the different groups of immune CEA.Tg mice, that were co-cultured with irradiated (2,000 rad) syngeneic CEA.Tg mouse splenocytes and soluble CEA (100–3.125 µg/mL). Proliferation was measured by ^{3}H-thymidine incorporation after 5 days of incubation at 37°C. Stimulation indices were calculated as follows: [cpm (antigen-stimulated cells)]/[cpm (unstimulated cells)]. Stimulation indices of splenic T cells isolated from untreated and control vaccinia virus (Wyeth)–vaccinated mice were approximately 1.0.

A striking example of this is seen in Figure 1, which shows that two injections of carcinoembryonic antigen (CEA) protein in adjuvant generated little, if any, of an immune response to CEA in a CEA-transgenic mouse. This would be expected because the host is seeing CEA as a self-antigen. However, when the rV virus containing the CEA transgene (designated rV-CEA) is administered one or two times, a strong CEA-specific T-cell response is elicited (13). The likely reason for this is that a strong inflammatory response is generated by the host against vaccinia proteins, which leads to an environment of cytokine production and T-cell proliferation. Although this situation is excellent for inducing immune responses to bystander transgene products, this same phenomenon leads to a limitation in the use of rV vectors. After one or two administrations of rV, the host mounts potent antivaccinia antibody and T-cell responses (15,16). This leads to a reduction in the ability of vaccinia to replicate in subsequent booster vaccines and, hence, to limited transgene expression. However, some clinical studies have shown that the administration of one or two vaccinations of an rV virus can elicit T-cell responses to the inserted transgene even in patients who previously received the smallpox vaccine (17,18). Several experimental studies and some clinical studies have demonstrated that rV viruses are best used for priming the immune response (19–22). Subsequent vaccinations can use

proteins, peptides, or replication-defective poxviruses, as well as other recombinant vectors (19–25).

MVA is a replication-defective poxvirus derived from vaccinia after 500 passages in chicken embryo cells. It has been used in many experimental studies and has been administered to more than 120,000 humans without apparent side effects (1). This virus has been molecularly characterized and has been found to have lost several genes involved in host-range determination and possible immune system suppression. Although MVA efficiently infects human cells and expresses both early and late genes, it is replication-defective and incapable of producing infectious progeny in mammalian cells. MVA-recombinant viruses have been shown to be highly immunogenic in both rodents and primates. To date, only a few experimental studies have used recombinant MVA as anticancer vaccines (26,27).

The avipoxviruses represent potentially attractive vectors for use in cancer vaccines. Although the immunogenicity of the inserted transgene may not be as potent as that of vaccinia virus, avipoxviruses such as fowlpox and canarypox can be administered numerous times to enhance immunogenicity (6,19,28). Because they are replication-defective, induction of any host immune responses should be inconsequential. Avipoxviruses are also distinguished from vaccinia in that the inserted transgene is expressed in infected cells for 14 to 21 days before the death of the cell. In a vaccinia-infected cell, the transgene is expressed for 1 to 2 days until cell lysis, and for approximately 1 week in the host until virus replication is arrested by host immune responses.

One of the advantages in using recombinant poxviruses as anticancer vaccines is the ability to insert large amounts of foreign DNA and multiple genes. To date, as many as seven genes have been inserted into vaccinia virus (29). Generally, poxvirus-based vaccines have been shown to be cost-effective, safe, easy to administer, and stable for long periods without special storage conditions. Other advantages include the following:

1. A wide host and cell-type range
2. Stability
3. Accurate replication
4. Efficient posttranslational processing of the inserted transgene
5. The tendency of recombinant gene products to be more immunogenic

Recombinant poxviruses can be used in several modalities in the development of cancer vaccines. The first modality involves the insertion of one or more tumor-associated antigen (TAA) genes into the vector, which can then be administered as conventional vaccine subcutaneously, by skin scarification, intramuscularly or, potentially, by the intravenous route. In addition to containing one or more TAAs, a recombinant poxvirus vector can also contain one or more costimulatory molecule genes or cytokine genes. Recombinant poxviruses can also be injected directly into the tumor containing TAA, cytokine, chemokine, or T-cell costimulatory genes. Another application of the use of recombinant poxviruses as anticancer vaccines is the infection *in vitro* of tumor cells that can subsequently be x-irradiated and administered to patients. It has also been demonstrated that one can infect professional APCs, such as dendritic cells, with recombinant poxviruses containing either tumor-antigen genes or costimulatory genes to sensitize tumor antigen-specific T lymphocytes *in vitro* (30,31).

EXPERIMENTAL STUDIES

The unique biologic properties of recombinant poxviruses have enabled development of two related strategies for designing cancer vaccines capable of inducing antitumor immunity. In an antigen-specific approach, one or more TAA-encoding genes that are associated with a certain cancer and that are known to elicit or are suspected of invoking immune responses in cancer patients are specifically engineered into the vector. The intent of this approach is to present these selected antigens to the immune system in a manner capable of inducing tumor-specific cellular responses.

Diversified Prime and Boost Protocols

A number of investigators have demonstrated the advantage of priming with vaccinia recombinants and boosting with immunogens such as recombinant protein, peptide, DNA, or recombinant avipoxvirus vectors to enhance immune responses in cancer vaccine models (19,20,23,32). The experimental studies that involved priming with rV and boosting with recombinant avipoxvirus also demonstrated that the host immune response to the transgene increased with continued booster vaccinations (19).

Delivery of Cytokines

Several studies have shown that recombinant poxviruses can efficiently deliver a wide range of cytokines and chemokines via traditional vaccination and tumor cell infection (33–38). Interleukin-12 (IL-12) has been expressed by rV virus and Avipoxviruses and found to be effective in the generation of antitumor immunity in two animal models (33–35). Additionally, the use of granulocyte-macrophage colony-stimulating factor (GM-CSF) as the transgene in tumors, which are used as a vaccine, has demonstrated that these modified tumor cells can enhance antitumor activity in several models (37–39).

Delivery of Costimulatory Molecules

T-cell activation has been shown to require at least two signals. The first signal is antigen-specific, is delivered through the T-cell receptor via the peptide/major histocompatibility complex, and causes the T cell to enter the cell cycle. The second, costimulatory signal is required for cytokine production and proliferation, and is mediated through ligand interaction on the surface of the T cell. Several molecules normally found on the surface of professional APC have been shown to be capable of providing the second signal critical for T-cell activation. These molecules include B7-1 (CD80), B7-2 (CD86), intercellular adhesion molecule-1 (ICAM-1, CD54), and leukocyte function–associated antigen-3 (LFA-3, human CD58/murine CD48) (40). Each of these molecules has been

inserted into poxvirus vectors, and each has been shown to efficiently mediate T-cell costimulation (40). Initial studies involved the use of B7-1 inserted into rV-B7-1 that was admixed before vaccination with rV-CEA (41). Although the single administration of rV-CEA inhibited tumor development to some extent, a more dramatic antitumor effect and CEA-specific T-cell response was seen when using the admixture. The power of the use of admixtures for replication-competent viruses, such as vaccinia, was also demonstrated in a tumor therapy model. In these studies, the admixture of rV-B7-1 and rV-MUC-1, when compared to the use of rV-MUC-1 alone, was shown to be extremely efficient in eliminating experimental lung metastases expressing the MUC-1 tumor antigen (42). Some studies have demonstrated that as long as the plaque-forming unit (pfu) levels in the admixture are sufficient to coinfect cells with both recombinants and the appropriate route is used, this methodology is just as efficient as using a vector containing both the tumor-antigen gene and the costimulatory molecule gene (43). Studies have also revealed enhanced antitumor effects using rV-B7-1, rV-B7-2, rV-ICAM-1, rV-LFA-3, and rV-CD70 in anticancer vaccines (44–47). The use of a costimulatory molecule and a TAA in replication-defective viruses most likely requires that both genes be in the same vector to guarantee coexpression of the TAA and costimulatory molecule on the same cell (40).

One of the major advantages in the use of recombinant poxvirus vaccines is the ability to insert multiple transgenes. Using retroviral vector infection of tumor cells and multiple drug selections, it has been shown that the insertion of two costimulatory molecule genes into tumors can produce additive or synergistic activation of T cells (48–51). Newly designed and developed poxvirus constructs are capable of expressing a *tri*ad of *co*stimulatory *m*olecules (B7-1, ICAM-1, and LFA-3, designated TRICOM) (40). Within 5 hours of infection, tumor cells infected with either recombinant fowlpox (rF)-TRICOM or rV-TRICOM were shown to express all three costimulatory molecules on the cell surface. Using Concanavalin A as a generic signal 1, a panel of tumor cells was created that expressed each of the three costimulatory molecules alone and together (as the TRICOM construct) to provide costimulatory signals. Both CD4+ and CD8+ T cells were isolated, and their ability to be stimulated was analyzed. The stratification of stimulator cell effects on proliferation was similar for both CD4+ and CD8+ T cells (Fig. 2). As can be seen, the TRICOM vector provided the most potent stimulation of both CD4+ and CD8+ T cells. Moreover, these effects were clearly synergistic, not additive. Tumor cells stimulated with rV-B7-1, rV-ICAM-1, or rV-LFA-3 to provide signal 2 were compared with TRICOM-stimulated cells. An evaluation of cytokine secretion by those cells revealed that IL-2 and interferon-γ production in CD4+ and CD8+ cells, respectively, was much higher for the TRICOM vector than for the single costimulatory molecule vectors. These studies demonstrated that poxviruses containing as many as three costimulatory molecules as transgenes can rapidly and efficiently activate T-cell populations to levels far greater than those achieved when any one or two of these costimulatory molecules are used. Previous toxicology studies analyzing the effects of multiple administrations of rV-B7-1 in mice revealed no toxicity, including no

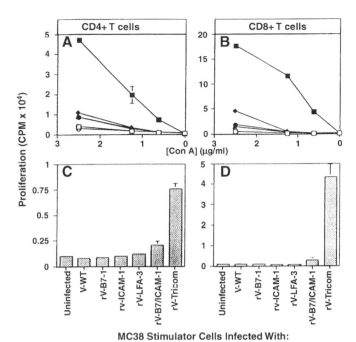

FIGURE 2. Effect of costimulation on specific T-cell populations. Murine CD4$^+$ (panel A) or CD8$^+$ T cells (panel B) were co-cultured with uninfected MC38 cells (open circle), or cells infected with wild-type vaccinia (V-WT) (open squares), recombinant vaccinia leukocyte function–associated antigen (rV-LFA-3) (closed triangles), rV-intercellular adhesion molecule-1 (rV-ICAM-1) (closed circles), rV-B7-1 (closed diamonds) or rV-TRICOM (*triad of costimulatory molecules*) (closed squares) at a 10:1 ratio for 48 hours in the presence of various concentrations of Con A. Panels C and D show the proliferative responses of purified CD4$^+$ and CD8$^+$ cells, respectively, when co-cultured in the presence of vector-infected MC38 stimulator cells at a low Con A concentration (0.625 μg/mL).

evidence of autoimmunity (52). Similar studies are ongoing using recombinant TRICOM-poxvirus vectors. The ability to achieve this new threshold of T-cell activation using vectors containing multiple costimulatory molecules has broad implications in the design and development of anticancer vaccines because there is overwhelming evidence that the vast majority of TAAs are weakly immunogenic.

Whole Tumor Cell Vaccines

Another strategy uses recombinant poxviruses in encoding and expressing one or more immunomodulating proteins (e.g., costimulatory molecules, cytokines, or chemokines) to stereotypically modify tumor cells *in vivo* or *ex vivo*. Although tumor cells may display TAAs on their surface, they usually do not elicit immune responses. One explanation is that, unlike APCs, tumor cells do not naturally express costimulatory molecules and, therefore, are unable to activate the immune system. To address this deficiency, recombinant poxviruses that express one or more costimulatory molecules can be used to infect tumor cells by direct injection into the tumor itself. Infection results in short-term, or transient, expression of the costimulatory molecules. In preclinical models, such expression has proven sufficient to activate immune responses directed against the antigens naturally present on the surface of tumor cells. Once activated, these immune responses may be capable of recognizing all

tumor cells of the same type, whether or not these tumor cells also express costimulatory molecules.

Many studies have revealed the efficacy of whole tumor cell vaccines to enhance antitumor activity in experimental models (37–39,44–47,53–56). Because this approach is not dependent on the identification of specific tumor antigens, it can be used for the treatment of multiple cancers, including those for which TAAs have not been identified. Advantages of this approach include

1. Efficient delivery of genes to the tumor cells by recombinant poxviruses.
2. Ability to phenotypically modify tumor cells *in vivo*, rather than only after surgical removal.
3. Capability of rapid, efficient *ex vivo* infection of tumor cells by recombinant poxviruses; cells can subsequently be x-irradiated and administered back to the patient.
4. The transient nature of the tumor modification. This is naturally limited by the immune system's eventual destruction of infected cells and by the fact that poxviruses do not insert their genetic material into the genome of the cells they infect.

In some cases, the vaccines consisted of live or x-irradiated tumor cells that were highly or moderately immunogenic (56). In other studies, tumor cells were shown to be weakly immunogenic or not immunogenic at all (i.e., the tumor cells would grow readily in the host, and vaccines consisting of x-irradiated tumor cells were not capable of inducing antitumor immunity). It is in these cases that the insertion and expression of transgenes such as cytokine genes and costimulatory molecule genes may make tumors more immunogenic. Insertion of costimulatory molecule genes is extremely attractive in the case of tumor vaccines because the vast majority of nonhematopoietic tumors do not express T-cell costimulatory molecules. To date, most whole tumor cell vaccines expressing a transgene via a vector have used retroviral vectors. Several studies have used poxvirus vectors to infect whole tumor cell vaccines. One study has compared for the first time the use of a poxvirus vector versus a retroviral vector to express the B7-1 costimulatory molecule transgene in both live and x-irradiated whole tumor cell vaccines (57). Both the recombinant retrovirus (R-B7) and the rV-B7 induced equivalent expression of B7 on the surface of the MC38 murine carcinoma cells slated to be used as a vaccine. Wild-type retrovirus (R-WT) and vaccinia virus (V-WT) were used as controls. Using live whole tumor cells as vaccine, cells transduced via recombinant retrovirus or rV virus expressing B7-1 equally induced protection against challenge with native MC38 tumor cells. On rechallenge with native tumor cells 40 days later, however, the R-B7 vaccine was shown to be less effective than the rV-B7 vaccine whole tumor cell. These experiments were also conducted using x-irradiated tumor cells as vaccine. Again, the rV-B7 vector-infected x-irradiated tumor cells were superior to the vaccine prepared with R-B7. Comparative studies have also been conducted in which x-irradiated tumor cell vaccines were administered to mice containing experimental lung metastases. In these therapy studies, all mice receiving x-irradiated native tumor cells developed more than 200 metastatic nodules in the lung, similar to

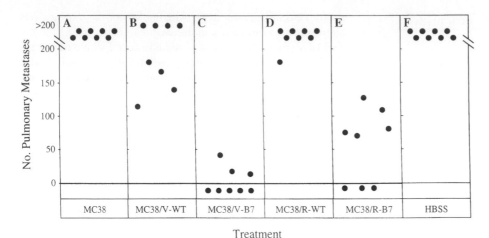

FIGURE 3. Treatment of lung metastases using x-irradiated whole tumor cell vaccines in mice that had been administered wild-type vaccinia (V-WT). On day 14, all mice received 1×10^7 plaque-forming units V-WT. Groups of eight mice were then inoculated intravenously with 1×10^6 native MC38 cells on day 0. On days 3, 10, and 17, mice received as vaccine x-irradiated MC38 tumor cells (panel A), or x-irradiated tumor cells previously infected with V-WT (panel B), V-B7 (panel C), R-WT (panel D), or R-B7 (panel E), or no tumor cells (HBSS buffer; panel F). On day 28, mice were sacrificed and lung metastases were counted.

the result seen in nonvaccinated mice. All mice receiving vaccine consisting of x-irradiated tumor cells infected with V-WT or R-WT also developed lung metastases. Mice receiving the x-irradiated rV-B7 tumor-cell vaccine experienced a statistically significant reduction in lung metastases compared to those receiving vaccine infected with R-WT. Similarly, mice receiving the x-irradiated rV-B7 tumor vaccine had a statistically significant reduction in the development of lung metastases compared to those receiving x-irradiated V-WT vaccine. Mice receiving the x-irradiated rV-B7 vaccine experienced a statistically significant reduction in lung metastases compared to mice receiving the x-irradiated vaccine infected with R-B7.

One of the concerns inherent in using an rV-based vaccine is that previous immunity—via the smallpox vaccine or poxvirus vaccinations, for example—would inhibit its effectiveness (15,19). To determine if earlier exposure to vaccinia would inhibit the antitumor efficacy of x-irradiated whole tumor cell vaccines with the rV-B7 vector, these studies were performed in mice that had received 10^7 pfu V-WT 17 days before vaccination. This dose and interval had been shown to lead to the development of substantial antivaccinia immune responses. As seen in Figure 3, the x-irradiated R-B7 tumor-cell vaccine was still statistically significant in its therapeutic effectiveness as compared to the retroviral vaccine. Indeed, in these types of whole tumor cell vaccines, there is no need for virus replication; therefore, there should be no inhibition of antitumor efficacy by antipoxvirus immune responses. Moreover, such immune responses may actually enhance the antitumor effect in this setting. This phenomenon formed the basis for the use of oncolysate, using extracts of vaccinia as vaccines (58). As previously pointed out, such preparations may have been less than optimal because no costimulatory molecules were present to provide the required second signal for enhanced T-cell activation. Studies have been reported in which anti-cytotoxic T lymphocyte A4 (CTLA4) monoclonal antibodies were used to inhibit growth of tumors in some murine models but not in others, particularly those tumors that are poorly immunogenic (59–61). The use of anti-CTLA4 monoclonal antibodies was shown to be ineffectual in the tumor model used in the studies (62).

Pros and cons exist in the use of any vector for anticancer vaccine applications. Advantages of using a retroviral vector in whole tumor cell vaccines include the following:

1. Stable integration
2. Transgene expression by all cells, if the cells are drug-selected and cloned
3. Proposed lack of immunogenicity

Most studies have used murine retroviruses in murine systems. It is not clear at this point if antiretroviral immunity in humans develops after administration of tumor cell vaccines containing retroviruses. There are several potential disadvantages in using a retroviral vector that do not exist when using poxvirus vectors in whole tumor cell vaccines. Poxviruses do not require a lengthy drug-selection or cloning process, because it has been shown that they can express the transgene efficiently in greater than 95% of cells within 5 hours (40,44). Moreover, unlike retroviruses, poxviruses do not require cell division to express transgenes. Although the use of retrovirus vectors is efficient for established tumor-cell lines that rapidly divide *in vitro* and *in vivo*, this is not the case for cells derived from human tumor biopsies or for human tumors *in situ*. For example, it is extremely difficult to propagate tumor cells from biopsies in cases of breast and colon carcinoma, and cells do not divide rapidly *in situ*. Perhaps the main advantage in using poxviruses in whole tumor cell vaccines is that one can insert multiple genes into a poxvirus vector, which is not possible for most other types of vectors. Vectors containing three or more costimulatory molecules possess great potential for this approach and clearly merit further investigation.

CLINICAL STUDIES

Poxviruses have been widely used as human vaccines. Vaccinia has been used in the worldwide eradication of smallpox. Recombinant avipoxviruses and rV viruses have also been used clinically to induce immunity to a range of viruses and other pathogens. These vaccines include: rV-HIV (11,21,24,25); ALVAC-HIV (7–10,63,64); rV-Japanese encephalitis virus (65); ALVAC-Japanese encephalitis virus (65); rV-malaria (29); rV-Epstein-Barr virus (66); and ALVAC-rabies (6). To date, few or no serious adverse effects stemming from the use of these vaccines have been reported. The use of recombinant poxviruses as anticancer vaccines is in a relatively early stage. Anticancer

TABLE 1. RECOMBINANT POXVIRUS ANTICANCER VACCINES: CLINICAL STUDIES

Immunogen	Immune Response
rV-CEA	CTL
ALVAC-CEA	CTL
rV-MUC-1	CTL
rV-MUC-1/IL-2	Studies ongoing
rV-PSA	Ab, Studies ongoing
rF-PSA	Studies ongoing
rV-HPV	CTL, Ab
rV-MART	Studies ongoing
rF-MART	Studies ongoing
rF-gp100	Studies ongoing
rV-CEA→ALVAC-CEA (3X)	CTL
ALVAC-CEA (3X)→rV-CEA	CTL
ALVAC-CEA-B7-1	Studies ongoing
ALVAC-B7-1	Studies ongoing
ALVAC-IL-12	Studies ongoing

Ab, antibody; ALVAC, *Avipoxvirus* group; CEA, carcinoembryonic antigen; CTL, cytotoxic T lymphocyte; HPV, human papillomavirus; IL, interleukin; PSA, prostate-specific antigen; rV, recombinant vaccinia.

recombinant poxvirus vaccines that are being evaluated clinically are listed in Table 1.

A phase 1 rV virus trial in cancer patients focused on the use of rV-CEA (67). Three dose levels were given to different cohorts, and each patient received three vaccinations. Peripheral blood mononuclear cells (PBMCs) from the advanced cancer patients who had received this vaccine yielded T cells that were analyzed for their ability to respond to a range of potential immunodominant epitopes of CEA. These studies identified a peptide (YLSGANLNL) designated CAP-1, which could be used to generate CEA-specific T cells from the PBMCs of vaccinated patients. No such T-cell lines could be generated using PBMCs from the same patients before vaccination. These studies elucidated the ability to generate a T-cell response to a self-antigen, such as CEA, using a recombinant poxvirus vector. The T-cell lines were shown to be capable of lysing (a) CEA peptide-pulsed targets, (b) autologous B cells that had been transduced with the CEA gene, and (c) colon cancer cells, as long as the tumor was expressing CEA and the appropriate major histocompatibility complex allele.

Phase 1 studies have also been carried out using the replication-defective ALVAC-CEA recombinant in advanced cancer patients (68). These studies also showed the generation of CEA-specific CTLs obtained from patients postvaccination. No such CTLs could be obtained before vaccination. These CTLs were shown to be capable of lysing allogeneic and autologous tumor cells. CTL responses were determined by classical precursor frequency studies. Ongoing studies involve the administration of ALVAC-CEA with recombinant GM-CSF at the injection site, as well as with low-dose IL-2 given postvaccination.

Studies were then carried out using diversified prime and boost protocols. In these studies, cohort A received a primary vaccination with rV-CEA followed by three vaccinations with ALVAC-CEA, and cohort B received three vaccinations of ALVAC-CEA followed by a single vaccination of rV-CEA. T-cell responses in both cohorts were measured using the enzyme-linked immunospot (ELISPOT) assay for interferon-γ produc-

tion in response to a CEA peptide. The CEA-specific T-cell responses of cohort A, in which rV-CEA was given as the primary vaccination, were shown to be statistically superior to those of cohort B. These clinical results were in agreement with preclinical studies showing the advantage of diversified prime and boost protocols. Studies have also been conducted using an rV virus containing sequences of the MUC-1 carcinoma-associated mucin and IL-2 in the same vector. These ongoing studies have resulted in the induction of anti-MUC-1 T-cell responses in vaccinated breast cancer patients with some early indications of antitumor effects (69). Another phase 1 trial focusing on a different portion of the MUC-1 gene in an rV virus has just been initiated in breast cancer patients (70).

Several studies using rV and avipoxviruses have been completed, and others are in progress in patients with melanoma. To date, however, these studies have not been as successful as those using modified melanoma peptides. Research is ongoing to insert modified melanoma-associated and carcinoma-associated genes into recombinant poxviruses (71–73).

Clinical studies are also ongoing with rV viruses containing the genes for human papillomavirus (HPV) (types 16 and 18), E6 and 27 genes (rV-HPV) (74,75). These vectors are being administered to patients with late-stage cervical carcinoma. Initial analysis indicated that HPV-specific antibody responses and CTL responses were being elicited by this vaccine. Clinical trials have also been conducted in which the human prostate-specific antigen (PSA) has been inserted into an rV virus (18). These studies have revealed that prostate cancer patients can generate a PSA-specific antibody responses after vaccination with rV-PSA, and PSA-specific T-cell responses (18,76).

Two clinical trials using ALVAC-CEA/B7-1 as a vaccine in patients with advanced cancer have been completed (77–79). These were the first clinical trials to use a recombinant poxvirus vector containing a costimulatory molecule gene and a TAA gene. Using the ELISPOT assay for interferon-γ production and analyzing PBMCs after less than 24 hours in culture, substantial increases in CEA-specific T cells were observed postvaccination compared to prevaccination. As a control, no changes in T-cell responses were observed to a Flu peptide from PBMCs obtained pre- and postvaccination. Clinical trials testing the direct administration of ALVAC-B7-1 or ALVAC-IL-12 into tumor lesions have just begun.

The phase 1 clinical results described previously in this section clearly demonstrate that recombinant poxviruses containing tumor-associated genes can be used to generate specific immune responses to a range of tumor antigens in a safe manner. Some phase 2 clinical studies using some of the modalities described (see under Experimental Studies) are just beginning; planning is under way for others.

FUTURE DEVELOPMENT OF RECOMBINANT POXVIRUS VACCINES

Considerable potential exists in the future development of recombinant poxvirus vaccines for cancer management. Virtually all of the clinical studies described have been carried out in patients with rather advanced cancers. These patients most likely have subtle but depressed immune responses, which have been exhibited two ways: (a) via downregulation of the ζ chain of the T-cell receptor and (b) in the cytokine profile of T cells obtained from advanced cancer patients (type 2 profile) compared to a type 1 profile from healthy individuals. Thus, the full potential of these vaccines has yet to be defined. The advantage of diversified prime and boost protocols using poxvirus recombinants has been demonstrated preclinically and in the clinic. It is not known, however, how many boosts using replication-defective avipoxviruses or MVAs are optimal.

Modification of tumor-associated immunodominant epitopes, such as those of gp100 and CEA, has been shown to enhance immune responses *in vitro* (72) and in patients (71,73,80). The use of recombinant poxviruses containing these modifications in tumor-antigen genes may enhance immune responses in patients. The use of cytokine genes as transgenes in recombinant poxviruses either alone or with tumor-antigen genes is currently being explored, as is the administration of recombinant cytokines such as GM-CSF and IL-2 in vaccine protocols containing recombinant poxviruses.

Perhaps the most intriguing advantage of using recombinant poxvirus vectors in anticancer vaccines is the ability to insert multiple transgenes; this can include the use of multiple tumor-antigen genes, cytokine genes, and/or T-cell costimulatory molecule genes. The belief that the vast majority of tumor-associated genes are weak immunogens supports this approach. Underscoring these vectors' significant potential as vaccines is the demonstration that recombinant poxviruses can efficiently express three T-cell costimulatory molecules in the same APC and activate T cells to levels not previously achievable with the use of any one or two of these molecules. Modes of application of pox vector–based vaccines potentially include direct administration into patients as a classical vaccine, infection of whole tumor cells either *in vitro* or *in situ*, or the *in vitro* infection of APCs such as dendritic cells to enhance the effectiveness of this approach.

REFERENCES

1. Moss B. Genetically engineered poxviruses for recombinant gene expression, vaccination and safety. *Proc Natl Acad Sci U S A* 1996;93:11341–11348.
2. Moss B, Carroll MW, Wyatt LS, et al. Host range restricted, non-replicating vaccinia poxvirus vectors as vaccine candidates. *Adv Exp Med Biol* 1996;397:7–13.
3. Paoletti E. Applications of pox virus vectors to vaccination: an update. *Proc Natl Acad Sci U S A* 1996;93:11349–11353.
4. Perkus ME, Tartaglia J, Paoletti E. Poxvirus-based vaccine candidates for cancer, AIDS, and other infectious diseases. *J Leukoc Biol* 1995;1:1–13.
5. Fernandez N, Duffour M-T, Perricaudet M, et al. Active specific T cell-based immunotherapy for cancer: nucleic acids, peptides, whole native proteins, recombinant viruses, with dendritic cell adjuvants or whole tumor cell-based vaccines. Principles and future prospects. Cytokines, *Cell Mol Ther* 1998;4:53–65.
6. Fries LF, Tartaglia J, Taylor J, et al. Human safety and immunogenicity of a canarypox-rabies glycoprotein recombinant vaccine: an alternative poxvirus vector system. *Vaccine* 1996;14:428–434.
7. Tubiana R, Gomard E, Fleury H, et al. Vaccine therapy in early HIV-1 infection using a recombinant canarypox virus expressing gp160MN (ALVAC-HIV): a double-blind controlled randomized study of safety and immunogenicity. *AIDS* 1997;11:819–820.
8. Egan MA, Pavlat WA, Tartaglia J, et al. Induction of human immunodeficiency virus type 1 (HIV-1)-specific cytolytic T lymphocyte responses in seronegative adults by a non-replicating, host-range-restricted canarypox vector (ALVAC) carrying the HIV-1MN env gene. *J Infect Dis* 1995;171:1623–1627.
9. Belshe RB, Gorse GJ, Mulligan ML, et al. Induction of immune responses to HIV-1 by canarypox virus (ALVAC) HIV-1 and gp120 SF-2 recombinant vaccines in uninfected volunteers. *AIDS* 1998;12:2407–2415.
10. Clements-Mann ML, Weinhold K, Matthews TJ, et al. Immune responses to human immunodeficiency virus (HIV) type 1 induced by canarypox expressing HIV-1MN gp120, HIV-1SF2 recombinant gp120, or both vaccines in seronegative adults. *J Infect Dis* 1998;177:1230–1246.
11. Graham BS, Belshe RB, Clements ML, et al. Vaccination of vaccinia-naïve adults with human immunodeficiency virus type 1 gp160 recombinant vaccinia virus in a blinded, controlled, randomized clinical trial. *J Infect Dis* 1992;166:244–252.
12. Irvine KJ, Schlom J. Comparison of a CEA-recombinant vaccinia virus, purified CEA, and an anti-idiotype antibody bearing the image of a CEA epitope in the treatment and prevention of CEA-expressing tumors. *Vaccine Res* 1993;2:79–94.
13. Kass E, Schlom J, Thompson J, et al. Induction of protective host immunity to carcinoembryonic antigen (CEA), a self-antigen in CEA transgenic mice, by immunizing with a recombinant vaccinia-CEA virus. *Cancer Res* 1999;59:676–683.
14. Bernards R, Destree A, McKenzie S, et al. Effective tumor immunotherapy directed against an oncogene-encoded product using a vaccinia virus vector. *Proc Natl Acad Sci U S A* 1987;19:6854–6858.
15. Demkowicz Jr WE, Littaua RA, Wang J, et al. Human cytotoxic T-cell memory: long-lived responses to vaccinia virus. *J Virol* 1996;2627–2631.
16. Stienlauf S, Shoresh M, Solomon A, et al. Kinetics of formation of neutralizing antibodies against vaccinia virus following re-vaccination. *Vaccine* 1999;17:201–204.
17. McAneny D, Ryan CA, Beazley RM, et al. Results of a phase I trial of a recombinant vaccinia virus that expressed carcinoembryonic antigen in patients with advanced colorectal cancer. *Ann Surg Oncol* 1996;3:495–500.
18. Sanda MG, Smith DC, Charles LG, et al. Recombinant vaccinia-PSA (PROSTVAC) can induce a prostate-specific immune response in androgen-modulated human prostate cancer. *Urology* 1999;53:260–266.
19. Hodge JW, McLaughlin JP, Kantor JA, et al. Diversified prime and boost protocols using recombinant vaccinia virus and recombinant non-replicating avian pox virus to enhance T-cell immunity and antitumor responses. *Vaccine* 1997;15:759–768.
20. Bei R, Kantor J, Kashmiri SV, et al. Enhanced immune responses and anti-tumor activity by baculovirus recombinant carcinoembryonic antigen (CEA) in mice primed with the recombinant vaccinia CEA. *J Immunother Emphasis Tumor Immunol* 1994;16:275–282.
21. Corey L, McElrath MJ, Weinhold K, et al. Cytotoxic T cell and neutralizing antibody responses to human immunodeficiency virus type 1 envelope with a combination vaccine regimen. *J Infect Dis* 1998;177:301–309.
22. Marshall JL, Richmond E, Pedicano J, et al. Phase I/II trial of Vaccinia-CEA and ALVAC-CEA in patients with advanced CEA-bearing tumors. Meeting Abstract, American Society of Clinical Oncology (ASCO), 35th Annual Meeting, Atlanta, Georgia, May 15–18, 1999.
23. Cole DJ, Wilson MC, Baron PL, et al. Phase I study of recombinant CEA vaccinia virus vaccine with post-vaccination CEA peptide challenge. *Hum Gene Ther* 1996;7:1381–1394.
24. Graham BS, Gorse GJ, Schwartz DH, et al. Determinants of antibody response after recombinant gp160 boosting in vaccinia-naïve volunteers primed with gp160-recombinant vaccinia virus. *J Infect Dis* 1994;170:782–786.
25. Montefiori DC, Graham BS, Kliks S, et al. Serum antibodies to HIV-1 in recombinant vaccinia virus recipients boosted with purified recombinant gp160. *J Clin Immunol* 1992;12:429–439.
26. Moss B, Carroll MW, Wyatt LS, et al. Host range restricted, non-

replicating vaccinia virus vectors as vaccine candidates. *Adv Exp Med Biol* 1996;397:1–13.

27. Carroll MW, Overwijk WW, Chamberlain RS, et al. Highly attenuated modified vaccinia virus Ankara (MVA) as an effective recombinant vector: a murine tumor model. *Vaccine* 1997;15:387–394.

28. Tartaglia J, Excler J-L, El Habib R, et al. Canarypox virus-based vaccine: prime-boost strategies to induce cell-mediated and humoral immunity against HIV. *AIDS Res Hum Retroviruses* 1998;14:S291–S298.

29. Ockenhouse CF, Sun PF, Lanar DE, et al. Phase I/IIa safety, immunogenicity, and efficacy trial of NYVAC-Pf7, a pox-vectored, multiantigen, multistage vaccine candidate for plasmodium falciparum malaria. *J Infect Dis* 1998;177:1664–1673.

30. Bronte V, Carroll MW, Goletz TJ, et al. Antigen expression by dendritic cells correlates with the therapeutic effectiveness of a model recombinant poxvirus tumor vaccine. *Proc Natl Acad Sci U S A* 1997;94:3183–3188.

31. Kim CJ, Prevette T, Cormier J, et al. Dendritic cells infected with poxviruses encoding Melan A sensitize T lymphocytes *in vitro*. *J Immunother* 1997;20:276–286.

32. Kahn M, Sugawara H, McGowan P, et al. CD4+ T-cell clones specific for the human p97 melanoma-associated antigen can eradicate pulmonary metastases from a murine tumor expressing the p97 antigen. *J Immunol* 1991;146:3235–3241.

33. Carroll MW, Overwijk WW, Surman DR, et al. Construction and characterization of a triple-recombinant vaccinia virus encoding B7-1, interleukin-12, and a model tumor antigen. *J Natl Cancer Inst* 1998;90:1881–1887.

34. Kawakita M, Rao GS, Ritchey JK, et al. Effect of canarypox virus (ALVAC)-mediated cytokine expression on murine prostate tumor growth. *J Natl Cancer Inst* 1997;89:428–436.

35. Puisieux I, Odin L, Poujol D, et al. Canarypox virus-mediated interleukin-12 gene transfer into murine mammary adenocarcinoma induces tumor suppression and long-term antitumoral immunity. *Hum Gene Ther* 1998;9:2481–2492.

36. Leong KH, Ramsay AJ, Boyle DB, et al. Selective induction of immune responses by cytokines coexpressed in recombinant fowlpox virus. *J Virol* 1994;68:8125–8130.

37. Qin H, Chatterjee SK. Cancer gene therapy using tumor cells infected with recombinant vaccinia virus expressing GM-CSF. *Hum Gene Ther* 1996;7:1853–1860.

38. McLaughlin JP, Abrams S, Kantor J, et al. Immunization with a syngeneic tumor infected with recombinant vaccinia virus expressing granulocyte-macrophage colony-stimulating factor (GM-CSF) induces tumor regression and long-lasting systemic immunity. *J Immunother* 1997;20:449–459.

39. Dranoff G, Jaffee E, Lazenby A, et al. Vaccination with irradiated tumor cells engineered to secrete murine granulocyte-macrophage colony-stimulating factor stimulates potent, specific, and long-lasting anti-tumor immunity. *Proc Natl Acad Sci U S A* 1993;90:3539–3543.

40. Hodge JW, Sabzevari H, Lorenz MGO, Yafal AG, Gritz L, Schlom J. A triad of costimulatory molecules synergize to amplify T-cell activation. *Cancer Res* 1999;59:5800–5807.

41. Hodge JW, McLaughlin JP, Abrams SI, et al. Admixture of a recombinant vaccinia virus containing the gene for the costimulatory molecule B7 and a recombinant vaccinia virus containing a tumor-associated antigen gene results in enhanced specific T-cell responses and antitumor immunity. *Cancer Res* 1995;55:3598–3603.

42. Akagi J, Hodge JW, McLaughlin JP, et al. Therapeutic antitumor response after immunization with an admixture of recombinant vaccinia viruses expressing a modified MUC-1 gene and the murine T-cell costimulatory molecule B7. *J Immunother* 1997;20:38–47.

43. Kalus RM, Kantor J, Gritz L, et al. The use of combination vaccinia vaccines and dual-gene vaccinia vaccines to enhance antigen-specific T-cell immunity via T-cell costimulation. *Vaccine* 1999;17:893–903.

44. Hodge JW, Abrams S, Schlom J, et al. Induction of antitumor immunity by recombinant vaccinia viruses expressing B7-1 or B7-2 costimulatory molecules. *Cancer Res* 1994;54:5552–5555.

45. Uzendoski K, Kantor JA, Abrams SI, et al. Construction and characterization of a recombinant vaccinia virus expressing murine intercellular adhesion molecule-1: induction and potentiation of antitumor responses. *Hum Gene Ther* 1997;8:851–860.

46. Lorenz MGO, Kantor JA, Schlom J, et al. Induction of antitumor immunity elicited by recombinant vaccinia virus expressing murine leukocyte function associated antigen-3 (LFA 3). *Hum Gene Ther* 1999;10:623–631.

47. Lorenz MGO, Kantor JA, Schlom J, et al. Antitumor immunity elicited by a recombinant vaccinia virus expressing CD70 (CD27L). *Hum Gene Ther* 1999;10:1095–1103.

48. Parra E, Wingren AG, Hedlund G, et al. The role of B7-1 and LFA-3 in costimulation of CD8+ T cells. *J Immunol* 1997;158:637–642.

49. Cavallo F, Martin-Fontecha A, Bellone M, et al. Co-expression of B7-1 and ICAM-1 on tumors is required for rejection and the establishment of a memory response. *Eur J Immunol* 1995;25:1154–1162.

50. Wingren AG, Parra E, Varga M, et al. T-cell activation pathways: B7, LFA-3, and ICAM-1 shape unique T-cell profiles. *Crit Rev Immunol* 1995;15:235–253.

51. Hellstrom KE, Chen L, Hellstrom I, et al. Costimulation of T cell-mediated tumor immunity: costimulation by CD48 and B7-1 induces immunity against poorly immunogenic tumors. *Cancer Chemother Pharmacol* 1996;38:S40–S41.

52. Freund YR, Mirsalis JC, Fairchild DG, et al. Immunization with a recombinant vaccinia vaccine containing B7-1 causes no significant immunotoxicity and enhances T cell-mediated cytotoxicity. *Int J Cancer* 2000;85:508–517.

53. Dunussi-Joannopoulos K, Weinstein HJ, Nickerson PW, et al. Irradiated B7-1 transduced primary acute myelogenous leukemia (AML) cells can be used as therapeutic vaccines in murine AML. *Blood* 1996;87:2938–2946.

54. Emtage PCR, Wan Y, Muller W, et al. Enhanced interleukin-2 gene transfer immunotherapy of breast cancer by coexpression of B7-1 and B7-2. *J Interferon Cytokine Res* 1998;18:927–937.

55. Gajewski TF, Fallarino F, Uyttenhove C, et al. Tumor rejection requires a CTLA-4 ligand provided by the host or expressed on the tumor. *J Immunol* 1996;156:2909–2917.

56. Chen L, McGowan P, Ashe S, et al. Tumor immunogenicity determines the effect of B7 costimulation on T cell-mediated tumor immunity. *J Exp Med* 1994;179:523–532.

57. Hodge JW, Schlom J. Comparative studies of a retrovirus versus a poxvirus vector in whole tumor-cell vaccines. *Cancer Res* 1999;59:5106–5111.

58. Wallack MK, Sivanandham M, Balch CM, et al. Surgical adjuvant active specific immunotherapy for patients with stage III melanoma: the final analysis of data from a phase III, randomized, double-blind, multicenter vaccinia melanoma oncolysate trial. *J Am Coll Surg* 1998;187:69–77.

59. Leach DR, Krummel MF, Allison JP. Enhancement of antitumor immunity by CTLA-4 blockade. *Science* 1996;271:1734–1736.

60. Greenfield EA, Nguyen KA, Kuchroo VK. CD28/B7 costimulation: a review. *Crit Rev Immunol* 1998;18:389–418.

61. Yang YF, Zou JP, Mu J, et al. Enhanced induction of antitumor T-cell responses by cytotoxic T lymphocyte-associated molecule-4 blockade: the effect is manifested only at the restricted tumor-bearing stages. *Cancer Res* 1997;57:4036–4041.

62. Mokyr MB, Kalinichenko T, Gorelik T, et al. Realization of the therapeutic potential of CTLA-4 blockade in low-dose chemotherapy-treated tumor-bearing mice. *Cancer Res* 1998;58:5301–5304.

63. Fleury B, Janvier G, Pialoux G, et al. Memory cytotoxic T lymphocyte responses in human immunodeficiency virus type 1 (HIV-1)-negative volunteers immunized with a recombinant canarypox expressing gp160 of HIV-1 and boosted with a recombinant gp160. *J Infect Dis* 1996;174:734–738.

64. Pialoux G, Excler JL, Riviere Y, et al. A prime-boost approach to HIV preventive vaccine using a recombinant canarypox virus expressing glycoprotein 160 (MN) followed by a recombinant glycoprotein 160 (MN/LAI). *AIDS Res Hum Retroviruses* 1995;11:373–381.

65. Konishi E, Kurane I, Mason PW, et al. Induction of Japanese encephalitis virus-specific cytotoxic T lymphocytes in humans by poxvirus-based JE vaccine candidates. *Vaccine* 1998;16:842–849.

66. Gu SY, Huang TM, Ruan L, et al. First EBV vaccine trial in humans using recombinant vaccinia virus expressing the major membrane antigen. *Dev Biol Stand* 1995;84:171–177.

67. Tsang KY, Zaremba S, Nieroda C, et al. Generation of human cytotoxic T cells specific for human carcinoembryonic antigen epitopes from patients immunized with recombinant vaccinia-CEA vaccine. *J Natl Cancer Inst* 1995;87:949–951.

68. Marshall JL, Hawkins MJ, Tsang KY, et al. Phase I study in cancer patients of replication-defective avipox recombinant vaccine that expresses human carcinoembryonic antigen. *J Clin Oncol* 1999;17:332–337.

69. Balloul JM, Acres RB, Geist M, et al. Recombinant MUC-1 vaccinia virus: a potential vector for immunotherapy of breast cancer. *Cell Mol Biol* 1994;40:S49–S59.

70. Akagi J, Nakagawa K, Egami H, et al. Induction of HLA-unrestricted and HLA-class-II-restricted cytotoxic T lymphocytes against MUC-1 from patients with colorectal carcinoma using recombinant MUC-1 vaccinia virus. *Cancer Immunol Immunother* 1998;47:21–31.

71. Clay TM, Custer MC, McKee MD, et al. Changes in the fine specificity of gp100(209-217)-reactive T cells in patients following vaccination with a peptide modified at an HLA-A2.1 anchor residue. *J Immunol* 1999;162:1749–1755.

72. Zaremba S, Barzaga E, Zhu M, et al. Identification of an enhancer agonist cytotoxic T lymphocyte peptide from human carcinoembryonic antigen. *Cancer Res* 1997;57:4570–4577.

73. Rosenberg SA, Yang JC, Schwartzentruber DJ, et al. Immunologic and therapeutic evaluation of a synthetic peptide vaccine for the treatment of patients with metastatic melanoma. *Nat Med* 1998;4:321–327.

74. Boursnell ME, Rutherford E, Hickling JK, et al. Construction and characterization of a recombinant vaccinia virus expressing human papillomavirus proteins for immunotherapy of cervical cancer. *Vaccine* 1996;14:1485–1494.

75. Borysiewicz LK, Fiander A, Nimako M, et al. A recombinant vaccinia virus encoding human papillomavirus types 16 and 18, E6 and E7 proteins as immunotherapy for cervical cancer. *Lancet* 1996;347:1523–1527.

76. Eder JP, Kantoff PW, Roper K, et al. A phase I trial of a recombinant vaccinia virus expressing prostate specific antigen in advanced prostate cancer. *Clin Cancer Res* 2000 (*in press*).

77. von Mehren M, Davies M, Rivera V, et al. Phase I trial with ALVAC-CEA B7.1 immunization in advanced CEA-expressing adenocarcinomas. Meeting Abstract, American Society of Clinical Oncology (ASCO), 35th Annual Meeting, Atlanta, Georgia, May 15–18, 1999.

78. Lee DS, Conkright W, Hörig HE, et al. Preliminary results of ALVAC-CEA-B7.1 phase I vaccine trial in patients with metastatic CEA-expressing tumors. Meeting Abstract, American Society of Clinical Oncology (ASCO), 35th Annual Meeting, Atlanta, Georgia, May 15–18, 1999.

79. Von Mehren M, Arlen P, Tsang KY, et al. Pilot study of a dual gene recombinant Avipox vaccine containing both CEA and B7.1 transgenes, in patients with recurrent CEA expressing adenocarcinomas. *Clin Cancer Res* 2000 (*submitted*).

80. Cormier JN, Salgaller ML, Prevette T, et al. Enhancement of cellular immunity in melanoma patients immunized with a peptide from MART-1/Melan A. *Cancer J Sci Am* 1997;3:37–44.

18.6

CANCER VACCINES: CLINICAL APPLICATIONS

Adenovirus and Other Viral Vaccines

BRUCE ROBERTS

The identification of tumor-associated antigens (TAAs) that are targets for cancer patient–derived immune effector cells has revolutionized the field of cancer immunotherapy. Clinicians are attempting to focus the immune system on these specific molecular targets in the hope that anti-TAA immune responses are sufficient to cause tumor cell elimination. Two strategies that use adenoviral vectors have been pursued to elicit anti-TAAs, and, thus, antitumor cell immune responses (Fig. 1). In one approach, tumor cells are used as the source of antigens, and adenoviral vectors are used to deliver immunomodulatory genes to tumors cells to enhance their immunogenicity. The use of tumor cells as the source of antigens favors the presentation of the full repertoire of TAAs to the immune system. Tumor cells, however, can elaborate immunosuppressive factors that can thwart one's efforts to use them to provoke immunity, and they may possess defects in antigen presentation that render them defective for the generation of immune responses. In an alternative approach, tumor antigen genes are delivered via adenoviral vectors to professional antigen-presenting cells (APCs), such as dendritic cells (DCs), to maximize presentation to the immune system. The efficiency of gene transfer to patients' APCs (as opposed to tumor cells) can be more predictable, and targeting of APCs favors optimal presentation of tumor antigens to the immune system. Drawbacks of this approach include the

Genetic Modification of Tumor Cells Using Adenovirus

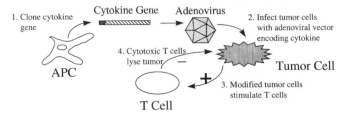

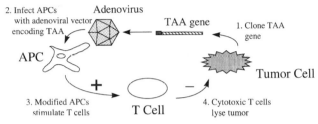

Genetic Modification of APCs Using Adenovirus

FIGURE 1. Adenovirus cancer vaccines. Adenoviral vectors encoding immunomodulatory genes can be used to enhance the immunogenicity of tumor cells, as shown in the top panel, whereas adenoviral vectors encoding tumor-associated antigens (TAAs) can be used to provoke anti-TAA immune reactivity, as shown in the bottom panel. (APC, antigen-presenting cell.)

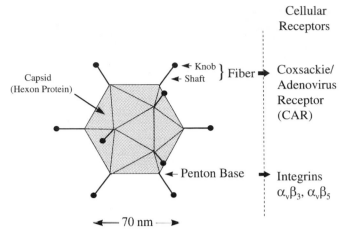

FIGURE 2. Adenoviral particle structure. This diagram illustrates the fiber and penton base proteins of the adenoviral particle that participate in the two-step infection of target cells via specific cellular receptors.

requirement for cloned antigens, of which few are available, and the limitations associated with generating a narrow, highly restricted immune response against a handful of TAAs.

This chapter reviews the properties and attributes of adenoviral vectors as they pertain to their use in immunotherapy. Comprehensive reviews of adenovirus and adenoviral vectors have appeared previously (1,2).

ADENOVIRUS FAMILY

Adenoviruses are nonenveloped icosahedral nucleocapsid particles of 70 nm in diameter, containing a linear double-stranded DNA genome of approximately 35 to 36 kilobase (kb) (1). Forty-one different human adenovirus serotypes have been classified into seven subgroups (A through G) based on a variety of criteria. Adenoviruses of subgroup C (serotypes 1, 2, 5, and 6) cause mild infections of the respiratory tract, whereas subgroups B and E viruses are associated with acute respiratory disease and subgroup D viruses are associated with keratoconjunctivitis. The majority of adenoviral vectors are based on the serotypes 5 and 2 viruses. Although one might imagine adenoviruses might exhibit a preferential tropism for epithelial cells based on the observed clinical symptoms in humans, adenoviral vectors can infect a variety of cell types.

The proteinaceous outer capsid of adenovirus consists of predominantly three structural proteins: a 120-kd hexon protein (720 copies per viral particle), a 85-kd penton base protein (60 copies per particle), and a 62-kd fiber protein (36 copies per particle). Of these structural proteins, the fiber and penton base proteins (Fig. 2) participate in the infection of target cells via a two-step process. The fiber protein, which extends from the corners of the icosahedral particle like an aerial, is thought to inter-

act first with a cellular fiber receptor, allowing the pentose base protein of the viral particle to engage a second cellular receptor (the $\alpha_v\beta_3$ or $\alpha_v\beta_5$ integrins). A cellular receptor (CAR) for the fiber protein, which also serves as a receptor for coxsackie virus, has been identified (3); however, the fact that target cells lacking CAR can be infected with adeovirus suggests other means of entry may exist.

Internalization of the adenoviral particle occurs via receptor-mediated endocytosis. Once inside a cell, a series of modifications of the outer capsid occurs, enabling the virus to escape from the endosome and gain entry to the nucleus. This feature of adenovirus enables it to infect dividing and nondividing cells, an attribute that makes adenovirus ideal for gene transfer. Once established within the nucleus, the double-stranded DNA of the adenoviral genome remains as a linear extrachromosomal element. The fact that adenovirus does not integrate into the host genome has been exploited as an important safety feature for gene therapy applications.

As with other viruses, the genome is divided into early and late transcription units (1). The E1a and E1b protein products encoded by the first of the four early transcription regions are master control proteins that participate in a number of regulatory functions, including transactivation of gene transcription within the other three early regions, as well as the late region. The E1 proteins also enable replication of the adenoviral genome in infected cells in part by the ability of E1a to bind the Rb tumor suppressor and E1b to bind p53. As a consequence of these interactions, the combination of the E1a and E1b genes can be oncogenic in rodent but not human cell lines.

The majority of adenoviral vectors generated for gene transfer purposes are deleted for the E1a and E1b products (2) for the following purposes:

1. To render the vectors' replication deficient
2. To eliminate the adenoviral genes associated with transformation of rodent cells
3. To eliminate the activation of late gene expression and the potential cytotoxicity of viral proteins

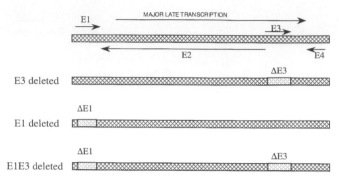

FIGURE 3. Adenoviral vector design. E1-, E3- or E1E3 deleted adenoviral vectors have been generated to create sufficient cloning capacity for the insertion of therapeutic genes. (Adapted from Graham FL, Prevec L. Manipulation of adenovirus vectors. In: Murray EJ, ed. *Methods in molecular biology.* Clifton, NJ: Humana, 1991:109–128.)

4. To provide cloning space for the insertion of transgenes into the genome (Fig. 3).

The availability of the 293 helper cell line harboring the E1 genes and able to provide in trans the E1 proteins, which are required for viral replication, enables the preparation of high-titer stocks of adenoviral vectors ($\sim 2 \times 10^{11}$ infectious units per mL, equivalent to 2×10^{12} particle per mL). An exception to this general design is one in which the E3 region of the genome is deleted and the transgene of interest cloned into the space created by the deletion (2). Because the E1 region can be retained, vectors can be replication competent. Thus, spread of vector from transduced cells to neighboring cells is possible.

An issue associated with first-generation adenoviral vectors is the generation of replication-competent adenovirus caused by the recombination of DNA sequences flanking the deleted E1 region with homologous DNA sequences contained within 293 cells. Thus, second-generation adenoviral vectors have been designed to remedy this problem. Because the protein IX gene, which lies immediately 3' of the E1b region, is a potential site for recombination, vectors deleted for this region have been constructed. Because the protein IX gene is required for stabilization and packaging of adenoviral genomes in excess of 100% of the size of the wild-type genome, protein IX–deleted vectors are restricted in terms of their cloning capacity, unless the protein IX product is provided in trans by a suitable helper cell line. An alternative solution involves translocation of the protein IX gene from its normal site to a novel site at the right-hand end of the genome within space created by deletion of the E4 region (4). The latter solution permits use of the existing 293 helper cell lines for vector production. In 1998, an alternative helper cell line was described, which contains the minimal sequences of the E1 region required for replication under the control of a phosphoglycerate kinase promoter. Thus, the possibility of homologous recombination between vector sequences and E1 sequences harbored by the helper cells is negligible (5).

The E3 region of the adenoviral genome encodes proteins whose normal role is to enable virus-infected cells to evade immune surveillance (1). Thus, the E3 19K protein binds to major histocompatibility complex (MHC) class I molecules and inhibits the presentation of MHC molecules on the cell surface, whereas the E3 14.7K protein is antagonistic to the actions of tumor necrosis factor–α. The expression of these genes is greatly diminished in E1-deleted vectors owing to the fact that the E1 products are required to transactivate E3 gene expression. Adenoviral vectors completely deleted for E3 genes have been constructed (2).

A variety of methodologies have been described to construct recombinant adenoviral vectors. In one approach, a linearized shuttle plasmid containing the transgene of interest is cotransfected with a restriction enzyme–digested viral DNA onto a suitable helper cell line (2). As arising viral plaques can be the desired recombinant or parental viral vectors, several rounds of time-consuming plaque purification may be required to obtain the desired recombinant. Using an alternative strategy, the entire viral genome is first assembled in a suitable host, such as *Escherichia coli*, and the complete viral DNA is then transfected onto helper cells to generate viral plaques. Theoretically, any plaques that arise should correspond to the desired recombinant, thus eliminating the need for plaque purification. The development of rapid cloning methods in the late 1990s involving the use of homologous recombination in bacteria to generate plasmids containing complete adenoviral genomes (6,7) has accelerated the process of obtaining clonally pure adenoviral preparations ready for large-scale production.

Genetic Modification of Antigen-Presenting Cells Using Adenoviral Vectors

Genetic modification of APCs affords several advantages when compared with other modes of TAA delivery for the following reasons:

1. The potential exists for a continuous supply of tumor antigen–derived peptides for presentation.
2. Intracellular expression of the tumor antigen gene favors entry of TAA-derived peptides into the class I pathway.
3. The potential exists for CD4 and CD8 T-cell epitopes of the same TAA to be presented by the same APC.
4. Coexpression of a TAA gene with accessory molecules that might enhance an immune response within an APC is possible.

An ideal vector for the delivery of tumor antigen genes should fulfill a number of criteria, including:

1. An ability to mediate efficient gene transfer to target cells without adversely affecting APC function or viability
2. Ease of manipulation of the vector genome
3. An ability to induce antigen-specific immune responses with minimal generation of immune responses directed toward the vector itself.

Adenoviral vectors have been found to meet the above criteria.

Adenoviral vectors can be potentially used to transduce a variety of APCs, but investigators have paid particular attention to DCs because they are considered to be the most potent APCs in the body (8). Gene transfer to human DCs via adenoviral vectors is of 2 to 3 orders of magnitude more efficient than electroporation or lipofection (9). Typically, at a multiplicity of infection (MOI) of 100 to 250, one can achieve as much as a 90% to 100% transduction of human (9,10) or murine (11–13) DCs *in vitro*, as judged by marker gene expression. A variety of factors may account for variations in reported efficiencies, including the quality of the adenoviral preparations, the culture conditions used to derive DCs, the source of the DCs, and the sensitivity of the assay used to assess the extent of gene transfer (14).

Monocyte-derived DCs are susceptible to adenovirus-mediated gene transfer and so are monocytes themselves (11,15). Adenoviral vector–transduced monocytes, however, have been reported to be inferior to transduced monocyte–derived DCs in their ability to induce a cytotoxic T lymphocyte (CTL) response and confer protective immunity (11). This observation is consistent with the observation that monocytes lack important costimulatory and adhesion molecules and are inferior to DCs as professional APCs (8).

No data is available regarding the efficiency of gene transfer to APCs *in vivo*. As subcutaneous (s.c.), intraperitoneal (i.p.), intravenous (i.v.), and intradermal (i.d.) administration of adenoviral vectors encoding antigens can induce potent antiantigen immune responses (Table 1), it is inferred that APCs of one sort or another can be transduced with adenoviral vectors *in vivo*. On the other hand, it is well documented that i.m., i.v., and s.c. injection of adenoviral vectors can achieve high degrees of gene transfer to muscle, liver, and fibroblasts *in vivo*. Thus, the potential for direct or indirect antigen presentation by these tissues exists.

Adenovirus-transduced cells have been shown to be able to present individual T-cell epitopes encoded by mini genes (14,16) or complete tumor antigen genes (17), and multiple epitopes encoded by complete tumor antigen genes (18) or concatamers of minigenes (19) to established T-cell lines *in vitro* in an MHC-restricted fashion. Transgene expression, and, thus, presentation have been shown to persist in adenovirus-transduced human DCs for at least 8 days *in vitro* with no signs of cytopathic effects (17).

As most adenoviral vectors used as cancer vaccines have been replication deficient, no provision exists for amplification of transgene copy number within virus-transduced target cells; however, chemical treatments can be used to augment gene expression, and, hence, antigen presentation. Tumor necrosis factor–α and sodium butyrate treatments have been reported to enhance tumor antigen gene expression in virus-transduced

cells, as judged by Northern or fluorescence-activated cell sorter analysis when transgene expression is regulated by a cytomegalovirus promoter (18). Furthermore, the susceptibility of adenovirus-transduced cells to lysis by established antigen-specific T cells can be enhanced by tumor necrosis factor–α or sodium butyrate treatment (18).

Adenoviral cancer vaccines have used the cytomegalovirus promoter to control tumor antigen gene expression, and no systematic examination of the effect of different promoters on the level or duration of TAA presentation has been undertaken. In the context of adenoviral vectors, however, the cytomegalovirus promoter has been shown to be active in APCs and capable of directing high levels of tumor antigen gene expression (17,18). The adenovirus E3 19K protein can potentially down-regulate cell surface presentation of MHC class I molecules in vector-transduced cells (1). Transactivation of gene expression within the E3 region by adenoviral E1 proteins greatly enhances the production of E3 proteins, but as adenoviral vectors used for cancer vaccines are deleted for E1 genes, expression of E3 gene products should be minimal. Although the E3 19K protein product can be detected in vector-transduced cells, levels are not sufficient to cause a detectable decrease in class I presentation (18), and a separate study has shown only modest reductions in total class I and HLA-A2 levels in adenovector-transduced DCs (17).

Adenovirus types 2 and 5 contain sequence motifs that block immune activation by stimulatory CpG motifs (20). Replication-deficient types 2 and 5 vectors, however, are deleted for the E1 region, which coincidentally harbors these immunosuppressive DNA sequences. Replication-competent adenoviral vectors, which retain E1 functions, have been generated (2) as antiviral vaccines. It remains to be determined to what degree these immunosuppressive sequences impinge on their ability to induce immune responses.

Adenoviral transduction appears to have little effect on the morphology or viability of DCs (10). Furthermore, adenoviral transduction does not appear to alter the levels of characteristic cell surface markers on human (9) or murine (11,13) DCs, as judged by fluorescence-activated cell sorter analysis. The function of DCs does not appear to be impaired as a consequence of exposure to adenoviral vectors, as transduced human (9) and murine (11,13) DCs are equivalent to nontransduced cells in a mixed lymphocyte reaction. Adenovirus-transduced murine DCs have been reported to exhibit reduced viability and

TABLE 1. SUMMARY OF PRECLINICAL STUDIES DEMONSTRATING THE EFFICACY OF *IN VIVO* INJECTION OF ADENOVIRUS

Transgene	Dose of Virus Administered	Route of Administration	Animal Model (Tumor Cell Type:Mouse Strain)	References
Polyoma middle T	10^7–10^9 PFU	i.m., i.p., s.c., i.v.	MMTV/Middle T transgenic mice (FVB/N)	13
P815A murine mastocytoma antigen	10^8–10^9 PFU	i.d., i.p., s.c., i.n., intratrachial	P815:DBA/2J	16
Human gp100	2×10^9 PFU	i.v.	B16:C57BL/6	18,28
Multiple epitopes	1×10^8 PFU	i.p., s.c., i.m.	A5E1A expressing tumor cells:B6	19
Escherichia coli β-galactosidase	10^6–10^9 IU	i.v., i.m., i.n.	CT26 expressing β-galactosidase: BALB/c	25
Murine gp75 (TRP-1)	10^9 PFU	i.d.	B16:C57BL/6	26
Human GA733 antigen	1.2×10^8 PFU	i.p.	CT26 expressing GA733: BALB/c	27

MMTV, mouse mammary tumor virus; PFU, plaque-forming units; TRP-1, tyrosinase-related protein.

impaired activity in a mixed lymphocyte reaction when MOIs of 200 or 500 are used (11). This report of adenovirus-induced cytotoxicity on murine DCs is at variance with a report that no loss in viability occurs when MOIs of as many as 10,000 are used to transduce human DCs (9). Differences in the quality of adenoviral preparations may account for this apparent discrepancy. Finally, transduced DCs have been shown to migrate to the spleen after i.v. injection (13), suggesting adenoviral infection does not alter the capacity of DCs to translocate from a site of injection to T-cell–rich regions.

The ability of adenoviral-transduced DCs to induce immune responses has been examined *in vitro*. DCs transduced with a wild-type adenovirus or a replication-deficient mutant deleted for the E1a protein induce proliferation of antiadenovirus CD4 and CD8 T-cell responses (21). Characterization of expanded T-cell populations supports the conclusion that class I and class II molecules of transduced DCs present adenoviral antigens to T cells (21). Human donor–derived DCs transduced with an adenovirus encoding human melan-A/MART-1 can be used to generate T cells reactive to the encoded TAA *in vitro* (17). A subsequent report has shown that human DCs transduced with the same adenoviral vector can stimulate CD4$^+$ and CD8$^+$ antigen-specific T cells from melanoma patients' peripheral blood mononuclear cells (PBMCs) *in vitro* (22). This observation suggests that antigen presentation via class I and class II pathways can occur in transduced DCs in accordance with earlier observations (21).

Little data is available regarding the relative potency of adenoviral vector–transduced DCs as compared with peptide-pulsed, RNA-pulsed, or protein-pulsed DCs in an instance in which immune responses are induced to a "standard" TAA. It has been reported, however, that DCs transduced with an adenovirus encoding a specific CTL epitope are more potent than peptide-pulsed cells in inducing peptide-specific T-cell reactivity *in vitro* and *in vivo* (14), whereas DCs transduced with an adenovirus encoding β-galactosidase are more potent than DCs pulsed with β-galactosidase protein in inducing CTLs *in vivo* (23). This may be owing to the fact that genetically modified DCs are predicted to have a continuous supply of TAAs. Thus, sustained presentation of TAA-derived peptides may be possible.

An ideal cancer vaccine should induce immune responses directed towards the encoded TAA and not towards the vector itself. Little antiadenoviral CTL reactivity is generated when transduced DCs are used to stimulate T cells *in vitro* (17,22) in spite of the fact that adenoviral proteins would be present in transduced DCs. CTL reactivity to adenoviral proteins, however, can be generated if DCs, transduced with an empty adenoviral vector devoid of a tumor antigen gene, are used as stimulators (17,21). Furthermore, it has been demonstrated that *de novo* gene expression is not required for the presentation of adenoviral antigens by transduced DCs (21). Little advantage may exist in using high MOIs to transduce DCs, as excess viral particles are available for uptake by DCs, and immune responses may be skewed in favor of an antiadenoviral response at the expense of a desired antitumor antigen response. In addition, these observations suggest competition for presentation may occur in adenovirus-transduced DCs.

Provided that TAA transgene expression is driven by a strong promoter within the vector, anti-TAA immune responses may be preferentially induced.

The ability of DCs to induce immune responses has been deliberately altered by transduction with an adenovirus encoding the T-cell attractant chemokine lymphotactin (24). The transduced DCs are more potent than unmodified DCs in inducing T-cell responses and conferring protective immunity when pulsed with a T-cell epitope peptide and administered subcutaneously. As most first-generation adenoviral vectors have a 6- to 8-kb cloning capacity (2), tumor antigen and immunomodulatory genes could be incorporated into the design of adenoviral vectors to create superior cancer vaccines.

Adenoviral vaccines have been administered via a variety of routes (see Table 1). Viruses administered intravenously (18,25), intramuscularly (25), intradermally (16,26), intranasally (25), or intraperitoneally (27) have been shown to induce protective immunity. Differences in vector design and choice of antigen prohibit attempts to deduce whether an optimum route of administration exists. In comparative studies using a single vector, however, investigators have reported variable levels of efficacy depending on the route of administration. Thus, i.m. delivery of an adenoviral vector encoding the model antigen polyoma middle T has been reported to be superior to i.p., s.c., or i.v. delivery, and whereas a dose of 10^7 plaque-forming units (PFU) given intramuscularly is sufficient to induce protective immune responses, higher doses are required to achieve comparable levels of protective immunity when other routes are used (13). i.d. injection of an adenoviral vector encoding a CTL epitope can induce antigen-specific T cells. i.p., s.c., intranasal or intratrachial administrations of vector are also effective in inducing immune responses (16). i.p. delivery of an adenoviral vector encoding multiple CTL epitopes in a string-of-beads fashion is as effective as s.c. or i.m. administration of the vector (19). Thus, it would appear that a variety of routes of administration may be suitable for direct *in vivo* immunization.

Direct injection of adenoviral vectors encoding TAAs or CTL epitopes has been shown to be an efficient means of inducing antigen-specific immunity. i.d. administration of an adenovirus encoding the minimal P1A epitope is sufficient to induce anti-P815A CTL reactivity (16). i.v. administration of an adenoviral vector encoding a model tumor antigen (β-galactosidase) has been shown to induce antigen-specific CTL activity in splenocytes of immunized animals (25). i.v. administration of an adenoviral vector encoding human gp100 stimulates the generation of B16-reactive CTLs (18) cross-reactive with the endogenous gp100 of the murine cells (28). Depletion of T-cell populations by administration of antibodies after adenovirus injection revealed that CD8$^+$ T cells are predominantly associated with the induced antitumor cell reactivity (18). i.p. delivery of an adenovirus encoding multiple epitopes can induce MHC-restricted epitope-specific T-cell reactivity in splenocytes (19). Anti-CD4 and anti-CD8 antibodies can impair the ability of an adenovector encoding murine tyrosinase–related protein-1 to confer protection from tumor cell challenge when given intradermally, suggesting that CD4 and CD8 T cells play important roles in adenovirus vector–induced immunity (26).

TABLE 2. SUMMARY OF PRECLINICAL STUDIES DEMONSTRATING THE EFFICACY OF ADENOVIRUS-TRANSDUCED DENDRITIC CELLS

Transgene	Dose of Transduced Dendritic Cells	Route of Administration	Animal Model (Tumor Cell Type/Mouse Strain)	Reference
Human MUC-1	5×10^5	i.v.	MC38 expressing human MUC-1:C57BL/6	11
Escherichia coli β-galactosidase	5×10^5	i.v.	MC38 expressing β-galactosidase:C57BL/6	11
	3×10^5	s.c.	CT26 expressing β-galactosidase:BALB/c	12
Polyoma middle T	$1 \times 10^5 - 4 \times 10^6$	i.v.	MMTV/Middle T transgenic mice (FVB/N)	13
Ovalbumin CTL epitope	3×10^5	i.p.	EL-4 expressing ovalbumin:C57BL/6	14
Human MART-1	5×10^5	i.v.	NFSA expressing human MART-1:C3H	29

CTL, cytotoxic T lymphocyte; MMTV, mouse mammary tumor virus; MUC-1, mucin1.

The ability of adenoviral vectors encoding tumor antigens to induce antigen-specific reactivity correlates with their ability to confer protection from tumor cell challenge. i.v. administration of an adenovirus encoding a model antigen can confer protection from an i.v. challenge with tumor cells engineered to express the model antigen (25). i.v. injection of an adenovirus encoding human gp100 can provide partial protection from s.c. (18) or i.v. (28) challenge with B16 tumor cells. Similarly, it has been reported that i.p. injection of an adenovirus encoding multiple defined epitopes can confer protection from subsequent challenge with tumor cells (19). Finally, i.d. administration of an adenoviral vector encoding murine tyrosinase–related protein-1 is able to reduce the number of lung metastases that develop after subsequent i.v. challenge with tumor cells (26).

The administration of APCs genetically modified *ex vivo* by adenoviral vectors intravenously (11,13,29) or subcutaneously (12) has been shown to confer protective immunity (Table 2). Administration of Ad/β-galactosidase–transduced murine DCs intravenously (11) or subcutaneously (12) can induce CTL reactivity in splenocytes and confer protective immunity from subsequent challenge with a tumor cell engineered to express β-galactosidase. In models that are perhaps more clinically relevant as they use human TAAs, murine DCs transduced with adenoviral vectors encoding the human tumor antigens MART-1 (29) or mucin 1 (11) can induce antigen-specific CTLs when given intravenously and confer protective immunity from subsequent challenge with tumor cell lines engineered to express the respective human tumor antigens.

In vitro antibody depletion studies have shown that CD4 and CD8 antigen–specific T cells are generated by adenovirus-transduced DCs (11). Administration of an established murine DC line transduced with an adenovirus encoding a minimal CTL epitope can confer protection from subsequent tumor cell challenge (14) in normal but not CD8 knockout mice, stressing the important role played by CD8 T cells. As stimulation of CD4 T responses may provide important "help" for CD8 T-cell responses, the fact that adenovirus–transduced DCs can present antigen via class I and class II pathways may have important implications for the induction of anticancer cell immune responses.

The majority of animal studies conducted have used models of prophylactic immunization to evaluate the efficacy of adenoviral vaccines. As patients with established disease are most likely to be the recipients of adenoviral vaccines, it is surprising, perhaps, that little has been reported regarding the efficacy of adenoviral vaccines in active treatment models of cancer. Immunization with an

adenoviral vector encoding a model antigen provides only partial protection from the development of lung metastases in an active treatment model; however, concurrent interleukin-2 (IL-2) treatment appears to greatly improve efficacy (25). i.v. administration of adenovirus-tranduced DCs 3 days after s.c. challenge with tumor cells can confer partial protection from tumor growth (29). The reduced efficacy of adenoviral vaccines in active treatment as compared with prophylactic models may be owing to a variety of factors, including the aggressive growth kinetics of the tumor cells used. One potential means to improve efficacy is to repeat dose. Weekly administrations of transduced DCs for 3 weeks has been shown to enhance the magnitude of the CTL response induced, but such is not the case when vector alone is administered intraperitoneally three times a week (14). In addition, dosing of transduced DCs at two separate time points post–tumor cell challenge is superior to providing a single dose in an active treatment model (29). Thus, repeat dosing and boosting of antigen-specific immune responses may be an essential component in the clinical application of adenoviral vaccines.

Adenoviral vectors have also been reported to induce antigen-specific humoral responses. i.p. delivery of an adenovirus encoding the CO17-1A/GA733 antigen can induce antigen-specific antibodies, as well as antigen-specific cytotoxic T cells (27) in a pretreatment model, and can confer protection from subsequent or concurrent challenge with tumor cells engineered to express the cognate antigen. i.m. injection of an adenovirus encoding the single-chain Fv of a B-cell lymphoma idiotypic (Id) protein can induce an anti-Id antibody response (30). Although the overall titer of the antibody response was lower than that induced by vaccination with recombinant Id protein alone, the type of response induced is qualitatively different in that immunoglobulin G_{2a} (IgG_{2a}) predominates over immunoglobulin G1 (IgG_1) (30). IgG_{2a} is associated with Th1 responses, whereas IgG_1 is associated with Th2 responses. Th1-directed immune responses have been associated with favorable antitumor effects, and adenoviral cancer vaccines may provide a useful means of inducing antitumor cell IgG_{2a} responses to complement CTL responses (30).

The types of immune responses induced by adenoviral vaccines are likely to be dependent on the nature of the tumor antigen gene used, but the route of viral vector administration may play a significant role, too. Although studies have reported that protective immunity can be induced by the administration of adenoviral vectors via a variety of routes, a systematic study of the types of immune responses induced (humoral versus cellu-

TABLE 3. SUMMARY OF PHASE 1 CLINICAL TRIALS WITH ADENOVIRAL VACCINES

Indication	Transgene	Number of Patients	Dose	Route of Administration	References
Melanoma	Human MART-1	16 without IL-2; 20 with IL-2	10^7–10^{11} IU	i.m., s.c.	31
Melanoma	Human gp100	Six without IL-2; 12 with IL-2	10^9–6×10^{10} IU	i.m.	31
Melanoma and breast cancer	IL-2	15 melanoma; eight breast cancer	10^7–10^{10} PFU	Intratumoral	56
Neuroblastoma	IL-2	Ten	10^4–10^7 transduced tumor cells/kg body weight	s.c.	55

IL-2, interleukin-2; PFU, plaque-forming units.

lar, CD4 versus CD8) as a function of route of administration has not been undertaken.

An exhaustive study of dose response has not been conducted for direct injection of virus or immunization with transduced DCs. i.d. administration of 10^8 or 10^9 PFU of an adenovirus encoding a minimal epitope is sufficient to induce CTLs; however, a dose of 10^7 PFU is ineffective (16). As few as 10^5 transduced DCs are sufficient to induce protective immunity (11,13). A dose in humans of 2.5×10^7 transduced DCs would be equivalent to 10^5 transduced DCs in the mouse (based on surface area), whereas a dose of 2.5×10^{10} PFU of virus for patients would be equivalent to 10^8 PFU in the mouse. Given that 5×10^8 DCs can be prepared from the apheresis product of one patient and doses of as many as 1×10^{11} PFU of an adenoviral vaccine have been administered to patients (31), it is technically possible to administer doses of adenovirus or adenoviral-transduced DCs that are predicted to be efficacious based on mouse model data to patients. Although *in vivo* and *ex vivo* application of adenoviral vaccines is feasible, it should be noted that transduced DCs have been reported to be more potent than injected virus in inducing protective immunity (13,14).

Ideally, one would like to use a gene transfer vector in a manner to minimize the induction of an antivector antibody response that might preclude repeat dosing, and an antivector T-cell response that might be counterproductive to the induction of the desired anti-TAA immune response. *In vivo* administration of adenoviral vectors can induce antiadenoviral antibodies and CTLs, but the degree to which these immune responses impinge on the ability of vector to act as a cancer vaccine has not been evaluated in a systematic manner. Weekly i.p. administrations of an adenoviral vector (but not of transduced DCs) can induce a strong antiadenoviral neutralizing antibody response (14). Although a preexisting antiadenovirus antibody response is sufficient to block the ability of vector to confer protective immunity when given intraperitoneally, it does not impair the ability of adenovirus-transduced DCs to induce immune responses (14). Prior exposure to adenovirus under conditions that are likely to induce antiadenovirus antibodies does not impinge on the ability of an adenoviral vector encoding a model tumor antigen to induce protective immunity when given intravenously, although the serum titers were not reported (25). Two i.p. injections of adenovirus induce an antiadenovirus antibody response that is sufficient to restrict the ability of an adenoviral vector encoding a minimal epitope to induce immunity when given intraperitoneally (16). Although the presence of antiadenovirus antibodies can apparently restrict or even eliminate the ability of adenoviral vectors encoding tumor or model antigens

to elicit immune responses when given intraperitonally or intravenously, it is not clear to what degree preexisting immunity impairs adenovirus-mediated gene transfer in patients.

A variety of strategies could be adopted to circumvent the potential limiting issue of neutralizing antiadenoviral antibodies. Investigators have shown that gene transfer can be achieved in the face of an antiadenoviral humoral response by sequential administration of human adenoviral vectors of different serotypes. Thus, efficient gene transfer via subgroup C adenoviral vector is possible in spite of prior exposure to subgroups E or D adenoviruses (32) or to a different subgroup C adenovirus (33), but not to the same subgroup C adenovirus (32,33). Although proof of principle has been demonstrated for this strategy in murine models, it may be impractical economically to produce multiple clinical grade adenoviral vectors of different serotypes encoding common tumor antigens to induce and boost antitumor immune responses in patients.

Little information is available regarding the *in vivo* generation of antiadenoviral CTLs after administration of adenoviral cancer vaccines. Numerous reports, however, have shown that the i.m., i.v., s.c., or i.p. administration of adenoviral vectors can induce antiadenoviral CTLs that can restrict the duration of transgene expression in transduced target tissues. Circumstances have been reported in which long-term expression of a transgene was achieved in spite of the presence of antiadenoviral CTLs. This may be in part owing to the site of gene expression or the nature of the transgene product, or both. DCs transduced with adenoviral vectors fail to induce significant antiadenovirus CTL reactivity *in vivo* (11,13) in accordance with *in vitro* observations (17). This suggests that little presentation exists of adenoviral antigens by transduced DCs when expression of the TAA gene within the adenoviral vector is controlled by a strong promoter.

Only two clinical trials have been conducted using adenoviral vectors encoding tumor antigens or epitopes (Table 3). In both instances, the recombinant vectors were administered subcutaneously or intramuscularly at least twice with or without concurrent high-dose IL-2 to stage IV, HLA-A2–positive melanoma patients (31). Doses up to 10^{11} IU (or approximately 10^{12} viral particles) were administered, and no signs of article-related toxicity were detected, including inflammation at the injection site or changes in blood chemistry parameters or liver enzymes. One of 16 patients receiving an adenoviral vector encoding human melan-A/MART-1 (Ad2/MART-1) alone experienced an objective clinical response, whereas 4 of 20 patients receiving the virus plus high-dose IL-2 experienced objective clinical responses. In a second study, none of six patients injected intramuscularly with an adenovirus encoding human gp100 (Ad2/gp100) alone experienced an objective clinical response, whereas 1 of 12 patients receiving the gp100 virus plus high-dose IL-2 had a response.

As a biopsy was not performed on the site of vector administration, it is not possible to assess the degree of transgene transfer to these patients after i.m. or s.c. injection of virus. Of 36 patients who received the Ad2/MART-1, 25 patients were evaluated for HLA-A2–restricted reactivity in PBMCs to an immunodominant MART-1 peptide (residues 27–35). Five of the 25 evaluable patients showed enhanced MART-1 peptide reactivity postimmunization. It was not possible to determine whether those patients who experienced an objective clinical response also had enhanced MART-1 peptide reactivity in PBMCs postimmunization. Of the 18 patients injected intramuscularly with the Ad2/gp100 virus, none showed enhanced HLA-A2–restricted reactivity in PBMCs to any of the three immunodominant gp100 peptides. As patients were injected with adenoviruses encoding the entire MART-1 or gp100 proteins, it is conceivable that immunity could have been generated to TAA-derived peptides other than those tested or via HLA molecules other than A2. This was not investigated because of technical limitations.

Serum titers of total and neutralizing antiadenoviral antibodies were investigated. Three general observations can be made:

1. No apparent correlation existed between the dose or route of adenovirus administration and the titers of antiadenoviral antibodies induced, although patients who received greater than or equal to 10^{10} IU of virus tended to have higher serum titers.
2. No apparent correlation existed between the level of total antiadenoviral antibodies and neutralizing antiadenoviral antibodies.
3. No apparent correlation existed between the serum titers of antiadenoviral antibodies and clinical responses.

Thus, all patients, including those who experienced clinical responses, exhibited serum antiadenoviral antibodies before s.c. or i.m. injection of vector. Serum neutralizing antibody titers remained unchanged from baseline levels in most patients when low doses (up to 10^9 IU) were administered, suggesting a therapeutic window may exist for the administration of adenoviral vectors that provokes a minimal antiadenovirus immune response.

Genetic Modification of Tumor Cells Using Adenoviral Vectors

The ideal features of a vector for genetic modification of tumor cells are largely the same as those cited in the previous section for modification of APCs with the exception that, although vector-induced cytopathic effects might jeopardize the use of genetically modified APCs, such effects are less of an issue for genetically modified tumor cells and could, in fact, be an asset. Because of the heterogeneity of tumor cells, variable efficiencies of adenovirus-mediated gene transfer have been reported, but, in general, a variety of human tumor types can be transduced. In the clinic, one could transduce tumor cells *ex vivo* at high multiplicities of infection to favor gene transfer. For *in vivo* administration, multiple intratumoral injections of accessible lesions on a repeated basis would favor the genetic modification of a high proportion of cells within a tumor.

A variety of transgenes, including cytokines, costimulatory molecules, and combinations thereof have been delivered to tumor cells in an attempt to enhance their immunogenicity (Table 4). More than any other cytokine, IL-2 has been evaluated for its ability to stimulate antitumor cell immune reactivity after adenoviral vector–mediated delivery of the gene to tumor cells. Tumor cells transduced *ex vivo* (34,35) or *in vivo* via intratumoral injection (35–39) with Ad/IL-2 are impaired in their ability to form tumors. Instances of regression of established tumors have been reported, but results are variable depending on the model, size of tumor, and dose of vector administered (35–38). IL-2 gene expression at the tumor site appears to be required, as delivery of the IL-2 gene to distal sites provides no benefit (35). Rejection of transduced tumor cells can lead to protection from subsequent challenge with unmodified parental tumor cells (35–37). Histologic evaluation of regressing tumors producing IL-2 indicates the presence of a cellular infiltrate predominated by T cells (35–37). Local expression of IL-2 in adeno-transduced tumor tissue, however, is not without its problems, as it has been reported to cause liver toxicity not unlike that seen with recombinant IL-2 protein. Thus, the therapeutic window may be narrow (38).

In an attempt to enhance the immunogenicity of tumor cells, investigators have transduced tumor cells with adenoviral vectors encoding the costimulatory molecule B7.1. This approach is supported by *in vitro* (40) data showing that human ovarian and cervical tumor cells transduced with an adenovirus encoding B7.1 are superior to unmodified tumor cells in their ability to stimulate the proliferation of PBMC-derived T cells. Intratumoral injection of Ad/B7.1 has been reported to be ineffective or partially effective in reducing established tumors (39,41,42). Thus, gene transfer of B7 in conjunction with cytokines has been explored. An adenoviral vector encoding both subunits of IL-12, as well as B7, is more effective than adenoviral vectors encoding IL-12 or B7 alone in causing regression of established tumors (41). Similarly, an adenovirus encoding B7 and IL-2 is more effective than adenoviral vectors encoding IL-2 or B7 alone, as judged by induction of tumor regression and tumor-reactive T cells (42).

After a seminal report that tumor cells genetically modified to express GM-CSF can induce protective immunity (43), investigators have used adenoviral vectors as an efficient means to deliver this particular cytokine to tumor cells *ex vivo* (44), as well as *in vivo* (45). The administration of Ad/GM-CSF–transduced tumor cells induces systemic immunity as characterized by antitumor cell CTL reactivity in splenocytes and confers protection from challenge with unmodified tumor cells (44). Histologic evaluation has indicated DC recruitment to the site of injected tumor cells (44). Intratumoral injection of Ad/GM-CSF can retard tumor formation; however, the coinjection of Ad/GM-CSF and an adenovirus encoding the 5FC-activating enzyme cytosine deaminase (CD) in conjunction with 5FC treatment can be synergistic (45). DC infiltrates have been observed whether Ad/GM-CSF or Ad/GM-CSF plus Ad/CD are injected into tumors, whereas antitumor CTL reactivity is more pronounced after combination therapy.

TABLE 4. SUMMARY OF PRECLINICAL MODEL STUDIES DEMONSTRATING THE EFFICACY AFTER GENETIC MODIFICATION OF TUMOR CELLS USING ADENOVIRAL VECTORS

Transgene	Gene Transfer Mode	Animal Model (Tumor Cell Type:Mouse Strain)	References
IL-2	*Ex vivo*	P815 mastocytoma:DBA/2;	34
		MMTV/Middle T transgenic mice (FVB/N)	35
	In vivo	MMTV/Middle T transgenic mice (FVB/N)	35
		P815 mastocytoma: DBA/2	36
		MH134 HCC:C3H	37
		FSA fibrosarcoma:C3H	38
		M-MSV fibrosarcoma:BALB/c	39
B7.1	*In vivo*	M-MSV fibrosarcoma:BALB/c	39
		MMTV/Middle T transgenic mice (FVB/N)	41,42
IL-12 and B7.1		MMTV/Middle T transgenic mice (FVB/N)	41
IL-2 and B7.1		MMTV/Middle T transgenic mice (FVB/N)	42
GM-CSF	*Ex vivo*	Lewis lung 3LL:C57BL/6	44
	In vivo	B16:C57BL/6	45
GM-CSF and *Escherichia coli* cytosine deaminase	*In vivo*	B16:C57BL/6	45
IL-12	*In vivo*	MCA-26 colon carcinoma:BALB/c	46
		MMTV/Middle T transgenic mice (FVB/N)	47,54
		MB49 bladder carcinoma: C57BL/6	48
		MC38 adenocarcinoma or MCA205 fibrosarcoma: C57BL/6	49
IL-4	*Ex vivo, In vivo*	MMTV/Middle T transgenic mice (FVB/N)	50
Interferon-α2b	*In vivo*	PC-3 or Hep3B:nude mice	51
IL-2 and HSV thymidine kinase	*In vivo*	MCA-26 colon carcinoma:BALB/c	52
		M-MSV fibrosarcoma:BALB/c	39
IL-2 and IL-12	*In vivo*	MMTV/Middle T transgenic mice (FVB/N)	53

GM-CSF, granulocyte-macrophage colony-stimulating factor; HSV, herpes simplex virus; IL, interleukin; M-MSV, mouse murine sarcoma virus; MMTV, mouse mammary tumor virus.

Some of the most promising results obtained involving adenoviral-transduced tumor cells as cancer vaccines involves the use of IL-12. IL-12 is a master control cytokine that is expressed by activated APCs, can induce interferon-γ levels, and can enhance Th1-type immune responses in conjunction with IL-2. Intratumoral injection of an adenovirus encoding both subunits of IL-12 (Ad/mIL-12) can inhibit tumor growth (46,47), and, in some cases, cause tumor regression, whereas injection of virus at a site distal to the tumor retards tumor growth but does not induce regression (48,49), suggesting that local delivery of IL-12 at the tumor site is essential for regression. A dose response has been reported in which intratumoral delivery of 10^9 PFU has been shown to be optimal, whereas 10^8 PFU induces only partial, transient regression, and 10^7 PFU is largely ineffective (48). Animals that have rejected injected tumors demonstrate antitumor cell reactivity characterized predominantly by CD8 T cells in the spleen (49), whereas *in vivo* administration of anti-CD4 or anti-CD8 antibodies has been shown to abrogate immune responses induced by intratumoral injection of Ad/IL-12 (48). Animals that reject injected tumors are protected from subsequent challenge with tumor cells (47–49), suggesting that systemic immunity is induced. Intratumoral injection of Ad/IL-12 has also been shown to cause concurrent regression of distal lung metastases (48). Histologic examination of injected tumors reveals a CD4 and CD8 T-cell infiltrate post injection (49), and injected animals can exhibit elevated levels of IL-12 and interferon-γ at the tumor site (47), as well as in the blood (48,49). Transient expression of the IL-12 transgene has been reported such that baseline levels of cytokine are detected 7 to 14 days post tumor injection (48).

Tumor cells transduced *ex vivo* with an adeno vector encoding IL-4 are impaired in their ability to cause tumors in mice (50), and histologic evaluation reveals the presence of an eosinophil infiltrate in tumor cells expressing IL-4. Intratumoral injection of Ad/IL-4 slows the growth of s.c. tumors or induces complete tumor regression, and "cured" animals are protected from subsequent challenge with unmodified tumor cells. Similarly, multiple intratumoral injections of an adenovirus encoding interferon-α2b has been reported to induce regression of s.c. tumors (51). As these experiments were conducted in athymic nude mice, no assessment of immunologic memory to the tumor was investigated.

Given the variable levels of efficacy achieved by adenovirus-mediated delivery of a single transgene to tumor cells, investigators have explored combination gene therapy. In a model in which an adenovirus encoding IL-2 had little benefit and an adenovirus encoding the ganciclovir prodrug-activating enzyme herpes simplex virus thymidine kinase had partial benefit. The intratumoral administration of both adenoviruses caused significant tumor destruction, induced potent antitumor cell reactivity as characterized by tumor reactive CD8+ T cells, and conferred protective immunity from subsequent tumor cell challenge (52). In other models, however, combination therapy with Ad/TK plus Ad/IL-2 has been reported to be no better than Ad/TK alone (39). Intratumoral coinjection of adenoviral vectors encoding IL-12 and IL-2 is superior to either vector alone, as judged by the frequency of observed complete regression of injected, as well as distal, tumors (53).

Preexisting immunity to an adenoviral vector could potentially reduce the efficiency of gene transfer to tumor cells after intratumoral injection of virus. Intratumoral gene transfer efficiency is reduced 2.4-fold in animals exhibiting preexisting antiadenoviral antibodies (54). This reduction in gene transfer efficiency, however, is insufficient to inhibit the ability of an adenovirus encoding IL-12 to cause regression of injected tumors and, thus, the induction of antitumor T-cell reactivity. No change in antiadenovirus antibody titers has been detected in patients receiving an s.c. injection of tumor cells previously transduced *ex vivo* with adenovirus, suggesting that an insufficient presentation of viral antigen exists in the transduced tumor cell vaccine (55). Thus, antiadenovirus antibodies may not be a limiting issue in the clinical application of adenoviral vectors for genetic modification of tumors *in vivo*.

A potential concern associated with using adenoviral vectors to deliver cytokine genes to tumor cells is that the induction of an antiadenovirus CTL response might detract from the desired antitumor cell immune response. It is well documented that the *in vivo* administration of adenovirus can induce CTLs; however, control experiments involving the intratumoral injection of adenoviral vectors encoding a marker gene, such as β-galactosidase, have shown that (a) the generation of antitumor cell CTL reactivity is not impaired by the introduction of adenovirus, and (b) the regression of injected tumors cannot be attributed to the action of antiadenovirus CTLs.

Clinical experiences with adenovirus vector–transduced tumor cells is limited. A study involving the intratumoral administration of a replication-deficient adenoviral vector encoding IL-2 into metastatic breast cancer or melanoma has been conducted (56), and an account of gene transfer to cutaneous plasmacytoma in one patient enrolled in this trial has appeared (57). A total of 23 patients (15 melanoma, 8 breast cancer) received intratumoral injections of 10^7 to 10^{10} PFU of the Ad/IL-2 virus with 18 patients receiving a single injection, four receiving two injections, and one patient receiving five injections. No grade 3 or 4 toxicities were noted in any of the patients; however, injection site–localized inflammation that resolved in 5 to 7 days was noted at all doses. Six patients experienced localized regression of injected tumors, but no partial or complete responses were noted. Eighteen of 22 injected tumor biopsies were positive for Ad/IL-2 vector, as judged by polymerase chain reaction 7 days after injection, whereas 62% of the samples were positive for IL-2 messenger RNA as judged by real-time polymerase chain reaction. Seventeen of 21 injected tumor samples showed an increase in lymphocyte infiltration predominated by CD8-positive T cells post injection. Serum titers of antiadenoviral antibodies increased in 16 patients evaluated, with more consistent and marked increases noted for viral doses of 5×10^9 PFU and higher. Nine of these 16 patients exhibited no neutralizing antiadenoviral antibodies in serum preinjection, and no change occurred for three of the nine patients post injection. Nine of the 16 patients demonstrated a significant increase in serum titers of antiadenoviral neutralizing antibodies, and, as above, more consistent increases were noted for viral doses of 5×10^9 PFU and higher. This study demonstrated the Ad/IL-2 vector is safe and relatively nontoxic, and extensive analysis of clinical samples revealed that no evidence existed for significant vector dissemination to organs or virus shedding, thus addressing potential safety concerns.

The s.c. administration of unirradiated autologous tumor cells transduced with an adenovirus encoding IL-2 to patients with advanced neuroblastoma has been reported (55). Of ten patients treated, five clinical responses were observed, including one complete response, one partial response, and three instances of stable disease. An evaluation of injection sites revealed the presence of a T-cell infiltrate, which varied from patient to patient, but was predominated by CD4+ T cells. All of the five patients who experienced a clinical response exhibited enhanced antineuroblastoma CTL reactivity.

Other Viral Vectors

Viral vectors based on herpes simplex virus and adenovirus-associated virus (AAV) have also been explored for immunotherapy of cancer in a limited number of studies. A replication-deficient herpes simplex viral vector encoding IL-2 can efficiently transduce tumor cells *in vitro*, and mice injected with irradiated, transduced tumor cells develop protective immunity and exhibit antitumor CTL activity (58). A replication-competent herpes simplex virus can inhibit tumor growth when injected intratumorally by cytotoxic viral replication, but inclusion of IL-12 within the vector enhances its antitumor effects and the generation of antitumor CTLs (59). Inhibition of tumor growth has been observed in immunocompetent but not immunodeficient animals. An AAV vector encoding an IL-12 fusion protein has been used to transduce acute myeloid leukemic blasts *in vitro* (60), whereas AAV vectors have been used to deliver IL-12 and the costimulatory molecule B7-2 to tumor cells *in vitro* (61), but no reports exist of *in vivo* efficacy. The observation that little information is available regarding the potential use of herpes simplex and AAV viral vectors for immunotherapy of cancer may be in part owing to the fact that production of sufficient quantities of replication-deficient forms of these vectors to support preclinical studies remains a challenge.

SUMMARY

Encouraging preclinical data has been obtained, suggesting that DCs genetically modified by adenoviral vectors encoding TAAs and intratumoral injection of adenoviral vectors encoding immunomodulatory factors can be efficacious. Although clinical experience with adenoviral vector vaccines is limited, new immunotherapy studies are planned using autologous DCs transduced with adenoviral vectors encoding melanoma antigens and intratumoral injection of adenoviral vectors encoding potent cytokines, such as IL-12. Combination gene therapy has been shown to be synergistic in the induction of antitumor cell immunoreactivity in preclinical studies; therefore, it is not unreasonable to imagine that future clinical trials will involve the concurrent genetic modification of APCs and of tumor cells to dampen immune evasion by tumor cells, thereby enabling more effective destruction by antitumor immune effector cells. As adenoviral vectors constitute an efficient means to genetically modify APCs and tumor cells, the clinical application of adenoviral vaccines holds great promise.

REFERENCES

1. Horwitz MS. Adenoviridae and their replications. In: Fields BN, Knipe DM, eds. *Virology*, 2nd ed. New York: Raven Press, 1990:1679–1721.
2. Graham FL, Prevec L. Manipulation of adenovirus vectors. In: Murray EJ, ed. *Methods in molecular biology*. Clifton, NJ: Humana, 1991:109–128.
3. Bergelson JM, Cunningham JA, Droguett G, et al. Isolation of a common receptor for Coxsackie B viruses and adenoviruses 2 and 5. *Science* 1997;275:1320–1323.
4. Hehir KM, Armentano D, Cardoza LM, et al. Molecular characterization of replication-competent variants of adenovirus vectors and genome modifications to prevent their occurrence. *J Virol* 1996;70:8459–8467.
5. Fallaux FJ, Bout A, van der Velde I, et al. New helper cells and matched early region 1-deleted adenovirus vectors prevent generation of replication-competent adenoviruses. *Hum Gene Ther* 1998;9:1909–1917.
6. Crouzet J, Naudin L, Orsini C, et al. Recombinational construction in Escherichia coli of infectious adenoviral genomes. *Proc Natl Acad Sci U S A* 1997;94:1414–1419.
7. He TC, Zhou S, da Costa LT, Yu J, Kinzler KW, Vogelstein B. A simplified system for generating recombinant adenoviruses. *Proc Natl Acad Sci U S A* 1998;95:2509–2514.
8. Steinman RM. The dendritic cell system and its role in immunogenicity. *Annu Rev Immunol* 1991;9:271–296.
9. Arthur JF, Butterfield LH, Roth MD, et al. A comparison of gene transfer methods in human dendritic cells. *Cancer Gene Ther* 1997;4:17–25.
10. Dietz AB, Vuk-Pavlovic S. High efficiency adenovirus-mediated gene transfer to human dendritic cells. *Blood* 1998;91:392–398.
11. Gong J, Chen L, Chen D, Kashiwaba M, Manome Y, Tanaka T, Kufe D. Induction of antigen-specific antitumor immunity with adenovirus-transduced dendritic cells. *Gene Ther* 1997;4:1023–1028.
12. Song W, Kong HL, Carpenter H, et al. Dendritic cells genetically modified with an adenovirus vector encoding the cDNA for a model antigen induce protective and therapeutic antitumor immunity. *J Exp Med* 1997;186:1247–1256.
13. Wan Y, Bramson J, Carter R, Graham F, Gauldie J. Dendritic cells transduced with an adenoviral vector encoding a model tumor-associated antigen for tumor vaccination. *Hum Gene Ther* 1997;8:1355–1363.
14. Brossart P, Goldrath AW, Butz EA, Martin S, Bevan MJ. Virus-mediated delivery of antigenic epitopes into dendritic cells as a means to induce CTL. *J Immunol* 1997;158:3270–3276.
15. Frey BM, Hackett NR, Bergelson JM, et al. High-efficiency gene transfer into *ex vivo* expanded human hematopoietic progenitors and precursor cells by adenovirus vectors. *Blood* 1998;91:2781–2792.
16. Warnier G, Duffour M-T, Uyttenhove C, Gajewski TF, Lurquin C, Haddada H, Perricaudet M, Boon T. Induction of a cytotoxic T-cell response in mice with a recombinant adenovirus coding for tumor antigen P815A. *Int J Cancer* 1996;67:303–310.
17. Butterfield LH, Jilani SM, Chakraborty NG, et al. Generation of melanoma-specific cytotoxic T lymphocytes by dendritic cells transduced with a MART-1 adenovirus. *J Immunol* 1998;161:5607–5613.
18. Zhai Y, Yang JC, Kawakami Y, et al. Antigen-specific tumor vaccines: development and characterization of recombinant adenoviruses encoding MART1 or gp100 for cancer therapy. *J Immunol* 1996; 156:700–710.
19. Toes REM, Hoeben RC, van der Voort EIH, et al. Protective antitumor immunity induced by vaccination with recombinant adenoviruses encoding multiple tumor associated cytotoxic T lymphocyte epitopes in a string-of-beads fashion. *Proc Natl Acad Sci U S A* 1997;94:14660–14665.
20. Krieg AM, Wu T, Weeratna R, et al. Sequence motifs in adenoviral DNA block immune activation by stimulatory CpG motifs. *Proc Natl Acad Sci U S A* 1998;95:12631–12636.
21. Smith CA, Woodruff LS, Kitchingman GR, Rooney CM. Adenovirus-pulsed dendritic cells stimulate human virus-specific T-cell responses *in vitro*. *J Virol* 1996;70:6733–6740.
22. Perez-Diez A, Butterfield LH, Li L, Chakraborty NG, Economou JS, Mukherji B. Generation of CD8+ and CD4+ T-cell response to dendritic cells genetically engineered to express the MART-1/Melan-A gene. *Cancer Res* 1998;58:5305–5309.
23. Sonderbye L, Feng S, Yacoubian S, Buehler H, Ahsan N, Mulligan R, Langhoff E. *In vivo* and *in vitro* modulation of immune stimulatory capacity of primary dendritic cells by adenovirus-mediated gene transduction. *Exp Clin Immunogenet* 1998;15:100–111.
24. Cao X, Zhang W, He L, et al. Lymphotactin gene-modified bone marrow dendritic cells act as more potent adjuvants for peptide delivery to induce specific antitumor immunity. *J Immunol* 1998;161:6238–6244.
25. Chen PW, Wang M, Bronte V, Zhai Y, Rosenberg SA, Restifo NP. Therapeutic antitumor response after immunization with a recombinant adenovirus encoding a model tumor-associated antigen. *J Immunol* 1996;156:224–231.
26. Hirschowitz EA, Leonard S, Song W, et al. Adenovirus-mediated expression of melanoma antigen gp75 as immunotherapy for metastatic melanoma. *Gene Ther* 1998;5:975–983.
27. Li W, Berencsi K, Basak S, et al. Human colorectal cancer (CRC) antigen CO17-1A/GA733 encoded by adenovirus inhibits growth of established CRC cells in mice. *J Immunol* 1997;159:763–769.
28. Zhai Y, Yang JC, Spiess P, et al. Cloning and characterization of the genes encoding the murine homologues of the human melanoma antigens MART-1 and gp100. *J Immunother* 1997;20:15–25.
29. Ribas A, Butterfield LH, McBride WH, et al. Genetic immunization for the melanoma antigen MART-1/melan-A using recombinant adenovirus-transduced murine dendritic cells. *Cancer Res* 1997;57:2865–2869.
30. Caspar CB, Levy S, Levy R. Idiotype vaccines for non-Hodgkin's lymphoma induce polyclonal immune responses that cover mutated tumor idiotypes: comparison of different vaccine formulations. *Blood* 1997;90:3699–3706.
31. Rosenberg SA, Zhai Y, Yang JC, et al. Immunizing patients with metastatic melanoma using recombinant adenoviruses encoding MART-1 or gp100 melanoma antigens. *J Natl Cancer Inst* 1998;90:1894–1900.
32. Mastrangeli A, Harvey B-G, Yao J, et al. "Sero-switch" adenovirus-mediated *in vivo* gene transfer: circumvention of anti-adenovirus vector administration by changing the adenovirus serotype. *Hum Gene Ther* 1996;7:79–87.
33. Mack CA, Song W-R, Carpenter H, et al. Circumvention of anti-adenovirus neutralizing immunity by administration of an adenoviral vector of an alternate serotype. *Hum Gene Ther* 1997;8:99–109.
34. Haddada H, Ragot T, Cordier L, Duffour MT, Perricaudet M. Adenoviral interleukin-2 gene transfer into P815 tumor cells abrogates tumorigenicity and induces antitumoral immunity in mice. *Hum Gene Ther* 1993;4:703–711.
35. Addison CL, Braciak T, Ralston R, Muller WJ, Gauldie J, Graham FL. Intratumoral injection of an adenovirus expressing interleukin 2 induces regression and immunity in a murine breast cancer model. *Proc Natl Acad Sci U S A* 1995;92:8522–8526.
36. Cordier L, Duffour MT, Sabourin JC, Lee MG, Cabannes J, Ragot T, Perricaudet M, Haddada H. Complete recovery of mice from a preestablished tumor by direct intratumoral delivery of an adenovirus vector harboring the murine IL-2 gene. *Gene Ther* 1995;2:16–21.
37. Huang H, Chen SH, Kosai K, Finegold MJ, Woo SL. Gene therapy for hepatocellular carcinoma: long-term remission of primary and metastatic tumors in mice by interleukin-2 gene therapy *in vivo*. *Gene Ther* 1996;3:980–987.
38. Toloza EM, Hunt K, Swisher S, et al. *In vivo* cancer gene therapy with a recombinant interleukin-2 adenovirus vector. *Cancer Gene Ther* 1996;3:11–17.
39. Felzmann T, Ramsey WJ, Blaese RM. Characterization of the antitumor immune response generated by treatment of murine tumors with recombinant adenoviruses expressing HSVtk, IL-2, IL-6 or B7-1. *Gene Ther* 1997;4:1322–1329.
40. Gilligan MG, Knox P, Weedon S, Barton R, Kerr DJ, Searle P, Young LS. Adenoviral delivery of B7-1 (CD80) increases the immunogenicity of human ovarian and cervical carcinoma cells. *Gene Ther* 1998;5:965–974.
41. Putzer BM, Hitt M, Muller WJ, Emtage P, Gauldie J, Graham FL. Interleukin 12 and B7-1 costimulatory molecule expressed by an adenovirus vector act synergistically to facilitate tumor regression. *Proc Natl Acad Sci U S A* 1997;94:10889–10894.
42. Emtage PC, Wan Y, Bramson JL, Graham FL, Gauldie J. A double recombinant adenovirus expressing the costimulatory molecule B7-1 (murine) and human IL-2 induces complete tumor regression in a murine breast adenocarcinoma model. *J Immunol* 1998;160:2531–2538.

43. Dranoff G, Jaffee E, Lazenby A, et al. Vaccination with irradiated tumor cells engineered to secrete murine granulocyte-macrophage colony-stimulating factor stimulates potent, specific, and long-lasting anti-tumor immunity. *Proc Natl Acad Sci U S A* 1993;90:3539–3543.

44. Lee CT, Wu S, Ciernik IF, Chen H, Nadaf-Rahrov S, Gabrilovich D, Carbone DP. Genetic immunotherapy of established tumors with adenovirus-murine granulocyte-macrophage colony-stimulating factor. *Hum Gene Ther* 1997;8:187–193.

45. Cao X, Ju DW, Tao Q, et al. Adenovirus-mediated GM-CSF gene and cytosine deaminase gene transfer followed by 5-fluorocytosine administration elicit more potent antitumor response in tumor-bearing mice. *Gene Ther* 1998;5:1130–1136.

46. Caruso M, Pham-Nguyen K, Kwong YL, et al. Adenovirus-mediated interleukin-12 gene therapy for metastatic colon carcinoma. *Proc Natl Acad Sci U S A* 1996;93:11302–11306.

47. Bramson JL, Hitt M, Addison CL, Muller WJ, Gauldie J, Graham FL. Direct intratumoral injection of an adenovirus expressing interleukin-12 induces regression and long-lasting immunity that is associated with highly localized expression of interleukin-12. *Hum Gene Ther* 1996;7:1995–2002.

48. Chen L, Chen D, Block E, O'Donnell M, Kufe DW, Clinton SK. Eradication of murine bladder carcinoma by intratumoral injection of a bicistronic adenoviral vector carrying cDNAs for the IL-12 heterodimer and its inhibition by the IL-12 p40 subunit homodimer. *J Immunol* 1997;159:351–359.

49. Gambotto A, Tuting T, McVey DL, et al. Induction of antitumor immunity by direct intratumoral injection of a recombinant adenovirus expressing interleukin-12. *Cancer Gene Ther* 1999;6:45–53.

50. Addison CL, Gauldie J, Muller WJ, Graham FL. An adenoviral vector expressing interleukin-4 modulates tumorigenicity and induces regression in a murine breast cancer model. *Int J Oncol* 1995;7:1253–1260.

51. Ahmed CMI, Sugarman BJ, Johnson DE, Bookstein RE, Saha DP, Nagabhushan TL, Wills KN. *In vivo* tumor suppression by adenovirus-mediated interferon alpha 2b gene delivery. *Hum Gene Ther* 1999;10:77–84.

52. Chen SH, Chen XH, Wang Y, Kosai K, Finegold MJ, Rich SS, Woo SL. Combination gene therapy for liver metastasis of colon carcinoma *in vivo*. *Proc Natl Acad Sci U S A* 1995;92:2577–2581.

53. Addison CL, Bramson JL, Hitt MM, Muller WJ, Gauldie J, Graham FL. Intratumoral coinjection of adenoviral vectors expressing IL-2 and IL-12 results in enhanced frequency of regression of injected and untreated distal tumors. *Gene Ther* 1998;5:1400–1409.

54. Bramson JL, Hitt M, Gauldie J, Graham FL. Pre-existing immunity to adenovirus does not prevent tumor regression following intratumoral administration of a vector expressing IL-12 but inhibits virus dissemination. *Gene Ther* 1997;4:1069–1076.

55. Bowman L, Grossmann M, Rill D, et al. IL-2 adenovector-transduced autologous tumor cells induce antitumor immune responses in patients with neuroblastoma. *Blood* 1998;92:1941–1949.

56. Stewart AK, Lassam NJ, Quirt IC, et al. Adenovector-mediated gene delivery of interleukin-2 in metastatic breast cancer and melanoma: results of a phase 1 clinical trial. *Gene Ther* 1999;6:350–363.

57. Stewart AK, Schimmer AD, Bailey DJ, et al. *In vivo* adenoviral-mediated gene transfer of interleukin-2 in cutaneous plasmacytoma [letter]. *Blood* 1998;91.1095–1097.

58. Tung C, Federoff HJ, Brownlee M, Karpoff H, Weigel T, Brennan MF, Fong Y. Rapid production of interleukin-2-secreting tumor cells by herpes simplex virus-mediated gene transfer: implications for autologous vaccine production. *Hum Gene Ther* 1996;7:2217–2224.

59. Toda M, Martuza RL, Kojima H, Rabkin SD. In situ cancer vaccination: an IL-12 defective vector/replication-competent herpes simplex virus combination induces local and systemic antitumor activity. *J Immunol* 1998;160:4457–4464.

60. Anderson R, Macdonald I, Corbett T, Hacking G, Lowdell MW, Prentice HG. Construction and biological characterization of an interleukin-12 fusion protein (Flexi-12): delivery to acute myeloid leukemic blasts using adeno-associated virus. *Hum Gene Ther* 1997; 8:1125–1135.

61. Maass G, Bogedain C, Scheer U, et al. Recombinant adeno-associated virus for the generation of autologous, gene-modified tumor vaccines: evidence for a high transduction efficiency into primary epithelial cancer cells. *Hum Gene Ther* 1998;9:1049–1059.

18.7

CANCER VACCINES: CLINICAL APPLICATIONS

Dendritic Cell Vaccines

RAMSEY M. DALLAL
ROBBIE MAILLIARD
MICHAEL T. LOTZE

In addition to granulocytes, lymphocytes, and mononuclear phagocytes, there is a fourth variety of adherent nucleated cell whose morphological features are quite distinct. . . . The cytoplasm of this large cell is arranged in pseudopods of varying length with form and number resulting in a variety of cell shapes ranging from bipolar elongate cells to elaborate stellate or dendritic ones. Most pseudopods are long, uniform in width, and have blunt terminations, but smaller spinous processes are also evident. The cytoplasm contains many large circular phase-dense granules as well as infrequent refractile granules, probably lipid. There is no morphological evidence of active endocytosis even if the cells are cultivated for several hours in high concentrations (40% volume/volume) of serum, conditions known to stimulate endocytosis in macrophages *in vitro*.

—Zanvil A. Cohn and Ralph M. Steinman (1973)

Identified in the early 1970s by Cohn and Steinman, dendritic cells (DCs) were named for their curious morphology with long dendritic processes. DCs were difficult to study and define until the development of modern culture techniques in the 1990s using recombinant cytokines. These strategies have been used to define the DCs' central role in antigen processing and presentation (1). In the mid-1990s, we have seen substantial refinement in our understanding of what is a family of cells and their potential application in treating disease in preclinical models, as well as in clinical protocols. We are beginning to understand the role of DCs, not only as antigen-presenting cells (APCs) capable of monitoring the internal milieu, but also as regulators of tissue repair, transplant rejection, and the initiation and maintenance of the inflammatory response (2,3). In addition to playing a role in regulating the initiation of the immune response (4), DCs appear to play a role in the maintenance of the immune response, providing signals for effector T-cell survival. Nonimmune roles as well are suggested by the finding that they produce proangiogeneic and antiangiogeneic hormones. The DC truly has a central role as the pacemaker of the immune system.

DCs not only serve in antigen presentation; they provide costimulation and cytokines to prevent apoptotic death for recruited effector T cells. A number of tumor types, including colorectal cancer and hepatoma and lung cancer (5–8), express Fas ligand (FasL). FasL, a molecule on the cell surface and counterreceptor for the Fas receptor, is expressed on virtually all mammalian cells, including activated T cells, and causes the induction of apoptosis in susceptible T cells. Thus, we have the seemingly paradoxic situation of tumors killing T cells instead of T cells killing tumors. For that reason, one goal of the tumor immunologist is the prevention of premature T-cell apoptotic death and the engagement of so-called T-cell futile cycles. DCs, by virtue of their expression of so-called costimulatory molecules, such as CD80 (B7.1) and CD86 (B7.2), and several "dendrikines," including interferon-α (IFN-α), interleukin-12 (IL-12), and IL-18, may be uniquely capable of preventing premature T-cell death, and, thus, becoming the mediators of T-cell survival.

The biologic therapist has five goals when seeking to treat cancer:

1. The induction of an effective cell-mediated T-cell response
2. The promotion of T-cell survival in the inhibitory milieu of the tumor microenvironment
3. The development of long-lived memory
4. Designing strategies to deliver T cells across the endothelial barrier
5. Regulating angiogenesis (9)

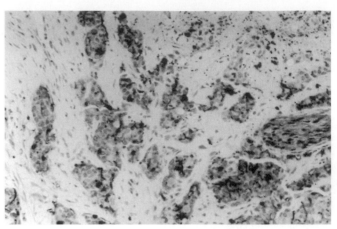

FIGURE 1. Pancreatic adenocarcinoma specimen demonstrates extensive infiltration of S100+ dendritic cells. Only 3 of 47 patients exhibited this degree of S100+ DC infiltration and lived 50, 34, and 3 months (group average, 18 months). (Dallal RM et al. *Unpublished data.*)

Just as chronic responses to microbial pathogens are maintained in part by retention of antigens in follicular, and, perhaps, other DCs, a durable T-cell response may require DC provision of survival factors, and, possibly, antigens at the site of tumor, as well as regulating the local vascular blood supply.

DC biology was initially related to cancer with the observation that DC numbers correlated with prognosis in numerous tumor types, including (a) various cancers from the lung, head, and neck; (b) breast, cervical, endometrial, esophageal, gastric, pancreatic, colon, and prostate cancer; and (c) Hodgkin's disease and mycosis fungoides (10–16) (Fig. 1, Table 1). These findings legitimize DC-based immunotherapy, for reversing DC dysfunction and paucity in cancer patients by genetic engineering, cytokine treatment, or the adoptive transfer of DCs may prove therapeutic. The use of DCs in cancer patients may lead to a long-lasting tumor response through efficient activation of specific T cells and the prevention of tumor-induced T-cell death (TICD). Our clinical immunotherapy regimes have combined receptor IL-2 therapy with the adoptive transfer of tumor-infiltrating lymphocytes or lymphokine-activated killer cells with mediocre results (17). Newer strategies involve the adoptive transfer of DCs primed with tumor antigens to elicit a specific, cell-mediated response (18). Promising murine results from our group and others have been brought to intriguing human trials, many of which are reporting responses. Furthermore, the administration of the dendropoietic cytokines FLT-3 ligand (FL), IL-12, or granulocyte macrophage colony-stimulating factors (GM-CSF) may enhance *in vivo* DC production, and, thereby, specifically enhance T-cell activation (19–21).

DENDRITIC CELLS

DCs appear to be central to the regulation, maturation, and maintenance of a cellular immune response to cancer. They are characterized by the presence of veils and long processes that are quite active, continually extending and retracting, which allows them to be highly mobile. DCs are the most potent APCs in

TABLE 1. RELATIONSHIP BETWEEN DENDRITIC CELL INFILTRATION AND PROGNOSIS IN MALIGNANCY

Tumor	Author (Year)	Dendritic Cell Infiltration
Arsenical skin	Yu (1992)	Less compared with normal skin
Basal cell	Bergfelt (1994)	Less in tumors
Basal cell	Bergfelt (1992)	? Improved
Breast	Wilson (1991)	? Improved prognosis
Bronchoalveolar	Tosi (1992)	No effect
Cervix	Morelli (1993)	Less in human papilloma virus + tumors
Cervix	Nakano (1992)	Improved
Cervix, stage III	Nakano (1993)	Marked improved prognosis
Cervix/penile	Morelli (1992)	Less with human papilloma virus infection
Cervix/human immunodeficiency virus	Spinillo (1993)	Less in acquired immunodeficiency syndrome
Endometrial	Coppola (1998)	Langerhans' infiltration favorable
Esophageal	Furihata (1992)	Marked improved prognosis
Esophageal	Imai (1993)	Direct relationship to grade
Gastric	Tsujitani (1992)	Marked improved prognosis
Gastric	Tsujitani (1995)	More in tumor draining lymph nodes
Gastric, stage III	Tsujitani (1993)	Marked improved prognosis
Hodgkin's disease	Alavaikko (1994)	Follicular dendritic dells improve prognosis
Lung	Zeid (1993)	Marked improved prognosis
Lung	Tazi (1993)	Related granulocyte-macrophage colony-stimulating factor production
Melanoma	Toriyama (1993)	Inverse with tumor thickness
Mycosis fungoides/SS	Meissner (1993)	Marked improved prognosis
Prostate	Bigotti (1991)	Improved prognosis
Pancreatic adenocarcinoma	Dallal et al., manuscript in prep.	Virtually no dendritic cells found
Skin tumors	Schreiner (1995)	Less in tumors
Tongue cancer	Goldman (1998)	Increased dendritic cells improved prognosis
Thyroid (papillary)	Willgeroth (1992)	No effect

humans; they express high levels of class I and class II major histocompatibility complex (MHC) costimulatory molecules and produce a variety of cytokines, including IL-1, IL-12, IL-18, and IFN-α (22,23). These cytokines stimulate T-helper type 1 (Th1) cells, thus promoting the cellular immune response. DCs are up to 100-fold more efficient in stimulating an allogeneic mixed lymphocyte reaction than other APCs. MHC products are 10 to 100 times higher on DCs than on monocytes or B cells, and DCs contain far more signal two–signaling molecules and T-cell adhesion molecules than other APCs. DCs take up antigen through a variety of pathways, including Fc receptors, mannose receptors, and fluid-phase macropinocytosis. So-called immature DCs take up apoptotic and necrotic cells, microbes, particulate antigens, and soluble proteins. After antigen capture and maturation, DCs apparently promote T-cell survival and selection. After encounter with the appropriate T cells and their subsequent expansion, DCs undergo an apoptotic death in the lymph node and can become targets for T cells or be engulfed by resident macrophages or DCs (24–26).

Dendritic Cell Origins

DCs constitute a rare but heterogeneous population phenotypically distinct from macrophages (CD14$^-$) and represent less than 1% of the entire circulating leukocyte population. They are lineage-negative cells that are distinct from T cells, B cells, natural killer (NK) cells, and monocytes. They include:

1. Langerhans' cells (LCs), located primarily in the skin and epithelial tissues

2. Interdigitating cells, located within T-cell–rich areas within secondary follicles
3. Lymphoid DCs, located in the germinal centers of lymphoid follicles (27)
4. Thymic DCs, a subtype of lymphoid-derived DCs located in the thymic medulla, where they are involved in T-cell selection
5. Veiled cells found in peripheral blood

Various surface markers can be used to identify and distinguish DCs (Table 2) from other cell types.

DCs are derived primarily from the bone marrow, as revealed by their expression of the common leukocyte antigen CD45 (28). Irradiated mice transplanted with allogeneic bone marrow demonstrate donor MHC on DCs located from the spleen and epidermis (29). These cells express CD13, CD33, and CD11, which are markers of myeloid derivation. The myeloid origin of DCs, however, is confusing. In Ikaros mutants, where all lymphoid precursors are lacking, only the LCs and DCs remain (30). Furthermore, nonprimitive progenitors for lymphoid cells and DCs can be distinct from those of myeloid, megakaryocytic, and erythroid cells, implying that the DC lineage may be more related to the lymphoid lineage than to the myeloid lineage (31).

LCs are located in the basal and suprabasal layers of the epidermis. LCs are myeloid progenitors from CD34$^+$ cells, which express the skin-homing cutaneous lymphocyte-associated antigen (CLA) (32). LCs express high amounts of CD1a and are associated with Birbeck granules. CD1a, an MHC-like molecule that associates with beta-2-microglobulin, presents mycobacterial lipids and glycolipids to T cells and some NK-T cells (33,34). LC precursors can differentiate into macrophages under the response

TABLE 2. CHART OF RELEVANT SURFACE MARKERS RELATED TO DENDRITIC CELLS

Surface Marker	Cell Expressing	Comments
CD1a,b,c,d	Cortical thymocytes, Langerhans' cells, some DCs, B cells (CD1c), intestinal epithelium (CD1d)	MHC class I–like molecules associated with beta-2-microglobulin. Presents glycolipids to $\gamma\delta$ T-cell receptor
CD4	Helper T cells, weakly positive in lymphoid DC subsets	Coreceptor for MHC class II molecules. Binds lck on cytoplasmic face of membrane.
CD8	Lymphoid DCs express α chain, cytotoxic T cells	Found in DCs with lymphoid origin. Coreceptor of MHC class I molecules
CD11b	Lymphoid DCs	αM subunit of integrin
CD11c	Myeloid DC cells	αX subunit of integrin CR4 (associated with CD18); binds fibrinogen
CD13	Myelomonocytic cells	Zinc metalloproteinase, cleaves N-terminal amino acids from MHC class II–bound peptides
CD14	Myelomonocytic cells	Receptor for complex of LPS and LPS binding protein
CD25	Activated T cells, B cells, monocytes	Interleukin-2 receptor α, marker for terminally differentiated DCs
CD32	Monocytes, granulocytes, B cells, eosinophils	Low affinity Fc receptor for aggregated Ig/immune complexes
CD33	Myeloid progenitor cells, monocytes	Involved in cell-cell adhesion
CD34	Hematopoietic precursors, capillary endothelium	Ligand for CD62 (L-selectin)
CD40	Mature B cells, DCs, activated monocytes	Receptor for CD40L on T cells
CD45	All hematopoietic cells except erythrocytes	Necessary for signaling through T-cell receptor
CD54	Numerous cell types, DCs	Enhances interaction between T cells and antigen-presenting cells
CD58	Numerous cell types	LFA-3 binds CD2, adhesion molecule
CD64	Monocytes, macrophages	High-affinity receptor for IgG
CD80	Resting monocytes, DCs	Interacts with CD28 to provide signal 2
CD83	Activated B cells, activated T cells, circulating DCs (veil cells)	Maturation marker DC; unknown function
CD86	B-cell subset	Interacts with CD28 to provide signal 2
CD102	Numerous	Intercellular adhesion molecule, binds CD11a/CD18 (LFA-1) and CD11b/CD18 (Mac-1) integrins
CDw116	Monocytes, eosinophils, endothelium	GM-CSFR α chain GM-CSFR cytokine receptor superfamily

DC, dendritic cell; GM-CSFR, granulocyte-macrophage colony-stimulating factor receptor; Ig, immunoglobulin; LFA, leukocyte function–associated antigen-3; LPS, lipopolysaccharide; MHC, major histocompatibility complex.

of macrophage colony-stimulating factor (35). Interstitial DCs and CD34-derived cells differ from LCs by lacking CLA, demonstrating higher antigen capture efficiency, and associating with germinal centers. Interstitial DCs are CD1a$^+$ and FXIIIa$^+$ (36). LCs and other DCs express E cadherin (37), α-6/β-1 integrin, chemokine receptors CCR 1, 2, 5, and 6, as well as the CXCR1 (38).

GM-CSF and tumor necrosis factor (TNF) stimulate growth and differentiation of DC progenitors into DC precursors (39). This differentiation can be enhanced by multiple cytokines, including c-kit, Flt-3 ligand (FL), tumor growth factor–β (TGF-β), IL-4, IL-13, and, in particular, TNF-α. Protein kinase C and nuclear factor κB (NFκB) activation seem central in this process (40). IκB phosphorylation releases NFκB in DCs and supports the survival and maturation of these cells. Although numerous agents, including TNF, IL-1, IL-17, lipopolysaccharide, various viruses, phorbol myristate acetate, oxidative agents, and mitogens, cause phosphorylation of IκB, which releases NFκB, the kinase responsible for this in DCs had been elusive. A potent dendropoietic cytokine, FL, induces massive (up to 300-fold) increases in the numbers of DCs in mice and humans. These DCs are functionally and phenotypically indistinct from IL-4/GM-CSF–derived DCs when tested *in vitro*.

When cultured with IL-4 and GM-CSF, peripheral blood monocytes can be induced without proliferation to differentiate into immature DCs (i.e., veiled cells high in costimulatory molecules, class II, CD40, and capable of stimulating a T-cell response at low concentrations) from CD14$^+$ monocytes (41). DCs also can be derived from CD34$^+$ hematopoietic progenitor

cells isolated from specific cell columns. Once incubated with IL-4, supercritical fluid (SCF), TNF-α, and GM-CSF, these CD34$^+$ cells proliferate 6 to 8 times and have the phenotype and function of immature DCs (42). Many debate the differences between the myeloid DCs derived directly from CD34$^+$ cells and CD14$^+$ cells. CD34$^+$ DCs may have a preferential capacity to activate CD8$^+$ T cells (43), and CD14-derived DCs elicit enhanced immunoglobulin M (IgM) production from B cells after coculture and addition of soluble CD40L and IL-2. Only the CD14-derived DCs secreted IL-10 after CD40 activation (44). In our early murine studies, we demonstrated that GM-CSF plus IL-4–cultured DCs were superior in their antitumor effects when compared with those derived from CD34 precursors cultured in GM-CSF alone or GM-CSF and TNF-α (45).

The understanding of the ontogeny and phylogeny of DCs has advanced considerably. It appears that the so-called myeloid DCs, those best defined in the early 1970s as separate and distinguishable from macrophages, are directly descended from a CD34$^+$, CD45RA$^+$, or CD10$^-$ progenitor or indirectly through a monocyte/macrophage–type cell. A second type of DC, a "lymphoid"-related DC first identified in the thymus and then in peripheral nodal tissue and peripheral blood, is believed to be most closely related to T cells, B cells, and NK cells. The individual roles of myeloid and lymphoid DCs have not been delineated. Lymphoid DCs might be involved in the maintenance of tolerance. Liu et al. propose two distinct DC phenotypes, DC1 and DC2. The human DC1, the conventional "myeloid" DC, plays a role in driving maturation of naïve CD4$^+$ cells into Th1-type cells. When maintained in IL-3 and soluble CD40L, DC2, the "lymphoid" DC, promotes Th2 differentiation (39). Conversely, some groups suggest that lymphoid DCs (which, in their model, produce IL-12) induce Th1 phenotype based on adoptive transfer of DCs in murine models (46). Both models suffer from somewhat protracted culture and isolation of cells; their legitimate role in negative and positive selection or generation of Th1 or Th2 cells requires additional study.

Thymic DCs presumably collect and present self antigen to developing T cells and initiate apoptosis (i.e., mediate negative selection) and the induction of self tolerance (47,48). They express many of the characteristic markers of DCs; in mice they are CD8α^+ and in humans they are CD4$^+$ (49,50). Thymic DCs (also known as *lymphoid* or *plasmacytoid DCs*) are bone marrow derived but have a relatively short life span, unlike follicular DCs. In the mouse, these cells are initially unresponsive to GM-CSF but respond to IL-3, FL, CD40L, TNF-α, IL-1, IL-7, and SCF (51). Thus, one classifies them as *lymphoid DCs* (52).

Thymic DCs, lymphoid DCs, and liver DCs differ from myeloid DCs in their appearance and function. By electron microscopy, these plasmacytoid cells have abundant endoplasmic reticulum but die rapidly in culture unless placed in culture with IL-3 and CD40 ligand. The major distinguishing characteristics of the DC2 from so-called DC1 or myeloid DCs is a failure to express CD1a, b, and c and a somewhat higher expression of CD1d. They express CD4 compared with only low-level expression on DC1s and fail to express high levels of CD11b, CD11c, CD13, or CD33. Their DC1s are CD45RO$^+$, whereas DC2s are CD45RA$^+$. DC1s express the GM-CSF receptor α chain, whereas DC2s express the IL-3 receptor α chain and produce a paucity of cytokines, including IL-8 (53). DC1s produce IL-1α, IL-1β, IL-6, IL-7, IL-12 (p35 and p40), IL-15, IL-18, TNF-α, TGF-β, macrophage colony-stimulating factor, and GM-CSF (54). Naïve T cells cocultured with DC1s produce INF-γ, whereas DC2s induce production of IL-4, IL-5, and IL-10 (55). Although one observes IFN-γ induction from naïve cells by DC2s, it is attenuated, especially in proportion to the amount of IL-4 produced (56).

NK T cells with characteristic T-cell receptor rearrangement (mouse, Vα14 and Vβ8; human, Vα24 and Vβ11) respond to myeloid DCs depending on IL-12 availability. When IL-12 is available, they become predominantly Th1-like and make IFN-γ and induce cytotoxic T lymphocytes (CTLs). In the absence of IL-12, NK-T cells become more Th2-like and produce IFN-γ and IL-4 (57).

Follicular DCs are found in the B-cell region of all secondary lymphoid tissue and exhibit typical dendritic morphology (58). Germinal centers contain rapidly proliferating B cells undergoing affinity maturation. They are involved in antigen presentation to B cells and memory B-cell development and lack phagocytic activity (59). They are particularly long lived and have the ability to capture antigen and present antigen for prolonged periods. Controversy exists as to whether follicular DCs have marked differences from other DCs (60).

Some have even suggested that neutrophils could also give rise to DCs by culturing CML blasts, which were CD65$^+$, MPO$^+$, and lactoferrin$^+$, and in 9 days of culture with GM-CSF, IL-4, and TNF-α. The blasts (class II$^+$, CD1a, b, c$^+$, CD40$^+$, MPO$^-$, lactoferrin$^-$) are consistent with a DC (61).

Murine CD19$^+$ pro-B cells develop into DCs with T-cell stimulatory properties when cultured in IL-1β, IL-3, IL-7, TNF-α, SCF, and FL. These pro-B cells acquired the DC-related markers CD11c and NLDC145/DEC-205, along with CD80, CD86, and a high density of MHC class II molecules. These marrow-derived DCs do not express CD4 or CD8α, markers related to thymic DCs (62).

Dendritic Cell Maturation

The concept of a stable and rigid DC phenotype oversimplifies the complex biology of DC maturation. DCs have multiple roles and dynamically shift phenotypes relative to their environment. The immature DC is an avidly phagocytic cell with moderate cytoplasmic veil formations. Typically, immature DCs are obtained by culturing the adherent layer of mononuclear cells with IL-4 and GM-CSF. IL-13, and, perhaps, IFN-α (Egawa S., *unpublished data*) can substitute for IL-4 in inducing DC formation (63,64). The mature DC is induced after interaction with bacterial products, such as lipopolysaccharide or saccharin, activated T cells expressing CD40L, apoptotic body uptake, monocyte-conditioned media (macrophage supernatant), and cytokines, including TNF-α or IL-1 (65–67). Mature DCs most notably express CD83, as well as the p55 actin–budling protein fascin (68,69). They develop extensive cytoplasmic veils, lack antigen-uptake capacity, express different cytokine genes, and display even higher levels of costimulatory molecules, as well as higher levels of class II MHC and CD40 (70). Antigen uptake promotes immature DCs to maturity and allows them to migrate into the lymph node and most efficiently activate a specific T-cell response. A terminally differentiated DC induced by a cytokine cocktail of prostaglandin E$_2$ (1 μg per mL), IL-1β (10 ng per mL), TNF-α (10 ng per mL), and IL-6 (1,000 U per mL) also exists, which displays even higher amounts of costimulatory molecules, as well as the IL-2 receptor α chain CD25 (Figs. 2–6) (71). These cells become unresponsive to CD40 ligation and do not produce IL-12 (72). Monocyte differentiation is reversible, as immature monocyte-derived DCs can reverse into a macrophage after cytokine withdrawal. Mature DCs cannot undergo this reversion. One reason some groups support adoptive transfer of mature DCs is that immature DCs may lose their efficiency for T-cell stimulation once removed from exogenously supplied cytokines.

Antigen Capture

Immature DCs are efficient at antigen uptake through several mechanisms, such as the engulfment of apoptotic bodies, macropinocytosis, and receptor-mediated endocytosis via mannose and Fc receptors (CD32 and CD64) (73–75). These antigens are then processed and complexed with MHC class II and can stimulate a T-helper response. Apoptotic bodies are internalized via binding to $\alpha_v\beta_5$, $\alpha_v\beta_3$, and CD36 (76). Macrophages are unable to efficiently present antigen from apoptotic cells in part because of the lack of $\alpha_v\beta_5$ associated with more rapid degradation of ingested material (77). Maturation also induces down-regulation in all of these receptors. $\alpha_v\beta_5$ is associated with a 180-kd protein downstream of CrK, DOCK180, which is a homologue of the *C. elegans* protein CED5, which confers slower degradation of antigen than $\alpha_v\beta_3$ (78,79).

Immature
IL-4
GM-CSF

Mature
Macrophage
Supernatant

Mature
(Terminally Differentiated)
Cytokine Cocktail

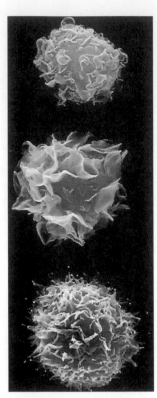

FIGURE 2. Scanning electron microscope appearance of dendritic cells at various states of maturity. (GM-CSF, granulocyte-macrophage colony-stimulating factor; IL-4, interleukin-4.)

The captured antigen is engulfed into the MHC class II compartments and relocalized to the cell surface, where the peptide-MHC complex can present to CD4$^+$ cells. How a CD8$^+$ cell is activated in an MHC class I–restricted manner from exogenous antigens is unclear; however, the occurrence of this *in vivo* cross-priming, especially when the antigen is an apoptotic body, is unique to DCs (80–82).

Dendritic Cell Migration

DCs traffic from the blood to the tissue, where they capture antigens and mature. They then migrate to the lymph nodes to present antigen to T and B cells. Complex regulation of chemokines and their receptors allow this process to proceed. *In vitro*–generated, monocyte-derived DCs express the chemokine receptors C5aR, CCR1, CCR2, CCR5, CCR6, CXCR1, CXCR2, and CXCR4. They migrate in response to the CC chemokines MCP-3, MCP-4, RANTES, MIP-1α, MIP-1β, and MIP-5 and to the CXC chemokines SDF-1 (83,84). Several adhesion molecules also participate in DC trafficking, such as CLA, CD44, and E-cadherin (85). DCs also possess metalloproteinases involved in matrix degradation, allowing for migration through basement membranes (86). Studies have shown that immature and mature DCs are not recruited by the same chemokines.

Immature DCs respond to many CC- and CXC-chemokines (MIP-1α, MIP-1β, MIP-5, MCP-3, MCP-4, RANTES, TECK, and SDF-1), and, in particular, to MIP-3α/LARC, which acts through CCR6, a receptor expressed predominantly on immature DCs and memory T cells (87). MIP-3α is inducible by several inflammatory stimuli like most other chemokines acting on immature DCs. In contrast, mature DCs have lost their responsiveness to most of these chemokines through receptor downregulation or desensitization, but acquired responsiveness to MIP-3β/ELC and 6Ckine/SLC as a consequence of CCR7 upregulation. The CCR7 ligands 6Ckine and macrophage inflammatory protein MIP-3β are selective chemoattractants for bone marrow–derived DCs at a potency 1,000-fold higher than their known activity on naïve T cells and play an important role the homing of DCs to lymphoid tissues (88).

Migration of DCs to draining lymph nodes occurs as a result of the downregulation of inflammatory chemokine receptors (89,90). Mature DCs cluster with T cells through various intercellular adhesion molecules that are upregulated on maturation as well, including CD102 (intracellular adhesion molecule-3), CD58 (leukocyte function–associated antigen–3), and CD54 (intracellular adhesion molecule–1) (91). The CX3C chemokine fractalkine is associated with DCs, and CD40 ligation increases expression by 2.5-fold. This molecule may also play a role in the interaction of mature DCs and T cells (92).

Perhaps the most facile means to contrast CD34-derived DCs and CD14 monocyte–derived DCs is by their chemokine

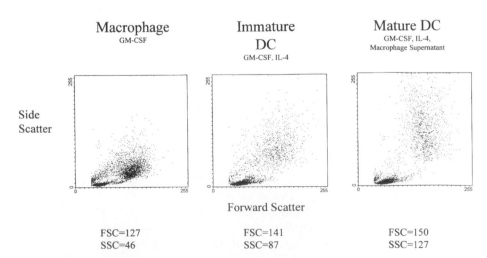

Macrophage
GM-CSF

Immature
DC
GM-CSF, IL-4

Mature DC
GM-CSF, IL-4,
Macrophage Supernatant

Side
Scatter

Forward Scatter

FSC=127
SSC=46

FSC=141
SSC=87

FSC=150
SSC=127

FIGURE 3. Dendritic cells (DCs) increase in size and internal complexity with maturation. (FSC, forward scatter; GM-CSF, granulocyte-macrophage colony-stimulating factor; IL-4, interleukin-4; SSC, side scatter.)

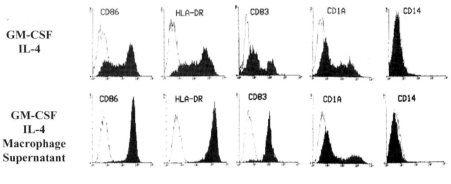

Relative Fluorescence Intensity

FIGURE 4. Phenotype of immature and mature dendritic cells. Note the increase in HLA-DR and CD83 with 48 hours incubation of macrophage supernatant. (GM-CSF, granulocyte-macrophage colony-stimulating factor; IL-4, interleukin-4.)

receptor expression and response to individual chemokines. CD34-derived DCs appear to respond preferentially to MIP-3α and not to MIP-1α or RANTES and conversely for monocyte-derived DCs. The CCR6 chemokine receptor appears to be on immature DCs, as well as memory T cells, responding to the chemokine MIP-3α. When culturing DCs from CD34⁺ cells, MIP-3α peaks at approximately days 7 to 10, decreasing considerably by day 13 with a concurrent increase in the expression of CCR7. Similarly, one can make this transition from CRC6 to CRC7 by culturing cells with CD40L stimulation.

T-Cell Priming

Activation of naïve T cells occurs only subsequent to priming by APCs containing high levels of antigen, costimulatory molecules, and proinflammatory cytokines. It requires 10 to 24 hours of engagement to become fully activated depending on the level of costimulatory molecules. Effector T cells, however, can become activated after triggering from fewer peptide-MHC complexes

within 1 hour. In an allogeneic mixed lymphocyte reaction, only one DC is needed for every 3,000 T cells. T cells become activated after reaching a threshold of antigen-MHC cross-linking of the T-cell receptor (TCR). The presence of costimulatory molecules and especially the duration of the signal can modify the threshold for activation. DCs provide high levels of adhesion molecules that enable prolonged TCR stimulation. Furthermore, proliferation and cytokine production require higher levels of TCR occupancy than the induction of cytotoxicity.

Effector T cells undergo activation-induced cell death (AICD) after prolonged TCR signaling in the absence of costimulation. Thus, DCs also serve to protect T cells from AICD. In general, tumor cells do not express CD80 or CD86. Furthermore, after CD40 ligation, DCs produce IL-12 and IL-18, potent stimulators of IFN-γ and the Th1 response (93–96). In the absence of a professional APC, anergy or apoptosis is induced. DCs are also involved in regulating and priming the humoral immune response, as they regulate B-cell growth and differentiation (97,98). DCs orchestrate Ig class switching

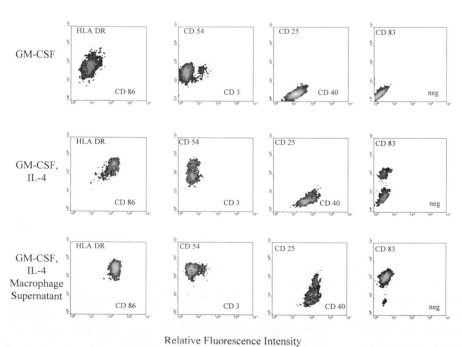

Relative Fluorescence Intensity

FIGURE 5. Phenotype of macrophages, immature dendritic cells, and mature dendritic cells. (GM-CSF, granulocyte-macrophage colony-stimulating factor; IL-4, interleukin-4.)

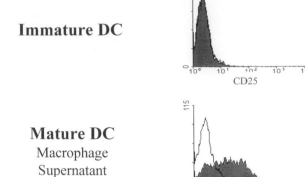

Immature DC

Mature DC
Macrophage
Supernatant

Mature DC
Cytokine Cocktail

Relative fluorescence intensity

FIGURE 6. Increasing expression of CD25 with dendritic cell (DC) maturation. Flow cytometry of 7-day granulocyte-macrophage colony-stimulating factor/interleukin-4–derived DC, after 48 hours macrophage supernatant and cytokine cocktail of prostaglandin E₂ (1 μg per mL), interleukin-1β (10 ng per mL), tumor necrosis factor–α (10 ng per mL), and interleukin-6 (1,000 U per mL).

of B cells, especially IgA2, thereby controlling mucosal immunity (99).

DENDRITIC CELLS AND THE TUMOR MICROENVIRONMENT

It is well demonstrated that the immune system can recognize and destroy tumor cells in humans and in animal models. Tumors, however, evade immune recognition through numerous mechanisms, including:

1. Downregulation of MHC molecule expression
2. Secretion of inhibitory hormones, such as TGF-β and IL-10
3. Upregulation of antiapoptotic proteins within the tumor, such as bcl-2
4. Diminished susceptibility to immune killing because of the inability to express or signal through Fas
5. Expression of apoptosis-inducing proteins, such as soluble and cellular FasL (100–103).

Tumors may also evade the immune system through tumor-induced DC apoptosis through regulation of bcl-2 and Bax expression (104).

Tumor-associated DCs undergo apoptotic death *in vivo*, and DCs isolated from tumor tissue showed significantly higher levels of apoptosis when compared with DCs isolated from spleen. CD40 ligation inhibits Fas-mediated apoptosis in human DCs (105). A variety of factors may negatively affect DC function in the tumor,

including prostaglandins, nitric oxide, IL-10, TGF-β, and various other poorly described tumor-suppressor products (106–109). Vascular endothelial growth factor alters the *in vitro* and *in vivo* development of DCs from bone marrow progenitors, in part by modifying NFκB production in bone marrow and mobilization into the nucleus (110,111). The initial notion that DCs are present within tumors to pick up tumor antigen and shuttle it to the lymph node to elicit the adaptive immune response may be a bit too simplistic. In fact, we and others have demonstrated the inability of tumor-derived DCs to express appropriate costimulatory molecules, class II MHC molecules, characteristic dendrites, and even mature dendrites from progenitors associated with their nominal "immunosuppressed state" (112–114).

Another means of DC-related tumor escape may reside with the macrophage. The tissue macrophage's major role is to eliminate apoptotic cells and debris. In the aberrant cytokine milieu of the tumor microenvironment, those macrophages that normally undergo a differentiation process to a DC may fail to become fully activated APCs. These cells may then become tolerogenic rather than immunogenic (115–117).

The failure of immunotherapy may be caused by this "counterattack" by the tumor against immune effector cells. We term apoptosis induced by the tumor on nonspecific T cells as *tumor-induced cell death* (118–120). To enhance the effectiveness of DC-based therapies, alternate approaches to delay AICD and TICD are being sought. An expected outcome of this approach is an enhanced quality and duration of an effective immune response. In addition, DCs that are not appropriately activated may induce a state of immune tolerance. Available literature suggests improved prognosis for cancer patients in relationship to tumor infiltration by DCs. This finding applies to a variety of tumor origins and suggests a positive therapeutic outcome if DCs are delivered to tumor sites. The dynamic relationship between tumor cells, DCs, and tumor-infiltrating lymphocytes within the tumor microenvironment are complex. Strategies that enhance DC number and prevent their premature apoptotic death at the tumor site could be therapeutic.

AICD, for example, is an apoptotic program that is induced after cognate antigen recognition in activated immune cells (121). This natural termination of an immune response is a powerful feedback mechanism that ensures removal of preactivated lymphocytes to avoid unwanted tissue injury and nominally returns the host to a state of homeostatic balance. Tumor cells, as well as normal cells, express molecules capable of modifying immunity. Unexpectedly, tumors cannot only induce AICD and eliminate presumably unnecessary specific effector lymphocytes but can also eliminate or induce anergy of other nonspecific T cells. TICD, which does not require cognate recognition, is a plausible means by which immune suppression is induced by tumor cells. The most frequently implicated mechanism mediating TICD is the Fas/FasL apoptotic pathway. Substantial criticism of the data associated with this premise has been presented given the difficulty in convincingly demonstrating this molecule on the cell surface.

Prevention of TICD may occur as a result of CD28 activation through the upregulation of bcl-xl, a member of the bcl-2 family of antiapoptotic proteins (122–124). IL-12 is protective of apoptotic death in activated T cells, making the presence of DCs, the major source of IL-12 at the tumor site, potentially critical for expansion and protection of antitumor immunity (125). DCs also express significant amounts of CD80 and CD86, the ligands for CD28 (and cytotoxic T lymphocyte antigen-4) (126). The central role of DCs in antigen presentation and in T-cell priming and protection makes their use in cancer therapy enticing. The lack of adequate antigen presentation of tumor antigen by host DCs may be overcome by DC-based immunotherapy (127). Two fundamental approaches exist in the use of DCs for therapy: delivering tumor antigen into the DC or delivering DCs into the tumor (Table 3).

DENDRITIC CELL–BASED CANCER THERAPY

Delivering Tumor Antigens onto Dendritic Cells

Pulsing synthetic peptides derived from known tumor antigen precursors, such as MART-1/Melan A, tyrosinase, carcinoembryonic antigen, HER2/NEU, or gp100, can load MHC complexes expressed on DCs (128–137). These peptides, however, only reside on the cell surface for a short period (hours) and are limited for use in patients who express an individual, specific MHC haplotype. Gene-based strategies do not require prior knowledge of the responder MHC haplotype or of the relevant MHC-restricted peptide epitope. Human DCs genetically engineered to express the melanoma antigens MART-1/Melan-A are able to generate MART-1 peptide–specific, class I–restricted CTLs in peripheral blood leukocyte cultures from normal donors (138).

Several disadvantages exist to the use of defined tumor antigen besides the overwhelming lack of known tumor rejection antigens for most human tumors. Where it has been tested most widely, the use of specific antigens benefit only a subpopulation of melanoma patients that express the relevant MHC allele, and even these patients may be prone to tumor resistance by mutations when a small repertoire of antigens are challenged. Furthermore, the ability to generate a CTL *in vitro* does not guarantee an effective immune response *in vivo*. DC-based strategies, which do not require prior knowledge of the responder MHC haplotype or of the relevant MHC-restricted peptide epitope, have also been developed using tumor itself as a source of antigen.

Multiple techniques have been described to load DCs with peptide when tumor rejection antigens are unknown. These range from "feeding" DCs tumor lysates (139,140), messenger RNA (141), acid-eluted peptides, apoptotic tumor, or creating tumor-DC fusion heteroconjugates (142,143). Coinsertion of known melanoma antigens with Th1 cytokines IL-12 or IFN-α enhances the magnitude of antigen-specific CTL reactivity in murine tumor models (144–147).

In 1998, tumor peptide–pulsed DC-derived exosomes (vesicles that contain high amounts of MHC, CD86, and peptide) were successfully used to prime specific CTLs *in vivo* and eradicate or suppress growth of established murine tumors (148). In a human chronic myeloid leukemia model, tumor cells incubated in GM-CSF, IL-4, and TNF-α differentiated into mature DCs capable of stimulating an autologous anti-chronic myelogenous leukemia CTL response.

Disadvantages of these techniques include the requirement for access to sufficient quantities of patient tumor and the possibility of autoimmune reactivity. We have observed vitiligo in

TABLE 3. POSSIBLE STRATEGIES FOR USING DENDRITIC CELL–BASED IMMUNOTHERAPY

Tumor Delivery into DCs
  Apoptotic bodies
  Tumor lysates
  Known tumor antigen
  RNA of known tumor antigen
  DNA of known tumor antigen
  RNA subtraction library
Tumor-DC fusion heteroconjugates
Tumor peptide–pulsed DC-derived exosomes
DCs Delivery into Tumor
Mobilization of DC *in vivo*
  GM-CSF and IL-4
  Flt-3 ligand
Autologous DC injection into tumor
Adoptive transfer of autologous DCs
Transduced with IL-12, GM-CSF

DC, dendritic cell; GM-CSF, granulocyte-macrophage colony-stimulating factor; IL, interleukin.

many patients successfully treated for melanoma with various IL-2–based strategies; one of our patients developed rheumatoid arthritis after a complete response to DC-based immunotherapy (149). A major limitation to fusion heteroconjugates is the requirement for a pure and proliferating neoplastic cell line.

The use of RNA, DNA, and subtractive hybridization strategies could allow the enrichment and easy amplification of tumor-specific RNA (150–153). The ease in generating large quantities of nucleic acids gives RNA-based vaccines an advantage over tumor lysates, especially if multiple restimulations are needed using a small tumor sample. Some have suggested that microdissection might also allow capture of only tumor cell–derived messenger RNA from fresh tumors, as a major limitation of using protein-encoded antigens derived from tumor is the availability of tumor and the contamination by normal tissue.

Viral and nonviral vectors have been used to modify human DCs (154,155). The validity of genetic approaches was first confirmed with the use of the gene gun with low-transfer efficiencies (1%–5%) (156). The use of viral vector is the mainstay of gene delivery with the use of retroviral vectors (157–159), adenoviral vectors (160), and poxviral vectors (161,162). Considering the potency of DC to elicit an immune response, viral coat proteins likely stimulate DC activation and serve as a source of immunogenic peptide.

DCs pulsed with acid-eluted peptides elicit an effective antitumor response in M05 melanoma, C3 sarcoma, Meth A sarcoma, and 3LL lung carcinoma murine models (163,164). Eighty percent of mice receiving the peptide-pulsed DC vaccine exhibited tumor regression or were tumor free, or both. Furthermore, DCs pulsed with class I MHC–restricted peptide antigen induced protective immunity to lethal challenge with tumor cells bearing those same antigens. In these models, DCs grown in GM-CSF and IL-4 showed improved antitumor activity when compared with those grown in GM-CSF and TNF-α or GM-CSF alone. Furthermore, the route of vaccination (intravenous, intraperitoneal, or subcutaneous) had no apparent effect on tumor resistance. Some animals were able to reject a chal-

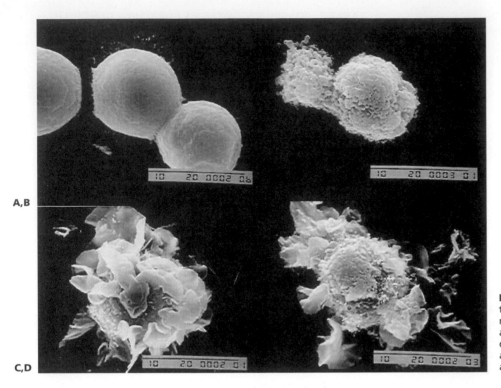

A,B

C,D

FIGURE 7. Dendritic cells engulfing apoptotic tumor. **A:** Scanning electron microscope image of normal adenocarcinoma cell. **B:** Apoptotic tumor after ultraviolet radiation. **C:** Normal immature dendritic cell. **D:** Dendritic cell after engulfing apoptotic tumor. (From Mailliard RB, Watkins S, and Lotze MT.)

lenge with an otherwise identical tumor that lacks the epitopes used in the original vaccination. This concept of epitope switching may play an important role in the induction of immunity in antigenically heterogeneous tumor populations.

The use of apoptotic bodies as a source of antigen has been proposed by Bender et al. (165–167). They demonstrated that DCs incubated with apoptotic macrophages infected with the influenza virus stimulated CTL activity significantly better than DCs incubated with influenza alone. We have used apoptotic bodies generated from ultraviolet radiation and NK-mediated death to generate potent antigen-bearing DCs to stimulate specific CTL activity (Figs. 7 and 8).

Human Trials

At least 30 separate clinical trials have been conducted using DCs, but, so far, only five reports have been published using antigen-

pulsed DCs in humans (Table 4). In 1995, Mukherji used adherent monocytes stimulated with GM-CSF only. These cells were pulsed with a nonapeptide epitope from MAGE-1 and injected intradermally and intravenously into melanoma patients with the appropriate MHC class I molecule (A1). Cytotoxic T cells were found at the site of immunization and at distant metastatic sites. No clinical response, however, was observed. Noting the limitations of single peptide vaccination, the same group, in 1998, reported 17 patients with melanoma treated again with monocytes stimulated with GM-CSF alone and tumor lysates. These patients were injected intradermally with as many as 107 cells. No patient developed substantial toxicity; only 13 patients completed the protocol. Three patients, however, had disease progression and one patient died of a myocardial infarction. Only one patient demonstrated disease regression, although varied biologic responses were noted. These studies were limited by the use of GM-CSF–stimulated macrophages as APCs instead of DCs (168).

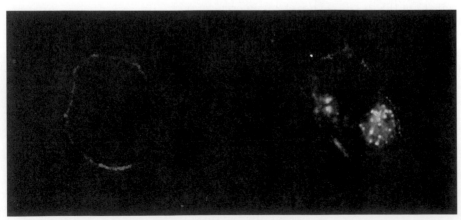

A,B

FIGURE 8. Fluorescent microscopy of dendritic cell engulfing apoptotic tumor. **A:** Immature dendritic cell stained with CD80. **B:** Tumor stained with membrane dye clearly visible within dendritic cell. Note: The intensity of micrograph B was significantly decreased, as the CD 80 staining was overwhelmingly bright. This demonstrates dendritic cell maturation with antigen uptake.

TABLE 4. CLINICAL TRIALS USING DENDRITIC CELL–BASED THERAPY

Author (Year)	Tumor Type	Method	Response
Mukherji (1995)	Melanoma	Monocytes + GM-CSF pulsed with single melanoma peptide	No clinical responses
Chakraborty (1998)	Melanoma	Monocyte + GM-CSF pulsed with tumor lysate	1 out of 13 with partial response
Hsu (1996)	B-cell lymphoma	DCs pulsed with idiotype protein	3 out of 4 with response
Nestle (1998)	Melanoma	DCs pulsed with tumor lysates or	Two complete and three partial responses out of 16
Holtl (1998)	Renal cell	Case report: Mature DCs pulsed with tumor lysate	A patient treated who had a significant response
Hall (1997)	Melanoma	Immature DCs pulsed with tumor lysates	One complete response and two partial responses
Tjoa (1999)	Prostate	DCs pulsed with two prostate-specific peptides	30% response rate; 58% of these were durable

DC, dendritic cell; GM-CSF, granulocyte-macrophage colony-stimulating factor.

In a promising study in 1996 by Hsu et al., four patients were adoptively transferred DCs for the treatment of B-cell lymphoma. DCs were isolated by leukapheresis and coculture with idiotypic Ig from autologous lymphoma. Patients were vaccinated four times intravenously, as well as given subcutaneous administration of idiotype protein. All patients developed measurable antitumor cellular immune responses and none developed significant side effects. One patient developed a complete tumor response and another, while having an ambiguous computed tomography scan, had no tumor by polymerase chain reaction analysis. A third patient had a partial regression (169).

In 1998, Nestle et al. reported the treatment of 16 patients with advanced melanoma with GM-CSF and IL-4–derived DCs pulsed with tumor lysates or a cocktail of melanoma peptide antigens depending on their MHC type. Two complete responses and three partial responses were noted (140). Murphy et al. treated patients with prostate cancer with autologous DCs and two HLA-A2–restricted prostate-specific membrane antigen peptides. They found that 30% of the evaluable patients were identified as partial responders. In addition, a 50% decrease of serum prostate-specific antigen or resolution of previously measurable lesions on imaging was detected. No significant side effects were noted other than rare, transient hypotension. In 1999, Tjoa et al. reported their follow-up on these patients. The average duration of response was 149 days in the metastatic group and 187 days for the local recurrence group. A majority of patients (58%) were still responsive at the end of the follow-up period, suggesting the durability of DC-based treatment strategies (170,171).

Finally, a report exists of a patient with renal cell carcinoma treated with mature DCs (CD83$^+$) pulsed with tumor lysates. This patient experienced a significant but incomplete reduction of his tumor burden (172).

These studies demonstrate the possibility of designing effective cancer therapy using DC strategies. More DC-based trials from our institute and others are planned. Understanding optimal routes of administration, optimal methods to load DCs, and the role of concurrent cytokine therapy may significantly improve early promising results.

Delivery of Dendritic Cells into Tumor

The delivery of DCs into tumor is an alternative approach in generating an antitumor response. This can be done most generally by applying DC-mobilizing cytokines, such as FL, or by direct injection of DCs after activation or transfection by relevant cytokine genes.

FL is a member of a small family of "fms-like tyrosine kinase signaling" growth factors, including macrophage colony-stimulating factor and the c-kit ligand that stimulate the proliferation of hematopoietic cells by binding to and activating distinct tyrosine kinase receptors (173–176). Expression of the FL receptor is restricted to the most primitive hematopoietic progenitor cells, and FL stimulates the proliferation *in vitro* and the expansion and mobilization *in vivo* of progenitor cells (177). FL as a single factor has little proliferative activity on these cells, but it synergizes with a wide range of other cytokines to stimulate proliferation of these cells (178). FL also mobilizes stem and progenitor cells to peripheral blood and stimulates the production of DCs from early progenitor cells (179–182). FL has been used in the generation of DCs *in vitro*. In murine systems, FL induces complete tumor regression in a substantial proportion of MCA-sarcoma in mice. In the remaining mice, decreased tumor growth was noted. Transferring CD8$^+$ cells from FL-treated mice into naïve irradiated mice conferred resistance to tumor challenge in these naïve mice (183). Antitumor activity in murine breast adenocarcinoma has also been reported (184).

FL is produced in Chinese hamster ovary cells with its transmembrane portion deleted. Normal individuals tolerate doses up to 100 µg per kg without difficulty with the exception of mild injection site discomfort and enlarged lymph nodes. Peripheral blood mononuclear cells (PBMCs) increased threefold, CD34$^+$ cell by 20-fold, colony-forming unit granulocyte macrophage by 80-fold, and monocytes tenfold, which, like DCs, developed a multilobulated appearance (185,186). After 14 days of treatment, approximately 14% of the PBMCs were DCs (approximately 1 million DCs per mL of blood). In the mouse, lymphoid DCs have an enhanced capacity to make IL-12 (compared with myeloid DCs), and were identified as DR$^+$, CD11c$^-$, IL-3 receptor$^+$, CD4$^+$, CD45RA$^+$. These lymphoid DCs constituted approximately 4% of the PBMCs, which is approximately a fourfold increase.

An alternative mobilization strategy involves the administration of IL-4 and GM-CSF systemically to mature macrophage progenitors into DCs. Animal models using the highly immunologic human papillomavirus–16-induced C3 sarcoma have demonstrated antitumor effects using this approach. Direct injection of DCs into tumor has achieved only modest success. In three different tumor models, this antitumor effect becomes substantial after transfection of these DCs with the gene encoding IL-12 (187). Also under investigation is the use of inducible promoters driving expression of cytokine genes only when DCs encounter antigen-specific T cells in nodal sites.

Other Cancer-Related Uses for Dendritic Cells

Tumor antigens capable of yielding target epitopes for T-cell reactivity have been identified in the setting of various human malignancies. A number of groups, including our own, are using DCs to generate T cells recognizing occult tumor antigens *ex vivo* or to expand T cells for therapy without direct identification of antigens.

DENDRITIC CELL GENERATION

Some data suggest that CD34–derived DCs are more potent at T-cell stimulation (188). We are conducting a trial, planned to conclude in 12 months, designed to assess these two types of DCs. As well, much debate as to the use of mature or immature DC immunotherapy exists. Although mature DCs would logically be more stimulatory than immature DCs in stimulating a specific CTL response, these cells appear to be incapable of eliciting antitumor responses in murine tumor models, whereas GM-CSF/IL-4 cultured cells elicit therapeutic effects. These differences may be owing to the loss of phagocytic capability or because of problems related to trafficking to appropriate lymphoid sites. Phenotypic or allostimulatory capacity cannot distinguish effective versus ineffective cells for use in clinical trials.

CD34+-derived DCs are generated in our institute from patients through a standard technique. Recombinant human G-CSF is given twice daily for 4 consecutive days at a dose of 8 µg per kg before collecting the mobilized PBMCs by leukapheresis. CD34+ cells are then isolated using the Isolex-50 or Isolex-300 magnetic cell separation system on whole, unmanipulated collections. These selected cells are washed, suspended at a concentration of 1×10^6 cells per mL, and AIM-V media plated in 10% human AB (or autologous) serum with SCF (10 ng per mL), GM-CSF (1,000 U per mL), IL-4 (1,000 U per mL), and TNF-α (10 ng per mL) is added. At day 7, only fresh IL-4 and GM-CSF are added, allowing the cells to differentiate into immature DCs by days 14 to 17 (189–194).

CD14+-derived DCs are generated by Ficoll separation of a patient leukapheresis collection. The mononuclear cell layer is then plated at a concentration of 1×10^7 cells per mL. After a 2-hour incubation, the nonadherent cells are removed and the remaining monocytes remain incubated for 1 week in serum-free AIM-V media with GM-CSF (1,000 U per mL) and IL-4 (1,000 U per mL) (195).

DENDRITIC CELL DELIVERY

One parameter that needs to be considered in adoptive approaches is the method of DC delivery. Many argue that subcutaneous injections are more efficacious than intravenous injections. Most of these studies have had nontherapeutic end points (196). We have noted comparable, and, perhaps, superior

effects with intravenous administration of DCs. Anecdotal information from Gerold Schuler (*personal communication*, 1997) suggest that patients on HLA-A2 peptide–pulsed DC protocols using mature DCs only responded clinically with tumor regression when their DCs were administered intravenously and not subcutaneously. DCs have also been given under ultrasound guidance directly into lymph nodes (140).

FUTURE STUDIES

Combinations of cytokines, such as FL, IL-2, IFN-α, or IL-12, seem likely to optimize DC-based clinical application via potent effects on DCs. Furthermore, these combined therapies would enhance T-cell survival given the high rate of spontaneous apoptotic death observed in T cells in the periphery of patients with a variety of neoplasms. It has taken more than 20 years to refine our approaches using T cells in the therapy of cancer. Although trials have not been able to predictably impact disease in patients with most tumor types, it is clear that clinical responsiveness is linked to enhanced T-cell immunity in many patients. Clearly, DCs play an important supportive role in promoting and maintaining antigen-specific T cells *in vivo*. In the future, DC-based strategies will likely become important components of biologic therapies for patients with cancer, and we are just beginning to determine the best means to use such cells.

REFERENCES

1. Steinman RM. The dendritic cell system and its role in immunogenicity. *Ann Rev Immunol* 1991;9:271–296.
2. Caux C, Liu Y-J, Banchereau J. Recent advances in the study of dendritic cells and follicular dendritic cells. *Immunol Today* 1995;16:2–5.
3. Banchereau J, Steinman RM. Dendritic cells and the control of immunity. *Nature* 1998;392:245–252.
4. Grabbe S, Beissert S, Schwarz T, Granstein RD. Dendritic cells as initiators of tumor immune responses: a possible strategy for tumor immunotherapy? *Immunol Today* 1995;16:117–121.
5. Hahne M, Rimoldi D, Schroter M, et al. Melanoma cell expression of fas (Apo-1/CD95) ligand: implications for tumor immune escape. *Science* 1996;274:1363–1366.
6. Niehans GA, Brumier T, Frizelle SP, et al. Human lung carcinomas express Fas ligand. *Cancer Res* 1997;57:1007–1012.
7. O'Connell J, O'Sullivan GC, Collins JK, Shanahan F. The Fas counterattack: Fas-mediated T cell killing by colon cancer cells expressing Fas ligand. *J Exp Med* 1996;184:1075–1082.
8. O'Connell J, Bennett MW, O'Sullivan GC, Collins JK, Shanahan F. The Fas counterattack: a molecular mechanism of tumor immune privilege. *Mol Med* 1997;3:294–300.
9. Numasaki M, Lotze MT, Tahara H. Interleukin 17 gene transfection into murine fibrosarcoma cell line MCA 205 increases tumorigenicity correlated with enhanced tumor microvascularity. *J Immunother* 20:399,1997.
10. Zeid NA, Muller HK. S100 positive dendritic cells in human lung tumors associated with cell differentiation and enhanced survival. *Pathology* 1993;25:338.
11. Furihata M, Ohtsuki Y, Ido E, et al. HLA-DR antigen- and S-100 protein-positive dendritic cells in esophageal squamous cell carcinoma—their distribution in relation to prognosis. *Virchows Arch* 1992;61:409.
12. Tsujitani S, Kakeji Y, Watanabe A, Kohnoe S, Maehara Y, Sugimachi K. Infiltration of dendritic cells in relationship to tumor invasion and lymph node metastasis in human gastric cancer. *Cancer* 1990;66:2012.

13. Giannini A, Bianchi S, Messerini L, et al. Prognostic significance of accessory cells and lymphocytes in nasopharyngeal carcinoma. *Pathol Res Pract* 1991;187:496.

14. Bigotti G, Coli A, Castagnola D. Distribution of Langerhans cells and HLA class II molecules in prostatic carcinomas of different histopathological grade. *Prostate* 1991;19(1):73–87.

15. Evans EM, Man S, Evans AS, Borysiewicz LK. Infiltration of cervical cancer tissue with human papillomavirus-specific cytotoxic T-lymphocytes. *Cancer Res* 1997;57(14):2943–2950.

16. Goldman SA, Baker E, Weyant RJ, Clarke MR, Myers IN, Lotze MT. Peritumoral CD1a-positive dendritic cells are associated with improved survival in patients with tongue carcinoma. *Arch Otolaryngol Head Neck Surg* 1998;124(6):641–646.

17. Rosenberg SA, Lotze MT, Yang JC, et al. Prospective randomized trial of high-dose interleukin-2 alone or in conjunction with lymphokine-activated killer cells for the treatment of patients with advanced cancer. *J Nat Cancer Inst* 1993;85(8):622–632.

18. Gilboa E, Nair SK, Lyerly HK. Immunotherapy of cancer with dendritic-cell-based vaccines. *Cancer Immunol Immunother* 1998;46(2):82–87.

19. Lotze MT. Getting to the source: dendritic cells as therapeutic reagents for the treatment of patients with cancer. *Ann Surg* 1997;226(1):1–5.

20. Lotze MT, Finn OJ. Current paradigms in cellular immunity: implications for immunity to cancer. *Immunol Today* 1990;11:190–193.

21. Lotze MT, Finn OJ. Cellular immunity and the immunotherapy of cancer. *J Immunother* 1993;14:79–87.

22. Inaba K, Inaba M, Witmer-Pack M, Hatchcock K, Hodes R, Steinman RM. Expression of B7 costimulator molecules on mouse dendritic cells. *Adv Exp Med Biol* 1995;378:65–70.

23. Guèry JC, Adorini L. Dendritic cells are the most efficient in presenting endogenous naturally processed self-epitopes to class-II-restricted cells. *J Immunol* 1995;154:536.

24. Cella M, Sallusto F, Lanzavecchia A. Origin, maturation and antigen presenting function of dendritic cells. *Curr Opin Immunol* 1997;9:10–16.

25. Palucka K, Banchereau J. Dendritic cells: a link between innate and adaptive immunity. *J Clin Immunol* 1999;19:12–25.

26. Austyn JM. The dendritic cell system and anti-tumour immunity. *In vivo* 1993;7:193–202.

27. Grouard G, Durand I, Filgueira L, Banchereau J, Liu YJ. Dendritic cells capable of stimulating T cells in germinal centres. *Nature* 1996;384:364–367.

28. Olweus J, BitMansour A, Warnke R, et al. Dendritic cell ontogeny: a human dendritic cell lineage of myeloid origin. *Proc Natl Acad Sci U S A* 1997;94:12551–12556.

29. Inaba K, Inaba M, Deguchi M, Hagi K, et al. Granulocytes, macrophages, and dendritic cells arise from a common major histocompatibility complex class II-negative progenitor in mouse bone marrow. *Proc Natl Acad Sci U S A* 1993;90:3038–3042.

30. Katz SI, Tamaki K, Sachs DH. Epidermal Langerhans cells are derived from cells originating in bone marrow. *Nature* 1979;282:324–326.

31. Galy A, Travis M, Cen D, Chen B. Human T, B, natural killer, and dendritic cells arise from a common bone marrow progenitor cell subset. *Immunity* 1995;3:459–473.

32. Strunk D, Egger C, Leitner G, Hanau D, Stingl G. A skin homing molecule defines Langerhans cell progenitor in human peripheral blood. *J Exp Med* 1997;185:1131–1136.

33. Porcelli SA, Segelke BW, Sugita M, Wilson IA, Brenner MB. The CD1 family of lipid antigen-presenting molecules. *Immunol Today* 1998;19:362–368.

34. Burdin N, Brossay L, Kronenberg M. Immunization with alpha-galactosylceramide polarizes CD1-reactive NK T cells towards Th2 cytokine synthesis. *Eur J Immunol* 1999;29(6):2014–2025.

35. Caux C, Vanbervliet B, Massacrier C, et al. CD34+ hematopoietic progenitors from human cord blood differentiate along two independent dendritic pathways in response to granulocyte macrophage colony-stimulating factor and TNF-alpha. *J Exp Med* 1996;184:695–706.

36. Gibran N, Nickoloff B, Holbrook K. Ontogeny and characterization of Factor XIIIa+ cells in developing human skin. *J Am Acad Dermatol* 1996;34(2):196–203.

37. Tang A, Amagai M, Granger LG, Stanley JR, Udey MC. Adhesion of epidermal Langerhans cells to keratinocytes mediated by E-cadherin. *Nature* 1993;361:82–85.

38. Lotze MT, Thomson AW. *Dendritic cells. Biology and clinical applications.* San Diego: Academic Press, 1999.

39. Romani M, Gruner S, Brang D, et al. Proliferating dendritic cell progenitors in human blood. *J Exp Med* 1994;180:83–93.

40. Davis TA, Saini AA, Blair PJ, et al. Porbol esters induce differentiation of human CD34+ hemopoietic progenitors to dendritic cells: evidence for protein kinase C-mediated signaling. *J Immunol* 1998;160:3689–3697.

41. Palucka KA, Taquet N, Sanchez-Chapuis F, Gluckman JC. Dendritic cells as the terminal stage of monocyte differentiation. *J Immunol* 1998;160:4587–4595.

42. Shortman K, Caux C. Dendritic cell development: multiple pathways to nature's adjuvants. *Stem Cells* 1997;15:409–419.

43. Ferlazzo G, Wesa A, Wei W-Z, Galy A. Dendritic cells generated either from CD34+ progenitor cells or from monocytes differ in their ability to activate antigen-specific CD8+ T cells. *J Immunol* 1999;163:3597–3604.

44. de Saint-Vis B, Fugier-Vivier I, Massacrier C, et al. The cytokine profile expressed by human dendritic cells is dependent on cell subtype and mode of activation. *J Immunol* 1998;160(4):1666–1676.

45. Mayordomo JI, Zitvogel L, Tjandrawan T, Lotze MT, Storkus WJ. Dendritic cells presenting tumor peptide epitopes stimulate effective anti-tumor CTL *in vitro* and *in vivo*. In: *Melanoma biology: experimental therapies.* Amsterdam: IOC Press, 1996.

46. Maldonado-Lopez R, De Smedt T, Pajak B, et al. Role of CD8alpha+ and CD8alpha– dendritic cells in the induction of primary immune responses *in vivo*. *J Leuk Biol* 1999;66(2):242–246.

47. Ardavin C, Wu L, Li CL, Shortman K. Thymic dendritic cells and T cells develop simultaneously in the thymus from a common precursor population. *Nature* 1993;362:761–763.

48. Kronin V, Vremec D, Winkel K, et al. Are CD8+ dendritic cells (DC) veto cells? The role of CD8 on DC in DC development and in the regulation of CD4 and CD8 T cell responses. *Int Immunol* 1997;9:1061–1064.

49. Winkel K, Sotzik F, Vremec D, Cameron PU, Shortman K. CD4 and CD8 expression by human and mouse thymic dendritic cells. *Immunol Lett* 1994;40:93–99.

50. Sotzik F, Rosenberg Y, Boyd AW, et al. Assessment of CD4 expression by early T precursors and dendritic cells in the human thymus. *J Immunol* 1994;152:3370–3377.

51. Saunders D, Lucas K, Ismaili J, Wu J, Maraskovsky E, Dunn A, Shortman K. Dendritic cell development in culture from thymic precursors in the absence of granulocyte/macrophage colony-stimulating factor. *J Exp Med* 1996;184:2185–2196.

52. Vremec D, Zorbas M, Scollay R, et al. The surface phenotype of dendritic cells purified from mouse thymus and spleen: investigation of the CD8 surface expression by a subpopulation of dendritic cells. *J Exp Med* 1992;176:47–58.

53. Olweus J, BitMansour A, Warnke R, et al. Dendritic cell ontogeny: a human dendritic cell lineage of myeloid origin. *Proc Nat Acad Sci U S A* 1997;94:12551–12556.

54. Schreiber S, Kilgus O, Payer E, et al. Cytokine pattern of Langerhans cells isolated from murine epidermal cell cultures. *J Immunol* 1992;149:3525–3534.

55. Rissoan MC, Soumelis V, Kadowaki N, et al. Reciprocal control of T helper cell and dendritic cell differentiation. *Science* 1999;283(5405):1183–1186.

56. Steinman RM, Inaba K. Myeloid dendritic cells. *J Leuk Biol* 1999;66(2):205–208.

57. Siegal FP, Kadowaki N, Shodell M, et al. The nature of the principal type 1 interferon-producing cells in human blood. *Science* 1999;284(5421):1835–1837.

58. Tew JG, Kosco MH, Burton GF, Szakal AK. Follicular dendritic cells as accessory cells. *Immunol Rev* 1990;117:185–211.

59. Petrasch S, Perez AC, Schmitz J, Kosco MH, Brittinger G. Antigenic

phenotyping of human follicular dendritic cells isolated from malignant and nonmalignant lymphatic tissue. *Eur J Immunol* 1990;20: 1013–1018.

60. Caux C, Vandervliet B, Massacrier C, et al. CD34+ hematopoietic progenitors from human cord blood differentiate along two independent dendritic cell pathways in response to GM-CSF+TNF alpha. *J Exp Med* 1996;184:695–706.

61. Boehmelt G, Madruga J, Dorfler P, Briegel K, Schwarz H, Enrietto PJ, Zenke M. Dendritic cell progenitor is transformed by a conditional v-Rel estrogen receptor fusion protein v-RelER. *Cell* 1995;80(2):341–352.

62. Bjorck P, Kincade PW. CD 19+ pro-B cells can give rise to dendritic cells *in vitro*. *J Immunol* 1998;161(11):5795–5799.

63. Sato K, Nagayama H, Tadokoro K, Juji T, Takahashi TA. Interleukin-13 is involved in functional maturation of human peripheral blood monocyte-derived dendritic cells. *Exp Hematol* 1999;27(2): 326–336.

64. Alters SE, Gadea JR, Holm B, Lebkowski J, Philip R. IL-13 can substitute for IL-4 in the generation of dendritic cells for the induction of cytotoxic T lymphocytes and gene therapy. *J Immunother* 1999;22(3):229–236.

65. Reddy A, Sapp M, Feldman M, Subklewe M, Bhardwaj N. A monocyte conditioned medium is more effective than defined cytokines in mediating the terminal maturation of human dendritic cells. *Blood* 1997;90(9):3640–3646.

66. Rovere P, Manfredi AA, Vallinoto C, et al. Dendritic cells preferentially internalize apoptotic cells opsonized by anti-beta2-glycoprotein I antibodies. *J Autoimmun* 1998;11(5):403–411.

67. Manfredi AA. Bystander apoptosis triggers dendritic cell maturation and antigen-presenting function. *J Immunol* 1998;161(9):4467–4471.

68. Ross R, Ross XL, Schwing J, Langin T, Reske-Kunz AB. The actin-bundling protein fascin is involved in the formation of dendritic processes in maturing epidermal Langerhans cells. *J Immunol* 1998;160(8):3776–3782.

69. Sonderbye L, Magerstadt R, Blatman RN, Preffer FT, Langhoff E. Selective expression of human fascin (p55) by dendritic leukocytes. *Adv Exp Med Biol* 1997;417:41–46.

70. Zhou U, Tedder TF. A distinct pattern of cytokine gene expression by human CD83+ blood dendritic cells. *Blood* 1995;86:3295–3301.

71. Jonuleit H, Kuhn U, Muller G, et al. Pro-inflammatory cytokines and prostaglandins induce maturation of potent immunostimulatory dendritic cells under fetal calf serum-free conditions. *Eur J Immunol* 1997;27(12):3135–3142.

72. Kalinski P, Schuitemaker JH, Hilkens CM, Wierenga EA, Kapsenberg ML. Final maturation of dendritic cells is associated with impaired responsiveness to IFN-gamma and to bacterial IL-12 inducers: decreased ability of mature dendritic cells to produce IL-12 during the interaction with Th cells. *J Immunol* 1999;162(6): 3231–3236.

73. Sallusto F, Celia M, Danieli C, Lanzavecchia A. Dendritic cells use macropinocytosis and the mannose receptor to concentrate macromolecules in the major histocompatibility complex class II compartment: downregulation by cytokines and bacterial products. *J Exp Med* 1995;182:389–400.

74. Fanger NA, Wardwell K, Shen U, Tedder TF, Guyre PM. Type I (CD64) and type II (CD32) Fc gamma receptor-mediated phagocytosis by human blood dendritic cells. *J Immunol* 1996;157:541–548.

75. Fanger NA, Voigtlaender D, Lui C, et al. Characterization of expression, cytokine regulation, and effector function of the high affinity IgG receptor Fc gamma RI (CD64) expressed on human blood dendritic cells. *J Immunol* 1997;158:3090–3098.

76. Albert ML, Pearce SF, Francisco UM, et al. Immature dendritic cells phagocytose apoptotic cells via alphavbeta5 and CD36, and cross-present antigens to cytotoxic T lymphocytes. *J Exp Med* 1998;188 (7):1359–1368.

77. Tarte K, Klein B. Dendritic cell based vaccine: a promising approach for cancer immunotherapy. *Leukemia* 1999;13:653–663.

78. Kiyokawa E, Hashimoto Y, Kurata T, Sugimura H, Matsuda M. Evidence that DOCK180 up-regulates signals from the CrkII-p130(Cas) complex. *J Biol Chem* 1998;273(38):24479–24484.

79. Wu YC, Horvitz HR. C. elegans phagocytosis and cell-migration protein CED-5 is similar to human DOCK180. *Nature* 1998; 392(6675):501–504.

80. Toujas U, Delcros J-G, Diez B, Gervois N, Semana G, Corradini G, Jotereau F. Human monocyte-derived macrophages and dendritic cells are comparably effective *in vitro* in presenting HLA class I-restricted exogenous peptides. *Immunology* 1997;91:635–642.

81. Watts C. Capture and processing of exogenous antigens for presentation on MHC molecules. *Ann Rev Immunol* 1997;15:821–850.

82. Albert ML, Sauter B, Bhardwaj N. Dendritic cells acquire antigen from apoptotic cells and induce class I-restricted CTUs. *Nature* 1998;392(6671):86–89.

83. Mohamadzadeh M, Poltorak AN, Bergstresser PR, Beutler B, Takashima A. Dendritic cells produce macrophage inflammatory protein-1γ, a new member of the CC chemokine family. *J Immunol* 1996;156:3102–3106.

84. Barratt-Boyes SM, Watkins SC, Finn OJ. *In vivo* migration of dendritic cells differentiated *in vitro*: a chimpanzee model. *J Immunol* 1997;158(10):4543–4547.

85. Barratt-Boyes SM, Watkins SC, Finn OJ. Migration of cultured chimpanzee dendritic cells following intravenous and subcutaneous injection. *Adv Exp Med Biol* 1997;417:71–75.

86. Kobayashi Y. Langerhans cells produce type IV collagenase (MMP-9) following epicutaneous stimulation with haptens. *Immunology* 1997;90:496–501.

87. Greaves DR, Wang W, Dairaghi DJ, et al. CCr6, a CC chemokine receptor that interacts with macrophage inflammatory protein 3 alpha and is highly expressed in human dendritic cells. *J Exp Med* 1988;186:837–844.

88. Kellermann SA, Hudak S, Oldham ER, Liu YJ, McEvoy UM. The CC chemokine receptor-7 ligands 6Ckine and macrophage inflammatory protein-3 beta are potent chemoattractants for *in vitro*- and *in vivo*-derived dendritic cells. *J Immunol* 1999;162(7):3859–3864.

89. Sozzani S, Allavena P, D'Amico G, et al. Cutting edge: differential regulation of chemokine receptors during dendritic cell maturation: a model for their trafficking properties. *J Immunol* 1998;161: 1083–1086.

90. Dieu MC, Vanbervliet B, Vicari A, et al. Selective recruitment of immature and mature dendritic cells by distinct chemokines expressed in different anatomic sites. *J Exp Med* 1998;188:373–386.

91. Dieu-Nosjean MC, Vicari A, Lebecque S, Caux C. Regulation of dendritic cell trafficking: a process that involves the participation of selective chemokines. *J Leuk Biol* 1999;66(2):252–262.

92. Papadopoulos EJ, Sassetti C, Saeki H, et al. Fractalkine, a CX3C chemokine, is expressed by dendritic cells and is up-regulated upon dendritic cell maturation. *Eur J Immunol* 1999;29(8):2551–2559.

93. Gardella S, Andrei C, Costigliolo S, Poggi A, Zocchi MR, Rubartelli A. Interleukin-18 synthesis and secretion by dendritic cells are modulated by interaction with antigen-specific T cells. *J Leukoc Biol* 1999;66(2):237–241.

94. Bennett SR, Carbone FR, Karamalis F, Flavell RA, Miller JF, Heath WR. Help for cytotoxic-T-cell responses is mediated by CD40 signaling. *Nature* 1998;393:478–480.

95. Cella M, Scheidegger D, Palmer-Lehmann K, Lane P, Uanzavecchia A, Alber G. Ligation of CD40 on dendritic cells triggers production of high levels of interleukin-12 and enhances T cell stimulator capacity: T-T help via APC activation. *J Exp Med* 1996;184:747–752.

96. Bianchi R, Grohmann U, Vacca C, Belladonna ML, Fioretti MC, Puccetti P. Autocrine IL-12 is involved in dendritic cell modulation via CD40 ligation. *J Immunol* 1999;163(5):2517–2521.

97. Dubois B, Bridon JM, Fayette J, et al. Dendritic cells directly modulate B cell growth and differentiation. *J Leukoc Biol* 1999;66(2): 224–230.

98. Fayette J, Durand I, Bridon JM, et al. Dendritic cells enhance the differentiation of naive B cells into plasma cells *in vitro*. *Scand J Immunol* 1998;48(6):563–570.

99. Fayette J, Dubois B, Vandenabeele S, et al. Human dendritic cells shew isotype switching of CD40-activated naïve B cells towards IgA1 and IgA2. *J Exp Med* 1997;185:1909–1918.

100. Hahne M, Rimoldi D, Schroter M, et al. Melanoma cell expression

of Fas (Apo-1/CD95) ligand: implications for tumor immune escape. *Science* 1996;274:1363–1366.

101. Griffith TS, Brunner T, Fletcher SM, Green DR, Ferguson TA. Fas ligand-induced apoptosis as a mechanism of immune privilege. *Science* 1995;270:1189–1192.

102. Alderson MR, Tough TW, Davis-Smith T, et al. Fas ligand mediates activation-induced cell death in human T lymphocytes. *J Exp Med* 1995;181:71–77.

103. Akbar AN, Salmon M. Cellular environments and apoptosis: tissue microenvironments control activated T-cell death. *Immunol Today* 1997;18:72–76.

104. Hawkins CJ, Vaux DL. The role of the Bcl-2 family of apoptosis regulatory proteins in the immune system. *Semin Immunol* 1997;9:25–33.

105. Bjorck P, Banchereau J, Flores-Romo U. CD40 ligation counteracts Fas-induced apoptosis of human dendritic cells. *Int Immunol* 1997;9(3):365–372.

106. Reichert TE, Rabinowich H, Johnson JT, Whiteside TU. Mechanisms responsible for signaling and functional defects. *J Immunother* 1998;21(4):295–306.

107. Devergne O, Hummel M, Koeppen H, et al. A novel interleukin-12 p40-related protein induced by latent Epstein-Barr virus infection in B lymphocytes. *J Virol* 1996;70:1143–1153.

108. Esway J, Shurin GV, Lotze MT, Barksdale EM. Creating immune privilege: neuroblastoma soluble factors cause apoptosis of Fas-sensitive targets. *J Immunother* 1997;20:402.

109. Qin Z, Noffz G, Mohaupt M, Blankenstein T. Interleukin-10 prevents dendritic cell accumulation and vaccination with granulocyte-macrophage colony-stimulating factor gene-modified tumor cells. *J Immunol* 1997;159(2):770–776.

110. Gabrilovich D, Ishida T, Oyama T, et al. Vascular endothelial growth factor inhibits the development of dendritic cells and dramatically affects the differentiation of multiple hematopoietic lineages *in vivo*. *Blood* 1998;92(11):4150–4166.

111. Oyama T, Ran S, Ishida T, et al. Vascular endothelial growth factor affects dendritic cell maturation through the inhibition of nuclear factor-KB activation in hemopoietic progenitor cells. *J Immunol* 1998;160:1224–1232.

112. Ishida T, Oyama T, Carbone DP, Gabrilovich DI. Defective function of Langerhans cells in tumor-bearing animals is the result of defective maturation from hemopoietic progenitors. *J Immunol* 1998;161(9):4842–4851.

113. Chaux P, Favre N, Bonnotte B, Moutet M, Martin M, Martin F. Tumor-infiltrating dendritic cells are defective in their antigen-presenting function and inducible B7 expression. A role in the immune tolerance to antigenic tumors. *Adv Exp Med Biol* 1997;417:525–528.

114. Gabrilovich DI, Corak J, Ciernik IF, Kavanaugh D, Carbone DP. Decreased antigen presentation by dendritic cells in patients with breast cancer. *Clin Cancer Res* 1997;3(3):483–490.

115. Enk AH, Jonuleit H, Saloga J, Knop J. Dendritic cells as mediators of tumor-induced tolerance in metastatic melanoma. *Int J Cancer* 1997;73:309–316.

116. Koppi TA, Tough-Bement T, Lewinsohn DM, Lynch DH, Alderson MR. CD40 ligand inhibits Fas/CD95-mediated apoptosis of human blood-derived dendritic cells. *Eur J Immunol* 1997;27(12): 3161–3165.

117. Watson GA, Lopez DM. Aberrant antigen presentation by macrophages from tumor-bearing mice is involved in the down-regulation of their T cell responses. *J Immunol* 1995;155:3124–3134.

118. Zeh HJ III, Salter RD, Lotze MT, Storkus WJ. Flow cytometric determination of peptide-class I complex formation. *Hum Immunol* 1994;39:79–86.

119. Walker PR, Saas P, Dietrich PY. Role of Fas ligand (CD95L) in immune escape: the tumor cell strikes back. *J Immunol* 1997;158:4521–4524.

120. O'Connell J, Bennett MW, O'Sullivan GC, Collins JK, Shanahan F. The Fas counterattack: a molecular mechanism of tumor immune privilege. *Mol Med* 1997;3:294–300.

121. Ju ST, Panka DJ, Cui H, et al. Fas(CD95)/FasL interactions required for programmed cell death after T-cell activation. *Nature* 1995;373:444–448.

122. Boise UH, Minn AJ, Noel PJ, et al. CD28 costimulation can pro-

mote T cell survival by enhancing the expression of Bcl-xl. *Immunity* 1995;3:87–98.

123. Boise UH, Gonzalez-Garcia M, Postema CE, et al. Bcl-x, a bcl-2-related gene that functions as a dominant regulator of apoptotic cell death. *Cell* 1993;74:597–608.

124. Daniel PT, Kroidl A, Cayeux S, Bargou R, Blankenstein T, Dörken B. Costimulatory signals through B7.1/CD28 prevent T cell apoptosis during target cell lysis. *J Immunol* 1997;159:3808–3815.

125. Williams NJ, Harvey JJ, Duncan I, Booth RF, Knight SC. Interleukin-12 restores dendritic cell function and cell-mediated immunity in retrovirus-infected mice. *Cell Immunol* 1998;183(2):121–130.

126. Caux C, Vanbervliet B, Massacrier C, et al. B70/B7-2 is identical to CD86 and is the major functional ligand for CD28 expressed on human dendritic cells. *J Exp Med* 1994;180:1841–1847.

127. Schuler G, Steinman RM. Dendritic cells as adjuvants for immune-mediated resistance to tumors. *J Exp Med* 1997;186(8):1183–1186.

128. Alters SE, Gadea JR, Philip R. Immunotherapy of cancer. Generation of CEA specific CTL using CEA peptide pulsed dendritic cells. *Adv Exp Med Biol* 1997;417:519–524.

129. Traversari C, Van der Bruggen P, Leuscher IF, et al. A nonapeptide encoded by human gene MAGE-1 is recognized on HLA-A1 by cytolytic T lymphocytes directed against tumor antigen MZ2-E. *J Exp Med* 1992;176:1453.

130. Kawakami Y, Eliyahu S, Sakaguchi K, et al. Identification of the immunodominant peptides of MART-1 human melanoma antigen recognized by the majority of HLA-A2-restricted tumor infiltrating lymphocytes. *J Exp Med* 1994;180:347.

131. Bakker AB, Marland G, de Boer AJ, et al. Generation of antimelanoma cytotoxic T lymphocytes from healthy donors after presentation of melanoma-associated antigen-derived epitopes by dendritic cells *in vitro*. *Cancer Res* 1995;55(22):5330–5334.

132. Liau LM, Black KL, Prins RM, et al. Treatment of intracranial gliomas with bone marrow-derived dendritic cells pulsed with tumor antigens. *J Neurosurg* 1999;90:1115–1124.

133. Bakker ABH, Schreurs MWJ, de Boer AJ, et al. Melanocyte lineage-specific antigen gp100 is recognized by melanoma derived tumor infiltrating lymphocytes. *J Exp Med* 1994;179:1005–1009.

134. Anichini A, Maccalli C, Mortarini R, et al. Melanoma cells and normal melanocytes share antigens recognized by HLA-A2-restricted cytotoxic T cell clones from melanoma patients. *J Exp Med* 1993;177:989.

135. Tjandrawan T, Maeurer MJ, Castelli C, Lotze MT, Storkus WJ. Autologous dendritic cells pulsed with MART-1, gp100, or tyrosinase peptides elicit antimelanoma CTL from both normal donor and cancer patient peripheral blood lymphocytes *in vitro*. *J Immunother* 1998;21:149–157.

136. Brossart P, Stuhler G, Flad T, et al. Her-2/neu-derived peptides are tumor-associated antigens expressed by human renal cell and colon carcinoma lines and are recognized by *in vitro* induced specific cytotoxic T lymphocytes. *Cancer Res* 1998;58(4):732–736.

137. Celluzzi CM, Mayordomo JI, Storkus WJ, Lotze MT, Falo LD. Peptide-pulsed dendritic cells induce antigen specific CTL-mediated protective tumor immunity. *J Exp Med* 1996;183:283–287.

138. Bakker AB, Marland G, de Boer AJ, et al. Generation of antimelanoma cytotoxic T lymphocytes from healthy donors after presentation of melanoma-associated antigen-derived epitopes by dendritic cells in vitro. *Cancer Res* 1995;55(22):5330–5334.

139. Chakraborty NG, Sporn JR, Tortora AF, et al. Immunization with a tumor-cell-lysate-loaded autologous-antigen-presenting-cell-based vaccine in melanoma. *Cancer Immunol Immunother* 1998;47:58–64.

140. Nestle FO, Alijagic S, Gilliet M, et al. Vaccination of melanoma patients with peptide- or tumor lysate pulsed dendritic cells. *Nat Med* 1998;4(3):328–332.

141. Ashley DM, Faiola B, Nair S, Hale LP, Bigner DD, Gilboa E. Bone marrow-generated dendritic cells pulsed with tumor extracts or tumor RNA induce antitumor immunity against central nervous system tumors. *J Exp Med* 1997;186:1177–1182.

142. Salgaller M, Lodge P. Use of cellular and cytokine adjuvants in the immunotherapy of cancer. *J Surg Oncol* 1998;68:122–138

143. Hart I, Colaco C. Immunotherapy. Fusion induces tumour rejection. *Nature* 1997;388:626–627.

144. Tuting T, Wilson CC, Martin DM, et al. Autologous human monocyte-derived dendritic cells genetically modified to express melanoma antigens elicit primary cytotoxic T cell responses *in vitro*: enhancement by contransfection of genes encoding the Th1-biasing cytokines IL-12 and IFN-alpha. *J Immunol* 1998;160:1139–1147.

145. Zitvogel L, Couderc B, Mayordomo JI, Robbins PD, Lotze MT, Storkus WJ. IL-12-engineered dendritic cells serve as effective tumor vaccine adjuvants *in vivo*. In: Lotze MT, Trinchieri G, Gately MK, Wolf SF, eds. Interleukin 12: cellular and molecular immunology of an important regulatory cytokine. *N Y Acad Sci* 1996;795:284–293.

146. Nishioka Y, Robbins PD, Lotze MT, Tahara H. Induction of systemic and therapeutic antitumor immunity using intratumoral injection of bone marrow-derived dendritic cells genetically engineered to express Interleukin-12 (IL-12). *Cancer Res* 1999;59(16):4035–4041.

147. Nishioka Y, Shurin M, Robbins PD, Storkus WJ, Lotze MT, Tahara H. Effective tumor immunotherapy using bone marrow-derived dendritic cells (DC)'s genetically engineered to express Interleukin 12. *J Immunother* 1997;20:419.

148. Zitvogel L, Regnault A, Lozier A, et al. Eradication of established murine tumors using a novel cell-free vaccine: dendritic cell-derived exosomes. *Nat Med* 1998;4:594–600.

149. Nishioka Y, Hirao M, Robbins PD, Uotze MT, Tahara H. Induction of systemic and therapeutic antitumor immunity using intratumoral injection of dendritic cells genetically modified to express interleukin 12. *Cancer Res* 1999;59(16):4035–4041.

150. Gong J, Chen D, Kashiwaba M, Kufe D. Induction of antitumor activity by immunization with fusions of dendritic and carcinoma cells. *Nat Med* 1997;3:558–561.

151. Manickan E, Kanangat S, Rouse RJD, Yu Z, Rouse BT. Enhancement of immune response to naked DNA vaccine by immunization with transfected dendritic cells. *J Leukoc Biol* 1997;61:125.

152. Boczkowski D, Nair SK, Snyder D, Gilboa E. Dendritic cells pulsed with RNA are potent antigen-presenting cells *in vitro* and *in vivo*. *J Exp Med* 1996;184(2):465–472.

153. Condon C, Watkins SC, Celluzzi CM, Thompson K, Falo UD. DNA-based immunization by *in vivo* transfection of dendritic cells. *Nat Med* 1996;2:1122–1128.

154. Tuting T, Baar J, Gambotto A, et al. Interferon-α gene therapy for cancer: retroviral transduction of fibroblasts and particle-mediated transfection of tumor cells are equally effective strategies for gene delivery in murine tumor models. *Gene Ther* 1997;4:1053–1060.

155. Davis ID, Lotze MT. Cytokine Gene Therapy. In: Thomson A, ed. *The cytokine handbook*, 3rd ed. London: Academic Press, 1997:823–854.

156. Tuting T, Storkus WJ, Lotze MT. Gene-based strategies for the immunotherapy of cancer. *J Mol Med* 1997;75(7):478–491.

157. Bello-Fernandez C, Matyash M, Strobl H, et al. Efficient retrovirus-mediated gene transfer of dendritic cells generated from CD34+ cord blood cells under serum-free conditions. *Hum Gene Ther* 1997;8:1651–1658.

158. Reeves ME, Royal RE, Lam JS, Rosenberg SA, Hwu P. Retroviral transduction of human dendritic cells with a tumor-associated antigen gene. *Cancer Res* 1996;56(24):5672–5677.

159. Brossart P, Goldrath AW, Butz EA, Martin S, Bevan MJ. Virus-mediated delivery of antigenic epitopes into dendritic cells as a means to induce CTL. *J Immunol* 1997;158:3270–3276.

160. Wan Y, Bramson J, Carter R, Graham F, Gauldie J. Dendritic cells transduced with an adenoviral vector encoding a model tumor-associated antigen for tumor vaccination. *Hum Gene Ther* 1997;8:1355–1363.

161. Kim CJ, Prevette T, Cormier J, et al. Dendritic cells infected with poxviruses encoding MART-1/Melan A sensitize T lymphocytes *in vitro*. *J Immunother* 1997;20(4):276–286.

162. Bronte V, Carroll MW, Goletz TJ, et al. Antigen expression by dendritic cells correlates with the therapeutic effectiveness of a model recombinant poxvirus tumor vaccine. *Proc Natl Acad Sci U S A* 1997;94(7):3183–3188.

163. Lotze MT, Shurin M, Davis I, Amoscato A, Strokus WJ. Dendritic cell based therapy of cancer. In: Ricciardi-Castognoli P, ed. *Dendritic cells in fundamental and clinical immunology*. New York: Plenum Press, 1997. [Au Q 8]

164. Frassanito MA, Mayordomo JI, DeUeo RM, Storkus WJ, Uotze MT, DeLeo AB. Identification of Meth A sarcoma-derived class I major histocompatibility complex-associated peptides recognized by a specific CD8+ cytolytic T lymphocyte. *Cancer Res* 1995;55:124–128.

165. Bender A, Albert M, Reddy A, et al. The distinctive features of influenza virus infection of dendritic cells. *Immunobiology* 1998;198(5):552–567.

166. Albert ML, Sauter B, Bhardwaj N. Dendritic cells acquire antigen from apoptotic cells and induce class I-restricted CTUs. *Nature* 1998;392(6671):86–89.

167. Rubartelli A, Poggi A, Zocchi MR. The selective engulfment of apoptotic bodies by dendritic cells is mediated by the alpha(v)beta3 integrin and requires intracellular and extracellular calcium. *Eur J Immunol* 1997;27(8):1893–1900.

168. Mukherji B, Chakraborty NG, Yamasaki S, et al. Induction of antigen-specific cytolytic T cells in situ in human melanoma by immunization with synthetic peptide pulsed autologous antigen presenting cells. *Proc Natl Acad Sci U S A* 1995;92:8078–8082.

169. Hsu FJ, Benike C, Fagnoni F, et al. Vaccination of patients with B-cell lymphoma using autologous antigen-pulsed dendritic cells. *Nat Med* 1996;2:52–58.

170. Murphy G, Tjoa B, Ragde H, Kenny G, Boynton A. Phase I clinical trial: T-cell therapy for prostate cancer using autologous dendritic cells pulsed with HLA-A20201-specific peptides from prostate-specific membrane antigen. *Prostate* 1996;29:371–380.

171. Tjoa BA, Simmons SJ, Bowes VA, et al. Evaluation of phase I/II clinical trials in prostate cancer with dendritic cells and PSMA peptides. *Prostate* 1998;36(1):39–44.

172. Holtl U, Rieser C, Papesh C, Ramoner R, Bartsch G, Thurenher M. CD83+ blood dendritic cells as a vaccine for immunotherapy of metastatic renal-cell cancer (letter). *Lancet* 1998;352:1358.

173. Lyman SD. Biology of Flt3 ligand and receptor. *Int J Hematol* 1996;62:63–73.

174. Lynch DH, Andreasen A, Maraskovsky E, Whitmore J, Miller RE, Schuh JC. Flt3 ligand induces tumor regression and antitumor immune responses *in vivo*. *Nat Med* 1997;3(6):625–631.

175. Brasel K, Escobar S, Anderberg R, de Vries P, Gruss HJ, Lyman SD. Expression of the flt3 receptor and its ligand on hematopoietic cells. *Leukemia* 1995;9(7):1212–1218.

176. Lynch DH. Induction of dendritic cells (DC) by Flt3 Ligand (FL) promotes the generation of tumor-specific immune responses *in vivo*. *Crit Rev Immunol* 1998;18(1-2):99–107.

177. McKenna HJ, Lyman SD. Biologic of Flt3 ligand, a novel regulator of hematopoietic stem and progenitor cells. In: Ikehara S, Takaku F, Good RA, eds. *Bone marrow transplantation: basic and clinical studies*. New York: Springer-Verlag New York, 1996. [Au Q 8]

178. Lotze MT, Hellerstedt B, Stolincki L, et al. The role of interleukin-2, interleukin-12 and dendritic cells in cancer therapy. *J Cancer Res* 1997:S109–S114.

179. Maraskovsky E, Brasel K, Teepe K, et al. Dramatic increases in the numbers of functionally mature dendritic cells in Flt3 ligand-treated mice: multiple dendritic cell subpopulations identified. *J Exp Med* 1996;184:1953–1962.

180. Peron JM, Esche C, Hunter O, Subbotin VM, Lotze MT, Shurin MR. Effective treatment of murine liver metastases using FLT3 ligand (FL) and IL-12. *J Immunother* 1997;20:400.

181. Hunter O, Haluszczak C, Subbotin VM, Lotze MT, Shurin MR. Administration of IL-12 and FLT3 ligand enhances murine dendritic cell generation. *J Immunother* 1997;20:401.

182. Haluszczak C, Lotze MT, Shurin MR. IL-12 and FLT3 ligand differentially stimulate lymphoid and myeloid dendropoiesis *in vivo*. *J Immunother* 1997;20:406.

183. Lynch DH, Andreasen A, Maraskovsky E, Whitmore J, Miller RE, Schuh JC. Flt3 ligand induces tumor regression and antitumor immune responses *in vivo*. *Nat Med* 1997;3(6):625–631.

184. Chen K, Braun S, Lyman S, et al. Antitumor activity and immunotherapeutic properties of Flt3-ligand in a murine breast cancer model. *Cancer Res* 1997;57:3511–3516.

185. Pulendran B, Lingappa J, Kennedy MK, et al. Development pathways of dendritic cells *in vivo*: distinct function, phenotype, and localization of dendritic cell subsets in FLT3 ligand-treated mice. *J Immunol* 1997;159:2222–2231.

186. Maraskovsky E, Brasel K, Teepe M, et al. Dramatic increase in the numbers of functionally mature dendritic cells in Flt3 ligand-treated mice: multiple dendritic cell subpopulations identified. *J Exp Med* 1996;184(5):1953–1962.

187. Nishioka Y, Hirao M, Robbins PD, Lotze MT, Tahara H. Induction of systemic and therapeutic antitumor immunity using intratumoral injection of dendritic cells genetically modified to express Interleukin-12. *Cancer Res* 1999;59:4035–4041.

188. Mortarini R, Anichini A, Di Nicola M, et al. Autologous dendritic cells derived from CD34+ progenitors and from monocytes are not functionally equivalent antigen-presenting cells in the induction of melan-A/Mart-1(27-35)-specific CTLs from peripheral blood lymphocytes of melanoma patients with low frequency of CTL precursors. *Cancer Res* 1997;57(24):5534–5541.

189. Young JW, Szabolcs P, Moore MAS. Identification of dendritic cell colony-forming units among normal human CD34+ bone marrow progenitors that are expanded by c-kit-ligand and yield pure dendritic cell colonies in the presence of granulocyte/macrophage colony-stimulating factor and tumor necrosis factor alpha. *J Exp Med* 1995;182:1111.

190. Bernhard H, Disis ML, Heimfeld S, Hand S, Gralow JR, Cheever MA. Generation of immunostimulatory dendritic cells from human CD34+ hematopoietic progenitor cells of the bone marrow and peripheral blood. *Cancer Res* 1995;55:1099–1104.

191. Esche C, Shurin MR, Haluszczak C, Peron JM, Lotze MT. Generation of human dendritic cells from CD34+ precursors for human clinical trials. *J Immunother* 1997;20:403.

192. Strunk D, Rappersberger K, Egger C, et al. Generation of human dendritic cells/Langerhans cells from circulating CD34+ hematopoietic progenitor cells. *Blood* 1996;87:1292–1302.

193. Siena S, Di Nicola M, Bregni M, et al. Massive *ex vivo* generation of functional dendritic cells from mobilized CD34+ blood progenitors for anticancer therapy. *Exp Hematol* 1995;23(14):1463–1471.

194. Lane TA, Ho AD, Bashey A, Peterson S, Young D, Law P. Mobilization of blood-derived stem and progenitor cells in normal subjects by granulocyte-macrophage- and granulocyte-colony-stimulating factors. *Transfusion* 1999;39(1):39–47.

195. Thurner B, Roder C, Dieckmann D, et al. Generation of large numbers of fully mature and stable dendritic cells from leukapheresis products for clinical application. *J Immunol Methods* 1999;223(1):1–15.

196. Barratt-Boyes SM, Watkins SC, Finn OJ. Migration of cultured chimpanzee dendritic cells following intravenous and subcutaneous injection. *Adv Exp Med Biol* 1997;417:71–75.

18.8

CANCER VACCINES: CLINICAL APPLICATIONS

Vaccines Against Carbohydrate Antigens on Glycolipids and Glycoproteins

PHILIP O. LIVINGSTON
GOVINDASWAMI RAGUPATHI

The most abundantly expressed antigens at the cell surface of cancer cells are carbohydrates. Although carbohydrate tumor antigens are not known to be recognized by T cells, they have been proven to be uniquely effective targets for antibody-mediated active and passive cancer immunotherapy in the adjuvant setting (see Chapter 16.5). If antibodies of sufficient titer can be induced against cell surface carbohydrate antigens to eliminate tumor cells from the blood and lymphatic system and to eradicate micrometastasis, as demonstrated in mice with antibodies against GD2 (1), this would dramatically alter our approach to treating the cancer patient. With continuing showers of metastasis no longer possible as a consequence of high levels of circulating antibodies, aggressive local therapies of already established metastasis might result in long-term control of even metastatic cancer. It is also possible that recognition of cell surface carbohydrate epitopes of glycolipids and glycoproteins could lead to:

1. Complement or other Fc-mediated inflammation
2. Decreased circulating tumor antigen as a consequence of high levels of antibodies

3. Improved antigen presentation by specifically immune B lymphocytes, facilitating T-lymphocyte immunity, as demonstrated in other systems (2–4)

This is the rationale for vaccines against carbohydrate antigens, but implementation has proven more difficult than initially contemplated.

LESSONS FROM INFECTIOUS DISEASE VACCINES AND EXPERIMENTAL AUTOIMMUNITY FOR OVERCOMING OBSTACLES TO THE DEVELOPMENT OF CANCER VACCINES

A variety of obstacles to the development of effective cancer vaccines exist, but the single greatest obstacle is the poor immunogenicity of tumor-associated antigens, including tumor carbohydrate antigens. They are poor immunogens because they are expressed on many or some normal tissues, and, consequently, are tolerated immunologically to a greater or lesser degree. With regard to induction of experimental autoimmunity, injection of free antigen before normally pathogenic immunization (5) results in protection from autoimmunity (strengthening of tolerance). Similarly, it is expected that the poor immunogenicity of tumor antigens is reinforced by the presence of growing tumor and increasing quantities of shed antigen. Tumor antigens are poor immunogens not just because they are tolerated immunologically, but also because they are surrounded by autoantigens. Even as potent viral or bacterial antigens have been progressively purified or synthesized as single antigenic epitopes, they have become progressively less immunogenic. This is caused by the loss of the highly immunogenic surrounding antigens that augment the immune response by serving as immunologic carrier and adjuvant and the source of activated helper T cells. In the absence of strong bystander immunogens, the conditions necessary for optimal B- and T-lymphocyte responses to tumor antigens, including cytokine production by helper T lymphocytes and recruitment and activation of professional antigen-presenting cells, does not occur. The immune system uses the foreign milieu of viral or bacterial antigens to provide help for the immune response against the individual antigens, and it takes advantage of the normal self milieu of autoantigens to make immunization against autoantigens more difficult.

To further complicate the selection of tumor antigens for preparation of cancer vaccines, not all viral or bacterial antigens are useful targets for vaccination (6,7), and some are counterproductive. The selection of viral or bacterial antigens for construction of vaccines against infectious diseases is assisted by identification of postinfection immune responses, which are associated with protection from subsequent exposures. This was one of the criteria for the selection of GM2 ganglioside as a target for immunotherapy of melanoma (8,9), but most tumor antigens are not sufficiently immunogenic to induce an immune response naturally. Consequently, selection of new cancer antigens for vaccine construction has been based on a more empiric approach.

The final obstacles to the development of clinically effective cancer vaccines are the functional and antigenic heterogeneity, which are inherent features of malignancies, and the genetically based heterogeneity of responsiveness in the human immune response. Consequently, significant variability exists in the immune response to vaccination with even the same antigen in the same vaccine in different patients.

Based on these considerations, the design of tumor vaccines aimed at inducing an antibody response must include:

1. Covalently conjugating tumor antigens to immunogenic foreign proteins for enhanced presentation to the immune system
2. The use of a potent immunologic adjuvant to further augment immunogenicity
3. Limiting reinforcement of tolerance by vaccinating early in the disease, preferably in the adjuvant setting
4. The use of polyvalent vaccines to overcome the issue of tumor and host heterogeneity

APPROACHES FOR AUGMENTING THE IMMUNOGENICITY OF CARBOHYDRATE ANTIGENS: RESULTS OF PRECLINICAL STUDIES

Antibody Induction

Of the various carbohydrate antigens, vaccines against gangliosides have been studied most intensively. Vaccination of mice with irradiated melanoma cells selected for GD3 expression plus adjuvants was able to induce low levels of immunoglobulin M (IgM) antibodies against GD3, but this could be accomplished more effectively and simply by immunizing with purified GD3 plus immunologic adjuvants. Although GD3 alone induced no response at all, GD3 adherent to *Salmonella* minnesota mutant R595 or liposomes containing monophosphoryl lipid A (MPL) induced moderate titers of IgM antibodies in most mice, higher titers than vaccines containing bacille Calmette-Guérin (BCG), alum, Freund's adjuvant, or a variety of other adjuvants (10). Attempts at augmenting the immunogenicity of GD3 by making minor structural modifications to the GD3 so it would be foreign and not recognized as self were unsuccessful (10,11). Although GD3 amide, GD3 lactone, GD3 gangliosidol, and GD3 acetylated at various sites induced higher titers of antibodies against themselves than GD3 did, these antibodies reacted with GD3 only weakly, no more strongly than antibodies induced by unmodified GD3. These findings supported tolerance to autoantigens, such as GD3, as the major obstacle to overcome in cancer vaccines against carbohydrate antigens and underscored the remarkable specificity of the antibody response.

Based on progress with conjugate vaccines against bacterial polysaccharide antigens, Helling systematically compared the immunogenicity of conjugate vaccines constructed with different carriers and adjuvants using GD3 as antigen (12). Keyhole limpet hemocyanin (KLH) was the best of the six immunogenic carrier molecules tested; the conjugation method was important, and a potent immunologic adjuvant was required. GD3 conjugated to KLH at the ceramide double bond and mixed with immunologic adjuvant QS-21 (which is a purified saponin fraction obtained from the bark of the *Quillaja saponaria* Molina tree) (13) was optimal, inducing higher titers of antibody, and, for the first time, consistent IgG antibodies. Simple mixture of GD3 and QS-21 or GD3, KLH, and QS-21 induced no antibodies. More recently, we have conducted similar experiments with or without conjugation using different carrier proteins and different adjuvants with two other ganglioside antigens, GD3 lactone (14) and fucosyl GM1 (15). In each case, antibodies against GD3 and fucosyl GM1 and against tumor cells expressing these antigens were highest when these gangliosides were conjugated to KLH and mixed with QS-21. The neutral glycolipids Globo H and Lewis^y (Le^y) have also been synthesized, conjugated to bovine serum albumen or KLH, and mixed with QS-21 or no adjuvant. Conjugation to KLH and mixture with QS-21 was optimal in each case, inducing antibodies in the mouse that reacted with, and mediated complement lysis of, tumor cells expressing these antigens (16,17).

This same vaccination approach against carbohydrate antigens Thomsen-Friedenreich antigen (TF), Tn, and sialyl Tn (sTn) expressed on mucins has proved optimal for antibody induction. TF antigen (Galβ1-3galNAc-O-serine/threonine), as it is naturally expressed in desialylated porcine submaxillary mucin, and synthetic TF-ceramide with or without various adjuvants were not immunogenic. TF-KLH with or without complete Freund's adjuvant or DETOX [containing monophosphoryl lipid A (MPL) and BCG cell wall skeletons] was moderately immunogenic (median IgM and IgG titers, 1/40), whereas TF-KLH plus QS-21 or SAF-m (a lipid base adjuvant containing pleuronic block copolymer L121) was highly immunogenic with a median IgM titer of 1/160 and a median IgG titer of 1/10,000 (18). Tn (GalNAcα-O-serine/threonine) conjugated to ovine serum albumin or to a short synthetic lipopeptide and sTn-KLH have been used successfully for antibody induction in mice (19–21). Tn dimers and trimers (clusters) and sTn (*N*-acetyl neuraminic acidα2-3GalNAcα-O-serine/threonine) trimers on a serine backbone [sTn(c)] have also been used in conjugate vaccines (20–22). Although sTn and sTn(c) vaccines induce high-titer antibodies against the immunizing sTn epitopes, ovine submaxillary mucin, and tumor cells, their specificities were distinct. Antibodies induced by sTn(c) react with sTn(c) but not with sTn monomers, and sTn monomer–induced antibodies do not react with sTn(c) (21). Because Tn(c) and sTn(c) may be preferentially expressed on tumors as opposed to normal tissues, these clustered vaccines have generated considerable interest.

Protection Against Tumor Challenge

Preclinical studies involving tumor challenge experiments with vaccines against carbohydrate antigens should more directly address the clinical relevance of vaccine-induced antibodies and be applicable to clinical trials in humans than vaccines against protein antigens. This is because carbohydrate antigens predominantly mediate antibody responses in the mouse and humans; assays for measuring these responses are available and have been shown to correlate to clinical outcome. Presentation by HLA or H2 antigens is not required. Three of the carbohydrate antigens that are of interest as human tumor antigens have been identified on murine cancers (Tn, TF, and GD2), and, in each case, immunization with synthetic conjugate (or glycoprotein) plus adjuvant has resulted in protection from tumor challenge (1,23,24).

Immunization with desialylated bovine or ovine submaxillary mucins (which contain large concentrations of Tn antigen) plus immunologic adjuvant DETOX resulted in protection from tumor recurrence in more than 50% of mice subsequently challenged with the syngenic mouse mammary tumor TA3-Ha (23). Protection from tumor challenge with TA3-Ha, which expresses large amounts of Tn and TF antigens, also resulted from immunization with a glycoconjugate vaccine containing synthetic TF antigen covalently attached to KLH and mixed with immunologic adjuvant DETOX (24). Protection from tumor growth was seen even if the intraperitoneal challenge was given first, followed by a low dose of cyclophosphamide (which had no detectable antitumor effect directly) plus immunization beginning 2 days after the tumor challenge. Comparable protection from intravenous tumor challenge with EL4 lymphoma cells (which express GD2) was induced by subcutaneous immunization with GD2-KLH glycoconjugate mixed with QS-21 administered before intravenous tumor challenge or beginning 1 day after tumor challenge (1). Complete protection from tumor outgrowth was also seen when vaccination was initiated on day 17, 1 day after foot amputation of a 16-day palpable EL4 footpad tumor. All untreated mice died of systemic metastasis within 30 days of foot amputation. The previously demonstrated consistent antibody induction in preclinical studies with a variety of carbohydrate conjugate vaccines and the demonstrated ability of Tn-KLH, TF-KLH, and GD2-KLH vaccines to prevent tumor recurrence in tumor models simulating the adjuvant setting provided significant motivation for testing these conjugate vaccines in the clinic.

CLINICAL TRIALS WITH CARBOHYDRATE ANTIGEN VACCINES

The availability of reliable serologic assays to serve as surrogate markers in clinical trials has greatly accelerated progress in developing consistently immunogenic vaccines against carbohydrate epitopes on gangliosides, neutral glycolipids, and mucins.

Gangliosides

Gangliosides are acidic glycosphingolipids that express sialic acid at one end and ceramide at the other. They have been long known as prominent components of the melanoma cell surface. Tai et al. immunized 26 patients with a mixture of three allogenic cell lines and demonstrated antibodies against GM2 in ten patients and antibody against GD2 in two patients (25). We induced antibody against GM2 in 0% to 80% of patients depending on the cell lines chosen for vaccine production (26). Using irradiated melanoma cells, these vaccines induced only moderate titers of IgM antibodies (median titer ~1/160) and no IgG antibodies. These vaccines were difficult to prepare consistently and to administer. We were able to induce antibodies against GD2 in only occasional patients, and no antibodies against GD3.

We have conducted a series of small clinical trials using purified GM2 for vaccine production (26) based on studies with GD3 in the mouse. The serologic results are summarized in

TABLE 1. PEAK GM2 ANTIBODY TITER AFTER ADJUVANT IMMUNIZATION OF STAGE III–IV MELANOMA PATIENTS

Vaccine	Total Patients Treated	IgM Antibodies		IgG Antibodies	
		Patients Responding	Median ELISA Titer	Patients Responding	Median ELISA Titer
GM2	5	0	0	0	0
GM2/R595	5	0	0	0	0
CY + GM2/R595	6	5	1/40	0	0
GM2/MPL Liposomes	6	1	0	0	0
GM2/Proteosomes	33	22	1/80	4	0
GM2/BCG	5	4	1/80	0	0
CY + GM2/BCG	58	50	1/160	6	0
CY + GM2-KLH	6	5	1/80	0	0
CY + GM2-KLH/BCG	6	4	1/160	1	0
CY + GM2-KLH/DETOX	6	5	1/160	0	0
CY + GM2-KLH/QS-21	9	9	1/640	8	1/160
GM2-KLH/QS-21	40	39	1/640	35	1/160

BCG, bacille Calmette-Guérin; CY, cyclophosphamide; ELISA, enzyme-linked immunosorbent assay; Ig, immunoglobulin; KLH, keyhole limpet hemocyanin; MPL, monophosphoryl lipid A.

Table 1. The results were similar to those obtained previously in the mouse with one exception. Lipid A (or MPL) containing adjuvants (including R595 and liposomes) but not BCG were highly effective in the mouse, whereas the reverse was true in humans. Although lipid A and MPL activate macrophages in mice and humans, they are B-cell mitogens only in the mouse. When it comes to weak immunogens, such as these autoantigens, is appears that more is required of an adjuvant than antigen-depot effect and macrophage activation, the two traditional roles of adjuvants. Lipid A performs this in the mouse because of its mitogenic activity, and BCG is able to fill this role in humans because of the exquisite sensitivity of the human immune system to *Mycobacterium tuberculosis* and related mycobacteria.

Ganglioside alone was not immunogenic, and GM2 conjugated to KLH without adjuvant or with BCG or DETOX was moderately immunogenic, similar to GM2 plus BCG (26). GM2 covalently conjugated to KLH and mixed with immunologic adjuvant QS-21 was consistently immunogenic. GM2-KLH plus QS-21 induced the highest and longest-lasting IgM titers against GM2 in patients, and, for the first time, consistent IgG antibodies as well. The IgG antibodies induced were of the IgG1 and IgG3 subclasses, and, like the IgM antibodies, were able to induce complement-mediated lysis of GM2-positive tumor cells (27,28). Although decreasing suppressor cell activity with low-dose cyclophosphamide was found to augment the antibody response to GM2/BCG (29), it did not further augment the response to GM2-KLH plus QS-21 (26). Two Phase 1 trials identified 100 μg of QS-21 as the optimal dose of adjuvant (29) and doses of GM2 between 10 and 70 μg as comparable (30). The GM2 dose of 30 μg was selected for future trials. Coadministration of high-dose interferon-α with GM2-KLH plus QS-21 was shown to be safe and to have no impact on anti-GM2 titers (31). Recently, patients treated with repeated GM2-KLH/QS-21 booster vaccinations at 3- to 4-month intervals have been shown to maintain anti-GM2 IgM and IgG antibody titers for at least 2 years, as shown in Figure 1.

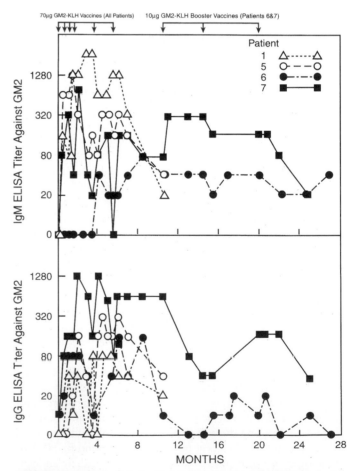

FIGURE 1. Immunoglobulin M (IgM) and IgG antibody titers in four representative melanoma patients after immunization with 6 or 9 GM2-keyhole limpet hemocyanin (KLH) plus QS-21 vaccinations. Arrows indicate dates of vaccinations. (ELISA, enzyme-linked immunosorbent assay.)

TABLE 2. COMPARISON OF SEROLOGIC RESPONSES AFTER IMMUNIZATION WITH OPTIMAL (KEYHOLE LIMPET HEMOCYANIN PLUS QS-21) CONJUGATE VACCINES AGAINST GLYCOLIPID ANTIGENS

| Antigen (30 mg) | No. Patients Treated | Median ELISA Titer | | | | FACS | | | | | | References |
| | | IgM | | IgG | | IgM | | IgG | | CDC | | |
		No. Pos	Titer	No. Pos	Titer	No. Pos	Median % Pos Cells	No. Pos	Median % Pos Cells	No. Pos	Median % Lysis (Target)	
GM2	13	13	640	12	160	13	82	11	42	13	58(A2394)	25,26
GD2	12	10	160	8	80							
GD3	12	1	80	1	80	0	—	0	—	0	—	12
GD3L	12	10	80	8	160	7	80	9	36	8	51(SKMEL28)	12
Fuc GM1	10	10	320	10	320	8	84	6	34	10	80(H4IIE)	35
Globo H	14	11	160	2	160	9	33	4	33	8	53(MCF7)	36,37
Le^y	12	8	320	2	80	8	64	0	—	5	39(MCF7)	47

CDC, complement-dependent cytotoxicity; ELISA, enzyme-linked immunosorbent assay; FACS, fluorescence-activated cell sorter; Ig, immunoglobulin; Le^y, Lewis^y; pos, positive.

Mixture with BCG and conjugation to KLH plus QS-21 have been used with other gangliosides. GD2/BCG and GD3/BCG were each used to immunize 12 patients. Antibodies against GD3 were not detected, and low-titer antibodies against GD2 were detected in only three patients (median titer, 1/40). GD3 congener/BCG vaccines were also tested and were not more effective in melanoma patients than they had been in the mouse (Table 2). GD3 lactones, GD3 amide, and GD3 acetylated in various locations plus BCG again induced antibodies against the synthetic immunizing gangliosides, which did not cross-react with natural GD3 or melanoma cells expressing GD3 (32,33). GD2 covalently conjugated to KLH plus QS-21 induced IgM antibodies in six of six patients (median titer, 1/160), but a GD3-KLH plus QS-21 vaccine was once again unable to induce antibodies against GD3 in 12 consecutive patients (26). The relative immunogenicity of these gangliosides in humans (GM2>GD2>GD3) is different than in the mouse (GD3>GD2>GM2), as a consequence of differential levels of tolerance resulting from the more extensive expression of GM2 in the liver and other normal tissues in the mouse, and the greater expression of GD3 on T lymphocytes (34) and normal stroma in humans.

Three additional trials with ganglioside-KLH plus QS-21 vaccines have been conducted. In the first trial, bivalent vaccines containing 30 μg of GM2 and increasing doses of GD2 (35) confirmed the immunogenicity of GD2 in this conjugate vaccine and identified 60 μg of GD2 as the optimal dose per vaccine. In the second trial, GD3 lactone-KLH was used in place of GD3-KLH, and, for the first time, antibodies against GD3 by enzyme-linked immunosorbent and immune stain assays and against GD3-expressing tumor cells by fluorescence-activated cell sorter and complement lysis assays were detected in 8 of 12 patients (14). In the third trial, ten patients with small-cell lung cancer in complete or partial remission after chemotherapy were immunized with fucosyl GM1-KLH plus QS-21 vaccines after completion of chemotherapy (36). Expression of fucosyl GM1 is restricted to small-cell lung cancer and occasional normal cells in the pancreas and spinal cord. High-titer antibodies against fucosyl GM1 were induced in all patients, demonstrating that fucosyl GM1 is as immunogenic as GM2 and significantly more

immunogenic than GD2 or GD3 (see Table 2). As with the GM2, GD2, and GD3 vaccines, antibody induction against fucosyl GM1 resulted in no demonstrable autoimmunity or other toxicity aside from that associated with QS-21, local erythema, and induration at vaccination sites lasting several days, and, in occasional patients, low-grade fever and malaise lasting as long as 36 hours (36).

Neutral Glycolipids

Globo H

Twenty patients with prostate cancer have been immunized with Globo H-KLH plus QS-21 vaccines containing 3, 10, 30, or 100 μg of Globo H (37,38). The 30-μg dose was selected as optimal for further trials. At this dose, all patients made IgM antibodies against Globo H (median peak titer, 1/1,280) and two patients made IgG antibodies with titers of 1/160 and 1/2,560. Inhibition studies with smaller carbohydrate molecules demonstrated that the antibody response was polyclonal with different antibodies in each serum recognizing at least several different epitopes on the Globo H molecule. Sera reacted with Globo H extracted from biopsy specimens of prostate cancer and breast cancer but not extracts of melanoma, which does not express Globo H. Reactivity with the cell surface of Globo H–positive cancer cells was demonstrated by strong flow cytometry reactions in four of five patients and strong complement-mediated cytotoxicity (more than 50% lysis) demonstrated in three of five patients as well. During 1999, nine breast cancer patients have been immunized with Globo H-KLH plus QS-21, and the results have been similar (see Table 2). All patients made IgM antibodies against Globo H (median titer, 1/320); these antibodies reacted against Globo H naturally expressed at the cell surface of breast cancer cells in six of nine patients, and strong complement lysis was seen with sera from five of nine patients.

Lewis^y

Twenty-four ovarian cancer patients who were free of grossly detectable disease after systemic and intraperitoneal chemother-

TABLE 3. COMPARISON OF THE SEROLOGIC RESPONSES TO IMMUNIZATION WITH TF, TN, AND STN-KLH CONJUGATE VACCINES IN CLINICAL TRIALS

| Vaccine Antigen (Dose µg) | Adjuvant | No. Patients Treated | ELISA | | | | References |
| | | | IgM | | IgG | | |
			No. Pos	Median Titer	No. Pos	Median Titer	
TF (100)	DETOX	10	9	640	9	640	41
TF (100)	NONE	6	1	40	0	0	42
TF (100)	DETOX	6	4	320	0	0	42
TF(c) (10,30)	QS-21	Pending					
STn	DETOX	85	83	256		64	43
STn (100)	DETOX	5	2	40	0	0	40
STn (100)	QS-21	5	4	80	3	40	40
STn(c) (30)	QS-21	9	9	1,280	8	1,280	46
Tn(c) (3,7,15)	QS-21	15	12	640	14	1,280	45

ELISA, enzyme-linked immunosorbent assay; FACS, fluorescence-activated cell sorter; Ig, immunoglobulin; pos, positive.

apy were vaccinated with Le^y-KLH plus QS-21 vaccines containing 3, 10, 30, or 60 µg of Le^y (39). IgG antibody responses against Le^y were restricted to one or two patients at each of the dose levels, but IgM responses were more common. The 10-µg and 30-µg doses resulted in more frequent and higher titer IgM antibody responses against Le^y. No patients had IgM antibodies by enzyme-linked immunosorbent assay or fluorescence-activated cell sorter before vaccination. Four of six patients at the 30-µg dose level developed enzyme-linked immunosorbent assay titers of at least 1/320 after immunization. Similarly, four of six patients developed strong IgM reactivity by fluorescence-activated cell sorter against the Le^y-positive ovarian cancer cell line OVCAR3. The percentage of positive cells for these four patients by flow cytometry was 40%, 45%, 84%, and 97%. No IgG reactivity was detected (see Table 2). Complement-dependent cytotoxicity (CDC) ranged between 21% and 62% for these six patients with four patients showing at least a tripling of the percentage of CDC from a median of 6% prevaccination to 39% after vaccination.

CARBOHYDRATE ANTIGENS ON MUCINS

The immunogenicity of TF, Tn, and sTn antigens has been studied in a series of small clinical trials. The chemical structures of these antigens and their expression on various cancers and normal tissues are described in Chapter 16.5.

TF and Tn

Pioneering trials by Springer were initiated in the mid-1970s with vaccines containing TF and Tn purified from natural sources and mixed with Typhoid vaccine as adjuvant (40). Springer described augmentation of natural levels of delayed-type hypersensitivity skin-test reactivity, induction of IgM antibodies, and a more favorable clinical outcome in vaccinated patients with breast cancer. O'Boyle used partially desialylated ovine submaxillary mucin (dOSM) containing Tn and sTn alone or mixed with BCG or

DETOX to immunize 20 colorectal cancer patients (41). dOSM alone was not immunogenic, but with BCG was slightly more immunogenic than with DETOX, inducing a median IgM antibody titer against Tn of 1/40 and against sTn and OSM of 1/160. OSM, dOSM, and porcine submaxillary mucin (expressing Tn and TF) have been widely used as *in vitro* targets mirroring clinical relevancy because TF, Tn, and sTn, although expressed significantly by cell lines growing *in vivo* and in tumor biopsy specimens, are not well expressed by cell lines growing *in vitro*. Ten ovarian cancer patients were immunized with two different doses of synthetic TF-KLH (100 or 500 µg) plus DETOX (42). Natural pretreatment IgM and IgG antibody titers against synthetic TF were increased by vaccination in nine of ten patients. The 100-µg dose of TF appeared more immunogenic than the 500-µg dose. Reactivity of these IgM and IgG antibodies against natural sources of TF antigen was also seen, although at lower titers than against the synthetic TF. In a separate trial, groups of colorectal carcinoma patients were immunized with TF-KLH alone or TF-KLH plus DETOX (43). Once again, the TF-KLH plus DETOX vaccine was more immunogenic than TF-KLH alone, and the increase in antibody titers against natural sources of TF was lower than against synthetic TF.

Studies in the mouse have demonstrated that Tn-serine trimers or clusters (c) but not single Tn epitopes were recognized by monoclonal antibodies that react with Tn on tumor cells (20). Consequently, prostate cancer patients have recently been immunized with Tn(c)-KLH plus QS-21 and TF(c)-KLH plus QS-21 vaccines. IgM and IgG antibody titers against OSM and dOSM were 10- to 100-fold higher than seen with the previous vaccines. Antibody reactivity demonstrated by flow cytometry against tumor cells expressing TF and Tn was seen for the first time (44). These results are summarized in Table 3.

sTn

A variety of sTn-KLH conjugate vaccines mixed with various immunologic adjuvants have been tested in clinical trials. Breast cancer patients have been immunized with sTn-KLH plus

DETOX in combination with low-dose cyclophosphamide (300 μg per meter^2 intravenously 3 days before immunization), and high-titer IgM and IgG antibodies (median titer, 1/1,024) against synthetic sTn were induced in most patients (45). IgM and IgG reactivity against ovine submaxillary mucin (OSM) was lower (1/64) but clearly present, and titers were twofold to fourfold lower in patients not pretreated with low-dose cyclophosphamide. In a separate trial, patients with colon cancer were immunized with sTn-KLH plus DETOX or QS-21 (without cyclophosphamide) in the adjuvant setting (43). Median IgM and IgG antibody titers against synthetic sTn were two- and eightfold higher (1/5,120, and 1/2,560), respectively, with QS-21 than with DETOX, but IgM and IgG titers against OSM were only 1/80 and 1/40. Although sTn-KLH plus QS-21 vaccines clearly augment natural IgM antibodies and induce IgG antibodies against mucins, they induce far higher titers of antibodies against synthetic sTn.

In 1997, breast cancer patients were immunized with sTn(c)-KLH plus QS-21 (46). For the first time, median IgM titers against synthetic sTn and OSM were the same (1/2,560–1/1,520) and IgG titers were 1/1,280 and 1/640. Consistent reactivity with sTn expressed at the cell surface of cancer cells was demonstrated for the first time by flow cytometry with these sera. These results are summarized in Table 3. They demonstrate that sTn(c) more closely resembles sTn, as it is expressed at the tumor cell surface, than individual sTn epitopes, and is therefore a better immunogen. A similar increase in relevant immunogenicity has been described using single sTn epitopes when they were packed more tightly onto the KLH surface (i.e., when sTn/KLH ratios were 2,000:1 or more) (43).

CLINICAL IMPACT OF IMMUNIZATION WITH CARBOHYDRATE ANTIGEN VACCINES

Vaccine-induced antibody responses against GM2 and sTn have been associated with a more favorable clinical course. A randomized trial with GM2/BCG was conducted in 122 stage III melanoma patients who were free of disease after resection of metastatic disease in regional lymph nodes (47). This trial was based on the previous demonstration that immunization with GM2/BCG induced IgM antibodies in 85% of patients and that the production of these antibodies correlated with a more favorable prognosis. Patients were randomized to receive five immunizations over a 6-month period with BCG alone (64 patients) or BCG with GM2 adherent to the BCG surface (58 patients). Fifty-seven patients had GM2 antibody, which was present naturally or vaccine induced, and these patients had a significantly increased disease-free ($p = .004$) and overall ($p = .02$) survival. Comparing the GM2/BCG and BCG groups, exclusion of all patients with preexisting GM2 antibodies (one patient in the GM2/BCG group and five patients in the BCG group) resulted in differences of 23% (from 27% of patients remaining disease free to 50%) in disease-free survival, and 14% in overall survival with a minimum follow-up of 50 months. When all patients in the two treatment groups were compared as randomized, these increases were 18% and 11%

for disease-free and overall survival in favor of vaccination with GM2/BCG, with neither difference achieving statistical significance. Antibody responses were predominantly IgM of moderate titer and short lived (returning to baseline within 2 months of the final immunization).

Correlation between vaccine-induced antibody responses and clinical course has also been seen after immunization with sTn-KLH plus DETOX (48). In a series of 113 patients with various types of epithelial cancers, the 51 patients with high antibody responses to OSM after vaccination survived significantly longer than the 62 patients with lower antibody responses. Antibody responses against KLH showed no such correlation. In a separate study, improved survival was also seen in 25 patients with advanced breast cancer who had a high antibody response to the sTn vaccine in combination with intravenous cyclophosphamide compared with 25 patients with a low antibody response who did not receive the intravenous cyclophosphamide (45). The median survival increased from 13.3 months in patients with low anti-sTn antibody titers compared with 26.5 months in those with high responses.

ONGOING TRIALS AND FUTURE DIRECTIONS

Randomized phase 3 clinical trials with GM2 and sTn conjugate vaccines are in progress. The trials with GM2-KLH plus QS-21 vaccines prepared by Progenics Pharmaceuticals, Inc. (Tarrytown, NY) are based on the higher-titer, longer-lasting antibodies against GM2 induced by the GM2-KLH vaccine compared with the previous GM2/BCG vaccine. Two randomized trials have been initiated. A trial comparing standard treatment (high-dose interferon) to GM2-KLH plus QS-21 vaccine is being conducted in patients with deep stage II primary melanomas (more than 4-mm depth) or stage III disease (lymph node metastasis) by the Eastern Cooperative Oncology Group, The Southwest Oncology Group, The North Central Treatment Group, Memorial Sloan-Kettering Cancer Center, and the Cancer and Leukemia Group B. Patient accrual was completed in September 1999. A second phase 3 trial was initiated in the latter half of 1998 in New Zealand, Australia, and subsequently in Europe and South America, comparing the same GM2 vaccine to placebo. A large, multicenter, randomized phase 3 trial with sTn-KLH plus DETOX prepared by Biomira Inc. (Edmonton, Alberta, Canada) was initiated late in 1998 in North America and Europe. The sTn-KLH plus DETOX vaccine (Theratope) is being compared with no treatment in patients with metastatic breast cancer who have had a complete or partial response to combination chemotherapy. This trial is based on the consistent immunogenicity, correlation of vaccine-induced antibody response to more favorable clinical outcome, and preclinical models for this vaccine (described above).

Although every indication exists that immunization with these single antigen vaccines may prove beneficial when administered in the adjuvant setting, in the long run polyvalent vaccines offer greater promise. As described above, we have induced consistent antibodies against GM2, fucosyl GM1, and sTn. Conjugate vaccines against GD3, GD2, Tn, TF, Globo H, and Le^y have induced antibody responses in 60% or more of patients. In most

TABLE 4. CARBOHYDRATE ANTIGENS FOR POLYVALENT VACCINE CONSTRUCTION OF PROVEN IMMUNOGENICITY IN MORE THAN 60% OF PATIENTS

Tumor	Antigens
Melanoma	GM2, GD2, GD3L
Neuroblastoma	GM2, GD2, GD3L
Sarcoma	GM2, GD2, GD3L
B-cell lymphoma	GM2, GD2
Small-cell lung cancer	GM2, Fucosyl GM1, Globo H
Breast	GM2, Globo H, TF(c)
Prostate	GM2, Tn(c), sTn(c), TF(c)
Lung	GM2, Globo H, Le^y
Colon	GM2, sTn(c), TF(c), Le^y
Ovary	GM2, Globo H, sTn(c), TF(c), Le^y
Stomach	GM2, Le^y

Le^y, Lewis^y.

cases, these antibodies have been demonstrated to react strongly with the cell surface of antigen-positive cancer cells, and this reactivity has induced strong complement-mediated cytotoxicity of antigen-positive tumor cells in the case of the glycolipid antigens. The known distribution of carbohydrate antigens on cancers and normal tissues was described in Chapter 16.5. Based on this distribution and the results of vaccination trials demonstrating consistent immunogenicity of each of these antigens conjugated to KLH plus QS-21 vaccines, polyvalent vaccines against the cell surface carbohydrate antigens of a variety of malignancies are planned. These malignancies and the antigens considered for inclusion in the polyvalent vaccines are listed in Table 4. Several antigens are conspicuously absent from this list because of a high risk of autoimmunity, including GM3, which is a melanoma ganglioside also extensively expressed in the liver, and Lewis^x and sialylated Lewis^x, which are epithelial cancer antigens that are also expressed on polymorphonucleocytes. Also Lewis^a, sialyl Lewis^a, and polysialic acid are omitted because they have not been tested. Phase 2 polyvalent vaccine trials against melanoma, sarcoma, prostate cancer, and ovarian cancer are planned to begin before the end of 2000, and a phase 3 trial is to be initiated in patients with breast cancer in the year 2001.

CONCLUSIONS

It is possible that improvements in our understanding of the requirements for optimal dendritic cell (and other professional antigen-presenting cell) activation and of the cascade of cytokines required for B-lymphocyte activation may result in more specific and powerful immunization approaches. The sequence of cytokines and other activities induced by potent adjuvants, such as QS-21, and carriers, such as KLH, however, may be impractical to imitate by administration of cytokines or genes coding these cytokines. In any case, the optimal approach for augmenting the antibody response against carbohydrate and peptide antigens at this time is conjugation to KLH and mixture with a potent adjuvant, such as QS-21.

The primary function of antibodies is the elimination of circulating viral or bacterial pathogens or toxins from the blood-stream, lymphatics, and interstitial spaces. Once induced, antibodies are ideally suited for eliminating circulating tumor cells and micrometastases from these spaces as well. Natural, tumor-induced and vaccine-induced antibodies against antigens expressed at the cancer cell surface have been correlated with an improved clinical outcome. In the mouse, passive administration of monoclonal antibodies and active induction of antibodies with cancer vaccines against cell surface carbohydrate antigens have resulted in prolonged survival and complete protection from tumor challenges administered before treatment, a setting similar to the adjuvant setting in humans. Carbohydrate antigens are the most abundant antigens at the cell surface of cancer cells, where they play important roles in cell-cell interactions, proliferation, and the metastatic process. They have been shown to be excellent targets for immune attack by antibodies against human cancers, especially in the adjuvant setting. Vaccines containing a variety of carbohydrate tumor antigens covalently attached to the immunogenic carrier protein KLH plus a potent immunologic adjuvant, such as QS-21, have been shown to induce antibodies against these antigens in cancer patients. These antibodies generally induce complement-mediated lysis and antibody-dependent cell-mediated cytotoxicity of antigen-positive tumor cells. Phase 3 clinical trials with GM2-KLH and sTn-KLH conjugate vaccines have already been initiated in the adjuvant or minimal disease setting in patients with melanoma and breast cancer. Phase 3 trials with polyvalent vaccines against several different antigens tailored for particular cancer types are planned for 2000 and 2001.

REFERENCES

1. Zhang H, Zhang S, Cheung NK, Ragupathi G, Livingston PO. Antibodies can eradicate cancer micrometastases. *Cancer Res* 1998;58:2844–2849.
2. Lin R-H, Mamula MJ, Hardin JA, Janeway CA Jr. Induction of autoreactive B cells allows priming of autoreactive T cells. *J Exp Med* 1991;173:1433–1439.
3. Serreze DV, Chapman HD, Varnum DS, et al. B lymphocytes are essential for the initiation of T cell-mediated autoimmune diabetes: analysis of a new "speed congenic" stock of NOD.Igμ^{null} mice. *J Exp Med* 1996;184:2049–2053.
4. Sopori ML, Donaldson LA, Savage SM. T Lymphocyte heterogeneity in the rat III. Autoreactive T cells are activated by B cells. *Cell Immunol* 1990;128:427–437.
5. Rose NR. Autoimmune disease. *Sci Am* 1981;244:80.
6. Norrby E, Enders-Ruckle G, Ter Meulen V. Differences in the appearance of antibodies to structural components of measles virus after immunization with inactivated and live virus. *J Infect Dis* 1975,132.262.
7. Oehen S, Hengartner H, Zinkernagel RM. Vaccination for disease. *Science* 1991;251:195–198.
8. Jones PC, Sze LL, Liu P, Morton DL, Irie RF. Prolonged survival for melanoma patients with elevated IgM antibody to oncofetal antigen. *J Natl Cancer Inst* 1981;66:249–263.
9. Livingston PO, Ritter G, Srivastava P, et al. Characterization of IgG and IgM antibodies induced in melanoma patients by immunization with purified GM2 ganglionic. *Cancer Res* 1989;49:7045–7050.
10. Ritter G, Boosfeld E, Calves MJ, Oettgen HF, Old LJ, Livingston PO. Antibody response after immunization with gangliosides GD3, GD3 lactones, GD3 amide and GD3 gangliosidol in the mouse. GD3 lactone I induces antibodies reactive with human melanoma. *Immunobiology* 1990;182:32–43.

11. Ritter G, Boosfeld E, Markstein E, et al. Biochemical and serological characteristics of natural 9-0-acetyl GD3 from human melanoma and bovine buttermilk and chemically O-acetylated GD3. *Cancer Res* 1990;50:1403–1410.

12. Helling F, Shang Y, Calves M, Oettgen HF, Livingston PO. Increased immunogenicity of GD3 conjugate vaccines: comparison of various carrier proteins and selection of GD3-KLH for further testing. *Cancer Res* 1994;54:197–203.

13. Kensil CR, Patel U, Lennick M, Marciani D. Separation and characterization of saponins with adjuvant activity from Quillaja saponaria Molina cortex. *J Immunol* 1991;146:431–437.

14. Ragupathi G, Meyers M, Adluri S, Howard L, Musselli C, Livingston PO. Induction of antibodies against GD3 ganglioside in melanoma patients by vaccination with GD3-lactone-KLH conjugate plus immunological adjuvant QS-21. *Int J Cancer* 2000;85:659–666.

15. Cappello S, Liu NX, Musselli C, Brezicka FT, Livingston PO, Ragupathi G. Immunization of mice with fucosyl-GM1-keyhole limpet hemocyanin conjugate results in antibodies against human small-cell lung cancer cells. *Cancer Immunol Immunother* 1999;48:483–492.

16. Ragupathi G, Park TK, Zhang S, et al. Immunization of mice with the synthetic hexasaccharide Globo H results in antibodies against human cancer cells. *Angewandte Chemie* 1997;36:125–128.

17. Kudryashov V, Kim IJ, Ragupathi G, Danishefsky SJ, Livingston PO, Lloyd KO. Immunogenicity of synthetic conjugates of Lewis Y oligosaccharide with protein in mice: towards the design of anti-cancer vaccines. *Cancer Immunol Immunother* 1998;45:281–290.

18. Livingston PO, Koganty R, Longenecker BM, Lloyd KO, Calves M. Studies on the immunogenicity of synthetic and natural Thomsen-Friedenreich (TF) antigens in mice: augmentation of the response by Quil A and SAF-m adjuvants and analysis of the specificity of the responses. *Vaccine Res* 1992;1:99–109.

19. Toyokuni T, Dean B, Cai S, Boivin D, Hakomori S, Singhal AK. Synthetic vaccines: synthesis of a dimeric Tn antigen-lipopeptide conjugate that elicits immune responses against Tn-expressing glycoproteins. *J Am Coll Surg* 1994;116:395–396.

20. Toyokuni T, Singhal AK. Recent progress in synthetic vaccines based on tumor-associated carbohydrate antigens. *Chem Soc Rev* 1995;24: 231–242.

21. Zhang S, Walberg LA, Ogata S, et al. Immune sera and monoclonal antibodies define two configurations for the sialyl Tn tumor antigen. *Cancer Res* 1995;55:3364–3368.

22. Ragupathi G, Koganty R, Qiu D, Lloyd K, Livingston PO. A novel and efficient method for synthetic carbohydrate conjugate vaccine preparation: synthesis of sialyl Tn-KLH conjugate using a 4-(4-N-maleimidomethyl) cyclohexane-1-carboxyl hydrazide (MMCCH) linker arm. *Glycoconj J* 1998;15:217–221.

23. Singhal AK, Fohn M, Hakomori S. Induction of Tn (a-N-acetyl-galactosamine-O-Serine/Threonine) antigen-mediated cellular immune response for active immunotherapy in mice. *Cancer Res* 1991;51:1406–1411.

24. Fung PYS, Madej M, Koganti R, Longenecker BM. Active specific immunotherapy of a murine mammary adenocarcinoma using a synthetic tumor-associated glycoconjugate. *Cancer Res* 1990;50:4308–4314.

25. Tai T, Cahan LD, Tsuchida T, Saxton RE, Irie RF, Morton DL. Immunogenicity of melanoma-associated gangliosides in cancer patients. *Int J Cancer* 1985;35:607.

26. Livingston PO. Approaches to augmenting the immunogenicity of melanoma gangliosides: from whole melanoma cells to ganglioside-KLH conjugate vaccines. *Immunol Rev* 1995;145:145–166.

27. Helling F, Zhang A, Shang A, et al. GM2-KLH conjugate vaccine: increased immunogenicity in melanoma patients after administration with immunological adjuvant QS-21. *Cancer Res* 1995;55:2783–2788.

28. Livingston PO, Zhang S, Walberg L, Ragupathi G, Helling F, Fleischer M. Tumor cell reactivity medicated by IgM antibodies in sera from melanoma patients vaccinated with GM2-KLH is increased by IgG antibodies. *Cancer Immunol Immunotherapy* 1997;43:324–330.

29. Livingston PO, Adluri S, Helling F, et al. Phase I trial of immunological adjuvant QS-21 with a GM2 ganglioside-KLH conjugate vaccine in patients with malignant melanoma. *Vaccine* 1994;12:1275–1280.

30. Chapman PB, Morrissey DM, Panageas KS, et al. Induction of antibodies against GM2 ganglioside by immunizing melanoma patients using GM2-KLH QS21 vaccine: a dose-response study. *Clin Cancer Res* (in press).

31. Chapman P, Morrissey D, Ibrahim J, et al. Eastern cooperative oncology group phase II randomized adjuvant trial of GM2-KLH + QS21 (GMK) vaccine ± high dose interferon-α2b (HD IFN) in melanoma (MEL). (In preparation).

32. Ritter G, Boosfeld E, Adluri R, et al. Antibodies response to immunization with ganglioside GD3 and GD3 congeners (lactones, amide and gangliosidol) in patients with malignant melanoma. *Int J Cancer* 1991;48:379–385.

33. Ritter G, Ritter-Boosfeld E, Adluri R, et al. Analysis of the antibody response to immunization with purified O-acetyl GD3 gangliosides in patients with malignant melanoma. *Int J Cancer* 1995;62:1–5.

34. Merritt WD, Taylor BJ, Der-Minassian V, Reaman GH. Coexpression of GD3 ganglioside with CD45RO in resting and activated human T lymphocytes. *Cell Immunol* 1996;173:131–148.

35. Chapman P, Meyers M, Williams L, et al. Immunization of melanoma patients (pts) with a bivalent GM2/GD2 ganglioside conjugate vaccine. *Am Assoc Clin Res Proc* 1998;39:2515.

36. Dickler MN, Ragupathi G, Liu NX, et al. Immunogenicity of the fucosyl-GM1-keyhole limpet hemocyanin (KLH) conjugate vaccine in patients with small-cell lung cancer. *Clin Cancer Res* 1999;5:2773–2779.

37. Slovin S, Ragupathi G, Adluri S, et al. Carbohydrate vaccines in cancer: immunogenicity of a fully synthetic Globo H hexasaccharide conjugate in man. *Proc Natl Acad Sci U S A* 1999;11:5710–5715.

38. Ragupathi G, Slovin S, Adluri R, et al. Induction of antitumor humoral response by a full synthetic Globo H hexasaccharide-based vaccine in human. *Angewandte Chemie* 1999;38:563–567.

39. Sabbatini P, Kudryashov V, Ragupathi G, et al. Immunization of ovarian cancer patients with a synthetic LewisY–protein conjugate vaccine: clinical and serological results. *Int J Cancer* (in press).

40. Springer GF, Desai PR, Tegtmeyer H, Spencer BD, Scanlon EF. Pan-carcinoma T/Tn antigen detects human carcinoma long before biopsy does and its vaccine prevents breast carcinoma recurrence. *Ann N Y Acad Sci* 1993;690:355–357.

41. O'Boyle KP, Zamore R, Adluri S, et al. Immunization of colorectal cancer patients with modified ovine submaxillary gland mucin and adjuvants induces IgM and IgG antibodies to sialylated Tn. *Cancer Res* 1992;52:5663–5667.

42. McLean GD, Bowen-Yacyshyn MB, Samuel J, et al. Active immunization of human ovarian cancer patients against a common carcinoma (Thomsen-Friedenreich) determinant using a synthetic carbohydrate vaccine. *J Immunother* 1992;11:292–301.

43. Adluri S, Helling F, Calves MJ, Lloyd KO, Livingston PO. Immunogenicity of synthetic TF and sTn-KLH conjugates in colorectal carcinoma patients. *Cancer Immunol Immunother* 1995;41:185–192.

44. Slovin SF, Ragupathi G, Olkiewicz K, et al. Tn-cluster (c) vaccine conjugate in biochemically relapsed prostate cancer (pc): results of a phase I trial studying KLH and PAM. *Am Assoc Clin Res Proc* (in press).

45. MacLean GD, Miles DW, Rubens RD, Reddish MA, Longenecker BM. Enhancing the effect of Theratope STn-KLH cancer vaccine in patients with metastatic breast cancer by pretreatment with low-dose intravenous cyclophosphamide. *J Immunother* 1996;19(4):309–316.

46. Dickler M, Gilewski T, Ragupathi G, et al. Vaccination of breast cancer patients (pts) with no evidence of disease (NED) with sialyl Tn cluster [sTn(c)]-keyhole limpet hemocyanin (KLH) conjugate plus adjuvant QS-21: preliminary results. *Proc Am Soc Clin Oncol* 1997;16:1572.

47. Livingston PO, Wong GYC, Adluri S, et al. Improved survival in AJCC stage III melanoma patients with GM2 antibodies: a randomized trial of adjuvant vaccination with GM2 ganglioside. *J Clin Oncol* 1994;13:1036–1044.

48. MacLean GD, Reddish MA, Koganty RR, Longenecker BM. Antibodies against mucin-associated sialyl-Tn epitopes correlate with survival of metastatic adenocarcinoma patients undergoing active specific immunotherapy with synthetic STn vaccine. *J Immunother* 1996;19(1):59–68.

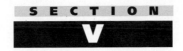

PRINCIPLES AND PRACTICE OF GENE THERAPY

BASIC PRINCIPLES OF GENE THERAPY

Basic Principles and Safety Considerations

KENNETH G. CORNETTA
MICHAEL J. ROBERTSON

Gene therapy can be defined as the transfer of genetic material with therapeutic intent. Gene transfer has become clinically feasible due to elucidation of the molecular basis for many diseases and improvement in techniques for manipulating genetic material in the laboratory. Gene therapy approaches would superficially appear to be best suited for the correction of inherited genetic diseases, such as hemoglobinopathies, immunodeficiency syndromes, and metabolic disorders. Indeed, clinical trials of gene therapy have been undertaken for adenosine deaminase (ADA) deficiency, cystic fibrosis, chronic granulomatous disease, and other genetic disorders. ADA deficiency, the first disease to be treated by gene transfer (1), illustrates characteristics considered to be ideal for successful gene therapy. ADA is a life-threatening disorder caused by mutations in a single human gene that has been cloned. The cells affected by the disease are readily obtainable for *ex vivo* manipulation and expression of the exogenous genetic material confers a selective advantage on the transduced cells. Moreover, precise regulation of transgene expression is not required, because elevated ADA levels do not appear to be harmful and levels as low as 5% of normal can correct the disease phenotype.

Although the inherited genetic diseases are an obvious target for gene therapy approaches, most gene-transfer clinical protocols submitted for regulatory review to date have involved patients with cancer. This reflects in part the inadequacy of conventional treatments for most advanced solid tumors; novel and potentially toxic treatments are considered justifiable in this situation. Moreover, malignant cells harbor genetic mutations that are believed to be responsible for the neoplastic phenotype and that may be amenable to correction through gene transfer approaches. Gene transfer techniques have facilitated the development of novel strategies for cancer therapy (Table 1). This chapter provides a brief summary of the gene transfer systems that are being used currently and then summarizes the safety and regulatory issues involved in producing clinical grade material for human gene therapy studies. It concludes with a discussion of several of these strategies.

GENE TRANSFER TECHNIQUES

The term gene therapy *vector* refers to a system designed to transfer exogenous genetic material (the *transgene*) into a target cell. The simplest systems are vectors composed of naked DNA, usually in the form of plasmid DNA. Plasmids are designed to contain the gene of interest and regulatory elements that enhance gene expression. Plasmid vectors are limited by low gene-transfer efficiency and are not well suited to systemic administration, as the DNA may be degraded before sufficient material is exposed to the target tissue. To address these limitations several viruses have been engineered to transport genetic material (Table 2). Each of these vectors has its advantages and disadvantages. The critical determinants for choosing a particular vector system for a specific application include: (a) host range and tissue specificity; (b) ability to transfer genes to dividing versus nondividing cells; (c) capacity to integrate in the host genome versus episomal maintainance; (d) effects on target-cell viability and potential *in vivo* toxicity; (e) potential to generate replication-competent virus; (f) immunogenicity; (g) ease of manipulation; and (h) the amount of exogenous DNA that can be accommodated.

SAFETY CONSIDERATIONS

General Principles and Regulatory Issues

To justify initiating a particular gene therapy clinical trial, investigators must present evidence that the proposed treatment is reasonably safe for patients. Safety must be evaluated on a number of levels. The possible side effects of transgene expression must be considered. For example, excessive production of factor VIII could cause abnormal clotting after successful factor-VIII gene transfer to patients with hemophilia. Furthermore, the manufacturing process itself must be scrutinized to insure pathogens or toxic materials have not been introduced during vector production and that the generated material has sufficient activity to confer the intended therapeutic benefit (2). Finally,

TABLE 1. SELECTED GENE TRANSFER APPROACHES FOR TREATMENT OF CANCER

Approach	Transgene	Target Cell	Goal
Cancer vaccine	Immunostimulatory molecules or defined tumor antigens[a]	Melanoma, renal cell cancer, other tumors	Stimulate antitumor immune response
Designer T cells	Chimeric T-cell receptor/anti-CEA antibody	Adenocarcinomas	Target effector–T cells to CEA-expressing tumors
Suicide gene	HSV-TK or cytosine deaminase	Mesothelioma, glioma, ovarian, colon, prostate cancer	Render tumor cells sensitive to ganciclovir or 5-fluorocytosine
Tumor-suppressor gene	Wild-type p53	Head and neck, lung, breast cancer	Inhibit proliferation, trigger apoptosis
Antisense	Antisense K-ras	Lung cancer	Inhibit oncogene expression
Myeloprotection	MDR-1, MGMT, DHFR	Hematopoietic stem and progenitor cells	Protect cells from cytotoxic therapy

CEA, carcinoembryonic antigen; DHFR, dihydrofolate reductase; HSV-TK, herpes simplex virus thymidine kinase; MDR-1, multidrug resistance gene 1; MGMT, methylguanine methyltransferase.
[a]Various immunostimulatory molecules (e.g., GM-CSF, IL-2, IL-4, IL-12, B7) and tumor antigens (e.g., MART-1, gp100, CEA, PSA) are under investigation.

the potential risks of the proposed vector system must be addressed; these are discussed more fully here.

In the United States, a variety of regulatory and advisory bodies function to evaluate the safety profile of materials used in clinical gene therapy studies (Fig. 1). An Institutional Review Board must approve and monitor any research study involving human subjects. The Institutional Review Board must assure that clinical trials are based on a reasonable hypothesis and pose no undue risk to subjects participating in the trial. Informed consent must be obtained from patients receiving investigational therapy. Guidelines for conducting Institutional Review Board activity and oversight are provided by the National Institutes of Health (NIH) Office for Protection from Research Risks.

The application of molecular biology techniques in laboratory and clinical settings has raised concern about potential misuse of recombinant genetic material. The Office of Recombinant DNA Activities (ORDA) was formed to oversee recombinant DNA research in the United States. ORDA has established guidelines dictating the containment measures that must be taken by investigators working with recombinant DNA. These are published in the Federal Register as the *NIH Guidelines for Research Involving Recombinant DNA Molecules* (July 5, 1994, 59 FR 34496; and an amendment effective April 29, 1999, published May 11, 1999, 64 FR 25361). The level of containment is determined by the organism from which the DNA is derived, the transgene that is to

be expressed, the amount of viral sequences retained in the vector, and the presence of replication-competent virus. Local Institutional Biosafety Committees (IBC) are charged with insuring that recombinant DNA work is performed in compliance with ORDA regulations. Clinical trials involving use of recombinant DNA must be approved by the local IBC and subsequently submitted to ORDA for consideration by the Recombinant DNA Advisory Committee (RAC) (see Fig. 1). Investigators are required to address the "Points to Consider in the Design and Submission of Protocols for the Transfer of Recombinant DNA Molecules into One or More Human Subjects" listed in Appendix M of the *NIH Guidelines for Research Involving Recombinant DNA Molecules* and to respond to a series of questions regarding vector design, proposed use, and safety risks. An expedited review may be given to those protocols that use previously approved vectors and targets. Novel applications are reviewed before the entire RAC. The charge of the RAC is to insure the clinical trial is scientifically based, considers the ethical implications of the proposed work, and poses no unacceptable health risks to study participants or the population at large.

Vectors to be used for clinical studies in the United States generally require approval by the U.S. Food and Drug Administration (FDA) (3,4). Because gene therapy applications have not yet been approved for general clinical use, investigators are required to submit an Investigational New Drug application

TABLE 2. CHARACTERISTICS OF VIRAL VECTORS

	Murine Retrovirus	Adenovirus	AAV	Herpes Virus	Human Lentivirus
Genome	RNA	ds DNA	ss DNA	ds DNA	RNA
Transgene size[a]	3–7	7–36	2.0–4.5	10–100	8–9
Titer[b]	10^6–10^7	10^{11}–10^{12}	10^6–10^9	10^4–10^{10}	10^6–10^9
Host cell proliferation[c]	Required	Not required	Improves efficiency	Not required	Improves efficiency
Stable integration	Yes	No	Occasional	No	Yes
Immunogenicity	Low	High	Low	Variable	Not well studied

ds, double-stranded; ss, single-stranded.
[a]Approximate size (in kilobases) of transgene that can be accommodated.
[b]Infectious units per mL.
[c]Relationship between host cell proliferation and transduction efficiency.

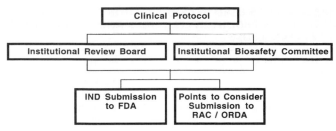

FIGURE 1. Review process for gene therapy protocols. Initial review of gene therapy protocols is performed at the local institutional committees that deal with human subjects and recombinant DNA work. After local approval, protocols are submitted, usually simultaneously, to the Recombinant DNA Advisory Committee (RAC) in the Office of Recombinant DNA Activities (ORDA), and to the U.S. Food and Drug Administration (FDA) in the context of an Investigational New Drug (IND) application.

(IND) that must be reviewed by the FDA before clinical trials are initiated. The FDA has thirty days to respond to an investigator after an IND submission. A hold can be placed on the trial if serious safety concerns are noted. If no concerns are raised, the investigator may begin the trial after the 30-day waiting period. The FDA does not approve vectors for routine clinical purposes but allows them to be used in clinical trials that are based on adequate data (5).

When evaluating an IND, the FDA addresses fundamental issues outlined in the *Code of Federal Regulations* (21 CFR 610, General Biological Products Standards). These include safety, identity, purity, potency, and efficacy. Review of gene therapy proposals is usually performed by the Center for Biologics Evaluation and Research (CBER) within the FDA (4). CBER reviews an IND for its preclinical safety data (toxicology) and manufacturing issues (identity, purity, and potency). Special emphasis is currently placed on safety because of the paucity of clinical efficacy data for gene therapy vectors. In an attempt to insure that the appropriate toxicology studies and an acceptable manufacturing process are identified before IND submission, the FDA encourages telephone conversation and offers the opportunity for a confidential pre-IND meeting early in the process of developing gene therapy clinical trials.

Toxicology studies attempt to determine the risks of vector administration. Safety issues to be addressed include: (a) toxicity of the vector alone (irrespective of the transgene), including its potential tumorigenicity; (b) toxicity of transgene expression *in vivo* that may not be apparent from *in vitro* studies; (c) occurrence and consequences of ectopic transgene expression in non-targeted tissues; (d) occurrence and consequences of immune responses to transgene or vector proteins; and (e) possibility of germ-line transduction. Preclinical toxicology studies should include doses equivalent to and higher than the intended human dose and, when appropriate, the toxic dose should be determined in animals (5). In general, some studies should be performed using the material intended for clinical use to detect contaminants introduced during the manufacturing process. The route of administration is generally the same as that intended for clinical use but studies evaluating other routes may be requested, in particular intravenous routes. Evaluations of animals used for toxicological studies may include blood chemistry evaluations and pathologic examination of organs. The

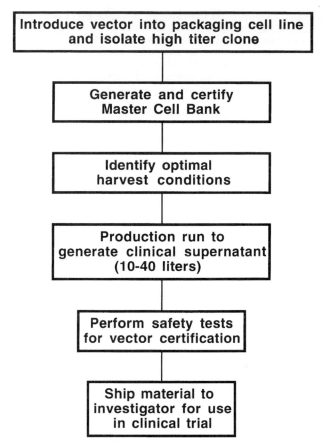

FIGURE 2. Clinical vector production. A schema for retroviral vector production used by the National Gene Vector Laboratory, illustrates the multistep process involved with generation and certification of clinical-grade material.

species required for proper toxicological evaluation may vary with the vector, transgene, route of administration, patient population, and the disease being treated. The cost of these studies can be quite substantial, especially when nonhuman primate studies are required. Early discussion with the FDA during development of a toxicology plan may prevent delays and added expenses due to inadequate data. Recognizing that the costs of toxicological studies are often prohibitive to most gene therapy investigators, the NIH National Centers for Research Resources (NCRR) has provided funds for toxicology studies through the National Gene Vector Laboratories (6). Funds are also available for support of toxicological studies through the National Cancer Institute Rapid Access to Intervention Development (RAID) program for cancer gene therapy protocols.

Proper manufacturing practices must be used for clinical grade vector production (Fig. 2). Production of many vectors, in particular viral vectors, requires unique methods for which specialized testing is needed to ensure adequate purity, potency and identity. Several publications by the FDA and NIH can assist investigators in the design of their production and certification processes (Table 3). For example, production of retroviral vectors requires generation of a vector producer cell line by stable integration of one or more copies of the vector genome into the chromosomes of specially designed packaging cells. In most cases, a clone is selected for its ability to produce vector particles

TABLE 3. "POINTS TO CONSIDER" DOCUMENTS AND FDA PUBLICATIONS ADDRESSING PRODUCTION OF GENE THERAPY VECTORS FOR CLINICAL USE

Guidance for Human Somatic Cell Therapy and Gene Therapy, 1998.

Points to Consider in the Manufacture and Testing of Monoclonal Antibody Products for Human Use, 1997.

Gene Therapy Resource Book, 1996.

Points to Consider in the Characterization of Cell Lines Used to Produce Biologicals, 1993.

Supplement to the Points to Consider in the Production and Testing of New Drugs and Biologicals Produced by Recombinant DNA Technology: Nucleic Acid Characterization and Genetic Stability, 1992.

Points to Consider in Human Somatic Cell Therapy and Gene Therapy, 1991.

Points to Consider in the Production and Testing of New Drugs and Biologicals Produced by Recombinant DNA Technology: Nucleic Acid Characterization and Genetic Stability, 1985.

TABLE 4. TESTS USED IN CERTIFICATION OF MURINE RETROVIRAL PRODUCER CELL LINES AND SUPERNATANT FOR CLINICAL USE

Master Cell Bank	Supernatant
Sterility	Sterility
Mycoplasma	Mycoplasma
RCR (eco, xeno, ampho, or GALV)	RCR (ampho)
Porcine virus	Porcine virus
Bovine virus	Bovine virus
Cell identity	Cell identity
Titer	Titer
In vivo virus assay	Endotoxin
MAP/LCM assay	General safety
In vitro virus assay	—
Vector sequence	—

ampho, amphotropic; eco, ecotropic; GALV, gibbon ape leukemia virus; LCM, lymphochoriomeningitis virus; MAP, murine antibody production; RCR, replication competent retrovirus; xeno, xenotropic.

at high titer. For most phase 1 clinical trials, such a clone is expanded to generate 100 to 200 vials of cells, which are cryopreserved and stored as the Master Cell Bank. Approximately 20 vials are used for certification assays (Table 4) and 10 archived per the *Code of Federal Regulations*. Extensive screening for replication-competent retrovirus is performed to detect recombination between vector and viral sequences within the cell line (1% of cells and 5% of the media must be screened). The use of fetal calf serum and porcine trypsin in the culture of these cells may require screening for bovine and porcine viruses. Because the packaging cell lines are of mouse origin various assays are used to detect contaminating murine pathogens. Sterility and *Mycoplasma* testing are similar to that performed on any product intended for human use and are described in the *Code of Federal Regulations* (21 CFR 610.12 and 610.30, respectively). Production and testing must also follow specific procedures for "Good Laboratory Practice" and "Good Manufacturing Practice" (21 CFR 58 and 21 CFR 210-211, respectively), including documentation and auditing procedures. The testing required for a particular vector varies significantly. For adenoviral vectors produced in human cell lines extensive screening of clinical material for human viruses is required during certification. Gene therapy is a rapidly changing technology. The requirements for toxicologic evaluation and certification continue to evolve as more sophisticated testing methods become available and further data regarding the performance of current producer cell lines and clinical toxicities are generated.

Once a Master Cell Bank is certified a vial of cells is thawed and expanded to generate the clinical grade supernatant. In the National Gene Vector Laboratory at Indiana University, the cells are propagated in roller bottles and approximately 10 to 20 L of material is harvested per run. Aliquots of cell-free supernatant are frozen and stored. Additional safety testing is performed on the supernatant (Table 4), and once complete, the material is shipped to the investigator.

The costs associated with generation of a high-titer clone and Master Cell Bank and production of an adequate volume (~20 to 40 L) of supernatant for a typical phase 1 study are in excess of $100,000 per retroviral vector. In general, production of supernatant is the least complicated and costly step in gener-

ating vector for clinical use. Certification testing in compliance with Good Manufacturing Practice and Good Laboratory Practice is the major cost of producing clinical material and is beyond the capability of most gene therapy investigators. To bridge the gap caused by the expense and effort required to produce this material, the NCRR has created the National Gene Vector Laboratories. This cooperative group of university-based production facilities generates clinical grade plasmid, retroviral, adenoviral, and adeno-associated virus (AAV)–based vectors. After successful review of a submitted application by an oversight committee, the clinical grade material for phase 1 and 2 trials are supplied to the investigator free of charge. To date, 63 clinical trials have been supported by the National Gene Vector Laboratories in fields ranging from cancer, human immunodeficiency virus infection, genetic disease, cardiology, and rheumatology.

SAFETY ISSUES WITH SPECIFIC VECTOR SYSTEMS

Retroviral Vectors

Retroviral vectors are similar to their parent murine leukemia viruses in causing little direct toxicity to the infected cell. It is therefore not anticipated that administration of retroviral vectors to patients results in immediate serious adverse events. The major safety concerns with the clinical use of retroviral vectors relate to two potential delayed toxicities: (a) development of secondary malignancy due to insertional mutagenesis caused by integration of viral sequences into the host cell genome; (b) infection by replication-competent retrovirus. The latter could be generated by homologous recombination *in vitro* during vector preparation in packaging cells or *in vivo* after infection of patient cells by replication-defective vector.

It is not known whether murine retroviruses are pathogenic for humans. Amphotropic murine retrovirus administered intravenously to immunocompetent or moderately immunosuppressed rhesus monkeys is cleared from the serum within 15 minutes. Primate serum is known to inactivate murine retroviruses, which probably explains this rapid viral clearance (7,8).

Despite rapid disappearance of retrovirus from the serum, peripheral blood mononuclear cells of these animals were infected at very low frequencies. However, such infection was not associated with viremia or clinical illness (8). Two studies have evaluated monkeys exposed to replication-competent retrovirus during periods of severe immunosuppression after autologous bone marrow transplantation. Donahue et al. (9) attempted gene transfer into rhesus monkeys by coculturing bone marrow with packaging cells producing vector and replication-competent retrovirus. Three of ten animals developed lethal lymphomas of T-cell origin, which resembled the disease produced in mice by infection with Moloney murine leukemia virus. Two viruses were detected within lymphoma cells of the monkeys. These retroviruses arose by recombination between vector sequences, packaging sequences, and endogenous murine retroviral genome sequences (10,11). In a retrospective study of four monkeys exposed to replication-competent retrovirus in a similar transplant model, animals were clinically well more than 6 years after retrovirus exposure (12). In both studies, monkeys with detectable antiviral antibodies did not develop lymphoma, whereas animals with disease failed to mount antibody responses and had persistent viremia. These findings indicate that murine retroviruses can be pathogenic in severely immunocompromised primates. Great care must be taken, therefore, to ensure that replication-competent retroviruses are not inadvertently administered to patients during gene therapy using retroviral vectors.

Two steps have been taken to decrease the chance of accidental exposure to replication-competent retrovirus. First, packaging cell lines and retroviral vectors have been specifically designed to decrease the likelihood that recombination generates replication-competent virus [(13,14); for a detailed review, 15]. Second, careful screening methods have been developed to test vector preparations for contamination by replication-competent retrovirus (16,17). Guidelines for testing vector preparations before clinical use have been published (18), and the related methodology continues to be refined (19).

The potential for *in vivo* recombination of vectors with human endogenous retroviral sequences (HERV) is also a concern with retroviral gene transfer. The human genome contains many HERV; however, known HERV have mutations that render them replication-defective (20–22). The risk of recombination between HERV and retroviral vectors appears low because murine-based vectors and HERV share little sequence homology and differ in enhancer, promoter, and transfer ribonucleic acid binding sites. Furthermore, the same regions of the viral genome that have been deleted in the construction of retroviral vectors are frequently deleted in HERV sequence. Thus, HERV would be unlikely to complement retroviral vectors even if homologous recombination between them occurs. The factors that limit complementation of retroviral vectors by HERV should also apply to human retroviruses such as HIV and the human T-cell leukemia viruses. This hypothesis is supported by the data of Martineau and colleagues (19), who studied samples obtained from 81 human immunodeficiency virus–infected patients participating in a retroviral gene therapy protocol. No evidence of replication-competent murine retrovirus could be detected by sensitive polymerase chain reaction (PCR) and enzyme-linked immunosorbent assays in more than 500 samples that were tested. It is also reassuring to note that none of the clinical gene therapy trials performed so far have detected patient exposure to replication-competent retrovirus or any malignancies arising as a consequence of insertional mutagenesis.

Other risks, largely of a theoretical kind, could be associated with the use of retroviral vectors for gene therapy. On rare occasions virions can inadvertently package helper-cell messenger RNA (mRNA). A more common event is the transfer of virus-like 30 elements (VL30) (23,24) or intracisternal A-type particles (IAP) (25,26) contained within retroviral packaging cell lines. There are approximately 200 copies of VL30 and 1,000 copies of IAP sequences per haploid genome. Nevertheless, packaging of retroviral vector sequences is at least 10,000 times more likely than packaging of VL30 or IAP sequences. VL30 sequences have been transmitted to monkeys developing lymphoma after exposure to replication-competent retrovirus, but VL30 RNA was not transcribed (11). Transfer of these sequences during retrovirus-mediated gene therapy is not likely to be of clinical significance because both VL30 and IAP genomes are defective and noninfectious (27–29).

Adenoviral Vectors

The safety of adenoviral vectors for human gene therapy has been less well characterized than that of retroviral vectors. Because adenoviral DNA is maintained episomally and rarely integrates into the host genome, the risk of insertional mutagenesis should be minimal (30,31). Indeed, adenoviruses have not been convincingly associated with any human malignancy. However, the risk of generating replication-competent adenovirus is not negligible for first-generation adenoviral vectors. Wild-type, replication-competent adenoviruses generally cause only mild upper respiratory infections in immunocompetent humans (30,31). Nevertheless, fatal systemic adenovirus infections can occur in immunocompromised patients (32,33). Moreover, replication-competent adenovirus could act as a helper to complement the replication of the recombinant virus. This could potentially allow the transgene-containing vector to be disseminated to the tissues of a treated patient and even to be transmitted to other persons. Thus, prudence dictates that recombinant vector material that is to be used in clinical trials must be suitably tested for the presence of replication-competent adenovirus. Several detection methods have been developed, including lysis of noncomplementing cell lines, Southern blot analysis, and PCR techniques (34).

Other Vectors

AAV typically is not pathogenic, and AAV vectors are generally believed to have a favorable safety profile. As is the case with retroviral vectors, however, integration of AAV sequences into the host genome carries a risk of insertional mutagenesis. Furthermore, production of AAV vectors has generally required the use of adenovirus, so the contamination of AAV vector stocks with replication-competent adenovirus is a potential safety concern. At the time of this writing, the FDA is organizing a symposium to discuss safety issues related to AAV vectors with the intention of developing a Master Drug File of preclinical and clinical data related to AAV vector administration. This file serves as a resource and reference for contributing investigators throughout the United States. It also supports IND applications involving AAV vector-based gene transfer that are submitted to the FDA. It has been proposed that the National Gene Vector Laboratory hold and administer this Master Drug File.

Because human lentiviruses can cause serious diseases, including the acquired immunodeficiency syndrome, substantial safety issues must be addressed with respect to the clinical use of lentivirus vectors. Several strategies are being pursued in attempts to improve the safety profile of these vectors. Production of vector by transient transfection using three-plasmid expression systems should greatly decrease the chance of recombination events that could result in generation of replication-competent virus. Deletion of accessory genes from lentivirus vectors does not prevent the transduction of nondividing cells (35,36) and should decrease the risk of toxicity. Development of self-inactivating lentivirus vectors may also enhance their safety (37,38), although similar murine retroviral vectors have not proven clinically useful (39). Most of the published studies regarding lentivirus vectors are concerned with vector design. Animal studies that examine the safety of administering various modified lentivirus vectors are generally lacking. Careful toxicology studies, particularly in nonhuman primates, are required before lentivirus vectors can be used in clinical trials.

ETHICAL ISSUES

The ethical issues surrounding genetic engineering were debated long before gene transfer became technically feasible. The major ethical issues involve three key areas: (a) the goal of gene transfers; (b) the patient population targeted for gene therapy; and (c) the effects of gene transfer on the human germ line.

Goal of Gene Transfer

At least three goals of clinical gene transfer can be envisioned: (a) disease treatment, for which the transferred genetic material is intended to correct a specific genetic defect or modify a disease state; (b) enhancement engineering, whereby a specific phenotype (such as short stature) in a healthy person is altered by single gene insertion; and (c) eugenics, whereby complex human traits (such as personality, intelligence, etc.) are manipulated through alterations in many genes.

Transfer of genetic material for the sole purpose of treating serious disease has not generally provoked major ethical objections from the religious, political, or scientific communities. Current gene therapy protocols have followed the guidelines proposed by Anderson and Fletcher in 1980 (40), which indicate that the ethical application of gene-transfer technology requires demonstration of satisfactory gene transfer and expression as well as acceptable safety in preclinical studies. Specifically, the transgene of interest should be transferred to a sufficient number of target cells and be expressed at high enough levels for an adequate period of time to be of clinical

benefit; transgene expression should not exceed levels that could be detrimental. Preclinical data should be available to predict the toxicity associated with vector administration and transgene expression, so that the risk-to-benefit ratio can be estimated.

Enhancement engineering has not been undertaken so far and remains an area of considerable ethical debate. The advantages and disadvantages of enhancement engineering are similar to those of enhancement procedures that do not involve gene transfer. It has been difficult to achieve consensus regarding a suitable distinction between enhancement procedures versus disease therapy. For example, what height should be used to distinguish short stature that is a normal variant from that which is a medical condition worthy of treatment? Should enhancement be distinguished from treatment using objective criteria (biochemical tests, nomograms, etc.) or social definitions of disability or disadvantage? Anderson has suggested that enhancement gene therapy may have a role in preventive medicine (41). For example, use of gene therapy to increase low-density lipoprotein (LDL) receptor levels and delay the onset of atherosclerosis in asymptomatic persons with familial hypercholesterolemia might be considered an acceptable form of enhancement engineering. Others would argue that this is not enhancement but treatment of a preclinical disease state. Precedent exists for gene therapy before the onset of symptomatic disease. Asymptomatic newborns with ADA deficiency have been treated with autologous cord blood cells transduced with retroviral vector expressing an intact ADA gene (42). Nevertheless, enhancement engineering has raised significant concerns about potential inappropriate use of gene transfer technology. Given known abuses with anabolic steroids, growth hormone, and other performance-enhancing medications, it is not unlikely that unapproved uses of gene therapy for enhancement purposes could be sought by patients or parents. These concerns are aggravated by the virtual absence of data on the long-term effects of gene therapy. If one accepts the premise that ethical gene therapy requires an appropriate risk-to-benefit ratio, better understanding of the long-term consequences of gene therapy is needed before it can be used as a means of enhancing physical or mental abilities.

Eugenics is essentially a subject for philosophic debate, due to the current paucity of data on the genetics of complex human traits. Some of the genetic factors that affect personality, intelligence, growth, and development have been identified, but the sophisticated understanding needed to meaningfully manipulate these traits is lacking. Nevertheless, the possibility of eugenics in the future provokes consideration of how the potential ability to alter complex human traits by genetic manipulation affects our notion of what it is to be human.

Patient Populations Chosen for Gene Therapy

Gene therapy is currently considered an investigational treatment. As is true of any clinical research, ethical conduct of gene therapy studies requires adequate protection of research subjects, including an obligation to obtain informed consent. It has been suggested that, in the early gene therapy clinical trials, the investigational nature of the treatment was not made sufficiently clear to patients (43). However, patients with cystic fibrosis who participated in a phase 1 study of gene therapy appear to have had a realistic understanding of their low probability of clinical benefit (44). There are insufficient data to address this issue rigorously at the present time, and further study is needed.

One of the most active areas of ethical debate in gene therapy is the use of gene transfer in fetuses. Heretofore, diagnosis of some genetic diseases *in utero* has been possible, but corrective treatment for affected fetuses has not been available; the only therapeutic intervention that could be undertaken was elective abortion. Gene therapy offers the possibility of *in utero* treatment and has raised complex ethical issues reviewed by Fletcher and Richter (45). Participation in a fetal gene therapy trial may be morally preferable to abortion because of its potential therapeutic benefit for the fetus and because it is a means of decreasing psychological trauma for the parents. Nevertheless, fetal therapy raises several difficult issues. What is the moral and legal status of the fetus, and does it have rights similar to a child or patient? If so, how are these rights balanced against the rights of the mother? A child may receive medical treatment against his or her parents' wishes when the state determines this to be in the best interest of the child. If effective *in utero* gene therapy becomes available, should the state intervene when a mother refuses treatment for the fetus? Anderson and Zanjani have recently submitted proposals for the treatment of alpha thalassemia and ADA deficiency to the RAC. Their intention is to define and address the ethical issues before submission of an actual clinical research protocol. It has been debated whether current technical limitations in gene transfer are such that any risk to the fetus and mother is unacceptable (46,47). The possibility of germ-line gene transfer, although believed to be remote with current technology, has been a major concern for critics of fetal gene therapy (47). Moreover, a wide range of religious and political opinions persists regarding the acceptability of manipulating fetal tissues. Vigorous debate on this issue continues.

Effects of Gene Transfer on the Human Germ Line

Gene therapy can be divided into somatic cell versus germ-line therapy. In somatic cell gene therapy, a transgene is targeted to somatic cells of an individual with the intention of correcting a disease state. The transgene is not transferred to reproductive tissues and, hence, cannot be passed on to subsequent progeny (i.e., the gene pool is unaffected). In germ-line gene therapy, the vector is capable of insertion into the reproductive tissues, thereby altering the gene pool and having consequences for subsequent generations.

All current applications of gene therapy are directed at somatic cells. Most political and religious groups have not objected to gene therapy that does not affect future progeny. In contrast, germ-line gene therapy has raised major medical and ethical concerns, and very few people have argued in its favor. From a medical perspective, we do not know how a transgene inserted into the human germ line could affect the growth and development of future offspring. Unregulated expression of a transgene could be beneficial in certain adult tissues but could have disastrous consequences for a developing fetus. Resulting abnormalities could cause significant morbidity and mortality in first-generation offspring. More subtle abnormalities could elude detection for sev-

eral generations, allowing dissemination of the deleterious genetic change in the general population. Furthermore, the vector backbone itself could have undesirable consequences and could not be eliminated from the germ line by currently available technology.

Unlike somatic-cell gene therapy, therefore, germ-line therapy requires a broader discussion of whether the risks (both foreseen and unexpected) are outweighed by potential benefit to society. Anderson has argued that germ-line gene therapy could be appropriate if three criteria are met (41). He suggests that sufficient experience with somatic gene therapy be available to gauge safety risks, that adequate animal studies be performed to ensure reproducibility and safety of the germ-line transfer procedure, and that there be public awareness and approval of the procedure. This view is not shared by many, for whom alteration of the gene pool is objectionable for scientific, ethical, or religious reasons. The RAC has stated that it "will not at present entertain proposals for germ-line alterations but will consider proposals involving somatic-cell gene transfer." Currently, most organizations that have considered this issue have recommended a moratorium on germ-line therapy, with continued discussion as the scientific and medical aspects of this approach mature.

In addition to the ethical issues discussed earlier, the development of gene therapy requires consideration of the socioeconomic implications of this new technology. If efficacy is established, gene therapy may prove to be one of the true revolutions in medicine. Nevertheless, the early development relies on free access to reagents (vectors) and support by government funding agencies for investigators in the academic community. Some of the most attractive applications for gene therapy are in genetic diseases that are rare but possess properties that make them ideal candidates for this approach. The rarity of such so-called orphan diseases makes them unattractive targets for investment of research resources by the pharmaceutical industry. Nevertheless, these orphan diseases offer an opportunity to improve gene transfer technology. Many believe that academic institutions are best suited for this initial research (48). How gene therapy approaches are developed by the pharmaceutical industry and how the new technology can be made available to patients in need, especially those in developing countries (49), are challenges as significant as the technical aspects of gene transfer.

GENE TRANSFER APPLICATIONS FOR CANCER THERAPY

Since the first human gene-transfer experiment in 1989 (50), several hundred clinical trials involving gene transfer have been initiated. These clinical trials can be classified into two major categories: (a) gene-marking studies, in which gene transfer is used to determine the fate of cells infused into patients; and (b) gene therapy studies, in which an exogenous gene is expressed in a targeted cell to alter its phenotype in a clinically beneficial way.

GENE MARKING STUDIES

The first human gene transfer clinical trial was a marking study performed by Rosenberg and colleagues to determine the fate of autologous tumor-infiltrating lymphocytes (TILs) after intravenous infusion (50). TILs are lymphocytes isolated from tumor-biopsy specimens and expanded for 4 to 8 weeks *in vitro* using recombinant human interleukin-2 (IL-2) (51,52). Intravenous infusion of expanded TILs together with high-dose bolus injections of IL-2 can induce objective tumor responses in patients with metastatic melanoma (52). The TIL gene-marking study demonstrated the safety of administering retrovirus vector–transduced cells to humans (50). No exposure of patients to replication-competent retrovirus was detected. This study also showed that adoptively transferred TILs can persist *in vivo* for several months and can home to sites of autologous tumor.

Gene-marking studies have also been used to investigate the biology of autologous hematopoietic stem-cell transplantation. Brenner and colleagues have unequivocally shown that neoplastic cells infused in autologous stem-cell products can contribute to relapse after high-dose therapy for acute leukemia and neuroblastoma (53,54). Similar studies have shown that leukemic cells in autografts contribute to relapse of chronic myelogenous leukemia after autologous transplantation (55). These gene-marking studies have also demonstrated that normal progenitor cells in the autografts contribute to long-term hematopoiesis after engraftment (55,56).

GENE THERAPY STUDIES

Gene-marking techniques represent a powerful new tool for addressing clinically relevant issues in cancer therapy. However, the remainder of this chapter focuses on the use of gene transfer with therapeutic intent. Some ongoing approaches to cancer therapy using gene-transfer technology are summarized in Table 1 and discussed here.

Stimulation or Enhancement of Antitumor Immunity

A major strategy for exploiting gene transfer techniques in cancer therapy involves attempts to promote antitumor immune responses. Preclinical studies have conclusively shown that the mammalian immune system can recognize and eliminate malignant tumor cells *in vivo* (57,58). Depending on the particular experimental system used, participation of helper effector T cells, cytotoxic T-lymphocytes (CTLs), natural killer (NK) cells, and other cell types has been implicated in the eradication of tumor cells in preclinical animal models. Clear understanding of the gene-transfer approaches for promoting antitumor immunity requires some knowledge of fundamental immunology.

Optimal activation of naïve CD4$^+$ T cells requires at least two major signals (59,60). Signal 1 is provided by ligation of the T-cell receptor (TCR) complex by specific antigenic peptide bound in the cleft of major histocompatibility complex–class II molecules. Signal 2, also known as *costimulation*, is provided by engagement of CD28 on the T-cell surface by members of the B7 family of costimulatory molecules on the surface of professional antigen-presenting cells (APCs). Although activated B cells and monocytes can function as APCs, the most potent known APCs for T-cell activation are

dendritic cells (61). Following activation and clonal expansion, activated CD4$^+$ T cells differentiate into helper effector cells of either the Th1 or Th2 phenotype (62,63). Th1 cells produce cytokines, such as IL-2, IFN-γ, and tumor necrosis factor (TNF), that stimulate monocytes and NK cells and promote the differentiation of activated CD8$^+$–T cells into CTLs. Thus, Th1 cells are crucial for the development of cell-mediated immune responses to intracellular pathogens and some neoplastic cells. In contrast, Th2 cells produce cytokines, such as IL-4, IL-5, IL-10, and IL-13, that promote humoral immunity and the recruitment and activation of eosinophils. Th2 cells are characteristically recruited during immune responses to helminths and other extracellular pathogens. Whether a CD4$^+$ T cell develops into a Th1 or Th2 effector cell appears to depend predominantly on the cytokine milieu present when the cell is activated and undergoing differentiation (62,63).

Activation of naïve CD8$^+$ T cells also requires two signals. Ligation of the T-cell receptor by peptide antigen/major histocompatibility complex–class-I complexes provides signal 1; the nature of signal 2 for CD8$^+$ T cells has not been fully elucidated but requires the presence of helper CD4$^+$ T cells. It appears that an important costimulatory ligand for CD8$^+$ T cells is transiently expressed on APCs after the latter interact with activated CD4$^+$ T cells (64–66). Induction of the costimulatory ligand requires interactions between CD40 on the APC and CD40 ligand transiently expressed on activated CD4$^+$ T cells. Differentiation of activated CD8$^+$ T cells into functional CTLs is promoted by cytokines produced by Th1–helper-effector cells (62,63).

Despite extensive preclinical data demonstrating the existence of antitumor immune responses *in vivo*, it is obvious that most patients with cancer have not mounted an effective immune response to their tumor. This could be due to defects in antigen presentation, costimulation, or differentiation of activated T cells into functional effector cells. Gene therapy strategies have been developed to address each of these possibilities.

Gene Transfer into Tumor Cells: Cancer Vaccines

A major gene transfer approach for cancer therapy is the introduction of genes into tumor cells to promote their immunogenicity. Extensive preclinical studies have shown that introduction of genes encoding immunostimulatory molecules can induce the rejection of malignant tumor cells (Table 5). For example, transduction of the B7-1 or B7-2 genes into murine tumor-cell lines does not affect their growth *in vitro* or in immunodeficient mice but markedly reduces their tumorigenicity in immunocompetent syngeneic mice (67–69). In contrast, syngeneic mice depleted of CD8$^+$ T cells fail to reject B7-transduced tumor cells, confirming the participation of CD8 T cells in tumor rejection. Immunocompetent mice that have rejected B7-transduced tumor cells can subsequently reject an implant of nontransduced tumor cells. This suggests that vaccination with B7-transduced tumor cells can elicit durable antitumor immunity. However, transduction of B7-1 or B7-2 into poorly immunogenic tumors does not stimulate effective immune responses (67,69). Thus, B7 gene transfer may not be optimal

TABLE 5. SELECTED PRECLINICAL STUDIES OF GENE-TRANSDUCED TUMOR CELLS

Author (Reference)	Cytokine Gene Transduced into Tumor Cells	Tumor Model	Reduction of Tumorigenicity[a]	Response in Established Tumors[b]	Induction of Durable Tumor Immunity[c]
Vieweg (73)	IL-2	MatLyLu prostate cancer	Yes	Yes	Yes
Golumbek (127)	IL-4	Renca renal cell cancer	Yes	Yes	Yes
Porgador (128)	IL-6	D122 lung cancer	Yes	Yes	Yes
Aoki (129)	IL-7	203 glioma	Yes	Not reported	Yes
Tahara (72)	IL-12	MCA207, 102 sarcoma	Yes	Yes	Yes
Gansbacher (130)	IFN-γ	CMS-5 sarcoma	Yes	No	Yes
Asher (131)	TNF-α	MCA205 sarcoma	Yes	No	Yes
Dranoff (71)	GM-CSF	B16 melanoma	Not evaluable	Yes	Yes
Chen (78)	Flt3 ligand	C3L5 breast cancer	Yes	Not reported	Yes
Townsend (68)	B7-1	K1735 melanoma	Yes	Not reported	Yes
Yang (69)	B7-2	P815 mastocytoma	Yes	Not reported	Yes

IL, interleukin.
[a]Effects of transducing gene on the ability of tumor cells to grow in syngeneic animals.
[b]Effects of vaccination with cytokine-transduced tumor cells on established nontransduced tumors.
[c]Ability to reject subsequent challenge with nontransduced tumors.

for cancer vaccine strategies involving poorly immunogenic human tumors.

An alternative approach is transduction of tumor cells with genes encoding cytokines (70). This approach allows high levels of cytokines to be produced in the vicinity of the transduced tumor cells, thus potentially avoiding the toxicities associated with systemic administration of pharmacologic doses of cytokines. Paracrine production of cytokines might also mimic more closely the situation that occurs during physiologic immune responses. Paracrine production of several cytokines using this approach has been shown to inhibit tumorigenicity and promote durable, specific antitumor immunity in preclinical models (see Table 5). Unlike B7 gene transfer, cytokine gene transfer has proved efficacious even in models using poorly immunogenic tumors (71,72). Furthermore, vaccination with tumor cells transduced with several cytokines can provoke the rejection of established, nontransduced tumors (72–74). These results raise the hope that cancer vaccine therapy could be used to treat patients with cancer.

The mechanisms by which vaccination with cytokine gene–transduced tumor cells stimulate tumor rejection and durable antitumor immunity have not been completely defined and are probably variable. IL-2 and IL-12 secreted by transduced tumor cells presumably directly stimulate immunologic effector cells, such as CD4+–T cells, CD8+–T cells, or NK cells (72,73). In some animal models, granulocyte-macrophage colony-stimulating factor (GM-CSF)–transduced tumor cells stimulate antitumor immunity more potently than tumor cells expressing several known immunostimulatory molecules (71,75). It is believed that paracrine production of GM-CSF leads to the recruitment and activation of professional APCs, and that presentation of tumor antigens by these activated APCs potently induces specific T-cell immune responses (71). Flt3 ligand strongly induces differentiation and expansion of dendritic cells *in vitro* and *in vivo* (76,77). Stimulation of dendritic cells may thus account in part for the efficacy of vaccination with Flt3 ligand-transduced tumor cells in a breast cancer model (78). Nevertheless, NK cells may also contribute to the elimination of

malignant tumors after vaccination with GM-CSF or Flt3 ligand gene-transduced cancer vaccines (74,79).

Many clinical trials of cancer vaccination using gene-transduced tumor cells have been initiated (Table 6). These clinical trials involve autologous or allogeneic tumor cells that have been transduced *in vitro* with genes encoding immunostimulatory cytokines or costimulatory molecules. Results of a phase 1 clinical trial of vaccination with irradiated, GM-CSF gene-transduced autologous melanoma cells have been published (80). Autologous tumor cells were successfully harvested and transduced with the GM-CSF gene using replication-incompetent retroviral vector for 29 of 33 patients. Delayed-type hypersensitivity reactions in response to intradermal injection of irradiated, nontransduced autologous melanoma cells occurred after vaccination in all 21 evaluable patients. These reactions were characterized by dense infiltration by T lymphocytes and eosinophils. Immune responses to metastatic lesions could be detected in 11 of 16 patients from whom metastases were resected after vaccination. These were characterized by diffuse infiltration of metastatic lesions by T cells and plasma cells, extensive necrosis of melanoma cells, and fibrosis. Antimelanoma IgG antibodies were detected after vaccination in the serum of seven patients who were tested. Minor objective tumor responses were observed in five patients. This study confirmed the feasibility and safety of administering irradiated, GM-CSF gene-transduced autologous tumor cells to patients with metastatic melanoma. Demonstration of antimelanoma immune

TABLE 6. CLINICAL TRIALS OF GENE-TRANSDUCED TUMOR CELLS

Tumor Cells	Transgene	Tumor Types
Autologous	IL-2, IL-4, IFN-γ, GM-CSF, B7-1	Melanoma, renal cell cancer, breast cancer, ovarian cancer, prostate cancer, lung cancer, neuroblastoma
Allogeneic	IL-2, B7-1	Melanoma, renal cell cancer, breast cancer

responses in treated patients supports further clinical evaluation of this vaccine strategy.

Although successful *in vitro* gene transfer into autologous tumor cells has been shown in several cancer vaccine studies, several limitations to this approach exist. Patients without readily accessible superficial metastases must undergo invasive surgical procedures to obtain autologous tumor. Furthermore, routine growth of autologous tumor cells *in vitro* has proved difficult for many common cancers. Several approaches have been taken to circumvent these problems. Use of allogeneic tumor-cell lines obviates the need to obtain autologous tumor samples for vaccine production. Moreover, these cell lines can be readily grown *in vitro*. Clinical trials of cancer vaccines based on allogeneic cell lines are in progress for melanoma, renal cell cancer, and breast cancer. Disadvantages of this approach include the potential hazards of exposing patients to allogeneic tumor-cell lines and possible lack of shared antigens between the cell lines and patients' autologous tumor cells. A different strategy for producing autologous tumor vaccines is *in vivo* injection of tumor masses with transgene-containing vectors. Clinical research protocols have been developed in which vectors encoding IL-2, IL-12, GM-CSF, IFN-γ, or B7-1 are injected into tumor masses *in situ*. Preliminary results of some of these trials have been reported (81–83). Although retrovirus vectors have been used in many of these clinical trials, adenoviral vectors may be better suited for this approach. Because prolonged expression of the transgene is not required, the failure of adenoviral vectors to stably integrate is not a problem. Unlike retroviral vectors, adenoviral vectors can efficiently transduce nondividing cells. Because the malignant cells in most macroscopic tumors are not actively dividing at any given time, it is expected that transgene expression in most primary tumors is higher after transduction using adenoviral as opposed to retroviral vectors. Furthermore, the intrinsic immunogenicity of adenoviral vectors may be advantageous in this setting (84). Adenoviral sequences could act as an adjuvant in stimulating specific antitumor immune responses. Moreover, adenoviral peptides could promote nonspecific destruction of the transduced tumor cells, leading to uptake of tumor-specific antigens by professional APCs. Several clinical studies of cancer vaccines produced by transduction of tumor cells with adenoviral vectors are being conducted (85–87).

Gene Transfer into Normal Cells: Cancer Vaccines

An alternative gene therapy strategy for generating cancer vaccines is transfer of vectors encoding tumor antigens. Although true "tumor-specific" antigens have not been clearly defined in humans, several tumor-associated antigens have been shown to be suitable targets for cancer vaccine approaches in preclinical models. Clinical studies of local or systemic injection of vectors encoding carcinoembryonic antigen, prostate specific antigen, and the melanoma-associated antigens MART-1 and gp100 are in progress (83,88). An advantage of this approach is its relative simplicity compared with generation of autologous tumor-cell vaccines. Furthermore, the antigenic stimulus is known, allowing monitoring of specific immune responses as a surrogate end

point. A theoretical disadvantage is that the antitumor immune response stimulated by this approach would be focused on a single antigen. Selection *in vivo* for antigen-loss variants could thus limit the efficacy of this approach. In contrast, autologous tumor-cell vaccines could potentially induce immune responses to multiple tumor antigens, some of which might be required for maintenance of the neoplastic phenotype.

Gene Transfer into Normal Cells: Adoptive Immunotherapy

Gene transfer can also be used to modify immune effector cells in attempts to promote antitumor immune responses. The Rosenberg group has introduced the TNF gene into TILs used for adoptive immunotherapy of cancer (89). High concentrations of TNF produced by transduced TIL that accumulates at tumor sites after intravenous injection could enhance the efficacy of TIL therapy. A different strategy for adoptive immunotherapy involves the transfer of chimeric TCR/antibody genes (90). Investigators have engineered chimeric genes that encode the variable regions of the immunoglobulin gene linked to the ζ chain of the TCR. Transduction of this gene into polyclonal T cells allows the latter to be triggered by cells that express the antigen recognized by the antibody encoded by the native immunoglobulin gene. Infusion of chimeric TCR/antibody gene-transduced T cells can successfully treat antigen-bearing tumor cells in preclinical models (91,92). Clinical trials of adoptive immunotherapy using chimeric TCR/antibody-transduced autologous T cells have been developed for patients with ovarian and colorectal cancer.

INTRODUCTION OF SUICIDE GENES

Suicide genes encode proteins that convert relatively nontoxic molecules into toxic species. For example, the herpes simplex virus thymidine kinase (HSV-TK) is about 1,000-fold more efficient than mammalian thymidine kinases at phosphorylating ganciclovir. Ganciclovir monophosphate can then be sequentially converted by mammalian thymidine kinases to ganciclovir triphosphate, which inhibits DNA polymerase and is thus toxic to cells. Systemic administration of ganciclovir after intratumoral injection of fibroblasts transduced with an HSV-TK retroviral vector can induce regression of gliomas in rats (93). Adjacent normal brain tissue exhibited no toxicity; this was expected, because normal brain tissue does not proliferate and therefore should not be susceptible to transduction by retroviral vectors. The efficacy of HSV-TK transduction of tumors followed by ganciclovir therapy has been confirmed in several preclinical models (94). Major tumor regression has been observed despite the observation that only a small fraction of tumor cells generally has been transduced with the HSV-TK gene. The nature of the "bystander effect" of transduced on nontransduced tumor cells appears to be complex and remains to be fully elucidated. Diffusion of phosphorylated ganciclovir species from transduced to nontransduced cells via gap junctions occurs *in vitro* (95) and may contribute to the bystander effect *in vivo*. However, some investigators have found that immune effector cells participate in the bystander effect *in vivo* (96,97). Indeed, preclinical studies have shown that HSV-TK gene therapy and immunostimulatory therapy can exert synergistic antitumor effects in murine models (97).

Clinical trials of HSV-TK suicide gene therapy have been initiated. Several investigators are conducting studies in which ganciclovir is given after the HSV-TK gene has been introduced into tumor cells *in vivo* using retroviral or adenoviral vectors. This approach is being tested in patients with brain tumors, mesothelioma, or ovarian cancer. The generally higher transduction efficiency of adenoviral vectors is a potential advantage for this approach (98). Moreover, the strong immunogenicity of adenoviral vectors might provoke immune destruction of transduced tumor cells and enhance the immunologic component of the bystander effect (84). However, increased toxicity could also occur due to destruction of normal tissues that have been transduced by the adenoviral vector. Retroviral vectors, which transduce only dividing cells, might thus be preferred for situations in which avoidance of adjacent normal tissue damage is particularly important (e.g., treatment of brain tumors).

An alternative strategy for suicide gene therapy involves transducing allogeneic immunocompetent cells with the HSV-TK gene before adoptive transfer. A majority of patients with chronic myelogenous leukemia in hematologic or cytogenetic relapse after allogeneic BMT who are given donor leukocyte infusions (DLI) achieves durable molecular remissions (99,100). DLI has also been successfully used to treat posttransplant Epstein-Barr virus (EBV)-related lymphoproliferative disorders (101). However, DLI is associated with a substantial risk of graft-versus-host disease (GVHD). Bonini has reported a study in which HSV-TK–transduced donor leukocytes were given to eight patients with relapsed leukemia or EBV-associated lymphoproliferative disease after BMT (102). Transduced cells could be detected in the bone marrow and peripheral blood of all but one patient for up to 12 months postinfusion and antitumor responses were observed in five patients. Two patients developed acute GVHD after DLI. PCR-detectable transgene-expressing cells and clinical signs of GVHD disappeared in both patients after administration of intravenous ganciclovir. A third patient developed chronic GVHD after DLI, which improved after ganciclovir therapy; transgene-expression cells were decreased but not eliminated by ganciclovir in this patient. Clinical trials are being conducted at several centers using HSV-TK–transduced donor leukocytes to treat malignancy relapse and certain infectious complications after bone marrow transplantation.

Another suicide gene under active investigation for cancer therapy is the cytosine deaminase gene (103,104). Cytosine deaminase converts the nontoxic fluoropyrimidine 5-fluorocytosine to 5-fluorouracil. 5-Fluorouracil is converted by endogenous cellular enzymes into fluorodeoxyuridine monophosphate, which inhibits thymidylate synthase activity, and fluorouridine triphosphate, which can be incorporated into RNA and interfere with RNA processing and transcription (105). Transduction of the cytosine deaminase gene renders tumor cells exquisitely sensitive to 5-fluorocytosine *in vitro* and *in vivo*. As with HSV-TK gene transfer, evidence exists that cytosine-deam-

inase gene transfer into tumor cells promotes antitumor immune responses (103).

Replacement of Defective Tumor-Suppressor Genes

Several tumor-suppressor genes, including p53, RB, APC, and WT1, were identified by their association with rare kindreds afflicted by hereditary cancers (106,107). However, it is now known that many common sporadic tumors harbor inactivating or recessive mutations in one or more tumor-suppressor genes. Gene transfer techniques can be applied to introduce wild-type copies of tumor-suppressor genes into malignant cells, thus potentially reversing the neoplastic phenotype. There has been considerable interest in targeting the p53-tumor suppressor gene for this approach. p53 mutations occur commonly in a variety of human cancers, including those of breast, lung, colon, prostate, bladder, and cervix (108). Transduction of a p53 transgene has been shown to inhibit tumor growth both *in vitro* and *in vivo* (109–113). Use of adenoviral vectors to deliver the p53 transgene to human tumors is being evaluated in phase 1 clinical trials (114). Objective responses of some tumors injected with the viral vector have been described. Preclinical studies also support gene replacement therapy using vectors encoding p21, p16, and RB (115,116). Given the relatively low gene transfer efficiencies achieved with currently available vectors, however, it is difficult to believe that tumor-suppressor gene therapy can be efficacious for bulky or disseminated cancers. Despite a possible bystander effect of gene therapy on nontransduced tumor cells, effective replacement of tumor-suppressor genes most likely requires technical advances in gene transfer efficiency.

Inhibition of Transforming Oncogenes

In contrast to tumor-suppressor genes, oncogenes promote neoplastic transformation by acquiring dominant or gain-of-function mutations. Excessive expression or dysregulated activity of the protein products of oncogenes is believed to contribute to the malignant phenotype (107,117). Thus, disruption of oncogene expression could be therapeutically beneficial. The antisense strategy includes several related approaches for achieving this goal. Antisense oligodeoxynucleotides are synthetic nucleotides that are complementary to short sequences of specific mRNAs (116,118). When successfully introduced into a cell, the antisense oligonucleotide can bind to the mRNA, preventing its translation and/or accelerating its degradation. Antisense oligonucleotides have been shown to efficiently inhibit *in vitro* the activity of several oncogenes. Moreover, antisense oligonucleotides specific for bcl/abl, c-myc, c-myb, and c-raf-1 have been shown to inhibit *in vivo* tumorigenesis in murine models (119–121). A major limitation of systemic antisense therapy is the rapid degradation of oligonucleotides *in vivo* and their inefficient uptake into potential target cells. Modifications of their phosphate backbone have rendered antisense oligonucleotides more resistant to digestion by nucleases. Antisense oligonucleotides have been conjugated to lipophils and incorporated into liposomes in attempts to enhance their delivery to target cells (118).

An alternative approach is to transduce cells with vectors encoding antisense RNA. Complementary DNA encoding antisense RNA can be delivered using any of the viral vectors systems described above. This approach has been used to successfully inhibit the expression of c-myc and K-ras *in vitro* and to reverse the transformed phenotype of cell lines *in vitro* and their tumorigenicity *in vivo* (122–125). Phase 1 clinical trials of retroviral vectors encoding antisense mRNA specific for K-ras are in progress (126).

CONCLUSION

The number of gene therapy clinical trials has increased exponentially since the results of the first gene-marking study were published in 1990 (50). Most of these clinical trials have involved patients with cancer. A variety of strategies are being developed that use gene-transfer technique for cancer therapy; however, unequivocal clinical benefit has yet to be shown in any gene therapy trial. Assessment of the therapeutic efficacy of gene transfer approaches requires longer follow-up and additional studies. Almost all gene therapy trials performed to date have been phase 1 studies that sought to evaluate safety and address issues regarding dose and schedule. Several gene therapy applications are poised to enter phase 2 studies that can begin to evaluate efficacy. Nevertheless, many of the phase 1 trials have demonstrated low gene transfer efficiencies. Thus, the value of extensive phase 2 testing is doubtful unless gene transfer efficiency can be substantially improved. Indeed, technical limitations currently represent the major obstacle to progress in gene therapy. These limitations are being addressed by ongoing basic research efforts, including the development of improved vector systems. As gene-transfer technology becomes more powerful and sophisticated, anticipated outcomes and ethical issues also need to be continually addressed (43).

Animal models of genetic diseases indicate that gene therapy has considerable potential. Preclinical tumor models have also been encouraging. However, translating successful approaches developed in animal models to human cancer therapy has proved notoriously difficult. Therefore, data from preclinical gene therapy studies must be viewed with caution. Nevertheless, gene-transfer techniques have made possible a variety of novel approaches for cancer treatment. Solutions to the technical challenges of gene delivery and expression should allow exploration of new therapeutic options for patients with cancer.

REFERENCES

1. Blaese RM. Treatment of severe combined immunodeficiency due to adenosine deaminase deficiency with autologous lymphocytes transduced with a human ADA gene. *Hum Gene Ther* 1990;1:327.
2. Ostrove JM. Safety testing programs for gene therapy viral vectors. *Cancer Gene Ther* 1994;1:125.
3. Epstein SL. Regulatory concerns in human gene therapy. *Human Gene Ther* 1991;2:243.
4. Kessler DA, Siegel JP, Noguchi PD, Zoon KC, Feiden KL, Woodcock J. Regulation of somatic-cell therapy and gene therapy by the Food and Drug Administration. *N Engl J Med* 1993;329:1169.
5. Epstein SL. The regulatory process and gene therapy. In: E Wickstrom, ed. *Clinical trials of genetic therapy with antisense DNA and DNA vectors.* New York: Marcel Dekker, 1998:89.
6. Advancing gene therapy from bench to bedside. *NCRR Reporter* 1998;22:15.
7. Banapour B, Sernatinger J, Levy JA. The AIDS associated retrovirus is not sensitive to lysis or inactivation by human serum. *J Virol* 1986;152:268.
8. Cornetta K, Moen RC, Culver K, et al. Amphotropic murine leukemia retrovirus is not an acute pathogen for primates. *Hum Gene Ther* 1990;1:15.
9. Donahue RE, Kessler SW, Bodine D, et al. Helper virus induction of T cell lymphoma in nonhuman primates after retroviral mediated gene transfer. *J Exp Med* 1992;176:1125.
10. Vanin EF, Kaloss M, Broscius C, Nienhuis AW. Characterization of replication-competent retroviruses from non-human primates with virus-induced T cell lymphomas and observations regarding the mechanism of oncogenesis. *J Virol* 1994;68:4241.
11. Purcell DFJ, Broscius CM, Vanin EF, Buckler CE, Nienhuis AW, Martin MA. An array of murine leukemia virus-related elements is transmitted and expressed in a primate recipient of retroviral gene transfer. *J Virol* 1996;70:887.
12. Cornetta K, Morgan RA, Gillio A, et al. No retroviremia or pathology in long-term follow-up of monkeys exposed to a murine amphotropic retrovirus. *Hum Gene Ther* 1991;2:215.
13. Mann R, Mulligan RC, Baltimore D. Construction of a retrovirus packaging mutant and its use to produce helper-free defective retrovirus. *Cell* 1983;33:153.
14. Watanabe S, Temin HM. Construction of a helper cell line for avian reticuloendotheliosis virus cloning vectors. *Mol Cell Biol* 1983; 3:2241.
15. Miller AD. Retrovirus packaging cells. *Hum Gene Ther* 1990;1:5.
16. Forestell SP, Dando JS, Bohnlein E, Rigg RJ. Improved detection of replication-competent retroviruses. *J Virol Methods* 1996;60:171.
17. Cornetta K, Nguyen N, Morgan RA, Muenchau DD, Hartley J, Anderson WF. Infection of human cells with murine amphotropic replication-competent retroviruses. *Hum Gene Ther* 1993;4:579.
18. Wilson CA, Ng T, Miller AE. Evaluation of recommendations for replication-competent retrovirus testing associated with use of retroviral vectors. *Hum Gene Ther* 1997;8:869.
19. Martineau D, Klump WM, McCormack JE, et al. Evaluation of PCR and ELISA assays for screening clinical trial subjects for replication-competent retrovirus. *Hum Gene Ther* 1997;8:1231.
20. Bonner TI, O'Connell C, Cohen M. Cloned endogenous retroviral sequences from human DNA. *Proc Natl Acad Sci U S A* 1982;79:4709.
21. Rabson AB, Hamagishi Y, Steele PE, Tykocinski M, Martin MA. Characteristics of human endogenous retroviral envelope RNA transcripts. *J Virol* 1985;56:176.
22. Repaske R, Steele PE, O'Neill RR, Rabson AB, Martin MA. Nucleotide sequence of a full-length human endogenous retroviral segment. *J Virol* 1985;54:764.
23. Courtney MG, Elder PK, Steffen DL, Getz MJ. Organization and expression of endogenous virus-like (VL30) DNA sequences in nontransformed and chemically transformed mouse embryo cells in culture. *Cancer Res* 1982;42:569.
24. Hatzoglou M, Hodgson CP, Mularo F. Efficient packaging of a specific VL30 retroelement by two cells which produce MoMLV recombinant retroviruses. *Hum Gene Ther* 1990;1:385.
25. Lueders KK, Kuff EL. Intracisternal A-particle genes: identification in the genome of Mus musculus and comparison of multiple isolates from a mouse gene library. *Proc Natl Acad Sci U S A* 1980;77:3571.
26. Ono M, Cole MD, White AT, Huang RC. Sequence organization of cloned intracisternal A-particle genes. *Cell* 1980;21:465.
27. Mietz JA, Grossman Z, Lueders KK, Kuff EL. Nucleotide sequence of a complete mouse intracisternal A-particle genome: relationship to known aspects of a particle assembly and function. *J Virol* 1987;6:3020.
28. Morgan RA, Cornetta K, Anderson WF. Application of polymerase chain reaction in retroviral-mediated gene transfer and the analysis of

gene-marked human TIL cells. *Hum Gene Ther* 1990;1:136.

29. Adams SE, Rathjen PS, Stanway CA, Fulton SM. Complete nucleotide sequence of a mouse VL30 retro-element. *Mol Cell Biol* 1988;8:2989.

30. Hitt MM, Addison CL, Graham FL. Human adenovirus vectors for gene transfer into mammalian cells. *Adv Pharmacol* 1997;40:137.

31. Leber SM, Yamagata M, Sanes JR. Gene transfer using replication-defective retroviral and adenoviral vectors. *Methods Cell Biol* 1996; 51:161.

32. Blanke C, Clark C, Broun ER, et al. Evolving pathogens in allogeneic bone marrow transplantation: increased fatal adenoviral infections. *Am J Med* 1995;99:326.

33. Shields AF, Hackman RC, Fife KH, Corey L, Meyers JD. Adenovirus infections in patients undergoing bone-marrow transplantation. *N Engl J Med* 1985;312:529.

34. Lochmuller H, Jani A, Huard J, et al. Emergence of early region 1-containing replication-competent adenovirus in stocks of replication-defective adenovirus recombinants (ΔE1+ΔE3) during multiple passages in 293 cells. *Hum Gene Ther* 1994;5:1485.

35. Reiser J, Harmison G, Kluepfel-Stahl S, Brady RO, Karlsson S, Schubert M. Transduction of nondividing cells using pseudotyped defective high-titer HIV type 1 particles. *Proc Natl Acad Sci U S A* 1996;93:15266.

36. Kim VN, Mitrophanous K, Kingsman SM, Kingsman AJ. Minimal requirement of a lentivirus vector based on human immunodeficiency virus type 1. *J Virol* 1998;72:811.

37. Miyoshi H, Blomer U, Takahashi M, Gage FH, Verma IM. Development of a self-inactivating lentivirus vector. *J Virol* 1998;72:8150.

38. Zufferey R, Dull T, Mandel RJ, et al. Self-inactivating lentivirus vector for safe and efficient *in vivo* gene delivery. *J Virol* 1998;72:9873.

39. Yu S-F, Ruden TV, Kantoff PW, et al. Self-inactivating retroviral vectors designed for transfer of whole genes into mammalian cells. *Proc Natl Acad Sci U S A* 1986;83:3194.

40. Anderson WF, Fletcher JC. Gene therapy in human beings: when is it ethical to begin? *N Engl J Med* 1980;303:1293.

41. Anderson WF. Human gene therapy: scientific and ethical considerations. *J Med Philos* 1985;10:275.

42. Kohn DB, Weinberg KI, Nolta JA, et al. Engraftment of gene-modified umbilical cord blood cells in neonates with adenosine deaminase deficiency. *Nat Med* 1995;1:1017.

43. King NMP. Rewriting the "points to consider": the ethical impact of guidance document language. *Hum Gene Ther* 1999;10:133.

44. Blair C, Kacser E, Porteous C. Gene therapy for cystic fibrosis: a psychosocial study of trial participants. *Gene Ther* 1998;5:218.

45. Fletcher JC, Richter G. Human fetal gene therapy: moral and ethical questions. *Hum Gene Ther* 1996;7:1605.

46. Schneider H, Coutelle C. In utero gene therapy: the case for. *Nat Med* 1999;5:256.

47. Billings PR. In utero gene therapy: the case against. *Nat Med* 1999;5:255.

48. Hillman AL. Gene therapy: socioeconomic and ethical issues. A roundtable discussion. *Hum Gene Ther* 1996;7:1139.

49. Sikora K. Gene therapy in the developing world. *Gene Ther* 1998;5:3.

50. Rosenberg SA, Aebersold P, Cornetta K, et al. Gene transfer into humans—immunotherapy of patients with advanced melanoma, using tumor infiltrating lymphocytes modified by retroviral gene transduction. *N Engl J Med* 1990;323:570.

51. Topalian SL, Muul LM, Solomon D, Rosenberg SA. Expansion of human tumor infiltrating lymphocytes for use in immunotherapy trials. *J Immunol Methods* 1987;102:127.

52. Rosenberg SA, Packard BS, Aebersold PM, et al. Use of tumor-infiltrating lymphocytes and interleukin-2 in the immunotherapy of patients with metastatic melanoma. A preliminary report. *N Engl J Med* 1988;319:1676.

53. Brenner MK, Rill DR, Moen RC, et al. Gene-marking to trace origin of relapse after autologous bone-marrow transplantation. *Lancet* 1993;341:85.

54. Rill DR, Santana VM, Roberts WM, et al. Direct demonstration that autologous bone marrow transplantation for solid tumors can

return a multiplicity of tumorigenic cells. *Blood* 1994;84:380.

55. Deisseroth AB, Zu Z, Claxton D, et al. Genetic marking shows that Ph+ cells present in autologous transplants of chronic myelogenous leukemia (CML) contribute to relapse after autologous bone marrow in CML. *Blood* 1994;83:3068.

56. Brenner MK, Rill DR, Holladay MS, et al. Gene marking to determine whether autologous marrow infusion restores long-term hemopoiesis in cancer patients. *Lancet* 1993;342:1134.

57. Boon T. Toward a genetic analysis of tumor rejection antigens. *Adv Cancer Res* 1993;60:177.

58. Roth C, Rochlitz C, Kourilsky P. Immune response against tumors. *Adv Immunol* 1994;57:281.

59. Schwartz RH. Costimulation of T lymphocytes: the role of CD28, CTLA-4, and B7/BB1 in interleukin-2 production and immunotherapy. *Cell* 1992;71:1065.

60. Reiser H, Stadecker MJ. Costimulatory B7 molecules in the pathogenesis of infectious and autoimmune diseases. *N Engl J Med* 1996;335:1369.

61. Banchereau J, Steinman RM. Dendritic cells and the control of immunity. *Nature* 1998;392:245.

62. Paul WE, Seder RA. Lymphocyte responses and cytokines. *Cell* 1994;76:241.

63. Abbas AK, Murphy KM, Sher A. Functional diversity of helper T lymphocytes. *Nature* 1996;383:787.

64. Ridge JP, Rosa FD, Matzinger P. A conditioned dendritic cell bridge between a CD4+ T-helper and a T-killer cell. *Nature* 1998; 393:474.

65. Schoenberger SP, Toes REM, van der Voort EIH, Offringa R, Melief CJM. T-cell help for cytotoxic T lymphocytes is mediated by CD40-CD40L interactions. *Nature* 1998;393:480.

66. Bennett SRM, Carbone FR, Karamalis F, Flavell RA, Miller JFAP, Heath WR. Help for cytotoxic-T-cell responses is mediated by CD40 signaling. *Nature* 1998;393:478.

67. Chen L, McGowan P, Ashe S, et al. Tumor immunogenicity determines the effect of B7 costimulation on T cell-mediated tumor immunity. *J Exp Med* 1994;179:523.

68. Townsend SE, Allison JP. Tumor rejection after direct costimulation of CD8+ T cells by B7-transfected melanoma cells. *Science* 1993;259:368.

69. Yang G, Hellstrom KE, Hellstrom I, Chen L. Antitumor immunity elicited by tumor cells transfected with B7-2, a second ligand for CD28/CTLA-4 costimulatory molecules. *J Immunol* 1995;154: 2794.

70. Vieweg J, Gilboa E. Considerations for the use of cytokine-secreting tumor cell preparations for cancer treatment. *Cancer Invest* 1995; 13:193.

71. Dranoff G, Jaffee E, Lazenby A, et al. Vaccination with irradiated tumor cells engineered to secrete murine granulocyte-macrophage colony stimulating factor stimulates potent, long-lasting anti-tumor immunity. *Proc Natl Acad Sci U S A* 1993;90:3539.

72. Tahara H, Zitvogel L, Storkus WJ, et al. Effective eradication of established murine tumors with IL-12 gene therapy using a polycistronic retroviral vector. *J Immunol* 1995;154:6466.

73. Vieweg J, Rosenthal FM, Bannerji R, et al. Immunotherapy of prostate cancer in the Dunning rat model: use of cytokine gene modified tumor vaccines. *Cancer Res* 1994;54:1760.

74. Braun SE, Chen K, Blazar BR, et al. Flt3 ligand anti-tumor activity in a murine breast cancer model: a comparison with GM-CSF and a potential mechanism of action *Human Gene Ther* 1999;10:2141.

75. Dunussi-Joannopoulos K, Dranoff G, Weinstein HJ, Ferrara JLM, Bierer BE, Croop JM. Gene immunotherapy in murine acute myeloid leukemia: granulocyte-macrophage colony-stimulating factor tumor cell vaccines elicit more potent antitumor immunity compared with B7 family and other cytokine vaccines. *Blood* 1998;91:222.

76. Maraskovsky E, Brasel K, Teepe M, et al. Dramatic increase in the numbers of functionally mature dendritic cells in Flt3 ligand-treated mice: multiple dendritic cell subpopulations identified. *J Exp Med* 1996;184:1953.

77. Strobl H, Bello-Fernandez C, Riedl E, et al. flt3 ligand in cooperation with transforming growth factor-β1 potentiates *in vitro* devel-

opment of Langerhans-type dendritic cells and allows single-cell dendritic cell cluster formation under serum-free conditions. *Blood* 1997;90:1425.

78. Chen K, Braun S, Lyman S, et al. Antitumor activity and immunotherapeutic properties of Flt3-ligand in a murine breast cancer model. *Cancer Res* 1997;57:3511.

79. Levitsky HI, Lazenby A, Hayashi RJ, Pardoll DM. *In vivo* priming of two distinct antitumor effector populations: the role of MHC class I expression. *J Exp Med* 1994;179:1215.

80. Soiffer R, Lynch T, Mihm M, et al. Vaccination with irradiated autologous melanoma cells engineered to secrete human granulocyte-macrophage colony-stimulating factor generates potent antitumor immunity in patients with metastatic melanoma. *Proc Natl Acad Sci U S A* 1998;95:13141.

81. Fong T, Nemunaitis J, Peters G, Ando D, Oldham F. Phase I trial of interferon-gamma retroviral vector administered intratumorally with multiple courses in patients with metastatic melanoma. *Proc Am Soc Clin Oncol* 1999;18:444a(abst).

82. Figlin R, Galanis E, Thompson J, Gillespie D. Direct gene transfer of a plasmid encoding the IL-2 gene (Leuvectin) as treatment for patients with metastatic renal cell carcinoma. *Proc Am Soc Clin Oncol* 1999;18:431a(abst).

83. Von Mehren M, Davey M, Rivera V, et al. Phase I trial with ALVAC-CEA B7.1 immunization in advanced CEA-expressing adenocarcinomas. *Proc Am Soc Clin Oncol* 1999;18:437a(abst).

84. Bromberg JS, Debruyne LA, Qin L. Interactions between the immune system and gene therapy vectors: bidirectional regulation of response and expression. *Adv Immunol* 1998;69:353.

85. Dranoff G, Salgia R. A phase I study of vaccination with autologous, lethally irradiated non-small cell lung carcinoma cells engineered by adenoviral mediated gene transfer to secrete human granulocyte-macrophage colony stimulating factor. *Hum Gene Ther* 1998;9:915.

86. Dranoff G, Soiffer R. A phase I study of vaccination with autologous, lethally irradiated melanoma cells engineered by adenoviral mediated gene transfer to secrete human granulocyte-macrophage colony-stimulating factor. *Hum Gene Ther* 1998;9:914.

87. Bowman L. Phase I study of chemokine and cytokine gene modified autologous neuroblastoma cells for treatment of relapsed/refractory neuroblastoma using an adenoviral vector. *Hum Gene Ther* 1998;9:2429.

88. Eder JP, Kantoff PW, Roper K, et al. A phase I trial of recombinant prostate specific antigen expressing vaccinia virus vaccine, PROST-VAC (rV-PSA) in advanced prostate cancer. *Proc Am Soc Clin Oncol* 1999;18:439a(abst).

89. Rosenberg SA. Gene therapy of patients with advanced cancer using tumor infiltrating lymphocytes transduced with the gene coding for tumor necrosis factor. *Hum Gene Ther* 1990;1:441.

90. Pelegrin M, Marin M, Noel D, Piechaczyk M. Genetically engineered antibodies in gene transfer and gene therapy. *Hum Gene Ther* 1998;9:2165.

91. Stancovski I, Schindler DG, Waks T, Yarden Y, Sela M, Eshhar Z. Targeting of T lymphocytes to Neu/HER2-expressing cells using chimeric single chain Fv receptors. *J Immunol* 1993;151:6577.

92. Hwu P, Yang JC, Cowherd R, Treisman J, Eshhar Z, Rosenberg SA. *In vivo* antitumor activity of T-cells redirected with chimeric antibody/T-cell receptor genes. *Cancer Res* 1995;55:3369.

93. Culver KW, Ram Z, Wallbridge S, Ishii H, Oldfield EH, Blaese RM. *In vivo* gene transfer with retroviral vector-producer cells for treatment of experimental brain tumors. *Science* 1992;256:1550.

94. Davis BM, Koc ON, Lee K, Gerson SL. Current progress in the gene therapy of cancer. *Curr Opin Oncol* 1996;8:499.

95. Bi WL, Parysek LM, Warnick R, Stambrook PJ. *In vitro* evidence that metabolic cooperation is responsible for the bystander effect observed with HSV tk retroviral gene therapy. *Hum Gene Ther* 1993;4:725.

96. Barba D, Hardin J, Sadelain M, Gage FH. Development of antitumor immunity following thymidine kinase-mediated killing of experimental brain tumors. *Proc Natl Acad Sci U S A* 1994;91:4348.

97. Chen S-H, Li-Chen XH, Wang Y, et al. Combination gene therapy for liver metastasis of colon carcinoma *in vivo*. *Proc Natl Acad Sci U S A* 1995;92:2577.

98. Smythe WR, Hwang HC, Amin KM, et al. Use of recombinant adenovirus to transfer herpes simplex virus thymidine kinase gene (HSVtk) gene to thoracic neoplasms: an effective *in vitro* drug sensitization system. *Cancer Res* 1994;54:2055.

99. Collins-Jr RH, Shpilberg O, Drobyski WR, et al. Donor leukocyte infusions in 140 patients with relapsed malignancy after allogeneic bone marrow transplantation. *J Clin Oncol* 1997;15:433.

100. Kolb H-J, Schattenberg A, Goldman JM, et al. Graft-versus-leukemia effect of donor lymphocyte transfusions in marrow grafted patients. *Blood* 1995;86:2041.

101. Papadopoulos EB, Ladanyi M, Emanuel D, et al. Infusions of donor leukocytes to treat Epstein-Barr virus-associated lymphoproliferative disorders after allogeneic bone marrow transplantation. *N Engl J Med* 1994;330:1185.

102. Bonini C, Ferrari G, Verzeletti S, et al. HSV-TK gene transfer into donor lymphocytes for control of allogeneic graft-versus-leukemia. *Science* 1997;276:1719.

103. Mullen CA, Coale MM, Lowe R, Blaese RM. Tumors expressing the cytosine deaminase suicide gene can be eliminated *in vivo* with 5-fluorocytosine and induce protective immunity to wild type tumor. *Cancer Res* 1994;54:1503.

104. Huber BE, Austin EA, Good SS, Knick VC, Tibbels S, Richards CA. *In vivo* antitumor activity of 5-fluorocytosine on human colorectal carcinoma cells genetically modified to express cytosine deaminase. *Cancer Res* 1993;53:4619.

105. Grem JL. Fluorinated pyrimidines. In: Chabner BA, Collins JM, eds. *Cancer chemotherapy: principles and practice*. Philadelphia: JB Lippincott Co, 1990:180.

106. Marshall CJ. Tumor suppressor genes. *Cell* 1991;64:313.

107. Bishop JM. Molecular themes in oncogenesis. *Cell* 1991;64:235.

108. Kirsch DG, Kastan MB. Tumor-suppressor p53: implications for tumor development and prognosis. *J Clin Oncol* 1998;16:3158.

109. Cheng J, Yee J-K, Yeargin J, Friedmann T, Haas M. Suppression of acute lymphoblastic leukemia by the human wild-type *p53* gene. *Cancer Res* 1992;52:222.

110. Cai DW, Mukhopadhyay T, Liu Y, Fujiwara T, Roth JA. Stable expression of wild-type *p53* in human lung cancer cells after retrovirus-mediated gene transfer. *Hum Gene Ther* 1993;4:617.

111. Fujiwara T, Grimm EA, Mukhopadhyay T, et al. Induction of chemosensitivity in human lung cancer cells *in vivo* by adenovirus-mediated transfer of the wild-type *p53* gene. *Cancer Res* 1994;54:2287.

112. Liu T-J, Zhang W-W, Taylor DL, Roth JA, Goepfert H, Clayman GL. Growth suppression of human head and neck cancer cells by the introduction of wild-type *p53* gene via a recombinant adenovirus. *Cancer Res* 1994;54:3662.

113. Clayman GL, El-Naggar AK, Roth JA, et al. *In vivo* molecular therapy with *p53* adenovirus for microscopic residual head and neck squamous carcinoma. *Cancer Res* 1995;55:1.

114. Nemunaitis J, Bier-Laning CM, Costenla-Figueiras M, Yver A, Dreiling LK. Three phase II trials of intratumoral injection with a replication-deficient adenovirus carrying the p53 gene (AD5CMV-P53) in patients with recurrent/refractory head and neck cancer. *Proc Am Soc Clin Oncol* 1999;18:431a(abst).

115. Bookstein R, Shew J-Y, Chen P-L, Scully P, Lee W-H. Suppression of tumorigenicity of human prostate carcinoma cells by replacing a mutated RB gene. *Science* 1990; 247:712.

116. Zhang WW. Antisense oncogene and suppressor gene therapy of cancer. *J Mol Med* 1996;74:191.

117. Cantley LL, Auger KR, Carpenter C, et al. Oncogenes and signal transduction. *Cell* 1991;64:281.

118. Narayan R, Akhtar S. Antisense therapy. *Curr Opin Oncol* 1996; 8:509.

119. Ratajczak MZ, Kant JA, Luger SM, Hijiya N, Zhang J, Zon G, Gewirtz AM. *In vivo* treatment of human leukemia in a *scid* mouse model with c-myb antisense oligodeoxynucleotides. *Proc Natl Acad Sci U S A* 1992;89:11823.

120. Skorski T, Nieborowska-Skorska M, Campbell K, et al. Leukemia treatment in severe combined immunodeficiency mice by antisense

oligodeoxynucleotides targeting cooperative oncogenes. *J Exp Med* 1995;182:1645.

121. Monia BP, Johnston JF, Geiger T, Muller M, Fabbro D. Antitumor activity of a phosphorothioate antisense oligodeoxynucleotide targeted against *c-raf* kinase. *Nat Med* 1996;2:668.

122. Mukhopadhyay T, Tainsky M, Cavender AC, Roth JA. Specific inhibition of K-*ras* expression and tumorigenicity of lung cancer cells by antisense RNA. *Cancer Res* 1991;51:1744.

123. Georges RN, Mukhopadhyay T, Zhang Y, Yen N, Roth JA. Prevention of orthotopic human lung cancer growth by intratracheal instillation of a retroviral antisense K-*ras* construct. *Cancer Res* 1993;53:1743.

124. Zhang Y, Mukhopadhyay T, Donehower LA, Georges RN, Roth JA. Retroviral vector-mediated transduction of K-*ras* antisense RNA into human lung cancer cells inhibits expression of the malignant phenotype. *Hum Gene Ther* 1993;4:451.

125. Sklar MD, Thompson E, Welsh MJ, et al. Depletion of c-*myc* with specific antisense sequences reverses the transformed phenotype in ras oncogene-transformed NIH 3T3 cells. *Mol Cell Biol* 1991;11:3699.

126. Stass SA, Mixson AJ. Oncogenes and tumor suppressor genes: thera-

peutic implications. *Clin Cancer Res* 1997;3:2687.

127. Golumbek PT, Lazenby AJ, Levitsky HI, et al. Treatment of established renal cancer by tumor cells engineered to secrete interleukin-4. *Science* 1991;254:713.

128. Porgador A, Tzehoval E, Katz A, et al. Interleukin 6 gene transfection into Lewis lung carcinoma tumor cells suppresses the malignant phenotype and confers immunotherapeutic competence against parental metastatic cells. *Cancer Res* 1992;52:3679.

129. Aoki T, Tashiro K, Miyatake S-I, et al. Expression of murine interleukin 7 in a murine glioma cell line results in reduced tumorigenicity *in vivo*. *Proc Natl Acad Sci U S A* 1992;89:3850.

130. Gansbacher B, Bannerji R, Daniels B, Zier K, Cronin K, Gilboa E. Retroviral vector-mediated γ-interferon gene transfer into tumor cells generates potent and long-lasting antitumor immunity. *Cancer Res* 1990;50:7820.

131. Asher AL, Mule JJ, Kasid A, et al. Murine tumor cells transduced with the gene for tumor necrosis factor-α: evidence for paracrine immune effects of tumor necrosis factor against tumors. *J Immunol* 1991;146:3227.

19.2

BASIC PRINCIPLES OF GENE THERAPY

Gene Transfer into Mammalian Cells

SUSAN A. ZULLO

NATASHA J. CAPLEN

RICHARD A. MORGAN

The methods used to transfer nucleic acid (oligonucleotides, RNA, or DNA) into mammalian cells, either *ex vivo* or *in vivo*, form the bases of all approaches to gene therapy, as this determines the efficiency and duration of the effect induced. The current methods used for gene transfer into mammalian cells can be described in two broad categories, physical–chemical or viral. Examples of the physical chemical approach include direct introduction of the DNA using injection, particle bombardment, or electroporation, calcium phosphate transfection, complexation with cationic lipids or polymer, or linkage to a specific ligand, and the use of the corresponding receptor. Virus-based gene delivery systems attempt to exploit aspects of the natural viral life cycle to elicit high-efficiency gene transfer. Viral vectors have been developed from many different viruses, from small RNA-based viruses to complex DNA viruses. Viral vectors are the most efficient vehicles for gene delivery because these make use of receptors or other interactions with the cell that have evolved over time. Current gene-delivery systems all have advantages and limitations for the treatment of various genetic and acquired diseases (Table 1). However, a method that would allow highly efficient and stable gene transfer to a wide range of cancer cells regardless of their state of proliferation in a safe and controllable, tissue-specific or inducible manner would be superior. This review gives an introduction to the different gene transfer systems currently being developed for gene transfer into mammalian cells.

TABLE 1. SUMMARY OF COMMONLY USED VECTORS

Gene Transfer System	Description	Advantages	Disadvantages	Vector and Insert Sizes
Retrovirus	Replicative defective vectors based on MoMLV	Extensively studied	Low titer	8–10 kb
	Most gene transfer conducted *ex vivo*	Stable integration into host-cell genome	Infection limited to dividing cells	8–10 kb
		Efficient gene transfer	Limited *in vivo*	
Adenoassociated virus	Naturally replication-defective	Long-term expression	Requires helper virus (adeno- or herpes simplex virus) for production	5 kb
	Can integrate into host cell genome	Potential for stable integration into host-cell genome	Limited insert size (<5 kb)	4.0–4.5 kb
	Site-specific integration (Chr19)	Infection of nondividing cells	Low titer	
Adenovirus	Replication-defective vectors based on adenovirus 2 or 5 (serotype C)	High titer	Immunogenic	36 kb
		Efficient entry into most cell types	Stimulation of T- and B-cell responses	7.5 kb except when utilizing "gutless" vectors
		High level of expression	Transient expression	
		Infection of nondividing cells		
Vaccinia virus	Naturally replication-competent	Efficient entry into most cell types	Immunogenic	187 kb
	Transient gene expression	High level of expression	Safety concerns in immunosuppressed patients	25 kb
		Infection of nondividing cells		
DNA/Protein liposome complexes	Complex of plasmid DNA and cationic lipid	No size constraints	Limited persistence	No limit
		No viral genes	Low efficiency of transfer	No limit
		No risk associated with random integration	Complexes highly heterogeneous and formulation dependent	
Naked DNA	Engineered bacterial plasmid	Easy to prepare	Inefficient entry and uptake in most cell types	No limit
		No size constraint	Limited persistence	No limit

MoMLV, Moloney murine leukemia virus.
The most commonly used gene transfer systems are briefly described including their advantages and disadvantages. In every system, the gene of interest is cloned into either the viral-vector genome or a modified bacterial plasmid.

PHYSICAL–CHEMICAL GENE TRANSFER APPROACHES

Naked DNA

Naked DNA in the form of an oligonucleotide or as a plasmid can be used to modulate endogenous gene expression or to express a new gene respectively. Oligonucleotides are short nucleic acid molecules (15 to 20 nucleotides) that can be based on DNA, RNA, or both. The direct intravenous administration of oligonucleotides has been exploited in a number of cancer clinical trials with the aim of transfecting cancer cells with an oligonucleotide that targets a specific cancer-related gene. The principal interaction exploited to produce a therapeutic effect is the alteration of gene expression by the hybridization of an oligonucleotide [with a sequence complementary to a messenger RNA (mRNA) transcript] to this mRNA target (1,2). The binding of the antisense oligonucleotide to the mRNA arrests translation and can induce the destruction of the specific mRNA. Targets of antisense oligonucleotides relevant to gene therapy for cancer include various growth factors associated with tumorigenesis; adhesion molecules; cytokines; and transcription factors and oncogenes, for example, *c-myb* and *bcr-abl*, respectively (3). Early *in vitro* studies used unmodified phosphodiester oligonucle-

otides; however, these molecules are highly susceptible to exonuclease degradation, and, thus, for *in vivo* application, a more stable molecule is required. Of the analogues produced, phosphorothioates-based oligonucleotides have been the most extensively studied and are currently in use in clinical trials in patients with acute myelogenous leukemia and myelodysplastic syndrome (4). However, further studies are necessary to evaluate the potential of these antisense oligonucleotides, as problems with *in vivo* delivery, production, and toxicity remain.

Another common application of the direct administration of naked DNA has been as part of a variety of vaccination strategies or other immunologically based cancer treatments. The DNA, encoding the gene or genes of interest, is usually incorporated into a plasmid. Plasmids are circular, double-stranded DNA (dsDNA) molecules found naturally in a wide variety of bacteria. Recombinant plasmids are modified natural plasmids from which unwanted or unnecessary DNA sequences have been removed; plasmid vectors are well characterized and can be relatively easily manipulated and purified using standard molecular biology techniques (5). The gene of interest is usually in the form of a complementary DNA that has been generated from the corresponding mRNA and thus contains only the appropriate coding information for that gene. Intramuscular injection of naked DNA expressing a given protein has been shown to elicit a protective immune response (both cellular and humoral) against the expressed protein in several animal models (6). It appears that the DNA is taken up by myocytes, which express the protein; the protein is then processed into peptides, which are taken up as antigens by antigen-presenting cells, leading to an immune response (7). An important component in the induction of this immune response appears to be the immunogenicity of the plasmid DNA itself. Plasmid DNA is produced in bacteria and thus carries a bacterial DNA methylation pattern, which differs from that seen in mammalian cells. This hypomethylated state of CpG motifs can yield a nonspecific immune response to the plasmid itself and is thus recognized as a foreign molecule by mammalian cells (8). Antitumor responses can be elicited by vaccination in several ways. One strategy is to coexpress tumor-associated molecules such as the carcinoembryonic antigen, which is expressed in a number of cancers including gastric, pancreatic, and colorectal, with genes encoding immunomodulating proteins such as the B7-1 costimulatory molecule (to increase antigen presentation) or granulocyte-macrophage colony-stimulating factor (9). Direct injection, and/or particle bombardment of plasmids expressing these molecules can induce a specific anticarcinoembryonic antigen and thus potentially an antitumor response. Another approach has been to generate DNA vaccines consisting of antiidiotypic single-chain antibody fragments that correspond to the immunoglobulin molecules expressed by malignant B-cell clones. This type of strategy has been used to protect against B-lymphoma (10) and more recently has been adapted to induce responses against both lymphoma and myeloma (11).

Cationic Lipids

Cationic liposomes are membranous lipid vesicles that enclose an aqueous volume and carry a net positive charge. The combination of plasmid DNA, which has a net negative charge, with the positively charged cationic lipids causes the formation of liposome complexes, or lipoplexes (12,13). Mammalian cells take up these lipoplexes by mechanisms that are still unknown. The initial interaction between the cell and the lipoplex is electrostatic; endocytosis, phagocytosis, pinocytosis, and direct fusion with the cell membrane may all play a role in lipoplex cell entry depending on the cell type. The DNA and the lipid appear to be closely associated, protecting at least a proportion of the DNA from enzyme digestion, allowing sufficient molecules to reach the nucleus. DNA likely needs to be released from lipoplexes before entry into the nucleus (14). Plasmid DNA is the most commonly transferred genetic material; however, RNA, antisense oligonucleotides, and DNA up to 150 kilobase (kb) in length have also been transferred using this technique (15,16).

Several different cell types have been transfected using a variety of different cationic lipid preparations including mixtures of dioleoyl phosphatidylethanolamine (DOPE) with DOTMA (lipofectin), DOTAP (Boehringer Mannheim, Indianapolis, IN), DMRIE (Vical, Inc., San Diego, CA), DC-Chol: DOPE (17), and GL67 (18). The determination of the optimal formulation of any given lipoplex is critical, as this can influence the level of gene transfer and expression obtained by several orders of magnitude. The most important variables to be considered are the ratio of the nucleic acid and the cationic lipid, the concentration of these components, and the total amount of DNA and lipid (19). Several cationic polymers have also been synthesized that have similar properties to cationic lipids when used as gene transfer agents. Examples of these include polyethylenimine and polyamido-amine polymers (20,21).

The first clinical attempt to genetically modify tumors *in situ* using lipoplexes involved the direct injection of an allogene coding the histocompatibility antigen HLA-B7 complexed with the cationic liposome DMRIE:DOPE. The aim was that the transient expression of the foreign antigen HLA-B7 on the cell surface of the tumor, in this case melanoma lesions, should induce a systemic antitumor immune reaction in the host (22). A few examples of other antitumor genes that have been transferred by lipid-mediated gene transfer include p53, tumor necrosis factor–α, and interferon-β. Although this strategy can yield very high transfer efficiencies *in vitro*, the *in vivo* levels are far less encouraging. Further applications of liposomes in cancer gene therapy require further improvements in gene transfer efficiency, gene expression, and specific targeting of the vectors by conjugating ligands specific for tumor surface antigens to lipid moieties.

Receptor-Mediated Gene Transfer

By linking various receptor-specific ligands to polycations such as protamine or polylysine that bind nucleic acids, DNA can be delivered to different cell types via a specific receptor. Receptor targets that have been used include the transferrin receptor and the asialoglycoprotein receptor, which is specific for liver cells (23–26). This strategy has an advantage compared with other methods in its potential for specific targeting to different cell types depending on the receptor-ligand combination used. However, the efficiency of transfer and the level of expression achieved using receptor-mediated transfer is relatively low because of lysosomal degradation of the introduced DNA; coinfection with inactivated adenovirus or addition of the drug chloroquine has been used to overcome this problem by enhancing lysosomal release (27). Mohr and colleagues have recently developed a system to target gene transfer to hepatocellular carcinoma cells *in vitro* using a novel monoclonal antibody, AF-20, conjugated to the gene delivery system (28).

VIRUS-MEDIATED GENE TRANSFER

Viral gene transfer vectors can be categorized on the basis of the fate of the introduced genetic material (Fig. 1). Retroviral- and lentiviral-mediated gene transfer results in the integration of the vector into the host genome (see Fig. 1A), whereas adenoviral-mediated gene transfer results in episomal maintenance of the vector (see Fig. 1B).

Retroviral Vectors

Retroviruses have an RNA genome that replicates by forming a DNA intermediate a provirus—that integrates randomly into

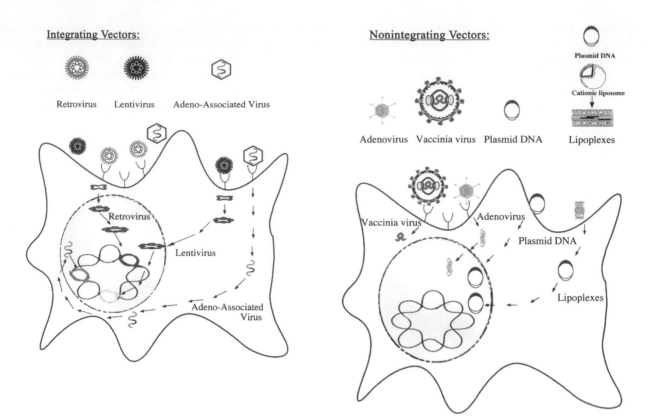

Integrating Vectors:

Retrovirus   Lentivirus   Adeno-Associated Virus

Nonintegrating Vectors:

Plasmid DNA

Cationic liposome

Adenovirus   Vaccinia virus   Plasmid DNA   Lipoplexes

Retrovirus

Lentivirus

Adeno-Associated Virus

Vaccinia virus   Adenovirus

Plasmid DNA

Lipoplexes

A   B

FIGURE 1. A: Integrating vectors. Virus particles bind to specific receptors on the surface of target cells. These vectors are internalized and their genome enters the cell. In the case of retroviruses, the single-stranded RNA genome is converted into double-stranded DNA by the reverse transcriptase enzyme encoded by the virus. The double-stranded DNA is taken up by the nucleus and integrates within the host genome as a provirus. The integration is random for retroviruses. Lentiviruses have a similar life cycle, whereas adenoassociated virus vectors do not replicate through an RNA intermediate. **B:** Nonintegrating vectors. Adenovirus bind to specific receptors on the surface of susceptible cells. These viruses are then adsorbed and internalized by receptor-mediated endocytosis. The viral genome enters the cytoplasm of the cell. The double-stranded DNA genome is taken up by the nucleus. In contrast to adenoviral vectors, vaccinia-based particles are found in the cytoplasm of cells. Nonviral based gene transfer of DNA results in episomal maintenance of plasmid DNA in the nucleus.

the host genome (29). Retroviruses have been shown to infect fibroblasts, epithelial cells, and hepatocytes, but have been used most extensively in the transduction of hematopoietic cells. Several vectors have been developed, but the most widely used are based on the Moloney murine leukemia virus (MoMLV) with the therapeutic gene of interest replacing the viral gene sequences, *gag*, *pol*, and *env*. Retroviral-mediated gene transfer is dependent on a two-component system, the packaging cell and viral vector. A packaging cell is a cell that contains a retroviral genome from which the signals for encapsidation of the viral genome into virus particles have been removed. The viral genome in the packaging cell line produces all of the proteins necessary for virus replication and assembly (*gag*, *pol*, and a variable *env*), but cannot create an infectious particle due to the lack of a transferable viral genome. A retroviral vector that contains a gene or genes of interest and a promoter complement the packaging cell genome in that it lacks all of the normal viral protein coding sequences but retains the encapsidation signals (30–37). The introduction of a gene expression cassette [the gene(s) of interest plus the necessary regulatory sequences] into the vector is usually performed with the retroviral vector in the form of a plasmid. Standard molecular biology techniques can be used to

clone the gene expression cassette between the two flanking long-terminal repeat sequences of the retroviral genome. Gene expression can be driven by the retroviral long-terminal repeat sequence or by the introduction of an exogenous promoter.

The first step in retrovirus production is the transfection of the retroviral vector-plasmid DNA into a packaging cell line. The vector DNA is transcribed into an RNA that can be packaged into retroviral particles that bud from the cell membrane. The medium into which the retrovirus is secreted is called the *retroviral vector supernatant*. When this infectious retroviral vector supernatant is added to cells, the viral particles bind to the cell and the retroviral vector RNA genome enters the cell. The retroviral genome is subjected to RNA-dependent reverse transcription that results in the production of a double-stranded DNA copy of the input viral RNA. Within the nucleus, the DNA copy is inserted into the host cell genome. It should be noted that reverse transcription and integration require cell division, and, although retroviral-mediated gene transfer is highly efficient, it is not effective for nondividing cells. Because the retroviral vector is replication-defective, this process is referred to as *transduction* rather than *infection*, as with a replication-competent virus (31).

The viral tropism of retroviruses is determined by the envelope glycoprotein. Modifications of the sequences encoding the envelope protein can be made within the packaging cell lines. Retroviruses can be classified by this tropism. Ecotropic viruses target murine and other rodent cells, whereas xenotropic viruses target nonrodent mammalian cells. Amphotropic viruses target mammalian cells including rodent cells. Other envelope sequences derived from the Gibbon ape leukemia virus and vesicular stomatitis virus G glycoprotein (VSV-G) have been used in virus production. Gibbon ape leukemia virus–based retroviruses predominantly infect primate cells, while VSV-G–derived viruses infect a wide range of vertebrate cells (38). Additionally, sequences such as those encoding epidermal growth factor or insulinlike growth factor have been fused to *env* in an attempt to produce viral particles that target specific cell types (39–41).

Theoretically, integration of the retroviral vector as a provirus should lead to maintenance of the transgene in the infected cells and transfer to any progeny; however, expression of the transgene can be transient, probably as a result of downregulation of transcription rather than gene loss (42). Other problems currently limiting their broader application include the potential that the random integration events may lead to transformation (insertional mutagenesis) or the possibility that replication-competent viruses may be formed through recombination or complementation by proteins expressed by other viruses and the inability of retroviruses to infect nondividing cells (43–45).

Because high levels of transduction can be achieved with retroviral vectors *ex vivo*, they have been used in cancer gene therapy for applications that can exploit this property. Gene transfer of an immunostimulatory molecule such as GM-CSF into tumor cells before infusion into patients either as a tumor cell vaccine or as tumor infiltrating lymphocytes have been efficacious (46,47). Vector producer cells have also been injected into patients with recurring gliomas for delivery of "suicide" genes (48).

Lentivirus Vectors

Lentivirus vectors based on the human immunodeficiency virus (HIV-1), equine infectious anemia virus, and feline immunodeficiency virus are the most recent additions to a growing list of gene transfer vectors (49). As with MoMLV-based vectors, these retroviruses are also comprised of an RNA genome. However, the major advantage to the use of these viruses is their ability to infect and stably integrate into nondividing cells. Most of the lentivirus vectors in use are based on the HIV-1 genome. To create a safe gene transfer vector based on this human pathogen, its genome was separated onto three different plasmids and mutated to produce replication-defective particles much less likely to recombine to form wild-type HIV-1. The first plasmid is the vector that contains an internally promoted transgene, the HIV-1 packaging signal, the *cis*-acting reverse transcriptase, and integration signals. The second plasmid expresses all of the HIV-1 proteins except for the envelope (*env*). The final plasmid encodes an envelope capable of pseudotyping the virus particles, most commonly VSV-G (50). Several studies both *in vitro* and *in vivo* have demonstrated successful gene transfer including transduction of nondividing hemopoietic cells at high efficiencies (up to 90%) and sustained gene expression in several target tissues of interest: liver (8 weeks), and muscle and brain (6 months) with no obvious immune response (51–54). The major drawback to the use of this vector is the safety concern that wild-type HIV-1 could be generated after administration of the vector system *in vivo*. This issue may be addressed by further deleting the HIV-1 genes and production of a packaging cell line (55).

Adenoassociated Viral Vectors

Adenoassociated virus (AAV) is a small, single-stranded DNA virus that may serve as a viable alternative to retrovirus in some instances. AAV is a defective human parvovirus in that it requires a helper virus for infection, usually an adenovirus or herpesvirus. In the absence of helper virus, the AAV genome (provirus) integrates into the host chromosomal DNA in a relatively site-specific manner and establishes latency, which has been maintained in cultured cells for more than 100 serial passages (56). As would be expected given its need for coinfection with adenovirus, AAV exhibits tropism for the airway (57,58). AAV vectors have also been successfully used to transfer genes into muscle and liver (59–61). AAV vectors containing a variety of different genes have been constructed and successfully shown to transfer and express genes both *in vitro* and *in vivo* regardless of the mitotic state of the target cell. A significant limitation exists, however, to the size of the insert that these vectors can accommodate [4.0 to 4.5 kilobase (kb)] and manipulation of the genome appears to disrupt the site-specific nature of the integration process (62). Also, the lack of packaging cell lines limits the production of relatively high-titer AAV vectors. AAV vectors can be used for a variety of cancer treatment approaches, delivery of antisense genes, "suicide" gene therapy by transfer of the herpes simplex virus thymidine kinase (HSV-*tk*) gene, and, recently, for the delivery of antiangiogenesis factors including angiostatin and endostatin (63,64).

Adenoviral Vectors

Adenoviruses are small, nonenveloped viruses. Their genome consists of a linear, dsDNA of approximately 36 kb in length, which codes for at least 30 different mRNA transcripts. The adenovirus (Ad) genome is organized into two groups of genes (early and late), depending on the role the protein products play in the life cycle of the virus (65). One of these genes, *E1a*, is of particular interest with respect to the development of adenoviral vectors. The deletion of this gene renders the adenovirus replication-deficient in many cell types. Other vectors have also been deleted in the *E3* gene (that encodes a polypeptide that influences immune recognition of the infected cell) (66). More recently, second-generation viruses have been developed that contain alterations in the *E2* gene, which further block expression of the Ad late genes, which encode the viral structural proteins (67). The deletion of these endogenous sequences allows for insertion of the DNA that is to be transfected, without affecting the ability of the virus to package the DNA into the viral capsid. The most commonly used recombinant adenoviruses are based on serotypes 2 (Ad2) and 5 (Ad5). The wild-type virus (Ad2/Ad5) is most commonly associated with respiratory illnesses in humans and believed to be nononcogenic. Adenoviruses infect nondividing cells, but expression is transient because the DNA does not integrate into the host genome but is maintained episomally. Replication-deficient viruses must be propagated in 293 cells, human embryonic kidney cells, which have an integrated fragment of adenovirus (left arm of Ad5) that expresses the *E1* functions *in trans* (68).

Adenoviral vectors have numerous advantages for use in gene therapy. Titers of the recombinant viruses can be as high as 10^{12} plaque-forming units per mL, depending on the transgene inserted within the deleted region. The therapeutic gene expression cassette may be as large as 8 kb of DNA (69) with recent studies describing vectors with capacities of up to nearly 34 kb following deletion of most of the Ad genome (70). These viral vectors are capable of efficiently transducing a broad range of target cells, both *in vitro* and *in vivo*, including endothelial cells, neurons and muscle, and, in particular, because of their natural tropism, several different cell types associated with the respiratory tract (71–74). Adenoviral vectors are strongly immunogenic, however, which may preclude repeat administration without immune modulation or utilization of alternate serotypes (75–77). Because of their ability to efficiently transduce a wide range of cells with a high level of transient transgene expression, adenoviral vectors have been used primarily for delivery of cytokines, costimulatory molecules, tumor-suppressor genes, and "suicide" genes, including HSV-*tk* and cytosine deaminase (CD) (78,79). Although treatment of an entire tumor mass is not likely, the two "suicide" gene therapy strategies make use of a phenomenon referred to as the *bystander effect*, in which genetically modified cells are toxic to surrounding unmodified cells, which become susceptible to the prodrug. Recently, combinations of these approaches have been used in an attempt to fully eradicate the tumor mass (80,81). Modifications to the adenoviral fiber protein, including inclusion of an RGD peptide, have also been applied to direct these vectors specifically to tumor cells (82,83).

Herpes Simplex Virus Vectors

Herpesviruses are a diverse family of large DNA viruses all capable of establishing lifelong latency (84). Gene delivery vectors based on HSV have two major advantages over other viral vectors. First, very large inserts can be accommodated and packaged within the HSV particle. For example, the full-length complementary DNA for huntingtin (approximately 10 kb) can be packaged in these virions (85). Second, HSV vectors have a natural tropism for cells in the central nervous system. This may allow for the tropism to be exploited for the delivery of HSV-*tk* gene to brain tumors (86,87). Several clinical trials are currently in discussion that would use this system. HSV vectors can be produced by use of a helper virus system or an amplicon system. The first approach is based on construction of viruses lacking either single or combinations of essential genes that can accommodate the insertion of at

least 40-kb DNA. By necessity, the debilitated recombinant viruses must be grown in cell lines expressing the deleted viral genes (88,89). The amplicon approach is based on defective HSV genomes, which arise spontaneously, by recombination. These are amplified during serial passages at high multiplicities of infection. The defective genomic subunit referred to as an *amplicon* consists of the terminal *a* sequence containing the packaging signal and an origin of viral replication but lacks both viral structural-protein sequences and sequences encoding proteins for viral-DNA synthesis and exocytosis. These proteins must be supplied for the amplicons to be made. Theoretically, amplicons could accommodate inserts as large as 150 kb. Amplicons are arranged from head-to-tail in virions and have been shown to efficiently express cellular genes incorporated into them (90,91). Tumor cells infected with HSV alone are destroyed during viral replication even without a transgene. HSV-*tk* is transferred to the cancer cells allowing for sensitivity to the prodrug ganciclovir. HSV vectors have also been used for the transfer of interleukins to glioma in mice and enhancement of *tk* delivery by addition of tumor necrosis factor–α both *in vitro* and *in vivo* (92,93). Although toxicity is not critical when treating cancer cells because the focus is usually on cell death, viral toxicity and transient expression limit gene-transfer strategies for HSV especially when used for central nervous system treatment. Deletion of a combination of the immediate-early genes including a transcriptional transactivation showed decreased cytotoxicity allowing for more efficient gene transfer and extended gene expression from HSV vectors and may be important for broader usage of HSV for gene transfer (94).

Epstein-Barr Virus Vectors

Epstein-Barr virus (EBV) is another member of the herpesvirus family that causes mononucleosis in its acute viral-replication state and polyclonal B-lymphoproliferative diseases in its latent infectious state. The latent replication origin, ORI-P, allows for viral replication in human cells without cell lysis. Episomal replication is only maintained in cells expressing EBV nuclear antigen (EBNA1) gene (95,96). This type of replication is the basis for EBV vectors for gene transfer. EBV-episomal vectors have been used recently to transfer the adenosine deaminase gene to CD34+ cells *in vitro* although the safety of using this system *in vivo* remains uncertain. An HSV/EBV hybrid has also been constructed that makes use of the EBV ORI-P element and EBNA1 that allows for replication and maintenance of the EBV genome as an extrachromosomal entity in dividing cells (97). This hybrid strategy, which can be efficiently packaged using an HSV-1–helper virus, may be useful in the treatment of dividing cells such as *in vivo* prodrug delivery to tumor cells.

Vaccinia Virus Vectors

Vaccinia virus is a member of the *Poxviridae* family and, like HSV, possesses a complex dsDNA genome, which contains 186 kb encoding more than 200 proteins. Most of the viral genes can be deleted and replaced by marker or therapeutic gene(s) except for the ITR sequences within the genome that are responsible for viral replication. Recombinant vectors are achieved by homologous recombination after transfection of vaccinia virus-infected cells with plasmid DNA constructs (98). This virus is replication-competent and cytopathic with a broad host range and the capability to infect both vertebrate and invertebrate hosts (99). The advantages of using vaccinia viruses for gene transfer include their ability to accommodate inserts of at least 25 kb allowing for large or multiple gene inserts; their ability to infect cells regardless of their mitotic state; and their cytoplasmic replication, which avoids any potential for chromosomal mutation on insertion (100). However, vaccinia has been widely used as a vaccine for smallpox, therefore, administration of vaccinia virus for gene transfer could be impaired by a robust host immune response. In contrast, this potential disadvantage (intrinsic antigenicity) can be exploited to elicit an immune response against tumor-associated antigens to activate an antitumor immunotherapeutic response *in vivo* (101). Vaccination of tumors with cytokines including IL-12 have also resulted in a high level of expression as well as inhibition of tumor growth as a result of the cytopathic nature of the vaccinia virus (102).

Hybrid Virus Vector Systems

Several groups have described hybrid viral strategies that attempt to use the advantages of the two parental vectors while limiting, or compensating for, the effect of their respective disadvantages. For example, adenoviral vectors have the ability to transduce a broad range of cell types including nondividing cells, but transgene expression is short lived (usually 21 to 28 days). In contrast, retroviral vectors based on MoMLV have the advantage of generating stable, long-term expression as a result of proviral integration, but they only transduce dividing cells. One system developed by Feng and coworkers consisted of two adenoviruses: one carrying a retroviral transcription unit encoding green fluorescent protein (GFP) and a second expressing retroviral *gag*, *pol*, and *env* functions was used to transduce ovarian tumor cells (SKOV3.pi) *in vivo*. Coinjection of both adenoviruses resulted in more efficient transduction of the tumor compared with administration of the adenovirus carrying the GFP vector alone (103). A second group used an adenovirus carrying a retroviral vector to generate high-titer retrovirus from retroviral packaging cells (104) and a series of transcomplementing adenoviruses expressing (a) a retroviral vector, (b) retroviral *gag* and *pol,* and (c) the VSV-G envelope. Administration of the transcomplementing adenoviruses to tumor cells *in vivo* lead to the generation of a retroviral vector, which could subsequently infect adjacent cells (105).

Other hybrids under development include retroviruses and Alphaviruses, which have the potential to include complex mammalian regulatory sequences, including intron and untranslated regions, because their replication bypasses the nucleus and takes place solely in the cytoplasm within an autocatalytic loop that has the potential to generate large amounts of transferred gene product such as a tumor-suppressor gene, "suicide" gene, or cytokine (106,107). Other Alphavirus vectors expressing either HSV-*tk* and targeted

TABLE 2. SUMMARY OF GENE TRANSFER VECTORS UTILIZED IN BOTH OPEN AND CLOSED CANCER-RELATED CLINICAL PROTOCOLS[a]

Gene Transfer Vector	Utilized in Number of Protocols
Viral vectors:	
Retrovirus	89
Adenovirus	46
Poxvirus (vaccinia, canarypox, fowlpox)	17
Herpes simplex virus	1
Nonviral vectors:	
Naked DNA	7
Cationic lipid	35
Other: RNA	1
Total	**196**

[a]Numbers reflect completed protocols at various review levels. Information provided by the National Institutes of Health, Office of Recombinant DNA Activities, Bethesda, MD. (As of February 10, 1999.)

reported and may prove to be useful for cancer gene therapy applications (108,109).

SUMMARY

The utilization of gene therapy in the arsenal of treatment strategies for cancer is still in the preliminary stages with optimal vector delivery systems and therapeutic genes for any given tumor still only an educated guess based on our understanding of carcinogenesis and gene transfer studies to date (Table 2). Current approaches to gene therapy for cancer are focused on introduction of genetic material for systemic antitumor immunity by expression of cytokines, costimulatory molecules, foreign histocompatibility genes, vaccine strategies, induction of susceptibility to a prodrug, expression of tumor-suppressor gene products, and downregulation of oncogenes often using antisense oligonucleotides (Table 3). For gene therapy to be a feasible alternative or addition to traditional clinical intervention, the therapeutic gene needs to be expressed at high levels and targeted specifically to tumor cells to minimize toxicity to normal cells. Targeting may be achieved by including inducible or tumor-specific promoters or by conjugating tumor-specific antigens to the vector. Clinical trials incorporating the individual patients' genetic mutations and antigenic determinants into the treatment protocol may allow for the efficient and specific gene transfer of therapeutic DNA, RNA, or oligonucleotides by a variety of vectors that, more likely than not, differ from cancer to cancer and possibly even patient to patient. Unfortunately, no gene transfer system exists that allows for specific targeting for metastatic cancer, or that can guarantee gene transfer to all cells for a localized tumor. A primary experimental difficulty impeding the success of gene transfer is the lack of an effective *in situ* gene delivery method that would allow for effective delivery to solid organs and tissues, accessibility to target cells, and potential treatment for dominant negative or pathologic gene products and storage diseases. Although a universal delivery system for all maladies seems unlikely, development of effective schemes for one or more specific diseases is an attainable clinical goal.

TABLE 3. SUMMARY OF GENE TRANSFER PROTOCOLS BY THERAPEUTIC APPROACH FOR CANCER-RELATED PROTOCOLS

Gene Therapy Strategies	Number of Protocols
Antisense	4
Chemoprotection	9
Immunotherapy: *in vitro* transduction	56
Immunotherapy: *in vivo* transduction	51
Prodrug/ HSV-*tk* and ganciclovir	28
Tumor-suppressor gene	18
Single chain antibody	2
Oncogene downregulation	3
Vector-directed cell lysis	2
Total	173

REFERENCES

1. Zamecnik PC, Stephenson ML. Inhibition of Rous sarcomavirus replication and transformation by a specific oligonucleotide. *Proc Natl Acad Sci U S A* 1978;75:280–284.
2. Zamecnik PC. History of antisense oligonucleotides. In: Agrawal S, ed. *Antisense therapeutics*. Totowa, NJ: Humana Press, 1996:1–11.
3. Gewirtz AM, Sokol DL, Ratajczak MZ. Nucleic acid therapeutics: state of the art and future prospects. *Blood* 1998;92:712–736.
4. Bishop MR, Iversen PL, Bayever E, et al. Phase I trial of an antisense oligonucleotide OL1p53 in hematologic malignancies. *J Clin Oncol* 1996;14:1320–1326.
5. Horn NA, Meek JA, Budahazi G, Marquet M. Cancer gene therapy using plasmid DNA: purification of DNA for human clinical trials. *Hum Gene Ther* 1995;6:565–573.
6. Donnelly JJ, Ulmer JB, Shiver JW, Liu MA. DNA vaccines. *Ann Rev Immunol* 1997;15:617–648.
7. Fu T, Ulmer J, Caulfield M, et al. Priming of cytotoxic T lymphocytes by DNA vaccines: requirement for professional antigen presenting cells and evidence for antigen transfer from myocytes. *Mol Med* 1997;3:362–371.
8. Sato Y, Roman M, Tighe H, et al. Immunostimulatory DNA sequences necessary for effective intradermal gene immunization. *Science* 1996;273:352–354.
9. Conry RM, Widera G, LoBuglio AF, et al. Selected strategies to augment polynucleotide immunization. *Gene Ther* 1996;3:67–74.
10. Syrengelas A, Chen T, Levy R. DNA immunization induces protective immunity against B-cell lymphoma. *Nat Med* 1996;2:1038–1041.
11. King C, Spellerberg M, Zhu D, et al. DNA vaccines with single-chain Fv fused to fragment C of tetanus toxin induce protective immunity against lymphoma and myeloma. *Nat Med* 1998;4:1281–1286.
12. Felgner PL, Gadek TR, Holm M, et al. Lipofection: a highly efficient, lipid-mediated DNA-transfection procedure. *Proc Natl Acad Sci U S A* 1987;84:7413–7417.
13. Felgner PL, Rinegold GM. Cationic liposome mediated transfection. *Nature* 1989;337:387–388.
14. Zabner J, Fasbender AJ, Moninger T, Poellinger KA, Welsh MJ. Cellular and molecular barriers to gene transfer by a cationic lipid. *J Biol Chem* 1995;270:18997–19007.
15. Chen M, Compton ST, Coviello VF, Green ED, Ashlock MA. Transient gene expression from yeast artificial chromosome DNA in mammalian cells is enhanced by adenovirus. *Nucleic Acids Res* 1997;25:4416–4418.
16. Kronenwett R, Steidi U, Kirsch M, Sczakiel G, Haas R. Oligodeoxyribonucleotide uptake in primary human hematopoietic cells is enhanced by cationic lipids and depends on the hematopoietic cell subset. *Blood* 1998;91:852–862.
17. Gao X, Huang L. A novel cationic liposome reagent for efficienttransfection of mammalian cells. *Biochem Biophys Res Commun* 1991; 179:280–285.
18. Lee ER, Marshall J, Siegel CS, et al. Detailed analysis of structures and formulations of cationic lipids for efficient gene transfer to the lung. *Hum Gene Ther* 1996;7:1701–1717.
19. Caplan NJ. Nucleic acid transfer using catatonic lipids. In: Kmiec E, ed. *Methods in molecular biology: gene targeting protocols*. Totowa, NJ: Humana Press, 2000:1–19.
20. Boussif O, Lezoualc'h F, Zanta MA, et al. A versatile vector for gene and oligonucleotide transfer into cells in culture and *in vivo*: polyethylenimine. *Proc Natl Acad Sci U S A* 1995;92:7297–7301.
21. Tang MX, Redemann CT, Szoka FC Jr. *In vitro* gene delivery by degraded polyamido-amine dendrimers. *Bioconjugate Chem* 1996; 7(6):703–714.
22. Nabel EG, Yang Z, Muller D, et al. Safety and toxicity of catheter gene delivery to the pulmonary vasculature in a patient with metastatic melanoma. *Hum Gene Ther* 1994;5:1089–1094.
23. Cotten M, Langle-Rouault F, Kirlappos H, et al. Transferrin-polycation-mediated introduction of DNA into human leukemic cells: stimulation by agents that affect the survival of transfected DNA or modulate transferrin receptor levels. *Proc Natl Acad Sci U S A* 1990;87:4033–4037.
24. Kawakami S, Yamashita F, Nishikawa M, Takakura Y, Hashida M. Asialoglycoprotein receptor-mediated gene transfer using novel galactosylated cationic liposomes. *Biochem Biophys Res Commun* 1998;252:78–83.
25. Plank C, Zatloukal K, Cotten M, Mechtler K, Wagner E. Gene transfer into hepatocytes using asialoglycoprotein receptor mediated endocytosis of DNA complexed with an artificial tetra-antennary galactose ligand. *Bioconjug Chem* 1992;3:533–539.
26. Wagner E, Zenke M, Cotten M, Beug H, Birnstiel ML. Transferrin-polycation conjugates as carriers for DNA uptake into cells. *Proc Natl Acad Sci U S A* 1990;87:3410–3414.
27. Curiel DT, Agarwal S, Wagner E, Cotten M. Adenovirus enhancement of transferrin-polylysine-mediated gene delivery. *Proc Natl Acad Sci U S A* 1991;88:8850–8854.
28. Mohr L, Schauer JI, Boutin RH, Moradpour D, Wands JR. Targeted gene transfer to hepatocellular carcinoma cells *in vitro* using a novel monoclonal antibody-based gene delivery system. *Hepatology* 1999;29:82–89.
29. Coffin JM. Retroviridae: the viruses and their replication. In: Fields BN, Knipe DM, Howley PM, eds. *Virology*. Philadelphia: Lippincott–Raven, 1996:1767–1848.
30. Cone RD, Mulligan RC. High-efficiency gene transfer into mammalian cells: generation of helper-free recombinant retrovirus with broad mammalian host range. *Proc Natl Acad Sci U S A* 1984;81:6349–6353.
31. Bunnell BA, Morgan RA. Retrovirus-mediated gene transfer. In: Adolph KW, ed. *Viral genome methods*. Boca Raton, FL: CRC Press, 1996:3–23.
32. Danos O, Mulligan RC. Safe and efficient generation of recombinant retroviruses with amphotropic and ecotropic host ranges. *Proc Natl Acad Sci U S A* 1988;85:6460–6464.
33. Markowitz D, Goff S, Bank A. A safe packaging cell line for gene transfer: separating viral genes on two different plasmids. *J Virol* 1988;62:1120–1124.
34. Miller AD. Retroviral vectors. *Curr Top Microbiol Immunol* 1992; 158:1–24.
35. Miller AD, Buttimore C. Redesign of retroviral packaging cell lines to avoid recombination leading to helper virus production. *Mol Cell Biol* 1986;6:2895–2903.
36. Miller AD, Garcia JV, Suhr NV, Lynch CM, Wilson C, Eiden MV. Construction and properties of retrovirus packaging cells based on gibbon ape leukemia virus. *J Virol* 1991;65:2220–2224.
37. Miller AD, Rosman GJ. Improved retroviral vectors for gene transfer and expression. *BioTechniques* 1989;7:980–990.
38. Miller AD. Cell-surface receptors for retroviruses and implications for gene transfer. *Proc Natl Acad Sci U S A* 1996;93:11407–11413.
39. Cosset FL, Morling FJ, Takeuchi Y, Weiss RA, Collins MK, Russell SJ. Retroviral retargeting by envelopes expressing an N-terminal binding domain. *J Virol* 1995;69:6314–6322.
40. Cosset FL, Russell SJ. Targeting retrovirus entry. *Gene Ther* 1996; 3:946–956.

41. Chadwick MP, Morling FJ, Cosset FL, Russell SJ. Modification of retroviral tropism by display of IGF-I. *J Mol Biol* 1999;285:485–494.

42. Challita P-M, Kohn DB. Lack of expression from a retroviral vector after transduction of murine hematopoietic stem cells is associated with methylation *in vivo. Proc Natl Acad Sci U S A* 1994;91;2567–2571.

43. Cornetta K, Morgan RA, Anderson WF. Safety issues related to retroviral-mediated gene transfer in humans. *Hum Gene Ther* 1991; 2:5–14.

44. Cornetta K, Morgan RA, Gillio A, et al. No retroviremia or pathology in long-term follow-up of monkeys exposed to a murine amphotropic retrovirus. *Hum Gene Ther* 1991;2:215–219.

45. Donahue RE, Kessler SW, Bodine D, et al. Helper virus induced T cell lymphoma in nonhuman primates after retroviral mediated gene transfer. *J Exp Med* 1992;176:1125–1135.

46. Dranoff G, Jaffee E, Lazenby A, et al. Vaccination with irradiated tumor cells engineered to secrete murine granulocyte-macrophage colony-stimulating factor stimulates potent, specific, and long-lasting anti-tumor immunity. *Proc Natl Acad Sci U S A* 1993;90:3539–3543.

47. Rosenberg SA, Aebersold P, Cornetta K, et al. Gene transfer into humans—immunotherapy of patients with advanced melanoma, using tumor-infiltrating lymphocytes modified by retroviral gene transduction. *N Engl J Med* 1990;323:570–578.

48. Oldfield EH, Ram Z, Culver KW, Blaese RM, DeVroom HL, Anderson WF. Gene therapy for the treatment of brain tumors using intra-tumoral transduction with the thymidine kinase gene and intravenous ganciclovir. *Hum Gene Ther* 1993;4:39–69.

49. Joag SV, Stephens EB, Narayan O. Lentiviruses. In: Fields BN, Knipe DM, Howley PM, eds. *Virology.* Philadelphia: Lippincott–Raven, 1996:1977–1996.

50. Naldini L, Blömer U, Gallay P, et al. *In vivo* gene delivery and stable transduction of non-dividing cells by a lentiviral vector. *Science* 1996;272:263–267.

51. Blömer U, Naldini L, Kafri T, Trono D, Verma IM, Gage FH. Highly efficient and sustained gene transfer in adult neurons with a lentivirus vector. *J Virol* 1997;71;6641–6649.

52. Kafri T, Blömer U, Peterson DA, Gage FH, Verma IM. Sustained expression of genes delivered directly into liver and muscle by lentiviral vectors. *Nat Genet* 1997;17:314–317.

53. Miyoshi H, Smith KA, Mosier DE, Verma IM, Torbett BE. Transduction of human CD34(+) cells that mediate long-term engraftment of NOD/SCID mice by HIV vectors. *Science* 1999;283:682–686.

54. Naldini L, Blömer U, Gage FH, Trono D, Verma I. Efficient transfer, integration, and sustained long-term expression of the transgene in adult rat brains injected with a lentiviral vector. *Proc Natl Acad Sci U S A* 1996;93:11382–11388.

55. Kafri T, van Praag H, Ouyang L, Gage FH, Verma IM. A packaging cell line for lentivirus vectors. *J Virol* 1999;73:576–584.

56. Berns KI. Paroviridae: the viruses and their replication. In: Fields BN, Knipe DM, Howley PM, eds. *Virology.* Philadelphia: Lippincott–Raven, 1996:2173–2198.

57. Flotte TR, Solow R, Owens RA, Afione S, Zeitlin PL, Carter BJ. Gene expression from adeno-associated virus vectors in airway epithelial cells. *Am J Respir Cell Mol Biol* 1992;7:349–356.

58. Flotte T, Carter B, Conrad C, et al. A phase I study of an adeno-associated virus-CFTR gene vector in adult CF patients with mild lung disease. *Hum Gene Ther* 1996;7:1145–1159.

59. Miao CH, Snyder RO, Schowalter DB, et al. The kinetics of rAAV integration in the liver. *Nat Genet* 1998;19:13–15.

60. Snyder RO, Miao C, Meuse L, et al. Correction of hemophilia B in canine and murine models using recombinant adeno-associated viral vectors. *Nat Med* 1999;5:64–70.

61. Song S, Morgan M, Ellis T, et al. Sustained secretion of human alpha-1-antitrypsin from murine muscle transduced with adeno-associated virus vectors. *Proc Natl Acad Sci U S A* 1998;95:14384–14388.

62. Muzyczka N. Use of adeno-associated virus as a general transduction vector for mammalian cells. *Curr Top Microbiol Immunol* 1992;158: 97–123.

63. Mizuno M, Yoshida J, Colosi P, Kurtzman G. Adeno-associated virus vector containing the herpes simplex virus thymidine kinase gene causes complete regression of intracerebrally implanted human glio-

64. Nguyen JT, Wu P, Clouse ME, Hlatky L, Terwilliger EF. Adeno-associated virus-mediated delivery of antiangiogenic factors as an antitumor strategy. *Cancer Res* 1998;58:5673–5677.

65. Shenk T. Adenoviridae: the viruses and their replication. In: Fields BN, Knipe DM, Howley PM, eds. *Virology.* Philadelphia: Lippincott–Raven, 1996:2111–2148.

66. Bett AJ, Haddara W, Prevec L, Graham FL. An efficient and flexible system for construction of adenovirus vectors with insertions or deletions in early regions 1 and 3. *Proc Natl Acad Sci U S A* 1994;91: 8802–8806.

67. Yang Y, Nunes FA, Berencsi K, Gönczöl E, Engelhardt JF, Wilson JM. Inactivation of *E2a* in recombinant adenoviruses improves the prospect for gene therapy in cystic fibrosis. *Nat Genet* 1994;7:362–369.

68. Graham FL, Smiley J, Russell WC, Nairn R. Characteristics of a human cell line transformed by DNA from human adenovirus type 5. *J Gen Virol* 1977;36:59–74.

69. Brody SL, Crystal RG. Adenovirus-mediated *in vivo* gene transfer. *Ann N Y Acad Sci* 1994;716:90–101.

70. Schiedner G, Morral N, Parks RJ, et al. Genomic DNA transfer with a high-capacity adenovirus vector results in improved *in vivo* gene expression and decreased toxicity. *Nat Genet* 1998;18:180–183.

71. Rosenfeld MA, Siegfried W, Yoshimura K, et al. Adenovirus-mediated transfer of a recombinant α_1-antitrypsin gene to the lung epithelium *in vivo. Science* 1991;252:431–434.

72. Lemarchand P, Jaffe HA, Danel C, et al. Adenovirus-mediated transfer of a recombinant human αl-antitrypsin cDNA to human endothelial cells. *Proc Natl Acad Sci U S A* 1992;89:6482–6486.

73. Le Gal La Salle G, Robert JJ, Berrard S, et al. An adenovirus vector for gene transfer into neurons and glia in the brain. *Science* 1993;259:988–990.

74. Ragot T, Vincent N, Chafey P, et al. Efficient adenovirus-mediated transfer of a human minidystrophin gene to skeletal muscle of *mdx* mice. *Nature* 1993;361:647–650.

75. Yang Y, Nunes FA, Berencsi K, Furth EE, Gönczöl E, Wilson JM. Cellular immunity to viral antigens limits E1-deleted adenoviruses for gene therapy. *Proc Natl Acad Sci U S A* 1994;91:4407–4411.

76. Wilson CB, Embree LJ, Schowalter D, et al. Transient inhibition of CD28 and CD40 ligand interactions prolongs adenovirus-mediated transgene expression in lung and facilitates expression after secondary vector administration. *J Virol* 1998;72:7542–7550.

77. Mack CA, Song W-R, Carpenter H, et al. Circumvention of anti-adenovirus neutralizing immunity by administration of an adenoviral vector of an alternate serotype. *Hum Gene Ther* 1997;8:99–109.

78. Moolten FL. Tumor chemosensitivity conferred by inserting herpes thymidine kinase genes: paradigm for a prospective cancer control strategy. *Cancer Res* 1986;46:5276–5281.

79. Mullen C, Kilstrup M, Blaese R. Transfer of the bacterial gene for cytosine deaminase to mammalian cells confers lethal sensitivity to 5-fluorocytosine; a negative selection system. *Proc Natl Acad Sci U S A* 1992;89:33–37.

80. Putzer BM, Bramson JL, Addison CL, et al. Combination therapy with interleukin-2 and wild-type p53 expressed by adenoviral vectors potentiates tumor regression in a murine model of breast cancer. *Hum Gene Ther* 1998;9:707–718.

81. Ju DW, Wang BM, Cao X. Adenovirus-mediated combined suicide gene and interleukin-2 gene therapy for the treatment of established tumor and induction of antitumor immunity. *J Cancer Res Clin Oncol* 1998;124:683–689.

82. Yoshida Y, Sadata A, Zhang W, Saito K, Shinoura N, Hamada H. Generation of fiber-mutant recombinant adenoviruses for gene therapy of malignant glioma. *Hum Gene Ther* 1998;9:2503–2515.

83. Dmitriev I, Krasnykh V, Miller CR, et al. An adenovirus vector with genetically modified fibers demonstrates expanded tropism via utilization of a coxsackievirus and adenovirus receptor-independent cell entry mechanism. *J Virol* 1998;72:9706–9713.

84. Roizman B, Sears AE. Herpes simplex viruses and their replication. In: Fields BN, Knipe DM, Howley PM, eds. *Virology.* Philadelphia: Lippincott–Raven, 1996:2231–2296.

85. Martindale D, Hackman A, Wieczorek A, et al. Length of hunting-tin and its polyglutamine tract influences localization and frequency of intracellular aggregates. *Nat Genet* 1998;18:150–154.

86. Breakefield XO, Kramm CM, Chiocca EA, Pechan PA. *Herpes simplex virus vectors for tumor therapy.* New York: Appleton & Lange, 1995.

87. Chamber R, Gillespie GY, Soroceanu L, et al. Comparison of genetically engineered herpes simplex viruses for the treatment of brain tumors in SCID mouse model of human malignant glioma. *Proc Natl Acad Sci U S A* 1995;92:1411–1415.

88. Glorioso JC, Bender MA, Goins WF, DeLuca N, Fink DJ. Herpes simplex virus as a gene-delivery vector for the central nervous system. In: Kaplitt MG, Loewy AD, eds. *Viral vectors: gene therapy and neuroscience applications.* New York: Academic, 1995:1–23.

89. Johnson PA, Yopshida K, Gage FH, Friedmann T. Effects of gene transfer into cultured CNS neurons with a replication-defective herpes simplex virus type 1 vector. *Mol Brain Res* 1992;12:95–102.

90. Geller A, Breakefield X. A defective HSV-1 vector expresses *Escherichia coli* beta-galactosidase in cultured peripheral neurons. *Science* 1988;241:1667–1669.

91. Geller A, Freese A. Infection of cultured central nervous system neurons with a defective herpes simplex virus 1 vector results in stable expression of *Escherichia coli* beta-galactosidase. *Proc Natl Acad Sci U S A* 1990;87:1149–1153.

92. Andreansky S, He B, van Cott J, et al. Treatment of intracranial gliomas in immunocompetent mice using herpes simplex viruses that express murine interleukins. *Gene Ther* 1998;5:121–130.

93. Moriuchi S, Oligino T, Krisky D, et al. Enhanced tumor cell killing in the presence of ganciclovir by herpes simplex virus type 1 vector-directed coexpression of human tumor necrosis factor-alpha and herpes simplex virus thymidine kinase. *Cancer Res* 1998;58:5731–5737.

94. Krisky DM, Wolfe D, Goins WF, et al. Deletion of multiple immediate-early genes from herpes simplex virus reduces cytotoxicity and permits long-term gene expression in neurons. *Gene Ther* 1998;5:1593–1603.

95. Kieff E. Epstein-Barr virus and its replication. In: Fields BN, Knipe DM, Howley PM, eds. *Virology.* Philadelphia: Lippincott–Raven, 1996:2343–2396.

96. Rickinson AB, Kieff E. Epstein-Barr virus. In: Fields BN, Knipe DM, Howley PM, eds. *Virology.* Philadelphia: Lippincott–Raven, 1996:2397–2446.

97. Wang S, Vos J-M. A hybrid herpesvirus infectious vector based on Epstein-Barr virus and herpes simplex virus type 1 for gene transfer into human cells *in vitro* and *in vivo. J Virol* 1996;70:8422–8430.

98. Moss B, Flexner C. Vaccinia virus expression vectors. *Ann Rev Immunol* 1987;5:305–324.

99. Moss B. Poxviridae: the viruses and their replication. In: Fields BN, Knipe DM, Howley PM, eds. *Virology.* Philadelphia: Lippincott–Raven, 1996:2637–2671.

100. Smith GL, Moss B. Infectious poxvirus vectors have a capacity for at least 25,000 base pairs of foreign DNA. *Gene* 1983;25:21–28.

101. McCabe BJ, Irvine KR, Nishimura MI, et al. Minimal determinant expressed by a recombinant vaccinia virus elicits therapeutic antitumor cytolytic T lymphocyte response. *Cancer Res* 1995;55:1741–1747.

102. Meko JB, Yim JH, Tsung K, Norton JA. High cytokine production and effective antitumor activity of a recombinant vaccinia virus encoding murine IL-12. *Cancer Res* 1995;55:4765–4770.

103. Feng M, Jackson WH, Goldman CK, et al. Stable *in vivo* gene transduction via a novel adenoviral/retroviral chimeric vector. *Nat Biotech* 1997;15:866–870.

104. Ramsey WJ, Caplen NJ, Li Q, Higginbotham JN, Shah M, Blaese RM. Adenovirus vectors as transcomplementing templates for the production of replication defective retroviral vectors. *Biochem Biophys Res Commun* 1998;246:912–919.

105. Caplen NJ, Higginbotham JN, Scheel JR, et al. Adeno-retroviral chimeric viruses as *in vivo* transducing agents. *Gene Ther* 1999;6:454–459.

106. Li KJ, Garoff H. Packaging of intron-containing genes into retrovirus vectors by alphavirus vectors. *Proc Natl Acad Sci U S A* 1998;95:3650–3654.

107. Wahlfors JJ, Xanthopoulos KG, Morgan RA. Semliki Forest virus-mediated production of retroviral vector RNA in retroviral packaging cells. *Hum Gene Ther* 1997;8:2031–2041.

108. Zhang J, Asselin-Paturel C, Bex F, et al. Cloning of human IL-12 p40 and p35 DNA into the Semliki Forest virus vector: expression of IL-12 in human tumor cells. *Gene Ther* 1997;4:367–374.

109. Iijima Y, Ohno K, Ikeda H, Sawai K, Levin B, Meruelo D. Cell-specific targeting of a thymidine kinase/ganciclovir gene therapy system using a recombinant Sindbis virus vector. *Int J Cancer* 1999;80:110–118.

GENE THERAPY: CLINICAL APPLICATIONS

Gene Therapy Using Lymphocyte Modification

PATRICK HWU

Adoptive immunotherapy, the transfer of T cells to patients, has produced relevant clinical results in several settings, including the use of tumor-infiltrating lymphocytes (TILs) in melanoma patients (1); donor lymphocytes (2) and cytomegalovirus-reactive T-cell clones (3) in allogeneic transplant patients with lymphoid malignancies; and Epstein-Barr virus (EBV)–reactive T cells in patients with transplant-related EBV lymphomas (4). The ability to efficiently gene-modify primary lymphocytes has created opportunities to confer new properties to adoptively transferred cells in an attempt to increase their efficacy or safety profile and to understand their biology *in vivo* (Table 1).

Initial studies used marker genes to follow transferred cells and their progeny *in vivo* to investigate the survival and trafficking of these cells after infusion. Following this, cytokine genes were introduced into lymphocytes in an attempt to improve their efficacy against tumor. More recently, receptor genes, using native T-cell receptor (TCR) alpha and beta chains or fusion proteins with antibody variable regions, have been used to alter T-cell specificity to allow the recognition of tumor targets. Finally, in the setting of allogeneic bone marrow transplantation (BMT) for lymphomas, donor T-cell infusions can be effective against the tumor but can induce life-threatening graft-versus-host disease (GVHD). Therefore, suicide genes have been used in donor lymphocytes in an attempt to increase their safety profile in this setting.

However, the use of gene-modified lymphocytes first requires a safe, efficient, and reliable method of stable gene transfer into primary T cells.

METHODS OF GENE TRANSFER INTO LYMPHOCYTES

Although many methods of gene transfer into mammalian cells exist, such as electroporation and calcium phosphate transfection, most do not allow efficient DNA transfer in primary lymphocytes. In contrast to gene transfer into tumor cells and many other cell types, which can be successfully performed using a variety of methods, the efficient expression of foreign DNA in lymphocytes presents unique problems and challenges, requiring a careful selection of the mode of gene transfer. Large numbers of T cells are required for adoptive therapy, and, consequently, a relatively efficient method of gene transfer is needed to allow the growth of an adequate number of transduced cells. These therapies are often used in patients with advanced malignancies; thus, the generation of cells must be performed in a timely fashion, underscoring the need for an efficient method of gene insertion. Finally, although several methods exist to genetically modify T-cell tumor lines or established, long-term T-cell clones, adoptive immunotherapy often requires the use of bulk populations of nontransformed, primary T-cell lines.

With these stringent requirements, traditional nonviral methods of gene transfer, such as electroporation, calcium phosphate transfection, and lipofection, are not adequate for the genetic modification of lymphocytes for use in adoptive therapy.

In the 1970s, however, the finding that tumor viruses transferred genetic material to transformed cells led to the idea of using these viruses as vectors for gene transfer. Since the mid-1980s, these viral vectors have been refined for use in high-efficiency gene transfer into many cell types in the absence of replication-competent virus. Although improvements in gene transfer and expression techniques are needed for optimal use in lymphocytes, viral vectors have enabled the study of genetic modification as a means to improve effector cells for adoptive therapy. The most important of these vectors have been derived from murine retroviruses.

RETROVIRAL VECTORS AND THE USE OF ALTERNATIVE ENVELOPE GENES

Retroviral virions each consist of two single strands of RNA (ssRNA) within a protein core, or capsid, surrounded by a lipid

TABLE 1. POTENTIAL GENE THERAPY APPROACHES TO IMPROVE LYMPHOCYTES USED IN ADOPTIVE IMMUNOTHERAPY

Gene	Rationale
TNF	Interfere with tumor blood supply
Chimeric antibody/T-cell receptor (variable region of monoclonal antibody plus T-cell signaling chain)	Alter recognition of T cell (non-MHC–restricted)
Alpha and beta chain of TCR that specifically recognizes tumor antigen	Alter recognition of T cell (MHC restricted)
Suicide genes	Enhance safety profile of donor lymphocytes
IL-2 receptor	Increase sensitivity to administered IL-2
Erythropoietin, IL-3, or GM-CSF receptors (or chimeras using IL-2 receptor cytoplasmic domains)	Substitute IL-2 dependence for a less toxic molecule
Adhesion and costimulatory molecules	Enhance lymphocyte ability to traffic to tumor sites or to become activated on contact with tumor
IL-2	Increase lymphocyte survival *in vivo*
MDR	Select antitumor lymphocytes *in vivo* with chemotherapy (e.g., Taxol)

GM-CSF, granulocyte-macrophage colony-stimulating factor; IL-2, interleukin-2; MDR, multi-drug resistance gene; MHC, major histocompatibility complex; TNF, tumor necrosis factor.

envelope. On binding of a protein on the retroviral envelope to a cell-surface receptor, the retrovirus enters the cell. During migration to the nucleus, the RNA is reverse-transcribed to DNA, which, on entering the nucleus, is integrated into the host genome. This integrated retroviral genome, termed the *provirus*, then uses host cell transcriptional machinery to express the proviral genes. This leads to the manufacture of structural viral proteins and enzymes necessary for production of further retroviral particles. Packaging of proviral-RNA transcript into newly forming virions (encapsidation) is dependent on a specific sequence termed ψ+ (5).

To modify the retroviral genome to safely introduce genes into mammalian cells, all structural genes are removed from the retrovirus and are replaced with the gene of interest. The encapsidation and replication signals, however, are retained. This replication-incompetent retroviral vector is then packaged into retroviral virions using cell lines (packaging cells) that contain helper-plasmid sequences encoding all of the viral proteins (Fig. 1). The helper sequences, consisting of the retroviral *gag/pol* and *env* genes, do not themselves contain the ψ+ sequence, and thus are not packaged into newly forming virions to produce replication-competent virus. However, retroviral vectors, which contain the ψ+ sequence followed by the gene of interest, are packaged into the retroviral virions on transfection into packaging cells. Because retroviral vectors do not contain any retroviral structural genes themselves, they can be used to safely transfer the gene of interest into target cells in the absence of wild-type, replication-competent retrovirus (5,6).

Retroviral packaging cells can use a variety of envelope genes from other viruses. Because the envelope protein is the primary determinant of the host range of the retrovirus, the particular envelope or pseudotype used can have a profound impact on transduction efficiencies (7). Table 2 lists a number of envelope genes along with their relative host ranges. The development of packaging cell lines using alternative envelope genes has resulted in significant advances in the ability to transduce pri-

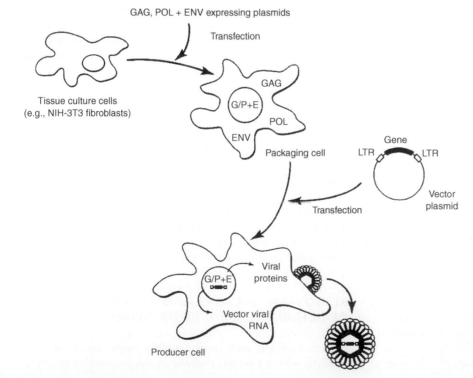

FIGURE 1. Production of retroviral vectors with packaging cells. The gene of interest is cloned into a retroviral vector and then transfected into a helper cell line, which provides the retroviral structural genes in *trans*. The retroviral structural genes cannot be packaged due to the absence of a packaging sequence (ψ), whereas the retroviral vector can be packaged, thereby producing a replication incompetent retrovirus. (LTR, long terminal repeat.) (From Eglitis MA, Anderson WF. Retroviral vectors for introduction of genes into mammalian cells. *Biotechniques* 1988:6;608–614, with permission.)

TABLE 2. ENVELOPES USED FOR RETROVIRAL VECTORS

Envelope Source	Host Range Includes
Ecotropic	Mouse, rat
Amphotropic	Human, mouse, rat, rabbit, cat, dog, monkey
GALV	Human, rat, rabbit, cat, dog, monkey (not mouse)
VSV-G	All

GALV, gibbon ape leukemia virus; VSV-G, vesicular stomatitis virus G glycoprotein.

mary lymphocytes. Retroviral vectors produced from the PG13 packaging cell line (8), which uses the gibbon ape leukemia virus envelope, are capable of transducing B cells (9) and T cells (10) with significantly higher efficiencies compared to those derived from amphotropic packaging cell lines. In one study, transduction of primary T cells was fourfold to 18-fold higher with PG13-packaged vectors compared to amphotropic PA317-packaged vectors (Table 3) (10). This was found to correlate with an eightfold to 19-fold higher expression of the gibbon ape leukemia virus envelope receptor (Pit-1) compared to the amphotropic receptor (Pit-2) in primary T cells (Table 4), although other factors besides receptor expression have been found to play a role in transduction efficiency (11). By combining the use of PG13-packaged vectors with a 1-hour centrifugation at 1,000 g, Bunnell et al. were able to obtain transduction efficiencies of primary T cells in the 40% range (12).

The vesicular stomatitis virus-G glycoprotein (VSV-G) can also be used to pseudotype retroviral vectors (13). Unlike other envelope proteins, the VSV-G protein confers enhanced physical stability to retroviral particles, allowing concentration with ultracentrifugation to titers of 10^9 or higher. VSV-G pseudo-

TABLE 3. COPY NUMBER OF TRANSDUCED NEO^R GENES IN TUMOR-INFILTRATING LYMPHOCYTES (TILS) AND PERIPHERAL BLOOD LYMPHOCYTES (PBLS)[a]

Experiment		PG13-NEO	PA317-NEO	Copy No. PG13-NEO / Copy No. PA317-NEO
1337 TII	1	0.72	0.04	18
	2	0.20	0.04	5
1143 TIL	1	1.11	0.16	7
	2	1.31	0.28	5
1495 TIL	1	0.63	0.09	7
	2	0.56	0.10	6
1475 TIL	1	0.71	0.04	18
	2	1.55	0.18	9
1102 TIL	1	0.39	0.06	7
	2	0.81	0.19	4
PBL 4353	—	0.19	0.03	6
PBL 4374	—	0.35	0.09	4
PBL 4376	—	0.25	0.04	6
PBL 4377	—	0.40	0.04	10
PBL 4378	—	0.70	0.06	12

Neo^R, neomycin resistance.
[a]Transduction efficiency was analyzed by competitive polymerase chain reaction assay.
From Lam JS, Cowherd R, Rosenberg SA, Hwu P. Improved gene transfer into lymphocytes using retroviruses that express the gibbon ape leukemia virus envelope. *Hum Gene Ther* 1996:7;1415–1422, with permission.

TABLE 4. COMPARISON OF PIT-1 TO PIT-2 MESSENGER RNA (MRNA) EXPRESSION IN TUMOR-INFILTRATING LYMPHOCYTES (TILS) AND PERIPHERAL BLOOD LYMPHOCYTES (PBLS)

Cell Line	mRNA (ng[a]) Pit-1	Pit-2	Pit-1 mRNA[b] / Pit-2 mRNA
1337 TIL	0.236	0.016	19
1143 TIL	0.093	0.009	8
1495 TIL	0.134	0.017	13
1475 TIL	0.215	0.013	14
1102 TIL	0.108	0.009	15
4353 PBL	0.116	0.013	11
4374 PBL	0.177	0.015	12
4376 PBL	0.173	0.015	13
4377 PBL	0.229	0.016	15
4378 PBL	0.162	0.012	14

Pit, gibbon ape leukemia virus envelope receptor.
[a]Per 20 µg of total RNA.
[b]Ratios were corrected for loading by multiplying by (β-actin$_{Pit-2}$ ÷ β-actin$_{Pit-1}$). The β-actin values were obtained by measuring radioactive counts per minute (β-emissions) of β-actin probe hybridized to Pit-2 and Pit-1 blots.
From Lam JS, Cowherd R, Rosenberg SA, Hwu P. Improved gene transfer into lymphocytes using retroviruses that express the gibbon ape leukemia virus envelope. *Hum Gene Ther* 1996:7;1415–1422, with permission.

typed retroviral vectors have a wide host range and have been used successfully to transduce primary T cells (14,15).

OTHER VIRAL VECTORS

Retroviral vectors offer the advantage of permanent integration within the host genome and the transfer of only the gene of interest without transferring other viral genes. Because of these properties, retroviral vectors have been the most widely used vectors for gene-therapy clinical protocols. However, in comparison to many other cell types, such as tumor cells and fibroblasts, retroviral transduction into lymphocytes results in lower transduction efficiencies and levels of gene expression. For these reasons, current efforts are focused on developing alternative vectors for use in lymphocytes.

These alternatives include vectors based on recombinant adenovirus (16), adenoassociated virus (AAV) (17), and poxviruses (18–21). All have advantages and disadvantages compared to retroviruses for gene transfer into lymphocytes, and their ultimate utility for this purpose is based on further study, as well as the particular goals and requirements of lymphocyte transduction with the specific gene of interest for a particular application.

Of these potential viral vectors for lymphocyte transduction, only AAV, like retroviruses, can permanently integrate the introduced gene into the target-cell genome. In contrast, gene transfer via adenoviral vectors or pox vectors is transient, and expression thus decreases as the cell divides. Pox vectors, however, have the capability of transducing cells with high efficiency, including lymphocytes (unpublished studies in our laboratory), compared to retroviral vectors. Adenoviral vectors appear to be capable of transducing lymphocytes with relatively high efficiency, compared to retroviruses, but gene expression has been low (preliminary studies from our laboratory). AAV vectors have not yet been fully tested in lymphocytes, partially due to the difficulty in producing high-titer, purified AAV vector stocks.

Because adenoviral, AAV, and retroviral vectors rely on eukaryotic or viral promoters, which require host transcriptional machinery, gene expression can be regulated by normal host mechanisms. Studies thus far of retroviral gene transfer into lymphocytes have revealed that levels of vector-derived transcript in transduced lymphocytes were significantly lower compared to that in transduced tumor cells (22). With the current cellular and viral promoters available, gene expression in primary lymphocytes is relatively low, compared to the abundant levels of expression observed in most other cell types. Therefore, the use of adenoviral, AAV, and retroviral vectors in lymphocytes is currently limited by the levels of gene expression obtainable from currently used promoters. Although this level of expression may be adequate for some applications, full utility of these vectors is realized only after new promoter or enhancer regions are identified, which allow improved expression in primary lymphocytes.

In contrast, poxviruses, such as vaccinia and fowlpox, contain genes that encode their own RNA polymerases, allowing transcription to occur in the target-cell cytoplasm independent of host cell transcriptional machinery. Consequently, foreign gene expression is significantly higher with poxviruses compared to other methods. However, vaccinia vectors are eventually toxic to host cells, and, in our experience, result in lymphocyte cell death within 72 hours. In contrast, fowlpox vectors have not been toxic to lymphocytes, while allowing high levels of gene expression in some cultures in preliminary experiments. As previously discussed, though, gene transfer is transient, and gene expression decreases as the cells divide (unpublished studies in our laboratory).

Thus, alternative viral vectors for gene transfer into lymphocytes are currently under study, and each have their own advantages and disadvantages. It is likely that some vectors are most amenable to a particular application while others are more useful for another application, depending, for example, on the levels and duration of gene expression required.

MARKING STUDIES

The introduction of foreign DNA into humans raised many safety issues concerning patients and the general public. The first gene-transfer study in humans, performed in the Surgery Branch of the National Cancer Institute, used a marker gene conferring neomycin resistance (Neo^R) to assess the safety and feasibility of transferring foreign genes into humans. The trial was performed using TILs retrovirally transduced with the replication-defective N2 vector containing the gene encoding the bacterial enzyme neomycin phosphotransferase (Fig. 2) (23,24). Sensitive S+/L– studies were performed to rule out the presence of replication-competent retrovirus. Ten patients were treated, and no safety or toxicity problems were detected from the gene transfer. Because a novel gene was introduced into TILs that could be distinguished from endogenous DNA, the survival and distribution of the TILs could be followed *in vivo*. Furthermore, as TILs proliferated *in vivo*, daughter cells would all be marked with the Neo^R gene as well. Using polymerase chain reaction analysis, which was capable of detecting 1:10,000 to 1:100,000

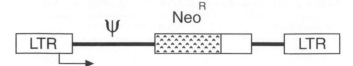

FIGURE 2. Schematic diagram of the LNL6 retroviral vector, which contains the gene for neomycin resistance. The vector is a derivative of the Moloney murine leukemia virus. (LTR, long terminal repeat; Neo^R, neomycin resistance.) (From Miller AD, Buttimore C. Redesign of retrovirus packaging-cell lines to avoid recombination leading to helper-virus production. *Mol Cell Biol* 1986:6;2895–2902, with permission.)

cells, peripheral blood and tumor cells were analyzed for presence of the Neo^R gene. Neo^R TILs were found in tumor biopsies up to 64 days and in peripheral blood up to 189 days after injection (Fig. 3) (24,25).

Since this initial study using Neo^R-marked TILs, other groups have also begun gene-marking studies using melanoma TILs (26,27), renal TILs (28), bone marrow stem cells (29,30), and anti-human immunodeficiency virus (HIV) cytotoxic T cells (31). Using gene-marked, EBV-specific cytotoxic T lymphocytes (CTLs) in immunocompromised patients, Heslop et al. found that EBV precursors could proliferate in response to *in vivo* or *ex vivo* viral challenge for as long as 18 months (Fig. 4) (32).

Researchers at the University of Washington in Seattle have used Neo^R-marked HIV type 1 (HIV-1), *gag*-specific CD8+ CTL clones to treat HIV-infected individuals (33). Using polymerase

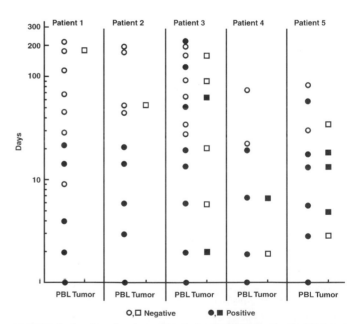

FIGURE 3. Results of polymerase chain reaction assays of peripheral blood mononuclear cells (*circles*) and tumor biopsy specimens (*squares*) obtained from patients at various intervals after the infusion of gene-transduced tumor-infiltrating lymphocytes. Open symbols denote negative results, and solid symbols positive results. All results were corroborated in at least two separate Southern blot assays. The assays were performed and assessed in a blinded fashion. (PBL, peripheral blood lymphocyte.) (From Rosenberg SA, Aebersold P, Cornetta K, et al. Gene transfer into humans—immunotherapy of patients with advanced melanoma, using tumor-infiltrating lymphocytes modified by retroviral gene transduction. *N Engl J Med* 1990:323;570–578, with permission.)

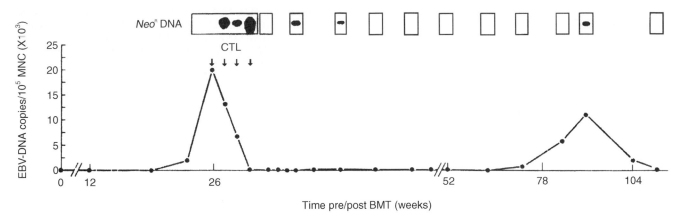

FIGURE 4. Recruitment of gene-marked, Epstein-Barr virus (EBV)–specific cytotoxic T lymphocytes (CTLs) by antigenic stimulation *in vivo*. DNA was obtained from peripheral blood mononuclear cells of a patient between 0 and 108 weeks after bone marrow transplantation (BMT) and divided into two portions. One was analyzed by polymerase chain reaction amplification using EBV-specific primers, whereas the second was amplified using neomycin-specific primers. The figure shows the relationship between levels of EBV-DNA and the presence of neomycin resistance (Neo^R)–marked, EBV-specific, gene-positive T cells. (MNC, mononuclear cells.) (From Heslop HE, Ng CY, Li C, et al. Long-term restoration of immunity against Epstein-Barr virus infection by adoptive transfer of gene-modified virus-specific T lymphocytes. *Nat Med* 1996:2;551–555, with permission.)

chain reaction amplification for the Neo^R gene followed by *in situ* hybridization with fluorescein-labeled Neo^R-specific oligonucleotides, the percentage of circulating transduced cells could be quantitated by flow cytometry. One day after cell infusion, 2.0% to 3.5% of CD8$^+$ cells circulating in the periphery were Neo^R positive. The frequency of Neo^R-modified CTLs was found to correlate inversely with the percentage of HIV-infected cells in the peripheral blood after cell infusion (Fig. 5). Additionally, Neo^R+ CTLs were found to accumulate in lymph node biopsies obtained 4 days after cell infusion (2.2% to 7.9%) compared to the concurrent percentages of Neo^R+ CTLs circulating in the periphery (0.5% to 0.7%). Neo^R+ CTL aggregates were found in the parafollicular regions of the lymph node near cells that were productively infected with HIV. This illustrates the utility of cell marking to determine not only the overall traffic and survival of infused cells, but also their microanatomic localization.

CYTOKINE GENES

Having demonstrated the safety and feasibility of using gene-modified cells in humans with marking protocols, the next step was to use this novel approach to increase the antitumor potency of TILs. In a gene therapy trial for cancer at the Surgery Branch of the National Cancer Institute, TILs were retrovirally transduced with the gene for tumor necrosis factor alpha (TNF-α). In a number of murine tumor models, systemic TNF-α has resulted in the dramatic regression of advanced disease (34–36). Humans, however, can tolerate only 2% of the systemic TNF dose (per weight) required in mice, due to dose-limiting hypotension (37–41). Impressive tumor regressions have been seen in patients treated locally with high concentrations of TNF given either as an intralesional injection (42,43) or as an isolated limb perfusion (44). Regressions of liver metastases have been seen in patients treated with TNF administered as an isolated hepatic perfusion (45). Therefore, tumor regressions are possible

when adequate local concentrations of TNF can be achieved. Because TILs have been demonstrated to accumulate at sites of tumor (46–48), the transduction of TILs with the TNF gene may allow high concentrations of TNF to be delivered locally in the absence of systemic toxicity (22).

TILs retrovirally transduced with the TNF-α complementary DNA (cDNA), using a bicistronic vector that also contained the neomycin resistance gene, was found to contain a high percentage of transduced cells within the population after selection in the neomycin analog G418 (22). Although Southern blot analyses of DNA from G418-selected TILs demonstrated that the foreign TNF gene was inserted in the genome with adequate efficiency, TNF gene expression was suboptimal. However, other cell types, such as fibroblasts and tumor cells, transduced with the identical retroviral vector produced high levels of TNF. Northern blot analyses demonstrated that transduced TILs had significantly lower levels of vector-derived transcript compared to transduced tumor (Table 5). Therefore, promoter or enhancer regions that direct higher levels of gene expression in primary lymphocytes should be identified to optimize this treatment strategy.

Besides TNF, other growth factors and their receptors may have utility when overexpressed in adoptively transferred lymphocytes. Interleukin-2 (IL-2) is a cytokine that signals T-cell growth. On T-cell stimulation, production of IL-2 and IL-2 receptor is upregulated, resulting in T-cell proliferation (49). Studies in murine tumor models have demonstrated that systemic IL-2 administration enhances the antitumor response from TILs (50) and have suggested that this is due to the ability of systemic IL-2 to maintain *in vivo* viability and to stimulate proliferation of the administered TILs. Marking studies using Neo^R-transduced TILs in cancer patients suggested that TILs were not detectable long after the discontinuation of systemic IL-2 treatment (24). The duration of IL-2 administration is limited in humans due to adverse reactions, such as hypotension. Thus, one possible approach to improve adoptive immunotherapy is to

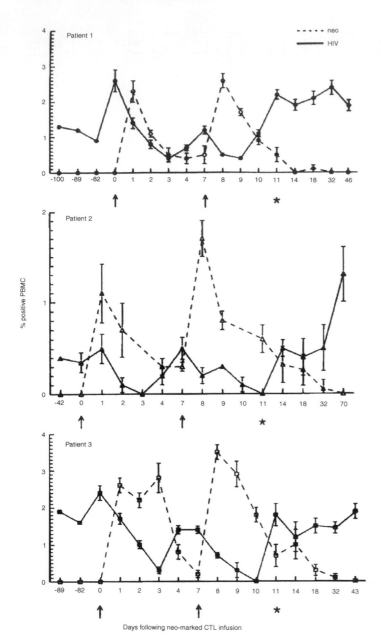

FIGURE 5. Temporal relationship between the percentage of human immunodeficiency virus (HIV)–specific CD8[+] T cells marked with neomycin (Neo[R]) resistance and the percentage of CD4[+] T cells expressing HIV-gag messenger RNA in peripheral blood mononuclear cells (PBMCs) of three patients collected before, during, and after adoptive transfer of Neo[R]-modified, HIV-specific cytotoxic T lymphocyte (CTL) clones. Up arrows (*horizontal axis*) indicate the days CTLs were infused. (From Brodie SJ, Lewinsohn DA, Patterson BK, et al. *In vivo* migration and function of transferred HIV-1–specific cytotoxic T cells [see comments]. *Nat Med* 1999;5;34–41, with permission.)

modify lymphocytes so that they can either sustain themselves through autocrine pathways or respond to alternative cytokines administered exogenously that have milder adverse reactions.

Potentially, insertion of the IL-2 gene into effector T cells could support continued growth *in vivo* without the need for exogenous IL-2. Yamada and colleagues (51) inserted the human IL-2 gene into the IL-2–dependent CTL line (CTLL) and found that the cells could grow *in vitro* in the absence of IL-2. Additionally, IL-2–transduced CTLL formed subcutaneous

TABLE 5. TRANSCRIPTION OF THE LTSN TUMOR NECROSIS FACTOR (TNF) VECTOR: A QUANTITATIVE COMPARISON BETWEEN TRANSDUCED TUMOR-INFILTRATING LYMPHOCYTES (TILS) AND TRANSDUCED TUMOR CELLS

Patient No.	% Full Length, 5'LTR-Generated, 4.0-kb TNF Transcript in TILs Compared to MEL-TNF tumor[a,b]
1102	0.8
1104	1.6
1118	6.4
1122	36.0
1126	3.9
1143.A	13.8
1144	10.8
1155	9.3
1160	3.9
1166	8.4
Mean (SEM)	9.5 (3.2)

LTR, long terminal repeat; LTSN, TNF-containing retroviral vector; MEL-TNF, TNF-transduced melanoma cell line; TNF, tumor necrosis factor.
[a]Transduced and selected TIL cultures were compared with a transduced, fully selected MEL-TNF.
[b]RNA probed with ^{32}P-labeled TNF complementary DNA (cDNA). All comparisons of RNA between TILs and tumor were corrected for loading differences via use of actin controls, background differences, and differences in percent of cells transduced. All values were quantitated directly via beta scope, and the correction factors were incorporated into the following formula:

corrected percentage of long terminal repeat-derived transcript (LTRDT) from tumor =

$$\frac{(LTRDT_{TIL} - Background_{TILNV})/(Actin_{TIL} - Background)}{(LTRDT_{tumor} - Background_{tumorNV})/(Actin_{tumor} - Background)} \times \frac{1}{T_{TIL}} \times 100\%$$

where T_{TIL} = calculated fraction of TIL transduced (compared to the 100% transduced MEL-TNF tumor line).
From Hwu P, Yannell, J, Kriegler M, et al. Functional and molecular characterization of TIL transduced with the TNF-alpha cDNA for the gene therapy of cancer in man. *J Immunol* 1993:150;4104–4115, with permission.

tumors in nude mice. Karasuyama et al. (52) introduced murine IL-2 cDNA into the IL-2–dependent murine T-cell line HT-2. The transfectants proliferated autonomously *in vitro*, and high IL-2–expressing clones developed tumors *in vivo*. Treisman et al. (53) introduced the IL-2 cDNA into the murine T helper cell line 14.1 (54), which is specific against sperm-whale myoglobin. The IL-2–transduced 14.1 cells proliferated autonomously in the absence of exogenous IL-2 and maintained specificity against sperm-whale myoglobin, as measured by specific release of murine interferon-γ.

One potential limitation in attempting to generalize this approach to primary, tumor-reactive T cells is that it might require the constitutive expression of the high-affinity IL-2 receptor. Normally, high-affinity IL-2 receptor expression is upregulated after T-cell stimulation with specific antigen (49). *In vivo*, tumor-reactive T cells could potentially interact with antigen, resulting in upregulation of IL-2 receptor. Alternatively, the concomitant introduction of the IL-2 receptor chain genes into T cells might be necessary.

Another approach toward maintaining T-cell viability *in vivo* is to introduce receptor genes responsive to alternative growth factors less toxic to patients than IL-2 (55). The IL-2 receptor is a member of the cytokine receptor superfamily, which includes the receptors for IL-3, IL-4, granulocyte-macrophage colony-stimulating factor (GM-CSF), IL-6, IL-7, erythropoietin (Epo), and granulocyte colony-stimulating factor (55). These receptors

Antibody

TCR

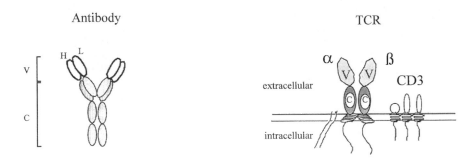

scFv- γ

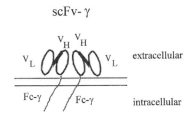

FIGURE 6. The chimeric immunoglobulin T-cell receptor (TCR) combines antibody-variable regions with T-cell signaling chains. In this diagram, a single-chain antibody (scFv) fragment derived from the variable regions of a monoclonal antibody is joined to the crystallizable fragment (Fc) receptor chain, although other signaling chains, such as the TCR-ζ chain, can be used for T-cell signal transduction.

share consensus sequences in their extracellular domains. Several are heteromultimeric, and some have been shown to share a common chain (56–59).

Kitamura et al. (60) expressed the human IL-3 receptor in murine IL-2–dependent CTLL-2 cells and found that the modified cells could proliferate in response to physiologic concentrations of human IL-3, in the absence of IL-2. Similarly, CTLL-2 cells transfected with the α and β subunits of the human GM-CSF receptor could proliferate in response to low concentrations of human GM-CSF. These results suggest that signal transduction from the IL-2, GM-CSF, and IL-3 receptors may share common components. However, conflicting reports exist on the ability of the erythropoietin receptor to induce proliferation in IL-2–dependent cells. Showers et al. (61) reported that Epo-R–transfected CTLL-2 cells could proliferate in response to Epo in the absence of IL-2, but a similar study by Yamamura et al. (62) failed to confirm this. Both studies, however, reported that an Epo-R–transfected IL-3–dependent cell line, Ba/F3, could proliferate in response to Epo alone. Thus, while similarities seem to exist in signal transduction between the IL-3 and Epo receptors, it is not clear whether the Epo and IL-2 receptors share such similarities.

Another strategy toward substituting IL-2 dependency for other ligands is the construction of chimeric receptors using the cytoplasmic domains of the IL-2 chains joined to the extracellular regions from another cytokine receptor. This would more likely ensure that signal transduction occurred along physiologic pathways consistent with normal IL-2 stimulation. One approach uses the extracellular domains from the GM-CSF receptor joined to the transmembrane and intracellular domains of the IL-2 receptor. Because CTLs produce GM-CSF but not IL-2 on activation, it is hoped that transfected cells proliferate on contact with antigen via an autocrine loop (63).

Applying these strategies to primary effector T cells has been difficult due to the limited expression of transgenes in these cells. Additionally, many cytokine receptors consist of two to three different chains, requiring the introduction of multiple genes, which has been difficult to accomplish with adequate efficiency in primary T cells.

Because of the possibility of tumor development with these approaches, the concomitant introduction of a suicide gene might be required. This would be especially important in those situations resulting in autocrine loops consisting of high constitutive production of both ligand and receptor. For example, the introduction of the IL-2 gene into T cells that constitutively express large amounts of high-affinity IL-2 receptor would more likely result in tumorigenic T cells than with T cells that only express high-affinity IL-2 receptors after T-cell stimulation.

RECEPTOR GENES THAT ALTER T-CELL SPECIFICITY

Chimeric Antibody and T-Cell Receptor Genes

Use of adoptive immunotherapy against many histologic types of cancer is limited by the difficulty in isolating and expanding specific antitumor T cells from these tumor types. However, monoclonal antibodies exist that bind to specific tumor types. By joining the antigen-binding variable regions of antibody genes with T-cell signaling chains, chimeric TCRs can be constructed to direct T-cell specificity (Fig. 6). T cells of undefined specificities could then be genetically modified with the appropriate chimeric receptor gene to confer antitumor activity. This approach has the potential to generalize the applicability of adoptive immunotherapy.

The first demonstration of an immunoglobulin (Ig)/TCR chimera was reported in 1987 by Kuwana et al. (64). Using a monoclonal antibody (MAb) against phosphorylcholine (PC), they joined the light chain variable (V_L) and heavy chain variable (V_H) region genes to the Cα- and Cβ-chain genes of the

TCR. Murine thymoma EL4 cells cotransfected with $V_LC\alpha/V_HC\beta$ or $V_LC\beta/V_HC\alpha$ gene combinations exhibited increased cytoplasmic calcium concentrations when stimulated with PC-positive bacteria. Similarly, Gross et al. (65) constructed Ig/TCR chimeric receptors using an MAb against trinitrophenyl (TNP). Jurkat (a human T-cell line) or MD.45 (a hybridoma cell line) cells transfected with $V_LC\alpha/V_HC\beta$ or $V_LC\beta/V_HC\alpha$ gene combinations exhibited specific IL-2 secretion or nonmajor histocompatibility complex–restricted cytolysis when cocultured with TNP-labeled cells. Similar studies were also performed by other groups (66,67) using antidigoxin or anti-PC MAb systems in EL-4 cells, Jurkat cells, and transgenic mice.

Although these initial approaches confirmed that chimeric Ig/TCR genes could be functional in select transformed T-cell lines, this strategy required the insertion of two genes. Because primary T cells used for adoptive immunotherapy are relatively difficult to genetically modify, the insertion of two separate genes is not ideal for a clinical approach. Therefore, Eshhar et al. (68) used a single-chain antibody (scFv) approach whereby the V_L and V_H domains are joined by a flexible linker (69–71). ScFv regions have been shown to exhibit similar specificities and affinities compared to normal antibody variable regions. The scFv gene was then joined to the TCR ζ chain or Fc receptor γ chain, both of which are closely related and capable of activating T cells when cross-linked (72–76). Thus, on a single gene, the scFv-γ/ζ design (see Fig. 6) provides both antigen recognition and T-cell signal transduction. ScFv-γ/ζ constructs derived from anti-TNP MAb were capable of redirecting MD.45-hybridoma cells against TNP-labeled targets (68).

Hwu et al. (77) demonstrated the feasibility of using this approach against human tumor, using gene-modified primary T cells. Melanoma-specific human TIL was gene-modified with scFv-γ receptor genes derived from MAb against TNP (Sp6) or ovarian cancer (MOv18). TIL retrovirally transduced with the ovarian cancer receptor gene (MOv-γ TIL) specifically lysed a human ovarian cancer line (IGROV-1) (Fig. 7). Similarly, Sp-γ and MOv-γ TIL specifically released GM-CSF when cocultured with the appropriate antigen. To assess the *in vivo* efficacy of such an approach, murine TILs derived from methylcholanthrene-induced colon carcinoma were retrovirally transduced with the MOv-γ receptor gene. Intraperitoneal MOv-TIL significantly increased survival in nude mice that had received IP human ovarian cancer cells 3 days before the TIL. Additionally, intravenous MOv-TIL significantly decreased the number of lung metastases in mice that 3 days before were given an irrelevant, syngeneic tumor transfected with the appropriate ovarian antigen gene (78).

Besides triggering direct T-cell activation with γ and ζ chains, antibody variable regions can be coupled to other signaling chains such as the intracellular portion of CD28, an important T-cell costimulatory receptor. This approach has been found to enhance T-cell survival and proliferation *in vitro* (79).

Most recently, the transduction of hematopoietic stem cells with chimeric receptor genes has been under investigation, as this may not only provide a stable supply of redirected T cells, but also granulocytes, macrophages, and natural killer cells, all of which may have significant antitumor activity on expression of chimeric receptor genes. Mice that received MOv-γ–trans-

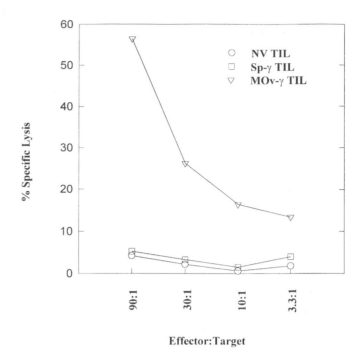

FIGURE 7. Transduction of tumor-infiltrating lymphocytes (TILs) with an antiovarian chimeric-receptor gene (MOv-γ) results in specific lysis against ovarian cancer cells. Nontransduced (NV), Sp-γ (anti-trinitrophenyl)–transduced, and MOv-γ–transduced TILs were studied for their ability to lyse the ovarian cancer cell line IGROV-1. All TILs, which were derived from melanoma, could lyse the autologous melanoma cell line (not shown), but the IGROV-1 ovarian cancer cell line was only lysed by MOv-γ–transduced TILs. (From Hwu P, Shafer GE, Treisman J, et al. Lysis of ovarian cancer cells by human lymphocytes redirected with a chimeric gene composed of an antibody variable region and the Fc-receptor gamma-chain. *J Exp Med* 1993:178;361–366, with permission.)

duced bone marrow cells exhibited significant antigen-specific antitumor activity *in vivo* (Fig. 8) (80).

These strategies have the potential of widely generalizing the use of adoptive immunotherapy. ScFv-γ/ζ receptors have been constructed against breast cancer using an anti-HER-2 MAb (81), colon cancer using an anti-GA733 MAb (82), and HIV using an anti-gp41 MAb (83). This strategy could be applied to a wide range of cancer histologies or infectious diseases for which appropriate MAb exist.

Native T-Cell Receptor Genes

T-cell specificity can also be altered by the introduction of genes encoding native TCR. The TCR consists of an α- and β-chain heterodimer that confers the ability to specifically recognize peptide and major histocompatibility complexes on antigen-presenting cells and target cells. TCRs derived from melanoma-specific CTLs have been identified, cloned, and characterized (84). Clay et al. (85) transduced primary lymphocytes with a TCR gene specific for the MART-1 melanoma tumor-rejection antigen. Because the TCR consists of two individual chains, a retroviral vector was constructed that used internal ribosomal entry sites (IRES sequences), which allow the translation of multiple genes from a single transcript (Fig. 9). Primary T cells transduced with this construct were capable of specifically recognizing tumor cells expressing the MART-1 melanoma tumor antigen in the context

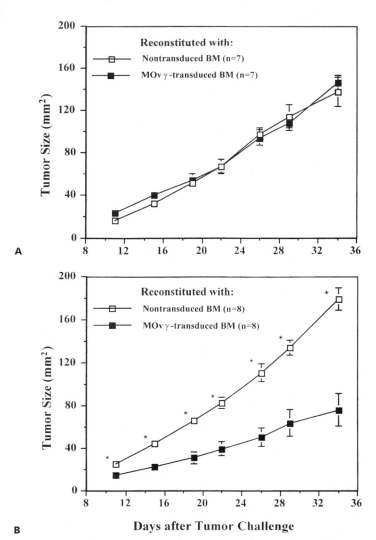

A

B

Days after Tumor Challenge

FIGURE 8. Tumor growth in MOv-γ–reconstituted mice. Ten months after bone marrow (BM) transplantation, MOv-γ– and control-reconstituted mice were subcutaneously inoculated with 1×10^5 24JK or 24JK-FBP tumor cells, the latter expressing the FBP tumor antigen recognized by MOv-γ. Tumor size was measured from day 11 to 34 after initial tumor inoculation twice a week in a blinded fashion, and expressed as square millimeter (mm^2) by multiplying 2 perpendicular diameters. **A:** Mice inoculated with 24JK tumor cells. **B:** Mice inoculated with 24JK-FBP tumor cells. The result represents one of two identical but independently executed experiments. Error bars are standard error of mean. Asterisks indicate differences are statistically significant (p_2 <0.005). (From Wang G. A T cell-independent antitumor response in mice with bone marrow cells retrovirally transduced with an antibody/Fc-gamma chain chimeric receptor gene recognizing a human ovarian cancer antigen. *Nat Med* 1998:4;168–172, with permission.)

SUICIDE GENES

Adoptively transferred T cells have been safely administered to many patients since 1988. However, in specific situations, the adoptively transferred cells may be toxic to the host, such as in

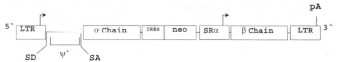

FIGURE 9. Retroviral construct encoding the α and β chains from a T-cell receptor recognizing the MART-1 melanoma antigen. The α chain is driven by the long terminal repeat (LTR) from the Moloney murine leukemia virus, whereas the β chain is driven from the SRα promoter. (IRES, internal ribosomal entry site; Neo[R], neomycin phosphotransferase gene; pA, polyadenylation signal; ψ+, packaging signal; SA, splice acceptor; SD, splice donor.) (From Clay TM, Custer M, Sachs J, et al. Efficient transfer of a tumor antigen-reactive TCR to human peripheral blood lymphocytes confers antitumor reactivity. *J Immunol* 1999:163:507–513, with permission.)

the treatment of immunocompromised HIV patients. In the setting of allogeneic BMT for hematologic malignancies, donor lymphocyte infusions can be highly effective against tumor and EBV-induced lymphoma, but may also incite GVHD. In an attempt to increase the therapeutic index of adoptively trans-

TABLE 6. LYSIS OF MART-1–POSITIVE CELLS BY T CELLS TRANSDUCED WITH A MART-1–SPECIFIC T-CELL RECEPTOR GENE

Clone	E:T Ratio	% Specific Lysis			
		T2+ Irrelevant	T2+ MART-1	888 MEL	888 A2 MEL
65-17	80:1	0	50	0	21
65-59	80:1	0	30	0	10
65-158	22:1	0	9	0	13
65-159	80:1	1	78	0	22
65-162	80:1	4	8	0	0
65-168	15:1	0	5	0	0
65-172	44:1	2	3	0	0
65-176	80:1	5	7	0	0
66-4	80:1	0	50	4	27
66-19	58:1	0	65	0	35
66-20	46:1	0	98	0	64
66-28	72:1	9	78	1	28
66-36	80:1	7	100	9	81
66-63	30:1	2	91	0	85
66-67	50:1	0	71	0	56
66-78	80:1	1	69	0	15
66-80	80:1	2	22	0	0
67-7	72:1	1	74	0	31
67-9	80:1	1	90	0	18
67-32	80:1	0	56	0	0
67-34	64:1	6	100	29	75
67-47	80:1	1	39	0	0
67-53	40:1	0	27	4	0
67-57	80:1	0	46	3	1
67-65	80:1	0	18	0	0
67-70	68:1	2	79	3	30
67-76	80:1	5	81	0	44
67-93	80:1	6	52	0	9
67-104	80:1	2	60	6	6

MEL, melanoma cell line.
Note: Peripheral blood mononuclear cells (PBMCs) from three normal donors (65,66,67) were transduced with a T-cell receptor (TCR) gene recognizing the MART-1 melanoma tumor antigen; 24 of 29 clones were specifically lytic against HLA-A2+ target cells pulsed with the MART-1 immunodominant peptide (range of lysis, 18% to 100%; mean, 64.5%), and 15 of 29 clones specifically lysed an A2+ melanoma cell line (range of lysis, 15% to 85%; mean, 42.1%).
From Clay TM, Custer M, Sachs J, et al. Efficient transfer of a tumor antigen-reactive TCR to human peripheral blood lymphocytes confers antitumor reactivity. *J Immunol* 1999:163;507–513, with permission.

of HLA-A2 (Table 6). As more TCRs recognizing specific tumor antigens are characterized and cloned, this strategy may generalize the use of adoptive immunotherapy, circumventing the need to isolate T cells with specific reactivities from individual patients.

TABLE 7. EFFECT OF GANCICLOVIR TREATMENT ON ELIMINATION OF HERPES THYMIDINE KINASE–MODIFIED DONOR LYMPHOCYTES AND ON GRAFT-VERSUS-HOST DISEASE (GVHD)

| Patient | GVHD (grade) | Proportion of Transduced Peripheral Blood Lymphocytes (%) | | Clinical Outcome of GVHD |
		Preganciclovir	24 h after ganciclovir	
1	Acute skin (II/III)	13.4	$<10^{-4}$	CR
2	Acute liver (III)	2.0	$<10^{-4}$	CR
8	Chronic lung, skin, gastrointestinal	11.9	2.8	PR

CR, complete remission of GVHD; PR, partial remission of GVHD.
Adapted from Bonini C, Ferrari G, Verzeletti S, et al. HSV-TK gene transfer into donor lymphocytes for control of allogeneic graft-versus-leukemia [see comments]. *Science* 1997;276:1719–1724.

ferred cells in these situations, suicide genes can be introduced into lymphocytes to specifically delete the transduced cells should they become toxic to patients *in vivo*. The gene for herpes thymidine kinase (hTK) has been used for this purpose, as it specifically sensitizes cells to the antiviral agent ganciclovir.

In one study using hTK-transduced donor lymphocytes, three of eight patients receiving donor lymphocytes after allogeneic BMT for hematologic malignancies developed acute or chronic GVHD. In these patients, ganciclovir administration significantly diminished the number of circulating hTK-transduced cells within 24 hours, resulting in complete or partial remissions of the GVHD (86) (Table 7).

In another study, anti-HIV CTLs were transduced with a fusion gene encoding hTK and the selectable marker hygromycin before administration in HIV-infected patients (87). Because HIV patients are immunocompromised, the CTLs could be eradicated with ganciclovir should the transduced cells become toxic. However, initial results of the trial revealed that the patients were developing cellular immune responses against the hTK-hygromycin fusion protein (Table 8), thus demonstrating that foreign genes, including selectable markers, can themselves become targets of the host immune response.

OVERVIEW AND SUMMARY

The ability to introduce foreign genes into T cells has opened exciting opportunities for enhancing the adoptive immunotherapy of cancer. For adoptively transferred lymphocytes to be most effective, they must survive and proliferate *in vivo*, recognize tumor cells, and respond with an adequate effector mechanism. Attempts are under way to improve on each of these steps through gene modification. The introduction into lymphocytes of the genes encoding IL-2, IL-2 receptor, or other growth-factor receptors or chimeras may lead to increased survival of lymphocytes *in vivo*. The use of chimeric-antibody/TCR genes or native α/β TCR genes may allow enhanced recognition of tumor *in vivo*. Additionally, this approach may enable the generation of tumor-specific lymphocytes against histologies from which specific antitumor lymphocytes are difficult to grow. Finally, the introduction of the gene for TNF may enhance T-cell effector function by enabling lymphocytes to deliver high concentrations of TNF to tumor sites, without causing systemic TNF toxicity.

For these approaches to succeed, progress is required in the development of vectors, resulting in enhanced transduction efficiencies and gene expression in primary T lymphocytes. Ultimately, vectors whose expression can be regulated *in vivo* may be of great clinical utility. In addition, further progress is needed toward the understanding and resolution of other primary challenges in improving the clinical outcome in patients receiving adoptively transferred T cells. For example, although it is known that adoptively transferred T cells can cause the regression of large tumor burdens in some patients, the percentage that traffic to and penetrate into the tumor is often small. A greater understanding of the adhesion molecules and intracellular signals that

TABLE 8. HyTK-SPECIFIC CYTOTOXIC T LYMPHOCYTE (CTL) RESPONSES BEFORE INITIATING AND 1 WEEK AFTER COMPLETING FOUR COURSES OF ADOPTIVE IMMUNOTHERAPY WITH HyTK-TRANSDUCED CD8$^+$ HUMAN IMMUNODEFICIENCY VIRUS–SPECIFIC CTL CLONES

| Patient | E/T | Preinfusion CTL response to HyTK | | Postinfusion CTL response to HyTK | |
| | | Target cell (% lysis) | | Target cell (% lysis) | |
		Mock	HyTK	Mock	HyTK
1	10:1	0	0	0	57
	5:1	0	0	0	35
2	5:1	0	0	0	0
3	5:1	4	0	6	65
	2.5:1	2	1	5	46
4	5:1	6	6	2	63
	2.5:1	3	2	1	58
5	10:1	1	0	3	66
	5:1	0	0	3	69
6	5:1	0	0	0	21
	2.5:1	0	0	0	13

HyTK, hygromycin–thymidine kinase fusion protein.
Note: Cryopreserved peripheral blood mononuclear cells obtained before therapy and 1 week after completing T-cell therapy were stimulated twice, 1 week apart at a responder to stimulator ratio of 2:1 with an aliquot of irradiated autologous HyTK-transduced T-cell clones. The cultures were assayed in a chromium (Cr) release assay at various effector to target ratios against ^{51}Cr-labeled control parental nontransduced autologous T cells or LCL targets designated as *mock* and against autologous HyTK-transduced CTLs or HyTK-transduced LCL targets designated *HyTK*.
Adapted from Riddell SR, Elliott M, Lewinsohn DA, et al. T-cell mediated rejection of gene-modified HIV-specific cytotoxic T lymphocytes in HIV-infected patients [see comments]. *Nat Med* 1996;2:216–223.

are necessary for T cells to mobilize into solid tumors may lead to improved abilities to genetically manipulate T cells to allow them to more effectively traffic to these sites.

REFERENCES

1. Rosenberg SA, Packard BS, Aebersold PM, et al. Use of tumor infiltrating lymphocytes and interleukin-2 in the immunotherapy of patients with metastatic melanoma. Preliminary report. *N Engl J Med* 1988;319:1676–1680.
2. Drobyski WR, Keever CA, Roth MS, et al. Salvage immunotherapy using donor leukocyte infusions as treatment for relapsed chronic myelogenous leukemia after allogeneic bone marrow transplantation: efficacy and toxicity of a defined T-cell dose. *Blood* 1993;82:2310–2318.
3. Walter EA, Greenberg PD, Gilbert MJ, et al. Reconstitution of cellular immunity against cytomegalovirus in recipients of allogeneic bone marrow by transfer of T-cell clones from the donor. *N Engl J Med* 1995;333:1038–1044.
4. Brenner MK, Rill DR, Heslop HE, et al. Gene marking after bone marrow transplantation. *Eur J Cancer* 1994;30A:1171–1176.
5. Miller AD. Retroviral vectors. *Curr Top Microbiol Immunol* 1992; 158:1–24X.
6. Morgan R, Anderson WF. Human Gene Therapy. *Annu Rev Biochem* 1993;62:191–217.
7. Miller AD. Cell-surface receptors for retroviruses and implications for gene transfer. *Proc Natl Acad Sci U S A* 1996;93:11407–11413.
8. Miller AD, Garcia JV, von Suhr N, Lynch CM, Wilson C, Eiden MV. Construction and properties of retrovirus packaging cells based on gibbon ape leukemia virus. *J Virol* 1991;65:2220–2224.
9. Bauer TR Jr, Miller AD, Hickstein DD. Improved transfer of the leukocyte integrin CD18 subunit into hematopoietic cell lines by using retroviral vectors having a gibbon ape leukemia virus envelope. *Blood* 1995;86:2379–2387.
10. Lam JS, Cowherd R, Rosenberg SA, Hwu P. Improved gene transfer into lymphocytes using retroviruses that express the gibbon ape leukemia virus envelope. *Hum Gene Ther* 1996;7:1415–1422.
11. Uckert W, Willimsky G, Pedersen FS, Blankenstein T, Pedersen L. RNA levels of human retrovirus receptors Pit1 and Pit2 do not correlate with infectability by three retroviral vector pseudotypes. *Hum Gene Ther* 1998;9:2619–2627.
12. Bunnell BA, Muul LM, Donahue RE, Blaese RM, Morgan RA. High-efficiency retroviral-mediated gene transfer into human and nonhuman primate peripheral blood lymphocytes. *Proc Natl Acad Sci U S A* 1995;92:7739–7743.
13. Yee JK, Friedmann T, Burns JC. Generation of high-titer pseudotyped retroviral vectors with very broad host range. *Methods Cell Biol* 1994;43(A):99–112.
14. Sharma S, Cantwell M, Kipps TJ, Friedmann T. Efficient infection of a human T-cell line and of human primary peripheral blood leukocytes with a pseudotyped retrovirus vector. *Proc Natl Acad Sci U S A* 1996;93:11842–11847.
15. Gallardo HF. Recombinant retroviruses pseudotyped with the vesicular stomatitis virus G glycoprotein mediate both stable gene transfer and pseudotransduction in human peripheral blood lymphocytes. *Blood* 1997;90:952–957.
16. Berkner KL. Expression of heterologous sequences in adenoviral vectors. *Curr Top Microbiol Immunol* 1992;158:39–66.
17. Muzyczka N. Use of adeno-associated virus as a general transduction vector for mammalian cells. *Curr Top Microbiol Immunol* 1992;158: 97–129.
18. Moss B. Vaccinia virus vectors. *Biotechnology* 1992;20:345–362.
19. Moss B. Poxvirus expression vectors. *Curr Top Microbiol Immunol* 1992;158:25–38.
20. Jenkins S, Gritz L, Fedor CH, O'Neill EM, Cohen LK, Panicali DL. Formation of lentivirus particles by mammalian cells infected with recombinant fowlpox virus. *AIDS Res Hum Retroviruses* 1991; 7:991 998.
21. Spehner D, Drillien R, Lecocq JP. Construction of fowlpox virus vectors with intergenic insertions: expression of the beta-galactosidase gene and the measles virus fusion gene. *J Virol* 1990;64:527–533.
22. Hwu P, Yannelli J, Kriegler M, et al. Functional and molecular characterization of TIL transduced with the TNFα cDNA for the gene therapy of cancer in man. *J Immunol* 1993;150:4104–4115.
23. Kasid A, Morecki S, Aebersold P, et al. Human gene transfer: characterization of human tumor-infiltrating lymphocytes as vehicles for retroviral-mediated gene transfer in man. *Proc Natl Acad Sci U S A* 1990;87:473–477.
24. Rosenberg SA, Aebersold P, Cornetta K, et al. Gene transfer into humans—immunotherapy of patients with advanced melanoma, using tumor-infiltrating lymphocytes modified by retroviral gene transduction. *N Engl J Med* 1990;323:570–578.
25. Rosenberg SA, Anderson WF, Blaese M, et al. The development of gene therapy for the treatment of cancer. *Ann Surg* 1993;218:455.
26. Favrot MC, Philip T. Treatment of patients with advanced cancer using tumor infiltrating lymphocytes transduced with the gene of resistance to neomycin. *Hum Gene Ther* 1992;3:533–542.
27. Lotze MT. The treatment of patients with melanoma using interleukin-2, interleukin-4 and tumor infiltrating lymphocytes. *Hum Gene Ther* 1992;3:167–177.
28. Miller AR, Skotzko MJ, Rhoades K, et al. Simultaneous use of two retroviral vectors in human gene marking trials: feasibility and potential applications. *Hum Gene Ther* 1992;3:619–624.
29. Brenner MK, Rill DR, Holladay MS, et al. Gene marking to determine whether autologous marrow infusion restores long-term haemopoiesis in cancer patients. *Lancet* 1993;342:1134–1137.
30. Bill DR, Santana VM, Roberts WM, et al. Direct demonstration that autologous bone marrow transplantation for solid tumors can return a multiplicity of tumorigenic cells. *Blood* 1994;84:380–383.
31. Riddell SR, Greenberg PD, Overell RW, et al. Phase I study of cellular adoptive immunotherapy using genetically modified CD8+ HIV-specific T cells for HIV seropositive patients undergoing allogeneic bone marrow transplant. The Fred Hutchinson Cancer Research Center and the University of Washington School of Medicine, Department of Medicine, Division of Oncology. *Hum Gene Ther* 1992;3:319–338.
32. Heslop HE, Ng CY, Li C, et al. Long-term restoration of immunity against Epstein-Barr virus infection by adoptive transfer of gene-modified virus-specific T lymphocytes. *Nat Med* 1996;2:551–555.
33. Brodie SJ, Lewinsohn DA, Patterson BK, et al. *In vivo* migration and function of transferred HIV-1-specific cytotoxic T cells [see comments]. *Nat Med* 1999;5:34–41.
34. Haranaka K, Satomi N, Sakurai A. Antitumor activity of murine tumor necrosis factor (TNF) against transplanted murine tumors and heterotransplanted human tumors in nude mice. *Int J Cancer* 1984;34:263–267.
35. Creasey A, Reynolds MT, Laird W. Cures and partial regression of murine and human tumors by recombinant human tumor necrosis factor. *Cancer Res* 1986;46:5687–5690.
36. Asher A, Mulé J, Reichert C, Shiloni E, Rosenberg SA. Studies on the anti-tumor efficacy of systemically administered recombinant tumor necrosis factor against several murine tumors *in vivo*. *J Immunol* 1987;138:963–974.
37. Feinberg B, Kurzrock R, Talpaz M, Blick M, Saks S, Gutterman J. A phase I trial of intravenously-administered recombinant tumor necrosis factor-alpha in cancer patients. *J Clin Oncol* 1988;6:1328–1334.
38. Moritz T, Niederle N, Baumann J, et al. Phase I study of recombinant human tumor necrosis factor alpha in advanced malignant disease. *Cancer Immunol Immunother* 1989;29:144–150.
39. Rosenberg SA, Lotze M, Yang J, et al. Experience with the use of high-dose interleukin-2 in the treatment of 652 cancer patients. *Ann Surg* 1989;210:474–485.
40. Sherman M, Spriggs D, Arthur K, Imamura K, Frei E, Kufe D. Recombinant human tumor necrosis factor administered as a five-day continuous infusion in cancer patients: phase I toxicity and effects on lipid metabolism. *J Clin Oncol* 1988;6(2):344–350.
41. Spriggs D, Sherman M, Michie H, et al. Recombinant human tumor necrosis factor administered as a 24-hour intravenous infu-

sion. A phase I and pharmacologic study. *J Natl Cancer Inst* 1988;80:1039–1044.

42. Bartsch H, Pfizenmaier K, Schroeder M, Nagel G. Intralesional application of recombinant human tumor necrosis factor alpha induces local tumor regression in patients with advanced malignancies. *Eur J Cancer Clin Oncol* 1989;25(2):287–291.

43. Kahn J, Kaplan L, Ziegler J, et al. Phase II trial of intralesional recombinant tumor necrosis factor alpha (rTNF) for AIDS associated Kaposi's sarcoma (KS). *Proc ASCO* 1989;8:4(abst).

44. Lienard D, Ewalenko P, Delmotte J, Renard N, Lejeune F. High-dose recombinant tumor necrosis factor alpha in combination with interferon gamma and melphalan in isolation perfusion of the limbs for melanoma and sarcoma. *J Clin Oncol* 1992;10(1):52–60.

45. Alexander HRJ, Bartlett DL, Libutti SK, Fraker DL, Moser T, Rosenberg SA. Isolated hepatic perfusion with tumor necrosis factor and melphalan for unresectable cancers confined to the liver. *J Clin Oncol* 1998;16:1479–1489.

46. Fisher B, Packard B, Read E, et al. Tumor localization of adoptively transferred indium-111 labeled tumor infiltrating lymphocytes in patients with metastatic melanoma. *J Clin Oncol* 1989;7:250–261.

47. Griffith KD, Read EJ, Carrasquillo JA, et al. *In vivo* distribution of adoptively transferred indium-111 labeled tumor infiltrating lymphocytes and peripheral blood lymphocytes in patients with metastatic melanoma. *J Natl Cancer Inst* 1989;81:1709–1717.

48. Pockaj BA, Sherry RM, Wei JP, et al. Localization of 111-Indium-labeled tumor infiltrating lymphocytes to tumor in patients receiving adoptive immunotherapy. *Cancer* 1994;73:1731–1737.

49. Waldmann TA. The multi-subunit interleukin-2 receptor. *Annu Rev Biochem* 1989;58:875–911.

50. Shu S, Chou T, Rosenberg SA. *In vitro* sensitization and expansion with viable tumor cells and interleukin-2 in the generation of specific therapeutic effector cells. *J Immunol* 1986;136:3891–3898.

51. Yamada G, Kitamura Y, Sonoda H, et al. Retroviral expression of the human IL-2 gene in a murine T cell line results in cell growth autonomy and tumorigenicity. *EMBO J* 1987;6:2705–2709.

52. Karasuyama H, Tohyama N, Tada T. Autocrine growth and tumorigenicity of interleukin 2-dependent helper T cells transfected with IL-2 gene. *J Exp Med* 1989;169:13–25.

53. Treisman J, Hwu P, Minamoto S, Shafer GE, Cowherd R, Morgan R, Rosenberg SA. Interleukin-2-transduced lymphocytes grow in an autocrine fashion and remain responsive to antigen. *Blood* 1995;85:139.

54. Berkower I, Kawamura H, Matis LA, Berzofsky JA. T cell clones to two major T cell epitopes of myoglobin: effect of I-A/I-E restriction on epitope dominance. *J Immunol* 1985;135:2628–2634.

55. Schreurs J, Gorman DM, Miyajima A. Cytokine receptors: a new superfamily of receptors. *Int Rev Cytol* 1992;137B:121–155.

56. Kondo M, Takeshita T, Higuchi M, et al. Functional participation of the IL-2 receptor gamma chain in IL-7 receptor complexes. *Science* 1994;263:1453–1454.

57. Russell SM, Keegan AD, Harada N, et al. Interleukin-2 receptor gamma chain: a functional component of the interleukin-4 receptor [see comments]. *Science* 1993;262:1880–1883.

58. Noguchi M, Nakamura Y, Russell SM, et al. Interleukin-2 receptor gamma chain: a functional component of the interleukin-7 receptor [see comments]. *Science* 1993;262:1877–1880.

59. Kondo M, Takeshita T, Ishii N, et al. Sharing of the interleukin-2 (IL-2) receptor gamma chain between receptors for IL-2 and IL-4 [see comments]. *Science* 1993;262:1874–1877.

60. Kitamura T, Miyajima A. Functional reconstitution of the human interleukin-3 receptor. *Blood* 1992;80:84–90.

61. Showers MO, Moreau JF, Linnekin D, Druker B, D'Andrea AD. Activation of the erythropoietin receptor by the Friend spleen focus-forming virus gp55 glycoprotein induces constitutive protein tyrosine phosphorylation. *Blood* 1992;80:3070–3078.

62. Yamamura Y, Kageyama Y, Matuzaki T, Noda M, Ikawa Y. Distinct downstream signaling mechanism between erythropoietin receptor and interleukin-2 receptor. *EMBO J* 1992;11:4909–4915.

63. Greenberg P, Watanabe K, Gilbert M, Nelson B, Riddell S. Reconstitution of viral immunity by the adoptive transfer of T cell clones modified by gene insertion. *J Cell Biochem* 1993;17E[Suppl]:187(abst).

64. Kuwana Y, Asakura Y, Utsunomiya N, et al. Expression of chimeric receptor composed of immunoglobulin-derived V regions and T-cell receptor-derived C regions. *Biochem Biophys Res Commun* 1987;149(3):960–968.

65. Gross G, Waks T, Eshhar Z. Expression of immunoglobulin-T-cell receptor chimeric molecules as functional receptors with antibody-type specificity. *Proc Natl Acad Sci U S A* 1989;86:10024–10028.

66. Becker MLB, Near R, Mudgett-Hunter M, et al. Expression of a hybrid immunoglobulin-T cell receptor protein in transgenic mice. *Cell* 1989;58:911–921.

67. Goverman J, Gomez SM, Segesman KD, Hunkapiller T, Laug WE, Hood L. Chimeric immunoglobulin-T cell receptor proteins form functional receptors: implications for T cell receptor complex formation and activation. *Cell* 1990;60:929–939.

68. Eshhar Z, Waks T, Gross G, Schindler D. Specific activation and targeting of cytotoxic lymphocytes through chimeric single chains consisting of antibody-binding domains and the gamma or zeta subunits of the immunoglobulin and T-cell receptors. *Proc Natl Acad Sci U S A* 1993;90:720–724.

69. Huston JS, Levinson D, Mudgett-Hunter M, et al. Protein engineering of antibody binding sites: recovery of specific activity in an anti-digoxin single-chain Fv analogue produced in Escherichia coli. *Proc Natl Acad Sci U S A* 1988;85:5879–5883.

70. Bird RE, Hardman KD, Jacobson JW, et al. Single-chain antigen-binding proteins. *Science* 1988;242:423–426.

71. Bird RE, Walker BW. Single chain antibody variable regions. *Trends Biotech* 1991;9:132–137.

72. Orloff D, Ra C, Frank SJ, Klausner RD, Kinet J-P. Family of disulfide-linked dimers containing the zeta and eta chains of the T-cell receptor and the gamma chain of Fc receptors. *Nature* 1990;347:189–191.

73. Letourneur F, Klausner RD. T-cell and basophil activation through the cytoplasmic tail of T-cell-receptor zeta family proteins. *Proc Natl Acad Sci U S A* 1991;88:8905–8909.

74. Romeo C, Amiot M, Seed B. Sequence requirements for induction of cytolysis by the T cell antigen/Fc receptor zeta chain. *Cell* 1992;68:889–897.

75. Romeo C, Seed B. Cellular immunity to HIV activated by CD4 fused to T cell or Fc receptor polypeptides. *Cell* 1991;64:1037–1046.

76. Irving BA, Weiss A. The cytoplasmic domain of the T cell receptor zeta chain is sufficient to couple to receptor-associated signal transduction pathways. *Cell* 1991;64:891–901.

77. Hwu P, Shafer GE, Treisman J, et al. Lysis of ovarian cancer cells by human lymphocytes redirected with a chimeric gene composed of an antibody variable region and the Fc receptor gamma chain. *J Exp Med* 1993;178:361–366.

78. Hwu P, Yang JC, Cowherd R, Treisman J, Eshhar Z, Rosenberg SA. *In vivo* antitumor activity of T-cells redirected with chimeric antibody/T-cell receptor genes. *Cancer Res* 1995;55:33–69.

79. Krause A. Antigen-dependent CD28 signaling selectively enhances survival and proliferation in genetically modified activated human primary T lymphocytes. *J Exp Med* 1998;188:619–626.

80. Wang G. A T cell-independent antitumor response in mice with bone marrow cells retrovirally transduced with an antibody/Fc-gamma chain chimeric receptor gene recognizing a human ovarian cancer antigen. *Nat Med* 1998;4:168–172.

81. Stancovski I, Schindler DG, Waks T, Yarden Y, Sela M, Eshhar Z. Targeting of T lymphocytes to Neu/HER2 expressing cells using chimeric single chain Fv receptors. *J Immunol* 1993;151:6577–6582.

82. Daly T, Royal RE, Kershaw M, et al. Recognition of human colon cancer by T cells transduced with a chimeric receptor gene. *Cancer Gene Ther* 1999 (*in press*).

83. Finer MH, Dull TJ, Qin L, Farson D, Roberts MR. kat: a high-efficiency retroviral transduction system for primary human T lymphocytes. *Blood* 1994;83:43–50.

84. Cole DJ, Weil DP, Shilyansky J, et al. Characterization of the functional specificity of a cloned T-cell receptor heterodimer recognizing the MART-1 melanoma antigen. *Cancer Res* 1995;55:748–752.

85. Clay TM, Custer M, Sachs J, Hwu P, Rosenberg SA, Nishimura M. Efficient transfer of a tumor antigen-reactive TCR to human peripheral blood lymphocytes confers anti-tumor reactivity. *J Immunol* 1999;163:507–513.

86. Bonini C, Ferrari G, Verzeletti S, et al. HSV-TK gene transfer into donor lymphocytes for control of allogeneic graft-versus-leukemia [see comments]. *Science* 1997;276:1719–1724.

87. Riddell SR, Elliott M, Lewinsohn DA, et al. T-cell mediated rejection of gene-modified HIV-specific cytotoxic T lymphocytes in HIV-infected patients [see comments]. *Nat Med* 1996; 2:216–223.

88. Eglitis MA, Anderson WF. Retroviral vectors for introduction of genes into mammalian cells. *Biotechniques* 1988;6:608–614.

89. Miller AD, Rosman GJ. Improved retroviral vectors for gene transfer and expression. *Biotechniques* 1989;7:980–988.

90. Miller AD, Buttimore C. Redesign of retrovirus packaging cell lines to avoid recombination leading to helper virus production. *Mol Cell Biol* 1986;6:2895–2902.

20.2

GENE THERAPY: CLINICAL APPLICATIONS

Gene Therapy Using Stem Cell Modification

ALBERT DEISSEROTH

JO HONG WON

LIXIN ZHANG

XUE YUEN PENG

TAKUMA FUJII

TAO WANG

X. Y. DAVID GUO

ALLON CANAAN

S. SHRIMDKANDADA

FRANK HSIEH

ANDRES CANOVA

If a genetic modification technique is to have a long-lasting effect on the disease process of a cancer-causing disorder during the lifetime of the affected individual, the genetic element must be introduced into a stem cell of the target tissue such that continued expression of the gene is ensured. The delivery of the gene to the target tissue must not diminish the self-renewal potential of the target cell. The properties of stem cells from all tissues studied thus far have provided obstacles to the implementation of genetic modification strategies. These obstacles include the low frequency of stem cells in any tissue, the quiescent or nondividing nature of most of these cells, the absence of methods with which to isolate and purify these cells before or after modification, and the lack of detailed knowledge about the types of receptors on the surface of these cells.

In the beginning, gene therapy studies were designed to use retroviral vectors to introduce the therapeutic transgenes into the DNA of the target stem cells to produce a durable modification of the phenotype of the cell (1). Genetic therapy strategies have since been expanded to include the use of adenoviral and adeno-associated viral vectors for the modification of the phenotype of a target cell and the introduction into tissues of vectors carrying therapeutic transcription units (2). In the case of the adeno-associated viral vector, the nucleic acid of the vector is stable in a nonintegrated form in the nondividing differentiated cells of a tissue (e.g., myotubes) for up to a year (2). The transcription unit is engineered so that the protein produced will be secreted into the systemic circulation for diseases arising from a protein that is missing from the bloodstream (2).

Initially, the studies of the use of genetic elements to correct constitutional or acquired disorders leading to unregulated growth focused on stem cells derived from primarily hematopoietic tissue. The target tissues have been expanded into stem cells from the central nervous system, connective tissue, bone, muscle cells, and liver cells. These efforts, which have had very limited success in delivering therapeutic genes to cells that exhibit indefinite self-renewal, have taught us indirectly about the biologic properties of stem cells in these tissues.

In this chapter, we discuss the development of genetic modification techniques for hematopoietic stem cells. This discussion includes a description of the vectors available, the systems used for delivering such vectors, the cell and animal models in which the success or failure of such gene delivery techniques are studied, and the clinical trials that have taught us much about the challenges to be overcome in this field.

PROPERTIES OF STEM CELLS

The frequency representation of stem cells in tissues is usually very low, approximately 1 per 10,000. This low level and the fact that the majority of the stem cells in any tissue have been found to be quiescent have frustrated attempts to isolate these cells and to characterize their immunophenotype and biologic properties. Indeed, controversy exists as to whether these cells can be brought into cycle without committing them to a program of differentiation that limits their self-renewal (3–5). Existing experimental evidence suggests that it is difficult to modify human hematopoietic stem cells with retroviral vectors without reducing their self-renewal capacity, but it may be possible with hematopoietic stem cells from the mouse (6–9).

It is not yet clear whether the stem cell compartment present at birth can be expanded during postnatal life. In the succession model of hematopoiesis—based on experimental evidence involving retroviral modification of mouse stem cells (6)—the number of stem cells present at birth is fixed and can never be expanded. During life, these stem cells are activated one by one, and the replication events that involve each, as they become active in cellular division, result in symmetric cellular divisions (both daughter cells are similar). These divisions are polarized in terms of increasing levels of maturation and decreasing capacity for self-renewal with succeeding replication events. In addition, the subsets of genes, which define the functional state of the differentiated tissue arising from the stem cell, or the lineages of cells that exist within the tissue, become activated during this process of sequential maturation.

In this model, the stem cell compartment resembles the ovary, which contains the lifetime allotment of eggs at birth. During life, these are used sequentially. If the same is true of hematopoietic tissue, then the bone marrow's staggering cell production (250 billion cells per day) arises from a hierarchical array of cells emanating from a small subset of stem cells available at birth. In addition, the progeny of these stem cells are actively replicating for only a finite period (several months).

An alternate hypothetical model of hematopoiesis from stem cells that accounts for the evolution of a hierarchical array of ever-expanding numbers of hematopoietic cells at increasing levels of maturation and differentiated phenotype and decreasing levels of self-renewal stipulates that both symmetric and asymmetric cellular divisions occur at all levels of maturation. The occurrence of the asymmetric cellular division produces one daughter cell that retains the undifferentiated phenotype of the mother cell and one daughter cell that acquires a new more mature or differentiated phenotype. This acquisition results in a change in maturation and gene expression as well as diminished capacity for self-renewal. In symmetric cellular division, in this model, both daughter cells retain the phenotype of the mother cell.

The mechanism that controls whether a symmetric or asymmetric division occurs in this latter model has been hypothesized to be either instructional (i.e., an extracellular signal, such as a growth factor that triggers the asymmetric division) or non-instructional (i.e., an intrinsic property of the genetic program). The intrinsic programming of an asymmetric cellular division could hypothetically be dependent on the number of replication events allowable at each stage of maturation, or a stochastic model, in which the majority of replication events are symmetric, and the infrequent asymmetric division occurs randomly. Another property of this model is that the number of symmetric replication events is in the majority at each stage, but the frequency of the asymmetric replication events increases as maturation proceeds.

The number of replication events a stem cell would undergo is far lower in the succession of hematopoiesis model. From a theoretical point of view, the probability of acquisition of somatic mutations from errors in DNA replication or exposure to mutagens increases dramatically when the number of replication events exceeds 1 billion.

The succession of hematopoiesis model, if true, would protect the organism from acquisition of mutations that lead to hematopoietic diseases such as myelodysplastic syndrome or leukemia but would also limit the potential for developing genetic therapy for cancer with a lifelong impact, through the use of stem cell modification.

The resolution of this question about this very basic property of stem cells might largely determine the potential for developing genetic therapy that involves insertion of vector DNA into the target cell DNA and thereby has a lifelong effect. In the dividing tissues, the genetic modification procedure must successfully modify a very early cell to have a lifelong impact. For the modification of tissues with no cellular division, or only scheduled intermittent cellular division, it is not necessary to modify a stem cell to ensure a change of the tissue cell phenotype with respect to the reversal of a disease process through genetic therapy. An example of this is provided by the work of Herzog and colleagues (2).

The proliferating tissues of the body (which would require genetic modification of stem cells) include the hematopoietic system, the endothelial vascular system, bone, all epithelial tissues (e.g., lung, breast, prostate, ovary, bladder, cervix, skin, gastrointestinal tissues), and those components of nondividing tissues that are turning over [i.e., the glial cells of the central nervous system, the fibrous or stromal cells of all epithelial and hematopoietic tissues, and the mesenchyme-derived cells that line all of the body cavities (the cerebrospinal fluid system, pleural space, peritoneal space, pericardial sac, and serosal surfaces of joint spaces)]. Tissues that are not replicating, and therefore could be used as small units from which a gene product could be released into the systemic circulation, include the liver, muscle, and neurons of the central nervous system. The muscle cells (nondividing myotubes) have been used to express therapeutic proteins in replacement strategies for constitutional disorders involving coagulation factors (2).

INDIRECT STEM CELL FINDINGS

Much more has been learned indirectly about stem cell properties, through the study of settings in which repopulation of tissue is undertaken. Repopulation involves the transfer of stem cells from one individual to another, and the study in this setting of chimeras and mosaicism in tissues (with respect to genetic or immunohistochemical markers), either in the steady state, or in transplantation experiments with or without genetic modification.

Unless a subset of stem cells has a selective competitive advantage, mixtures of stem cells with polymorphic markers (made so that the ratio of two variants is different in each of a series of sequential independent transplant experiments) retain the frequency that exists at the time of transplant throughout the lifetime of the animal. This principle results in mosaicism in tissues with respect to properties such as X-chromosome condensation and produces mixtures of hematopoietic cells, which may differ with respect to the ratio of different surface immunophenotypic markers, for which no selective pressure exists. This principle also leads to mixtures of hematopoietic cells that are genetically modified or not modified (marked) after a gene marking experiment (see Retroviral Vectors).

The number of receptors on stem cells that can be used for engaging viruses is very low in the early stages of cell maturation (10). As discussed later, this presents a significant obstacle in delivery of the gene therapy vectors to stem cells, because the number of surface molecules involved in viral binding or uptake into cells is very low or nonexistent on the stem cells. The current approach to this problem is to pseudo-type the retroviral vectors (11); to create targeting bifunctional antibody molecules for targeting the vectors to the stem cells (12); to engineer the surface-binding virus-binding coat proteins, so that they will selectively bind to the plasma membrane receptors unique to cells at the earliest stages of maturation (13); or to construct chimeric vectors that use the adeno-associated vector infection to deliver to the target cell a receptor transcription unit that enables the retroviral vector to infect the target cell (14). These steps accomplish two things:

1. The vector becomes competent to bind and to be taken up into the target stem cell.

2. The vectors are not sequestered from the stem cells by binding to the vast excess of more differentiated cells that are irrelevant for self-renewal in a specific tissue.

Chimeras of adenoviral and retroviral vectors have also been constructed to combine the best of both vectors and to circumvent the restriction that the distribution of the amphotropic receptor imposes on retroviral vectors (15).

For long-term modification of early hematopoietic cells—the viral vectors derived from the retrovirus and adeno-associated virus (vectors capable of generating integrant vector transgenes)—the vector must be able to traffic the viral complementary DNA (cDNA; in the case of retroviral vectors) or DNA (in the case of adeno-associated vectors) into the nucleus, where it can be integrated in the nondividing cell. This has been a problem, because unlike DNA viruses, which traffic DNA into the nucleus of the nondividing cell, the retroviral vector is incapable of trafficking its cDNA through the nuclear membrane into the nucleus. Thus, to integrate the cDNA of a retroviral vector into host cell chromosomal DNA, the cell must pass through S phase and mitosis, in which the nuclear membrane

disappears, thereby allowing the retroviral cDNA access to the host chromosomal DNA. There, the retroviral LTRs can mediate the integration of the vector cDNA. Thus, the frequency of integrants of vector cDNA in stem cells is very low, due to (a) lack of binding of the vector to the target stem cell and (b) inability of the vector cDNA to pass through the nuclear membrane of the nondividing stem cell (the majority of stem cells). The recent strategy to avoid this obstacle has been to use the human immunodeficiency virus–associated vectors in which the long terminal repeats (LTRs) and viral proteins can traffic the cDNA of the vector through the intact nuclear membrane of the nondividing cell to generate integrants (16).

Once integrated into the chromosomal DNA of the host cell, the retroviral genome encounters another problem: extinction of expression of the vector transgenes. This problem reflects the fact that a mechanism to limit the expression of vector transgenes is in place in embryonic and early undifferentiated stem cells. One strategy to overcome this obstacle was to change the transcriptional regulatory elements of the retroviral vectors to those of the mouse embryonic stem cell retroviruses (17). These elements are not subject to the extinction mechanism to the degree observed in the Maloney retroviral vectors.

Thus, as the biology of the stem cell has become more fully understood, strategies have been developed to attempt circumvention of these intrinsic limitations of the stem cell.

VECTOR DELIVERY SYSTEMS

Several different viruses have been used to engineer safety-modified delivery vehicles. Each of these has advantages and disadvantages for the specific properties of the stem cell, some of which were discussed in the previous sections. In this section, the complementary discussion is undertaken: how the properties of the various viruses produce advantages or disadvantages for genetic modification of the stem cell.

Retroviral Vectors

The retroviral vector, which is used for gene therapy, is usually derived from murine RNA tumor or leukemia viruses and consists of two identical sequences called long terminal repeats (LTRs) at the 3' and 5' boundary of the vector, which contain transcriptional regulatory elements, elements for replication, and elements for integration of the vector cDNA into the host chromosomal genome. The *gag*, *pol*, and *env* genes, normally found between the LTRs, have been removed from the retroviral vector, but the packaging sequences necessary for assembly of the retroviral vector in a packaging cell line that carries the *gag*, *pol*, and *env* genes as integrants remains near the 5' LTR. The recombinant vector carries the therapeutic transcription unit under the control of the retroviral LTR, or an independent promoter. The capacity of this vector is 7 kilobase (kb).

The ligands on the envelope proteins of the retroviral vectors exhibit species-specific tropisms that depend on the distribution of the receptors that bind to them on mammalian cells (Table 1).

Orlic and colleagues (10) showed that expression of the amphotropic receptor on stem cells was prohibitively low, which

TABLE 1. RETROVIRAL VECTOR LIGANDS FOR MAMMALIAN CELL RECEPTORS

Receptor	Functions	Species
Ecotrophic	Amino acid transporter	Mouse
Amphotropic	Phosphate channel	Mouse, dog, human
Gibbon ape leukemia virus	Phosphate channel	Dog, nonhuman primate, and human

has led to attempts to make the retroviral vector more sensitive to retroviral gene therapy vectors by pseudo-typing the vectors with the Gibbon ape leukemia virus envelope ligand or with the vesicular stomatitis virus G protein (11). The receptors for both of these ligands are highly represented on the surface of the stem cell.

Other workers have attempted to target the vector to the stem cell by using bispecific antibodies (12), re-engineering the ligands available on the envelope protein of the retroviral vector, or by replacing the amino-terminal end of the amphotropic receptor ligand by ligands present on the surface of the producer cell (13). These vectors are chimeric for the wild-type amphotropic ligand and the recombinant ligand. Kasabara et al. (13) have succeeded in placing the c-kit receptor ligand and the ligand for the erythropoietin receptor on the end of the amphotropic ligand on the retroviral vector.

As outlined above, the retroviral vector is incapable of delivering its cDNA into the nucleus of the nondividing stem cell, because this virus does not produce any protein that can traffic the cDNA of the retroviral vector into the nucleus. Two approaches have been taken to circumvent this problem:

1. Many workers have attempted to promote the integration of retroviral transgenes into the chromosomal DNA of the stem cells by exposing the stem cells to late-acting growth factors, such as granulocyte-macrophage colony-stimulating factor and interleukin-3 (IL-3) and IL-6, in the presence of serum and stem cell factor (18,19). Although this has increased the transduction frequency of the stem cells with retroviral transgenes, exposure to late-acting growth factors in the presence of serum and supercritical fluid has reduced the reconstitution and self-renewal capacity of the stem cell in the transplantation setting (20). This reduction has resulted in only transient engraftment with vector-modified cells in the post-transplant animal and in clinical marking trials (21–24). To circumvent this serum-induced decrement in engraftment, workers have shifted to serum-free conditions for the stem cell modification setting; conditions in which the replication of the stem cell can occur in the absence of conditions that limit the self-renewal properties of these vectors (25,26).

2. Some researchers have switched to the lentiviral vector, the cDNA of which can penetrate the intact mammalian nuclear membrane (16). This method has led to the successful modification of hematopoietic stem cells as well as nondividing muscle cells and central nervous system neurons, which are also nondividing. This technique is discussed in greater detail later, under Lentiviral Vectors.

The low titer sometimes found with retroviral vectors has been addressed by a vertical flow transduction device developed by Palsson et al. (27). The passage of an entire volume of suspended vector particles increases the number of particles to which the target cell is exposed and results in an increase in the transduction frequency.

Another problem is that the amphotropic and other ligands involved in the engagement of the retroviral vector with the target cell membrane are unstable in the serum-containing medium at 37°C. These vector ligands are stable for only 2 hours in the presence of complement-containing serum. This issue is sidestepped by using antibodies to protect this ligand or by carrying out the transduction in serum-free medium or in the presence of complement inactivators.

Adeno-Associated Viral Vectors

The adeno-associated virus is a defective DNA virus that requires helper functions to be provided by the adenovirus. It is a small vector (7 kb) that has identical sequences called *inverted terminal repeats* (ITRs), which are located at the 5' and 3' ends of the vector. The *rep* and *cap* genes, which are normally located between the ITRs, are no longer present in the recombinant adeno-associated vector, and in their place is the therapeutic transcription unit under the control of its own transcriptional promoter. Until recently, the *cap* and *rep* genes were placed on a separate plasmid and cotransfected into the producer cell line along with the plasmid carrying the recombinant adeno-associated vector bearing the therapeutic transcription unit. In addition, infection of the producer cell line with wild-type adenovirus would be required to provide the helper functions required for replication. The expression of the *rep* and *cap* genes and the adenoviral infection were both toxic to the producer cell, thus requiring multiple sequential rounds of production. This problem has been solved with the cloning of the adenoviral vector helper functions.

Despite the limitations of small capacity (5 kb of DNA) and the requirement for target stem cell replication for integration of the transcription unit carried by the vector, the adeno-associated viral vector has been useful because its nucleic acid is retained for long periods in the cytoplasm of cells, where the transcription unit can be expressed without integration of the adeno-associated viral vector DNA for long periods. Early on, the adeno-associated vector was used to transfer replacement transcription units for single-gene defects of hematopoietic cells (28,29). If the target cell is nondividing, a stable pattern of transgene expression from the episome without integration is observed. One example was the use of the adeno-associated vector to deliver the gene for hemophilia B to myotubes, from which the transgene can be expressed and the protein product released into the bloodstream for up to 1 year at levels that prevent spontaneous bleeding (2). The adeno-associated vector is of potential value, but its use in hematopoietic stem cells has not yet resulted in stable expression in early hematopoietic cells.

Adenoviral Vectors

The adenoviral vector is a 38-kb DNA virus that is nonpathogenic for normal immunocompetent individuals due to the very robust immune (both cellular and humoral) response it generates. Among immunoincompetent individuals, however, this virus is very dangerous, and infection can result in loss of life. The vector has a wide host range, which depends on the binding of the fibrillar protein to the Coxsackie virus-associated receptor, which is widely distributed on the surface of most mammalian cells. After binding, viral uptake depends on the presence of certain integrin receptors (alpha-V, beta-3, or beta-5) on the surface of the target cell, which interact with the penton proteins of the virus (located at the base of the fibrillar protein) (30). Once taken up and released from the endosome, the adenoviral DNA is transported through the intact nuclear membrane into the nucleus, where the DNA is transcribed into RNA and ultimately translated into protein in the cytoplasm.

The adenoviral vector used for genetic therapy has been rendered nonreplicative by removal of the *E1A* and *E1B* genes (and in some instances the *E3* gene) of the virus. The transgene expression lasts 14 days. The vector evokes an immune response that destroys the cells in which the virus transgene is being expressed and this limits to 2 weeks the period during which the transgene is expressed. This vector is not integrated into host chromosomal DNA. On the basis of work in several laboratories (31,32), it appears that the integrin receptors required for viral uptake are not represented on the earliest of the hematopoietic stem cells, which are therefore resistant to infection by this virus. During the induction of maturation of the earliest hematopoietic stem cells, when it is exposed in the presence of serum to the hematopoietic growth factors stem cell factor, IL-3, and IL-6, the integrin receptors necessary for viral infection appear on the cell surface as the stem cell matures and the vector transgenes are expressed within the cell (32). This maturation, which is necessary for the expression of the integrin receptors required for viral entry into the stem cell, reduces the self-renewal potential of the genetically modified stem cell, thus leading only to short-term effects. Thus, the adenoviral vector is not now a candidate for the delivery of transgenes to hematopoietic stem cells because of the absence of the receptors necessary for its uptake.

Several investigators have made use of bifunctional antibodies or re-engineering of the fibrillar protein of the vector that mediates initial binding to target cells to deliver the vector to specific types of cells (33,34). It has not yet been possible to modify the penton protein so that its specificity for the alpha-V, beta-3, and beta-5 integrins can be changed. Other investigators are studying ways of using cationic lipids to promote the uptake of viral genomes (both adenoviral and adeno-associated vectors) in order to broaden the host range of vectors for hematopoietic stem cells (35).

Lentiviral Vectors

One of the most exciting breakthroughs in the attempt to develop methods to deliver genetic elements to the hematopoietic stem cell has been the engineering of lentiviral vectors, which have the capacity to deliver their cDNA, once generated in the cytoplasm of nondividing cells, through the intact nuclear membrane of the nondividing cell, to the nucleus, where the vector cDNA is integrated into the target cell. This

vector has been stripped of its replicative machinery and envelope protein. To produce the vector, a three-way transfection of the recombinant vector carrying the therapeutic gene with its own promoter, another plasmid with the replication cassette for the virus, and a third plasmid carrying the envelope pseudo-type envelope protein system is carried out. Miyoshi et al. (16) have shown that this vector is competent to modify nondividing myotubes, neurons, and hematopoietic cells. A performance analysis of this vector system, using animal models in which the repopulating capability of cells modified by this vector can be tested, is under way in many laboratories.

The potential clinical utility of this vector will depend on the results of ongoing experiments to determine its safety in humans.

Gutless Adenoviral Vectors

In an attempt to decrease the cellular immune response (which limits the adenoviral vector transgenes' duration of expression) and to increase the capacity of the adenoviral vectors for domains of the mammalian chromosome (which are extensive), Schneider and coworkers (36) have reported the construction of the so-called gutless adenoviral vectors. These vectors are useful only for nondividing cells, because they are replication incompetent.

Episomal Nonviral Vectors

Proteins produced by certain DNA viruses, such as the E2 protein (37) of the human papillomavirus (HPV) or the EBNAI protein (38) of the Epstein-Barr virus (EBV), that tether the episomal DNA to the mammalian chromosomal proteins have been identified. This tethering protects viral DNA from nuclease destruction and preserves equal partitioning of the DNA between daughter cells in dividing cells. The E2 protein plays this role in the latent HPV infection of germinal epithelial cells (37). The E2 protein connects the long control region of the episomal DNA origin of replication of HPV with chromosomal proteins. The EBNAI protein connects the chromosomal proteins and the ORI-P promoter of the EBV episome (38), which contains the origin of replication of the EBV episomal DNA.

Banerjee et al. (38) have explored the use of vectors carrying the ORI-P of EBV and EBNAI to tether therapeutic expression vectors to the mammalian chromosome. This technique results in retention of therapeutic expression plasmids carrying the origin of replication of EBV in cells expressing the EBNAI EBV protein for months. An advantage of this type of vector is the almost unlimited capacity (150 kb), which allows the introduction of entire regions into the vector in a way that ensures correct and natural expression driven by elements such as the long control region. Because the expression vectors express their transgenes without being integrated into the chromosomal DNA, the transgenes are not subject to the usual variation in the levels of expressions of integrated transcription units that arise from the presence of negative regulatory transcriptional elements in the vicinity of an integration site. Banerjee et al. (38) succeeded in using such vectors to reverse the phenotype of cells from Fanconi's anemia patients. Others have used such elements to maintain the entire beta-globin developmental gene cassette.

ADJUNCTS TO VECTOR AND NONVECTOR GENE DELIVERY SYSTEMS

Vertical Flow Transduction Systems

Bernhard Palsson and his co-workers (27) have reported the development of a filtration transduction system in which suspensions of retroviral vector particles produced at low concentrations can be pulled through a membrane on which the target cells can be distributed, bringing the entire population of vector particles into contact with the target cells. Otherwise, the 0.3-mm thick diffusion path limits the number of particles that can reach the target cells. The more dilute the vector preparation, the more unlikely it is that any vector particle will connect with a target cell because of the very short diffusion path of a very large particle such as a vector. Thus, in a static transduction system, most of the viral particles produced go to waste. The vertical flow transduction system is of tremendous advantage for increasing the probability that a viral particle will encounter a rare target such as the stem cell.

Concentration Systems

Because of the instability of the retroviral envelope, it is very difficult to concentrate the retroviral vector without decreasing the number of functional infectious particles. In contrast, the adenoviral vector can be concentrated by physical means (i.e., cesium gradient centrifugation) without loss of activity.

Centrifugation Transduction

Increases in the transduction frequency have been observed when mixtures of target cells and supernatants of retroviral vectors are subjected to centrifugation. The mechanism through which this adjunct works is unknown.

Engineering of the Binding Proteins

To reduce the loss of the delivery vector to cells that are irrelevant to the goal of engraftment or repopulation, the binding proteins have been engineered so that the vector will bind only to the target cell (13). Doing so increases the effective ratio of infectious particles to target cells.

Conditional Replication Competency

Another potential solution to the huge number of target cells—conditional replication competency within the target cell population—has been accomplished by Heise et al. (39). Two of the problems in gene therapy vector design include reaching the very-low-frequency cells and the loss of the vectors due to binding to irrelevant cells. The solution to both of these problems is to confer replication competency on the vector. Thus, even if the frequency of collision and infection of a vector particle with the target cell is one in a million, as long as one collision occurs, the infected cell could release more particles for infection of other cells. Unfortunately, with a particle that has the capability of integrating into the chromosomal DNA of the target cell, the probability of an adverse event due to integration mutagenesis becomes an issue. Thus, all of the work on conditionally replication-competent vectors is targeted to adenoviral vectors rather than retroviral vectors.

Cationic Lipid Complexes

The coating of nucleic acid, which is a highly charged molecule, with molecules that are not repelled by the plasma membrane, such as cationic lipids, may promote the entry of nucleic acid carrying a gene or transcription unit (35). The lipid delivery systems are intrinsically less directed than a vector. To compensate for this, liposomal delivery vehicles have been coated with polyethylene glycol to reduce the rate of nonspecific binding to any plasma membrane.

Gene Gun

Another physical means of delivering genetic material is to accelerate small particles that carry nucleic acid so that these particles penetrate the skin surface and are deposited in cells. This delivery method, although unaccompanied by the risks of a viral vector, is less efficient than lipid complexes or vectors.

Serum-Free Transduction Systems

The recent development of culture systems that preserve the self-renewal capacity of the stem cell is a breakthrough. Several laboratories have demonstrated that serum-free, chemically defined culture media can support stem cell replication without reducing their self-renewal capacity (25,26). Thus, the *in vitro* triggering of a replication event need not necessarily result in the commitment of the cell to maturation and a reduction of the stem cells' self-renewal capacity. These media will be used in future attempts to create conditions that lead to the modification of stem cells by retroviral vectors and other vectors that require integration of the vector nucleic acid for expression of the transgene.

Microinjection

DNA can be injected intranuclearly into the target cell, but the number of such injection events falls far below the number of cells needed to produce a biologically significant event in tissue unless the transgene confers a selective advantage for the modified cell. An example is the adenosine deaminase transgene that produces a protein of relevance for the correction of a disease state and confers a selective advantage on the target cell.

Recombinant Fibronectin Systems

One of the most important developments in the field of retroviral vector–mediated modification of suspension cells is the use of a recombinant fragment of fibronectin that binds both the hematopoietic stem cells (via the alpha-1, beta-5 integrin receptor) and the vectors used for genetic modification. Hanenberg et al. (40) have succeeded in using plates coated with a recombinant fragment of the fibronectin molecule. These plates have been used in a clinical trial of the multidrug resistance gene-1 (MDR-1) retroviral vectors and have shown transduction of the hematopoietic cells at levels ranging from 20% to 50% (41). These fragments are of use in that they bring the vector and target cells together. The use of the fibronectin fragment increases the frequency of the transduction of the suspension cells in that they become monolayer cells. In addition, the effective titer of the vector is increased, because the vectors become concentrated on the bottom surface of the plate, thereby increasing the effective concentration of the viral particles in the target cells' vicinity. These monolayer systems are in wide use, and the aggregate impact of these studies will soon be recognized.

MODEL SYSTEMS FOR EVALUATION OF STEM CELL MODIFICATION

Because the stem cell cannot be isolated, the success of a genetic stem cell modification transduction experiment can only be measured indirectly, usually by the progeny of the stem cell. Often the duration of the genetic modification in a proliferating population is the criterion used to determine whether a stem cell has been modified. If a stem cell population is known to evolve into separate lineages, then the representation of the genetic element in all of the progeny, which develop into the independent lineages, is a measure of the stem cell modification. Both cell culture systems and animal models are used in the measurement of the success of a genetic modification experiment.

Usually, the duration of the cells that contain the genetic modification is a criterion of the immaturity of the cell that has been modified. The distribution of the transgenes into all of the lineages that arise from the differentiation of the stem cell is also a criterion of success. The systems used to measure such success are described below. All of these systems are designed to determine the number of replication events modified cells can carry out after modification.

Long-Term Marrow Culture Systems

In long-term marrow culture systems, genetic modification is carried out on a population of enriched cells in the most immature cells of that tissue (42). The cells are placed into culture in a system that supports the continued proliferation of the cells. Aliquots are taken from the cultures weekly, and the number of differentiated clonogenic progenitors growing in suspension are determined. The longer the genetically modified clonogenic progenitors persist in the culture, the earlier the cell was modified. These cultures are usually carried out for 5 to 6 weeks. The use of the long-term bone marrow culture (43) or simply stromal monolayers (44) has produced increments in transduction frequency. The use of genetically modified stromal layers has also increased the transduction frequency into clonogenic progenitor cells (45,46), but the effect on the persistence of genetically marked progeny of long-term repopulating cells in animal transplantation systems has not been definitively shown.

Transplantation Systems in Small and Large Immunocompetent Animals

The ultimate measure of the stem cell is its ability to reconstitute an entire organism. Thus, in stem cell modification experiments, the ability to modify a population of cells enriched in the immature cells without reducing the stem cells' ability to reconstitute

an organism into which they have been transplanted is the ultimate measure of the quality of the stem cell modification conditions. In a mouse transplantation experiment, the mouse cells are exposed to conditions designed to promote the introduction of the genetic element into the target stem cell population. Then these cells are infused into a lethally irradiated recipient that is isogenic with the donor of the stem cells. The length of time the genetically modified cells persist in the infused animal is a measure of success of the genetic modification (8,47–50). To truly test the self-renewal capability of the modified cells, the marrow or hematopoietic cells of an animal that has been lethally irradiated and transplanted with a modified population are collected and infused into a second lethally irradiated recipient. This is called the *serial transplant*. Because one-tenth of the total number of stem cells from the original donor are taken for the initial transplant, exhaustion of the stem cell pool can occur within a small number of serial transplants. This is known as *stressing the self-renewal capability* of the modified cells. Similar models have been developed for dogs (8) and primates.

Xenotransplantation Systems

Nonobese Diabetic Mouse X-Linked Severe Combined Immunodeficiency Disease Mice

The measurement of the replicative potential of a population of mouse hematopoietic cells after a genetic modification procedure is directly informative about the properties of the mouse hematopoietic stem cell, but the results of these experiments do not necessarily apply to human hematopoietic stem cells. Thus, it is necessary to test the proliferative potential of human hematopoietic stem cell in animal models. The laboratory of John Dick (51) was the first to establish that human hematopoietic cells could be maintained in the immunodeficient recipient animals.

Fetal Sheep Model

Porada and colleagues (52) have shown that the injection of human hematopoietic cells into fetal sheep *in utero* results in the engraftment of human hematopoietic cells for the lifetime of the sheep. That species barriers can be transcended has provided a powerful model of the assessment of the replication potential of human stem cells. Porada et al. (52) have shown that the incubation of stem cells *in vitro* in serum-free medium can be carried out without reducing the engraftment potential of human hematopoietic cells beyond 2 years. In comparison, incubation of human hematopoietic cells in serum-containing medium results in exhaustion of human hematopoiesis in 1 to 2 years. Genetic modification has been carried out in this model (51).

MARKING STUDIES OF MARROW AND PERIPHERAL BLOOD CELLS

When genetic therapy studies began, the first question posed was whether vectors could be used to deliver transgenes into somatic cells such that transgenes would be integrated into the chromosomal DNA of the target cell.

The answer from several years of very systematic studies is unequivocally yes; it is possible to deliver transgenes to target cells (7–9). But the full answer is that it depends on the type of cell, the conditions used for the transduction, the vector backbone used, and the transcriptional regulatory elements in the vector.

In the beginning, murine leukemia and sarcoma viruses were used as the basis on which the vectors (Maloney murine sarcoma virus and Harvey sarcoma virus) were built. Because the RNA of the vector, which is converted into cDNA in the cytoplasm, cannot pass through the intact nuclear membrane, these cells are capable of integrating their transgenes into chromosomal DNA of dividing cells only. Thus, for the vector's cDNA to integrate, the cell must divide. In contrast, the cDNA of lentiviral vectors can pass through the intact nuclear membrane into the nondividing cell and be integrated (16).

Another factor limited the utility of retroviral vectors as they were originally built: The receptors on the surface membrane of the target cells for the ligand on the envelope of the retrovirus are not found on the surface of immature cells. Thus, although the virus can infect mature cells, the percentage of early or immature cells that can be infected by the retroviral vector is very low—if not nonexistent (10).

Finally, the duration of expression of the retroviral transgenes, once integrated into the target cell DNA, is sometimes short-lived owing to the tendency of stem cells to methylate the transcriptional regulatory elements of the vector, whereas this is less likely to happen in more mature cells.

Thus, when the first studies of *ex vivo* marking of hematopoietic cells collected from donors were carried out, the transduction conditions used were designed to stimulate a replication event in the target cells by adding exogenous hematopoietic growth factors and fetal bovine serum to the culture medium. This type of transduction design often used a preincubation of the cells in serum-containing medium and then exposure of the cell to recombinant growth factors followed by 2 days of incubation in the presence of growth factors, serum, and the vector supernatant. Finally, the cells were incubated in the absence of the vector for an additional day to promote integration.

In general, the incidence of the marking was 10% to 20% in the clonogenic progenitors before transplantation of the vector-exposed cells into the recipient animals or patients, but the percentage of cells that were vector-positive after transplantation was low in all of these experiments (7,9,53,54). Some investigators tried to increase the level of the integration in the transduced population by sorting out the transduced cells physically or by marker resistance selection.

The first two marking trials to be published were carried out with leukemia cells (7–9), using a short incubation that would merely deliver the vector inside the hematopoietic cells, without eliciting a replication event *ex vivo*. In both cases—one in childhood acute myelogenous leukemia (7) and the other in adult chronic myelogenous leukemia (9)—the transgenes were detectable in the leukemia cells as well as in normal cells at a rate of 1% to 5% after transplantation of the cells into the intensively treated recipients. When long-term follow-up was available, the transgenes were detectable in all lineages (7). The transgenes continued to be detectable for up to 5 years but at low frequency (7). These studies indicated that retroviral vectors could transduce stem cells

but at low frequency. Later trials using serum-containing medium and more prolonged incubation in breast cancer patients or acute myelogenous leukemia patients undergoing autografts showed even lower posttransplant frequency of marked cells (53,54). A comparison was made of short-term exposure of hematopoietic cells to vector supernatants (4 to 6 hours) with longer exposure (2 to 4 days), but no difference between these two methods was identified (55). Unfortunately, the vast majority of the cells transduced were not the immature stem cells but the more mature cells with limited self-renewal capacity. The level of genetic modification and the duration of this marking was higher in clinical conditions in which the progeny of the modified stem cells has a selective advantage, as in the adenosine deaminase gene replacement studies (56); whether this was due to the *in vivo* selection, the use of cord blood, or the optimization of *in vitro* modification (57) is not known. Much higher levels of genetic marking were achieved with lymphocytes in the adenosine deaminase replacement studies (58).

Chemotherapy Protection

On the basis of the results of the gene marking trials, which showed that a low level of modification could be achieved, three groups [National Institutes of Health, Columbia University, and the University of Texas M. D. Anderson Cancer Center (47–50)] tested the hypothesis that the presence of the MDR-1 chemotherapy resistance gene in the vector could be used to select cells that were positive for the vector MDR-1 transcription unit. MDR-1 codes for an adenosine triphosphate–dependent membrane pump protein (*p*-glycoprotein) that transports alkaloids out of the modified cells, thus protecting them from chemotherapy. Normally, *p*-glycoprotein is expressed at high levels in early hematopoietic precursors, but the expression levels fall as hematopoietic cells mature, resulting in levels that are insufficient to protect more mature cells. All three of these trials were based on animal model data in the mouse that showed evidence for success in the transduction of the hematopoietic target cell and presence of ample levels of the vector-positive cells posttransplant (47–50). In addition, one of the trials showed that the delivery of chemotherapy posttransplant resulted in an increase in the level of the transduced cells, which carried a gene the product of which could confer resistance to the conditions of selection (47).

When these strategies were applied to clinical trials in human patients (21–24), the results fell far short of the high expectations that were held for the therapy on the basis of early experience in mouse models (47–50). In contrast to that experience (47–50), in the clinical trials, only very short-term engraftment could be measured posttransplant and the level of vector-positive cells was very low in patients after transplant (21–24).

A recent discussion of the reasons for these results has been published (59). All of the trials used transduction conditions that involved at least 4 days of incubation in medium supplemented with serum, late-acting hematopoietic growth factors (e.g., IL-3), and stem cell factor. These conditions were used to trigger a replication event in the cells infected with the retroviral vectors that carried the chemoprotection gene (i.e., the MDR-1 gene), which coded for the ATP dependent membrane *p*-glycoprotein.

The presence of stem cell factor and IL-3 in serum has been reported after the initiation of human MDR-1 trials to induce maturation of the early hematopoietic cells (20). The level of posttransplantation chemotherapy delivered to patients was very low, thus failing to provide a selective advantage for the modified cells. The titers of the retroviral vectors were low. Finally, the transcriptional regulatory elements of the vectors were subject to silencing in the stem cells. Thus, these early trials were subject to several problems:

1. The transduction conditions were such that the early stem cells would lose their reconstitution capability.
2. The vectors used could not infect the stem cell.
3. The vectors used carried transgenes that could be extinguished in the stem cells.
4. Only dividing cells (which excludes most of early stem cells) would take up the vector and integrate it into the chromosomal DNA.

In the present era, the feasibility of transducing hematopoietic cells with vectors carrying chemotherapy resistance genes is being addressed once again. These studies use vectors exhibiting higher titers and higher doses of posttransplantation chemotherapy (24). Improved conditions for the *in vitro* transduction, using the fibronectin recombinant fragment, which brings the stem cells and the vector physically together are being used (41). In the future, other modifications in the vectors, such as the lentiviral vectors, or retroviral vectors of the Maloney or Harvey types that can be pseudo-typed so that the infectivity of the stem cells can be increased, and with transcriptional regulatory elements that are not extinguished in stem cells, will be studied as well. This direction of research with MDR-1 may be complicated by the report in a mouse model of myelodysplastic syndrome after MDR-1 modification (60). However, many other chemotherapy protection transgenes are currently being investigated.

Chemotherapy Sensitization

In addition to being used for chemotherapy protection, vectors have been used to selectively sensitize tumor cells that contaminate collections of autografts to the effects of chemotherapy (62–64). Because adenoviral vectors are so efficient in infecting epithelial cells, they have been used to carry chemotherapy sensitization genes into the neoplastic cells that contaminate autografts. A wide selection of chemotherapy sensitization genes is available for modification of the target epithelial cells. Herpesvirus thymidine kinase was used first to selectively sensitize breast cancer cells to the effects of chemotherapy (61). Herpesvirus thymidine kinase can catalyze the phosphorylation of antiviral agents, such as ganciclovir, that are not phosphorylated mammalian cell thymidine kinase. These vectors have proved very efficient in producing the death of cells infected with the adenoviral vector. A limitation of the herpesvirus thymidine kinase/ganciclovir system is that the incorporation of the ganciclovir, once phosphorylated by the viral thymidine kinase, depends on cellular division. So once again, the vector effect depends on the target cell dividing. This restriction is significant, because the majority of epithelial neoplastic cells are nondividing. Investigators have attempted to circumvent this limitation by exploiting what is called the *bystander effect*, which is based

on the transfer of the vector transgene product from infected to uninfected cells. The herpesvirus thymidine kinase system has been much more useful in vectors used to modify lymphocytes to prevent graft-versus-host disease because the lymphocytes can be stimulated to divide and incorporate the retroviral vectors efficiently without diminishing the proliferative potential of these cells. Moreover, the modified cells can be selected, either physically with a surface tag or by growth selection under antibiotic negative selection. Other investigators have attempted to use adenoviral vectors carrying the *p53* or *Bcl-X* short transcription units for selective reduction of the neoplastic cells that contaminate hematopoietic cells in autografts (62,63).

A second transgene, cytosine deaminase, is being used to sensitize neoplastic cells, which contaminate hematopoietic autografts to the effects of chemotherapy (31). Cytosine deaminase is a bacterial gene (64) that catalyzes the conversion of a nontoxic precursor, 5-fluorocytosine, into a chemotherapy agent, 5-fluorouracil. The levels of phosphorylated 5-fluorouracil inside epithelial cells are so high that sufficient incorporation into RNA occurs such that the processing of messenger RNA is disrupted and eventually even the nondividing cells die of protein starvation (65). Hirschowitz et al. (66) have used such vectors in normal volunteers as well as in patients with colon cancer that had metastasized to the liver. Early hematopoietic stem cells cannot be infected by adenoviral vectors because the vector requires the presence of the $\alpha v\beta 3$ integrin receptor, which is not present on early hematopoietic stem cells. Thus, selectivity of action can be engineered into therapeutic approaches based on these vectors.

Current efforts involve engineering of the fibrillar protein of the adenoviral vector so that it will bind to hematopoietic cells. Bispecific antibodies are also being used to deliver adenoviral vectors to hematopoietic stem cells (12). Finally, adenoviral vectors, which are conditionally replication-competent in cells of different epigenotypes (39), are being developed so that these vectors can be used to modify the hematopoietic stem cell. This strategy is sometimes based on the introduction of transcriptional promoters that are specific for the regulatory environments of different tissues (67).

Vector Targeting

Phage display screening has been used to collect all of the immunoglobulin genes circulating in cancer patients and to use panning or sequential negative selection of these populations of phage to produce phage clones that bear immunoglobulin genes specific for particular types of tumor cells (68). In fact, it is possible to derive human single-chain immunoglobulin antibody molecules that are specific for tumor cells and not reactive for normal cells (68). The specificities to which these antibody molecules are reactive are often glycoprotein modifications of commonly expressed tumor cells that are specific for the tumor cell on the basis of glycosylation. The utility of such single-chain antibody molecules for targeting vectors to the target cell is only now being evaluated.

One of the most troublesome problems with vector-mediated gene delivery of all kinds is that vectors bind to normal cells, and the number of normal nontarget cells often vastly exceeds the number of target cells, whether they be normal or abnormal. To render genetic therapy more specific and to increase the frequency of vector-modified cells, attempts to genetically engineer the vector envelope proteins in the case of retroviral vectors or to engineer the fibrillar proteins of adenoviral vectors have been carried out with significant success. In the case of retroviral vectors, the ligand on the retroviral vector surface that engages the amphotropic receptor of the mammalian cell has been engineered so that it presents ligands for lineage and stage-specific hematopoietic receptors for growth factors. Kasabara et al. (13) have introduced the amino-terminal end of erythropoietin at this position. His vectors have been shown to transduce specifically erythroid precursors. In addition, this same group has placed the ligand that engages the stem cell factor receptor, c-kit, and this vector transduces early but not late hematopoietic cells (13). Although this work has been successful as a feat of genetic engineering, the utility of these vectors has been limited by other weaknesses of the retroviral vector: primarily the restriction of transduction to dividing cells and the loss of expression in stem cells owing to methylation inhibition of the vector transcriptional regulatory units, and the continued expression of the wild-type receptor ligand.

Attempts to target adenoviral vectors are more complex than for retroviral vectors because the fibrillar protein—the first point of contact between the adenoviral vector and its receptor on the surface of the mammalian cell—is a trimer of fibrillar proteins and even small changes in the backbone structure of this protein can destabilize its trimeric nature. However, many of the experimental approaches for this re-engineering have been very successful. Such engineering efforts that involve the adenoviral vector are more useful than the retroviral vector because the adenoviral vector can express its transgene in nondividing cells as an episome and because the virus has a wide host range in terms of infection. The targeting of the adenoviral vector to the stem cell thus becomes a priority to avoid its being consumed by binding to irrelevant cells and thereby unavailable to target cells.

The most successful and active group in this regard is led by David Curiel (12,33,34). This group has used bispecific antibody molecules to deliver the vector to specific target cells. One end of the molecule engages the end of the fibrillar protein, called the *knob protein*, and the other end of the bispecific antibody engages an antigen or receptor on the surface of the target cell.

This effort is still evolving, and some groups are using functional screening with adenoviral vectors that have reporter genes (e.g., the green fluorescent protein) and libraries of random amino acid peptides that are inserted into the knob of the fibrillar protein to select adenoviral vectors that will bind selectively to any cell, even when the cell-specific antigen is not known. Another challenge is to make the adenoviral vector conditionally replication-competent within the target cell so that all of the members of a population of cell in a tissue or in a tumor nodule will be infected by the vector.

Gene Replacement Studies for Hematopoietic Disorders

One dream of genetic therapy is to develop strategies that will replace missing genes, in single-gene constitutional disorders,

resulting in reversal of the abnormal phenotype of a disease process. This goal has been elusive because the insertion of transcription units into the chromosomal DNA was originally thought to be a requisite step in this process. This focus on integration of transcription units has limited the success of replacement strategies because the stem cells in a tissue, which must be modified to produce a correction of the abnormal phenotype that has a lifelong impact, are nondividing. Thus, the retroviral vector is unable to affect these cells, and the change of phenotype has often been only short term.

The adeno-associated adenoviral vector has also been studied as a means for the introduction of transcription units into chromosomal DNA. Unfortunately, the same restriction that has limited the utility of the retroviral vectors—the inability to modify a nondividing cell—also applies to the adeno-associated vector. The adenoviral vector DNA can maintain itself in the cytoplasm and nucleus of a nondividing cell for months, if not years (2). This discovery has led to preclinical animal model data showing that the gene for hemophilia B can persist in the cytoplasm of cells infected with the adeno-associated vector transcription units for more than a year. This persistence results in the release of factor IX into the systemic circulation in quantities sufficient to reverse the abnormal phenotype of this disorder (spontaneous bleeding into the joint spaces) in a strain of hemophilia dogs. This finding, reported by Herzog et al. (2), has led to the initiation of clinical trials of this strategy in human patients. The strategy involved the injection of the infectious but replication-incompetent vector into the nondividing myotubes of dogs. The transcription unit was engineered with signal sequences that result in the secretion of the protein produced from the transcription unit into the systemic circulation. This breakthrough is a validation of the paradigm of genetic therapy via vector-mediated delivery. Achievement of this success followed years of unsuccessful trials with both retroviral and adeno-associated vectors, which have clarified the limitations of each and the needs of transcription units within modified cells.

Publication of the successful reduction to practice of a lentiviral vector that carries a reporter gene has signaled a new direction in strategies for the modification of hematopoietic stem cells (16). In theory, this modification will lead to the reversal of the abnormal phenotype members of specific lineages of hematopoietic cells or to the use of hematopoietic cells as vehicles with which to correct abnormalities in any tissue that involve a protein product released into the systemic circulation. The issue to be addressed experimentally is the safety of these vectors. The envelope proteins necessary to the vectors' infection and destruction of the cellular immune response that leads to acquired immunodeficiency syndrome have been removed from the vectors in order to safely modify these vectors. The genes that code for viral products essential to completion of the viral life cycle have also been removed. This removal has not necessarily solved all of the safety concerns that arise from the fear that recombinant vectors may recombine with wild-type vectors in individuals whose infection with wild-type acquired immunodeficiency syndrome viruses may be undetectable at the time of vector introduction. In an attempt to further reduce the probability that these vectors could recombine and produce a replication-competent recombinant, most of the sequences in the recombinant safety modified vector, which are homologous to the wild-type vector, have been removed. These are called *third-generation lentiviral safety modified vectors*.

Very early in the field of genetic therapy, experiments showed that the clones of retroviral integrants that dominate the marrow hematopoietic cells would change with time. This finding suggested that a succession of stem cells that are active at any given time persist in terms of proliferation and generation of progeny in the lineages of the bone marrow. This sequential model predicts that the genetic modification of a stem cell at a given time, with a given pattern of expression, may not persist for more than 6 months—only to be replaced by another cohort of stem cells that could display another pattern of expression because the integration sites are random within the genome and the level of transcriptional activity in each of these regions is different. This issue of sequential stem cell activation (sequential versus continuous) has not been resolved, and the outcome of current experiments designed to resolve this question will determine the strategies necessary to ensure that expression of a transcription unit is reliable and unchanging over a period of months to years. Alternatively, if it turns out that the progeny to cells that are modified persist only for a short time and the majority of the stem cells are inaccessible to gene therapists, the gene modification may have to be repeated every 6 months. The level of success at each of the six monthly intervals may determine the feasibility of using multiple sequential modifications for the maintenance of a corrected phenotype of a single-gene defect.

Because endothelial cells line the vessels of the body and because they have been shown to arise from a stem cell precursor that shares the stromal cell as a common precursor, the use of the endothelial cell or the common precursor cell has emerged as a major goal of gene therapy. The vector systems that have been used include retroviral and adenoviral vectors. The endothelial cells have been used as targets for cancer vaccine therapy because they are the first to come into contact with injected vectors. Phage display libraries have been used with intravenous injection in mouse models to show that the molecules presented in the endothelial surface of different tissues are specific for each of these tissues. The identities of the molecules in each of these different tissues are just now being elucidated. When these molecules are identified, the feasibility of targeting therapy to specific tissues will increase. Even before the identification of these specificities, strategies are being pursued that involve insertion into the hinge region of the fibrillar protein of a library of random amino acid dodecapeptides, which can target the vectors to any cell.

GENERAL ISSUES TO BE RESOLVED

Many issues must be resolved before genetic therapy is successful for hematopoietic stem cells. As outlined, one issue is the pattern of activation of stem cells in the bone marrow. If it is found that the majority of stem cells are inaccessible to the modification of genes at any given time or that a succession of active stem cells exist in hematopoietic tissue, then the genetic modification will have to be administered repeatedly to cells with short-term self-renewal capacity.

If the use of lentiviral vectors that integrate into the chromosomal DNA of nondividing cells is successful, a single genetic modification may have a lifelong impact, provided transgene expression can be maintained. To achieve lifelong expression, the transcrip-

tional regulatory elements of viruses, such as the mouse embryonic stem cell virus, that continue to be expressed in transduced stem cells and embryonic cells for prolonged periods will be used.

If the adenoviral vectors can be engineered to be conditionally replication-competent, with a very low background in non-target cells, these vectors can be used to treat single-gene defects affecting hematopoietic cells, provided the immune response to the adenoviral proteins can be prevented.

Finally, many genes need to be expressed only for a short time. The expression of a therapeutic gene must be regulated developmentally. The gene may be required to be expressed intermittently so that it can respond to changes in the systemic circulation in a way that is integrated into the systemic response to external stimuli. The level of the gene expression may also be important. Nowhere has this proved to be more of a problem than in the case of the globin genes. To avoid the ineffective erythropoiesis seen in thalassemia, the balance between alpha- and the nonalpha-globin genes must be absolute. Because the tissue-specific regulators of these genes are located both near and far from the genes that are regulated, it has been difficult to engineer vectors that are suitable for the correction of globin gene defects. The ability to engineer complex regulatory elements that are tissue-specific and that respond to factors in trans in a physiologic way is a major priority for the future.

ACKNOWLEDGMENTS

The authors recognize the support of the Ensign Professorship at the Yale University School of Medicine. In addition, the following entities have provided support to Albert Deisseroth during the past several years: the George and Barbara Bush Leukemia Research Fund, the National Institutes of Health Grants NCI 49639 and 55164, U.S. Army Grant (BCRP BC 980260), support from the Susan B. Komen Foundation, support from the Donaghue Foundation, support from the Cure for Lymphoma Foundation, support from the Lymphoma Foundation of America, support from the Hull Foundation, and support from the Yale Cancer Center.

REFERENCES

1. Miller AD, Miller DG, Garcia JV, et al. Use of retroviral vectors for gene transfer and expression. *Methods Enzymol* 1993;217:581.
2. Herzog RW, Yang EYH, Conto LB, et al. Long term correction of canine hemophilia by gene transfer of blood coagulation factor IX mediated by AAV. *Nat Med* 1999;5:56.
3. Sekhar M, Yu JM, Soma T, Dunbar CE. Murine long-term repopulating ability is compromised by *ex vivo* culture in serum-free medium despite preservation of committed progenitors. *J Hematother* 1997;6(6):543–549.
4. Bodine DM, Karlsson S, Nienhuis AW. Combination of interleukins 3 and 6 preserves stem cell function in culture and enhances retrovirus-mediated gene transfer into hematopoietic stem cells. *Proc Natl Acad Sci U S A* 1989;86:8897.
5. Conneally E, Cashman J, Petzer A, Eaves C. Expansion *in vitro* of transplantable human cord blood stem cells demonstrated using a quantitative assay of their lympho-myeloid repopulating activity in nonobese diabetic SCID/SCID mice. *Proc Natl Acad Sci U S A* 1997;94:9836.
6. Lemischka IR, Raulet DH, Mulligan RC. Developmental potential

and dynamic behavior of hematopoietic stem cells. *Cell* 1986;45:917.

7. Brenner MK, Rill DR, Holladay MS, et al. Gene marking to determine whether autologous marrow infusion restores long-term hematopoiesis in cancer patients. *Lancet* 1993;342:1134.

8. Keim HP, Darovsky B, Von Kalle C, et al. Long-term persistence of canine hematopoietic cells genetically marked by retrovirus vectors. *Hum Gene Ther* 1996;7:89.

9. Deisseroth AB, Zu Z, Claxton D, et al. Genetic marking shows that Ph+ cells present in autologous transplants of CML contribute to relapse after autologous bone marrow in CML. *Blood* 1994;83:3068.

10. Orlic D, Girard LJ, Anderson SM, et al. Identification of human and mouse hematopoietic stem cell populations expressing high levels of mRNA encoding retrovirus receptors. *Blood* 1998;91:3247.

11. Yang Y, Vanin EF, Whitt M, et al. Inducible high level production of infectious murine leukemia retroviral vector particles pseudotyped with vesicular stomatitis virus G envelope protein. *Hum Gene Ther* 1995;6:1203.

12. Rogers BE, Douglas JT, Ahlem C, Buchsbaum DJ, Frincke J, Curiel DT. Use of a novel cross-linking method to modify adenovirus tropism. *Hum Gene Ther* 1997;4:1387.

13. Kasabara N, Dozy AM, Kan YW. Tissue specific targeting of retroviral vectors through ligand-receptor interactions. *Science* 1994;266:1373.

14. Bertran J, Miller JL, Yang Y, et al. Recombinant adeno-associated virus-mediated high-efficiency, transient expression of the murine cationic amino acid transporter (ecotropic retroviral receptor) permits stable transduction of human HeLa cells by ecotropic retroviral vectors. *J Virol* 1996;70:759.

15. Fen M, Jackson Jr WH, Goldman CK, et al. Stable *in vivo* transudation via a novel adenoviral/retroviral chimeric vector. *Nat Biotechnol* 1997;15:866.

16. Miyoshi H, Smith KA, Mosier D, Verma IM, Torgbett BE. Transduction of human CD34+ cells that initiate long-term engraftment of NOD/SCIEN mice by HIV vectors. *Science* 1999;283:682.

17. Baum C, Hegewisch-Becker S, Eckert HG, Stocking C, Ostsertag W. Novel retroviral vectors for efficient expression of the multidrug resistance (MDR-1) gene in early hematopoietic cells. *J Virol* 1998;69:7541.

18. Dunbar CE, Seidel NE, Doren S, et al. Improved retroviral gene transfer into murine and Rhesus peripheral blood or bone marrow repopulating cells primed *in vivo* with stem cell factor and granulocyte colony stimulating factor. *Proc Natl Acad Sci U S A* 1996;93:11871.

19. Tisdale JF, Hanazono Y, Selklers SE, et al. *Ex vivo* expansion of genetically marked rhesus peripheral blood progenitor cells results in diminished long-term repopulating ability. *Blood* 1998;92:1131.

20. Yonemura Y, Ku H, Hirayama F, Souza LM, Ogawa M. Interleukin-3 or interleukin-1 abrogates the reconstituting ability of hematopoietic stem cells. *Proc Natl Acad Sci U S A* 1996;93:4040.

21. Hanania EG, Giles RE, Kavanagh J, et al. Results of MDR-1 vector modification trial indicate that granulocyte/macrophage colony forming unit cells do not contribute to post transplant hematopoietic recovery following intensive systemic therapy. *Proc Natl Acad Sci U S A* 1996;93:15346.

22. Hesdorffer C, Ayello JK, Ward MAK, et al. Phase I trial of retroviral mediated transfer to the human MDR-1 gene as marrow chemoprotection in patients undergoing high dose chemotherapy in autologous stem cell transplantation. *J Clin Oncol* 1998;16:165.

23. Rahman Z, Kavanagh J, Champlin R, et al. Chemotherapy immediately following autologous stem cell transplantation in patients with advanced breast cancer. *Clin Cancer Res* 1998;4:2717.

24. Cowan KH, Mosacow JA, Huang H, et al. Paclitaxel chemotherapy following autologous stem cell transplantation and engraftment of hematopoietic cells transduced with a retrovirus containing the multidrug resistance cDNAs (MDR-1) in metastatic breast cancer patients. *Clin Cancer Res* 1999;5:1619–1628.

25. Miller CJ, Eaves CJ. Expansion *in vitro* of murine hematopoietic stem cells with transplantable lympho-myeloid reconstituting ability. *Proc Natl Acad Sci U S A* 1997;94:13648.

26. Brown RL, Fen SX, Dusting SKI, Lie Q, Fischer R, Patched M. Serum-free culture conditions for cells capable of producing long-term survival in lethally irradiated mice. *Stem Cells* 1997;15:237.

27. Chuck AS, Palsson BO. Consistent and high rates of gene transfer can be obtained using flow through transduction which raises transduction

frequencies with retroviral vectors. *Hum Gene Ther* 1996;7:743.

28. Podaskoff G, Wong Jr KK, Chatterjee S. Efficient gene transfer into nondividing cells by adeno-associated virus-based vectors. *J Virol* 1994;68:5656.

29. Miller JL, Donahue RE, Sellers SE, Samulski RJ, Young NS, Nienhuis AW. Recombinant adeno-associated virus (rAAV)-mediated expression of a human gamma-globin gene in human progenitor-derived erythroid cells. *Proc Natl Acad Sci U S A* 1994;91:10183.

30. Wickham TJ, Mathias P, Cheresh DA, Nemerov G. Multiple adenovirus serotypes use alpha V integrins for infection. *J Virol* 1993;68:6811.

31. Garcia-Sanchez F, Pizzorno G, Fu SQ, et al. Cytosine deaminase adenoviral vector and 5-Fluorocytosine selectively reduces breast cancer cells one million fold when they contaminate hematopoietic cells: a potential purging method for autologous transplantation. *Blood* 1988;92:672.

32. Neering SJ, Harhy SF, Minamoto DE, Spratt 3, Jordan DT. Transduction of primitive human hematopoietic cells with recombinant adenovirus vectors. *Blood* 1996;87:1147.

33. Dimtriev I, Krasnhykh V, Miller CR, et al. An adenovirus vector with genetically modified fibers demonstrates expanded tropism via utilization of a coxsackievirus and adenovirus receptor-independent cell entry mechanism. *J Virol* 1998;72:9706.

34. Douglas JT, Rogers BE, Rosenfeld ME, Michael SI, Feng M, Curiel DT. Targeted gene delivery by tropism-modified adenoviral vectors. *Nat Biotechnol* 1996;14:1574.

35. Lebkowski JS, McNally MN, Okarma TB, et al. Adeno-associated virus: a vector system for efficient introduction and integration of DNA into a variety of mammalian cell types. *Mol Cell Biol* 1988;8:3988.

36. Schneider G, Morral N, Parks R, et al. Genomic DNA transfer with a high capability adenovirus results in improved *in vivo* gene expression and decreased toxicity. *Nat Genet* 1998;18:180.

37. Lehman CW, Botchan MR. Segregation of viral plasmids depends on tethering to chromosomes and is regulated by phosphorylation. *Proc Natl Acad Sci U S A* 1998;95:4338.

38. Banerjee S, Livanos E, Vos JMH. Therapeutic gene delivery in human lympho-blastoid cells by engineered non-transforming infectious Epstein-Barr virus. *Nat Med* 1995;12:1303.

39. Heise C, Sampson-Johannes A, Williams A, McCormick F, Von Hoff DD, Kirn DH. ONYX-015, an E1B gene attenuated adenoviral vector, causes tumor specific cytolysis and antitumoral efficacy that can be augmented by standard chemotherapeutic agents. *Nat Med* 1997;3:639.

40. Hanenberg H, Hashino K, Konishi H, Hock RA, Kato I, Williams DA. Optimization of fibronectin-assisted retroviral gene transfer into human CD34+ cells. *Hum Gene Ther* 1997;8:2193.

41. Abnonour R, Einhorn L, Hall K, et al. Improved MDR-1 Gene Transfer into long term repopulating cells of patients undergoing autologous transplantation for germ cell tumors. *J Clin Oncol* 1999;18:439.

42. Dexter TM, Allen TD, Lajtha LG. Conditions controlling the proliferation of haemopoietic stem cells *in vitro*. *J Cell Physiol* 1977;91:335.

43. Hughes PF, Eaves CJ, Hogge DE, Humphries RKI. High efficiency gene transfer to human hematopoietic cells maintained in long-term culture. *Blood* 1989;74:1915.

44. Moore KA, Deisseroth AB, Reading CL, Williams DE, Belmont JW. Stromal support enhances cell free retroviral vector transduction of human bone marrow long term culture initiating cells. *Blood* 1992;79:1393.

45. Nolta JA, Hanley MB, Kohn DB. Sustained human hematopoiesis of marrow stroma expressing human interleukin-3: analysis of gene transduction of long lived progenitors. *Blood* 1994;43:3041.

46. Toksoz D, Zsebo KM, Smith DA, et al. Support of human hematopoiesis in long term bone marrow cultures by murine stromal cells selectively expressing the membrane bound and secreted forms of the human homologue of the steel gene product, stem cell factor. *Proc Natl Acad Sci U S A* 1992;89:7350.

47. Sorrentino B, Brandt SJ, Bodine D, et al. Selection of drug resistant bone marrow cells *in vivo* after retroviral transfer of human MDR-1. *Science* 1992;257:99.

48. Podda S, Ward M, Himelstein A, et al. Transfer and expression of the human multiple drug resistance gene into live mice. *Proc Natl Acad Sci U S A* 1992;89:9676.

49. Hanania EG, Deisseroth A. Serial transplantation shows that early hematopoietic precursor cells are transduced by MDR-1 retroviral vector in a mouse gene therapy model. *Cancer Gene Ther* 1994;1:24.

50. Hanania EG, Fu SQ, Roninson I, Zu Z, Deisseroth AB. Resistance to taxol chemotherapy produced in mouse marrow cells by safety modified retroviruses containing a human MDR-1 transcription unit. *Gene Ther* 1995;2:279.

51. Bhatia M, Bonnet D, Murdoch B, Gan OI, Dick JE. A newly discovered class of human hematopoietic progenitor cells: the SCID repopulating cell. *Nat Med* 1998;4:1038.

52. Porada CD, Tran N, Eglites M, et al. In utero gene therapy: transfer and long term expression of the bacterial NEO gene in sheep after direct injection of retroviral vectors in pre immune fetuses. *Hum Gene Ther* 1998;9:157.

53. Dunbar CE, Cottler-Fox M, O'Shaughnessy JA, et al. Retrovirally marked CD34 enriched peripheral blood and bone marrow cells contribute to long term engraftment after autologous transplantation. *Blood* 1995;85.3048.

54. Cornetta K, Srour EF, Moore A, et al. Retroviral gene transfer in autologous bone marrow transplantation for adult acute leukemia. *Hum Gene Ther* 1996;7:1323.

55. Emmons RV, Doren S, Zujewskik J, et al. Retroviral gene transduction of adult peripheral blood or marrow derived CD34+ cells for six hours without growth factors or on autologous stroma does not improve marking efficiency assessed *in vivo*. *Blood* 1997;89:4040.

56. Nolta JA, Smogorzewska EM, Kohn DB. Analysis of optimal conditions for retroviral mediated transduction of primitive human hematopoietic cells. *Blood* 1995;86:101.

57. Kohn DB, Weinberg KI, Nolta JA, et al. Engraftment of gene modified umbilical cord blood cells in neonates with adenosine deaminase deficiency. *Nat Med* 1995;1:1017.

58. Bordigon C, Motarangelo LK, Nobili N, et al. Gene therapy in peripheral blood lymphocytes and bone marrow for ADA-immuno-deficient patients. *Science* 1995;270:470.

59. Deisseroth AB. Clinical trials involving multidrug resistance transcription units in retroviral vectors. *Clin Cancer Res* 1999;5:1607.

60. Bunting KD, Galipeau J, Topham D, Benaim E, Sorrentino BP. Transduction of murine bone marrow cells with MDR-1 vector enables *ex vivo* stem cell expansion, but the expanded grafts cause myeloproliferative syndrome in transplanted animals. *Blood* 1998;92(7):2269–2279

61. Chen L, Pulshipher M, Chen D, Sieff C, Elias A, Fine HA, Kufe DW. Selective transgene expression for detection and elimination of contaminating carcinoma cells in hematopoietic stem cell sources. *J Clin Invest* 1996;98:2539.

62. Seth P, Brinkmann UY, Schwartz GN, et al. Adenovirus mediated gene transfer to human breast tumor cells: an approach for cancer gene therapy and bone marrow purging. *Cancer Res* 1996;56:1346.

63. Clarke MF, Apel U, Benedict MNA, et al. A recombinant BCL-Xshort adenovirus selectively induces apoptosis in cancer cells but not in normal cells. *Proc Natl Acad Sci U S A* 1995;92:11024.

64. Mullen CA, Kilstrug M, Blaese RM. Transfer of the bacterial gene for cytosine deaminase to a mammalian cell confers lethal sensitivity to 5-FC: a negative selection system. *Proc Natl Acad Sci U S A* 1992; 56:1346.

65. Armstrong RD, Lewis M, Stern SG, Cadman EC. Acute effect of 5FU on cytoplasmic and nuclear dihydrofolate reductase mRNA metabolism. *J Biol Chem* 1986;261:72366.

66. Hirschowitz EA, Ohwada A, Pascal WR, Russi TJ, Crystal RG. *In vivo* adenovirus mediated gene transfer of the E. Coli cytosine deaminase gene to human colon carcinoma derived tumors induces chemosensitivity to 5FC. *Hum Gene Ther* 1995;6:1055.

67. Chung I, Schwartz P, Crystal RG, Pizzorno GP, Leavitt J, Deisseroth A. Use of L-plastin promoter to develop an adenoviral system that confers transgene expression in ovarian cancer cells but not in normal mesothelial cells. *Cancer Gene Ther* 1999;6:99.

68. Wang B, Chen YB, Ayalon O, Bender J, Garen A. Human single-chain Fv immunoconjugates targeted to a melanoma associated chondroitin sulfate proteoglycan mediate specific lysis of human melanoma cells by natural killer cells and complement. *Proc Natl Acad Sci U S A* 1999;96:1627.

20.3

GENE THERAPY: CLINICAL APPLICATIONS

Suicide Gene Therapy

DAVID L. BARTLETT
J. ANDREA MCCART

Gene therapy for cancer can be divided into indirect (e.g., vaccines) and tumor-directed approaches. The tumor-directed approach requires vectors that specifically express genes in tumor cells in order to mediate their own death. Cell death can be immunologically mediated, as in the case of cytokine gene expression, or secondary to apoptosis, as in the case of tumor suppressor gene replacement. Another tumor-directed method is the expression of an enzyme that converts a systemically delivered, nontoxic prodrug into a toxic agent within the cell. *Suicide gene therapy* has become synonymous with this enzyme/prodrug approach, which is also known as *gene-directed enzyme/prodrug therapy*. This technique requires that a gene encoding an enzyme normally not present in human cells be targeted to cancer cells and allow high expression of the enzyme within the cancer cells. The prodrug must be nontoxic and taken up into the cancer cell after systemic delivery, where it is converted into a toxin. The toxin should kill the cancer cell expressing the gene as well as surrounding cells not expressing the gene (bystander effect).

The herpes simplex virus thymidine kinase type 1 (*HSV-tk*) gene was initially called a *suicide gene* by Plautz et al. (1) when it was included in a retrovirus intended for long-term replacement gene therapy. If the retrovirus was inserted into the genome such that malignant transformation occurred, the transformed cells and resultant tumor could be eliminated with the nontoxic prodrug ganciclovir (GCV), which in the presence of *HSV-tk* is converted into the toxic metabolite ganciclovir triphosphate. This "suicide" system was designed to enhance the safety of clinically utilized retroviruses. Previously, Moolten (2) demonstrated that the *HSV-tk* system could eliminate tumors that were stably transfected with the *HSV-tk* gene. His intention was to create tissue mosaicism for drug sensitivity, ensuring that any tumor arising clonally could be eliminated without affecting a large percentage of normal cells in the organ. This concept was then expanded into an active cancer therapy by Huber et al. (3). They achieved hepatoma-specific cytotoxicity using a retrovirus containing the α-fetoprotein promoter controlling expression of the varicella zoster virus thymidine kinase (*VZV-TK*) gene, followed by exposure to the nontoxic prodrug 6-methoxypurine arabinonucleoside (ara-M). *VZV-TK* converted ara-M to ara-M monophosphate in hepatoma cells, resulting in cytotoxicity.

The enzyme/prodrug strategy has many theoretical advantages over other forms of cancer gene therapy. As opposed to vaccine approaches, suicide gene therapy does not depend on the host's immune system and tumor immunogenicity, which to date have not been reliably understood, controlled, or manipulated. Suicide gene therapy should be applicable to all histologies, and the bystander effect allows surrounding cells not expressing the gene to be killed, unlike suppressor gene replacement strategies or antisense oncogene strategies, which would not be expected to have a bystander effect. Another advantage of the enzyme/prodrug approach is that the toxic effect is not seen until the prodrug is delivered. Therefore, prodrug delivery acts as a controllable switch for activation of the system. This allows *in vitro* expansion of viruses expressing these genes without concern for host cell toxicity. It also allows a buildup of enzyme within the tumor *in vivo* before prodrug delivery, which should improve potency and lead to an enhanced bystander effect.

Limitations to this form of therapy include (a) the potential toxicity to surrounding normal cells, as the converted toxin is generally not specific for tumor cells, and (b) a significant percentage of cells within a tumor must express the gene of interest, requiring a highly efficient vector. A number of enzyme/prodrug systems have been described and are summarized in this chapter. In addition, a review of published clinical trials using suicide genes is included.

SUICIDE GENE VECTORS

The ideal suicide gene vector provides highly efficient, tumor-specific gene delivery and expression. The advantage of suicide gene therapy over other forms of gene therapy (correcting inborn errors of metabolism) is that gene expression can be transient. Gene expression must only last long enough to mediate the death of the cell. The disadvantage is the need for a highly efficient and specific vector, such that the majority of cells within a tumor express the gene of interest. Whereas many suicide gene systems function efficiently *in vitro*, the main limitation to clinical application is the poor efficiency of current vectors *in vivo*. Achieving even 1% to 2% transduction efficiency *in vivo* with a systemically delivered vector is beyond the capability of most current vectors. Nevertheless, vector development is progressing at a rapid pace, and the technological feasibility of an efficient, tumor-specific vector exists.

The most commonly studied vectors for tumor-directed gene therapy include viruses, plasmid DNA delivered via liposomes, and protein/DNA complexes. Characteristics of these vectors are summarized in Table 1. Originally, Huber et al. (3) described the use of retroviruses expressing a suicide gene under the control of a tissue-specific promoter as described above. A nonreplicating retrovirus can safely provide long-term gene expression via integration into the host genome and theoretically provides some tumor specificity because it can only transduce dividing cells. Retroviral integration into the genome could be oncogenic, but this is of minimal concern in the setting of transient gene expression for cancer therapy. Unfortunately, retroviruses are relatively inefficient and difficult to produce in high titers for clinical studies. In addition, only a small percentage of cells within a tumor are dividing at any one time, greatly limiting the *in vivo* transduction efficiency. These limitations led to the injection of retroviral producer cells into tumors, which release retroviruses over a long period, and should improve the chance of stable integration of the gene of interest into tumor cells. Culver et al. (4) demonstrated dramatic growth inhibition of gliomas in rats after injection of 3×10^6 murine fibroblasts producing a retrovirus expressing *HSV-tk* followed by systemic GCV. Although conceptually appealing, this method requires that producer cells be evenly distributed throughout the tumor and survive immunologic clearance in order for prolonged release of retroviruses.

Attention was then turned toward more efficient vectors, which do not require dividing cells for successful gene delivery. The most studied vector in this regard has been the adenovirus. Adenovirus has many advantages over other vectors, including its abilities to grow in high titers [10^{12} plaque-forming units (PFUs) per mL], to infect and express genes in nondividing cells of multiple histologies, and to create a safe nonreplicating virus by deletion of early genes. Smythe et al. (5) demonstrated *in vitro* efficacy of an adenovirus expressing *HSV-tk* in pleural mesothelioma. Chen et al. (6) initially reported the use of adenovirus to express the *HSV-tk* gene as an intratumoral treatment for experimental gliomas in nude mice, demonstrating dramatic inhibition of tumor growth. Since then, many articles have described successes with intratumoral injections of adenoviruses expressing suicide genes in animal models, and numerous clinical trials have been instituted.

TABLE 1. GENERAL CHARACTERISTICS OF COMMONLY STUDIED VECTORS FOR SUICIDE GENE THERAPY

Vector	Efficiency of Gene Transfer	Potential Tumor Targeting	Potential Tumor-Specific Gene Expression	Potential Tumor-Specific Amplification	Lack of Preformed Immunity	Nonimmunogenic (Multiple Dosing)	Production Efficiency/ Quantity
Viral							
Retrovirus	−	+	+	−	+	−	−
Adenovirus	±	+	+	+	±	−	+
Herpes	+	−	+	+	±	−	+
Vaccinia	+	±	−	+	−	−	+
Nonviral							
Naked DNA	−	−	+	−	+	+	+
Liposomes	−	+	+	−	+	+	+
Protein-DNA complex	−	+	+	−	+	+	+
Other							
Endothelial cells	−	+	−	+	+	±	±
Bacteria	−	+	−	+	±	−	+

+, favorable; −, unfavorable; ±, neither favorable nor unfavorable.
Note: Vectors are rated as favorable or unfavorable relative to the other vectors.

Although it demonstrates improved *in vivo* transduction efficiencies compared to retroviruses, the adenovirus has many limitations. Cell infection occurs via the coxsackievirus and adenovirus receptor (CAR) (7), which is variably present in different tumor and host tissues (8). Cell lines with low levels of CAR may not achieve more than 10% transduction efficiency under ideal conditions *in vitro* and worse *in vivo*. Chen et al. (6) showed that a stereotactic injection of 10^8 PFU of adenovirus into 0.4-mm^2 intracerebral tumors resulted in an antitumor response. Larger tumors, such as those encountered in patients, would require multiple injections of much larger quantities of virus, and this may not be feasible. Intravenous injection of adenovirus is not a reasonable option because it leads to infection of normal tissues that have the CAR receptor (e.g., normal mouse hepatocytes), leading to unacceptable toxicity. A strong immune response to the viral proteins and preformed circulating antibodies in 98% of adults further limits the expected magnitude and duration of gene expression (9). Adenoviral efficiency can be improved through CAR-independent infection and tumor-specific replication as discussed under Tumor-Specific Targeting.

Other viruses that have been studied as suicide gene vectors include the replication-competent herpesvirus and vaccinia virus.

A replicating virus should allow enhancement of gene expression throughout a tumor. The infection of a cell with a single virus particle can lead to the release of thousands of progeny viruses, which will infect surrounding cells and slowly spread throughout the tumor (until eliminated by the host's immune system). Although a replicating virus leads to the death of infected cells, concomitant expression of a suicide gene could lead to bystander killing of noninfected cells, thus increasing the chance of a significant tumor response before immunologic clearance of the vector (Fig. 1). The safety of a replicating vector is a major concern, but genetically altering the virus to allow tumor-specific replication should prevent systemic host infection. The addition of a suicide gene may also improve the safety of a replicating vector either by causing cell death before the virus has a chance to replicate or by directly inhibiting viral DNA replication. Herpes simplex virus is a large DNA virus with efficient uptake resulting in high levels of gene expression. Although the wild-type vector is able to cause latent infections of nerve cells, specific mutations in the genome can prevent this (ICP34.5 mutation). This vector appears to be more efficient for *in vivo* gene transfer than a nonreplicating adenovirus. Vaccinia is a large DNA virus that infects multiple cell types and undergoes cytoplasmic replication using proteins syn-

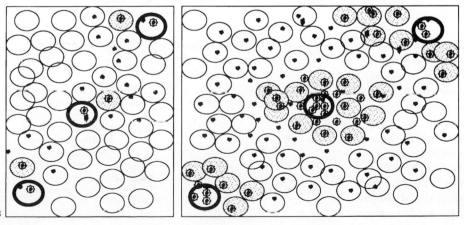

FIGURE 1. Schematic representation of the *In vivo* bystander zone with a nonreplicating **(A)** and replicating **(B)** vector. A replicating vector leads to a higher number of cells expressing the gene and, therefore, an improved bystander zone. Note that *in vivo*, the diffusible toxin may readily enter the bloodstream and diffuse away from the tumor microenvironment. Thick-walled circles indicate blood vessels; shaded cells indicate infected cells; dense particles represent toxins.

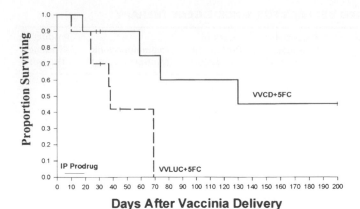

Days After Vaccinia Delivery

FIGURE 2. Survival of athymic (C57BL6) mice injected intratumorally (subcutaneous MC38 tumor) with a lethal dose of replicating vaccinia virus (VVLUC, control expressing luciferase; VVCD, expressing cytosine deaminase) followed by treatment with intraperitoneal (i.p.) 5-fluorocytosine (5-FC) for 14 days. All animals died from viral toxicity (not tumor). The VVCD-treated animals show prolonged survival, demonstrating protection from virus toxicity by prodrug conversion and presumed inhibition of viral DNA synthesis and replication by 5-fluorouracil.

thesized and packaged by the virus itself, resulting in very high *in vitro* and *in vivo* efficiency. The cytosine deaminase (CD) suicide gene system can inhibit viral replication *in vitro* and prolong survival *in vivo* after a lethal injection of replicating vaccinia virus (Fig. 2).

The immune response to viral vectors remains a significant obstacle to successful gene therapy. Although the development of viruses that evade the immune system has been proposed, these vectors would theoretically be unsafe in the general population. *In vivo* recombination events could lead to an ubiquitously infectious virus that cannot be eliminated by the host. Reversible immunosuppression—as a means of allowing gene expression long enough to provide an antitumor response, followed by immune recovery to eliminate the vector and ensure the safety of the host—may be an alternative.

Plasmid DNA delivered by liposomes and protein/DNA complexes have undergone significant improvements to enhance transfection efficiency (10). These approaches have the benefit of an almost unlimited delivery capability, including repeated dosing without immunologic clearance. Nevertheless, the *in vivo* efficiency remains unsatisfactory and may never surpass that of a virus that has evolved solely for the purpose of expressing genes within host cells. The main limitation appears to be inefficient mechanisms of uptake and escape of the DNA from the cellular endosomal shunt (11). As liposomes become more complex, incorporating proteins that bind to cell surface receptors and enhance efficiency, the disadvantages associated with viral therapy become more pronounced (12,13). With continued technological modifications, an artificial system may have many potential advantages over viral vectors.

Other vectors for suicide gene therapy have been proposed, such as the delivery of cells carrying suicide genes to tumors, without the tumors themselves expressing the genes. By delivering a prodrug that is converted within the transduced cells, surrounding tumor cells may also be killed owing to the bystander effect. This system would require a diffusible toxin. One exam-

ple is endothelial cells, which seem to track to tumors when injected systemically (14). Bacteria such as salmonella and clostridium may also be an option (15). Although these vectors are mostly of theoretical interest at this time, they highlight the versatility and utility of an effective enzyme/prodrug system.

TUMOR-SPECIFIC TARGETING

Vector targeting has been achieved by controlling gene transcription, viral infectivity, or viral replication. Many tissue- and tumor-specific transcriptional regulatory sequences have been described (Table 2). Using genetic sequences that control the expression of therapeutic genes in cancer cells is an ideal way to take advantage of the genetic differences between tumor and normal cells. These transcriptional regulatory sequences consist of classical promoter regions (where initiation of transcription occurs) and enhancer elements that recruit polymerases to the promoter in a cell-specific manner. Many tissue-specific promoters sacrifice promoter strength for specificity and are unable to express therapeutic genes at a clinically useful level. Enhancer elements, often included as multiple repeats, can markedly upregulate gene expression while maintaining specificity (16). Siders et al. (17) demonstrated high levels of gene expression specifically in melanoma cells using the tyrosinase promoter coupled to a dimer of the tyrosinase-enhancer element. This technique allowed efficient transcriptional targeting of mela-

TABLE 2. SPECIFIC PROMOTERS FOR SUICIDE GENE THERAPY

Promoter	Specificity
Tissue-specific	
Prostate-specific antigen, kallikrein 2	Prostate/prostate cancer
Tyrosinase	Melanocytes/melanoma
Albumin, hepatitis B virus core promoter	Liver/hepatoma
Growth hormone	Pituitary/pituitary cancer
Osteocalcin	Bone/osteosarcoma
Myelin basic protein, glial fibrillary acidic protein	Glial cells/glioblastoma multiforme
Thyroglobulin	Thyroid/thyroid cancer
CD11	Leukocytes/lymphoma
B-casein	Mammary/breast cancer
Surfactant	Bronchoalveolar/lung cancer
mck	Myogenic cells/rhabdomyosarcoma
kdr, tir, e-selectin	Endothelial cells/tumor vasculature
Tumor-specific	
α-Fetoprotein	Oncofetal/hepatoma
Carcinoembryonic antigen	Oncofetal/colon cancer
MUC-1	MUC-1 producing tumors
erbB-2	ErbB-2 expressing tumors
grp 78/BiP	Stress inducible glucose regulated/tumor-specific
pax3 DNA binding, site prs-9	Alveolar rhabdomyosarcoma
Secretory leukoprotease inhibitor	Carcinomas
Hexokinase type II	Glycolysis regulator/tumor-specific

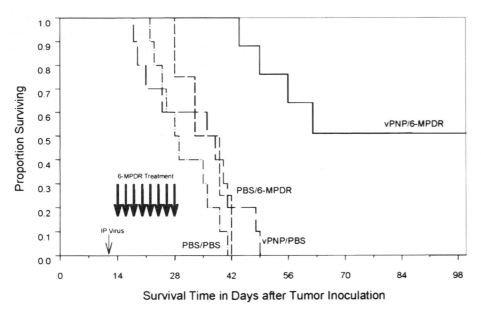

FIGURE 3. Survival in athymic (C57BL6) mice with hepatic metastases (intrasplenic MC38 injection) after intraperitoneal (IP) delivery of a thymidine kinase–deleted vaccinia virus expressing purine nucleoside phosphorylase (PNP), followed by systemic therapy with 6-methylpurine deoxyriboside (6-MPDR). Treatment animals survived significantly longer than controls, with 50% long-term cures. All deaths were due to hepatic replacement with tumor. No viral deaths were noted at this dose. PBS, phosphate buffered saline. (Adapted from Puhlmann M, Gnant M, Brown CK, et al. Thymidine kinase deleted vaccinia virus expressing purine nucleoside phosphorylase as a vector for tumor directed gene therapy. *Hum Gene Ther* 1999;10:649–657.)

noma cells. Many transcriptional regulatory signals are active at low levels in normal cells or are specific for a tissue or cell type. For example, the tyrosinase promoter is specific for all melanin-producing cells in the body. This may lead to unacceptable toxicity if melanin-producing retinal cells are destroyed. The most appealing promoters are those that are specific for tumor cells, such as oncofetal antigen promoters (α-fetoprotein, carcinoembryonic antigen) or specific for genes upregulated in transformed cells such as the E2F-1 transcription factor. Parr et al. (18) demonstrated that the E2F-1 promoter mediated high levels of marker gene expression specifically in cancer cells *in vivo* and could eradicate established gliomas when used to express a toxic gene. Promoters active in nonessential tissues (e.g., prostate-specific promoters) are also useful, where ablation of the normal tissue will have minimal side effects.

Altering viral coat proteins to allow specific binding to tumor cell surface antigens or receptors is another means of targeting that is actively being investigated. This includes the expression of antitumor single-chain antibody fragments on the viral coat that will target tumor antigens, as well as the expression of peptides that act as ligands for tumor-specific receptors. Altering the viral coat can enhance viral uptake into otherwise resistant tumor cells, as well as potentially inhibit infection of normal cells. Martin et al. (19) incorporated a single-chain antibody (ScFv), directed against high-molecular-weight melanoma-associated antigen (HMWMAA), into the retroviral envelope and demonstrated preferential infection of melanoma cells. Dmitriev et al. (20) showed that incorporation of an Arg-Gly-Asp–containing peptide, specific for the αvβ3-integrin, into the HI loop of the fiber knob coat protein of adenovirus resulted in CAR-independent infection and increased infectivity by two to three orders of magnitude in otherwise resistant cells.

Perhaps the most important step towards a clinically relevant vector for suicide gene therapy has been the development of viruses that specifically replicate in tumor cells. Adenovirus has been engineered for this purpose. The adenovirus E1B 55-kd gene product is considered essential for viral replication and acts

by binding *p53* and preventing cellular apoptosis, a natural antiviral response. It was believed that deleting the *E1B* gene in adenovirus would limit replication to *p53*-mutant cancer cells (or cells with other downstream mutations in the apoptotic pathway), in which apoptosis was already blocked. Bischoff et al. (21) demonstrated *in vitro* specificity for *p53*-mutant tumor cell lines with this vector and significant tumor regression *in vivo*. Other investigators have subsequently questioned the mechanism for this specificity (22–24). Nevertheless, this replication-selective virus was shown to have an antitumor effect and is currently being investigated as an oncolytic virus in clinical trials. Wildner et al. (25) demonstrated that the inclusion of the *HSV-tk* gene in this replication-specific virus led to an improved antitumor response with GCV treatment compared to a control replicating virus.

Another means of engineering a tumor-specific replication competent adenovirus is by using tissue-selective promoters to express essential viral genes. Rodriguez et al. (26) created an adenovirus expressing the essential *E1A* gene under the control of the prostate-specific antigen enhancer and promoter. They achieved prostate-specific viral replication, which resulted in tumor regression when injected intratumorally.

The herpes simplex virus has also been genetically altered to achieve tumor-specific replication. Deletion of genes, such as thymidine kinase, ribonucleotide reductase, and neurovirulence factor (ICP 34.5 gene), which are essential for nucleotide synthesis and viral replication in nondividing cells, allows tumor-specific replication with decreased toxicity (27). The addition of a suicide gene should further enhance the antitumor response over that of a replicating virus. We have been interested in exploring the vaccinia virus as a suicide gene vector because of its remarkable efficiency as a cytoplasmic virus. We have found that a TK-deleted vaccinia virus selectively replicates in tumor tissue *in vivo* when injected systemically and can lead to a survival advantage and some cures when combined with the *CD*/5-fluorocytosine (5-FC) or purine nucleoside phosphorylase (*PNP*)/6-methylpurine deoxyriboside (6-MPDR) systems in a murine model of hepatic metastases (28,29) (Fig. 3).

BYSTANDER EFFECT

The bystander effect of an enzyme/prodrug gene therapy system is essential for the killing of surrounding tumor cells that do not express the gene of interest. This is the most significant advantage of suicide gene therapy over other forms of tumor-directed gene therapy (e.g., tumor suppressor gene replacement). Once a prodrug is converted to a toxin within a tumor cell, that toxin can affect surrounding cells through one of three mechanisms: (a) free diffusion through the cell membrane, (b) intercellular transport via gap junctions (13), or (c) delivery in apoptotic vesicles for phagocytosis.

The advantage of freely diffusible toxins is that cell-to-cell contact is not required, and cells at a distance may be exposed to the toxin. The disadvantage is the higher potential for toxicity to normal cells. For example, PNP converts 6-MPDR into the highly potent and diffusible toxin 6-methylpurine (6-MP). The *in vivo* efficacy of the *PNP*/6-MPDR system is limited by systemic toxicity of the converted prodrug, and the therapeutic window seems narrow. The bystander effect of toxins requiring intercellular communications (e.g., the *HSV-tk*/GCV system) has the advantage of being safe for surrounding normal cells, but the antitumor effect can be quite variable depending on the concentration of gap junctions. Tumor cells may lose these communications as they become less differentiated. Mesnil et al. (30) demonstrated that HeLa cells lacked both gap junctions and a bystander effect using the *HSV-tk*/GCV system. By transfecting with a gene-encoding connexin 43 (a gap junction protein), a bystander effect could be elucidated (30). Both the connexin 43 gene and a suicide gene could be transferred in a single vector to optimize the bystander effect, but the complexity of this system may decrease efficiency.

Cells undergoing toxin-mediated apoptosis may theoretically have a bystander effect by transferring toxins via apoptotic vesicles, which are phagocytosed by surrounding cells. This has been visualized *in vitro* by cell-to-cell transfer of fluorescent-labeled compounds (31). The *in vivo* significance of this phenomenon is unknown.

In vitro studies are ideal for demonstrating a bystander effect, where the mixing of different ratios of transduced cells expressing the gene of interest with untransduced cells allows determination of the percentage of transduced cells required to kill the entire cell population. The zone of cells affected by the converted toxin *in vitro* (bystander zone) may have no correlation to the zone of cells that will be exposed *in vivo*. *In vitro* studies allow an even distribution of the gene throughout the cells, and the converted toxin is released into the supernatant that continually bathes surrounding cells. This will not be the case for most *in vivo* gene transfer, in which toxins will preferentially diffuse into the bloodstream and be taken away from the tumor microenvironment, increasing systemic toxicity while limiting the *in vivo* bystander zone.

Other factors that may be responsible for a bystander effect *in vivo* that are not seen *in vitro* include (a) immunologic/cytokine-mediated effect and (b) toxicity to vascular endothelial cells resulting in an ischemic effect. *In vivo* therapy with the *HSV-tk*/GCV system has resulted in hemorrhagic necrosis of the tumor within 24 hours of prodrug administration. This dramatic effect is not consistent with cytotoxicity from converted prodrug, suggesting a cytokine-mediated hemorrhagic necrosis such as that seen with tumor necrosis factor. This inconsistency suggests that the inflammatory response to toxin-mediated cell death may result in a cytokine cascade that causes coagulative necrosis of the tumor (32). Melcher et al. (33) demonstrated that a toxin-mediated necrotic cell death uniquely results in heat shock protein release and an inflammatory response.

An *in vivo* virus-mediated oncolysate may also act as a potent vaccine. The *in vivo* destruction of cells leads to efficient uptake and presentation of tumor antigens by immune effector cells. Evidence supports an improved antitumor effect in an immune-competent mouse compared to a T cell–deficient mouse, using the *HSV-tk*/GCV system, even though gene expression should be higher and more prolonged in the immune-deficient mouse (34). Cytotoxic T cells appear to be responsible for bystander killing and immune memory (35). It is possible that distant uninfected tumor may be responsive to immune destruction if tumor-specific cytotoxic T cells are generated. These cytotoxic T cells may also protect against the growth and development of metastatic disease. The application of this observation to humans is not clear. In an attempt to enhance the *in vivo* bystander effect, investigators have combined suicide gene systems with cytokine genes to enhance the immune response (36,37).

It is theoretically possible that damage to vascular endothelium from diffusion of a converted prodrug or from direct gene transfer to endothelial cells may lead to vascular thrombosis and ischemic necrosis. This would lead to a higher percentage of tumor cell death than could be explained by the *in vitro* bystander effect. Diffusible toxins may have some advantage because gap junctions between tumor cells and endothelial cells are unlikely.

Many techniques to improve the bystander effect have been tested. For some systems, expression of the enzyme on the cell surface by the addition of a secretory leader sequence and transmembrane domain may enhance the bystander effect. This method ensures improved access of the enzyme to the prodrug, allows extracellular conversion of the prodrug, and facilitates diffusion of the converted toxin. Marais et al. (38) demonstrated that the carboxypeptidase G2 (CPG2) enzyme could function as a cell surface protein.

SUICIDE GENE SYSTEMS

The various suicide gene systems are summarized in Table 3.

Herpes Simplex Virus Thymidine Kinase

The prototypical suicide gene system is the *HSV-tk*/GCV system. *HSV-tk* phosphorylates nucleoside analogs (GCV/acyclovir) into their monophosphate and triphosphate forms, which are incorporated into DNA during cell division, leading to cell death. Moolten (2) first demonstrated in 1986 that transfection of the *HSV-tk* gene into sarcoma cells rendered them sensitive to the cytotoxic effects of GCV. Since then, numerous studies have demonstrated the efficacy of the system. Many strategies for delivering the *HSV-tk* gene have been used, including liposomal

TABLE 3. ENZYME/PRODRUG SYSTEMS

Enzyme	Prodrug	Active Drug
Herpes simplex virus thymidine kinase	Ganciclovir	Ganciclovir triphosphate
Varicella-zoster virus thymidine kinase	(E)-5-(2-bromovinyl)-2'-deoxyuridine (BVDU)	BVDU triphosphate
Cytosine deaminase	5-Fluorocytosine	5-Fluorouracil
Purine nucleoside phosphorylase	6-Methylpurine deoxyriboside	6-Methylpurine
β-lactamase	7-(4-Carboxybutanamido)-cephalosporin mustard	Phenylenediamine mustard
Carboxypeptidase G2	4-[(2-Chloroethyl)(2-mesyloxyethyl)amino] ben-zoyl-L-glutamic acid (CMDA)	4-[(2-Chloroethyl)(2-mesyloxyethyl)amino] ben-zoic acid (CJS11)
Cytochrome P450-2B1	Cyclophosphamide/ifosfamide	Acrolein + phosphoramide mustard
Escherichia coli nitroreductase	CB1954 (5-aziridin-1-yl-2-4-dinitrobenzamide)	5-Aziridin-1-yl-4-hydroxylamino-2-nitrobenzamide
Xanthine-guanine phosphoribosyl transferase	6-Thioxanthine	6-Thioxanthine monophosphate
β-Glucuronidase	Epirubicin-glucuronide	Epirubicin
Thymidine phosphorylase	5'-Deoxy-5-fluorouridine	5-Fluorouracil
Deoxycytidine kinase	Cytosine arabinoside	Cytosine arabinoside monophosphate
Carboxylesterase	7-Ethyl-10-[4-(1-piperidino)-1-piperidino] car-bonyloxycamptothecin (CPT-11)	7-Ethyl-10-hydroxycamptothecin (SN-38)
Linamarase/β-glucosidase	Linamarin/amygdalin	Cyanide
Carboxypeptidase A	Methotrexate-phenylalanine	Methotrexate
Cytochrome P450-4B1	2-Aminoanthracene, 4-ipomeanol	Unknown alkylating agents

transfections (39), retroviral transductions (40,41), and adenoviral infections (5,42–46). One advantage of this system is that only dividing cells are affected, so systemic toxicity is minimal. Another advantage is that GCV has been shown to be safe in humans and is readily available.

In vitro treatment of glioma cells with a nonreplicating adenovirus carrying *HSV-tk* was cytotoxic to cells in the presence of GCV at multiplicities of infection above 150 (42). Smythe et al. (6) demonstrated that 10% to 20% of mesothelioma cells expressing the *HSV-tk* gene were able to sensitize 70% to 80% of cells to GCV, indicating a fairly significant bystander effect in these cells. Although GCV triphosphate is unable to freely diffuse across the cell membrane, a variable bystander effect is seen. Several investigators have studied this phenomenon because a strong bystander effect is thought to be essential *in vivo* when tumor cell transduction is inefficient. The *in vitro* bystander effect for the *HSV-tk* system is thought to be mediated by gap junctions that allow transport of GCV triphosphate between cells (47). The observation that cell lines with relatively few gap junctions had minimal bystander effects (47–49) led to the upregulation of a gap junction protein (connexin 43) in a glioma cell line that increased the bystander effect *in vitro* and *in vivo* as discussed above, under Bystander Effect.

Several *in vivo* studies have demonstrated the potential therapeutic utility of this system. Subcutaneous sarcomas in Balb/C mice, retrovirally transduced with the *HSV-tk* gene, demonstrated a complete response after treatment with intraperitoneal (i.p.) GCV (40). Hepatic metastases transduced *in vivo* with a retrovirus expressing *HSV-tk* were treated with twice-daily injection of GCV for 5 days. This led to a significant inhibition of tumor growth compared to that seen in control subjects (41), with some complete regressions. Nonreplicating recombinant adenovirus carrying the *HSV-tk* gene has been used in many tumor models. Mice with intracerebral gliomas were injected intratumorally with adenovirus carrying *HSV-tk* and then received i.p. GCV twice daily for 6 days. This resulted in a 23-fold decrease in tumor size compared to that seen in control subjects and two complete regressions. No toxicity to the sur-

rounding normal brain was found (42). Similar adenoviral/ *HSV-tk*/GCV systems have effectively treated experimental ovarian cancer (44), head and neck cancer (43), breast cancer (45), and melanoma (46). No systemic toxicity from the converted prodrug has been demonstrated.

Varicella Thymidine Kinase

Varicella zoster virus is a virus in the Herpesviridae family whose TK gene shares 28% homology with the *HSV-tk* gene and has a different substrate specificity (50). Several prodrugs have been tested for activity in a suicide gene system using *VZV-TK*, including GCV, acyclovir, (E)-5-(2-bromovinyl)-2'-deoxyuridine (BVDU) (50), and others (51).

Breast cancer cells retrovirally transfected with *VZV-TK*, or controls, were treated with GCV, acyclovir, or BVDU. In nontransduced controls, toxicity was minimal owing to the prodrugs. In transduced cell lines sensitivity to GCV or acyclovir was minimally increased but sensitivity to BVDU was extreme (400- to 2,000-fold over that of parental cells) (50). Fifty percent of glial cells were needed to express the *VZV-TK* in order to see a global cytotoxic effect. The bystander effect was dependent on the cell line tested rather than the *VZV-TK*/BVDU system itself (50) and may be a reflection of the number of intercellular gap junctions, similar to the *HSV-tk* system.

Subcutaneously injected cells expressing the *VZV-TK* gene were similarly sensitive to BVDU. Significant dose-dependent growth inhibition was seen after eight daily i.p. injections of BVDU, although no complete regressions were seen (50). No systemic toxicity from the converted prodrug was found.

Cytosine Deaminase

CD is a bacterial enzyme that deaminates cytosine to uracil and 5-FC to 5-fluorouracil (5-FU) (52,53). Because it is not normally present in mammalian cells, the CD gene is useful in suicide gene systems. Transfer of the CD gene to mammalian tumor cells allows local conversion of 5-FC to 5-FU, which inhibits both RNA and DNA synthesis and leads to cell death (52,53). 5-FU is an effective chemotherapy agent and has selectivity for dividing cells. It is standard therapy for various gastrointestinal and breast cancers. The prodrug 5-FC is well tolerated by humans and has been used in antifungal therapy.

Several methods to selectively transfer the CD gene to tumor cells have been used, including plasmid transfections (52,54,55), retroviral transduction (35,52,56,57), adenoviral infection (58–62), vaccinia infection (29,62), and antibody conjugates (63).

In vitro studies have demonstrated the ability to sensitize tumor cells to 5-FC by expression of the *CD* gene (52,54, 50,51). The ability of 5-FU to diffuse through the cell membrane makes this an attractive system because of the bystander effect. When 20% of the cells expressed the *CD* gene, 60% to 80% cytotoxicity was seen after 4 days (54,57). The detection of 5-FU in the supernatants of CD-transduced cells suggests that direct cell-to-cell contact (as in the TK systems) is not needed for a bystander effect (54,57).

Subcutaneous tumors retrovirally transduced with the *CD* gene showed significant growth inhibition, which was further improved with earlier treatment and higher doses of 5-FC (36,56). The use of viruses to deliver the *CD* gene to subcutaneous xenografts has also been successful with significant growth inhibition (58) or tumor regression (60,62) when injected intratumorally. Intrahepatic (59) or intravenous (61) delivery of an adenovirus carrying the *CD* gene inhibited tumor growth after 5-FC administration with no systemic toxicity from the prodrug or its metabolites. Intravenous delivery of an antibody-CD conjugate followed by i.p. 5-FC led to high tumor levels of 5-FU compared to that in other organs. This may be an additional method for achieving high tumor levels of 5-FU without systemic toxicity (63).

Purine Nucleoside Phosphorylase

PNP is an enzyme involved in the purine salvage pathway. Both prokaryotic and eukaryotic enzymes exist, but they use unique substrates (64). Only *Escherichia coli* PNP can convert adenosine and adenosine analogs and has a tenfold higher activity against purine arabinosides (64), allowing the system to be used in enzyme-prodrug therapy. *E. coli* PNP converts the prodrug 6-MPDR to the toxic metabolite 6-MP, which is highly toxic to tumor cells via inhibition of both RNA and protein synthesis. Although this prodrug is well tolerated in animals, it has not been used in humans. Fludarabine is another substrate for this enzyme that has been used in humans for the treatment of hematologic malignancies and is associated with systemic toxicity at high doses.

In vitro studies have shown greater than 90% cytotoxicity in multiple cell types by day 5 after *PNP* gene transfer (16,65,66). These studies highlight several advantages of the *PNP* system:

1. The conversion from 6-MPDR to 6-MP is very efficient with minimal measurable prodrug in cell supernatants by day 3 (16).
2. Because 6-MP inhibits both RNA and protein synthesis, it does not require cell proliferation to have an effect.
3. 6-MP is freely diffusible across cell membranes, leading to a strong bystander effect. Complete cytotoxicity was seen *in*

vitro when as little as 2% of cells expressed the *PNP* gene (66), illustrating the potency of the system.

In vivo studies have shown efficacy of this system in nude mice. Parker et al. (67) showed significant regression of subcutaneous tumors, retrovirally transduced to express the *PNP* gene, when treated with 6-MPDR for 3 days. In addition, no toxicity due to systemic 6-MP was seen for this dosing regimen. Puhlmann et al. (28) showed efficacy in a hepatic metastases model using a replicating vaccinia virus to deliver the *PNP* gene. Nude mice with hepatic metastases were treated with i.p. vaccinia virus carrying the *PNP* gene, followed by either weekly or every other daily injections of 6-MPDR. Both groups had a significant prolongation of survival with a 30% and 50% cure rate, respectively. No evidence of toxicity from the converted prodrug was seen with this dosing regimen, but significant hepatic toxicity was seen at higher doses, presumably owing to the potency and diffusibility of 6-MP (28). This system is ultimately limited by systemic toxicity of the converted prodrug, requiring careful prodrug dosing.

β-Lactamase

β-Lactamase is a bacterial enzyme that confers resistance to β-lactam antibiotics by cleavage of the amide bond in the β-lactam ring (68). The synthesis of nontoxic prodrugs, consisting of cephalosporins conjugated to chemotherapy agents, has allowed the system to be used for suicide gene therapy because the conjugated prodrug is similarly cleaved, releasing active drug. Several prodrugs have been synthesized for this system including cephalosporin-doxorubicin (C-Dox), 7-(4-carboxybutanamido)-cephalosporin mustard (CCM), cephalosporin–mitomycin C, cephalosporin-paclitaxel, and cephalosporin-carboplatinum (68–70). Tumor-specific antibodies conjugated to the β-lactamase enzyme have allowed tumor-targeted activation of the various prodrugs (69,70,73–76).

In vitro studies showed that treatment of melanoma cells with an antibody/β-lactamase conjugate, followed by the prodrugs C-Dox and CCM, led to a four- and 30-fold increase, respectively, in the sensitivity of cells to the prodrugs, although some nonspecific prodrug toxicity was seen (69). Subcutaneous melanoma xenografts in nude mice treated weekly with antibody/β-lactamase and C-Dox showed tumor regression that eventually progressed (69). In contrast, similar treatments using CCM led to complete long-term regression in 80% of the mice. Although some neurologic toxicity was seen with C-Dox, no systemic toxicity from the CCM was seen (69). Similar studies using antibody/β-lactamase/C-Dox to treat xenografts of breast and colon carcinoma cells showed tumor growth inhibition in both histologies with minimal toxicity (73), although no complete regressions were seen. Finally, nude mice with subcutaneous melanoma xenografts were treated using a single-chain antibody/β-lactamase fusion protein in combination with CCM. Complete tumor regressions, in the majority of animals treated with CCM 12 hours after delivery of the fusion protein, were seen with no evidence of systemic toxicity (75). Although this system has not been studied in a gene delivery approach, the β-lactamase protein is extremely versatile and should be functional in this context.

Carboxypeptidase G2

CPG2 is a bacterial enzyme that catalyzes the hydrolytic cleavage of folates and methotrexate to pteroates and L-glutamic acid (77,78). Similar cleavage releases active alkylating agents from prodrugs synthesized with a glutamic acid group blocking the enzyme's function (77,78). Various methods of tumor-specific expression of CPG2 have been studied, including antibody targeting (78–80) and stable transfection (38), suggesting it would be a good enzyme for use in a suicide gene system.

Stable transfection of colon and ovarian carcinoma cell lines with CPG2 resulted in a 16- to 95-fold increase in sensitivity to the prodrug 4-[(2-chloroethyl)(2-mesyloxyethyl) amino] benzoyl-L-glutamic acid (38). One hundred percent cytotoxicity was seen when 3.7% to 12.0% of the cells expressed CPG2 (38). *In vivo* studies have used tumor-specific monoclonal antibodies conjugated to CPG2 as a means of enzyme delivery (78–80). A nude mouse model of human choriocarcinoma showed significantly increased survival when treated with anti–human chorionic gonadotropin antibody/CPG2 conjugates, followed by only three doses of prodrug 72 hours later (78). Subcutaneous colon carcinoma xenografts had significant growth delay when treated with antibody/CPG2 conjugate followed by prodrug, although the tumors subsequently regrew (80). Minimal toxicity to the prodrug and its metabolites was seen.

Cytochrome P450-2B1

Cytochrome P450-2B1 (CYP2B1) is a naturally occurring liver enzyme necessary in the conversion of cyclophosphamide and ifosfamide to their 4-hydroxy derivatives (81,82). These metabolites are unstable and further degrade to become the toxic metabolites acrolein and phosphoramide mustard, which cause protein and DNA alkylation, respectively (82). Because tumor levels of the enzyme are low (82), these chemotherapeutic agents are normally metabolized in the liver, leading to systemic toxicity before a maximal tumor response. Use in a suicide gene system allows upregulation of CYP2B1 expression in tumor cells, leading to local conversion of cyclophosphamide and ifosfamide and potentially less systemic toxicity. This system is appealing because it may enhance the effect of agents that have already shown to be effective in cancer therapy and for which a safety profile has already been defined.

In vitro studies demonstrated that glioma cells (81,82) and breast cancer cells (83), stably transfected with the CYP2B1 gene, acquired sensitivity to cyclophosphamide and ifosfamide (81–83). This sensitivity was blocked by the CYP2B1 inhibitor metyrapone (82,83). A significant bystander effect was seen when 20% to 50% of the cells expressed the CYP2B1 gene (82,83), and this persisted in co-culture experiments, suggesting that direct cell contact is not needed for this effect.

Several studies (81–83) have shown enhanced sensitivity of subcutaneous tumors (glioma, breast cancer) retrovirally transduced with CYP2B1 (*ex vivo*) to cyclophosphamide. In one study, this led to complete inhibition of tumors in 95% of animals after a single i.p. injection of cyclophosphamide (82). Inoculation of retroviral producer cells or replication-deficient adenovirus expressing the CYP2B1 gene into intracerebral gliomas led to prolonged survival after one dose of i.p. cyclophosphamide (84). No notable toxicity from the cyclophosphamide conversion was found at the doses studied.

Finally, Chase et al. (85) were able to show that intratumoral injection of a CYP2B1-expressing herpes simplex virus and cyclophosphamide had an enhanced oncolytic effect compared to the virus alone.

Nitroreductase

Initial studies of the alkylating agent CB1954 showed promise in a rat Walker tumor model; however, human trials were disappointing (86). Subsequently it was shown that the human equivalent of rat DT diaphorase was inefficient at converting CB1954 to its active metabolite, the 4-hydroxylamino derivative that causes DNA cross-linking and cell death (86). The identification of a bacterial enzyme with similar activity (87)—E. coli nitroreductase (NTR)—led to its use in suicide gene systems (88–90), in which tumor-specific expression of the bacterial enzyme would render tumor cells uniquely sensitive to CB1954.

In vitro studies have shown a ten- to 100-fold increase in sensitivity of pancreatic, colonic (88), and mammary (90) cell tumor lines to CB1954 when transfected with plasmids expressing the NTR gene. Retroviral transduction led to a 17- to 500-fold increase insensitivity to CB1594, which correlated with the amount of NTR produced by the cells (88). Cell mixing experiments demonstrated a significant *in vitro* bystander effect if 30% of the cells express the gene. Transgenic mice engineered to express a CD2/NTR transgene in T cells and thymocytes had much smaller spleens and thymuses and a significantly increased level of apoptosis in these organs 5 days after treatment with CB1954 (89). Clark et al. (90) showed that transgenic mice expressing NTR under the control of the β-lactoglobulin promoter, had increased levels of ntr mRNA and protein in mammary glands compared to other tissues, and treatment with CB1954 resulted in disrupted mammary glands with increased apoptosis. Nonspecific toxicity from the prodrug or converted active drug was not seen.

Xanthine-Guanine Phosphoribosyl Transferase

Traditionally, the E. coli xanthine-guanine phosphoribosyl transferase (GPT) gene has been used for positive selection in a purine salvage pathway (91) as it catalyzes the conversion of xanthine, hypoxanthine, and guanine to their respective monophosphates. Cells that express the GPT gene can use xanthine as a purine analog in the presence of mycophenolic acid and hypoxanthine, which inhibit the mammalian pathway. Conversely, GPT has been used to selectively sensitize tumor cells to 6-thioxanthine (6-TX) (92,93) as it is incorporated into this purine synthesis pathway. Mroz and Moolten (93) showed that retrovirally transducing the GPT gene into sarcoma cells conferred an 86-fold increased sensitivity to 6-TX. Tamiya et al. (92) showed that glioma cells were sensitive to 6-TX at an

LD50 of 2.5 μ*M* when transduced with *GPT*. Untransfected cells were minimally sensitive at 50 μ*M*. As well, a significant bystander effect (75% cytotoxicity) was seen when 10% of the cells expressed *GPT*. This effect was abrogated when the cells were separated, suggesting that cell-to-cell contact was required (92). Syngeneic Balb/C mice injected subcutaneously with a transduced sarcoma cell line showed complete regression in 95% of the animals after 5 days of treatment with 6-TX. A 10% treatment mortality due to toxicity of the converted prodrug was seen and was eradicated with an alternate-day dosing schedule (93). Nude mice subcutaneously injected with transduced glioma cells showed a significant inhibition of tumor growth when treated with i.p. 6-TX for 10 days at a reduced dose, with no treatment toxicity (92). In the same study, nude mice with transduced intracerebral gliomas showed prolonged survival after 6-TX treatment. In another study (94), similar subcutaneous tumor inhibition was seen, and regrowth was correlated with loss of the retrovirally expressed *GPT* gene after 3 weeks. In this study, survival after intracerebral tumor injection was prolonged by 6-TX, in the presence of the *GPT* gene. Pathologic evaluation of these brains did not show any neurotoxicity from the 6-TX treatment (94).

β-Glucuronidase

β-Glucuronidase (GUS) is a glycosidase normally present in low amounts in normal human tissues (95) and slightly higher levels in tumor tissues (96,97). GUS hydrolyses inactive glucuronide conjugates into active drugs (98). Several glucuronide prodrugs have been described for use in a GUS suicide gene system, including conjugates of epirubicin (95), daunorubicin (90), *p*-hydroxyaniline mustard (99), and doxorubicin (100). Although these prodrugs are nontoxic in animals, they have not been used in humans.

GUS has been conjugated to monoclonal antibodies (95,98–100) to increase tumor-specific expression. Haisma et al. (95) used the anti–pan carcinoma antibody (323/A3) conjugated to GUS and demonstrated equivalent activity of the antibody-GUS/epirubicin-glucuronide to epirubicin alone *in vitro*, demonstrating activation of the prodrug. Similar effects were seen for the daunorubicin prodrug (98). A single-chain antibody against the pan carcinoma antigen conjugated to GUS was also effective against an ovarian cell line treated with a doxorubicin-glucuronide prodrug (100). *In vivo* treatment of a rat hepatoma model of ascites, with a hepatoma cell–specific antibody conjugated to GUS, resulted in long-term cure of rats when treated with three i.p. injections of the *p*-hydroxyaniline glucuronide prodrug (99). Minimal toxicity of prodrug conversion was noted despite the presence of native GUS in some tissues (99).

Other Suicide Gene Systems

Several other suicide gene systems have been described. Thymidine phosphorylase, which catalyzes the reversible phosphorolytic cleavage of thymidine, deoxyuridine, and their analogs, has been used to convert the prodrug 5'-deoxy-5-fluorouridine to 5-FU (101). Cytosine arabinoside (ara-C) requires phosphoryla-

tion by deoxycytidine kinase (dCK) to form its active metabolite. Delivery of dCK to glioma cells sensitized them to treatment by ara-C (102). Overexpression of a rabbit carboxylesterase was shown to sensitize human cells to 7-ethyl-10-[4-(1-piperidino)-1-piperidino]-carbonyloxycamptothecin (CPT-11) by its conversion to an active metabolite (SN38) (103). Both β-glucosidase (104) and the plant equivalent linamarase (105) have been shown to hydrolyse amygdalin and linamarase, respectively, to cyanide. This hydrolysis leads to tumor-specific toxicity when delivered via antibody targeting (104) or retroviral transduction (105), with no noted systemic toxicity (105).

Bovine carboxypeptidase A has been shown to cleave the amide bond of a methotrexate-phenylalanine prodrug, yielding free methotrexate (106). This enzyme was conjugated to a monoclonal antibody for tumor-specific delivery, and *in vitro* studies showed that ovarian carcinoma cells became sensitive to the methotrexate-phenylalanine prodrug in the presence of carboxypeptidase A (106). Finally, a novel rabbit cytochrome P450 isoenzyme (CYP4B1) has been shown to convert the prodrugs 2-aminoanthracene and 4-ipomeanol into toxic alkylating agents (107). Glioma cells stably transfected with *CYP4B1* showed increased sensitivity to 2-aminoanthracene and 4-ipomeanol *in vitro* and *in vivo* compared to controls. A strong bystander effect was seen, with 70% to 80% cytotoxicity when 1% of the cells expressed the *CYP4B1* gene (107).

COMPARISON OF SUICIDE GENE SYSTEMS

Few studies have compared the efficacy and bystander effects of the different suicide gene systems. The use of different promoters and different delivery systems (plasmid, retroviral, adenoviral) makes head-to-head comparisons necessary. Trinh et al. (108) compared the *HSV-tk*/GCV and *CD*/5-FC systems. Plasmids containing each gene under the control of the cytomegalovirus promoter were stably transfected into cells and rendered the cells sensitive to their respective prodrugs. Prodrug treatment resulted in complete regression of all subcutaneous xenografts when 100% of the cells expressed either *HSV-tk* or *CD*. However, when only 10% of cells in the tumors expressed *HSV-tk*, only a slight inhibition of growth was seen after treatment with GCV. In contrast, when only 4% of cells expressed the *CD* gene, 60% of tumors had a complete response to 5-FC. The inability of GCV to diffuse readily from cell to cell is one likely explanation for this difference; different cell lines may show different results (108).

Hoganson et al. (109) compared the efficacy of *HSV-tk*/GCV, *CD*/5-FC, and *DCK*/ara-C against lung adenocarcinoma cell lines. Stable transduction of cell lines with retroviruses expressing the suicide genes under the control of the CMV promoter showed that both *HSV-tk* and *CD* could confer sensitivity to GCV and 5-FC, respectively. However, only the *CD* system demonstrated a bystander effect with 60% growth inhibition by day 7 when only 10% of the cells expressed the gene. Transduction with *DCK* did not improve sensitivity of the cell lines to ara-C (109).

Nishihara et al. (110) retrovirally transduced thyroid carcinoma cell lines with the *HSV-tk*, *CD*, *NTR*, or *DCK* genes under the control of a long-terminal-repeat promoter. *HSV-tk/*GCV demonstrated the best therapeutic index (IC50 parental cells/IC50 transduced), ranging from 31 to 120 depending on the cell line, whereas *DCK/*ara-C had minimal effect compared to control (therapeutic index: 1.2 to 1.5). Comparison of *in vitro* bystander effects indicated that the *CD/*5-FC system (90% growth inhibition when 20% of cells expressed *CD*) was superior to both *NTR/*CB1954 (90% inhibition when 50% of cells expressed *NTR*) and *HSV-tk/*GCV (90% inhibition when 80% of cells expressed *HSV-tk*). This effect was not assessed *in vivo* (110).

In summary, although the cytotoxicity of the *HSV-tk/*GCV system was equal or better than other systems studied, the *in vitro* bystander effect was minimal. Although this may not predict *in vivo* results, a suicide gene system with a strong bystander effect is needed for cancer treatment *in vivo*, given the poor transduction efficiencies of current vectors.

COMBINED MODALITIES

Because of the limitations inherent in vector systems and limited therapeutic results from suicide gene systems *in vivo*, modifications have been tested that combine different modalities for an enhanced tumor response. These modifications include combining suicide gene therapy with conventional chemotherapy and radiotherapy, combining multiple suicide genes, and combining oncolytic viruses with suicide genes. As the systems become more complicated, it will be increasingly difficult to assess whether the advantages of the gene therapy approach are real compared to systemically delivered agents.

Double suicide gene systems have been included in a single vector as a means of enhancing response, and these systems have the theoretical advantage of more potent killing of infected cells and cells within the bystander zone. Aghi et al. (111) demonstrated synergistic *in vivo* activity of combined *HSV-tk/*GCV and *CD/*5-FC systems in stable transfectants. Graham and Prevec (112) created a *CD-TK* fusion gene that demonstrated enhanced cytotoxicity after delivery of both GCV and 5-FC. Both the *HSV-tk/*GCV and *CD/*5-FC systems have been shown to enhance radiation sensitivity of experimental tumors (113,114). Rogulski et al. (115) demonstrated marked improvement in cure rates *in vivo* when radiation was added to *CD-TK* fusion gene therapy.

The combination of a replicating oncolytic virus with a suicide gene system may have significant therapeutic potential. The suicide gene may extend the zone of necrosis beyond that the virus alone could accomplish. Wildner et al. (116) demonstrated that a tumor-specific replicating adenovirus (E1b M$_r$ 55,000 deleted) expressing *HSV-tk* achieved superior tumor response *in vivo* after addition of GCV, compared to the oncolytic effect of the virus alone. Freytag et al. (117) combined an oncolytic adenovirus (E1b M$_r$ 55,000 deleted) with the *CD-TK* fusion gene and radiotherapy to achieve marked *in vivo* efficacy. Puhlmann et al. (28) demonstrated a 50% cure rate using a systemically administered replication-competent vaccinia virus expressing PNP followed by 6-MPDR for disseminated hepatic metastases in a murine model (see Fig. 3).

CLINICAL TRIALS

Animal models are often insufficient and inappropriate for investigating gene therapy with viral vectors. Tissue selectivity of viruses may be completely different in humans compared to animal models. In addition, the immune response to the vector is different in humans, making it difficult to extrapolate gene expression data from animal experiments. The strong immune response in humans may change the toxicity profile predicted from animal experiments, because tissue inflammation from the immune response may mediate more toxicity than virus-mediated cell death. Preformed antibodies from prior exposure to viruses may greatly limit gene expression in patients and may also result in unexpected toxicities. Therefore, vectors and suicide genes need to be studied in humans. The clinical trials to date have been essential for initiating our understanding of these vectors, despite having demonstrated minimal therapeutic effect.

Knowing the limitations of current vectors, clinical trials have studied the intratumoral injection or regional administration of viruses into the peritoneal or pleural cavity. The true clinical applicability of these systems is limited, and local injection of a vector for gene delivery and conversion of a prodrug ultimately needs to be compared to local injection of the toxic agent. Some theoretical advantages to local gene therapy exist. Intracellular toxin formation may be more potent than extracellular delivery. Cells resistant to topical 5-FU may be sensitive to intracellular production of 5-FU via conversion of 5-FC. Tumor-specific viral replication and tissue-specific gene expression may help prevent toxicity in the normal cells surrounding the tumor, which may be affected by direct local injection of toxic agents. This is especially important for brain tumors, in which minimizing toxicity to normal cells is essential for acceptable morbidity. Appropriately, patients with brain tumors have been among the first investigated with this strategy.

Regardless of the ultimate clinical utility, local injection of vectors has been an important first step toward the clinical use of suicide genes for cancer therapy. Of 300 proposed gene therapy trials, approximately 10% involve the use of suicide genes, and the majority use the *HSV-tk/*GCV system (Table 4). The first clinical gene therapy trial using a suicide gene was proposed by Freeman (118) and approved in 1991. It consisted of infusing *HSV-tk-*transduced ovarian cancer cells into the peritoneal cavity for the bystander treatment of ovarian cancer. Because this was a tumor confined to the peritoneal cavity, it allowed a regional approach to vector delivery. This therapy relied on the transduced tumor cells intermixing with the tumor cells present in the peritoneal cavity and then killing them by virtue of the bystander effect after prodrug delivery. The first patient was treated in 1993. The results of this trial have not been published to date.

Ram et al. (119) investigated the *HSV-tk* system for malignant brain tumors. Murine retroviral producer cells, which generated retroviruses expressing *HSV-tk*, were injected into brain tumors. Fifteen patients were treated using computed tomography–guided stereotactic injections of varying doses of cells (2.5 $\times 10^8$ to 1×10^9 cells) in linear tracts 3 to 6 mm apart within the tumor, followed in 7 days by intravenous GCV (5 mg per kg b.i.d.) for 14 days. Five lesions in four patients had at least a

TABLE 4. CLINICAL PROTOCOLS OF SUICIDE GENE THERAPY

Investigators	Institution	Tumor	Vector	Suicide Gene
S. M. Freeman et al.	University of Rochester	Ovarian	Ovarian cancer cells	TK
E. Oldfield et al.	National Institutes of Health	Brain tumors	Retroviral producer cells	TK
K. Culver et al.	Iowa Methodist Medical Center	Brain tumors	Retroviral producer cells	TK
C. Raffel et al.	Childrens Hospital Los Angeles	Astrocytomas	Retroviral producer cells	TK
L. E. Kun et al.	St. Jude Children's Research Hospital	Pediatric brain tumors	Retroviral producer cells	TK
E. H. Oldfield et al.	National Institutes of Health	Leptomeningeal carcinomas	Retroviral producer cells	TK
S. L. Eck et al.	University of Pennsylvania	Brain tumors	Adenovirus	TK
S. M. Albelda et al.	University of Pennsylvania	Pleural mesothelioma	Adenovirus	TK
R. Grossman et al.	Baylor College of Medicine	Brain tumors	Adenovirus	TK
M. Fetell et al.	Multiple institutions	Glioma	Retroviral producer cells	TK
C. Link et al.	Iowa Methodist Medical Center	Ovarian	Retroviral producer cells	TK
N. C. Munshi et al.	University of Arkansas	Bone marrow transplant	Donor leukocytes	TK
R. G. Crystal et al.	New York Hospital	Hepatic metastases	Adenovirus	CD
R. D. Alvarez et al.	University of Alabama	Ovarian	Adenovirus	TK
P. T. Scardino et al.	Baylor College of Medicine	Prostate	Adenovirus	TK
C. J. Link et al.	Multiple institutions	Bone marrow transplant	Donor lymphocytes	TK
B. W. O'Malley et al.	Johns Hopkins University	Head and neck cancers	Adenovirus	TK
G. R. Harsh IV et al.	Harvard Medical School	Glioma	Retrovirus	TK
M. W. Sung et al.	Mount Sinai Medical Center	Hepatic metastases	Adenovirus	TK
B. Maria et al.	Multiple institutions	Glioblastoma	Retroviral producer cells	TK
F. Lieberman et al.	Mount Sinai Medical Center	Glioblastoma	Adenovirus	TK
S. J. Hall et al.	Mount Sinai Medical Center	Prostate	Adenovirus	TK
W. N. Rom et al.	Multiple institutions	Small cell lung	Adenovirus	TK
W. I. Bensinger et al.	Multiple institutions	Bone marrow transplant	Donor mononuclear cells	TK
D. Klatzmann et al.	Hôpital Pitie-Salpetriere	Melanoma	Retroviral producer cells	TK
C. Bordignon et al.	The San Raffaele Hospital	Bone marrow transplant	Donor lymphocytes	TK
D. Klatzmann et al.	Hôpital Pitie-Salpetriere	Glioblastoma	Retroviral producer cells	TK
P. Tiberghien et al.	Laboratoire d'Histocompatibilité et Thera-peutique Immuno Moleculaire	Bone marrow transplant	Donor lymphocytes	TK

CD, cytosine deaminase; TK, thymidine kinase.
Data from Human gene marker/therapy clinical protocols. *Hum Gene Ther* 1999;10:1043–1092.

partial response, including two complete responders. The responding lesions were all small (average volume, 1.4 mL). Two patients suffered neurologic deficits from intratumoral hemorrhage as a result of the injections, two had worsening seizures, and one had new seizures. Up to 14 injections per tumor were given. Retroviral producer cell antibodies were detected in 10 of 15 patients. Two tumors were resected before GCV treatment, revealing *HSV-tk* mRNA by *in situ* hybridization in cells immediately adjacent to the injection tracts, including some endothelial cell transduction. Overall, the percentage of cells expressing the gene was low and probably explains the minimal response. This trial was followed by four similar trials by different investigators.

Klatzmann et al. (120) reported results from murine retroviral producer cells (M11) injected into the surgical cavity margins after surgical debulking for recurrent glioblastomas in 12 patients. The cells were injected tangentially and orthogonally at 1-cm intervals along the tumor margin to a maximum depth of 1.5 cm. The number of injections ranged from 15 to 55, and the number of cells injected ranged from 7.1 to 9.8×10^6. Three patients had easily controlled hemorrhage at the time of injections. GCV (5 mg per kg) was given twice daily for 14 days, beginning 7 days after injection of the producer cells. It is difficult to assess safety and efficacy in an adjuvant trial, because complications are common after aggressive surgery alone, and it is difficult to predict the outcome from surgical resection alone.

Nevertheless, they concluded the therapy was both safe and efficacious with a 25% 4-month disease-free survival rate.

Klatzmann et al. (121) also reported a similar trial of retroviral producer cells injected into cutaneous melanoma nodules. Toxicity was limited to inflammatory skin reactions at the injection site and fever after repeated injections. The gene could be demonstrated in tumor nodules by polymerase chain reaction in three of six patients, and none of the injected lesions had objective responses.

Investigators from the University of Pennsylvania first used intratumoral injection of adenovirus expressing the *HSV-tk* gene for the treatment of brain tumors, and intrapleural injection for the treatment of mesothelioma. Sterman et al. (122) reported the results of a phase 1 clinical trial in malignant mesothelioma. Twenty-one patients were treated with intrapleural administration of adenovirus expressing *HSV-tk* followed by 2 weeks of systemic therapy with GCV (5 mg per kg b.i.d.). The viral dose was escalated from 1×10^9 PFU to 1×10^{12} PFU without reaching dose-limiting toxicity. Side effects included fever (100° to 102°F 6 to 12 hours after viral injection), anemia, transient liver enzyme elevations, and bullous skin eruptions. A temporary systemic inflammatory response was noted at the highest dose, manifested by hypotension immediately after vector delivery. The toxicity seemed to be related to an inflammatory response to the adenovirus and not to prodrug conversion. Immune manipulation may improve this inflammatory reaction. Subsequently, they have pretreated patients with high-dose steroids to improve viral tolerance. Although gene expression from the pleural tumor was detectable by polymerase chain reaction in 11 of 20 posttreatment biopsies, overall the percentage of transduced cells was low and limited to the tumor surface. The success of gene transfer did not correlate with the titer of pre-existing adenoviral antibodies, but it did correlate with the viral dose.

Other histologies that have been treated with intratumoral or regional administration of *HSV-tk*-expressing adenoviral vectors include head and neck cancers, hepatocellular cancers, hepatic metastases, lung cancer, ovarian cancer, and prostate cancer. Crystal et al. (123) were the first to use the *CD*/5-FC system in a clinical trial, giving intratumoral injections of adenoviruses expressing the *CD* gene into hepatic metastases from colorectal cancer. Other studies using *CD* for breast cancer are under way.

A practical use for suicide genes in cancer management is the stable transduction of donor lymphocytes with *HSV-tk* in patients undergoing allogeneic bone marrow transplantation. This technique allows treatment of graft-versus-host disease by killing the donor cells responsible for the problem with delivery of GCV. It has been tested in clinical trials (124). Theoretical limitations of this therapy include the possible increased immunogenicity of the transduced cells, which may have a negative impact on engraftment.

CONCLUSIONS

The concept of genetic manipulation of tumor cells to mediate their own death is exciting and can be envisioned as an effective cancer treatment. Although numerous methods are effective *in vitro*, the limitation *in vivo* is inefficient gene delivery to tumor cells. The almost unlimited ability to genetically engineer viruses should eventually allow the development of an efficient vector that is tumor-specific and safe for the patient and the environment. Although nonviral vectors ultimately may be more useful than viruses, they are currently less efficient. When the ideal vector is created, it will be important to perform *in vivo* comparisons of suicide gene systems to demonstrate which has the largest bystander zone with acceptable systemic toxicity. The combination of an efficient, specific vector and a potent suicide gene system should lead to a significant therapeutic response.

Perhaps the biggest obstacle to effective suicide gene therapy will be the immune system, which will either result in the inability to express genes in a large enough population of tumor cells or will mediate unacceptable toxicity due to the inflammatory response to the vector. Immunologic manipulation of the patient may be required to allow the level and duration of gene expression necessary to achieve a tumor response. All of these technological advances appear within reach, making the future of suicide gene therapy very promising.

REFERENCES

1. Plautz G, Nabel EG, Nabel GJ. Selective elimination of recombinant genes *in vivo* with a suicide retroviral vector. *The New Biologist* 1991, 3:709–715.

2. Moolten FL. Tumor chemosensitivity conferred by inserted herpes thymidine kinase genes: paradigm for a prospective cancer control strategy. *Cancer Res* 1986;46:5276–5281.

3. Huber BE, Richards CA, Krenitsky TA. Retroviral-mediated gene therapy for the treatment of hepatocellular carcinoma: an innovative approach for cancer therapy. *Proc Natl Acad Sci U S A* 1991;15:8039–8043.

4. Culver KW, Ram Z, Wallbridge S, Hiroyuki I, Oldfield E, Blaese RM. *In vivo* gene transfer with retroviral rector-producer cells for treatment of experimental brain tumors. *Science* 1992;256:1550–1552.

5. Smythe WR, Hwang HC, Amin KM, et al. Use of recombinant adenovirus to transfer the herpes simplex virus thymidine kinase (*HSVtk*) gene to thoracic neoplasms: an effective *in vitro* drug sensitization system. *Cancer Res* 1994;54:2055–2059.

6. Chen SH, Shine HD, Goodman JC, Grossman RG, Woo SL. Gene therapy for brain tumors: regression of experimental gliomas by adenovirus-mediated gene transfer *in vivo*. *Proc Natl Acad Sci U S A* 1994;91:3054–3057.

7. Bergelson JM, Cunningham JA, Droguett G, et al. Isolation of a common receptor for Coxsackie B viruses and adenoviruses 2 and 5. *Science* 1997;275:1320–1323.

8. Hemmi S, Geertsen R, Mezzacasa A, Peter I, Dummer R. The presence of human coxsackievirus and adenovirus receptor is associated with efficient adenovirus-mediated transgene expression in human melanoma cell cultures. *Hum Gene Ther* 1998;9:2363–2373.

9. Rosenberg SA, Zhair Y, Yang JC, et al. Immunizing patients with metastatic melanoma using recombinant adenoviruses encoding MART-1 or gp100 melanoma antigens. *J Natl Cancer Inst* 1998;90:1894–1900.

10. Budker V, Gurevich V, Hagstrom JE, Bortzov F, Wolff JA. pH-sensitive, cationic liposomes: a new synthetic virus-like vector. *Nat Biotechnol* 1996;14:760–764.

11. Wivel NA, Wilson JM. Methods of gene delivery. *Hematol Oncol Clin North Am* 1998;12:483–501.

12. Goren D, Horowitz AT, Zalipsky S, Woodle MC, Yarden Y, Gabizon A. Targeting of stealth liposomes to erbB-2 (Her/2) receptor: *in vitro* and *in vivo* studies. *Br J Cancer* 1996;74:1749–1756.

13. Hart SL, Arancibia-Carcamo CV, Wolfert MA, et al. Lipid-mediated enhancement of transfection by a nonviral integrin-targeting vector. *Hum Gene Ther* 1998;9:575–585.

14. Ojeifo JO, Forough R, Paik S, Maciag T, Zwiebel JA. Angiogenesis-directed implantation of genetically modified endothelial cells in mice. *Cancer Res* 1995;55:2240–2244.

15. Fox ME, Lemmon MJ, Mauchline ML. Anaerobic bacteria as a delivery system for cancer gene therapy: *in vitro* activation of 5-fluorocytosine by genetically engineered clostridia. *Gene Ther* 1996;3:173–178.

16. Park BJ, Brown CK, Hu Y, et al. Augmentation of melanoma-specific gene expression using a tandem melanocyte-specific enhancer results in increased cytotoxicity of the purine nucleoside phosphorylase gene in melanoma. *Hum Gene Ther* 1999;10:889–898.

17. Siders WM, Halloran PJ, Fenton RG. Transcriptional targeting of recombinant adenoviruses to human and murine melanoma cells. *Cancer Res* 1996;56:5638–5646.

18. Parr MJ, Manome Y, Tanaka T, et al. Tumor-selective transgene expression *in vivo* mediated by an E2F-responsive adenoviral vector. *Nat Med* 1997;3:1145–1149.

19. Martin F, Kupsch J, Takeuchi Y, Russell S, Cosset FL, Collins M. Retroviral vector targeting to melanoma cells by single-chair antibody incorporation in envelope. *Hum Gene Ther* 1998;9:737–746.

20. Dmitriev I, Krasnykh V, Miller CR, et al. An adenovirus vector with genetically modified fibers demonstrates expanded tropism via utilization of a coxsackievirus and adenovirus receptor-independent cell entry mechanism. *J Virol* 1998;72:9706–9713.

21. Bischoff JR, Kirn DH, Williams A, et al. An adenovirus mutant that replicates selectively in p53-deficient human tumor cells [see comments]. *Science* 1996;274:373–376.

22. Hall AR, Dix BR, O'Carroll SJ, Braithwaite AW. p53-dependent cell death/apoptosis is required for a productive adenovirus infection. *Nat Med* 1998;4:1068–1072.

23. Goodrum FD, Ornelles DA. p53 status does not determine outcome of E1B 55 kilodalton mutant adenovirus lytic infection. *J Virol* 1998;72:9479–9490.

24. Turnell AS, Grand RJ, Gallimore PH. The replicative capacities of large E1B-null group A and group C adenoviruses are independent of host cell p53 status. *J Virol* 1999;73:2074–2083.

25. Wildner O, Blaese RM, Morris JC. Therapy of colon cancer with oncolytic adenovirus is enhanced by the addition of herpes simplex virus-thymidine kinase. *Cancer Res* 1999;59:410–413.

26. Rodriguez R, Schuur ER, Lim HY, Henderson GA, Simons JW, Henderson DR. Prostate attenuated replication competent adenovirus (ARCA) CN706: a selective cytotoxic for prostate-specific antigen-positive prostate cancer cells. *Cancer Res* 1997;57:2559–2563.

27. Kramm CM, Chase M, Herrlinger U, et al. Therapeutic efficiency and safety of a second- generation replication-conditional HSV1 vector for brain tumor gene therapy. *Hum Gene Ther* 1997;8:2057–2068.

28. Puhlmann M, Gnant M, Brown CK, Alexander HR, Bartlett DL. Thymidine kinase deleted vaccinia virus expressing purine nucleoside phosphorylase as a vector for tumor directed gene therapy. *Hum Gene Ther* 1999;10:649–657.

29. Gnant M, Puhlmann M, Alexander HR Jr, Bartlett DL. Systemic administration of a recombinant vaccinia virus expressing the cytosine deaminase gene and subsequent treatment with 5-fluorocytosine leads to tumor specific gene expression and cures of established liver metastases. *Cancer Res* 1999 (*in press*).

30. Mesnil M, Piccoli C, Tiraby G, Willecke K, Yamasaki H. Bystander killing of cancer cells by herpes simplex virus thymidine kinase gene is mediated by connexins. *Proc Natl Acad Sci U S A* 1996; 93:1831–1835.

31. Cantor AM, Rigby CC, Beck PR, Mangion D. Neurofibromatosis, phaeochromocytoma, and somatostatinoma. *Br Med J* 1982;285: 1618–1619.

32. Ramesh R, Marrogi AJ, Munshi A, Abboud CN, Freeman SM. *In vivo* analysis of the "bystander effect": a cytokine cascade. *Exp Hematol* 1996;24:829–838.

33. Melcher A, Todryk S, Hardwick N, Ford M, Jacobson M, Vfile RG. Tumor immunogenicity is determined by the mechanism of cell death via induction of heat shock protein expression. *Nat Med* 1998;4:581–587.

34. Gagandeep S, Brew R, Green B. Prodrug-activated gene therapy: involvement of an immunological component in the "bystander effect." *Cancer Gene Ther* 1999;3:83–88.

35. Consalvo M, Mullen CA, Modesti A, et al. 5-fluorocytosine-induced eradication of murine adenocarcinomas engineered to express the cytosine deaminase suicide gene requires host immune competence and leaves an efficient memory. *J Immunol* 1995;154:5302–5312.

36. Chen S-H, Chen SHL, Wang Y, et al. Combination gene therapy for liver metastasis of colon carcinoma *in vivo*. *Proc Natl Acad Sci U S A* 1995;92:2577–2581.

37. Mullen CA, Petropoulos D, Lowe RM. Treatment of microscopic pulmonary metastases with recombinant autologous tumor vaccine expressing interleukin 6 and *Escherichia coli* cytosine deaminase suicide genes. *Cancer Res* 1996;56:1361–1366.

38. Marais R, Spooner RA, Light Y, Martin J, Springer CJ. Gene-directed enzyme prodrug therapy with a mustard prodrug/carboxypeptidase G2 combination. *Cancer Res* 1996;56:4735–4742.

39. Aoki K, Yoshida T, Matsumoto N, et al. Gene therapy for peritoneal dissemination of pancreatic cancer by liposome-mediated transfer of herpes simplex virus thymidine kinase gene. *Hum Gene Ther* 1997; 8:1105–1113.

40. Moolten FL, Wells JM. Curability of tumors bearing herpes thymidine kinase genes transferred by retroviral vectors. *J Natl Cancer Inst* 1990;82:297–300.

41. Caruso M, Panis Y, Gagandeep S, Houssin D, Salzmann J-L, Klatzmann D. Regression of established macroscopic liver metastases after *in situ* transduction of a suicide gene. *Proc Natl Acad Sci U S A* 1993;90:7024–7028.

42. Chen S-H, Shine HD, Goodman JC, Grossman RG, Woo SLC. Gene therapy for brain tumors: regression of experimental gliomas by adenovirus-mediated gene transfer *in vivo*. *Proc Natl Acad Sci U S A* 1994;91:3054–3057.

43. O'Malley BW, Chen S-H, Schwartz MR, Woo SLC. Adenovirus-mediated gene therapy for human head and neck squamous cell cancer in a nude mouse model. *Cancer Res* 1995;55:1080–1085.

44. Rosenfeld ME, Wang M, Siegal GP, et al. Adenoviral-mediated delivery to herpes simplex virus thymidine kinase results in tumor reduction and prolonged survival in a SCID mouse model of human ovarian carcinoma. *J Mol Med* 1996;74:455–462.

45. Kwong Y-L, Chen S-H, Kosai K, Finegold MJ, Woo SLC. Adenoviral-mediated suicide gene therapy for hepatic metastases of breast cancer. *Cancer Gene Ther* 1996;3:339–344.

46. Bonnekoh B, Greenhalgh DA, Bundman DS, et al. Adenoviral-mediated herpes simplex virus-thymidine kinase gene transfer *in vivo* for treatment of experimental human melanoma. *J Invest Dermatol* 1996;106:1163–1168.

47. Dilber MS, Abedi MR, Christensson B, et al. Gap junctions promote the bystander effect of herpes simplex virus thymidine kinase *in vivo*. *Cancer Res* 1997;57:1523–1528.

48. McMasters RA, Saylors RL, Jones KE, Hendrix ME, Moyer MP, Drake RR. Lack of bystander killing in herpes simplex virus thymidine kinase-transduced colon cell lines due to deficient connexin43 gap junction formation. *Hum Gene Ther* 1998;9:2253–2261.

49. Yang L, Chiang Y, Lenz H-J, et al. Intercellular communication mediates the bystander effect during herpes simplex thymidine kinase/ganciclovir-based gene therapy of human gastrointestinal tumor cells. *Hum Gene Ther* 1998;9:719–728.

50. Grignet-Debrus C, Calberg-Bacq C-M. Potential of Varicella zoster virus thymidine kinase as a suicide gene in breast cancer cells. *Gene Ther* 1997;4:560–569.

51. Degrève B, Andrei G, Izquierdo M, et al. Varicella-zoster virus thymidine kinase gene and antiherpetic pyrimidine nucleoside analogues in a combined gene/chemotherapy treatment for cancer. *Hum Gene Ther* 1997;4:1107–1114.

52. Mullen CA, Kilstrup M, Blaese RM. Transfer of the bacterial gene for cytosine deaminase to mammalian cells confers lethal sensitivity to 5-fluorocytosine: a negative selection system. *Proc Natl Acad Sci U S A* 1992;89:33–37.

53. Austin EA, Huber BE. A first step in the development of gene therapy for colorectal carcinoma: cloning, sequencing, and expression of *Escherichia coli* cytosine deaminase. *Mol Pharmacol* 1993;43:380–387.

54. Rowley S, Lindauer M, Gebert JF, et al. Cytosine deaminase gene as a potential tool for the genetic therapy of colorectal cancer. *J Surg Oncol* 1996;61:42–48.

55. Tiraby M, Cazaux C, Baron M, Drocourt D, Reynes J-P, Tiraby G. Concomitant expression of *E. coli* cytosine deaminase and uracil phosphoribosyltransferase improves the cytotoxicity of 5-fluorocytosine. *FEMS Microbiol Lett* 1998;167:41–49.

56. Mullen CA, Coale MM, Lowe R, Blaese RM. Tumors expressing the cytosine deaminase suicide gene can be eliminated *in vivo* with 5-fluorocytosine and induce protective immunity to wild type tumor. *Cancer Res* 1994;54:1503–1506.

57. Kuriyama S, Samui K, Sakamoto T, et al. Bystander effect caused by cytosine deaminase gene and 5-fluorocytosine *in vitro* is substantially mediated by generated 5-fluorouracil. *Anticancer Res* 1998;18: 3399–3406.

58. Hirschowitz EA, Ohwada A, Pascal WR, Russi TJ, Crystal RG. *In vivo* adenovirus-mediated gene transfer of the *Escherichia coli* cytosine deaminase gene to human colon carcinoma-derived tumors induces chemosensitivity to 5-fluorocytosine. *Hum Gene Ther* 1995;6:1055–1063.

59. Ohwada A, Hirschowitz EA, Crystal RG. Regional delivery of an adenovirus vector containing the *Escherichia coli* cytosine deaminase gene to provide local activation of 5-fluorocytosine to suppress the growth of colon carcinoma metastatic to liver. *Hum Gene Ther* 1996;7:1567–1576.

60. Kanai F, Lan K-H, Shiratori Y, et al. *In vivo* gene therapy for α-fetoprotein-producing hepatocellular carcinoma by adenovirus-mediated transfer of cytosine deaminase gene. *Cancer Res* 1997;57:461–465.

61. Topf N, Worgall S, Hackett NR, Crystal RG. Regional "pro-drug" gene therapy: intravenous administration of an adenoviral vector expressing the E. coli cytosine deaminase gene and systemic administration of 5-fluorocytosine suppresses growth of hepatic metastasis of colon carcinoma. *Gene Ther* 1998;5:507–513.

62. McCart JA, Puhlmann M, Lee J, Libutti SK, Alexander HR, Bartlett DL. Anti-tumor activity of a thymidine kinase (TK)-detected vac-

cinia virus. *Soc Surg Oncol* 1999;62:24(abst).

63. Wallace PM, MacMaster JF, Smith VF, Kerr DE, Senter PE, Cosand WL. Intratumoral generation of 5-fluorouracil mediated by an anti-body-cytosine deaminase conjugate in combination with 5-fluorocy-tosine. *Cancer Res* 1994;54:2719–2723.

64. Mao C, Cook WJ, Zhou M, Koszalka GW, Krenitsky TA, Ealick SE. The crystal structure of *Escherichia coli* purine nucleoside phospho-rylase: a comparison with the human enzyme reveals a conserved topology. *Structure* 1997;5:1373–1383.

65. Sorscher EJ, Peng S, Bebok Z, Allan PW, Bennett LL Jr, Parker WB. Tumor cell bystander killing in colonic carcinoma utilizing the *Escherichia coli* DeoD gene to generate toxic purines. *Gene Ther* 1994;1:233–238.

66. Hughes BW, Wells AH, Bebok Z, et al. Bystander killing of mela-noma cells using the human tyrosinase promoter to express the Escherichia coli purine nucleoside phosphorylase gene. *Cancer Res* 1995;55:3339–3345.

67. Parker WB, King SA, Allan PW, et al. In vivo gene therapy of cancer with E. coli purine nucleoside phosphorylase. *Hum Gene Ther* 1997;8:1637–1644.

68. Siemers NO, Yelton DE, Bajorath J, Senter PD. Modifying the specific-ity and activity of the *Enterobacter cloacae* P99 β-Lactamase by mutagen-esis within an M13 phase vector. *Biochemistry* 1996;35:2104–2111.

69. Kerr DE, Schreiber GJ, Vrudhula VM, et al. Regressions and cures of melanoma xenografts following treatment with monoclonal anti-body β-lactamase conjugates in combination with anticancer pro-drugs. *Cancer Res* 1995;55:3558–3563.

70. Vrudhula VM, Svensson HP, Senter PD. Immunologically specific acti-vation of a cephalosporin derivative of mitomycin C by monoclonal antibody β-Lactamase conjugates. *J Med Chem* 1997;40:2788–2792.

71. Rodrigues ML, Carter P, Wirth C, Mullins S, Lee A, Blackburn BK. Synthesis and β-Lactamase mediated activation of a cephalosporin-taxol prodrug. *Chem Biol* 1995;2:1–5.

72. Hanessian S, Wang J. Design and synthesis of a cephalosporin-car-boplatinum prodrug activatable by a β-lactamase. *Can J Chem* 1993;71:906.

73. Meyer DL, Law KL, Payne JK, et al. Site-specific prodrug activation by antibody-β-Lactamase conjugates: preclinical investigation of the efficacy and toxicity of doxorubicin delivered by antibody directed catalysis. *Bioconjugate Chem* 1995;6:440–446.

74. Rodrigues ML, Presta LG, Kotts CE, et al. Development of a humanized disulfide-stabilized anti-p185^HER2^Fv-β-Lactamase fusion protein for activation of a cephalosporin doxorubicin prodrug. *Cancer Res* 1995;55:63–70.

75. Siemers NO, Kerr DE, Yarnold S, et al. Construction, expression, and activities of L49-sFv-β-Lactamase, a single-chain antibody fusion protein for anticancer prodrug activation. *Bioconjugate Chem* 1997;8:510–519.

76. Svensson HP, Frank IS, Berry KK, Senter PD. Therapeutic effects of monoclonal antibody-β-Lactamase conjugates in combination with a nitrogen mustard anticancer prodrug in models of human renal cell carcinoma. *J Med Chem* 1998;41:1507–1512.

77. Springer CJ, Antonio P, Bagshawe KD, Searle F, Bisset GMF, Jarman M. Novel prodrugs which are activated to cytotoxic alkylating agents by carboxypeptidase G2. *J Med Chem* 1990;33:677–681.

78. Springer CJ, Bagshawe KD, Sharma SK, et al. Ablation of human choriocarcinoma xenografts in nude mice by antibody-directed enzyme prodrug therapy (ADEPT) with three novel compounds. *Eur J Cancer* 1991;27:1361–1366.

79. Blakey DC, Burke PJ, Davies DH, et al. ZD2767, an improved sys-tem for antibody directed enzyme prodrug therapy that results in tumor regression in colorectal tumor xenografts. *Cancer Res* 1996;56:3287–3292.

80. Stribbling SM, Martin J, Pedley RB, Boden JA, Sharma SK, Springer CJ. Biodistribution of an antibody-enzyme conjugate for antibody-directed enzyme prodrug therapy in nude mice bearing a human colon adenocar-cinoma xenograft. *Cancer Chemother Pharmacol* 1997;40:277–284.

81. Wei MX, Tamiya T, Chase M, et al. Experimental tumor therapy in mice using the cyclophosphamide-activating cytochrome P450 2B1 gene. *Hum Gene Ther* 1994;5:969–976.

82. Chen L, Waxman DJ. Intratumoral activation and enhanced chemo-therapeutic effect of oxazaphosphorines following cytochrome P-450

gene transfer: development of a combined chemotherapy/cancer gene therapy strategy. *Cancer Res* 1995;55:581–589.

83. Chen L, Waxman DJ, Chen D, Kufe DW. Sensitization of human breast cancer cells to cyclophosphamide and ifosfamide by transfer of a liver cytochrome P450 gene. *Cancer Res* 1996;56:1331–1340.

84. Manome Y, Wen PY, Chen L, et al. Gene therapy for malignant glio-mas using replication incompetent retroviral and adenoviral vectors encoding the cytochrome P450 2B1 gene together with cyclophos-phamide. *Gene Ther* 1996;3:513–520.

85. Chase M, Chung RY, Chiocca EA. An oncolytic viral mutant that delivers the *CYP2B1* transgene and augments cyclophosphamide chemotherapy. *Nat Biotechnol* 1998;16:444–448.

86. Boland MP, Knox RJ, Roberts JJ. The differences in kinetics of rat and human DT diaphorase result in a differential sensitivity of derived cell lines to CB 1954 (5-(aziridin-1-YL)-2,3-dinitrobenza-mide). *Biochem Pharmacol* 1991;41:867–875.

87. Anlezark GM, Melton RG, Sherwood RF, Coles B, Friedlos F, Knox RJ. The bioactivation of 5-(aziridin-1-yl)-2,4-dinitrobenzamide (CB1954)—I. *Biochem Pharmacol* 1992;44:2289–2295.

88. Green NK, Youngs DJ, Neoptolemos JP, et al. Sensitization of colorec-tal and pancreatic cancer cell lines to the prodrug 5-(aziridin-1-yl)-2,3-dinitrobenzamide (CB1954) by retroviral transduction and expression of E.coli nitroreductase gene. *Cancer Gene Ther* 1997;4:229–238.

89. Drabek D, Guy J, Craig R, Grosveld F. The expression of bacterial nitroreductase in transgenic mice results in specific cell killing by the prodrug CB1954. *Gene Ther* 1997;4:93–100.

90. Clark AJ, Iwobi M, Cui W, et al. Selective cell ablation in transgenic mice expressing *E. coli* nitroreductase. *Gene Ther* 1997;4:101–110.

91. Mulligan RC, Berg P. Selection for animal cells that express the *Escherichia coli* gene coding for xanthine-guanine phosphoribosyl-transferase. *Proc Natl Acad Sci U S A* 1981;78:2072–2076.

92. Tamiya T, Ono Y, Wei MX, Mroz PJ, Moolten FL, Chiocca EA. *Escherichia coli gpt* gene sensitizes rat glioma cells to killing by 6-thioxanthene or 6-thioguanine. *Cancer Gene Ther* 1996;3:155–162.

93. Mroz PJ, Moolten FL. Retrovirally transduced *Escherichia coli gpt* genes combine selectability with chemosensitivity capable of mediat-ing tumor eradication. *Hum Gene Ther* 1993;4:589–595.

94. Ono Y, Ikeda K, Wei MX, Harsh GRI, Tamiya T, Chiocca EA. Regression of experimental brain tumors with 6-Thioxanthine and *Escherichia coli gpt* gene therapy. *Hum Gene Ther* 1997;8:2043–2055.

95. Haisma HJ, Boven E, van Muijen M, de Jong J, van der Vijgh WJF, Pinedo HM. A monoclonal antibody-β-glucuronidase conjugate as activator of the prodrug epirubicin-glucuronide for specific treat-ment of cancer. *Br J Cancer* 1999;66:474–478.

96. Bosslet K, Czech J, Hoffman D. A novel one-step tumor-selective prodrug activation system. *Tumor Targeting* 1995;1:45–50.

97. Schumacher U, Adam E, Zangemeister-Wittke U, Gossrau R. His-tochemistry of therapeutically relevant enzymes in human tumours transplanted into severe combined immunodeficient (SCID) mice: nitric oxide synthase-associated diaphorase, β-D-glucuronidase and non-specific alkaline phosphatase. *Acta Histochem* 1996;98:381–387.

98. Houba PHJ, Leenders RGG, Boven E, Scheeren JW, Pinedo HM, Haisma HJ. Characterization of novel anthracycline prodrugs acti-vated by human β-glucuronidase for use in antibody-directed enzyme prodrug therapy. *Biochem Pharmacol* 1996;52:455–463.

99. Chen B-M, Chan L-Y, Wang S-M, Wu M-F, Chern J-W, Roffler SR. Cure of malignant ascites and generation of protective immunity by monoclonal antibody-targeted activation of a glucuronide prodrug in rats. *Int J Cancer* 1997;73:392–402.

100. Haisma HJ, Brakenhoff RH, vd Meulen-Muileman I, Pinedo HM, Boven E. Construction and characterization of a fusion protein of single-chain anti-carcinoma antibody 323/A3 and human β-glucu-ronidase. *Cancer Immunol Immunother* 1998;45:266–272.

101. Patterson AV, Zhang H, Moghaddam A, et al. Increased sensitivity to the prodrug 5'-deoxy-5-fluorouridine and modulation of 5-fluoro-2'-deoxyuridine sensitivity in MCF-7 cells transfected with thymi-dine phosphorylase. *Br J Cancer* 1995;72:669–675.

102. Manome Y, Wen PY, Fine HA. Viral vector transduction of the human deoxycytidine kinase cDNA sensitizes glioma-cells to the cytotoxic effects of cytosine-arabinoside *in vitro* and *in vivo*. *Nat Med* 1996;2:567–573.

103. Danks MK, Morton CL, Pawlik CA, Potter PM. Overexpression of a rabbit liver carboxylesterase sensitizes human tumor cells to CPT-11. *Cancer Res* 1989;58:20–22.

104. Syrigos KN, Rowlinson-Busza G, Epenetos AA. *In vitro* cytotoxicity following specific activation of amygdalin by β-glucosidase conjugated to a bladder cancer-associated monoclonal antibody. *Int J Cancer* 1998;78:712–719.

105. Cortés ML, de Felipe P, Martín V, Hughes MA, Izquierdo M. Successful use of a plant gene in the treatment of cancer *in vivo*. *Gene Ther* 1998;5:1499–1507.

106. Perron M-J, Page M. Activation of methotrexate-phenylalanine by monoclonal antibody-carboxypeptidase. a conjugate for the specific treatment of ovarian cancer *in vitro*. *Br J Cancer* 1996;73:281–287.

107. Rainov NG, Dobberstein K-U, Sena-Esteves M, et al. New prodrug activation gene therapy for cancer using cytochrome P450 4B1 and 2-aminoanthracene/4-ipomeanol. *Hum Gene Ther* 1998;9:1261–1273.

108. Trinh QT, Austin EA, Murray DM, Knick VC, Huber BE. Enzyme-prodrug gene therapy: comparison of cytosine deaminase/5-fluorocytosine *versus* thymidine kinase-ganciclovir enzyme/prodrug systems in a human colorectal carcinoma cell line. *Cancer Res* 1995;55:4808–4812.

109. Hoganson DK, Batra RK, Olsen JC, Boucher RC. Comparison of the effects of three different toxin genes and their levels of expression on cell growth and bystander effect in lung adenocarcinoma. *Cancer Res* 1996;56:1315–1323.

110. Nishihara E, Nagayama Y, Narimatsu M, et al. Treatment of thyroid carcinoma cells with four different suicide gene/prodrug combinations *in vitro*. *Anticancer Res* 1998;18:1521–1526.

111. Aghi M, Kramm CM, Chou T-C, Breakefield XO, Chiocca EA. Synergistic anticancer effects of ganciclovir/thymidine kinase and 5-fluorocytosine/cytosine deaminase gene therapies. *J Natl Cancer Inst* 1998;90:370–380.

112. Graham FL, Prevec L. Glioma cells transduced with an *Echerichia coli CS/HSV-1 TK* fusion gene exhibit enhanced metabolic suicide and radiosensitivity. *Hum Gene Ther* 1997;8:73–85.

113. Kim JH, Kim SH, Brown SL, Freytag SO. Selective enhancement by an antiviral agent of the radiation-induced cell killing of human glioma cells transduced with *HSV-tk* gene. *Cancer Res* 1994;54:6053–6056.

114. Khil M, Kim JH, Mullen CA, Kim SH, Freytag SO. Radiosensitization by 5-fluorocytosine of human colorectal carcinoma cells in culture transduced with cytosine deaminase gene. *Clin Cancer Res* 1996;2:53–57.

115. Rogulski KR, Zhang K, Kolozsvary A, Kim JH. Pronounced antitumor effects and tumor radiosensitization of double suicide gene therapy. *Clin Cancer Res* 1997;3:2081–2088.

116. Wildner O, Blaese RM, Morris JC. Therapy of colon cancer with oncolytic adenovirus is enhanced by the addition of herpes simplex virus-*thymidine kinase*. *Cancer Res* 1999;59:410–413.

117. Freytag SO, Rogulski KR, Paielli DL, Gilbert JD, Kim JH. A novel three-pronged approach to kill cancer cells selectively: concomitant viral, double suicide gene, and radiotherapy. *Hum Gene Ther* 1998;9:1323–1333.

118. Freeman SM. Gene transfer for the treatment of cancer. *Hum Gene Ther* 1995;6:927–939.

119. Ram Z, Culver KW, Oshiro EM, et al. Therapy of malignant brain tumors by intratumoral implantation of retroviral vector-producing cells. *Nat Med* 1997;3:1354–1361.

120. Klatzmann D, Valéry CA, Bensimon G, et al. A Phase I/II study of herpes simplex virus type 1 thymidine kinase "suicide" gene therapy for recurrent glioblastoma. *Hum Gene Ther* 1998;9:2595–2604.

121. Klatzmann D, Chérin P, Bensimon G, et al. A Phase I/II dose-escalation study of herpes simplex virus type 1 thymidine kinase "suicide" gene therapy for metastatic melanoma. *Hum Gene Ther* 1998;9:2585–2594.

122. Sterman DH, Treat J, Litzky LA, et al. Adenovirus-mediated herpes simplex virus thymidine kinase—ganciclovir gene therapy with localized malignancy: results of a phase I clinical trial in malignant mesothelioma. *Hum Gene Ther* 1998;9:1083–1092.

123. Crystal RG, Hirschowitz E, Dale J, et al. Phase I study of direct administration of a replication deficient adenovirus vector containing the *E. coli* cytosine deaminase gene to metastatic colon carcinoma of the liver in association with the oral administration of the pro-drug 5-fluorocytosine. *Hum Gene Ther* 1997;8:985–1001.

124. Bordignon C, Notarangelo LD, Nobili N. Gene therapy in peripheral blood lymphocytes and bone marrow for ADA-immunodeficient patients. *Science* 1995;270:470–475.

20.4

GENE THERAPY: CLINICAL APPLICATIONS

Gene Therapy Using Direct *In Vivo* Gene Injection

BINGLIANG FANG
JACK A. ROTH

Gene therapy was originally envisioned as a technique for restoring the expression of normal genes in inherited monogenic disorders, such as adenosine deaminase deficiency and cystic fibrosis. However, the clinical application of gene therapy has focused on cancer with the attempts to use genes as anticancer agents and immunostimulants. In this chapter, the applications of gene therapy using intratumoral injection for local-regional tumor control and induction of an antitumor immune response are reviewed.

GENE TRANSFER VECTORS

Gene transfer vectors are agents that constitute or contain therapeutic genes for delivery into target cells. A vector can be naked DNA or RNA, DNA or RNA attached to other agents (e.g., peptides or liposomes), or a virus particle containing a therapeutic gene. Several different delivery systems [reviewed elsewhere (1,2)] have been developed, but there are still no perfect universal vectors. Here, we briefly discuss the vectors used in direct *in vivo* injection. Readers who are interested in recent developments in vector and gene delivery technology are encouraged to consult other chapters on the basic aspects of gene therapy.

Viral Vectors

Adenovirus

Adenovirus is one of most popular vectors in the field of gene therapy because of its ease of production and high *in vivo* transduction efficiencies. It is also widely used for direct *in vivo* injection. Usually, adenoviral vectors are constructed by replacing the E1 region with an expression cassette of the desired transgene (3). The vectors are generated and propagated in packaging cells, such as 293, that provide E1 functions in trans (4). However, it is possible to generate adenoviral vectors containing only the replication origin and packaging signal. In this case, a helper virus is required for vector production (5). For efficient production of vectors, the vector genome should be between 27 and 37 kilobases long (75% to 104% of the wild-type viral genome) (6,7).

In vivo administration of adenoviral vector has been shown to result in the highly efficient delivery of genes to a variety of tissues (8–10) and to induce complete phenotypic corrections of genetic disorders in mice (11,12), rabbits (13,14), and dogs (15). This vector system has also been extensively used for *in vivo* cancer gene therapy both preclinically and clinically (16–18) [see Roth and Cristiano (19) for review]. In most cases, constructing adenoviral vectors is quite straightforward (3). However, constructing vectors that express highly proapoptotic or cytotoxic genes may become problematic. For example, constructing an adenoviral vector that would express high levels of Fas ligand, *BAX*, or *BAK* proved to be difficult because of the high apoptotic activities of the proteins (20). Yet, we have demonstrated that this obstacle can be overcome by using a *GAL4* gene regulatory system along with adenovirus-mediated gene codelivery (21). The synthetic *GAL4*-responsive promoter, which consists only of *GAL4*-binding sites and a TATA box, has extremely low basal transcriptional activities in the absence of its transactivator but 10^4- to 10^6-fold higher activity in its presence both *in vitro* and *in vivo* (22). Constructing adenoviral vectors that contain a *BAX* or *BAK* gene driven by this minimal promoter is straightforward, and the transgene expression can be efficiently induced by coinfecting cells with a vector expressing a transactivating protein, the GAL4/VP16 fusion protein (21).

Extensive efforts have been made to develop novel adenoviral vectors by (a) modifying the adenoviral genome to inactivate viral gene expression (23–28) or (b) modifying viral proteins to enhance transduction efficiency in refractory cells or enhance targeting (29–34). Other strategies for improving direct *in vivo* gene delivery with adenoviral vectors have also been tried. One involves modulating the host immune response to adenoviral vector to prolong transgene expression and offset the effect of humoral immune response. It has been demonstrated that transgene expression is prolonged in newborn or immunocompromised mice and in animals treated with immunosuppressive agents (12,35,36) or agents such as anti-CD4 antibody or CTLA4-Ig that block activation of the immune system around the time of vector administration (37). Improving efficiency in repeated administration of adenoviral vectors has also been attempted. For example, concurrent administration of interleukin-12 (IL-12) or high-dose cyclophosphamide can reportedly inhibit the development of neutralizing antibodies (38,39). Treating animals with low-dose etopside can suppress the formation of neutralizing antibodies and enhance intratumoral transgene expression in immunized animals, suggesting that repeated adenovirus-mediated gene therapy may be achievable in cancer patients concomitantly receiving certain chemotherapeutic agents (40).

Adeno-Associated Virus

Use of adeno-associated virus (AAV) as a vector for gene transfer and gene therapy has been comprehensively reviewed (41–43). AAV vectors have been used to transduce a wide range of cell types *in vitro*, including respiratory epithelial cells, bone marrow, and lymphocyte-derived cells. *In vivo* transduction in lung and brain has been observed in rodents and nonhuman primates. A phase 1 human trial of gene therapy for cystic fibrosis using an AAV vector is currently underway.

The advantages of using AAV as a vector for gene therapy include (a) its ability to infect nonreplicating cells and to be integrated into the host genome so that the therapeutic gene will persist in transduced cells and (b) its lack of viral coding sequences, which therefore avoids the immune response elicited by expression of vector proteins in transduced cells. Disadvantages are (a) the labor intensiveness of vector production and (b) the low efficiency of transduction owing in part to the vector's single-stranded genome. Conversion of the single-stranded DNA into double-stranded DNA before expression of the transgene is a limiting step in AAV-mediated gene transfer (44). Nonetheless, AAV is exceptional at transducing muscle tissue, as shown by the high level of stable transgene expression achieved in mouse muscle after intramuscular injection of purified vector (45). More recently, it was shown that a relatively high level of transgene expression in liver could be achieved by portal vein injection of vectors (46,47). When transduced, AAV vector genomes either remain as a head-to-tail circularized episomal monomer and concatemer in transduced cells or are integrated randomly into the host genome as concatemers (48).

Retrovirus

Retroviral vectors have been extensively used for *ex vivo* gene delivery and are the most useful vector for stably integrating foreign DNA into target cells. They are not efficient for direct *in vivo* injection because of inactivation by host complement (49). Efforts are under way to improve *in vivo* transduction efficiency of retroviral vectors. For example, vectors produced in packaging cells of human origin may escape complement inactivation (50). Modifying the viral envelope for targeted delivery [for review, see Schnierle and Groner (51)], producing higher titers of vector, and generating lentivirus-based vectors capable of transducing nondividing cells are also under intensive studies (52,53).

Other Viral Vectors

Vaccinia Virus

Vaccinia virus is a member of the poxvirus family, which is unique in that its viral DNA replication and RNA transcription occur exclusively in the cytoplasm. Several attributes of poxviruses have led to their extensive use as expression vectors, including their capacity for carrying large amounts of DNA and their wide range of hosts (54,55). Because the vector's RNA is transcribed in the cytoplasm, therapeutic gene expression requires either poxvirus promoters or bacteriophage RNA polymerases and cognate promoters. Thus far, this vector has been used in clinical trials to deliver genes encoding tumor antigens (e.g., melanoma antigen, carcinoembryonic antigen, prostate-specific antigen), interleukins (e.g., IL-1β, IL-12), and costimulatory molecule B7 (56–58).

Replication-Competent Viruses

Until recently, viral gene expression and viral replication were believed to pose safety concerns in gene therapy. Therefore, most efforts in developing viral vectors for gene therapy were directed at removing or inactivating viral genes and generating packaging cell lines that could produce high titers of vectors with minimal likelihood of generating replication-competent viruses. Nevertheless, the destructive effect of virus replication could also be beneficial as long as the replication was limited to tumor cells. On this basis, a replication-competent adenovirus, herpes simplex virus, and reovirus have been tested for use in treating cancers (59–62). Adenovirus with a mutation in E1B region has been reported to replicate specifically in *p53*-mutated tumors (59) and may be useful for cancer therapy because *p53* is the most frequently mutated gene identified in human cancers (63). However, studies indicate that lytic infection of cells with E1B-mutated adenovirus does not depend on *p53* status and that *p53* may play a necessary part in mediating cellular destruction via a productive adenovirus infection (64,65).

Nonviral Vectors

Naked DNA

Naked DNA (i.e., purified plasmids) can be introduced into cells in a variety of physical or chemical ways. The physical techniques for *in vivo* gene delivery include direct injection and injection by *gene gun* (high-velocity bombardment of tissues with DNA attached to gold particles). Direct injection of DNA vectors into muscles can result in sustained, albeit low, expression of introduced genes (66,67). In other tissues, how-

ever, DNA uptake after direct injection is minimal. Nevertheless, studies showed that high levels of transgene expression can be achieved in liver and lung if plasmid DNA can be retained in these organs for a prolonged time (68,69). Direct injection of plasmid DNA expressing a tumor antigen has also been used in clinical trials of cancer vaccination (58). Delivery by gene gun can induce gene expression in skin, liver, and tumor models (70).

DNA-Carrier Complexes

Liposomes are the most popular nonviral vectors for gene delivery [for review, see Gao and Huang (71); Lee and Huang (72)]. Liposomes, when combined with DNA of any size, form a lipid-DNA complex that can be delivered to many cell types. They are also actively used in clinical trials for *in vivo* and *ex vivo* delivery of genes encoding cytokines, immunostimulatory molecules, and adenoviral E1A genes. Successful intravenous gene delivery via liposomes has been reported in animals (73,74). At present, most liposomes are prepared from biodegradable cationic lipids, although preparing them from anionic or neutral lipids has been proposed (72). Incorporating neutral lipids into cationic liposomes has been shown to increase vector stability after systemic administration. Mechanical extrusion of liposomes has also been reported to increase transduction efficiency (75). In general, however, the expression of genes introduced via liposomes remains low and transient. Peptides have also been exploited for gene delivery. For efficient gene delivery, a peptide should be (a) capable of binding to DNA, (b) efficiently internalized by cells, (c) capable of disrupting the endosomal membrane, and (d) capable of carrying DNA to the nucleus. Peptides that bind specifically to certain cell-surface molecules may be useful for targeted gene delivery.

GENES FOR ANTICANCER THERAPY

With the progress in mapping, cloning, and functionally characterizing the human genome and genomes of other organisms, a growing number of established and potential anticancer genes are being identified and tested. In fact, it is virtually impossible to list here all the genes that might be used for cancer gene therapy. For this chapter, however, we have classified genes used in cancer gene therapy into four categories according to their targets: (a) genes targeted to tumor cells, (b) genes targeted to the immune system, (c) genes targeted to tumor microenvironments or tumor vasculature, and (d) genes targeted to normal, nonmalignant cells. Such classification is arbitrary because some genes may affect more than one class of target. For example, IL-12 is used to augment antitumor immunity, yet it has a strong effect on tumor angiogenesis. *p53* promotes apoptosis of tumor cells, suppresses angiogenesis by downregulating vascular endothelial growth factor (VEGF) expression, and has also been proposed as a target for a tumor vaccine. These genes are potential targets for gene therapy approaches. Clinical trials completed or in progress using these approaches are summarized in Table 1.

TABLE 1. WORLDWIDE CLINICAL TRIALS FOR CANCER GENE THERAPY WITH DIRECT INTRATUMORAL INJECTION

Principal Investigator	Protocol	Target Cell	Vector	Delivery Vehicle	No. of Patients Entered	Evidence of Gene Expression[a]	No. and Type of Response[b]	Adverse Reactions[c]
Immunotherapy/cytokine								
A. E. Chang (Univ. of Michigan Medical Center, Ann Arbor, MI)	Immunotherapy for cancer by direct gene transfer into tumors	Melanoma cells	HLA-B7, 2-micro-globulin	Lipid	10	Y	NA	None
	Phase 2 study of immunotherapy of metastatic cancer by direct gene transfer	Cancer cells	HLA-B7, 2-micro-globulin	Lipid	0	NA	NA	NA
R. A. Figlin (UCLA Medical Center, Los Angeles, CA)	Immunotherapy of metastatic cancer by direct gene transfer	Renal cell carcinoma cells	Allovectin-7	Lipid	8	NA	NA	NA
	HLA-B7 as an immunotherapeutic agent in renal cancer with IL-2 therapy	Renal cell carcinoma cells	Allovectin-7	Lipid	6	NA	3 SD	NA
J. L. Gluckman (Univ. of Cincinnati, Cincinnati, OH)	Allovectin-7 in the treatment of squamous cell carcinoma of the head and neck	Squamous cell carcinoma	Allovectin-7	Lipid	3	NA	1 PR 2 MR	None
A. L. Harris (Churchill Hospital, Oxford, UK)	Cancer therapy for metastatic melanoma	Melanoma cells	pTyrIL-2/ pTyr-Gal	Plasmid	7	Y	None	None
E. Hersh (Arizona Cancer Center, Tucson, AZ)	Study of gene transfer of *IL-2* gene	Tumor cells	Leuvectin	Lipid	24	Y	NA	NA
	Study of gene transfer of *HLA-B7* gene	Tumor cells	Allovectin-7	Lipid	14	Y	1 CR	NA
H. K. Lyerly (Duke Univ., Durham, NC)	Autologous human IL-2 lipofection gene-modified tumor cells in patients with refractory or recurrent metastatic breast cancer	Metastatic breast cancer cells	IL-2	Lipid	0	NA	NA	NA
G. J. Nabel[145] (Univ. of Michigan Medical Center, Ann Arbor, MI)	Immunotherapy of malignancy by *in vivo* gene transfer into tumors	Melanoma cells	HLA-B7, 2-micro-globulin	Lipid	5	Y	1 PR	None
J. Rubin (Mayo Clinic, Rochester, MN)	Study of immunotherapy of advanced colorectal carcinoma by direct gene transfer into hepatic metastases	Colorectal carcinoma cells	HLA-B7	Lipid	0	NA	NA	NA
H. Silver (BC Cancer Center, Vancouver, BC, Canada)	Immunotherapy by direct gene transfer	Melanoma/ renal/lymphoma cells	VCL-1005-201	Lipid	5	NA	NA	NA
	Intralesional transfection with plasmid HLA-B7 in melanoma	Melanoma cells	VCL-1005	Lipid	7	Y	NA	NA
N. J. Vogelzang (Univ. of Chicago Medical Center, Chicago, IL)	Immunotherapy of metastatic renal cell carcinoma by direct gene transfer: phase 2 study in renal, colon, breast	Renal cancer cells	Allovectin-7 (HLA-B7)	Lipid	14	Y	None	Injection pain
	Immunotherapy of metastatic cancer by direct gene transfer	Cancer cells	Allovectin-7	Lipid	4	Y	None	NA
Drug sensitivity								
S. M. Albelda (Univ. of Pennsylvania Medical Center, Philadelphia, PA)	Gene therapy for malignant mesothelioma with *HSV-tk*	Malignant mesothelioma cells	H5.01ORSV TK	Adenovirus	10	Y	None	Fever, abnormal liver function

(continued)

TABLE 1. (CONTINUED)

Principal Investigator	Protocol	Target Cell	Vector	Delivery Vehicle	No. of Patients Entered	Evidence of Gene Expression[a]	No. and Type of Response[b]	Adverse Reactions[c]
R. G. Crystal (Cornell Medical Center, New York, NY)	Administration of replication-deficient adenovirus vector containing the *Escherichia coli* cytosine deaminase gene to metastatic colon carcinoma of the liver with 5-fluorocytosine	Liver cells	AdCVcD.10	Adenovirus	1	NA	NA	None
D. Curiel (Univ. of Alabama, Birmingham, AL)	Adenovirus intraperitoneal *HSV-tk* for ovarian and extraovarian cancer	Ovarian cancer cells	AdTK	Adenovirus	0	NA	NA	NA
S. L. Eck (Univ. of Pennsylvania, Philadelphia, PA)	Recombinant adenovirus for CNS malignancy	Glioblastoma/astrocytoma cells	H5.01ORSVTK	Adenovirus	2	NA	None	None
M. R. Fetell (Columbia-Presbyterian Medical Center, New York, NY)	Stereotactic injection of *HSV-tk* vector producer cells for recurrent malignant glioma	Glioma cells	G1TK1SvNa.7	Retrovirus	2	NA	None	NA
G. Finocchiaro (Inst. Nazionale Neurologico C. Besta, Milan, Italy)	Gene therapy of glioblastoma with *HSV-tk*	Glioblastoma cells	HSV-tk	Retrovirus	0	NA	NA	NA
R. G. Grossman (Baylor College of Medicine, Houston, TX)	*HSV-tk* for CNS tumors	Brain tumor cells	adv. RSV-tk	Adenovirus	0	NA	NA	NA
M. Izquierdo (Univ. Autonoma de Madrid, Madrid, Spain)	Gene therapy of glioblastoma with *HSV-tk*	Glioblastoma cells	p tk zip Neo[R]	Retrovirus	9	N	1 PR 1 MR	Fever
D. Klatzmann (Hôpital Pitie-Salpetrie, Paris, France)	Gene therapy for metastatic melanoma with *HSV-tk*	Melanoma cells	pm TK	Retrovirus	7	Y	NA	None
	Gene therapy for glioblastoma with *HSV-tk*	Glioblastoma cells	pM-TK	Retrovirus	13	NA	NA	None
L. E. Kun (St. Jude Children's Research Hospital, Memphis, TN)	Stereotactic injection of *HSV-tk* producer cells for progressive or recurrent primary supratentorial pediatric brain tumors	Neoplastic glial cells	G1Tksv Na.7	Retrovirus	2	NA	1 MR	Increased local edema
C. J. Link (Human Gene Therapy Research Inst., Des Moines, IA)	*HSV-tk* treatment of refractory or recurrent ovarian cancer	Ovarian carcinoma cells	LTKOSN	Retrovirus	0	NA	NA	NA
L. Mariani (Neurochirugische Klinik Inselspital, Bern, Switzerland)	Gene therapy for glioblastoma with *HSV-tk*	Glioblastoma cells	G1TK1sv Na.7	Retrovirus	6	NA	NA	None
N. H. Mulder (Academisch Ziekenhuis Groningen, Groningen, Netherlands)	Gene therapy of glioblastoma with *HSV-tk*	Glioblastoma cells	G1TK1sv Na.7	Retrovirus	3	N	1MR	Seizures, abducens paresis, confusion

(continued)

TABLE 1. (CONTINUED)

Principal Investigator	Protocol	Target Cell	Vector	Delivery Vehicle	No. of Patients Entered	Evidence of Gene Expression[a]	No. and Type of Response[b]	Adverse Reactions[c]
E. H. Oldfield (National Inst. of Health, NINDS, Bethesda, MD)	Gene therapy of brain tumors with *HSV-tk*	Malignant glial tumors	G1Tk1svNa	Retrovirus	20	Y	2 CR 3 PR	Intratumoral hemorrhage
C. Raffel (Mayo Clinic, Rochester, MN)	Gene therapy for recurrent pediatric malignant astrocytomas with *in vivo* tumor transduction with *HSV-tk*	Astrocytoma cells	HSV-tk	Retrovirus	0	NA	NA	NA
J. C. Van Gilder (Univ. of Iowa Hospital, Iowa City, IA)	Gene therapy for glioblastoma with *HSV-tk*	Glioblastoma cells	HSV-tk	Retrovirus	14	NA	NA	NA
S. Yla-Herttuala (Univ. of Kopio, Kopio, Finland)	Gene therapy for glioma with *HSV-tk*	Glioma cells	Retrovec-tk	Retrovirus	0	NA	NA	NA
Tumor suppressor/antisense								
G. L. Clayman (M. D. Anderson Cancer Center, Houston, TX)	Modification of tumor suppressor gene expression in HNSCC with an adenovirus expressing wild-type *p53*	HNSCC	Ad5CMV-*p53*	Adenovirus	17	NA	NA	None
N. Habib[146,147] (Hammersmith Hospitals NHS Trust, London, UK)	*p53* DNA injection in colorectal liver metastases	Colorectal liver metastases	pC53/SN3	Plasmid	6	Y	None	Fever
	p53 DNA injection in hepatocellular carcinoma	Hepatocellular carcinoma cells	pC53/SN3	Plasmid	8	Y	1 CR 2 PR 1 MR	Fever
J. Holt (Vanderbilt Univ. Medical School, Nashville, TN)	Retroviral antisense c-fos RNA for metastatic breast cancer	Breast cancer cells in effusions	XM6:anti-fos	Retrovirus	1	N	None	None
J. Holt (National Inst. of Health, Bethesda, MD)	*BRCA1* retroviral gene therapy for ovarian cancer	Ovarian cancer cells	LXN-BRCA1	Retrovirus	2	N	None	None
G. N. Hortobagyi (M. D. Anderson Cancer Center, Houston, TX)	*E1A* gene therapy for metastatic breast or epithelial ovarian cancer that overexpresses HER-2/neu	Breast cancer	*E1A* gene	Lipid	0	NA	NA	NA
J. A. Roth[148] (M. D. Anderson Cancer Center, Houston, TX)	Modification of oncogene and tumor suppressor gene expression in NSCLC	Lung cancer cells	ITR*p53*/IT-rasK-ras	Retrovirus	9	Y	1 CR 2 PR 3 SD	None
M. Steiner (Univ. of Tennessee, Memphis, TN)	Treatment of advanced prostate cancer by *in vivo* transduction with prostate-targeted retroviral vectors expressing antisense c-myc RNA	Prostate cancer cells	XM6	Retrovirus	0	NA	NA	NA
S. G. Swisher[149] (M. D. Anderson Cancer Center, Houston, TX)	Modification of tumor suppressor gene expression and induction of apoptosis in NSCLC with adenovirus vector expressing wild-type *p53* and cisplatin	Lung cancer cells	Ad5CMV-*p53*	Adenovirus	7	Y	NA	None

(continued)

TABLE 1. (CONTINUED)

Principal Investigator	Protocol	Target Cell	Vector	Delivery Vehicle	No. of Patients Entered	Evidence of Gene Expression[a]	No. and Type of Response[b]	Adverse Reactions[c]
	Adenoviral vector expressing wild-type *p53* administered intralesionally as an adjunct to radiation therapy in NSCLC	Lung cancer cells	Ad5CMV-*p53*	Adenovirus	12	NA	NA	NA
A. Venook (Univ. of California, San Francisco, San Francisco, CA)	Adenovirus expressing *p53* via hepatic artery infusion for primary and metastatic liver tumors	Primary and metastatic liver cancers	rAD/*p53*	Adenovirus	0	NA	NA	NA

CR, complete response; HNSCC, head and neck squamous cell carcinoma; *HSV-tk*, herpes simplex virus thymidine kinase; IL-2, interleukin 2; MR, minor response; N, no; NA, not available; NSCLC, non–small-cell lung cancer; PR, partial response; SD, stable disease; Y, yes.

[a] *In vivo* or in target cell.

[b] All principal investigators were asked to use the following response criteria: CR was defined as disappearance of all clinical evidence of tumor in the treated area for local treatment or for all lesions for systemic treatment without the appearance of new lesions for at least 4 weeks. Patients evaluable for a less-than-complete response were those having a bidimensionally measurable tumor. PR was defined as a ≥50% reduction in the sum of the products of the diameters of the measurable disease, including the treated lesion for local treatment or all lesions for systemic therapy. MR was defined as a 25% to <50% reduction in the sum of the products of the diameters of the measurable lesion. Patients were designated as having progressive disease if they showed a ≥25% increase in the size of their disease or if they developed unequivocal new lesions during treatment, and as having stabilization if they had any tumor change that did not meet the criteria described here.

[c] Related to gene transfer.

From Recombinant DNA Advisory Committee (RAC) Data Management Report; The RAC & Worldwide Gene Therapy Report, TMC Development, Paris, France; Herrmann E. Clinical application of gene transfer. *J Mol Med* 1996;74:213–221; and Sobol RE, Scanlan KJ, eds: *Internet book of cancer gene therapy*. Stamford, CN: Appleton & Lange, 1995, with permission. Survey forms were sent to all cancer gene-therapy protocol principal investigators with results tabulated and verified by each investigator as of June 19, 1996.

Genes Targeted to Tumor Cells

Genes targeted to tumor cells include those that kill tumor cells or change the biologic properties of malignant cells. Among these are genes that activate anticancer prodrugs, genes that interrupt tumorigenic processes, genes that are cytotoxic or proapoptotic and promote cell death directly, and genes that change biologic properties (e.g., invasiveness and metastasis) of malignant cells.

Prodrug Activation

Genes that encode enzymes capable of converting nontoxic prodrugs into highly toxic metabolites have been extensively tested in cancer gene therapy on the premise that their actions will limit the toxic metabolites locally to tumor sites, thereby remarkably reducing the systemic side effects of chemotherapy. Genes that might be used this way have been reviewed by Connors (76). The most commonly explored prodrug-activating gene is the thymidine kinase gene of the herpes simplex virus type 1 (*HSV-tk*). *HSV-tk* converts the nucleoside analog ganciclovir to its monophosphate form by phosphorylation. This monophosphate is subsequently modified into its toxic triphosphate form by endogenous cellular enzymes and then incorporated into nascent DNA, thus causing chain termination and cell death. The rate of monophosphorylation of ganciclovir by endogenous cellular thymidine kinase is, however, three orders of magnitude lower than that of *HSV-tk*. Because phosphorylated ganciclovir cannot pass through the plasma membrane, it accumulates within the cell, resulting in enhanced anticancer activity. The untransduced neighboring cells are also killed by the so-called bystander effect. The underlying mechanisms are not fully understood.

Another prodrug-activating system involves the use of the fungal or bacterial gene encoding the enzyme cytosine deaminase. Cytosine deaminase, which is not found in mammalian cells, converts the antifungal drug 5-fluorocytosine (5-FC) into the anticancer drug 5-fluorouracil (5-FU) through deamination. The transfer of the cytosine deaminase gene into mammalian cells renders them selectively sensitive to 5-FC. A bystander effect has also been observed in this system: Released 5-FU can diffuse to nearby tumor cells and pass through their cell membranes.

A third prodrug-activating system involves a bacterial nitroreductase that catalyzes CB1954 reduction, thus generating a 4-hydroxylamine metabolite. This molecule then reacts with thioesters, such as acetyl CoA, to produce a highly cytotoxic difunctional alkylating agent capable of cross-linking DNA and 10,000 times more cytotoxic than its parental prodrug (77). Again, a bystander effect for CB1954 when activated by nitroreductase has been reported. Unlike *HSV-tk*, however, the anticancer activity of the CB1954 nitroreductase system does not require cells to be in S phase, thus suggesting that this prodrug may be used to eliminate nondividing neoplastic cells.

Intratumoral implantation of murine fibroblasts that express the *HSV-tk* gene was done in 15 patients with progressive growth of recurrent malignant brain tumors (78). Gene transfer was limited but some antitumor activity was noted in five patients.

Tumor Suppressors and Antioncogenes

So far, *p53* is the most extensively tested tumor suppressor gene used for cancer gene therapy, both in research and clinic. The *p53* gene is the most frequently mutated gene in human cancers (63,79), and its absence or inactivation of wild-type *p53* may con-

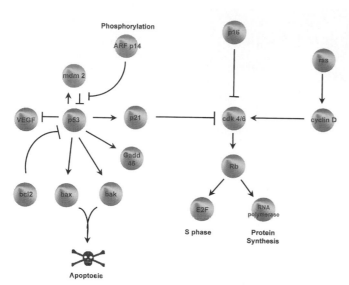

FIGURE 1. Molecular pathways in oncogenesis. This figure shows the interrelationships between tumor suppressor genes, oncogenes, and other genes regulating cell-cycle progression and apoptosis. These genes and their pathways represent potentially important targets for gene replacement strategies.

tribute to malignant transformation. Theoretically, then, replacement of a functional copy of the tumor suppressor gene in cells with a homozygous loss of function could restore normal growth and proliferation pathways. The need to correct all genetic lesions in every malignant cell with a gene-based drug may seem daunting, especially given that no currently available technique can deliver a therapeutic gene or its product to all tumor cells; however, studies undertaken in our laboratory and subsequently by others have shown that it may not be necessary to reverse all the genetic changes in a cancer cell to have a therapeutic effect. Indeed, the restoration of wild-type *p53* expression in cells with mutant or deleted *p53* is sufficient to cause apoptosis or growth arrest despite the presence of multiple genetic abnormalities present in such cells (19). Moreover, other studies have shown that the presence of a wild-type *p53* gene may sensitize tumor cells to chemotherapy and radiation therapy (80). For instance, one study demonstrated that introducing the wild-type *p53* gene could enhance tumor cell sensitivity to cisplatin and other agents (18).

Besides *p53*, other tumor suppressor genes are being rapidly added to the list of candidate genes for cancer gene therapy. The genes most frequently abnormal in terms of mutations or absence of expression include genes regulating the cell cycle, tumor suppressor genes, and oncogenes (Fig. 1). Among them are the retinoblastoma (*RB*), von Hippel-Lindau, breast cancer (*BRCA1*), mutated in multiple advanced cancers 1/phosphatase and tensin homologue (*MMAC1/PTEN*), *p16*, *E2F*, and fragile histidine triad (*FHIT*) genes. Clinical trials with *BRCA1* and *RB* have already been initiated. Although the classification of *E2F* and *FHIT* as tumor suppressor genes remains controversial, *in vitro* and *in vivo* studies have demonstrated that they cause apoptosis of tumor cells and inhibit tumor growth after their adenovirus-mediated transfer into tumor cells (81–83). However, introducing *FHIT* gene to cultured normal human bronchial epithelial cells did not induce apoptosis (83).

While research into restoring the functions of tumor suppressor genes continues, so does fervent research into inactivating activated oncogenes. Three members of the ras family of oncogenes—H-*ras*, K-*ras*, and N-*ras*—are among the most commonly activated oncogenes in human cancers and thus excellent therapeutic targets. The *RAS* genes encode a protein with GTPase activity that localizes to the inner surface of the plasma membrane. A single mutation in the genes is sufficient to render the gene product transforming. Several strategies have been designed to combat these gain-of-function mutations, including ones using antisense nucleotides, ribozymes (84,85), and intracellular single-chain antibodies (86). *In vivo* gene therapy with K-*ras*, c-*fos*, and c-*myc* antisense nucleotides and a single-chain antibody to erbB-2 are currently under clinical trials (58).

Clinical Studies with Tumor Suppressor Gene p53

Local control of the primary tumor is an under appreciated problem in oncology. For example, up to one-third of patients with non–small cell lung cancer (NSCLC) die only from progression of the local tumor, and in patients undergoing radiation therapy, local control is achieved less than 20% of the time (87). Furthermore, improved local control has translated into improved survival (88).

Intratumoral injection has been most widely studied with viral vectors expressing the wild-type *p53* gene. In our initial human study, nine patients with NSCLC received a retroviral vector containing the wild-type *p53* gene under the control of a beta-actin promoter (15). All patients had failed other treatments and had tumors documented as having a *p53* mutation. Because transduction via retrovirus was known to yield low titers of the transduced gene, the vector was injected into the tumor on 5 consecutive days, using either a bronchoscope or, in the case of chest wall lesions, percutaneous needle.

Regression of the injected lesion was seen in three patients, whereas stabilization of disease was seen in three others (Fig. 2). In one patient who died of a progressive kidney metastasis, no evidence of viable tumor at the treated site was found on autopsy 4 months after injection. One patient had progressive primary disease, and two were inevaluable (one was intolerant of the general anesthetic and did not complete treatment, and one died within 3 weeks of treatment). Polymerase chain reaction (PCR), *in situ* hybridization studies, or both of posttreatment biopsies before evaluation of treatment effects from eight patients showed that tumor cells had indeed integrated vector DNA sequences, in up to 20% of cells in certain areas of tumor. An important finding was that terminal deoxynucleotidyltransferase–mediated dUTP-biotin nick end labeling (TUNEL) staining (which detects DNA nicking and therefore indicates apoptosis) of posttreatment biopsy samples increased after treatment, compared with the pretreatment baseline.

No side effects attributable to the *p53*-vector sequences occurred in any patient, although bronchoscopy-related complications occurred in three patients. We found no evidence of retroviral sequences in DNA extracted from lymphocytes, sputum samples, or various nontumor tissues obtained at autopsy on three patients. These results thus confirmed a high safety profile, successful delivery of normal *p53* sequences to tumor cells, and a biologic effect of the transduced gene.

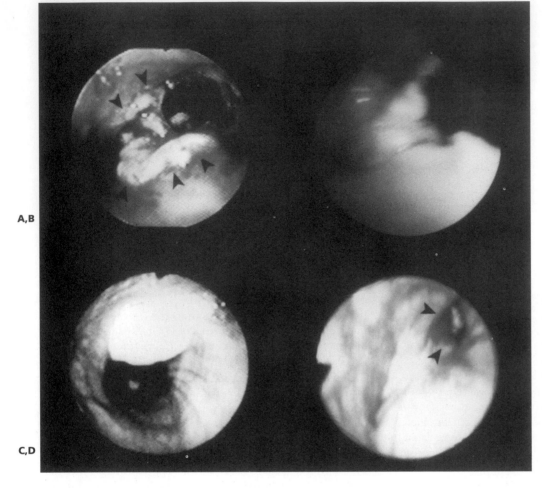

A,B

C,D

FIGURE 2. Pretreatment **(A,C)** and 30-day posttreatment **(B,D)** bronchoscopic images of patients 1 **(A,B)** and 5 **(C,D)**. **A:** The lesion is situated in the left mainstem bronchus on the division of the upper and lower lobes; biopsies showed squamous cell carcinoma (*arrowheads*). **B:** Left mainstem bronchus 30 days after ITRp53A injection; five independent biopsies showed absence of viable tumor cells. **C:** Adenocarcinoma obstructing the right upper lobe orifice. **D:** Right upper lobe orifice (*arrowheads*) 30 days after treatment; biopsies in this region showed residual

These promising results have been supported by a two-arm study in which a wild-type *p53* gene was given to 52 patients with NSCLC, using an adenovirus vector. Patients received adenovirus *p53* (Ad-*p53*) either alone or preceded by cisplatin (CDDP) (80 mg per m^2 over 2 hours, 3 days before *p53* injection). (CDDP was chosen because of the preclinical studies that had shown a synergistic effect with *p53* gene replacement.) *p53* treatment was given as a single intratumoral injection, either bronchoscopically or under computed tomographic guidance, once per month for up to 6 months. Most patients had received previous chemotherapy, in some cases with cisplatin, and all had progressive tumor growth on conventional therapy before entry into the study.

As with the study using the retroviral vector, both clinical and laboratory evidence of *p53* expression was seen. Ad-*p53* alone (26 evaluable patients) mediated two partial responses and stabilization of disease in 16 patients (Fig. 3). Progression-free survival was increased with a higher dose of Ad-*p53*. Ad-*p53*/CDDP (23 evaluable patients) mediated a partial response in two patients previously treated with CDDP. One additional patient achieved a partial response but did not have the required follow-up documentation to confirm the response. Progression-free survival was prolonged with Ad-*p53*/CDDP as compared to Ad-*p53* alone. A majority of patients also had evidence of vector DNA by vector-specific PCR of posttreatment biopsies. DNA extracted from 18 of 21 evaluable tumors from patients receiving

Ad-*p53* alone showed vector-specific adenoviral sequences. All tested tumors above 10^6 plaque-forming units (PFU) showed evidence of adenoviral sequences by DNA-PCR. Vector-specific mRNA *p53* sequences were detected by reverse transcriptase-PCR in 12 of 26 specimens with adequate RNA. *p53* transgene expression was noted in nine of 16 patients (56%) treated at doses above 10^9 PFU as opposed to only three of 10 patients (30%) treated with 10^9 PFU or less. Transgene expression of *p53* occurred after initial and subsequent treatments at all dose levels above 10^6 PFU. The mean pretreatment apoptotic index was 3.6 ± 1.0% (mean ± SEM) with 95% confidence intervals of 1.5% to 5.8% for patients receiving Ad-*p53* alone. Eleven of 24 evaluable patients fell outside the 95% confidence intervals with apoptotic indices of 7% to 87% in posttreatment tumor biopsies. No consistent change in inflammatory cell infiltration was seen after Ad-*p53* treatment in posttreatment tumor biopsies, suggesting that nonspecific inflammation or immune-mediated effects were not responsible for the antitumor effects noted.

Although antiadenovirus antibodies were detected in all patients after one treatment, subsequent treatments were not accompanied by anaphylaxis or other toxicities except transient fever. Perhaps surprising, despite high levels of serum antiadenovirus antibody, *p53* transgene expression occurred in the tumor cells and clinical responses were maintained. Of 12 patients receiving endobronchial injections with an obstructed airway, six showed opening of the airway. Vector-related adverse

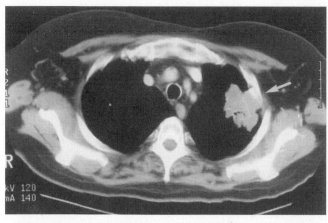
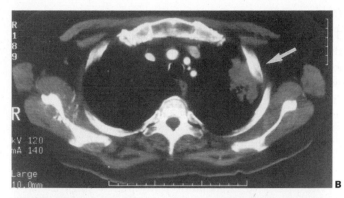
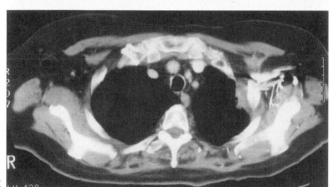
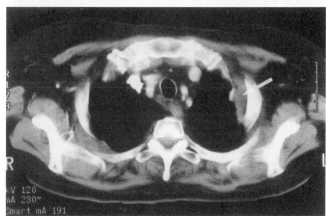

FIGURE 3. Pretreatment **(A)**, 1 month posttreatment **(B)**, 8 months posttreatment **(C)**, and 16 months posttreatment **(D)** computed tomographic scans of patient after six courses of 10^9 plaque-forming units of adenovirus *p53* (Ad-*p53*). **A:** Recurrent left upper lobe adenocarcinoma (*white arrow*), which progressed after 66 Gy of external beam radiation therapy and six courses of Taxol/carboplatin. **B:** Tumor regression (*white arrow*) after one course of Ad-*p53* treatment. **C:** Tumor regression (*white arrow*) after six courses of Ad-*p53* gene therapy. **D:** Stable tumor (*white arrow*) 18 months after beginning treatment with Ad-*p53*. No viable tumor was demonstrated during the last 4 months of therapy (14 sequential percutaneous biopsies), and the patient was observed off all treatment for 12 months without evidence of tumor progression. (Reprinted with permission from Swisher SG, Roth JA, Nemunaitis J, et al. Adenoviral-mediated *p53* gene transfer in advanced non–small cell lung cancer. *J Natl Cancer Inst* 1999;91:763–771.)

events were minimal. No grade 4 toxicity was seen, and grade 3 vector-related toxicity was limited to one incident of nausea after Ad-*p53* injection. Toxicity related to CDDP was not increased when Ad-*p53* was added.

Even though these studies corrected only one of the many genetic abnormalities present in NSCLC, the evidence suggests an antitumor effect based directly on *p53*-mediated apoptosis, as shown in both the retroviral *p53* and Ad-*p53* trials. The two trials provided no evidence for the contrary view that tumor stabilization and regression resulted from a nonspecific immune reaction. In the adenovirus-*p53* study, vector DNA was detected by PCR in the majority of patients, but fewer patients showed evidence of gene expression. Detection of gene expression after transfer of wild-type *p53 in vivo* is difficult because successful transfer and expression of wild-type *p53* in a tumor may destroy evidence of gene expression if apoptosis is induced and the cells die. However, in those patients in whom serial gene expression could be quantitated by immunohistochemistry, it was clear that expression of the transgene occurred despite the presence of high titers of anti-adenovirus antibody. It is possible that serum antibodies have little effect because of poor penetration into solid tumors, as a result

of high interstitial fluid pressure. It is not known whether suppression of the antiadenovirus immune response would further enhance the levels of transgene expression in the tumor. In any case, repeated intratumoral injections of Ad-*p53* appear safe despite increases in antiadenovirus antibodies.

Similar results were observed in 33 patients with incurable recurrent local or regionally metastatic head and neck squamous cell carcinoma receiving intratumoral injections with or without tumor resection (75). In 17 patients evaluable for response, two showed tumor regression greater than 50%, six showed stable disease for up to 3.5 months, and one resectable patient had a complete response. There was no dose-limiting toxicity up to 10^{11} PFU, and no serious adverse events occurred.

Clinical trials reported in abstract form have confirmed the safety and efficacy of Ad-*p53* gene replacement for recurrent ovarian carcinoma (89). A total of 37 women who had received an average of 12 pretreatment chemotherapy cycles (range, 5 to 37) were treated with intraperitoneal doses of Ad-*p53* ranging from 7.5×10^{10} to 7.5×10^{13} particles as a single dose for 5 consecutive days. Reduction in CA125 levels were observed in over half of the patients.

Proapoptotic and Cytotoxic Genes

The importance of apoptosis in tumorigenesis and antitumor therapy has been recognized. Emerging evidence suggests that many antitumor therapies function by inducing apoptosis in tumor cells (90–92). Because they vary in their susceptibility to apoptosis induction, tumor cells may respond to chemotherapy or radiation therapy by undergoing apoptosis, whereas normal cells merely undergo cell-cycle arrest. This important difference provides a therapeutic window of opportunity. A major mode of cellular resistance to antitumor therapy may be insensitivity to apoptosis induction (90,93,94).

Genes involved in apoptotic pathways have been reviewed (91,92,95). In addition, strategies using tumor suppressor genes and antioncogenes have similarly been used to manipulate genes involved in the apoptotic pathway to elicit antitumor effects directly or to sensitize tumor cells to other therapeutics. For example, introducing the gene for Fas or Fas ligand or for a single-chain antibody to Bcl-2 resulted in tumor cell killing or tumor regression in animal models (96–98). Accumulating evidence also suggests that the status of *BAX* gene expression correlates with clinical outcomes of cancer patients (99–106). More recently, it has been shown that overexpression of *BAX* reduces efflux and therefore enhances the intracellular accumulation of the chemotherapeutic agent paclitaxel (104). Nevertheless, constructing viral vectors that express highly apoptosis-inducing genes may prove difficult because of the potential toxic effect on packaging cells. As mentioned above, this problem can be solved by using the *GAL4* gene regulatory system, and adenovirus-mediated gene codelivery.

Genes That Alter Malignant Behaviors

The penetration of basement membranes by malignant cells is the critical event in tumor invasion and metastasis. It is known that cellular protease (e.g., metalloproteinases and serine proteases) activities must be elevated for tumor cells to cross the basement membrane and subsequently metastasize. Therefore, proteins that inhibit these proteases' activities (e.g., the tissue inhibitor of metalloproteinase, plasminogen activator inhibitors, and serpins) may be used as therapeutic agents for cancer treatment (107,108). Proteins involved in cell-cell or cell-extracellular matrix adhesion [e.g., immunoglobulins, integrins, cadherins, selectins, and hyaluronic acid receptors and their ligands (e.g., CD44)] have been found to be involved in the metastatic process [extensively reviewed in Guenthert and Birchmeier (109)]. They can also be the targets of cancer gene therapy, as the metastatic process can be disrupted by manipulation of these molecules. For example, the urokinase-type plasminogen activator receptor (u-PAR) on the surface of tumor cells binds to u-PA released from surrounding cells. This u-PAR/u-PA complex focuses proteolytic activity onto the tumor cell surface by converting the plasma protein plasminogen into the serine protease plasmin. In addition, overexpression of u-PAR in breast cancer cells results in increased tumor invasion and metastasis (110). The use of an adenoviral vector expressing antisense u-PAR sequences for cancer gene therapy is currently under testing in experimental tumor models.

Genes Targeted to the Immune System

It has long been believed that tumor cells themselves contain specific antigens. Thus, the immune system should be able to detect and eliminate malignant cells in the body. However, in many cases, tumor-specific antigens are too weak to elicit a helper T-cell response or a cellular cytotoxic response, and immune anergy ensues. Moreover, in the majority of malignancies aroused in immunocompetent hosts, tumor cells have devised stratagems to escape immune surveillance. Transforming growth factor β1, for example, is secreted by several tumor types and has immunosuppressive properties (111). Low or absent expression of class I major histocompatibility complex (MHC) molecules may lead to inadequate presentation of antigens on tumor cells (112–114).

Consequently, for several decades, great effort has been directed toward developing a strategy of cancer immunotherapy and testing various immunomodulatory agents for their ability to increase immune responses against malignancies. It is now known that to elicit an anticancer immune response requires three synergistic components: (a) tumor antigens bound with HLA molecules for presentation to the immune system, (b) costimulatory signals for efficient antigen presentation, and (c) cytokines or growth factors for the recruitment and proliferation of tumor-reactive lymphocytes. Therefore, genes that encode various cytokines, costimulatory molecules, allogenic antigens, and tumor-associated antigens are currently being intensively tested for their ability to augment tumor-specific immune responses (115–117). It is foreseeable that the identification of tumor rejection antigens and the characterization of the critical components of the afferent and efferent limbs of the immune response that are defective in cancer patients will remain important topics of research (118–121).

At present, most protocols of cancer immune gene therapy involve the delivery of genes directly into tumor cells, although the introduction of genes into lymphocytes or antigen-presenting cells (APCs), mainly dendritic cells, is also being tested. The rationale for intratumoral delivery of cytokines, costimulatory molecules, and antigens is that local delivery of the cytokines will limit their systemic toxicity and that tumor cells may function as APCs if costimulatory molecules are present in them (122,123). New insights into the molecular biology of antigen processing and presentation have revealed that dendritic cells play a critical role in the induction of primary, cell-mediated immune responses (124–126). Moreover, T-cell priming can occur only in the context of MHC-peptide complexes expressed by host APCs but not by immunized tumor cells (127). However, antigen can be transferred from cells expressing the antigen to the APCs, a process triggered by inflammatory reactions that cause the degradation and release of antigen from the dying cells. This process is called *cross-priming* or *indirect presentation*. Cytokines or costimulatory molecules delivered to tumor cells are believed to enhance the transfer of tumor antigens to APCs. Thus, *ex vivo* gene delivery to cultured autologous APCs such as dendritic cells or direct *in vivo* gene delivery to APCs may be more efficient in stimulating cellular antitumor immunity (125,126). Despite these promising approaches, however, a variety of important issues remain to be addressed, including the heterogeneity of tumor cells, the alteration of the biologic properties or gene expression in metastatic versus parental tumor cells, and the suppressed expression in tumor cells of MHC molecules essential for their recognition by the immune system.

Introduction of a gene encoding a foreign class I major histocompatibility protein can trigger an immune response to the foreign antigen. This in turn can generate a cytolytic T-cell response against nontransduced tumor cells by increasing the local immune response. In one clinical trial, the *HLA-B7* gene in DNA-liposome complexes was injected to the tumors of melanoma patients who were *HLA-B7* negative. Recombinant HLA-B7 protein was shown in tumor biopsies from all five patients. Immune responses to *HLA-B7* and autologous tumors were detected. An increase in the frequency of *HLA-B7*–reactive cytotoxic lymphocytes was detected after treatment. Tumor-specific cytotoxic lymphocytes were detected in posttreatment lymphocytes originating either from peripheral blood or the tumor. One of five patients showed regression of injected and uninjected nodules (128).

Genes Targeted to Tumor Vasculature

Depriving tumor cells of nutrients by blocking or reducing the blood flow to tumors has already been explored in experimental tumor models and achieved by direct occlusion of the tumor vasculature or by inhibition of angiogenesis in tumors (129,130). Therapeutic approaches that target the tumor vasculature rather than the tumor cells themselves hold great promise for a broad spectrum of and high capacity for antitumor activity. Such approaches, while damaging only a single vessel, might kill millions of tumor cells.

Angiogenesis, a complex process involving cell-cell and cell-matrix interactions, is essential for the growth and metastasis of solid tumors. This process is strictly controlled by a redundant system of pro- and antiangiogenic paracrine peptide molecules [reviewed by Fan et al. (131), Norrby (132), Augustin (130)]. The balance between these positive and negative regulators of angiogenesis in the local tumor environment is important for the homeostasis of microvessels. It is now known that tumor cells can secrete proangiogenic paracrine factors and thus stimulate endothelial cells to form new blood vessels.

Of the more than 20 proangiogenesis peptides identified so far, VEGF and placenta growth factor have been shown to directly influence the behavior of endothelial cells. VEGF is also abundantly secreted by tumor cells, and its expression is upregulated by hypoxia, a microenvironmental condition that exists preferentially in solid tumors. Cellular *p53* status and c-src activity also influence VEGF expression (133,134). Introducing the wild-type *p53* gene into tumor cells suppressed VEGF expression and inhibited angiogenesis in experimental tumors (135), whereas using antisense or soluble receptor molecules to block the functions of VEGF and other angiogenic factors reportedly suppressed tumor growth in animal models (136,137).

Genes encoding antiangiogenesis peptides have also been used to suppress angiogenesis in tumors. Of these, the IL-12 gene has already entered clinical trials. A potent immune system modulator, IL-12 also significantly inhibits angiogenesis and upregulates the expression of E-cadherin, a metastasis suppres-

sor. Other angiogenic inhibitors that have shown therapeutic promise are angiostatin and endostatin (138–140). For instance, introducing angiostatin complementary DNA into tumors established in mice inhibits angiogenesis, tumor growth, and metastasis in certain animal tumor models.

Genes Targeted to Normal Cells

Systemic chemotherapy is currently one of the most effective and widely used forms of antitumor treatment. Its efficacy is limited, however, by the destructive effects that can be inflicted on normal tissues before doses sufficient to achieve efficient tumor killing are reached. Indeed, this acute toxicity most often manifests itself as myelosuppression. Autologous bone marrow replacement has been successfully used to combat this acute hemopoietic toxicity. However, as autologous bone marrow replacement is used more and more, the frequency of therapy-related malignancies will probably also rise because of the presence of malignant cells in the transplants.

Alternatively, hematopoietic stem cells and early progenitors can be protected by augmenting their resistance to the toxic and mutagenic effects of antitumor agents. This may be accomplished by transferring appropriate drug-resistance genes into hematopoietic cells *ex vivo* and then transplanting the cells back into the patient. Thus far, drug-resistance genes have been tested for their ability to protect normal cells from the toxic effects of conventional doses of chemotherapy. The first such study attempted to enhance marrow protection during chemotherapy by transferring the multiple-drug resistance gene *MDR1* into normal bone marrow and blood-derived stem cells (141,142). Other genes that have been tested for the same purpose include the DNA repair protein *O*-methylguanidine-DNA-methyltransferase, which protects hematopoietic cells from nitrosourea-induced toxicity (143), and methotrexate-resistant dihydrofolate reductase, which protects against methotrexate toxicity (144).

There are, however, at least two problems with this strategy of drug resistance. First, the current technology is limited to bone marrow only, so the toxic effects in unprotected nonhematologic cells may limit the dose of chemotherapy. Second, the cancer cells in bone marrow may be transduced with the drug-resistance gene, resulting in a drug-resistant relapsed tumor. Thus, to avoid the transduction of malignant cells, hemopoietic stem cells are isolated by CD34 column fractionation before they are treated with a drug-resistant vector.

REFERENCES

1. Blaese M, Blankenstein T, Brenner M, et al. Vectors in cancer therapy: how will they deliver? *Cancer Gene Ther* 1995;2:291–297.
2. Ross G, Erickson R, Knorr D, et al. Gene therapy in the United States: a five-year status report. *Hum Gene Ther* 1996;7:1781–1790.
3. Graham FL, Prevec L. Manipulation of adenovirus vectors. In: Murray EJ, ed. *Methods in molecular biology.* Clinton, NJ: The Humana Press Inc, 1991;109–128.
4. Graham FL, Smiley J, Russell WC, et al. Characteristics of a human cell line transformed by DNA from human adenovirus type 5. *J Gen Virol* 1977;36:59–74.
5. Parks RJ, Chen L, Anton M, et al. A helper-dependent adenovirus vector system: removal of helper virus by Cre-mediated excision of

the viral packaging signal. *Proc Natl Acad Sci U S A* 1996;93: 13565–13570.

6. Bett AJ, Prevec L, Graham FL. Packaging capacity and stability of human adenovirus type 5 vectors. *J Virol* 1993;67:5911–5921.

7. Parks RJ, Graham FL. A helper-dependent system for adenovirus vector production helps define a lower limit for efficient DNA packaging. *J Virol* 1997;71:3293–3298.

8. Li QT, Kay MA, Finegold M, et al. Assessment of recombinant adenoviral vectors for hepatic gene therapy. *Hum Gene Ther* 1993;4:403–409.

9. Rosenfeld MA, Siegfried W, Yoshimura K, et al. Adenovirus-mediated transfer of a recombinant a1-antitrypsin gene to the lung *in vivo*. *Science* 1991;252:431–434.

10. Stratford-Perricaudet LD, Makeh I, Perricaudet M, et al. Widespread long-term gene transfer to mouse skeletal muscles and heart. *J Clin Invest* 1992;90:626–630.

11. Fang B, Eisensmith RC, Li XH, et al. Gene therapy for phenylketonuria: phenotypic correction in a genetically deficient mouse model by adenovirus-mediated hepatic gene transfer. *Gene Ther* 1994;1:247–254.

12. Stratford-Perricaudet LD, Levrero M, Chasse JF, et al. Evaluation of the transfer and expression in mice of an enzyme-encoding gene using a human adenovirus vector. *Hum Gene Ther* 1990;1:241–256.

13. Kozarsky KF, McKinley DR, Austin LL, et al. *In vivo* correction of low density lipoprotein receptor deficiency in the Watanabe heritable hyperlipidemic rabbit with recombinant adenoviruses. *J Biol Chem* 1994;269:13695–13702.

14. Li J, Fang B, Eisensmith RC, et al. *In vivo* gene therapy for hyperlipidemia: phenotypic correction in Watanabe rabbits by hepatic delivery of the rabbit LDL receptor gene. *J Clin Invest* 1995;95:768–773.

15. Kay MA, Landen CN, Rothenberg SR, et al. *In vivo* hepatic gene therapy: complete albeit transient correction of factor IX deficiency in hemophilia B dogs. *Proc Natl Acad Sci U S A* 1994;91:2353–2357.

16. Chen SH, Shine HD, Goodman JC, et al. Gene therapy for brain tumors: regression of experimental gliomas by adenovirus-mediated gene transfer *in vivo*. *Proc Natl Acad Sci U S A* 1994;91:3054–3057.

17. Cordier L, Duffour MT, Sabourin JC, et al. Complete recovery of mice from a pre-established tumor by direct intratumoral delivery of an adenovirus vector harboring the murine IL-2 gene. *Gene Ther* 1995;2:16–21.

18. Fujiwara T, Grimm EA, Mukhopadhyay T, et al. Induction of chemosensitivity in human lung cancer cells *in vivo* by adenoviral-mediated transfer of the wild-type p53 gene. *Cancer Res* 1994;54: 2287–2291.

19. Roth JA, Cristiano RJ. Gene therapy for cancer: what have we done and where are we going? [Review]. *J Natl Cancer Inst* 1997;89:21–39.

20. Larregina AT, Morelli AE, Dewey RA, et al. FasL induces Fas/Apo1-mediated apoptosis in human embryonic kidney 293 cells routinely used to generate E1-deleted adenoviral vectors. *Gene Ther* 1998;5:563–568.

21. Kagawa S, Pearson SA, Ji L, et al. A binary adenoviral vector system for expressing high levels of the proapoptotic gene bax. *Gene Ther* 2000;7:75–79.

22. Fang B, Ji L, Bouvet M, et al. Evaluation of GAL4/TATA *in vivo*: induction of transgene expression by adenovirally mediated gene codelivery. *J Biol Chem* 1998;273:4972–4975.

23. Gorziglia MI, Kadan MJ, Yei S, et al. Elimination of both E1 and E2 from adenovirus vectors further improves prospects for *in vivo* human gene therapy. *J Virol* 1996;70:4173–4178.

24. Lieber A, He CY, Kirillova I, et al. Recombinant adenoviruses with large deletions generated by cre-mediated excision exhibit different biological properties compared with first-generation vectors *in vitro* and *in vivo*. *J Virol* 1996;70:8944–8960.

25. Mitani K, Graham FL, Caskey CT, et al. Rescue, propagation, and partial purification of a helper virus-dependent adenovirus vector. *Proc Natl Acad Sci U S A* 1995;92:3854–3858.

26. Wang Q, Jia X-C, Finer MH. A packaging cell line for propagation of recombinant adenovirus vectors containing two lethal gene-region deletions. *Gene Ther* 1995;2:775–783.

27. Schiedner G, Morral N, Parks RJ, et al. Genomic DNA transfer with a high-capacity adenovirus vector results in improved *in vivo* gene expression and decreased toxicity. *Nat Genet* 1998;18:180–183.

28. Fang B, Koch PE, Roth JA. Diminishing adenovirus gene expression and viral replication by promoter replacement. *J Virol* 1997;71: 4798–4803.

29. Wickham TJ, Tzeng E, Shears LL II, et al. Increased *in vitro* and *in vivo* gene transfer by adenovirus vectors containing chimeric fiber proteins. *J Virol* 1997;71:8221–8229.

30. Dmitriev I, Krasnykh V, Miller CR, et al. An adenovirus vector with genetically modified fibers demonstrates expanded tropism via utilization of a coxsackievirus and adenovirus receptor-independent cell entry mechanism. *J Virol* 1998;72:9706–9713.

31. Douglas JT, Rogers BE, Rosenfeld ME, et al. Targeted gene delivery by tropism-modified adenoviral vectors. *Nat Biotechnol* 1996;14: 1574–1578.

32. Stevenson SC, Rollence M, Marshall-Neff J, et al. Selective targeting of human cells by a chimeric adenovirus vector containing a modified fiber protein. *J Virol* 1997;71:4782–4790.

33. Wickham TJ, Roelvink PW, Brough DE, et al. Adenovirus targeted to heparan-containing receptors increases its gene delivery efficiency to multiple cell types. *Nat Biotechnol* 1996;14:1570–1574.

34. Wickham TJ, Segal DM, Roelvink PW, et al. Targeted adenovirus gene transfer to endothelial and smooth muscle cells by using bispecific antibodies. *J Virol* 1996;70:6831–6838.

35. Dai Y, Schwarz EM, Gu D, et al. Cellular and humoral immune responses to adenoviral vectors containing factor IX gene: tolerization of both factor IX and vector antigens allows for long term expression. *Proc Natl Acad Sci U S A* 1995;92:1401–1405.

36. Fang B, Eisensmith RC, Wang H, et al. Gene therapy for hemophilia B: host immunosuppression prolongs the therapeutic effect of adenovirus-mediated factor IX expression. *Hum Gene Ther* 1995;6:1039–1044.

37. Kay M, Holterman S, Meuse L, et al. Long-term hepatic adenovirus-mediated gene expression in mice following CTLA4-Ig administration. *Nat Genet* 1995;11:191–197.

38. Jooss K, Yang Y, Wilson JM. Cyclophosphamide diminishes inflammation and prolongs transgene expression following delivery of adenoviral vectors to mouse liver and lung. *Hum Gene Ther* 1996;7:1555–1566.

39. Yang Y, Trinchieri G, Wilson JM. Recombinant IL-12 prevents formation of blocking IgA antibodies to recombinant adenovirus and allows repeated gene therapy to mouse lung. *Nat Med* 1995;1:890–893.

40. Bouvet M, Fang B, Ekmekcioglu S, et al. Suppression of the immune response to an adenovirus vector and enhancement of intratumoral transgene expression by low-dose etoposide. *Gene Ther* 1998;5:189–195.

41. Berns KI, Giraud C. Current topics in microbiology and immunology. In: Berns KI, Giraud C, eds. Adeno-associated virus (AAV) in gene therapy. Berlin: Springer-Verlag New York, 1996.

42. Flotte TR, Carter BJ. Adeno-associated virus vectors for gene therapy [Review]. *Gene Ther* 1995;2:357–362.

43. Muzyczka N. Use of adeno-associated virus as a general transduction vector for mammalian cells [Review]. *Curr Top Microbiol Immunol* 1992;158:97–129.

44. Fisher KJ, Gao GP, Weitzman MD, et al. Transduction with recombinant adeno-associated virus for gene therapy is limited by leading-strand synthesis. *J Virol* 1996;70:520–532.

45. Fisher KJ, Jooss K, Alston J, et al. Recombinant adeno-associated virus for muscle directed gene therapy. *Nat Med* 1997;3:306–312.

46. Snyder RO, Miao CH, Patijn GA, et al. Persistent and therapeutic concentrations of human factor IX in mice after hepatic gene transfer of recombinant AAV vectors. *Nat Genet* 1997;16:270–276.

47. Xiao W, Berta SC, Lu MM, et al. Adeno-associated virus as a vector for liver-directed gene therapy. *J Virol* 1998;72:10222–10226.

48. Duan D, Sharma P, Yang J, et al. Circular intermediates of recombinant adeno-associated virus have defined structural characteristics responsible for long-term episomal persistence in muscle tissue. *J Virol* 1998;72:8568–8577.

49. Bartholomew RM, Esser AF, Muller-Eberhard HJ. Lysis of oncornaviruses by human serum. Isolation of the viral complement (C1) receptor and identification as p15E. *J Exp Med* 1978;147:844–853.

50. Rigg RJ, Chen J, Dando JS, et al. A novel human amphotropic packaging cell line: high titer, complement resistance, and improved safety. *Virology* 1996;218:290–295.

51. Schnierle BS, Groner B. Retroviral targeted delivery [Review]. *Gene Ther* 1996;3:1069–1073.

52. Naldini L, Blomer U, Gallay P, et al. *In vivo* gene delivery and stable transduction of nondividing cells by a lentiviral vector. *Science* 1996;272:263–267.

53. Poeschla E, Corbeau P, Wong-Staal F. Development of HIV vectors for anti-HIV gene therapy [Review]. *Proc Natl Acad Sci U S A* 1996;93:11395–11399.

54. Binns MM, Smith GL. *Recombinant poxviruses.* Ann Arbor, MI: CRC Press, 1992.

55. Moss B. Vaccinia virus: a tool for research and vaccine development [Review]. *Science* 1991;252:1662–1667.

56. Hodge JW, Abrams S, Schlom J, et al. Induction of antitumor immunity by recombinant vaccinia viruses expressing B7-1 or B7-2 costimulatory molecules. *Cancer Res* 1994;54:5552–5555.

57. Peplinski GR, Tsung K, Whitman ED, et al. Construction and expression in tumor cells of a recombinant vaccinia virus encoding human interleukin-1 beta. *Ann Surg Oncol* 1995;2:151–159.

58. Cusack JC Jr, Tanabe KK. Cancer gene therapy. *Surg Oncol Clin North Am* 1998;7:421–469.

59. Bischoff JR, Kirn DH, Williams A, et al. An adenovirus mutant that replicates selectively in p53-deficient human tumor cells. *Science* 1996;274:373–376.

60. Boviatsis EJ, Park JS, Sena-Esteves M, et al. Long-term survival of rats harboring brain neoplasms treated with ganciclovir and a herpes simplex virus vector that retains an intact thymidine kinase gene. *Cancer Res* 1994;54:5745–5751.

61. Yoon SS, Carroll NM, Chiocca EA, et al. Cancer gene therapy using a replication-competent herpes simplex virus type 1 vector. *Ann Surg* 1998;228:366–374.

62. Coffey MC, Strong JE, Forsyth PA, et al. Reovirus therapy of tumors with activated Ras pathway. *Science* 1998;282:1332–1334.

63. Hollstein M, Sidransky D, Vogelstein B, et al. *p53* mutations in human cancers. *Science* 1991;253:49–53.

64. Hall AR, Dix BR, O'Carroll SJ, et al. P53-Dependent cell death/apoptosis is required for a productive adenovirus infection. *Nat Med* 1998;4:1068–1072.

65. Goodrum FD, Ornelles DA. p53 status does not determine outcome of E1B 55-kilodalton mutant adenovirus lytic infection. *J Virol* 1998;72:9479–9490.

66. Wolff JA, Malone RW, Williams P, et al. Direct gene transfer into mouse muscle *in vivo*. *Science* 1990;247:1465–1468.

67. Wolff JA, Williams P, Acsadi G, et al. Conditions affecting direct gene transfer into rodent muscle *in vivo*. *Biotechniques* 1991;11:474–485.

68. Zhang G, Vargo D, Budker V, et al. Expression of naked plasmid DNA injected into the afferent and efferent vessels of rodent and dog livers. *Hum Gene Ther* 1997;8:1763–1772.

69. Song YK, Liu F, Liu D. Enhanced gene expression in mouse lung by prolonging the retention time of intravenously injected plasmid DNA. *Gene Ther* 1998;5:1531–1537.

70. Cheng L, Ziegelhoffer PR, Yang NS. *In vivo* promoter activity and transgene expression in mammalian somatic tissues evaluated by using particle bombardment. *Proc Natl Acad Sci U S A* 1993;90:4455–4459.

71. Gao X, Huang L. Cationic liposome-mediated gene transfer [Review]. *Gene Ther* 1995;2:710–722.

72. Lee RJ, Huang L. Lipidic vector systems for gene transfer. *Crit Rev Ther Drug Carrier Syst* 1997;14:173–206.

73. Zhu N, Liggitt D, Liu YL, et al. Systemic gene expression after intravenous DNA delivery into adult mice. *Science* 1993;261:209–211.

74. Templeton NS, Lasic DD, Frederik PM, et al. Improved DNA: liposome complexes for increased systemic delivery and gene expression. *Nat Biotechnol* 1998;15:647–652.

75. Clayman GL, El-Naggar AK, Lippman SM, et al. Adenovirus-mediated p53 gene transfer in patients with advanced recurrent head and neck squamous cell carcinoma. *J Clin Oncol* 1998;16:2221–2232.

76. Connors TA. The choice of prodrugs for gene directed enzyme prodrug therapy of cancer. *Gene Ther* 1995;2:702–709.

77. Knox RJ, Friedlos F, Boland MP. The bioactivation of CB 1954 and its use as a prodrug in antibody-directed enzyme prodrug therapy (ADEPT). *Cancer Metastasis Rev* 1993;12:195–212.

78. Ram Z, Culver KW, Oshiro EM, et al. Therapy of malignant brain tumors by intratumoral implantation of retroviral vector-producing cells. *Nat Med* 1997;3:1354–1361.

79. Vogelstein B. Cancer. A deadly inheritance. *Nature* 1990;348:681–682.

80. Lowe S, Ruley H, Jacks T, et al. p53-dependent apoptosis modulates the cytotoxicity of anticancer agents. *Cell* 1993;74:957–967.

81. Hunt KK, Deng J, Liu TJ, et al. Adenovirus-mediated overexpression of the transcription factor E2F-1 induces apoptosis in human breast and ovarian carcinoma cell lines and does not require *p53*. *Cancer Res* 1997;57:4722–4726.

82. Fueyo J, Gomez-Manzano C, Yung WK, et al. Overexpression of E2F-1 in glioma triggers apoptosis and suppresses tumor growth *in vitro* and *in vivo*. *Nat Med* 1998;4:685–690.

83. Ji L, Fang B, Yen N, Fong K, Minna JD, Roth JA. Induction of apoptosis and inhibition of tumorigenicity and tumor growth by adenovirus vector-mediated *FHIT* gene overexpression. *Cancer Res* 1999;59:3333–3339.

84. Birikh KR, Heaton PA, Eckstein F. The structure, function and application of the hammerhead ribozyme [Review]. *Eur J Biochem* 1997;245:1–16.

85. Stull RA, Szoka Jr FC. Antigene, ribozyme and aptamer nucleic acid drugs: progress and prospects [Review]. *Pharm Res* 1995;12:465–483.

86. Marasco WA. Intrabodies: turning the humoral immune system outside in for intracellular immunization [Review]. *Gene Ther* 1997;4:11–15.

87. Le Chevalier T, Arriagada R, Quoix E, et al. Radiotherapy alone versus combined chemotherapy and radiotherapy in nonresectable non-small-cell lung cancer: first analysis of a randomized trial in 353 patients. *J Natl Cancer Inst* 1991;83:417–423.

88. Schaake-Koning C, van den Bogaert W, Dalesio O, et al. Effects of concomitant cisplatin and radiotherapy on inoperable non-small cell lung cancer. *N Engl J Med* 1992;326:524–530.

89. Buler RE, Pegram M, Runnebaum I, et al. A phase I study of gene therapy with recombinant intraperitoneal p53 in recurrent ovarian cancer. *Cancer Gene Ther* 1998;5:S25(abst).

90. Fisher DE. Apoptosis in cancer therapy: crossing the threshold. *Cell* 1994;78:539–542.

91. Thompson CB. Apoptosis in the pathogenesis and treatment of disease. *Science* 1995;267:1456–1462.

92. Hetts SW. To die or not to die: an overview of apoptosis and its role in disease [Review]. *JAMA* 1998;279:300–307.

93. Lotem J, Sachs L. Regulation by bcl-2, c-myc, and p53 of susceptibility to induction of apoptosis by heat shock and cancer chemotherapy compounds in differentiation-competent and -defective myeloid leukemic cells. *Cell Growth Differ* 1993;4:41–47.

94. Miyashita T, Reed JC. Bcl-2 oncoprotein blocks chemotherapy-induced apoptosis in a human leukemia cell line. *Blood* 1993;81:151–157.

95. Staunton MJ, Gaffney EF. Apoptosis: basic concepts and potential significance in human cancer [Review]. *Arch Pathol Lab Med* 1998;122:310–319.

96. Weller M, Malipiero U, Rensing-Ehl A, et al. Fas/APO-1 gene transfer for human malignant glioma. *Cancer Res* 1995;55:2936–2944.

97. Piche A, Grim J, Rancourt C, et al. Modulation of Bcl-2 protein levels by an intracellular anti-Bcl-2 single-chain antibody increases drug-induced cytotoxicity in the breast cancer cell line MCF-7. *Cancer Res* 1998;58:2134–2140.

98. Arai H, Gordon D, Nabel EG, et al. Gene transfer of Fas ligand induces tumor regression *in vivo*. *Proc Natl Acad Sci U S A* 1997;94:13862–13867.

99. Krajewski S, Blomqvist C, Franssila K, et al. Reduced expression of proapoptotic gene BAX is associated with poor response rates to combination chemotherapy and shorter survival in women with metastatic breast adenocarcinoma. *Cancer Res* 1995;55:4471–4478.

100. Binder C, Marx D, Binder L, et al. Expression of Bax in relation to Bcl-2 and other predictive parameters in breast cancer. *Ann Oncol* 1996;7:129–133.

101. Kapranos N, Karaiosifidi H, Valavanis C, et al. Prognostic significance of apoptosis related proteins Bcl-2 and Bax in node-negative breast cancer patients. *Anticancer Res* 1997;17:2499–2505.

102. Tai YT, Lee S, Niloff E, et al. BAX protein expression and clinical outcome in epithelial ovarian cancer. *J Clin Oncol* 1998;16:2583–2590.

103. Strobel T, Swanson L, Korsmeyer S, et al. BAX enhances paclitaxel-induced apoptosis through a p53-independent pathway. *Proc Natl Acad Sci U S A* 1996;93:14094–14099.

104. Strobel T, Kraeft SK, Chen LB, et al. BAX expression is associated with enhanced intracellular accumulation of paclitaxel: a novel role for BAX during chemotherapy-induced cell death. *Cancer Res* 1998;58:4776–4781.

105. Sakakura C, Sweeney EA, Shirahama T, et al. Overexpression of bax enhances the radiation sensitivity in human breast cancer cells. *Surg Today* 1997;27:90–93.

106. Sakakura C, Sweeney EA, Shirahama T, et al. Overexpression of bax sensitizes breast cancer MCF-7 cells to cisplatin and etoposide. *Surg Today* 1997;27:676–679.

107. Schmitt M, Harbeck N, Thomssen C, et al. Clinical impact of the plasminogen activation system in tumor invasion and metastasis: prognostic relevance and target for therapy. *Thromb Haemost* 1997;78:285–296.

108. Wojtowicz-Praga SM, Dickson RB, Hawkins MJ. Matrix metalloproteinase inhibitors [Review]. *Invest New Drugs* 1997;15:61–75.

109. Guenthert U, Birchmeier O. Attempts to understand metastasis formation. In: Anonymous, ed. Current topics in microbiology and immunology. Berlin: Springer-Verlag, 1996.

110. Andreasen PA, Kjoller L, Christensen L, et al. The urokinase-type plasminogen activator system in cancer metastasis: a review. *Int J Cancer* 1997;72:1–22.

111. Torre-Amione G, Beauchamp RD, Koeppen H, et al. A highly immunogenic tumor transfected with a murine transforming growth factor type beta 1 cDNA escapes immune surveillance. *Proc Natl Acad Sci U S A* 1990;87:1486–1490.

112. Blanchet O, Bourge JF, Zinszner H, et al. Altered binding of regulatory factors to HLA class I enhancer sequence in human tumor cell lines lacking class I antigen expression. *Proc Natl Acad Sci U S A* 1992;89:3488–3492.

113. Elliott BE, Carlow DA, Rodricks A-M, et al. Perspectives on the role of MHC antigens in normal and malignant cell development. *Adv Cancer Res* 1989;53:181–245.

114. Gattoni-Celli S, Kirsch K, Timpane R, et al. Beta 2-microglobulin gene is mutated in a human colon cancer cell line (HCT) deficient in the expression of HLA class I antigens on the cell surface. *Cancer Res* 1992;52:1201–1204.

115. Tuting T, Storkus WJ, Lotze MT. Gene-based strategies for the immunotherapy of cancer. *J Mol Med* 1997;75:478–491.

116. Resser JR, Carbone DP. Immunotherapy of head and neck cancer. *Curr Opin Oncol* 1998;10:226–232.

117. Lindauer M, Stanislawski T, Haussler A, et al. The molecular basis of cancer immunotherapy by cytotoxic T lymphocytes. *J Mol Med* 1998;76:42–47.

118. Ferrone S. Human tumor-associated antigen mimicry by anti-idiotypic antibodies. Immunogenicity and clinical trials in patients with solid tumors [Review]. *Ann N Y Acad Sci* 1993;690:214–224.

119. Gattoni-Celli S, Cole DJ. Melanoma-associated tumor antigens and their clinical relevance to immunotherapy [Review]. *Semin Oncol* 1996;23:754–758.

120. Lanzavecchia A. Identifying strategies for immune intervention [Review]. *Science* 1993;260:937–944.

121. Rosenberg SA. The immunotherapy of solid cancers based on cloning the genes encoding tumor-rejection antigens [Review]. *Annu Rev Med* 1996;47:481–491.

122. Allison JP, Hurwitz AA, Leach DR. Manipulation of costimulatory signals to enhance antitumor T-cell responses [Review]. *Curr Opin Immunol* 1995;7:682–686.

123. Pardoll DM. Paracrine cytokine adjuvants in cancer immunotherapy [Review]. *Annu Rev Immunol* 1995;13:399–415.

124. Stingl G, Bergstresser PR. Dendritic cells: a major story unfolds. *Immunol Today* 1995;16:330–333.

125. Morse MA, Lyerly HK. Immunotherapy of cancer using dendritic cells. *Cytokines Cell Mol Ther* 1998;4:35–44.

126. Lotze MT, Shurin M, Davis I, et al. Dendritic cell based therapy of cancer. *Adv Exp Med Biol* 1997;417:551–569.

127. Huang AY, Golumbek P, Ahmadzadeh M, et al. Role of bone marrow-derived cells in presenting MHC class I-restricted tumor antigens. *Science* 1994;264:961–965.

128. Nabel GJ, Nabel EG, Yang ZY, et al. Direct gene transfer with DNA-liposome complexes in melanoma—expression, biologic activity, and lack of toxicity in humans. *Proc Natl Acad Sci U S A* 1993;90:11307–11311.

129. Huang X, Molema G, King S, et al. Tumor infarction in mice by antibody-directed targeting of tissue factor to tumor vasculature. *Science* 1997;275:547–550.

130. Augustin HG. Antiangiogenic tumour therapy: will it work? *Trends Pharmacol Sci* 1998;19:216–222.

131. Fan TP, Jaggar R, Bicknell R. Controlling the vasculature: angiogenesis, anti-angiogenesis and vascular targeting of gene therapy. *Trends Pharmacol Sci* 1995;16:57–66.

132. Norrby K. Angiogenesis: new aspects relating to its initiation and control. *APMIS* 1997;105:417–437.

133. Mukhopadhyay D, Tsiokas L, Sukhatme VP. Wild-type p53 and v-Src exert opposing influences on human vascular endothelial growth factor gene expression. *Cancer Res* 1995;55:6161–6165.

134. Rak J, Filmus J, Finkenzeller G, et al. Oncogenes as inducers of tumor angiogenesis. *Cancer Metastasis Rev* 1995;14:263–277.

135. Bouvet M, Ellis LM, Nishizaki M, et al. Adenovirus-mediated wild-type p53 gene transfer downregulates vascular endothelial growth factor expression and inhibits angiogenesis in human colon cancer. *Cancer Res* 1998;58:2288–2292.

136. Saleh M, Stacker SA, Wilks AF. Inhibition of growth of C6 glioma cells *in vivo* by expression of antisense vascular endothelial growth factor sequence. *Cancer Res* 1996;56:393–401.

137. Lin P, Buxton JA, Acheson A, et al. Antiangiogenic gene therapy targeting the endothelium-specific receptor tyrosine kinase Tie2. *Proc Natl Acad Sci U S A* 1998;95:8829–8834.

138. O'Reilly MS, Boehm T, Shing Y, et al. Endostatin: an endogenous inhibitor of angiogenesis and tumor growth. *Cell* 1997;88:277–285.

139. Cao Y, O'Reilly MS, Marshall B, et al. Expression of angiostatin cDNA in a murine fibrosarcoma suppresses primary tumor growth and produces long-term dormancy of metastases. *J Clin Invest* 1998;101:1055–1063.

140. Tanaka T, Cao Y, Folkman J, et al. Viral vector-targeted antiangiogenic gene therapy utilizing an angiostatin complementary DNA. *Cancer Res* 1998;58:3362–3369.

141. Pastan I, Gottesman MM, Ueda K, et al. A retrovirus carrying an MDR1 cDNA confers multidrug resistance and polarized expression of P-glycoprotein in MDCK cells. *Proc Natl Acad Sci U S A* 1988;85:4486–4490.

142. Sorrentino BP, Brandt SJ, Bodine D, et al. Selection of drug-resistant bone marrow cells *in vivo* after retroviral transfer of human MDR1. *Science* 1992;257:99–103.

143. Moritz T, Mackay W, Glassner BJ, et al. Retrovirus-mediated expression of a DNA repair protein in bone marrow protects hematopoietic cells from nitrosourea-induced toxicity *in vitro* and *in vivo*. *Cancer Res* 1995;55:2608–2614.

144. May C, Gunther R, Mcivor RS. Protection of mice from lethal doses of methotrexate by transplantation with transgenic marrow expressing drug-resistant dihydrofolate-reductase activity. *Blood* 1995;86:2439–2448.

145. Nabel EG, Yang Z, Muller D, et al. Safety and toxicity of catheter gene delivery to the pulmonary vasculature in a patient with metastatic melanoma. *Hum Gene Ther* 1994;5:1089–1094.

146. Habib NA, Ding S-F, El-Masry R, et al. Contrasting effects of direct p53 DNA injection in primary and secondary liver tumours. *Tumor Targeting* 1995;1:295–298.

147. Habib NA, Ding SF, El-Masry R, et al. Preliminary report: the short term effects of direct p53 DNA injection in primary hepatocellular carcinomas. *Cancer Detect Prev* 1996;20(2):103–107.

148. Roth JA, Nguyen D, Lawrence DD, et al. Retrovirus-mediated wild-type p53 gene transfer to tumors of patients with lung cancer. *Nat Med* 1996;2:985–991.

149. Swisher SG, Roth JA, Nemunaitis J, et al. Adenoviral-mediated p53 gene transfer in advanced non-small cell lung cancer. *J Natl Cancer Inst* 1999;91:763–771.

20.5

GENE THERAPY: CLINICAL APPLICATIONS

Antisense Oligodeoxynucleotides

IRINA LEBEDEVA
C. A. STEIN

A major problem with the use of cytotoxic and biologic agents in the treatment of human cancer is the lack of specificity. Many systemic targets other than those critical to the growth and reproduction of the malignant cell may be attacked during the clinical course of treatment; this inevitably leads to systemic toxicity to the patient, and in turn leads to a diminution in drug dose, dose intensity, and therapeutic efficacy.

It is the idea of specificity of treatment that provides the impetus to use antisense oligonucleotides as therapeutic agents. In one of several possible antisense approaches, the idea of specificity is embodied in the ability of messenger RNA (mRNA) to bind to its complement via Watson-Crick base pair formation. In theory, if the protein that results from the translation of any mRNA is necessary for cellular growth and division and if the translation of that mRNA into protein can be blocked, then cellular reproduction can also be blocked (Fig. 1). (It should be noted that the selection of mRNA that is necessary changes over time. What was thought necessary in the early 1990s is now perhaps not entirely so because of a greater appreciation of the redundancy of intracellular pathways.) It had been long postulated that one way to inhibit translation of mRNA into protein would be to anneal to it a short, sequence-complementary oligodeoxynucleotide (oligo) (1). It was believed, and may well be true in some cases, that the resulting mRNA-DNA hybrid would then be impervious to ribosomal read-through; this oligo would thus cause cessation of protein synthesis. Because, by convention, the mRNA strand is the sense strand, the oligo is known as the *antisense strand*. Because an oligo of more than 15 to 17 nucleotides in length would have a unique sequence relative to the entire human genome, absolute specificity would, in theory, be assured. These were the assumptions that directed antisense research over the past 15 years. This research has, indeed, led to several human clinical therapeutic trials and the approval by the U.S. Food and Drug Administration of the antisense oligonucleotide fomivirsen, which is active in the treatment of cytomegalovirus retinitis (2). Many other trials have not been successful, which cannot be too surprising given the novelty of this technology.

Some of the first antisense experiments were performed by Stevenson and Zamecnik (3,4) who manually synthesized a series of phosphodiester oligomers complementary to the terminal reiterated sequences of the Rous sarcoma virus mRNA. They found that reverse transcriptase activity was drastically decreased in the supernatants of infected chick embryo fibroblast cells, but lack of a convenient synthetic method made further work difficult. Soon thereafter, a major advance in oligo synthetic chemistry was made by Caruthers (5) and his coworkers, who developed the phosphoramidite method of oligonucleotide synthesis. The method made possible the synthesis of oligonucleotides of virtually any length with only ~1% product loss during each coupling step of monomer to the growing chain. Automation quickly followed, leading to several generations of so-called gene machines. These machines have made oligo synthesis almost routine for many laboratories; their industrial counterparts are capable of synthesizing grams of material at a time.

Over the past 15 years, a large amount of effort has gone into solving problems resulting from certain structural features of DNA. The simplest class of oligonucleotide that can be synthesized contains a phosphodiester linkage at each phosphorus atom, and is called *normal* or *phosphodiester DNA*. A major problem with the use of this type of oligonucleotide is that ubiquitous intra- and extracellular nucleases rapidly and completely digest them. Digestion appears to occur predominantly from the 3' to 5' direction (6), although endonuclease digestion (at internal sites) probably occurs in at least some human tumor cell lines. Digestion may be vitiated by heat inactivation of the serum at 65°C but not eliminated. Also, it should be remembered that the concentration of an n-mer oligo on a per base basis is n times the molar concentration of the oligo. Complete digestion of a phosphodiester oligomer, therefore, yields large quantities of nucleotide monophosphates that may have significant biologic activity, as has been pointed out by Vaerman et al. (7). For example, deoxyadenosine monophosphate, a product of phosphodiester oligonucleotide digestion, can be transformed into dATP. This molecule can inhibit ribonucleotide reductase, which is necessary to synthesize deoxyribonucleotides from ribonucleotides. Additionally, deoxyadenosine triphosphate can form a complex with the proteins Apaf-1 and procaspase

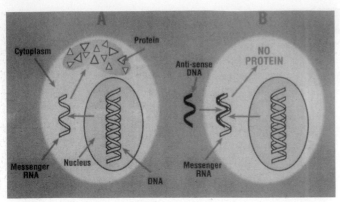

FIGURE 1. A schematic representation of the basis of antisense oligode-oxynucleotide-mediated inhibition of gene expression. The flow of genetic information in untreated cells **(A)** is from DNA to RNA to protein. When the cells are treated with oligodeoxynucleotides complementary to a specific messenger RNA **(B)**, the oligodeoxynucleotides hybridize to messenger RNA and cause inhibition of protein synthesis. In theory, the size and the sequence of the oligodeoxynucleotide exert specificity. [From Sharma HW, Narayanan R. The therapeutic potential of antisense oligonucleotides. *Bioessays* 1995;17(12):1055–1063, with permission.]

9 (8), which appears to initiate the intracellular apoptotic process. Control oligonucleotides without the same proportions of bases may produce entirely different results. Therefore, molecules that contain only phosphodiester linkages cannot be used as antisense oligomers.

Since 1980, significant effort has been expended to develop nuclease-resistant oligonucleotides. Spearheading these efforts were P. Miller and P. Ts'o at Johns Hopkins, who synthesized methylphosphonate oligonucleotides (9,10), and W. Stec and G. Zon (11), who, based on earlier work of F. Eckstein and colleagues (12), synthesized phosphorothioate oligonucleotides. In the methylphosphonate oligonucleotide, a methyl group replaces one of the nonbridging oxygen atoms at phosphorus. If a methylphosphonate linkage is placed at each phosphorus, the result is nuclease indigestibility but also net loss of the negative charge. These uncharged methylphosphonate oligonucleotides are significantly less soluble than their charged congeners, which may result in formulation difficulties with some methylphosphonate oligonucleotides and the need for using high concentrations (>50 μ*M*) to achieve biologic effects. Methylphosphonate oligonucleotides have been shown to block translation of a mutated Ha-ras allele in transformed NIH 3T3 fibroblasts without affecting the wild-type allele (13), but there have been relatively few other successful antisense experiments published using methylphosphonate oligonucleotides at the time of this writing. This may be due to one serious drawback to the tissue culture or *in vivo* applications of methylphosphonate oligonucleotides and to uncharged oligomers in general. Methylphosphonate oligonucleotides and other nonanionic antisense oligonucleotides, such as peptide nucleic acids, do not act as substrates for ribonuclease (RNase) H activity.

As of this writing, RNase H activity appears to be the major driving force behind what is experimentally observed as antisense inhibition of protein translation. The enzyme is ubiquitous; its function is to cleave the RNA strand of an mRNA-DNA duplex. The oligomer can then dissociate from the cleaved mes-

sage and interact with another uncleaved target, in effect making antisense oligonucleotides catalytic. Although this hypothesis is attractive and probably true, it has never been rigorously proven to be so in mammalian cells. If true, though, it would seem to indicate that the antisense effect must take place in the nucleus, because that is where the majority of the RNase H activity is located. Evidence that tends to support this view is that in the absence of oligonucleotide carriers (e.g., cationic lipids, polyamines), nuclear localization of fluorescent oligomer does not occur, and neither does antisense activity (except perhaps under certain circumstances.

RNase H does not require 100% complementarity of oligo with mRNA to cleave the mRNA strand. In fact, it is generally believed that only a six-base region of complementarity may be necessary (14). This fact creates an unusual set of counterintuitive problems. It is accepted that the higher the melting temperature of the DNA-mRNA duplex, the more likely that translation will be inhibited. However, if increased Tm is obtained by lengthening the oligomer, the phenomenon of irrelevant cleavage appears. *Irrelevant cleavage* refers to the RNase H cleavage (14,15) of nontargeted duplexes and is due to the minimal cleavage requirements of RNase H. Thus, if a six-base region of complementarity is all that is required for cleavage, then the longer the antisense oligonucleotide, the more six-base motifs are contained within it, and thus the more cleavage of nontargeted mRNAs bearing that motif theoretically occur. However, if the oligomer is too short, the Tm may be too low for optimal hybridization. Each of these difficulties seems to be minimized at a length of approximately 18- to 20-mer, which appears to be the optimum length for an antisense oligonucleotide.

We have encountered irrelevant cleavage in some of our recent studies on the antisense oligonucleotide inhibition of protein kinase C-α (PKC-α) protein expression (16). The earliest work with these oligonucleotides was performed by Dean and colleagues (17), who evaluated two 20-mer phosphorothioate oligomers, Isis 3521 and Isis 3522. The former is targeted to the 3' UTR of the mRNA and the latter to the initiation codon region. In our work (16), PKC-α, but not PKC-α, -β1, -δ, or -ε protein, and mRNA expression were more than 80% (n = 13) inhibited by both. However, Isis 3521 also inhibited (>90%) PKC-ζ protein and mRNA expression, which Isis 3522 did not. This may be accounted for by irrelevant cleavage, as there is an 11-base contiguous complementarity between Isis 3521 and the PKC-ζ mRNA, but only a four-base complementarity between it and Isis 3522 (Fig. 2). Similarly, we have identified several antisense oligonucleotides that target the bcl-xL mRNA in prostate cancer cells that also, presumably because of complementarity and irrelevant cleavage, eliminate bcl-2 protein expression as well. These oligonucleotides are modified at the C5 position of each pyrimidine in the molecule by a propyne residue, which dramatically increases the Tm of the DNA-mRNA (18,19) and hence irrelevant cleavage as well. Such molecules may find clinical application, because it is difficult to believe that downregulation of only a single intracellular target, given the redundancy in intracellular pathways, is sufficient to kill a single cell, much less a collection of the heterogeneous cancer cells typically found in patients. In fact, in the experiments described, synchronous downregulation of bcl-xL and bcl-2 does inhibit cellular prolif-

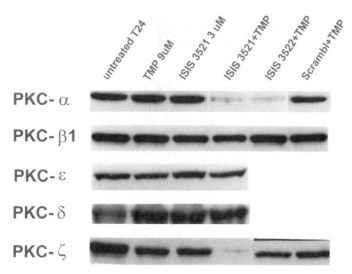

FIGURE 2. Regulation of protein kinase C (PKC) isoform expression by complexes of phosphorothioate oligonucleotides with tetra meso(4-methylpyridyl)porphine (TMP) in the T24 bladder-carcinoma cell line. The phosphorothioate oligonucleotide ISIS 3521 directed against the PKC-α messenger RNA (mRNA) causes irrelevant cleavage of the PKC-ζ mRNA. Western blots of total protein lysate stained with the corresponding monoclonal antibodies are shown. (MAb, monoclonal antibodies, mRNA, messenger RNA.) (From Benimetskaya L, Takle O, Vilenchik M, et al. Cellular delivery of antisense oligodeoxynucleotides by a novel cationic porphyrin vehicle. *Nucleic Acids Res* 1998;26:5310–5317, with permission.)

can be slowly digested. The rate of digestion seems to be dependent on sequence (phosphorothioate and phosphodiester linkages 5' to purines are stable), and on the stereochemistry at phosphorus. [The oligonucleotide phosphorothioate-linkage is chiral (i.e., has the property of handedness). The two enantiomers are named Rp and Sp. The Rp stereoisomer is digested as rapidly as a phosphodiester linkage, whereas the Sp linkage is digested more slowly.] Intracellular digestion can lead to the release of nucleotide monophosphorothioates, which may also be growth inhibitory in some cell lines. In other lines, these molecules may actually be growth stimulatory, with SdG monophosphorothioate being perhaps the most active (24). However, evidence demonstrating that this set of events actually occurs *in vivo* is currently lacking. Phosphorothioate oligonucleotides may act as substrates for RNase H activity when hybridized to their complement, but they can also bind to human RNase H in a nonsequence-specific manner and can competitively inhibit the binding of the enzyme to its DNA-mRNA substrate (25). This type of behavior implies that there may only be a narrow intracellular concentration range in which phosphorothioate oligonucleotides are active antisense agents in at least some human cells.

Several other types of oligonucleotides are nuclease resistant and may act as antisense agents (Fig. 3). Oligoribonucleotides, when modified at the 2'-O position on the ribose moiety with a methyl or other alkyl group, become nuclease resistant and may be useful as antisense agents. They also dramatically increase the Tm of the mRNA-DNA duplex although they are not substrates for RNase H activity (26). They are finding use now as a member of novel chimeric oligonucleotides (27,28), which contain a central core of phosphorothioate linkages to preserve RNase H activity flanked at the 3' and 5' termini by 2'-O-methylribonucleotides to block nuclease digestion and increase Tm. This strategy also probably increases irrelevant cleavage. The phosphate backbones may be removed entirely and replaced with polyamide structures to which the nitrogenous bases are linked (29). These so-called peptide nucleic acids (PNAs) hybridize extremely well to their targets, but are not highly soluble in physiologic saline, are not internalized well by cells, and are in general not useful as antisense oligonucleotides. Many efforts are underway to attempt to expand the range of utility of PNAs to take advantage of their duplex-stabilizing ability, mostly by incorporating them into chimeric oligomers.

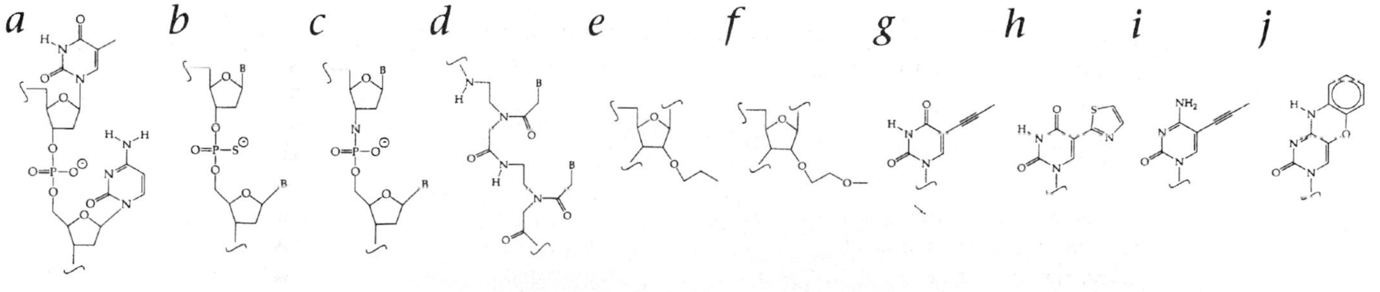

eration to some extent, but does not lead to extensive apoptosis. However, the prostate cancer cells do become sensitized to the proapoptotic effects of several chemotherapeutic agents, including paclitaxel (Taxol), mitoxantrone, and etoposide.

Perhaps the most important modification made to generate nuclease-resistant oligo substitutes a sulfur atom for a nonbridging oxygen atom at each phosphorus, producing a phosphorothioate oligo. The use of these molecules as antisense agents has been reviewed several times (20,21). The substitution retains the net charge and the property of aqueous solubility, but phosphorothioate oligonucleotides hybridize with their complementary mRNAs with lower Tm relative to phosphodiester oligonucleotides. Phosphorothioate oligonucleotides are nuclease resistant both *in vitro* (22) and *in vivo* (23), but in fact

a b c d e f g h i j

FIGURE 3. Modifications of antisense oligonucleotides: (a) an unmodified 5'-TpC-3' dimer; (b) phosphorothioate linkage; (c) N3'-P5' phosphoroamidate linkage; (d) peptide nucleic acid linkage; (e) 2'-O-propyl ribose; (f) 2'-methylethoxy ribose; (g) C-5 propynyl U; (h) C-5 thiazole U; (i) C-5 propynyl C; (j) phenoxazine C. (From Wagner RW. The state of art in antisense research. *Nat Med* 1995;1:1116–1118, with permission.)

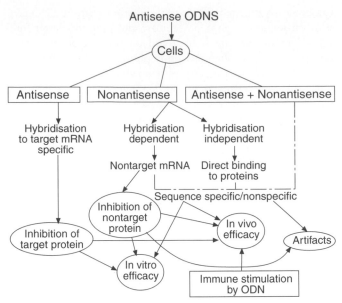

Antisense ODNS

FIGURE 4. A current view of the mechanisms of action of antisense oligodeoxynucleotides (ODNs). Antisense ODN action is complex and involves multiple mechanisms. Multiple controls are needed to rule nonsequence specificity of an ODN. Nonspecific components can mimic specific effects in biologic assays, making interpretation difficult. It is highly likely that specific and nonspecific components coexist in any given antisense ODN experiment. (mRNA, messenger RNA.) (From Sharma HW, Narayanan R. The therapeutic potential of antisense oligonucleotides *Bioessays* 1995;17(12):1055–1063, with permission.)

Oligonucleotides may also be useful in the targeting of individual cellular genes at the DNA level. This is because a polypyrimidine oligo can bind in the major groove of the DNA to form a triple helix. Binding of the oligo to the double helix is a consequence of so-called Hoogsteen base pairing and is stable in the presence of divalent cations for CG...C and TA...T triplets. *In vivo* transcription of the interleukin-2a receptor (30) and of c-myc (31) by targeting of the genomic promoter region has been thus accomplished by the use of triplex-forming phosphodiester oligonucleotides in what has been termed *antigene therapy*. Imaginative variants of the triple helix approach, using the formation of regions of contiguous triplex helix and duplex formation by a single mRNA-targeted phosphodiester oligo or hairpin oligonucleotides forming triple helices with single-strand regions of mRNA, have also been proposed, but at the present time little *in vivo* data is available for evaluation.

INTERPRETATION OF DATA: THE PROBLEM OF NONSEQUENCE SPECIFICITY

It is not possible to interpret literature data in which antisense effects are purportedly documented without an understanding of the effects of the oligo, which confound this antisense interpretation (Fig. 4). This is especially true of phosphorothioate oligonucleotides, for which nonsequence specificity is a major problem.

This nonsequence specific inhibitory activity highlights one of the most significant problems with the use of chemically modified oligonucleotides. This activity, due to the polyanionic

backbone of the oligo, is particularly pronounced for phosphorothioate oligonucleotides. This is reflected in the fact that the binding of a phosphorothioate oligo to a protein usually occurs with a dissociation constant (K_d) that is one to three orders of magnitude lower than that of the isosequential phosphodiester oligo. These values of K_d can lie in the low nanomolar range (32,33) and may approach the affinity of the oligo-bound protein for its natural ligand, whereupon a nonspecific biologic effect of the phosphorothioate oligo can be observed. Such nonsequence specificity of the phosphorothioates has resulted in dose-limiting clinical toxicity in several trials.

It appears that the high-affinity protein binding of phosphorothioate oligomers is specific for heparin-binding proteins (34,35), and in that sense, these antisense oligonucleotides are heparin-mimetics. Nanomolar affinity binding can be observed for basic fibroblast growth factor and other members of the fibroblast growth factor family. Binding can also easily be observed to the proangiogenic vascular endothelial growth factor (VEGF); to platelet-derived growth factor; and to a wide variety of other heparin-binding proteins, including CD4,[32] laminin, and fibronectin [thus dramatically affecting cellular adhesion (36)], Mac-1 (CD11b/CD18), both α and β subunits (37), and to heparin-binding proteins that are cell-surface receptors, including epidermal growth factor receptor (EGFR) (but not EGF, which is not heparin binding), and the VEGF receptor flk-1 (38). The interaction of phosphorothioates with heparin-binding proteins appears to be completely independent of stereochemistry at phosphorus (39). Binding to EGFR (38), however, has curious biologic consequences; the binding of the cognate ligand EGF is inhibited and receptor phosphorylation blocked by phosphorothioate oligonucleotides in a length- and concentration-dependent manner. On the other hand, in the absence of the cognate ligand, receptor autophosphorylation is stimulated. Observations of this kind point out the potential difficulties in data interpretation if cells are treated with naked oligonucleotide (i.e., without a carrier) at high concentration (>10–20 μm). Under these conditions, the biologic activity of phosphorothioate oligonucleotides exclusive of Watson-Crick hybridization is so extensive that the cellular context in which any event is observed cannot be the same as in the untreated cell.

INTERPRETATION OF RESULTS: THE G-QUARTET PROBLEM

It has been shown that certain sequence motifs are overrepresented in reports of oligonucleotides that produce antisense effects (40). These include the GG, GGG, and GGC motifs, which are present at a frequency of 9.9%, 3.4%, and 3.1%, respectively, in a series of successful antisense oligonucleotides. Some sequence motifs occurring at a low frequency in mRNA are found more often in antisense oligonucleotides. For example, the sequence GACG, with an overall frequency of occurrence in mRNA of 0.41%, is present in 10% of 206 evaluated antisense oligonucleotides.

Another sequence motif that appears rather frequently is four contiguous guanosine residues. The trouble arises because this motif has a tendency to form higher order structures; in one such structure, four individual strands interact to form a tetra-plex (41,42). (Thus, DNA can exist in single-stranded, duplex, triplex, and tetraplex forms.) The tetraplex is held together by Hoogsteen base-pair formation between guanosine residues, and the cavity formed has a high affinity for and is stabilized by monovalent cations, although they are not absolutely required for tetraplex formation. Other higher order structures, such as duplexes, can also be formed by Hoogsteen base-pair formation between two identical strands or between nonidentical strands that contain the G-quartet motif. Furthermore, no rules at present define the orientation of the strands in either a duplex or tetraplex. In the latter, for example, all strands may be parallel, or three may be parallel and one antiparallel, or two may be parallel and two antiparallel, etc., leading to a bewildering variety of compounds that all may potentially be in equilibrium with each other in solution. Additionally, the ability of any G-tetrad containing oligo to form tetraplexes depends to some extent on the flanking sequences, but even more so on its position within the molecule. G-tetrads found at or near (probably within three to four bases of) either the 3' or 5' molecular termini can form extremely stable tetraplexes that occasionally can dissociate under strenuous conditions (43). Such species can easily be observed on sodium dodecyl sulfate-polyacrylamide gel electrophoresis (SDS-PAGE) slab gels because they migrate slowly in an electric current. When the four contiguous G are in the center of the molecule, however, tetraplexes may form that dissociate in slab gels but can still be observed by their characteristic migration via capillary gel electrophoresis (44). This is what is observed with the antisense c-myc codon 2–9 18-mer phosphorothioate oligo that has been used in several studies since 1988.

A problem with the use of this type of molecule is that a sense control would not contain four contiguous G, but a four contiguous C residue, which does not have the same ability to form higher order species as the four contiguous Gs. Furthermore, scrambled sequences are not controls if the integrity of the G-quartet is not maintained, or if the four contiguous Gs are not placed in the same position in the control as in the antisense molecule. To further complicate the picture, tetraplexes appear to have increased nonsequence specificity versus the single-stranded form, probably related, at least in part, to charge density (43).

The net effect of all of these caveats is to make the use of four contiguous Gs containing oligonucleotides for antisense purposes problematic and not recommended. In 1997, we performed a series of experiments to show that, depending on the target, such oligonucleotides may mimic antisense activity but are actually related solely to the presence of higher-order structures, such as duplexes and tetraplexes (43). The target was one of the proteins composing the nuclear transcriptional regulatory factor nuclear factor kappa B, p65, or RelA. A 20-mer phosphorothioate oligo at 20 µm had been shown to downregulate RelA protein expression in a variety of cell types both in tissue culture and in xenografted tumors (45). However, this oligo contained the sequence 5' GAGGGG...., which was shown to form stable tetraplexes and other less well-defined higher-order structures. The ability of the monomer to form tetraplexes was eliminated by the substitution of 7-deazagua-

nosine for guanosine at a single position in the G-tetrad. This blocks Hoogsteen base-pair formation while only minimally decreasing (0.5°C) the Tm of Watson-Crick duplex. This substituted molecule does not produce antisense activity, suggesting that what was observed with the original molecule was not due to antisense at all but rather due to a nonspecific effect of the tetraplex. Because of problems of this type, and the fact that commonly used techniques such as SDS-PAGE may erroneously not identify tetraplexes or other higher-order structures, it is probably best not to use molecules containing this motif in any antisense experiments.

INTERPRETATION OF RESULTS: THE NUMBERS PARADOX

An additional seldom-spoken paradox further adds to the quandaries of interpretation of literature-derived data (46). As demonstrated in carefully constructed studies, it has been the almost universal observation that for every eight or so oligomers tested against any one particular target, only one is active. In fact, the ratio of one success in eight tested seems to be the best such attained; 1 success in 12 or, or even 1 in 15 seems to be more common. Tu et al. (47) culled 2,026 reports of successful antisense inhibition from the biomedical literature. Data include:

1. 1,655 (81.7%) citations tested one antisense oligonucleotide only
2. An additional 248 (12.2%) tested two or three
3. Another 81 (3.9%) evaluated from four to nine
4. Only 42 (2.1%) examined more than 10

Thus, 93.9% of the experiments were successful using less than three tested oligonucleotides (and the great majority used only one), when detailed studies by scientists experienced in the field have conclusively shown that at the best only one in eight antisense oligonucleotides (12.5%) is successful. (Success often meant cell death. Phosphorothioates can produce cell death by many mechanisms.) This could mean that the published literature represents a selection bias—that, in fact, perhaps eight times more than 1,655 (equaling 13,240) unique oligomers were evaluated, the literature reporting only the 12.5% positive results. This may in part account for the discrepancy, but it cannot be the only explanation, because certain sequence motifs are highly overrepresented in this group of successful experiments. The other possibility is that some, if not many, of the 1,655 citations do not represent an antisense observation, but combinations of antisense plus nonsequence specificity, or antisense plus cytotoxicity (which may promote antisense efficacy by promoting endosomal leakage of sequestered oligomer), coupled in some cases with G-quartet effects. But without in-depth evaluation, it may be difficult to sort all this out in any given paper after the passage of some years.

None of the preceding discussion should imply that obtaining antisense results is not possible. It assuredly is possible (at least within certain confidence intervals), but doing so requires that certain rules be followed, as in any other area of science. Given here are a series of such rules that we have derived empirically from our own work and that of countless others over the past decade. We believe that if closely adhered to, they provide a good chance that almost any target can be downregulated by an antisense approach. This does not mean that the level of the target is the only level altered by treatment with antisense oligonucleotides, and in that sense we doubt very much that anything approaching absolute specificity exists. However, this point may or may not be of significance depending on the outcome desired by the experimentalist. Over the past several years, the antisense biotechnology field has significantly progressed in its understanding of how to conduct meaningful experiments that do not conflate an antisense effect and non–sequence-specific behavior (48). An initial set of guidelines were published in 1994 (49) but have not been updated to reflect experience.

Antisense Rules: Guidelines To Experimental Design

1. At the present time, the best and most readily commercially available oligonucleotides have the phosphorothioate backbone (see 2). Do not use unprotected phosphodiesters, as the mononucleotide products of enzymatic digestion may cause problems (e.g., inhibition of cellular growth). dG-methylphosphonate may be the most toxic, at least in some cases. Obtain the oligomers from a reputable manufacturer. Never store oligonucleotides in water. The pH of such a solution falls in an acidic urban environment, leading to depurination and strand cleavage. Instead, they should be stored between pH 7.5 and 8.0 in buffer, such as tris-ethylenediaminetetraacetic acid, at −20°C (although they survive almost indefinitely at 4°C).

2. Nonsequence specificity must be minimized. The lower the concentration of oligonucleotide used in the experiment, the better. Phosphorothioate 3' and 5' endcapped oligomers (three phosphorothioates per terminus, the remainder of the linkages' phosphodiester) preserve RNase H activity and diminish sulfur content, and thus nonsequence specificity. C5-propyne substitution at one or more pyrimidine residues in the oligomer, or 2'-O-methyl–RNA substitution may increase Tm and potentiate the antisense effect. Use these judiciously, however, as irrelevant cleavage also probably increases, and the C5-propyne residues may be toxic, especially *in vivo*.

3. To find an active oligomer, randomly generate a panel of 30–40 oligomers by walking along mRNA. For every eight to ten oligonucleotides tested, probably just one is active. (This can be an expensive way of doing things, but at the moment, there is little other choice. However, it is possible that the TCCC motif may promote activity because RNase H prefers purine cleavage site mRNA.) mRNA-folding programs are not predictive of active molecules and have little or no value in selecting target sites because they cannot account for local, critical microenvironments at the mRNA level. The other oligomers that are not active can be thought of as controls for the backbone. The more control oligomers used, the more likely that an observed effect represents true antisense.

4. Demonstrate inhibition of the target protein by Western blotting and of the mRNA by Northern blotting or by reverse transcriptase-polymerase chain reaction. However, it is possible

that some antisense activity can occur via steric blockade (28), and thus mRNA levels do not change. This is especially true for 2'-O-methyloligoribonucleotides, which are not substrates for RNase H activity. However, for deoxyribonucleotide oligomers that are all-phosphorothioate, or chimerics (also known as *gapmer*) containing either phosphorothioate or phosphodiester linkages or both, the general consensus is that target mRNA levels should decrease in the presence of an active antisense oligonucleotide because of RNase-H activity.

Question of Appropriate Controls

5. A sense-oligomer control is not necessary, and a total random-mer (mixture of bases at each position) is not an appropriate control. The other oligonucleotides that are active can be used to determine specificity by examining their effects on proteins that are related to the target (e.g., one with an approximately equal half-life that is in the same family). Do not use actin as a control protein if your target has a half-life of only a few hours. The evaluation of the expression of other genes with significant sequence homology may be important to evaluate the extent of irrelevant cleavage. Remember, the more control oligomers tested, the more assurance that the result is specific (arbitrary minimum of two). The use of oligonucleotides with two different backbones, each producing the identical antisense effect, is usually convincing. An additional control is to attempt to antisense knockout your gene in an over-expressing line. If the cells are rescued from the antisense effect, your case is strengthened, but still not proved.

6. Another useful control is to introduce the target gene with one or more mutations in the region complementary to the antisense molecule. Lack of inhibition suggests a true antisense effect, but does not prove it if the rate of transcription and hence the copy number of the mRNA is high. An additional control is to clone your gene in the antisense orientation into an expression vector. Successful suppression of translation of the transfected gene, with the identical biologic activity as seen with the antisense oligomers, is always convincing. Because of high-order mRNA structure, however, the antisense strand may not be able to invade the sense strand, and the method may fail.

Cellular Delivery of Antisense Oligonucleotides

7. Do not treat cells with naked phosphorothioate oligonucleotides, although exceptions to this rule may exist. As mentioned, phosphorothioates are highly nonspecifically active at the cell membrane, with concentrations as low as 2 μm causing defined effects.

8. Deliver oligonucleotides with a carrier. Many are commercially available, including Lipofectin, LipofectACE, Cytofectin (serum stable), Starburst dendrimers of many generations, cationic porphyrins, and others. Remember that antisense may be caused by the summation of effects of the carrier plus the oligomer, as the carriers dissociate from the oligomer intracellularly. You must optimize the molar ratios and concentrations for each carrier and cell line, and probably oligomer sequence as well.

And Watch Out for . . .

9. When possible, avoid active oligomers with the CpG motif. Depending on the sequence context, they can be highly immune stimulating (50). This can be a problem in xenograft models (if it is your eventual plan to use them) because of immune-mediated graft rejection. However, methylation at C5 of cytidine eliminates immune stimulation.

10. Do not treat cells with oligonucleotides containing G-quartets until verified by capillary gel-electrophoresis that higher-order structures are not present in solution.

11. Finally, do not attempt to correlate an observed biologic effect with antisense efficacy (e.g., do not say that an antisense effect is causative of inhibition of proliferation or cell death, as especially the phosphorothioates are intrinsically too biologically active. Rather, demonstrate downregulation of protein expression by Western blotting and target mRNA levels by Northern blot, and make no other claims.

12. These rules are subject to change and augmentation as the field advances.

CELLULAR UPTAKE OF ANTISENSE OLIGODEOXYNUCLEOTIDES

The success of oligonucleotides as antisense agents depends on their efficient delivery to the cytoplasm and the nucleus. Phosphorothioate oligonucleotides are taken up by a wide range of cells *in vitro* (51). In many cases, internalization is a calcium-dependent process (52) and is slowed by metabolic inhibitors, such as deoxyglucose, cytochalasin B, and sodium azide (53). Oligonucleotide internalization in tissue culture depends predominantly on the two processes of adsorptive endocytosis and fluid-phase endocytosis (pinocytosis). The adsorptive process has two components; initial binding to the cell surface and internalization (33,53). Supporting the importance of adsorptive endocytosis is the fact that oligonucleotides that adsorb well to the cell surface (e.g., phosphodiesters and phosphorothioates) tend to be internalized to a much higher degree than those that do not (methylphosphonates and peptide nucleic acids) (54). Uptake is also influenced by temperature, cell type, cell culture conditions, media, sequence (to a small extent), and length of the oligonucleotide (55). The existence of an oligonucleotide receptor mediating active transport has been postulated (51,53), but a purified or cloned receptor protein, or both, is still not available to date, except for Mac-1, which has been shown to be an oligonucleotide-binding and -internalization protein in human polymorphonuclear leukocytes (37). The predominant mechanism of uptake is concentration dependent: At an oligomer concentration less than 1 μm, uptake occurs by the relatively efficient process of adsorptive endocytosis (56,57). Uptake occurring via fluid-phase endocytosis is less efficient at higher oligonucleotide concentrations.

Regardless of the mechanism of the uptake, the bulk of the internalized oligomer is trapped, at least initially, in an intracellular vesicle (54). However, this compartment is useless for antisense activity. Here, antisense oligonucleotides are sequestered from their ultimate targets in the nucleus and cytoplasm and are directly exposed to degradative enzymes. If oligonucleotides can escape from the endosomal/lysosomal compartment into cytoplasm, it appears they are rapidly translocated to the nucleus (58).

Delivery Facilitated by Carriers

Enhanced delivery of oligodeoxynucleotides to cells has been achieved by linking them to hydrophobic moieties, such as peptides (59–61), cholesterol (62), or poly-L-lysine. The targeted transfer of antisense oligonucleotides can also be achieved by using small synthetic peptides that are specific to cellular receptors (63). Additionally, sugar moieties, such as lactose or mannose, can be bound to the polycation poly-L-lysine, forming complexes that can bind to sugar receptors expressed on various target cells (64,65). Covalent linking of hydrophobic molecules to the 3'-position of the oligomer decreases degradation by nucleases and increases intracellular internalization, probably by an interaction between the complex and the cell membrane (66,67). However, the hydrophobic groups may dramatically reduce the melting temperature of the hybrid of oligonucleotide with its target mRNA and may interfere with the intracellular distribution of the oligonucleotide conjugate. Linkers susceptible to cleavage by intracellular internalization have been designed and include disulfide and carboxyester bonds [e.g., acyloxyalkyl esters of phosphorothioate oligodeoxynucleotides (68) and S-alkyl-phosphorothioates (69)].

Delivery by Cationic Lipids and Liposomes

Encapsulation of oligonucleotides into liposomes has been used to increase their delivery across membranes (70). Liposomes are spheric structures consisting of multiple phospholipid bilayers. They are arranged to create hydrophobic layers alternating with hydrophilic layers or can consist of a single phospholipid bilayer encasing an aqueous core. Antisense sequences can either be partitioned into the hydrophobic layers [if a hydrophobic moiety such as cholesterol is conjugated to the oligonucleotide (71)] or be dissolved in the aqueous layers. Additionally, the lipid protects the oligonucleotide from serum or lysosomal nucleases. Liposomes can be targeted by attached antibodies to specific cell surface markers (72).

Alternatively, cationic lipids such as Lipofectin or Cytofectin are frequently used as delivery vectors. This class of transfection agents contains positively charged amine groups that interact directly with the negatively charged phosphate residues of the oligonucleotide. These complexes result in efficient delivery to the cytoplasm and nucleus, presumably via destabilization of endosomal membranes (73–75). Attempts have been made to modify the lipids by adding ligands of such cellular receptors as folate, providing a targeted delivery to tumor cells (76,77). Other modifications include the use of peptide or protein residues, and antibodies directed against antigens expressed on the target cells (78–80). However, one disadvantage of the use of cationic lipids is that significant cellular toxicity of the oligonucleotide-lipid complex has been observed.

Another approach is the delivery of oligonucleotides adsorbed to polyalkylcyanoacrylate (81,82), methylmethacrylate (83), or polynanoparticles (D-, L-lactose) (84). However, cyanoacrylate-based nanoparticles have significant cytotoxicity. Some improvement in toxicity has been achieved using novel polymers, such as methylmethacrylate. Water-soluble macromolecular carrier systems, such as polyamine-poly(ethylene glycol) copolymers (85) and N-(2-hydroxypropyl)methacrylamide polymer (86) have shown great potential for oligonucleotide delivery. They exhibit little or no binding to cell surfaces, little immunogenicity, and are captured by cells via fluid-phase endocytosis. Cationic porphyrins (16,87), and Starburst dendrimers (88) are also efficient for oligonucleotide delivery in tissue culture.

Our ability to specifically inhibit gene expression in tissue culture has dramatically increased because there are several approaches available for the exogenous delivery of oligonucleotides. However, oligonucleotide delivery *in vivo* may not require them. In animal studies, several provocative reports have suggested that oligodeoxynucleotides can penetrate cells in at least some tissues in the absence of cationic lipids (89–91). More recently, though, these results too have been called into question (92).

CLINICAL TRIALS OF ANTISENSE OLIGONUCLEOTIDES IN CANCER

Despite mechanistic questions and delivery issues, there have been definite successes in antisense technology. Problems have existed with the interpretation of earlier results, and nonantisense effects of oligodeoxynucleotides continue to emerge. However, convincing demonstrations of specific antisense effects have been achieved using highly controlled assays. The first Investigational New Drug application for an antisense oligonucleotide was filed with the U.S. Food and Drug Administration in late 1991 (92). Since that time, antisense oligonucleotides complementary to selected targets, such as *c-Myc* (93), *c-Myb* (94), *c-Raf* (95), PKC-α (96), prekallikrein activator (97,98), *H-ras* (26,99), and bcl-2 (100,111), have been studied extensively in *in vitro* and *in vivo* models and are currently being evaluated in human clinical trials. All antisense oligonucleotides in human clinical trials are phosphorothioates except for that targeting prekallikrein activator, which is a mixed-backbone oligonucleotide (phosphorothioate oligodeoxynucleotide containing regions of 2'-O-methyloligoribonucleotides).

Preclinical and Clinical Toxicology

The animal pharmacokinetics and toxicology of the phosphorothioates appear to be a result of the chemical structure of the oligonucleotides and not the specific antisense sequence (101–103). To date, pharmacokinetic and toxicologic data obtained in animals are surprisingly similar among phosphorothioates of widely differing sequences directed against disparate gene products (104). Phosphorothioates appear to be distributed predominantly to liver, kidney, spleen, and lymph nodes, with lesser amounts being found in heart, pancreas, lungs, bone marrow, and virtually none in the central nervous system (105–107). The elimination half-life of phosphorothioates from tissue compartments may be two- to threefold longer than that found in the plasma, which is 24 to 72 hours (108).

A major toxicity of the phosphorothioates is due to oligonucleotide activation of complement (109). Other problems include their binding to thrombin resulting in a transient coagulopathy. Additionally, the immunostimulatory effects of DNA (bacterial DNA and phosphorothioate oligonucleotides containing the CpG motif are mitogenic to lymphocytes and stimulate cytokine release) should be appreciated (50). These effects are dependent not only on the CpG motif, but on the flanking sequences as well. When optimized, sufficient immunostimulation can be observed in rodents to warrant developing these molecules as vaccine adjuvants.

An antiproliferative effect may require continued exposure to the antisense drug; therefore, antisense drugs might have to be administered orally for maximum effect. However, the compounds presently in trial are not orally bioavailable due to their size, charge, and acid lability.

Therapeutic Applications

Because the ultimate effect of antisense oligonucleotides on the time to disease progression, the time to metastasis, or survival may require months or years to determine, in some cases the evolution of these agents may depend on the measurement of pharmacokinetic, molecular, or biologic end points (110). This has been accomplished with varying degrees of success in the experiments described in the following paragraphs (Table 1).

The bcl-2 proto-oncogene is derived from t(14;18) chromosomal translocation (111). Overproduction of bcl-2 protein is seen in one-half or more of human malignancies and has been suggested to be a poor prognostic marker in some cases (112). Increased bcl-2 expression is also known to inhibit apoptosis and to be associated with resistance to multiple chemotherapeutic agents in both cell culture and tumors *in vivo* (113).

Several groups have explored the antitumor activity *in vitro* of oligonucleotides directed against bcl-2 (114,115). G3139, an 18-mer phosphorothioate oligonucleotide directed against the first six codons of the human bcl-2 mRNA, significantly reduced bcl-2 protein expression and cell viability of DoHH2 lymphoma cells. G3139 was administered to severe combined immunodeficiency disease (SCID)-hu mice inoculated with lymphoma xenografts (116). Disease-free survival in treated mice appeared to be related to dose and to the duration of the infusion. G3139 doses of 1, 5, and 10 mg per kg, cured 0%, 50%, and 100% of the mice, respectively.

The preliminary results of a clinical trial G3139 have been published. Nine patients with bcl-2-positive, relapsed, stage-IV non-Hodgkin's lymphoma were treated in the United Kingdom (117). The phosphorothioate oligonucleotide was tolerated in doses up to 73.6 mg per m^2 per day. The authors found that in some treated patients, antisense therapy led to an improvement in symptoms. In two patients, this was accompanied by biochemical and computed transaxial tomography scan evidence of tumor response. In two patients, the number of circulating lymphoma cells decreased during treatment. Bcl-2 protein levels in lymphocyte and bone marrow samples were measured in five patients and

TABLE 1. ONGOING CLINICAL TRIALS (1998) USING ANTISENSE OLIGONUCLEOTIDES (OLIGOS) IN ONCOLOGIC THERAPEUTICS

Gene Target	Name of the Oligo	Sponsor	Backbone	Size	Disease/Trial Phase	Method of Delivery	Reference
Bcl-2	G3139	Genta and Memorial Sloan-Kettering Cancer Center	PS	18-mer	Non-Hodgkin's lymphoma/phase 1	Systemic, s.c.	118
					Prostate cancer/phase 1–2a		119
c-myb	LR-3001	A. Gewirtz and Lynx	PS	24-mer	CML/phase 1	Systemic, i.v.	124
					AML/phase 1–2	*Ex vivo* purging of bone marrow	125
bcr abl		Lynx	PS	26-mer	CML advanced phase/pilot	*Ex vivo* purging of bone marrow	133,134
p53 exon	OL(1)p53	J. Armitage and Lynx	PS	20-mer	AML and myelodysplastic syndrome/phase 1	Systemic, i.v.	135
						Ex vivo purging of bone marrow and peripheral blood stem cells	138
PKC-α	CGP64128 A (ISIS 3521)	ISIS/Novartis	PS	20-mer	Variety of solid tumors (ovarian, prostate, breast, brain, colon, lung) and melanoma phase 1–2a	Systemic, i.v.	142–144
PKA-1	GEM 231	Hybridon	PS with 2'-O-Me modifications of a backbone	18-mer	Refractory solid tumors/phase 1	Systemic, i.v.	99
c-raf kinase	CGP69846 A (ISIS 5132)	ISIS/Novartis	PS	20-mer	Variety of solid tumors (ovarian, prostate, breast, pancreas, colon, lung)/phase 1–2	Systemic, i.v.	146,147
Ha-ras	ISIS 2503	ISIS	PS	20-mer	Variety of solid tumors/phase 1	Systemic, i.v.	100

AML, acute monocytic leukemia; CML, chronic myelogenous leukemia; PKA-1, protein kinase A, type 1; PKC-α, protein kinase C-α.

decreased in two. It is possible that at higher doses or with more prolonged administration a more significant molecular response would be seen. In preparation for potential clinical trials in patients with hematologic and solid tumors, the National Cancer Institute is evaluating the combination of G3139 and cytotoxic agents in preclinical systems to improve the activity of the antisense agent (118). However, it is still unclear if the sequence of G3139 is optimal. Based on other *in vitro* studies, a bcl-2–directed phosphorothioate oligonucleotide of different sequence demonstrated higher efficiency in assays of viability in a small-cell lung cancer cell line (119).

Downregulation of the c-myb proto-oncogene with antisense oligonucleotides has been shown to be efficient *in vitro* and *in vivo* (120). However, the data also indicate that some of the results of the inhibition of cellular proliferation by the *c-myb*–directed oligonucleotide are not sequence specific (121,122). A phosphorothioate oligonucleotide targeting the *c-myb* gene was evaluated as a marrow-purging agent for different groups of nine and 18 chronic- or accelerated-phase patients with chronic myelogenous leukemia (CML) or other refractory leukemias (123,124). The clinical benefits of treatment were uncertain, although some patients demonstrated marked, sustained, hematologic improvement with virtual

normalization of their blood counts. The toxicity of the oligonucleotide treatment was minimal.

The BCR-ABL fusion gene is found in CML (125). The bcr-abl transcript provides a tumor-specific target potentially susceptible to suppression by antisense oligonucleotides. Inhibition of the growth of antisense-treated leukemic cells was observed in several experiments (126). A 26-mer phosphorothioate oligonucleotide directed against the b2a2 breakpoint junction of the bcr-abl transcript completely inhibited the growth of a Philadelphia chromosome-positive cell line, BV173 (127,128). Treatment with this oligonucleotide also increased duration of life of SCID mice implanted with BV173 cells. However, it is possible that the observed inhibition was due to nonsequence specific interactions (129,130), as the oligonucleotides failed to reduce cellular bcr-abl protein levels (131).

A phosphorothioate oligonucleotide specific for the b2a2 junction has been used for the *in vitro* purging of bone marrow cells. A patient with CML was engrafted with the purged marrow cells and was reported to be in a complete hematologic remission at 9 months posttreatment (132). In another group of patients treated with bcr-abl antisense oligodeoxynucleotides, hematopoietic reconstitution of reinfused cells with low toxicity was observed (133). However, Kirkland et al. have investigated purging strategies with phosphodiester and phosphorothioate oligomers and have been unable to show specific inhibition of CML chronic phase progenitors (126). Although effective antisense strategies might be developed, perhaps by combining antisense with other purging agents such as mafosfamide, trials of single-agent antisense purging with BCR-ABL oligomers may be premature in light of the currently available data.

A phase 1 trial using an antisense oligonucleotide [(OL(1)p53) targeted to p53 in 16 patients with refractory acute myeloid leukemia] produced no responses, but treatment-related toxicities attributed to the oligonucleotide were minimal (134). The results of this study are difficult to interpret because in eight patients the p53 status was unknown and was wild type in seven of the other eight. Because p53 can be a proapoptotic protein and its elimination may lead to cell proliferation, the rationale for this trial was unclear (135). It is also possible that the suppression of p53 expression by OL(1)p53, as observed in tissue culture, can be explained by the nonspecific, nonantisense, antiproliferative activity of this molecule (107,136). In further experiments, transplantation of autologous bone marrow cells treated with OL(1)p53 resulted in successful recovery of circulating neutrophils after high-dose therapy in patients with acute myelogenous leukemia or myelodysplastic syndrome (137).

Another promising molecular target for inhibitors of protein phosphorylation is represented by the PKC gene family. PKC is a family of serine-threonine kinases that include at least 11 distinct isozymes and regulate a variety of cellular responses, including proliferation, differentiation, and apoptosis (138). Existing inhibitors of PKC either lack selectivity for the enzyme or demonstrate PKC selectivity but lack isoform specificity. The antisense approach offers an opportunity to circumvent these problems and to knock out target gene expression by a highly selective and sequence-specific mechanism. CGP 64128A (ISIS 3521) is a 20-mer phosphorothioate oligodeoxynucleotide targeted against the 3'-UTR of human PKC-α that specifically inhibits the expression of human PKC-α mRNA and protein m (IC$_{50}$ of 150 nm) in human cancer cells (139,140). Most important, CGP 64128A has been demonstrated to be a true isoform-specific inhibitor of PKC-α (140). GSP 64128A caused partial regression of a pelvic mass in a patient with ovarian cancer and stabilization of a rising carcinoembryonic antigen in a patient with colon cancer in a phase 1 trial (141,142). All observed side effects were believed to represent nonspecific phosphorothioate class effects, and no toxic events attributable to sequence-specific effects have been observed in human trials. No molecular correlations of drug action were presented in a published abstract. Currently, ISIS 3521 is in phase 2 clinical trial as an antitumor agent (143).

The raf proto-oncogene encodes a serine-threonine kinase that is activated by the *ras*- protein as part of the mitogen-activated protein-kinase signaling cascade (144). Mutations of *ras* or *raf* genes that result in their constitutive activation have been identified and elevated. Aberrant expression of these gene products has been reported in many human tumors. Monia et al. screened 34 phosphorothioate oligonucleotides against the human c-*raf* mRNA and found a potent sequence-specific inhibitor of c-*raf* mRNA expression *in vitro* and *in vivo* (91).

This oligonucleotide, ISIS 5132 (also known as *CGP 69846A*), entered phase 1 clinical trials for solid tumors in early 1996: It is administered as a 2-hour infusion three times weekly or as a 21-day continuous infusion (145,146). However, it has been suggested that the use of c-*raf*-1 antisense oligodeoxynucleotides could be limited by their toxicity to normal cells, as c-*raf*-1 is a critical component for cellular proliferation and differentiation. Despite this potential problem, preliminary results using an antisense oligodeoxynucleotide complementary to murine c-*raf*-1 failed to show any oligodeoxynucleotide-associated toxicities in normal mice, suggesting that oligodeoxynucleotides might be preferentially effective in tumors. It is also possible that other members of the *raf* family might compensate for c-*Raf*-1 activity in normal cells.

Antisense oligonucleotide ISIS 2503 demonstrated potent and specific activity against Ha-ras mRNA, but had no effect on the expression of K-ras or G3PDH in a variety of cell lines (147). On the basis of its isoform selectivity and antitumor activity in xenograft models (148) this oligomer also is entering phase 1 clinical trials for the treatment of solid tumors (100).

In the past 5 years, there has been a dramatic increase in the understanding of the ways in which antisense oligonucleotides function. The first antisense drug has been approved for cytomegalovirus retinitis; several more are currently in clinical trials. The most optimal clinical uses for these molecules are unknown, but for best results in a cancer indication it seems likely that they should be used in association with cytotoxic agents. In this context, they undoubtedly are an important addition to the growing armamentarium of anticancer drugs.

REFERENCES

1. Belikova AM, Zarytova VF, Grineva NI. Synthesis of ribonucleosides and diribonucleoside phosphates containing 2-chloroethylamine and nitrogen mustard residues. *Tetrahedron Lett* 1967;37:3357–3362.
2. Stix G. Shutting down a gene. Antisense drug wins approval. *Sci Am* 1998;279:46–50.
3. Zamecnik PC, Stephenson ML. Inhibition of Rous sarcoma virus replication and cell transformation by a specific oligodeoxynucleotide. *Proc Natl Acad Sci U S A* 1978;75:280–284.
4. Stephenson ML, Zamecnik PC. Inhibition of Rous sarcoma viral RNA translation by a specific oligodeoxyribonucleotide. *Proc Natl Acad Sci U S A* 1978;75:285–288.
5. Caruthers M. Gene synthesis machines: DNA chemistry and its uses. *Science* 1985;230:281–285.
6. Eder P, DeVine R, Dagle J, et al. Substrate specificity and kinetics of degradation of antisense oligonucleotides by a 3' exonuclease in plasma. *Antisense Res Dev* 1991;1:141–151.
7. Vaerman J, Moureau P, Deldime F, et al. Antisense oligodeoxyribonucleotides suppress hematologic cell growth through stepwise release of deoxyribonucleotides. *Blood* 1997;90:331–339.
8. Liu X, Kim C, Yang J, et al. Induction of apoptotic program in cell-free extracts: requirement for dATP and cytochrome c. *Cell* 1996;86:147–157.
9. Miller P. Antisense oligonucleotide methylphosphonates. In: Murray J, ed. *Antisense RNA and DNA*. New York: Wiley-Liss, 1992:241–253.
10. Miller PS, Ts'o P. A new approach to chemotherapy based on molecular biology and nucleic acid chemistry. Matagen (masking tape for gene expression). *Anticancer Drug Des* 1987;2:117–128.
11. Stec WJ, Zon G, Egan W, et al. Automated solid-phase synthesis, separation and stereochemistry of phosphorothioate analogues of oligodeoxyribonucleotides. *J Am Chem Soc* 1984;106:6077–6079.

12. Eckstein F. Nucleoside phosphorothioates. *Annu Rev Biochem* 1985;54:367–402.

13. Chang E, Miller P, Cushman C, et al. Antisense inhibition of ras p21 expression that is sensitive to a point mutation. *Biochemistry* 1991; 30:8283–8286.

14. Tidd D. Ribonuclease H-mediated antisense effects of oligonucleotides and controls for antisense experiments. In: Stein C, Krieg A. *Applied antisense oligonucleotide technology*. New York: Wiley-Liss, 1998:161–172.

15. Giles R, Ruddell C, Spiller D, et al. Single base discrimination for ribonuclease H-dependent antisense effects within intact human leukaemia cells. *Nucleic Acids Res* 1995;23:954–961.

16. Benimetskaya L, Takle O, Vilenchik M, et al. Cellular delivery of antisense oligodeoxynucleotides by a novel cationic porphyrin vehicle. *Nucleic Acids Res* 1998;26:5310–5317.

17. Dean N, McKay R. Inhibition of protein kinase C-expression in mice after systemic administration of phosphorothioate antisense oligodeoxynucleotides. *Proc Natl Acad Sci U S A* 1994;91: 11762–11766.

18. Moulds C, Lewis J, Froehler B, et al. Site and mechanism of antisense inhibition by C-5 propyne oligonucleotides. *Biochem* 1995;34:5044–5053.

19. Flannagan WM, Wagner R. The development of C-S propyne oligonucleotides as inhibitors of gene function. In: Stein C, Krieg A. *Applied antisense oligonucleotide technology*. New York: Wiley-Liss, 1998:175–191.

20. Stein CA, Cohen J. Phosphorothioate oligodeoxynucleotide analogues. In: Cohen J, ed. *Oligodeoxynucleotides: antisense inhibitors of gene expression*. London: Macmillan, 1989:97–117.

21. Stein C, Tonkinson J, Yakubov L. Phosphorothioate oligonucleotides. *Pharmacol Ther* 1991;52:365–384.

22. Stein CA, Subashinge C, Shinozuka K, et al. Physico-chemical properties of phosphorothioate oligodeoxynucleotides. *Nucleic Acids Res* 1988;16:3209–3221.

23. Crooke S. Therapeutic applications of oligonucleotides. *Annu Rev Pharmacol Toxicol* 1992;32:329–376.

24. Koziolkiewicz M, Stec W, Stein CA. Unpublished observations.

25. Gao WY, Storm C, Egan W, et al. Cellular pharmacology of phosphorothioate homooligodeoxynucleotides in human cells. *Mol Pharmacol* 1993;43:45–50.

26. Monia BP, Johnston JF, Ecker DJ, et al. Selective inhibition of mutant Ha-ras mRNA expression by antisense oligonucleotides. *J Biol Chem* 1992;267:19954–19962.

27. Schmitz JC, Agrawal S, Chu E. Repression of human thymidylate synthase mRNA translation by antisense 2'-O-methyl oligoribonucleotide. *Antisense Nucleic Acid Drug Dev* 1998;8:371–378.

28. Altmann KH, Fabbro D, Dean NM, et al. Second-generation antisense oligonucleotides: structure-activity relationships and the design of improved signal-transduction inhibitors. *Biochem Soc Trans* 1996; 243:630–637.

29. Nielsen PE, Egholni M, Berg RH, et al. Sequence selective recognition of DNA by strand displacement with a thymine-substituted polyamide. *Science* 1991;252:1497–1500.

30. Grigoriev M, Praseuth D, Robin P, et al. A triple helix-forming oligonucleotide intercalator conjugate acts as a transcriptional repressor via inhibition of NF-κB binding to interleukin-2 receptor α-regulatory sequence. *J Biol Chem* 1992;267:3389–3395.

31. Postel EH, Flint SJ, Kessler DJ, et al. Evidence that a triplex-forming oligodeoxyribonucleotide binds to the c-myc promoter in HeLa cells, thereby reducing c-myc mRNA levels. *Proc Natl Acad Sci U S A* 1991;88:8227–8231.

32. Yakubov L, Khaled Z, Zhang L-M, et al. Oligodeoxynucleotides interact with recombinant CD4 at multiple sites. *J Biol Chem* 1993;268:18818–18823.

33. Stein CA, Tonkinson JL, Zhang L-M, et al. Dynamics of the internalization of phosphodiester oligodeoxynucleotides in HL60 cells. *Biochemistry* 1993;32:4855–4861.

34. Guvakova MA, Yakubov LA, Vlodavsky I, et al. Phosphorothioate oligodeoxynucleotides bind to basic fibroblast growth factor, inhibit its binding to cell surface receptors, and remove it from low affinity binding sites on extracellular matrix. *J Biol Chem* 1995; 270:2620–2627.

35. Fennewald SM, Rando RF. Inhibition of high affinity basic fibroblast growth factor binding by oligonucleotides. *J Biol Chem* 1995;270:21718–21721.

36. Khaled Z, Benimetskaya L, Khan I, et al. Multiple mechanisms may contribute to the cellular antiadhesive effects of phosphorothioate oligodeoxynucleotides. *Nucleic Acids Res* 1996;24:737–745.

37. Benimetskaya L, Loike J, Khaled Z, et al. Mac-1 (CD11b/CD18) is a cell surface oligodeoxynucleotide binding protein. *Nat Med* 1997; 3:414–420.

38. Rockwell P, O'Connor W, King K, et al. Cell surface perturbations of the EGF and VEGF receptors by phosphorothioate oligodeoxynucleotides. *Proc Natl Acad Sci U S A* 1997;94:6523–6528.

39. Benimetskaya L, Tonkinson J, Koziolkiewicz M, et al. Binding of phosphorothioate oligodeoxynucleotides to basic fibroblast growth factor, recombinant soluble CD4, laminin and fibronectin is P-chirality independent. *Nucleic Acids Res* 1995;23:4239–4245.

40. Smetsers I, Boezeman J, and Mensink C. Bias in nucleotide composition of antisense oligonucleotides. *Antisense Nucleic Acid Drug Dev* 1996;6:63–67.

41. Cheong C, Moore PB. Solution structure of an unusually stable RNA tetraplex containing G- and U-quartet structures. *Biochemistry* 1992;31:8406–8414.

42. Wang Y, Patel DJ. Solution structure of a parallel-stranded G-quadruplex DNA. *J Mol Biol* 1993;234:1171–1183.

43. Benimetskaya L, Berton M, Kolbanovsky A, et al. Formation of a G-tetrad and higher order structures correlates with biological activity of the RelA (NF-kappaB p65) "antisense" oligodeoxynucleotide. *Nucleic Acids Res* 1997;25:2648–2456.

44. Vilenchik M, Stein CA. Unpublished results.

45. Perez JR, Li YL, Stein CA, et al. Sequence-independent induction of Sp1 transcription factor activity by phosphorothioate oligonucleotides. *Proc Natl Acad Sci U S A* 1994;91:5957–5961.

46. Stein CA. Keeping the biotechnology of antisense in context. *Nat Biotechnol* 1999;17:209.

47. Tu G, Cao Q, Zhou F, et al. Tetranucleotide GGGA motif in primary RNA transcripts. *J Biol Chem* 1998;273:25125–2513.

48. Stein CA. How to design an antisense oligodeoxynucleotide experiment: a consensus approach. *Antisense Nucleic Acid Drug Dev* 1998;8:129–132.

49. Stein CA, Krieg A. Problems in interpretation of data derived from *in vitro* and *in vivo* use of antisense oligodeoxynucleotides [Editorial]. *Antisense Res Dev* 1994;4:67–69.

50. Krieg AM. The CpG motif: implications for clinical immunology. *Bio Drugs* 1998;105:341–346.

51. Loke SL, Stein CA, Zhang XH, et al. Characterization of oligonucleotide transport into living cells. *Proc Natl Acad Sci U S A* 1989;86:3474–3478.

52. Wu-Pong S, Weiss T, Hunt CA. Calcium-dependent cellular uptake of a c-myc antisense oligonucleotide. *Cell Mol Biol* 1994;40:843–850.

53. Yakubov LA, Deeva EA, Zarytova VF, et al. Mechanism of oligonucleotide uptake by cells: involvement of specific receptors? *Proc Natl Acad Sci U S A* 1989;86:6454–6458.

54. Tonkinson JL, Stein CA. Patterns of intracellular compartmentalization, trafficking and acidification of 5'-fluorescein labeled phosphodiester and phosphorothioate oligodeoxynucleotides in HL60 cells. *Nucleic Acids Res* 1994;22:4268–4275.

55. Crooke RM, Graham MJ, Cooke ME, et al. *In vitro* pharmacokinetics of phosphorothioate antisense oligonucleotides. *J Pharmacol Exp Ther* 1995;275:462–473.

56. Beltinger C, Saragovi HU, Smith RM, et al. Binding, uptake, and cellular trafficking of phosphorothioate-modified oligonucleotides. *J Clin Invest* 1995;95:1814–1823.

57. Gezelowitz DA, Neckers LM. Analysis of oligonucleotide binding, internalization, and intracellular trafficking utilizing a novel radiolabeled crosslinker. *Antisense Res Dev* 1992;2:17–25.

58. Stein CA. Controversies in the cellular pharmacology of oligodeoxynucleotides. *Antisense Nucleic Acid Drug Dev* 1997;7:207–209.

59. Bongartz JP, Aubertin AM, Mithaud PG, et al. Improved biological activity of antisense oligonucleotides conjugated to a fusogenic pep-

tide. *Nucleic Acids Res* 1994;22:4681–4688.

60. Midoux P, Kichler A, Boutin V, et al. Membrane permeabilization and efficient gene transfer by a peptide containing several histidines. *Bioconjugate Chem* 1998;9:260–267.

61. Chaloin L, Vidal P, Lory P, et al. Design of carrier peptide—oligonucleotide conjugates with rapid membrane translocation and nuclear localization properties. *Biochem Biophys Res Commun* 1998;243:601–608.

62. Svinarchuk FP, Konevetz DA, Pliasunova OA, et al. Inhibition of HIV proliferation in MT-4 cells by antisense oligonucleotide conjugated to lipophilic groups. *Biochimie* 1993;75:49–54.

63. Bachmann AS, Surovoy A, Jung G, et al. Integrin-receptor-targeted transfer peptides for efficient delivery of antisense oligodeoxynucleotides. *J Mol Med* 1998;76:126–132.

64. Midoux P, Mendes C, Legrand A, et al. Specific gene transfer mediated by lactosylated poly-L-lysine into hepatoma cells. *Nucleic Acids Res* 1993;21:871–878.

65. Lemaitre M, Bayard B, Lebleu B. Specific antiviral activity of a poly(L-Lysine)-conjugated oligodeoxyribonucleotide sequence complementary to vesicular stomatitis virus N protein mRNA initiation site. *Proc Natl Acad Sci U S A* 1987;84:648–652.

66. Clarenc JP, Degols G, Leonetti JP, et al. Delivery of antisense oligonucleotides by poly(L-lysine) conjugation and liposome encapsulation. *Anticancer Drug Des* 1993;8:81–94.

67. Pichon C, Freulon I, Midoux P, et al. Cytosolic and nuclear delivery of oligonucleotides mediated by an amphiphilic anionic peptide. *Antisense Nucleic Acid Drug Dev* 1997;7:335–343.

68. Iyer RP, Yu D, Agrawal S. Prodrugs of oligonucleotides: the acyloxy esters of oligodeoxyribonucleoside phosphorothioates. *Biorg Chem* 1995;23:1–21.

69. Barber I, Rayner B, Imbach JL. The prooligonucleotide approach. I. Esterase-mediated reversibility of dithymidine S-alkyl-phosphorothioates to dithymidine phosphorothioates. *Bioorg Med Chem* 1995;5:563–568.

70. Juliano RL, Akhtar S. Liposomes as a drug delivery system for antisense oligonucleotides. *Antisense Res Dev* 1992;2:165–176.

71. Oberhauser B, Wagner E. Effective incorporation of 2'-O-methyl-oligoribonucleotides into liposomes and enhanced cell association through modification with thiocholesterol. *Nucleic Acids Res* 1992;20:533–538.

72. Zelphati O, Imbach JL, Signoret N, et al. Antisense oligonucleotides in solution or encapsulated in immunoliposomes inhibit replication of HIV-1 by several different mechanisms. *Nucleic Acids Res* 1994;22:4307–4314.

73. Bennett CF, Chiang M-Y, Chan H, et al. Cationic lipids enhance cellular uptake and activity of phosphorothioate antisense oligonucleotides. *Molec Pharmacol* 1992;41:1023–1033.

74. Capaccioli S, Di Pasquale G, Mini E, et al. Cationic lipids improve antisense oligonucleotide uptake and prevent degradation in cultured cells and in human serum. *Biochem Biophys Res Commun* 1993;197:818–825.

75. Zelphati O, Szoka FC Jr. Intracellular distribution and mechanism of delivery of oligonucleotides mediated by cationic lipids. *Pharm Res* 1996;13:1367–1372.

76. Gottschalk S, Cristiano RJ, Smith LC, Woo SLC. Folate receptor-mediated DNA delivery into tumor-cells—potosomal disruption results in enhanced gene-expression. *Gene Ther* 1994;1:185–191.

77. Lee RJ, Huang L. Folate targeted, anionic liposome-entrapped poly-lysine-condensed DNA for tumor cell-specific gene-transfer. *J Biol Chem* 1996;271;8481–8487.

78. Chaudhiri G. Scavenger receptor-mediated delivery of antisense mini-exon phosphorothioate oligonucleotide to *Leishmania*-infected macrophages. Selective and efficient elimination of the parasite. *Biochem Pharmacol* 1997;53:385–391.

79. Wang S, Lee RJ, Cauchon G, et al. Delivery of antisense oligodeoxyribooligonucleotides against the human epidermal growth factor receptor into cultured KB cells with liposomes conjugated to folate via polyethylene glycol. *Proc Natl Acad Sci U S A* 1995;92:3318–3322.

80. Zelphati O, Zon G, Lesennan L. Inhibition of HIV-1 replication in cultured cells with antisense oligonucleotides encapsulated in immunoliposomes. *Antisense Res Dev* 1993;3:323–338.

81. Zobel H-P, Kreuter J, Werner D, et al Cationic polyhexylcyanoacrylate nanoparticles as carriers for antisense oligonucleotides. *Antisense Res Dev* 1997;7:483–493.

82. Schwab G, Chavany C, Duroux I, et al. Antisense oligonucleotides adsorbed to polyalkylcyanoacrylate nanoparticles specifically inhibit mutates Ha-ras-mediated cell proliferation and tumorigenicity in nude mice. *Proc Natl Acad Sci U S A* 1994;91:10460–10464.

83. Tondelli L, Ricca A, Laus M, et al. Highly efficient cellular uptake of c-myb antisense oligonucleotides through specifically designed polymeric nanospheres. *Nucleic Acids Res* 1998;26:5425–5431.

84. Maruyama A, Ishihara I, Kim JS, et al. Nanoparticle DNA carrier with poly(L-lysine) grafted polysaccharide copolymer and poly(D,L-lactic acid). *Bioconjug Chem* 1997;8:735–742.

85. Vinogradov S, Bronich T, Kabanov AV. Self-assembly of polyamine-poly(ethylene glycol) copolymers with phosphorothioate oligonucleotides. *Bioconjugate Chem* 1998;9:805–812.

86. Wang L, Kristensen J, Ruffner DE. Delivery of antisense oligonucleotides using HPMA polymer: synthesis of a thiol polymer and its conjugation to water-soluble molecules. *Bioconjugate Chem* 1998;9:749–757.

87. Takle GB, Thierry AR, Flynn SM, et al. Delivery of oligoribonucleotides to human hepatoma cells using cationic lipid particles conjugated to ferric protoporphyrin IX (heme). *Antisense Nucleic Acid Drug Dev* 1997;7:177–185.

88. Kukowska-Latallo JF, Bielinska AU, Johnson J, et al. Efficient transfer of genetic material into mammalian cells using Starburst polyamidoamine dendrimers. *Proc Natl Acad Sci U S A* 1996;93:4897–4902.

89. McKay R, Dean MN. Inhibition of protein kinase C-α expression in mice after systemic administration of phosphorothioate. *Proc Natl Acad Sci U S A* 1994;91:1762–1766.

90. Plenat F. Animal models of antisense oligonucleotides: lessons for use in humans. *Mol Med Today* 1996;2:250–257.

91. Monia BP, Johnston IF, Geiger T, et al. Antitumor activity of a phosphorothioate antisense oligodeoxynucleotide targeted against C-*raf* kinase. *Nat Med* 1996;2:668–675.

92. Black LE, Degeorge JJ, Cavagnaro JA, et al. Regulatory considerations for evaluating the pharmacology and toxicology of antisense drugs. *Antisense Res Dev* 1993;3:399–404.

93. Calabretta B, Skorski T. Targeting c-myc in leukemia. *Anticancer Drug Des* 1997;12:373–381.

94. Gewirtz AM. Antisense oligonucleotide therapeutics for human leukemia. *Curr Opin Hematol* 1998;5:59–71.

95. Monia BP. First and second generation antisense inhibitors targeted to human c-*raf* kinase: *in vitro* and *in vivo* studies. *Anticancer Drug Des* 1997;12:327–339.

96. Geiger T, Muller M, Dean NM, et al. Antitumor activity of a PKC-α antisense oligonucleotide in combination with standard chemotherapeutic agents against various human tumors transplanted into nude mice. *Anticancer Drug Des* 1998;13:35–45.

97. Nesterova M, Cho-Chung YS. A single-injection protein-kinase A-directed antisense treatment to inhibit tumor growth. *Nat Med* 1995;1:528–533.

98. Tortora G, Caputo R, Damiano V, et al. Synergistic inhibition of human cancer cell growth by cytotoxic drugs and mixed backbone antisense oligonucleotide targeting protein kinase A. *Proc Natl Acad Sci U S A* 1997;94:12586–12591.

99. Cowsert LM. *In vitro* and *in vivo* activity of antisense inhibitors of ras: potential for clinical development. *Anticancer Drug Des* 1997;12:359–371.

100. Cotter FE, Johnson P, Hall P, et al. Antisense oligonucleotides suppress B-cell lymphoma growth in a SCID-hu mouse model. *Oncogene* 1994;9:3049–3055.

101. Henry SP, Monteith D, Bennett F, et al. Toxicological properties of chemically modified antisense inhibitors of PKC-alpha and C-*raf* kinase. *Anticancer Drug Des* 1997;12:409–420.

102. Monteith DK, Henry SP, Howard RB, et al. Immune stimulation—a class effect of phosphorothioate oligodeoxynucleotides in rodents. *Anticancer Drug Des* 1997;12:421–432.

103. Sarmiento UM, Perez JR, Becker JM. *In vivo* toxicological effects of rel A antisense phosphorothioates in CD-1 mice. *Antisense Res Dev* 1994;4:99–107.

104. Srinivasan SK, Tewary HK, Iversen PL. Characterization of binding sites, extent of binding, and drug interactions of oligonucleotides with albumin. *Antisense Res Dev* 1995;5:271–277.

105. Agrawal S, Zhang X, Lu Z, et al. Absorption, tissue distribution and *in vivo* stability in rats of a hybrid antisense oligonucleotide following oral administration. *Biochem Pharmacol* 1995;50:571–576.

106. Iversen PL, Copple BL, Tewary HK. Pharmacology and toxicology of phosphorothioate oligonucleotides in the mouse, rat, monkey and man. *Toxicol Lett* 1995;82–83:425–430.

107. Saijo Y, Perlaky L, Wang H, et al. Pharmacokinetics, tissue distribution, and stability of antisense oligodeoxynucleotide phosphorothioate ISIS 3466 in mice. *Oncol Res* 1996;6:243–249.

108. Zhang R, Diasio RB, Lu Z, et al. Pharmacokinetics and tissue distribution in rats of an oligodeoxynucleotide phosphorothioate (GEM 91) developed as a therapeutic agent for human immunodeficiency virus type-I. *Biochem Pharmacol* 1995;49:929–939.

109. Galbraith WM, Hobson WC, Giglas PC, et al. Complement activation and hemodynamic changes following intravenous administration of phosphorothioate oligonucleotides in the monkey. *Antisense Res Dev* 1994;4:201–207.

110. Boral AL, Dessain S, Chabner BA. Clinical evaluation of biologically targeted drugs: obstacles and opportunities. *Cancer Chemother Pharmacol* 1998,42[Suppl]:S3–S21.

111. Hockenbery D, Nunez G, Milliman C, et al. Bcl-2 is an inner mitochondrial membrane protein that blocks programmed cell death. *Nature* 1990;348:334–336.

112. Reed IC. Regulation of apoptosis by bcl-2 family proteins and its role in cancer and chemoresistance. *Curr Opin Oncol* 1995;7:541–546.

113. Miyashita T, Reed JC. Bcl-2 gene transfer increases relative resistance of S49.1 and Wehi7.2 lymphoid cells to cell death and DNA fragmentation induced by glucocorticoids and multiple chemotherapeutic drugs. *Cancer Res* 1992;52:5407–5411.

114. Reed JC, Stein C, Subashinge C, et al. Antisense-mediated inhibition of bcl-2 proto-oncogene expression and leukemic cells growth and survival: comparisons of phosphodiester and phosphorothioate oligodeoxynucleotides. *Cancer Res* 1990;50:6575–6579.

115. Smith MR, Abubakr Y, Mohammad R, et al. Antisense oligodeoxyribonucleotide down-regulation of bcl-2 gene expression inhibits growth of the low-grade non-Hodgkin's lymphoma cell line WSU-FSCCL. *Cancer Gene Ther* 1995;2:207–212.

116. Cotter FE, Johnson P, Hall P, et al. Antisense oligonucleotides suppress B-cell lymphoma growth in a SCID-hu mouse model. *Oncogene* 1994;9:3049–3055.

117. Webb A, Cunningham D, Cotter F, et al. BCL-2 antisense therapy in patients with non-Hodgkin lymphoma. *Lancet* 1997;349:1137–1141.

118. Ho PTC, Parkinson DR. Antisense oligonucleotides as therapeutics for malignant diseases. *Semin Oncol* 1997;24:187–202.

119. Ziegler A, Luedke GH, Fabbro D, et al. Induction of apoptosis in small cell lung cancer cells by an antisense oligodeoxynucleotide targeting the bcl 2 coding sequence. *J Natl Cancer Inst* 1997;89:1027–1036.

120. Gewirtz AM. The c-myb proto-oncogene: a novel target for human gene therapy. *Cancer Treat Res* 1996;84:93–112.

121. Burgess IL, Fisher EF, Ross SL, et al. The antiproliferative activity of c-myb and c-myc antisense oligonucleotides is caused by a nonantisense mechanism. *Proc Natl Acad Sci U S A* 1995;92:4051–4055.

122. Castier Y, Chemla E, Nierat J, et al. The activity of c-myb antisense oligonucleotide to prevent intimal hyperplasia is nonspecific. *J Cardiovasc Surg* (Torino) 1998;39:1–7.

123. Luger SM, Ratajczak MZ, Stadtmauer EA, et al. Autographing for chronic myelogenous leukemia (CML) with c-myb antisense oligodeoxynucleotide purged bone marrow: a preliminary report. *Blood* 1994;84[Suppl 1]:151a(abst).

124. Gewirtz AM, Luger S, Sokol D, et al. Oligodeoxynucleotide therapeutics for human myelogenous leukemia: interim results. *Blood* 1996;88[Suppl 1]:270a(abst).

125. Daley GQ, Van Etten RA, Baltimore D. Induction of chronic myelogenic leukemia in mice by the p210$^{bcr-abl}$ gene of the Philadelphia chromosome. *Science* 1990;247:824–830.

126. Kirkland MA, O'Brien SG, McDonald C, et al. BCR-ABL antisense purging in chronic myeloid leukaemia. *Lancet* 1993;342:614.

127. Szczylik C, Skorski T, Malaguamera L, et al. Inhibition of *in vitro* proliferation of chronic myelogenous leukemia progenitor cells by c-myb antisense oligodeoxynucleotides. *Folia Histochem Cytobiol* 1996;34:129–134.

128. Skorski T, Nieborowska-Skorska M, Nicolaides NC, et al. Suppression of Philadelphia 1 leukemia cell growth in mice by BCR-ABL antisense oligodeoxynucleotide. *Proc Natl Acad Sci U S A* 1994;91:4504–4508.

129. O'Brien SG, Kirkland MA, Melo JV, et al. Antisense BCR-ABL oligomers cause non-specific inhibition of chronic myeloid leukemia cell lines. *Leukemia* 1994;8:2156–2162.

130. Bergan RC, Kyle E, Connell Y, et al. Inhibition of protein-tyrosine kinase activity in intact cells by the aptameric action of oligodeoxynucleotides. *Antisense Res Dev* 1995;5:33–38.

131. Smetsers TFCM, van de Locht LTF, Pennings AH, et al. Phosphorothioate BCR-ABL antisense oligonucleotides induce cell death, but fail to reduce cellular bcr-abl protein levels. *Leukemia* 1995;9:118–130.

132. De Fabritius P, Amadori S, Petti MC, et al. *In vitro* purging with BCR-ABL antisense oligodeoxynucleotides does not prevent haematologic reconstitution after autologous bone marrow transplantation. *Leukemia* 1995;9:662–664.

133. De Fabritius P, Petti MC, Montefusco E, et al. BCR-ABL antisense oligonucleotide *in vitro* purging and autologous bone marrow transplantation for patients with chronic myelogenous leukemia in advanced phase. *Blood* 1998;91(9):3156–3162.

134. Bishop MR, Iversen PL, Bayever E, et al. Phase I trial of an antisense oligonucleotide OL(1)53 in hematologic malignancies. *J Clin Oncol* 1996;14:1320–1326.

135. Lowe SW, Bodis S, McClatchey, et al. p53 status and the efficacy of cancer therapy *in vivo*. *Science* 1994;266:807–810.

136. Bayever E, Haines KM, Iversen PL, et al. Selective cytotoxicity to human leukemic myeloblasts produced by oligodeoxyribonucleotide phosphorothioates complementary to p53 nucleotide sequences. *Leuk Lymphoma* 1994;12:223–231.

137. Bishop MR, Jackson ID, Tarantolo SR, et al. *Ex vivo* treatment of bone marrow with phosphorothioate oligonucleotide OL(1)p53 for autologous transplantation in acute myelogenous leukemia and myelodysplastic syndrome. *J Hematother* 1997;6(5):441–446.

138. Basu A. A potential of protein kinase C as a target for anticancer treatment. *Pharm Ther* 1993;59:257–280.

139. Dean NM, McKay R, Condon TP, et al. Inhibition of protein kinase C-α expression in human A549 cells by antisense oligonucleotides inhibits induction of intercellular adhesion molecule 1 (ICAM-1) mRNA by phorbol esters. *J Biol Chem* 1994;269:16416–16424.

140. Dean NM, McKay R, Miraghia L, et al. Inhibition of growth of human tumor cell lines in nude mice by an antisense oligonucleotide inhibitor of PKC-α expression. *Cancer Res* 1996;15:3499–3507.

141. Nemunaitis J, Eckhardt G, Dorr A, et al. Phase I evaluation of CGP 64128A, an antisense inhibitor of protein kinase C-α (PKC-α), in patients with refractory cancer. *Proc Am Soc Clin Oncol* 1997;16:870(abst).

142. Sikic BI, Yuen AR, Halsey J, et al. A phase I trial of an antisense oligonucleotide targeted to protein kinase C-α (ISIS 3521) delivered by 21 day continuous intravenous infusion. *Proc Am Soc Clin Oncol* 1997;16:741(abst).

143. Dean NM, Lemonidis K, McKay R, et al. The use of antisense oligonucleotides to inhibit expression of isozymes of protein kinase C. In: Stein CA, Krieg A, eds. *Applied antisense oligonucleotide technology*. New York: Wiley-Liss, 1998:193–205.

144. Daum G, Eisenmann-Tappe I, Fries HW, et al. The ins and outs of *raf* kinases. *Trends Biochem Sci* 1994;19:474–480.

145. Holmlund J, Nemunaitis J, Schiller J, et al. Phase I trial of c-*raf* antisense oligonucleotide ISIS 5132 (CGP 69846 A) by 21-day continuous intravenous infusion (CIV) in patients with advanced cancer. *Proc Am Soc Clin Oncol* 1998;17:811(abst).

146. O'Dwyer PJ, Stevenson JP, Gallagher M, et al. Phase I/pharmacokinetic/pharmacodynamic trial of raf-1 antisense oligodeoxynucleotide (ISIS 5132, CGP 69846 A). *Proc Am Soc Clin Oncol* 1998;17:810(abst).

147. Chen G, Oh S, Monia BP, et al. Antisense oligonucleotides demonstrate a dominant role of c-Ki-RAS proteins in regulating the proliferation of diploid human fibroblasts. *J Biol Chem* 1996;271:28259–28265.

PRINCIPLES AND PRACTICE OF ANTIANGIOGENIC THERAPY

21

ANTIANGIOGENESIS: BASIC PRINCIPLES AND PRECLINICAL MODELS

MICHAEL S. O'REILLY

In 1971, Folkman proposed that tumor growth was dependent on angiogenesis based on his studies of tumor growth in isolated perfused organs (1). Historically, the increased vascularity of malignant tissue as compared to normal tissue had been often noted. However, this hyperemia had been assumed to result from the dilation of preexisting host vessels in response to tumor necrosis and metabolic byproducts from the tumor cells. Neovascularization in association with a tumor was merely assumed to be a byproduct of inflammation and was not considered important. Thus, Folkman's proposal that a tumor was dependent on the endothelial cell was widely criticized. However, numerous lines of direct evidence have now clearly established that the growth and expansion of tumors and their metastases is dependent on angiogenesis (2).

Several factors that stimulate angiogenesis have been identified and described (3). These include the fibroblast growth factors (FGFs) such as acidic and basic FGF (aFGF, bFGF) (4), vascular endothelial cell growth factor/vascular permeability factor (VEGF/VPF) (5,6), hepatocyte growth factor/scatter factor (7), transforming growth factor beta (8,9), proliferin (10), erythropoietin (11), and several others. Numerous inhibitors of angiogenesis have also been described, and the discovery and characterization of these inhibitors has become an area of intense focus. Many of the first angiogenesis inhibitors to be described were substances with other functions whose antiangiogenicity were discovered incidentally. Other substances have been developed that are selective angiogenesis inhibitors. More recently, strategies have been developed that have led to the discovery of highly specific inhibitors of angiogenesis.

With the discovery of angiogenic factors, the field of angiogenesis research has grown rapidly, and new applications of angiogenesis have arisen. This chapter identifies some themes that appear to be emerging based on the discovery and characterization of angiogenesis inhibitors.

ANGIOGENESIS IS REGULATED BY BOTH STIMULATORS AND INHIBITORS

Angiogenesis, the growth of new capillary blood vessels from preexisting vessels, is a fundamental process that is required for a wide variety of physiologic and pathophysiologic processes.

Examples of physiologic processes that require angiogenesis include wound healing, tissue repair, reproduction, growth, and development (12). For angiogenesis to occur, an increased production of stimulatory factors and/or a decreased production or generation of inhibitors is necessary. Angiogenesis is therefore regulated by a complex balance (Fig. 1) of stimulators and inhibitors (13,14). Endothelial cells are normally quiescent, and years may pass between cell divisions (15). Under physiologic conditions that require neovascularization, angiogenesis is a tightly regulated process, and the balance in favor of stimulation is generally short-lived. However, in malignant angiogenesis the process is sustained and requires the continued production of stimulators by tumor and stromal cells in excess of inhibitors (16,17). Many disease states both arise and are maintained by the persistence of angiogenesis and the loss of normal regulatory mechanisms (17,18). These include cancer; ophthalmologic disorders, such as ocular neovascularization in patients with diabetes or macular degeneration; arthritis and other inflammatory disorders; psoriasis; and many others (17,19). Furthermore, a number of differences between malignant and physiologic angiogenesis are becoming apparent (20). In malignant angiogenesis induced by a cancer, endothelial cells are not returned to their normal state of quiescence, and angiogenic vessels appear markedly disordered relative to their physiologic counterparts (21). Malignant angiogenesis is often characterized by a distorted architecture, the lack of pericytes and other support cells (22), impaired and/or intermittent flow (23–25), the presence of plasma proteins that function as a neostroma (26,27), and increased permeability (28). Thus, strategies that target angiogenesis have clear clinical implications for a variety of conditions, both neoplastic and nonneoplastic, and the study of angiogenesis helps in the understanding of a number of disease states.

Before the onset of angiogenesis, tumor growth is limited by perfusion, and preangiogenic tumors remain in an *in situ* stage in which tumor volume is limited to a few cubic millimeters (1,14,29,30). For a tumor to grow beyond this prevascular stage, neovascularization is needed to produce new vessels that are required to perfuse the tumor with nutrients and oxygen and for the removal of metabolic catabolites (Fig. 2). However, the endothelial cells also produce a number of paracrine growth factors that are stimulatory for tumor growth (31,32). The tumor

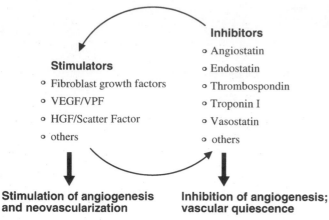

FIGURE 1. Angiogenesis is regulated by a balance of stimulators and inhibitors. The capillary endothelial cell is normally maintained in a state of quiescence by a variety of endogenous inhibitors that prevent angiogenesis. However, if factors that stimulate angiogenesis are produced in excess of the inhibitory factors, neovascularization can occur. Under physiologic conditions, this balance is precisely regulated. However, under pathophysiologic conditions, angiogenesis is poorly regulated and disordered due to the continued production of stimulators in excess of the inhibitors. (HGF, human growth factor; VEGF/VPF, vascular endothelial growth factor/vascular permeability factor.)

cells also produce or induce the production of factors such as VEGF that prevent apoptosis, induce Bcl-2 expression, and are important for endothelial cell survival (33,34). A tumor's growth is dependent on both its endothelial cells and its malignant cells, each of which produce factors that stimulate the other. Angiogenesis, therefore, provides both a perfusion effect and a paracrine effect to a growing tumor (see Fig. 2), and a circuit is established in which tumor cells and endothelial cells continue to drive each other. These observations led Folkman to propose a two-compartment model of malignancy consisting of endothelial cell and tumor cell populations (35).

Much of the focus of angiogenesis research has centered on the concept that the growth of all solid tumors is dependent on angiogenesis. Neovascularization is critical in the dissemination and progression of both primary and metastatic disease (Fig. 3). Leukemia has also been shown to be dependent on angiogenesis (36). As with physiologic angiogenesis, the neovascularization of solid tumors and their metastases is also regulated by the balance of stimulators and inhibitors (see Fig. 1). However, tumors

require that this imbalance be sustained. The studies of Bouck and her colleagues (37,38) support a model in which the net balance of the stimulators and inhibitors of angiogenesis controls tumor growth. To promote angiogenesis, tumor cells produce a number of stimulatory factors, such as VPF and VEGF, and bFGF and aFGF. However, Bouck and her colleagues have further demonstrated that when hamster cells are transformed to an angiogenic phenotype, they must also downregulate the production of angiogenesis inhibitors during the transition to an angiogenic phenotype. They found that transformed hamster cells upregulate the production of angiogenesis stimulators but must also downregulate the production of thrombospondin, an angiogenesis inhibitor, to form angiogenic lesions. Thrombospondin production is under the regulation of the wild-type p53 tumor-suppressor gene (39).

PRECLINICAL MODELS USED IN THE EVALUATION OF ANGIOGENESIS INHIBITORS

In Vitro Angiogenesis Assays

To prove his hypothesis that tumor growth was dependent on angiogenesis, Folkman developed methods to isolate and grow capillary endothelial cells, which are still in use today (40). Their isolation and characterization allowed the field of angiogenesis to progress and has led to the discovery of a number of inhibitors and stimulators of angiogenesis. The process of angiogenesis requires endothelial cell proliferation, migration, and invasion. Numerous *in vitro* systems that model events critical for angiogenesis *in vivo* using endothelial cells from a variety of species and tissues have been described. Using these assays, compounds can be screened for evidence of angiogenic activity (4,41).

The *in vitro* proliferation of endothelial cells provides a powerful tool for the study of angiogenesis. In our laboratory, we routinely use primary cultures of capillary endothelial cells derived from bovine adrenal tissue. Because angiogenesis typically occurs at the level of the capillary, the use of capillary endothelial cells would seem of more relevance to the study of angiogenesis. However, several groups also study angiogenesis using large vessel endothelial cells derived from human umbilical veins, bovine aorta, and a variety of other sources. Proliferation of endothelial cells can be determined directly by cell count or indirectly by the quantitation of DNA synthesis or mitosis, or

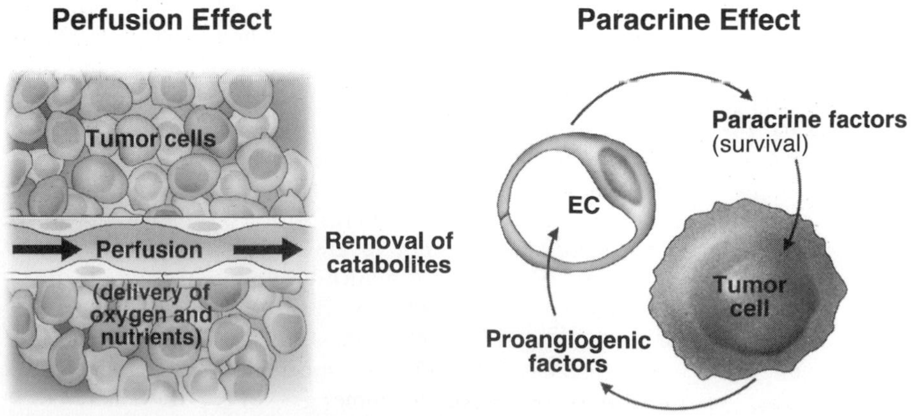

Perfusion Effect   Paracrine Effect

FIGURE 2. The angiogenic response has both a perfusion and a paracrine effect. For a malignancy to grow beyond the size of 1 to 2 mm³, it must stimulate angiogenesis. The newly formed capillaries provide the growing tumor with nutrients and oxygen and remove catabolites (perfusion effect). For the tumor cell to induce angiogenesis, it must produce and induce factors that can activate the capillary endothelial cell. The activated endothelial cell, in turn, produces a number of paracrine factors that are needed for tumor cell survival. The resultant circuit drives both cell populations (the paracrine effect) and promotes tumor expansion. (EC, endothelial cell.)

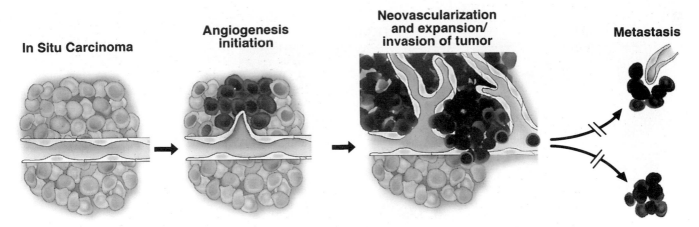

FIGURE 3. Angiogenesis in primary and metastatic tumor growth. Angiogenesis is required for growth of both primary and metastatic tumors. Within a primary tumor, heterogeneity of the angiogenic phenotype may exist, and angiogenesis may initially be limited to distinct regions of the tumor (*black circles*). As the malignancy of the tumor progresses, angiogenesis and tumor growth and invasion accelerates. Metastatic cells can then escape from the tumor to target organs. Once established, a metastasis must induce angiogenesis to grow (*upper lesion*). If a metastasis cannot induce angiogenesis in the target tissue, it may persist as a dormant lesion and is limited by perfusion (*lower lesion*).

both. Alternatively, the internalization of magnetic microbeads by capillary endothelial cells (42) (the microbead assay) can be used to detect soluble pro- and antiangiogenic factors. If a stimulator of angiogenesis is applied to the cells, the beads are distributed evenly among daughter cells during division. In contrast, the intracellular beads are retained in the presence of inhibitors. Endothelial cell migration is also required for angiogenesis, and a number of migration assays have been developed. Chemokinetic assays that use colloidal gold and chemotactic assays using the modified Boyden chamber have been developed (43). Alternatively, the ability of endothelial cells to grow into a wound made in a monolayer has also been used to assess migration.

Angiogenesis requires multiple coordinated steps, and assays that focus on only one aspect, such as proliferation or migration, may not reflect the whole process. The ability of endothelial cells in culture to form tube-like structures that resemble capillaries has been described as a model of *in vitro* angiogenesis (44). The formation of endothelial tubes or cords allows for the study of angiogenesis in a model that seems to parallel capillary development [reviewed by Montesano (45) and Williams (46)]. For example, endothelial cells form capillary-like structures in type-1 collagen gels (47) that can be dissociated and disrupted by the addition of 16K prolactin (48) or mediated by laminin domains (49). Several different *in vitro* angiogenesis models have been described to assess tube formation in two dimensions on tissue culture plates coated with gelatin or in three dimensions in collagen or fibrin gels (29,47,50–53) or into Matrigel (49). The aortic ring model, in which a circumferential section of a rat aorta is placed in a gel, has also been used and allows for the study of several aspects of angiogenesis (54).

Although useful for the screening of materials for their potential ability to regulate angiogenesis, *in vitro* assays have several limitations. The ability to inhibit endothelial cell proliferation, migration, and tube formation *in vitro* may not reflect the potency of an angiogenesis *in vivo*, and the results obtained in a tube assay may be difficult to interpret. Furthermore, many

substances, such as transforming growth factor-beta and tumor necrosis factor-alpha are potent inhibitors of the *in vitro* proliferation of endothelial cells yet stimulate angiogenesis *in vivo* (8,55). Quantitative assays are therefore needed to screen compounds for angiogenic activity. Currently, our laboratory typically uses a variety of *in vitro* assays in combination to characterize angiogenesis inhibitors.

In Vivo Angiogenesis Assays

Chicken Chorioallantoic Membrane Assay

The chicken chorioallantoic membrane (CAM) has been used extensively in the characterization of angiogenic factors (56). Using the CAM assay, some of the first angiogenesis inhibitors, such as protamine (57) and angiostatic steroids (58) were discovered. With the CAM assay, substances can be tested for their ability to regulate spontaneous angiogenesis on the developing 6-day-old CAM or induced angiogenesis on the established 10-day-old CAM. Human angiostatin potently inhibits angiogenesis in the developing CAM, leaving a large avascular zone (Fig. 4). Inhibition of angiogenesis on the 6-day-old CAM from human angiostatin was dose-dependent (59). The CAM can also be used to screen for evidence of inflammation or toxicity from the test substance.

One of the limits of the original CAM assay is the lack of quantitation. To allow for more precise quantitation in the CAM assay, Nguyen and her colleagues (60) modified the CAM assay by placing a collagen gel sandwiched between nylon mesh directly onto the developing CAM. The number of vessels into the collagen gel can then be quantitated by counting the number of capillary loops.

In Dr. Folkman's laboratory, the CAM assay typically is used as the first *in vivo* system to test potential angiogenesis inhibitors identified using *in vitro* models. Although it is rare for a substance that does not work in the CAM assay to prove to be

a

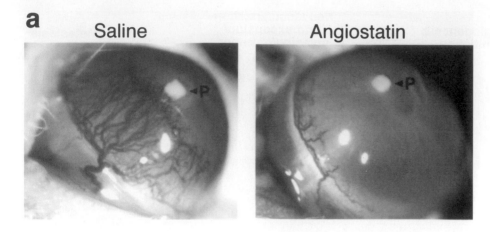

Saline   Angiostatin

b

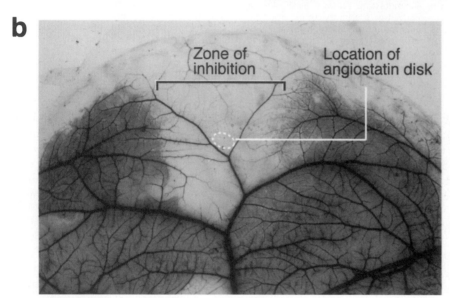

Zone of inhibition   Location of angiostatin disk

FIGURE 4. Inhibition of angiogenesis by angiostatin. **A:** Mouse corneal angiogenesis assay. A pellet (P) containing sucrose octasulfate, Hydron, and basic fibroblast growth factors (80 to 100 ng per pellet) was placed into a corneal micropocket. Mice received subcutaneous injections of human native angiostatin (50 mg per kg) or vehicle every 12 hours starting 48 hours before implantation. In control eyes, neovascularization is evident and vessels have extended into the pellet (P) within 6 days. In contrast, there is a potent inhibition of angiogenesis in mice treated with angiostatin. **B:** Chick chorioallantoic membrane (CAM) assay. Recombinant mouse angiostatin in a methylcellulose disc was applied to a developing CAM. After 48 hours, a large zone of angiogenesis inhibition that persisted for several days was observed.

an angiogenesis inhibitor, many substances that inhibit angiogenesis in the CAM assay do not inhibit angiogenesis in more advanced *in vivo* systems. Thus, the CAM assay is used primarily as a first screen in our group.

Disc Angiogenesis Assays

To quantitate angiogenesis in a variety of animal models, techniques have been developed in which a matrix or polymer is injected or implanted, or both, into a test animal. In many cases, a factor that stimulates angiogenesis is added to the disc. Test substances can be added to the disc or the animal can be treated systemically. Several methods have been described, including a polyvinyl alcohol foam surrounded by Millipore filters (61), polyurethane sponges inserted with a pellet containing bFGF or other angiogenesis stimulators (62), gelatin-impregnated sponges, and encapsulated tumor cells.

A tumor-derived extract of basement membrane, called *Matrigel* (63), is liquid at cold temperatures and reconstitutes into a gel when injected into animals. The addition of heparin and angiogenic factors induces angiogenesis *in vivo* that can be quantitated by microvessel count or by hemoglobin content. A

variety of inhibitors and stimulators of angiogenesis have been tested in this model using systemic or local delivery.

Corneal Angiogenesis Assays

The cornea is normally avascular and therefore is useful in the study of angiogenesis. Several methods have been developed in which angiogenesis is induced in the cornea. Initially, test tissues, such as a section of tumor, were placed into a corneal micropocket in rabbit (64), rat (65), or mouse (66) eye and tumor-derived angiogenesis stimulators would induce an angiogenic response. More recently, angiogenic factors, such as bFGF or VEGF/VPF, have been placed in sustained-release polymers for implantation into corneal micropockets in the mouse, rat, and rabbit. The mouse corneal assay provides a powerful tool for the screening of angiogenesis inhibitors against a defined angiogenic response (67). Substances can then be screened for the ability to inhibit angiogenesis by adding them to the pellet or by systemic therapy (68). The inhibition of angiogenesis can then be quantitated as a function of the length of the vessels and the circumferential area of the cornea involved. The systemic administration of angiostatin, for example, inhibited angiogenesis by greater than 90% in a mouse corneal angiogenesis assay using bFGF (see Fig. 4A) or VEGF/VPF as a mitogen. In normal mice, new capillary vessels grew from the corneal limbus and across the cornea in response to the sustained-release of bFGF from the pellet within 3 days. Within 6 days of implantation, the new vessels had grown across the cornea and into the pellet. In contrast, in mice treated with angiostatin, there was a virtually complete absence of corneal neovascularization in response to the bFGF pellet.

To provide a more accurate quantitation of angiogenesis in corneal assays, computerized image analysis of the angiogenesis in the cornea has been used to precisely calculate the vessel density.

Primate Model of Ocular Angiogenesis

Rodent models have been used extensively in the study of angiogenesis and allow for substances to be screened for their ability to inhibit angiogenesis by local or systemic administration. However, the use of a primate model offers advantages over the rodent models but is technically more difficult and more costly. A model of iris neovascularization in the monkey that is clinically and histologically similar to human disease was first developed by Virdi and Hayreh (69). The model has since been modified by Miller and her colleagues (70,71) and provides an effective method to screen angiogenesis inhibitors. Using a series of laser bursts directed at the retina of the monkey, the central retinal veins are occluded. Retinal ischemia and hypoxia is produced and results in the expression and production VEGF/VPF that causes both retinal and iris neovascularization within 5 to 10 days of laser treatment (72). The degree of neovascularization can then be assessed by slit-lamp examination and fluorescein angiography. Interferon-α (IFN-α), for example, has been shown to be an inhibitor of angiogenesis in this system (71) and is now being used clinically to treat malignant angiogenesis (73).

Experimental and Spontaneous Metastasis Models

The metastatic process involves multiple steps in which tumors' cells must invade locally, penetrate through stomal tissues and into a vessel wall, enter into the circulation, adhere to the endothelium at a target site, extravasate, and invade into a target tissue. Angiogenesis is critical for the metastatic process to begin and for metastases to grow (74,75) (see Fig. 3). To grow, metastatic tumor cells must induce an angiogenic phenotype on the vascular endothelial cells of the tissues they invade. However, metastases that do not induce angiogenesis may persist for prolonged intervals as dormant lesions that cuff preexisting host vessels (O'Reilly et al., *unpublished*). The dependence of the growth of metastases on angiogenesis has led to the development of several assays using experimental, in which tumor cells are delivered to the target organ by intravenous injection, or spontaneous metastases from different tumors.

One model of spontaneous metastatic disease was developed in our laboratory and led to the discovery of angiostatin (59). Metastases of a variant of Lewis lung-carcinoma remain dormant until the primary tumor is removed. Angiogenesis inhibi-

tors can be screened in this system for their ability to prevent the growth of spontaneous metastases.

Tumor Growth on the Chicken Chorioallantoic Membrane

The CAM allows for the growth of a variety of tumors. Typically, 10-day-old embryos in which the CAM is fully developed are used, and tumor fragments or suspensions are implanted. This system has been used extensively in several laboratories for the characterization of antiangiogenic and antivascular agents. For example, in the Cheresh laboratory, this model was used to demonstrate that antagonists of the integrin αvβ3 could disrupt angiogenesis and induce tumor regression (76) and that PEX, a metalloproteinase fragment, can potently inhibit tumor angiogenesis (77).

Primary Tumor Growth (Transplantable Models)

The dependence of the growth of solid tumors on angiogenesis allows for the study of the efficacy for angiogenesis inhibitors. The use of microvascular corrosion casting provides a method to determine the vascular patterns of transplantable tumors (78). This method has been used for several different tumor xenografts in mice and demonstrated that tumor cells may induce characteristic vascular networks (21).

By determining the ratio of the volume of treated over control tumors, different inhibitors can be compared for their ability to inhibit the growth of transplantable rodent tumors in syngeneic mice. TNP-470, which was first named AGM-1470 and is a synthetic analogue of the antibiotic fumagillin (41), has been used to treat a wide variety of transplantable tumors in animal models and potently inhibits tumor growth and angiogenesis. However, TNP-470 only selectively inhibits angiogenesis, is generally only cytostatic, and only rarely leads to tumor regressions (79). In a compelling series of experiments, Christofferson and his colleagues found that treatment with TNP-470 *in vivo* induced differentiation of neuroblastoma xenografts (80). TNP-470, like IFN-α, has also been shown to inhibit the growth of hemangiomas (81,82). In fact, TNP-470 has now been tested on more than 60 different transplantable tumors in rodents (Folkman, *personal communication*, 1999) and, as of this writing, all tumors tested thus far respond to therapy with TNP-470.

Systemic therapy with angiostatin has also been shown to inhibit the growth of subcutaneous and orthotopic malignant gliomas (83); hemangioendotheliomas (84); lung carcinomas (85); and human breast, colon, and prostate (Fig. 5) xenografts (86) in mice. As with TNP-470, a tumor that does not respond to angiostatin therapy has not been identified, suggesting that strategies that target the endothelial cell directly may be useful against a wide variety of neoplasms.

Stable Transfection of Angiogenesis Inhibitors into Tumor Cell Lines

As an alternative to systemic therapy, tumor cells can be transfected with the gene corresponding to an angiogenesis inhibitor and the cells then injected into mice. Tumor growth can then be

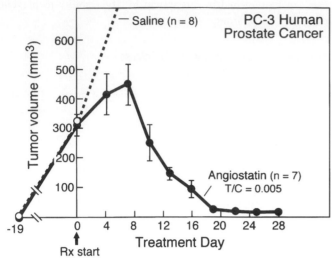

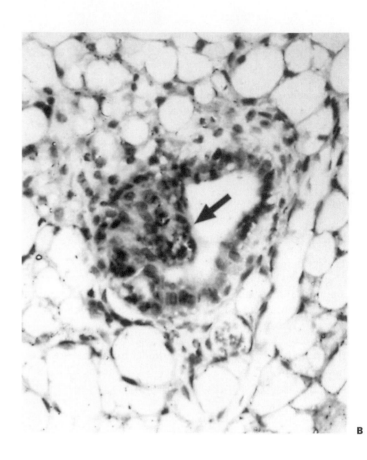

FIGURE 5. Treatment of PC-3 human prostate carcinoma in mice with human angiostatin. **A:** Severe combined immunodeficiency mice were implanted with human prostate carcinoma and treated with human angiostatin (50 mg per kg every 12 hours) or vehicle alone. All of the mice treated with vehicle alone (*dotted line*) had rapidly growing tumors. Tumors in mice treated with angiostatin (*solid line*) were inhibited but still grew for the first 8 days of therapy. However, with continued angiostatin therapy, all tumors regressed to small and pale lesions that did not grow for as long as angiostatin was administered. **B:** Histology of PC-3 human prostate carcinoma treated with angiostatin. Sections were stained with hematoxylin and eosin. The angiostatin-treated tumor regressed to a lesion (*arrow*) limited to four to eight cell layers in diameter surrounded by fat and fibrotic tissue. Immunohistochemistry revealed blocked angiogenesis and a high proliferation of the tumor cells balanced by high apoptosis.

compared to the appropriate vector controls. Cao and his colleagues transfected an aggressive murine fibrosarcoma (T241) with a complementary DNA of murine angiostatin and observed an 80% inhibition of primary tumor growth (87). Furthermore, metastases in 70% of mice implanted with the angiostatin-transfected tumors remained in a state of dormancy after primary tumor resection. The dormant metastases appeared as avascular cuffs around the normal lung capillaries and exhibited a high rate of proliferation balanced by apoptosis. The pattern was similar to the pattern seen in tumors treated systemically with angiostatin (59) and defines the dormant state that can be induced by angiogenesis inhibition (30). Steeg and her colleagues transfected human breast carcinoma cells with thrombospondin-1 (88) and saw a significant inhibition of tumor growth in immunocompromised mice and a decreased microvessel density. The stable transfection of thrombospondin-1 into transformed endothelial cells restored a normal phenotype to these cells *in vitro* and suppressed tumorigenesis *in vivo* (89). Furthermore, thrombospondin-1 transfection almost completely blocked angiogenesis and tumor growth of human skin carcinomas injected subcutaneously in mice (90). In this study, thrombospondin deposition in the matrix around the transfected tumors hindered blood vessel penetration into the tumor. The authors also noted that proliferation of growing and suppressed tumors was virtually identical. Although they did not measure tumor cell apoptosis, they did note increased necrotic cell death in the dormant tumors that were overexpressing thrombospondin. Thus, the induction of tumor dormancy by thrombospon-

din may be similar to the pattern of dormancy seen with angiostatin, endostatin, and other angiogenesis inhibitors.

Mouse and Human Chimeric Models of Tumor Growth

In an attempt to study the effect of angiogenesis inhibitors on human endothelium in an *in vivo* tumor model, human skin can be grafted onto an immunocompromised mouse. Human tumors implanted onto the skin graft induce an angiogenic phenotype of the dermal microvascular endothelial cells in the graft (91). The growth of human tumors with angiogenic vessels made up of human endothelial cells in a murine model can then be studied. For example, LM609 antibodies directed against the integrin $\alpha v \beta 3$ were able to block angiogenesis and tumor growth of a human breast cancer implanted into a human skin graft in a severe combined immunodeficiency mouse/human chimeric model (91). Analysis of the neovessels in the tumors showed that they were made up of human endothelial cells.

Transgenic Models

Although useful in the study of angiogenesis inhibitors in the treatment of malignancy, transplantable tumor models, even with orthotopic implantation, are somewhat limited. In an attempt to develop models of tumor growth that would be more analogous to the development of cancer in patients, transgenic models were developed in which animals develop spontaneous tumors. Transgenic models allow for the study of cancer arising from physiologically normal cells that progress through multiple stages of carcinogenesis [reviewed by Hanahan and Folkman (14)]. Transgenic mice that carry knockouts of tumor suppressor genes or dominant oncogenes have been developed and are being used widely. In addition to allowing for the study of the effect of angiogenesis inhibitors and other therapies on both the development and growth of malignancy, such models have allowed the switch to the angiogenic phenotype to be studied. In these models, tumors develop in distinct stages that are substantially similar to the development of human cancer. Using oncogenes with tissue-specific promoters, Hanahan and his colleagues have developed three distinct transgenic mouse models of tumor development and have extensively characterized the angiogenic switch (14). In one model, referred to as the *RIP-Tag transgenic mouse*, the SV40-T antigen oncogene is expressed by pancreatic-islet beta cells and induces the formation of solid tumors by 12 to 16 weeks of age. Angiogenesis appears in a subset of hyperplastic islets before the onset of tumor formation (29). In other transgenic models, bovine papillomavirus oncogenes induce the multistage development of fibrosarcomas from dermal cells (92) or targeted expression of human papillomavirus type 16 oncogenes to epidermal basal cells induces the development of squamous cell carcinomas (93). Studies of these and other transgenic models have defined angiogenesis as a rate-limiting step in tumor development (14).

The RIP-Tag transgenic mouse has been used to test the efficacy of several angiogenesis inhibitors in the prevention of tumor development and progression after the switch to the angiogenic phenotype. Mice were treated with a combination of the angiogenesis inhibitors TNP-470, minocycline, and IFN-α and IFN-β before the development of malignant tumors. Although tumor formation was not prevented, pancreatic islet tumor volume and capillary density was reduced by 90% and 40%, respectively (94). Tumor-cell proliferation was not substantially different between treated and control tumors, but tumor cell apoptosis was doubled in the treated tumors. The effect of monotherapy with the angiogenesis inhibitors TNP-470 (AGM-1470), BB-94 (batimastat), angiostatin, or endostatin was studied in the RIP1-TAG2 model of pancreatic islet cell carcinogenesis (95). The experiments were designed to study the effect of angiogenesis suppression in the prevention of the switch to the angiogenic phenotype, in the growth of small tumors, or in the treatment of large end-stage lesions. The different angiogenesis inhibitors had varying efficacy depending on the stage of carcinogenesis being targeted. BB-94, angiostatin, and endostatin significantly prevented the angiogenic switch, whereas TNP-470 did not. However, only TNP-470 or angiostatin and endostatin administered in combination was able to induce significant tumor regression. All of the compounds were efficacious in the intervention trial. These results suggest that combinations of angiogenesis inhibitors that target different angiogenic pathways may have improved efficacy as compared to monotherapy.

Immunohistochemistry of Tumors and Microvessel Density

Tumor tissue can be analyzed by immunohistochemistry to quantitate the microvessel density of the treated and control tumors. A variety of antibodies, such as antifactor-VIII–related antigen and von Willebrand's factor or anti-PECAM-1/CD31, directed against the endothelial cell have been used (96–98). Clinically, microvessel density has been studied extensively and has been shown to have prognostic value for a wide variety of tumors (99). In animal models, a decrease in microvessel density can often be seen in tumors treated with angiogenesis inhibitors. However, the results can be difficult to interpret. In some cases, if the tumor shrinks in direct proportion to the number of endothelial cells, there would not be an apparent difference in the microvessel density of the tumor.

The studies of Holmgren et al. (30) demonstrated a new mechanism to explain tumor dormancy brought about by angiogenesis suppression. Dormancy was the result of a balance of apoptosis to proliferation of tumor cells, which arises after the suppression of angiogenesis. Treatment with an angiogenesis inhibitor is not only associated with decreased neovascularization, but also with a three- to fivefold increase in apoptosis, and an increase in tumor cell apoptosis may be a hallmark of angiogenesis suppression. Thus, immunohistochemistry to study microvessel density, tumor-cell proliferation, and apoptosis of tumor and endothelial cells can be useful to define an antiangiogenic effect.

ANGIOGENESIS INHIBITORS CAN BE MOBILIZED BY MALIGNANT TUMORS

Angiostatin Provides a Mechanism for Concomitant Resistance

A new class of endogenous-specific angiogenesis inhibitors has been discovered by studying the different patterns of metastatic presentation. Fifty percent of all cancer patients have metastases (74). These patients can be grouped into five clinical presentations (17) based on the pattern of growth of metastases in relation to the primary tumor. In one of these metastatic patterns, a primary tumor can inhibit the growth of its metastases. For example, the resection of a primary tumor can, in up to 10% of cases (Brem, *personal communication*, 1999), lead to the rapid growth of previously undetected distant metastases. A number of experimental models (in animals) of the inhibition of tumor growth by tumor mass have been described [reviewed by Gorelik (100,101)] and the phenomenon has been referred to as *concomitant resistance* [reviewed by Prehn (102,103)]. In the laboratory of Judah Folkman, I developed a model of the concomitant resistance in which a variant of Lewis lung carcinoma completely suppresses the growth of its metastases (59). We proposed that a primary tumor produces an excess of stimulators of angiogenesis that result in neovascularization in its own vascular bed. As a result, the primary tumor can grow. However, we further proposed that some primary tumors might also produce inhibitors of angiogenesis that accumulate in the circulation in excess of the stimulators and thereby inhibit angiogenesis in the vascular bed of a metastasis or secondary tumor. Angiostatin, a fragment of plasminogen, was purified from the urine of these tumor-bearing mice (59). Angiostatin potently inhibits endothelial cell proliferation and migration *in vitro* and induces endothelial cell apoptosis (104,105) on a variety of endothelial cell types and induces the activation of focal adhesion kinase (105). Adenosine triphosphate synthase on the surface of endothelial cells has been described as a receptor for angiostatin (106). *In vivo* (see Figs. 4 and 5), angiostatin potently inhibits angiogenesis and tumor growth (59,86). Fragments of plasminogen that include at least the first three kringles and up to all five of the kringles have angiostatin activity (85,107–111). Angiostatin therapy induces a state of harmless dormancy of malignant tumors without toxicity.

The Discovery of Endostatin

In other models of concomitant resistance, a primary tumor suppresses the growth of one or several secondary tumors (101,112,113). We noted that a murine hemangioendothelioma inhibits the growth of satellite nodules by endostatin (114), a 20-kd carboxyl-terminal fragment of collagen XVIII. Endostatin is a specific inhibitor of endothelial cell proliferation and has no obvious effect on resting endothelial cells or on a variety of non-endothelial cells (114). The crystal structure of human and mouse endostatin have been determined (115,116). Endostatin was shown to induce endothelial cell apoptosis and a marked reduction in Bcl-2 and Bcl-XI antiapoptotic protein (117) and to inhibit migration and proliferation and cause G1 arrest of endothelial cells stimulated with bFGF or VEGF (118). In our report of the discovery of endostatin, we showed that systemic administration of endostatin to tumor-bearing mice resulted in regression of tumors to a microscopic size (114). A dormant state, defined by a balance of proliferation and apoptosis of the tumor cells without evidence of toxicity, can be maintained for as long as endostatin is administered. Using several recombinant endostatins, Sukhatme's laboratory has since shown similar efficacy against human renal cancer xenografts in mice (119).

Restin, a C-terminal fragment of collagen XV that is homologous to collagen XVIII, has also been shown to be antiangiogenic (120). As with endostatin (119), restin was able to potently inhibit the growth of human renal cell carcinoma xenografts. Currently, several groups are studying fragments derived from other collagens to elucidate their role in angiogenesis.

Vasostatin, a potent and specific angiogenesis inhibitor, is an N-terminal fragment of calreticulin that was purified from the supernatant of Epstein-Barr virus–immortalized cell lines. The generation of vasostatin, along with IP-10 and Mig, is in part responsible for angiogenesis suppression and tumor regression induced by Epstein-Barr virus–immortalized cells.

A Method to Detect Angiogenesis Inhibitors Produced by Human Tumors

To determine if human tumors might also produce inhibitors of angiogenesis, a corneal angiogenesis assay in mice bearing human tumor xenografts has been used. Several human tumors inhibited angiogenesis in this assay (121). Evidence of a circulating inhibitor of angiogenesis associated with human prostate cancer has also been described in an intravital microscope study in mice (122). Furthermore, the inhibition of the growth of experimental B16F10 melanoma metastases by a human fibrosarcoma (HT1080) was shown to be due to the inhibition of

angiogenesis by thrombospondin-1 derived from the primary tumor cells (123).

We have developed a method to screen human tumors for the production of angiogenesis inhibitors. The ability of a primary tumor on the flank of an immunocompromised mouse to inhibit the growth of a similar implant on the opposite flank suggests that a tumor might be generating an angiogenesis inhibitor (124a). While studying the inhibition by a human small cell lung cancer model in this model system, we discovered that the cleaved conformation of antithrombin III has potent antiangiogenic and antitumor activity. The intact native molecule did not have this effect. As with angiostatin and endostatin, the inhibitory activity was specific for endothelial cells.

ANGIOGENESIS INHIBITORS

A number of factors that inhibit angiogenesis have been discovered [reviewed by Auerbach and Auerbach (124)], and the specificity of these agents is becoming an important distinction. Thrombospondin, an endogenous inhibitor of angiogenesis, has already been discussed earlier in this chapter. Many of the first angiogenesis inhibitors were discovered incidentally. Fumagillin, whose analogue TNP-470 is in clinical trial, for example, was discovered from a fungal contaminant that was noted to inhibit endothelial cells (41). More recently, Robert D'Amato developed a profile of potential side effects of angiogenesis inhibition and screened known drugs for these characteristics. In this fashion, the antiangiogenic potentials of thalidomide (125) and 2-methoxyestradiol (126) were discovered. For thalidomide, the drug must be metabolized to become antiangiogenic (68,125,127). A long list of agents that inhibit angiogenesis, including somatostatin analogues, such as octreotide (128), carboxyaminotriazole (129), spironolactone (130), and captopril (131), have since been identified. The goal of this section, however, is not to provide a list of all of the substances that have been described as angiogenesis inhibitors in the literature. Rather, I attempt to give examples of different classes of angiogenesis inhibitors and to develop the concept of angiogenesis inhibition.

Proteolytic Fragments That Inhibit Angiogenesis

Several endogenous inhibitors have been described that are fragments of proteins with distinct functions. One of the first such fragments to be described is a 16-kd fragment of the hormone prolactin (48,132) produced from intact prolactin in the pituitary. Native and recombinant 16K prolactin maintain biologic activity as prolactin agonists but, unlike intact prolactin, also inhibit endothelial proliferation and capillary tube formation *in vitro* and angiogenesis *in vivo*. N-terminal fragments of the human prolactin and growth hormone family and the intact molecules have been found to have opposing effects on angiogenesis (133). Recombinant N-terminal fragments of prolactin, growth hormone, placental lactogen, and growth hormone variant all inhibit angiogenesis possibly by blocking the activation of MAPK downstream of bFGF and VEGF (134) or by increased expression of plasminogen activator inhibitor-1 in capillary endothelial cells. A dual role in angiogenesis has also been described for proliferin, which is angiogenic, and prolif-erin-related peptide, which is antiangiogenic, in the placenta (10). The association between stimulatory and inhibitory effects on angiogenesis within the same molecules may provide an effi-cient means of regulating physiologic angiogenesis.

Furthermore, a plasmin-derived internal fragment of the angiogenesis-inhibitor platelet factor 4 (135) is up to 50-fold more potent than the intact molecule (136). Synthetic frag-ments of murine epidermal growth factor (137), fragments of laminin (49,138), and peptides derived from thrombospondin (37,139,140) all inhibit endothelial cell proliferation and angio-genesis. A 29-kd plasmin-derived fragment of fibronectin (141), the prothrombin kringle-2 domain (142), and a fragment of SPARC (143) can inhibit the proliferation of endothelial cells *in vitro.*

When taken together with the discovery of angiostatin (59), fragments of plasminogen, and endostatin (114) (a fragment of collagen XVIII), a theme has emerged in which endogenous inhibitors of angiogenesis arise from larger proteins with distinct and varied functions. If common proteases or similar cleavage patterns, or both, are found, a new general mechanism of pro-teolytic events regulating the vascular system may be revealed.

Protease Inhibitors Can Be Antiangiogenic

Increased protease activity is a critical step in both angiogenesis and tumor progression. Furthermore, the extracellular matrix and its components play a critical role in angiogenesis (144,145). Matrix metalloproteinases (MMPs) have a prominent role in the progres-sion of malignancy [reviewed by Liotta (146), Stetler-Stevenson (147), and Moses (148)]. Furthermore, the activity of MMPs in the urine of cancer patients may have prognostic value (149). The pres-ence of metalloproteinases in cartilage may in part explain its resis-tance to angiogenesis (150). Troponin I has been identified as a potent inhibitor of angiogenesis found in cartilage (151).

A family of endogenous proteins, the tissue inhibitors of the metalloproteinase family, has been shown to inhibit angiogenesis (150,152,153). However, the difficulties associated with the development of proteins for clinical use have led to the discovery of small molecules that can inhibit MMP activity. Many of the first agents used were tetracycline derived and include minocy-cline and, more recently, COL-3. Other agents, such as marim-astat and batimastat, target the incorporation of zinc into the MMP catalytic site of MMPs (154). More recently, selective inhibitors, such as BAY 12-9566 and AG3340 and several others (155,156), have been developed to selectively target only those MMPs that are important for tumor growth and angiogenesis.

Plasmin is also important in the outgrowth of capillaries in the angiogenic response (157). The serpin plasminogen activa-tor inhibitor-1 has been shown to inhibit angiogenesis, possibly by blocking the interaction of αvβ3 with vitronectin (158). Taken together with our discovery that antithrombin III, another serpin, can also inhibit angiogenesis (O'Reilly et al., submitted), these findings suggest that other serpins involved in the coagulation system may have effects on the endothelial cell.

TABLE 1. REGULATION OF ANGIOGENESIS BY FACTORS DERIVED FROM THE CLOTTING SYSTEM[a]

Coagulation-derived factors
  Antiangiogenic
    Kininogen fragment
    Prothrombin kringle 2
    Plasminogen kringles (angiostatin)
    Antithrombin (antiangiogenic conformation)
    Plasminogen activator inhibitor-1
  Proangiogenic
    Thrombin
    Plasmin
    Tissue factor
    Urokinase
    Tissue-type plasminogen activator
Platelet-derived factors
  Antiangiogenic
    Platelet factor 4
    Thrombospondin
    Fibronectin fragments
  Proangiogenic
    Vascular endothelial cell growth factor/vascular permeability factor
    Platelet-derived growth factor
    Transforming growth factor-β
    Platelet-derived endothelial cell growth factor

[a]A number of factors derived from the coagulation and fibrinolytic systems can stimulate or inhibit angiogenesis. Many of the endogenous inhibitors are generated by the proteolytic degradation of these factors. Furthermore, many clotting factors have direct and indirect roles in the stimulation of angiogenesis and are involved with the capillary endothelial cell sprouting and invasion. Platelets also function to regulate angiogenesis, and their activation can lead to the release of both stimulators and inhibitors of angiogenesis.

Furthermore, the degradation of plasminogen by plasminogen activators in the presence of sulfhydryl donors can mobilize angiostatin (110,159). Thus, the regulation of plasminogen activation has both a stimulatory and inhibitory role in angio-genesis (Table 1).

The inhibition of protease activity may therefore offer both a direct antitumor effect and an antiangiogenic effect in the treat-ment of cancer. However, in a small population of cancer patients there may be a potential disadvantage to administering a metalloproteinase inhibitor. As has been described, many of the endogenous inhibitors of angiogenesis are generated by the cleavage of other proteins by metalloproteinases and other enzymes (109,159–163). In these patients, the level of endoge-nous angiogenesis inhibitors could potentially decrease and need to be replaced.

Agents That Target Angiogenic Factors and Their Receptors

Most of the known angiogenesis factors bind to and are regu-lated by heparin, and many of the first agents designed to target these factors were heparin like. Examples include pentosan polysulfate, tecogalan sodium, suramin derivatives (164), squalamine, and several others. However, the disadvantage of this strategy is the lack of specificity of these agents.

Angiogenesis is regulated by a variety of stimulators of the process that interact with growth factor receptors. Strategies that target these receptors, either directly or indirectly, have been developed. One strategy involves directly blocking the binding of the growth factor to its target receptor using antibodies or small molecule inhibitors. Alternatively, the signaling of the growth factor receptor can be blocked. These strategies offer great potential. However, one theoretical concern is the development of resistance by the tumor by the production of multiple stimulators of angiogenesis.

IFN-α and IFN-β (165) have been shown to inhibit angiogenesis and work by downregulation of the expression of bFGF (166). The antiangiogenic activity of IFN requires sustained levels of the drug, and its use is limited by the toxicity seen when it is given in high dose. However, Fidler and colleagues have demonstrated that human prostate cancer cells transfected with IFN-β were significantly inhibited when implanted orthotopically and subcutaneously *in vivo* due to angiogenesis inhibition and activation of host effector cells (167).

Soluble receptors for angiogenic factors may play a role in the regulation of angiogenesis. Circulating soluble receptors for Flt-1 (168), a receptor for VEGF, and binding proteins for fibroblast growth factors (169) have been described. Their function is not known, but they may serve to limit the levels of angiogenic factors in the circulation and counteract the elevated levels of angiogenic factors seen in cancer patients (170).

Antisense targeting of angiogenic factors or their receptors, such as VEGF/VPF (171) and bFGF (172), can be used to inhibit angiogenesis and tumor growth. Furthermore, strategies that use monoclonal antibodies or soluble receptors to angiogenic factors, such as bFGF (173), VEGF/VPF (174–178), and Tie2 (179), can potently inhibit a wide variety of tumors and angiogenesis. A variety of agents have also been produced that target autophosphorylation or the downstream signals of receptor tyrosine-kinase activity (180). By selectively targeting the endothelial cell, these strategies have shown significant antitumor efficacy.

The interaction of endothelial cells with the extracellular matrix is critical for angiogenesis. Agents that target the binding of endothelial integrins have been studied (181). Integrin αvβ3, for example, was shown to be preferentially expressed by angiogenic blood vessels (76), and antagonists trigger endothelial cell apoptosis, are anti-vascular, and potently inhibit angiogenesis and tumor growth (76,91). Strategies that target αvβ3 and other related integrins, including antibodies and small molecules, are currently the focus of intense research.

A new class of ligands for the receptor tyrosine-kinase Tie2, which is expressed almost exclusively by endothelial cells, have been described (182,183). These molecules, angiopoietin-1 and angiopoietin-2, function in the regulation of angiogenesis and vascular development (184). Angiopoietin-1 recruits pericytes to newly formed capillary sprouts and may help stabilize newly formed capillaries (185), whereas angiopoietin-2 may antagonize the process.

USE OF ANGIOGENESIS INHIBITORS IN COMBINATION WITH OTHER MODALITIES

A malignant tumor has been described as having at least two distinct cell populations (35). Classically, therapies have primarily targeted the tumor cell component, and strategies have been optimized for the delivery of these agents to target only the tumor cells. Thus, although cytotoxic agents can inhibit angiogenesis, when they are given at their maximal tolerated dose, their antiangiogenic effect may not be sustained. By targeting both the endothelial cell population of a tumor and the tumor cell population, improved efficacy should be possible.

Angiogenesis Inhibitors Combined with Chemotherapeutics

Teicher and her colleagues were among the first to show a synergistic effect between cytotoxic agents and antiangiogenic therapy. A combination of the angiogenesis inhibitors tetrahydrocortisol (186), beta-cyclodextrin tetradecasulfate (187), and minocycline (188) given with a variety of cytotoxic agents significantly increased the growth delay of Lewis lung carcinoma xenografts as compared to antiangiogenic or cytotoxic monotherapy (189). Furthermore, the formation and growth of lung metastasis was reduced in all mice, and 40% of the mice treated with combination therapy remained clinically disease-free for longer than 120 days. In a similar set of experiments, a combination of TNP-470 (AGM-1470) and minocycline were given to mice bearing Lewis lung carcinoma (190). A similar improvement in efficacy when angiogenesis inhibitors and cytotoxic agents were combined was demonstrated. A synergistic effect between the combination of TNP-470 with chemotherapy was also seen for murine mammary carcinomas (191) and human pancreatic carcinoma (192). Other angiogenesis inhibitors, such as protamine, when combined with carmustine in the treatment of rat gliomas (193) improved efficacy. Furthermore, by targeting a chemotherapeutic agent directly to the tumor endothelium using homing peptides identified by phage display (20), antitumor efficacy was markedly enhanced.

Angiogenesis Inhibitors and Ionizing Radiation

It had long been assumed that an angiogenesis inhibitor would impair the effect of ionizing radiation by inducing tumor hypoxia. However, Teicher and her colleagues observed that antiangiogenic therapy with a combination of TNP-470 (41) and minocycline improved tumor oxygenation and the antitumor effect of radiation therapy (194). More recently, Weichselbaum and colleagues demonstrated a synergistic effect when angiostatin and ionizing radiation were combined for a variety of transplantable tumors in mice (195,196). The studies were designed using low doses of both modalities and large established murine Lewis lung carcinoma or human glioblastomas, squamous cell carcinomas, or prostate carcinomas. The sequencing of the two modalities was also critical, and the concurrent administration of the radiation and antiangiogenic therapies produced the best efficacy (196). The antitumor effect of hyperthermia is also enhanced by the combination with antiangiogenic therapy with TNP-470 (197,198).

Gene Therapy

Angiogenesis inhibitors often require extended time to begin to work and can induce stasis of tumor growth followed by dormancy after prolonged therapy. They may also require extended therapy for maximal efficacy. Thus, gene therapy may be an attractive strategy for the delivery of an angiogenesis inhibitor [reviewed by Folkman (199), and Kong and Crystal (200)]. Several angiogenesis inhibitors, including angiostatin (201–203), endostatin (204), a truncated VEGF receptor (205), and Tie2 (206), have been delivered using gene therapy. In these studies, a potent inhibition of angiogenesis and tumor growth without evidence was observed. These studies suggest that gene therapy may provide a platform for the therapeutic delivery of angiogenesis factors.

Angiogenesis Inhibition and Immunotherapy

The use of angiogenesis inhibitors may also provide a platform for immunotherapy. The combination of angiogenesis suppression by an alpha-v antagonist and an antibody-cytokine fusion protein induced the complete regression of spontaneous metastases (207). Regressions were not seen with the two modalities when they were administered separately. Furthermore, some molecules may induce both an antiangiogenic and an immunomodulatory response. This is true of interleukin-12, which inhibits angiogenesis indirectly by up regulating IFN-γ (208) that then induces IFN-inducible protein 10 and MIG-1. IFN-γ has since been found to inhibit angiogenesis by the upregulation of IP-10 and MIG. Both are potent inhibitors of angiogenesis and tumor growth (209–211). The potent efficacy of interleukin-12 against a wide variety of tumors may be explained by the combination of its effects on the immune system to induce a tumoricidal effect and its antiangiogenic effect.

TUMOR DORMANCY BY ANGIOGENESIS SUPPRESSION

Initially, angiogenesis inhibitors were expected to be cytostatic only in the treatment of malignant tumors. However, studies of concomitant resistance that led to the discovery of angiostatin and endostatin showed that angiogenesis inhibitors could maintain metastases in a state of dormancy (30,59,114). The mechanism of tumor dormancy induced by angiogenesis suppression was studied by Holmgren et al. and is defined by a dynamic equilibrium between proliferation and apoptosis of tumor cells regulated by the capillary endothelial cell (30). Subsequently, angiostatin has caused regression of established human primary carcinomas (see Fig. 5), growing in mice to microscopic dormant foci in which tumor-cell proliferation was balanced by apoptosis in the presence of blocked angiogenesis (86). This pattern has since been termed *dormancy therapy* and constitutes a novel anticancer strategy in which malignant tumors are regressed by prolonged blockade of angiogenesis. The mechanism of the induction of dormancy and increased tumor-cell apoptosis by angiogenesis suppression remains unknown. Angiogenesis blockade may result in a loss of endothelial-derived paracrine factors needed by the tumor cells. The lack of toxicity seen with angiogenesis inhibition demonstrates the advantage of antitumor therapy directed against the endothelial compartment.

USE OF ANGIOGENESIS INHIBITORS TO BYPASS DRUG RESISTANCE

Acquired drug resistance is a major problem in the treatment of cancer, and the emergence of resistance depends in part on the genetic instability and heterogeneity of tumor cells. In contrast, endothelial cells are genetically stable, homogenous, and have a low mutation rate. Therefore, antiangiogenic therapy that is directed against angiogenic endothelial cells should not induce significant drug resistance. Kerbel first proposed the hypothesis that antiangiogenic therapy could be a strategy to circumvent acquired drug resistance in cancer therapy (212). In a series of preliminary studies, drug resistance was not seen in mice bearing Lewis lung carcinomas treated with TNP-470, a selective angiogenesis inhibitor that inhibits tumor growth (213). However, these studies were limited by the lack of specificity of the agents being tested.

We therefore treated mice bearing Lewis lung carcinoma, T241 fibrosarcoma, or B16F10 melanoma with endostatin, a potent angiogenesis inhibitor (214). Mice were treated with cycled endostatin therapy, and mice were treated systemically with endostatin until tumors had regressed for each cycle. Tumors were then allowed to regrow, and endostatin therapy was resumed. The rate of tumor regression induced by endostatin was essentially the same in all cycles with endostatin. No resistance to therapy was seen even after repeated cycles. We have since observed a similar lack of resistance with other tumors. These experiments show that drug resistance does not develop in response to treatment with a specific inhibitor of angiogenesis.

In a surprising finding, after repeated treatment cycles of endostatin, tumors entered a state of self-sustained dormancy and did not recur after discontinuation of therapy. An unexpected finding is that repeated cycles of antiangiogenic therapy are followed by prolonged tumor dormancy without further therapy. Histologic sections of the primary site revealed a residual tumor of microscopic size that has the same pattern of dormancy as was first defined by Holmgren et al. (30), and the tumors were hypovascular. Some microscopic tumors were mildly infiltrated by leukocytes, and others contained focal necrosis. Although the mechanism of self-sustained dormancy is unknown, it illustrates the powerful control exerted by the vascular endothelial cell population over the tumor cell population. Furthermore, the self-sustained dormancy may be analogous to the cancer patient who has recurrent diseases after a prolonged period of disease-free survival.

Drug resistance may not be a general property of angiogenesis inhibitors. It may be reasonable to assume that angiogenesis inhibitors that specifically or selectively target vascular endothelial cells are less likely to induce resistance than inhibitors that target a tumor-derived mediator of angiogenesis (214). As cells arise that produce other angiogenic factors, the tumor itself may acquire resistance. However, tumors could potentially become resistant to a specific angiogenesis inhibitor should they generate a degrading enzyme. Given that resistance to an angiogenesis inhibitor has not been observed, however, these concerns may not be realized.

INTEGRATION OF ANGIOGENESIS AND OTHER PHYSIOLOGIC PROCESSES

As discussed in this chapter, angiogenesis is a complex process dependent on the balance of inhibitors and stimulators of the process. Numerous lines of evidence now suggest that angiogenesis is regulated in synchrony with other physiologic processes. For example, several factors involved in the coagulation cascade are also critical in the induction and maintenance of the angiogenic response (see Table 1). Tissue factor, for example, can induce angiogenesis by upregulating VEGF/VPF and downregulating the angiogenesis inhibitor thrombospondin-2 (215). Furthermore, platelets sequester VEGF, and their activation may induce angiogenesis by its release (216). Plasma protein forms a neostroma for tumor growth, but these same factors may provide a substrate for the enzymatic mobilization of angiogenesis inhibitors. A general process in which components of the clotting system play a major role in the regulation of angiogenesis has been proposed by Judah Folkman (35). This hypothesis is supported by the presence of potent inhibitors of angiogenesis within proteins such as plasminogen (59), thrombospondin, platelet factor 4 (135), kininogen (217), prothrombin, and antithrombin III (O'Reilly et al., *submitted*). Furthermore, several associations between angiogenesis and the nervous system have emerged. Human neourpilin-1, a receptor for the collapsin and semaphorin family of proteins that mediates neuronal cell guidance, has been found to also be an isoform specific receptor for VEGF165 (218). Furthermore, the ephrin-B2 and its receptor Eph-B4 (219), which are involved in neuronal development, have been shown to play a major role in the embryonic development of arteries and veins. A close association between angiogenesis and other systems may allow for the precise regulation and integration of angiogenesis with physiologic processes.

SUMMARY AND FUTURE DIRECTIONS

Since its beginning in the 1970s, the field of angiogenesis research has grown dramatically and has broadened the understanding of a number of physiologic and pathophysiologic processes. In addition to cancer, a number of other pathologic conditions, including atherosclerosis (220), arthritis (221), ectopic bone formation (222), and ocular neovascularization (71), can also be treated with angiogenesis inhibitors. Antiangiogenic agents should have far-reaching applications in a variety of clinical settings and have the potential to improve efficacy and diminish toxicity in a variety of diseases. In the future, it may be reasonable to combine chemotherapy, radiation therapy, immunotherapy, and emerging modalities with antiangiogenic therapy and to then continue antiangiogenic therapy if needed. If tumor eradication is not possible, then angiogenesis inhibitors may be able to serve as gate keepers to induce and maintain tumors in a state of harmless dormancy and prevent tumor expansion. Clinical trials with a number of antiangiogenic agents have begun or are due to begin shortly. However, a great deal of effort is still required even after antiangiogenic agents become available to learn how to use them to their full potential.

ACKNOWLEDGMENTS

I would like to thank Dr. Judah Folkman for his guidance, teaching, and ideas and for his superb role as a mentor. The field of angiogenesis would not have advanced so far were it not for his persistence and efforts. The figures for this manuscript were designed by Advanced Medical Graphics (Boston, MA).

REFERENCES

1. Folkman J. Tumor angiogenesis: therapeutic implications. *N Engl J Med* 1971;285;1182–1186.
2. Folkman J. What is the evidence that tumors are angiogenesis dependent? *J Natl Cancer Inst* 1990;82:4–6.
3. Folkman J, Klagsburn M. Angiogenic factors. *Science* 1987;235: 442–447.
4. Shing Y, Folkman J, Sullivan R, et al. Heparin-affinity: purification of a tumor-derived capillary endothelial cell growth factor. *Science* 1984;223:1296–1299.
5. Senger DR, Galli SJ, Dvorak AM, Perruzzi CA, Harvey VS. Tumor cells secrete a vascular permeability factor that promotes accumulation of ascites fluid. *Science* 1983;219:983–985.
6. Ferrara N, Henzel WJ. Pituitary follicular cells secrete a novel heparin-binding growth factor specific for vascular endothelial cells. *Biochem Biophys Res Commun* 1989;161:851–858.
7. Grant DS, Kleinman HK, Goldberg ID, et al. Scatter factor induces blood vessel formation *in vivo*. *Proc Natl Acad Sci U S A* 1993;90: 1937–1941.
8. Roberts AB, Sporn MB, Assoian RK, et al. Transforming growth factor type-beta: rapid induction of fibrosis and angiogenesis *in vivo* and stimulation of collagen formation *in vitro*. *Proc Natl Acad Sci U S A* 1986;83:4167–4171.
9. O'Mahony CA, Albo D, Tuszynski GP, Berger DH. Transforming growth factor-beta1 inhibits generation of angiostatin by human pancreatic cancer cells. *Surgery* 1998;124:388–393.
10. Jackson D, Volpert O, Bouck N, Linzer D. Stimulation and inhibition of angiogenesis by placental proliferin and proliferin-related protein. *Science* 1994;266:1581–1585.
11. Ribatti D, Presta M, Vacca A, et al. Human erythropoietin induces a pro-angiogenic phenotype in cultured endothelial cells and stimulates neovascularization *in vivo*. *Blood* 1999;93:2627–2636.
12. Folkman J, Shing Y. Angiogenesis. *J Biol Chem* 1992;267: 10931–10934.
13. Iruela-Arispe ML, Dvorak HF. Angiogenesis: a dynamic balance of stimulators and inhibitors. *Thromb Haemost* 1997;78:672–677.
14. Hanahan D, Folkman J. Patterns and emerging mechanisms of the angiogenic switch during tumorigenesis. *Cell* 1996;86:353–364.
15. Hobson B, Denekamp J. Endothelial proliferation in tumors and normal tissues: continuous labeling studies. *Br J Cancer* 1984;49:405–413.
16. Folkman J. In: Mendelsohn J, Howley PM, Israel MA, Liotta LA, eds. *The Molecular Basis of Cancer*. Philadelphia: WB Saunders, 1995:206–232.[Au: 22]
17. Folkman J. Angiogenesis in cancer, vascular, rheumatoid and other disease. *Nat Med* 1995;1:27–31.
18. Folkman J. The vascularization of tumors. *Sci Am* 1976;234:58–73.
19. Folkman J. Clinical applications of angiogenesis research. *N Engl J Med* 1995;333:1757–1763.
20. Arap W, Pasqualini R, Ruoslahti E. Cancer treatment by targeted drug delivery to tumor vasculature in a mouse model. *Science* 1998;279:377–380.
21. Konerding MA, Malkusch W, Klapthor B, et al. Evidence for characteristic vascular patterns in solid tumours: quantitative studies using corrosion casts. *Br J Cancer* 1999;80:724–732.
22. Orlidge A, D'Amore P. Inhibition of capillary endothelial cell growth by pericytes and smooth muscle cells. *J Cell Biol* 1987;105:1455–1462.
23. Jain RK, Baxter LT. Mechanisms of heterogeneous distribution of monoclonal antibodies and other macromolecules in tumors: signifi-

cance of elevated interstitial pressure. *Cancer Res* 1988;48:7022–7032.

24. Jain RK. Determinants of tumor blood flow: a review. *Cancer Res* 1988;48:2641–2658.

25. Jain RK. Delivery of novel therapeutic agents in tumors: physiological barriers and strategies. *J Natl Cancer Inst* 1989;81:570–576.

26. Dvorak HF, Nagy JA, Dvorak JT, Dvorak AM. Identification and characterization of the blood vessels of solid tumors that are leaky to circulating macromolecules. *Am J Pathol* 1988;133:95–109.

27. Dvorak HF. Tumors: wounds that do not heal. *N Engl J Med* 1986;315:1650–1659.

28. Gerlowski LE, Jain RK. Microvascular permeability of normal and neoplastic tissues. *Microvasc Res* 1986;31:288–305.

29. Folkman J, Watson K, Ingber D, Hanahan D. Induction of angiogenesis during the transition from hyperplasia to neoplasia. *Nature* 1989;339:58–61.

30. Holmgren L, O'Reilly MS, Folkman J. Dormancy of micrometastases: balanced proliferation and apoptosis in the presence of angiogenesis suppression. *Nat Med* 1995;1:149–153.

31. Hamada J, Cavanaugh PG, Lotan O, Nicolson GL. Separable growth and migration factors for large-cell lymphoma cells secreted by microvascular endothelial cells derived from target organs for metastasis. *Br J Cancer* 1992;66:349–354.

32. Nicosia RF, Tchao R, Leighton J. Interactions between newly formed endothelial channels and carcinoma cells in plasma clot culture. *Clin Exp Metastasis* 1986;4:91–104.

33. Alon T, Hemo I, Itin A, et al. VEGF acts as a survival factor for newly formed retinal vessels and has implications for retinopathy of prematurity. *Nat Med* 1995;1:1024–1028.

34. Nor JE, Christensen J, Mooney DJ, Polverini PJ. VEGF-mediated angiogenesis is associated with enhanced endothelial cell survival and induction of Bcl-2 expression. *Am J Pathol* 1999;154:375–384.

35. Folkman J. Tumor angiogenesis and tissue factor. *Nat Med* 1996;2:167–168.

36. Perez-Atayde AR, Sallan SE, Tedrow U, et al. Spectrum of tumor angiogenesis in the bone marrow of children with acute lymphoblastic leukemia. *Am J Pathol* 1997;150:815–821.

37. Good DJ, Polverini PJ, Rastinejad F, et al. A tumor suppressor-dependent inhibitor of angiogenesis is immunologically and functionally indistinguishable from a fragment of thrombospondin. *Proc Natl Acad Sci U S A* 1990;87:6624–6628.

38. Rastinejad F, Polverini PJ, Bouck NP. Regulation of the activity of a new inhibitor of angiogenesis by a cancer suppressor gene. *Cell* 1989;56:345–355.

39. Dameron KM, Volpert OV, Tainsky MA, Bouck N. Control of angiogenesis in fibroblasts by p53 regulation of thrombospondin-1. *Science* 1994;265:1582–1584.

40. Folkman J, Haudenschild CC, Zetter BR. Long-term culture of capillary endothelial cells. *Proc Natl Acad Sci U S A* 1979;76:5217–5221.

41. Ingber D, Fujita T, Kishimoto S, et al. Synthetic analogues of fumagillin that inhibit angiogenesis and suppress tumor growth. *Nature* 1990;348:555–557.

42. Gao Y, Ji R, Folkman J. Microbead assay: a novel assay that detects endothelial cell proliferation and inhibition. *Lab Invest* 1998;78:1029–1030.

43. Blood CH, Zetter BR. Tumor interactions with the vasculature: angiogenesis and tumor metastasis. *Biochim Biophys Acta* 1990;1032:89–118.

44. Folkman J, Haudenschild C. Angiogenesis in vitro. *Nature* 1980;288:551–556.

45. Montesano R. Regulation of angiogenesis in vitro. *Eur J Clin Invest* 1992;22:504–515.

46. Williams S. Angiogenesis in three-dimensional cultures. *Lab Invest* 1993;69:491–493.

47. Montesano R, Orci L, Vassali P. In vitro rapid organization of endothelial cells into capillary-like networks is promoted by collagen matrices. *J Cell Biol* 1983;97:1648–1652.

48. Clapp C, Martial JA, Guzman RC, Rentier-Delrue F, Weiner RI. The 16-kilodalton N-terminal fragment of human prolactin is a potent inhibitor of angiogenesis. *Endocrinology* 1993;133:1292–1299.

49. Grant DS, Tashiro K, Segui-Real B, et al. Two different laminin domains mediate the differentiation of human endothelial cells into capillary-like structures in vitro. *Cell* 1989;58:933–943.

50. Pepper MS, Ferrara N, Orci L, Montesano L. Potent synergism between vascular endothelial growth factor and basic fibroblast growth factor in the induction of angiogenesis in vitro. *Biochem Biophys Res Commun* 1992;189:824–831.

51. Montesano R, Vassali JD, Baird A, Guillemin R, Orci L. Basic fibroblast growth factor induces angiogenesis in vitro. *Proc Natl Acad Sci U S A* 1986;83:7297–7301.

52. Ingber DE, Folkman J. Mechanochemical switching between growth and differentiation during fibroblast growth factor-stimulated angiogenesis in vitro: role of extracellular matrix. *J Cell Biol* 1989;109:317–330.

53. Goto F, Goto K, Weindel K, Folkman J. Synergistic effects of vascular endothelial growth factor and basic fibroblast growth factor on the proliferation and cord formation of bovine capillary endothelial cells within collagen gels. *Lab Invest* 1993;69:508–517.

54. Nicosia RF, Ottinett A. Growth of microvessels in serum-free matrix culture of rat aorta—a quantitative assay of angiogenesis in vitro. *Lab Invest* 1990;63:115–122.

55. Leibovich SJ, Polverini PJ, Shepard HM, et al. Macrophage-induced angiogenesis is mediated by tumour necrosis factor-a. *Nature* 1987;329:630–632.

56. Auerbach R, Kubai L, Knighton D, Folkman J. A simple procedure for the long-term cultivation of chicken embryos. *Dev Biol* 1974;41:391.

57. Taylor S, Folkman J. Protamine is an inhibitor of angiogenesis. *Nature* 1982;297:307–312.

58. Crum R, Szabo S, Folkman J. A new class of steroids inhibits angiogenesis in the presence of heparin or a heparin fragment. *Science* 1985;230:1375.

59. O'Reilly MS, Holmgren L, Shing Y, et al. Angiostatin: a novel angiogenesis inhibitor that mediates the suppression of metastases by a Lewis lung carcinoma. *Cell* 1994;79:315–328.

60. Nguyen M, Shing Y, Folkman J. Quantitation of angiogenesis and antiangiogenesis in the chick embryo chorioallantoic membrane. *Microvasc Res* 1994;47:31–40.

61. Fajardo LF, Kowalski J, Kwan HH, Prionas SD, Allison AC. The disc angiogenesis system. *Lab Invest* 1988;58:718–724.

62. Kusaka M, Sudo K, Fujita T, et al. Potent anti-angiogenic action of AGM-1470: comparison to the fumagillin parent. *Biochem Biophys Res Commun* 1991;174:1070–1076.

63. Passaniti A, Taylor RM, Pili R, et al. A simple, quantitative method for assessing angiogenesis and antiangiogenic agents using reconstituted basement membrane, heparin, and fibroblast growth factor. *Lab Invest* 1992;67:519–528.

64. Gimbrone MA, Cotran R, Leapman S, Folkman J. Tumor growth and neovascularization: an experimental model using the rabbit cornea. *J Natl Cancer Inst* 1974;52:413–427.

65. Fournier GA, Lutty GA, Watt S, Fenselau A, Patz A. A corneal micropocket assay for angiogenesis in the rat eye. *Invest Ophthalmol Vis Sci* 1981;21:351–354.

66. Muthukkaruppan V, Auerbach R. Angiogenesis in the mouse cornea. *Science* 1979;28:1416–1418.

67. Kenyon BM, Voest EE, Chen CC, et al. A model of angiogenesis in the mouse cornea. *Invest Ophthalmol Vis Sci* 1996;37:1625–1632.

68. Kenyon BM, Browne F, D'Amato RJ. Effects of thalidomide and related metabolites in a mouse corneal model of neovascularization. *Exp Eye Res* 1997;64:971–978.

69. Virdi PS, Hayreh SS. Ocular neovascularization with retinal vascular occlusion: association with experimental retinal vein occlusion. *Arch Ophthalmol* 1982;100:331–341.

70. Miller JW, Stinson WG, Gregory WA. Phthalocyanine photodynamic therapy of experimental iris neovascularization. *Ophthalmology* 1991;98:1711–1719.

71. Miller JW, Stinson WG, Folkman J. Regression of experimental iris neovascularization with systemic alpha-interferon. *Ophthalmology* 1993;100:9–14.

72. Adamis AP, Shima DT, Tolentino MJ, et al. Inhibition of vascular endothelial growth factor prevents retinal ischemia-associated iris

neovascularization in a nonhuman primate. *Arch Ophthalmol* 1996;114:66–71.

73. White CM, Sondheimer HM, Crouch EC, Wilson H, Fan LF. Treatment of pulmonary hemangiomatosis with recombinant interferon alfa-2a. *N Engl J Med* 1989;320:1197–1200.

74. Fidler IJ, Ellis LM. The implications of angiogenesis for the biology and therapy of cancer metastasis. *Cell* 1994;79:185–188.

75. Rak JW, St Croix BD, Kerbel RS. Consequences of angiogenesis for tumor progression, metastasis and cancer therapy. *Anticancer Drugs* 1995;6:3–18.

76. Brooks PC, Stromblad S, Sanders LC, et al. Integrin avb3 antagonists promote tumor regression by inducing apoptosis of angiogenic blood vessels. *Cell* 1994;79:1157–1164.

77. Brooks PC, Silletti S, von Schalscha IL, Friedlander M, Cheresh DA. Disruption of angiogenesis by PEX, a noncatalytic metalloproteinase fragment with integrin binding activity. *Cell* 1998;92:391–400.

78. Less JR, Skalak TC, Sevick EM, Jain RK. Microvascular architecture in a mammary carcinoma: branching patterns and vessel dimensions. *Cancer Res* 1991;51:265–273.

79. Wassberg E, Christofferson R. Angiostatic treatment of neuroblastoma. *Eur J Cancer* 1997;33:2020–2023.

80. Wassberg E, Hedborg F, Skoldenberg E, Stridsberg M, Christofferson R. Inhibition of angiogenesis induces chromaffin differentiation and apoptosis in neuroblastoma. *Am J Pathol* 1999;154:395–403.

81. Liekens S, Verbeken E, Vandeputte M, DeClercq E, Neyts J. A novel animal model for hemangiomas: inhibition of hemangioma development by the angiogenesis inhibitor TNP-470. *Cancer Res* 1999;59:2376–2383.

82. O'Reilly MS, Brem H, Folkman J. Treatment of murine hemangioendotheliomas with the angiogenesis inhibitor AGM-1470. *J Pediatr Surg* 1995;30:325–330.

83. Kirsch M, Strasser J, Allende R, et al. Angiostatin suppresses malignant glioma growth *in vivo. Cancer Res* 1998;58:4654–4659.

84. Lannutti BJ, Gately ST, Quevedo ME, Soff GA, Paller AS. Human angiostatin inhibits murine hemangioendothelioma tumor growth *in vivo. Cancer Res* 1997;57:5277–5280.

85. Wu Z, O'Reilly MS, Folkman J, Shing Y. Suppression of tumor growth with recombinant murine angiostatin. *Biochem Biophys Res Commun* 1997;236:651–654.

86. O'Reilly MS, Holmgren L, Chen CC, Folkman J. Angiostatin induces and sustains dormancy of human primary tumors in mice. *Nature Med* 1996;2:689–692.

87. Cao Y, O'Reilly MS, Marshall B, et al. Expression of angiostatin cDNA in a murine fibrosarcoma suppresses primary tumor growth and produces long term dormancy of metastases. *J Clin Invest* 1998; 101:1055–1063.

88. Weinstat-Saslow DL, Zabrenetzky VS, VanHoutte K, et al. Transfection of thrombospondin 1 complementary DNA into a human breast carcinoma cell line reduces primary tumor growth, metastatic potential and angiogenesis. *Cancer Res* 1994;54:6504–6511.

89. Sheibani N, Frazier WA. Thrombospondin 1 expression in transformed endothelial cells restores a normal phenotype and suppresses their tumorigenesis. *Proc Natl Acad Sci U S A* 1995;92:6788–6792.

90. Bleuel K, Popp S, Fusenmg NE, Stanbridge EJ, Boukamp P. Tumor suppression in human skin carcinoma cells by chromosome 15 transfer or thrombospondin-1 overexpression through halted tumor vascularization. *Proc Natl Acad Sci U S A* 1999;96:2065–2070.

91. Brooks PC, Stromblad S, Klemke R, et al. Antiintegrin avb3 blocks human breast cancer growth and angiogenesis in human skin. *J Clin Invest* 1995;96:1815–1822.

92. Hanahan D. Heritable formation of pancreatic beta-cell tumors in transgenic mice harboring recombinant insulin/simian virus 40 oncogenes. *Nature* 1985;315:115–122.

93. Arbeit J, Munger K, Howley P, Hanahan D. Progressive squamous epithelial neoplasia in K14-HPV16 transgenic mice. *J Virol* 1994;68:4358–4368.

94. Parangi S, O'Reilly M, Christofori G, et al. Antiangiogenic therapy of transgenic mice impairs de novo tumor growth. *Proc Natl Acad Sci U S A* 1996;93:2002–2007.

95. Bergers G, Javaherian K, Lo K, Folkman J, Hanahan D. Effects of angiogenesis inhibitors on multistage carcinogenesis in mice. *Science* 1999;284:808–812.

96. Charpin C, Devictor B, Bergeret D, et al. CD31 quantitative immunocytochemical assays in breast carcinomas—correlation with current prognostic factors. *Am J Clin Pathol* 1995;103:443–448.

97. Fox SB, Leek RD, Weekes MP, et al. Quantitation and prognostic value of breast cancer angiogenesis: comparison of microvessel density, Chalkley count, and computer image analysis. *J Pathol* 1995;177:275–283.

98. Weidner N. Current pathologic methods for measuring intratumoral microvessel density within breast carcinoma and other solid tumors. *Breast Cancer Res Treat* 1995;36:169–180.

99. Weidner N. Intratumor microvessel density as a prognostic factor in cancer. *Am J Pathol* 1995;147:9–19.

100. Gorelik E, Segal S, Feldman M. On the mechanism of tumor concomitant immunity. *Int J Cancer* 1981;27:847–856.

101. Gorelik, E. Concomitant tumor immunity and the resistance to a second tumor challenge. *Adv Cancer Res* 1983;39:71–120.

102. Prehn RT. The inhibition of tumor growth by tumor mass. *Cancer Res* 1991;51:2–4.

103. Prehn RT. Two competing influences that may explain concomitant tumor resistance. *Cancer Res* 1993;53:3266–3269.

104. Lucas R, Holmgren L, Garcia I, et al. Multiple forms of angiostatin induce apoptosis in endothelial cells. *Blood* 1998;92:4730–4741.

105. Claesson-Welsh L, Welsh M, Ito N, et al. Angiostatin induces endothelial cell apoptosis and activation of focal adhesion kinase independently of the integrin-binding motif RGD. *Proc Natl Acad Sci U S A* 1998;95:5579–5583.

106. Moser TL, Stack MS, Asplin I, et al. Angiostatin binds ATP synthase on the surface of human endothelial cells. *Proc Natl Acad Sci U S A* 1999;96:2811–2816.

107. Cao Y, Ji RW, Davidson D, et al. Kringle domains of human angiostatin. *J Biol Chem* 1996;271:29461–29467.

108. Cao R, Wu HL, Veitonmaki N, et al. Suppression of angiogenesis and tumor growth by the inhibitor K1-5 generated by plasmin-mediated proteolysis. *Proc Natl Acad Sci U S A* 1999;96:5728–5733.

109. Gately S, Twardowski P, Stack MS, et al. The mechanism of cancer-mediated conversion of plasminogen to the angiogenesis inhibitor angiostatin. *Proc Natl Acad Sci U S A* 1997;94:10868–10872.

110. Gately S, Twardowski P, Stack MS, et al. Human prostate carcinoma cells express enzymatic activity that converts human plasminogen to the angiogenesis inhibitor angiostatin. *Cancer Res* 1996;56:4887–4890.

111. Sim BK, O'Reilly MS, Liang H, et al. A recombinant human angiostatin protein inhibits experimental primary and metastatic cancer. *Cancer Res* 1997;57:1329–1334.

112. Gorelik E. Resistance of tumor-bearing mice to a second tumor challenge. *Cancer Res* 1983;43:138–145.

113. Ruggierro RA, Bustuoabad OD, Cramer P, Bonfil RD, Pasqualini CD. Correlation between seric antitumor activity and concomitant resistance in mice bearing nonimmunogenic tumors. *Cancer Res* 1990;50:7159–7165.

114. O'Reilly MS, Boehm T, Shing Y, et al. Endostatin: an endogenous inhibitor of angiogenesis and tumor growth. *Cell* 1997;88:277–285.

115. Hohenester E, Sasaki T, Olsen BR, Timpl R. Crystal structure of the angiogenesis inhibitor endostatin at 1.5 A resolution. *EMBO J* 1998;17:1656–1664.

116. Ding Y, Javaherian K, Lo KM, et al. Zinc dependent dimers observed in crystals of human endostatin. *Proc Natl Acad Sci U S A* 1998;95:10443–10448.

117. Dhanabal M, Ramchandran R, Volk R, et al. Endostatin induces endothelial cell apoptosis. *J Biol Chem* 1999;274:11721–11726.

118. Dhanabal M, Volk R, Ramchandran R, Simons M, Sukhatme V. Cloning, expression, and in vitro activity of human endostatin. *Biochem Biophys Res Commun* 1999;258:345–352.

119. Dhanabal M, Ramchandran R, Volk R, et al. Endostatin: yeast production, mutants, and antitumor effect in renal cell carcinoma. *Cancer Res* 1999;59:189–197.

120. Ramchandran R, Dhanabal M, Volk R, et al. Antiangiogenic activity of restin, NC10 domain of human collagen XV: comparison to endostatin. *Biochem Biophys Res Commun* 1999;255:735–739.

121. Chen C, Parangi S, Tolentino MJ, Folkman J. A strategy to discover circulating angiogenesis inhibitors generated by human tumors. *Cancer Res* 1995;55:4230–4233.

122. Sckell A, Safabakhsh N, Dellian M, Jain RK. Primary tumor size-dependent inhibition of angiogenesis at a secondary site: an intravital microscopic study in mice. *Cancer Res* 1998;58:5866–5869.

123. Volpert O, Lawler J, Bouck NP. A human fibrosarcoma inhibits systemic angiogenesis and the growth of experimental metastases via thrombospondin-1. *Proc Natl Acad Sci U S A* 1998;95:6343–6348.

124. Auerbach W, Auerbach R. Angiogenesis inhibition: a review. *Pharmac Ther* 1994;63:265–311.

124a. O'Reilly MS, Pirie-Shepherd S, Lane WS, Folkman J. Antiangiogenic activity of the cleaved conformation of the serpin antithrombin. *Science* 1999 (submitted).

125. D'Amato RJ, Loughnan MS, Flynn E, Folkman J. Thalidomide is an inhibitor of angiogenesis. *Proc Natl Acad Sci U S A* 1994;91: 4082–4085.

126. D'Amato RJ, Lin CM, Flynn E, Folkman J, Hamel E. 2-Methoxyestradiol, an endogenous mammalian metabolite, inhibits tubulin polymerization by interacting at the colchicine site. *Proc Natl Acad Sci U S A* 1994;91:3964–3968.

127. Bauer KS, Dixon SC, Figg WD. Inhibition of angiogenesis by thalidomide requires metabolic activation, which is species-dependent. *Biochem Pharm* 1998;55:1827–1834.

128. Danesi R, Agen C, Benelli U, et al. Inhibition of experimental angiogenesis by the somatostatin analogue octreotide acetate (SMS 201-995). *Clin Cancer Res* 1997;3:265–272.

129. Kohn EC, Alessandro R, Spoonster J, Wersto RP, Liotta LA. Angiogenesis: role of calcium-mediated signal transduction. *Proc Natl Acad Sci U S A* 1995;92:1307–1311.

130. Klauber N, Browne F, Anand-Apte B, D'Amato RJ. New activity of spironolactone: inhibition of angiogenesis *in vitro* and *in vivo*. *Circulation* 1996;94:2566–2571.

131. Volpert OV, Ward WF, Lingen MW, et al. Captopril inhibits angiogenesis and slows the growth of experimental tumors in rats. *J Clin Invest* 1996;98:671–679.

132. Ferrara N, Clapp C, Weiner RI. The 16K fragment of prolactin specifically inhibits basal or FGF stimulated growth of capillary endothelial cells. *Endocrinology* 1991;129:896–900.

133. Struman I, Bentzien F, Lee H, et al. Opposing actions of intact and N-terminal fragments of human prolactin/growth hormone family members on angiogenesis: an efficient mechanism for the regulation of angiogenesis. *Proc Natl Acad Sci U S A* 1999;96:1246–1251.

134. D'Angelo G, Struman I, Martial J, Weiner RI. Activation of mitogen-activated protein kinases by vascular endothelial growth factor and basic fibroblast growth factor in capillary endothelial cells is inhibited by the antiangiogenic factor 16-kDa N-terminal fragment of prolactin. *Proc Natl Acad Sci U S A* 1995;92:6374–6378.

135. Maione TE, Gray GS, Petro J, et al. Inhibition of angiogenesis by recombinant human platelet factor-4 and related peptides. *Science* 1990;247:77–79.

136. Gupta SK, Hassel T, Singh JP. A potent inhibitor of endothelial cell proliferation is generated by proteolytic cleavage of the chemokine platelet factor 4. *Proc Natl Acad Sci U S A* 1995;92:7799–7803.

137. Nelson J, Allen WE, Scott WN, et al. Murine epidermal growth factor (EGF) fragment (33-42) inhibits both EGF- and laminin-dependent endothelial cell motility and angiogenesis. *Cancer Res* 1995;55:3772–3776.

138. Sakamato N, Iwahana M, Tanaka NG, Osaka Y. Inhibition of angiogenesis and tumor growth by a synthetic laminin peptide, CDPGYIGSA-NH$_2$. *Cancer Res* 1991;51:903–906.

139. Tolsma SS, Volpert OV, Good DJ, et al. Peptides derived from two separate domains of the matrix protein thrombospondin-1 have antiangiogenic activity. *J Cell Biol* 1993;122:497–511.

140. Dawson DW, Volpert OV, Pearce SF, et al. Three distinct D-amino acid substitutions confer potent antiangiogenic activity on an inactive peptide derived from a thrombospondin-1 type 1 repeat. *Mol Pharmacol* 1999;55:332–338.

141. Homandberg GA, Williams JE, Grant DBS, Eisenstein R. Heparin-binding fragments of fibronectin are potent inhibitors of endothelial cell growth. *Am J Pathol* 1985;120:327–332.

142. Lee T, Rhim Y, Kim SS. Prothrombin kringle-2 domain has a growth inhibitory activity against basic fibroblast growth factor-stimulated capillary endothelial cells. *J Biol Chem* 1998;273:28805–28812.

143. Sage EH, Bassuk JA, Vost JC, Folkman MJ, Lane TF. Inhibition of endothelial cell proliferation by SPARC is mediated through a Ca (2+)-binding EF-hand sequence. *J Cell Biochem* 1995;57:127–140.

144. Ingber DE, Folkman J. How does extracellular matrix control capillary morphogenesis? *Cell* 1989;58:803–805.

145. Vlodavsky I, Korner G, Ishai-Michaeli R, et al. Extracellular matrix-resident growth factors and enzymes: possible involvement in tumor metastasis and angiogenesis. *Cancer Metastasis Rev* 1990;9:203–226.

146. Liotta LA, Stetler-Stevenson WG, Steeg PS. Cancer invasion and metastasis: positive and negative regulatory elements. *Cancer Invest* 1991;9:543–551.

147. Stetler-Stevenson WG. Matrix metalloproteinases in angiogenesis: a moving target for therapeutic intervention. *J Clin Invest* 1999;103: 1237–1241.

148. Moses MA. The regulation of neovascularization by matrix metalloproteinases and their inhibitors. *Stem Cells* 1997;15:180–189.

149. Moses MA, Wiederschain D, Loughlin KR, et al. Increased incidence of matrix metalloproteinases in urine of cancer patients. *Cancer Res* 1998;58:1395–1399.

150. Moses MA, Sudhalter J, Langer R. Identification of an inhibitor of neovascularization from cartilage. *Science* 1990;248:1408–1410.

151. Moses MA, Wiederschain D, Wu I, et al. Troponin I is present in human cartilage and inhibits angiogenesis. *Proc Natl Acad Sci U S A* 1999;96:2645–2650.

152. Anand-Apte B, Pepper MS, Voest E, et al. Inhibition of angiogenesis by tissue inhibitor of metalloproteinase-3. *Invest Ophthalmol Vis Sci* 1997;38:817–823.

153. Takigawa M, Nishida Y, Suzuki F, et al. Induction of angiogenesis in chick yolk-sac membrane by polyamines and its inhibition by tissue inhibitors of metalloproteinases (TIMP and TIMP-2). *Biochem Biophys Res Commun* 1990;171:1264–1271.

154. Davies B, Brown PD, East N, et al. A synthetic MMP inhibitor decreases tumor burden and prolongs survival of mice bearing human ovarian carcinoma xenografts. *Cancer Res* 1993;53:2087.

155. Lozonschi L, Sunamura M, Kobari M, et al. Controlling tumor angiogenesis and metastasis of C26 murine colon adenocarcinoma by a new matrix metalloproteinase inhibitor, KB-R7785, in two tumor models. *Cancer Res* 1999;59:1252–1258.

156. Maekawa R, Maki H, Yoshida H, et al. Correlation of antiangiogenic and antitumor efficacy of BPHA, an orally active, selective matrix metalloproteinase inhibitor. *Cancer Res* 1999;59;1231–1235.

157. Mignatti P, Rifkin DB. Plasminogen activators and matrix metalloproteinases in angiogenesis. *Enz Prot* 1996;49:117–137.

158. Stefansson S, Lawrence DA. The serpin PAI-1 inhibits cell migration by blocking integrin avb3 binding to vitronectin. *Nature* 1996;383: 441–443.

159. Stathakis P, Fitzgerald M, Matthias LJ, Chesterman CN, Hogg PJ. Generation of angiostatin by reduction and proteolysis of plasmin. *J Biol Chem* 1997;272:20641–20645.

160. Cornelius LA, Nehring LC, Harding E, et al. Matrix metalloproteinases generate angiostatin: effects on neovascularization. *J Immunol* 1998;161:6845–6852.

161. Patterson BC, Sang QXA. Angiostatin-converting enzyme activities of MMP-7 and MMP-9. *J Biol Chem* 1997;272:28823.

162. O'Mahony CA, Seidel A, Albo D, et al. Angiostatin generation by human pancreatic cancer. *J Surg Res* 1998;77:55–58.

163. Dong Z, Kumar R, Yang X, Fidler IJ. Macrophage-derived metalloelastase is responsible for the generation of angiostatin in lewis lung carcinoma. *Cell* 1997;88:801–810.

164. Danesi R, Del Bianchi S, Soldani P, et al. Suramin inhibits bFGF-induced endothelial cell proliferation and angiogenesis in the CAM. *Br J Cancer* 1993;68:932–938.

165. Brouty-Boye D, Zetter BR. Inhibition of cell motility by interferon. *Science* 1980;206:516–518.

166. Singh RK, Gutman M, Bucana CD, Sanchez R, Llansa N. Interferons a and b down-regulate the expression of basic fibroblast growth

factor in human carcinomas. *Proc Natl Acad Sci U S A* 1995;92: 4562–4566.

167. Dong Z, Greene G, Pettaway C, et al. Suppression of angiogenesis, tumorigenicity, and metastasis by human prostate cancer cells engineered to produce interferon-beta. *Cancer Res* 1999;59:872–879.

168. Kendall RL, Thomas KA. Inhibition of VEGF activity by an endogenously encoded soluble receptor. *Proc Natl Acad Sci U S A* 1993;90:10705–10709.

169. Hanneken A, Ying W, Ling N, Baird A. Identification of soluble forms of the fibroblast growth factor receptor in blood. *Proc Natl Acad Sci U S A* 1994;91:9170–9174.

170. Nguyen M, Watanabe H, Budson AE, Richie JP, Folkman J. Elevated levels of the angiogenic peptide basic fibroblast growth factor in urine of bladder cancer patients. *J Natl Cancer Inst* 1993;85:241–242.

171. Millauer B, Shawver LK, Plate KH, Risau W, Ullrich A. Glioblastoma growth inhibited *in vivo* by a dominant-negative Flk-1 mutant. *Nature* 1994;367:576–579.

172. Wang Y, Becker D. Antisense targeting of bFGF and FGF receptor-1 in human melanomas blocks intratumoral angiogenesis and tumor growth. *Nature Med* 1997;3:887–893.

173. Hori A, Sasada R, Matsutani E, et al. Suppression of solid tumor growth by immunoneutralizing monoclonal antibody against human basic fibroblast growth factor. *Cancer Res* 1991;51:6180–6184.

174. Kim KJ, Li B, Winer J, et al. Inhibition of vascular endothelial growth factor-induced angiogenesis suppresses tumor growth *in vivo*. *Nature* 1993;362:841–844.

175. Asano M, Yukita A, Matsumoto T, Kondo S, Suzuki H. Inhibition of tumor growth and metastasis by an immunoneutralizing monoclonal antibody to human VEGF/VPF. *Cancer Res* 1995;55:5296–5301.

176. Goldman CK, Kendall RL, Cabrera G, et al. Paracrine expression of a native soluble VEGF receptor inhibits tumor growth, metastasis, and mortality rate. *Proc Natl Acad Sci U S A* 1998;95:8795–8800.

177. Lin P, Sankar S, Shan S, et al. Inhibition of tumor growth by targeting tumor endothelium using a soluble VEGF receptor. *Cell Growth Differ* 1998;9:49–58.

178. Borgstrom P, Bourdon MA, Hillan KJ, Sriramarao P, Ferrara N. Neutralizing anti-vascular endothelial growth factor antibody completely inhibits angiogenesis and growth of human prostate carcinoma micro tumors *in vivo*. *Prostate* 1998;35:1–10.

179. Lin P, Polverini P, Dewhirst M, et al. Inhibition of tumor angiogenesis using a soluble receptor establishes a role for Tie2 in pathologic vascular growth. *J Clin Invest* 1997;100:2072–2078.

180. Shawver LK, Schwartz DP, Mann E, et al. Inhibition of PDGF-mediated signal transduction and tumor growth by SU101. *Clin Cancer Res* 1997;3:1167–1177.

181. Eliceiri BP, Cheresh DA. The role of av integrins during angiogenesis: insights into potential mechanisms of action and clinical development. *J Clin Invest* 1999;103:1227–1230.

182. Suri C, Jones PF, Patan S, et al. Requisite role of angiopoietin-1, a ligand for the TIE2 receptor, during embryonic angiogenesis. *Cell* 1996;87:1153–1155.

183. Davis S, Aldrich TH, Jones PF, et al. Isolation of angiopoietin-1, a ligand for the TIE2 receptor, by secretion-trap expression cloning. *Cell* 1996;87:1153–1155.

184. Asahara T, Chen D, Takahashi T, et al. Tie2 receptor ligands, angiopoietin-1 and angiopoietin-2, modulate VEGF-induced postnatal neovascularization. *Circ Res* 1998;83:233–240.

185. Papapetropoulos A, Garcia-Cardena G, Dengler TJ, et al. Direct actions of angiopoietin-1 on human endothelium: evidence for network stabilization, cell survival, and interaction with other angiogenic growth factors. *Lab Invest* 1999;79:213–223.

186. Folkman J, Langer R, Linhardt R, Haudenschild C, Taylor S. Angiogenesis inhibition and tumor regression caused by heparin or a heparin fragment in the presence of cortisone. *Science* 1983;221:719–725.

187. Folkman J, Weisz PB, Joullie MM, Li WW, Ewing WR. Control of angiogenesis with synthetic heparin substitutes. *Science* 1989;243: 1490–1493.

188. Tamargo RJ, Bok RA, Brem H. Angiogenesis inhibition by minocycline. *Cancer Res* 1991;51:672–675.

189. Teicher BA, Sotomayon EA, Huang ZD. Antiangiogenic agents potentiate cytotoxic cancer therapies against primary and metastatic

disease. *Cancer Res* 1992;52:6702–6704.

190. Teicher BA, Holden SA, Ara G, Sotomayor E, Huang ZD. Potentiation of cytotoxic cancer therapies by TNP-470 alone and with other antiangiogenic agents. *Int J Cancer* 1994;57:1–6.

191. Teicher BA, Holden SA, Dupuis NP, et al. Potentiation of cytotoxic therapies by TNP-470 and minocycline in mice bearing EMT-6 mammary carcinoma. *Breast Cancer Res Treat* 1995;36:227–236.

192. Shishido T, Yasoshima T, Denno R, et al. Inhibition of liver metastasis of human pancreatic carcinoma by angiogenesis inhibitor TNP-470 in combination with cisplatin. *Jap J Cancer Res* 1998;89:963–999.

193. Arrieta O, Guevara P, Reyes S, et al. Protamine inhibits angiogenesis and growth of C6 rat glioma; a synergistic effect when combined with carmustine. *Eur J Cancer* 1998;34:2101–2106.

194. Teicher BA, Dupuis N, Kusomoto T, et al. Antiangiogenic agents can increase tumor oxygenation and response to radiation therapy. *Rad Oncol Invest* 1995;2:269–276.

195. Mauceri HJ, Hanna NN, Beckett MA, et al. Combined effects of angiostatin and ionizing radiation in antitumor therapy. *Nature* 1998;394:287–291.

196. Gorski DH, Mauceri HJ, Salloum RM, et al. Potentiation of the antitumor effect of ionizing radiation by brief concomitant exposures to angiostatin. *Cancer Res* 1998;58:5686–5689.

197. Ikeda S, Akagi K, Shiraishi T, Tanaka Y. Enhancement of the effect of an angiogenesis inhibitor on murine tumors by hyperthermia. *Oncol Reports* 1998;5:181–184.

198. Nishimura Y, Murata R, Hiraoka M. Combined effects of angiogenesis inhibitor (TNP-470) and hyperthermia. *Br J Cancer* 1996;73: 270–274.

199. Folkman J. Antiangiogenic gene therapy. *Proc Natl Acad Sci U S A* 1998;95:9064–9066.

200. Kong H, Crystal RG. Gene therapy strategies for tumor angiogenesis. *J Natl Cancer Inst* 1998;90:273–286.

201. Tanaka T, Gao Y, Folkman J, Fine HA. Viral vector-targeted antiangiogenic gene therapy utilizing an angiostatin complementary cDNA. *Cancer Res* 1998;58:3362–3369.

202. Griscelli F, Li H, Bennaceur-Griscelli A, et al. Angiostatin gene transfer: inhibition of tumor growth *in vivo* by blockage of endothelial cell proliferation associated with mitosis arrest. *Proc Natl Acad Sci U S A* 1998;95:6367–6372.

203. Liu Y, Thor A, Shtivelman E, et al. Systemic gene delivery expands the repertoire of effective antiangiogenic agents. *J Biol Chem* 1999;274:13338–13344.

204. Blezinger P, Wang J, Gondo M, et al. Systemic inhibition of tumor growth and tumor metastases by intramuscular administration of endostatin gene. *Nat Biotechnol* 1999;17:343–348.

205. Kong HL, Hecht D, Song W, et al. Regional suppression of tumor growth by *in vivo* transfer of a cDNA encoding a secreted form of the extracellular domain of the Flt-1 VEGF receptor. *Hum Gene Ther* 1998;9:823–833.

206. Lin P, Buxton JA, Acheson A, et al. Antiangiogenic gene therapy targeting the endothelium-specific receptor tyrosine kinase Tie2. *Proc Natl Acad Sci U S A* 1998;95:8829–8834.

207. Lode HN, Moehler T, Xiang R, et al. Synergy between an antiangiogenic integrin alpha v antagonist and an antibody-cytokine fusion protein eradicates spontaneous tumor metastases. *Proc Natl Acad Sci U S A* 1999;96:1591–1596.

208. Voest EE, Kenyon BM, O'Reilly MS, et al. Inhibition of angiogenesis *in vivo* by interleukin 12. *J Natl Cancer Inst* 1995;87:581–586.

209. Angiolillo AL, Sgadari C, Taub DD, et al. Human interferon-inducible protein 10 is a potent inhibitor of angiogenesis *in vivo*. *J Exp Med* 1995;182:155–162.

210. Sgadari C, Angiolillo AL, Cherney BW, et al. Interferon-inducible protein-10 identified as a mediator of tumor necrosis *in vivo*. *Proc Natl Acad Sci U S A* 1996;93:13791–13796.

211. Arenberg DA, Kunkel SL, Polverini PJ, et al. Interferon-gamma-inducible protein 10 (IP-10) is an angiostatic factor that inhibits human non-small cell lung cancer (NSCLC) tumorigenesis and spontaneous metastases. *J Exp Med* 1996;184:981–992.

212. Kerbel RS. Inhibition of tumor angiogenesis as a strategy to circumvent acquired resistance to anti-cancer therapeutic agents. *Bioessays*

1991;13:31–36.

213. Brem H, Goto F, Budson A, Saunders L, Folkman J. Minimal drug resistance after prolonged antiangiogenic therapy with AGM-1470. *Surg Forum* 1994;XLV:674–677.

214. Boehm T, Folkman J, Browder T, O'Reilly MS. Antiangiogenic therapy of experimental cancer does not induce acquired drug resistance. *Nature* 1997;390:404–407.

215. Zhang Y, Deng Y, Luther T, et al. Tissue factor controls the balance of angiogenic and antiangiogenic properties of tumor cells in mice. *J Clin Invest* 1994;94:1320–1327.

216. Pinedo HM, Verheul HM, D'Amato RJ, Folkman J. Involvement of platelets in tumor angiogenesis? *Lancet* 1998;352:1775–1777.

217. Colman RW, Lin Y, Johnson D, Mousa SA. Inhibition of angiogenesis by peptides derived from kininogen. *Blood* 1998;92[Suppl]:174a.

218. Soker S, Takashima S, Miao HQ, Neufeld G, Klagsbrun M. Neuropilin-1 is expressed by endothelial and tumor cells as an isoform-spe-cific receptor for vascular endothelial growth factor. *Cell* 1999;92:735–745.

219. Wang HU, Chen Z, Anderson DJ. Molecular distinction and angiogenic interaction between embryonic arteries and veins revealed by ephrin-B2 and its receptor Eph-B4. *Cell* 1998;93:741–753.

220. Moulton KS, Heller E, Konerding MA, et al. Angiogenesis inhibitors endostatin or TNP-470 reduce intimal neovascularization and plaque growth in apolipoprotein E-deficient mice. *Circulation* 1999;99:1726–1732.

221. Oliver SJ, Cheng TP, Banquerigo ML, Brahn E. Suppression of collagen-induced arthritis by an angiogenesis inhibitor, AGM-1470, in combination with cyclosporin: reduction of VEGF. *Cell Immunol* 1995;166:196–206.

222. Mori S, Yoshikawa H, Hashimoto J, et al. Antiangiogenic agent (TNP-470) inhibition of ectopic bone formation. *Bone* 1998;22:99–105.

22

ANTIANGIOGENESIS: CLINICAL APPLICATIONS

STEVEN K. LIBUTTI
JAMES M. PLUDA

The concept of treating cancer by attacking the tumor's blood supply is one that has recently received increased attention. However, the observation that growing tumors are critically dependent on the in-growth of host neovasculature is one that was made in the 1940s. In a series of elegant experiments using transparent chambers made in tissue flaps, Drs. Algire and Chalkley, working at the National Cancer Institute, demonstrated that the tumor vasculature originated from the host and was required by the tumor for it to grow larger than a few millimeters (1). The importance of this observation and its therapeutic implications was elucidated by Judah Folkman over 25 years later, when he recognized that tumors secrete molecules, which he termed *tumor angiogenesis factors*, that recruited blood vessels into the growing tumor (2). In this landmark paper, the concept of tumor dormancy—that is, arresting the tumor at the size of several millimeters by blocking its ability to recruit blood vessels—was born.

Antiangiogenesis as a therapeutic modality is directed at preventing the recruitment or growth of a vascular supply, which is critical for continued tumor enlargement, invasion, and metastasis. This chapter describes some of the evidence supporting the notion that tumor growth is angiogenesis dependent. Additionally, it outlines issues related to the selection of angiogenesis inhibitors for clinical use. It also describes novel clinical trial designs for angiogenesis inhibitors and emerging methods for measuring end points of response. Last, it discusses the agents that are currently in clinical trials, the agents that are in preclinical development, and the clinical development of antiangiogenic gene therapy.

BACKGROUND

Several clinical observations have supported the importance of tumor vascularity to the malignant phenotype. Weidner and colleagues were the first to report that tumor vascular density may be predictive for the risk of metastases, disease-free survival, and overall survival (3). Since then, there have been an increasing number of reports of similar observations in a growing number of tumors, including breast cancer, prostate cancer, gas-

tric cancer, and colon cancer (3,4). Lu and colleagues have also reported that there may be an inverse relationship between tumor microvascular density and the rate of tumor-cell apoptosis (5). Circulating factors known to induce angiogenesis, such as vascular endothelial growth factor (VEGF) and basic fibroblast growth factor (bFGF), have also been reported to correlate with extent of disease, clinical status, and survival (6,7). Inhibitors of angiogenesis have been shown to suppress tumor growth *in vivo* but have little or no effect on tumor cell proliferation *in vitro* (8–11). Thus, it appears that the development of a blood supply is important not only for the growth of the primary tumor but also for invasion and distant spread.

During the growth of a tumor mass, tumor cells are rarely shed into the circulation before the onset of active neovessel formation (12). However, once angiogenesis commences, the number of tumor cells shed into the circulation correlates directly with the density of tumor blood vessels. These tumor cells access the circulation based on an important property of tumor neovessels. Newly forming vessels in the tumor bed are "leaky" and contain fragmented basement membranes (13). This disruption in endothelial cell barrier function allows malignant cells to more easily enter the circulation, where they can travel to distant sites and establish metastatic deposits. Their growth at these distant sites is also critically dependent on angiogenic activity. The action of collagenases is necessary for both angiogenesis and the invasion of tumor cells (14). Several stages are important for tumor growth and metastases, and many of these are reliant on the formation of tumor vessels. Thus, attacking the formation of tumor vasculature can theoretically inhibit both the growth of the primary tumor and the ability of that tumor to metastasize.

The endothelial cell is an attractive target for anticancer therapy. Unlike tumor cells, which are transformed and rapidly dividing, host endothelial cells are normal and respond to mitogens secreted by the tumor. Therefore, endothelial cells are not dividing at as rapid a rate as tumor cells and do not possess the genetic instability of tumor cells. This is important, as this makes it extremely difficult for endothelial cells to develop genetic mutations associated with resistance to the therapies directed against them. This phenomenon makes antiangiogenic therapy particularly attractive, because theoretically it would be extremely difficult for tumors to generate escape mechanisms.

The environment in which it is growing can dramatically alter the endothelial cell's phenotype. The expression of surface molecules such as receptors and integrins can change in response to various cytokines or environmental changes such as hypoxia (15,16). To develop therapies directed against tumor vasculature, it is critical to understand the unique features of the endothelial cell.

Endothelial cells lining the vasculature of normal tissues exist in a quiescent or resting state. They provide a homeostatic barrier, which prevents the uncontrolled extravasation of intravascular components and inhibits coagulation (17). When a tumor begins to grow in a region of normal tissue, factors are released from the tumor cells, which elicit responses from the surrounding endothelium and result in vascular invasion into the tumor (18). Not all tumor cells, however, are capable of stimulating this response. The ability to release these important angiogenic factors and the conversion within the tumor cell from a nonangiogenic to an angiogenic inducer has been referred to as the *angiogenic switch* (19).

Most tumors arise without angiogenic activity and switch when a critical subset of cells acquires the angiogenic phenotype (19). The switch is associated with increased production of angiogenic factors by the tumor such as VEGF and bFGF. Avascular tumors, which are in a dormant or inactive state, have a balance between tumor cell proliferation and apoptotic cell death (20,21). As tumor cells begin to induce angiogenesis, there is a decrease in the incidence of cell death by apoptosis within the tumor itself (21). The factors involved in the regulation of the angiogenic switch are being elucidated. An understanding of these mechanisms is critical in the further development of antiangiogenic therapies for use in the clinic.

A careful balance exists between those stimulatory factors that potentiate neovessel development and those factors that serve to suppress the angiogenic response. Several potential stimulatory mechanisms, which may lead to the potentiation of tumor-associated angiogenesis, have been described previously (19–21). However, there are also events that lead to a loss of inhibition that can shift the balance in favor of angiogenesis. The loss of tumor-suppressor gene function, such as mutations in p53, can lead to a decreased production of angiogenesis inhibitors like thrombospondin (22). Mutations in the von Hippel-Lindau tumor-suppressor gene may lead to a loss of control of VEGF expression, resulting in increased VEGF production (23,24). Tumors arising in this familial cancer syndrome are notable for their increased vascularity and increased production of VEGF by both Northern and Western blot analysis. Studies have further demonstrated that mutations in the ras oncogene may also upregulate VEGF expression (25). Taken as a whole, the important factors involved in the angiogenic switch can be grouped by those that activate angiogenesis and those that inhibit it. To maintain equilibrium between new vessel development and growth and control of pathologic or neoplastic vascular invasion, these activators and inhibitors must be carefully balanced. With respect to tumor growth, invasion, and metastasis, it may be possible to exploit this balance and tip it in favor of angiogenesis inhibition.

SELECTION OF ANGIOGENESIS INHIBITORS FOR CLINICAL DEVELOPMENT

Ideally, an antiangiogenic agent should possess several properties. It is important to keep these properties in mind when planning strategies for the development of this class of agent. The angiogenesis inhibitor should have specificity for a particular step, aspect, or component of the neovascularization process. By selecting critical steps important for neovascular formation, a broad spectrum of antitumor activity can be achieved. The ideal agent should demonstrate a lack of resistance developed by the tumor. Therapies directed against the endothelial cell might have advantages over therapies directed against the tumor cell due to the inability of the endothelial cell to develop resistant clones. However, agents directed against a single angiogenic molecule or isolated step in the angiogenic process may potentially be defeated by the tumor if the tumor cells are able to produce another factor that achieves the same result but circumvents the block by the agent. The ideal agent should be relatively nontoxic, particularly because these agents may need to be administered for a prolonged period (26). They should also be able to synergize with other cancer therapies. Because the target of antiangiogenic therapy is the tumor vasculature, combining these agents with more traditional chemotherapies or radiation directed against the tumor cell might be a strategy that maximizes the efficacy of each therapy (27–29).

The selection of agents for further clinical development is based on the preclinical data generated in the laboratory. This makes it important to understand the mechanism of action of the agent and whether the assay that is chosen to determine the activity of a compound is appropriate for the agent being tested. Several assays are routinely used in the laboratory to assess the degree of antiangiogenic activity of a given compound (Table 1). Endothelial cell functional assays generally measure proliferation, migration, invasion, and capillary tube formation (30). Bovine capillary endothelial cells are commonly used in proliferation assays as are human umbilical vein endothelial cells, lung microvascular endothelial cells, and dermal microvascular endothelial cells. These same cells can be used in migration, invasion, and capillary tube formation assays. By making use of the basement membrane material Matrigel as an artificial extracellular matrix, cells can grow and organize as they might *in vivo*. One must be careful, however, in the interpretation of the results of these assays, as there are

TABLE 1. PRECLINICAL ANGIOGENESIS ASSAYS

In vitro
  Endothelial cell proliferation
  Endothelial cell migration
  Endothelial cell invasion
  Capillary tube formation
  Rat aortic ring assay
In vivo
  Corneal micropocket
  Chicken chorioallantoic membrane
  Matrigel implantation
  Sponge implantation
  Rat dorsal air sac

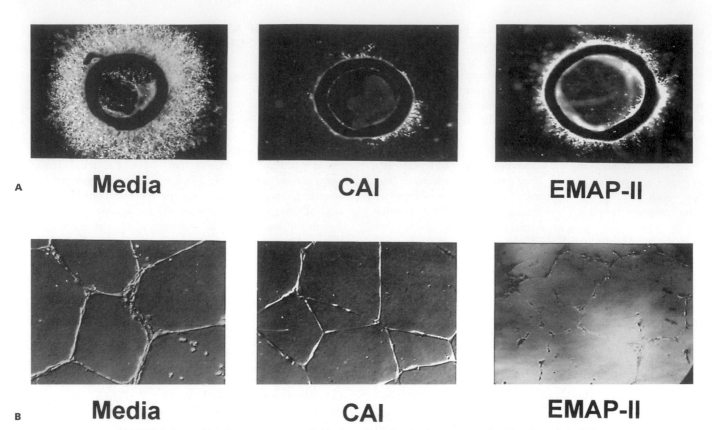

A **Media** **CAI** **EMAP-II**

B **Media** **CAI** **EMAP-II**

FIGURE 1. Several *in vitro* assays are available that allow for the assessment of antiangiogenic activity of agents as they are being evaluated for further development. Panel **(A)** illustrates the use of the rat aortic ring assay, which is used to measure angiogenic activity. Rat aorta is sectioned and placed in Matrigel containing either media alone or media containing various inhibitors of angiogenesis. The amount of vessel outgrowth from the aortic ring can be determined. Panel **(B)** illustrates the use of a tube-forming assay. Endothelial cells are plated on Matrigel and assayed for their ability to form tubes, which appear as a lattice or matrix on phase-contrast microscopy. Agents, which perturb this tube formation, can be analyzed. Both of these assays can be semi-quantified using image-processing software. (CAI, carboxyamido-triazole; EMAP-II, endothelial monocyte-activating polypeptide II.)

differences between the types of endothelial cells and the individual endothelial cells' behavior on various extracellular matrixes (Berger et al., *manuscript in preparation*). Additionally, there may be species specificity for the activity of a compound. Also, a compound may require metabolic activation. In this circumstance, the parent compound may be inactive in *in vitro* assays but extremely active *in vivo*.

The rat aortic ring assay is a useful *in vitro* assay for measuring the inhibition of angiogenesis (31). Circular sections of the rat aorta are placed in Matrigel with or without an angiogenic stimulus such as bFGF. Over 5 to 8 days, an arborization of vessels can be seen emanating from the central aortic disc. In the presence of an inhibitor of angiogenesis, this arborization of vessels is impaired to varying degrees (Fig. 1). This assay is readily reproducible and easy to interpret. However, one must be certain of the species specificity and metabolic activation of the compound being tested.

For example, thalidomide has been shown to inhibit angiogenesis in preclinical models (32). However, when thalidomide was administered at similar doses orally in mice it had no antiangiogenic activity. Furthermore, when thalidomide is placed on rat aortic rings, there is no inhibition of neovessel formation. In contrast, when thalidomide was mixed with a preparation of

human hepatocytes, there was potent activity in the rat aortic ring assay. Combining thalidomide with murine hepatocytes demonstrated no effect (33). This observation underscores the importance of species specificity and metabolism in the activation and subsequent efficacy of various agents.

Several *in vivo* angiogenesis assays exist for preclinical use. The corneal micropocket assay and the chicken chorioallantoic membrane (CAM) assay are standard screening assays that can demonstrate potent inhibition of neovessel formation (34–38). Matrigel can also be implanted in subcutaneous pockets in mice with or without angiogenic stimulatory molecules. Animals can then be given systemic treatment with putative antiangiogenic agents, and the degree of vascular invasion into the Matrigel can be assessed. These assays rely on either microscopic examination of explanted Matrigel or on actual hemoglobin content determinations from the Matrigel. The level of hemoglobin directly correlates with the amount of vascular ingrowth into the Matrigel implant.

Once an agent has demonstrated activity consistent with the inhibition of vascular growth, the next step is to ascertain whether the agent has an effect on tumor growth. A variety of models exist for measuring the antitumor effects of antiangiogenic agents in the preclinical setting. Tumor xenograft models may be used involving human tumors grown in immunodeficient mice. Alternatively, mouse tumors may be implanted into syngeneic mice. Additionally, a number of models for tumor metastases in either the liver or lung have been characterized. However, a growing body of literature suggests that there are differences in the microvasculature in various models and that testing an agent for activity against subcutaneously implanted tumors may not be a true representation of whether that agent inhibits tumor growth in the tissue of origin. In an attempt to examine more potentially relevant models, researchers are using orthotopic tumor models, in which the tumor cells are placed directly into the organ of origin. An example would be colon cancer cells injected into the colon (39). Another approach uses spontaneous tumor models based on the formation of organ-specific tumors in transgenic mice (40–42).

Once an agent has demonstrated antitumor activity, experiments exploring the appropriate route and schedule of administration should be performed. The route of administration often depends on the physical properties of the agent. Oral dosing is preferable, but many agents are not orally bioavailable. The solubility of a compound may have an effect on whether it can be administered intravenously or via a subcutaneous injection. The pharmacokinetics of a compound also influence the schedule of administration. However, it is important to keep in mind that the biologic half-life of a compound may in fact have a greater effect on schedule than its pharmacologic half-life. For example, a compound with a pharmacologic half-life measured in minutes need not be administered on a frequent or continuous schedule if its biologic half-life is several days. Finally, the toxicity of a compound must be ascertained. This can have a profound influence on the route and schedule of administration.

CLINICAL TRIAL DESIGNS FOR ANGIOGENESIS INHIBITORS

Antiangiogenic agents currently under development have been thought to be static drugs inhibiting tumor growth rather than causing tumors to regress. Many have had relatively little toxicity, which is important given the potential need for long-term administration. The end points typically used in early clinical trial designs evaluating cytotoxic agents may not apply to antiangiogenic agents. New paradigms for the clinical development of antiangiogenic agents need to be developed. This includes end points other than toxicity as the determinant of drug doses and schedules from phase 1 trials. This may influence the way in which decisions are made to move drugs on to phase 2 and phase 3 clinical trials.

Trial designs analyzing various routes of administration, including oral, subcutaneous injection, and intravenous delivery, are important. Whether these agents should be given as a bolus or more likely as continuous low-dose therapy can be determined by measuring pharmacologic end points as well as early biologic and clinical responses. Given the potential for prolonged administration, traditional end points such as toxicology should be examined and expanded to include long-term toxicity data.

Route of administration and pharmacokinetics are determined for an agent in phase 1 trials. Traditional phase 2 trials generally occur after the maximum tolerated dose. The phase 2 trial is generally directed at a single histologic type of cancer with the end point being tumor response. Given the theoretical possibility that antiangiogenic agents work across a variety of tumor histologies, because the endothelium is the target, certain modifications of the traditional phase 2 trial may be necessary.

A modified phase 2 trial may take a variety of forms. Because appropriate historical controls for cytotoxic agents may not be available, trials with a concurrent control arm may be useful. For example, one could conduct a two-armed randomized trial between an antiangiogenic agent and either no therapy or standard therapy. These trials may not be empowered to give a definitive answer with regard to the superiority of one agent over another as would be derived from a large-scale phase 3 trial. However, a carefully designed randomized phase 2 trial may allow one to eliminate agents as being less than promising. Alternatively, various doses or routes of administration could be randomized against each other with the same agent to better delineate the most efficacious regimen for use in larger phase 3 studies. The end points to these trials can also vary from the traditional measures of response.

Time to progression and progression-free survival as well as prolongation of survival can be determined by randomizing an agent against an appropriate concurrent control arm. In some cases, a decreased rate of progression may be strong enough evidence to suggest moving a particular agent into further study. Once promising agents have been selected from these phase 2 designs, definitive phase 3 studies can be performed. These studies can be random assignment trials comparing antiangiogenic agents to placebo controls using prolongation of survival, time to progression, progression-free survival, and overall response rate as end points. Trials may also compare standard chemotherapeutic agents with chemotherapy plus the antiangiogenic agent. These combination therapy trials may demonstrate synergy that was predicted from preclinical data. The overall goal of the design of clinical trials for antiangiogenic agents should be to exploit the fact that the agents studied to date have relatively mild side effects and, therefore, modified phase 1 and phase 2 trials may be the most efficient for early clinical evaluations.

END POINT MEASURES

The traditional end points used to define the efficacy of anticancer therapies in clinical trials have been response rate, time to progression, disease-free survival, and overall survival. Response rates are generally determined by standard established criteria based on the measurements of the perpendicular diameters of index-tumor lesions. The most commonly used imaging modalities are computed tomography and magnetic resonance imaging (MRI). These radiographic measures of the changes in tumors are limited to an assessment of the tumor's physical dimensions. In their most often used formats, these imaging modalities give no information on the physiologic changes that are occurring within the tumor and the tumor microenvironment.

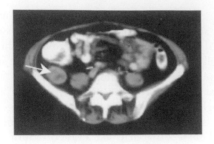

CT SCAN

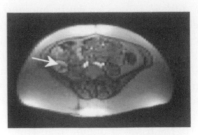

Dynamic MRI

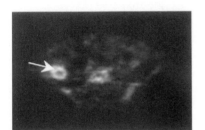

¹⁸FDG-PET

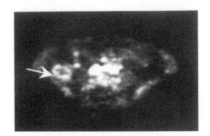

¹¹CO Blood volume image

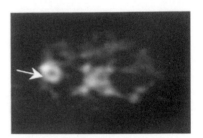

H₂¹⁵O blood flow image

FIGURE 2. A variety of functional imaging studies are available to assess the degree of vascularity of tumors as well as changes in tumor metabolism. Illustrated here are five images obtained from a patient with a retroperitoneal mass (*arrow*) using a variety of imaging modalities. (^{11}CO, radiolabeled carbon monoxide; CT, computed tomography; ^{18}FDG-PET, radiolabeled fluorodeoxyglucose positron emission tomography; H$_2$^{15}O, radiolabeled water; MRI, magnetic resonance imaging.)

Several early clinical trials of antiangiogenic agents relied on these standard radiographic imaging techniques that have become commonplace in the evaluation of chemotherapeutics. Many of these antiangiogenic agents demonstrated static activity in that their use resulted in the stabilization of disease with few documented tumor regressions. These results, however, may hide some important effects of these novel treatment strategies and may result in the loss of important information regarding the biology of the tumor's response. To address this issue, several functional imaging modalities are being developed.

Functional imaging attempts to visualize changes in aspects of tumor metabolism, oxygen consumption, blood flow, and receptor expression. With respect to antiangiogenic imaging, several challenges must be overcome. Methods that allow for the quantification of changes in tumor vasculature must be identified. These methods must be validated against standard methods of measuring vascular density such as microvessel counting. They also must be shown to have a meaningful correlation with actual clinical activity of the agents being tested. Finally, one must be able to compare the results of these functional imaging studies with the more traditional scans and the patient's ultimate outcome. A variety of imaging techniques are under study as possible functional measures for antiangiogenic therapies (43).

Positron emission tomography (PET) can be used to assess a variety of aspects of the biologic response to antiangiogenic agents. Depending on the radiopharmaceutical used, assessments of changes in tumor metabolism, tumor blood flow, and tumor blood volume can be made before, during, and after therapy with antiangiogenic agents (Fig. 2). Several studies have shown that malignant lesions demonstrate elevated glycolysis when compared to normal tissues (44,45). By using the radiolabeled glucose analog (18-F) fluorodeoxyglucose (FDG) investigators have documented increased uptake of FDG in cancer tissues (46,47). PET scanning with ^{18}FDG has been used to image a variety of malignant neoplasms, including breast cancer, head and neck tumors, lung cancer, lymphoma, melanoma, ovarian tumors, bone cancers, and colorectal carcinomas.

The mechanism whereby ^{18}FDG is selectively accumulated in neoplastic tissue is based not only on increased uptake of FDG and conversion to FDG-6-phosphate, but also on the inability of neoplastic cells to further metabolize FDG-6-phosphate. This molecule is therefore trapped in the cells, facilitating accurate imaging. As the blood flow to a tumor is decreased, the supply of oxygen and nutrients should be decreased as well. This may result in a shift from aerobic to anaerobic metabolism, and this also may impact on glucose metabolism of the tumor cells. Therefore, ^{18}FDG-PET may demonstrate changes in the tumor during the course of antiangiogenic therapy that may not be appreciated on conventional imaging (43).

If an agent is designed to inhibit new vessel formation and to decrease the overall vascularity of a tumor, it follows that the blood flow to the tumor and the total blood volume in the tumor should change. PET has been used in a variety of clinical settings to measure both blood flow and blood volume (48–50). Much of this work has been done in the heart and the brain to measure normal physiologic parameters. These techniques have been applied to the study of neoplastic tissue (51–55). Using the radiopharmaceuticals $H_2^{15}O$ (radiolabeled water) and ^{11}CO (radiolabeled carbon monoxide), assessments of blood flow and blood volume can be made. Accurate quantification of myocardial blood flow (in absolute units of mL per minute per g of tissue) has been performed as well as quantification of blood flow to the liver, cerebral blood flow, and metabolism. With regard to neoplasms, investigators have shown changes in the blood flow to tumors in the brain in response to angiotensin-2 using such techniques (54).

Use of ^{11}CO, which is an excellent red blood cell label (attaching to hemoglobin), permits quantitative measurement of red blood cell volume in tissues. Both radiolabeled water and radiolabeled carbon monoxide can be easily administered. Radiolabeled water can be delivered intravenously, and its short half-life and rapid clearance allows for short imaging times. Radiolabeled carbon monoxide is administered by inhalation and, although it binds tightly to red cells, it, too, has a relatively short half-life. By combining the information obtained using these two agents, accurate assessments of blood flow and blood volume have been obtained (56–64). Both of these agents are well tolerated, and the small volume of water (<10 cc per injection) has little physiologic effect. The sensitivity of the PET scanner is such that the amount of radiolabeled carbon monoxide that is administered is many orders of magnitude below that needed to produce any deleterious physiologic effect.

In addition to PET scanning, dynamic MRI is also a promising new technique (43,65). Dynamic enhanced MRI involves the rapid administration of a gadolinium-based contrast agent followed by ultrafast analysis of signal intensity. Patterns of MRI contrast uptake within tumors correlate within microvascular density (66). Some variability has been noted in the strength of this correlation, but it should be possible in individual subjects to monitor changes in microvascular density using dynamic enhanced MRI. This is particularly true for the early phases of enhancement after injection when the agent is principally intravascular and has not yet leaked into the interstitial space. Early studies have concentrated on MRI mammography in which differences in enhancement patterns have been shown to be predictors of the malignancy of a lesion (67–71). Still others have investigated the role of dynamic contrast-enhanced MRI in uterine cervical cancer, myocardium, and liver metastases (72–74). The development of contrast agents that remain in the intravascular space and do not leak into interstitial tissues may further improve the sensitivity of dynamic MRI for the quantification of microvascular density.

Using image-processing algorithms established for the detection of malignancy for MRI, it may be possible to assess changes in perfusion and microvessel density over time in lesions being treated with agents that inhibit angiogenesis. Comparative quantification can be used to assess changes in tumor microvascular density. Diffusion-weighted MRI allows an assessment of net perfusion and diffusion and is widely used in the assessment of cerebrovascular accidents. This technique may also reflect tumor perfusion, as diffusion would be expected to decrease as the flow decreases. Therefore, the activity of antiangiogenic agents as measured by their ability to decrease microvascular density and therefore tumor blood flow and blood volume may be accurately assessed by these advanced functional imaging techniques.

There are several potential biologic markers that can also be used as end points in assessing the efficacy of antiangiogenic agents. Circulating angiogenic-related factors, such as VEGF and bFGF, can be measured in the urine, serum, and plasma of patients before and during therapy. Changes in these levels may be predictive of ultimate tumor responses (75,76). If tumor tissue is accessible for biopsy, a variety of assays can be performed.

Microvessel density as a determinant of the angiogenic index can be followed while patients are on therapy. Proliferation and migration assays can be performed on tumor cells, tumor-associated endothelial cells, or both (30). Apoptosis assays [TUNEL (*in situ* DNA nick end labeling)] can be performed on fresh tissues and interpreted for both the tumor cells and the endothelial cells. The production and subsequent activity of angiogenesis-associated factors, whether they are stimulatory or inhibitory, can be measured (77,78). The expression of endothelial cell surface receptors can also be determined as can their level of phosphorylation or activation, or both (15,79).

With the advent of DNA microarray technology, the upregulation or downregulation of important genes related to tumor growth or vascular development can be rapidly screened for from small quantities of biopsy material (80). Using laser-capture microdissection, tumor cells and endothelial cells can be separated and analyzed independently (81). These powerful new techniques can be used to ascertain the processes involved in the mechanism of antiangiogenic action. Newer automated systems can screen thousands of genes at a time.

Although the ultimate end point desired is the prolongation of survival and inhibition of tumor progression, the trials needed to assess these end points often require hundreds of patients, taking years to accomplish. In the early development of antiangiogenic agents, these end points, although an important ultimate goal, may represent an unrealistic challenge. Using surrogate end points and advanced imaging techniques, more rapid screening of novel antiangiogenic agents may be accomplished.

ANTIANGIOGENIC AGENTS CURRENTLY IN CLINICAL TRIALS

The number of clinical trials evaluating antiangiogenic agents increased significantly in the late 1990s. Table 2 lists the agents currently being evaluated in the clinic along with their putative mechanism of action, the trial type, and the tumor histologies being accrued. This list is evolving and may not be complete. We discuss several of these agents in detail to provide examples of the different types of compounds currently under clinical investigation.

Trinitrophenyl-470

Fumagillin is an antibiotic derived from the fungus *Aspergillus fumigatus Fresenius*. Fumagillin was initially shown to be an inhibitor of angiogenesis in a variety of assays, including the CAM assay and the dorsal, air-sac assay in the mouse. However,

TABLE 2. ANTIANGIOGENIC AGENTS CURRENTLY IN CLINICAL TRIALS

Agent	Mechanism of Action	Trial Type	Histologies	Sponsor
TNP-470	Inhibits endothelial cell growth; synthetic analogue of fumagillin	Phase 1, 2	Adult cancers, pediatric solid tumors, lymphomas, leukemias	TAP Pharmaceuticals, Deerfield, IL
Thalidomide	Unknown, possible modulation of TNF-α VEGF	Phase 1, 2, 3	Kaposi's sarcoma, prostate, lung, breast, glioblastoma, colon, renal, myeloma	Celgene, Warren, NJ
CAI	Inhibitor of calcium influx	Phase 1, 2, 3	Ovarian, non–small-cell lung, renal cancer	NCI, Bethesda, MD
Suramin	Unknown, effects are at multiple sites	Phase 1, 2, 3	Prostate	Parke-Davis, Morris Plains, NJ
Squalamine lactate, MSI-1256F	Inhibits sodium-hydrogen exchange; extracted from dogfish shark liver	Phase 1	Adult cancers	Magainin Pharmaceuticals, Plymouth Meeting, PA
Combretastatin A-4 (CA4P)	Induces apoptosis in proliferating endothelial cells	Phase 1, 2, 3	Adult cancers	Oxigene, Boston, MA
Neovastat	Naturally occurring MMP inhibitor	Phase 1, 2, 3	Adult solid tumors, non–small-cell lung cancer	Aeterna, Sainte-Foy, Quebec
COL-3	Derivative of tetracycline, synthetic MMP inhibitor	Phase 1, 2	Solid tumors	Novartis, East Hanover, NJ
Marimastat	Synthetic MMP inhibitor	Phase 3	Pancreas, non–small-cell lung, breast	British Biotech, Annapolis, MD
AG3340	Synthetic MMP inhibitor	Phase 3	non–small-cell lung, prostate	Agovron, La Jolla, CA
Bay 12-9566	Synthetic MMP inhibitor	Phase 3	Lung and pancreatic	Bayer, West Haven, CT
Vitaxin	Humanized antibody to $\alpha v \beta 3$ integrin on ECs	Phase 1	Adult solid tumors	Ixsys, Inc., La Jolla, CA
EMD121974	Inhibits/blocks $\alpha v \beta 3$ and $\alpha v \beta 5$	Phase 1	Adult solid tumors	Merke KCgaA, Darmstadt, Germany
Anti-VEGF antibody	Monoclonal humanized antibody to VEGF	Phase 1, 2, 3	Lung, breast, prostate, colorectal, renal cell	Genentech, South San Francisco, CA
Interferon-α	Inhibits production of bFGF and VEGF	Phase 1, 2	Solid tumors	Available commercially
SU5416	Blocks signaling of VEGF receptor	Phase 1	Adult solid tumors and Kaposi's sarcoma	Sugen, Redwood City, CA
SU6668	Blocks signaling of VEGF, FGF, and EGF receptors	Phase 1	Adult solid tumors	Sugen, Redwood City, CA
PTK 787/ZK 22584	Blocks VEGF receptor signaling	Phase 1, 2	Glioblastoma, Kaposi's sarcoma, von Hippel-Lindau's	Novartis, East Hanover, NJ
Interleukin-12	Upregulates expression of interferon-γ and IP10	Phase 1, 2	Solid tumors and Kaposi's sarcoma	Genetics Institute, Cambridge, MA
IM862	Unknown	Phase 3	Kaposi's sarcoma	Cytran, Kirkland, WA
Platelet factor 4	Inhibits endothelial cell growth	Phase 2	Adult solid tumors	Repligen, Cambridge, MA
ZD0101	Bacterial toxin that binds new blood vessels and induces inflammation	Phase 2	Adult solid tumors	Zeneca Pharmaceuticals, Wilmington, DE
CM 101	Induction of host response to tumor vasculature	Phase 1	Solid tumors	Carbomed, Brentwood, TN
AE-941	Inhibits MMPs and angiogenesis (mechanism unknown)	Phase 1, 2	Lung cancer, solid tumors	Aeterna, Sainte-Foy, Quebec
PNU-145156E-a	Sulfonated distamycine A derivative lowers AT III levels	Phase 1	Solid tumors	Pharmacia & Upjohn, Milan, Italy
Endostatin	Unknown	Phase 1	Solid tumors	NLI, Bethesda, MD and Eutremed, Rockville, MD

AT, Antithrombin III; bFGF, basic fibroblast growth factor; CAI, carboxyamido-triazole; ECs, Endothelial cells; EGF, epidermal growth factor; FGF, fibroblast growth factor; IP10, interferon inducible protein 10; MMPs, matrix metalloproteinases; TNF-α, tumor necrosis factor-α; TNP-470, trinitrophenyl-470; VEGF, vascular endothelial growth factor.

fumagillin is extremely toxic, and, therefore, potent nontoxic analogues were sought. Trinitrophenyl-470 (TNP-470) is one such analogue of this natural product (82,83). A variety of preclinical studies were performed using TNP-470 *in vivo* with tumor-bearing animals. These studies demonstrated reductions in the size and number of both primary tumors as well as experimentally induced metastases (84). Based on favorable preclinical data, TNP-470 entered into clinical trials.

Early phase 1 trials were conducted in patients with recurrent squamous cell carcinoma of the cervix, androgen-independent prostate cancer, and human immunodeficiency virus (HIV)–associ-

ated Kaposi's sarcoma (82,85–87). Taken as a whole, the results of these phase 1 trials indicated that when the drug was given as a 1-hour infusion every other day or on a Monday, Wednesday, and Friday schedule, the dose-limiting toxicity was neurocerebellar, and the maximum tolerated dose was 50 to 60 mg per m^2 per dose. A 4-hour infusion weekly also had as its dose-limiting toxicity neurocerebellar manifestations. The 120-hour (5-day) continuous infusion every 3 weeks is still an ongoing study. Based on the tolerated doses demonstrated in the phase 1 trials, phase 2 trials were performed in glioblastoma multiforme, advanced pancreatic carcinoma, cervical cancer, and renal cell carcinoma. The trial performed for renal cell carcinoma used a dose of 60 mg per m^2 as a 1-hour infusion given three times per week. Thirty-three patients were enrolled in this trial, of which 20 were evaluable. There was one partial response (PR), five (25%) patients had stable disease for longer than 16 weeks, and the dose-limiting toxicity included two patients with central nervous system toxicity, one patient with fatigue, and one death from gastrointestinal hemorrhage after only one dose (88). TNP-470 may be limited in its efficacy as a single agent. Ongoing studies are evaluating extended duration of infusion and alternate formulations. Combination studies with cytotoxic agents are currently under way. Preclinical data has demonstrated that the addition of TNP-470 to paclitaxel and carboplatin results in increased antitumor activity and efficacy (89).

Thalidomide

Thalidomide was first developed in the 1950s as an oral sedative. It had been extensively studied in preclinical animal models and showed little or no toxicity (82). In 1961, a connection was made between thalidomide and babies born with malformed limbs to mothers using the drug as a sleeping pill (90). Further clinical use of the drug was halted at that time. The experience with thalidomide is an important example of the differences across species in the metabolism of various agents. Mice lack the enzymes necessary in their livers to metabolize thalidomide down to its derivative products, which are metabolically active. The absence of toxicity in the preclinical models is therefore understandable.

Thalidomide is an immunomodulatory drug that has the ability to downregulate the expression of tumor necrosis factor-α (TNF-α) messenger RNA (91). Thalidomide's immunomodulatory properties led to its use in the treatment of patients with erythema nodosum leprosum that is a complication of lepromatous leprosy. Thalidomide is currently U.S. Food and Drug Administration approved for this use. Treatment of severe ulcers associated with Behçet's disease and HIV infection as well as chronic graft-versus-host disease and tuberculosis with thalidomide is also under evaluation (92).

Thalidomide has been shown in preclinical models to prevent the development of neovascularization (93,94). The exact mechanism of this action is not yet known. Several metabolites of thalidomide are active. There is some speculation that modulation of VEGF levels as well as TNF-α may be the important targets. Preclinical models have also demonstrated that thalidomide can result in antitumor activity against murine colon cancer (95). The observation that thalidomide inhibits neovessel formation may, in fact, be related to the mechanism of teratogenicity that was seen in children born with malformed limbs (32). Based on the preclinical data indicating the effectiveness of thalidomide at inhibiting tumor neovessel formation and based on its ease of dosing as an oral agent, thalidomide was moved into clinical trials.

A phase 1 trial has been conducted in patients with acquired immunodeficiency syndrome (AIDS)–associated Kaposi's sarcoma (96). The trial accrued 12 patients (all homosexual or bisexual males) with a mean age of 31 years. Four dose levels were evaluated: 200, 300, 400, and 600 mg per day. Thalidomide was continued until toxicity or disease progression. Dose-dependent somnolence developed in all patients, and resulted in therapy being discontinued in two of three patients at the 600-mg per day dose.

Other toxicities consisted of skin rash (one patient receiving 300 mg), fever (one patient receiving 300 mg), headache (one patient receiving 600 mg), dry mouth (one patient receiving 300 mg), and peripheral neuropathy (one patient receiving 400 mg per day after 4 months). Although the main end point was toxicity, all patients were evaluable for response. Two PRs were seen, and seven patients had stable disease. Median time to progression was 4 months, and survival was 4 to 18 months. The maximum tolerated dose was defined as 600 mg per day in this patient population (96).

Similar results were seen in a phase 1 and 2 trial of thalidomide in patients with advanced cancers (97). This trial accrued 60 patients with a variety of histologies, including melanoma, breast, colon, mesothelioma, renal cell, and glioblastoma. The maximum tolerated dose was 500 mg per day. Overall, two patients had a PR, with ten patients having stable disease (97).

In a phase 2 trial of patients with metastatic melanoma, renal cell, ovarian, and breast cancers, thalidomide was given at a dose of 100 mg per day and was well tolerated. Of the 48 patients enrolled, ten had stable disease whereas three had differential responses (98). In this trial, stable disease was associated with stable or falling serum and urine VEGF levels. Those patients who progressed had rising VEGF levels detected in the urine and serum (98). This study illustrates the potential utility of secondary end point measures in evaluating the activity of antiangiogenic agents.

A randomized two-arm phase 2 study examining two doses of thalidomide, 200 mg per day versus 600 mg per day, has been conducted in patients with androgen-independent prostate cancer. This study has been completed, and it appears that the 200 mg per day dose may have equal efficacy to the 600 mg per day dose and fewer side effects (WD Figg, *personal communication*, 1999). The response rates and pharmacokinetic data are pending.

A trial has opened at the National Cancer Institute studying thalidomide in doses up to 300 mg per day randomized against a placebo for the treatment of patients after the resection of colorectal cancer metastases. The end point for this trial is disease-free survival. Other trials looking at glioblastoma multiforme, recurrent head and neck carcinoma, multiple myeloma, and hormone-sensitive prostate carcinoma are under way.

Squalamine Lactate

Squalamine lactate (MSI-1256F) is an amino sterol isolated from the dogfish shark liver. Its mechanism of action appears to be the inhibition of the sodium-hydrogen exchanger NHE3. Preclinical data demonstrated inhibition of endothelial cell proliferation. Two phase 1 clinical trials have been conducted (99,100).

A 5-day continuous infusion every 3 weeks was evaluated using the continual reassessment method of dose escalation and the accrual of a single patient at dose levels with minimal toxicity (99). To date, 12 patients received 26 courses at doses ranging from 6 to 255 mg per m^2 per day. No dose-limiting toxicities have occurred. Toxicities that were not dose limiting included nausea, fatigue, and anorexia. No response data were reported (99).

A second continuous-infusion trial was performed in 16 patients with a variety of tumor types, including lung, ovarian, melanoma, breast, colon, renal cell and soft tissue sarcoma (100). Doses were escalated from 6 to 538 mg per m^2 per day. Dose-limiting toxicity was encountered in the two patients who received 538 mg per m^2 per day and consisted of grade 3 elevations of transaminases. Other non–dose-limiting toxicities included fatigue, nausea, anorexia, myalgia, and lip numbness. No objective tumor responses were noted, and 14 patients have had disease progression (100).

Carboxyamido-Triazole

Carboxyamido-triazole (CAI) is an agent with cytostatic and antiproliferative properties. It has been shown to have antiinvasive and antiangiogenic activity (101–103). CAI selectively inhibits non–voltage-gated calcium influx and thereby modulates the elements involved in invasion and angiogenesis (104). As endothelial cells adhere to and spread on extracellular matrix proteins, an increase in intracellular calcium is seen. This can be inhibited by CAI exposure (104). CAI was evaluated in clinical trials using two formulations administered orally.

A polyethylene glycol (PEG)–400 solution or gelatin capsule containing the PEG-400 CAI solution was used (105). Patients with advanced refractory cancers were entered on the study and assessed for toxicity, pharmacokinetics, and response (105–107). Patients experienced mild or moderate nausea and vomiting that became compliance limiting in these trials. Using an every-other-day dosing schedule, one patient experienced reversible grade 3 sensory neuropathy, and one patient developed neutropenia (105). Based on these phase 1 data, the recommended phase 2 dose and formulation was 150 mg per m^2 per day in the PEG-400 liquid formulation. Disease stabilization was observed in 49% of the patient cohort, which lasted from 2 to 7 months. Patients had ovarian cancer, melanoma, colorectal cancer, pancreatic or biliary cancer, and lung cancer (105). To improve the tolerance to the agent, a phase 1 trial was conducted using a micronized formulation of CAI in patients with refractory solid tumors (105).

Twenty-one patients with refractory solid tumors were enrolled in this study. Patients received a test dose followed 1 week later by daily administration of CAI and the encapsulated-micronized formulation at doses of 100 to 350 mg per m^2. Patients remained on CAI until disease progression or dose-limiting toxicity. All 21 patients were assessed for toxicity, and 18 were evaluable for pharmacokinetics and response. Fifty percent of the patients demonstrated grade I and II gastrointestinal side effects. Dose-limiting toxicity was observed at the dose of 350 mg per m^2 per day, which consisted of reversible grade 2 and 3 cerebellar ataxia and confusion. One minor response was observed in a patient with renal cell carcinoma, and another nine patients had disease stabilization. The micronized formulation was thought to have a better toxicity profile and a similar frequency of disease stabilization. It was easier to administer, and the dose of 350 mg per m^2 per day was selected for further phase 2 investigations (105). Currently, a phase 2 trial evaluating orally administered CAI for patients with persistent or refractory epithelial-ovarian cancer or primary peritoneal cancers is under way as well as a phase 3 trial for non–small-cell lung cancer (NSCLC).

Inhibitors of Vascular Endothelial Growth Factor and Basic Fibroblast Growth Factor

VEGF and bFGF are important endothelial cell mitogens. The influence of these factors on the host vasculature leads to the invasion of vessels into the tumor and the formation of tumor neovasculature. This allows for tumor growth, invasion, and metastases. Therefore, inhibition of these cytokines either by preventing their production or interfering with their binding to receptors may have an impact on inhibiting tumor angiogenesis. Several strategies are being evaluated in clinical trials specifically directed against VEGF and bFGF.

Rhu Monoclonal Antibody Against Vascular Endothelial Growth Factor

A humanized, murine, monoclonal antibody (MAb) against VEGF has been developed and is currently being evaluated in a variety of clinical studies. RhuMAb VEGF has been designed to bind free-circulating VEGF and, therefore, decrease the levels of VEGF available to initiate the neovascular process. A phase 1 trial was conducted using RhuMAb VEGF as a single agent in adult patients (108). Doses were escalated from 0.1 to 10 mg per kg intravenously delivered over 90 minutes. Patients were treated on day 0, day 28, day 35, and day 42. Twenty-five patients were enrolled in the trial, 24 of whom completed all four doses. Toxicity was evaluated and grade 1 or 2 toxicity was seen in more than 20% of the patients. Three patients experienced tumor-related hemorrhage. Other toxicities noted were headache, asthenia, fever, nausea and vomiting, cough and dyspnea, and skin rash. Thirteen patients demonstrated stabilization of disease at 72 days after therapy. Pharmacokinetic analysis demonstrated linear pharmacokinetics at doses greater than or equal to 0.3 mg per kg with a mean terminal half-life of 17 days. No neutralizing antibodies to RhuMAb VEGF were seen (108).

Based on these results, several phase 2 trials have been initiated using RhuMAb VEGF as either a single agent or in combination with chemotherapy. Currently, there are trials with RhuMAb VEGF as a single agent for metastatic breast cancer, hormone-refractory prostate cancer, and renal cell carcinoma. RhuMAb VEGF is also being evaluated in combination with chemotherapy in patients with stage III and IV NSCLC and patients with previously untreated metastatic colon cancer.

Interferon-α

Interferon-α (IFN-α) decreases the production of proangiogenic cytokines such as bFGF (109). It has been gaining increasing popularity as an antiangiogenic agent, having been used successfully to treat life-threatening pulmonary hemangioma (18,110). Chronic low-dose administration of IFN-α was used to induce remission in 10 of 20 patients with life- or sight-threatening hemangiomas or tissue-destructive hemangiomas (111). IFN-α has been evaluated as a single agent in trials for hairy cell leukemia, chronic myelogenous leukemia, Kaposi's sarcoma, and squamous cell carcinoma (82). IFN-α has been used in combination with interleukin-2 (IL-2) and 5-fluorouracil (5-FU) in the treatment of metastatic renal cell cancer.

Forty-seven patients with metastatic renal cell cancer were treated using recombinant IL-2 and recombinant IFN-α subcutaneously in combination with intravenous 5-FU. Patients received an average of 2.4 cycles, and toxicity of grades 2 to 3 were observed in 24 and 17 patients, respectively. Nine major responses (seven complete and two partial) for an objective response rate of 19.1% were seen (112).

Clearly, an evaluation of a triple-drug combination such as this cannot discern the contribution of each individual agent because there was no randomization against a comparative arm. However, toxicity appeared to be acceptable. IFN-α has also been used in combination with TNP-470 in preclinical models and has shown an additive effect (82). IFN-α is being evaluated in a phase 2 pilot study for patients with progressive hairy cell leukemia after splenectomy. Additionally, this agent is being used in a trial treating recurrent unresectable meningiomas and malignant meningiomas. A pegulated formulation of IFN-α is being used in a phase 1 and 2 study in patients with solid tumors (113). In addition to measuring response, the ability to measure circulating serum levels of bFGF as well as levels of bFGF in the urine of patients on IFN-α represents a potentially important surrogate end point for these trials.

SU-5416

The agent SU-5416 is a synthetic compound that selectively inhibits the signaling of the VEGF receptor 2 (KDR) receptor tyrosine kinase (114). SU-5416 was shown to inhibit VEGF-dependent mitogenesis of human endothelial cells without having an effect on a variety of tumor cells *in vitro*. In mouse models, systemic administration of SU-5416 at nontoxic doses led to the inhibition of growth of subcutaneously implanted tumors. Furthermore, this antitumor effect was accompanied by a pale appearance of the tumors consistent with antiangiogenic activity (114).

A phase 1 single-agent trial was conducted in 12 patients using a biweekly infusion of doses ranging from 4.4 to 15 mg per m^2 per day. Tumor types included colon, breast, lung, prostate, and Kaposi's sarcoma. Toxicities have included pain and burning at the injection site, shortness of breath, cough, fatigue, and allergic reaction (115). No response data were reported in this study.

Several phase 2 and phase 3 trials are planned in a variety of tumor histologies, including Kaposi's sarcoma, colorectal, renal cell, prostate, head and neck, glioma, melanoma, and myeloma. Some of these trials plan to evaluate combination therapy with other antiangiogenic agents, such as thalidomide and IFN-α, or chemotherapy with 5-FU, leucovorin, cisplatin, and doxorubicin.

Vitaxin

Although VEGF and bFGF are important angiogenic stimulatory molecules and appear to be critical in the angiogenic response, there are other potential targets on endothelial cells for which novel therapeutic strategies have been developed. The endothelial cell-surface integrin $\alpha v \beta 3$ has been shown to be important for endothelial cell attachment to the basement membrane and inhibition of endothelial cell apoptosis (18,116). By targeting $\alpha v \beta 3$ and preventing its binding to the extracellular matrix, it is hypothesized that endothelial cells are not able to properly adhere and align themselves. The cells then undergo programmed cell death. Evidence supporting this hypothesis has been demonstrated in preclinical studies. Based on these data, a

recombinant humanized murine monoclonal antibody has been developed against $\alpha v \beta 3$. This agent, vitaxin, is currently being evaluated in a phase 1 trial for adult solid tumors.

Twelve patients have been enrolled in this phase 1 trial and have received doses ranging from 0.1 to 2 mg per kg given once a week for 6 weeks. Several patients had infusion-associated fever, but no other significant side effects were noted. Of 12 evaluable patients, there was one PR (sarcoma), six patients with stabilization of disease, and five patients with progressive disease (116). Based on its favorable toxicity profile, vitaxin is being readied for a phase 2 trial.

Interleukin-12

IL-12 has been shown to interfere with neovascularization by its induction of IFN-γ and IFN inducible protein 10 (IP10) (117). IP10 has inhibitory effects on tumor vasculature. IP10 does not act on cell growth or on migration and attachment but rather it acts to interfere with formation of tube-like structures and may inhibit bFGF-induced neovascularization *in vivo* (18,118). In a study performed *in vivo* using a NSCLC model, intratumor injection of IP10 for a period of 8 weeks resulted in significant inhibition of tumor growth, tumor-associated angiogenic activity, and neovascularization. IP10 may prove to be a useful antiangiogenic agent in its own right.

A phase 1 trial of intravenous, recombinant, human IL-12 was conducted in patients with advanced malignancies. Patients were eligible for the trial if they had refractory tumors, normal organ function, and a Karnovsky performance status of greater than 70%. Recombinant IL-12 was given by intravenous bolus once as an inpatient and then after a 2-week rest period once daily for 5 days every 3 weeks as an outpatient. Forty patients were enrolled in the trial, including 20 with renal cancer, 12 with melanoma, and five with colon cancer. Twenty-five patients had received earlier systemic therapy. Common toxicities were fever and chills, fatigue, nausea, vomiting, and headache. Dose-limiting toxicity included oral stomatitis and liver function test abnormalities that occurred in three of four patients at the 1 μg per kg dose level. The 500 ng per kg dose level was determined to be the maximum tolerated dose. Biologic effects included dose-dependent increases in circulating IFN γ without any detectable changes in other factors such as TNF-α. An objective tumor response was observed in two patients, one with metastatic renal cell carcinoma and one with melanoma. Four additional patients completed six 21-day treatment cycles with stable disease. Of note, of the 14 patients treated at the maximum tolerated dose (six renal, four melanoma) no responses were seen (119).

A pilot dose-finding trial was conducted in patients with AIDS-associated Kaposi's sarcoma (120). Doses of 100 ng per kg (five patients), 300 ng per kg (six patients), and 500 ng per kg (four patients) of subcutaneous IL-12 were administered twice a week. The main toxicities noted were reversible neutropenia, hepatotoxicity, and constitutional symptoms at the initiation of dosing. Only three patients were removed from the trial for toxicity. No responses were seen at the 100 ng per kg dose. Of the nine remaining patients with evaluable disease, four had PRs (three patients at the 300 ng per kg dose and one patient at the 500 ng per kg dose). Overall, the drug appeared to be well tolerated in this patient population.

Matrix Metalloproteinase Inhibitors

Tumor angiogenesis and tumor invasion are two critically interdependent activities. Factors important to each may be critical targets for anticancer therapy. For tumor cells to spread through tissues, gain access to the circulation, and establish distant sites of metastases, they must be able to digest the substance present in the basement membrane and extracellular matrix. Matrix metalloproteinases (MMPs) are therefore extremely important to the tumor's ability to invade and spread. Inhibitors of MMPs may have activity not only on the growth of the primary tumor but also on its ability to metastasize.

MMPs are a family of stromal proteases that have a zinc ion within their active site and share strong structural and sequence homology. They are involved in the normal remodeling of the supporting interstitium during tissue morphogenesis and wound healing (18). MMPs are secreted by tumor cells and endothelial cells and are involved in extracellular matrix degradation. Tumor cells use MMPs to break down and remodel tissue matrices during metastatic spread, and endothelial cells use MMPs for vascular invasion into surrounding tissue, including the tumor. Several inhibitors of MMPs have been developed and are entering clinical trials.

Marimastat

Marimastat is a synthetic inhibitor of MMPs that specifically inhibits MMP-1, MMP-2, MMP-7, and MMP-9 (121). A pilot escalating dose study of oral marimastat has been performed in patients with recurrent colorectal cancer. In these patients, an examination of serologic response was made by measurement of carcinoembryonic antigen (CEA) levels. This study assessed the safety and tolerability of 4 weeks of administration of marimastat and determined a dose range that produced detectable serologic effects (121). Patients were recruited by the criteria of a serum CEA level greater than 5 ng per mL and rising by more than 25% over a 4-week screening period. Patients were treated for 28 days and entered into a continuation protocol if a serologic response or clinical benefit was observed. A biologic effect was defined as a CEA value on day 28, no greater than on day 0; a partial biologic effect was defined as a rise in CEA over the 28-day treatment period of less than 25%.

Of the patients recruited, 63 completed the 28-day treatment period and 55 were eligible for CEA analysis. The median rates of rise of CEA fell significantly during the treatment period when patients received twice-daily marimastat. No effect was seen with the once-daily regimen. Toxicities were mainly musculoskeletal and occurred in a dose- and time-dependent fashion. The occurrence of musculoskeletal side effects defined 25 mg twice a day as the upper-limit dose range for continuous use (121). This trial used a surrogate marker (CEA levels) as a means of rapidly evaluating the potential efficacy of an agent in a relatively short period.

A phase 1 and 2 study of marimastat combined with captopril and dalteparin (Fragmin) has been completed (122). Seven-

teen patients were enrolled representing a variety of tumor types, including renal, colorectal and prostate cancer. The dose of marimastat administered was 10 mg orally twice a day. In addition to toxicity, the trial assessed response rates and changes in circulating cytokines such as VEGF (122). Toxicities attributed to marimastat included altered taste, musculoskeletal pain, and myalgia or arthralgia. One patient had a PR. VEGF levels fell in five patients (122).

A dose-finding study using marimastat for patients with pancreatic cancer has been performed (123). A total of 64 patients were enrolled in the trial; all had advanced pancreatic cancer that had failed earlier therapy. Patients received doses of marimastat ranging from 10 to 150 mg daily administered orally. The end points of the trial were safety, tolerance, and changes in the rate of rise of CA 19-9 (a tumor marker) as a surrogate marker for disease progression (123). Overall, marimastat was well tolerated. Dose-limiting toxicity included joint pain and stiffness; doses of 5, 10, and 25 mg twice a day were found to be acceptable. A reduced rate of rise in CA 19-9 was found at all three of these doses, and the median survival was 160 days with a 1-year survival of 21% (123).

Marimastat was evaluated in combination with carboplatin and paclitaxel and was well tolerated (124). In this study, 22 patients with NSCLC were treated, and 50% achieved a PR (124). Several other trials are ongoing evaluating marimastat alone or in combination with chemotherapy or radiation therapy (125,126). Of particular note are two randomized phase 3 trials, one evaluating marimastat in patients with breast cancer and the other in patients with small-cell lung cancer. As these trials mature, the potential role for marimastat may become more fully elucidated.

AG3340

The compound AG3340 is a selective inhibitor of MMPs 2, 3, 9, and 14 (29). MMPs 2, 3, 9, and 14 are associated with tumor angiogenesis, invasion, and metastasis. AG3340 has been evaluated in a human malignant glioma model in severe combined immunodeficient (SCID) mice (127). Animals were treated with daily intraperitoneal injections of AG3340 or a control and tumor volumes were measured over 31 days. Animals receiving AG3340 had a 78% reduction in tumor volume and survived 40 days longer (71 versus 31 days) than animals receiving a negative control (127). No significant toxicity was appreciated.

A phase 1 study of AG3340 in combination with paclitaxel and carboplatin for patients with advanced solid tumors has been completed (29). Fifteen patients were enrolled and received a regimen consisting of chemotherapy administered on day 1 of a 21-day cycle (carboplatin AUC = 5 mg per minute per mL and paclitaxel 200 mg per m^2) and AG3340 administered at a dose of 25 mg orally twice a day starting on day 15 and continuing thereafter. The majority of toxicities seen were attributable to one or the other chemotherapeutic agents. Toxicities specific to AG3340 were seen in two patients and were notable for one case of an alteration in taste and a grade 2 myalgia. Overall, the regimen was well tolerated. Of the 15 patients enrolled, 13 remain on study with stable disease while two have terminated the treatment due to disease progression (29). Further follow-up is needed to evaluate patients for response.

COL-3

Another synthetic MMP inhibitor is the derivative of tetracycline designated COL-3 (128). COL-3 has been shown to downregulate MMP-2 and MMP-9 expression. Several phase 1 studies of COL-3 are ongoing. One is a phase 1 trial of COL-3 in patients with advanced solid tumors being conducted at the San Antonio Cancer Institute with end points being the definition of maximum tolerated dose, identification of dose-limiting toxicity, and definition of pharmacokinetics and pharmacodynamics. A phase 1 study of COL-3 in patients with HIV-related Kaposi's sarcoma is being conducted by the AIDS-Associated Malignancies Clinical Trials Consortium. In addition to standard phase 1 end points, this trial is also designed to evaluate the effect of COL-3 on CD4 and CD8 cell counts and on serum levels of MMP-2 and MMP-9 as surrogate markers. Serum from these patients is also being evaluated for antiangiogenic activity using *in vitro* assays. A phase 1 study of oral COL-3 in patients with refractory-metastatic solid tumors or lymphoma is also being conducted at the National Cancer Institute. This trial is designed to assess the effects of serum from patients being treated with COL-3 on bioassays designed to measure antiangiogenic activity, as well as toxicity and pharmacolcinetics.

Bay 12-9566

Bay 12-9566 is a nonpeptide biphenyl compound that inhibits MMP-2 and MMP-9 predominantly (129). Preclinical studies demonstrated inhibition of tumor growth, invasion, and metastasis with prolonged administration and led to the initiation of several clinical trials (129–132). In a phase 1 trial, 20 patients with solid tumors received daily doses ranging from 100 to 1,600 mg per day. A variety of schedules were used, including once a day, twice a day, three times a day, and four times a day dosing. Doses of 400 mg three times a day and 400 mg four times a day were notable for toxicities, including grade 3 hyperbilirubinemia, grade 2 thrombocytopenia, and grade 2 nausea each leading to dose reductions. Overall, the agent was well tolerated (129).

In another phase 1 study, 29 patients were treated with doses up to 1,200 mg per day (131). The tumor types were varied and included colon, ovarian, breast, renal, and soft tissue sarcoma. The main toxicities were dose-related thrombocytopenia and transient elevations of transaminases. These were for the most part mild and not dose limiting. No significant musculoskeletal toxicities occurred. No response data were noted; however, patients tolerated therapy for up to 10 months, indicating that chronic administration may be possible (131).

Bay 12-9566 has also been studied in combination with paclitaxel and carboplatin (132). A total of 19 patients were treated in one of three cohorts: (a) paclitaxel + Bay 12-9566, (b) paclitaxel + carboplatin + Bay 12-9566, and (c) carboplatin + Bay 12-9566. All patients received Bay 12-9566 at a dose of 800 mg orally twice a day starting on day 8 of therapy. Toxicities were

seen mainly in patients who had been heavily pretreated with chemotherapy. Most toxicity was attributable to carboplatin or paclitaxel. Overall, the regimen was well tolerated. Pharmacokinetic data indicated that Bay 12-9566 did not significantly alter the plasma concentration or clearance of the chemotherapeutic agents (132). Based on these initial studies, several phase 3 trials have opened utilizing Bay 12-9566 alone or in combination with chemotherapy.

ANTIANGIOGENIC AGENTS ON THE VERGE OF CLINICAL TRIALS

Given the rapidity with which the field of angiogenesis research is growing, there is no doubt that by the time this chapter appears in print, several more agents will be added to those currently being evaluated in clinical trials. There are some notable ones, for which preclinical data has matured enough that they are likely to appear in clinics in the near future. This section briefly describes these agents, the targets of their action, and their likelihood for further clinical development.

Angiostatin

Angiostatin was isolated from the urine of mice bearing the murine Lewis lung carcinoma based on its ability to inhibit endothelial cell proliferation *in vitro* (10). It was further characterized by its ability to inhibit metastatic lesions from Lewis lung carcinoma when exogenously administered. Structural analysis of angiostatin demonstrated that it comprises the first four kringles of plasminogen (10). Some reports indicate that smaller fragments of the molecule may be all that are required for its antiangiogenic effect (133). Angiostatin can act in a paracrine or endocrine manner and is generated by tumor media proteolysis of plasminogen.

Although the mechanism of action of angiostatin is not completely understood, some work has demonstrated that angiostatin binds to the cell surface of endothelial cells and may, in fact, bind the alpha subunit of adenosine triphosphate synthase (134). This binding may inhibit adenosine triphosphate synthase, which may be an important mediator of endothelial cell proliferation. Angiostatin has also been shown to induce apoptosis in endothelial cells (135).

Several preclinical studies of angiostatin have demonstrated the effectiveness of this agent in inhibiting the growth of tumors across a variety of histologies and in a variety of models. No significant toxicity has been seen to date (136). Given its broad spectrum of activity and favorable toxicity profile, angiostatin is currently being readied for phase 1 clinical trials.

Endostatin

Endostatin is another antiangiogenic molecule identified by Folkman and his coworkers using a similar strategy to that used for the isolation of angiostatin (11). Endostatin was purified from the urine of mice bearing a murine hemangioendothelioma and was found to be a 20-kd protein identical to the C-terminal fragment of collagen XVIII (11). Systemic administration of endostatin specifically inhibits endothelial cell proliferation and is a potent inhibitor of angiogenesis. Endostatin has been shown to induce apoptosis selectively in endothelial cells. *In vivo* animal studies have shown that endostatin is able to inhibit the growth of metastases. It also results in regression or almost total obliteration of primary tumors with repeated treatment (11). Furthermore, it has been shown that mice bearing Lewis lung carcinoma, T241 fibrosarcoma, or B16 410 melanoma, did not develop resistance with multiple administrations of endostatin (137). Like angiostatin, endostatin has been shown to have broad activity against a variety of histologies in a number of different tumor models. None of these early preclinical models have demonstrated toxicity from repeat administrations of endostatin. Given its favorable toxicity profile and efficacy in preclinical models, three phase 1 clinical trials are in progress.

2-Methoxyestradiol

The endogenous estrogen metabolite 2-methoxyestradiol (2-ME) is a potent inhibitor of endothelial cell proliferation and invasion *in vitro* (138–140). Although its mechanism of action has not been completely elucidated, it does not appear to exert its effects through the estrogen receptor (139). Furthermore, it does not require heparin or sulfated cyclodextrins for its activity, unlike the angiostatic steroids of corticoid structure (141). The compound may interfere with a basic proliferation-associated cellular event, as its antiproliferative effects are not restricted to endothelial cells (139). Inhibition of cell growth was seen in several normal lines as well as a variety of tumor lines (139). Oral administration of 2-ME, 100 mg per kg per day, to mice bearing subcutaneous Meth-A sarcoma or B16 melanoma resulted in the inhibition of tumor growth with no apparent signs of toxicity (139). Quantification of tumor neovasculature demonstrated a marked reduction in the treated animals compared to controls (139).

The antiangiogenic effects of 2-ME were also evaluated in a corneal neovascularization assay (138). An oral dose of 150 mg per kg inhibited bFGF- and VEGF-induced neovascularization in mice by 39% and 54%, respectively (138). In a mouse model of human breast cancer, severe combined immunodeficient (SCID) mice bearing a subcutaneously implanted estrogen receptor–negative human breast cancer were treated with 75 mg per kg per day of 2-ME for 29 days (138). This resulted in a 65% reduction in tumor volume compared to controls without significant toxicity (138).

The activity of 2-ME against endothelial cells and tumor cells may involve an initiation of apoptotic cell death (140). Human pancreatic carcinoma cells when exposed to 2-ME demonstrated an increase in apoptotic cell death as well as a prolonged S phase after 48 hours of exposure (140). An inhibition of lung metastases was also demonstrated using this same cell line in nude mice (140). The ability to administer 2-ME orally as well as its low toxicity and broad activity make it an attractive agent for further clinical development.

RGD Peptides

RGD peptides, an exciting group of agents that bind specifically to receptors or integrins expressed on the endothelial cell surface, are being readied for use in clinical trials. These are peptides that contain an arginine, glycine, and aspartic acid residue. One such class of agents has a specific amino acid motif that selectively binds to the $\alpha v \beta 3$ subunit, which is expressed on the antiluminal surface of endothelial cells. Using a phage display library, Arup and coworkers identified a 3-amino acid motif (RGD) which binds avidly to $\alpha v \beta 3$ (142). Preclinical data demonstrated that conjugating chemotherapeutics, such as doxorubicin, to an RGD-containing peptide motif resulted in targeted delivery of a chemotherapeutic agent to tumor neovasculature (142). This type of targeted delivery to neovasculature can be exploited not only for therapeutic agents but also for the imaging of developing vessels. One could either radiolabel RGD-containing peptides or conjugate contrast agents, such as gadolinium, to these motifs, allowing the use of gamma cameras or MRI to visualize tumor vasculature. Other potential targets for surface binding on endothelial cells include the Tie receptors (Tie 1 and Tie 2), tissue factor, and VEGF receptors (18).

Thrombospondin

Thrombospondin is a 420-kd glycoprotein, which binds the CD36 receptor (143,144). Thrombospondin is a multifunctional matrix protein released from alpha granules of activated platelets in response to thrombin and influences the growth and function of a variety of normal and neoplastic epithelial and mesenchymal cell types (18). Thrombospondin is a binding inhibitor of plasmin as determined by loss of amidolytic activity, loss of ability to degrade fibrinogen, and decreased lysosomes in fibrin plate assays (145). Thrombospondin may be involved in tumor inhibition through a vascular means, as studies have shown that it functions by overriding the effects of VEGF (146). It has also been shown to inhibit bFGF-induced angiogenesis in the rat cornea model (147). Preclinical models are still being studied to determine the role of thrombospondin in the inhibition of tumor growth and metastases.

Endothelial Monocyte-Activating Polypeptide II

Endothelial monocyte-activating polypeptide II (EMAP-II) was isolated from the supernatant of the Meth-A fibrosarcoma based on its ability to induce tissue factor upregulation on the surface of endothelial cells (148,149). EMAP-II is a processed protein that is first synthesized in a pro-form of 34 kd and then cleaved at an interleukin converting enzyme–like cleavage site to a mature 22-kd form. Purified, recombinant, mature EMAP-II activates endothelial cells and results in elevation of cytosolic-free calcium concentrations, release of von Willebrand's factor, induction of tissue factor, and expression of E-selectin and P-selection (150).

EMAP-II was first studied with regard to its ability to render previously resistant tumors sensitive to the antitumor effects of TNF-α. Intratumoral injection of recombinant EMAP-II into a resistant mouse-mammary carcinoma (as well as B16 melanoma and a human fibrosarcoma) rendered these tumors sensitive to subsequent systemic injections of TNF (17). Further studies demonstrated that retroviral transduction of a human melanoma resistant to TNF, with the complementary DNA (cDNA) for EMAP-II, resulted in a conversion of the phenotype to a TNF-sensitive one (151).

The mechanism by which EMAP-II renders tumor vasculature sensitive to TNF-α appears to be through the upregulation of TNF-receptor I on endothelial cells (152,153). Cell lines transduced with EMAP-II are sensitive to TNF *in vivo*, although their *in vitro* sensitivity to TNF is unchanged. All of this evidence taken as a whole points to EMAP-II as a potent inducer of endothelial cell functions.

In addition to its upregulation of E-selectin, P-selectin, tissue factor, and TNF–receptor 1 on endothelial cells, EMAP-II appears to be a potent inhibitor of endothelial cell proliferation and neovascular formation. Early work demonstrated that recombinant EMAP-II inhibited neovessel formation in the CAM assay (ML Kayton, SK Libutti, *unpublished data*). Preliminary data using recombinant EMAP-II suggested that it might have an effect on endothelial cell apoptosis and neovessel growth in a subcutaneous Matrigel assay (154). Recombinant EMAP-II is being evaluated in preclinical animal models studying its antitumor effects as well as its toxicity.

DEVELOPMENT OF ANTIANGIOGENIC GENE THERAPY

A number of the antiangiogenic agents described thus far are naturally occurring proteins or cleavage products thereof. These proteins can be difficult to produce recombinantly due to instability and sensitivity to changes in environmental factors such as freezing and thawing. Preclinical and clinical studies have indicated that it may be necessary to deliver antiangiogenic agents chronically to maintain long-term inhibition of primary tumor growth as well as to prevent the growth of micrometastases. Thus, to achieve adequate local tissue levels, high doses may need to be delivered systemically for prolonged periods. For example, effective doses of endostatin in murine models range from 10 to 100 mg per kg per day depending on whether murine or human recombinant endostatin is used (155). It may be difficult to produce large enough quantities of these recombinant materials to keep up with demand if they prove to be efficacious antitumor agents. Gene delivery strategies are an attractive alternative to exogenous dosing.

By engineering vectors that carry the coding sequence for an antiangiogenic protein, one can target specific sites in the host and allow the host to produce chronic levels of the antiangiogenic agent either regionally, where the tumor is growing, or systemically to prevent the growth of distant microscopic disease. This strategy has been attempted using several different gene-delivery vectors as well as a variety of genes encoding antiangiogenic agents (156–160). The approach has been to select a vector, such as an adenovirus, retrovirus, or liposome; construct an expression system carrying the gene of interest; and deliver that gene to the host.

Using an adenoviral vector to deliver a recombinant Tie 2–soluble receptor that blocked activation of the Tie 2 receptor on endothelial cells, Lin and his colleagues demonstrated that a single intravenous injection of this construct resulted in high circulating levels of the soluble receptor protein for up to 8 days (157). Growth of two different primary tumors was inhibited, and neovascularization and growth of lung metastases were

almost completely abrogated (157). Using a cDNA coding for DNA complementary to angiostatin, Tanaka and associates demonstrated that retroviral and adenoviral vectors could be used to inhibit endothelial cell growth *in vitro* and angiogenesis *in vivo*. This technique mediated the inhibition of tumor-associated angiogenesis, resulting in increased apoptotic tumor cell death, leading to inhibition of tumor growth (158).

Plasminogen activator inhibitor type I has been used in an adenovirus-mediated gene-transfer model and demonstrated the *in vivo* inhibition of metastasis of an intraocular melanoma in a murine model (159). The use of this adenoviral vector resulted in transduction of more than 95% of human and murine uveal melanoma cells in the eyes of nude mice. A 50% reduction in the number of animals developing liver metastases was seen. Intravenous injection of the adenovirus plasminogen activator inhibitor type I construct resulted in transduction of normal liver cells, culminating in the reduction in the incidence of metastases and prolongation of survival (159).

The cDNA coding for angiostatin, endostatin, and an antisense messenger RNA species against VEGF have been used to create a recombinant adenoassociated virus by Nguyen and his colleagues at the Beth Israel Deaconess Medical Center (160). Although this study was an *in vitro* study, they were able to demonstrate measurable levels of antiangiogenic protein production in the supernatant of transfected cells. Concentrated supernatant demonstrated antiangiogenic activity in an endothelial cell proliferation assay.

Using a unique signal sequence attached to the cDNA coding for endostatin, an adenoviral vector was created that efficiently transfected cells in culture. Measurements of endostatin in the cell supernatant from cells infected with signal-sequence endostatin had detectable levels, whereas the endostatin construct without a signal sequence showed only intracellular levels of the molecule without secretion into the supernatant (161). Furthermore, when this adenoviral construct was injected systemically into immunocompromised mice, significantly increased circulating levels of endostatin could be detected in the serum up to 3 µg per mL at 4 days. Tumor growth was inhibited in nude mice bearing a subcutaneous colon cancer (162).

The main hurdle to antiangiogenic gene therapy is finding vector systems that deliver the gene efficiently, resulting in sustained and effective levels of gene production without toxicity to the host from either the vector itself or the protein being produced. To date, viral vectors have been limited by their immunogenicity, often resulting in neutralization of the virus (163). With the introduction of new vector systems, such as liposomes and other synthetic carriers, effective clinical gene therapy may become a reality.

Although there are currently no open clinical trials utilizing antiangiogenic gene therapy, the number of preclinical studies is increasing rapidly. As the hurdles to gene therapy are overcome, many of these strategies become viable ones for evaluation in the clinic.

SUMMARY AND CONCLUSIONS

The focus of anticancer therapies has, for the better part of this century, been on attacking the tumor cell directly. Since the

1970s, this has been shifting to other aspects of the tumor host interaction. The relationship between tumors and their vasculature is a prime example of the tumor-host interface that can be an important target for antitumor strategies. The interest in antiangiogenic therapy has increased dramatically.

We have summarized the strategies for bringing agents from the bench to the bedside and highlighted those agents that are currently being evaluated in clinical trials. Emerging techniques in noninvasive imaging and in the ability to measure surrogate end points dramatically improves the ability to assess the biologic activity of this novel class of therapeutics and aid in their development. By using novel methods of gene therapy, exciting new advances may be on the horizon. Through the study of the relationship between the tumor and its blood supply, more is learned about how tumors invade and spread, helping to develop new methods to combat them.

ACKNOWLEDGMENTS

We would like to thank Barbara Owen and Sudhen Desai for their help with the preparation of the manuscript and Adam Berger and Steve Bacharach for their help with the figures.

REFERENCES

1. Algire GH, Chalkley HW, Legallais FY, Park HD. Vascular reactions of normal and malignant tissues *in vivo*. I. Vascular reactions of mice to wounds and to normal and neoplastic transplants. *J Natl Cancer Inst* 1945:73–85.
2. Folkman J. Tumor angiogenesis: therapeutic implications. *N Engl J Med* 1971;285:1182–1186.
3. Weidner N, Folkman J, Pozza F, et al. Tumor angiogenesis: new significant and independent prognostic indicator in early-stage breast carcinoma. *J Natl Cancer Inst* 1992;84:1875–1887.
4. Weidner N, Folkman J. Tumoral vascularity as a prognostic factor in cancer. *Important Adv Oncol* 1996:167–190.
5. Lu C, Tanigawa N. Spontaneous apoptosis is inversely related to intratumoral microvessel density in gastric carcinoma. *Cancer Res* 1997;57:221–224.
6. Nguyen M, Watanabe H, Budson AE, Richie JP, Hayes DF, Folkman J. Elevated levels of an angiogenic peptide, basic fibroblast growth factor, in the urine of patients with a wide spectrum of cancers. *J Natl Cancer Inst* 1994;86:356–361.
7. Linderholm B, Tavelin B, Grankvist K, Henriksson R. Vascular endothelial growth factor is of high prognostic value in node-negative breast carcinoma. *J Clin Oncol* 1998;16:3121–3128.
8. Ingber D, Fujita T, Kishimoto S, et al. Synthetic analogues of fumagillin that inhibit angiogenesis and suppress tumour growth. *Nature* 1990;348:555–557.
9. Yamaoka M, Yamamoto T, Ikeyama S, Sudo K, Fujita T. Angiogenesis inhibitor TNP-470 (AGM-1470) potently inhibits the tumor growth of hormone-independent human breast and prostate carcinoma cell lines. *Cancer Res* 1993;53:5233–5236.
10. O'Reilly MS, Holmgren L, Shing Y, et al. Angiostatin: a novel angiogenesis inhibitor that mediates the suppression of metastases by a Lewis lung carcinoma. *Cell* 1994;79:315–328.
11. O'Reilly MS, Boehm T, Shing Y, et al. Endostatin: an endogenous inhibitor of angiogenesis and tumor growth. *Cell* 1997;88:277–285.
12. Liotta LA, Kleinerman J, Saidel FM. The significance of hematogenous tumor cell clumps in the metastatic process. *Cancer Res* 1976;36:889.
13. Dvorak HF, Nagy JA, Dvorak JT, Dvorak AM. Identification and characterization of the blood vessels of solid tumors that are leaky to circulating macromolecules. *Am J Pathol* 1988;133:95–109.
14. Liotta LA, Steeg PS, Stetler-Stevenson WG. Cancer metastasis and angiogenesis: an imbalance of positive and negative regulation. *Cell* 1991;64:327–336.
15. Guo WX, Ghebrehiwet B, Weksler B, Schweitzer K, Peerschke EI. Up-regulation of endothelial cell binding proteins/receptors for complement component C1q by inflammatory cytokines. *J Lab Clin Med* 1999;133:541–550.
16. Liu J, Razani B, Tang S, Terman BI, Ware JA, Lisanti MP. Angiogenesis activators and inhibitors differentially regulate caveolin-1 expression and caveolae formation in vascular endothelial cells. Angiogenesis inhibitors block vascular endothelial growth factor-induced down-regulation of caveolin-1. *J Biol Chem* 1999;274:15781–15785.
17. Marvin MR, Libutti SK, Kayton M, et al. A novel tumor-derived mediator that sensitizes cytokine-resistant tumors to tumor necrosis factor. *J Surg Res* 1996;63:248–255.
18. Desai SB, Libutti SK. Tumor angiogenesis and endothelial cell modulatory factors. *J Immunother* 1999:186–211.
19. Hanahan D, Folkman J. Patterns and emerging mechanisms of the angiogenic switch during tumorigenesis. *Cell* 1996;86:353–364.
20. Folkman J, Watson K, Ingber D, Hanahan D. Induction of angiogenesis during the transition from hyperplasia to neoplasia. *Nature* 1989;339:58–61.
21. Holmgren L, O'Reilly MS, Folkman J. Dormancy of micrometastases: balanced proliferation and apoptosis in the presence of angiogenesis suppression. *Nat Med* 1995;1:149–153.
22. Dameron KM, Volpert OV, Tainsky MA, Bouck N. Control of angiogenesis in fibroblasts by p53 regulation of thrombospondin-1. *Science* 1994;265:1582–1584.
23. Chan CC, Vortmeyer AO, Chew EY, et al. VHL gene deletion and enhanced VEGF gene expression detected in the stromal cells of retinal angioma. *Arch Ophthalmol* 1999;117:625–630.
24. Maxwell PH, Wiesener MS, Chang GW, et al. The tumour suppressor protein VHL targets hypoxia-inducible factors for oxygen-dependent proteolysis. *Nature* 1999;399:271–275.
25. Rak J, Mitsuhashi Y, Bayko L, et al. Mutant ras oncogenes upregulate VEGF/VPF expression: implications for induction and inhibition of tumor angiogenesis. *Cancer Res* 1995;55:4575–4580.
26. Pluda JM. Tumor-associated angiogenesis: mechanisms, clinical implications, and therapeutic strategies. *Semin Oncol* 1997;24:203–218.
27. Herbst RS, Takeuchi H, Teicher BA. Paclitaxel/carboplatin administration along with antiangiogenic therapy in non-small-cell lung and breast carcinoma models. *Cancer Chemother Pharmacol* 1998;41: 497–504.
28. Evans WK, Latreille J, Batist G, et al. AE-941, an inhibitor of angiogenesis: rationale for development in combination with induction chemotherapy/radiotherapy in patients with non small-cell lung cancer (NSCLC). *Proc Am Soc Clin Oncol* 1999(abst).
29. D'Olimpio J, Hande K, Collier M, Michelson G, Clendeninn PN. Phase I study of the matrix metalloproteinase inhibitor AG3340 in combination with paclitaxel and carboplatin for the treatment of patients with advanced solid tumors. *Proc Am Soc Clin Oncol* 1999;18:(abst).
30. Murohara T, Witzenbichler B, Spyridopoulos I, et al. Role of endothelial nitric oxide synthase in endothelial cell migration. *Arterioscler Thromb Vasc Biol* 1999;19:1156–1161.
31. Nicosia RF, Ottinetti A. Growth of microvessels in serum-free matrix culture of rat aorta. A quantitative assay of angiogenesis *in vitro*. *Lab Invest* 1990;63:115–122.
32. D'Amato RJ, Loughnan MS, Flynn E, Folkman J. Thalidomide is an inhibitor of angiogenesis. *Proc Natl Acad Sci U S A* 1994;91:4082–4085.
33. Bauer KS, Dixon SC, Figg WD. Inhibition of angiogenesis by thalidomide requires metabolic activation, which is species-dependent. *Biochem Pharmacol* 1998;55:1827–1834.
34. Parsons-Wingerter P, Lwai B, Yang MC, et al. A novel assay of angiogenesis in the quail chorioallantoic membrane: stimulation by bFGF and inhibition by angiostatin according to fractal dimension and grid intersection. *Microvasc Res* 1998;55:201–214.
35. Schlatter P, Konig MF, Karlsson LM, Burri PH. Quantitative study of intussusceptive capillary growth in the chorioallantoic membrane (CAM) of the chicken embryo. *Microvasc Res* 1997;54:65–73.
36. Cruz A, Rizzo V, DeFouw DO. Microvessels of the chick chorio-

allantoic membrane uniformly restrict albumin extravasation during angiogenesis and endothelial cytodifferentiation. *Tissue Cell* 1997;29:277–281.

37. Auerbach R, Arensman R, Kubai L, Folkman J. Tumor-induced angiogenesis: lack of inhibition by irradiation. *Int J Cancer* 1975;15:241–245.

38. Phillips P, Kumar S. Tumour angiogenesis factor (TAF) and its neutralization by a xenogeneic antiserum. *Int J Cancer* 1979;23:82–88.

39. Killion JJ, Radinsky R, Fidler IJ. Orthotopic models are necessary to predict therapy of transplantable tumors in mice. *Cancer Metastasis Rev* 1998;17:279–284.

40. Bergers G, Javaherian K, Lo KM, Folkman J, Hanahan D. Effects of angiogenesis inhibitors on multistage carcinogenesis in mice. *Science* 1999;284:808–812.

41. Hanahan D, Christofori G, Naik P, Arbeit J. Transgenic mouse models of tumour angiogenesis: the angiogenic switch, its molecular controls, and prospects for preclinical therapeutic models. *Eur J Cancer* 1996;32A:2386–2393.

42. Parangi S, O'Reilly M, Christofori G, et al. Antiangiogenic therapy of transgenic mice impairs de novo tumor growth. *Proc Natl Acad Sci U S A* 1996;93:2002–2007.

43. Libutti SK, Choyke P, Carrasquillo JA, Bacharach S, Neumann RD. Methods to monitor responses to antiangiogenic agents using noninvasive imaging tests. *Cancer J Sci Am* 1999;5:252–256.

44. Conti PS, Lilien DL, Hawley K, Keppler J, Grafton ST, Bading JR. PET and [18F]-FDG in oncology: a clinical update. *Nucl Med Biol* 1996;23:717–735.

45. DiChiro G. Positron emission tomography using [18F]fluorodeoxyglucose in brain tumors: a powerful diagnostic and prognostic tool. *Invest Radiol* 1986;22:360–371.

46. Pounds TR, Valk PE, Haseman MK. Whole-body PET-FDG imaging in the diagnosis of recurrent colorectal cancer. *J Nucl Med* 1995;36:1573–1581.

47. Ito K, Kato T, Tadokoro M. Recurrent rectal cancer and scar: differentiation with PET and MR imaging. *Radiology* 1992;182:549–552.

48. Schelbert HR. Blood flow and metabolism by PET. *Cardiol Clin* 1994;12:303–315.

49. Brudin LH, Rhodes CG. Regional structure-function correlations in chronic obstructive lung disease measured with positron emission tomography. *Thorax* 1992;47:914–921.

50. Cross SJ, Lee HS. Assessment of left ventricular regional wall motion with blood pool tomography: comparison of ^{11}CO PET with 99Tcm SPECT. *Nucl Med Commun* 1994;15:283–288.

51. Leenders KL. Pet-blood-flow and oxygen-consumption in brain tumors. *J Neurooncol* 1994;22:269–273.

52. Mineura K, Sasajima T. Blood flow and metabolism of central neurocytome—a positron emission tomography study. *Cancer* 1995;76:1224–1232.

53. Sagar SM, Klassen GA. Tumor blood-flow measurement and manipulation for therapeutic gain. *Cancer Treat Rev* 1993;19:299–349.

54. Tomura N, Kato T. Increased blood flow in human brain-tumor after administration of angiotensin-II-demonstration by PET. *Comput Med Imaging Graph* 1993;17:443–449.

55. Kahn D, Weiner GJ, Hichwa RD. Positron tomographic measurement of bone marrow blood flow to the pelvis and lumbar vertebrae in young normal adults. *Blood* 1994;83:958–963.

56. Iida H, Kanno I, Takahashi A. Measurement of absolute myocardial blood flow with H2O-15 and dynamic positron emission tomography. *Circulation* 1988;78:104–115.

57. Herrero P, Markham J, Bergmann SR. Quantitation of myocardial blood flow with H2O-15 and positron emission tomography: assessment and error analysis. *J Comput Assist Tomogr* 1989;13:862–873.

58. Frackowiak RSJ, Lenzi F, Jones T, Heather JD. Quantitative measurement of regional cerebral blood flow and oxygen metabolism in man using 0-15 and PET: theory, procedure and normal values. *J Comput Assist Tomogr* 1980;4:727–736.

59. Bacharach SL, Carson RE. Whither water? [editorial comment]. *J Nucl Med* 1994;35:567–568.

60. Iida H, Rhodes CG. Use of the left ventricular time-activity curve as a noninvasive input function in dynamic oxygen-15-water positron emission tomography. *J Nucl Med* 1992;33:1669–1677.

61. Huang S-C, Carson RE. Quantitative measurement of local cerebral blood flow in humans by positron computed tomography and ^{15}O-water. *J Cereb Blood Flow Metab* 1983;3:141–153.

62. Huang S-C, Carson RE. Measurement of local blood flow distribution volume with short-lived isotopes: a general input technique. *J Cereb Blood Flow Metab* 1982;2:99–108.

63. Iida H, Kanno I. Error analysis of a quantitative cerebral blood flow measurement using H2^{15}O autoradiography and positron emission tomography, with respect to the dispersion of the input function. *J Cereb Blood Flow Metab* 1986;6:536–545.

64. Iida H, Rhodes C. Use of the left ventricular time-activity curve as a noninvasive input function in dynamic oxygen-15-water positron emission tomography. *J Nucl Med* 1992;33:1669–1677.

65. Kim H, Waluch V, Presant CA, Wolf W. Noninvasive *in vivo* measurement of human tumor blood flow (TBF) using dynamic enhanced MRI (DEMRI): implication for drug delivery and for angiogenesis (AG). *Proc Am Soc Clin Oncol* 1999;18:(abst).

66. van Dijke CF, Brasch RC, Roberts TP, et al. Mammary carcinoma model: correlation of macromolecular contrast-enhanced MRI image characterizations of tumor microvasculature and histologic capillary density. *Radiology* 1996;198:813–818.

67. Stomper PC, Winston JS, Herman S, Klippenstein DL, Arredondo MA, Blumenson LE. Dynamic echo-planar imaging of the breast: experience in diagnosing breast carcinoma and correlation with tumor angiogenesis. *Radiology* 1997;205:837–842.

68. Stomper PC, Winston JS, Herman S, Klippenstein DL, Arredondo MA, Blumenson LE. Angiogenesis and dynamic MRI imaging gadolinium enhancement of malignant and benign breast lesions. *Breast Cancer Res Treat* 1997;45:39–46.

69. Buadu LD, Murakami J, Murayama S, et al. Breast lesions: correlation of contrast medium enhancement patterns on MRI images with histopathologic findings and tumor angiogenesis. *Radiology* 1996;200:639–649.

70. Buckley DL, Drew PJ, Mussurakis S, Monson JR, Horsman A. Microvessel density of invasive breast cancer assessed by dynamic Gd-DTPA enhanced MRI. *J Magn Reson Imaging* 1997;7:461–464.

71. Buadu LD, Murakami J, Murayama S, et al. Patterns of peripheral enhancement in breast masses: correlation of findings on contrast medium enhanced MRI with histologic features and tumor angiogenesis. *J Comput Assist Tomogr* 1997;21:421–430.

72. Hawighorst H, Knapstein PG, Weikel W, Knopp MV. Angiogenesis of uterine cervical carcinoma characterization by pharmacokinetic magnetic resonance parameters and histological microvessel density with correlation to lymphatic involvement. *Cancer Res* 1997;57:4777–4786.

73. Pearlman JD, Hibberd MG, Chuang ML, et al. Magnetic resonance mapping demonstrates benefits of VEGF-induced myocardial angiogenesis. *Nat Med* 1995;10:1085–1089.

74. Brasch R, Pham C, Shames D, et al. Assessing tumor angiogenesis using macromolecular MRI imaging contrast media. *J Magn Reson Imaging* 1997;7:68–74.

75. Salven P, Manpaa H, Orpana A, Alitalo K, Joensuu H. Serum vascular endothelial growth factor is often elevated in disseminated cancer. *Clin Cancer Res* 1997;3:647–651.

76. Salven P, Orpana A, Joensuu H. Leukocytes and platelets of patients with cancer contain high levels of vascular endothelial growth factor. *Clin Cancer Res* 1999;5:487–491.

77. Nguyen M. Angiogenic factors as tumor markers. *Invest New Drugs* 1997;15:29–37.

78. Salven P, Perhoniemi V, Tykka H, Maenpaa H, Joensuu H. Serum VEGF levels in women with a benign breast tumor or breast cancer. *Breast Cancer Res Treat* 1999;53:161–166.

79. Nguyen M, Corless CL, Kraling BM, et al. Vascular expression of E-selectin is increased in estrogen-receptor-negative breast cancer: a role for tumor-cell-secreted interleukin-1 alpha. *Am J Pathol* 1997;150:1307–1314.

80. Kurian KM, Watson CJ, Wyllie AH. DNA chip technology. *J Pathol* 1999;187:267–271.

81. Dean-Clower E, Vortmeyer AO, Bonner RF, Emmert-Buck M,

Zhuang Z, Liotta L. Microdissection-based genetic discovery and analysis applied to cancer progression. *Cancer J from Sci Am* 1997;3:259–265.

82. Gradishar WJ. An overview of clinical trials involving inhibitors of angiogenesis and their mechanism of action. *Invest New Drugs* 1997;15:49–59.

83. Dezube BJ, Von Roenn JH, Holden-Wiltse J, et al. Fumagillin analog in the treatment of Kaposi's sarcoma: A Phase I AIDS Clinical Trial Group Study. *J Clin Oncol* 1998;16:1444–1449.

84. Yanase T, Tamura M, Fujita K, Kodama S, Tanaka K. Inhibitory effect of angiogenesis inhibitor TNP-470 on tumor growth and metastasis of human cell lives *in vitro* and *in vivo*. *Cancer Res* 1993;53:2566–2570.

85. Pluda JM, Wyvill K, Figg WD, et al. A Phase I study of angiogenesis inhibitor, TNP-470 (AGM-1470) administered to patients with HIV-associated Kaposi sarcoma. *Proc Am Soc Clin Oncol* 1994;13:(abst).

86. Ski A, Gutterman J, Ebui C, et al. Phase I trial of the angiogenesis inhibitor TNP-470 (AGM-1470) in patients with androgen independent prostate cancer. *Proc Am Soc Clin Oncol* 1994;13:(abst).

87. Kudelka A, Edwards C, Freedman R, et al. A Phase I study of the toxicity pharmacokinetics, and activity of TNP-470 administered to patients with advanced or recurrent squamous cell cancer of the cervix. *Proc Am Soc Clin Oncol* 1995;14:281(abst).

88. Stadler WM, Shapiro CL, Sosmann J, Clark J, Vogelzang NJ, Kuzel T. A multi-institutional study of the angiogenesis inhibitor TNP-470 in metastatic renal cell carcinoma (RCC). *Proc Am Soc Clin Oncol* 1998;17:310a(abst).

89. Herbst RS, Takeuchi H, Teicher BA. Paclitaxel/carboplatin administration along with antiangiogenic therapy in non-small-cell lung and breast carcinoma models. *Cancer Chemother Pharmacol* 1998;41:497–504.

90. Mellin GW, Katsenstein M. The saga of thalidomide. *N Engl J Med* 1962;264:1184–1193.

91. Moreira AL, Sampaio EP, Zmuidzinas A, Frindt P, Smith KA, Kaplan G. Thalidomide exerts its inhibitory action on tumor necrosis factor alpha by enhancing mRNA degradation. *J Exp Med* 1993;177:1675–1680.

92. Gunzler V. Thalidomide in human immunodeficiency virus (HIV) patients. A review of safety considerations. *Drug Saf* 1992;7:116–134.

93. Or R, Feferman R, Shoshan S. Thalidomide reduces vascular density in granulation tissue of subcutaneously implanted polyvinyl alcohol sponges in guinea pigs. *Exp Hematol* 1998;26:217–221.

94. Kenyon BM, Browne F, D'Amato RJ. Effects of thalidomide and related metabolites in a mouse corneal model of neovascularization. *Exp Eye Res* 1997;64:971–978.

95. Ching LM, Browne WL, Tchernegovski R, Gregory T, Baguley BC, Palmer BD. Interaction of thalidomide, phthalimide analogues of thalidomide and pentoxifylline with the anti-tumour agent 5,6-dimethylxanthenone-4-acetic acid: concomitant reduction of serum tumour necrosis factor-alpha and enhancement of anti-tumour activity. *Br J Cancer* 1998;78:336–343.

96. Politi P, Reboredo G, Losso M, Vujacich C, Schwartsmann G, Lewi D. Phase I trial of thalidomide (T) in AIDS-related Kaposi sarcoma (KS). *Proc Am Soc Clin Oncol* 1998;17:41a(abst).

97. Marx GM, Levi JA, Bell DR, et al. A Phase VII Trial of Thalidomide as an Antiangiogenic Agent in the Treatment of Advanced Cancer. *Proc Am Soc Clin Oncol* 1999;18:454a(abst).

98. Eisen T, Boshoff C, Vaughan MM, et al. Anti-angiogenic treatment of metastatic melanoma, renal cell, ovarian and breast cancers with thalidomide: a phase II study. *Proc Am Soc Clin Oncol* 1998;17:441a(abst).

99. Patnaik A, Rowinsky E, Hammond L, et al. A Phase I and pharmacokinetic (PK) study of the unique angiogenesis inhibitor, squalamine lactate (MSI-1256F). *Proc Am Soc Clin Oncol* 1999;18:162a(abst).

100. Bhargava P, Trocky N, Marshall J, et al. A Phase I safety, tolerance and pharmacokinetic study of rising dose, rising duration continuous infusion of MSI-1256F (Squalamine Lactate) in patients with advanced cancer. *Proc Am Soc Clin Oncol* 1999;18:162a(abst).

101. Kohn EC, Liotta LA. L651582: a novel antiproliferative and antimetastasis agent. *J Natl Cancer Inst* 1990;82:54–60.

102. Kohn EC, Sandeen MA, Liotta LA. *In vivo* efficacy of a novel inhibitor of selected signal transduction pathways including calcium, arachidonate, and inositol phosphates. *Cancer Res* 1992;52:3208–3212.

103. Kohn EC, Alessandro R, Spoonster J, Wersto RP, Liotta LA. Angiogenesis: role of calcium-mediated signal transduction. *Proc Natl Acad Sci U S A* 1995;92:1307–1311.

104. Alessandro R, Masiero L, Liotta LA, Kohn EC. The role of calcium in the regulation of invasion and angiogenesis. *In Vivo* 1996;10:153–160.

105. Kohn EC, Figg WD, Sarosy GA, et al. Phase I trial of micronized formulation carboxyamidotriazole in patients with refractory solid tumors: pharmacokinetics, clinical outcome, and comparison of formulations. *J Clin Oncol* 1997;15:1985–1993.

106. Kohn EC, Reed E, Sarosy G, et al. Clinical investigation of a cytostatic calcium influx inhibitor in patients with refractory cancers. *Cancer Res* 1996;56:569–573.

107. Figg WD, Cole KA, Reed E, et al. Pharmacokinetics of orally administered carboxyamido-triazole, an inhibitor of calcium-mediated signal transduction. *Clin Cancer Res* 1995;1:797–803.

108. Gordon MS, Talpaz M, Margolin K, et al. Phase I trial of recombinant humanized monoclonal anti-vascular endothelial growth factor (anti-VEGF MAb) in patients (pts) with metastatic cancer. *Proc Am Soc Clin Oncol* 1998;17:210a(abst).

109. Dinney CP, Bielenberg DR, Perrotte P, et al. Inhibition of basic fibroblast growth factor expression, angiogenesis, and growth of human bladder carcinoma in mice by systemic interferon-alpha administration. *Cancer Res* 1998;58:808–814.

110. White CW, Sondheimer HM, Crouch EC, Wilson H, Fan LL. Treatment of pulmonary hemangiomatosis with recombinant interferon alfa-2a. *N Engl J Med* 1989;320:1197–1200.

111. Ezekowitz RA, Mulliken JB, Folkman J. Interferon alfa-2a therapy for life-threatening hemangiomas of infancy. *N Engl J Med* 1992;326:1456–1463.

112. Samland D, Steinbach F, Reiher F, Schmidt U, Gruss A, Allhoff EP. Results of immunochemotherapy with interleukin-2, interferon-alpha2 and 5-fluorouracil in the treatment of metastatic renal cell cancer. *Eur Urol* 1999;35:204–209.

113. Bukowski R, Ernstoff M, Gore M, et al. Phase I study of polyethylene glycol (PEG) interferon alpha-2B (PEG INTRON) in patients with solid tumors. *Proc Am Soc Clin Oncol* 1999;18:446a(abst).

114. Fong TA, Shawyer LK, Sun L, et al. SU5416 is a potent and selective inhibitor of the vascular endothelial growth factor receptor (Flk-1/KDR) that inhibits tyrosine kinase catalysis, tumor vascularization, and growth of multiple tumor types. *Cancer Res* 1999;59:99–106.

115. Rosen LS, Kabbinavar F, Rosen P, Mulay M, Quigley S, Hannah AL. Phase I trial of SU5416, a novel angiogenesis inhibitor in patients with advanced malignancies. *Proc Am Soc Clin Oncol* 1998;17:218a(abst).

116. Gutheil JC, Campbell TN, Pierce PR, et al. Phase I study of vitaxin, an anti-angiogenic humanized monoclonal antibody to vascular integrin $\alpha v \beta 3$. *Proc Am Soc Clin Oncol* 1998;17:215a(abst).

117. Voest EE, Kenyon BM, O'Reilly MS, Truitt G, D'Amato RJ, Folkman J. Inhibition of angiogenesis *in vivo* by interleukin 12. *J Natl Cancer Inst* 1995;87:581–586.

118. Angiolillo AL, Sgadari C, Tosato G. A role for the interferon-inducible protein 10 in inhibition of angiogenesis by interleukin-12. *Ann NY Acad Sci* 1996;795:158–167.

119. Atkins MB, Robertson MJ, Gordon M, et al. Phase I evaluation of intravenous recombinant human interleukin 12 in patients with advanced malignancies. *Clin Cancer Res* 1997;3:409–417.

120. Pluda JM, Wyvill K, Little R, et al. A pilot/dose-finding study of interleukin 12 (IL-12) administered to patients (pts) with AIDS-associated Kaposi's Sarcoma (KS). *Proc Am Soc Clin Oncol* 1999;18:547a(abst).

121. Primrose JN, Bleiberg H, Daniel F, et al. Marimastat in recurrent colorectal cancer: exploratory evaluation of biological activity by measurement of carcinoembryonic antigen. *Br J Cancer* 1999;79:509–514.

122. Jones PH, Elliott M, Dobbs N, et al. Phase VII study of combination antiangiogenesis therapy with marimastat, captopril and Fragmin. *Proc Am Soc Clin Oncol* 1999;18:447a(abst).

123. Rosemurgy A, Harris J, Langleben A, Casper E, Goode S, Rasmussen H. Marimastat in patients with advanced pancreatic cancer: a dose-finding study. *Am J Clin Oncol* 1999;22:247–252.

124. Anderson I, Supko J, Eder J, et al. Pilot pharmacokinetic study of mari-

mastat (MAR) in combination with carboplatin (C)/paclitaxel (T) in patients with metastatic or locally advanced inoperable non-small-cell lung cancer (NSCLC). *Proc Am Soc Clin Oncol* 1999;18:187a(abst).

125. Adams M, Thomas H. A Phase I study of the matrix metalloproteinase inhibitor, marimastat, administered concurrently with carboplatin, to patients with relapsed ovarian cancer. *Proc Am Soc Clin Oncol* 1998;17:217(abst).

126. O'Reilly S, Mani S, Ratain MJ, et al. Schedules of 5FU and the matrix metalloproteinase inhibitor marimastat (MAR): a phase I study. *Proc Am Soc Clin Oncol* 1998;17:217a(abst).

127. Price A, Shi Q, Morris D, et al. Marked inhibition of tumor growth in a malignant glioma tumor model by a novel synthetic matrix metalloproteinase inhibitor AG3340. *Clin Cancer Res* 1999;5:845–854.

128. McGarvey ME, Tulpule A, Cai J, et al. Emerging treatments for epidemic (AIDS-related) Kaposi's sarcoma. *Curr Opin Oncol* 1998;10: 413–421.

129. Rowinsky E, Hammond L, Aylesworth C, et al. Prolonged administration of BAY 12-9566, an oral non peptidic biphenyl matrix metalloproteinase (MMP) inhibitor: a phase I and pharmacokinetic (PK) study. *Proc Am Soc Clin Oncol* 1998;17:216a(abst).

130. Grochow L, O'Reilly S, Humphrey R, et al. Phase I and pharmacokinetic study of the matrix metalloproteinase inhibitor (MMPI), Bay 12-9566. *Proc Am Soc Clin Oncol* 1998;17:213a(abst).

131. Goel R, Hirte H, Major P, et al. Clinical pharmacology of the metalloproteinase (MMP) and angiogenesis inhibitor Bayer 12-9566 in cancer patients. *Proc Am Soc Clin Oncol* 1999;18:160a(abst).

132. Tolcher A, Rowinsky EK, Rizzo J, et al. A phase I and pharmacokinetic of the oral matrix metalloproteinases inhibitor Bay 12-9566 in combination with paclitaxel and carboplatin. *Proc Am Soc Clin Oncol* 1999;160a(abst).

133. Kost C, Benner K, Stockmann A, Linder D, Preissner KT. Limited plasmin proteolysis of vitronectin. Characterization of the adhesion protein as morpho-regulatory and angiostatin-binding factor. *Eur J Biochem* 1996;236:682–688.

134. Moser TL, Stack MS, Asplin I, et al. Angiostatin binds ATP synthase on the surface of human endothelial cells. *Proc Natl Acad Sci U S A* 1999;96:2811–2816.

135. Lucas R, Holmgren L, Garcia I, et al. Multiple forms of angiostatin induce apoptosis in endothelial cells. *Blood* 1998;92:4730–4741.

136. Zetter BR. Angiogenesis and tumor metastasis. *Annu Rev Med* 1998;49:407–424.

137. Boehm T, Folkman J, Browder T, O'Reilly MS. Antiangiogenic therapy of experimental cancer does not induce acquired drug resistance. *Nature* 1997;390:404–407.

138. Klauber N, Parangi S, Flynn E, Hamel E, D'Amato NA. Inhibition of angiogenesis and breast cancer in mice by the microtubule inhibitors 2-methoxyestradiol and taxol. *Cancer Res* 1997;81–86.

139. Fotsis T, Zhang Y, Pepper M, et al. The endogenous oestrogen metabolite 2-methoxyoestradiol inhibits angiogenesis and suppresses tumor growth. *Nature* 1999;368:237–239.

140. Schumacher G, Kataoka M, Roth JA, Mukhopadhyay T. Potent antitumor activity of 2-methoxyestradiol in human pancreatic cancer cell lines. *Clin Cancer Res* 1999;5:493–499.

141. Crum R, Szabo S, Folkman J. A new class of steroids inhibits angiogenesis in the presence of heparin or a heparin fragment. *Science* 1985;230:1375–1378.

142. Arap W, Pasqualini R, Ruoslahti E. Cancer treatment by targeted drug delivery to tumor vasculature in a mouse model. *Science* 1998;279(5349):377–380.

143. Lawler J, Derick LH, Connolly JE, Chen JH, Chao FC. The structure of human platelet thrombospondin. *J Biol Chem* 1985;260:3762–3772.

144. Silverstein RL, Baird M, Rowe SK, Yesner LM. Sense and antisense cDNA transfection of CD36 (glycoprotein 4) in melanoma cells. Role of CD36 as a thrombospondin receptor. *J Biol Chem* 1992; 267:16607–16612.

145. Hogg PJ, Stenflo J, Mosher DF. Thrombospondin is a slow tight-binding inhibitor of plasmin. *Biochemistry* 1992;31:265–269.

146. Volpert OV, Dameron KM, Bouck N. Sequential development of an angiogenic phenotype by human fibroblasts progressing to tumorigenicity. *Oncogene* 1997;14:1495–1502.

147. Good DJ, Polverini PJ, Rastinejad F, et al. A tumor suppressor-dependent inhibitor of angiogenesis is immunologically and functionally indistinguishable from a fragment of thrombospondin. *Proc Natl Acad Sci U S A* 1990;87:6624–6628.

148. Clauss M, Murray JC, Vianna M, et al. A polypeptide factor produced by fibrosarcoma cells that induces endothelial tissue factor and enhances the procoagulant response to tumor necrosis factor/cachectin. *J Biol Chem* 1990;265:7078–7083.

149. Kao J, Ryan J, Brett G, et al. Endothelial monocyte-activating polypeptide II. A novel tumor-derived polypeptide that activates host-response mechanisms. *J Biol Chem* 1992;267:20239–20247.

150. Kao J, Houck K, Fan Y, et al. Characterization of a novel tumor-derived cytokine. Endothelial-monocyte activating polypeptide II. *J Biol Chem* 1994;269:25106–25119.

151. Wu PC, Alexander HR, Huang J, et al. *In vivo* sensitivity of human melanoma to tumor necrosis factor (TNF)-alpha is determined by tumor production of the novel cytokine endothelial-monocyte activating polypeptide II (EMAP-II). *Cancer Res* 1999;59:205–212.

152. Berger AC, Alexander HR, Wu PC, et al. Tumor necrosis factor receptor I (p55) is upregulated on endothelial cells by exposure to the tumor-derived cytokine endothelial monocyte activating polypeptide II (EMAP-II). *Cytokine* 2000 (*in press*).

153. Wu PC, Berger AC, Huang J, et al. *In vivo* tumors that overexpress endothelial monocyte-activating polypeptide II demonstrate upregulation of tumor necrosis factor receptor p55 on tumor neovasculature. *Surg Forum* 1998;XLIX:436–438.

154. Schwarz M, Brett J, Li J, Hayward J, Allen L, Kitterman J. Endothelial monocyte-activating polypeptide (EMAP) II, a novel antiangiogenic protein, suppresses tumor growth and induces apoptosis in endothelial cells. *Circ Suppl* 1995;92(abst).

155. Sim BKL, Fogler WE, Zhou XH, et al. Potent inhibition of experimental metastases and primary tumors by recombinant human Endostatin that is suitable for human use. *Proc Am Assoc Cancer Res* 1999;40:620(abst).

156. Kong HL, Crystal RG. Gene therapy strategies for tumor antiangiogenesis. *J Natl Cancer Inst* 1998;90:273–286.

157. Lin P, Buxton JA, Acheson A, et al. Antiangiogenic gene therapy targeting the endothelium-specific receptor tyrosine kinase Tie2. *Proc Natl Acad Sci U S A* 1998;95:8829–8834.

158. Tanaka T, Cao Y, Folkman J, Fine HA. Viral vector-targeted antiangiogenic gene therapy utilizing an angiostatin complementary DNA. *Cancer Res* 1998;58:3362–3369.

159. Ma D, Gerard RD, Li XY, Alizadeh H, Niederkorn JY. Inhibition of metastasis of intraocular melanomas by adenovirus-mediated gene transfer of plasminogen activator inhibitor type 1 (PAI-1) in an athymic mouse model. *Blood* 1997;90:2738–2746.

160. Nguyen JT, Wu P, Clouse ME, Hlatky L, Terwilliger EF. Adeno-associated virus-mediated delivery of antiangiogenic factors as an antitumor strategy. *Cancer Res* 1998;58:5673–5677.

161. Feldman AL, Restifo NP, Alexander HR, Bartlett DL, Hwu P, Libutti SK. The 18 amino acid E3/19K adenoviral signal sequence allows secretion of endostatin from cells infected with adenovirus carrying the endostatin gene. *Proc Am Soc Gene Ther* 1999;22a(abst).

162. Feldman AL, Restifo NP, Alexander HR, et al. Antiangiogenic gene therapy of cancer utilizing a recombinant adenovirus to elevate systematic endostatin levels in mice. *Cancer Res* 2000;60 (*in press*).

163. Gnant MFX, Puhlmann M, Alexander HR Jr, Bartlett DL. Systemic administration of a recombinant vaccinia virus expressing the cytosine deaminase gene and subsequent treatment with 5-fluorocytosine leads to tumor specific gene expression and prolongation of survival in mice. *Cancer Res* 1999;59:3396–3403.

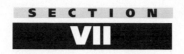

EVOLVING APPROACHES
TO BIOLOGIC THERAPY

23

DELIVERY OF BIOLOGIC MOLECULES
AND CELLS TO TUMORS

RAKESH K. JAIN

To be successful, a therapeutic agent must satisfy two requirements: It must be effective in the *in vivo* microenvironment, and it must reach target cells *in vivo* in optimal quantities (1). Extraordinary advances in molecular biology and biotechnology have helped researchers identify novel targets and develop a vast array of therapeutic agents including the biologic agents described in this book.

These agents can be divided into three categories: molecules, particles, and cells. In chemotherapy, the therapeutic agent can be injected as a molecule or incorporated in a particle (e.g., a liposome). In gene therapy, it can be a molecule, a viral or nonviral particle, or a genetically engineered cell. Similarly, for immunotherapy, molecules such as antibodies, particles such as liposomes, or cells such as activated lymphocytes can be used.

When any of these agents is injected into a patient, the material is distributed throughout the body via the circulatory system. It then arrives in the blood vessels of the tumor and moves across the vessel walls and through the interstitial compartment to reach the cancer cells. To be effective, the therapeutic agent must cross these barriers and successfully reach targets in optimal quantities. Unfortunately, tumors develop in ways that hinder each of these steps (Fig. 1) (2,3).

This chapter explores the current understanding of these physiologic barriers to delivery and effectiveness, as well as some strategies to overcome or exploit them.

DISTRIBUTION THROUGH VASCULAR SPACE

The chaotic blood supply of tumors is the first barrier encountered by a blood-borne agent. The tumor blood supply consists of vessels recruited from the preexisting network of the host vasculature and vessels resulting from the angiogenic response of host vessels to cancer cells (4,5). Movement of molecules and cells through the vasculature is governed by the vascular morphology (i.e., the number, length, diameter, and geometric arrangement of various blood vessels) and the rate of blood flow (6–10).

Although the tumor vasculature originates from the host vasculature and the mechanisms of angiogenesis are similar (4,10–12), its organization may be completely different depending on the tumor type, its growth rate, and its location. The fractal

dimensions and minimum path lengths of tumor vasculature are different from those of normal host vessels (7,9,12,13). The architecture and blood flow are different not only among various tumor types but also among a tumor and its metastases (5,14). For example, unlike normal tissue, in which red blood cell velocity depends on vessel diameter, no such dependence is seen in tumors (15–17). Furthermore, the red blood cell velocity may be an order of magnitude lower in some tumors compared to the host vessels (Fig. 2). The temporal and spatial heterogeneity in tumor blood flow may, in part, be a result of elevated geometric and viscous resistance in tumor vessels (18–21), coupling between high vascular permeability and elevated interstitial fluid pressure (8,22), vascular remodeling by intussusception (11), and solid stress generated by proliferating cancer cells (23,24).

Based on perfusion rates, four regions can be recognized in a tumor: (a) an avascular, necrotic region; (b) a seminecrotic region; (c) a stabilized microcirculation region; and (d) an advancing front (25) (see Fig. 1A). Intratumoral blood flow distributions in spontaneous animal and human tumors are now being investigated using nuclear magnetic resonance, positron emission tomography, and functional computed tomography (26–29). Although limited, these results are in concert with the transplanted tumor studies: Blood flow rates in necrotic and seminecrotic regions of tumors are low, whereas those in nonnecrotic regions are variable and can be substantially higher than in surrounding (contralateral) host normal tissues (30). Considering these spatial and temporal heterogeneities in blood supply along with variations in the vascular morphology at both microscopic and macroscopic levels, it is not surprising that the spatial distribution of therapeutic agents in tumors is heterogeneous and that the average uptake decreases, in general, with an increase in tumor weight.

METABOLIC MICROENVIRONMENT

The temporal and spatial heterogeneities in blood flow lead to a compromised metabolic microenvironment in tumors, which decreases the effectiveness of some therapies. To quantify the spatial gradients of key metabolites, two optical techniques have

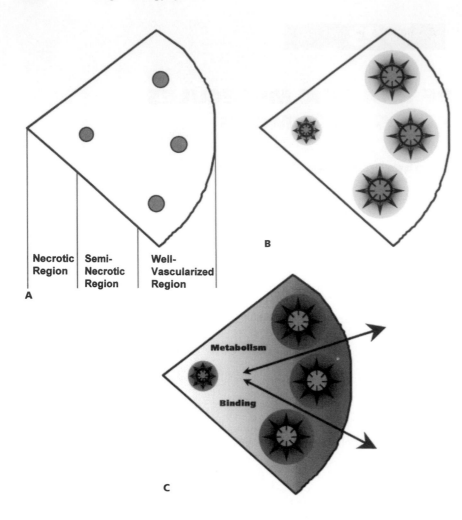

Necrotic Region **Semi-Necrotic Region** **Well-Vascularized Region**

A

B

Metabolism

Binding

C

FIGURE 1. Physiologic barriers that a blood-borne molecule encounters before it reaches a cancer cell in a solid tumor. **A:** Schematic of a heterogeneously perfused tumor showing well-vascularized periphery; a seminecrotic intermediate zone; and an avascular, necrotic central region. Note that immediately after intravenous injection, the molecules are delivered to perfused regions only. **B:** Low interstitial pressure in the periphery permits adequate extravasation of fluid and macromolecules. **C:** These macromolecules move toward the center by the slow process of diffusion. In addition, interstitial fluid oozing from tumor carries macromolecules with it by convection into the normal tissue. Note that the interstitial movement may be further retarded by binding. Products of metabolism may be cleared rapidly by blood. (Adapted from Jain RK. Delivery of novel therapeutic agents in tumors: physiological barriers and strategies. *J Natl Cancer Inst* 1989:81:570–576.)

been adapted: fluorescence ratio-imaging microscopy and phosphorescence quenching microscopy (31–35). As shown in Figure 3, pH and PO_2 decrease as the distance increases from tumor vessels leading to acidic and hypoxic regions in tumors. Coupled with the use of cells selected for impaired glycolytic and oxidative pathways, these methods have provided novel insight into pH regulation in tumors (36). Although low PO_2 and pH are detrimental to some therapies (e.g., radiation), they might enhance the effect of certain drugs, if the drug could be delivered in adequate quantities in those regions (37–39).

To gain further insight into tumor metabolism, two powerful approaches have been combined: magnetic resonance spectroscopy and tissue-isolated tumors. The former allows measurement of the energy level in tumors, whereas the latter allows control of the supply of individual substrates (e.g., glucose, oxygen) to the tumor. Using this combined approach, it has been shown that solid tumors depend more on glucose than oxygen to maintain their adenosine triphosphate level (40).

TRANSPORT ACROSS THE MICROVASCULAR WALL

The vessel wall is the second barrier to therapeutic agents. Once a blood-borne molecule has reached an exchange vessel, it

extravasates, by diffusion, convection, and—to some extent—presumably by transcytosis (41). Diffusive flux is proportional to the vascular permeability [P (measured in centimeters per second)], surface area of the exchange vessel [S (measured in square centimeters)], and the difference between the plasma and interstitial concentrations. Convection is proportional to the rate of fluid leakage from the vessel. Fluid flux, in turn, is proportional to the hydraulic conductivity [L_p (measured in centimeters per milligrams of mercury)], surface area of the exchange vessel, and the difference between the vascular and interstitial hydrostatic pressures. Thus, the transport of a molecule across tumor vessels is governed by two transport parameters (vascular permeability and hydraulic conductivity), the surface area for exchange, and the transvascular concentration and pressure gradients.

Vascular permeability and hydraulic conductivity of tumors in general are significantly higher than that of various normal tissues (16,41–47), and hence, these vessels may lack permselectivity (48) (Fig. 4). Positively charged molecules have a higher permeability (49). Despite increased overall permeability, not all blood vessels of a tumor are leaky (see Fig. 4). Even the leaky vessels have a finite pore size, which has been measured in a variety of human and rodent tumors (50). Our hypothesis is that the large pore size in tumors represents wide interendothelial junctions (50,51). Not only does the vascular permeability vary from one tumor to the

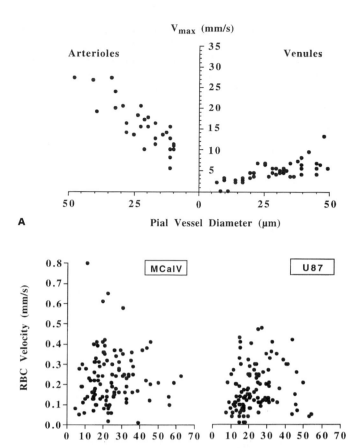

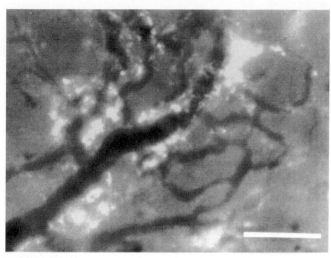

FIGURE 4. Heterogeneous extravasation of 90-nm diameter liposomes from LS174T tumor vessels, 48 hours after injection. Note that some vessels are leaky, indicated by the brighter fluorescence for rhodamine, while others are not. Extravasated liposomes do not diffuse far from blood vessels. (Adapted from Yuan F, Salehi HA, Boucher Y, et al. Vascular permeability and microcirculation of gliomas and mammary carcinomas transplanted in rat and mouse cranial windows. *Cancer Res* 1994;54:4564–4568.)

FIGURE 2. Blood velocity as a function of vessel diameter in normal pial vessels **(A)** a murine mammary carcinoma (MCaIV) and a human glioma (*U87*) xenograft on the pial surface **(B)**. Note that in normal microcirculation, blood velocity depends on vessel diameter, whereas in tumors no such dependence exists. Furthermore, the blood velocity in tumor vessels is about an order of magnitude lower than in host vessels. (RBC, red blood cell; V_{max}, maximal velocity.) (Adapted from Yuan F, Salehi HA, Boucher Y, et al. Vascular permeability and microcirculation of gliomas and mammary carcinomas transplanted in rat and mouse cranial windows. *Cancer Res* 1994;54:4564–4568.)

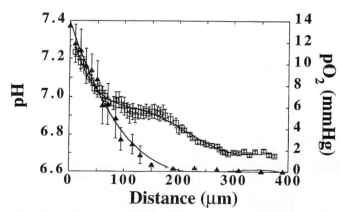

FIGURE 3. Spatial gradients of metabolites in tumors: pH (□) and Po_2 (▲). Distance from the vessel wall, in microns, is shown on the x-axis, with zero being the vessel wall. (Adapted from Helmlinger G, Yuan F, Dellican M, Jain RK. Interstitial pH and pO_2 gradients in solid tumors *in vivo*: simultaneous high-resolution measurements reveal a lack of correlation. *Nat Med* 1997;3:177–182.)

next, but within the same tumor it varies both spatially and temporally, and during tumor growth, regression, and relapse (41,52). The local microenvironment plays an important role in controlling vascular permeability. For example, a human glioma (HGL21) is fairly leaky when grown subcutaneously in immunodeficient mice, but it exhibits blood–brain barrier properties in the cranium. Such site-dependent differences have been noted for other tumors in other orthotopic sites (17). Our working hypothesis is that the host-tumor interactions control the production and secretion of cytokines associated with permeability changes [e.g., vascular permeability factor (VPF)/vascular endothelium growth factor (VEGF) and its inhibitors] (53,54). A better understanding of the molecular mechanisms of permeability regulation in tumors is likely to yield strategies for improved drug delivery (55).

If tumor vessels are indeed leaky to fluid and macromolecules, then what leads to the poor extravasation of these agents in various regions of tumors? As shown by us and others (56–69), experimental and human tumors exhibit high interstitial fluid pressure (Table 1). Furthermore, the uniformly high pressure drops precipitously to normal values in the tumor's periphery or in the peritumor region (57,70,71). This may lower fluid extravasation in the high-pressure regions, especially because the osmotic and hydrostatic pressures are also equal between the intravascular and extravascular spaces (58,72,73). Because the transvascular transport of macromolecules in normal tissues occurs primarily by convection (41,74), convective transport of macromolecules in the center of tumors may be less than in the tumor periphery (42,70,71). Additionally, the average vascular surface area per unit of tissue weight decreases with tumor growth; hence, reduced transvascular exchange would be expected in large tumors compared with small tumors (6,70).

TABLE 1. INTERSTITIAL FLUID PRESSURE IN NORMAL AND NEOPLASTIC TISSUES

Tissue Type	N	Mean (mm Hg)	Range (mm Hg)
Normal skin	5	0.4	–1.0–3.0
Normal breast	8	0.0	–0.5–3.0
Head and neck carcinomas	27	19.0	1.5–79.0
Cervical carcinomas	26	23.0	6.0–94.0
Lung carcinomas	26	10.0	1.0–27.0
Metastatic melanomas	14	21.0	0.0–60.0
Metastatic melanomas	12	14.5	2.0–41.0
Breast carcinomas	13	29.0	5.0–53.0
Breast carcinomas	8	15.0	4.0–33.0
Brain tumors[a]	17	7.0	2.0–15.0
Brain tumors[a]	11	1.0	–0.5–8.0
Colorectal liver metastasis	8	21.0	6.0–45.0
Lymphomas	7	4.5	1.0–12.5
Renal cell carcinoma	1	38.0	—

[a]Patients were treated with antiedema therapy.

TRANSPORT THROUGH INTERSTITIAL SPACE AND LYMPHATICS

Once a molecule has extravasated, it moves through the third barrier—the interstitial space—by diffusion and convection (64). Diffusion is proportional to the concentration gradient in the interstitium, and convection is proportional to the interstitial fluid velocity (u_i, measured in centimeters per second). The latter, in turn, is proportional to the pressure gradient in the interstitium. Just as the interstitial diffusion coefficient (D, measured in square centimeters per second) relates the diffusive flux to the concentration gradient, the interstitial hydraulic conductivity (K, measured in square centimeters per millimeter of mercury times seconds) relates the interstitial velocity to the pressure gradient (64). Values of these transport coefficients are determined by the structure and composition of the interstitial compartment as well as by the physicochemical properties of the solute molecule (75–82).

Using fluorescence recovery after photobleaching, we have found D of various molecules to be about one-third that in water (83) and similar to that in the host tissue (76). Similarly, the value of K for a human colon carcinoma xenograft (LS174T) measured using two different methods (69,84) was found to be higher than that of a hepatoma (81), which in turn was higher than that of the liver. Given these relatively high values of D and K, why do exogenously injected macromolecules not distribute uniformly in tumors? Two reasons exist for this apparent paradox.

The time constant for a molecule with diffusion coefficient D to diffuse across distance L is approximately $L^2/4D$. For diffusion of immunoglobulin G (IgG) in tumors, this time constant is approximately 1 hour for a 100-μm distance, days for a 1-mm distance, and months for a 1-cm distance. So, for a 1-mm tumor, diffusional transport would take days, and for a 1-cm tumor, it would take months. If the central vessels have collapsed completely owing to cellular proliferation (23) and interstitial matrix rearrangement, no delivery of macromolecules by blood flow to this necrotic center will occur (24). Binding may further retard the transport in tumors (83,85–91). The role of binding-site-barrier is clearly illustrated in Figure 5, which compares the rate of fluorescence recovery of a photobleached spot in tumor tissue injected with a nonspecific versus specific IgG. In addition to the heterogeneity in D in tumors, the most unexpected result of these photobleaching studies was the large extent (30% to 40%) of nonspecific binding (83).

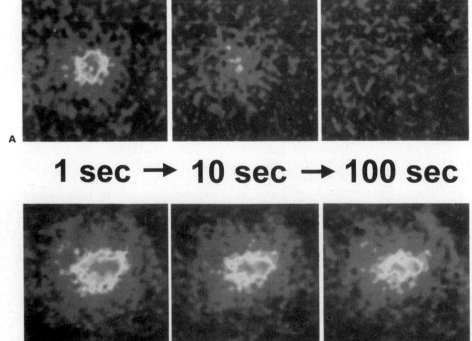

1 sec → 10 sec → 100 sec

FIGURE 5. Role of binding in the interstitial transport in tumors, measured using fluorescence recovery after photobleaching. **A:** Recovery of a photobleached spot is complete in approximately 100 seconds for a nonspecific monoclonal antibody. **B:** Recovery is incomplete for an antibody against carcinoembryonic antigen, present on the surface of many carcinoma cells. (Adapted from Berk DA, Yuan F, Leunig M, Jain RK. Direct *in vivo* measurement of targeted binding in a human tumor xenograft. *Proc Natl Acad Sci U S A* 1997;94:1785–1790.)

As mentioned, interstitial fluid pressure is high in the center of tumors and low in the periphery and surrounding tissue (57,70,71). Therefore, one would expect interstitial fluid motion from the tumor's periphery into the surrounding normal tissue (see Fig. 1). In various animal and human (xenograft) tumors studied to date, 6% to 14% of plasma entering the tumor has been found to leave from the tumor's periphery (41,92). This fluid leakage leads to a radial outward interstitial fluid velocity of 0.1 to 0.2 µm per second at the periphery of 1 cm tissue-isolated tumor (41). [The radial outward velocity is likely to be an order of magnitude lower in a tumor grown in the subcutaneous tissue or muscle (70).] A macromolecule at the tumor periphery has to overcome this outward convection to diffuse into the tumor. The relative contribution of this mechanism of heterogeneous distribution of antibodies in tumors may be smaller than the contribution of heterogeneous extravasation owing to elevated pressure and necrosis (70).

In most normal tissues, extravasated macromolecules are taken up by the lymphatics and brought back to the central circulation. Because of the lack of functional lymphatics within the tumor, the fluid and macromolecules oozing from the tumor surface must be picked up by the peritumor host lymphatics (6). To characterize the transport into and within the lymphatic capillaries, we have developed a mouse tail model (93). We have measured uptake and transport in this model using a macroscopic approach (residence time distribution analysis) and a microscopic approach (fluorescence recovery after photobleaching) (94,95). Concerted efforts towards uncovering mechanisms of lymphangiogenesis (96) and understanding changes in lymphatic transport in the presence of a tumor (97) are needed. Preliminary studies suggest that lymphatics are collapsed in tumors owing to stress exerted on them by proliferating cancer cells (97).

TRANSPORT OF CELLS

Cells may face additional barriers beyond those encountered by molecules and particles (e.g., liposomes) in tumors. When a cell enters a blood vessel, it may continue to move with flowing blood, collide with the vessel wall, adhere transiently or stably, and finally extravasate. These interactions are governed by local hydrodynamic forces and adhesive forces. The former are determined by the vessel diameter and blood velocity, and the latter by the expression, strength, and kinetics of bond formation between adhesion molecules and by surface area of contact (98,99). Deformability of cells affects both types of forces. Despite their importance in cell-based immunotherapy and gene therapy, the determinants of cell transport in tumors have not been examined extensively.

Using intravital microscopy, rolling of endogenous leukocytes has been shown to be generally low in tumor vessels, whereas stable adhesion (≥30 seconds) is comparable between normal and tumor vessels (100). On the other hand, both rolling and stable adhesion are nearly zero in angiogenic vessels induced in collagen gels by basic fibroblast growth factor (bFGF) or VEGF/VPF, two of the most potent angiogenic factors (101). Whether the latter is due to a low flux of leukocytes into angiogenic vessels, downregulation of adhesion molecules

in these immature vessels, or both is currently under investigation. The age of the animal also plays an important role in leukocyte-endothelium interactions (102).

To gain further insight into the type of cells that adhere to tumor vessels, the localization of interleukin-2 (IL-2) activated natural killer (A-NK) cells was examined in normal and tumor tissues in mice using positron emission tomography (103,104). After systemic injection, these cells localized primarily in the lungs immediately after injection, and an undetectable number of cells arrived in the tumor (103). These findings were consistent with previous work on the deformability of these cells using micropipet aspiration technique, in which IL-2 activation was demonstrated to make these cells rigid and predict their mechanical entrapment in the lung microcirculation (105,106). Constitutive expression of certain adhesion molecules in the lung vasculature also facilitates their localization in the lungs (107).

One approach to reduce lung entrapment is to reduce the rigidity of these cells (108). Instead, to circumvent the lung, A-NK cells were injected into the blood supply of tumors, and A-NK cells, both xenogenic and syngeneic, adhered to blood vessels in three different tumor models (104,109,110). These results also supported the hypothesis that the endogenous cells that adhere to tumor vessels after systemic IL-2 injection are mostly activated lymphocytes (111).

To determine the adhesion molecules involved in the A-NK cell adhesion to tumor vessels, two *in vitro* approaches were used. In the first approach, the tumor vasculature was simulated *in vitro* by incubating human umbilical vein endothelial cells (HUVECs) in the tumor interstitial fluid (collected using a micropore chamber) (37,112–114). Using fluorometry, the expression of relevant adhesion molecules on the HUVEC monolayers was quantified (115). To determine the relative contributions of these molecules in adhesion under physiologic flow conditions, the flow chamber was used (116). Using appropriate antibodies, it was found that molecules upregulated on HUVECs include intercellular adhesion molecule–1 and vascular cell adhesion molecule–1, which bind to CD18 and VLA-4 on A-NK cells. Sporadic upregulation of E-selectin was also observed. The role of these molecules *in vivo* was confirmed by treating A-NK cells with antibodies against CD18 and VLA-4 before injecting them into the arterial supply of tumors. As in *in vitro* studies, blocking these adhesion molecules nearly eliminated the adhesion of A-NK cells to tumor vessels (114).

What leads to the upregulation of these molecules in the tumor vasculature? It was already known that these molecules can be upregulated by tumor necrosis factor–α and a protein of 90-kd molecular weight (p90) secreted by some neoplastic cells (98,117,118) and downregulated by transforming growth factor–β (119–121). What was unknown was whether other molecules present in the tumor milieu also induce this upregulation. Because tumor growth and metastasis are angiogenesis dependent, the two most potent angiogenic molecules—bFGF and VEGF/VPF—were investigated (4,107,122). It was found that VEGF can mimic tumor interstitial fluid and upregulate these molecules (123,124). bFGF, on the other hand, exhibited no effect when used alone, but abrogated the upregulation induced by VEGF or tumor necrosis factor–α (114). These findings were in concert with earlier reports that bFGF retards the trans-

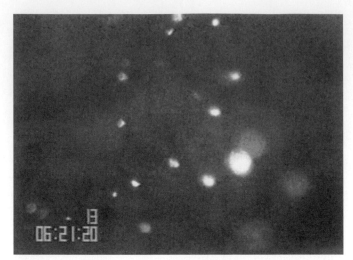

FIGURE 6. Heterogeneous adhesion of interleukin-2–activated natural killer cells to the tumor vasculature. (Adapted from Melder RJ, Salehi HA, Jain RK. Localization of activated natural killer cells in MCaIV mammary carcinoma grown in cranial windows in C3H mice. *Microvasc Res* 1995;50:35–44.)

migration of lymphocytes across endothelial monolayer (125) and reduces adhesion of endothelial cells to collagen at low cell density (126). The findings also offer a possible explanation for heterogeneous leukocyte-endothelium interactions in tumors: bFGF may have downregulated adhesion molecules in these tumors (Fig. 6). Further efforts are now needed to defining interactions between angiogenic and adhesion molecules using various *in vitro* and *in vivo* approaches, including genetically engineered mice (107,123,127,128).

PHARMACOKINETIC MODELING: SCALE-UP FROM MOUSE TO HUMAN

Thus far, each of the steps in the delivery of molecules and cells to and within solid tumors has been analyzed. Can this information be integrated into a unified framework? Some success has been realized in this endeavor, using physiologically based pharmacokinetic modeling. This approach, pioneered by two chemical engineers—K. Bischoff and R. L. Dedrick—in the 1960s, has been applied successfully to describe and scale up the biodistribution of low-molecular-weight agents (129–131). This approach has been extended to macromolecules and cells (132–136).

In this approach, a mammalian body is represented by a number of physiologic compartments that are interconnected anatomically. The volume and rate of blood flow to each of these compartments, or organs, are known or can be measured. The parameters that characterize transport across the subcompartments (i.e., vascular, interstitial, and cellular) and the metabolism of various agents are not generally known and cannot be easily measured. Our philosophy has been to use as many measured parameters as possible and estimate the remaining parameters by fitting the model to the murine biodistribution data. By scaling up the parameters using well-defined scale-up laws (130), the biodistribution in human patients is predicted and compared with clinical data. Discrepancies between predictions and actual data

assist in identification of interspecies differences and force reevaluation of the model assumptions. This is an evolutionary process: As the understanding of underlying physiology and biochemistry improves, the relevant parameters are modified and the model is refined further. The model is useful not only for designing murine experiments and clinical trials but also in identifying the sensitive parameters that need careful measurement and analysis. If detailed spatial information about a tissue or organ is needed, researchers develop a distributed parameter model for that organ (e.g., tumor) (6,70,85,86,132,133,137–139). Although simple in principle, this cyclic approach of analysis and synthesis has served as a useful paradigm for developing a deeper understanding of drug and cell distribution in normal and malignant tissues. The sophistication of these models is likely to improve with the understanding of underlying principles (7).

BENCH TO BEDSIDE

The physiologic factors that contribute to the heterogeneous delivery of therapeutic agents to tumors include heterogeneous blood supply, interstitial hypertension, relatively long transport distances in the interstitium, and cellular heterogeneities (see Fig. 1). How can these physiologic barriers be exploited or overcome? Can the findings about these barriers move from the bench to the bedside? Two strategies with the potential to improve the detection and treatment of solid tumors in patients are described here.

As mentioned, all solid tumors in patients exhibit interstitial hypertension (see Table 1), provided the patient has not received any antiedema treatment (61). It has been confirmed that interstitial fluid pressure rises quite steeply in the tumor boundary (55,71). This knowledge has been used to improve the design of the needle used by radiologists to localize tumors for surgical excision (140). Needle placement in a tumor can be facilitated by placing a pressure sensor in the needle. Because tumors begin to exhibit interstitial hypertension almost from the onset of angiogenesis (73), this needle may be able to help in localizing early disease. The same concept may be useful in optimizing location and infusion pressure of needles used in intratumoral infusion of therapeutic agents (84) and for monitoring response to therapy (68).

Several physical (e.g., radiation, heat) and chemical (e.g., vasoactive drugs) agents may lead to an increase in tumor blood flow or vascular permeability (14,24,41,141–146) or lower pH (37,39). Another approach may be based on increasing the interstitial transport rate of molecules by increasing K or D enzymatically (81,84,92) or using multistep approaches (133,147–149). Several physical and chemical agents have been used to lower interstitial fluid pressure in tumors (15,24,150–156). Because microvascular and interstitial pressures in tumors are approximately equal, any change in one is rapidly followed by a similar change in the other, and thus the convective enhancement disappears rapidly (58,157–159). By developing a mathematical model for solid tumors, we have calculated theoretically and confirmed experimentally that the time constant of pressure transmission across the tumor vasculature is approximately 10 seconds (157). During such a short time, the convective enhancement is calculated to be very small (approximately 1%). However, if the vascular pressure is increased repeatedly and the transvascular transport is unidirectional or if the molecule binds avidly in the extravascular region, then in principle, drug delivery to solid tumors can be increased significantly (160).

In contrast, the physiologic barriers discussed here may be less of a problem for (a) radioimmunodetection; (b) treating leukemias, lymphomas, and small tumors (e.g., micrometastases) in which the physiologic barriers are not yet fully established; (c) treatment of adequately perfused, low-pressure regions of large tumors for debulking; and (d) treatment with antibodies or other agents directed against the host cells (e.g., tumor endothelial cells, fibroblasts) or the subendothelial matrix. These physiologic barriers may also pose fewer problems for treatment with a molecule or cell that has nearly 100% specificity for cells in the tumor. Until such selective molecules or cells are developed, methods are urgently needed to overcome or exploit these physiologic barriers in tumors. It is hoped that an improved understanding of transport in tumors will contribute to the development of such strategies (1,3,161).

ACKNOWLEDGMENTS

I thank Carol Lyons for typing this manuscript, Gerald Koenig for his help with the references, Lance Munn for his help with the figures, and Yves Boucher for help with Table 1. Research described here was primarily supported by grants from the National Cancer Institute, the National Science Foundation, and the National Foundation for Cancer Research.

This is an updated version of an article published as "1995 Whitaker Lecture: Delivery of Molecules, Particles and Cells to Solid Tumors," in the *Annals of Biomedical Engineering* (1996;24:457–473). The author thanks the Biomedical Engineering Society for allowing him to reproduce parts of this article.

REFERENCES

1. Jain RK. The next frontier of molecular medicine: delivery of therapeutics. *Nat Med* 1998;4:655–657.
2. Jain RK. Barriers to drug delivery in solid tumors. *Sci Am* 1994;271:58–65
3. Jain RK. 1996 Landis Award Lecture: Delivery of molecular and cellular medicine to solid tumors. *Microcirculation* 1997;4:1–23.
4. Folkman J. Tumor angiogenesis. In: Mendelsohn PM, Howley MAP, eds. *The Molecular Basis of Cancer.* Philadelphia: WB Saunders, 1995:206–232.
5. Jain RK. Determinants of tumor blood flow: a review. *Cancer Res* 1988;48:2641–2658.
6. Baxter LT, Jain RK. Transport of fluid and macromolecules in tumors. II. Role of heterogeneous perfusion and lymphatics. *Microvasc Res* 1990;40:246–263.
7. Baish JW, Gazit Y, Berk DA, Nozue M, Baxter LT, Jain RK. Role of tumor vascular architecture in nutrient and drug delivery: an invasion percolation model. *Microvasc Res* 1996;51:327–346.
8. Baish JW, Netti PA, Jain RK. Transmural coupling of fluid flow in microcirculatory network and interstitium in tumors. *Microvasc Res* 1997;53:128–141.
9. Gazit Y, Berk DA, Leunig M, Baxter LT, Jain RK. Scale-invariant

10. Less JR, Skalak TC, Sevick EM, Jain RK. Microvascular architecture in a mammary carcinoma: branching patterns and vessel dimensions. *Cancer Res* 1991;51:265–273.
11. Patan S, Munn LL, Jain RK. Intussusceptive microvascular growth in solid tumors: a novel mechanism of tumor angiogenesis. *Microvasc Res* 1996;51:260–272.
12. Baish JW, Jain RK. Cancer, angiogenesis and fractals. *Nat Med* 1998;4:984.
13. Gazit Y, Baish JW, Safabakhsh N, Leunig M, Baxter LT, Jain RK. Fractal characteristics of tumor vascular architecture: significance and implications. *Microcirculation* 1997;4:395–402.
14. Jain RK, Ward-Hartley KA. Tumor blood flow: characterization, modifications and role in hyperthermia. *IEEE Trans Sonics Ultrasonics* 1984;31:504–526.
15. Leunig M, Yuan F, Menger MD, Boucher Y, Goetz AE, Messmer K, Jain RK. Angiogenesis, microvascular architecture, microhemodynamics, and interstitial fluid pressure during early growth of human adenocarcinoma LS174T in SCID mice. *Cancer Res* 1992;52:6553–6560.
16. Yuan F, Salehi HA, Boucher Y, Vasthare US, Tuma RF, Jain RK. Vascular permeability and microcirculation of gliomas and mammary carcinomas transplanted in rat and mouse cranial windows. *Cancer Res* 1994;54:4564–4568.
17. Fukumura D, Yuan F, Monsky WL, Chen Y, Jain RK. Effect of host microenvironment on the microcirculation of human colon adenocarcinoma. *Am J Pathol* 1997;150:679–688.
18. Sevick EM, Jain RK. Geometric resistance to blood flow in solid tumors perfused ex vivo: effects of tumor size and perfusion pressure. *Cancer Res* 1989;49:3506–3512.
19. Less JR, Posner MC, Skalak T, Wolmark N, Jain RK. Geometric resistance to blood flow and vascular network architecture in human colorectal carcinoma. *Microcirculation* 1997;4:25–33.
20. Sevick EM, Jain RK. Viscous resistance to blood flow in solid tumors: effect of hematocrit on intratumor blood viscosity. *Cancer Res* 1989;49:3513–3519.
21. Sevick EM, Jain RK. Effect of red blood cell rigidity on tumor blood flow: increase in viscous resistance during hyperglycemia. *Cancer Res* 1991;51:2727–2730.
22. Netti PA, Roberge S, Boucher Y, Baxter LT, Jain RK. Effect of transvascular fluid exchange on arterio-venous pressure relationship: implication for temporal and spatial heterogeneities in tumor blood flow. *Microvasc Res* 1996;52:27–46.
23. Helmlinger G, Netti PA, Lichtenbeld HC, Melder RJ, Jain RK. Solid stress inhibits the growth of multicellular tumor spheroids. *Nat Biotechnol* 1997;15:778–783.
24. Griffon-Etienne G, Boucher Y, Brekken C, Suit HD, Jain RK. Taxane-induced apoptosis decompresses blood vessels and lowers interstitial pressure in tumors. *Cancer Res* 1999;59:3776–3782.
25. Endrich B, Reinhold HS, Gross JF, Intaglietta M. Tissue perfusion inhomogeneity during early tumor growth in rats. *J Natl Cancer Inst* 1979;62:387–395.
26. Eskey CJ, Wolmark N, McDowell CL, Domach MM, Jain RK. Residence time distributions of various tracers in tumors: implications for drug delivery and blood flow measurement. *J Natl Cancer Inst* 1994;86:293–299.
27. Eskey CJ, Koretsky AP, Domach MM, Jain RK. 2H-nuclear magnetic resonance imaging of tumor blood flow: spatial and temporal heterogeneity in a tissue-isolated mammary adenocarcinoma. *Cancer Res* 1992;52:6010–6019.
28. Hamberg LM, Kristjansen PE, Hunter GJ, Wolf GL, Jain RK. Spatial heterogeneity in tumor perfusion measured with functional computed tomography at 0.05 microliter resolution. *Cancer Res* 1994;54:6032–6036.
29. Shtern F, Wingfield D. Report of joint conference on quantitative in vivo functional imaging in oncology. *Academic Radiology* 1999;6:S259–S300.
30. Vaupel P, Jain RK. *Tumor blood supply and metabolic microenvironment: characterization and therapeutic implications.* Stuttgart, Germany: Gustav Fischer Publications, 1991.

31. Dellian M, Helmlinger G, Yuan F, Jain RK. Fluorescence ratio imaging and optical sectioning: effect of glucose on spatial and temporal gradients. *Br J Cancer* 1996;74:1206–1215.

32. Helmlinger G, Yuan F, Dellian M, Jain RK. Interstitial pH and pO2 gradients in solid tumors *in vivo*: simultaneous high-resolution measurements reveal a lack of correlation. *Nat Med* 1997;3:177–182.

33. Martin GR, Jain RK. Fluorescence ratio imaging measurement of pH gradients: calibration and application in normal and tumor tissues. *Microvasc Res* 1993;46:216–230.

34. Martin GR, Jain RK. Noninvasive measurement of interstitial pH profiles in normal and neoplastic tissue using fluorescence ratio imaging microscopy. *Cancer Res* 1994;54:5670–5674.

35. Torres-Filho IP, Leunig M, Yuan F, Intaglietta M, Jain RK. Noninvasive measurement of microvascular and interstitial oxygen profiles in a human tumor in SCID mice. *Proc Natl Acad Sci U S A* 1994;91:2081–2085.

36. Helmlinger G, Sckell A, Dellian M, Jain RK. Acid production in variant, glycolysis-deficient and parental tumors *in vivo*: evidence for a role of the pentose cycle, 1999 (Submitted).

37. Jain RK, Shah SA, Finney PL. Continuous noninvasive monitoring of pH and temperature in rat Walker 256 carcinoma during normoglycemia and hyperglycemia. *J Natl Cancer Inst* 1984;73:429–436.

38. Nozue M, Lee I, Manning JM, Manning LR, Jain RK. Oxygenation in tumors by modified hemoglobins. *J Surg Oncol* 1996;62:109–114.

39. Ward KA, Jain RK. Response of tumours to hyperglycaemia: characterization, significance and role in hyperthermia. *Int J Hyperthermia* 1988;4:223–250.

40. Eskey CJ, Koretsky AP, Domach MM, Jain RK. Role of oxygen vs. glucose in energy metabolism in a mammary carcinoma perfused *ex vivo*: direct measurement by 31P NMR. *Proc Natl Acad Sci U S A* 1993;90:2646–2650.

41. Jain RK. Transport of molecules across tumor vasculature. *Cancer Metastasis Rev* 1987;6:559–593.

42. Lichtenbeld HC, Yuan F, Michel CC, Jain RK. Perfusion of single tumor microvessels: application to vascular permeability measurement. *Microcirculation* 1996;3:349–357.

43. Dvorak HF, Brown LF, Detmar M, Dvorak AM. Vascular permeability factor/vascular endothelial growth factor, microvascular hyperpermeability, and angiogenesis. *Am J Pathol* 1995;146:1029–1039.

44. Gerlowski LE, Jain RK. Microvascular permeability of normal and neoplastic tissues. *Microvasc Res* 1986;31:288–305.

45. Sevick EM, Jain RK. Measurement of capillary filtration coefficient in a solid tumor. *Cancer Res* 1991;51:1352–1355.

46. Yuan F, Leunig M, Berk DA, Jain RK. Microvascular permeability of albumin, vascular surface area, and vascular volume measured in human adenocarcinoma LS174T using dorsal chamber in SCID mice. *Microvasc Res* 1993;45:269–289.

47. Yuan F, Leunig M, Huang SK, Berk DA, Papahadjopoulos D, Jain RK. Microvascular permeability and interstitial penetration of sterically stabilized (stealth) liposomes in a human tumor xenograft. *Cancer Res* 1994;54:3352–3356.

48. Yuan F, Dellian M, Fukumura D, et al. Vascular permeability in a human tumor xenograft: molecular size-dependence and cut-off size. *Cancer Res* 1995;55:3752–3756.

49. Dellian M, Yuan F, Trubetskoy VS, Torchilin VP, Jain RK. Vascular permeability in a human tumor xenograft: molecular charge dependence. *Br J Cancer* 2000 (*in press*)

50. Hobbs S, Monsky W, Yuan F, et al. Regulation of transport pathways in tumor vessels: role of tumor type and microenvironment. *Proc Natl Acad Sci U S A* 1998;95:4607–4612.

51. Hashizume H, Baluk P, Morikawa S, et al. Openings between defective endothelial cells explain tumor vessel leakiness. *Am J Pathol* 2000 (*in press*).

52. Jain RK, Safabakhsh N, Sckell A, Chen Y, Benjamin LA, Yuan F, Keshet E. Endothelial cell death, angiogenesis, and microvascular function following castration in an androgen-dependent tumor: role of VEGF. *Proc Natl Acad Sci U S A* 1998;95:10820–10825.

53. Fukumura D, Xavier R, Sugiura T, et al. Tumor induction of VEGF promoter activity in stromal cells. *Cell* 1998;94:715–725.

54. Jain RK, Munn LL. Leaky vessels? Call Ang1! *Nat Med* 2000;6:131–132.

55. Yuan F, Chen Y, Dellian M, Safabakhsh N, Ferrara N, Jain RK. Time-dependent changes in vascular permeability and morphology in established human tumor xenografts induced by an anti-VEGF/VPF antibody. *Proc Natl Acad Sci U S A* 1996;93:14765–14770.

56. Arbit E, Lee J, DiResta G. Interstitial hypertension in human brain tumors: possible role in peritumoral edema formulation. In: Nagai H, Kamiya K, Ishi S, eds. *Intracranial pressure*. Vol. IX. Tokyo: Springer-Verlag New York, 1994:609–614.

57. Boucher Y, Baxter LT, Jain RK. Interstitial pressure gradients in tissue-isolated and subcutaneous tumors: implications for therapy. *Cancer Res* 1990;50:4478–4484.

58. Boucher Y, Jain RK. Microvascular pressure is the principal driving force for interstitial hypertension in solid tumors: implications for vascular collapse. *Cancer Res* 1992;52:5110–5114.

59. Boucher Y, Lee I, Jain RK. Lack of general correlation between interstitial fluid pressure and pO_2 in tumors. *Microvasc Res* 1995;50:175–182.

60. Boucher Y, Kirkwood JM, Opacic D, Desantis M, Jain RK. Interstitial hypertension in superficial metastatic melanomas in humans. *Cancer Res* 1991;51:6691–6694.

61. Boucher Y, Salehi H, Witwer B, Harsh GR, Jain RK. Interstitial fluid pressure in intracranial tumors in patients and in rodents: effect of anti-edema therapy. *Br J Cancer* 1997;75:829–836.

62. Curti BD, Urba WJ, Alvord WG, et al. Interstitial pressure of subcutaneous nodules in melanoma and lymphoma patients: changes during treatment. *Cancer Res* 1993;53:2204–2207.

63. Gutmann R, Leunig M, Feyh J, et al. Interstitial hypertension in head and neck tumors in patients: correlation with tumor size. *Cancer Res* 1992;52:1993–1995.

64. Jain RK. Transport of molecules in the tumor interstitium: a review. *Cancer Res* 1987;47:3039–3051.

65. Less JR, Posner MC, Boucher Y, Borochovitz D, Wolmark N, Jain RK. Interstitial hypertension in human breast and colorectal tumors. *Cancer Res* 1992;52:6371–6374.

66. Nathanson SD, Nelson L. Interstitial fluid pressure in breast cancer, benign breast conditions, and breast parenchyma. *Ann Surg Oncol* 1994;1:333–338.

67. Roh HD, Boucher Y, Kalnicki S, Buchsbaum R, Bloomer WD, Jain RK. Interstitial hypertension in carcinoma of uterine cervix in patients: possible correlation with tumor oxygenation and radiation response. *Cancer Res* 1991;51:6695–6698.

68. Znati CA, Karasek K, Faul C, et al. Interstitial fluid pressure changes in cervical carcinomas in patients undergoing radiation therapy: a potential prognostic factor. 2000 (Submitted).

69. Znati CA, Boucher Y, Rosenstein M, Turner D, Watkins S, Jain RK. Effect of radiation on the interstitial matrix and hydraulic conductivity of tumors. 2000 (Submitted).

70. Baxter LT, Jain RK. Transport of fluid and macromolecules in tumors. I. Role of interstitial pressure and convection. *Microvasc Res* 1989;37:77–104.

71. Jain RK, Baxter LT. Mechanisms of heterogeneous distribution of monoclonal antibodies and other macromolecules in tumors: significance of elevated interstitial pressure. *Cancer Res* 1988;48:7022–7032.

72. Stohrer M, Boucher Y, Stangassinger M, Jain RK. Oncotic pressure in human tumor xenografts. 2000 (Submitted).

73. Boucher Y, Leunig M, Jain RK. Tumor angiogenesis and interstitial hypertension. *Cancer Res* 1996;56:4264–4266.

74. Rippe B, Haraldsson B. Fluid and protein fluxes across small and large pores in the microvasculature: applications of two-pore equations. *Acta Physiol Scand* 1987;131:411–428.

75. Berk DA, Yuan F, Leunig M, Jain RK. Fluorescence photobleaching with spatial Fourier analysis: measurement of diffusion in light-scattering media. *Biophys J* 1993;65:2428–2436.

76. Chary SR, Jain RK. Direct measurement of interstitial convection and diffusion of albumin in normal and neoplastic tissues by fluorescence photobleaching. *Proc Natl Acad Sci U S A* 1989;86:5385–5389.

77. Johnson ME, Berk DA, Jain RK, Deen WM. Diffusion and partitioning of proteins in charged agarose gels. *Biophys J* 1995;68:1561–1568.

78. Johnson ME, Berk DA, Jain RK, Deen WM. Hindered diffusion in agarose gels: test of effective medium mode. *Biophys J* 1996;70:

1017–1026.

79. Johnson ME, Berk DA, Blankschtein D, Golan DE, Jain RK, Langer R. Lateral diffusion of small compounds in human stratum corneum and model lipid bilayer systems. *Biophys J* 1996;71:2656–2668.

80. Nugent LJ, Jain RK. Extravascular diffusion in normal and neoplastic tissues. *Cancer Res* 1984;44:238–244.

81. Swabb EA, Wei J, Gullino PM. Diffusion and convection in normal and neoplastic tissues. *Cancer Res* 1974;34:2814.

82. Pluen A, Jain RK, Berk DA. Diffusion of macromolecules in agarose gels: comparison of linear and globular configurations. *Biophys J* 1999;77:542–552

83. Berk DA, Yuan F, Leunig M, Jain RK. Direct *in vivo* measurement of targeted binding in a human tumor xenograft. *Proc Natl Acad Sci U S A* 1997;94:1785–1790.

84. Boucher Y, Brekken C, Netti PA, Baxter LT, Jain RK. Intratumoral infusion of fluid: estimation of hydraulic conductivity and compliance and implications for the delivery of therapeutic agents. *Br J Cancer* 1998;78·1442–1448.

85. Baxter LT, Jain RK. Transport of fluid and macromolecules in tumors. Ill. Role of binding and metabolism. *Microvasc Res* 1991;41:5–23.

86. Baxter LT, Jain RK. Transport of fluid and macromolecules in tumors. IV. A microscopic model of the perivascular distribution. *Microvasc Res* 1991;41:252–272.

87. Juweid M, Neumann R, Paik C. Micropharmacology of monoclonal antibodies in solid tumor: direct experimental evidence for a binding site barrier. *Cancer Res* 1992;52:5144.

88. Kaufman EN, Jain RK. Quantification of transport and binding parameters using fluorescence recovery after photobleaching: potential for *in vivo* applications. *Biophys J* 1990;58:873–885.

89. Kaufman EN, Jain RK. Measurement of mass transport and reaction parameters in bulk solution using photobleaching: reaction limited binding regime. *Biophys J* 1991;60:596–610.

90. Kaufman EN, Jain RK. Effect of bivalent interaction upon apparent antibody affinity: experimental confirmation of theory using fluorescence photobleaching and implications for antibody binding assays. *Cancer Res* 1992;52:4157–4167.

91. Kaufman EN, Jain RK. *In vitro* measurement and screening of monoclonal antibody affinity using fluorescence photobleaching. *J Immunol Methods* 1992;155:1–17.

92. Jain RK. Delivery of novel therapeutic agents in tumors: physiological barriers and strategies. *J Natl Cancer Inst* 1989;81:570–576.

93. Leu AJ, Berk DA, Yuan F, Jain RK. Flow velocity in the superficial lymphatic network of the mouse tail. *Am J Physiol* 1994;267: H1507–H1513.

94. Berk DA, Swartz MA, Leu AJ, Jain RK. Transport in lymphatic capillaries: II. Microscopic velocity measurement with fluorescence recovery after photobleaching. *Am J Physiol* 1996;270:H330–H337.

95. Swartz MA, Berk DA, Jain RK. Transport in lymphatic capillaries: I. Macroscopic measurements using residence time distribution theory. *Am J Physiol* 1996;270:H324–H329.

96. Jeltsch M, Kaipainen A, Joukov V, et al. Hyperplasia of lymphatic vessels in VEGF-C transgenic mice. *Science* 1997;276:1423–1425.

97. Padera T, Kadambi A, Yun C-O, Jain RK. Molecular and functional evaluation of initial lymphatics in a murine sarcoma. 2000 (Submitted).

98. Melder RJ, Munn LL, Yamada S, Ohkubo C, Jain RK. Selectin and integrin mediated T lymphocyte rolling and arrest on TNFα-activated endothelium is augmented by erythrocytes. *Biophys J* 1995;69:2131–2138.

99. Munn LL, Melder RJ, Jain RK. Role of erythrocytes in leukocyte-endothelia interactions: mathematical model and experimental validation. *Biophys J* 1996;71:466–478.

100. Fukumura D, Salehi H, Witwer B, Tuma RF, Melder RJ, Jain RK. TNFα-induced leukocyte-adhesion in normal and tumor vessels: effect of tumor type, transplantation site and host. *Cancer Res* 1995;55:4824–4829.

101. Dellian M, Witwer BP, Salehi HA, Yuan F, Jain RK. Quantitation and physiological characterization of bFGF and VEGF/VPF induced vessels in mice: effect of microenvironment on angiogenesis. *Am J Pathol* 1996;149:59–71.

102. Yamada S, Melder RJ, Leunig M, Ohkubo C, Jain RK. Leukocyte-

rolling increases with age. *Blood* 1995;86:4707–4708.

103. Melder RJ, Brownell AL, Shoup TM, Brownell GL, Jain RK. Imaging of activated natural killer cells in mice by positron emission tomography: preferential uptake in tumors. *Cancer Res* 1993;53: 5867–5871.

104. Melder RJ, Elmaleh D, Brownell AL, Brownell GL, Jain RK. A method for labeling cells for positron emission tomography (PET) studies. *J Immunol Methods* 1994;175:79–87.

105. Sasaki A, Jain RK, Maghazachi AA, Goldfarb RH, Herberman RB. Low deformability of lymphokine-activated killer cells as a possible determinant of *in vivo* distribution. *Cancer Res* 1989;49:3742–3746.

106. Melder RJ, Jain RK. Kinetics of interleukin-2 induced changes in rigidity of human natural killer cells. *Cell Biophys* 1992;20:161–176.

107. Jain RK, Koenig GC, Dellian M, Fukumura D, Munn LL, Melder RJ. Leukocyte-endothelial adhesion and angiogenesis in tumors. *Cancer Metastasis Rev* 1996;15:195–204.

108. Melder RJ, Jain RK. Reduction of rigidity in human activated natural killer cells by thioglycollate treatment. *J Immunol Methods* 1994;175:69–77.

109. Melder RJ, Salehi HA, Jain RK. Localization of activated natural killer cells in MCaIV mammary carcinoma grown in cranial windows in C3H mice. *Microvasc Res* 1995;50:35–44.

110. Sasaki A, Melder RJ, Whiteside TL, Herberman RB, Jain RK. Preferential localization of human adherent lymphokine-activated killer cells in tumor microcirculation. *J Natl Cancer Inst* 1991;83:433–437.

111. Ohkubo C, Bigos D, Jain RK. Interleukin-2 induced leukocyte adhesion to the normal and tumor microvascular endothelium *in vivo* and its inhibition by dextran sulfate: implications for vascular leak syndrome. *Cancer Res* 1991;51:1561–1563.

112. Gullino P. Techniques in tumor pathophysiology. In: Busch H, ed. *Methods in cancer research*. New York: Academic Press, 1970:45–92.

113. Jain RK, Wei J, Gullino PM. Pharmacokinetics of methotrexate in solid tumors. *J Pharmacokinet Biopharm* 1979;7:181–194.

114. Melder RJ, Koenig GC, Witwer BP, Safabakhsh N, Munn LL, Jain RK. During angiogenesis, vascular endothelial growth factor and basic fibroblast growth factor regulate natural killer cell adhesion to tumor endothelium. *Nat Med* 1996;2:992–997.

115. Munn LL, Koenig GC, Jain RK, Melder RJ. Kinetics of adhesion molecule expression and spatial organization using targeted sampling fluorometry. *Biotechniques* 1995;19:622–631.

116. Munn LL, Melder RJ, Jain RK. Analysis of cell flux in the parallel plate flow chamber: implications for cell capture studies. *Biophys J* 1994;67:889–895.

117. Jallal B, Powell J, Zachweija J, et al. Suppression of tumor growth *in vivo* by local and systemic 90K level increase. *Cancer Res* 1995;55:3223–3227.

118. Melder RJ, Koenig GC, Munn LL, Jain RK. Adhesion of activated natural killer cells to TNF-alpha treated endothelium under physiological flow conditions. *Nat Immunol* 1997;15:154–163.

119. Gamble JR, Vadas MA. Endothelial adhesiveness for blood neutrophils is inhibited by transforming growth factor-beta. *Science* 1988;242:97–99.

120. Gamble JR, Vadas MA. Endothelial cell adhesiveness for human T lymphocytes is inhibited by transforming growth factor-beta. *J Immunol* 1991;146:1149–1154.

121. Gamble JR, Khew-Goodall Y, Vadas MA. Transforming growth factor-beta inhibits E-selectin expression on human endothelial cells. *J Immunol* 1993;150:4494–4503.

122. Fidler IJ. Modulation of the organ microenvironment for treatment of cancer metastasis. *J Natl Cancer Inst* 1995;87:1588–1592.

123. Detmar M, Brown LF, Schoen MP, et al. Increased microvascular density and enhanced leukocyte rolling and adhesion in the skin of VEGF transgenic mice. *J Invest Dermatol* 1998;3:1–6.

124. Sckell A, Safabakhsh N, Dellian M, Jain RK. Primary tumor size-dependent inhibition of angiogenesis at a secondary site: an intravital microscopic study in mice. *Cancer Res* 1998;58:5866–5869.

125. Kitayama J, Nagawa J, Yasuhara H. Suppressive effect of basic fibroblast growth factor on transendothelial emigration of CD4(+) T-lymphocyte. *Cancer Res* 1994;54:4729–4733.

126. Hoymng JB, Williams SK. Effects of basic fibroblast growth factor on human microvessel endothelial cell migration on collagen I corre-

lates with adhesion and is cell density dependent. *J Cell Physiol* 1996;168:294–304.

127. Yamada S, Mayadas T, Yuan F, et al. Rolling in P-selectin deficient mice is reduced but not eliminated in the dorsal skin. *Blood* 1995;86:3487–3492.

128. Koenig GC, Chen Y, Melder RJ, Jain RK. Basic FGF inhibits inducible CAMs on endothelial cells through PLCγ, PLD, and PKC signaling. 2000 (Submitted).

129. Jain RK. Transport phenomena in tumors. *Adv Chem Eng* 1994;20:129–200.

130. Dedrick RL. Animal scale-up. *J Pharmacokinet Biopharm* 1973;1:435–461.

131. Gerlowski LE, Jain RK. Physiologically based pharmacokinetic modeling: principles and applications. *J Pharm Sci* 1983;72:1103–1127.

132. Baxter LT, Zhu H, Mackensen DG, Butler WF, Jain RK. Biodistribution of monoclonal antibodies: scale-up from mouse to man using a physiologically based pharmacokinetic model. *Cancer Res* 1995; 55:4611–4622.

133. Baxter LT, Zhu H, Mackensen DG, Jain RK. Physiologically based pharmacokinetic model for specific and nonspecific monoclonal antibodies and fragments in normal tissues and human tumor xenografts in nude mice. *Cancer Res* 1994;54:1517–1528.

134. Zhu H, Melder RJ, Baxter LT, Jain RK. Physiologically based kinetic model of effector cell biodistribution in mammals: implications for adoptive immunotherapy. *Cancer Res* 1996;56:3771–3781.

135. Zhu H, Baxter LT, Jain RK. Potential and limitations of radioimmunodetection and radioimmunotherapy with monoclonal antibodies: evaluation using a physiologically based pharmacokinetic model. *J Nucl Med* 1997;38:731–741.

136. Zhu H, Jain RK, Baxter LT. Tumor pretargeting for radioimmunodetection and radioimmunotherapy: evaluation using a physiologically based pharmacokinetic model. *J Nucl Med* 1998;39:65–76.

137. Jain RK, Wei J. Dynamics of drug transport in solid tumors: distributed parameter model. *J Bioeng* 1977;1:313–329.

138. Jain RK. Effect of inhomogeneities and finite boundaries on temperature distribution in a perfused medium with application to tumors. *Trans ASME J Biomech Eng* 1978;100:235–241.

139. Jain RK. Transient temperature distributions in an infinite perfused medium due to a time-dependent, spherical heat source. *Trans ASME J Biomech Eng* 1979;101:82–86.

140. Jain RK, Boucher Y, Stacey-Clear A, Moore R, Kopans D. Method for locating tumors prior to needle biopsy. U.S. Patent #5,396,897, 1995.

141. Dudar TE, Jain RK. Differential response of normal and tumor microcirculation to hyperthermia. *Cancer Res* 1984;44:605–612.

142. Fukumura D, Yuan F, Endo M, Jain RK. Role of nitric oxide in tumor microcirculation: blood flow, vascular permeability, and leukocyte-endothelial interactions. *Am J Pathol* 1997;150:713–725.

143. Gerlowski LE, Jain RK. Effect of hyperthermia on microvascular permeability to macromolecules in normal and tumor tissues. *Int J Microcirc Clin Exp* 1985;4:363–372.

144. Kristensen CA, Nozue M, Boucher Y, Jain RK. Reduction of interstitial fluid pressure after TNF-α treatment of human melanoma xenografts. *Br J Cancer* 1996;74:533–536.

145. Kristensen CA, Roberge S, Jain RK. Effect of tumor necrosis factor-alpha on vascular resistance, nitric oxide production, glucose and oxygen consumption in perfused, tissue-isolated human melanoma xenografts. *Clin Cancer Res* 1997;3:319–324.

146. Fukumura D, Jain RK. Role of nitric oxide in angiogenesis and microcirculation in tumors. *Cancer Metastasis Rev* 1998;17:77–89.

147. Yuan F, Baxter LT, Jain RK. Pharmacokinetic analysis of two-step approaches using bifunctional and enzyme-conjugated antibodies. *Cancer Res* 1991;51:3119–3130.

148. Baxter LT, Jain RK. Pharmacokinetic analysis of the microscopic distribution of enzyme-conjugated antibodies and prodrugs: comparison with experimental data. *Br J Cancer* 1996;73:447–456.

149. Baxter LT, Yuan F, Jain RK. Pharmacokinetic analysis of the perivascular distribution of bifunctional antibodies and haptens: comparison with experimental data. *Cancer Res* 1992;52:5838–5844.

150. Znati CA, Rosenstein M, Boucher Y, Epperly MW, Bloomer WD, Jain RK. Effect of radiation on interstitial fluid pressure and oxygenation in a human colon carcinoma xenograft. *Cancer Res* 1996;56:964–968.

151. Kristjansen PE, Boucher Y, Jain RK. Dexamethasone reduces the interstitial fluid pressure in a human colon adenocarcinoma xenograft. *Cancer Res* 1993;53:4764–4766.

152. Lee I, Boucher Y, Jain RK. Nicotinamide can lower tumor interstitial fluid pressure: mechanistic and therapeutic implications. *Cancer Res* 1992;52:3237–3240.

153. Lee I, Boucher Y, Demhartner TJ, Jain RK. Changes in tumour blood flow, oxygenation and interstitial fluid pressure induced by pentoxifylline. *Br J Cancer* 1994;69:492–496.

154. Lee I, Demhartner TJ, Boucher Y, Jain RK, Intaglietta M. Effect of hemodilution and resuscitation on tumor interstitial fluid pressure, blood flow, and oxygenation. *Microvasc Res* 1994;48:1–12.

155. Leunig M, Goetz AE, Dellian M, et al. Interstitial fluid pressure in solid tumors following hyperthermia: possible correlation with therapeutic response. *Cancer Res* 1992;52:487–490.

156. Leunig M, Goetz AE, Gamarra F, Zetterer G, Messmer K, Jain RK. Photodynamic therapy-induced alterations in interstitial fluid pressure, volume and water content of an amelanotic melanoma in the hamster. *Br J Cancer* 1994;69:101–103.

157. Netti PA, Baxter LT, Boucher Y, Skalak R, Jain RK. Time dependent behavior of interstitial pressure in solid tumors: implications for drug delivery. *Cancer Res* 1995;55:5451–5458.

158. Zlotecki RA, Baxter LT, Boucher Y, Jain RK. Pharmacologic modification of tumor blood flow and interstitial fluid pressure in a human tumor xenograft: network analysis and mechanistic interpretation. *Microvasc Res* 1995;50:429–443.

159. Zlotecki RA, Boucher Y, Lee I, Baxter LT, Jain RK. Effect of angiotensin II induced hypertension on tumor blood flow and interstitial fluid pressure. *Cancer Res* 1993;53:2466–2468.

160. Netti PA, Hamberg LM, Babich JW, et al. Enhancement of fluid filtration across tumor vessels: implications for delivery of macromolecules. *Proc Natl Acad Sci U S A* 1999;96:3137–3142.

161. Jain RK. Delivery of molecular medicine to solid tumors. *Science* 1996;271:1079–1080.

24

FLT-3 AND FLT-3 LIGAND

EUGENE MARASKOVSKY
STEWART D. LYMAN
CHARLES R. MALISZEWSKI
DAVID H. LYNCH

Interaction of cell surface receptors with their specific protein ligands is the major mechanism by which cells communicate with, and respond in a coordinated fashion to, their immediate microenvironment. For instance, cytokines and related growth factors such as the interleukins (ILs) and colony-stimulating factors (CSFs) bind to distinct families of receptors and elicit unique patterns of biologic activities. The receptor tyrosine kinases represent a family of cell surface receptors that play an important role in regulating the survival, growth, and differentiation of hematopoietic cells. In this chapter, we focus on one such receptor, tyrosine kinase, *fms*-like tyrosine kinase 3 (Flt-3), and the biologic effects of interactions with its cognate ligand, Flt-3 ligand (FL).

DISCOVERY AND CHARACTERIZATION OF THE FLT-3 TYROSINE KINASE RECEPTOR

Flt-3 was isolated independently by two groups looking for novel members of the tyrosine kinase receptor family (1–3). The name is derived from the fact that the receptor is structurally related to another tyrosine kinase receptor known as *c-fms* (1). The receptor has also been referred to as *fetal liver kinase 2* (flk-2) (3) and *stem cell kinase-1* (Stk-1) (4).

Both mouse (1,000 amino acids) and human (993 amino acids) Flt-3 contain numerous potential sites for N-linked glycosylation in their extracellular domains (2–5), and carbohydrates are attached at one or more of these sites (6). The predicted size of the protein backbone is approximately 110 kd; however, anti-Flt-3 antibodies immunoprecipitate two proteins of 130 to 143 kd and 155 to 160 kd (6–8). Pulse-chase analysis showed that the larger protein arises from the smaller protein (6), most likely as a result of glycosylation processing. Consistent with this interpretation is the finding that only the 158-kd species is found on the cell surface (6). There do not appear to be any O-linked sugars on the protein (9). The binding affinity of human FL for Flt-3 on human myeloid leukemia cells has been estimated to be kd = 200 to 500 pm (10), and only high-affinity binding sites are seen. Although the mechanistic details are unknown, it is thought that a dimer of FL causes dimerization of Flt-3, which results in signal transduction.

The human Flt-3 genomic locus is approximately 100 kilobases (kb) in size (11). The exon:intron structure of the entire receptor has been reported to contain 24 exons (12), but only the portion of the gene encoding the C-terminal domain has been published (13). The gene encoding human Flt-3 maps to chromosome 13q12 (1), near the Flt tyrosine-kinase receptor locus. The Flt-3 and Flt genes are linked (14) in a head-to-tail fashion and are separated by approximately 150 kb (11). There have been no reports of any genetic defects associated with either Flt-3 or its ligand.

The mouse Flt-3 gene maps to chromosome 5 at the G region (1). The mouse Flt-3 gene (14) is located less than 350 kb from the mouse Flt tyrosine-kinase receptor (15) but is separated from the clustered c-*kit*, platelet-derived growth factor A, and Flf-1/KDR receptors, which are also on chromosome 5.

In addition to the full-length species, only one other isoform of Flt-3 has been described. This isoform is missing the fifth of the five immunoglobulin-like regions in the extracellular domain of the protein. This isoform results from the skipping of two exons during transcription (16). This alternative isoform is present at lower levels than the wild-type receptor, although it binds FL and is phosphorylated as a result of this binding. The fifth immunoglobulin-like domain of Flt-3 is therefore apparently not required for either ligand binding or receptor phosphorylation. The physiologic significance of this isoform of Flt-3 is presently unknown. A soluble version of Flt-3 has not yet been identified in human serum.

CLONING OF THE LIGAND FOR THE FLT-3

A soluble form of mouse Flt-3 was used by two groups to clone its cognate mouse ligand via expression cloning (17) or protein purification strategy (18). Once the mouse FL complementary DNA (cDNA) had been isolated, it was used in cross-species hybridization experiments to isolate cDNA encoding the human gene (18,19). The mouse and human FL proteins are 72% identical at the amino acid level. No restriction in species specificity has been observed with regard to the biologic activities of FL. The mouse and human FL proteins are both fully

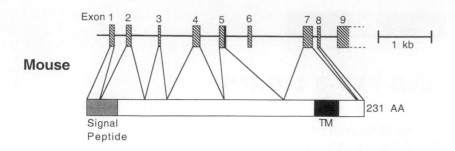

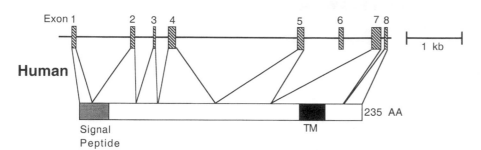

FIGURE 1. Structure of mouse and human Flt-3 ligand (FL) genomic locus and the encoded proteins. Exons and introns are drawn to the same scale for both mouse and human loci. The human FL locus is larger than the mouse locus as a result of having larger introns (23). The sequence information encoding the transmembrane form of FL is contained within exons 1 to 5 plus 7 and 8; an alternatively spliced exon 6 is used to generate a soluble form of FL protein. (AA, amino acids; kb, kilobase; TM, transmembrane.)

active on cells bearing either the mouse or human receptor (20). Furthermore, the human FL protein has been found to stimulate mouse, cat, rabbit, and nonhuman primate cells.

The FL protein is clearly ancestrally related to both macrophage CSF (M-CSF) (also known as *CSF-1*) as well as the c-*kit* ligand (KL) (17,18). All three proteins are type 1 transmembrane proteins with short cytoplasmic domains. They share a number of conserved cysteine residues, and all three proteins bind to tyrosine kinase receptors with five immunoglobulin-like domains in their extracellular region (the receptors are also ancestrally related). Finally, their genomic exon:intron structures are similar (21), and all three proteins are involved in regulating hematopoiesis. An extensive comparison of the biologic activities of FL and KL has been published (22).

The genomic loci encompassing the coding regions of mouse and human FL are approximately 4.0 kb and 5.9 kb, respectively, and comprise eight exons (21) (Fig. 1). The sizes of the individual FL exons are well conserved between species, whereas the intron sizes are much more variable. The human FL gene maps to chromosome 19q13.3–13.4 (23,24). This region is syntenic with mouse chromosome 7, which is where the mouse FL gene maps (17).

The primary translation product of the FL gene is a type 1 transmembrane protein (see Fig. 1). The mouse and human proteins contain 231 and 235 amino acids, respectively. The first 27 (mouse) or 26 (human) amino acids constitute a signal sequence, followed by a 161 (mouse) or 156 (human) amino acid extracellular domain, a 22 (mouse) or 23 (human) amino acid transmembrane domain, and a 21 (mouse) or 30 (human) amino acid cytoplasmic tail. The cytoplasmic domains of mouse and human FL are only 52% identical, and therefore are much more divergent than the extracellular domains. The mouse and human FL proteins each contain two potential sites for N-linked glycosylation.

Multiple isoforms of both mouse and human FL have been identified by analysis of cDNA clones and by polymerase chain reaction (17–19,23). The biologic significance of these isoforms is presently unknown. The predominant isoform of human FL is the transmembrane protein, which is biologically active on the cell surface (17–19). This isoform is also found in the mouse, but it is not the most abundant isoform in that species (see below). The transmembrane FL protein can be proteolytically cleaved to generate a soluble form of the protein that is also biologically active (17). The exact site in the FL amino acid sequence where cleavage takes place has not been identified, and the protease responsible for this cleavage is also unknown.

The most abundant isoform of mouse FL (21) is a 220 amino acid form that is membrane associated, but is not a transmembrane protein (18,23). This isoform results from a failure to splice an intron out of the messenger RNA (mRNA). This leads to a change in the reading frame, which terminates in a stretch of hydrophobic amino acids that serve to anchor the protein in the membrane (19). This isoform is also missing the spacer and tether regions that contain the proteolytic cleavage site present in the transmembrane isoform. As a result, the membrane-associated isoform is resistant to proteolytic cleavage, although it is biologically active on the cell surface (23). This membrane-associated isoform has not been identified in any human FL cDNA examined.

A third FL isoform identified in both mouse (23) and human (21) tissues arises as the result of an alternatively spliced sixth exon. This exon introduces a stop codon near the end of the extracellular domain, and thereby generates a soluble, biologically active protein, which appears to be relatively rare compared to other isoforms (21). Another method of generating soluble FL in humans is to splice out the transmembrane domain (19), but the relative abundance of this isoform has not been quantitated in any species.

As noted above, a soluble, biologically active form of FL can also be generated by proteolytic cleavage of the transmembrane protein. It is unclear what factors regulate the proteolytic cleavage of FL, and what, if any, physiologic processes are affected by this form of the protein. It is unknown if the protease that generates a soluble, biologically active form of FL is the same one that generates soluble forms of M-CSF and KL (17,18,25).

EXPRESSION OF FLT-3 ON CELL LINES, PRIMARY CELLS, AND LEUKEMIAS

Knowing the expression pattern of Flt-3 is one of the keys to understanding the function of FL. Flt-3 is expressed on only a limited number of cell types. In contrast, numerous studies have shown that FL is widely expressed in a variety of tissues. Among mouse cell lines examined, no Flt-3 expression is seen on myeloid, macrophage, erythroid, megakaryocyte, or mast cell lines (26,27), nor on most early B cell lines, but it has been reported on several mature B cell lines (27). In contrast, most human pre-B cell lines do express Flt-3 (28,29). Additionally, Flt-3 expression has been seen on only one mouse pro-T cell line, but not on any mature mouse T cell lines (26,27).

Numerous studies have been published demonstrating expression of Flt-3 on a limited range of human cell lines. Flt-3 is found on a high percentage of human myeloid and monocytic cell lines (27–29), in contrast to what is observed among mouse cell lines (26,27). Although a few megakaryocytic cell lines are positive, no Flt-3 expression has been detected on myeloma, erythroid, or erythroblastic cell lines (27–29). Among lymphoid cell lines, pro-B as well as pre-B lines are Flt-3 positive, whereas natural killer (NK) cells, Hodgkin's, and T cell lines are negative (27–29).

Flt-3 expression in the hematopoietic system appears to be predominantly restricted to the progenitor/stem cell compartment. Flt-3 expression in mouse bone marrow (BM) is restricted to blast cells, monocytes, and a small fraction of lymphocytes (30). Nucleated mouse erythroid cells lack Flt-3 expression (30). Initial studies indicated that Flt-3 mRNA is expressed by mouse B and T cells from thymus, spleen, and peripheral blood (PB) (2). However, later studies of mature mouse B and T cells suggest that these do not express Flt-3 (30,31). Thus, the initial findings were likely due to a small fraction of contaminating Flt-3-positive cells, such as more primitive B- and T-cell progenitors.

No expression of Flt-3 mRNA has been reported on mature lymphohematopoietic cells fractionated from human PB (4), on B cells, T cells, monocytes, or granulocytes (32), or on megakaryocytes (33). However, in other studies, monocytes and granulocytes have been shown as weakly positive at the mRNA and cell surface expression level (5,34).

Expression of Flt-3 in primary leukemias has also been widely investigated (35). Most adult acute myelogenous leukemia (AML) samples from all French-American-British (leukemia classification system) (FAB) classes are positive for Flt-3 expression (7,32,36–39). All B-lineage acute lymphoid leukemia (ALL) samples examined are Flt-3 positive (32,36,37), as are most hybrid (also known as *mixed* or *biphenotypic*) leukemia samples (32). The greatest variability reported in Flt-3 expression is on T-lineage ALL, which have been reported as being all negative (36), having a small percentage positive (37), or having approximately one-half of the samples positive (32). In contrast, both T-cell and B-cell lymphomas are negative for Flt-3 expres-

sion (32). Tandem in-frame duplications in the juxtamembrane region of human Flt-3 have been reported to be associated with leukocytosis (40), leukemic transformation (41), and shorter disease-free survival in childhood AML (42). Almost all chronic or accelerated phase chronic myelogenous leukemia (CML) samples are negative for Flt-3 expression (32,37). However, approximately two thirds of the samples from CML patients in blast crisis are Flt-3 positive (32,37).

RESPONSIVENESS OF PRIMARY LEUKEMIA CELLS TO FLT-3 LIGAND

Whether Flt-3 or its ligand plays a causal role in the development of human leukemias has not been determined. A large percentage of AML cells from children (36) and adults (38,39) proliferate in response to FL. To put this in context, however, it should be noted that these same AML samples proliferate in response to a number of other growth factors as well. Within groups of children or adults, some FAB subtypes show a greater response compared to others (36,39). Because not enough samples of each FAB subtype have been analyzed, it is unclear whether there is a difference in the FL responsiveness of Flt-3-positive AML samples from children and adults. As a result, Flt-3 expression on AML samples is simply not predictive of FL responsiveness.

As mentioned previously, all B-lineage ALL and some T-lineage ALL samples express Flt-3. However, only a small percentage of B-lineage ALL samples proliferates in response to FL (36). One study showed that pediatric T-lineage ALL samples did not proliferate in response to FL, but these samples were all negative for Flt-3 expression (36). In a separate study on a variety of ALLs, several Flt-3-positive samples proliferated in FL (43). However, the majority of samples failed to proliferate in FL, even though they were Flt-3 positive (43). Flt-3 expression is therefore not predictive for proliferation of ALL cells to FL *in vitro*.

EXPRESSION OF FLT-3 LIGAND

The FL gene is widely expressed in mouse and human tissues, including both hematopoietic and nonhematopoietic tissue types (18,19,23). Highest levels of FL mRNA on human tissue Northern blots are in PB mononuclear cells, but the ligand is also expressed in almost every tissue that has been examined (17–19). However, it should be pointed out that similar studies of FL protein expression have not been performed. Mouse developmental *in situ* hybridization studies have not yet been done with FL, although it would be interesting to see how the distribution of FL would compare to Flt-3 (44).

HUMAN SERUM AND PLASMA LEVELS OF FLT-3 LIGAND

Serum levels of FL in normal individuals average less than 100 pg per mL, which is the limit of detection of the enzyme-linked immunosorbent assay (45). FL levels are not elevated in a variety of anemias that predominantly affect only the erythroid lineage (45). In contrast, serum levels of FL are highly elevated in patients with hematopoietic disorders that specifically affect the stem cell compartment. Thus, a majority of patients with Fanconi anemia or acquired aplastic anemia have highly elevated levels of FL (up to 10 ng per mL) (45). Cancer patients treated with chemotherapy or radiation, or both, also have elevated levels of FL (46).

The simplest interpretation of these data is that the loss of functional stem/progenitor cells leads to the loss of a negative regulator of FL production that is made by the stem and progenitor cells. FL concentrations in blood then become elevated (to a physiologically relevant level) as part of a compensatory hematopoietic response to drive the proliferation of the remaining stem and progenitor cells. In this regard, serum concentrations of FL were found to return to normal levels in a Fanconi anemia patient treated with a cord blood transplant (45). A similar outcome has also been achieved in patients with acquired aplastic anemia after either BM transplant or immunosuppressive therapy (46). These data suggest that restoration of stem cells in these patients is associated with a return of FL serum concentrations to those measured in normal, healthy individuals, and that FL serum levels may be a surrogate marker for stem cell activity or content in BM.

FLT-3 LIGAND IS A REGULATOR OF HEMATOPOIETIC CELL DEVELOPMENT

The restricted expression of Flt-3 on primitive hematopoietic stem and progenitor cells suggested that the ligand (FL) might play a role in hematopoietic cell development. FL weakly stimulates proliferation or colony formation of hematopoietic progenitor cells (HPCs) when used as a single cytokine *in vitro* (17,18). In addition, FL weakly supports the survival of primitive HPCs, which remain responsive to cytokines, which can induce growth and differentiation (30,47–49). In contrast, FL displays synergistic effects on hematopoietic cell growth and differentiation when combined with other ILs and CSFs (30,50–52), as well as with receptors for thrombopoietin and granulocyte CSF (G-CSF) receptor (53), in promoting the colony growth of both primitive and committed progenitors. The use of *in vitro* assays has demonstrated that FL affects the growth of primitive multipotent HPCs as well as myeloid and lymphoid-committed progenitors (54). FL alone does not significantly support the *ex vivo* expansion of progenitor cells but does increase their survival *in vitro* (55). It also synergizes with several growth factors, including various combinations of IL-1, IL-3, IL-6, IL-11, G-CSF, KL, or erythropoietin, to potentiate the *ex vivo* expansion of colony forming units (22,50,51,55,56). However, long-term culture-initiating cells, which represent the most primitive human progenitors, can be expanded with FL alone (47,57), and this can be further augmented when combined with IL-3 and KL (57). Mackarechtschian and colleagues (58) also demonstrated a major effect of FL on the most primitive HPCs when examining mice deficient in Flt-3. Although these animals were viable and healthy, they displayed a defect in their primitive stem cells as measured in long-term competitive

repopulation assays and by their potential to reconstitute both the lymphoid and myeloid compartments when transferred to irradiated recipients (58).

ONTOGENY AND FUNCTION OF DENDRITIC CELLS

Dendritic cells (DCs) are rare, hematopoietically derived leukocytes that form a cellular network involved in immune surveillance, antigen (Ag) capture, and presentation (59). DCs are predominantly found in the T-cell dependent areas of lymphoid tissue (59), as well as in other tissues and organs. Immature processing-type DCs are located at body surfaces and in the interstitial spaces of most tissues where they can acquire Ags in the local microenvironment. In the presence of maturation-inducing stimuli, such as cellular necrosis due to tissue damage, proinflammatory cytokines [e.g., IL-1β, tumor necrosis factor–α (TNF-α), IL-6, and interferon-α (IFN-α)], or bacterial products, DCs exhibit elevated expression of adhesion (e.g., LFA-1, -2, -3, and intercellular adhesion molecule-1, -2, -3) and costimulatory molecules (e.g., CD40, CD80, and CD86) and begin the transformation from cells specializing in Ag capture and processing to more potent, terminally differentiated, stimulators of T-cell immunity (60–64). During this process, DCs migrate to the T-cell areas in draining lymphoid tissues under the influence of chemokines and other homing interactions, where they present captured Ags as processed peptides [in association with major histocompatibility complex (MHC)–encoded molecules] to rare Ag-specific T cells (65). On activation by DCs, T cells upregulate expression of CD40L, which in turn binds to CD40 on DCs and ultimately results in the augmentation of their Ag-presenting function. CD40L also induces DCs to secrete IL-12 (66,67), which has been shown to regulate IFN-γ production by T cells (68).

In addition to their localization in T-cell areas, a subset of DCs has also been identified in the B-cell–dependent germinal centers (69) and suggests a role for germinal center DCs in B-cell maturation (70). In addition to their capacity for processing and presenting foreign or altered self-Ags to induce immunity (59), certain DC subsets are believed to negatively regulate T-cell immunity (71–74). Furthermore, there is emerging evidence that DCs may regulate the cytokine repertoire of T cells during the induction of immunity (75–78). Thus, DCs are emerging as key regulators of lymphocyte-mediated immune responses.

The most rapidly evolving aspect of DC biology is the striking diversity of phenotypes that have been described from *in vitro* and *in vivo* studies in both mouse and humans. Although the number of seemingly distinct DC subsets appear to be growing, however, the developmental relationships between these distinct DC subsets remain largely undefined. More important, the functional differences between these distinct DC phenotypes are relatively unclear. DCs can be derived from at least two ontogenically distinct pathways: the myeloid and lymphoid pathways (79). The relationship of DCs to the myeloid lineage is based mainly on *in vitro* experimentation showing that DCs can be generated from BM or cord blood progenitors, as well as PB mononuclear cells, using a combination of granulocyte-macrophage CSF (GM-CSF) and other cytokines such as TNF-α (83–87), IL-4 (84,85), and KL (86,87). In contrast, certain DC subsets can arise from the most immature T-cell precursors, which can also generate NK and B cells, but not cells of the myeloid lineage (65,88–90). Unlike myeloid-related DCs, DCs derived from the putative lymphoid-committed precursors have been shown to express high levels of the CD8α homodimer (80,90,91) and do not require GM-CSF for *in vitro* development (89,92). Differences between these two subsets of DCs are supported by the fact that mice treated with a polyethylene glycol–modified form of murine GM-CSF display increased numbers of myeloid-related DCs in both spleen and other lymphoid tissues, whereas no significant increases in the CD8α⁺ lymphoid-related DC subset were observed (77). The increased levels of GM-CSF present in GM-CSF–expressing transgenic mice does not significantly increase the number of DCs in lymphoid tissue (93). Furthermore, mice deficient in the GM-CSF receptor-β chain show only marginal decreases in the numbers of DCs in the lymphoid tissues, suggesting that growth factors other than GM-CSF are important for DC generation *in vivo* (94).

The efficiency with which DCs initiate and regulate lymphocyte-mediated immunity has led to the study of DCs as cellular vaccine adjuvants for the immunotherapy of cancer or infectious disease (95,96). Numerous studies in mouse models have demonstrated efficacy of DC-based immunization protocols for generation of antitumor responses (95,96). Despite promising results from mouse models, the use of DCs as vaccine vectors for immunotherapy is limited by the extremely small numbers of DCs found in human PB and the uncertainty as to which *in vitro*–generated DC subset generates the most appropriate T-cell immunity *in vivo*. In this regard, the preferential use by most clinical groups of only one type of DC precursor (i.e., monocyte) in clinical studies may not necessarily provide the diversity in Ag-presenting cell–derived signals that can result in the generation of effective and long-lasting T-cell immunity (97). The use of cytokines, which increase the number of DCs *in vivo* without altering subset diversity, may obviate many of the potential problems surrounding current DC-based immunotherapy strategies.

FLT-3 LIGAND STIMULATES DENDRITIC CELL DEVELOPMENT IN MICE

Daily subcutaneous injections of mammalian cell–expressed recombinant human FL for 10 days resulted in a dramatic increase in the numbers of hematopoietic progenitors in the BM, PB, and spleen (98,99). Examination of the effects of systemic FL on more mature, lineage-committed cells indicated that the FL-mediated expansion and mobilization of BM progenitors was accompanied by an increase in myeloid lineage cells, early B lymphocytes, and NK cells (data not shown), but there was no apparent effect on T lymphocytes or erythroid or megakaryocyte-lineage cells (98,99). A significant increase in MHC class II⁺ Thy-1⁻ CD8α⁺ cells was also observed in the PB of FL-treated mice, a phenotype consistent with DCs. Under normal conditions, DCs constitute only a small percentage of total spleen cells (<1%) and require enzymatic digestion to be

released from the stroma (100). In FL-treated mice, however, approximately 20% of spleen cells coexpress MHC class II and the DC marker, CD11c (101). These MHC class II⁺ CD11c⁺ DCs express low levels of surface CD86, are morphologically indistinguishable from the rare DCs that can be extracted from the spleens of untreated mice (control DCs), and can be separated into three subpopulations using CD11b expression [CD11b⁻, CD11b^dull and CD11b^bright (101)]. A proportion of the CD11b⁻ and CD11b^dull subsets express the lymphoid-related DC marker, CD8α, whereas the CD11b^bright subset is CD8α⁻ and expressed myeloid-related DC markers such as F4/80 and 33D1 (102). These observations indicate that systemic treatment of mice with FL expands both myeloid- and CD8α⁺ lymphoid-related DCs *in vivo*.

Daily injections of mice with FL results in a 17-fold increase in the absolute number of DCs in the spleen, a fourfold increase in the lymph nodes (LNs) and sixfold increase in the PB by day 9 (101). Increased numbers of DCs could be detected as early as day 5 in the spleen and by day 7 in LNs and PB (101). The FL-mediated DC expansion was transient and reversible as DC numbers returned to basal levels within 7 days after cessation of growth factor administration (101). FL-generated DCs were as efficient as control DCs at stimulating the proliferation of allogeneic T cells or of Ag-specific T cells in *in vitro* assays (101). Furthermore, FL-generated spleen DCs were as efficient as control DCs at generating Ag-specific T cells *in vivo* after being pulsed with Ag *ex vivo* (77,101). Elevated numbers of DCs were detected in both lymphoid- and nonlymphoid tissue in FL-treated mice, including the BM, gut-associated lymphoid tissue, liver, LNs, lung, PB, peritoneal cavity, spleen, and thymus (101). Of particular interest is the elevated numbers of DCs in the gut-associated lymphoid tissue, lung, and PB, which are sites amenable to vaccine delivery in clinical immunotherapy regimens.

MECHANISM OF FLT-3 LIGAND–MEDIATED DENDRITIC CELL DEVELOPMENT AND IMMUNE CONSEQUENCES

The mechanism(s) by which FL influences DC generation *in vivo* and *in vitro* is not completely understood. It is unlikely that FL treatment simply causes the mobilization of existing mature DCs from other sites into the lymphoid tissue. First, Flt-3 is not detected on mature DCs (as assessed by flow cytometry), and mature DCs do not proliferate when cultured in FL alone (as assessed either by microphysiometric analysis of cytoplasmic pH changes or by thymidine incorporation of proliferating cells). Second, elevated numbers of DCs have been detected in multiple organs and tissues in FL-treated mice, indicating that there is a generalized expansion of DCs throughout these animals. Third, the effects of FL on the expansion of DCs from BM progenitors, its described effects on primitive progenitors *in vitro*, and the potent effects of FL on hematopoiesis *in vivo* suggest that FL expands the primitive progenitor cell pool in the BM and other organs, whereas other signals potentiate and induce DC maturation *in vivo*. In this way, FL may facilitate the terminal development of a primitive, FL-sensitive, rapidly expanding progenitor population into functionally mature DCs.

TABLE 1. ANALYSIS OF PROLIFERATION AND GENERATION OF DENDRITIC CELLS FROM *IN VITRO*–CULTURED CD34⁺ BONE MARROW PROGENITORS

Growth Factor Conditions	Total Number of Cultured Cells ($\times 10^{-6}$)	Percent CD1A⁺, HLA-DR⁺, CD86⁺ Cells	Total Number of CD1A⁺, HLA-DR⁺, CD86⁺ Cells ($\times 10^{-6}$)
GM-CSF, IL-4, TNF-α	6.0 ± 0.8	48.3 ± 12.3	2.9 ± 0.9
+ FL	48.5 ± 1.6	46.2 ± 10.2	22.4 ± 1.6

FL, Flt-3 ligand; GM-CSF, granulocyte-macrophage colony-stimulating factor; IL-4, interleukin-4; TNF-α, tumor necrosis factor-α.
Data are derived from the mean $\pm$ SD of five experiments. Cultures were initiated with 1×10^6 CD34⁺ cells.

DENDRITIC CELL DEVELOPMENT IN FLT-3 LIGAND–DEFICIENT MICE

The importance of FL for DC generation from progenitors is further highlighted by examination of mice rendered genetically deficient in FL. McKenna and colleagues have reported that FL$^{-/-}$ mice show a significant reduction in leukocyte cellularity in the BM, PB, LN, and spleen, but not in the thymus. Furthermore, the absolute numbers of primitive BM progenitors, BM-myeloid cells, and B cells are significantly reduced. The absolute number of NK cells in the spleen of FL-deficient mice is also dramatically reduced (103). Additionally, these animals display deficient DC development and reduced numbers of mature DCs in the peripheral lymphoid tissues. Although both myeloid-related and CD8α^+ lymphoid-related DCs were reduced, a significantly greater reduction in CD8α^+ lymphoid-related DCs was observed. The residual splenic DCs present in these mice are functionally normal with respect to their capacity to stimulate the proliferation of alloreactive T cells *in vitro*, suggesting that FL is not essential for optimal DC functional maturation *in vivo*, but is required for DC expansion from the progenitor pool.

FLT-3 LIGAND STIMULATES *In Vitro* DENDRITIC CELL DEVELOPMENT FROM HUMAN CD34⁺ BONE MARROW PROGENITORS

The importance of FL in DC development *in vitro* is further supported by studies showing that FL can increase the absolute numbers of mature myeloid-related DCs generated in serum containing culture systems from CD34⁺ BM progenitors using GM-CSF, IL-4, TNF-α, and KL (97,104,105). Transforming growth factor–β has also been shown to enhance *in vitro* DC development in serum-free culture systems (106). Regardless of the cytokine combinations used, these *in vitro*-generated DCs express high levels of CD1a and CD13 and are positive for HLA-DR, CD80, and CD86. The addition of FL to GM-CSF, IL-4, and TNF-α–containing cultures enhanced the total expansion of CD34⁺ BM progenitors by eightfold (Table 1). However, no significant change was observed in the percentage of progeny coexpressing CD1a, HLA-DR, and CD86 relative to cells generated in the absence of FL. As a result, the enhanced expansion of the starting progenitor pool translated into an eightfold increase in the absolute numbers of DCs. Sorted CD1a⁺, HLA-DR⁺, CD86⁺ DCs from FL-containing cultures were as efficient at stimulating the proliferation of alloreactive T

cells or processing and presenting tetanus toxoid to autologous tetanus toxoid–specific T cells as DCs generated in the absence of FL (103). This suggests that the addition of FL into these cultures enhances the expansion of the cultured cells, but has little effect on the proportion of cells that differentiate into DCs or on their functional development.

FLT-3 LIGAND STIMULATES DENDRITIC CELL DEVELOPMENT IN HUMANS

DCs represent a minor fraction (<1%) of PB mononuclear cells (PBMCs) (<1%) in humans and can be distinguished from other mature cell lineage by their characteristic dendritic morphology; the lack of surface expression of CD3, CD14, CD19, and CD56; and high expression of CD1b/c, CD4, CD11c, CD33, and HLA-DR. Additionally, a DC precursor subset lacking CD11c expression and expressing high levels of surface IL-3 receptor-α (CD11c⁻ DC) and previously referred to as the *plasmacytoid T cell* has been identified in lymphoid tissue and PB (107,108).

The effect of FL treatment on expansion of DC has been examined in a randomized, placebo-controlled, double-blind study. Twenty healthy human volunteers received daily subcutaneous doses of either placebo or FL at five dose levels (10, 25, 50, 75, or 100 µg per kg per day) for 14 consecutive days. Each dose group consisted of three FL-treated individuals and one placebo control. Samples of PB were collected every 2 days for 21 days and analyzed by flow cytometry for changes in the distribution of various leukocyte populations. FL treatments were well tolerated by all subjects at all doses tested compared to the placebo controls, and resulted in increased numbers of white blood cells (WBCs), PBMCs, and CD14⁺ monocytes, but not lymphocytes (109). PBMCs lacking the monocyte marker CD14, but expressing CD11c, were rare in the blood of both placebo-treated individuals (Fig. 2A). After 14 days of FL treatment, however, approximately 14% of PBMCs expressed CD11c, but not CD14 (see Fig. 2A). This population of cells was determined to be DCs lacking surface expression of the mature-lineage markers CD3, CD14, CD19, CD56 (Lin-) and expressing CD33 or HLA-DR (110). FL treatment also increased the proportion of the CD11c⁺CD14± monocyte fraction.

FL-generated CD11c⁺CD14⁻ PBMCs were CD1a⁻ but CD1b/c⁺ and were CD11b⁺, CD40⁻, CD80⁻, CD83⁻, CD86⁻, and HLA-DR⁺ (Fig. 2B), a phenotype consistent with blood DCs. The expression of CD11b and low-to-undetectable levels

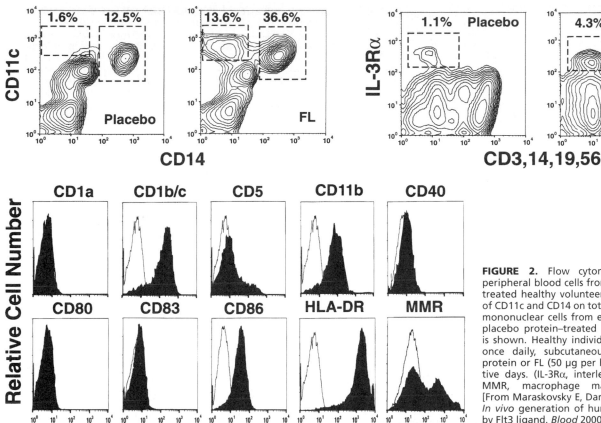

FIGURE 2. Flow cytometric analysis of peripheral blood cells from Flt-3 ligand (FL)–treated healthy volunteers. The distribution of CD11c and CD14 on total peripheral blood mononuclear cells from either FL-treated or placebo protein–treated healthy volunteers is shown. Healthy individuals were injected once daily, subcutaneously, with placebo protein or FL (50 μg per kg) for 14 consecutive days. (IL-3Rα, interleukin-3 receptor-α; MMR, macrophage mannose receptor.) [From Maraskovsky E, Daro E, Roux ER, et al. *In vivo* generation of human dendritic cells by Flt3 ligand. *Blood* 2000 (*in press*).]

of CD40, CD80, CD83, and CD86 suggests that the CD11c$^+$ DCs are not fully mature (62,66,111–113). These CD11c$^+$ DCs represent a heterogenous population, as they can be further subdivided on the basis of CD5 and macrophage mannose receptor expression (see Fig. 2B). FL was also able to increase the numbers of CD11c$^-$ IL-3 receptor-α$^+$ DCs (Fig. 2C), representing the plasmacytoid DC subpopulation. When cultured in IL-3 and CD40L, these cells develop into functional DCs. Furthermore, once matured, these DCs appear to differentially regulate IL-4–, IL-5–, and IL-10–secreting T cells compared to CD11c$^+$ DCs, which induce IFN-γ–secreting T cells (78). The CD11c$^+$ DCs are efficient stimulators of Ag-specific T cells *in vitro* (110). Finally, as is the situation in mice, FL-mediated DC expansion in humans is transient and reversible, resolving to baseline levels within 2 weeks after cessation of treatment (110).

FLT-3 LIGAND ENHANCES ANTIGEN PRESENTATION *IN VIVO* TO INDUCE IMMUNITY OR TOLERANCE

It seems reasonable to hypothesize that the expansion of distinct DC subpopulations *in vivo* should result in a more robust or sensitive immune response to antigenic challenge. FL has been tested as a cytokine adjuvant for either the tolerization or immunization of mice to soluble Ag (77,114,115). Depending on the route of Ag administration, FL pretreatment could either enhance the level of tolerance induced against an orally admin-

istered Ag or prevent tolerance and amplify the degree of immunization against a systemically administered Ag. In a model of oral tolerance, mice fed high doses of soluble ovalbumin are tolerant to a subsequent challenge with the same Ag. In contrast, when fed low doses of Ag, normal mice are rendered immune to that Ag. Mice fed low doses of Ag and simultaneously treated with FL are rendered tolerant, however, suggesting that FL-mediated expansion of DCs can alter the immune response outcome for orally administered Ag (114). In contrast, mice administered with tolerizing doses of soluble ovalbumin by a systemic route during FL treatment exhibited an augmented immune response to the Ag, indicating that induction of systemic tolerance was prevented by FL administration (115).

Some results have also demonstrated that distinct DC subsets generated with FL are capable of differentially regulating the quality and class of immune response generated in mice (76,77). The data indicate that the CD8α$^+$ lymphoid-related DC subset, which produces the highest levels of inducible IL-12, generates a predominantly IFN-γ–secreting, Ag-specific T-cell repertoire *in vivo*. In contrast, the myeloid-related DC subset generates a mixture of IL-4 and IFN-γ–secreting T-cell effectors. These reports not only emphasize the importance of the route of vaccination and how critical the repertoire of Ag-presenting cells present at the site of Ag entry is, but also emphasize how FL administration can alter the balance of a developing immune response by expanding the numbers of DCs in those same sites. However, conclusions as to which DC subset influences particular immune responses requires further evaluation, as demonstrated by others (78,116).

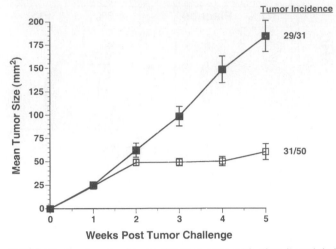

FIGURE 3. Treatment of tumor-bearing mice with Flt-3 ligand (FL) induces tumor regression. Groups of mice (five mice per group) were injected intradermally with 5×10^5 viable B10.2 tumor cells, followed by 19 daily injections with either control buffer (■) or FL (□), and tumor sizes monitored over the ensuing 5-week period. The mean tumor size of only those mice bearing detectable tumors is plotted, and the number of tumor-bearing mice per number challenged is noted. (Data from Lynch DH, Andreasen A, Maraskovsky E, Whitmore J, Miller RE, Schuh JCL. Flt3 ligand induces tumor regression and anti-tumor immune responses *in vivo. Nat Med* 1997;3:625–631.)

FLT-3 LIGAND CAN INDUCE IMMUNE-MEDIATED ANTI-TUMOR ACTIVITY *IN VIVO*

As noted earlier, repeated administration of FL leads to the generation of comparatively larger numbers of DCs *in vivo*. Knight et al. noted that transfer of relatively low numbers of DCs into tumor-bearing mice had a significant inhibitory effect on the growth of a mouse sarcoma *in vivo* (117). Results from a number of studies in humans have also shown a correlation between the numbers of DCs infiltrating a tumor and clinical prognosis (118–121). In addition, culture-derived DCs pulsed with either tumor Ags or peptides from a tumor Ag have been shown to induce a protective antitumor immune response *in vivo* (122).

These observations led us to hypothesize that by enhancing the numbers of DCs *in vivo* we would also enhance the generation of T-cell responses to tumors. To address this hypothesis, C57BL/10 (B10) mice were intradermally injected with B10.2 tumor cells, a methylcholanthrene-induced fibrosarcoma of B10 origin, followed by systemic administration of FL (10 μg per day) over a 19-day period. Compilation of results from six independent experiments comparing tumor growth in mice treated with FL to tumor growth in control mice demonstrated that the tumors grew at similar rates in both groups of mice over the first 2.0 to 2.5 weeks, followed by a decrease in mean tumor size in FL-treated mice (Fig. 3). Complete tumor regression was observed in 38% (19 of 50) of FL-treated mice compared to 3% (1 of 30) control mice ($p <0.0001$, using Fisher's exact test). Additionally, the rate of tumor growth in FL-treated mice was significantly reduced compared to control mice (the mean tumor sizes of the two groups at week 5 post tumor challenge

TABLE 2. EFFECT OF THE NUMBER OF FLT-3 LIGAND (FL) TREATMENTS ON TUMOR REGRESSION *IN VIVO*[a]

Cytokine Treatment	No. of Treatments	No. TBA/No. Challenged[b]	Mean Tumor Size (mm²)[c]
Control buffer	19	10/10	182.5 ± 31
FL	4	9/10	199 ± 32.5
FL	7	9/10	101 ± 20
FL	10	10/15	71.5 ± 11
FL	14	4/15	82 ± 27
FL	19	3/15	40 ± 17.5

[a]Composite results from three independent experiments.
[b]Number of tumor-bearing animals per number challenged 5 weeks after tumor implantation.
[c]Mean tumor size of only those mice bearing tumors at the termination of the experiment at week 5.
Data from Rosnet O, Mattel MG, Marchetto S, Birnbaum D. Isolation and chromosomal localization of a novel FMS-like tyrosine kinase gene. *Genomics* 1991;9:380–385.

was 60 ± 11 mm² in FL-treated mice versus 185 ± 15 mm² in control mice; $p <0.0001$ by analysis of variance).

The observed beneficial effects of FL treatment were found to be not only dose-dependent, but also dependent on the length of time over which FL is administered. As noted earlier, although as few as nine daily injections of FL result in the production of maximal numbers of DCs in the periphery, the absolute number of these cells decreases rapidly on cessation of such treatments and returns to baseline levels within 7 days (101). As might be expected, mice treated for short periods (4 or 7 days) showed only limited benefit with regard to their ability to mount effective tumor immune responses *in vivo* (123). However, groups of mice treated for 14 or 19 days manifested similar responses in that there was a higher proportion of complete tumor regressions compared to that of untreated mice (Table 2), and the rate of tumor growth in the remaining mice was significantly reduced compared to the control group ($p <0.0001$). Mice treated with FL for 10 days showed an intermediate response in that there was only a slight increase in the number of complete regressions, but a clear decrease in tumor size compared to controls. It is also of interest that this time course of treatment corresponds to the kinetics of DC generation *in vivo*—that is, 9 days of FL treatment results in higher numbers of DCs in spleen than 5 or 7 days of treatment. Indeed, only modest increases in the numbers of DCs from LN or PB were detected after 7 days of treatment (101), and this was substantially increased after an additional 2 days of treatment. These data suggest a pivotal role for DCs in the generation of antitumor immune responses after FL treatment.

Histologic analysis of tumors revealed a substantial difference in both the quantity and quality of cells infiltrating the tumors of FL-treated mice compared to those of control mice. In control mice, the tumors became progressively larger and showed both superficial and central necrosis over time. A thin infiltrate composed of lymphocytes, plasma cells, infrequent granulocytes, and fibroblasts bordered the tumors in these mice (Fig. 4A). In addition to the cellular infiltrate found in control mice, the tumors in FL-treated mice were surrounded by an extensive infiltrate of mononuclear cells with large, vesiculated, and, often, folded

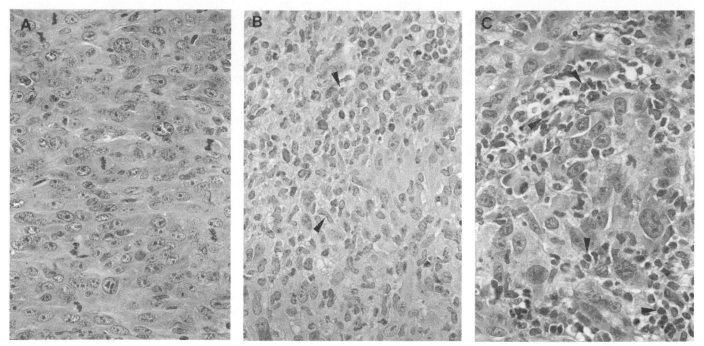

FIGURE 4. High-power views of histologic sections from subcutaneous B10.2 fibrosarcomas obtained from mice treated for 2 weeks with either a control buffer **(A)**, or Flt-3 ligand (FL) **(B)**, or 2 weeks after cessation of treatment with FL **(C)**. (Data from Lynch DH, Andreasen A, Maraskovsky E, Whitmore J, Miller RE, Schuh JCL. Flt3 ligand induces tumor regression and anti-tumor immune responses *in vivo*. *Nat Med* 1997;3:625–631.)

nuclei (Fig. 4B). Although this infiltrate was also present in control mice, the infiltrate was more pronounced, extended deeper into the tumor tissue, and was associated with destruction of tumor cells in FL-treated mice with visible tumor regression.

The morphology of the mononuclear cell infiltrate in the tumors from FL-treated mice at week 2 is consistent with DC or myeloid precursors, or both, and immunohistochemical staining has shown a clear increase in the numbers of CD86+ cells. Some flow cytometric analyses indicate that FL treatment of tumor-bearing mice induces a similar array of DCs within the tumor mass as seen in peripheral lymphoid tissues, including both myeloid- and lymphoid-related DCs, suggesting that these subsets may also be actively involved in the induction of antitumor immune responses *in vivo*.

It is important to point out that the nature of the cellular infiltrates in tumors of FL-treated mice is substantially different at weeks 4 and 5, with a pronounced shift toward lymphocytes (Fig. 4C). It seems likely that the lymphocytic infiltrates seen in those tumors in FL-treated mice that have only been partially rejected by week 5 after tumor inoculation are tumor-reactive effector cells that are actively involved in the destruction of tumor cells and may be responsible for the decrease in tumor growth rates in those mice that have not completely rejected the tumor challenge. Similar results have also been obtained with breast cancer cells transduced with a cDNA expressing FL (124). Injection of these cells into mice leads not only to their rejection, but also to the subsequent rejection of freshly transplanted, untransduced, breast cancer cells.

The conclusion that tumor rejection is associated with the generation of a cognate T-cell mediated immune response is supported by the finding that those mice that had rejected the tumor challenge subsequent to treatment with FL were immune to a rechallenge with the same tumor, but not to unrelated tumors. Phenotypic analysis of cells mediating tumor rejection *in vivo* clearly demonstrated that FL treatment of tumor-bearing mice promotes the generation of Thy1+, CD4−CD8+ effector cells, which play a pivotal role in tumor rejection *in vivo* (123).

Data have also been obtained in several other tumor models, demonstrating that FL treatment of mice with preexisting tumors results in complete tumor rejection in a high proportion of cases, and significant decreases in tumor growth rates are seen in a majority of cases in which no rejections are observed (125–128). This effect was influenced by both the size of the tumor when FL treatments were begun and the dose of FL per treatment (Fig. 5). The results demonstrated that increasing the amount of FL used from 10 μg per day to 30 μg per day significantly enhanced both the number of tumor rejections observed and the degree of growth inhibition in mice with tumors established up to 7 days previously (123). Finally, although the data also demonstrated that increasing the dose of FL to 30 μg per day did not increase the rejection frequency in tumors established 10 to 14 days previously, there was a clear dose-dependent reduction rate of tumor growth ($p = 0.0041$).

An unexpected finding from our studies was that, in addition to induction of cognate immune responses to tumor Ags, FL treatment of tumor-bearing mice also induces a non-T cell–mediated mechanism that can substantially decrease the rate of tumor growth *in vivo*. This conclusion is based on the fact that the rate of tumor growth in B6 (severe combined immunodefi-

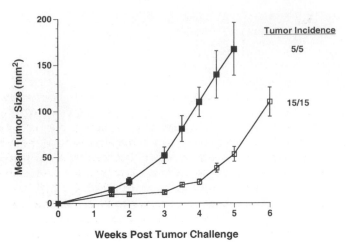

FIGURE 5. Flt-3 ligand (FL) treatment induces a nonimmunologic mechanism that slows tumor growth *in vivo*. B6 (severe combined immunodeficiency disease) mice were intradermally injected with B10.2 tumor cells followed by 19 daily treatments with either control buffer (■) or FL (□). Mean tumor size of only those mice bearing tumor and the number of tumor-bearing animals/the number challenged at the termination of the experiment is shown. (Data from Lynch DH, Andreasen A, Maraskovsky E, Whitmore J, Miller RE, Schuh JCL. Flt3 ligand induces tumor regression and anti-tumor immune responses *in vivo. Nat Med* 1997;3:625–631.)

ciency disease) mice relative to that of control mice declined dramatically during FL treatment (Fig. 6). After cessation of FL treatment, the rate of tumor growth gradually increased until it equaled that of control mice. Preliminary histologic evaluation of tumors in severe combined immunodeficiency disease mice suggests that FL treatment induces a similar cellular infiltrate of monocytes and myeloid precursor cells, as seen in immunologically intact mice. The infiltrates disappeared on cessation of FL treatment. Thus, the potential role of nonmyeloid DCs in mediating a nonspecific tumoricidal function must also be considered. An additional possibility is a role for NK cells in the nonimmunologic mechanism of the inhibition of tumor growth, because these cells are also elevated (approximately tenfold) in mice after FL treatment (129). Indeed, both Peron et al. (127) and Fernandez et al. (125) have also shown that induction of innate immune mechanisms by treatment with FL leads to decreases in tumor burden. The effects of FL in these settings

seems to be primarily due to the generation of increased numbers of NK cells from hematopoietic progenitors and not activation of mature NK cells (129). This concept is further supported by the results of McKenna et al. (103) who found that there is a nearly complete absence of NK cells in FL gene knockout mice, but that NK cells could be generated by a 10-day course of treatment with FL.

In conclusion, the data demonstrate that systemic administration of FL to tumor-bearing mice can have dramatic effects on tumor regression *in vivo*. FL treatment resulted in complete tumor rejection in a high proportion (approximately 40%) of the mice tested and led to a dramatic decrease of tumor growth rate in the remaining mice. Both of these events are associated with the development of an effective antitumor immune response mediated by CD8+ T cells. The data also indicate that FL treatment induces a non-T cell–mediated mechanism that can inhibit tumor growth *in vivo*. Collectively, these data suggest that FL may prove to be an important cytokine in the treatment of cancer *in situ*, either alone or in combination with other therapeutic strategies.

POTENTIAL THERAPEUTIC USES OF FLT-3 LIGAND

Data on the systemic effects of FL in humans indicate that FL has a good safety profile with only minor adverse events (109). This is consistent with animal data showing that no adverse events were detected during short courses of FL treatment *in vivo*. Because FL acts synergistically with several cytokines it is also possible to envision its use in combination with cytokines that affect both primitive and differentiated hematopoietic cells.

Stem Cell Mobilization

FL may prove to be useful in mobilizing or expanding stem and progenitor cells *in vivo*. These stem cells can be used in either autologous or allogenic stem cell transplantation of cancer patients after high-dose chemotherapy. FL has been shown to stimulate the expansion and mobilization of stem and progenitor cells in animal models and nonhuman primates (99,130). The use of FL in combination with a second cytokine, such as

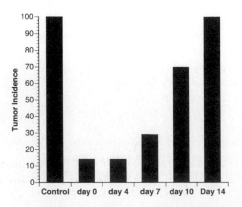

Day of Flt3L Treatment Initiation

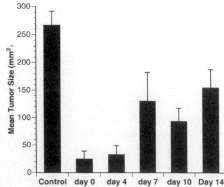

FIGURE 6. Flt-3 ligand (FL) treatment of mice with established tumors induces tumor regression. Mice were intradermally injected with 5 × 10⁵ viable B10.2 tumor cells, followed by 19 daily injections with either control buffer on day 0 or FL (30 mg per injection) beginning day 0, 4, 7, 10, or 14 (as indicated). Tumor incidence and size at week 6 of the experiment are shown. (Data from Lynch DH, Andreasen A, Maraskovsky E, Whitmore J, Miller RE, Schuh JCL. Flt3 ligand induces tumor regression and anti-tumor immune responses *in vivo. Nat Med* 1997;3:625–631.)

G-CSF or GM-CSF, appears to increase the number of stem cells mobilized *in vivo* (109,131–135).

Ex Vivo Stem Cell Expansion

One clinical modality being extensively investigated is the area of *ex vivo* stem cell expansion. The generation of sufficient numbers of autologous or HLA-matched, primitive stem/progenitor cells *in vitro* may become an effective way of reducing the number of BM harvests or leukaphereses required for stem cell reconstitution, thereby enabling repetitive cycles of high-dose chemotherapy to be performed on cancer patients. Furthermore, because contaminating tumor cells in autologous stem cell harvests can contribute to tumor relapse (136,137), selective *ex vivo* expansion of stem or progenitor cells may also reduce or eliminate these tumor cells (138). FL as a single factor is able to maintain human BM–derived colony forming unit-GM and high-proliferative potential *ex vivo* for 3 to 4 weeks, and this can be further enhanced when combined with factors such as IL-1, IL-3, IL-6, and EPO (47,57). Furthermore, long-term culture-initiating cells, which represent the most primitive human hematopoietic progenitors, can also be expanded *in vitro* with FL alone and this can be further augmented when combined with IL-3 and KL (57). It is unclear, however, whether *ex vivo* expansion protocols for human progenitor or stem cells contain sufficient numbers of pluripotent long-term repopulating cells (LTRCs) to provide long-lasting cellular reconstitution in cancer patients. In this regard, the predominant function of stem cell grafts in current high-dose chemotherapy regimens is to provide efficient short-term reconstitution. Long-term reconstitution in current procedures may be significantly facilitated by endogenous stem cells, which survive the high-dose chemotherapy rather than from the stem cell transplant itself. However, for multicycled chemotherapy regimens, it is crucial that the stem cell harvests contain LTRCs for long-lasting engraftment and cellular recovery in cancer patients (138,139).

FL has been found to be efficient at stimulating the production of progenitor cells from CD34$^+$CD38$^-$ progenitors cultured *in vitro* on stroma for up to 56 days (140). Furthermore, FL was required for the generation of LTRC from CD34$^+$ BM progenitors cultured in IL-3, IL-6, and KL before transfer into immune-deficient mice (141) and was found to act on myeloid as well as multipotent BM progenitors expressing differing levels of c-kit (142). A promising combination of factors for the *ex vivo* expansion of cord blood stem and progenitor cells is the combination of FL and thrombopoietin, which has been shown to expand these cells over a 5-month period (143). FL is currently being evaluated by several groups for its clinical potential in *ex vivo* stem cell expansion.

Gene Therapy

Hematopoietic stem cells are considered excellent candidates for gene therapy due to their extensive capacity for self-renewal and to generate large numbers of progeny that can be widely distributed throughout the body. Furthermore, stem cells can be readily isolated from BM, mobilized PB, or cord blood and can therefore be easily manipulated *in vitro* (128). Although gene transfer into mouse LTRC has been successfully performed with high efficiency (144,145), such studies on human stem cells have been rather disappointing (56,146). The use of retroviruses for integrating into host cell DNA is currently the most widely used in gene therapy protocols that target stem cells. However, a limitation of retroviral vectors is that they are inefficient at integrating into quiescent stem cells, which therefore requires that these stem cells be induced into cell cycle during gene transduction. FL has been shown to efficiently trigger cell cycle in stem cells, this being more efficient than that seen with later-acting factors such as IL-3 or IL-6 (56,147). Furthermore, FL appears to better preserve the pluripotent capacity of stem cells (i.e., their self-renewal and engrafting potential) than either KL or later-acting cytokines and KL (56).

Immunotherapy

Although mouse models suggest that DCs can be used as cellular vectors for tumor immunotherapy (95,96), the feasibility of this strategy requires in-depth clinical evaluation. The extremely small numbers of DCs found in the PB of cancer patients, the functional competence of these DCs in light of impaired DC function in cancer patients (96,148), and the uncertainty as to which DC subsets are the most appropriate for the induction of immunity *in vivo* underscore the need for further research into DC development and functional heterogeneity. Clinical trials currently examining the safety and efficacy of using DCs to deliver tumor Ag vaccines *in vivo* are primarily targeting the monocyte-derived DC subset (96). Functional distinctions between monocyte-derived DC and other DC subsets have been reported and suggest that they are not equivalent in their capacity to stimulate T- and B-cell responses (78,97,149). These studies emphasize how understanding the functional heterogeneity of DC subsets is essential for their appropriate use in immunotherapy. In this respect, the most successful immunotherapy strategies are likely those that maintain the diversity of DC subsets or those that can specifically target their distinct functional characteristics *in vivo*.

The ability of FL to expand the numbers of DCs *in vivo* for immunotherapy offers an alternative strategy to the use of *in vitro*–generated DCs. First, FL treatment of healthy volunteers generated functionally competent DC subsets and DC precursors *in vivo* in the presence of inhibitory serum factors (such as M-CSF). Second, both myeloid-related and lymphoid-related DC subsets are expanded in FL-treated mice (101,102,150), and in humans, both CD11c$^+$ and CD11c$^-$ DC (and subsets therein) have been increased in FL-treated individuals. The ability to expand a diverse repertoire of DC subsets may bypass many of the issues regarding which type of *in vitro*–generated DC population is most appropriate for the generation of clinically effective immunity *in vivo*. Finally, FL has been shown to generate effective T cell– and NK cell–mediated antitumor responses in tumor-bearing mice, suggesting that FL may augment antitumor immunity *in vivo* (123,126). Thus, FL may be an important cytokine for augmenting immunotherapy of cancer.

Of great interest is the capacity of FL to generate functionally competent DCs in cancer patients. Clinical studies using FL in cancer patients are currently under way. By increasing the numbers of DCs in the circulation, the uptake and presentation of endogenous tumor Ag may be augmented as may the direct immunization of cancer patients with antitumor vaccines. Alternatively, transient *ex vivo* manipulation of specific FL-expanded blood DC subsets with tumor vaccines before their reinfusion into cancer patients can be examined in greater detail. Finally, FL can also be used to increase the number of circulating DC precursors (e.g., CD34$^+$ cells, monocytes, or myeloid precursors), that can be differentiated *in vitro* into mature DCs for vaccine delivery.

The stage is now set for testing the feasibility of DC-mediated immunotherapy. The identification of which FL-generated DC subset is most appropriate for the induction of effective T cell–mediated immunity, the identification of their distinct ontogenic derivation, and whether FL can generate functionally competent DCs in cancer patients may result in the effective use of FL in the modulation of the immune responses.

ACKNOWLEDGMENTS

The authors wish to acknowledge the contributions of our many colleagues at Immunex who have contributed to this work, including Ken Brasel, Hilary McKenna, Bali Pulendran, Elizabeth Daro, Robert Miller, Eileen Roux, Mark Teepe, Laurent Galibert, and Doug Williams. We would also like to thank Anne Aumell for her excellent editorial work on this manuscript.

REFERENCES

1. Rosnet O, Mattel MG, Marchetto S, Birnbaum D. Isolation and chromosomal localization of a novel FMS-like tyrosine kinase gene. *Genomics* 1991;9:380–385.
2. Rosnet O, Marchetto S, deLapeyriere O, Bimbaum D. Murine *Flt3*, a gene encoding a novel tyrosine kinase receptor of the PDGFR/CSF1R family. *Oncogene* 1991;6:1641–1650.
3. Matthews W, Jordan CT, Wiegand GW, Pardoll D, Lemischka IR. A receptor tyrosine kinase specific to hematopoietic stem and progenitor cell-enriched populations. *Cell* 1991;65:1143–1152.
4. Small D, Levenstein M, Kim E, et al. STK-1, the human homolog of Flk-2/Flt-3, is selectively expressed in CD34$^+$ human bone marrow cells and is involved in the proliferation of early progenitor/stem cells. *Proc Natl Acad Sci U S A* 1994;91:459–463.
5. Rosnet O, Schiff C, Pebusque M-J, et al. Human *FLT3/FLK2* gene: cDNA cloning and expression in hematopoietic cells. *Blood* 1993;82:1110–1119.
6. Lyman SD, James L, Zappone J, Sleath PR, Beckmann MP, Bird T. Characterization of the protein encoded by the Flt3 (FLK2) receptor-like tyrosine kinase gene. *Oncogene* 1993;8:815–822.
7. Rosnet O, Buhring H-J, Marchetto S, et al. Human FLT3/FLK2 receptor tyrosine kinase is expressed at the surface of normal and malignant hematopoietic cells. *Leukemia* 1996;10:238–248.
8. Rose C, Rockwell P, Yang JQ, Pytowski B, Goldstein NI. Isolation and characterization of a monoclonal antibody binding to the extracellular domain of the flk-2 tyrosine kinase receptor. *Hybridoma* 1995;14:453–459.
9. Maroc N, Rottapel R, Rosnet O, et al. Biochemical characterization and analysis of the transforming potential of the FLT3/FLK2 receptor tyrosine kinase. *Oncogene* 1993;8:909–918.
10. Turner AM, Lin NL, Issarachai S, Lyman SD, Broudy VC. FLT3 receptor expression on the surface of normal and malignant human

11. Imbert A, Rosnet O, Marchetto S, Ollendorff V, Birnbaum D, Pebusque MJ. Characterization of a yeast artificial chromosome from human chromosome band 13q12 containing the FLT1 and FLT3 receptor-type tyrosine kinase genes. *Cytogenet Cell Genet* 1994;67:175–177.
12. Wang Z, Kim E, Chinault AC, Civin CI, Small D. Genomic organization of the human Stk-1 (Flt3/FLK2) gene. *Blood* 1996;88:111b.
13. Agnes F, Shamoon B, Dina C, Rosnet O, Birnbaum D, Galibert F. Genomic structure of the downstream part of the human *FLT3* gene: exon/intron structure conservation among genes encoding receptor tyrosine kinases (RTK) of subclass III. *Gene* 1994;145:283–288.
14. Rosnet O, Stephenson D, Mattei M-G, Marchetto S, Shibuya M, Chapman VM, Birnbaum D. Close physical linkage of the *FLT1* and *FLT3* genes on chromosome 13 in man and chromosome 5 in mouse. *Oncogene* 1993;8:173–179.
15. Shibuya M, Yamaguchi S, Yamane A, Ikeda T, Tojo A, Matsushime H, Sato M. Nucleotide sequence and expression of a novel human receptor-type tyrosine kinase gene (Flt) closely related to the fms family. *Oncogene* 1990;5:519–524.
16. Lavagna C, Marchetto S, Birnbaum D, Rosnet O. Identification and characterization of a functional murine FLT3 isoform produced by exon skipping. *J Biol Chem* 1995;270:3165–3171.
17. Lyman SD, James L, Vanden Bos T, et al. Molecular cloning of a ligand for the Flt3/flk-2 tyrosine kinase receptor: a proliferative factor for primitive hematopoietic cells. *Cell* 1993;75:1157–1167.
18. Hannum C, Culpepper J, Campbell D, et al. Ligand for FLT3/FLK2 receptor tyrosine kinase regulates growth of hematopoietic stem cells and is encoded by variant RNAs. *Nature* 1994;368:643–648.
19. Lyman SD, James L, Johnson L, et al. Cloning of the human homologue of the murine Flt3 ligand: a growth factor for early hematopoietic progenitor cells. *Blood* 1994;83:2795–2801.
20. Lyman SD, Brasel K, Rousseau AM, Williams DE. The Flt3 ligand: a hematopoietic stem cell factor whose activities are distinct from steel factor. *Stem Cells* 1994;12:99–107.
21. Lyman SD, Stocking K, Davison B, Fletcher F, Johnson L, Escobar S. Structural analysis of human and murine Flt3 ligand genomic loci. *Oncogene* 1995;11:1165–1172.
22. Lyman SD, Jacobsen SEW. c-*kit* ligand and Flt3 ligand: stem/progenitor cell factors with overlapping yet distinct activities. *Blood* 1998;91:1101–1134.
23. Lyman SD, James L, Escobar S, et al. Identification of soluble and membrane-bound isoforms of the murine Flt3 ligand generated by alternative splicing of mRNAs. *Oncogene* 1995;10:149–157.
24. McClanahan T, Culpepper J, Campbell D, et al. Biochemical and genetic characterization of multiple splice variants of the Flt3 ligand. *Blood* 1996;88:3371–3382.
25. Cerretti DP, Wignall J, Anderson D, et al. Human macrophage-colony stimulating factor: alternative RNA and protein processing from a single gene. *Mol Immunol* 1988;25:761–770.
26. Rossner MT, McArthur GA, Allen JD, Metcalf D. Fms-like tyrosine kinase 3 catalytic domain can transduce a proliferative signal in FDC-P1 cells that is qualitatively similar to the signal delivered by c-Fms. *Cell Growth Differ* 1994;5:549–555.
27. Brasel K, Escobar S, Anderberg R, de Vries P, Gruss H-J, Lyman SD. Expression of the Flt3 receptor and its ligand on hematopoietic cells. *Leukemia* 1995;9:1212–1218.
28. Da Silva N, Hu ZB, Ma W, Rosnet O, Birnbaum D, Drexler HG. Expression of the FLT3 gene in human leukemia-lymphoma cell lines. *Leukemia* 1994;8:885–888.
29. Meierhoff G, Dehmel U, Gruss H-J, et al. Expression of Flt3 receptor and Flt3-ligand in human leukemia-lymphoma cell lines. *Leukemia* 1995;9:1368–1372.
30. Rasko JEJ, Metcalf D, Rossner MT, Begley CG, Nicola NA. The Flt3/flk-2 ligand: receptor distribution and action on murine haemopoietic cell survival and proliferation. *Leukemia* 1995;9:2058–2066.
31. Wasserman R, Li YS, Hardy RR. Differential expression of the blk and ret tyrosine kinases during B lineage development is dependent on Ig rearrangement. *J Immunol* 1995;155:644–651.
32. Birg F, Courcoul M, Rosnet O, et al. Expression of the *FMS/KIT-like* gene *FLT3* in human acute leukemias of the myeloid and lymphoid

hematopoietic cells. *Blood* 1996;88:3383–3390.

lineages. *Blood* 1992;80:2584–2593.

33. Ratajczak MZ, Ratajczak J, Ford J, Kregenow R, Marlicz W, Gewirtz AM. FLT3/FLK-2 (STK-1) Ligand does not stimulate human megakaryopoiesis *in vitro*. *Stem Cells* 1996;14:146–150.

34. Rappold I, Ziegler BL, Köhler I, et al. Functional and phenotypic characterization of cord blood and bone marrow subsets expressing FLT3 (CD135) receptor tyrosine kinase. *Blood* 1997;90:111–125.

35. Drexler HG. Expression of FLT3 receptor and response to FLT3 ligand by leukemic cells. *Leukemia* 1996;10:588–599.

36. McKenna HJ, Smith FO, Brasel K, et al. Effects of Flt3 ligand on acute myeloid and lymphocytic leukemic blast cells from children. *Exp Hematol* 1996;24:378–385.

37. Carow CE, Levenstein M, Kaufmann SH, et al. Expression of the hematopoietic growth factor receptor FLT3 (STK-1/FLK2) in human leukemias. *Blood* 1996;87:1089–1096.

38. Stacchini A, Fubini L, Severino A, Sanavio F, Aglietta M, Piacibello W. Expression of type III receptor tyrosine kinases FLT3 and KIT and responses to their ligands by acute myeloid leukemia blasts. *Leukemia* 1996;10:1584–1591.

39. Piacibello W, Fubini L, Sanavio F, et al. Effects of human FLT3 ligand on myeloid leukemia cell growth: heterogeneity in response and synergy with other hematopoietic growth factors. *Blood* 1995;86:4105–4114.

40. Kiyoi H, Naoe T, Yokota S, et al. Internal tandem duplication of *FLT3* associated with leukocytosis in acute promyelocytic leukemia. *Leukemia* 1997;11:1447–1452.

41. Horiike S, Yokota S, Nakao M, et al. Tandem duplications of the *FLT3* receptor gene are associated with leukemic transformation of myelodysplasia. *Leukemia* 1997;11:1442–1446.

42. Iwaj T, Yokota S, Nakao M, et al. Internal tandem duplication of the FLT3 gene and clinical evaluation in childhood acute myeloid leukemia. The Children's Cancer and Leukemia Study Group, Japan. *Leukemia* 1999;13:38–43.

43. Eder M, Hemmati P, Kalina U, et al. Effects of Flt3 ligand and interleukin-7 on *in vitro* growth of acute lymphoblastic leukemia cells. *Exp Hematol* 1996;24:371–377.

44. deLapeyriere O, Naquet P, Planche J, et al. Expression of Flt3 tyrosine kinase receptor gene in mouse hematopoietic and nervous tissues. *Differentiation* 1995;58:351–359.

45. Lyman SD, Seaberg M, Hanna R, et al. Plasma/serum levels of Flt3 ligand are low in normal individuals and highly elevated in patients with Fanconi anemia and acquired aplastic anemia. *Blood* 1995;86:4091–4096.

46. Wodnar-Filipowicz A, Lyman SD, Gratwohl A, Tichelli A, Speck B, Nissen C. Flt3 ligand level reflects hematopoietic progenitor cell function in multilineage bone marrow failure. *Blood* 1996;88:4493–4499.

47. Gabbianelli M, Pelosi E, Montesoro E, et al. Multi-level effects of Flt3 ligand on human hematopoiesis: expansion of putative stem cells and proliferation of granulomonocytic progenitors/monocytic precursors. *Blood* 1995;86:1661–1670.

48. Jacobsen SEW, Veiby OP, Myklebust J, Okkenhaug C, Lyman SD. Ability of Flt3 ligand to stimulate the *in vitro* growth of primitive murine hematopoietic progenitors is potently and directly inhibited by transforming growth factor-β and tumor necrosis factor-α. *Blood* 1996;87:5016–5026.

49. Veiby OP, Jacobsen FW, Cui L, Lyman SD, Jacobsen SEW. The Flt3 ligand promotes the survival of primitive hemopoietic progenitor cells with myeloid as well as B lymphoid potential. Suppression of apoptosis and counteraction by TNF-alpha and TGF-beta. *J Immunol* 1996;157:2953–2960.

50. Hudak S, Hunte B, Culpepper J, et al. FLT3/FLK2 ligand promotes the growth of murine stem cells and the expansion of colony-forming cells and spleen colony-forming units. *Blood* 1995;85:2747–2755.

51. Jacobsen SEW, Okkenhaug C, Myklebust J, Veiby OP, Lyman SD. The FLT3 ligand potently and directly stimulates the growth and expansion of primitive murine bone marrow progenitor cells *in vitro*: synergistic interactions with interleukin (IL) 11, IL-12, and other hematopoietic growth factors. *J Exp Med* 1995;181:1357–1363.

52. Muench MO, Roncarolo MG, Menon S, et al. FLK-2/FLT-3 ligand regulates the growth of early myeloid progenitors isolated from human fetal liver. *Blood* 1995;85:963–972.

53. Ku H, Hirayama F, Kato T, et al. Soluble thrombopoietin receptor (Mpl) and granulocyte colony-stimulating factor receptor directly stimulate proliferation of primitive hematopoietic progenitors of mice in synergy with steel factor or the ligand for Flt3/FLK2. *Blood* 1996;88:4124–4131.

54. Lyman SD, Maraskovsky E, McKenna HJ. Flt3 ligand. In: Thomson AW, ed. *The cytokine handbook*. San Diego: Academic Press, 1998:728–752.

55. McKenna HJ, de Vries P, Brasel K, Lyman SD, Williams DE. Effect of Flt3 ligand on the *ex vivo* expansion of human CD34⁺ hematopoietic progenitor cells. *Blood* 1995;86:3413–3420.

56. Koller MR, Oxender M, Brott DA, Palsson BO. Flt-3 ligand is more potent than c-kit ligand for the synergistic stimulation of *ex vivo* hematopoietic cell expansion. *J Hematother* 1996;5:449–459.

57. Petzer AL, Hogge DE, Landsdorp PM, Reid DS, Eaves CJ. Self-renewal of primitive human hematopoietic cells (long-term-culture-initiating cells) *in vitro* and their expansion in defined medium. *Proc Natl Acad Sci U S A* 1996;93:1470–1474.

58. Mackarehtschian K, Hardin JD, Moore KA, Boast S, Goff SP, Lemischka IR. Targeted disruption of the *flk2/flt3* gene leads to deficiencies in primitive hematopoietic progenitors. *Immunity* 1995;3:147–161.

59. Steinman RM. The dendritic cell system and its role in immunogenicity. *Annu Rev Immunol* 1991;9:271–296.

60. Bender A, Sapp M, Schuler G, Steinman RM, Bhardwaj N. Improved methods for the generation of dendritic cells from non-proliferating progenitors in human blood. *J Immunol Methods* 1996;196:121–135.

61. Romani N, Reider D, Heuer M, et al. Generation of mature dendritic cells from human blood. An improved method with special regard to clinical applicability. *J Immunol Methods* 1996;196:137–151.

62. Jonuleit H, Kuhn U, Muller G, et al. Pro-inflammatory cytokines and prostaglandins induce maturation of potent immunostimulatory dendritic cells under fetal calf serum-free conditions. *Eur J Immunol* 1997;27:3135–3142.

63. Luft T, Pang KC, Thomas E, et al. Type I IFNs enhance the terminal differentiation of dendritic cells. *J Immunol* 1998;161:1947–1953.

64. Winzler C, Rovere P, Rescigno M, et al. Maturation stages of mouse dendritic cells in growth factor-dependent long-term cultures. *J Exp Med* 1997;185:317–328.

65. Caux C, Bancherau J. *In vitro* regulation of dendritic cell development and function. In: Whetton A, Gordon J, eds. *Blood cell biochemistry: hemopoietic growth factors and their receptors*. New York: Plenum Publishing, 1996:263–301.

66. Cella M, Scheidegger D, Palmer-Lehmann K, Lane P, Lanzavecchia A, Alber G. Ligation of CD40 on dendritic cells triggers production of high levels of interleukin-12 and enhances T cell stimulatory capacity: T-T help via APC activation. *J Exp Med* 1996;184:747–752.

67. Koch F, Stanzl U, Jennewein P, et al. High level IL-12 production by murine dendritic cells: upregulation via MHC class II and CD40 molecules and downregulation by IL-4 and IL-10. *J Exp Med* 1996;184:741–746.

68. Trinchieri G. Interleukin-12: a proinflammatory cytokine with immunoregulatory functions that bridge innate resistance and antigen-specific adaptive immunity. *Annu Rev Immunol* 1995;13:251–276.

69. Grouard G, Durand I, Filgueira L, Bancherau J, Liu Y-J. Dendritic cells capable of stimulating T cells in germinal centres. *Nature* 1996;384:364–367.

70. Dubois B, Massacrier C, Vanbervliet B, et al. Critical role of IL-12 in dendritic cell-induced differentiation of naive B lymphocytes. *J Immunol* 1998;161:2223–2231.

71. Inaba M, Inaba K, Hosono M, et al. Distinct mechanisms of neonatal tolerance induced by dendritic cells and thymic B cells. *J Exp Med* 1991;173:549–559.

72. Matzinger P, Guerder S. Does T-cell tolerance require a dedicated antigen-presenting cell? *Nature* 1989;338:74–76.

73. Mazda O, Watanabe Y, Gyotoku J-I, Katsura Y. Requirement of dendritic cells and B cells in the clonal deletion of Mls-reactive T cells in the thymus. *J Exp Med* 1991;173:539–547.

74. Süss G, Shortman K. A subclass of dendritic cells kills CD4 T cells via Fas/Fas ligand–induced apoptosis. *J Exp Med* 1996;183:1789–1796.

75. Macatonia SE, Hsieh C-S, Murphy KM, O'Garra A. Dendritic cells and macrophages are required for Th1 development of CD4$^+$ T cells from αβ TCR transgenic mice: IL-12 substitution for macrophages to stimulate IFN-γ production is IFN-γ-dependent. *Int Immunol* 1993;5:1119–1128.

76. Maldonado-López R, De Smedt T, Michel P, et al. CD8α$^+$ and CD8α$^-$ subclasses of dendritic cells direct the development of distinct T helper cells *in vivo*. *J Exp Med* 1999;189:587–592.

77. Pulendran B, Smith JL, Caspary G, et al. Distinct dendritic cell subsets differentially regulate the class of immune response *in vivo*. *Proc Natl Acad Sci U S A* 1999;96:1036–1041.

78. Rissoan MC, Soumelis V, Kadowaki N, et al. Reciprocal control of T helper cell and dendritic cell differentiation. *Science* 1999;283:1183–1186.

79. Steinman RM, Pack M, Inaba K. Dendritic cells in the T-cell areas of lymphoid organs. *Immunol Rev* 1997;156:25–37.

80. Inaba K, Steinman RM, Pack MW, et al. Identification of proliferating dendritic cell precursors in mouse blood. *J Exp Med* 1992;175:1157–1167.

81. Inaba K, Inaba M, Romani N, et al. Generation of large numbers of dendritic cells from mouse bone marrow cultures supplemented with granulocyte/macrophage colony-stimulating factor. *J Exp Med* 1992;176:1693–1702.

82. Inaba K, Inaba M, Deguchi M, et al. Granulocytes, macrophages, and dendritic cells arise from a common major histocompatibility complex class II-negative progenitor in mouse bone marrow. *Proc Natl Acad Sci U S A* 1993;90:3038–3042.

83. Caux C, Dezutter-Dambuyant C, Schmitt D, Bancnereau J. GM-CSF and TNF-α cooperate in the generation of dendritic Langerhans cells. *Nature* 1992;360:258–261.

84. Sallusto F, Lanzavecchia A. Efficient presentation of soluble antigen by cultured human dendritic cells is maintained by granulocyte/macrophage colony-stimulating factor plus interleukin-4 and downregulated by tumor necrosis factor α. *J Exp Med* 1994;179:1109–1118.

85. Romani N, Gruner S, Brang D, et al. Proliferating dendritic cell progenitors in human blood. *J Exp Med* 1994;180:83–93.

86. Young JW, Szabolcs P, Moore MAS. Identification of dendritic cell colony-forming units among normal human CD34$^+$ bone marrow progenitors that are expanded by c-*kit*-ligand and yield pure dendritic cell colonies in the presence of granulocyte/macrophage colony-stimulating factor and tumor necrosis factor α. *J Exp Med* 1995;182:1111–1120.

87. Szabolcs P, Moore MAS, Young JW. Expansion of immunostimulatory dendritic cells among the myeloid progeny of human CD34$^+$ bone marrow precursors cultured with c-*kit* ligand, granulocyte-macrophage colony-stimulating factor, and TNF-α. *J Immunol* 1995;154:5851–5861.

88. Ardavin C, Wu L, Li CL, Shortman K. Thymic dendritic cells and T cells develop simultaneously in the thymus from a common precursor population. *Nature* 1993;362:761–763.

89. Galy A, Travis M, Cen D, Chen B. Human T, B, natural killer, and dendritic cells arise from a common bone marrow progenitor cell subset. *Immunity* 1995;3:459–473.

90. Wu L, Li C-L, Shortman K. Thymic dendritic cell precursors: relationship to the T lymphocyte lineage and phenotype of the dendritic cell progeny. *J Exp Med* 1996;184:903–911.

91. Vremec D, Zorbas M, Scollay R, et al. The surface phenotype of dendritic cells purified from mouse thymus and spleen: investigation of the CD8 expression by a subpopulation of dendritic cells. *J Exp Med* 1992;176:47–58.

92. Saunders D, Lucas K, Ismaili J, et al. Dendritic cell development in culture from thymic precursor cells in the absence of granulocyte/macrophage colony-stimulating factor. *J Exp Med* 1996;184:2185–2196.

93. Metcalf D, Shortman K, Vremec D, Mifsud S, Di Rago L. Effects of excess GM-CSF levels on hematopoiesis and leukemia development in GM-CSF/*max* 41 double transgenic mice. *Leukemia* 1996;10: 713–719.

94. Vremec D, Shortman K. Dendritic cell subtypes in mouse lymphoid organs. Cross-correlation of surface markers, changes in incubation, and differences among thymus, spleen, and lymph nodes. *J Immunol* 1997;159:565–573.

95. Young JW, Inaba K. Dendritic cells as adjuvants for class I major histocompatibility complex-restricted antitumor immunity. *J Exp Med* 1996;183:7–11.

96. Schuler G, Steinman RM. Dendritic cells as adjuvants for immune-mediated resistance to tumors. *J Exp Med* 1997;186:1183–1187.

97. Mortarini R, Anichini A, Di Nicola M, et al. Autologous dendritic cells derived from CD34$^+$ progenitors and from monocytes are not functionally equivalent antigen-presenting cells in the induction of melan-A/Mart-1$_{27-35}$-specific CTLs from peripheral blood lymphocytes of melanoma patients with low frequency of CTL precursors. *Cancer Res* 1997;57:5534–5541.

98. Brasel K, McKenna HJ, Charrier K, Morrissey P, Williams DE, Lyman SD. Mobilization of peripheral blood progenitor cells with Flt3 ligand. *Blood* 1995;86:463a.

99. Brasel K, McKenna HJ, Morrissey PJ, et al. Hematologic effects of flt3 ligand *in vivo* in mice. *Blood* 1996;88:2004–2012.

100. Crowley M, Inaba K, Witmer-Pack M, Steinman RM. The cell surface of mouse dendritic cells: FACS analyses of dendritic cells from different tissues including thymus. *Cell Immunol* 1989;118:108–125.

101. Maraskovsky E, Brasel K, Teepe M, et al. Dramatic increase in the numbers of functionally mature dendritic cells in Flt3 ligand-treated mice: multiple dendritic cell subpopulations identified. *J Exp Med* 1996;184:1953–1962.

102. Pulendran B, Lingappa J, Kennedy MK, et al. Developmental pathways of dendritic cells *in vivo*. Distinct function, phenotype and localization of dendritic cell subsets in FLT3 ligand-treated mice. *J Immunol* 1997;159:2222–2231.

103. McKenna HJ, Stocking K, Miller RE, et al. Targeted disruption of the flt3 ligand gene results in mice with deficient hematopoiesis affecting multiple lineages including dendritic cells and natural killer cells. *Blood* 2000 (*in press*).

104. Siena S, Di Nicola M, Bregni M, et al. Massive *ex vivo* generation of functional dendritic cells from mobilized CD34$^+$ blood progenitors for anticancer therapy. *Exp Hematol* 1995;23:1463–1471.

105. Maraskovsky E, Roux E, Tepee M, et al. The effect of Flt3 ligand and/or c-*kit* ligand on the generation of dendritic cells from human CD34$^+$ bone marrow. *Blood* 1995;86:420a.

106. Strobl H, Bello-Fernandez C, Riedl E, et al. flt3 ligand in cooperation with transforming growth factor-beta1 potentiates *in vitro* development of Langerhans-type dendritic cells and allows single-cell dendritic cell cluster formation under serum-free conditions. *Blood* 1997;90:1425–1434.

107. Grouard G, Rissoan M-C, Filgueira L, Durand I, Bancnereau J, Liu Y-J. The enigmatic plasmacytoid T cells develop into dendritic cells with interleukin (IL)-3 and CD40-ligand. *J Exp Med* 1997;185:1101–1111.

108. Olweus J, A BitMansour, Warnke R, et al. Dendritic cell ontogeny: a human dendritic cell lineage of myeloid origin. *Proc Natl Acad Sci U S A* 1997;94:12551–12556.

109. Lebsack ME, McKenna HJ, Hoek JA, et al. Safety of FLT3 ligand in healthy volunteers. *Blood* 1997;90:751a.

110. Maraskovsky E, Daro E, Roux ER, et al. In vivo generation of human dendritic cells by Flt3 ligand. *Blood* 2000 (*in press*).

111. Caux C, Massacrier C, Vanbervliet B, et al. Activation of human dendritic cells through CD40 cross-linking. *J Exp Med* 1994;180: 1263–1272.

112. Sallusto F, Celia M, Danieli C, Lanzavecchia A. Dendritic cells use macropinocytosis and the mannose receptor to concentrate macromolecules in the major histocompatibility complex class II compartment: downregulation by cytokines and bacterial products. *J Exp Med* 1995;182:389–400.

113. Reddy A, Sapp M, Feldman M, Subklewe M, Bhardwaj N. A monocyte conditioned medium is more effective than defined cytokines in mediating the terminal maturation of human dendritic cells. *Blood* 1997;90:3640–3646.

114. Viney JL, Jones S, Chiu HH, et al. Mucosal addressin cell adhesion molecule-1: a structural and functional analysis demarcates the integrin binding motif. *J Immunol* 1996;157:2488–2497.

115. Puiendran B, Smith JL, Jenkins M, Schoenborn M, Maraskovsky E, Maliszewski CR. Prevention of peripheral tolerance by a dendritic cell growth factor: Flt3 ligand as an adjuvant. *J Exp Med* 1998;188:2075–2082.

116. Smith AL, de St Groth BF. Antigen-pulsed CD8α$^+$ dendritic cells generate an immune response after subcutaneous injection without homing to the draining lymph node. *J Exp Med* 1999;189:593–598.

117. Knight SC, Hunt R, Dore C, Medawar PB. Influence of dendritic cells on tumor growth. *Proc Natl Acad Sci U S A* 1985;82:4495–4497.

118. Tsujitani S, Kakeji Y, Watanabe A, Kohnoe S, Maehara Y, Sugimaghi K. Infiltration of S-100 protein positive dendritic cells and peritoneal recurrence in advanced gastric cancer. *Int Surg* 1992;77:238–241.

119. Nakano T, Oka K, Sugita T, Tsunemoto H. Antitumor activity of Langerhans cells in radiation therapy for cervical cancer and its modulation with SPG administration. *In Vivo* 1993;7:257–263.

120. Alavaikko MJ, Blanco G, Aine R, et al. Follicular dendritic cells have prognostic relevance in Hodgkin's disease. *Am J Clin Pathol* 1994;101:761–767.

121. Zeid NA, Muller HK. S100 positive dendritic cells in human lung tumors associated with cell differentiation and enhanced survival. *Pathology* 1993;25:338–343.

122. Mayordomo JI, Zorina T, Storkus WJ, et al. Bone marrow-derived dendritic cells pulsed with synthetic tumour peptides elicit protective and therapeutic antitumour immunity. *Nat Med* 1995;1:1297–1302.

123. Lynch DH, Andreasen A, Maraskovsky E, Whitmore J, Miller RE, Schuh JCL. Flt3 ligand induces tumor regression and anti-tumor immune responses *in vivo*. *Nat Med* 1997;3:625–631.

124. Chen K, Braun SE, Wiebke E, et al. Retroviral-mediated gene transfer of the Flt3 ligand into murine breast cancer cells prevents tumor growth *in vivo*. *Blood* 1995;86[Suppl l]:244a.

125. Fernandez NC, Lozier A, Flament C, et al. Dendritic cells directly trigger NK cell functions: cross-talk relevant in innate anti-tumor immune responses *in vivo*. *Nat Med* 1999;5:405–411.

126. Chen K, Braun S, Lyman S, et al. Antitumor activity and immunotherapeutic properties of Flt3-ligand in a murine breast cancer model. *Cancer Res* 1997;57:3511–3516.

127. Peron JM, Esche C, Subbotin VM, Maliszewski C, Lotze MT, Shurin MR. FLT3-ligand administration inhibits liver metastases: role of NK cells. *J Immunol* 1998;161:6164–6170.

128. Esche C, Subbotin VM, Maliszewski C, Lotze MT, Shurin MR. FLT3 ligand administration inhibits tumor growth in murine melanoma and lymphoma. *Cancer Res* 1998;58:380–383.

129. Shaw SG, Maung AA, Steptoe RJ, Thomson AW, Vujanovic NL. Expansion of functional NK cells in multiple tissue compartments of mice treated with Flt3-ligand: implications for anti-cancer and antiviral therapy. *J Immunol* 1998;161:2817–2824.

130. Winton EF, Bucur SZ, Bray RA, et al. The hematopoietic effects of recombinant human (rh) Flt3 ligand administered to non-human primates. *Blood* 1995;86:424a.

131. Winton EF, Bucur SZ, Bond LD, et al. Recombinant human (rh) Flt3 ligand plus rhGM-CSF or rhG-CSF causes a marked CD34$^+$ cell mobilization to blood in rhesus monkeys. *Blood* 1996;88[Suppl 1]:642a.

132. Brasel K, McKenna HJ, Charrier K, Morrissey P, Williams DE, Lyman SD. Flt3 ligand synergizes with granulocyte-macrophage colony-stimulating factor or granulocyte colony-stimulating factor to mobilize hematopoietic progenitor cells into the peripheral blood of mice. *Blood* 1997;90:3781–3788

133. Sudo Y, Shimazaki C, Ashihara E, et al. Synergistic effect of FLT-3 ligand on the granulocyte colony-stimulating factor-induced mobilization of hematopoietic stem cells and progenitor cells into blood in mice. *Blood* 1997;89:3186–3191.

134. Papayannopoulou T, Nakamoto B, Andrews RG, Lyman SD, Lee MY. *In vivo* effects of Flt3/Flk2 ligand on mobilization of hematopoietic progenitors in primates and potent synergistic enhancement with granulocyte colony-stimulating factor. *Blood* 1997;90:620–629.

135. Pless M, Wodnar-Filipowicz A, John L, et al. Synergy of growth factors during mobilization of peripheral blood precursor cells with recombinant human Flt3-ligand and granulocyte colony-stimulating factor in rabbits. *Exp Hematol* 1999;27:155–161.

136. Rill DR, Santana VM, Roberts WM, et al. Direct demonstration that analogous bone marrow transplantation for solid tumors can return a multiplicity of tumorigenic cells. *Blood* 1994;84:380–383.

137. Deisseroth AB, Zu Z, Claxton D, et al. Genetic marking shows that Ph+ cells present in autologous transplants of chronic myelogenous leukemia (CML) contribute to relapse after autologous bone marrow in CML. *Blood* 1994;83:3068–3076.

138. Emerson SG. *Ex vivo* expansion of hematopoietic precursors, progenitors, and stem cells: the next generation of cellular therapeutics. *Blood* 1996;87:3082–3088.

139. Lange W, Henschler R, Mertelsmann R. Biological and clinical advances in stem cell expansion. *Leukemia* 1996;10:943–945.

140. Shah AJ, Smogorzewska EM, Hannum C, Crooks GM. Flt3 ligand induces proliferation of quiescent human bone marrow CD34$^+$CD38$^-$ cells and maintains progenitor cells *in vitro*. *Blood* 1996;87: 3563–3570.

141. Dao MA, Hannum CH, Kohn DB, Nolta JA. FLT3 ligand preserves the ability of human CD34$^+$ progenitors to sustain long-term hematopoiesis in immune-deficient mice after *ex vivo* retroviral-mediated transduction. *Blood* 1997;89:446–456.

142. Sonoda Y, Kimura T, Sakabe H, et al. Human FLT3 ligand acts on myeloid as well as multipotential progenitors derived from purified CD34$^+$ blood progenitors expressing different levels of c-*kit* protein. *Eur J Haematol* 1997;58:257–264.

143. Piacibello W, Sanavio F, Garetto L, et al. Extensive amplification and self-renewal of human primitive hematopoietic stem cells from cord blood. *Blood* 1997;89:2644–2653.

144. Luskey BD, Rosenblatt M, Zsebo K, Williams DA. Stem cell factor, interleukin-3, and interleukin-6 promote retroviral-mediated gene transfer into murine hematopoietic stem cells. *Blood* 1992;80:396–402.

145. Correll PH, Colilla S, Dave HP, Karlsson S. High levels of human glucocerebrosidase activity in macrophages of long-term reconstituted mice after retroviral infection of hematopoietic stem cells. *Blood* 1992;80:331–336.

146. Brenner MK, Rill DR, Holladay MS, et al. Gene marking to determine whether autologous marrow infusion restores long-term haemopoiesis in cancer patients. *Lancet* 1993;342:1134–1137.

147. Ohishi K, Katayama N, Itoh R, et al. Accelerated cell-cycling of hematopoietic progenitors by the *flt3* ligand that is modulated by transforming growth factor-β. *Blood* 1996;87:1718–1727.

148. Gabrilovich DI, Corak J, Ciernik IF, Kavanaugh D, Carbone DP. Decreased antigen presentation by dendritic cells in patients with breast cancer. *Clin Cancer Res* 1997;3:483–490.

149. Caux C, Massacrier C, Vanbervliet B, et al. CD34$^+$ hematopoietic progenitors from human cord blood differentiate along two independent dendritic cell pathways in response to granulocyte-macrophage colony-stimulating factor plus tumor necrosis factor α: II. Functional analysis. *Blood* 1997;90:1458–1470.

150. Shurin MR, Pandharipande PP, Zorina TD, et al. FLT3 ligand induces the generation of functionally active dendritic cells in mice. *Cell Immunol* 1997;179:174–184.

25

CTLA-4 BLOCKADE IN TUMOR IMMUNOTHERAPY

JAMES P. ALLISON
ARTHUR A. HURWITZ
ANDREA VAN ELSAS
EUGENE KWON
TIMOTHY SULLIVAN
BARBARA FOSTER
NORMAN GREENBERG

T-CELL ACTIVATION IS REGULATED BY STIMULATORY, COSTIMULATORY, AND INHIBITORY SIGNALS

Advances in the understanding of the mechanisms that regulate T-cell activation allow the rational design of new strategies for immunotherapy of tumors. It has been known for some time that engagement of the T-cell antigen receptor is by itself not sufficient for full T-cell activation—a second costimulatory signal is required for induction of interleukin-2 production, proliferation, and differentiation to effector function of naïve T cells. Abundant data indicate that the primary source of this costimulation is mediated by engagement of CD28 on the T-cell surface by members of the B7 family on the antigen-presenting cell (1). Expression of B7 has been shown to be limited to professional antigen-presenting cells (APCs); specialized cells of the hematopoietic lineage, including dendritic cells, activated macrophages, and activated B cells. It has been suggested that this sharply defined restriction of B7 expression is a fail-safe mechanism for maintenance of peripheral T-cell tolerance ensuring that T-cell activation can only be stimulated by appropriate antigen-presuming cells (2). The fact that tumor cells do not express B7 is one factor that contributes to their poor capacity to elicit immune responses (3,4). The demonstration that induction of expression of B7 on many tumor cells by transfection, transduction, or other mechanisms can heighten tumor immunogenicity led to some great interest to pursue this as an approach to tumor immunotherapy. However, the utility of B7 expression as a vaccination approach is limited by several factors:

1. B7+ tumor cell vaccines are only effective when the tumor cells have a high degree of inherent immunogenicity.
2. Although B7+ vaccines have been shown in many cases to be effective in inducing protective immune responses, there has

been only limited utility inducing responses to previously established tumors.
3. Inactivation of tumor cells by radiation has been shown to destroy the immunoenhancing activity of the B7 gene product (5,6).

In the late 1990s, it has become apparent that costimulation is even more complex than originally thought. After activation, T cells express a close homologue to CD28, cytotoxic T lymphocyte-associated antigen 4 (CTLA-4), that binds members of the B7 family with a much higher affinity than CD28 (7). Although there was initially some controversy as to the role of CTLA-4 in regulating T-cell activation, it has become clear that CTLA-4 downregulates T-cell responses (8). This was initially suggested by *in vitro* observations that (a) blockade of CTLA-4/B7 interactions with antibody-enhanced T-cell responses, (b) the cross-linking of CTLA-4 along with CD3 and CD28 inhibited T-cell responses, and (c) the administration of antibodies to CTLA-4 *in vivo* enhanced response of mice to peptide antigens or superantigens (9–12).

The most convincing demonstration of the downregulatory role of CTLA-4 came from examination of deficient mice (13–15). CTLA-4 knockout mice have apparently spontaneously activated T cells beginning at approximately a week after birth, followed by rampant lymphoproliferation and lymphadenopathy. These mice die by approximately 3 weeks of age, either as a result of polyclonal T-cell expansion and tissue destruction or as a result of toxic shock resulting from lymphokine production by the T cells. Because thymocyte differentiation and selection proceed normally in CTLA-4–deficient mice, the rampant T-cell expansion that occurs in the mice indicates that CTLA-4 plays a critical role in downregulating T-cell responses in the periphery (16).

It is unclear from the phenotype of CTLA-4–deficient mice whether the T-cell expansion that occurs is a result of a failure of the mice to regulate expansion of T cells responding to environmental antigens or as a result of initiation of responses in T cells that would not have been activated in the presence of CTLA-4. Support for the former idea has been based on the assumption that because it is detectable only after T-cell activation, CTLA-4 could not be operative in the early stages of T-cell responses. However, we have shown that CTLA-4 cross-linking can inhibit many aspects of T-cell activation at stages at which expression of a protein is not readily apparent (17). This has led us to propose that CTLA-4 may serve as an attenuator of T-cell responses that effectively raise the threshold of costimulatory and perhaps antigen receptor–mediated signals that are necessary to achieve full activation of naïve T cells (8,18). This suggests that CTLA-4 may contribute to the maintenance of peripheral T-cell tolerance by damping signals resulting from chance encounters of self-reactive T cells with tissue-specific antigens in the absence of high levels of B7 (19). This scenario does not exclude the possibility that after its induction to maximal levels CTLA-4 could not also contribute to termination of ongoing responses. Whether one or both of these proves to be the case, the fact that CTLA-4 plays an important and obvious role in downregulation of T-cell responses has led us to explore the possibility of manipulation of the signaling pathway to develop new strategies for enhancing immunotherapeutic approaches to cancer.

In this review, we present evidence suggesting a role for CTLA-4 in maintaining peripheral tolerance and avoiding autoimmunity, and the evidence suggesting that CTLA-4 blockade can serve as a powerful approach to tumor immunotherapy.

INHIBITORY SIGNALS MEDIATED BY CTLA-4 MAY PLAY A ROLE IN PERIPHERAL TOLERANCE

The fact that we and others have shown that administration of CTLA-4 antibody-enhanced T-cell response to peptides and super antigens *in vivo* led us to explore the effects of CTLA-4 blockade in several models of autoimmunity. One model that has been examined extensively is experimental autoimmune encephalomyelitis (EAE), a murine model of multiple sclerosis. This disease is characterized by TH1-CD4+ responses that are antigens in the central nervous system (CNS), either myelin-basic protein or proteolipid protein. Immunization of certain susceptible strains of mice, such as SJL or PLJ with peptides derived from these proteins, leads to a cycling progressing and remitting paralysis accompanied by infiltration of the CNS with autoreactive T cells. We and others have shown that administration of CTLA-4 antibodies during either immunization or during active disease can exacerbate the severity of both clinical and histopathologic signs of disease and prolong it, confirming again the ability of CTLA-4 blockade to enhance and perhaps sustain T-cell responses (20–22).

More recently, we have sought to address the role of CTLA-4 during induction of EAE-like syndromes in normally resistant mice on immunization with CNS tissues. For example, we have found that immunization of Balb/c mice with homogenized syngeneic spinal cord emulsified in complete Freund's adjuvant does not lead to T-cell infiltration of the CNS nor to clinical manifestation of EAE. However, similar immunization together with anti–CTLA-4 leads to extensive CNS infiltration and to

clinical signs of EAE (Hurwitz and Allison, manuscript in preparation). Although our work on the basis for this effect is continuing, the explanation that we favor is that CTLA-4 lowers the threshold of activation, allowing responses of self-reactive T cells and the breaking of peripheral tolerance. These data support the notion that CTLA-4 may play a role in the maintenance of peripheral tolerance.

CTLA-4 BLOCKADE AND TUMOR IMMUNOTHERAPY

Our initial studies with CTLA-4 blockade focused on moderately immunogenic tumors in which we had found induction of B7 expression to be partially effective in reducing tumorigenicity. We sought to determine whether CTLA-4 blockade would enhance rejection of the B7-transfected tumor. Colon carcinoma 51Blim10 cells transfected with B7 grow for approximately 2 weeks before being slowly rejected. Injection of anti-CTLA-4 antibodies in the first week after implantation led to rapid rejection of the tumors by all of the mice. This was not unexpected, because administration of anti–CTLA-4 had been shown to increase T-cell responses *in vivo* (12). However, a more startling finding was made in the treatment of wild-type tumors that did not express B7. We found that administration of CTLA-4 after tumor implantation again resulted in tumor rejection (23). Similar results were found with the fibrosarcoma SA1N. In both these tumors, we found that rechallenge of the mice as late as 4 months after initial rejection of the tumor resulted in protection against tumor growth. We also found administration of the antibodies could be delayed as late as two weeks or until the tumors had reached a size of approximately 150 mm^2. For SAIN, complete tumor rejection was again accomplished in more than 80% of the animals even when started after prolonged tumor growth.

These studies were subsequently extended to a panel of tumors including those listed in Table 1. These tumors can be divided into three groups:

1. Tumors that are sensitive to anti–CTLA-4–induced rejection. In these tumors, we regularly obtained complete eradication and long-lasting immunity.
2. The second group consisted of tumors whose growth was significantly slowed by CTLA-4 blockade but in which rejection was only rarely obtained.
3. The third group typified by mammary carcinoma SM1 and the melanoma B16BL6, was largely resistant to the effects of anti–CTLA-4. For these tumors, we observed a slight retardation of tumor growth but did not succeed in obtaining tumor rejection.

The defining property seems to be the inherent immunogenicity of the tumors. Tumors that were susceptible to CTLA-4 blockade tended to be those that were also rejected on induction of B7 expression and included those shown to be immunogenic by the capacity of irradiated cells to protect mice against subsequent challenge with a tumor. Tumors resistant to CTLA-4 blockade, SM1 and B16BL6, were considered to be nonimmu-

TABLE 1. ANTI–CTLA-4 IN COMBINATION IMMUNOTHERAPY

	Treatment			
	Vaccine	Anti–CTLA-4	Tumor Rejection	Autoimmunity
SM-1	GM-SM-1	–	No effect	—
—	GM-SM-1	+	Yes	Not examined
B16 melanoma	GM-B16	–	Occasional	—
—	GM-B16	+	Yes	Vitiligo
Prostate adenocarcinoma in TRAMP mice	TRAMP	–	No effect	—
—	TRAMP	+	Diminished incidence and severity[a]	—
—	GM-TRAMP	–	No effect	—
—	GM-TRAMP	+	Diminished incidence and severity[a]	Prostatitis

GM, granulocyte-macrophage; TRAMP, transgenic adenocarcinoma of mouse prostate.
[a]Significant decrease in incidence of primary tumor 8 weeks after treatment of transgenic mice.

nogenic by the opposite criteria, such as the immunization of mice with irradiated tumor cells did not lead to protection nor did the induction of B7 lead to tumor rejection. Having demonstrated that CTLA-4 blockaded by itself was sufficient to achieve rejection of immunogenic tumors, we turned our attention to developing strategies to obtain rejection of the resistant, presumably poorly immunogenic or nonimmunogenic tumors.

CTLA-4 CAN BE EFFECTIVE IN COMBINATION IMMUNOTHERAPY OF POORLY IMMUNOGENIC TUMORS

SM1 Mammary Carcinoma

We chose granulocyte-macrophage colony-stimulating factor (GM-CSF)–transduced tumor cell vaccines as a first approach for evaluation of CTLA-4 as a component of combination immunotherapy because it had been previously shown that immunization with GM-CSF expressing B16 melanoma cells could lead to protection against subsequent challenge (24). However, vaccination with GM-CSF cells alone had not been found to lead to rejection of preestablished tumor (25). We initially tried combination therapy for treatment of the poorly immunogenic mammary carcinoma SM1 (26). We found that neither irradiated SM1 cells, irradiated GM-CSF–transfected SM1 cells (GM-SM1), nor anti-CTLA-4 given alone beginning on the day of tumor implantation had any significant effect on tumor growth. The combination of irradiated SM1 cells with anti-CTLA-4 slightly slowed tumor growth but did not lead to rejection. However, vaccination with GM-SM1 cells followed by anti-CTLA-4 regularly resulted in complete tumor rejection.

B16 Melanoma

The B16 melanoma is an extremely aggressive tumor model, characterized by a low median lethal dose and high capacity for metastasis. These features made this model a compelling one in which to assess the effectiveness of CTLA-4 blockade as a component of immunologic treatment (27). We found that neither CTLA-4 blockade nor immunization with irradiated B16 cells

alone or in combination had significant effects on tumors of subcutaneous implants of B16BL6, even when administered beginning on the day of implantation. Vaccination on the same day of tumor implantation with irradiated B16 cells transduced to express GM-CSF (GM-B16) resulted in a slight retardation of the rate of tumor growth, but rejection was only rarely obtained. However, vaccination with GM-B16 together with administration of anti-CTLA-4 antibodies prevented outgrowth of tumors in virtually all mice. Similarly, complete eradication of tumors was regularly obtained when initiation of the combination therapy was delayed until day 4 (in 68 of 85, or 80%, of treated mice). Tumor-free mice were found to be resistant to rechallenge 4 months later, indicating that rejection was accompanied by the induction of potent immunologic memory. Finally, we also found that the combination therapy was capable of protecting mice from death due to pulmonary metastases induced by intravenous injection of the B16 subline F10.

The mechanism of protection elicited by the anti–CTLA-4 combination therapy appears to differ from that in previously reported studies of prophylactic immunization with GM-CSF/ B16. Prophylaxis by GM/B16 has been shown to be mediated largely, if not exclusively, by CD4[+] T cells and their cytokines (25). In contrast, we found that rejection of preestablished tumors by the combination immunotherapy was not effected by depletion of CD4[+] T cells. The basis for this difference remains to be established. One possibility is that CTLA-4 blockade may lower the threshold of signaling needed for activation of CD8 to a level sufficient for full activation even in the absence of CD4[+] helper T-cell licensing of APCs by CD40 ligand and CD40 interactions (28–31). The cellular and molecular requirements for effectiveness of the combination immunotherapy are currently under investigation.

One important limitation observed in these studies was that the effectiveness of treatment began to wane after approximately a week of tumor growth. When treatment was begun on day 8 after tumor implantation, the rate of tumor growth was slowed considerably, but complete eradication was obtained in only a minority of animals (<20%). After 12 days, tumor growth was significantly delayed, but complete regression was not obtained. This is in stark contrast to our results with the more immunogenic tumors, where anti–CTLA-4 alone was capable of inducing regression in some models even after weeks of tumor growth. The basis for the limited period of effectiveness in the B16 system is not clear at present. It is possible that it is a consequence of the extreme aggressiveness and lethality of this inherently metastatic tumor line. It has also been shown that many tumors can downregulate T-cell responses, including induction of antigen-specific nonresponsiveness (31). Whether this is the case for the B16 melanoma remains to be determined and is an area of active investigation.

One striking phenomenon that developed in the majority of mice that had undergone tumor rejection was progressive depigmentation of the fur beginning at approximately 1 month after tumor rejection. Depigmentation is accompanied by infiltration of the skin with mononuclear cells along with the loss of normal melanocytes in the affected areas. The depigmentation is reminiscent of the vitiligo observed in those melanoma patients showing clinical responses in the immunotherapy trials carried out by Rosenberg and his colleagues (32). Normal melanocyte gene products have been shown to be frequent targets of anti-melanoma responses in human patients (33). There have been several examples of the induction of depigmentation or protection against challenge, or both, with B16 melanoma in mice after immunization with peptides derived from the murine equivalents of normal melanocyte antigens (34–39). However, the responses obtained have been shown to be sufficient to obtain rejection of established tumors. The effectiveness of CTLA-4 blockade in obtaining both tumor rejection and progressive depigmentation may reflect a more efficient mobilization of a larger spectrum of T cells reactive with normal melanocyte-associated antigens.

These results taken together establish

1. That combination immunotherapy with CTLA-4 blockade can be used to obtain eradication of this poorly immunogenic transplantable tumor.
2. That the immune response is at least in part directed to normal melanocyte-specific gene products, resulting in tissue-specific autoimmunity.

CTLA-4 Blockade Can Be Effective in Immunotherapy of Primary Prostatic Adenocarcinoma

It is clear that experiments using transplantable tumors can provide extremely valuable insight into immunologic principles and the rational design of immunotherapeutic strategies. However, the use of transplantable models raises several issues concerning the relevance of the specifics of data obtained to ultimate clinical application. One of these issues is that ectopic sites of tumor implantation are often used; most models use subcutaneous inoculation. This may be less of an issue for melanoma lines, but the skin is richly endowed with APCs for the initiation of immune responses and may not reflect what occurs in other tissues. Additionally, other organ sites may not be readily accessible to lymphocytes, and it is also possible that tumor growth might provide additional barriers such as interstitial pressure that would further compromise access. Finally, the

use of transplantable tumors with long histories of passage raises questions of genetic drift in both the tumor and mouse host as sources of new antigenic differences.

To avoid at least some of these problems, we have used the transgenic adenocarcinoma of mouse prostate (TRAMP) (40). In these mice, the androgen-regulated rat probasin promoter drives expression of the SV40-Tag oncogene in prostatic epithelium. We found that CTLA-4 blockade was sufficient to obtain partial or complete remission of early passage cell lines (TC1 and TC2) derived from these mice in nontransgenic syngeneic hosts (41,42). We then explored the use of CTLA-4 blockade in the treatment of primary cancer in the transgenic mice. Male TRAMP mice have developed a series of cellular changes beginning at puberty that closely reflect prostate carcinogenesis in man, including hyperplasia, frank neoplasia, and, finally, invasive adenocarcinoma (40). Mice were treated at 14 to 16 weeks of age, when most would be expected to bear early adenocarcinoma, with irradiated TRAMP (TC) cells and GM-CSF–expressing TRAMP cells (GM-TC) with anti–CTLA-4 or control hamster antibodies. We found that anti-CTLA-4 given along with the tumor cell vaccines resulted in a significant reduction in both tumor incidence and severity as determined by histopathologic analysis of prostatic tissue 8 weeks after treatment (43). Treatment of the mice with the vaccines or anti–CTLA-4 alone had no effect on tumor incidence. However, tumor incidence was significantly reduced in mice receiving either cell vaccine along with anti–CTLA-4. The effect was most pronounced in mice treated with anti–CTLA-4 and GM-TC at 14 weeks, in which the incidence was only 15% compared with 75% in control mice. We also observed a reduction in the severity of the tumors as indicated by clinical grading. Mice treated with the GM-TC vaccine alone had a mean score of 5.3, whereas those treated with GM-TC and anti–CTLA-4 had a score of 3.5. We also observed that the prostates of mice treated with GM-TC and anti–CTLA-4 showed extensive inflammation marked by accumulation of mononuclear cells, presumably lymphocytes, in the interductal spaces. There was no significant inflammation in the prostates of mice in the groups vaccinated in the absence of anti–CTLA-4. Together these results suggest that combination immunotherapy using CTLA-4 blockade can decrease incidence and severity of primary tumors in this transgenic model. This is a particularly significant finding given the aggressive nature of the transgene whose expression is presumably leading to the transformation of essentially all epithelial cells in the prostate.

One issue that arises from this work is whether the transgene product itself, the viral T antigen, is itself the target for immunologic responses. We thought this improbable because T-antigen expression cannot be detected by highly sensitive reverse transcriptase polymerase chain reaction technique in the TRAMP cell lines used for immunization, nor were these cell lines susceptible to cytolysis by T-cell lines specific for H2B-restricted epitopes of SV40 Tag [(42), and S. Tevethian, *personal communication*, 1999]. To address this question more directly, however, we immunized nontransgenic BL6 mice with the GM-TC vaccine with or without anti–CTLA-4. We observed that a month after vaccination in the presence of anti–CTLA-4 there was a marked infiltration of the normal prostate with mononuclear cells along with large-scale destruction of epithelium. These results indicate that the immune response elicited by the combination treatment protocol was not limited to the viral oncogene, but is at least in part due to induction of T cells reactive with normal prostate-associated antigens.

Taken together, these results demonstrate for the first time that the immunotherapeutic approach can be effective or at least partially effective in the treatment of primary cancer in this mouse model. Additionally, the immune response is directed at least in part to normal prostate tissue-specific antigens. We think that this finding is particularly important because there is a paucity of data on immune responses directed against normal prostatic tissue. Identification of the target antigens of this autoimmune prostatitis should allow the development of specific targets for the immunologic treatment of prostate cancer.

CTLA-4 BLOCKADE IN THE INDUCTION OF AUTOIMMUNITY AND TUMOR IMMUNITY

The data outlined in the previous sections have demonstrated that manipulation of signals involved in regulation of T-cell activation can be used effectively in the therapy of these experimental tumors. Consistent with our finding in autoimmune models, one of the consequences of the successful therapy of tumors seems to be the induction of tissue-specific autoimmunity. It should be stressed that in mice in that we have observed tissue-specific effects, there is no evidence of systemic autoimmune disease or of any other factors that detract from the general health of the animal. The immune responses seem to be limited to targets with which the animals are being vaccinated. Thus, we believe that these strategies offer considerable promise in the treatment of human cancers, at least of tissues that are not essential for survival such as prostate, melanocyte, breast, ovary, and testicle. In collaboration with others, we have produced a panel of antibodies reactive with human CTLA-4 for clinical trial evaluation of its therapeutic potential. These trials should begin in the year 2000.

ACKNOWLEDGMENT

The work described here was supported in part by a grant from the National Cancer Institute.

REFERENCES

1. Lenschow DJ, Walunas TL, Bluestone JA. CD28/B7 system of T cell costimulation. *Ann Rev Immunol* 1996;14:233–258.
2. Schwartz RH. Costimulation of T lymphocytes: the role of CD28, CTLA-4, and B7/BB1 in interleukin-2 production and immunotherapy. *Cell* 1992;71:1065–1068.
3. Chen L, Ashe S, Brady WA, et al. Costimulation of antitumor immunity by the B7 counterreceptor for the T lymphocyte molecules CD28 and CTLA-4. *Cell* 1992;71:1093–1102.
4. Townsend S, Allison JP. Tumor rejection after direct costimulation of CD8[+] T cells by B7-transfected melanoma cells. *Science* 1993;259: 368–370.
5. Allison JP, Hurwitz AA, Leach DR. Manipulation of costimulatory signals to enhance antitumor T-cell responses. *Curr Opin Immunol* 1995;7:682–686.
6. Townsend SE, Su FW, Atherton JM, Allison JP. Specificity and longevity of antitumor immune responses induced by B7-transfected tumors. *Cancer Res* 1994;54:6477–6483.
7. Linsley PS, Brady W, Urnes M, Grosmaire LS, Damle NK, Ledbetter JA. CTLA-4 is a second receptor for the B cell activation antigen B7. *J Exp Med* 1991;174:561–569.
8. Thompson CB, Allison JP. The emerging role of CTLA-4 as an immune attenuator. *Immunity* 1997;7:445–450.
9. Walunas TL, Lenschow DJ, Bakker CY, et al. CTLA-4 can function as a negative regulator of T cell activation. *Immunity* 1994;1:405–413.
10. Krummel MF, Allison JP. CD28 and CTLA-4 have opposing effects on the response of T cells to stimulation. *J Exp Med* 1995;182:459–465.
11. Kearney ER, Walunas TL, Karr RW, et al. Antigen-dependent clonal expansion of a trace population of antigen-specific CD4[+] T cells *in vivo* is dependent on CD28 costimulation and inhibited by CTLA-4. *J Immunol* 1995;155:1033–1036.
12. Krummel MF, Sullivan TJ, Allison JP. Superantigen responses and costimulation: CD28 and CTLA-4 have opposing effects on T cell expansion *in vitro* and *in vivo*. *Int Immunol* 1996;8:519–523.
13. Waterhouse P, Penninger JM, Timms E, et al. Lymphoproliferative disorders with early lethality in mice deficient in CTLA-4. *Science* 1995;270:985–988.
14. Tivol EA, Borriello F, Schweitzer AN, Lynch WP, Bluestone JA, Sharpe AH. Loss of CTLA-4 leads to massive lymphoproliferation and fatal multiorgan tissue destruction, revealing a critical negative regulatory role of CTLA-4. *Immunity* 1995;3:541–547.
15. Chambers CA, Sullivan TJ, Allison JP. Lymphoproliferation in CTLA-4-deficient mice is mediated by costimulation-dependent activation of CD4+ T cells. *Immunity* 1997;7:885–895.
16. Chambers CA, Cado D, Truong T, Allison JP. Thymocyte differentiation occurs normally in the absence of CTLA-4. *Proc Natl Acad Sci U S A* 1997;94:9296–9301.
17. Krummel MF, Allison JP. CTLA-4 engagement inhibits IL-2 accumulation and cell cycle progression upon activation of resting T cells. *J Exp Med* 1996;183:2533–2540.
18. Chambers CA, Krummel MF, Boitel B, et al. The role of CTLA-4 in the regulation and initiation of T cell responses. *Immunol Rev* 1996;153:27–46.
19. Allison JP, Chambers C, Hurwitz A, et al. A role for CTLA-4-mediated inhibitory signals in peripheral T cell tolerance. In: Bock GR, Goode JA, eds. *Immunological tolerance, Vol. 215. Novartis Foundation Symposium*. New York: Wiley-Liss, 1998:92–102.
20. Karandikar NJ, Vanderlugt CL, Walunas TL, Miller SD, Bluestone JA. CTLA-4: a negative regulator of autoimmune disease. *J Exp Med* 1996;184:783–788.
21. Perrin PJ, Scott D, Quigley L, et al. Role of B7:CD28/CTLA-4 in the induction of chronic relapsing experimental allergic encephalomyelitis. *J Immunol* 1995;154:1481–1490.
22. Hurwitz AA, Sullivan TJ, Krummel MF, Sobel RA, Allison JP. Specific blockade of CTLA-4/B7 interactions results in exacerbated clinical and histologic disease in an actively induced model of experimental allergic encephalomyelitis. *J Neuroimmunol* 1997;73:57–62.
23. Leach D, Krummel M, Allison JP. Enhancement of antitumor immunity by CTLA-4 blockade. *Science* 1996;271:1734–1736.
24. Dranoff G, Jaffee E, Lazenby A, et al. Vaccination with irradiated tumor cells engineered to secrete GM-CSF stimulates potent, specific, and long lasting anti-tumor immunity. *Proc Natl Acad Sci U S A* 1993;90:3539–3543.
25. Levitsky HI, Lazenby A, Hayashi RJ, Pardoll DM. *In vivo* priming of two distinct antitumor effector populations: the role of MHC class I expression. *J Exp Med* 1994;179:1215–1224.
26. Hurwitz AA, Yu TF, Leach DR, Allison JP. CTLA-4 blockade synergizes with tumor-derived GM-CSF for treatment of an experimental mammary carcinoma. *Proc Natl Acad Sci U S A* 1998;95:10067–10071.
27. van Elsas A, Hurwitz AA, Allison JP. Combination immunotherapy of B16 melanoma using anti-cytotoxic T lymphocyte-associated

antigen 4 (anti-CTLA-4) and granulocyte-macrophage colony-stimulating factor (GM-CSF) producing vaccines induces rejection of subcutaneous and metastatic tumors accompanied by autoimmune depigmentation. *J Exp Med* 1999;190:355–356.

28. Schoenberger SP, Toes RE, van der Voort EI, Offringa R, Melief CJ. T-cell help for cytotoxic T lymphocytes is mediated by CD40-CD40L interactions [see comments]. *Nature* 1998;393:480–483.

29. Ridge JP, Di Rosa F, Matzinger P. A conditioned dendritic cell can be a temporal bridge between a CD4+ T-helper and a T-killer cell [see comments]. *Nature* 1998;393:474–478.

30. Bennett SR, Carbone FR, Karamalis F, Flavell RA, Miller JF, Heath WR. Help for cytotoxic-T-cell responses is mediated by CD40 signaling. *Nature* 1998;393:478–480.

31. Staveley-O'Carroll K, Sotomayor E, Montgomery J, et al. Induction of antigen-specific T cell anergy: an early event in the course of tumor progression. *Proc Natl Acad Sci U S A* 1998;95:1178–1183.

32. Rosenberg SA, White DE. Vitiligo in patients with melanoma: normal tissue antigens can be targets for cancer immunotherapy. *J Immunother Emph Tumor Immunol* 1996;19:81–84.

33. Rosenberg S. A new era for cancer immunotherapy based on the genes that encode cancer antigens. *Immunity* 1999;10:281–287.

34. Weber LW, Bowne WB, Woichok JD, et al. Tumor immunity and autoimmunity induced by immunization with homologous DNA. *J Clin Invest* 1998;102:1258–1264.

35. Naftzger C, Takechi Y, Kohda H, Hara I, Vijayasaradhi S, Houghton AN. Immune response to a differentiation antigen induced by altered antigen: a study of tumor rejection and autoimmunity. *Proc Natl Acad Sci U S A* 1996;93:14809–14814.

36. Overwijk WW, Tsung A, Irvine KE, et al. gp100/pmel 17 is a murine tumor rejection antigen: induction of "self"-reactive tumoricidal T cells using high-affinity, altered peptide ligand. *J Exp Med* 1998;188:277–286.

37. Overwijk WW, Lee DS, Surman DR, et al. Vaccination with a recombinant vaccinia virus encoding a "self" antigen induces autoimmune vitiligo and tumor cell destruction in mice: requirement for CD4+ T lymphocytes. *Proc Natl Acad Sci U S A* 1999;96: 2982–2987.

38. Bloom MB, Perry-Lalley D, Robbins PF, et al. Identification of tyrosinase-related protein 2 as a tumor rejection antigen for the B16 melanoma. *J Exp Med* 1997;185:453–459.

39. Hara I, Takechi Y, Houghton AN. Implicating a role for immune recognition of self in tumor rejection: passive immunization against the brown locus protein. *J Exp Med* 1995;182:1609–1614.

40. Greenberg NM, DeMayo F, Finegold MJ, et al. Prostate cancer in a transgenic mouse. *Proc Natl Acad Sci U S A* 1995;92:3439–3443.

41. Foster BA, Gingrich JR, Kwon ED, Madias C, Greenberg NM. Characterization of prostatic epithelial cell lines derived from transgenic adenocarcinoma of the mouse prostate (TRAMP) model. *Cancer Res* 1997;57:3325–3330.

42. Kwon ED, Hurwitz AA, Foster BA, et al. Manipulation of T cell costimulatory and inhibitory signals for immunotherapy of prostate cancer. *Proc Natl Acad Sci U S A* 1997;94:8099–8103.

43. Hurwitz AA, Foster BA, Kwon ED, et al. Immunotherapy of primary prostate cancer in a transgenic model using a combination of CTLA-4 blockade and tumor cell vaccine. *Cancer Res* 2000 (*in press*).

INDEX

Note: Page numbers followed by *f* indicate figures; page numbers followed by *t* indicate tables.